Wilkins' Clinical Practice of the Dental Hygienist

Fourteenth Edition

Linda D. Boyd, RDH, RD, EdD

Professor
Associate Dean, Graduate Studies
Forsyth School of Dental Hygiene,
Massachusetts College of Pharmacy & Health Sciences
Boston, Massachusetts

Lisa F. Mallonee, RDH, RD, LD, MPH

Professor
Interim Associate Dean, Office of Academic Affairs
Texas A&M University School of Dentistry
Dallas, Texas

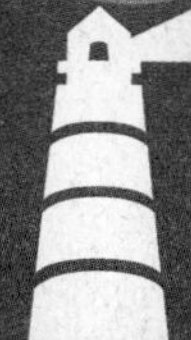

JONES & BARTLETT
LEARNING

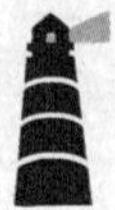

World Headquarters
Jones & Bartlett Learning
25 Mall Road
Burlington, MA 01803
978-443-5000
info@jblearning.com
www.jblearning.com

Jones & Bartlett Learning books and products are available through most bookstores and online booksellers. To contact Jones & Bartlett Learning directly, call 800-832-0034, fax 978-443-8000, or visit our website, www.jblearning.com.

Substantial discounts on bulk quantities of Jones & Bartlett Learning publications are available to corporations, professional associations, and other qualified organizations. For details and specific discount information, contact the special sales department at Jones & Bartlett Learning via the above contact information or send an email to specialsales@jblearning.com.

26423-4

Production Credits
Vice President, Product Management: Marisa R. Urbano
Vice President, Content Strategy and Implementation: Christine Emerton
Director, Product Management: Matthew Kane
Product Manager: Bill Lawrensen
Director, Content Management: Donna Gridley
Manager, Content Strategy: Carolyn Pershouse
Content Strategist: Ashley Malone
Director, Project Management and Content Services: Karen Scott
Manager, Program Management: Kristen Rogers
Manager, Project Management: Jackie Reynen
Project Manager: John Coakley
Program Manager: Alex Schab
Senior Digital Project Specialist: Angela Dooley
Marketing Manager: Mark Adamiak
Content Services Manager: Colleen Lamy
Vice President, Manufacturing and Inventory Control: Therese Connell
Composition: S4Carlisle Publishing Services
Cover Design: Kristin E. Parker
Text Design: Kristin E. Parker
Senior Media Development Editor: Troy Liston
Rights & Permissions Manager: John Rusk
Rights Specialist: Maria Leon Maimone
Cover Image (Title Page, Part Opener, Chapter Opener): © Flavio Coelho/Moment/Getty Images
Printing and Binding: LSC Communications

Library of Congress Cataloging-in-Publication Data
Names: Boyd, Linda D., author. | Mallonee, Lisa F., author.
Title: Wilkins' clinical practice of the dental hygienist / Linda D. Boyd, Lisa F. Mallonee.
Other titles: Clinical practice of the dental hygienist
Description: Fourteenth edition. | Burlington, Massachusetts : Jones & Bartlett Learning, [2023] | Includes bibliographical references and index.
Identifiers: LCCN 2022035729 | ISBN 9781284255997 (hardcover)
Subjects: MESH: Dental Prophylaxis | Dental Hygienists | Outline
Classification: LCC RK60.5 | NLM WU 18.2 | DDC 617.6/01--dc23/eng/20230206
LC record available at https://lccn.loc.gov/2022035729

6048

Printed in the United States of America
26 25 24 23 10 9 8 7 6 5 4 3 2 1

Tribute

The first edition of Dr. Esther Wilkins's *Clinical Practice of the Dental Hygienist* was published in 1959. Before that, the "book" was provided for Esther's students at the University of Washington as a series of individually copied, topic-related handouts, organized as the book is today, using an easy-to-read outline format. Over the next 60 years, Esther wrote and supervised the revision through 12 editions (an average of one new edition every 5 years!).

Anyone who worked with Esther on any of those editions understands the effort and energy she put into making the book as up-to-date and evidence based as possible. Even in that very first edition, every chapter contained a list of references to support the information in that chapter. A look through any of those previous editions reveals how current Esther's thinking was as she updated each edition. Anyone fortunate enough to be invited to visit Esther in her condo overlooking Boston Common will tell you that her home office was bursting with textbooks and copies of thousands of journal articles, stacked on every available surface and poking out of overfilled file cabinets. Such was her commitment to understanding the current science related to dental hygiene practice. Those of us who worked with her over the years can tell you about her attention to detail and insistence that everything be perfect as we submitted chapter manuscripts for publication.

The editorial and contributor teams who have revised the two new editions since Esther is no longer here to guide us are proud to say that we have done our best to carry forward the integrity, attention to detail, and dedication to the science and art of dental hygiene practice that was Esther's vision for this book.

Dedication

The 14th edition of *Wilkins' Clinical Practice of the Dental Hygienist* is dedicated to all past and present students who have studied from the preceding editions. Gratitude is expressed to their faculty in the many different dental hygiene programs around the world, for their leadership in, and devotion to, dental hygiene education.

A very special recognition goes to the students of the first 10 classes in dental hygiene at the University of Washington in Seattle for who used the original "mimeographed" syllabus. They are remembered with much appreciation because their need for text study material made this book possible in the first place.

Gratitude to my husband, who has supported me tirelessly on my academic journey, and to my grandmother, Fay Nelson, who instilled a love of learning. Special thanks to my professional mentors who recognized my potential even when I did not: Dr. John Chirgwin, Dr. Carole Palmer, and last, but never least, Dr. Esther Wilkins. Dr. Wilkins is the wind beneath our wings as educators and dental hygienists! Never forget all she has done for our profession!

—Linda D. Boyd

To my husband Scott and our children, Harper and Layne, who provide me with daily inspiration, love, and support in all that I do. To Dr. Esther Wilkins—it is an honor to play an integral role in moving your legacy for the profession of dental hygiene forward. A special thanks goes to all who have provided mentorship throughout my career, to my School of Dentistry dental hygiene family that provide a constant source of encouragement, and to my students—past, present, and future—who motivate me to be a voice for the dental hygiene profession and continually evolve to reach new heights.

—Lisa F. Mallonee

Brief Contents

SECTION IX Patients with Special Needs 837

Contents

SECTION VI Implementation: Prevention 437

CHAPTER 29 The Patient with Orthodontic Appliances 527

CHAPTER 30 Care of Dental Prosthesis 539

Preface

Dental hygienists are oral healthcare specialists who have professional goals centered on the prevention and/or control of oral disease and the maintenance of oral and general health. As primary healthcare professionals, dental hygienists can apply their knowledge and skills in a wide variety of areas related to clinical practice, education, research, public health, and advocacy for health promotion and disease prevention. Dental hygienists collaborate with dentists and members of other health professions to provide oral health care that links with total body health care. An expanding emphasis on the effect of oral health on systemic health challenges requires dental hygienists to widen their scope of practice.

Objectives

Objectives of the 14th edition include:

- To help prepare the beginning dental hygiene student to recognize the requirements of evidence-based dental hygiene practice.
- To develop skills and knowledge for entry into the profession.
- To help when studying for licensure board examinations; the condensed outline form aids in making review easier.
- To update professional hygienists who are already in practice to recognize changes in practice and the responsibility to apply evidence-based scientific approaches to patient care.

The Text Plan

Highlights

Highlights of *Wilkins' Clinical Practice of the Dental Hygienist*, 14th edition include the following:

- Chapters have been extensively updated with the best available evidence, edited, and reorganized to minimize redundancy.
- Key words are highlighted in each chapter and available in a comprehensive glossary at the end of the textbook.
- Chapter 5, Transmissible Diseases, had major updates, with the addition of a section on airborne transmission, coronavirus, and new tables for hepatitis and human herpes viruses.
- Chapter 6, Exposure Control: Barriers for Patient and Clinician, has new information on respiratory protection.
- Chapter 7, Infection Control: Clinical Procedures, has new information on engineering controls and ventilation, particularly those related to aerosol-generating procedures.
- Chapter 11, Medical History, includes a revised medical history sample with updated tables containing a new column for follow-up questions related to medical, dental, and psychosocial history to help guide students in how to ask questions to gather additional information.
- Chapter 25, Protocols for Prevention and Control of Dental Caries, includes updates from the 2021 evidence-based caries management practical guidelines.
- Chapter 32, The Patient with Nicotine Use Disorders, has additional updates related to electronic nicotine delivery systems (ENDS).
- Chapter 34, Fluorides, has updated content on silver diamine fluoride (SDF), including indications for use and application.
- Chapter 35, Sealants, has updated evidence to support the content in the chapter.
- Chapter 39, Nonsurgical Periodontal Therapy and Adjunctive Therapy, has been updated based on the most recent practice guidelines for treatment of Stage I-III periodontal disease.
- Chapter 47, The Pediatric Patient, has updated content regarding AAPD and CAMBRA recommendations for children younger than 6 years.
- Chapter 59, The Patient with a Substance-Related Disorder, underwent major updates throughout, but special attention was paid to opioid and marijuana use.

Organization of the Text

As in past editions, sections of *Wilkins' Clinical Practice of the Dental Hygienist* are sequenced to conform to the Dental Hygiene Process of Care. There are nine sections in the 14th edition, six of which are specifically identified by name with the recognized components of the Process of Care. They are *assessment*, *dental hygiene diagnosis*, *care planning*, *implementation*, *evaluation*, and *documentation*.

The text opens with chapters devoted to an introduction to the profession of dental hygiene and chapters related to preparation for practice. They include infection control and ergonomic health for the clinical practitioner and patient. The final, and largest, section, Section IX, applies the process of care to patients with special needs.

The nine major sections are:

- Section I: Orientation to Clinical Dental Hygiene Practice
- Section II: Preparation for Dental Hygiene Practice
- Section III: Documentation
- Section IV: Assessment
- Section V: Dental Hygiene Diagnosis and Care Planning
- Section VI: Implementation: Prevention
- Section VII: Implementation: Treatment
- Section VIII: Evaluation
- Section IX: Patients with Special Needs

Supplementary information is available online:

- American Dental Hygienists' Association Code of Ethics for Dental Hygienists
- National Dental Hygienists' Association Code of Ethics
- Canadian Dental Hygienists Association Dental Hygienists' Code of Ethics
- International Federation of Dental Hygienists' Code of Ethics

Features of This Edition

All chapters have been updated and many have been extensively revised. Each chapter includes the following features:

- Detailed **outline format** for the text makes it easier for the student to identify and understand important information they need to know for clinical practice.
- **Chapter Outlines** at the opening of each chapter can help readers locate material within the chapter at any time.
- **Learning Objectives** at the beginning of each chapter guide the student in studying the chapter.
- **Key Words** are bolded throughout the chapter to indicate these words are included in an alphabetized listing in the glossary.
- **Factors to Teach the Patient** boxes help students to select topics from the chapter that need special emphasis while teaching patients oral self-care.
- **Documentation** brings the clinical care of a patient full cycle. Example documentation for a variety of patients, written using the SOAP notes format outlined in Chapter 10, can increase students' awareness of the necessary components and significance of such notes in the permanent record of each patient.

Additional Resources

Digital Connections

Wilkins' Clinical Practice of the Dental Hygienist, 14th edition includes additional resources for both instructors and students that are available online.

Instructors

Approved adopting instructors will be given access to the following additional resources:

- Test bank
- Slides in PowerPoint format
- Lesson plans
- Image bank of images and tables from the book
- Answers to Workbook Exercises

Students

The following additional student resources are available online:

- Audio pronunciation glossary for select clinical terms
- Appendices
- Videos
- Flashcards
- TestPrep
- Learning Objectives
- Workbook

See the inside front cover of this text for more details.

Individualized Review

Customized practice quizzing with Navigate TestPrep for *Wilkins' Clinical Practice of the Dental Hygienist* remediates to the text. This powerful tool offers students practice tests, detailed rationales, and data dashboards.

Acknowledgments

A text of the size and scope of *Wilkins' Clinical Practice of the Dental Hygienist* is the work of many contributors. Comments and suggestions come from teachers, students, and practitioners from around the world, as the book has been translated into a variety of languages. Any suggestions are welcomed and considered in making future revisions.

Recognition for Our Contributors

We start with recognition and appreciation to our contributors for their efforts to incorporate the most current evidence to the revision of their chapter(s).

Other Appreciation

Appreciation is expressed to the following:

Tammy Marshall-Paquin Many thanks to the tireless efforts to update and improve on the ancillary materials for students and instructors for the 14th edition.

Marcia Williams of Santa Fe, New Mexico. Many illustrations have been the work of our talented artist. Her personal interest and patience in preparing new drawings, revising previous ones, and adding color to enhance the line drawings are acknowledged with sincere gratitude.

Our Readers. Finally, we would like to express our appreciation to our readers over the years: students, teachers, and practicing dental hygienists. Send us your comments and suggestions. As stated in the first edition, it is hoped that through greater understanding of each patient's oral and general health needs, more complete and effective dental hygiene services can be rendered.

—Linda Boyd and Lisa Mallonee

Contributors

Jaymi-Lyn Adams, RDH, MS
Assistant Professor, Forsyth School of Dental Hygiene
Massachusetts College of Pharmacy & Health Sciences University
Worcester, Massachusetts

Jessica August, RDH, CDA, MSDH
Director, Dental Programs
Portland Community College
Portland, Oregon

Linda D. Boyd, RDH, RD, EdD
Professor and Associate Dean
Forsyth School of Dental Hygiene
Massachusetts College of Pharmacy and Health Sciences University
Boston, Massachusetts

Danielle Collins, CDA, RDH, MS
Adjunct Clinical Faculty
Forsyth School of Dental Hygiene
Massachusetts College of Pharmacy & Health Sciences University
Compliance Officer III
Massachusetts Department of Public Health-Bureau of Substance Addiction Services
Boston, Massachusetts

Jane Cotter, BSDH, MS, CTTS, FAADH
Associate Professor
Texas A&M School of Dentistry
Dallas, Texas

Jennifer Cullen, RDH, BSDH, MPH
Director, Dental Hygiene Degree Completion Program
Division of Dental Hygiene, Department of Periodontics and Oral Medicine
University of Michigan School of Dentistry
Ann Arbor, Michigan

Heather Doucette, DipDH, BSc, MEd
Associate Professor
School of Dental Hygiene
Dalhousie University
Halifax, Nova Scotia

Lori J. Giblin-Scanlon, RDH, MS, DHSc
Professor and Associate Dean, Clinical Programs
Forsyth School of Dental Hygiene
Massachusetts College of Pharmacy & Health Sciences University
Boston, Massachusetts

S. Kim Haslam, DipDH, BA, MEd
Assistant Professor
School of Dental Hygiene
Dalhousie University
Halifax, Nova Scotia, Canada

Heather Hessheimer, RDH, MSDH
Assistant Professor
Department Dental Hygiene
University of Nebraska Medical Center-College of Dentistry
Lincoln, Nebraska

Laura Howerton, RDH, MS
Retired Educator
The Ohio State University, Columbus, Ohio
University of North Carolina, Chapel Hill, North Carolina
Wake Technical Community College
Raleigh, North Carolina

Michelle Hurlbutt, RDH, MSDH, DHSc
Associate Professor and Dean
Dental Hygiene Program
West Coast University
Anaheim, California

Susan J. Jenkins, RDH, PhD
Professor
Forsyth School of Dental Hygiene
Massachusetts College of Pharmacy & Health Sciences University
Boston, Massachusetts

Evie F. Jesin, RRDH, BSc
Professor
School of Dental Health
George Brown College
Toronto, Ontario, Canada

Lisa B. Johnson, RDH, MSDH, DHSc
Assistant Professor
Health Sciences, School of Arts and Sciences
Massachusetts College of Pharmacy and Health Sciences
Boston, Massachusetts

Faizan Kabani, RDH, MHA, MBA, PhD
Euless, Texas

Robin L. Kerkstra, RDH, MSDH
Assistant Professor
Dental Hygiene Program
University of New Haven
New Haven, Connecticut

Dana E. Kleckler, RDH, BS
Saint Clair Shores, Michigan

Lisa M. LaSpina, RDH, MS, DHSc
Associate Professor
Forsyth School of Dental Hygiene
Massachusetts College of Pharmacy & Health Sciences University
Boston, Massachusetts

Lory A. Libby, RDH, MSDH
Assistant Professor
Forsyth School of Dental Hygiene
Massachusetts College of Pharmacy & Health Sciences University
Boston, Massachusetts

Wendy Male, MBA, BDSc, RDH
Associate Dean
Diagnostics & Allied Health, School of Health Sciences, College of New Caledonia
Prince George, British Columbia, Canada
Edmonton, Alberta, Canada

Lisa F. Mallonee, RDH, RD, LD, MPH
Professor, Interim Associate Dean for Academic Affairs and Graduate Program Director
Texas A&M School of Dentistry
Dallas, Texas

Kelley M. Martell, RDH, BSDH, MSDH
Department Chair-Interdisciplinary Science/Allied Health
Mount Wachusett Community College
Gardner, Massachusetts

Catherine A. McConnell, RDH, BDSc, MEd
Clinic Coordinator
Dental Hygiene Department
John Abbott College
Sainte-Anne-de-Bellevue, Quebec, Canada

Jill C. Moore, RDH, BSDH, MHA, EdD
Director of Doctoral Health Sciences Program
University of New Haven
New Haven, Connecticut

Lisa J. Moravec, RDH, MSDH
Associate Professor, West Division Site Coordinator
Department Dental Hygiene
University of Nebraska Medical Center-College of Dentistry
Gering, Nebraska

Debra November-Rider, RDH, MSDH
Adjunct Assistant Professor
Forsyth School of Dental Hygiene
Massachusetts College of Pharmacy & Health Sciences University
Boston, Massachusetts

Uhlee (Yuri) Oh, RDH, BS, DHSc
Assistant Professor
Forsyth School of Dental Hygiene
Massachusetts College of Pharmacy & Health Sciences University
Boston, Massachusetts

Kristeen Perry, RDH, DHSc
Assistant Professor
Forsyth School of Dental Hygiene
Massachusetts College of Pharmacy & Health Sciences University
Boston, Massachusetts

Lori Rainchuso, RDH, MS, DHSc
Professor, Doctor of Health Sciences Program
School of Arts & Sciences
Massachusetts College of Pharmacy & Health Sciences University
Worcester, Massachusetts

Heather Reid, RDH, MS
Assistant Professor
Department of Dental Hygiene
Clayton State College
Morrow, Georgia

Erin E. Relich, RDH, BSDH, MSA
Punta Gorda, Florida

Irina Smilyanski, RDH, MS, DHSc
Associate Professor
Forsyth School of Dental Hygiene
Massachusetts College of Pharmacy & Health Sciences University
Worcester, Massachusetts

Amy N. Smith, RDH, EdD, MPH
Assistant Professor
Department of Dental Hygiene
Perimeter College-Georgia State University
Dunwoody, Georgia

Katherine Soal, RDH, MSDH
Professor
Department of Dental Hygiene
Quinsigamond Community College
Worcester, Massachusetts

Salima Thawer, MPH, BSc, RDH
Director of Regulatory Affairs
College of Registered Dental Hygienists of Alberta
Edmonton, Alberta, Canada

Naquilla Thomas, RDH, EdD
Assistant Professor and Chair
Department of Dental Hygiene
Clayton State College
Morrow, Georgia

Carol Tran, BOH, PhD
Oral Health Therapist, Private Practice
Queensland, Australia
Associate Professor, Head of Course for Oral Health
Central Queensland University
Rockhamptom, Australia

Marsha A. Voelker, CDA, RDH, MS
Graduate Faculty
Old Dominion University College of Health Sciences
Norfolk, Virginia

Mary Vu, RDH, MS
Clinical Assistant Professor
Texas A&M School of Dentistry
Dallas, Texas

Lisa Welch, RDH, EdD
Associate Professor
Department of Dental Hygiene
Utah Tech University
George, Utah

Denise Zwicker, BDH, MEd
Senior Instructor
Faculty of Dentistry School of Dental Hygiene
Dalhousie University
Halifax, Nova Scotia, Canada

Reviewers

Brenda A. Alberts, RDH, CDA
Northcentral Technical College

Jenna Allen-Coan, BA, RDH, MEd
Fresno City College

Marija Cahoon, RDH, MS
NYC College of Dentistry

Bridget Fitzhugh, BBA, BS, RDH
University of Arkansas for Medical Sciences

Cheri Hilenski, RDH, BS
Lorain County Community College

Jackie Kollasch, RDH, BA, MS, CDA
Des Moines Area Community College

Tracy Kuny, LSD, MSEd
Century College

Deb Merrigan, RDH, BSDH
Century College

Cathleen Sparks, RDH, BSDH
Rochester Community and Technical College

Maureen Strauss, CDA, RDH, MS
Middlesex Community College

Barbara T. Varnadore, CRDH, CDA, MSDH
Pensacola State College

Donna Winterberry, CRDH, RN, BSN, BASDH, MSDH
Pensacola State College

SECTION I

Orientation to Clinical Dental Hygiene Practice

Introduction for Section I

Professional dental hygiene practice is not defined solely by the clinical duties traditionally associated with private practice dental care settings. The professional roles, responsibilities, and ethical standards of the dental hygienist encompass both traditional clinical practice and alternative dental hygiene practice settings.

The dental hygienist is:

- An educated and licensed primary healthcare provider who fills numerous roles to contribute to better oral health.
- Concerned with the general health and well-being of both individual patients and population groups.
- Skilled in accessing, understanding, and analyzing the validity of current health information.

The Professional Dental Hygienist

The professional dental hygienist is dedicated to:

- A dental hygiene process of care that meets standards for clinical dental hygiene practice.
- Ethical standards and core values outlined in professional codes of ethics to dental hygiene practice in every setting.
- Evidence-based, best-practice dental hygiene interventions.
- Communication approaches to build rapport with individuals and groups of all ages and across cultures.
- Patient education strategies to motivate positive health behavior changes.
- Healthcare interventions, supported by current research, which take into consideration the unique needs and requirements of each patient.

Standard of Care and the Dental Hygiene Process of Care

- The American Dental Hygienists' Association *Standards for Clinical Dental Hygiene Practice*[1] and the Federation of Dental Hygiene Regulators of Canada *Entry-to-Practice Canadian Competencies for Dental Hygienists*[2] outline criteria for competency in dental hygiene care, as illustrated by the components of the Dental Hygiene Process of Care.
- The Dental Hygiene Process of Care is the basis for providing preventive, educational, and therapeutic dental hygiene services that meet accepted standards of patient care.
- The process explains the series of interrelated steps the dental hygienist follows to provide clinical patient care (**Figure I-1**).

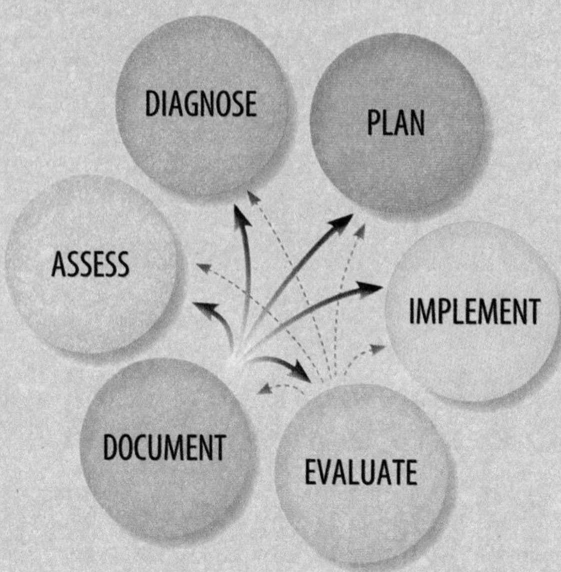

Figure I-1 The Dental Hygiene Process of Care

- The overall process is explained in Chapter 1. Each step in the process is described more completely throughout the sections of the text.

Ethical Applications

- Basic ethical concepts are described in the introduction to each section of the text.
- Reference charts are included to summarize ethical information.

References

1. American Dental Hygienists' Association. *Standards for Clinical Dental Hygiene Practice*. Chicago, IL: American Dental Hygienists' Association; 2016. https://www.adha.org/resources-docs/2016-Revised-Standards-for-Clinical-Dental-Hygiene-Practice.pdf. Accessed March 3, 2019.
2. Federation of Dental Hygiene Regulators of Canada (FDHRC). *Entry-to-Practice Canadian Competencies for Dental Hygienists*. https://www.fdhrc.ca/wp/competency-project/. Accessed April 21, 2022.

CHAPTER 1

The Professional Dental Hygienist

Linda D. Boyd, RDH, RD, EdD
Lisa F. Mallonee, RDH, RD, LD, MPH
Charlotte J. Wyche, RDH, MS
Esther M. Wilkins, BS, RDH, DMD

CHAPTER OUTLINE

LEARNING OBJECTIVES

After studying this chapter, the student will be able to:

1. Identify and define key terms and concepts related to the professional dental hygienist.
2. Describe the scope of dental hygiene practice.
3. Identify and describe the components of the dental hygiene process of care.
4. Identify and apply components of the dental hygiene code of ethics.
5. Explain interprofessional collaboration and the role of the dental hygienist.
6. Explain legal, ethical, and personal factors affecting dental hygiene practice.
7. Apply concepts in ethical decision making.

The American Dental Hygienists' Association (**ADHA**) defines the professional **dental hygienist** as *a primary care oral health professional* and the Federation of Dental Hygiene Regulators of Canada defines dental hygienists as *autonomous health professionals* who[1–3]:

- Have graduated from an accredited dental hygiene program in an institution of higher education.
- Are licensed or registered in dental hygiene to provide education, assessment, research, administrative, diagnostic, preventive, and therapeutic services.
- Work in collaboration with the dental team, health care team, and communities to improve the public's oral health.
- Support overall health through the promotion of optimal oral health and oral disease prevention.

History of the Dental Hygiene Profession

- In the early part of the 20th century, Dr. Alfred C. Fones, a dentist in Bridgeport, Connecticut, realized that most children already had dental decay by the time they reached his dental chair.
- He trained his assistant, Irene Newman, to demonstrate the value of prevention of dental decay and prophylaxis.[4]
- The name "dental hygienist" evolved because Fones felt that this term would create an association with the prevention, rather than the treatment, of oral disease.[4]
- **Box 1-1** provides a timeline of major events in the development of the **profession** of dental hygiene.
- **Figure 1-1** illustrates how the appearance of the clinical dental hygienist has changed as the profession has changed and grown.

Scope of Dental Hygiene Practice

- In the first textbook for dental hygienists, Dr. Alfred C. Fones, the "father of dental hygiene," emphasized education as the most important role in the practice of dental hygiene. He wrote:

  The dental hygienist must regard herself as the channel through which the knowledge of the dental profession is to be disseminated. The greatest service she can perform is the slow and painstaking education of the public in mouth hygiene and the allied branches of general hygiene. The education and training of dental hygienists does not aim to produce mechanical operators. An unlimited field of educational and preventive service is open to the dental hygienist who regards herself primarily as a hygienist and educators.[4]
- While the role of education and prevention is still primary, dental hygiene has changed and the scope of practice has developed and broadened from Dr. Fones' original concept.

Box 1-1 The Development of the Profession of Dental Hygiene: A Timeline

1910–1919	■ Irene Newman, Dr. Fones' assistant, became: • Licensed as the first dental hygienist. • The first president of an organized dental hygiene society in Connecticut. ■ Graduates from the first dental hygiene school, created by Dr. Fones, began working in public schools. ■ A dental hygienist was employed outside of a public school setting, in New Haven Hospital.

1920–1929	■ Licensed dental hygienists began to practice in numerous states, including Hawaii. ■ The American Dental Hygienists' Association (ADHA): • Was incorporated in Detroit, Michigan, in 1927. • Began publication of the *Journal of the ADHA*.
1930–1939	■ Dental hygienists continued working in schools, began making home visits, and most found positions in private dental practices. ■ Transportation was provided to Forsyth Dental Infirmary from Boston schools and children visiting the clinic received oral prophylaxis and oral health instruction from dental hygiene students. ■ ADHA and American Dental Association recommended minimum high school graduation as one requirement for dental hygiene licensure. ■ University of Michigan offered the first baccalaureate degree in dental hygiene.
1940–1949	■ ADHA recommended: • Changing a 1-year program to a 2-year course of study for dental hygiene licensure. • The term "registered dental hygienist" as the official credential for the profession. ■ Minimum standards for dental hygiene programs were adopted. ■ Dr. Frank Lamons wrote the first dental hygienist oath, to be used in graduation exercises. ■ Grand Rapids, Michigan, became the first city to add fluoride to its drinking water.
1950–1959	■ All states granted licensure for dental hygienists. ■ Minimum education standards for dental hygiene education were set and the accreditation process for dental hygiene programs began. ■ Sigma Phi Alpha, the dental hygiene honor society, was founded. ■ ADHA membership restrictions based on race, creed, or color were removed. ■ The first edition of the *Clinical Practice of the Dental Hygienist* textbook by Esther M. Wilkins, BS, RDH, DMD was published in 1959.
1960–1969	■ The first National Dental Hygiene Board Examination was implemented. ■ The first Regional Board Examination (North East) was given. ■ The first dental hygiene master's degree program began at Columbia University in New York. ■ ADHA bylaws were amended to allow for male dental hygienist members.
1970–1979	■ The first International Symposium on Dental Hygiene, organized and funded by the ADHA, was held in Italy. ■ The Forsyth Experiment, a groundbreaking investigation, proved conclusively that appropriately trained dental hygienists are safely and cost-effectively able to provide a defined set of restorative services. ■ Some state practice acts expanded to include administration of local anesthesia by dental hygienists. ■ Continuing education guidelines were drafted. ■ Dental hygienists began to serve on some state boards of dental examiners.
1980–1989	■ Washington was the first state with unsupervised dental hygiene practice in hospitals, nursing homes, and other specified settings. ■ Colorado allowed unsupervised practice for dental hygienists in all settings. ■ ADHA advocated for baccalaureate as the minimum degree for entry into the dental hygiene profession. ■ On the basis of research about the transmission of bloodborne infectious diseases, dental hygiene clinicians began wearing gloves during all procedures.
1990–1999	■ Occupational Safety and Health Administration's rules on occupational exposure to bloodborne pathogens were implemented; use of gloves and face masks during dental hygiene procedures became standard practice. ■ The *Dental Hygiene Process: Diagnosis and Care Planning* textbook was published, establishing a standard for clinical dental hygiene practice. ■ The National Center for Dental Hygiene Research was established. ■ New Mexico became the first state to allow: • Self-regulation of the profession by a dental hygiene committee. • Dental hygiene practice under a collaborative agreement with a dentist rather than supervision. ■ California created the Registered Dental Hygienist in Alternative Practice, allowing dental hygienists to provide unsupervised oral care to special populations in alternative settings.

(continues)

Box 1-1 The Development of the Profession of Dental Hygiene: A Timeline *(continued)*

2000–2010	■ The U.S. Department of Health and Human Services published *Oral Health in America: A Report of the Surgeon General*, which highlighted the relevance of oral health to general health. ■ U.S. Centers for Disease Control and Prevention published *Guidelines for Infection Control in Dental Health Setting.* ■ Development of the mid-level oral health provider was explored. • The ADHA adopted policy to develop the Advanced Dental Hygiene Practitioner (**ADHP**). • Dental Health Aide Therapists began providing dental care on tribal land in Alaska. • Minnesota passed the first law in the United States allowing dental hygienists to be further licensed as dental therapists using ADHP competencies. ■ Master-level dental hygiene programs increased in number. ■ Many states implemented "direct access" policies that allowed dental hygienists in at least some settings to initiate dental hygiene care: • Based on their assessment of the patient's needs. • Without the specific authorization of a dentist.
2011–2020 and Beyond—Focus on the Future	■ In 2013, ADHA celebrated 100 years of dental hygiene at the 90th ADHA Annual Session meeting in Boston. ■ Dental hygiene degree completion programs and online education opportunities continue to expand. ■ Opportunities for alternative setting and autonomy in dental hygiene practice continue to expand. ■ The dental hygiene profession affirmed and pursues its commitment to: • Optimal oral health as an essential component of general health. • Access to safe, effective, oral health services for all people. • Collaborative, interprofessional partnerships and coalitions for oral health.

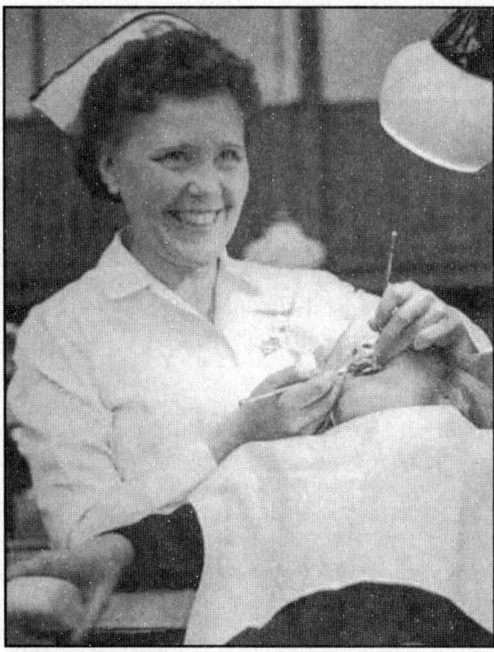

A

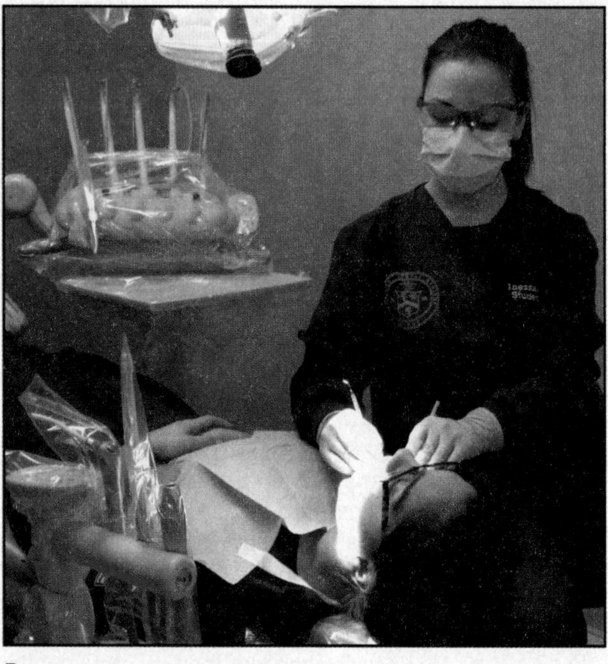

B

Figure 1-1 There is More Difference Than Just a Uniform, but Over Time the Dental Hygienist's Commitment to Safe and Effective Patient Care Remains. **A:** The dental hygienist providing patient care in the 1930s dressed in a starched white uniform and cap (as nurses also did) to indicate their commitment to cleanliness and good care. **B:** The dental hygienist of today protects self and patient from cross-infection by donning personal protective equipment and surface barriers during patient care.

I. Roles of the Dental Hygienist

- Various roles of licensed dental hygienists include the following[5]:
  - Education.
  - Assessment.
  - Diagnosis.
  - Prevention.
  - Nonsurgical therapy.
  - Research.
  - Administration.
  - Entrepreneur.
- Dental hygienists support oral health through their work in many settings, including[1,2,5]:
  - General and specialty dental practices.
  - Public health programs.
  - Research centers.
  - Educational institutions.
  - Hospital and residential care facilities.
  - Federal programs, including the military.
  - Dental corporate industries.
- Within the wide span of dental hygiene practice areas, dental hygienists may serve in a variety of capacities.
- Areas of responsibility in this variety of roles are defined in **Table 1-1**.

II. Supervision and Scope of Practice

- The professional dental hygienist is responsible to provide only those services allowed within the scope of practice outlined within each state, province, country, or territory dental hygiene practice act.[1,6]
- The type of **supervision** by a dentist required for delivery of dental hygiene services is also

Table 1-1 Professional Roles of the Dental Hygienist

Role	Description	Example Employment Settings and Positions
Clinician	Provide direct patient care in collaboration with other health professionals	▪ Private dental practices and community-based clinics ▪ Hospitals and long-term care facilities ▪ Schools
Corporate	Employment in a company that supports oral health through promotion of oral health products and services	▪ Product sales and research ▪ Corporate educator or administrator
Public health	Enhance access to care in community health programs funded by government or nonprofit organizations	▪ Clinician in: • Community clinics • Government health service • School sealant programs ▪ Oral health program administrator
Researcher	Conduct studies to test new procedures, products, or theories for accuracy and effectiveness	▪ Universities ▪ Corporations ▪ Government agencies
Educator	Use educational theory and methodology to educate competent oral health professionals or provide continuing education for licensed providers	▪ Dental hygiene program clinical or classroom instruction ▪ Corporate educator
Administrator	Apply organizational skills, communicate objectives, identify and manage resources, and evaluate and modify health or education programs	▪ Program director in clinical, educational, or corporate settings
Entrepreneur	Initiate or finance new oral health–related enterprises	▪ Practice management or product development ▪ Consulting ▪ Independent clinical practice ▪ Professional speaker or writer

Data from American Dental Hygienists' Association. Career Center: Career Paths. http://www.adha.org/professional-roles. Accessed March 27, 2022.

Box 1-2 Types of Supervision in Dental Hygiene Practice[8–10]

- **Direct supervision:** The dentist needs to be present.
- **Personal supervision:** The dentist needs to authorize, be present, and check work before dismissal of patient.
- **General supervision:** The dentist has authorized the procedure for a patient of record but need not be present when the authorized procedure is carried out by a licensed dental hygienist. The procedure is carried out in accordance with the dentist's diagnosis and treatment plan.
- **Direct access supervision:** The dental hygienist can provide appropriate services without specific authorization. This type of supervision is usually limited to preventive services provided in specified public health settings.
- **Collaborative practice:** The dental hygienist may practice without supervision with a collaborative agreement between a licensed dentist and a dental hygienist.
- **Indirect supervision:** The dentist must authorize procedure and be in the office while the services are performed.
- **Remote supervision:** The supervising dentist is not on-site. Communication between collaborating oral health practitioners is provided through use of current technologies. Sometimes referred to as teledentistry-assisted, affiliated dental hygiene practice.
- **Independent practice:** The dental hygienist can provide services within the scope of dental hygiene practice in any setting and without authorization or supervision by a dentist.

Data from American Dental Hygienists' Association. Dental hygiene practice acts overview: permitted functions and supervision levels by state. Revised January 2019. http://www.adha.org/resources-docs/7511_Permitted_Services_Supervision_Levels_by_State.pdf. Accessed February 15, 2019. Catlett A. A comparison of dental hygienists' salaries to state dental supervision levels. *J Dent Hyg*. 2014;88(6):380-385. Summerfelt FF. Teledentistry-assisted, affiliated practice for dental hygienists: an innovative oral health workforce model. *J Dent Educ*. 2011;75(6):733-742.

determined by individual practice acts in each state, province, country, or territory.

- Types of supervision commonly used for dental hygiene practice are defined in **Box 1-2**.
- Many states have enacted **collaborative practice** legislative initiatives and adopted practice rules that allow dental hygienists to provide care autonomously for underserved populations in specifically designated public health settings.[7]

Box 1-3 Three Categories of Preventive Services

- **Primary prevention:** Measures carried out before disease occurs to prevent disease or injury. *Examples:* Sealants placed in deep grooves and pits to prevent caries; oral hygiene education; fluoridation of community water supplies; nutrition education on sugar-sweetened beverage consumption to reduce caries risk and obesity in children.
- **Secondary prevention:** Treatment of early disease to prevent further progression of potentially irreversible conditions that, if not arrested, can lead eventually to extensive rehabilitative treatment or even loss of teeth. *Examples:* Removal of all calculus and dental biofilm while debriding a root surface in a relatively shallow periodontal pocket to prevent continued attachment loss and the formation of a deep pocket; remineralization therapy; sealants on noncavitated caries.
- **Tertiary prevention:** Methods to replace lost tissues and to rehabilitate the oral cavity to a level where function is as near normal as possible after secondary prevention has not been successful. *Examples:* Replacement of a missing tooth using a fixed partial denture or implant and therefore restoring function; restorations; crowns; bone and tissue grafts.

III. Types of Clinical Services

The clinical responsibilities of the dental hygienist are divided into preventive, educational, and therapeutic services. Clinical and educational activities are inseparable and overlap as patient care is planned and accomplished.

- *Preventive services* are the methods employed by the clinician and/or patient to promote and maintain oral health.
  - Prevention is an essential component of dental hygiene practice.
  - The three categories of preventive services are defined in **Box 1-3**.
- *Educational services* are strategies developed for an individual or a group to promote behavior change to make healthy lifestyle choices.
  - Educational aspects of dental hygiene service permeate the entire patient care system.
  - Educate patients and the public about the growing body of evidence related to the

association between oral and systemic disease to highlight the need to manage oral health for overall wellness.
    - Create a partnership with the patient for success of both preventive and therapeutic services.
- *Therapeutic services* are clinical treatments designed to arrest or control disease and maintain oral tissues in health.
    - Dental hygiene treatment services are an integral part of the patient's overall treatment plan.
    - Periodontal debridement, along with the steps in posttreatment care, is a part of the therapeutic phase in the treatment of periodontal infections.

IV. Patient Education

- Clinical services, both dental and dental hygiene, have limited long-range probability of success if the patient does not understand the need to take responsibility in daily oral self-care and regular appointments for professional care.
- Educational and clinical services, therefore, are mutually dependent and inseparable in the total **dental hygiene care** of the patient.
- Scientific information about the prevention of oral disease and association with systemic disease continues to emerge.
- There is a growing awareness of the need for dental hygiene care and the value of preventive services provided by the dental hygienist.

V. Dental Hygiene Specialties

- Entry-level dental hygiene programs prepare students for basic clinical dental hygiene practice.[2,11]
- **Continuing education** can help build skills in advanced periodontal instrumentation.
- Private practice orthodontics, pediatric dentistry, and periodontics specialties tend to value dental hygienists as partners in prevention.
- Educational institutions offer dental hygiene associate degree programs, bachelor's degree programs, bachelor's degree completion programs, and master's degree programs.
- Bachelor and advanced degrees enhance the ability of dental hygienists to pursue opportunities outside of clinical practice.[11–13]
- Dental hygienists earn masters or doctoral degrees in a variety of areas, such as:
    - Dental hygiene education.
    - Health behavior and education.
    - Public health and health policy.
    - Nutrition and dietetics.
    - Business and administration.
    - Law.
- A dental hygienist interested in specialty areas of practice can take advantage of many learning opportunities to enhance knowledge and skills.
    - Many continuing education opportunities exist for learning in all areas of dental hygiene practice.
    - In other special areas, short-term courses have been developed, such as instruction in the care of patients with disabilities.
- In-service training may be available in long-term care institutions, hospitals, and skilled nursing facilities.
- Other dental hygienists have learned to practice in a specialty through private study, special conferences, and personal experience.

VI. Alternative Practice Settings

- In 2021, 42 states allowed dental hygienists to provide **direct access** care (**Figure 1-2**).[14]
- In Canada, dental hygiene is self-regulated and has different legislation in each province/territory regarding the scope of practice and level of autonomy.[15]
- Direct access dental hygienists work in a variety of community settings including, but not limited to:
    - Schools.
    - Public health settings.
    - Head Start settings.
    - WIC (women, infants, and children) clinics.
    - Nursing home facilities.
    - Free clinics.
    - Community centers.
- Direct access means the dental hygienist can plan and initiate treatment based on patient assessment without specific authorization of the dentist.
    - Each state, province/territory, and country practice act varies as to the scope of practice and level of supervision by a dentist.
- Dental hygiene care in alternative practice settings is further described in Chapter 4.

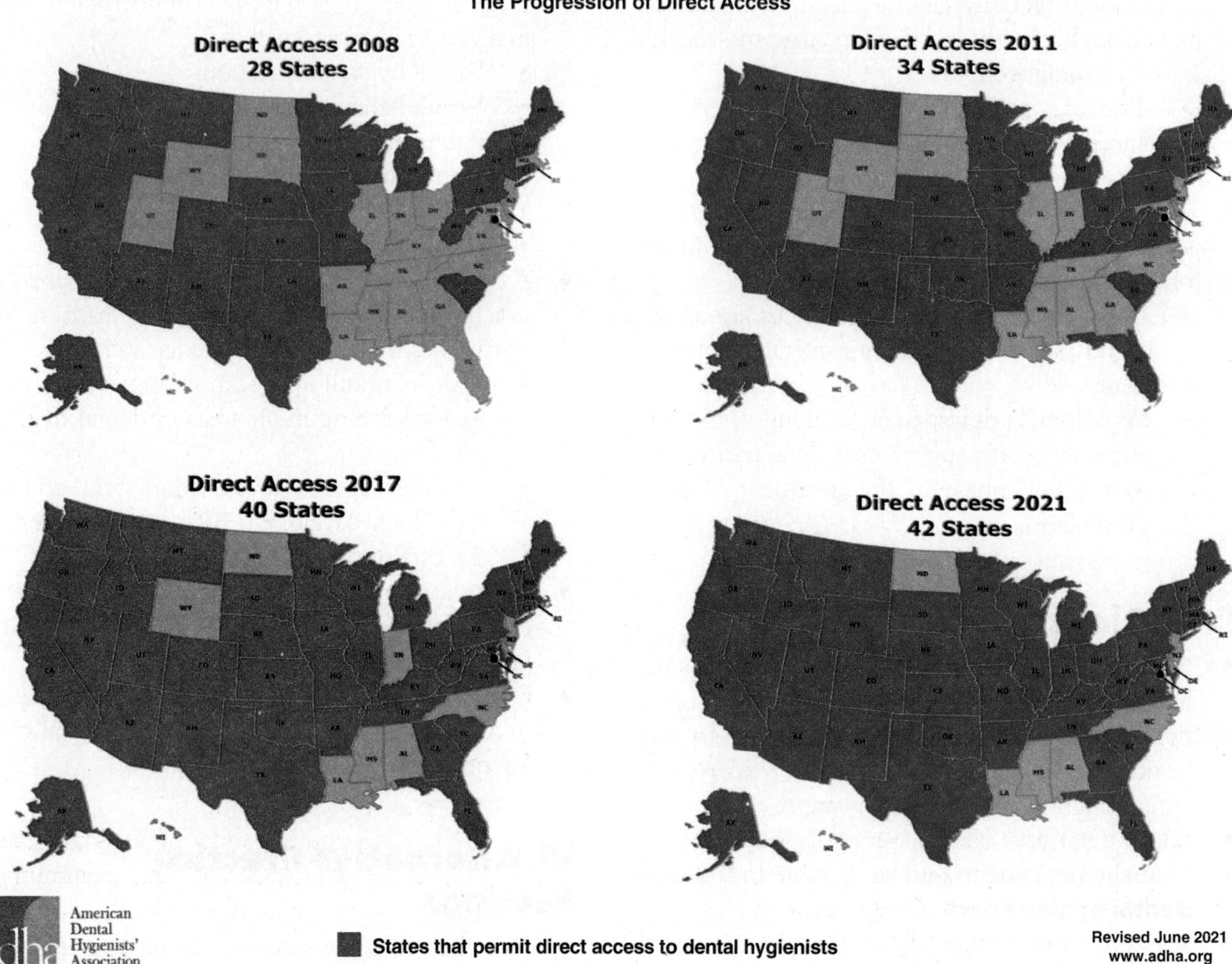

Figure 1-2 American Dental Hygienists' Association (ADHA) Direct Access. Maps of the United States to show the changes in the number and location of states with direct access since 2008

Reproduced from American Dental Hygienists' Association. The Progression of Direct Access. https://www.adha.org/resources-docs/ADHA_Progression_of_Direct_Access_2021.pdf

VII. Advanced Practice Dental Hygiene

- The current dental care model leaves many low-income individuals, at-risk populations, and those living in rural areas and inner cities without access to dental care.[16–18]
- Several mid-level dental provider models with a variety of names have emerged to address basic restorative and preventive care, particularly to children and, in some states/countries, to adults.
  - Internationally, the **dental therapist** was first introduced in 1921 in New Zealand and is now found in 54 countries.[19]
  - In 1949, Forsyth Dental Infirmary began an experiment to train New Zealand–type dental nurses, but it was stopped because of pressure from the American Dental Association.[20]
  - In 1971–1972, the Forsyth Experiment (more commonly known as the Rotunda Experiment) began training dental hygienists in basic restorative dentistry and local anesthesia.[21]
  - From 1971 to 1976, the University of Iowa and the University of Kentucky both trained dental hygienists with advanced skills in restorative dentistry.[22,23]
  - A Dental Health Aide Therapist (DHAT) was introduced in tribal villages in Alaska in 2006.[24] As of 2022, the DHAT model has also been authorized for pilots in Oregon, Idaho, Montana, New Mexico, and Washington tribal communities.[17]

A. Advanced Dental Hygiene Practitioner or Advanced Dental Therapist

- A 2009 Pew Report[25] first recognized that creating new mid-level oral healthcare providers, such as the Advanced Dental Hygiene

Practitioner proposed by the ADHA, could enhance access to oral health services for underserved populations.

- In 2009, the state of Minnesota approved the development of a master's-level degree program for advanced dental therapists (ADTs), which required applicants to be licensed dental hygienists holding a bachelor's degree. The University of Minnesota School of Dentistry (SOD) also developed a bachelor's dental therapy program and applicants were not required to be licensed dental hygienists.[26,27]
  - In 2016, the University of Minnesota SOD program evolved into a master's degree–level ADT program due to employers' preference for the dual licensure for dental hygiene and dental therapy.[28]
- These providers are dual licensed as a dental hygienist and dental therapist in Minnesota to provide preventive and basic restorative dental services[26,27]:
  - Directly to underserved populations.
  - Via a collaborative management agreement with a supervising dentist.
- Research findings suggest the safety and efficacy of restorative care provided by mid-level dental providers.[29,30] In addition, dental therapists expand access to under- and uninsured patients as well as diverse populations.[17]
- The Commission on Dental Accreditation (CODA) developed accreditation standards for dental therapy programs in 2015.[25]
- A variety of oral health stakeholder groups in many states continue to explore legislation to create new workforce models to increase access to quality oral health care for all individuals.[26–29]
- As of 2022, only an Alaska DHAT program has received CODA accreditation.[31] The Minnesota dental therapy programs were still under the authority of the Minnesota Board of Dentistry in 2020 and seeking CODA accreditation.[28]
- Other states that have passed dental therapy legislation, as of 2022, include the following[17]:
  - Maine passed legislation for a dental hygiene therapist in 2014, no educational programs available.
  - Vermont passed legislation in 2016, educational program under development.
  - Arizona, Connecticut, and Michigan passed legislation in 2018.
  - Nevada passed legislation in 2019.
  - Oregon passed legislation in 2021 following a pilot authorized in 2020.

B. Clinical Role of ADTs

- In addition to the traditional process of care performed by dental hygienists, the dental therapist has the following scope of practice[32]:
  - Caries removal, placement, and finishing of composite/resin and amalgam restorations.
  - Placement of space maintainers.
  - Fabrication and placement of stainless steel crowns and temporary crowns.
  - Pulpotomy.
  - Pulp vitality testing.
  - Simple extractions of erupted primary teeth.
  - Other duties may be specified in the state's scope of practice.
- ADT practice under a collaborative agreement with a dentist and patients who need more advanced care are referred.

C. Impact of ADTs

- The first dental therapists graduated in Minnesota in 2011.
- Initial impacts of this provider as part of the dental team include the following[17,33,34]:
  - An increase in the number of patients served in mobile dental clinics and community health centers, particularly the underserved and special populations.
  - Reduction in waiting times for patients to receive services.
  - Decreased travel time for patients because preventive and restorative care can be provided during the same appointment.
  - Possible reduction in emergency room use for dental care.
  - Increased productivity of the dental team.
  - Improved patient satisfaction.

VIII. Interprofessional Collaborative Patient Care

- In many situations, dental hygienists provide clinical patient care as a member of a dental team.
- In a growing number of facilities, dental hygienists provide care in collaboration with an interprofessional team of healthcare providers to meet the needs of patients with complex medical problems.
- Four **competency** domains necessary for participating in **interprofessional collaborative practice**, developed by a group of medical and dental professional associations, are explained in **Box 1-4**.[35]

- Based on the work of the interprofessional education collaborative, most medical and dental **accreditation** standards contain a standard related to the competency domains.[35]

IX. Advocacy for Oral Health

- The professional dental hygienist is an active advocate for oral health in both personal and professional situations.
- The dental hygienist who is an advocate for oral health:
  - Influences legislators, health agencies, and other organizations to bring available resources together to improve access to care.
  - Analyzes barriers to change and helps develop mechanisms to effect change.
  - Implements and evaluates health policy and programs that promote health for individuals, families, or communities.
  - Promotes lifestyle changes that contribute to oral health.

Box 1-4 Four Competency Domains for Interprofessional Collaborative Practice

Competency 1: Values/Ethics for Interprofessional Practice

Work with individuals of other professions to maintain a climate of mutual respect and shared values.

Competency 2: Roles/Responsibilities

Use the knowledge of one's own role and those of other professions to appropriately assess and address the healthcare needs of patients and to promote and advance the health of populations.

Competency 3: Interprofessional Communication

Communicate with patients, families, communities, and professionals in health and other fields in a responsive and responsible manner that supports a team approach to the promotion and maintenance of health and the prevention and treatment of disease.

Competency 4: Teams and Teamwork

Apply relationship-building values and the principles of team dynamics to perform effectively in different team roles to plan, deliver, and evaluate patient/population-centered care and population health programs and policies that are safe, timely, efficient, effective, and equitable.

Reproduced from Interprofessional Education Collaborative Expert Panel. Core Competencies for Interprofessional Collaborative Practice: 2016 Update. Washington, DC: Interprofessional Education Collaborative; 2016. https://www.ipecollaborative.org/resources.html. Accessed February 15, 2019.

- Examples of oral health advocacy activities include:
  - Joining other dental hygiene professionals to meet with legislators and public officials to encourage the inclusion of dental services in healthcare legislation.
  - Making public statements that support the oral health value of optimal fluoridation in community water systems when a community is considering defluoridation.

Objectives for Professional Practice

I. Overall Goals

- Overall professional goals of the dental hygiene profession relate to **health promotion** and disease prevention.
- The goal of each dental hygienist is *to aid individuals and groups in attaining and maintaining optimum oral health*. Other professional objectives are related to this primary goal.
- A dental hygienist's self-assessment is essential to attain goals for service to each patient and community.
- Personal and professional goals are outlined and reviewed frequently for continued self-improvement.

II. Personal Goals

- Exemplify the highest degree of professional **ethics** and conduct.
- Demonstrate interpersonal relationships that assure oral health information is presented effectively.
- Apply a continuing process of self-evaluation throughout professional life.
- Recognize the need for lifelong learning to acquire updated knowledge through reading professional literature and enrolling in continuing education programs.
- Maintain membership and active participation in the local, national, and international dental hygiene professional associations.

III. Clinical Practice Goals

- Maintain current knowledge and effective application of standard precautions for infection control in clinical practice.
- Apply evidence-based knowledge and understanding of the basic and clinical sciences to:
  - Associations between oral disease and a variety of systemic conditions.

- Recognition of oral conditions.
- Prevention and management of oral diseases.
- Patient education and clinical procedures.

- Tailor care planning and interventions according to individual needs.
- Utilize motivational interviewing to engage the patient in becoming an active participant in their care to bring about lasting behavioral changes to support optimal oral health.

Standards for Clinical Dental Hygiene Practice

- The primary purpose of standards for clinical practice is to guide dental hygiene practitioners in the development of a clinical relationship with their patients.[2,3]
- A secondary purpose is to educate the public, other healthcare providers, and policy makers about the profession of dental hygiene and the scope of dental hygiene practice.
- The six components of the **dental hygiene process of care** provide:
    - The foundation for clinical decision making and dental hygiene practice.
    - The framework for organizing the sections in this text.

Dental Hygiene Process of Care

- The dental hygiene process of care includes assessment, **dental hygiene diagnosis**, care or treatment planning, implementation, evaluation, and documentation, as illustrated in **Figure 1-3**.[2,32,36]
- The procedures of evaluation and documentation are integrated within each of the components in the process of care.
- As a process, the procedures performed are continual in nature and may overlap or occur simultaneously.

I. Purposes of the Dental Hygiene Process of Care

- To provide a framework to individualize the process of care for each patient.
- To identify the risk factors to aid in prevention and/or management of oral disease through dental hygiene interventions.

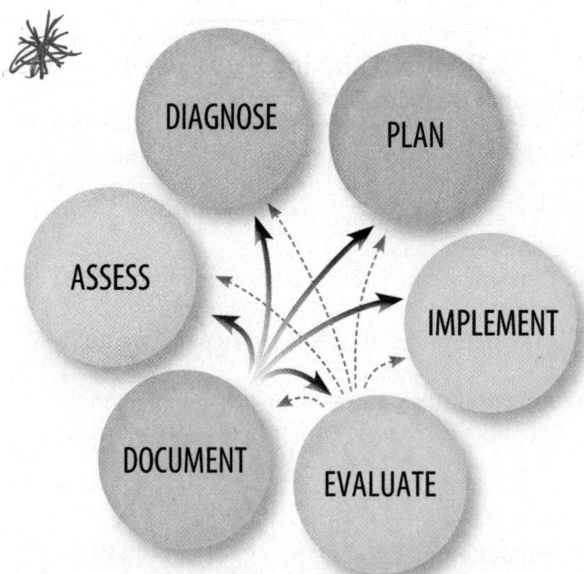

Figure 1-3 The Six Interrelated Components of the Dental Hygiene Process of Care. The steps in the process are followed one after another in a cycle, beginning with assessment. Evaluation and documentation are each linked to all of the other steps

II. Assessment

- The assessment phase is the first component of the dental hygiene process of care.
- This phase provides a foundation for patient care by collecting both subjective and objective data.
- Chapters 11–21 in this textbook are devoted to the assessment component of the dental hygiene process of care.

III. Dental Hygiene Diagnosis

- Dental hygiene diagnostic statements:
    - Employ the use of critical thinking to interpret assessment data, as indicated in **Box 1-5**.
    - Identify the health behaviors of each patient as well as the actual or potential oral health problems within the scope of practice for dental hygienists.
    - Provide the basis on which the **dental hygiene care plan** is designed, implemented, and evaluated.
    - Justify the treatment proposed to the patient.
- Chapter 22, Dental Hygiene Diagnosis, provides more information.

IV. The Dental Hygiene Care Plan

- Dental hygiene care planning is the selection of strategies and interventions that meet the needs of the patient in attaining oral health.

Box 1-5 Critical Thinking Skills Used to Interpret Clinical Data

- **Information gathering:** Pertinent information is gathered from the clinical assessments as well as from the patient to identify individual characteristics.
- **Classification:** Involves sorting of information into specific categories such as general systemic, oral soft tissue, periodontal, dental, and oral hygiene.
- **Interpretation:** Relies upon critical thinking to identify significance. The cognitive processes of analysis, synthesis, inductive reasoning, and deductive reasoning are the basis for determining a diagnosis.
- **Validation:** An attempt to verify the accuracy of data interpretation. Validation can assist in recognizing errors, isolating discrepancies, and identifying the need for additional information.

- The dental hygiene care plan is presented:
  - To the dentist for integration with the comprehensive dental care plan.
  - To the patient to develop understanding of the interventions needed and appointment requirements.
  - To the patient to obtain informed consent for treatment.
- Chapter 23 describes care planning and provides a template for the development of a written dental hygiene care plan.

V. Implementation

- The implementation phase in the dental hygiene process of care is the activation of the care plan.
- Further discussion of the concepts and procedures associated with implementation of dental hygiene preventive and treatment interventions is presented in Chapters 24–43.

VI. Evaluation

- The evaluation phase determines whether a specific area of a patient needs to be treated again, referred, or placed on a continuing care schedule.
- Evaluation of dental hygiene care is detailed in Chapter 44.
- Development of continuing care protocols is described in Chapter 45.

VII. Documentation

- The documentation of dental hygiene care:
  - Details all assessment data, diagnosis, care plan, treatments, patient education, and evaluation in a condensed, consistent format.
  - Represents a chronologic history of the patient's total care.
- Details for documentation are described in Chapter 10 and examples of documentation for a variety of dental hygiene interventions can be found at the end of each chapter.

Dental Hygiene Ethics

- The ethics of a profession provide the general standards of right and wrong that guide the behavior of the members in that profession.
- The members of a profession[37]:
  - Have extensive specialized education.
  - Possess mastery of a complex body of knowledge from study and research.
  - Provide services important for the common good of society; for example, dental hygienists provide preventive, educational, and therapeutic services that protect and enhance the overall health of the public.
  - Maintain an organization of members that sets professional standards.
  - Exercise autonomy and judgment in self-regulation.
  - Adhere to their professional code of ethics.

The Code of Ethics

- Describes professional conduct.
- Outlines responsibilities and duties of each member toward patients, colleagues, and society in general.

I. Purposes of the Code of Ethics

- To increase the awareness of, and sensitivity to, ethical situations in practice.
- To define a standard of conduct that will give each individual a strong sense of ethical consciousness in professional practice as well as in all phases of life.

II. Dental Hygiene Codes

- The Codes of the ADHA, the National Dental Hygienists' Association, the Canadian Dental Hygienists' Association, and the International Federation of Dental Hygienists can be accessed online.

- Each dental hygienist is responsible for the study and application of the codes of the particular associations in which memberships are held.

Core Values

Core values are selected principles of ethical behavior that are considered central to the code of a profession.

I. Core Values in Professional Practice

- The core values of the profession of dental hygiene are listed and defined in **Box 1-6** and in the ADHA Code of Ethics.
  - The core values are only part of the Code of Ethics for Dental Hygienists and students are encouraged to read the complete document at www.adha.org/bylaws-ethics.
- The complete ADHA Code of Ethics includes the following[38]:
  - Basic Beliefs.
  - Fundamental Principles.
  - Core Values.
  - Standards of Professional Responsibility.

II. Personal Values

- Value development begins at an early age and is influenced by familial, social, and economic factors.
- Personal values are guiding principles in one's life.[39]
- Members of a health profession can benefit from periodic self-assessment of individual values, attitudes, and responsibilities as they relate to professional practice.

III. Patient Centered

- Patient-centered care, or putting the patient first, is essential.
- Dental hygienists are ethically, morally, and legally responsible to provide oral care for all patients without discrimination.
- Ethical decision making and professional behavior should be reflected in every aspect of dental hygiene practice.

IV. Lifelong Learning: An Ethical Duty

- To ensure optimal care for each patient.
- To maintain competency.
- To learn scientific advances from new research.
- To provide evidence-based patient care.
- To apply consistent ethical reasoning.
- To ensure fulfillment of each patient's **rights**.

Box 1-6 Core Values in Professional Dental Hygiene Practice

Individual autonomy and respect for human beings
People have the right to be treated with respect. They have the right to informed consent prior to treatment, and they have the right to full disclosure of all relevant information so that they can make informed choices about their care.

Confidentiality
We respect the confidentiality of patient information and relationships as a demonstration of the value we place on individual autonomy. We acknowledge our obligation to justify any violation of a confidence.

Societal trust
We value patient trust and understand that public trust in our profession is based on our actions and behavior.

Nonmaleficence
We accept our fundamental obligation to provide services in a manner that protects all patients and minimizes harm to them and others involved in their treatment.

Beneficence
We have a primary role in promoting the well-being of individuals and the public by engaging in health promotion/disease prevention activities.

Justice/fairness
We value justice and support the fair and equitable distribution of healthcare resources. We believe all people should have access to high-quality, affordable oral health care.

Veracity
We accept our obligation to tell the truth and expect that others will do the same. We value self-knowledge and seek truth and honesty in all relationships.

Reproduced from American Dental Hygienists' Association. Bylaws and Code of Ethics. Chicago, IL: ADHA; Adopted June 2021:34-35. https://www.adha.org/bylaws-ethics. Accessed April 16, 2022.

Ethical Applications

A dental hygienist may be involved in a variety of **moral**, ethical, and legal situations as part of the daily routine. In ethics, a problem situation is considered either an **ethical issue** or an **ethical dilemma**.

I. Ethical Issue

- More clearly defined than a dilemma.
- A common problem wherein a solution is grounded in the governing practice act, recognized laws, or accepted standards of care based on the standard rules of practice.

II. Ethical Dilemma

- A problem that may involve two morally correct choices or courses of action.
- May not have a single answer and, depending on the choice, the outcomes can differ.

III. Models for Resolution of an Issue or a Dilemma

- There are a number of models for resolution of an ethical issue or dilemma, and all include elements of the following[40,41]:
  - Identify the facts of the issue or dilemma.
  - Identify who is involved in the issue or dilemma.
  - List options or alternatives to resolve the dilemma.
  - Rank and choose the best option or alternative to resolve the dilemma while trying to balance the various aspects of the ADHA Code of Ethics, such as individual autonomy, beneficence, nonmaleficence, autonomy, and justice/fairness.[34]
- An ethical decision-making model that can be used by the dental hygienist to resolve an ethical issue or dilemma in a clinical setting is detailed in **Box 1-7**.[35]

IV. Summary: The Final Decision

- Many factors can be used to solve a dilemma.
- All dental healthcare providers involved in the decision process can participate in a follow-up evaluation of the action taken.
- Questions to ask once a decision has been made include:
  - Is the decision/action that is selected morally defensible?
  - Can the choice to solve the dilemma be defended?
- A professional dental hygienist may need to defend it to the patient, the dentist, members of the dental team, a state board, or even a court of law.
- Most importantly, the decision must be defensible based on standards of practice established for the dental and dental hygiene profession.

Legal Factors in Practice

- The law must be studied and respected by each dental hygienist practicing within the state, province, or country.
- Although the various practice acts have certain basic similarities, differences in scope and definition exist.

Box 1-7 A Model for Resolution of an Ethical Issue or Dilemma

Step 1: Information	Gather information on the patient's medical, dental, and social history related to the situation.
Step 2: Identification	Assess whether this is an ethical issue or whether it is an issue best addressed by other resources.
Step 3: Clarification	Do the practitioner and patient understand the information relevant to the situation? What are the patient's rights? Is there a conflict of interest? Does an outside source need to be consulted?
Step 4: Assessment	Generate options or alternatives based on the patient situation and preferences. Consider the core values of the ADHA Code of Ethics to assess benefits and risks related to the alternatives. Collaboration with the patient and possibly other healthcare providers is part of the process of assessment of the alternatives.
Step 5: Recommendation	Choose the best alternative and obtain informed consent from the patient.
Step 6: Documentation	Document the recommendation in the patient record. Follow-up.

Data from Enck G. Six-step framework for ethical decision making. *J Health Serv Res Policy.* 2014;19(1):62-64.

- Terminology varies, but each practice act regulates the patient services delivered by the licensed dental hygienist.
  - It is the responsibility of each dental hygienist to stay current with changes to the practice act.
- Active engagement with the state dental hygiene association will aid in keeping the dental hygienist up to date.

Professionalism

- Each dental hygienist represents the entire profession to the patient, other healthcare professionals, and the community.
- Components of professionalism include[42]:
  - Competence: Acquire and maintain a high level of knowledge through lifelong learning, clinical expertise, and professional behavior for provision of patient care.
  - Fairness: Demonstrate consistency and equity when dealing with others. Promote equal access to care for the public.
  - Integrity: Be honest, do the right thing, and demonstrate strong moral principles.
  - Responsibility: Accountability for one's actions in accordance with the ADHA Code of Ethics.
  - Respect: Value and honor others' feelings, rights, abilities, etc.
  - Service-mindedness: Act for the benefit of the patients and public, and approach those served with compassion.
- The World Health Organization defines **health** as a state of physical, mental, and social well-being.[43] As healthcare providers, we must serve as a model for our patients.
- Basic components of self-care include a range of daily routine habits, health maintenance, and disease prevention behaviors. These components include the following:
  - *General physical needs* include personal hygiene, sleep, nutrition. Nutrition is discussed in Chapter 33.
- Routine examinations annually, including tests for hearing, sight, and certain communicable diseases.
- Immunizations recommended for healthcare providers. (See Chapter 5.)
- The maintenance of a healthy mouth models for the patient the value the dental hygienist places on prevention and control of oral disease.
- *Physical activity* helps with weight control, maintaining mental health, prevention of chronic disease, strengthening bone and muscle, managing stress, and even improving daily activity performance.[44]
- Recommendations for adults are for at least 150 minutes/week of moderate-intensity aerobic activity in addition to muscle strengthening activities at least 2 days/week.
- *Mental health*: The mental health of the dental hygienist is reflected in interpersonal relationships and the ability to inspire confidence through a display of professional and emotional maturity.
- Stress management helps to improve and manage mental health.[43]
- Avoid risky behaviors such as tobacco use, excessive alcohol use, illicit drug use, and risky sexual practices to prevent adverse effects and chronic diseases such as cardiovascular disease.[43]

Factors to Teach the Patient

- The role of the dental hygienist as a **co-therapist** with each patient, with the dentist, and with members of other health professions.
- The moral and ethical nature of being a dental hygiene professional.
- The scope of service of the dental hygienist as defined by the state practice act.
- The interrelationship of educational and clinical services in dental hygiene patient care.
- The shared responsibility of the patient for their oral health and how it can be improved and maintained.

References

1. Federation of Dental Hygiene Regulators of Canada. The dental hygiene profession in Canada. https://www.fdhrc.ca/wp/the-dental-hygiene-profession-in-canada/. Accessed March 27, 2022.
2. Federation of Dental Hygiene Regulators of Canada (FDHRC). *Entry-to-Practice Canadian Competencies for Dental Hygienists*. Dental Hygiene Regulators of Canada (FDHRC); 2021:34. https://www.fdhrc.ca/wp/competency-project/. Accessed January 15, 2022.
3. American Dental Hygienists' Association. *2016 Revised Standards for Clinical Dental Hygiene Practice*. Published June 2016. https://www.adha.org/resources-docs/2016-Revised-Standards-for-Clinical-Dental-Hygiene-Practice.pdf. Accessed December 11, 2021.

4. Fones AC. The origin and history of the dental hygienists. *J Dent Hyg*. 2013;87(Suppl 1):58-62.
5. American Dental Hygienists' Association. Career paths. https://www.adha.org/professional-roles. Accessed March 27, 2022.
6. American Dental Hygienists' Association. Scope of practice. https://www.adha.org/scope-of-practice. Accessed March 27, 2022.
7. American Dental Hygienists' Association. Direct access. https://www.adha.org/direct-access. Accessed April 16, 2022.
8. Summerfelt FF. Teledentistry-assisted, affiliated practice for dental hygienists: an innovative oral health workforce model. *J Dent Ed*. 2011;75(6):733-742.
9. Catlett A. A comparison of dental hygienists' salaries to state dental supervision levels. *J Dent Hyg*. 2014;88(6):380-385.
10. American Dental Hygienists' Association. *Dental Hygiene Practice Act Overview. Permitted Functions and Supervision Levels by State*. Published online March 2021. https://www.adha.org/resources-docs/7511_Permitted_Services_Supervision_Levels_by_State.pdf. Accessed April 16, 2022.
11. Battrell A, Lynch A, Steinbach P, Bessner S, Snyder J, Majeski J. Advancing education in dental hygiene. *J Evid Based Dent Pract*. 2014;14:209-221.e1.
12. DeRosa Hays R, Moglia Willis S. The baccalaureate as the minimum entry-level degree in dental hygiene. *J Dent Hyg*. 2021;95(6):46-53.
13. Jones-Teti J, Boyd LD, LaSpina L. Career paths and satisfaction of dental hygienists holding master's and doctoral degrees. *J Dent Hyg*. 2021;95(6):54-62.
14. American Dental Hygienists' Association. Direct access 2019: 42states.https://www.adha.org/resources-docs/7524_Current_Direct_Access_Map.pdf. Accessed January 30, 2021.
15. Canadian Dental Hygienists Association. *Dental Hygiene Profession in Canada*. Published online May 2021. https://files.cdha.ca/profession/Regulatory_Authority_chart_0521_FINAL.pdf. Accessed April 16, 2022.
16. National Research Council, Institute of Medicine, Board on Health Care Services, Board on Children, Youth, and Families, Committee on Oral Health Access to Services. *Improving Access to Oral Health Care for Vulnerable and Underserved Populations*. National Academies Press; 2012.
17. Mertz E, Kottek A, Werts M, Langelier M, Surdu S, Moore J. Dental therapists in the United States: health equity, advancing. *Med Care*. 2021;59(Suppl 5):S441-S448.
18. US Department of Health and Human Services, National Institutes of Health, National Institute of Dental. *Oral Health in America: Advances and Challenges*. US Department of Health and Human Services; 2021. https://www.nidcr.nih.gov/sites/default/files/2021-12/Oral-Health-in-America-Advances-and-Challenges.pdf. Accessed April 16, 2022.
19. Nash DA, Friedman JW, Mathu-Muju KR, et al. A review of the global literature on dental therapists. *Community Dent Oral Epidemiol*. 2014;42(1):1-10.
20. American Dental Association. Massachusetts dental nurse bill rescinded. *J Am Dent Assoc*. 1950;41:371.
21. Lobene RR. *The Forsyth Experiment: An Alternative System for Dental Care*. Harvard University Press; 1979. https://www.hup.harvard.edu/catalog.php?isbn=9780674310353. Accessed April 16, 2022.
22. Spohn EE, Chiswell LR, Davison DD. *The University of Kentucky Experimental Expanded Duties Dental Hygiene Project*. Lexington, KY: College of Dentistry, University of Kentucky; 1976:54.
23. Sisty NL, Henderson WG, Paule CL, Martin JF. Evaluation of student performance in the four-year study of expanded functions for dental hygienists at the University of Iowa. *J Am Dent Assoc*. 1978;97(4):613-627.
24. Wetterhall S, Bader JD, Burrus BB, Lee JY, Shugars DA. *Evaluation of the Dental Health Aide Therapist Workforce Model in Alaska*. Published online 2010. http://www.npaihb.org/download/authoring_project/native_dental_therapy_initiative/Alaska-DHAT-Program-Evaluation-Final-10-25-10-1.pdf. Accessed July 18, 2022.
25. Pew Center of the States, National Academy for State Health Policy, W.K. Kellogg Foundation. *Help Wanted: A Policy Maker's Guide to New Dental Providers*. Dental Therapy Resources. https://dentaltherapyresourceguide.wkkf.org/resources/resource/help-wanted-a-policy-makers-guide-to-new-dental-providers/. Accessed April 16, 2022.
26. American Dental Hygienists' Association. *The History of Introducing a New Provider in Minnesota: A Chronicle of Legislative Efforts 2008-2009*. Published online September 2015. https://www.adha.org/resources-docs/75113_Minnesota_Story.pdf. Accessed April 16, 2022.
27. Gwozdek AE, Tetrick R, Shaefer HL. The origins of Minnesota's mid-level dental practitioner: alignment of problem, political and policy streams. *J Dent Hyg*. 2014;88(5):292-301.
28. Self K, Brickle C. Dental therapy education in Minnesota. *Am J Public Health*. 2017;107(Suppl 1):S77-S80.
29. Mathu-Muju KR. Dental therapists provide technically competent clinical care when performing irreversible restorative procedures. *J Evid Based Dent Pract*. 2014;14(1):25-27.
30. Phillips E, Shaefer HL. Dental therapists: evidence of technical competence. *J Dent Res*. 2013;92(7 Suppl):11S-15S.
31. Commission on Dental Accreditation, American Dental Association. Search for dental programs: dental therapy. https://coda.ada.org/en/find-a-program/search-dental-programs#t=us&sort=%40codastatecitysort%20ascending&f:@programnamesubl_coveofacets_1=[Dental%20Therapy]. Accessed April 16, 2022.
32. Commission on Dental Accreditation, American Dental Association. Current accreditation standards. https://www.ada.org/en/coda/current-accreditation-standards. Accessed April 16, 2022.
33. Minnesota Board of Dentistry. *Early Impacts of Dental Therapists in Minnesota*. Minnesota Department of Health; 2014:42. https://mn.gov/boards/assets/2014DentalTherapistReport_tcm21-45970_tcm21-313376.pdf. Accessed April 16, 2022.
34. Langlier M, Surdu S, Moore J. *The Contributions of Dental Therapists and Advanced Dental Therapists in the Dental Centers of Apple Tree Dental in Minnesota*. Center for Health Workforce Studies, School of Public Health, SUNY; 2020. https://www.chwsny.org/our-work/reports-briefs/the-contributions-of-dental-therapists-and-advanced-dental-therapists-in-the-dental-centers-of-apple-tree-dental-in-minnesota/. Accessed April 16, 2022.
35. Interprofessional Education Collaborative. Core competencies for interprofessional collaborative practice: 2016 update. Published online 2016. https://www.ipecollaborative.org/core-competencies. Accessed July 18, 2022.
36. American Dental Hygienists' Association. *Dental Hygiene Diagnosis*. Published online September 2015. https://www.adha.org/resources-docs/Diagnosis-Position-Paper.pdf. Accessed April 16, 2022.

37. Cruess SR, Johnston S, Cruess RL. "Profession": a working definition for medical educators. *Teach Learn Med.* 2004; 16(1):74-76.
38. American Dental Hygienists' Association. Bylaws & code of ethics. Published online June 2021. https://www.adha.org/bylaws-ethics. Accessed April 16, 2022.
39. Sagiv L, Roccas S, Cieciuch J, Schwartz SH. Personal values in human life. *Nat Hum Behav.* 2017;1(9):630-639.
40. Enck G. Six-step framework for ethical decision making. *J Health Serv Res & Policy.* 2014;19(1):62-64.
41. American College of Dentists. Resources: Facilitating discussion of ethics dilemmas. Dental Ethics. Published 2021. https://www.dentalethics.org/resources/. Accessed April 16, 2022.
42. American Dental Education Association. ADEA Statement on Professionalism in Dental Education. Published 2009. https://www.adea.org/Pages/Professionalism.aspx. Accessed April 17, 2022.
43. World Health Organization. Health and well-being. https://www.who.int/data/gho/data/major-themes/health-and-well-being. Accessed April 17, 2022.
44. U.S. Department of Health and Human Services. *Physical Activity Guidelines for Americans,* 2nd ed.; 2018:118. https://health.gov/sites/default/files/2019-09/Physical_Activity_Guidelines_2nd_edition.pdf. Accessed April 17, 2022.

CHAPTER 2

Evidence-Based Dental Hygiene Practice

Faizan Kabani, RDH, PhD

CHAPTER OUTLINE

LEARNING OBJECTIVES

After studying this chapter, the student will be able to:

1. Explain evidence-based practice and its importance in clinical dental hygiene care.
2. Discuss various approaches to research, including the strength of evidence each provides.
3. Describe a systematic approach that can be used to find credible scientific literature.
4. Describe skills needed for analyzing evidence-based health information.

One of the main goals of clinical dental hygiene practice is to improve and maintain the patient's oral health. Clinical problems occur daily and require interventions based on current, valid, and reliable **evidence** to improve the patient's overall well-being.

- The evidence-based clinician relies on established **best practices** to guide their decision-making processes.
- **Evidence-based decision making (EBDM)** is a process of making decisions that are grounded

in the best available research, professional experience, and factors related to each patient's **context**, including needs and preferences.[1]

Evidence-Based Practice

I. Definition

- An interprofessional approach to clinical care where the clinician, in consultation with the patient, uses the best **scientific evidence** available to make decisions about clinical interventions needed to promote health.[2]
- **Evidence-based practice (EBP)** is the practical application of EBDM across diverse clinical and nonclinical professions. In health care, an interprofessional EBP approach incorporates the knowledge and expertise from diverse professions (i.e., collaboration among medical, dental, and research) to provide the best quality of care to patients.
- EBP assists dental hygienists in formulating a plan for objective, effective, and scientifically sound interventions that meet patient needs and provide positive health outcomes.
- EBP involves three major elements[3] (**Figure 2-1**):
  - Clinically relevant scientific evidence.
  - Sensitivity to patient's needs and preferences.
  - Healthcare professionals' clinical expertise.

II. Purposes

- To answer clinical questions quickly and efficiently.
- To resolve problems in patient care using current evidence.
- To improve patients' health outcomes and overall well-being.

III. The Need for EBP

A professional dental hygienist understands the following concepts and embraces the role of the evidence-based practitioner.

- Patients frequently search for health information on the Internet and other readily available sources.
- Patients:
  - Expect clinicians to be knowledgeable on the latest developments in health care.
  - Value practitioners who can discuss and help them evaluate the relevance, **validity**, and **reliability** of information obtained elsewhere.
  - Demand healthcare providers who remain current with evidence-based information on the most up-to-date oral health practices, techniques, technologies, and products.

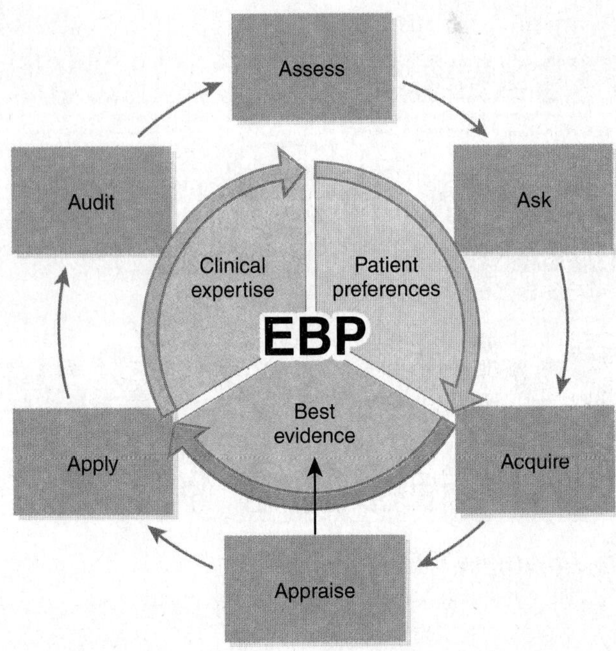

Figure 2-1 Evidence-Based Practice (EBP) Model for Dental Hygiene

Courtesy of Cathy J. Thompson, PhD, RN, CCNS, CNE.

- There are differences in practice procedures:
  - Clinicians are not consistently knowledgeable about all new and emerging therapies.
  - There may be inconsistencies between what is taught in dental hygiene schools and procedures tested by regional examination boards for licensure.
- Information management:
  - The amount of published evidence-based research continues to increase annually.
  - Clinicians need to be good consumers of current scientific literature and focus on higher levels of evidence to guide their decision making.

IV. EBP Model for Dental Hygiene Practice

The EBP model for dental hygiene care involves interaction among three primary components,[4] as illustrated in Figure 2-1.

- *Best available research evidence*. Review of relevant, current, and high-quality clinical research that identifies best-practice treatment choices.
- *Patient preferences or values*. Consider, respect, and evaluate the patient's needs, wants, expectations, and personal context (i.e., cultural, religious, capabilities, health status, and demographics).

- *Clinical expertise.* The dental hygienist's clinical skill and expertise enhance their ability to identify the patient's health, risks, needs, and potential for various interventions.

V. Skills Needed for Evidence-Based Dental Hygiene Practice

Implementing **evidence-based dental hygiene (EBDH) practice** into everyday clinical practice is an ethical responsibility for the dental hygienist. Identifying and using scientific evidence to support treatment and preventive interventions and recommendations require the dental hygienist to:

- *Understand EBDH practice.* Study a tutorial (examples listed in **Box 2-1**) to learn more about EBP.
- *Follow a systematic approach.* Develop a step-by-step approach by asking questions related to clinical practice to ensure success.
- *Read and understand research.* Recognize valid and reliable information. Determine strengths and limitations of publications, journal articles, research methods, study designs, and **biostatistics**.
- *Be computer literate.* Develop the skill to search for scientific literature in an effective and efficient manner. Practice critical thinking skills to evaluate information found online.
- *Embrace self-directed learning.* Develop a plan for continuing education and reading of professional literature that will help to maintain current knowledge.

Box 2-1 Evidence-Based Tutorials and Learning Opportunities

- Duke University: https://guides.mclibrary.duke.edu/ebptutorial
- Boston University Medical Campus: www.bumc.bu.edu/medlib/resources/tutorials/ebmebd-tutorials/
- University of Massachusetts Medical School: https://libraryguides.umassmed.edu/c.php?g=499783&p=3421956
- University of North Carolina at Chapel Hill: www.hsl.unc.edu/Services/Tutorials/EBM/welcome.htm
- University of Illinois at Chicago: http://researchguides.uic.edu/ebm
- The Cochrane Collaboration: https://training.cochrane.org/essentials
- PubMed Tutorial: www.nlm.nih.gov/oet/ed/pubmed/pubmed_in_ebp/index.html

- *Be a resource for others.* Help patients and colleagues identify and value scientific support for clinical recommendations.

A Systematic Approach

Dental hygienists should follow a systematic approach when identifying and selecting scientific evidence related to a particular patient's healthcare needs. The "6 As" approach includes *Assess, Ask, Acquire, Appraise, Apply*, and *Audit*.[3] **Figure 2-2** illustrates a step-by-step procedure that aids the dental hygienist in developing these crucial skills.

I. Assess: Determine the Clinical Issue

- The dental hygienist first completes an assessment of the patient or population.
- Next step is to identify what the clinical issue or problem is for the patient or population.
- Purpose is to clarify the clinical issue or problem.

II. Ask: Develop a Research Question

- Asking the right **research question** is fundamental and critical to the EBP model.
- Research questions should be focused and not be too broad or too narrow.
- A researchable question includes four parts, referred to as PICO. Examples of PICO questions related to dental hygiene practice can be found in **Table 2-1**.
- Good research questions should also adhere to the FINER criteria.
- Include important patient demographics (i.e., age, sex, race, and ethnicity).

A. PICO Criteria[5]

- *Patient problem or population (P):* What are the most important issues the patient or population of interest is facing?
- *Intervention (I):* What are you planning to do to address the patient's or population of interest's issues?
- *Comparison (C):* What is the main alternative being suggested? Compare the alternative with the standard intervention for the patient or population of interest.
- *Outcome (O):* What is the desired measurable outcome, accomplishment, improvement, or effect from the proposed intervention on the patient or the population of interest?

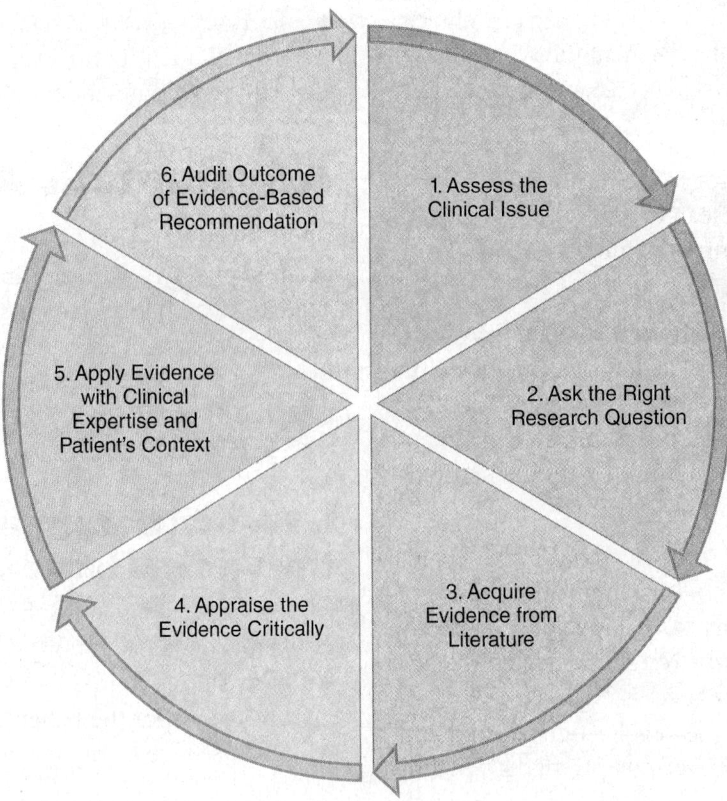

Figure 2-2 Systematic Steps in Evidence-Based Dental Hygiene Practice

Alper BS, Haynes RB. EBHC pyramid 5.0 for accessing preappraised evidence and guidance. *BMJ Evid Based Med*. 2016;21(4):123-125.

Table 2-1 Example of Clinical and Public Health–Related PICO Questions

Scenario	PICO Question
Mr. Ali is a 65-year-old Asian American who presents for his periodontal maintenance appointment. He reports a chief complaint of dental hypersensitivity when drinking cold beverages. He currently uses a generic, over-the-counter fluoridated toothpaste. He is wondering if there is any particular active ingredient he should consider when purchasing a toothpaste.	For a patient with concerns of dental hypersensitivity, will a toothpaste with potassium nitrate be more effective at reducing hypersensitivity than a toothpaste with traditional fluoride? ▪ **Patient/problem:** Patient reports chief complaint of dental hypersensitivity ▪ **Intervention:** Toothpaste with potassium nitrate as active ingredient ▪ **Comparison:** Traditional toothpaste with fluoride as active ingredient ▪ **Outcome:** Reduction in dental hypersensitivity
Mrs. Nisa Rumi is a 35-year-old African-American superintendent of a predominately Medicaid-based school district. She reports there is a dental caries epidemic in one of her elementary school's first-grade classrooms. Your dental office currently volunteers in an annual fluoride varnish program to help address dental caries. Mrs. Nisa Rumi mentions that she has heard from one of her principals about placement of dental sealants as another way to address the dental caries epidemic. She is wondering which route, placement of fluoride varnish or dental sealants, best helps to address the dental caries epidemic in her school district.	For a population experiencing a dental caries epidemic, will placement of dental sealants be as effective (or more effective) as application of fluoride varnish to help reduce dental caries? ▪ **Population/problem:** Dental caries epidemic in first-grade classroom of a predominately Medicaid-based school district ▪ **Intervention:** Placement of dental sealants ▪ **Comparison:** Application of fluoride varnish ▪ **Outcome:** Reduction in dental caries epidemic

Research about comparative cost is in addition to the literature review.

B. FINER Criteria[5]

- *Feasibility (F):* Are the necessary resources available to conduct the research study?
- *Interesting (I):* Is the research interesting, self-motivating, and/or intriguing?
- *Novel (N):* Is the research innovative? Does the research aim to address significant gaps in the literature?
- *Ethical (E):* Does the research align within ethical and legal standards/requirements?
- *Relevant (R):* Does the research advance the body of scientific knowledge in the particular healthcare field?

III. Acquire: Search for Scientific Evidence

- Select appropriate resources and conduct a thorough **literature review**. Scientific articles are available through library databases and by using appropriate search engines. Focus the literature review toward current and higher levels of evidence publications (**Figure 2-3**).

A. Types of Information Sources

- Primary sources are original accounts of events and/or publications. Primary sources are significant because they provide unfiltered access to an original record of thought and/or achievement during a specific period in history. Examples of primary sources include narratives, speeches, autobiographies, government documents, patents, raw data sets, and experimental research reports.
- Secondary sources are published materials that synthesize and/or analyze original sources. Examples of secondary sources include biographies, literature reviews, and nonexperimental scholarly articles.
- Tertiary sources are published materials that provide overviews of particular topics with information gathered from multiple sources. Examples of tertiary sources include encyclopedias, textbooks, and websites.

B. Types of Publications

The sources for obtaining scientific information are growing daily. Knowing how to determine the validity

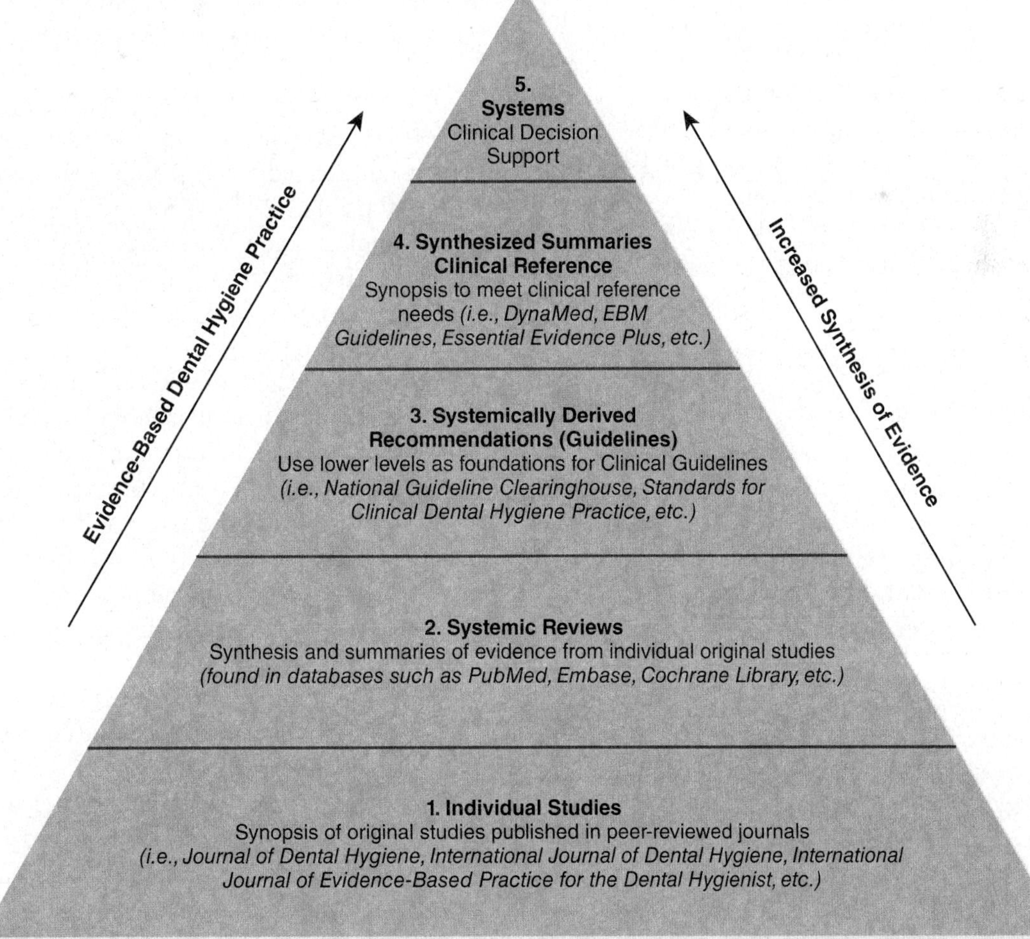

Figure 2-3 Strength of Evidence Resources

and reliability of information is critical for selecting successful patient care strategies and interventions. Refer to **Box 2-2** for a checklist of questions to ask when considering the validity and/or reliability of a publication.

- Textbooks
  - Generally accepted as credible basic-level resources.
  - Drawn-out publication processes can make textbooks become outdated quickly.
- Commercial-based journals/magazines
  - Often free and based on product and/or service sponsorships.
  - Potentially written by in-house staff members without professional credentials.
  - Some articles summarize recent research that may contain selective reference citations, but not include all available scientific evidence.
- Professional journals
  - Produced by professional organizations. Membership dues payment is required, or receiving publications is a benefit of being a member.
  - Part or all of the publication is devoted to scientific studies. Most contain articles with supporting reference citations.
- Peer-reviewed (refereed) publications
  - Subject matter experts (SMEs) critically examine all components of submitted manuscripts before recommending for or against publication.
  - Contributing author(s) must revise the manuscript and address all significant concerns or answer questions expressed by the reviewing SMEs before receiving approval for publication.
  - The **peer review** process helps assure the validity, reliability, and objectivity of published journal articles.
  - Peer-reviewed journals usually list all review board members and their respective credentials in each issue of the journal.

Box 2-2 Questions to Ask When Considering the Validity of a Publication

- Who is sponsoring?
- Is there an editorial review board?
- Are the journal articles peer-reviewed?
- What are the credentials of the contributors?
- Are there advertisements? How many?
- Are there good-quality production standards?
- Is the manuscript preparation information included?
- What type of articles are included? (Informational? Opinion/editorial? Case reports? Scientific study?)

C. Online Information

- The Internet continues to evolve as an avenue for people to search for health-related information.
- American adults are increasingly using online resources to diagnose either themselves or others.[6]
- Many popular search engines lead to newspaper and magazine articles or websites that may not provide science-based and/or research-supported information.
  - Search engines cannot assure the validity, accuracy, and objectivity of information.
  - Search engines display only fractions of all available resources on a specific topic.
- Search engines can also provide access to more valid and reliable websites that offer a variety of health information. Be familiar with the credibility level of various domain names:
  - Highest credibility: Governmental sources (.gov) and educational sources (.edu).
  - Moderate credibility: Organizational sources (.org) and institutional sources (.net).
  - Lowest credibility: Commercial sources (.com).
- Use the C.R.A.P. test for determining the credibility of information found online[7]:
  - Currency: Consider when the source was published and if the information is still current or relevant today. For example, websites with outdated information should be avoided.
  - Reliability: Consider the credibility and applicability of the information. For example, reliable information will come from websites that are peer-reviewed, are published by dependable organizations, and provide references to substantiate their claims.
  - Authority: Consider the reputation of the author. For example, authors of an information source, whether individuals or organizations, should hold appropriate academic and professional credentials.
  - Purpose: Consider the intent of the website. For example, sources may have the intent to inform, educate, entertain, persuade, or provide satirical information.
- Refer to **Box 2-3** for questions to ask when assessing information found on the Internet.

Box 2-3 **Questions to Ask When Assessing Information Found on the Internet**

- Who are the authors? What are their qualifications?
- Is the source peer-reviewed or edited?
- What is the domain name and source (i.e., .gov, .edu, .org, .net, .com, .mil)?
- Does the site have any affiliated biases?
- Does the author list sources or citations?
- Is the information verifiable elsewhere?
- Does the site reflect a particular bias or viewpoint?
- Are obvious errors in spelling or grammar present?
- Who is the website targeting as their audience?
- When was the website created and last updated/revised?
- Are the links current, good, and helpful? Are any links dead?
- Is the site comprehensive?
- Is the site easy to read?
- Are the site and material well organized?

- Search engines and databases devoted to specific professional literature provide access to information from scholarly articles in biomedical and other health-related journals.
- Some governmental agencies and nongovernmental associations specifically help people find credible health-related information on the web. These include:
  - HealthFinder.[8]
  - MedlinePlus.[9]
  - Medical Library Association.[10]
- Accrediting organizations provide certification aimed at assuring accurate and objective health information on the Internet.
  - Health on the Net Foundation.[11]
  - URAC Health Website Accreditation Program.[12]

Sites that display a symbol of accreditation from these organizations have met specific guidelines intended to assure the quality of health information they provide.

D. Biomedical Databases

- Refer to **Box 2-4** for a list of some valid and reliable **biomedical databases** to use when searching for evidence-based information related to oral health and patient care.
- The MEDLINE database is the U.S. National Library of Medicine's (NLM) main scientific database.[13]
- MEDLINE provides access to articles from more than 5,600 scientific journals, including PubMed and the Cochrane Collaboration database.

Box 2-4 **Databases for Locating Biomedical Information**

- MEDLINE (PubMed), www.ncbi.nlm.nih.gov/pubmed/: A service of the U.S. National Library of Medicine that includes over 16 million citations from MEDLINE and other life science journals for biomedical articles dating back to the 1950s; includes links to full-text articles and related resources.
- CINAHL (Cumulative Index to Nursing and Allied Health Literature), www.ebscohost.com/nursing/products/cinahl-databases/the-cinahl-database: A bibliographic database that includes abstracts of nursing and allied health articles.
- Cochrane Library (The Cochrane Collaboration), www.cochrane.org/: An international nonprofit and independent organization; produces and disseminates systematic reviews of healthcare interventions and promotes the search for evidence in the form of clinical trials and other studies of interventions.
- Database of Promoting Health Effectiveness Reviews (DoPHER), http://eppi.ioe.ac.uk/webdatabases4/Intro.aspx?ID=9: A database focused on covering systematic and nonsystematic reviews of effectiveness in health promotion and public health worldwide.
- ADA's EBD Website (The American Dental Association's Evidence-Based Dentistry), http://ebd.ada.org: A dental informatics resource; provides practitioners with access to current scientific information that is easy to comprehend and that can be quickly reviewed at the point of care.
- National Institutes of Health, http://health.nih.gov: An encyclopedia of health topics.
- Agency for Healthcare Research and Quality, www.ahrq.gov/: Subsidiary of the U.S. Department of Health and Human Services; aims to produce evidence to make health care safer, higher quality, more accessible, equitable, and affordable.

- MEDLINE indexes all published records using the NLM Medical Subject Headings (MeSH) format. MeSH enable researchers to connect search terms with keywords linked with each publication.[13]
- When journal articles or the abstract for a specific article is displayed, PubMed also provides:
  - The complete citation in NLM format.
  - In some cases, a link to the full text of the article.
  - Links to access "related citations."
- Systematic and effective MEDLINE searches include:
  - Use of the "related citations" link.
  - Checking the references listed in journal articles for additional relevant citations.

Box 2-5 Basic MEDLINE Literature Search Techniques Using the PubMed Search Engine

- A text or key word search locates articles that have the relevant terms in the title, abstract, or body of an article.
- A medical subject heading search locates articles indexed in the database by specific headings.
- A clinical queries search locates articles related to three specific clinical research categories: clinical studies, systematic reviews, and medical genetics.

- Using a combination of search techniques results in more efficient and effective searches.
- Refer to **Box 2-5** for basic MEDLINE literature searching techniques using the PubMed search engine.

E. The Cochrane Collaboration Database

- Global, independent, network working to promote access to credible and unbiased health information for both practitioners and patients.[14]
- Produces high-quality, systematic reviews and other synthesized research evidence to support clinical decision making.
- Each review article includes:
  - Complete scientifically written and well-supported analysis of search methods, data collection, and findings.
  - Plain language summary of results for non-healthcare providers.
- Has a searchable database for a large number of health-related topics, including oral health.

IV. Appraise: Clinically Evaluate Evidence

Once literature on a particular topic is acquired, it is necessary for the dental hygienist to evaluate the validity, reliability, and overall credibility of the information before providing professional recommendations/interventions.

A. Critically Evaluate the Evidence for Currency

- Determine if the evidence is current, outdated, or classic literature.
  - Current scientific literature is typically published within 5 years and provides relatively up-to-date knowledge on a given topic.
  - Outdated scientific literature is typically published more than 5 years ago and provides relatively older/dated knowledge on a given topic.
  - Classic scientific literature refers to original, historical, or early groundbreaking evidence that was seminal to the development of new understandings or knowledge on a given topic.
  - Noncurrent scientific literature should be referenced in the absence of current literature or when classic literature is needed/essential in communicating key messages.

B. Critically Evaluate the Evidence for Validity

- Determine if the study logically follows all steps of the research process.
- Determine if the focus of the study relates to the patient's or population's concerns.
- Determine if there are major concerns with internal validity.
- Determine if objectivity was maintained or if bias was introduced.
- Determine if the study has an adequate sample size.
- Determine if the most appropriate measurement scale and/or index was used.
- Determine if there are major concerns with external validity.
- Can the evidence be generalized to other similar patients or populations?

C. Critically Evaluate the Evidence for Clinical Value

- Analyze which specific **variables** the researchers used in their study.
  - Dependent variable: Also termed as the *outcome variable*. A value that depends on other interventions and what researchers aim to predict or explain. For example, the amount of biofilm left on a tooth after brushing.
  - Independent variable: Also termed as the intervention variable. Manipulating variable intended to create an effect on the dependent variable. For example, the different types of toothbrushes used to reduce biofilm left on a tooth.
  - Extraneous variables: Factors not directly involved between the dependent and independent variable but have an altering effect on the overall relationship. Extraneous variables further subdivide into control and

confounding variables. For example, a person's age, sex, race, ethnicity, socioeconomic status, and/or the extent of oral hygiene instruction provided on proper brushing techniques can influence the overall relationship between the type of intervention used and observed outcome/result.

- Analyze both **descriptive statistics** and **inferential statistics** for significance and relevance to the current problem in question.[15]
- Analyze the difference between **statistical significance** and **clinical significance**.
  - Statistical significance refers to the likelihood that a relationship between two or more variables is due to something other than chance.
  - Clinical significance refers to the practical relevance and importance among multiple therapies. In other words, clinical significance focuses on whether the significant probability of a particular therapy has a noticeable effect on a patient or population.
  - Researchers typically use ≤0.05 as the prespecified **probability value (*p*-value)** to determine statistical significance. In this scenario, there is a less than 5% probability that the statistically significant difference between multiple variables occurred due to chance.
  - Researchers also report data using **confidence intervals** to identify minimum and maximum values for probability.
- Evaluate whether treatment outcomes are beneficial enough to justify treatment.
- Evaluate if researchers provide rational arguments for using results in clinical practice.
- Determine the availability and affordability of treatment to patients or populations.

V. Apply: Integrate and Apply Evidence

- Integrate and apply evidence with clinical expertise and the patient's preferences.
- Consider the patient or population's circumstances and the clinician's ability to help obtain potential results.
- Document interventions in the patient's chart as part of clinical progress notes.

VI. Audit: Evaluate Outcomes

- Determine whether:
  - Application of the EBP model successfully helped the patient.
  - There is a need for additional research strategies and information.
  - There is a need for a modification in the original outcome goal.
- Begin the EBP process again if patient outcome is not successful and/or when a new problem arises.

Approaches to Research

- It is critical for dental hygienists to be aware of different approaches to and types of research designs, particularly when reading published literature to inform clinical EBP.[14]
- The dental hygienist can also conduct and/or participate in original research investigations.
- Depending on the clinical/public health problem and/or focused research question, dental hygienists can engage with research using a critical, objective, and methodical EBP approach.

I. Research Designs

- Qualitative research
  - Purpose is to understand and subjectively interpret complex social interactions.
  - Sample sizes are typically smaller and not randomly selected.
  - Data are collected and reported through participant observations, interviews, open-ended questions, field notations, and narrative reflections.
- Quantitative research
  - Purpose is to test hypotheses, view causal or correlational relationships, and make predictions.
  - Sample sizes are typically larger and randomly selected.
  - Data are collected and reported as quantifiable numbers and/or statistics.
- Mixed-methods research
  - Purpose is to combine the best of both qualitative and quantitative research approaches.
  - Sample sizes and random selection may vary.
  - Data are collected and reported as both qualitative insight and quantitative analysis.

II. Research Types

- Descriptive
  - Typically the first step in classifying and organizing information.
  - Focused on describing facts of people, places, and time.

- Helps identify basic relationships that further studies need to examine.
- Examples include case studies, natural observations, and population surveys.

- Correlational
  - Intended to predict and measure the relationship(s) among multiple variables.
  - Determine the type and strength of relationships among multiple variables.
  - Focuses on preventing the **post hoc fallacy** (i.e., correlation does not mean causation).
  - Examples include case–control studies, cohort studies, observations, population surveys, and cross-sectional and longitudinal studies.
- Quasi-experimental
  - Similar to the experimental approach minus the random assignment.
  - Researchers have lesser control than on true experimental designs.
  - Examples include correlational studies and results of case studies.
- Experimental
  - Intended to test cause and effect between variables.
  - Includes randomized assignment of study participants.
  - Experimental group receives intervention; control group does not receive intervention.
  - Examples include randomized controlled trials (RCTs).
- Review
  - Synthesizes relevant information on a particular research topic.
  - Intended to summarize and evaluate scientific literature.
  - Examples include critical review, narrative review, systematic review, and meta-analysis.

III. Evidence Sources

- Primary research refers to original studies including individual experimental and nonexperimental studies. Examples of primary research studies include RCTs, cohort studies, and case–control studies.
- Secondary research refers to existing studies used for purposes (i.e., reviews on previously conducted research). Examples of secondary research studies include systematic reviews, meta-analysis, and **clinical practice guidelines.**

IV. Levels of Evidence

The **levels of evidence pyramid** illustrates the hierarchy of research designs and strength of various scientific evidence.[16] The pyramid layout provides a visual representation of the number of studies published in literature; in particular, researchers conduct more lower-level than higher-level studies. Higher-level evidence provides the strongest basis for establishing clinical practice guidelines. **Figure 2-4** organizes the levels of evidence as follows.

A. Meta-Analysis and Systematic Reviews

- Highest levels of evidence.
- Meta-analysis, referred to as the platinum standard, is an advanced, analytical-based, literature

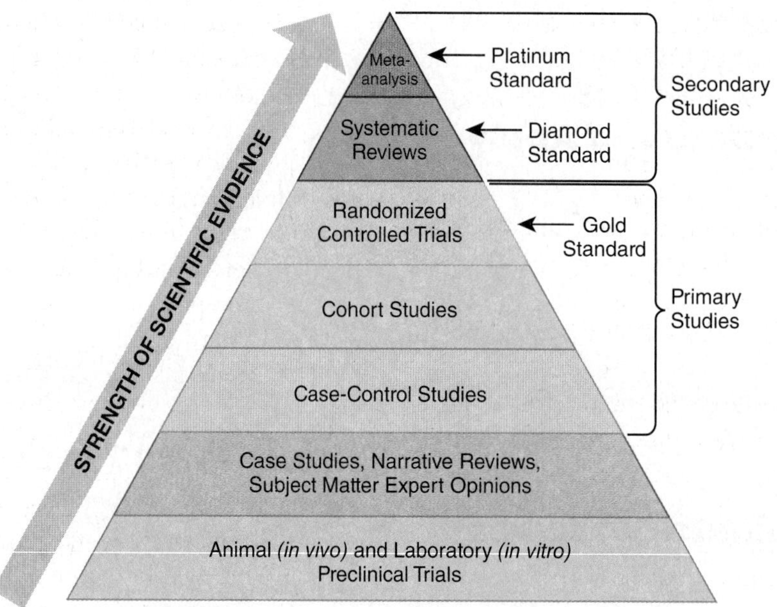

Figure 2-4 Levels of Scientific Evidence Pyramid

review that follows a systematic process with explicit inclusion and exclusion criteria.

- Researchers perform statistical testing on all studies included in the final analysis.
- Through statistical testing, meta-analysis can potentially transform *gold-standard* randomized controlled studies into an even stronger "platinum standard" evidence base.
- Systematic reviews, referenced to as the diamond standard, are advanced, descriptive-based, literature reviews that follows a methodological approach with explicit inclusion and exclusion criteria.
- Researchers produce a summary of all relevant studies based on preestablished criteria.
- Advantages of systematic reviews include that they:
  - Reduce bias.
  - Include only clinically relevant information.
  - Follow strict protocols.
  - Require prior determination of search methods.
  - Focus on specific clinical questions.
  - Have evaluation criteria.
  - Evaluate the strength of available evidence.
- A meta-synthesis best describes a systematic review of qualitative studies.

B. Randomized Controlled Clinical Trials: The "Gold-Standard" Clinical Study

- A **randomized controlled clinical trial** is a planned experiment that tests the efficacy or effectiveness of an exposure.
- They include random assignment/allocation of patients into one of at least two treatment groups.
- Researchers can reduce bias in RCTs by incorporating single-blinded, double-blinded, or triple-blinded protocols in their experiments.
- The double-blinded protocol in RCTs is the current gold-standard approach.

C. Cohort Studies and Case–Control Studies

- Cohort studies follow the same subject group from the present to a specified point in the future. This research design compares a group with exposure against a group without an exposure.
- Case–control studies explore into the past to identify common factors between two groups, one with an exposure and the other without an exposure.
  - The case group refers to the treatment, intervention, or exposure group.
  - The control group refers to the group that either received the standard care (i.e., positive control group) or received no treatment/placebo (i.e., negative control group).

D. Case Studies, Case Reports, and Narrative Reviews

- Case reports are professional articles that describe the diagnostic, preventive, and therapeutic services rendered to one patient with an unusual or complex condition.
- Case studies are in-depth analyses and descriptions of a series of cases of an unusual or complex condition.
- Narrative reviews are basic, descriptive-based literature reviews that synthesize information on a particular topic without a methodological approach.

E. Editorials and SME Opinions

- Editorials are articles in a newspaper or magazine that express the opinion of its editor or publisher.
- SME opinions are beliefs or conclusions held with confidence by experts in a particular field or topic but not substantiated by positive knowledge or proof.

F. Preclinical Trials (In Vitro and In Vivo)

- Preclinical, or nonclinical, research precedes trials involving **human subjects**.
- Purpose is to collect data to support safety of new treatment.
- In vitro trials refer to experimental testing completed through test tubes and other similar equipment in the laboratory.
- In vivo trials refer to experimental testing completed through the body of a nonhuman living organism (i.e., animal studies).

V. Time Intervals

- Prospective: A prospective study observes for outcomes, such as the development of a disease, between the present and some defined point in the future. These exposures are attributed as either risk or protective factors in the development of any given outcome.
- Retrospective: A retrospective study observes established outcomes, such as an existing disease,

but examines by exploring potential risk or protective factors between a specified timeframe in the past.
- Cross-sectional: Cross-sectional studies examine several different samples at one specified point in time (i.e., provide a snapshot). Can include annual surveys, single interventions, etc.
- Longitudinal: Longitudinal studies examine the same sample over an extended period (i.e., several points in time). Results from longitudinal studies can indicate potential causality claims.

Ethics in Research

- Research ethics focuses on the responsibility of researchers to conduct nonbiased research, report accurate results, and protect the rights of individuals participating as research subjects.[17]
- Bioethics is a subdivision concerned with the ethical implications of health-related research and its application on human health and well-being.[17]
  - Over the years, several unethical research studies (i.e., Tuskegee Syphilis Study) occurred due to unregulated policies.
  - The *Nuremberg Code* (1947), *Declaration of Helsinki* (1964), and the *Belmont Report* (1979) were substantial milestones in the field of bioethics.
- Although many dental hygienists may not actively fulfill the role of a researcher, each can look for evidence ensuring that researchers followed ethical principles when reading the report of a research study.
- Refer to Chapter 1 and Section Introductions throughout the text for basic ethical principles and decision-making guidelines.

I. Ethical Standards

The same ethical theories and ethical principles that guide professional interactions of the dental hygienist with patients, dental colleagues, other healthcare providers, and community members can apply when conducting research.[17] These include:

- Respect for persons (autonomy): Obligation to respect others and that they should be able to make their own informed decisions.
- Beneficence (protecting patients from harm): Obligation to "above all, do no harm." Focusing on maximizing benefits and minimizing harm.
- Justice (integrity and fairness): Obligation to give each person their due.

II. Ethical Research Involving Human Subjects

The term *human subjects* refers to people who participate in clinical trials. Examples of dental hygiene–related human subjects research include studies on extracted teeth, discarded gingiva, other tissues, saliva, blood, urine, etc., as long as they are from living individuals.

Ethical standards in research protect individuals who participate as research subjects, with regard to their rights to:

- Self-determination.
- Privacy.
- Anonymity and confidentiality.
- Fair treatment.
- Protection from discomfort and harm.
- Understanding the risks and benefits of participating in the study.
- **Informed consent**.

III. Informed Consent for Research

- Informed consent is the process of adequately explaining the research to prospective subjects and ensuring that they understand what will happen to them, especially the associated risks and benefits.
- All study participants need to volunteer and sign a standardized written consent form.
- Discussion of informed consent is included within the research proposal and includes:
  - A statement that the study involves research.
  - An explanation of the purposes of the research.
  - The expected duration of the subject's participation in the research.
  - A step-by-step description of the procedures.
  - Identification of any procedures that are experimental.
  - A confidentiality statement assuring the participant of anonymity.
  - Refusal to participate will involve "no penalty or loss of benefits to which the subject is otherwise entitled."
  - The subject may withdraw from the research at any time.

IV. Institutional Review Board

- Federal mandate requires that research proposals undergo evaluation by an appropriately designated **Institutional Review Board (IRB)**.
- The IRB is an independent board within the institution that reviews research proposals submitted

by researchers. The group can require modifications before approving research or disapprove research based on its review.

- The purpose of IRB review is to protect the rights and welfare of human subject volunteers in research, in accordance with the policies of the Department of Health and Human Services.
- Published research articles often include an IRB preapproval statement before conducting the study.

Documentation

Include the following factors in the patient's chart record when dental hygienists use current research findings from credible evidence sources to plan recommendations and/or interventions:

- Specify the issue that the patient inquired about during the appointment.
- List any limiting personal patient factors (i.e., disabilities, religious/cultural preferences).
- Articulate professional, evidence-based recommendations/interventions provided to the patient.
- **Box 2-6** provides an example of a completed evidence-based patient progress note.

Factors to Teach the Patient

- A result from one study does not necessarily provide the best answer. Take into consideration the type of study, patient's needs and preferences, and several other factors before making a decision about best-practice interventions.
- Research methods, study design, source of information, and many other factors can affect the validity, reliability, and usefulness of health-related information.
- A statistical significance cited in a study does not necessarily mean that it is the best clinical decision for a patient.

Box 2-6 Example Documentation: Providing an Evidence-Based Recommendation

- **S**—A patient with a chief complaint of dental hypersensitivity when drinking cold beverages presents for routine periodontal maintenance appointment. He inquires about active ingredients he should consider when purchasing a toothpaste to help mitigate his dental hypersensitivity.
- **O**—This patient's clinical attachment levels have decreased due to generalized gingival recession. Exposure of dentinal tubules places patient at higher risk for experiencing hypersensitivity.
- **A**—Review of scientific literature (P = experiencing dental hypersensitivity, I = toothpaste with potassium nitrate, C = toothpaste with fluoride, O = reduction in experience of dental hypersensitivity). Evidence found that toothpaste with potassium nitrate has successful clinical outcomes of reduced dental hypersensitivity. (Marto CM, Paula AB, Nunes T, et al. Evaluation of the efficacy of dentin hypersensitivity treatments – A systematic review and follow-up analysis. *J Oral Rehabil.* 2019;46:952-990.)
- **P**—Gave patient both verbal and written instructions on the importance of using toothpaste with potassium nitrate to reduce experience of dental hypersensitivity. American Dental Association's "Preventing and treating tooth sensitivity" educational pamphlet downloaded from the Internet and given to patient: www.ada.org/~/media/ADA/Publications/Files/FTDP_Sept2013_2.pdf?la=en

Next Step: Patient will bring new toothpaste to his next 3-month periodontal maintenance appointment. At next appointment, assess dental hypersensitivity.

Signed: ______________________, RDH
Date: ______________________

References

1. Opsahl A, Nelson T, Madeira J, Wonder AH. Evidence-based, ethical decision-making: using simulation to teach the application of evidence and ethics in practice. *Worldviews Evid Based.* 2020;17(6):412-417.
2. Draaisma E, Maggio LA, Bekhof J, Debbie A, Brand PLP. Impact of deliberate practice on evidence-based medicine attitudes and behaviours of health care professionals. *Perspect Med Educ.* 2021;10:118-124.
3. Duke University Medical Center Library. Introduction to EBP. Published 2020. https://guides.mclibrary.duke.edu/ebptutorial. Accessed August 4, 2021.
4. Center for Evidence-Based Dentistry, American Dental Association. About EBD. https://ebd.ada.org/en/about. Accessed August 4, 2021.
5. Dhir SK, Gupta P. Formulation of research question and composing study outcomes and objectives. *Indian Pediatr.* 2021;58(6):584-588.
6. Agency for Healthcare Research & Quality (ARHQ). *Strategy 6D: Internet Access for Health Information and Advice.* Published 2020. https://www.ahrq.gov/cahps/quality-improvement/improvement-guide/6-strategies-for-improving/access/strategy6d-internet.html. Accessed August 4, 2021.

7. University Writing Center, Texas A&M University. Evaluating scholarly sources. https://writingcenter.tamu.edu/Students/Writing-Speaking-Guides/Alphabetical-List-of-Guides/Citing-Documenting/Evaluating-Scholarly-Sources. Accessed August 3, 2021.
8. U.S. Department of Health and Human Services, Office of Disease Prevention and Health Promotion. MyHealthfinder. https://health.gov/myhealthfinder/. Accessed August 4, 2021.
9. National Library of Medicine. Health information. https://medlineplus.gov/. Published 2021. Accessed August 4, 2021.
10. Medical Library Association. For health consumers and patients. Published 2021. https://www.mlanet.org/p/cm/ld/fid=397. Accessed August 4, 2021.
11. Health on the Net Foundation. Our commitment to reliable health and medical information on the internet. Published 2020. http://www.hon.ch/home1.html. Accessed August 4, 2021.
12. URAC. Health web site. Published 2021. https://www.urac.org/. Accessed August 4, 2021.
13. U.S. National Library of Medicine. MEDLINE overview. Published 2021. https://www.nlm.nih.gov/medline/medline_overview.html. Accessed August 4, 2021.
14. Cochrane. What is Cochrane? Published 2021. http://www.cochrane.org/. Accessed August 4, 2021.
15. Torres D, Normando D. Biostatistics: essential concepts for the clinician. *Dental Press J Orthod*. 2021;26(1):e21spe1.
16. University of North Carolina Health Sciences Library. Evidence based dentistry. Published 2020. https://guides.lib.unc.edu/evidence-based-dentistry. Accessed August 4, 2021.
17. Council for International Organizations of Medical Sciences. *International Ethical Guidelines for Health-related Research Involving Humans*. Geneva, Switzerland; 2016. https://cioms.ch/wp-content/uploads/2017/01/WEB-CIOMS-EthicalGuidelines.pdf. Accessed July 18, 2022.

CHAPTER 3

Effective Health Communication

Salima Thawer, RDH, MPH

CHAPTER OUTLINE

LEARNING OBJECTIVES

After studying this chapter, the student will be able to:

1. Discuss the skills and attributes of effective health communication.
2. Identify factors that influence health communication.
3. Explain how the patient's age, culture, and health literacy level affect health communication strategies.
4. Identify communication theories relevant to effective health communication and motivational interviewing.
5. Use communication strategies to enhance the ability to provide patient-centered health information, motivate positive changes in health behaviors, and achieve improved health outcomes.
6. Implement good communication skills, in the context of dental hygiene care, to help patients embrace healthy behaviors of all types that allow them to attain and maintain oral health.

Types of Communication

- **Communication** is a process that involves at least two, and sometimes multiple, individuals.
- The sender, who intends to communicate some specific concept, encodes and then transmits a message to at least one receiver, who decodes the message.
- This process can then reverse itself and the receiver becomes the sender of a return message that may or may not provide direct **feedback** to the original message that was sent.
- The effectiveness of the communication depends on how closely the **encoding** and **decoding** match.
- All communication is either **verbal** or **nonverbal**. Each can be subdivided into **vocal** and **nonvocal**.

I. Verbal

- A form of communication based on language or words.
- Vocal communication is spoken language.
- Nonvocal communication is based on signs or signals that express language concepts, and include writing, Braille, and sign language.

II. Nonverbal

- Messages expressed by body language or **affect** can influence or interfere with a healthcare provider's ability to communicate, perhaps even more than the verbal method used.
- Nonverbal, vocal factors include:
  - Vocal qualifiers (volume, pitch, tempo, and cadence).
  - Vocal characterizers (crying, laughing).
- Nonverbal, nonvocal factors include:
  - Body position (posture or use of social space).
  - Movement of body parts such as hands or arms.
  - Eye movements and facial expression.
  - Appearance (grooming and dress).

III. Media Communication

- **Media communication** refers to the use of tools or technology to convey information.
- Media communication can be directed to:
  - An individual recipient (e.g., written care plan provided for an individual patient).
  - A wider, more diverse target audience (e.g., patient education brochures developed by a professional association or health information on the Internet).
- Public health efforts to enhance the health of populations are based on a community-based media approach to providing quality health information.
- Exposure to commercial media efforts, such as television, magazine, or social media advertisements for various products, have an astonishing effect on the health-related choices made by targeted audiences.[1]

Health Communication

- The ultimate goal of health communication is to persuade behavior change that will support optimum health.
- Healthy People 2030 health communication objectives[2] related to direct patient care include:
  - Increase of **health literacy** skills.
  - Good communication, including clear explanations and checking for patient understanding.
  - Shared decision making between patients and providers.
  - Accurate, accessible, and actionable personal health information, self-management tools, and resources.

I. Skills and Attributes of Effective Health Communicators

- Healthcare providers who most effectively deliver preventive interventions demonstrate the following during patient interactions[3]:
  - Expertise and knowledge in health and prevention.
  - Understanding of learning/behavior change theories and principles of good communication.
  - Relationship-building skills.
  - Interview and role-modeling skills.
  - Assessment for readiness to change behaviors.
  - Attention to the patient's attitudes and beliefs.
  - Personal attributes of confidence and flexibility.
- **Motivational interviewing** is an approach to patient counseling based on development and use of the listed skills. See Chapter 24 for more information.
- The use of "**plain language**" in both verbal and written health communication can improve patients' understanding of, and response to, health messages.[4]
- Plain language does not "dumb down" or "talk down" to the patient, but rather provides information in a clear and to-the-point manner, using words the patient can understand.

II. Attributes of Effective Health Information

- Recommendations made by a health educator are more likely to be effective if the patient perceives the information to be[5]:
  - Evidence based, accurate, balanced, and reliable.
  - Consistent with information from other sources.
  - Culturally and linguistically appropriate.
  - Delivered in an easily understood and accessible way.
  - Provided when the patient is most ready to receive it.
  - Repeated and reinforced over time.
- Health information is often received from a variety of sources, some of which may be biased, incomplete, or conflicting.[6] Sources of health information may include:
  - Mainstream media (e.g., TV, newspapers).
  - Educational institutions (e.g., schools).
  - Interactions with other people (e.g., family, friends, colleagues).
  - Web-based resources.
  - Social media.
  - Health professionals.
  - Product labels and pamphlets.

III. Barriers to Effective Health Communication

- It is rare that every message coded and transmitted by a sender is decoded and understood with complete accuracy by the receiver.
- Multiple factors that can affect the way health messages are understood are described in **Table 3-1**.
- Many of the factors listed in the table overlap in their description; more than one barrier may exist and have an effect on any attempt at communication.
- All of the factors listed can provide a barrier to communication, in either direction, between the clinician and the patient.
- Dental hygienists who strive to develop good listening skills, enhance their ability to assess a patient's needs, and approach each individual with empathy and respect can go far toward overcoming the barriers to effective health communication.

Table 3-1 Barriers to Effective Health Communication

Barrier	Description
Cultural	Differences in social norms or perceptions related to differences in gender, age, language, socioeconomic class, or ethnic background
Interpersonal	Discomfort related to perceptions about the individual; appearance causes distraction; individuals do not see "eye to eye" or relate well to each other
Attitudinal	Lack of sensitivity or respect; over- or underconfidence displayed by either patient or clinician
Physical	Distractions related to the physical environment; noise levels; face-to-face positioning not used
Physiologic	Inability to hear, see, touch, or vocalize as required to communicate
Psychosociologic	Emotional factors such as fear or pain cause distraction
Insufficient knowledge	Either the clinician is not well informed and cannot provide sufficient information or the patient has low health literacy and cannot understand the information provided
Lack of access to knowledge	Inability to access media or use technology to find information
Lack of interest	Patient is not ready to engage in health behavior change; clinician is experiencing "burn out" or disinterest in patient education
Information overload	Too much information on too many topics is provided at one time; no written reinforcement is provided
Poor communication skills	Either the patient or the clinician is not able to respond or provide feedback to messages received; clinician uses "jargon" or professional terminology that the patient does not understand

IV. Web-Based Health Messages

- There has been an explosion of health-related websites and an increasing number of patients of all ages who access Internet-based health information.
- Patients bring information they find on the Internet or via social media to the attention of their healthcare providers.
- Healthcare providers are responsible for keeping up-to-date on Internet sources of information to respond to questions patients may bring to a health education discussion.
- Healthcare providers may also be the creators and distributors of web-based health information (e.g., websites, digital tools). Considerations should be made to ensure that information is easy for patients to access and understand.
- The U.S. Department of Health and Human Services, Office of Disease Prevention and Health Promotion offers a guide and tips to assist in creating user-friendly websites and digital tools (available from: https://health.gov/healthliteracyonline/).
- The dental hygienist can help patients determine reliability and credibility of websites as well as provide recommendations for high-quality resources for patients searching for additional information. (See Chapter 2.)

V. Factors That Influence Health Communication

- Communication skills of the caregiver and effectiveness of the health information can affect:
  - The ability of healthcare providers to influence health behaviors.
  - The ability of patients and populations to take advantage of new knowledge provided by the health messages.
- Other factors that influence health communication include:
  - Health literacy of the patient or population receiving the health message.
  - The age and communication preferences of individuals receiving information.
  - The social and economic ability of the targeted individuals to take advantage of recommendations contained in the health messages.
  - The cultural background and health-related cultural norms of the individual receiving the message.
  - **Cultural sensitivity** and the ability to establish **cultural rapport** of individuals providing the health messages.

Health Literacy

- Healthy People 2030 acknowledges that health literacy consists of two key parts:
  - The capabilities of an individual.
  - An organization's ability to improve accessibility and comprehensibility of health information.[7]
- Patients need to be able to locate, understand, and use health information and services to inform the decisions they make regarding their health.
- Organizations and clinicians need to assess and promote health literacy of patients.

I. Personal Health Literacy

- A large part of an educated population may have low personal health literacy; often, these are the patients with the highest treatment needs and the greatest barriers to receiving health information.
- Populations particularly vulnerable to low or limited health literacy include[6]:
  - Older adults.
  - Immigrant populations.
  - Minority populations.
  - People who speak little or no English.
  - People with low levels of education (i.e., less than high school).
  - Individuals living below the poverty level.
- Low health literacy is associated with less use of healthcare services and resources and, ultimately, with poorer health outcomes.[8]
- The level of a patient's health literacy depends on not only the reading level, but also the complex interaction of cognitive and psychosocial skills.[9]

II. Organizational Health Literacy

- To enhance communication with all patients regardless of oral health literacy level[10–12]:
  - Assess health literacy level and provide an individualized approach for every patient.
  - Ensure a clinic environment that is helpful and user friendly by providing clear directions, visible and clearly written signs or universal symbols, and color-coded maps where necessary.
  - Encourage patients to write down and bring questions about their oral health to each appointment.
  - Provide forms (e.g., health history, informed consent) that are written in plain language. Provide help if required in completing forms.

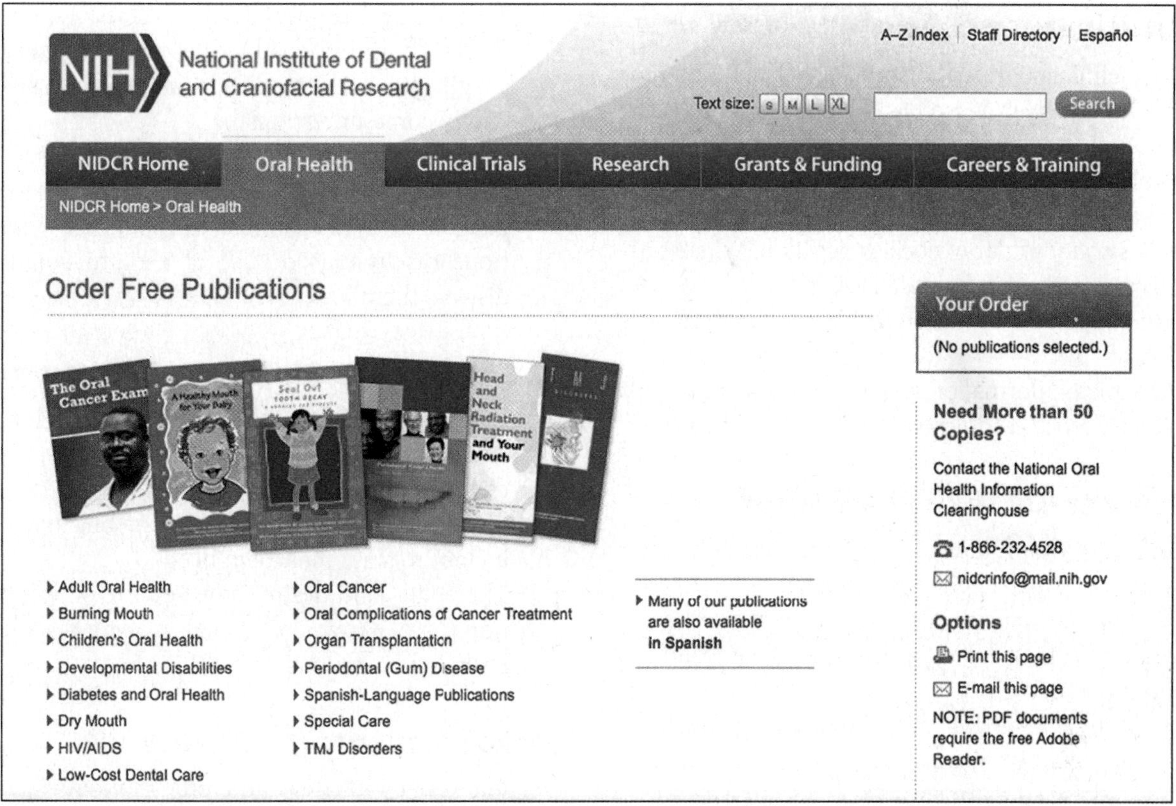

Figure 3-1 The U.S. Department of Health and Human Services, National Institutes of Health, provides free patient education materials on a variety of oral health topics at the National Institute of Dental and Craniofacial Research website: https://catalog.nidcr.nih.gov/. Accessed September 28, 2021

National Institutes of Health, and are available for free from the National Institute of Dental and Craniofacial Research website at: https://catalog.nidcr.nih.gov/. Accessed September 28, 2021.

- Build on the patient's current knowledge base to encourage healthy decision making.
- Provide written patient education materials that use plain language and avoid materials that use professional jargon or provide complex explanations.
- Excellent "plain language" oral health patient education publications have been developed by the U.S. Department of Health and Human Services and are available for free on the National Institute of Dental and Craniofacial Research website (see **Figure 3-1**).
- Use visual aids such as drawings or photographs for education materials when appropriate.
- Monitor to determine understanding of all forms and education materials. The "teach-back" method of asking patients to explain instructions to be followed is a helpful approach.

Communication Across the Life Span

- Irrespective of the patient's age, building rapport is key to effective health communication.

Box 3-1 Tips for Establishing Rapport with Patients of All Ages

- Listen more than talk, especially at the beginning of a conversation.
- Practice attentive listening rather than multitasking during conversations.
- Sit eye to eye with the patient rather than with the patient in a reclined position or standing/sitting taller than the patient.
- Convey a nonjudgmental attitude and reinforce an atmosphere of respect and valuing of the individual, even if the behavior is not acceptable.
- Maintain a calm, unhurried demeanor.
- Use a normal tone of voice and vocabulary that is appropriate and does not talk down to the patient.
- Look for clues, share your thoughts and observations, and ask questions.
- Do not jump to conclusions.
- Link information to activities of daily living to help provide context for recommendations.

- Tips for establishing rapport with patients of all ages are found in **Box 3-1.**
- Key points related to specific age groups are discussed in the subsequent sections.

I. Children and Adolescents

- The clinician must consider the health literacy of the caregiver as well as the child or adolescent patient.
- Build rapport with children and adolescents, treat them with respect, and involve them in discussions about their own health decisions where possible, based on individual factors.[13]
- Some age-appropriate communication strategies follow.
- Complete information about the oral health needs of children and adolescents is found in Chapter 47.

A. Infants (Birth to 12 Months)[14]

- Infants communicate primarily through their senses of touch, sight, and hearing.
- Techniques the clinician can use to communicate with an infant during a dental hygiene examination include:
  - Interact playfully with a receptive infant by mimicking facial expressions, rocking, and talking softly or singing.
  - Encourage an adult who is familiar with the infant to distract and comfort the child.
  - Wait until the infant is calm to approach closely.

B. Toddlers and Preschoolers (Ages 1–2 Years and 3–5 Years)[14]

- Although dependent on adults for their care, most children appreciate and respond to being approached directly.
- Development of a sense of self enhances the need to assert independence and maintain control over any situation.
- Offer encouragement and gentle hints or engage in "parallel" actions to demonstrate, rather than directly assist, to promote success in age-appropriate self-care tasks.
- Calmly distract or direct toward an alternative behavior to counter defiance or inappropriate behavior.
- To effectively control unwanted behavior, state specifically what the child is expected to do rather than criticize.
- Ask simple, specifically focused questions to help the child remember past experiences.
- To overcome the limited ability to process auditory information and short attention span, provide brief, truthful, and simple instructions and responses to questions.
- Toddlers are beginning to converse in short sentences, but if the adult becomes impatient or abrupt, the child may feel frustrated or ashamed and become unresponsive.
- Children of this age understand more than they are given credit for but often misinterpret language that is not familiar to them; therefore, serious discussions or use of certain words may distress them.

C. School-Age Children (6–11 Years)[14]

- The ability to understand serious events logically and comprehend how it will impact themselves is developing.
- More aware of the needs of others but may be reluctant to state their own needs.
- The ability and desire to respond to simple questions can allow the dental hygienist to assess knowledge and misconceptions.

D. Adolescents (12–21 Years)[14,15]

- Marked by intense and often extreme feelings about situations and persons in their world.
- Strongly independent and desire to have their viewpoint considered in a respectful and nonjudgmental manner.
- Tendency to withdraw or become hostile if they feel they are misunderstood.
- Actively engage them using a straightforward and interactive approach that explains and then solicits input into a discussion on topics that interest the adolescent. This is most effective to build rapport and establish trust.
- Adolescents expect their privacy and confidentiality to be respected. Be upfront about the confidentiality agreement and situations in which information about them would be shared and with whom.
- Confidentiality laws, which vary among jurisdictions, can help determine what behavior-related information the dental hygienist discusses with a parent or guardian. Anything that is an immediate safety issue (such as thoughts of suicide) is reported immediately.
- To develop a rapport and a trusting relationship with an adolescent patient:
  - Address the adolescent directly even when parent/guardian is present.
  - Ensure the adolescent has the opportunity to ask and answer questions independently (privately) as well as with parents/guardians.

II. Older Adults[16,17]

- Providing effective health education for aging patients who are experiencing a communication difficulty requires respect for the needs of the individual and responding to functional ability or limitations.
- Age-related communication difficulties can include:
  - Visual or hearing impairment.
  - Decreased ability to remember or formulate language.
  - Health conditions and related medications that may alter cognitive abilities.
- Strategies for communicating with older individuals experiencing communication difficulty are listed in **Box 3-2.**
- Oral health considerations related to aging are discussed in Chapter 48.

A. Physical and Cognitive Changes

- Cognitive disabilities are more likely to be present as an individual ages and to interfere with understanding health-related information.
- Communication disorders such as **dysarthria** and **aphasia** are associated with conditions that are more common in an aging population.
- Sensory loss (particularly hearing loss) can provide challenges in interpersonal communication.
- Physiologic changes may occur in speech patterns, including voice tremor, pitch, loudness, and speaking rate.

Box 3-2 Strategies for Effective Communication with Older Adults

- Identify each individual's communication barriers (such as cognitive impairments) and modify the communication approach appropriately.
- Avoid patronizing "elderspeak" and respect the patient's level of competence and independence.
- Suggest that the patient write down questions ahead of time.
- Practice attentive listening and avoid rushing the patient.
- Face the patient and maintain eye contact; remove masks during conversations.
- Speak slowly, clearly, and loud enough for the patient to hear.
- Use simple, patient-appropriate language.
- Present one idea at a time.
- Use visual aids, teach-back techniques, and repetition of key messages.
- Provide a written summary or follow-up for key messages.

B. Communication Predicament[17-19]

- Healthcare providers often use an inappropriate overmodification of speech and language when addressing older patients.
- This "baby talk" or "elderspeak" approach to communication does not enhance comprehension and can be perceived as patronizing or demeaning.
- *Accommodative speech* refers to use of a high-pitched tone of voice, a "singsong" cadence, and relatively simplistic language when addressing an older adult.
- The use of terms of endearment (honey, sweetie, dearie) and nicknames or diminutive forms of a patient's name can reflect a lack of respect for the individual as an adult person.
- The use of plural pronouns ("Are we ready for our appointment?") can imply that the patient cannot act alone or make independent decisions.

Social and Economic Aspects of Health Communication

- Social and economic factors, sometimes referred to as "**social determinants of health**," are the circumstances in which people are born, grow up, live, work, play, and age.[20]
- These factors:
  - Influence the ability of individuals and communities to receive and act upon health messages from healthcare providers or public health media.
  - Are responsible for unfair and avoidable differences in health status seen within and among populations.[20,21]
- Oral health professionals have a responsibility to address the needs of individuals in the context of their environment and experience when providing oral health education.[21–23]

Cultural Considerations

- Sociocultural differences can impede communication between the dental hygienist and patient.[24]
- Culturally sensitive delivery of dental hygiene services can make a positive difference in oral health outcomes.[24]
- A cultural awareness checklist is found in **Box 3-3**.

Box 3-3 A Checklist to Enhance Cultural Awareness during Patient Care

- Examine and recognize any personal bias that may affect communication when working with patients from a different **culture**.
- Conduct all patient assessments with cultural sensitivity in mind.
- Assess to determine the patient's cultural identification and, if necessary, research to identify implications for dental hygiene practice.
- Determine language barriers, identify patient's preferred method of communication, and regularly double-check to assure comprehension.
- Identify religious and health-related beliefs, views, or misconceptions that may influence dental hygiene interventions.
- Identify and address cultural dietary considerations.
- Double-check verbal and nonverbal signs routinely to determine the level of the patient's trust of healthcare providers.

Data from Seibert PS, Stridh-Igo P, Zimmerman CG. A checklist to facilitate cultural awareness and sensitivity. *J Med Ethics*. 2002;28(3):143-146.

I. Culture and Health

A. Effects of Culture on Health Status

- The increasing diversity of racial and ethnic communities and linguistic groups in North America influences the delivery of oral health services.
- Health disparities related to racial, ethnic, and socioeconomic background exist in the healthcare system.[25]
- Ignoring culture can lead to negative health consequences and/or poor clinical outcomes because culture and language can influence:
  - Beliefs and behaviors related to health, healing, and wellness.
  - Perceptions of illness, diseases, and their causes.
  - Attitudes of patients toward accessing health services or toward healthcare providers.
  - Attitudes and behaviors of providers who may have learned a set of values that are different from those of their patients.

B. Culturally Effective Oral Care[24]

- **Culturally effective health care** is patient centered and "responsive to diverse cultural health beliefs and practices, preferred languages, health literacy, and other communication needs."[26]
- Sensitivity to the effects of culture on healthcare delivery is "critical to reducing health disparities and improving access to high-quality health care."[27]
- Meeting each patient's individual oral care needs is the hallmark of dental hygiene practice.
- The ability to provide effective oral health education and dental hygiene services for culturally diverse patients requires assessing, being sensitive to, and respecting each patient's cultural differences.
- Culturally effective dental hygiene care respects each patient's health beliefs, practices, values, customs, and traditions in the plan for dental hygiene care.

II. Cross-Cultural Communication

- Communication with patients from other cultures is enhanced when the dental hygienist develops knowledge about and avoids stereotyping traditional behaviors and values of a patient's cultural group.
- Knowing general principles can enhance communication.

A. Nonverbal Communication

- There are culturally related differences in nonverbal communication.[28] These may include variations in, and acceptability related to:
  - Facial expressions.
  - Eye contact.
  - Hand gestures.
  - Body posture.
  - Personal space and touch.
- To communicate successfully, the dental hygienist will:
  - Be careful when interpreting facial expressions.
  - Follow the patient's lead for making eye contact.
  - Use hand and arm gestures with caution.
  - Follow the patient's lead for touching or personal space.

B. Language Proficiency

- Simplify language as much as possible without speaking down to the patient.
- Eliminate professional jargon.
- Use pictures, diagrams, and demonstrations to help increase understanding.
- Provide "plain language" health information or publications in the patient's primary language to reinforce and support compliance with oral health recommendations.

C. Using an Interpreter

- When the patient's skills in the dominant language are not sufficient to assure informed consent or compliance with recommendations, a professional interpreter can be used to enhance communication.
- A professional interpreter will have proficiency in both languages as well as an ability to convey complex information completely and accurately.
- Family members or friends are not the same as a professional interpreter.
- Informal interpreters could hinder health communication[29] and are more likely to modify important information or interject their own opinions, beliefs, or prejudices.
- It is particularly inadvisable to ask children to interpret sensitive health information.
- Focus on and direct all communication to the patient, with pauses to allow the interpreter to translate.

D. Family Decision Making

- In many cultures, an individual's health concern is considered to be a family concern.
- Involvement of certain family members in the treatment planning process may be a key factor in determining recommendations and assuring compliance.
- Sensitivity is needed when family members or children, even older children, are involved in the discussion.

III. Attaining Cultural Competence

- Achieving **cultural competence** in providing health care is a process[30] that requires a commitment to cultural awareness, a motivation to engage in cultural encounters, and an ongoing acquisition of cultural knowledge and communication skills.
- The dental hygienist who strives to become adept at providing culturally effective care:
  - Values (and not simply tolerates) diversity.
  - Conducts honest self-assessment to determine how personal health beliefs, traditions, and biases influence the ability to relate to culturally different individuals.
  - Actively acquires knowledge about patients' health beliefs, behaviors, and cultural norms.
  - Is nonjudgmental regarding cultural traditions and beliefs.
  - Avoids **stereotypes**.
  - Routinely adapts delivery of dental hygiene care in a way that reflects understanding of each patient's diversity and unique oral health needs.

IV. Cultural Competence and the Dental Hygiene Process of Care

- Respect for each patient's cultural differences, healthcare practices, health beliefs, and values can be integrated into all areas of the dental hygiene process of care.[31]

A. Assessment

- The ability to collect accurate, complete assessment data is key to providing dental hygiene interventions that meet patient needs.
- Culturally effective nonverbal communication and listening skills help build trust and patient rapport that can facilitate the transfer of essential personal health information.
- Skillful, nonjudgmental questioning can help elicit culture-specific data such as health beliefs and values, as well as avoid misunderstandings about a patient's culturally related health practices.
- Asking permission before touching a patient during the extra- and intraoral examination procedures can avoid problems with cultural differences in personal space.

B. Diagnosis

- A dental hygiene diagnosis is predicated on a clear understanding of the patient's history, medical status, symptoms, and current treatment modalities.
- The culturally competent dental hygienist will prepare diagnostic statements that take into consideration:
  - Culture-specific health risks that are related to oral status.
  - Cultural practices that may impact the patient's oral health status.

C. Planning

- The dental hygiene care plan formulates oral health goals that meet the needs of each individual patient realistically.
- The goals identified in the plan are based on a synthesis of needs determined by the dental hygienist and those expressed by the patient.

- A culturally sensitive dental hygiene care plan respects and takes into consideration the patient's current health practices and beliefs.
- With the patient's input, the plan may be devised to accept, modify, or eliminate current culturally relevant healthcare practices.
- The plan is sensitive to the practices, products, or substances that the patient's culture prohibits, such as mouthrinses containing alcohol for patients in some cultures.
- A culturally and linguistically sensitive approach to communicating the dental hygiene care plan can facilitate informed consent for dental hygiene interventions.

D. Implementation

- Culturally appropriate communication can enhance the patient's cooperation during treatment.
- Knowledge of culturally determined expressions of pain and discomfort during treatment can help the dental hygienist determine appropriate pain control measures.
- Language-appropriate instructions before, during, and after each procedure can enhance patient compliance with treatment.
- "Plain language" or translated oral health materials can enhance patient compliance with recommendations.

E. Evaluation

- A dental hygienist who is sensitive to cultural differences evaluates treatment success on the basis of goals determined in a previously prepared culturally relevant care plan.
- Feedback provided for the patient respects culturally diverse beliefs and values related to oral health.
- Self-evaluation regarding the cultural effectiveness of the practitioner's approach can provide insight for planning modifications to the patient's continuing care plan.

Interprofessional Communication

- Interprofessional collaboration is changing the way health care is delivered and to improve health outcomes.[32]
- Teamwork is a vital skill that relies on collaboration among a variety of healthcare providers who have responsibility for complex aspects of an individual patient's care.
- Sufficient and ongoing communication is a major factor in developing a collaborative practice workforce that strengthens healthcare systems, provides high-quality care, and supports positive patient outcomes.[33,34]
- The ability to communicate with other health professionals in a manner that supports a team approach to patient care requires competency in the following skills[33]:
  - Select effective communication tools and techniques, including information systems and communication technologies.
  - Organize and express information in a form that is easily understood by providers in other health disciplines.
  - Demonstrate active listening; encourage others to share ideas and opinions.
  - Provide timely, sensitive, and instructive feedback to other members of the team.
  - Be open to receiving feedback in a respectful and positive manner.
  - Use respectful language when in a difficult situation or a professional conflict.
  - Recognize how one's own communication style contributes to the interprofessional relationship.
  - Consistently communicate the importance of teamwork in patient-centered care.
- Continuous efforts to enhance interprofessional communication are necessary to improve the quality of patient care.[34,35]

Communication with Caregivers

- Young children and many patients with disabling conditions rely on someone else to help with or provide daily self-care regimens.
- In this situation, the dental hygienist communicates with the caregiver or parent as well as the patient.
- In a group conversation, keep the primary focus on the patient by maintaining eye contact and directing comments/questions to the patient, if appropriate, as well as the caregiver.

- Assess patient needs and caregiver relationships carefully to determine the extent of the caregiver's role in daily self-care.
- Encourage the caregiver to allow the patient to maintain as much independence as possible.

Documentation

When documenting communication aspects of a patient visit, the following factors are included:

- Patient's age, gender, and ethnicity.
- Factors or observations related to health literacy level.
- Cultural characteristics that can affect communication or delivery of dental hygiene care.
- Significant factors such as patient hearing loss, need to communicate with caregiver, use of an interpreter, and description of specific modifications made to accommodate those factors.
- An example of documentation for communication aspects of a patient visit is found in **Box 3-4**.

Factors to Teach the Patient

- The importance of communicating accurate and complete information about health status, needs, and concerns to optimize dental hygiene care that will be provided.
- Willingness and motivation to incorporate homecare recommendations is a key element for successful oral health outcomes.

Box 3-4 Example Documentation: Communication Aspects of a Patient Visit

- **S**—Following an initial data collection appointment, a 65-year-old African-American male presents for a second appointment to receive and discuss his complex treatment plan. Patient has significant hearing loss and does not use a hearing aid but reads lips during casual conversation. He prefers to ask complex questions and receive answers by writing on a notepad.
- **O**—Written dental hygiene care plan and dental treatment plans have been developed and are ready to be presented for patient consent.
- **A**—Patient understanding is necessary for documenting informed consent.
- **P**—Sequential presentation of each written component of the dental hygiene care plan and dental treatment plan. Additional appointment time scheduled so all questions can be answered in writing, as the patient prefers. Following the presentation of each component of the plan, the patient was asked to summarize or restate in writing to demonstrate that he understood what was discussed. At the end of the discussion, the patient wrote on his notepad that all of his questions were answered. Treatment Consent form was signed and dated.

Next Step: Begin implementation of phase 1 of dental hygiene care plan.

Signed: ______________________, RDH

Date: ______________________

References

1. Russell SJ, Croker H, Viner RM. The effect of screen advertising on children's dietary intake: a systematic review and meta-analysis. *Obes Rev*. 2018;20(4):554-568.
2. Healthy People 2030. Health communication.Washington, DC: U.S. Department of Health and Human Services. https://health.gov/healthypeople/objectives-and-data/browse-objectives/health-communication. Accessed August 29, 2021.
3. Burke LE, Fair J. Promoting prevention: skill sets and attributes of health care providers who deliver behavioral interventions. *J Cardiovasc Nurs*. 2003;18(4):256-266.
4. Plain language. National Institutes of Health. https://www.nih.gov/institutes-nih/nih-office-director/office-communications-public-liaison/clear-communication/plain-language. Accessed August 29, 2021.
5. European Centre for Disease Prevention and Control. What is health communication? https://www.ecdc.europa.eu/en/health-communication/facts. Accessed August 29, 2021.
6. U.S. Department of Health and Human Services, Office of Disease Prevention and Health Promotion. *National Action Plan to Improve Health Literacy*. Washington, DC: U.S. Department of Health and Human Services; 2010. https://health.gov/sites/default/files/2019-09/Health_Literacy_Action_Plan.pdf. Accessed August 29, 2021.
7. Santana S, Brach C, Harris L, et al. Updating health literacy for Healthy People 2030: defining its importance for a new decade in public health. *J Public Health Manag Pract*. 2021;27:S258-S264.

8. Berkman ND, Sheridan SL, Donahue KE, Halpern DJ, Crotty K. Low health literacy and health outcomes: an updated systematic review. *Ann Intern Med*. 2011;155(2):97-107.
9. Bröder J, Okan O, Bauer U, et al. Health literacy in childhood and youth: a systematic review of definitions and models. *BMC Public Health*. 2017;17(1):361.
10. Horowitz AM, Kleinman DV. Oral health literacy: the new imperative to better oral health. *Dent Clin North Am*. 2008;52(2):333-344, vi. 1
11. Horowitz AM, Kleinman DV. Creating a health literacy-based practice. *J Calif Dent Assoc*. 2012;40(4):331-340.
12. National Library of Medicine. An introduction to health literacy. https://new.nnlm.gov/guides/intro-health-literacy. Accessed September 28, 2021.
13. Bell J, Condren M. Communication strategies for empowering and protecting children. *J Pediatr Pharmacol Ther*. 2016;21(2):176-184.
14. Deering C, Cody D. Communicating with children and adolescents. *Am J Nurs*. 2002;102(3):34-41.
15. Daley AM, Polifroni EC, Sadler LS. "Treat me like a normal person!" A meta-ethnography of adolescents' expectations of their health care providers. *J Pediatr Nurs*. 2017;36:70-83.
16. Yorkston KM, Bourgeois MS, Baylor CR. Communication and aging. *Phys Med Rehabil Clin N Am*. 2010;21(2):309-319.
17. Stein PS, Aalboe JA, Savage MW, Scott AM. Strategies for communicating with older dental patients. *J Am Dent Assoc*. 2014;145(2):159-164.
18. Brown A, Draper P. Accommodative speech and terms of endearment: elements of a language mode often experienced by older adults. *J Adv Nurs*. 2003;41(1):15-21.
19. Williams K, Kemper S, Hummert ML. Enhancing communication with older adults: overcoming elderspeak. *J Gerontol Nurs*. 2004;30(10):17-25.
20. World Health Organization. Social determinants of health. https://www.who.int/health-topics/social-determinants-of-health#tab=tab_1. Accessed September 30, 2021.
21. Williams DM, Sheiham A, Watt RG. Oral health professionals and social determinants. *Br Dent J*. 2013;214(9):427.
22. Lee JY, Divaris K. The ethical imperative of addressing oral health disparities: a unifying framework. *J Dent Res*. 2014; 93(3):224-230.
23. Watt RG, Williams DM, Sheiham A. The role of the dental team in promoting health equity. *Br Dent J*. 2014;216(1):11.
24. Cadoret CA, Garcia RI. Health disparities and the multicultural imperative. *J Evid Based Dent Pract*. 2014;14:160-170.
25. Agency for Healthcare Research and Quality. *2019 National Healthcare Quality and Disparities Report*. Reviewed June 2021. https://www.ahrq.gov/research/findings/nhqrdr/nhqdr19/index.html. Accessed September 30, 2021.
26. U.S. Department of Health and Human Services, Office of Minority Health. *National Standards for Culturally and Linguistically Appropriate Services (CLAS) in Health and Health Care*. https://www.thinkculturalhealth.hhs.gov/assets/pdfs/EnhancedNationalCLASStandards.pdf. Accessed September 30, 2021.
27. National Institutes of Health. Clear communication: cultural respect. Reviewed July 7, 2021. https://www.nih.gov/institutes-nih/nih-office-director/office-communications-public-liaison/clear-communication/cultural-respect. Accessed September 30, 2021.
28. Lorié Á, Reinero DA, Phillips M, Zhang L, Riess H. Culture and nonverbal expressions of empathy in clinical settings: a systematic review. *Patient Educ Couns*. 2016;100(3):411-424.
29. Au M, Taylor E, Gold M. *Improving Access to Language Services in Health Care: A Look at National and State Efforts*. Washington: Mathematica Policy Research, Inc; 2009. https://www.imiaweb.org/uploads/pages/464.pdf. Accessed October 1, 2021.
30. Campinha-Bacote J. The process of cultural competence in the delivery of healthcare services: a model of care. *J Transcult Nurs*. 2002;13(3):181-184.
31. Fitch P. Cultural competence and dental hygiene care delivery: integrating cultural care into the dental hygiene process of care. *J Dent Hyg*. 2004;78(1):11-21.
32. Reeves S, Pelone F, Harrison R, Goldman J, Zwarenstein M. Interprofessional collaboration to improve professional practice and healthcare outcomes. *Cochrane Database Syst Rev*. 2017;(6):CD000072.
33. Interprofessional Education Collaborative. *IPEC Core Competencies for Interprofessional Collaborative Practice: 2016 Update*. https://ipec.memberclicks.net/assets/2016-Update.pdf. Accessed October 2, 2021.
34. Kishimoto M, Noda M. The difficulties of interprofessional teamwork in diabetes care: a questionnaire survey. *J Multidiscip Healthcare*. 2014;7:333-339.
35. Hepp SL, Suter E, Jackson K, et al. Using an interprofessional competency framework to examine collaborative practice. *J Interprof Care*. 2014;10:1-7.

CHAPTER 4

Dental Hygiene Care in Alternative Settings

Jennifer Cullen, RDH, MPH
Lisa F. Mallonee, RDH, MPH, RD, LD

CHAPTER OUTLINE

LEARNING OBJECTIVES

After studying this chapter, the student will be able to:

1. Identify and define key terms and concepts related to oral health care in alternative settings.
2. Identify materials necessary for providing dental hygiene care in alternative settings.
3. Plan and document adaptations to dental hygiene care plans and oral hygiene instructions for the patient who is residence-bound, bedridden, unconscious, or terminally ill.

Alternative Practice Settings

- Increasing attention is being paid to the oral health needs of individuals who are not able to access oral health services in a traditional dental practice setting.[1]
- Individuals confined to hospitals, **hospice**, institutions, **skilled nursing** or **long-term care** facilities, or private homes:
  - Experience barriers accessing routine dental services.
  - Receive inadequate oral care from caregivers.
  - Are likely to have poor oral health status and diminished quality of life.
  - May need special adaptations for oral care.
- Most states now have laws that allow direct access to dental hygiene services through **collaborative practice** or varying levels of supervision in certain public health settings.[2]
- An important role for the dental hygienist is to **triage** and ensure optimum use of available dental care resources.
  - Key words and definitions related to caring for patients in alternative settings are found in the glossary.

I. Barriers to Access

In addition to universal barriers such as cost and fear, providing care in alternative settings can also address unique barriers faced by this population.[3,4]

- Barriers to access for the residence-bound population may include:
  - Limited mobility.
  - Lack of suitable transportation.
  - Often inaccessible physical environment of dental offices.
  - Few on-site dental clinics in residential facilities.
  - Limited availability of general and specialty practitioners who provide home-based services.
  - Limited availability of direct access allied oral health providers.
  - Limited or nonexistent federal/state insurance coverage for dental services for adults and older adults.[5]

II. Eliminating Barriers

- Many services are delivered to **residence-bound (homebound)** individuals by home health agencies.
- Certain allied health professionals, such as a **nurse practitioner (NP)**, oversee programs that provide direct medical services for patients.
- New models of healthcare delivery, such as **teledentistry**, use Web-based communication tools to enhance collaboration between on-site and supervising health team members and facilitate communication between providers and remote patients.
- The National Network for Oral Health Access Teledentistry User's Guide provides an overview and practical tools for providers.[6]
- Current public health programs in numerous states allow dental hygienists to provide direct access care for certain underserved populations.
- Direct access care providers can address access issues related to shortage of dentists, limited availability of safety net options for low-income populations, and need for care in nontraditional settings.[7,8]
- Several direct access oral health provider models are currently being explored; some models are based on increased scope of practice for dental hygienists who have received additional education and certification.[9]

III. Portable Delivery of Care

For patients who cannot be transported to a dental treatment room, dental and dental hygiene services can be provided in a variety of surroundings using mobile equipment.

- Dental hygiene care:
  - Can be provided in any setting within the limits of state practice acts.
  - Particularly lends itself to care for residence-bound individuals because most dental hygiene treatments can be completed with manual instruments.

Residence-Bound Patients

- Potential residence-bound patients are listed in **Box 4-1**.
- The individual who is residence-bound may be:
  - Limited in one or more **ADL/IADL (activities of daily living/instrumental activities of daily living)**. (See Chapter 22.)

Box 4-1 Potential Residence-Bound Patients

Frail elderly
Severely medically compromised
Critically ill patient or **terminally ill patient**
Physically or developmentally disabled
Chronically ill
Cognitively impaired

- An American Society of Anesthesiologists' classification of III or higher. (See Chapter 22.)
- At increased risk of serious complications from communicable diseases.
- **Functional dependence** on caregivers.

- Instruction in personal oral preventive procedures has particular significance for comfort and quality of life, as well as the systemic health of these individuals.

I. Private Homes

- Individuals who are residence-bound might live:
  - Alone or with a partner, a spouse, a friend, family members, or other caregivers.
  - In a private, traditional neighborhood residence.
- A variety of home-based healthcare and **custodial care** services are often utilized.

II. Residential Facilities

Studies indicate individuals residing in nursing homes generally have poor oral health status, do not receive adequate daily oral care, and cannot adequately access routine dental services.[3,10,11]

- Residential facilities can include:
  - Skilled nursing or long-term care, including memory loss care.
  - Rehabilitation centers that provide temporary support for patients.
  - Independent and assisted living facilities for seniors or disabled individuals.
  - Group homes that serve adults of all ages with physical, mental, or other medical **disability**.
- Federal regulations:
  - Require residential facilities that receive Medicaid or Medicare funding to contract with qualified dental personnel.
  - Do not require skilled nursing facilities to cover the costs of dental care.
  - Require facilities to assist residents in obtaining certain services (**Box 4-2**).
- State regulations vary significantly:
  - Regarding the provision of dental services for both Medicaid-eligible and Medicaid-ineligible individuals.[13]
  - In terms of frequency of examinations or elements included in routine or emergency care.
  - In terms of requiring facilities contract with a dentist to advise on policies and education.

Box 4-2 Services for Residents at Facilities That Receive Medicaid or Medicare Funding

Federal regulations require a facility receiving Medicaid or Medicare funding to help residents obtain the following services[12]:

- Comprehensive assessment of dental status.
- Routine as well as emergency dental services.
- Transportation to and from dental appointments.
- Prompt referral to a dentist for lost or damaged dentures.
- Supplies related to oral health (e.g., toothbrush, dental floss) at no cost to the individual.

III. Community-Based Settings

Community-based settings for alternative dental hygiene practice may include:

- Senior/adult day programs and aggregate meal sites.
- Work/activity centers for disabled individuals.
- Medical practices.
- Homeless shelters and transitional housing programs.
- Churches.
- Elementary and secondary schools (some already provide school-based medical care). (See Chapter 35.)
- Head Start and day care centers.

Dental Hygiene Care

I. Common Oral Problems and Conditions

Residence-bound patients often experience compromised daily oral care and/or infrequent routine dental care.[10,11] Oral complications due to chronic disease, treatments, and medications can result in further pain and dysfunction.[14,15]

- Studies have found the following problems and conditions are frequently identified on clinical examination[10,11,14,15]:
  - Periodontal infections.
  - Difficulty biting and chewing.
  - Dental caries, especially root caries.
  - Toothache/pain and abscess/swelling.
  - Trauma, fractured/loose teeth, or dental restorations.
  - Lost fillings/crowns.
  - Angular cheilosis.
  - Clenching/bruxism.
  - Xerostomia.
  - Candidiasis infection.
  - General oral soreness (mucositis).
  - Denture problems.
- **Table 4-1** identifies strategies for the prevention and management of select conditions.

Table 4-1 Strategies for Prevention and Management: Residence-Bound, Critically Ill, and Terminally Ill Patients

Common Problems	Strategies for Planning Dental Hygiene Care (Based on Assessment of Individualized Patient Needs)
Barriers to professional oral care	■ Assess and triage patient needs ■ Provide dental hygiene care ■ Refer/facilitate access for dental treatment
Inadequate biofilm removal	■ Assess patient activities of daily living, emotional status, and knowledge related to ability to perform self-care regimens ■ Educate about the role of biofilm in oral and systemic disease ■ Provide oral hygiene aids or develop adaptive measures to facilitate self-care ■ Train caregivers, as necessary, to provide daily oral care
Increased risk for dental caries	■ Identify/treat/prevent xerostomia ■ Provide professional and/or home fluoride application ■ Provide dietary analysis ■ Educate about reducing intake of fermentable carbohydrates ■ Educate about effective plaque biofilm removal ■ Engage caregivers, as necessary, to limit food/drink that promotes caries
Increased risk for periodontal infections	■ Provide dental hygiene care ■ Educate about the relationship between oral disease and systemic health ■ Provide oral hygiene aids or develop adaptive measures to facilitate self-care ■ Train caregivers, as necessary, to provide daily oral care
Inadequate nutritional intake	■ Assess for oral pain or inadequate chewing function that may be affecting the patient's nutritional intake ■ Severe weight loss can compromise denture fit and overall health ■ Consult with staff nutritionist, if available, in the patient's residential setting ■ Educate patient or caregivers, as necessary, regarding oral status and potential for compromised nutritional status
Oral pain/ dysfunction	■ Provide oral examination to identify oral/mucosal lesions ■ Document and follow-up on patient complaints of oral pain ■ Collaborate with patient's healthcare or palliative care team to advocate for dental needs ■ Train caregivers, as necessary, to provide regular oral inspection and record observations
Trauma	■ Monitor patient for signs of abuse and neglect ■ Monitor/educate about potential for facial/oral trauma during a fall ■ Educate about protocols for oral injury emergency care
Xerostomia*	■ Identify medications with a potential for causing xerostomia ■ Eliminate the use of oral products with alcohol, glycerin, or lemon ■ Educate about using sips of water or ice chips to relieve dryness ■ Use atomizer to help control the volume of water to avoid pooling or aspiration ■ Encourage use of over-the-counter saliva substitutes ■ Recommend use of candies or gums that do not contain sucrose ■ Train caregiver, as necessary, to identify/treat signs and symptoms
Candidiasis (and other oral infections)*	■ Educate about increased risk with use of prolonged antibiotic therapy ■ Educate about signs and symptoms of infections ■ Recommend topical or systemic antifungal treatment ■ Educate about effect of oral infections on systemic health ■ Train caregivers, as necessary, to identify/treat signs and symptoms
General oral soreness (mucositis)*	■ Monitor and document active lesions ■ Educate about daily inspection of tissues and need for immediate care to avoid secondary infections ■ Select saline mouthrinses, wax- or water-based lubricants, or topical anesthetics for comfort care
Denture problems*	■ Inspect denture or prosthesis and adjacent soft tissue ■ Educate about exacerbation of oral problems/lesions due to ill-fitting denture ■ Educate about impact of weight loss on fit of denture ■ Educate about accumulation of pathogenic biofilm on unclean denture ■ Soft reline material and proper daily care may address acute issues ■ Denture-induced lesions are described in Chapter 30

*Bhavana S, Lakshmi CR, Mpv P, et al. Palliative dental care. *J Clin Diagn Res.* 2014;8(6):1-6. Jucan AC, Saunders RH. Maintaining oral health in palliative care patients. *Ann Longterm Care.* 2015;23(9):15–20.

II. Significance of Oral Health to Overall Health

A growing body of evidence supports the interdependent relationship between oral health and systemic conditions.[16]

- Residence-bound patients have additional challenges:
  - Physical and cognitive limitations can compromise daily personal oral care abilities.
  - Oral pain/discomfort/dysfunction can compromise nutritional status.
  - Pain, including oral pain, can exacerbate negative behaviors in the cognitively impaired patient.
  - Oral health status and oral cleanliness can affect patient self-esteem, quality of life, and ability to communicate with family and caregivers.

III. Objectives of Care

The objectives of dental hygiene care of residence-bound individuals will vary according to the patient's situation and needs.

- A dental hygienist providing care in a residential setting may:
  - Provide intraoral/extraoral screening to triage and refer patients who need treatment by a dentist or specialist.
  - Assist in preventing further complication of the patient's health status by identifying oral infections and other problems.
  - Provide routine screening to detect lesions that may be pathologic, particularly those that may be early cancer.
  - Provide dental hygiene treatment and education interventions to prevent dental caries and periodontal infections.
  - Customize adaptive oral care practices that consider patients' and/or caregivers' unique needs. (See Section IX.)
  - Provide **palliative care** for the individual with a shortened life span.
  - Participate in the patient's care as a member of the healthcare team.
  - Contribute to the patient's general well-being and quality of life.

IV. Preparation for the Residential Visit

When providing patient care in any situation, the rule is "know before you go." The following steps will help prepare for a homebound patient visit.

A. Understanding the Patient

- Review the patient's medical history. (Hint: Provide the medical history form in advance for patient to complete and return.)
  - Monitor medication lists carefully, especially when the patient takes multiple prescription or over-the-counter preparations.
- Arrange telephone call or teledentistry communication to:
  - Clarify responses or ask questions about medical history.
  - Prescreen patient for signs/symptoms of potential exposure to communicable disease.
- Consider specific characteristics and problems associated with the patient's age, chronic medical condition, medications, mental health status, or physical/cognitive limitations.
  - Section IX reviews considerations for a variety of individuals with special needs.
- Determine precautions necessary for the individual patient's care and safety.
- Arrange with a dentist or attending physician when premedication or other prescription is required.
- Determine need for local anesthesia.

B. Instruments and Equipment

- Routine dental hygiene care can often be provided using manual instruments and without the need for powered equipment.
- Several dental equipment companies (listed in **Box 4-3**) manufacture portable dental delivery units, suctions, X-ray units, and autoclaves.
- Covered plastic tubs or boxes, labeled "clean" or "contaminated," are useful for carrying materials.
- The Organization for Safety, Asepsis, and Prevention (OSAP) provides infection control guidelines for safe delivery of oral care outside the dental office.[17]
- Additional equipment and supplies that can be transported by the clinician to the patient's residence are listed in **Box 4-4**.

C. Appointment Time

- Arrange the dental hygiene visit during a time when the patient is usually awake.
- Coordinate with patient or caregiver to assure visit is scheduled around nursing care and meals.

D. Practice Management

- Dental hygienists providing **direct access** services in a residential setting may be working as

Box 4-3 Commercial Sources for Portable Equipment

Dental Delivery Systems

A-Dec, Inc.

Website: www.a-dec.com
Toll-free phone: (800) 547-1883

Aseptico

Website: www.aseptico.com
Toll-free phone: (866) 244-2954

ASI Dental Specialties

Website: https://asidental.com/
Toll-free phone: (800) 566-9953

Bell Dental

Website: www.belldental.com
Toll-free phone: (800) 920-4478

DNTLworks Equipment Corporation

Website: www.dntlworks.com
Toll-free phone: (800) 847-0694

Safari Dental, Inc.

Website: www.safaridental.com
Toll-free phone: (800) 567-0013

Hand-Held X-Ray System

Dexis

Website: www.dexis.com
Toll-free phone: (888) 88-DEXIS

Autoclave

SciCan

Website: www.scican.com
Toll-free phone: USA: (800) 221-3046

Illuminated Loupes

Orascoptic

Website: www.orascoptic.com
Toll-free phone: (800) 369-3698

PeriOptix, Inc.

Website: www.perioptix.com
Toll-free phone: (800) 445-0345

Suction Toothbrushes

Sage Products, Inc.

Website: www.sageproducts.com
Toll-free phone: (800) 323-2220

HIMS Lifestyle Innovation

Website: https://hims-inc.com/
Phone: (512) 837-2000

Trademark Medical

Website: www.trademarkmedical.com
Toll-free phone: (800) 325-9044

a volunteer, employee, independent contractor, and/or business owner.[18] In these cases, the dental hygienist may need to consider the following factors:

- Individual state, province, or territorial practice acts[20]: Educational requirements, direct access scope of services, practice settings, referral methods.
- Provider claim submission: Procedures for billing for services provided by a dental hygienist (Health Insurance Portability and Accountability Act: National Provider Identifier number and Healthcare Provider Taxonomy code).
- Payment/reimbursement methods[21]: Private insurance, state/federal programs, facility or agency funds, public/private grants.
- Tax codes and policies: Self-employed individuals, business owners.

V. Approach to Patient

The dental hygienist may find approaching a relatively helpless, disabled, or ill person to be difficult. In addition, patients with cognitive disorders or impairments, such as dementia, can exhibit resistance to personal care.[22,23]

A. Communication

- Clinician empathy and understanding, as well as good interpersonal and communication skills, can help project a caring attitude toward the patient and put a vulnerable patient at ease.
- An overly caring attitude may not contribute to development of a cooperative patient relationship; a gentle but firm approach is most successful.
- Direct communication with the patient is most appropriate; however, communication with a caregiver may be necessary.

B. Personal Factors

- Establishment of rapport with the patient may depend on whether it was the patient or caregiver who requested/arranged for the appointment.
- Cooperation may depend on the patient's attitude toward the illness or disability.
- Residence-bound adults dependent on others for care can be at increased risk for abuse, neglect, and exploitation. (See Chapter 14.)
  - Be alert to the signs and symptoms.
  - Protocols for mandatory reporting vary by state.

Box 4-4 Instruments and Equipment to Provide Dental Hygiene Care for Residence-Bound Patients

Personal Protective Equipment

- See Chapter 6

Patient Education/Oral Hygiene Instruction Materials

- Toothbrushes, floss, interdental aids, tongue cleaner
- Denture brush, if needed
- Samples of adaptive aids for demonstration
- Hand mirror
- Written or printed patient education materials
- See Section IX for additional ideas on adaptive practices

Sterile Instruments

- Selection of hand instruments and other items required for patient care (i.e., mouth prop/bite block, sharpening stone, lip retractors)
- Are transported:
  - Before use in the sealed packages in which they were sterilized
  - After use in special plastic containers labeled for contaminated instruments

Disposable Items—Prepared in "Single Treatment" Packages That Are Convenient to Open and Use at Bedside

- Patient bib
- 2 × 2 gauze
- Cotton rolls/applicators
- Lubricant for patient lips

Additional Equipment

- Emesis basin (kidney-shaped basin facilitates the rinsing process)
- Portable headrest (attached to wheelchair or straight back chair to provide head support during treatment)
- A large plastic drape (helpful if patient's coordination is limited during rinsing)

Pharmaceuticals

- Pretreatment mouthrinse (only for patients who can spit)
- Disclosing agent
- Fluoride varnish topical fluoride preparation (varnish)
- **Silver diamine fluoride**[19]

Lighting

- Dental loupe systems with light-emitting diode (LED) headlight offer a direct light source and magnification (**Figure 4-1A**)
- Alternatively, a common LED headlamp is a convenient and inexpensive form of light (**Figure 4-1B**)
- Lighted mouth mirror
- Photography spotlight or gooseneck lamp with narrow, concentrated beam and adequate wattage to facilitate visibility

Miscellaneous Items—Usually Available at the Patient's Home

- Large towels (for covering pillows)
- Pillows (firm enough to assist in maintaining patients' head in stationary position)
- Hospital bed (can be adjusted to position patient most effectively)
- Wheelchair or chair with high back for head support
- Container for prostheses
- Power toothbrush

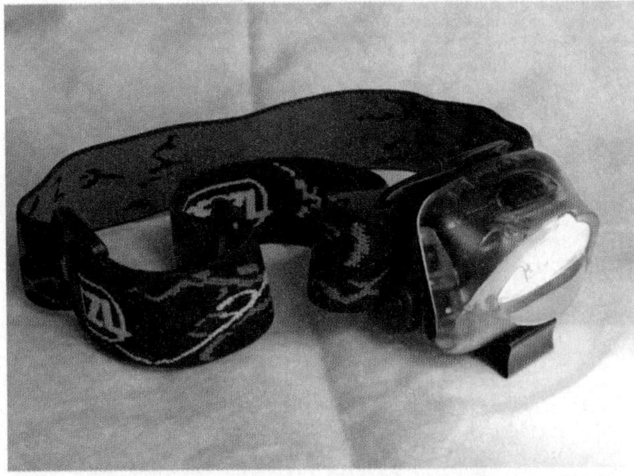

A

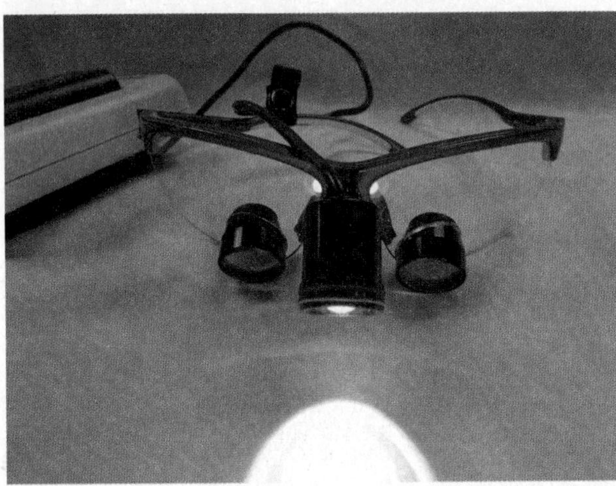

B

Figure 4-1 Lighting. **A.** A small light-emitting diode (LED) light with an attached headband, sometimes called a "camping" headlamp. **B.** Safety glasses with loupes and an attached LED headlamp. With either lighting system, the beam can be adjusted so that it is focused directly into the patient's oral cavity.

- Prolonged illness, suffering, the effects of inactivity, and monotonous confinement can contribute to **depression**.
  - A patient who is depressed may require extra attention to communication. (See Chapter 58.)
- Caring for the cognitively impaired or mentally ill patient can present unique challenges. (See Chapters 48 and 58.)

C. *Suggestions for General Procedure*

- For the safety of the patient, clinician, and others, limit the number of people in the workspace to those essential for patient care and procedural support.
- It may be helpful to request the primary caregiver be present to assist as needed and to demonstrate the current method of daily oral care.
- Introduce each step slowly to the patient. Do not make the patient feel rushed.
- Listen attentively; socializing is one of the best ways to establish rapport.
- Plan multiple appointments when extensive scaling is required to:
  - Avoid tiring the patient.
  - Observe tissue response.
  - Provide encouragement and follow-up education in biofilm control procedures.

VI. Treatment Location

Ingenuity is needed to arrange patient positioning to provide access for treatment as well as maintain comfort for both the patient and the clinician (**Figure 4-2**).

A. *Patient in Bed*

- *Hospital bed*: Adjust to lift patient's head to desirable height.
- *Ordinary bed, sofa, or cushioned chair*: Use firm pillows to support and stabilize the patient's head.
- *Small patient*: Positions for biofilm control described in Chapter 51 and shown in Figure 51-12 may be applicable during treatment.

B. *Patient in Wheelchair*

- Kitchen or a large bathroom can provide access to water and counter space.
- A portable headrest can be attached to the back of a straight chair or wheelchair. (See Chapter 51.)
- A straight chair or wheelchair can be backed against a wall to provide a stable headrest.

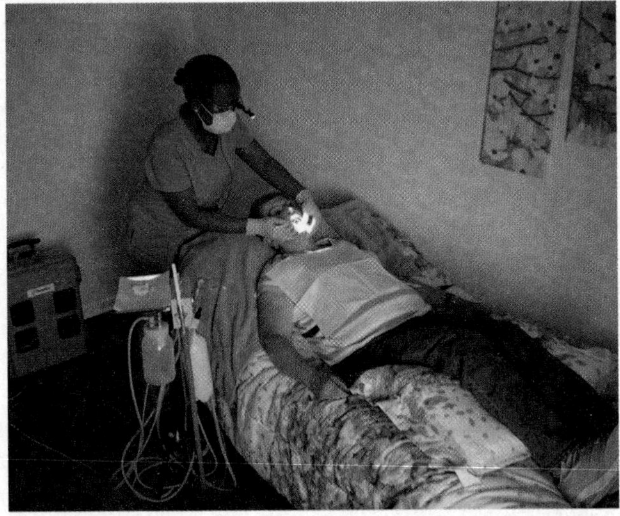

Figure 4-2 A Dental Hygiene Student Provides Patient Care Using a Headlamp and a Portable Dental Unit

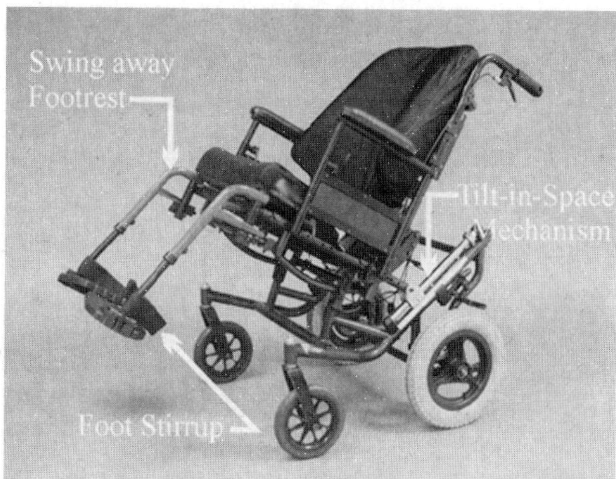

Figure 4-3 A Wheelchair That Is Designed to Tilt Back, Providing Comfort and Easy Access for Dental Care.

Reproduced from Frontera WR. *DeLisa's Physical Medicine and Rehabilitation*. 5th ed. Philadelphia, PA: Wolters Kluwer Health; 2010.

- Some wheelchairs tilt or slightly recline to facilitate patient positioning for care (**Figure 4-3**).
- A firm pillow can be inserted between the chair back and the patient's head to provide a cushioned resting surface.

VII. Additional Considerations

In addition to navigating patient treatment in an alternative setting, the unique needs of the residence-bound patient, and practice management matters, additional considerations may include:

- The role of the caregiver. Whether professional, family, or friend, the caregiver should be included in the care assessment, planning, and treatment according to the patient preferences and as much as they are able/willing.
- The role of communicable diseases. Residential settings can be less structured or controlled than clinical settings. Caring for vulnerable, enclosed populations requires multilayer precautions to limit the spread of disease. See interventions in Chapter 5.
- Identify threats to infection control and develop strategies to minimize risk of disease transmission. (See Chapters 5 and 6.)
- Keep up-to-date with recommended immunizations and screenings for healthcare workers.[24]
- Comply with local, state, and federal regulations to ensure sufficient protections.
- Initial assessment of the environment, patient needs, and business agreement can be discussed via virtual or face-to-face communication before treatment is planned or rendered.

VIII. Assessment and Care Planning

As in any patient care setting, dental hygiene interventions are provided using the dental hygiene process of care.

- Comprehensive patient assessment provides the basis for dental hygiene diagnosis.
- The dental hygiene diagnosis provides the foundation for planning treatment and prevention strategies that meet individualized patient needs.
- Follow-up appointments for maintenance and ongoing evaluation of the patient's oral condition determine whether treatment goals are met.
- Also, the direct access provider refers the patient to a dentist or specialist when warranted.

IX. Strategies for Prevention and Management

Table 4-1 identifies special considerations for developing a personalized prevention and management plan for residence-bound individuals.

- Additional strategies for preventing poor oral status can include:
  - Training caregivers.
  - Collaborating with members of **interprofessional healthcare teams**.

The Critically Ill or Unconscious Patient

Maintenance of oral cleanliness for the acutely ill or unconscious patient requires special procedures and approaches.

- When the patient's illness or injury involves the oral cavity, the advice and recommendations of the attending physician and/or oral surgeon are followed.
- Effective oral care can reduce the risk of pneumonia by preventing debris and microorganisms in the mouth from being aspirated, particularly in patients who have received mechanical breathing assistance.[16,25,26] (See Chapter 60.)
- The role of the dental hygienist is to evaluate and prioritize the patient's immediate oral care needs and provide appropriate curative or palliative oral care as needed.
  - Be familiar with the nature of the patient's chronic condition(s).

- Observe the health status of the soft and hard oral tissues.
- Address oral pain and infection first.
- Determine what type of services will improve or maintain the patient's oral health status without causing undue stress

I. Instructions for Caregivers

Personal oral care procedures for the unconscious or disabled patient must be accomplished by a caregiver.

- Assess caregiver's willingness and ability to provide daily oral care for the patient.
- Encourage and empower caregivers to provide daily oral care.
  - Include hands-on demonstration and practice.
  - For caregivers at a facility, this may include conducting an oral health in-service eduction program along with hands-on training.

A. Patients Who Are Edentulous or Dentulous

- Use appropriate precautions when placing fingers in the mouth to avoid injury from unintentional biting.
- A mouth prop can be placed in one side of the mouth while the other side is being retracted and cleaned.
- Gently brush or wipe all surfaces of the mouth (lips, teeth, gingiva, tongue, and oral mucosa) to remove biofilm at least twice a day. This will also prevent **sordes**.
  - A soft toothbrush or gauze-wrapped finger can be used to wipe the soft tissue.
  - A power toothbrush used with a very light touch or a suction toothbrush may be more efficient and effective on the hard tissue.

B. Patients with Removable Prosthesis

- If dentures or other removable prostheses are present, remove before providing oral care.
  - Often hospital policy requires removal of dentures when a patient is unconscious.
- When the dentures are removed:
  - Instruct the caregiver to clean and mark them. (See Chapter 30.)
  - Instruct the caregiver to change the water or liquid denture cleaner daily to prevent bacterial growth.
- Procedure for removing dentures is described in Chapter 30.

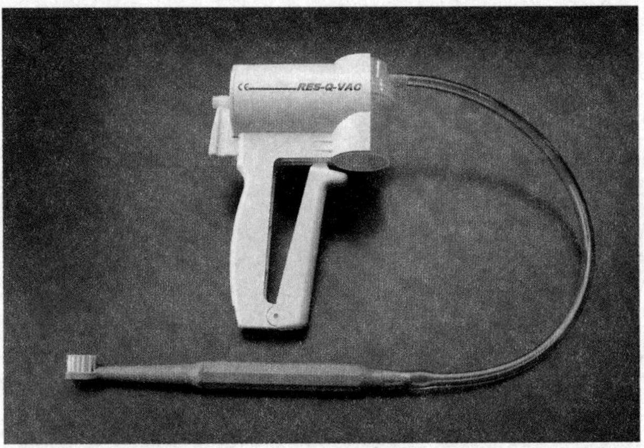

Figure 4-4 Commercial Suction Toothbrush. Plak-Vac/Res-Q-Vac combination features the Plak-Vac oral suction evacuator brush with the Res-Q-Vac hand-powered suction system.

Trademark Medical, St. Louis, MO.

II. Toothbrush with Suction Attachment

A specialized, single-use toothbrush is often used with patients who have difficulty swallowing or spitting.

- Tubing is connected from the end of a hollow toothbrush handle to an aspirator outlet or portable suction unit (**Figure 4-4**).
- During caregiver training, procedure for use is demonstrated and included in an oral care procedures manual.
- See **Box 4-5** for instructions on how to use a suction toothbrush.

The Terminally Ill Patient

The major difference in providing dental hygiene care for a terminally ill patient is a focus on short-term palliative care rather than long-term preventive care.[27]

- Terminal illness is no excuse for neglect of oral cleanliness; daily personal oral hygiene care is essential.
- Emphasis is on symptom relief and a clean oral environment, which can:
  - Enhance the patient's sense of dignity.
  - Improve quality of life.[14]
- The dental hygienist is in an ideal position to be a member of an interdisciplinary palliative care team.

I. Objectives of Care

The role of the dental hygienist is to provide oral care that emphasizes patient comfort more than preventive or restorative aspects of care. This may include:

- Providing relief of painful or aggravating symptoms of oral disease or lesions.

Box 4-5 Procedure for Use of Suction Toothbrush

- Prepare the patient.
- Although not able to respond in a usual manner, the patient may be aware of what is going on.
- Tell patient that the teeth are going to be brushed, and thereafter maintain a one-way conversation despite patient's inability to respond verbally.
- Turn patient on their side and place a pillow against the back for support.
- Place a small towel behind the patient's head and an emesis basin under patient's chin.
- Follow routine infection control and personal protective equipment guidelines.
- Attach toothbrush to suction outlet and lay brush on towel near patient's mouth.
- Place a rubber bite block on one side of the patient's mouth between the posterior teeth. Floss tied to the bite block can be fastened to patient's clothing with a safety pin.
- Dip brush in nonalcoholic, fluoridated mouthrinse or chlorhexidine; do not use toothpaste.
- Turn on suction.
- Gently retract lip and carefully apply the appropriate toothbrushing procedures; apply suction over each tooth surface with particular care at each interproximal area. Remoisten brush frequently.
- Move bite block to opposite side of mouth and continue brushing procedure.
- After brushing, place brush in a cup of clear water and allow water to be sucked through to clear and clean the tube.
- Remove bite block, wipe patient's lips, and apply a water-based lubricant.
- Rinse and disinfect toothbrush; sterilize bite block.

- Preventing aspiration of debris and oral microorganisms and reduce risk for pneumonia.
- Providing a "clean mouth" environment to reduce malodor and improve appearance and enhance personal interaction with caregivers and family members.
- Educating patients and caregivers about the importance of daily oral care.
- Helping develop standardized protocols for daily oral care as an integral part of the patient's overall palliative care treatment plan.

II. General Mouth Care Considerations

Poor oral hygiene is a common problem among terminally ill patients. Attention to mouth care and management of pain are essential components of providing end-of-life care.

A. Cleanliness

- Gentle but thorough daily cleaning of teeth, tongue, and oral mucosa is necessary.
- Provide oral care in any way the patient will allow, using soft toothbrush, gauze, or cloth.
- Dentifrice or other oral products are not necessary, but can add a refreshing flavor that the patient may like. Use caution as some products can cause irritation or create a burning sensation on already fragile tissues.
- Be mindful of the patient's limited swallowing function or spitting ability.

B. Common Oral Conditions

- Xerostomia: Common among terminally ill individuals due to medications, dehydration, or mouth breathing.[28] Work with palliative care team to minimize medications that increase xerostomia.[29]
- Candidiasis infection: Oral cultures of *Candida albicans* were found in as many as 79% of terminally ill patients. In immunocompromised individuals, the infection can become life threatening.[28]
- General oral soreness (mucositis): Approximately 75% of hospice patients examined in one study had evidence of pathologic changes in the oral mucosa, and 42% reported soreness of the oral mucosa.[28]
- Denture problems: More than 70% of hospice patients who wore dentures reported having some kind of difficulty wearing their dentures.[28]

C. Visual Inspection

- Frequent inspection of the patient's mouth is necessary to identify oral lesions that can cause discomfort or lead to serious infection.
- Use loupes with illumination, penlight or small flashlight, and soft handle of toothbrush to examine the oral cavity.

Documentation

Key concepts for documenting dental hygiene care provided in alternative settings include:

- Description of location where treatment is provided.
- Description of the patient's current health status and functional ability, particularly related to ability to provide self-care.
- Notation of whether or not caregiver assistance is needed/available for daily oral care.
- Summary of oral health assessment data.

- Specific recommendations/education for oral care techniques and adjunct oral hygiene aids.
- Details of dental hygiene interventions/services provided.
- Recommendations for follow-up care and referrals made.
- A sample documentation can be found in **Box 4-6**.

Factors to Teach the Patient

- Good oral health contributes to good general health and better quality of life.
- Dental caries is preventable through effective daily oral care and limited consumption of sugary food and drink, especially between meals.
- How to use customized adaptive oral care aids to facilitate patient's independence.

Factors to Teach the Caregiver

- Consider personal safety of caregiver and patient: environment, biting, infection control.
- Care for the patient's natural teeth and gums.
- Evaluate and address unique patient needs, adapt care as needed. (See Section IX.)
- Care for the patient's removable and nonremovable prostheses. (See Chapter 30.)
- Offer food and drink that are not cariogenic.
- How to use a suction toothbrush, power brush, or other device to assist with better oral care for the patient.

Box 4-6 Example Documentation: Bedside Oral Care for Patient in a Nursing Home

- **S**—Routine nursing home visit for continuing care. The 89-year-old female patient is confined to a hospital bed, comfortable and alert; arm strength notably weakened since last visit and she is distressed that she can no longer support her own toothbrush for daily oral care. Nurse aide caregiver has been trying to assist but doesn't know how. Patient states: "Every time she tries to brush my teeth she chokes me or hurts my gums."
- **O**—Excessive dental biofilm noted on facial surfaces of maxillary molars.
- **A**—Patient can no longer perform oral self-care independently, causing increased risk of oral infection and subsequent increased risk of systemic effects. Caregiver needs training to provide efficient, effective, and comfortable intraoral brushing.
- **P**—Discussed benefits of daily oral biofilm removal. Demonstrated effective oral care. Assured both patient and caregiver that oral care can be provided without discomfort. Demonstrated and supervised caregiver providing bedside oral care and biofilm removal with soft, child-sized toothbrush.

Next steps: Follow-up visit scheduled with patient and caregiver in 2 weeks.

Signed:______________________, RDH

Date: ______________________

References

1. National Research Council. *Improving Access to Oral Health Care for Vulnerable and Underserved Populations*. Washington, DC: The National Academies Press; 2011.
2. American Dental Hygienists' Association. Advocacy: practice issues: direct access. http://www.adha.org/direct-access. Accessed September 1, 2021
3. Smith BJ, Ghezzi EM, Manz MC, et al. Perceptions of oral health adequacy and access in Michigan nursing facilities. *Gerodontology*. 2008;25(2):89-98.
4. El-Yousfi S, Jones K, White S, et al. A rapid review of barriers to oral healthcare for vulnerable people. *Br Dent J*. 2019(227); 143-151.
5. Willink A, Schoen C, Davis K. Dental care and Medicare beneficiaries: access gaps, cost burdens, and policy options. *Health Affairs*. 2016;35(12):2241-2248.
6. National Network for Oral Health Access. *Teledentistry Learning Collaborative Teledentistry User Guide*. NNOHA Teledentistry Users Guide_Final August 2021.pdf. Accessed February 4, 2022.
7. Rodriguez TE, Galka AL, Lacy ES, et al. Can midlevel dental providers be a benefit to the American public? *J Health Care Poor Underserved*. 2013;24(2):892-906.
8. Langelier M, Baker B, Continelli T. Expanded scopes of practice for dental hygienists associated with improved oral health outcomes for adults. *Health Affairs*. 2016;35(12):2207-2215.
9. Langelier M, Baker B, Continelli T. *Development of a New Dental Hygiene Professional Practice Index by State*. Rensselaer, NY: Oral Health Workforce Research Center, Center for Health Workforce Studies, School of Public Health, SUNY Albany; 2016:152.
10. Sifuentes AMF, Lapane KL. Oral health in nursing homes: what we know and what we need to know. *J Nurs Homes Res Sci*. 2020;6:1-5.
11. Chen X, Clark JJ, Naorungroj S. Oral health in nursing home residents with different cognitive statuses. *Gerodontology*. 2013;30(1):49-60.
12. U.S. Government Printing Office. Electronic code of federal regulations (Title 42: Public Health, Part 483—requirements for

states and long term care facilities, Subpart B, Section 483.55, dental services). http://www.ecfr.gov/cgi-bin/text-idx?c=ecfr;sid=b97291f05d23f16ffa8e711922642bcc;rgn=div5;view=text;node=42%3A5.0.1.1.2;idno=42;cc=ecfr. Accessed Sep 1, 2021.

13. Centers for Medicare and Medicaid Services. Medicaid: dental care. https://www.medicaid.gov/medicaid/benefits/dental/index.html. Accessed September 1, 2021.
14. Fischer DJ, Epstein JB, Yao Y, et al. Oral health conditions affect functional and social activities of terminally ill cancer patients. *Support Care Cancer*. 2014;22(3):803-810.
15. Mercadante S, Aielli F, Adile C, et al. Prevalence of oral mucositis, dry mouth, and dysphagia in advanced cancer patients. *Support Care Cancer*. 2015;23(11):3249-3255.
16. Linden GJ, Lyons A, Scannapieco FA. Periodontal systemic associations: review of the evidence. *J Clin Periodontol*. 2013; 84(40 suppl):S8-S19.
17. Organization for Safety, Asepsis and Prevention. OSAP Resources. https://www.osap.org/resources. Accessed September 1, 2021.
18. Naughton D. Expanding oral care opportunities: direct access care provided by dental hygienists in the United States. *J Evid Based Dent Pract*. 2014;14 suppl:171-182.
19. Horst J, Ellenikiotis H, Milgrom PM. UCSF protocol for caries arrest using silver diamine fluoride: rationale, indications, and consent. *J Calif Dent Assoc*. 2016;44(1):16-28.
20. American Dental Hygienists' Association. Scope of practice. http://www.adha.org/scope-of-practice. Accessed July 14, 2017.
21. American Dental Hygienists' Association. Reimbursement. https://www.adha.org/reimbursement. Accessed September 1, 2021.
22. Jablonski R, Therrien B, Mahoney EK, et al. An intervention to reduce care-resistant behaviors in persons with dementia during oral hygiene: a pilot study. *Spec Care Dentist*. 2011;31(3):77-88.
23. Ahn H, Horgas AL. Disruptive behaviors in nursing home residents with dementia: management approaches. *J Clin Outcomes Manag*. 2013;20(12):566-576.
24. National Center for Immunization and Respiratory Diseases. Recommended vaccines for healthcare workers. https://www.cdc.gov/vaccines/adults/rec-vac/hcw.html. Accessed February 4, 2022.
25. Shi Z, Xie H, Wang P, et al. Oral hygiene care for critically ill patients to prevent ventilator-associated pneumonia. *Cochrane Database Syst Rev*. 2013;(8):CD008367.
26. Quinn B, Baker DL, Cohen S, et al. Basic nursing care to prevent nonventilator hospital-acquired pneumonia. *J Nurs Scholarsh*. 2014;46(1):11-19.
27. Bhavana S, Lakshmi CR, Mpv P, et al. Palliative dental care. *J Clin Diagn Res*. 2014;8(6):1-6.
28. Venkatasalu MR, Murang ZR, Ramasamy DTR, Dhaliwal JS. Oral health problems among palliative and terminally ill patients: an integrated systematic review. *BMC Oral Health*. 2020;20(1):79.
29. Jucan AC, Saunders RH. Maintaining oral health in palliative care patients. *Ann Longterm Care*. 2015;23(9):15-20.

SECTION II

Preparation for Dental Hygiene Practice

Introduction for Section II

Preparation for dental hygiene care is centered on the use of standard precautions for infection control to ensure the comfort and safety of patients, dental personnel, and others who come in contact with the environment of the clinic or office.

- Health services facilities, including dental facilities, must be places for prevention and management of disease, not for increasing risk of disease or discomfort following inadequate precautionary measures and habits of the professional personnel.
- The responsibility of the entire team is to develop and maintain work practices for all appointments that will:
  - Prevent direct or indirect cross-infection between dental personnel and patients and from one patient to another.
  - Maintain comfort for both the patient and the oral health provider.
- Chapters in this section:
  - Provide specific information about the chain of infection and the microorganisms that can be transmitted in the dental setting when standard precautions are not observed.
  - Describe specific materials and procedures necessary for safe clinical practice.
  - Place emphasis on the ergonomic factors of patient positioning; body posture; and hand, wrist, and arm positions to maintain practitioner comfort and prevent musculoskeletal problems.

The Dental Hygiene Process of Care

- Preparation for clinical practice does not form a specific step in the Dental Hygiene Process of Care (**Figure II-1**); however, practices described in this section protect the patient and the practitioner and are part of all the components of the process.

Ethical Applications

- A dental hygienist may be involved in a variety of moral, ethical, and legal situations during all professional actions related to the process of care.
- A goal of preparation for dental hygiene practice is to increase awareness of, and sensitivity to, potential ethical situations.
- Basic core values and principles, as outlined in the various dental hygiene codes of ethics, are applied in every phase of the dental hygiene appointment.
- Basic core values in dental hygiene are identified as selected principles of ethical behavior that can be considered integral to the code of the dental hygiene profession.
- Ethical principles contained in the codes clarify the standards of judgment that professionals will follow.
- Ethical principles are combined with philosophical theories when making a decision.
- An overview of the core values with definitions and applications is found in **Table II-1**.

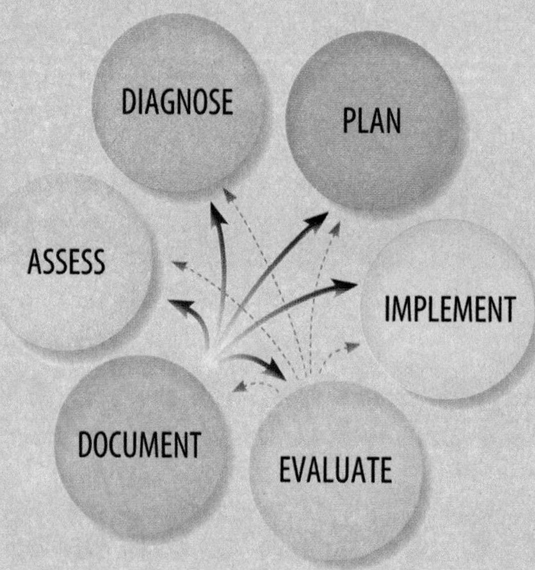

Figure II-1 The Dental Hygiene Process of Care

Table II-1 Dental Hygiene Core Values

Ethical Principle/Core Value	Explanation	Application Examples
Autonomy	Patient's right to self-determination and making choices for care.	Educate the patient before obtaining informed consent.
Beneficence	Performing services for the good of the patient.	Apply standards of infection control for all patients.
Nonmaleficence	Removing or preventing harm during the treatment process.	Individualize biofilm control and perform subgingival debridement.
Justice	Fair treatment for all patients.	Follow acceptable standards and provide access to care for all patients.
Confidentiality	Protection of sensitive information.	Follow HIPAA Security standards for protected patient information and records.
Veracity	Truth-telling.	Develop trust between patient and provider to obtain the medical history.
Fidelity	Keeping promises.	Help a fearful patient feel comfortable by using local anesthesia or nitrous oxide.

CHAPTER 5

Infection Control: Transmissible Diseases

Katherine Soal, RDH, MSDH

CHAPTER OUTLINE

LEARNING OBJECTIVES

After studying this chapter, the student will be able to:

1. Apply the concept of standard precautions and transmission-based precautions to the process of dental hygiene care.
2. Describe the infectious disease process and prevention of disease transmission.
3. Describe and identify transmissible diseases that may pose a risk to patients and dental healthcare personnel.
4. Evaluate the oral healthcare needs of each patient with transmissible disease(s).

For healthcare providers, **infection** and **communicable** disease can lead to illness, disability, and loss of work time. In addition, patients, family members, and community contacts may be exposed, may become ill, and lose productive time or suffer permanent aftereffects.

- In oral healthcare practice, the objective is to protect patients, **dental healthcare personnel (DHCP)**, and others who may become exposed to **infectious agents** in the clinical environment.
- Facilities must operate under an organized system for training of DHCP along with strict adherence to standard precautions, transmission-based precautions, safe injection practices, and sharps safety.
- All DHCP are responsible for preventing direct and/or indirect cross-contamination and disease transmission between DHCP and patients, and from patient to patient.

Infectious Agents

I. Definition

- Infectious agents are organisms that are capable of producing infection or infectious disease and include bacteria, viruses, fungi, protozoa, helminths, and prions.
- Each infectious agent has specific characteristics that produce specific reactions in an infected individual and can be pathogenic (disease producing) or nonpathogenic.
- Nonpathogenic agents may have pathogenic outcomes in susceptible individuals.
- Human response to infectious agents varies with the status of the host immune system and the pathogenicity of the invading agent.

II. Infectious Microorganisms

A. Bacteria

- Microscopic living organisms, composed of a single cell, found in every habitat and environment.
- Some diseases caused by bacteria can be treated with antibiotic medications, while others can be prevented through vaccination.
- Examples: *Streptococcus pyogenes* (strep throat) is treated with antibiotics and *Clostridium tetani* (tetanus) is prevented by vaccination.

B. Viruses

- **Viruses** are microscopic organisms that are generally considered to be nonliving as they can only replicate within a host cell.
- Some diseases caused by viruses can be treated with antiviral medications, while others can be prevented through vaccination.
- Examples: Herpes simplex 1 (HSV-1) can be treated, but not cured, with antivirals, and hepatitis B (HBV) is prevented through vaccination.

C. Fungi

- Can be single-celled or complex multicellular living organisms.
- Diseases caused by fungi can be treated with antifungal agents. There are no vaccines available to prevent fungal infections.
- Example: *Candida albicans* is treated with antifungal medications.

D. Protozoa, Helminths, and Prions

- Protozoa are single-celled organisms causing parasitic infections.
- Example: Mosquitoes transmit *Plasmodium* species to humans, causing malaria.
- Helminths are multicellular invertebrates that cause parasitic infections.
- Example: The roundworm *Trichinella spiralis* is transmitted to humans, causing trichinosis.
- Prions are misfolding proteins transmitted to humans by infected meat products that prompt normal proteins to misfold, causing neurodegenerative diseases such as Creutzfeldt-Jakob disease (CJD) and bovine spongiform encephalitis (BSE).

III. Immunity and Vaccines

Immunity to a disease occurs when the immune system develops **antibodies** in order to eliminate the infectious agent (**antigen**).[1]

A. Passive Immunity

- Protection transferred from one animal or person to another.
- Provides immediate but temporary immunity.
  - Examples: Antibodies passed from a mother to her infant, intravenous transfusion of immunoglobulin IgG to prevent hepatitis B after exposure.

B. Active Immunity

- Protection acquired in the body by having the disease and recovering, or by vaccination.
- Protection takes time to develop and can provide life-long immunity.

- Examples: A child who contracts measles and recovers, or a child who receives the measles vaccination and does not suffer the disease symptoms.

C. Vaccines

- Products that provide immunity by stimulating the immune system to produce antibodies to a specific infectious agent.
- Administered enterally (oral) or parentally (injection or nasal).
- The more similar a vaccine is to the infectious agent, the better the immune response to the vaccine.
- Live attenuated vaccines contain a weakened form of the infectious agent and can provide lifelong immunity.
    - Examples: Measles, mumps, and rubella (MMR) and varicella vaccines.
- Inactivated vaccines contain whole or partial inactive infectious agents manipulated to elicit an immune response.
- Immunity from inactivated vaccines may not last. Multiple doses and booster vaccinations may be necessary.
    - Examples: Poliomyelitis and hepatitis A virus (HAV) vaccines.

D. Messenger RNA Vaccines

- Some vaccines use messenger ribonucleic acid (mRNA) instead of live attenuated or inactivated virus.[1,2]
- mRNA vaccines work by taking a "message" to cells that prompts them to make a specific protein, which is then recognized by the immune system as an antigen.
- The immune system then makes antibodies against the specific protein, which in the case of SARS-CoV-2, is one of the spike proteins found on the surface of the virus.
- When the specific virus enters the body, the immune system recognizes the protein and sends antibodies to destroy the protein, which in turn destroys the virus.
- mRNA vaccines only deliver the message to make the protein. They cannot enter the cell nucleus or interact with, alter, or damage deoxyribonucleic acid (DNA).

E. Significance

- The World Health Organization lists 27 vaccine-preventable diseases, of which 20 can be life threatening, and diseases that were once common are now at an all-time low after extensive and decades-long vaccination programs.[3]
- Vaccines are the most effective way to prevent many serious infectious diseases and have dramatically reduced the number of deaths and disabilities attributed to disease.
    - Example: The measles vaccination averted 23 million deaths between 2010 and 2018.[3]
- Childhood diseases such as measles, mumps, rubella, and varicella can have serious consequences if contracted during adulthood, pregnancy, old age, or while immunocompromised.
- Vaccinations can prevent infection-related cancers, have eradicated smallpox, and have nearly eliminated polio worldwide.[3]

IV. Variants and Treatment Resistance

- All microorganisms are capable of replicating and evolving to survive.
- When infectious agents replicate, they can develop **mutations**, which are changes in their DNA or RNA caused by errors in replication or by stress from the host immune system, vaccines, and medications.
- Mutations allow the infectious agents to develop mechanisms that can evade the immune system and vaccines, and develop resistance to drugs used to treat the diseases they cause.
- When enough mutations have occurred, a new **variant** of the infectious agent emerges that can be more infectious, **drug resistant**, and difficult to treat.
- When a variant has developed distinct biologic characteristics that differ from the original version, it is called a new **strain**.

Microorganisms of the Oral Cavity

I. Origin

- In utero, the oral cavity is sterile, but after birth microorganisms are transmitted to the infant from the mother, other family members, and caretakers.[4,5]
- As the infant grows, there is continuing introduction of diverse microorganisms that colonize the oral cavity, forming complex oral biofilms.[4,5]
- The microbiota of the average adult harbors 50 to 100 billion bacteria, represented by over 700 different organisms.

II. Infection Potential

- Intact mucous membranes of the oral cavity provide some protection against infection.
- **Pathogenic**, potentially pathogenic, or nonpathogenic microorganisms may be permanently or transitorily present in the oral cavity of each patient.
- Patients may be **carriers** of certain diseases but show no signs or symptoms (**asymptomatic carrier**).

III. Cross-Contamination

- Spread of microorganisms from one source to another: person to person, or person to an inanimate object and then to another person.
- Recognition of possible transfer of transmissible diseases provides the basis for planning a system of disinfection, sterilization, and management of instruments, equipment, and environment.
- Disease transmission within a dental facility may occur because of inappropriate work practices, such as:
  - Careless handwashing and/or unhygienic personal habits.
  - Inadequate sterilization and handling of sterile instruments and materials.
  - Inadequate or inappropriate personal protective equipment (PPE), ventilation, and overall infection control practices.

Precautions

I. Standard Precautions

- **Standard precautions** represent a minimum standard of care to both protect DHCP and prevent DHCP from transmitting infectious agents among themselves and their patients.[6,7]
- Apply to all patients and procedures.
- Apply to contact with the following:
  - Blood.
  - Saliva.
  - All body fluids, secretions, and excretions (except sweat), regardless of whether they contain blood.
  - Nonintact (broken) skin.
  - Mucous membranes.

II. Transmission-Based Precautions

- **Transmission-based precautions** are to be used in addition to standard precautions when a patient has or is suspected of having a disease that can spread through contact, droplet, or airborne routes.[6,7,8]
- Droplet precautions
  - Intended to prevent disease transmission from close respiratory or mucous membrane contact with respiratory secretions transmitted through airborne droplets (sneezing, coughing, talking).
  - Examples: *Bordetella pertussis*, influenza virus, SARS-CoV-2.
- Contact precautions
  - Intended to prevent disease transmission from direct or indirect contact with the patient or patient's environment.
  - Examples: Vancomycin-resistant enterococci, methicillin-resistant *Staphylococcus aureus* (MRSA).
- Airborne precautions
  - Intended to prevent transmission of diseases that remain infectious while suspended in the air over long distances.
  - Special air handling and ventilation required.
  - Examples: *Legionella pneumophila, Mycobacterium tuberculosis*, SARS-CoV-2, and measles.
- Sharps precautions
  - Intended to prevent bloodborne pathogen transmission by **percutaneous** sharps injury.
  - Examples: Hepatitis B virus (HBV), hepatitis C virus (HCV), and human immunodeficiency virus (HIV).

The Infectious Process

I. Essential Features for Disease Transmission

A chain of events is required for the spread of an infectious agent. The six essential links are shown in **Figure 5-1** and described here.

- An *infectious agent* such as:
  - Bacteria, viruses, fungi, protozoa.
  - Each infectious agent has its own specific reaction in an infected host.
- A *reservoir* where the infectious agents are found in their own essential environment, which may be instruments, a dental unit waterline, respiratory secretions, and blood.
  - For example, a dental unit waterline is a potential reservoir for *L. pneumophila*, and lungs are reservoirs for *M. tuberculosis*.
- A *port of exit* or mode of escape from the reservoir.

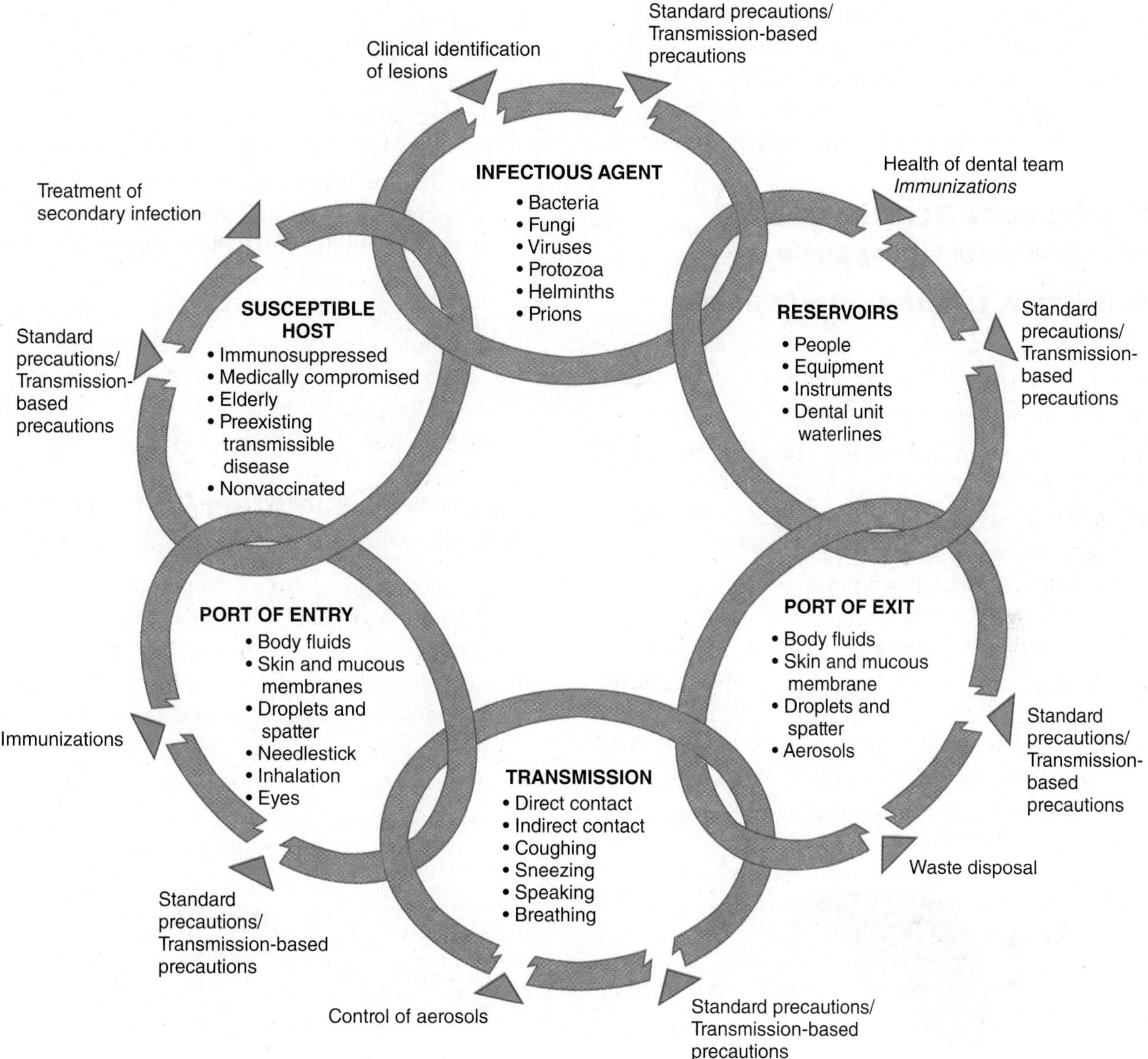

Figure 5-1 Interventions to Break the Chain of Disease Transmission. A break in the chain of six major links is required to stop the spread of an infectious agent. Standard precautions and transmission-based precautions are applied to interrupt the chain.

- Infectious agents exit from their reservoir(s) through various modes, such as coughing, sneezing, speaking, bleeding periodontium, sharps use, or in water from a contaminated waterline.
- Aerosol generating procedures (AGPs) facilitate the aerosolization of infectious agents from their respective reservoirs.

- A *mode of transmission*
  - May be direct as in person to person by respiratory aerosols, or indirect by contaminated hands or a percutaneous sharps injury.
  - Transmission by aerosol may be direct from the respiratory tract of one person to the oral cavity of the receiving host by coughing, sneezing, or speaking, or indirect by transfer to hands or instruments and then to the receiving host.
- A *port of entry* or mode of entry of the infectious agent into the new host.
  - Modes of entry may be similar to modes of exit.
  - The respiratory tract, eyes, mucous membranes, nonintact periodontium or skin, or percutaneous sharps injury.
- A **susceptible host** that does not have immunity or defense to the invading infectious agent, such as:
  - A patient taking an immunosuppressant drug to control autoimmune diseases, prevent solid organ transplant rejection, and as cancer chemotherapy.

- A patient who has not had or has not maintained recommended vaccinations, or does not seroconvert after vaccination.
- A patient who is medically compromised, elderly, or has preexisting transmissible disease.

II. Airborne Transmission of Infectious Diseases

A. Aerosol, Droplets, and Spatter

All dental procedures produce contamination in the form of aerosols that become airborne with the potential to transmit infectious diseases.[9,10]

- An aerosol is a solid or liquid particle suspended in air.
- Aerosol particles range in size from 1 to 100 μm and are classified according to size.[9-11]
  - Droplet nuclei: <5 μm.
  - Droplets: 5–100 μm.
  - Spatter: >100 μm.
- Particles up to 200 μm are capable of being inhaled.
- Aerosolized droplet nuclei can be inhaled deep into the lungs. *M. tuberculosis* and SARS-CoV-2 have been found in aerosols <5 μm.[10] (**Figure 5-2**).
- Particles <100 μm can travel up to 4 m when produced by coughing and up to 2 m when produced by speaking.[11,12]
- Spatter remains airborne a relatively short time because of size and weight, then drops or spatters in a ballistic pattern where it may be visible, particularly after it has landed on skin, hair, clothing, or environmental surfaces where gross contamination can result.
- Spatter may come in direct contact with mucous membranes of the eyes, nose, and mouth.
- Larger spatter particles can be trapped higher in the respiratory tract and may be coughed or sneezed out.

B. Aerosol-Generating Procedures (AGPs)

- All dental procedures produce aerosols directly through AGPs and indirectly when the patient coughs, sneezes, and speaks.[11]
- AGPs include use of sonic and ultrasonic scalers, air polishing, high- and low-speed handpieces, and air/water syringes.[9,11]
- Almost any dental procedure, such as taking radiographs and impressions or performing intra-

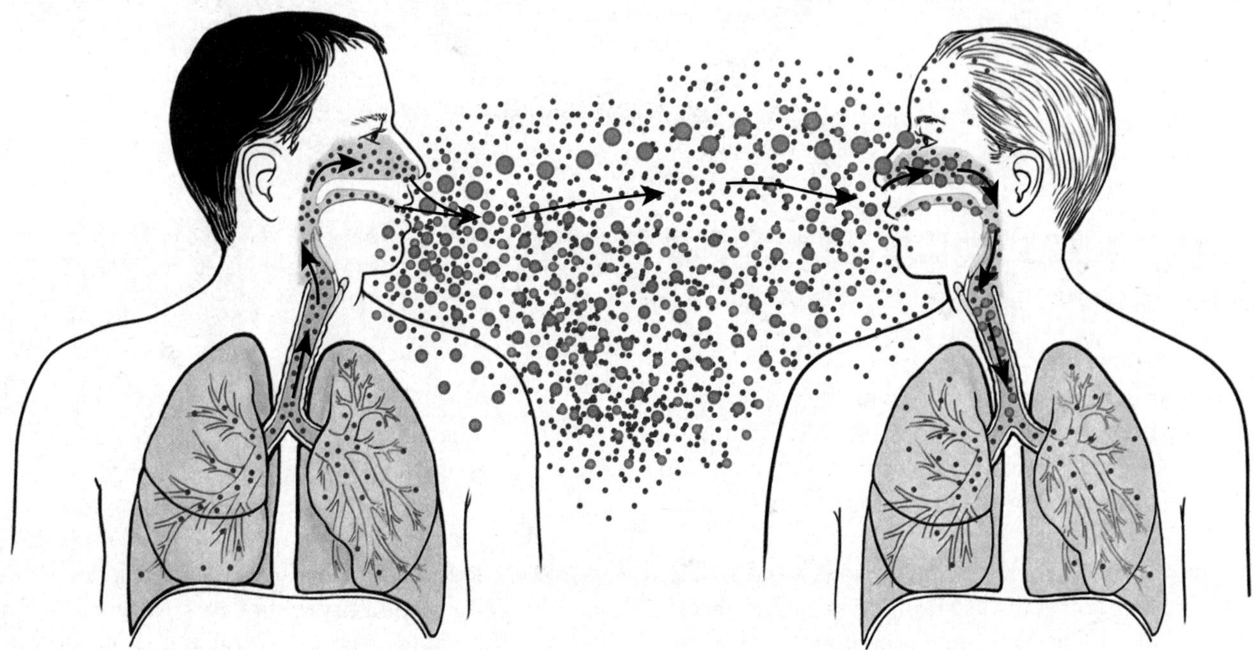

Figure 5-2 Many Potentially Pathogenic Microorganisms Are Disseminated by Aerosols and Spatter

oral examinations, can result in the production of aerosolized particles, especially if the patient coughs or gags.[11]

- Aerosols and spatter may contain:
  - Single or clumps of infectious agents such as *Staphylococcus* and *Streptococcus* species, *M. tuberculosis*, and viruses.
  - Tooth and restoration fragments, tissue, saliva, biofilm, blood, sputum, oil from hand pieces, and water from dental unit waterlines.[9]
- Concentration and distribution of aerosols and spatter:
  - Aerosols and spatter are in greater concentration close to the site of instrumentation.
  - Aerosols travel with air currents and may move from room to room.
  - Distribution of aerosols is influenced by temperature, humidity, and ventilation.[12]
  - Spatter can be transferred to all areas of the dental office by contact transfer and can result in self-inoculation if a patient or DHCP touches their own eyes or mucous membranes with contaminated hands.[12]
  - Aerosols and spatter can settle in dust particles, which can then be sources of contamination.
  - When doors are opened and closed and people pass in and out, dust is set into motion and can settle on instruments, working surfaces and equipment, or people.
  - *C. tetani* (tetanus) and enteric bacteria are among the infectious agents that may travel in dust in and around dental treatment areas.

III. Bloodborne Transmission of Infectious Diseases

A. Bloodborne Pathogens

- Bloodborne pathogens are microorganisms that can be transmitted to anyone exposed to contaminated body fluids.
- In dentistry, exposure to bloodborne pathogens is an occupational hazard that can have serious life-altering and life-threatening consequences.
- All dental procedures expose DHCP to potentially infectious body fluids, including blood and saliva.
- Blood may not always be visible in saliva.
- There are 20 bloodborne pathogens known to cause disease, of which three—HBV, HCV, and HIV—are of most concern to DHCP.[13]
- Only HBV has a vaccine that is recommended for all healthcare workers. There are no vaccines currently available for HCV and HIV.[13]

B. Transmission Routes of Bloodborne Pathogens

- Bloodborne pathogens can be transmitted by accidental percutaneous injury; contact with cuts, abrasions, or eyes; and mucocutaneous exposure to infected blood.
- Percutaneous injury to DHCP occurs when a sharp object pierces the skin.
- Examples of dental sharps that can cause injury include dental anesthetic needles, burs, endodontic files, scalpels, suture needles, scalers, and curets.
- Sharps injury can also occur during instrument processing and sterilization procedures.
- Sharps safety is of paramount importance in the dental office and is regulated by federal and state authorities.
- See Chapter 36 for additional information on sharps management.

A. General Precautions

- All dental procedures have the potential to transmit infectious diseases.[7]
- Procedures must be carefully monitored for all patients with or without a known communicable disease.
- All DHCP must observe strict adherence to standard and transmission-based precautions.[12]
- Dental facilities must have written infection control and safety protocols, and provide appropriate training of DHCP.[7]

B. Control of Airborne Disease Transmission

- Installation of air-control methods to supply clean air, adequate ventilation, filtration, and relative humidity in the operatory area.
- Management of AGPs to control the production and dissemination of potentially contaminated aerosols by[9,11]:
  - Use of high-volume extraoral suction during all procedures.
  - Use of high-volume intraoral evacuation with ultrasonic instrumentation and air polishing.
  - Use manual instrumentation as much as possible on patients with known or suspected infectious disease.
  - Use a rubber dam and high-volume evacuation for sealants and other applicable procedures.
  - Oral biofilm removal by patient prior to beginning of procedure.

- Routine preprocedural rinsing with antiseptic or antimicrobial mouthrinse such as chlorhexidine gluconate 0.12% can reduce the numbers of microorganisms contained in aerosols.[14]
    - Swish vigorously to force mouthrinse between teeth for at least 30 seconds to 2 minutes before expectorating.

C. Control of Bloodborne Disease Transmission

- Strict adherence to sharps safety protocols.[13]
- Appropriate use of safety-engineered devices such as safety syringes and needle recapping devices.
- Immediate and appropriate disposal of contaminated disposable sharps.
- Use of puncture-resistant gloves when handling contaminated instruments.

D. Clean Water

- Dental waterlines can harbor biofilm reservoirs for microorganisms such as *Legionella, Mycobacterium, and Pseudomonas* species.
- Water that meets Environmental Protection Agency regulatory standards for drinking water (less than 500 **CFU** [colony-forming units]/mL of heterotrophic water bacteria) must be used.[7]
- Flushing of waterlines for at least 20–30 seconds between patients can reduce cross-contamination with **planktonic** microorganisms.
- Flushing of waterlines will not affect or remove bacterial biofilms from the inside of dental waterlines.
- Additional methods to prevent and treat dental waterline biofilm are needed to assure treatment water quality.[7]
    - Self-contained water systems with in-line water filters and antiretraction devices to prevent backflow.
    - Regular water quality testing and chemical treatments to maintain safe waterlines.

E. Protection of Clinician

- Use PPE. See Chapter 6.
- Check and maintain personal immunizations.
- Education and training in the signs, symptoms, and transmission of infectious agents.
- Postexposure management for sharps injuries.
- Do not treat a patient who is infectious unless absolutely necessary.

F. Protection of Patient

- Use protective eyewear to prevent direct spatter and aerosols to face and eyes.
- DHCP must not treat patients if they themselves have transmissible disease signs and symptoms.

G. Maintain and Review Infection Control Protocols

- Utilize official guidelines from the Centers for Disease Control and Prevention (**CDC**), state public health agencies, and the Occupational Safety and Health Administration (OSHA).
- Follow recommendations described in Chapters 6 and 7.

Transmissible Diseases of Concern to DHCP

- Pathogens are often present without producing any discernable signs or symptoms, a fact of particular importance to the total consideration of prevention of disease transmission.
- Selected pathogens of concern to DHCP and their disease manifestations, mode of transfer, **incubation period**, and communicability periods are provided in **Table 5-1**.
- Viral hepatitis, human herpesviruses, human papillomavirus, HIV, MRSA, and SARS-CoV-2 are covered elsewhere in this chapter. See Chapter 60 for *M. tuberculosis*.

Coronavirus Disease

- Severe acute respiratory syndrome coronavirus-2 (SARS-CoV-2) is a strain of coronavirus that infects humans, causing coronavirus disease 2019 (COVID-19).
- SARS-CoV-2 is a critically serious occupational hazard for DHCP due to close proximity to patients and disease transmission vectors.

I. Transmission and Symptoms

- Transmission occurs directly via airborne droplets inhaled into the lungs, and direct and indirect contact of infectious droplets on mucous membranes and eyes.[15]
- COVID-19 infections can range from asymptomatic infection to death.
- A wide range of symptoms appear 2–14 days after exposure and can vary in severity.

Table 5-1 Transmissible Diseases of Concern to DHCP

Infectious Agent	Disease or Condition	Route or Mode of Transmission	Incubation Period	Communicable Period	Vaccine
Adenoviruses (Over 50 types)	Cold or flu-like symptoms, (fever, sore throat) Conjunctivitis Acute pneumonia Acute bronchitis Gastroenteritis	Direct and indirect contact, airborne droplet	2 d to 2 wk	During first few days of symptoms	Types 4 and 7, military use only
Non-polio enteroviruses (NPEVs) 71 types including coxsackieviruses, echoviruses, rhinoviruses	Hand-foot-and-mouth disease Encephalitis Respiratory disease	Fecal–oral Direct and indirect contact, airborne droplet	3–10 d	3 d after exposure to 10 d after symptoms develop	No
Poliovirus types 1, 2, 3	Poliomyelitis	Direct contact, saliva, airborne droplet Fecal–oral	7–14 d	As long as virus is secreted, most infectious 7–10 d before and after onset of symptoms	Yes
Rotaviruses	Diarrhea Gastroenteritis	Fecal–oral Direct or indirect contact	2 d	Onset of symptoms up to 10 d	Yes
Influenza viruses (A, B, C)	Influenza	Direct contact, nasal discharge, airborne droplets	Average 7–67 hr Type A average 34 hr Type B average 14 hr	1 d before symptoms Peaks 1–2 d after Can last for 7 d	Yes
Measles virus (*Morbillivirus*)	Rubeola (measles)	Direct contact, saliva, airborne droplet	7–18 d (average 10 d) to fever, 14 d to rash	Few days before fever to 4 d after rash appears	Yes
Rubella virus (*Togavirus*)	Rubella (German measles) Congenital rubella syndrome	Direct contact, nasopharyngeal secretions, airborne droplet, maternal infection	13–20 d	From 1 wk before to 5 d after rash appears Highly communicable Infants shed virus for months after birth	Yes
Group A streptococci (beta-hemolytic) *Streptococcus pyogenes*	Streptococcal sore throat Scarlet fever Impetigo Erysipelas Cellulitis Toxic shock syndrome Wound infections	Direct contact, airborne droplet	1–5 d (average 2 d)	14–21 d, untreated Many nasal oropharyngeal carriers	No

(continues)

Table 5-1 Transmissible Diseases of Concern to DHCP (continued)

Infectious Agent	Disease or Condition	Route or Mode of Transmission	Incubation Period	Communicable Period	Vaccine
Candida albicans	Candidiasis	Secretions, excretions (oral, skin, vaginal)	Variable 2–5 d for "thrush" in children	While lesions are present	No
Streptococcus pneumoniae	Pneumonia Pneumococcal pneumonia	Direct and indirect contact	1–3 d Not well determined	While virulent organisms are discharged	Yes
Mycobacterium tuberculosis See Chapter 60	Tuberculosis	Airborne droplet, sputum, saliva	3–8 wk, occasionally 12 wk Latency decades or indefinite	As long as viable bacilli are discharged in sputum	BCG (Bacille Calmette-Guérin) has limited efficacy, approximately 15 y

- Typical symptoms include cough, fever, shortness of breath, difficulty breathing, headaches, muscle aches, sore throat, **anosmia** (loss of smell) and **ageusia** (loss of taste), congestion, nausea, vomiting, and diarrhea.[15]
- Severe symptoms include respiratory distress and failure, chest pain, mental confusion, and hypoxia.[15]

II. Post-COVID-19 Syndrome

- Post-COVID-19 syndrome (PCS), also known as long COVID-19, is characterized by multiple persistent symptoms extending beyond 12 weeks after acute COVID-19 infection.[16,17]
- PCS symptoms include neurologic and cognitive problems, fatigue, respiratory problems, persistent anosmia and ageusia, and a wide range of problems with multiple organs.[17]
- PCS is more severe in patients with preexisting diseases such as diabetes, cardiovascular disease, obesity, and cancer.[17]

III. Role of the Oral Cavity

- The oral cavity plays an important role in the transmission of SARS-CoV-2, as high viral loads have been detected in saliva and oral tissues.[18,19]
- High viral load in saliva has been associated with the severity of COVID-19 symptoms.[18]
- Oral epithelial cells, tongue, tonsils, and salivary glands can be directly infected by the virus and have been reported as viral replication sites.[19]
- A wide variety of COVID-19 oral manifestations have been reported and include glossitis, hyposalivation, **sialadenitis**, multiple variations of mucosal lesions, trigeminal neuralgia, candidiasis, necrotizing periodontal diseases, and gingivitis.[20]
- Oral manifestations may be directly attributable to COVID-19 or a result of an **opportunistic infectious agent** such as candidiasis and human herpesviruses (HHVs).[20]

IV. Relation to Periodontal Infections

- Direct and indirect associations of periodontitis and severity of COVID-19 symptoms have been reported.
- Severe periodontitis in COVID-19 patients has been implicated in higher risk of hospital admission, pneumonia, ventilator-assisted breathing, and death.[21,22]
- Associations between periodontitis and COVID-19 severity and outcomes continue to be investigated, along with the impact of other comorbidities such as diabetes, obesity, autoimmune conditions, and other chronic diseases.[21,22]

Viral Hepatitis

- Hepatitis is inflammation of the liver, which can be caused by viruses.
- The viruses that cause hepatitis are HAV, HBV, HCV, hepatitis D virus (HDV), and hepatitis E virus (HEV).[23]
- Acute hepatitis can lead to liver failure.
- Chronic hepatitis can lead to cirrhosis and increased risk for liver cancer.

Table 5-2 Viral Hepatitis

Hepatitis Virus Type	HAV	HBV	HCV	HDV	HEV
Modes of transmission	Fecal-oral Ingestion of contaminated food or water Close contact Sexual contact	Percutaneous, mucosal, nonintact skin exposure to blood and body fluids Sexual contact Perinatal Shared injection drug equipment Contaminated sharps exposure Remains infectious on inanimate objects for 7 d	Percutaneous, mucosal, nonintact skin exposure to blood and body fluids Sexual contact Perinatal Shared injection drug equipment Contaminated sharps exposure Tattooing needles	HDV only occurs as coinfection or superinfection with HBV Percutaneous, mucosal, nonintact skin exposure to blood and body fluids Sexual contact Perinatal Shared injection drug equipment Contaminated sharps exposure	Fecal-oral Ingestion of contaminated food or water
Incubation period	15–50 d Average: 28 d	60–150 d Average: 90 d	14–182 d Average: 14–84 d	Co-infection with HBV: 45–160 d Average: 90 d Superinfection with HBV: 2-8 wk	15–60 d Average: 40 d
Signs and symptoms	Fever, fatigue, loss of appetite, nausea, vomiting, abdominal pain, jaundice, joint pain, clay-colored stool, dark urine. Diarrhea with HAV. HEV may be asymptomatic.				
Carrier state	No	Yes	Yes	Yes	No
Vaccine	Yes	Yes	No	HBV vaccine	Yes (China)

- **Table 5-2** lists the five types of viral hepatitis, modes of transmission, incubation periods, sign and symptoms, carrier state, and availability of vaccines.[23]

I. Significance

- Viral hepatitis is a critical occupational hazard for DHCP because of the close association with infected body fluids, especially saliva and blood.
- HBV and HCV are of particular significance to all healthcare workers and directly impact the practice of dental hygiene and patient care.
- HBV and HCV are considered to be bloodborne pathogens and can be readily transmitted via percutaneous sharps exposure.
- DHCP must adhere to standard precautions, safe injection practices, and sharps handling.
- All healthcare providers, including DHCP, should be vaccinated against HBV and have their immunity checked postvaccination.
- There is no vaccination for HCV.
- DHCP must be tested for HBV and HCV after potential exposure.
- **Table 5-3** lists hepatitis B abbreviations and interpretation of serologic tests.[23]

Human Herpesvirus Diseases

- Human herpesviruses (HHVs) are **endemic** worldwide, with over 95% of the adult population infected.
- HHV diseases are a significant public health problem due to lack of effective therapeutics and vaccines.
- There are nine herpesviruses that are known to infect humans. These nine types are listed in **Table 5-4**, with abbreviations and some of the infections they cause.

Table 5-3 Hepatitis B Abbreviations and Interpretation of Serologic Tests

Term	Test Abbreviation	Significance
Hepatitis B surface antigen	HBsAg	Protein on surface of HBV. Presence indicates person is infectious, regardless of whether the infection is acute or chronic. HbsAg is used to make HBV vaccine.
Total hepatitis B core antibody	Anti-HBc	Indicates previous or ongoing infection in an undefined time frame. Does not develop in persons whose immunity to HBV is from vaccine. Anti-HBc generally persists for life and is not a serologic marker for acute infection.
Hepatitis B surface antibody	Anti-HBs	Presence indicates recovery and immunity against reinfection. Can occur in response to HBV vaccine.
IgM antibody to hepatitis B core antigen	IgM anti-HBc	Indicates recent (<6 mo) HBV infection and acute disease status.

Testing for HBV and disease status is determined by combining several of the above tests and interpreting the collective results.

Testing Group	Results	Collective Interpretation
HBsAg	Negative	Susceptible
Anti-HBc	Negative	
Anti-HBs	Negative	
HBsAg	Negative	Immune due to infection (not vaccination)
Anti-HBc	Positive	
Anti-HBs	Positive	
HBsAg	Negative	Immune due to vaccination
Anti-HBc	Negative	
Anti-HBs	Positive	
HBsAg	Positive	Acute infection
Anti-HBc	Positive	
IgM anti-HBc	Positive	
Anti-HBs	Negative	
HBsAg	Positive	Chronic infection
Anti-HBc	Positive	
IgM anti-HBc	Negative	
Anti-HBs	Negative	
HBsAg	Negative	Four possible interpretations: 1. Resolved infection 2. Resolving acute infection 3. Low-level chronic infection 4. False-positive anti-HBc; therefore susceptible
Anti-HBc	Positive	
Anti-HBs	Negative	

Table 5-4 Human Herpes Viruses

<table>
<tr><th>Herpes Virus Number</th><th>Name of Virus and Abbreviation</th><th>Primary Infection Diseases</th><th>Latency Site</th><th>Reactivation Diseases</th><th colspan="2">Implicated and/or Associated Diseases</th></tr>
<tr><td>(HHV-1)</td><td>Herpes simplex virus, type 1 (HSV-1)</td><td>Herpetic gingivostomatitis</td><td>Trigeminal ganglion</td><td>Herpes labialis
Herpetic whitlow
Herpetic conjunctivitis</td><td>Oral cancer</td><td rowspan="2">HSV-1 and HSV-2 have been implicated in aseptic encephalitis and an increased risk of acquiring HIV and transmission</td></tr>
<tr><td>(HHV-2)</td><td>Herpes simplex virus, type 2 (HSV-2)</td><td>Genital herpes</td><td>Thoracic, lumbar, and sacral dorsal root ganglia</td><td>Recurrent genital herpes</td><td>Cervical cancer
Neonatal HSV</td></tr>
<tr><td>(HHV-3)</td><td>Varicella–zoster virus (VZV)</td><td>Varicella (chicken pox)</td><td>Sensory neurons</td><td>Herpes zoster (shingles)</td><td colspan="2">Varicella: Secondary bacterial skin infections, pneumonia, meningoencephalitis, kidney, liver, and bleeding complications
Zoster: Postherpetic neuralgia, secondary skin infections and scarring, and ocular and neurologic conditions</td></tr>
<tr><td>(HHV-4)</td><td>Epstein–Barr virus (EBV)</td><td>Infectious mononucleosis</td><td>Lymphocytes</td><td>Oral hairy leukoplakia in immunocompromised</td><td colspan="2">Burkitt's lymphoma, lymphoepithelial cysts of parotid gland, lymphatic cancers, nasopharyngeal cancers, periapical lesions, periodontal disease severity, rapidly progressing periodontitis</td></tr>
<tr><td>(HHV-5)</td><td>Human cytomegalovirus (CMV)</td><td>Mononucleosis, fever, hepatitis</td><td>Lymphocytes</td><td>Asymptomatic infections except in immunocompromised</td><td colspan="2">Periapical pathosis and increased severity of periodontal diseases
Immunosuppressed persons: CMV retinitis, neurologic deficiencies, pneumonia, encephalitis
Congenital infection: preterm and low birth weight (PLBW), microcephaly, seizures, intellectual and physical disabilities, vision and hearing loss</td></tr>
<tr><td>(HHV-6A)</td><td>Herpes lymphotropic virus (HLV-6A)</td><td>Asymptomatic infection acquired after HHV-6B infection</td><td>Lymphocytes</td><td rowspan="2">Asymptomatic infections except in immunocompromised</td><td colspan="2" rowspan="2">Hashimoto's thyroiditis, multiple sclerosis, immune system suppression, seizure disorders, encephalitis, infertility, drug-induced hypersensitivity syndrome (with HHV-7)</td></tr>
<tr><td>(HHV-6B)</td><td>Herpes lymphotropic virus (HLV-6B)</td><td>Roseola infantum (exanthema subitum or sixth disease)
Infantile fever
Seizures</td><td>Lymphocytes</td></tr>
<tr><td>(HHV-8)</td><td>Kaposi's sarcoma-related virus (KSHV or KS)</td><td>Asymptomatic in immunocompetent
Lymphadenopathy and rapid progression to Kaposi's sarcoma in immunocompromised</td><td>Lymphocytes</td><td>Asymptomatic infections except in immunocompromised</td><td colspan="2">Lymphoproliferative diseases
Multicentric Castleman's disease</td></tr>
</table>

I. General Characteristics

- HHVs produce diseases with wide-ranging primary, latent, and recurrent manifestations.[24]
- All HHVs except VZV are transmitted via saliva, mucosal and skin lesions, and genital secretions. VZV is transmitted via respiratory aerosols and contact with skin lesions.
- HHVs infect and replicate in epithelial cells of the oropharynx, genitals, and skin.
- After primary infection, HHVs remain in the body and establish life-long latent infections in sensory neurons or lymphocytes.[24]
- Latent HHV infection may become reactivated to produce **recurrent infection** after certain stimuli such as stress, trauma, sunlight, illness, or when the body's immunity is significantly lowered.
- HHVs are implicated in several types of cancers.[25]
- HHV infections are more frequent and severe in immunocompromised patients.

II. Relation to Periodontal Infections

- HHVs have been detected in periodontal pockets and may represent a coinfection with periodontal pathogens.[26]
- Herpes virus–positive periodontitis lesions involving cytomegalovirus (CMV) and Epstein–Barr virus (EBV) have higher levels of major periodontal pathogenic bacteria.[26,27]
- A coinfection of CMV and EBV is associated with more severe periodontitis.[26,27]
- CMV, EBV, and HSV-1 have a significant association with rapidly progressing periodontitis.[26,27]
- Although other HHVs have been detected in periodontal pockets, they have not shown any association with the initiation, progression, or severity of periodontal diseases.

III. Clinical Management for HHVs

- Professional terminology such as "herpes" may cause alarm with patients. Use terms such as "fever blisters" or "cold sores" to ensure patient understanding.
- Trauma to the oral area during a dental or dental hygiene appointment may trigger a herpetic recurrence.[28,29]
- Postpone appointment if patient has an active vesicular lesion.
- Explain the contagious nature of the disease[28,29]:
  - Prodromal stage can be the most transmissible to other patients and clinicians.
  - Limit personal contact with others while the lesion is active, especially saliva transfer and sharing of objects such as cosmetics, lip products, utensils, and drink containers.
  - Stress the importance of meticulous hygiene in limiting autoinfection through touching the lesion and then touching other susceptible body areas such as eyes and genitals. Auto-reinfection can also occur via lip moisturizing products and ointments used to treat the lesions.
  - Autoinoculation possible from instrumentation that can splash viruses to the patient's eye or extend the lesion to the nose.
  - Irritation to the lesions can prolong the course and increase severity of infection.

A. HHV-1 (HSV-1)

HHV-1, also known as HSV-1 is widespread, and it is estimated that between 50% and 90% of people worldwide are affected.

- **Primary infection** of HSV-1 manifests as primary herpetic gingivostomatitis and usually occurs in children but may occur at any age, especially in the immunocompromised.
  - Many cases of primary infection with HSV-1 are asymptomatic or mild and isolated to marginal and attached gingiva.[29]
  - Symptoms of clinical disease may vary from mild to severely debilitating.
  - Gingivostomatitis and pharyngitis are the most frequent manifestations, with fever, malaise, widespread oral ulcers and severe pain often interfering with the ability to eat, and lymphadenopathy for 2–7 days.
- **Latent infection** of HSV-1 occurs in the trigeminal nerve ganglion.[24]
- Recurrent infection of HSV-1 manifests as herpes labialis, herpetic whitlow, and ocular herpes. Genital herpes infection with HSV-1 is increasing in prevalence.[30]
- Herpes labialis (cold sore, fever blister) is common and often occurs at the vermillion border of the lower lip.[29]
  - Prodromal symptoms occur 6 to 24 hours before the lesion appears with pain, burning, slight stinging, or sensations of localized warmth and erythema of the affected epithelium with slight swelling.

- A group of vesicles form that coalesce, rupture, and eventually crust over.
- Lesions are infectious; the shedding virus may lead to autoinfection of the eye, mucous membranes, or fingers and infection of other people.
- Healing may take up to 10 days.

- Herpetic whitlow[31]
  - Herpetic whitlow is caused by HSV-1 or HSV-2 entering skin abrasions around a fingernail.
  - Chronic herpetic whitlow may be a manifestation of HIV infection.
  - Herpetic whitlow was once common among DHCP; standard precautions have almost eliminated the incidence among DHCP.
- Ocular/ophthalmic herpes[24,30]
  - Ocular herpes can be a primary or recurrent infection of HSV-1 or HSV-2 and may lead to blindness.
  - Transmission can occur from splashing saliva or fluid from a vesicular lesion directly into an unprotected eye.
  - Prevent ocular herpetic infection by using standard precautions, including eye protection for both clinician and patient.

B. HHV-2 (HSV-2)

- HHV-2, also known as HSV-2, is commonly known as genital herpes, but it also occurs as oral and perioral infections.[28]
- Neonatal herpes is a serious disease that can cause delayed mental development, blindness, neurologic problems, and death to newborns infected during childbirth.
  - Obstetricians may recommend delivery by cesarean section to women with active genital herpes to avoid transmission to the infant.
- Antiviral therapy can suppress HSV-2 lesions.

C. HHV-3 (VZV)

- HHV-3, also known as varicella–zoster virus (VZV).
- Primary infection of VZV causes varicella (chicken pox) infection.[32]
  - Extremely contagious and primarily childhood disease transmitted via respiratory aerosols and direct or indirect skin contact with discharge from vesicles and respiratory tract.
  - Can be life threatening to adults, immunocompromised patients, pregnant women, and newborns.
  - Two doses of the varicella vaccine are recommended, with the first dose at 12–15 months old and the second between 4 and 6 years old.
- VZV reactivation causes herpes zoster (shingles) infection[32]
  - VZV reactivates and spreads to skin along peripheral nerves, causing a painful vesicular rash lasting from 2 to 4 weeks.
  - Risk factors for zoster include increasing age, HIV infection, physical trauma or surgery, cancer, transplants, and immunosuppressive medications.
  - A shingles vaccine is available and is recommended for all adults 50 years and older.

D. HHV-4 (EBV)

- HHV-4 also known as Epstein–Barr virus (EBV).
- Primary infection with EBV causes infectious mononucleosis.[33]
  - EBV is common among teenagers and young adults, and is commonly spread through saliva even when the patient has no symptoms of disease.
  - May also be spread via sexual contact, organ transplants, and blood transfusions.
  - Prevention: Minimize contact with saliva by frequent handwashing, avoiding drinking from a common container; standard precautions by DHCP.
  - EBV remains latent but manifests as oral hairy leukoplakia in those with HIV and severe immunocompromise.[34]

E. HHV-5 (CMV)

- HHV-5. Also known as cytomegalovirus (CMV).[35]
  - Transmitted by direct contact with infected body fluids, via sexual contact, solid organ and bone marrow transplants, and blood transfusions.
  - CMV infections are widespread, with the most severe disease developing in infants infected in utero and in immunocompromised patients.

F. HHV-6A and HHV-6B

- HHV-6A and HHV-6B are considered to be distinct viral species rather than variants of the same species.[36]
- HHV-6A[36]
  - Acquired after HHV-6B infection as an asymptomatic primary infection.
  - Possible risk factor in accelerating HIV infection.

- HHV-6B[36]
  - Primary infection with HHV-6B occurs in 100% of humans by the age of 3 and is known as roseola infantum, exanthem subitem, or sixth disease.
  - HHV-6B has been found in endodontic abscesses and in the adenoids and tonsils of children with upper respiratory symptoms.

G. HHV-7

- Often found with HHV-6 and is implicated in a range of diseases and conditions.[36]
- Along with HHV-6B, it is a causative agent in roseola infantum.
- Some persons infected with HHV-7 are asymptomatic.

H. HHV-8

- HHV-8 is also known as Kaposi's sarcoma–associated herpesvirus.[25]
- Although HHV-8 is generally considered to be sexually transmitted, oral mucosa and saliva are the primary sites of **viral shedding** and infection transmission.
- Primary infection may be asymptomatic in healthy patients.
- HIV increases the risk of HHV-8 infection and those infected with HHV-8 after being infected with HIV are at significantly greater risk for rapid progression to Kaposi's sarcoma (KS).[25]

Human Papillomavirus

- There are over 200 numbered viruses considered to be human papillomaviruses (HPVs).[37]
- HPVs are very common sexually transmitted infections that are mostly asymptomatic and cleared by the immune system.
- Some HPV infections persist and are oncogenic (cancer causing).[15,37]
- Most types of HPV infect epithelial tissues of the skin, causing common warts.
- Approximately 40 types infect mucosal epithelium and are categorized as high- and low-risk HPVs.
- Low-risk HPV types 6 and 11 are considered non-oncogenic and cause recurrent respiratory papillomatosis and anogenital warts.[25,37]
- Oropharyngeal lesions caused by types 6 and 11 are benign squamous cell papillomas typically occurring on the palate, tongue, and lips.[37]
- High-risk HPV types 16, 18, 31, 33, 45, 52, and 58 are considered oncogenic and are known to cause cervical, vaginal, penile, anal, rectal, and oropharyngeal cancers.[25]
- HPV-16–associated oropharyngeal cancers typically develop near the base of the tongue and in the tonsils.[37]
- Periodontal pockets are a reservoir for oral HPV infections and may be associated with periodontitis.[38]
- The CDC recommends HPV vaccination for[39]:
  - All children aged 11–12 years, with two doses 6–12 months apart.
  - Everyone through age 26 years, with three doses over 6 months for those aged 15 years and older.
  - Vaccination is not recommended for those older than 26 years.

HIV/AIDS Infection

- HIV attacks the body's immune system, specifically the CD4$^+$ T lymphocyte cells (T-cells), which renders the immune system ineffective against opportunistic infections (OIs).[40]
- OIs such as *Pneumocystis carinii* pneumonia, tuberculosis, KS, HIV wasting syndrome, toxoplasmosis, all HHVs, and candidiasis take advantage of a weakened immune system to manifest severe disease signs and symptoms.[40]
- A weakened immune system under attack from OIs signals the last stage of HIV infection, known as acquired immunodeficiency syndrome (AIDS).
- Globally, over 36 million lives have been lost to HIV infection, and in 2020, an estimated 37.7 million people were living with HIV with an additional 1.5 million acquiring HIV.
- No effective cure currently exists, but HIV-infected individuals can have a near-normal life expectancy with antiretroviral therapy (ART).[40]
- Etiology and history of HIV[40]
  - A type of chimpanzee in West Africa has been identified as the source of HIV, which was transmitted to humans through contact with infected blood as a result of hunting the chimpanzees for meat.
  - The virus may have jumped species as far back as the late 1800s and has been present in the United States since the mid- to late 1970s.
  - There are two types of HIV:
    - HIV-1 causes the majority of infections and is **pandemic**.
    - HIV-1 is more infectious and virulent than HIV-2.
    - HIV-2 is generally confined to West Africa.

I. Transmission

- HIV is transmitted by direct contact with infected blood, semen, pre-seminal fluid, rectal fluids, vaginal fluids, and breast milk that enter the bloodstream through mucous membranes, breaks in the skin, or injection.[40]
- Persons with a high viral load are more likely to transmit HIV.[40]
- Common modes of HIV transmission include[40]:
  - **Parenteral**:
    - Sharing needles or other injection equipment used to prepare and/or inject illicit drugs, hormones, silicone, and steroids.
  - Sexual:
    - All unprotected insertive and receptive oral, anal, penile, and vaginal contact can transmit HIV, with anal and vaginal sexual contact having the highest risk.
    - Presence of another sexually transmitted disease (STI) such as gonorrhea, syphilis, HPVs, HHVs, hepatitis, and chlamydia increases risk of contracting and transmitting HIV.
- Less common and rare modes of HIV transmission[40]:
  - Deep open-mouthed kissing with the presence of open sores and bleeding gingivae.
  - All forms of oral sex, including fellatio, cunnilingus, and anal rimming.
  - Although now rare and preventable due to HIV medications, the virus can be transmitted in utero across the placenta, during vaginal birth, and breastfeeding.
  - Receiving contaminated blood transfusions, blood products, organ and tissue transplants.
  - Contact with broken skin, wounds, and mucous membranes by blood and/or blood-contaminated body fluids.
  - Prechewed food contaminated with infected blood.
  - Human bites with severe skin damage.
  - Breaches in or inadequate infection control and accidental needlestick injuries.
  - HIV is not transmitted by saliva, sweat, tears, insect bites, or social contact.

II. HIV Testing for Diagnosis and Staging of Infection

- HIV tests are very accurate but cannot detect the virus immediately after infection.
- Laboratory tests to determine HIV infection include[40,41]:
  - Nucleic acid tests (NATs) detect HIV and provide a viral load count.
  - Antigen/antibody tests detect HIV antibodies and antigens.
  - Antibody tests detect the presence of HIV antibodies.
- Self-administered HIV testing[40,41]:
  - Home Access HIV-1 Test System® involves a finger stick to obtain a blood sample that is then sent anonymously to a licensed lab. Results can be obtained as fast as the next day.
  - OraQuick In-Home HIV Test® involves obtaining a swab of oral fluids and using the kit to perform the test at home. Results are available in 20 minutes; however, 1 in 12 test false-negative for HIV due to the lower levels of antibodies in oral fluids.
- CD4 T lymphocyte and viral load counts[40,41]:
  - The CD4 T lymphocyte counts and viral load counts are done to estimate, at one point in time, the health of the immune system and help evaluate a person's risk of serious illness from OIs.
  - The tests provide data to evaluate over time but do not indicate health of the person, how they feel, or predict the future course of disease.
  - CD4 T lymphocyte count[41]:
    - Measures the number of CD4 T lymphocytes in 1 mm^3 of blood, which provides data to evaluate the HIV-compromised immune system, progression of infection, and efficacy of HIV medications.
    - A normal CD4 T lymphocyte count is 500–1,500 cells/mm^3 of blood in a non–HIV-infected adult.
    - $CD4^+$ T-cells can also be represented as a percentage of all white blood cells, with 32–68% considered normal in a non–HIV-infected adult.
    - A CD4 T lymphocyte count below 200 cells/mm^3 or a CD4 below 14% indicates a person is at risk for OIs.
  - Viral load count[41]:
    - Measures the amount of HIV in 1 mm^3 of blood, which provides data to evaluate potential damage to the immune system, efficacy of HIV medications, and drug resistance of the virus.
    - Viral suppression is when the viral load count is below 200 copies of HIV/mm^3 and the virus can be suppressed to the

point where it becomes undetectable in a blood test.
  - ART drugs must be taken by strict regimen to achieve viral suppression.

Stages of HIV Infection

- Stage 1: Acute HIV infection[41]
  - Within 2–4 weeks after infection, the person may experience flu-like symptoms lasting a few weeks; some may be asymptomatic.
  - During this time, the viral load is very high and the person is highly infectious.
  - No AIDS-defining OIs are present.
  - CD4 T lymphocyte count ≥500 cells/mm^3 or ≥29%.
- Stage 2: Clinical latency[33]
  - Also known as asymptomatic or chronic infection, which can last 10 years or longer, although some infections will progress to stage 3 faster.
  - HIV medications can maintain an infected person at this stage for decades.
  - HIV is active, replicating at a slow rate, and is still transmissible however, those with a low viral load are less likely to transmit the virus.
  - No AIDS-defining OIs are present.
  - CD4 T lymphocyte counts are 200–499 cells/mm^3 or 14–28%.
- Stage 3: AIDS[41]
  - CD4 T lymphocyte counts below 200 cells/mm^3 or <15% and emergence of OIs is necessary for an AIDS diagnosis.
  - The immune system is damaged and poorly functioning, which allows OIs to emerge and progress unchecked by the immune system.
  - The viral load is very high and without treatment, people may only survive 3 years.
  - Symptoms include fever, sweats, chills, swollen lymph nodes, weight loss, muscle wasting, and weakness.

III. HIV-Associated Oral Lesions

- DHCP are in a unique position to identify HIV-associated oral lesions, as they affect over one-third of those with HIV and are often the earliest manifestations of infection.
- Analysis of oral findings, their severity, and patient-provided information may offer insight into recognition and diagnosis of HIV infection and HIV/AIDS-related oral manifestations.[42]
- There are 24 different HIV-associated oral lesions, some of which are more prevalent indicators of HIV infection and potential markers of disease progression and severity.[43]
- The etiology of oral lesions associated with HIV/AIDS is listed in **Table 5-5**.
- ART has changed the overall prevalence and pattern of HIV-related oral manifestations.[42,43]

A. Consistently Encountered HIV-Associated Oral Lesions

- HIV-associated oropharyngeal candidiasis (HIV-OC)[42,43,44]
  - OC is the most prevalent OI in HIV/AIDS and can present as erythematous candidiasis, pseudomembranous candidiasis, and angular cheilitis.
  - Although *Candida albicans* is the most common **pathogen**, HIV-OC often involves several *Candida* species in complex biofilms.
  - HIV-OC treatment is further complicated by increasing resistance to antifungal medications and systemic dissemination.

Table 5-5 Etiology of Oral Lesions Associated with HIV/AIDS

Fungal Infections	Viral Infections	Bacterial Infections
Candida albicans *Candida glabrata* *Candida tropicalis* *Candida parapsilosis* *Candida krusei* *Candida dubliniensis* Cryptococcosis Histoplasmosis Paracoccidioidomycosis Penicilliosis Aspergillosis	Herpes simplex 1 (HHV-1) Herpes simplex 2 (HHV-2) Herpes zoster (HHV-3) Epstein–Barr (HHV-4) CMV (HHV-5) KS (HHV-8) Human papillomavirus (HPV)	*Mycobacterium tuberculosis* (TB) *Mycobacterium avium intracellulare* Periodontal infections Linear gingival erythema (LGE) Necrotizing periodontal diseases (NPD)

- HIV-associated oral hairy leukoplakia[34]
  - Associated with reactivation of latent EBV HHV-4.
  - Affects over 50% of HIV/AIDS patients, is asymptomatic and nononcogenic, and does not require treatment unless symptoms arise.
- Herpes simplex virus
  - Associated with reactivation of HHV-1 and HHV-2 (see prior section on HHV-1 and HHV-2).
  - Presents painful, deep blistering lesions, and fever may be manifest.
- Kaposi's sarcoma
  - KS is caused by HHV-8 (see prior section on HHV-8) and is the most common HIV-associated oral malignancy.
  - Lesions vary in color from purple to brown and black and are mostly found on the hard palate, attached gingivae, and dorsum of the tongue. They may be multifocal and progress rapidly, with larger lesions posing a risk of ulceration, secondary infection, and extensive periodontal destruction.
  - Oral bacteria and bacterial by-products are under investigation as triggers for progression of HHV-8 to KS in HIV patients.[45]
- HIV-related oral ulcers[43,46]
  - Oral ulcerations may occur in relation to another HIV-associated oral condition.
  - They may present as aphthous ulcers, erythema multiforme–like lesions, and nonspecific ulcerations not associated with bacterial, fungal, or viral origins.
  - HIV-related oral ulcers are frequently more painful and longer lasting, and may be influenced by poor oral health and malnutrition.
- Non-Hodgkin lymphoma[47]
  - Associated with reactivation of latent EBV HHV-4 and is 60 times more prevalent in HIV-infected persons.
  - 25% of lesions are in the oral cavity and present as growths and ulcerations affecting gingiva, palatal tissues, and alveolar mucosa.
- Periodontal and gingival manifestations of HIV[48]
  - Periodontal infections associated with HIV infection tend to show more severe symptoms and progress more rapidly.
  - Patients with well-managed HIV infection and who maintain a high level of personal and professional oral care may present with healthier periodontal tissues.
- Linear gingival erythema (LGE)[48,49]
  - Presents as a band of fiery red tissues extending 2–3 mm from the gingival margin that do not respond to traditional treatment.
  - *Candida* species have been implicated in the etiology of LGE.[43]
  - If left untreated, LGE may progress to more severe periodontitis and/or necrotizing periodontal diseases.
- Necrotizing periodontal diseases (NPDs)[50]
  - Necrotizing periodontal diseases are severe inflammatory diseases strongly associated with immune system impairment and are not isolated to those with HIV infection.
  - Risk factors for NPDs include smoking, poor oral hygiene, stress, malnutrition, and immunocompromise.
  - Other signs and symptoms may include pseudomembranous gingiva, regional lymphadenopathy, and fever.
  - All NPDs are varying stages of the same disease with the same microflora. See Chapter 19.

B. Less-Prevalent HIV-Associated Oral Lesions

- HHV-3 (herpes zoster; shingles) manifests as blisters and/or crusted lesions on the head, face, and neck.[42]
- HHV-5 (CMV) causes ulceration of oral mucosa and spreads to the gastrointestinal tract.[51]
- HPV lesions generally occur intraorally but may manifest in the HIV patient as papillomatous lesions or mucosal tags in the labial commissures.[37,42]
- Non-*Candida* fungal infections such as cryptococcosis, histoplasmosis, paracoccidioidomycosis, penicilliosis, and aspergillosis.
- *M. tuberculosis* is estimated to cause 13% of AIDS-related deaths and in advanced cases can manifest as oral lesions that may extend into paranasal sinuses.
- *M. avium intracellulare* infection is rare but may cause oral lesions.
- Intramucosal hemorrhages.
- Melanotic hyperpigmentation of oral mucosa.
- Salivary gland disease, swelling of salivary glands, and severe xerostomia.

C. Impact of ART on HIV-Associated Oral Lesions

- ART has reduced the prevalence of HIV-associated oral lesions with KS, candidiasis, LGE, and oral hairy leukoplakia being the most responsive.[43,46]

- As the viral load declines and CD4 T lymphocyte counts improve with ART, there is a corresponding improvement in immune system function, which can prompt a strong inflammatory response resulting in immune reconstitution inflammatory syndrome (IRIS).[44]
- Paradoxical IRIS is the worsening of an existing infection and unmasking IRIS is the appearance of a new infection.
- The oral lesions most typically associated with IRIS are KS, oral candidiasis, HPV, salivary gland disease, ulcers, and oral hairy leukoplakia.[44]
- Patients who are undergoing immune reconstitution may present with an exaggerated and atypical level of inflammation that requires more frequent care with a focus on prevention of oral candidiasis and HHVs.[42]

IV. Prevention and Treatment of HIV Infection

- Until a vaccine is available, HIV prevention depends on community health education that is focused on awareness of risk, modes of transmission, and preventive measures necessary to halt HIV transmission, especially in high-risk groups.
- Dental personnel who are well informed with accurate, current information can provide competent care for HIV-infected patients and give support to community health programs.
- Antiretroviral medications do not cure HIV and treatment usually requires a combination of several different medications, sometimes combined into one pill.[52]
- Medications must be taken on a strict regimen, and compliance may be problematic due to side effects, dose scheduling, illness, depression, fear of others finding out, and being unable to afford medications.
- Preexposure prophylaxis (PrEP) is a combination of two HIV medications taken to prevent HIV infection in high-risk individuals.[52]
- Consistent use of PrEP reduces risk of sexually contracting HIV by 99% and by 74% for injection drug users.
- Postexposure prophylaxis (PEP) is the use of antiretroviral drugs within 72 hours of a high-risk exposure to stop HIV **seroconversion**.[52]
- PEP may be prescribed to DHCP after possible exposure to HIV.
- HIV treatment for prevention is the use of antiretroviral drugs in those with HIV, to reduce the viral load to below 200 copies/mL of blood (viral suppression). Over time and with consistent use of the drug therapy, the viral load can be reduced to undetectable levels (undetectable viral load).[41,52]
- A person with an undetectable viral load has effectively no risk of transmitting HIV through sexual contact, injection drug use, or perinatal transmission from mother to child.[41,52]
- **Table 5-6** lists commonly prescribed Food and Drug Administration (FDA)–approved medications to treat and manage HIV.[41,52]

V. Dental Hygiene Management

- Legal and psychosocial considerations
  - The dental hygienist may be the first to suspect HIV infection when oral manifestations and symptoms are recognized.[42–44,46]
  - All persons with HIV infection are protected by the Americans with Disabilities Act and DHCP are ethically and legally obligated to treat HIV-positive or at-risk patients.
  - Use language that does not stigmatize or judge the HIV-positive patient in regard to their sexual orientation, gender identity, sexual and/or drug behaviors, and other medical and/or social behaviors.
  - DHCP must maintain strict patient confidentiality and realize the patient may be infected through no fault of their own.
  - Encourage HIV testing for at-risk patients and adherence to ART for those who are infected.
  - Assisting HIV-infected patients in maintaining their oral health can significantly improve their quality of life by reducing pain and susceptibility to OIs.
  - Pain and oral manifestations may be caused by the disease or medications.
  - Adverse effects of ART may include nausea and vomiting, which can be severe enough to contribute to dental caries and dental erosion.
  - Emphasize meticulous personal oral care and frequent professional periodontal therapy. Fluoride varnish needs to be included in the preventive oral hygiene program for all ages.

Methicillin-Resistant *Staphylococcus aureus*

- *S. aureus* is normally found on healthy human skin and mucous membranes and can cause serious infection if it enters the bloodstream or subcutaneous tissues.

Table 5-6 FDA-Approved HIV Medications

Drug Category and Action	Generic Name	Brand Name
Nucleoside reverse transcriptase inhibitors (NRTIs) Inhibit reverse transcriptase enzyme that HIV uses to replicate	abacavir (ABC)	Ziagen
	emtricitabine (FTC)	Emtriva
	lamivudine (3TC)	Epivir
	tenofovir disoproxil fumarate (TDF)	Viread
	zidovudine (AZT, ZDV)	Retrovir
Nonnucleoside reverse transcriptase inhibitors (NNRTIs) Binds to and alters reverse transcriptase enzyme that HIV uses to replicate	doravirine (DOR)	Pifeltro
	efavirenz (EFV)	Sustiva
	etravirine (ETR)	Intelence
	nevirapine (NVP)	Viramune
	rilpivirine (RPV)	Edurant
Protease inhibitors (PIs) Inhibit HIV protease enzyme that HIV uses to replicate	atazanavir (ATV)	Reyataz
	darunavir (DRV)	Prezista
	fosamprenavir (FOS-APV, FPV)	Lexiva
	ritonavir (RTV)	Norvir
	saquinavir (SQV)	Invirase
	tipranavir (TPV)	Aptivus
Fusion inhibitor Inhibits HIV entering CD4 cells	enfuvirtide (T-20)	Fuzeon
CCR5 antagonist Blocks CCR5 receptors to prevent HIV entering macrophages and T-cells	maraviroc (MVC)	Selzentry
Integrase strand transfer inhibitors (INSTIs) Inhibit HIV integrase enzyme that HIV uses to replicate	cabotegravir (CAB)	Vocabria
	dolutegravir ((DTG)	Tivicay
	raltegravir (RAL)	Isentress
Attachment inhibitor Inhibits an HIV protein, which prevents HIV entering CD4 cells	fostemsavir (FTR)	Rukobia
Postattachment inhibitor Antibody attaches to T-cells to prevent HIV entry	ibalizumab-uiyk (IBA)	Trogarzo
Pharmacokinetic enhancer (PK) Increases effectiveness of HIV medications	cobicistat (COBI)	Tybost
Preexposure prophylaxis (PrEP) Combination of two NRTIs	tenofovir disoproxil fumarate (TDF) and emtricitabine (FTC)	Truvada
	tenofovir alafenamide (TAF) and emtricitabine (FTC)	Descovy

- Methicillin-resistant *S. aureus* (MRSA) is a strain of *S. aureus* that is difficult to treat because it is resistant to many antibiotic therapies.[53,54]
- MRSA is transmitted by direct and indirect contact, and can be endemic in hospitals and institutions.[53,54]

- It is associated with infective endocarditis, acute osteomyelitis, bacteremia, septicemia, cellulitis, conjunctivitis, pneumonia, and toxic shock syndrome.[53]
- Persons may be a carrier of MRSA and spread the infection to others even if they do not have signs or symptoms of infection.
- Risk factors for acquisition of MRSA include prolonged hospital stay, intensive care stay, prolonged antimicrobial therapy, and surgical procedures.[53,54]

Documentation

Suggested documentation for the patient with an infectious disease includes the following:

- If the patient is under treatment for an infectious condition, note the patient's medication, its purpose, adverse effects, effects on oral health, and patient adherence to medication(s).
- Record all consultations and referrals with other healthcare personnel.
- Record results of specific laboratory tests (CD4 counts, viral load counts, antibody/antigen, biopsy results) that potentially affect dental hygiene treatment; note those values at each appointment.
- **Box 5-1** provides a sample Progress Note.

Factors to Teach the Patient

- Reasons for postponing an appointment when a herpes lesion ("fever blister" or "cold sore") is present on the lip.
- Importance of not touching or using lip products on the herpetic lesion because of self-inoculation to fingers or eyes.
- How microorganisms can transfer infection to other people through the air, by touching another person, or touching a contaminated object.
- Importance of keeping the medical history up to date by informing of additional exposures and immunizations to communicable diseases for self and family members.
- Importance of oral health to overall systemic health.
- Preparation for a dental or dental hygiene appointment by thorough mouth cleaning with toothbrush and dental floss, followed by a preprocedural mouthrinse to lower the bacterial count and thus lessen aerosol contamination in the treatment room.

Box 5-1 Example Documentation: Patient with Candidiasis and Immunosuppression

- **S**—52-year-old female presents for regular periodontal maintenance appointment with chief complaint of sore, red, and cracked labial commissures and a sore throat. Medical history indicates patient is a type I diabetic with a history of poor glycemic control and a corresponding HbA1c of 9.4, deteriorating vision, and had a kidney transplant 3 years ago. Current medications are insulin, cyclosporine, azathioprine, furosemide, omeprazole, and atorvastatin. Patient states she has not been diligent with her oral homecare and often forgets to take out her maxillary denture at night.
- **O**—Extraoral exam reveals bilateral erythema and fissuring of the labial commissures with areas of crusting, cracking, and bleeding. Intraoral exam reveals a red oropharynx and several large white plaques 6–8 mm in diameter under the denture. Saliva flow is difficult to stimulate. Oral hygiene: Generalized moderate supragingival dental biofilm. Gingival tissues: Generalized moderate to severe marginal erythema, with enlarged and fragile margins. Radiographic examination: Evidence of progressive horizontal bone loss #23–26 and new vertical bone loss #2, 3, 12, 14, 15, 19, and 31. Periodontal examination: All teeth exhibiting grade I–II+ mobility, periodontal probing postponed.
- **A**—Clinical impression: Oropharyngeal candidiasis exacerbated by poor glycemic control and immunosuppressive medications with possible disseminated systemic involvement. Limited clinical exam reveals progressive periodontitis likely exacerbated by poor glycemic control, immunosuppression, and poor oral hygiene.
- **P**—Discussed etiology and significance of *Candida* infection, risks of disseminated disease, and role of diabetes and immunosuppression. Discussed condition of her periodontium and pressing need to address as soon as her systemic health is showing improvement. Advised patient to remove denture at night and improve homecare. Referred patient to her physician for immediate evaluation and treatment of candidiasis, improving glycemic control, and consideration for antibiotic prophylaxis prior to subgingival examination and treatment.

Signed: ______________________, RDH

Date: ____________

References

1. Centers for Disease Control and Prevention. *Epidemiology and Prevention of Vaccine-Preventable Diseases*. Washington, DC: Public Health Foundation; 2021:1-7.
2. Centers for Disease Control and Prevention. Understanding mRNA COVID-19 vaccines. Atlanta, GA: National Center for Immunization and Respiratory Diseases, Division of Viral Diseases; 2021. https://www.cdc.gov/coronavirus/2019-ncov/vaccines/different-vaccines/mRNA.html?s_cid=11344:mrna%20vaccines:sem.ga:p:RG:GM:gen:PTN:FY21. Accessed September 19, 2021.
3. World Health Organization. WHO Immunization agenda 2030: a global strategy to leave no one behind. Published April 1, 2020. https://www.who.int/publications/m/item/immunization-agenda-2030-a-global-strategy-to-leave-no-one-behind. Accessed September 19, 2021.
4. Gomez A, Nelson KE. The oral microbiome of children: development, disease, and implications beyond oral health. *Microb Ecol*. 2017;73(2):492-503. doi:10.1007/s00248-016-0854-1
5. Krishnan K, Chen T, Paster BJ. A practical guide to the oral microbiome and its relation to health and disease. *Oral Dis*. 2017;23(3):276-286.
6. Centers for Disease Control and Prevention. Summary of infection prevention practices in dental settings: basic expectations for safe care. Atlanta, GA: U.S. Department of Health and Human Services; 2016. https://www.cdc.gov/oralhealth/infectioncontrol/summary-infection-prevention-practices/index.html. Accessed September 19, 2021.
7. Centers for Disease Control and Prevention. *Guidelines for Infection Control in Dental Health-Care Settings*. Atlanta, GA: U.S. Department of Health and Human Services; 2003. https://www.cdc.gov/mmwr/PDF/rr/rr5217.pdf. Accessed September 19, 2021.
8. Centers for Disease Control and Prevention. Guideline for isolation precautions: preventing transmission of infectious agents in healthcare settings. Atlanta, GA: Healthcare Infection Control Practices Advisory Committee; 2007. https://www.cdc.gov/infectioncontrol/guidelines/isolation/index.html. Accessed September 19, 2021.
9. Han P, Li H, Walsh LJ, et al. Splatters and aerosols contamination in dental aerosol generating procedures. *Applied Sciences*. 2021;11(4):1914.
10. Santarpia JL, Herrera VL, Rivera DN, et al. The size and culturability of patient-generated SARS-CoV-2 aerosol. *J Expo Sci Environ Epidemiol*. 2021;1-6.
11. Johnson IG, Jones RJ, Gallagher JE, et al. Dental periodontal procedures: a systematic review of contamination (splatter, droplets and aerosol) in relation to COVID-19. *BDJ Open*. 2021;7(1):15.
12. Locke L, Dada O, Shedd JS. Aerosol transmission of infectious disease and the efficacy of personal protective equipment (PPE): a systematic review. *J Occup Environ Med*. 2021;10:1097.
13. Shenoy ES, Weber DJ. Occupational health update: evaluation and management of exposures and postexposure prophylaxis. *Infect Dis Clin North Am*. 2021;35(3):735-754.
14. Mohd-Said S, Mohd-Dom TN, Suhaimi N, et al. Effectiveness of pre-procedural mouthrinses in reducing aerosol contamination during periodontal prophylaxis: A systematic review. *Front Med (Lausanne)*. 2021;8:600769.
15. Centers for Disease Control and Prevention. Symptoms of COVID-19. Atlanta, GA: National Center for Immunization and Respiratory Diseases, Division of Viral Diseases; 2021. https://www.cdc.gov/coronavirus/2019-ncov/symptoms-testing/symptoms.html. Accessed September 19, 2021.
16. Pierce JD, Shen Q, Cintron SA, Hiebert JB. Post-COVID-19 Syndrome. *Nurs Res*. 2022;71(2):164-174.
17. Anaya JM, Rojas M, Salinas ML, et al. Post-COVID syndrome. A case series and comprehensive review. *Autoimmun Rev*. 2021;20(11):102947.
18. Marchesan JT, Warner BM, Byrd KM. The "oral" history of COVID-19: primary infection, salivary transmission, and post-acute implications. *J Periodontol*. 2021;10.1002/JPER.21-0277.
19. Huang N, Pérez P, Kato T, et al. SARS-CoV-2 infection of the oral cavity and saliva. *Nat Med*. 2021;27(5):892-903.
20. Sharma P, Malik S, Wadhwan V, Gotur Palakshappa S, Singh R. Prevalence of oral manifestations in COVID-19: A systematic review. *Rev Med Virol*. 2022;e2345.
21. Gupta S, Mohindra R, Singla M, et al. The clinical association between periodontitis and COVID-19. *Clin Oral Investig*. 2021;1-14.
22. Mancini L, Americo LM, Pizzolante T, Donati R, Marchetti E. Impact of COVID-19 on periodontitis and peri-implantitis: A Narrative Review. *Front Oral Health*. 2022;3:822824.
23. Centers for Disease Control and Prevention. Viral hepatitis. Atlanta, GA: Division of Viral Hepatitis; 2021. https://www.cdc.gov/hepatitis/index.htm. Accessed September 19, 2021.
24. Cohen JI. Herpesvirus latency. *J Clin Invest*. 2020;130(7):3361-3369.
25. Hatano Y, Ideta T, Hirata A, et al. Virus-driven carcinogenesis. *Cancers*. 2021;13(11):2625.
26. Chen C, Feng P, Slots J. Herpesvirus-bacteria synergistic interaction in periodontitis. *Periodontol 2000*. 2020;82(1):42-64.
27. Luan X, Zhou X, Fallah P, et al. MicroRNAs: harbingers and shapers of periodontal inflammation. *Semin Cell Dev Biol*. 2021;S1084-9521(21)00139-7.
28. Whitley R, Baines J. Clinical management of herpes simplex virus infections: past, present, and future. *F1000Res*. 2018;7:F1000.
29. Crimi S, Fiorillo L, Bianchi A, et al. Herpes virus, oral clinical signs and QoL: systematic review of recent data. *Viruses*. 2019;11(5):463.
30. Rathbun MM, Szpara ML. A holistic perspective on herpes simplex virus (HSV) ecology and evolution. *Adv Virus Res*. 2021;110:27-57.
31. Shoji K, Saitoh A. Herpetic whitlow. *New Eng J Med*. 2018;378(6):563.
32. Centers for Disease Control and Prevention. *Epidemiology and Prevention of Vaccine-Preventable Diseases*. Washington, DC: Public Health Foundation; 2021:329-345.
33. Rostgaard K, Balfour HH Jr, Jarrett R, et al. Primary Epstein-Barr virus infection with and without infectious mononucleosis. *PLoS One*. 2019;14(12):e0226436.
34. Alramadhan SA, Bhattacharyya I, Cohen DM, Islam MN. Oral hairy leukoplakia in immunocompetent patients revisited with literature review. *Head Neck Pathol*. 2021;15(3):989-993.
35. Centers for Disease Control and Prevention. Cytomegalovirus (CMV) and congenital CMV infection. Atlanta, GA: Division of Viral Diseases; 2021. https://www.cdc.gov/cmv/clinical/overview.html. Accessed September 19, 2021.
36. Komaroff AL, Zerr DM, Flamand L. Summary of the 11th international conference on human herpesviruses-6A, -6B, and -7. *J Med Virol*. 2020;92(1):4-10.

37. Dable C, Nicolli E. Manifestations of human papillomavirus in the head and neck. *Med Clin North Am*. 2021;105(5):849-858.
38. Shigeishi H, Sugiyama M, Ohta K. Relationship between the prevalence of oral human papillomavirus DNA and periodontal disease. *Biomed Rep*. 2021;14(5):40.
39. Centers for Disease Control and Prevention. *Epidemiology and Prevention of Vaccine-Preventable Diseases*. Washington, DC: Public Health Foundation; 2021:165-178.
40. Centers for Disease Control and Prevention. HIV basics. Atlanta, GA: Division of HIV/AIDS prevention; 2021. https://www.cdc.gov/hiv/basics/index.html. Accessed September 19, 2021.
41. Centers for Disease Control and Prevention. HIV treatment and care. Atlanta, GA: Division of HIV/AIDS prevention; 2021. https://www.cdc.gov/hiv/clinicians/treatment/treatment-clinicians.html#anchor_1530102113214. Accessed September 19, 2021.
42. Indrastiti RK, Wardhany II, Soegyanto AI. Oral manifestations of HIV: can they be an indicator of disease severity? (A systematic review). *Oral Dis*. 2020;26 Suppl 1:133-136.
43. Tappuni AR. The global changing pattern of the oral manifestations of HIV. *Oral Dis*. 2020;26 Suppl 1:22-27.
44. Patil S, Majumdar B, Sarode SC, Sarode GS, Awan KH. Oropharyngeal in HIV-infected patients-an update. *Front Microbiol*. 2018;9:980.
45. Markazi A, Meng W, Bracci PM, McGrath MS, Gao SJ. The role of bacteria in KSHV infection and KSHV-induced cancers. *Cancers*. 2021;13(17):4269.
46. Khoury ZH, Meeks V. The influence of antiretroviral therapy on HIV-related oral manifestations. *J Natl Med Assoc*. 2021;113(4):449-456.
47. Navarro JT, Moltó J, Tapia G, Ribera JM. Hodgkin lymphoma in people living with HIV. *Cancers*. 2021;13(17):4366.
48. Ryder MI, Shiboski C, Yao TJ, Moscicki AB. Current trends and new developments in HIV research and periodontal diseases. *Periodontol 2000*. 2020;82(1):65-77.
49. Balaji TM, Varadarajan S, Sujatha G, et al. Necrotizing periodontal diseases in human immunodeficiency virus-infected patients receiving highly active antiretroviral therapy: a review. *Dis Mon*. 2021;67(9):101168.
50. Papapanou PN, Sanz M, Buduneli N, et al. Periodontitis: consensus report of workgroup 2 of the 2017 world workshop on the classification of periodontal and peri-implant diseases and conditions. *J Periodontol*. 2018;89(suppl 1):S173–S182.
51. Royston L, Isnard S, Lin J, Routy JP. Cytomegalovirus as an uninvited guest in the response to vaccines in people living with HIV. *Viruses*. 2021;13(7):1266.
52. Shin YH, Park CM, Yoon CH. An overview of human immunodeficiency virus-1 antiretroviral drugs: general principles and current status. *Infect Chemother*. 2021;53(1):29-45.
53. Tigabu A, Getaneh A. *Staphylococcus aureus*, ESKAPE bacteria challenging current health care and community settings: a literature review. *Clin Lab*. 2021;67(7).
54. Lena P, Ishak A, Karageorgos SA, Tsioutis C. Presence of methicillin-resistant *Staphylococcus aureus* (MRSA) on healthcare workers' attire: A systematic review. *Trop Med Infect Dis*. 2021;6(2):42.

CHAPTER 6

Exposure Control: Barriers for Patient and Clinician

Jaymi-Lyn Adams, RDH, MS
Lori J. Giblin-Scanlon, RDH, MS, DHSc

CHAPTER OUTLINE

LEARNING OBJECTIVES

After studying this chapter, the student will be able to:

1. Identify and define key terms and concepts related to exposure control, clinical barriers, and latex sensitivity.
2. Explain the rationale and techniques for exposure control.
3. Identify the criteria for selecting effective barriers.
4. Explain the rationale, mechanics, and guidelines for hand hygiene.
5. Identify and describe the clinical manifestations and management of latex sensitivity.

Infection Control

- Exposure control refers to all procedures during clinical care necessary to provide top-level protection from exposure to infectious agents for members of the dental team and their patients.
- Dental healthcare personnel (DHCP) have a professional obligation to serve *all* patients with comprehensive oral care, including patients with known or unknown communicable diseases.
- DHCP must regularly consult with state and local health department recommendations and requirements, which may vary depending on community level rates of transmission of a disease.[1]

I. Standard Precautions

- The practice of *standard precautions* is utilized for everyone and means the body fluids of all patients are treated as if they were infectious.
  - Use of personal protective equipment (PPE): Gloves, masks or respirators, protective eyewear or face shield, hair coverings, and gowns.
  - An organized system for exposure control: Proper management of needles and sharps is needed.
  - A written exposure control plan is prepared to serve as a guide for the entire team.[1] The written plan can be the basis for training new personnel.
  - Consistency among DHCP is necessary to maintain standards of asepsis and to prevent **cross-contamination**.
  - As new research and commercial products become available and adopted for use, the written protocol for cleaning and disinfection must be revised.
  - Using the protocol and transferring the objectives and overall aims to the clinical setting are the responsibilities of each member of the dental team.
  - Physical barriers and other requirements of the protocol provide safety for both the DHCP and the patients.
- Review specific recommendations from the Centers for Disease Control and Prevention (CDC).

Personal Protection for the Dental Team

The continuing health and productivity of DHCP depend to a large degree on individuals' efforts to maintain themselves in a high standard of good health.

- Loss of work time, personal suffering, long-term systemic effects, and even exclusion from continued practice are possible results from transmissible disease infection.
- The only safe procedure is to practice defensively at all times, with specific precautions for personal protection.
- All clinical staff members need to be aware of the signs and symptoms of diseases that are occupational hazards for clinical dental and dental hygiene practitioners.
- Seek early diagnosis and treatment of a seemingly minor condition that could be the initial symptom of a more serious transmissible disease.

I. Immunizations

Dental personnel in a hospital setting are subject to the rules and regulations for all hospital employees. Policies often require certain **immunizations** or proof of antibodies for new employees.

- In private dental practices, individual initiative is required to maintain standards of safety for all dental team members relative to immunizations.
- Immunizations recommended for healthcare workers include[2]:
  - Hepatitis B
  - Influenza
  - MMR (measles, mumps, rubella)
  - Tetanus, diphtheria, pertussis
  - Varicella–Zoster
  - Meningococcal
  - Coronavirus disease 2019 (COVID-19)
- General recommendations on immunizations are reviewed annually by the Advisory Committee on Immunization Practices (ACIP).[2]
- At the time of employment, it is reasonable for a dentist employer to request a record of current immunizations, as well as specific tests, such as for tuberculosis.
- The needs differ in different climates, countries, and locations. Persons changing work location, or traveling for participation in dental hygiene programs, need to investigate specific precautions.

II. Maintain Records

- Records for personal immunizations should be regularly updated.
- Obtain tests promptly when exposed to certain infectious diseases and seek prophylactic immunization as indicated and available.

- Keep confidential written records of immunizations, boosters, and reimmunizations; plan for regular follow-up.
- When the status of current immunizations is known, time is saved by not needing a titer before initiating passive immunizations when accidental exposure occurs.

Clinical Attire

The clinical apparel of clinicians is vulnerable to **contamination** from splash, spatter, aerosols, and patient contact.

- Standard clothing, such as scrubs and street clothes, is not intended to protect against hazardous materials and is not considered protective clothing.
- The recommended clinical attire is designed and cared for in a manner that protects exposure from infectious materials in splatter or aerosols and minimizes cross-contamination.[1]
- Clinical attire and shoes are not to be worn outside the clinical practice setting. When clinical attire is worn outside, contamination can be carried from, and brought into, the treatment area.

I. Protective Clothing

- Protective clothing, such as gowns or jackets, is designed to be worn over clinical attire to protect skin and prevent cross-contamination from blood and other potentially infectious materials (**Figure 6-1**).[3]
- Gowns and jackets are expected to be clean and maintained as free as possible from contamination.
- The gown or jacket is closed at the neck and fastened in back.
- The fabric is disposable or reusable, stain and fluid resistant, can be washed commercially, and withstands washing with bleach.
- The garment must cover the knees when the clinician is seated during treatment.
- Long sleeves with fitted cuffs permit protective gloves to extend over the cuffs.[3]
- Gloved hands, prepared for patient treatment, are kept from touching objects or being placed in pockets.
- In addition, a washable or a disposable apron may be used over the gown or laboratory coat when clinical procedures involving blood, spatter, or aerosols are performed.
- If soaked or soiled by infectious materials, change protective clothing immediately.
- When protective clothing is removed, turn inside out to prevent exposure to infectious material.

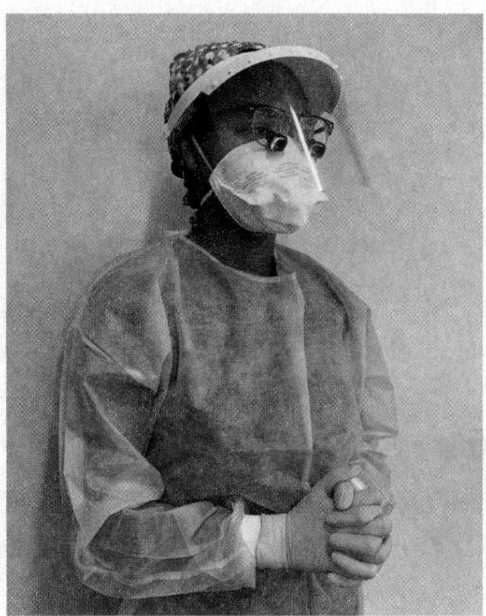

Figure 6-1 Protective Clothing: Disposable Gown Worn Over Clinical Attire

Courtesy of Susan Jenkins, RDH, MS.

II. Hair and Head Covering

- Hair is worn off the shoulders and fastened back away from the face.
  - Because the hair is exposed to contamination, an appropriate head cover is advised when performing **aerosol generating procedures (AGPs)** like using an ultrasonic scaler or air-powder polishing instruments.
- Facial hair needs to be covered with a face mask and face shield.

Use of Surgical Masks and Respiratory Protection

Basic personal **barrier protection** is composed of surgical mask, protective eyewear, and gloves.

- The use of the surgical mask is described first because it needs to be positioned first when preparing for clinical care procedures.
- The protective eyewear is placed second. After that, **hand hygiene** is performed before gloving.[3,4]

I. Aerosols

- Dispersion of particles of debris, polishing agents, calculus, and water, all of which are contaminated by the patient's oral flora, occurs regularly during treatment procedures.
- Aerosols are created following the use of a handpiece, prophylaxis angle, or a power-driven ultrasonic scaler.

- Particles can spread on the face, protective eyewear, uniform, and the barrier placed over the patient for protection from the spray.
- The CDC developed interim guidelines for providing care during the COVID-19 pandemic.[4] The most recent update advises DHCP avoid AGPs *only* for patients with suspected or confirmed infection with SARS-CoV-2.[1,4]
- The CDC recommends the use of high-evacuation suction and four-handed dentistry during AGPs.[1]

II. Mask Efficiency

A. Criteria: Essential Characteristics

See **Box 6-1** for a list of characteristics of an ideal mask.

- Filtration (measured in bacterial filtration efficiency [BFE]):
  - Surgical masks have a loose fit and provide a physical barrier from liquids such as splashes and large-particle droplets.[3]
  - The American Society for Testing and Materials uses a standard test method for evaluating the BFE of medical face masks. The BFE is a measurement of the masks' resistance to bacteria.
  - Use a surgical mask that will cover the nose and mouth with >95% BFE.[3]
  - Airborne droplets smaller than 5 μm in size can reach the alveoli of the lower respiratory tract and may potentially cause infection.[5]
  - Droplet nuclei (*Mycobacterium tuberculosis*) range from 0.5 to 1 μm and are a risk in healthcare settings.[6]
- Fit: Proper fit over face is vital to protect against inhaling droplet nuclei from aerosols.[7]
- Comfort: Degree of comfort with minimal interference with breathing encourages compliance in wearing.[7]

Box 6-1 Characteristics of an Ideal Mask

1. No contact with the wearer's nostrils or lips
2. Has a high bacterial filtration efficiency rate
3. Fits snugly around the entire edges of the mask
4. No fogging of eyewear
5. Convenient to put on and remove
6. Made of material that does not irritate skin or induce allergic reaction
7. Does not collapse during wear or when wet
8. No interference with breathing

III. Use of a Mask

- Adjust the mask and position eyewear before performing hand hygiene.
- Use a new mask for each patient.
  - Change mask each hour during routine procedures or more frequently when it becomes wet.
- Keep the mask on after completing a procedure while still in the presence of aerosols.
  - Particles 1–5 μm can remain suspended for extended periods and, when inhaled, can effectively penetrate the small bronchi and pulmonary alveoli.[5]
  - Removal of a mask in the treatment room immediately following the use of AGPs permits direct exposure to airborne organisms.
- Mask removal
  - Grasp side elastic or tie strings to remove (**Figure 6-2**).
  - Never handle the outside of a contaminated mask with gloved or bare hands.
  - Never place the mask under the chin.

IV. Use of a Respirator

- Particulate **respirator**
  - Heavy-duty protective device designed with a tight fit to filter airborne particles.
  - Use a National Institute for Occupational Safety and Health–certified respirator (e.g., N95, N99, or N100) for potentially infectious patients (active tuberculosis or suspected COVID-19), when ventilation is poor, and for

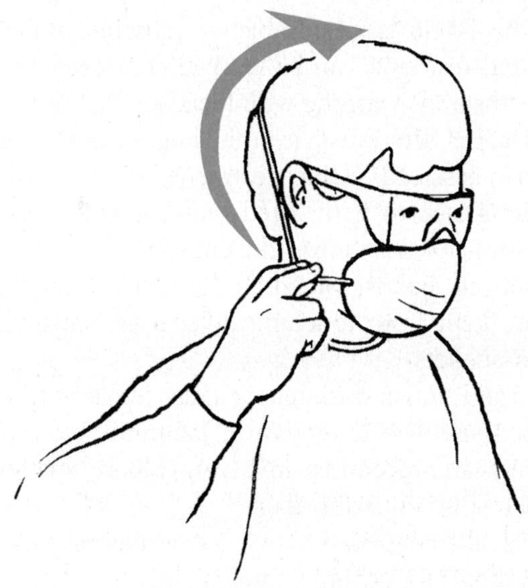

Figure 6-2 Removal of Mask. Handle only by the elastic or tie strings, carefully avoiding the contaminated mask.

procedures likely to produce droplet spatter or aerosols of oral or respiratory fluids.[1]
    - Before wearing a respirator, DHCP must receive medical clearance, undergo a fit test, and be trained in proper use and disposal.[8,9]
    - The CDC recommends that DHCP who work in communities with moderate to substantial community transmission of SARS-CoV-2 use N95 (or equivalent) during AGPs.[1]

V. Respiratory Hygiene

- Implement respiratory hygiene protocols for patients or anyone who presents in a dental setting with signs or symptoms of a respiratory illness such as coughing, sneezing, or runny nose.[1,10] Post signs to inform patients with symptoms of respiratory illness to cover their mouth and nose when sneezing or coughing.[10]
- Interim guidance from the CDC during a pandemic: Patients and DHCP should wear a cloth face covering or mask at all times while in the dental setting.[4]
- Tissues and receptacles with no touch technology for disposal should be available.[10]
- Offer methods for hand hygiene (sinks with soap and disposable towels or alcohol-based rub).[10]

Use of Protective Eyewear

Eye protection for the dental team members and patients is necessary to prevent physical injuries and infections of the eyes.[3]

- Severe and disabling eye accidents and infections have been reported.[11,12]
- Eye involvement may lead to pain, discomfort, loss of work time, and, in certain instances, permanent injury.
- Accidents can occur at any time, and as with most accidents, they occur when least prepared for or expected.
- Eye infections can follow the accidental dropping of an instrument on the face or the splashing of various materials from a patient's oral cavity into the eye.
- Contamination can be introduced from saliva, biofilm, carious material, pieces of old restorative materials during cavity preparation, bacteria-laden calculus during scaling, and any other microorganisms contained in aerosols or spatter.
- Careful, deliberate techniques and instrument management, with evacuation and other procedures for the control of oral fluids, contribute to the prevention of accidents and infections of the eyes.
- All measures described for the prevention of airborne disease transmission by aerosols and spatter apply to eye protection.

I. Indications for Use of Protective Eyewear

A. Dental Team Members

- Protective eyewear is worn for all procedures.
- Dental personnel who do not require corrective lenses for vision should wear protective eyewear with clear lenses.

B. General Features of Acceptable Eyewear

- Sufficient eye coverage, with side shields, to protect around the eye.[3]
- Shatterproof; made of strong, sturdy plastic.
- Lightweight.
- Flexible and with rounded smooth edges to prevent discomfort.
- Easily disinfected.
    - Smooth surface areas prevent accumulation of infectious material.
    - Disinfectant used cannot damage or distort the frames or lenses.
- A clear or lightly tinted lens, rather than a very dark lens, permits the dental team members to watch the patient's reactions and maintain contact and response.
- Desirable but not required: scratch-resistant, antifog, and antistatic.

C. Types of Eyewear

Many styles, including regular eyeglass shapes and those described as follows, have been used.

- Goggles: Shielding on all sides of the glasses may give the best protection, provided they fit closely around the edges.[13] Goggle-style coverage is necessary for protection during laboratory work.
- Eyewear with side shields (**Figure 6-3A**): A side shield can provide added protection, but does not protect from splashes or droplets as well as goggles.[13] For the member of the dental team who depend on a prescription lens, separate side shields are available that can be connected to the temples.
- Eyewear with curved frames (**Figure 6-3B**): When the sides of the eyewear are curved back, they

may provide a protection somewhat similar to that offered by those with the side shield.

- Disposable glasses are available that are made of antiultraviolet flexible plastic (**Figure 6-3C**).
- Dental loupes (**Figure 6-3D**): Designed to protect the eyes and magnify the oral cavity. When they are designed with a light or flip-up, do not touch during clinical procedures.

D. Face Shield

- A clinician needs to wear a face shield over a regular mask when an aerosol-producing handpiece, ultrasonic scaler, or air polishing equipment is used.[3]

E. Protective Eyewear for Patients

- Protective eyewear is essential for each patient at each appointment. The patient may need to be educated about the reasons for wearing protective eyewear.
- Patients with their own prescription lenses may prefer to wear them, but for the safety of the patient's glasses, the use of the protective eyewear with side shields provided in the office or clinic is preferred.
- Protection against glare. Certain patients may request tinted lenses or prefer to wear their own sunglasses when their eyes are especially sensitive to the dental light.
- Child-sized sunglasses.

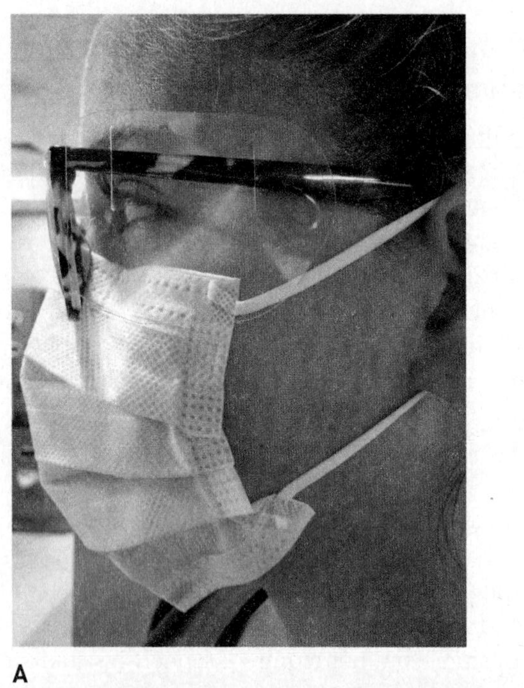

A

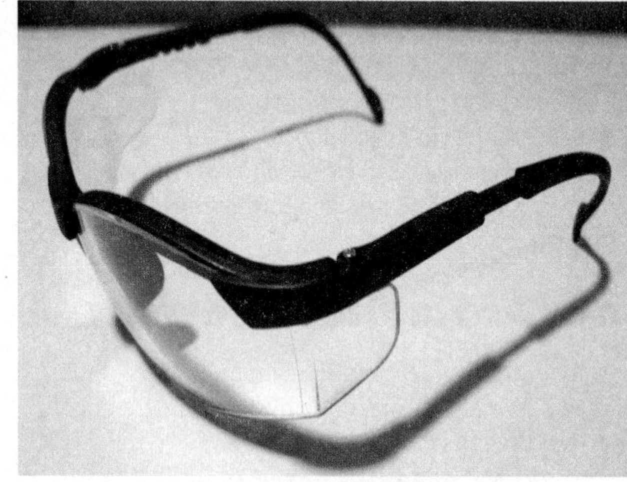

B

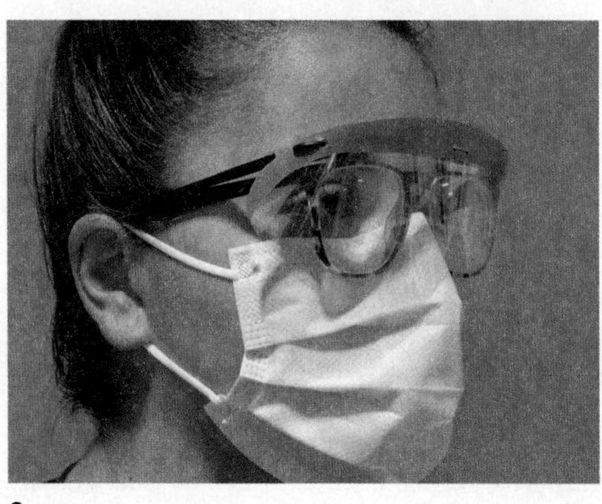

C

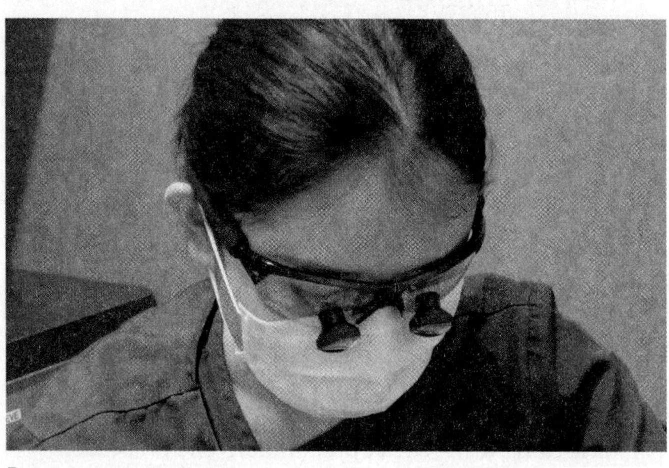

D

Figure 6-3 Protective Eyewear. Protective cover for both patient and clinician may be goggles-style **(A)** glasses with side shields, **(B)** safety glasses, **(C)** disposable eyewear, and **(D)** loupes.

Courtesy of Susan Jenkins, RDH, MS.

II. Suggestions for Clinical Application

A. Contact Lenses

- Dental team members and patients who wear contact lenses always need to wear protective eyewear over them during dental and dental hygiene procedures.[13]

B. Care of Protective Eyewear

- Contaminated eye protection must be cleaned with an approved disinfectant and rinsed thoroughly. Air-dry.
- Check periodically for scratches on the lens and replace appropriately.

C. Eye Wash Station

- Occupational Safety and Health Administration requires that facilities for flushing or washing of the eyes be provided in the immediate work environment.[14]
- Eye wash station equipment needs to be attached to a sink not used by clinicians for patient preparation.
- Eye wash stations must not be connected to regular faucets unless the hot water source is turned off permanently.

Hand Care

- In the infectious process of disease transmission, the hands may serve as a *means of transmission* of the blood, saliva, and dental biofilm from a patient.[3,15]
- The hands, especially under the fingernails, may serve as a *reservoir* for microorganisms.
- Skin breaks in the hands may serve as a *port of entry* for potentially pathogenic microorganisms.[3]
- By caring properly for the hands, using effective hand-hygiene procedures, and following the basic rules for gloving, primary cross-contamination can be controlled.
- A conscious effort is made to keep the gloved hands from touching objects other than the instruments and disinfected parts of the equipment prepared for the immediate patient.

I. Bacteriology of the Skin

- Resident bacteria[16]:
  - Many relatively stable bacteria inhabit the surface epithelium or deeper areas in the ducts of skin glands or depths of hair follicles; ultimately, they are shed with the exfoliated surface cells or with excretions of the skin glands.
  - Resident bacteria tend to be less susceptible to destruction by disinfection procedures.
- Transient bacteria[16]:
  - Transient bacteria reflect continuous contamination by routine contacts; some bacteria are pathogens.
  - They may be washed away or, in the event that a skin break exists, may cause an autogenous infection.
  - Transient bacteria can typically be removed by washing with soap and water or with 60–95% ethanol- or isopropanol-based hand rubs used as directed by the manufacturer.

II. Hand Care

A. Fingernails

- Maintain clean, smoothly trimmed, short fingernails with well maintained cuticles to prevent breaks where microorganisms can enter.
- Effects of short nails:
  - Make handwashing more effective to reduce microorganisms harbored under the nails.[17]
  - Prevent cuts from long nails in disposable gloves.
  - Allow greater dexterity during instrumentation.
  - Decrease chance of patient discomfort or injury.

B. Artificial Nails

- Artificial nails or extenders are more likely to harbor pathogens and are not recommended for clinicians.[16,18]
- Wearing rings and nail polish is not recommended because chipped nail polish and skin under the ring may harbor bacteria.[3,19]

C. Wristwatch and Jewelry

- Remove hand and wrist jewelry at the beginning of the day.
- Microorganisms can become lodged in crevices of rings, watchbands, and watches.[19,20]

D. Gloves

- After handwashing, put on gloves. Never expose open skin lesions or abrasions to a patient's oral tissues and fluids.
- After glove removal, wash hands to remove microorganisms.

Hand-Hygiene Principles

I. Rationale

- Effective and frequent hand hygiene can reduce the overall bacterial flora of the skin and prevent cross-contamination to surfaces and patients.[16]
- It is impossible to sterilize the skin, but every attempt is made to minimize the bacterial flora.

II. Purposes

Hand hygiene, including handwashing, hand antisepsis, or surgical hand antisepsis, is critical for reducing the bacterial flora of the hands. The chosen method is dependent on the procedure and the degree of contamination.

- An effective hand hygiene procedure can be expected to accomplish the following[3]:
  - Remove surface dirt and eliminate transient bacteria.
  - Reduce resident flora.

III. Facilities

- Sink
  - Use a sink with a foot pedal or electronic control for water flow to avoid contamination to/from faucet handles.
  - For a regular sink, turn on water at the beginning and leave on through the entire procedure. Turn faucets off with the towel after drying hands.
  - Clean around sink rim with disinfectant. The sink must be of sufficient size so that contact with the inside of the wash basin can be avoided. A sink cannot be sterilized and can become highly contaminated.
  - Prevent contamination of clothing by not leaning against the sink.
  - Use a separate area and sink reserved for instrument washing.
- Soap
  - Use a liquid or foam soap.
  - Apply from a foot- or knee-activated or electronically controlled dispenser to avoid contamination to and from a hand-operated dispenser or cake soap. Rinsing is a necessary part of the handwashing procedure.
- Towels
  - Obtain a disposable towel from a dispenser that requires no contact except with the towel itself, which hangs down, or a hands-free automatic dispenser.
  - Cloth towels are not recommended.

Methods of Hand Hygiene

Hand hygiene is considered the single most important procedure for the prevention of cross-contamination (**Box 6-2**).[16,21]

I. Indications

- Before and after treating each patient (before glove placement and after glove removal).
- Before regloving after removing gloves that are torn, cut, or punctured.
- After touching inanimate objects that may be contaminated with blood or saliva with ungloved hands.
- When hands are visibly soiled.
- Before leaving the treatment room.

II. Descriptions

A. Routine Handwash

Handwashing sufficient for routine dental examinations and nonsurgical dental procedures includes the following[3,16,21]:

- Wet hands with water; apply liquid, nonantimicrobial soap (plain soap); avoid hot water.
- Rub hands together for at least 15 seconds; cover all surfaces of fingers, hands, and wrists.
- Interlace fingers and rub to cover all sides.
- Rinse under running water; dry thoroughly with disposable towels.
- Turn off faucet with the towel.
- The procedure should take at least 40–60 seconds.

B. Antiseptic Handwash

- Water and liquid **antimicrobial soap** (e.g., chlorhexidine, iodine and iodophors, chloroxylenol [para-chloro-meta-xylenol, PCMX], triclosan).[3]
- To remove or destroy transient microorganisms and reduce resident flora.
  1. Preliminary steps[16]:
     - Remove watch and jewelry from hands.
     - Fasten hair back securely.
     - Put on protective eyewear and mask before handwashing to prevent contamination of washed hands ready for gloving.
     - Use cool water; hot water can increase risk for dermatitis.
  2. Handwashing procedure[16]
     - Lather hands, wrists, and forearms quickly with liquid antimicrobial soap.
     - Rub all surfaces vigorously; interlace fingers and rub back and forth with pressure for 15–20 seconds.

Box 6-2 Hand-Hygiene Methods and Indications[3,16,21]

Method	Agent	Purpose	Duration (minimum)	Indication
Routine handwash	Water and nonantimicrobial soap (e.g., plain soap)	Remove visible soil or debris and transient microorganisms	40–60 sec	▪ When visibly soiled ▪ Before and after touching a patient ▪ Before glove placement and after glove removal ▪ After touching any surface or object likely to be contaminated ▪ Before leaving the dental operatory or the dental laboratory
Antiseptic handwash	Water and antimicrobial soap (e.g., chlorhexidine, iodine and iodophors, chloroxylenol (para-chloro-meta-xylenol, PCMX), triclosan)	Remove or destroy transient microorganisms and reduce resident flora	15 sec	
Antiseptic hand rub	Alcohol-based hand rub	Remove or destroy transient microorganisms and reduce resident flora	Rub hands until the agent is dry	Use an alcohol-based hand rub as the preferred means for routine hand antisepsis unless visibly soiled
Surgical antisepsis	Water and antimicrobial soap (e.g., chlorhexidine, iodine and iodophors, chloroxylenol [PCMX], triclosan)	Remove or destroy transient microorganisms and reduce resident flora (persistent effect)	2–5 min	Before donning sterile surgeon's gloves for surgical procedures

Data from Kohn WG, Collins AS, Cleveland JL, et al. Guidelines for infection control in dental health-care settings--2003. *MMWR Recomm Rep.* 2003;52(RR-17):1-61; Boyce JM, Pittet D, Healthcare Infection Control Practices Advisory Committee, HICPAC/SHEA/APIC/IDSA Hand Hygiene Task Force. Guideline for hand hygiene in health-care settings. Recommendations of the Healthcare Infection Control Practices Advisory Committee and the HICPAC/SHEA/APIC/IDSA Hand Hygiene Task Force. *MMWR Recomm Rep.* 2002;51(RR-16):1-45, quiz CE1-4; World Health Organization. Surgical Hand Preparation: State-of-the-Art. World Health Organization; 2009. https://www.ncbi.nlm.nih.gov/books/NBK144036/. Accessed September 18, 2021.

- Rinse thoroughly, running the water from fingertips down the hands. Keep water running.
- Use paper towels for drying, taking care not to recontaminate.

C. Antiseptic Hand Rub

An **antiseptic** hand rub is used to remove or destroy transient microorganisms and reduce resident flora with the following procedure[3,21]:

- Wash visibly soiled hands before use.
- Decontaminate hands with an (60–95% ethanol or isopropanol) alcohol-based hand rub.
- Apply the product (follow manufacturer's directions for amount to use) to the palm of one hand, and vigorously rub hands together until dry.

D. Surgical Antisepsis[3] (Also Called Surgical Scrub)

- Water and antimicrobial liquid soap (e.g., chlorhexidine, iodine and iodophores, chloroxylenol [PCMX], triclosan).
- To remove or destroy transient microorganisms and reduce resident flora with a persistent or prolonged effect that inhibits proliferation or survival of microorganisms.

- Each hospital or oral surgery clinic has rules and regulations for surgical antisepsis. These will be posted over the sinks.
- The minimum duration of a surgical antisepsis is 2–6 minutes.
  1. Preliminary steps[21]
     - Remove watch and jewelry. Place hair and beard coverings and make sure hair is completely covered.
     - Put on protective eyewear and mask.
  2. Handwashing procedure[16]
     - Remove debris under fingernails with a nail cleaner under running water.
     - Apply antimicrobial soap to hands and forearms to remove gross surface dirt.
     - Lather vigorously with strong rubbing motions on each side of hands, wrists, and forearms along with interlacing fingers and thumbs.
     - Duration is 2–6 minutes or as directed by the manufacturer instructions.
     - Rinse thoroughly from fingertips across hands and wrists. Hold hands higher than elbows throughout the procedure. Leave water running.
     - Hold hands up and clasped together. Proceed to dressing area for gowning and gloving.

Gloves and Gloving

Wearing gloves is a standard practice to protect both the patient and the clinician from cross-contamination.

I. Criteria for Selection of Treatment/Examination Gloves

A. Safety Factors

- Effective barrier; evidence from manufacturer of quality control standards.
- Impermeable to patient's saliva, blood, and bacteria.
- Strength and durability to resist tears and punctures.
- Impervious to materials routinely used during clinical procedures.
- Nonirritating or harmful to skin; use nonlatex gloves when the patient or clinician is allergic.
- Length: Glove cuff extends to provide coverage over cuff of long sleeve.

B. Ergonomic Choice Factors

- Fit hand well; no interference with motion.
- Tactile sense not decreased.
- No tightness over palm or between thumb and index finger.

II. Types of Gloves

- Material
  - Latex.
  - Nonlatex: neoprene, block copolymer, vinyl, *N*-nitrile.
- For patient care
  - Nonsterile single-use examination/treatment: latex, nonlatex.
  - Presterilized single-use surgical: latex, nonlatex.
- Utility gloves
  - Heavy duty: latex, nonlatex (puncture resistant for clinic cleanup).
  - Plastic: Food handler's glove to wear as overglove.

III. Procedures for Use of Gloves

- Mask and eyewear placement
  - Place mask and protective eyewear before performing hand hygiene and gloving.
  - Prevent the need for manipulating the mask around the face and hair after washing the hands.
- Pregloving hand hygiene
  - Use an antiseptic handwash or hand rub before gloving.
  - Hands must be dried thoroughly to control moisture inside glove and discourage growth of bacteria.
- Glove placement
  - Always glove and deglove in front of the patient; a patient may need assurance that gloves are new and used only for that appointment.
  - Place gloves over the cuff of long-sleeved clinic gown to provide complete protection of arms from exposure to contamination.
- Avoiding contamination
  - Keep gloved hands away from face, hair, clothing (pockets), cell phone, patient records, clinician's stool, and all parts of the dental equipment that have not been disinfected and/or covered with a barrier.
- Torn, cut, or punctured glove
  - Remove immediately, perform hand hygiene, and put on new gloves.
- Removal of gloves
  - Develop a procedure whereby gloves can be removed without contaminating the hands from the exposed external surfaces of the gloves.

- **Figure 6-4** illustrates one system for glove removal.
- Perform hand hygiene promptly after glove removal. Organisms on the hands multiply rapidly inside the warm, moist environment of the glove, even when no external contamination has occurred.

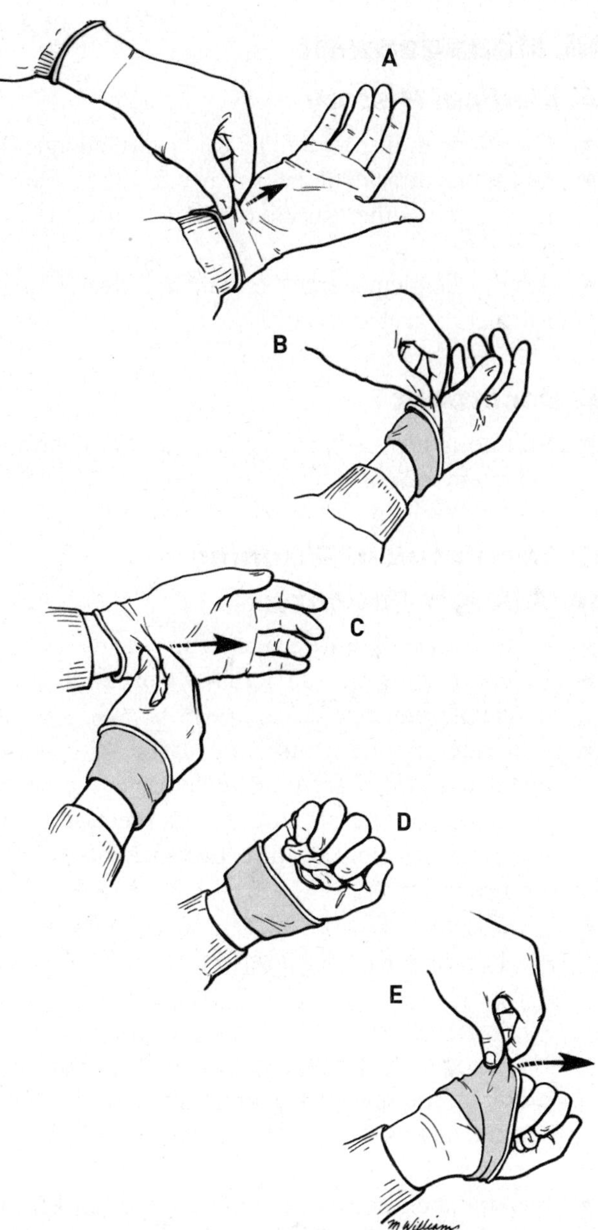

Figure 6-4 Steps for Removal of Gloves. **A:** Use left fingers to pinch right glove near edge to fold back. **B:** Fold edge back without contact with clean inside surface. **C:** Use right fingers to contact outside of left glove at the wrist to invert and remove. **D:** Bunch glove into the palm. **E:** With ungloved left hand, grasp inner noncontaminated portion of the right glove to peel it off, enclosing the other glove as it is inverted.

IV. Factors Affecting Glove Integrity

- Length of time worn
  - New pair for each patient is the basic requirement.
  - There is no optimal time for changing gloves during a procedure. Gloves can develop defects in 30 minutes to 3 hours due to minute tears.[3]
- Complexity of the procedure
  - Certain procedures are more likely to promote perforations, especially when sharp instruments are involved.
- Packaging of the gloves
  - Gloves in a new box are tightly packed and can be torn when removed so use care in removing them.
- Size of glove
  - When too long, the extra material at the fingertips can get caught, torn, or in the way; picking up small objects is difficult, especially sharp instruments.
- Pressure of time
  - Stress; working too fast increases the risk of glove damage.
- Storage of gloves
  - Keep in cool, dark place; exposure to heat, sun, or fluorescent light increases potential for deterioration and perforations.
- Agents used
  - Certain chemicals react with the glove material; for example, petroleum jelly, alcohol, and products made with alcohol tend to break down the glove integrity.
- Hazards from the hands
  - Long fingernails and rings can cause tears or perforations in the gloves.

Latex Hypersensitivity

Patients and clinicians may have or may develop sensitivity to natural rubber latex (NRL). Symptoms of a hypersensitive reaction range from a dermatitis to a life-threatening anaphylactic shock.[3] The only available treatment for **latex allergy** is avoiding all contact.

- Latex sensitivity is due to the protein **allergens** and to additives used when the commercial latex is prepared.
- Latex allergens occur in any equipment or product used that contains NRL.

- Gloves are the most frequently used item that contains latex.
- Equipment listed in **Box 6-3** may contain NRL. However, many of the items are also made of alternative materials. When the label on a product does not list the contents, the manufacturer can be contacted to identify latex-free items.

I. Clinical Manifestations

- Methods of exposure
    - Direct exposure to latex products.
    - **Aeroallergen** inhalation of the allergen when the powder (cornstarch) from the gloves becomes airborne.
    - Mucosal contact.
- Type I hypersensitivity (immediate reaction)
    - Urticaria: hives.
    - Dermatitis: rash, itching occurs in 5 minutes to 2 hours.[22]
    - Nasal problems: sneezing, itchy nose, runny nose.
    - Eyes: watery, itchy.
    - Respiratory reaction: breathing difficulty, asthma-like wheezing, coughing.
    - Drop in blood pressure: shock.
    - Anaphylaxis.
- Type IV hypersensitivity (delayed reaction)
    - Contact dermatitis develops 8 hours to 5 days after contact.[22]

II. Individuals at High Risk for Latex Sensitivity

- Have had frequent exposure to latex products.
    - **Occupational exposure**: Healthcare personnel who wear latex gloves regularly for patient care or those who have worked in a rubber manufacturing plant.
    - Multiple medical surgeries or treatments requiring placement of rubber tubes or drains. Examples: genitourinary anomalies, spina bifida.
- Have other documented allergies
    - Examples: food allergies (avocado, banana, kiwi fruit, chestnuts, papaya, peanuts).

Box 6-3 Equipment That May Contain Latex

- Bite blocks
- Blood pressure cuff
- Gloves
- Goggles
- Lead apron cover
- Masks (elastic head band)
- Mixing bowl
- Nitrous oxide nosepiece and tubing rubber dam
- O ring (on ultrasonic insert)
- Orthodontic elastics
- Rubber polishing cup
- Stethoscope
- Stopper in anesthesia carpule
- Suction adapter

III. Management

A. Medical History

- Questions in history will reveal known allergies.
- Questions directed to latex may not suffice. Questions about other specific products need to be asked.
- Advise allergic patients to obtain and wear a medical alert bracelet or necklace.

B. Document

- All information is carefully recorded for continuing reference.

C. Appointment Planning for Allergic Patient

- Treatment in a latex-free environment.
- Whenever possible, use nonlatex gloves and other nonlatex products.[23]
- Schedule appointments early in the day when powdered gloves are used: Before glove powder contaminates the air throughout the facility or outerwear of clinical attire becomes laden with airborne latex.
- Clean clinical areas:
    - Person preparing room must wear nonlatex gloves.
    - Wipe all surfaces to remove allergen.
- No latex in the treatment room: Use nonlatex products for high-risk patients (whether or not specific latex sensitivity has been known and reported in the history).
- Prepare latex-free carts: Materials and gloves, for use when seeing high-risk patients, can be readied in advance.[22]

D. Emergency Treatment Equipment and Drugs Ready

- Inform the entire dental team of appointment.
- Have a latex-free emergency cart available.[23]
- Be alert for an emergency.

Documentation

Documentation needs to record the following:

- Irregularities related to personal protection that could have influenced the procedures of a routine appointment.
- How the special needs were taken care of for a patient with an allergy to latex.
- Information in medical alert that patient is sensitive to latex.

A sample progress note may be found in **Box 6-4**.

Factors to Teach the Patient

- Need for the patient's complete history for the protection of both the patient and the professional person.
- Purposes for use of barriers (face mask, protective eyewear, and gloves) by the clinician for the benefit of the patient.
- Importance of eye protection.
- Significance of hand hygiene in the control of disease transmission (everywhere, not only dental office or clinic).

Box 6-4 Example Documentation: Patient with a Latex Sensitivity

- **S**—Initial appointment for new patient to our practice. She reports sensitivity to latex gloves.
- **O**—History form and questions completed. Informed patient that the office is latex free. Radiographs taken, risk assessment, caries examination, and periodontal assessment. Pocket depths 5–6 mm in the area of #30–31 with bleeding on probing, all other areas 3 mm or less. Plaque score 30%.
- **A**—Patient has a history of skin reactions when latex gloves are used. Careful attention to avoiding use of products containing latex. Localized Stage III, Grade A periodontitis between #30 and #31.
- **P**—Review of oral self-care with attention to optimal biofilm removal #30–31. Localized nonsurgical periodontal therapy with local anesthetic with prophylaxis full mouth. Applied 5% sodium fluoride varnish due to moderate caries risk.

Signed: ______________________________, RDH

Date: ______________________________

References

1. Centers for Disease Control and Prevention (CDC) Healthcare Infection Control Practices Advisory Committee. Core infection prevention and control practices for safe healthcare delivery in all settings–recommendations of the HICPAC. Published September 10, 2021. https://www.cdc.gov/hicpac/recommendations/core-practices.html. Accessed September 17, 2021.
2. Centers for Disease Control and Prevention (CDC). ACIP vaccine recommendations. Published January 13, 2021. https://www.cdc.gov/vaccines/hcp/acip-recs/index.html. Accessed September 17, 2021.
3. Kohn WG, Collins AS, Cleveland JL, et al. Guidelines for infection control in dental health-care settings--2003. *MMWR Recomm Rep*. 2003;52(RR-17):1-61.
4. Centers for Disease Control and Prevention (CDC). Interim infection prevention and control guidance for dental settings during the coronavirus disease 2019 (COVID-19) pandemic. Published February 11, 2020. https://www.cdc.gov/coronavirus/2019-ncov/hcp/dental-settings.html. Accessed August 28, 2021.
5. Sosnowski TR. Inhaled aerosols: their role in COVID-19 transmission, including biophysical interactions in the lungs. *Curr Opin Colloid Interface Sci*. 2021;54:101451.
6. Jensen PA, Lambert LA, Iademarco MF, Ridzon R, CDC. Guidelines for preventing the transmission of *Mycobacterium tuberculosis* in health-care settings, 2005. *MMWR Recomm Rep*. 2005;54(RR-17):1-141.
7. Bradford Smith P, Agostini G, Mitchell JC. A scoping review of surgical masks and N95 filtering facepiece respirators: learning from the past to guide the future of dentistry. *Saf Sci*. 2020;131:104920.
8. Food and Drug Administration. N95 respirators, surgical masks, face masks, and barrier face coverings. FDA. Published September 15, 2021. https://www.fda.gov/medical-devices/personal-protective-equipment-infection-control/n95-respirators-surgical-masks-face-masks-and-barrier-face-coverings. Accessed September 17, 2021.
9. Occupational Health and Safety Administration. 1910.134 - Respiratory Protection. Published June 8, 2011. https://www.osha.gov/laws-regs/regulations/standardnumber/1910/1910.134. Accessed September 17, 2021.
10. Centers for Disease Control and Prevention (CDC). Respiratory hygiene/cough etiquette in healthcare settings. Published April 17, 2019. https://www.cdc.gov/flu/professionals/infectioncontrol/resphygiene.htm. Accessed September 17, 2021.
11. Revankar VD, Chakravarthy Y, Naveen S, Aarthi G, Mallikarjunan DY, Noon AM. Prevalence of ocular injuries, conjunctivitis and musculoskeletal disorders–related issues as occupational hazards among dental practitioners in the city of Salem: a randomized cross-sectional study. *J Pharm Bioallied Sci*. 2019;11(Suppl 2):S335-S337.

12. Ajayi YO, Ajayi EO. Prevalence of ocular injury and the use of protective eye wear among the dental personnel in a teaching hospital. *Niger Q J Hosp Med*. 2008;18(2):83-86.
13. Centers for Disease Control and Prevention (CDC), National Institute for Occupational Safety and Health. Eye safety: eye protection for infection control. Published May 18, 2020. https://www.cdc.gov/niosh/topics/eye/eye-infectious.html. Accessed September 17, 2021.
14. Occupational Safety and Health Administration. 1910.151 - Medical services and first aid. Published June 18, 1998. https://www.osha.gov/laws-regs/regulations/standardnumber/1910/1910.151. Accessed September 18, 2021.
15. Resende KKM, Neves LF, de Rezende Costa Nagib L, Martins LJO, Costa CRR. Educator and student hand hygiene adherence in dental schools: a systematic review and meta-analysis. *J Dent Educ*. 2019;83(5):575-584.
16. Boyce JM, Pittet D, Healthcare Infection Control Practices Advisory Committee, HICPAC/SHEA/APIC/IDSA Hand Hygiene Task Force. Guideline for hand hygiene in health-care settings. Recommendations of the Healthcare Infection Control Practices Advisory Committee and the HICPAC/SHEA/APIC/IDSA Hand Hygiene Task Force. *MMWR Recomm Rep*. 2002;51(RR-16):1-45.
17. Rayan GM, Flournoy DJ. Microbiologic flora of human fingernails. *J Hand Surg*. 1987;12(4):605-607.
18. Hedderwick SA, McNeil SA, Lyons MJ, Kauffman CA. Pathogenic organisms associated with artificial fingernails worn by healthcare workers. *Infect Control Hosp Epidemiol*. 2000;21(8):505-509.
19. Arrowsmith VA, Taylor R. Removal of nail polish and finger rings to prevent surgical infection. *Cochrane Database Syst Rev*. 2014;2014(8):CD003325.
20. Greenshield K, Chavez J, Nial KJ, Baldwin K. Examining bacteria on skin and jewelry since the implementation of hand sanitizer in hospitals. *Am J Infect Control*. 2020;48(11):1402-1403.
21. World Health Organization. *Surgical Hand Preparation: State-of-the-Art*. World Health Organization; 2009. https://www.ncbi.nlm.nih.gov/books/NBK144036/. Accessed September 18, 2021.
22. Muller BA. Minimizing latex exposure and allergy: how to avoid or reduce sensitization in the healthcare setting. *Postgrad Med*. 2003;113(4):91-98.
23. National Institute for Occupational Safety and Health. *Preventing Allergic Reactions to Natural Rubber Latex in the Workplace*. National Institute for Occupational Safety and Health; 1997:16. https://www.cdc.gov/niosh/docs/97-135/pdfs/97-135.pdf?id=10.26616/NIOSHPUB97135. Accessed September 22, 2021.

CHAPTER 7

Infection Control: Clinical Procedures

Lory A. Libby, RDH, MSDH

CHAPTER OUTLINE

LEARNING OBJECTIVES

After studying this chapter, the student will be able to:

1. Describe the basic considerations for safe infection control practices.
2. Explain methods for cleaning and sterilizing instruments.
3. Describe procedures to prepare, clean, and disinfect the treatment area.
4. Explain process for managing hypodermic needles and occupational postexposure management.
5. List types of waste disposal and explain how each type is handled.

Infection Control

The success of a planned system for control of disease transmission depends on the cooperative effort of each member of the dental team.

- The aim is to provide the highest level of **infection control** to ensure a safe environment for both patients and the clinical team.
- The presence of specific disease-producing organisms is rarely known; therefore, application of protective, preventive procedures is needed before, during, and following *all* patient appointments.

I. Objectives

The following are guidelines necessary to prevent the transmission of infectious agents and eliminate cross-contamination:

- Reduction of available pathogenic microorganisms to a level at which the normal resistance mechanisms of the body can prevent infection.
- Elimination of cross-contamination by breaking the chain of infection. (See Chapter 5.)
- Application of standard and transmission-based precautions by treating each patient as if all human blood and body fluids are infectious.[1]

II. Engineering Controls and Ventilation

Though there are guidelines from the Centers for Disease Control and Prevention (CDC) for ventilation practices in hospitals, none exist for the dental setting. The CDC does, however, provide recommendations for maintaining a healthy system as well as patient distancing and **de-densification** of dental office space.[2]

III. Ventilation

- General ventilation practices
  - Vents should be free from clutter to allow free movement of air.
  - Air should flow from a *"clean to less clean"* direction.[2]
  - Filters should be changed regularly according to manufacturer's directions.
  - Keep vents cleaned and maintained.[2]
  - It is recommended to consult with a professional to help determine the highest filtration available for the existing heating, ventilation, and air conditioning (HVAC) system.[2]
- Ventilation should be run continuously during business hours and for 2 hours after closing.[2]
- Portable high efficiency particulate air (HEPA) filter.
  - Always place these units near the patient's chair, ensuring the dental provider is not positioned in the zone of air flow to or from the unit.[2]
- **Upper-room ultraviolet germicidal irradiation (UVGI)** units can be used in conjunction with ventilation units. The units are installed near the ventilation vents to aid in the inactivation of microorganisms through ultraviolet light.[3]
- The bathroom exhaust fan should run continuously until the end of day.[2]

- Patient placement
  - Individual treatment rooms are best to prevent the spread of pathogens.[2]
  - Open floor plans ideally should[2]:
    - Position patients 6 feet apart.
    - Provide physical barriers between patient chairs.
    - Position patients parallel to the direction of the air flow (**Figure 7-1**).
    - Place the patient's head near the air return vents whenever possible.
    - Whenever possible, position the patient's head away from open hallways, especially if aerosol generating procedures (AGPs) are being performed.
- Patient scheduling
  - Schedule patient appointments appropriately, allowing time for cleaning and disinfection and to allow for de-densification of the dental office.
  - Implement policies that allow only patients in the building whenever possible; visitors should wait outside the office.

IV. Basic Considerations for Safe Practice

When developing a safe practice routine, the **sterilization** and disinfection of patient care items are categorized into the following:

- *Critical items*: These items will come into contact with soft tissue and bone and run the highest risk of disease transition. These items should be disposable or sterilized using a heat sterilizer.[1] Examples of these are surgical instruments, scalers, probes, needles, and scalpel blades.
- *Semi-critical items*: These items come into contact with intact mucous membranes. Semi-critical items have a lower risk of transmitting disease than do critical items; however, these should also be disposable or be processed using heat sterilization.[4,5] If these items are heat sensitive, they should be processed using a high-level **disinfectant**.[3] Examples of these include mouth mirrors and impression trays.
- *Noncritical items*: These items could potentially come into contact with intact skin and pose the lowest risk of disease transmission.[4,5]

Treatment Room Features

A partial list of notable features is included here and illustrated in **Figure 7-2**. The objective is to have materials, shapes, and surface textures to facilitate the effective use of infection control measures.

I. Contact Surfaces

Contact surfaces can sometimes be referred to as noncritical items and consist of instruments and surfaces that may come into contact with intact skin.[6,7] These surfaces can potentially be contaminated by spray or splatter or hand contact by a dental healthcare personnel. Contact

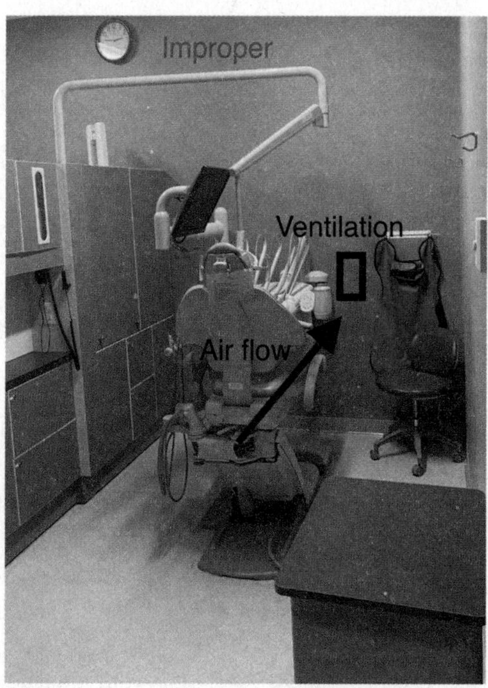

A

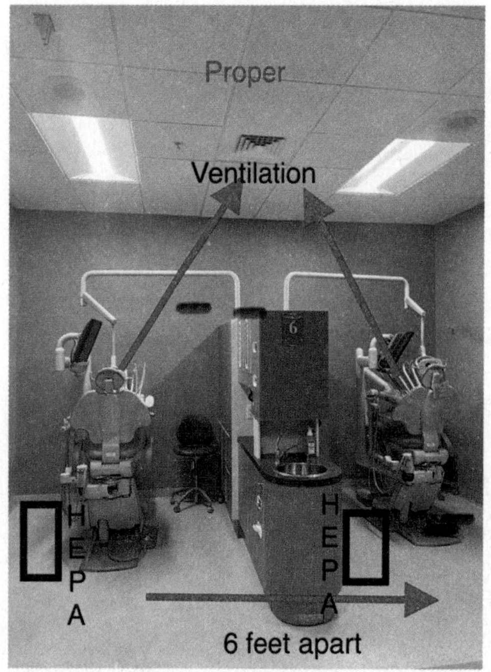

B

Figure 7-1 Ventilation. **A:** Improper unit placement. **B:** Proper unit placement.

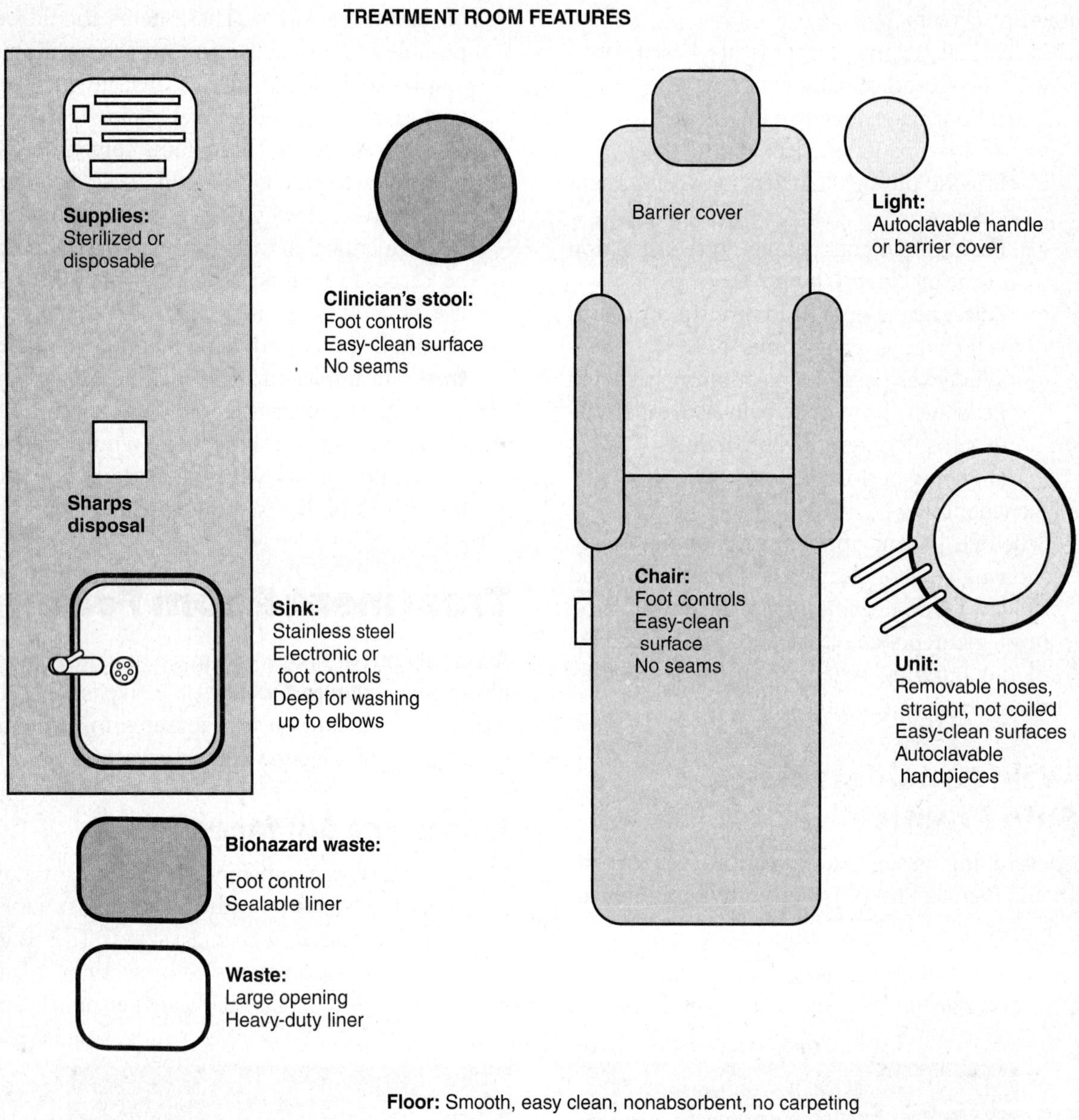

Figure 7-2 Optimal Treatment Room Features

surfaces can be disinfected using an **Environmental Protection Agency (EPA)-registered** hospital disinfectant but should be covered with a barrier whenever possible. Examples of these surfaces include light switches, draw handles, faucets, pens, pencils, doorknobs, and telephones, as well as the following standard features of a dental treatment room.[7,8]

A. The Unit

- Designed for easy cleaning and disinfection, with smooth, uncluttered surfaces.
- Removable hoses that can be cleaned, disinfected, and covered.
- Syringes with autoclavable tips or fitted with disposable tips.

B. Dental Chair

- Foot-operated controls.
- Surface and seamless finish of easily cleaned plastic material that withstands chemical disinfection without damage.
- Cloth upholstery to be avoided.

C. Light

- Removable handle for sterilization or disposable barrier cover.

D. Clinician's Chair

- Smooth, plastic seat cover that is easily disinfected with a minimum of seams and creases.

E. Radiographic Equipment

- Constructed of a smooth material for easy disinfection or disposable barrier cover.

II. Housekeeping Surfaces

Housekeeping surfaces consist of surfaces such as floors, wall, sinks, bathrooms, or any surface that poses no risk of disease transmission in dental care settings.[2] The CDC recommends these areas be cleaned using detergent and water or an EPA-registered hospital disinfectant/detergent.[6]

A. Floor

- No cloth carpeting.
- Smooth floor covering, easily cleaned, nonabsorbent.

B. Sink

- Smooth material (stainless steel).
- Wide and deep enough for effective handwashing without splashing or touching sides.
- Automatic water faucets and soap dispensers with electronic hand-, knee-, or foot-operated controls.

C. Waste

- Most waste is disposed of with usual waste.
- The receptacle should have an opening large enough to prevent contact with sides when material is deposited.
- Heavy-duty plastic bag liner to be sealed tightly for disposal.
- Separate container for sharps disposal.
- Small **biohazard** receptacle near treatment area to receive contaminated gauze and other waste, for disposal in large waste container clearly marked for **contaminated waste**.

Instrument Processing Center

The successful practice of standard and transmission-based precautions to prevent cross-contamination depends on the development of, and strict adherence to, a planned program for both critical and semi-critical instrument management. The processing center is used for care, cleaning, packaging, sterilizing, and storage of instruments. The center should be separated into respective areas of sterilized and contaminated instruments. It should be centrally located and apart from the treatment rooms.[6]

I. Supplies

All critical and semi-critical supplies should be sterilizable or disposable.

- A good rule is to learn the most effective, safe system and then to follow it without exception.
- A specific routine is easier for the entire dental team to follow, and peer review should be built in.
- The basic steps in the recirculation of instruments from the time an appointment procedure is completed until the instruments are sterilized and ready for use in a continuing clinical appointment are shown in the flowchart in **Figure 7-3**. Each of the steps is described in the following sections.

Precleaning Procedures

There are three basic methods for precleaning to remove any organic or inorganic debris from instruments before sterilization: manual scrubbing, washer/thermal disinfector, and ultrasonic processing.[7]

I. Manual Scrubbing

- The use of automated devices is the preferred method of instrument cleaning. Manual scrubbing

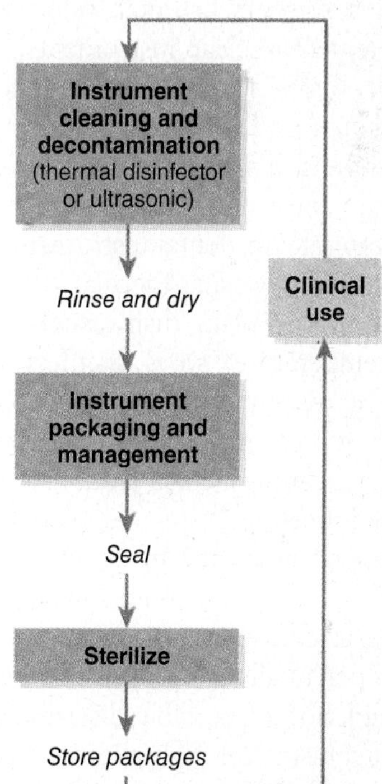

Figure 7-3 Recirculation of Instruments. Flowchart shows step-by-step process. At the completion of treatment, instruments are cleaned, packaged, sterilized, and stored. They are kept sealed until the patient appointment begins.

is not a recommended cleaning method. However, if manual scrubbing is necessary, the following precautions are essential[6]:

- Wear heavy-duty gloves, protective eyewear, and mask.
- Dismantle instruments with detachable parts. Open jointed instruments.
- Use detergent and scrub with a long-handled brush under running water; hold the instruments low in the sink. Scrubbing one instrument at a time minimizes risk of puncture injury.
- Brush with strokes away from the body; be careful not to splash and contaminate the surrounding area.
- Rinse thoroughly.
- Air-dry resting on paper towels to avoid saturation of the sterilization package.

- Care of brushes
    - Color-code instrument brushes to distinguish from hand wash brushes.
    - Soak and wash contaminated brushes in detergent; rinse thoroughly and sterilize.

II. Instrument Washer/Thermal Disinfector

- Instrument washers use high-velocity hot water and a detergent to clean instruments.
    - Some models are equipped to dry the instruments.
    - Household dishwashers may look similar to instrument washers but are different and not appropriate for dental instruments.[8]
- The instrument washer/thermal disinfector also differs from the plain dishwasher by having a higher temperature, so it disinfects as well as cleans the instruments (**Figure 7-4A**).[4] Benefits from the use of washer/thermal disinfector and ultrasonic cleaning versus manual scrubbing include the following[5]:
    - Increased efficiency in obtaining a high degree of cleanliness for improved disinfection.
    - Reduced danger to clinician from direct contact with potentially pathogenic microorganisms.
    - Elimination of possible dissemination of microorganisms through release of aerosols and droplets, which can occur during the scrubbing process.
- Disinfection allows the instruments in cassettes to be handled with gloves while packaging.

III. Ultrasonic Processing

An ultrasonic processor removes debris from instruments using acoustic energy waves transmitted in liquid, disrupting the attachment of debris from an object.[6,7]

- Ultrasonic cleaning before sterilization is safer than manual cleaning. Manual cleaning of instruments is a dangerous, difficult, and time-consuming procedure.
- Ultrasonic equipment should be maintained and used according to manufacturer's guidelines (**Figure 7-4B**).
- *Ultrasonic processing is not a substitute for sterilization; it is only a cleaning process to remove debris.*

A. Procedure

- Guard against overloading; the solution must contact all surfaces. Instruments need to be completely immersed.
- Dismantle instruments with detachable parts. Open jointed instruments.
- Use the time recommended by the manufacturer's instructions.
- Drain, rinse, and air-dry.

B. Indications for Thorough Drying

- When sterilizing by dry heat or chemical vapor, nonstainless steel instruments or carbon steel require pre-dip in rust inhibitor before steam autoclaving; water on instruments dilutes the anti-rust solution.

Instrument Packing and Management System

Instrument management systems can prevent **contamination** of newly sterilized instruments. The system should:

- Provide a means of organizing instrument packets for different procedures.
- Assure instruments are sterilized and ready for immediate use on opening.
- Provide a means of storing instrument packets.

I. Instrument Arrangement

- Each package is dated and marked for identification of contents: for example, *Adult Prophylaxis; Examination.*

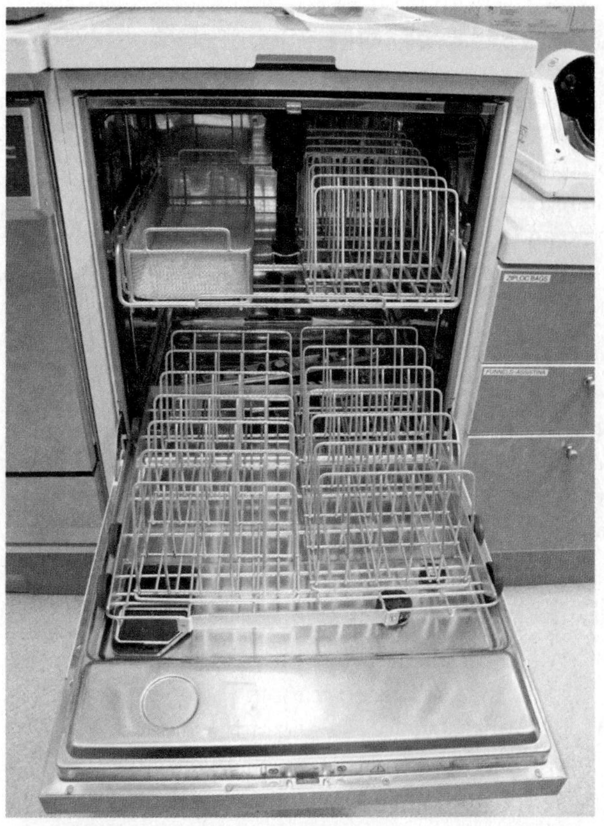

A

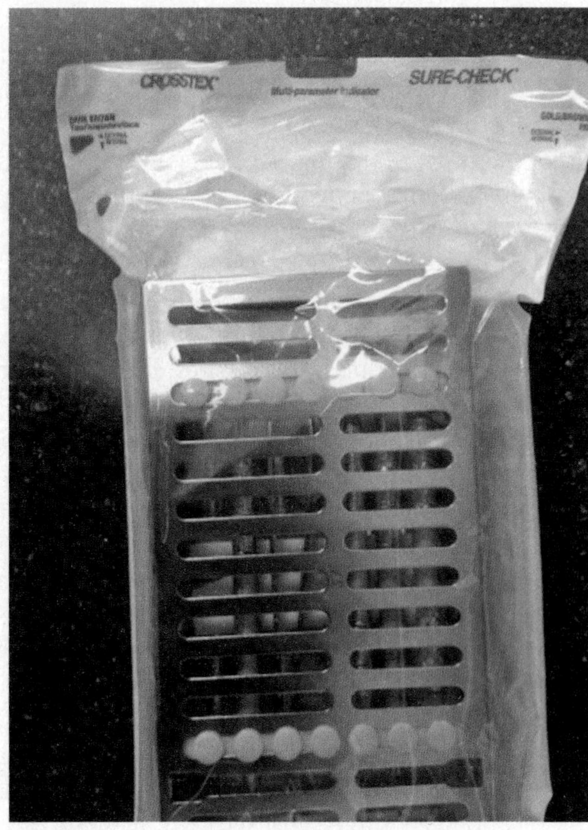

C

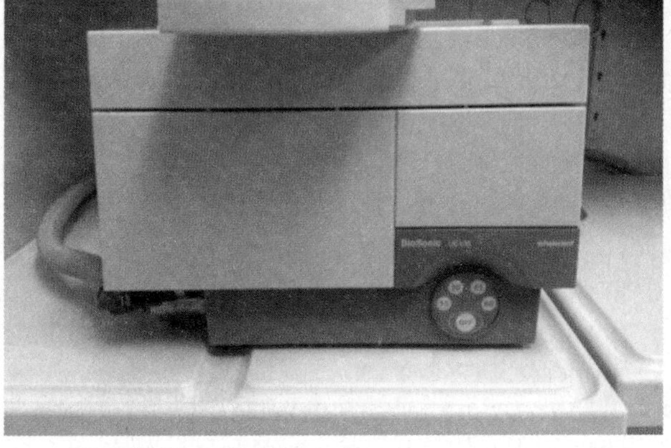

B

Figure 7-4 **A:** Instrument washer. **B:** Ultrasonic processor. **C:** Instrument cassette in a sterilization pouch.

- Clear packages that self-seal and permit instrument identification without special labeling can be used (**Figure 7-4C**).
- Instruments can be organized into tray systems, dental storage containers, or cassettes customized based on various dental hygiene procedures such as an initial exam of an adult patient, child patient, or periodontal maintenance patient.
- Instruments and accessories held in one unit provide a sterile environment for instruments during treatment.
- After the treatment, they serve as packaging for the process of cleaning, disinfection, and sterilization.

II. Preparation

- Cassettes can be wrapped or packaged, and single instruments are packaged.
  - Each method of sterilization has specific requirements, and the manufacturers' recommendations must be followed.

- The packaging material permits the steam or chemical vapor to pass through the contents and maintains sterility during transport and storage.
- Sturdy wrapping is necessary to prevent punctures or tears that break the chain of **asepsis** and require a repeat of the process.

- Seal
  - Pins, paper clips, or other types of metal fasteners are not used to seal packages because they may create holes for the entry of microorganisms.
  - **Chemical indicator** tape is used unless the package is self-seal and the wrap has built-in indicators (**Figure 7-5**).
  - The change of color on the indicator confirms the autoclave reached a designated temperature required for penetration. This is not a confirmation of sterilization, but an indication the device is working properly.[4]
  - When using indicator tape, distinct black stripes will appear. A lighter color change may be a warning signal the autoclave function needs to be checked.
  - The striped indicator tape is left on the sealed package and thereby serves to identify those packages ready for use. Packages are kept completely sealed until unwrapped in front of the patient.

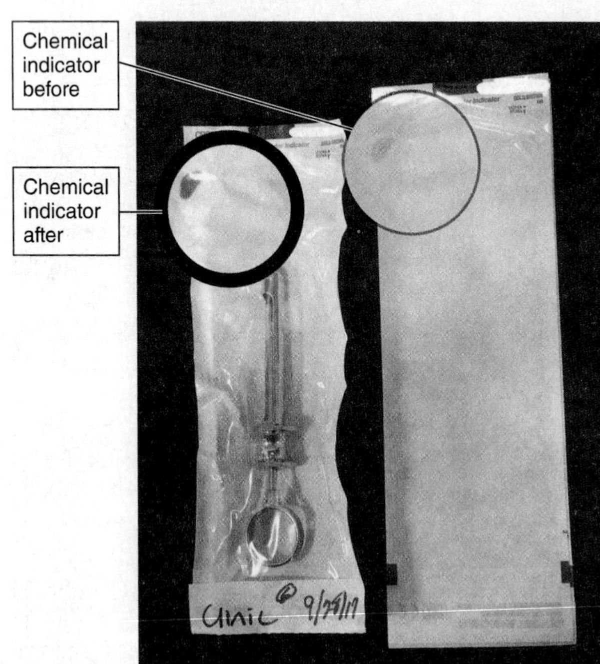

Figure 7-5 Built-in Chemical Indicator Before and After Sterilization

Sterilization

Sterilization is accomplished with equipment cleared by the U.S. Food and Drug Administration (**FDA**). Sterilizing equipment should be used according to the manufacturer's specifications. All of the methods listed here are described in the following sections. **Table 7-1** summarizes the operating requirements of each.

I. Approved Methods

- Steam under pressure (autoclave).
- Dry heat.
- Chemical vapor.
- Immediate-use steam sterilization (flash).
- Chemical (cold) sterilization—not recommended.

II. Selection of Method

- All materials and items cannot be treated by the same system of sterilization.
- The method for sterilization selected provides complete destruction of all microorganisms, viruses, and spores, yet must not damage the instruments and other materials.
- Incomplete sterilization frequently results from inadequate preparation of the materials to be sterilized (cleaning all debris, packaging), misuse of the equipment (overloading, timing, temperature selection), or inadequate maintenance.[7,9]

III. Tests for Sterilization

- Sterilization is the process by which all forms of life are destroyed. That definition provides the rationale for testing whether a sterilizer is working properly.[7,9]
- Three tests are used: an external and an internal chemical indicator and a **biologic monitor**.

Table 7-1 Comparison of Methods for Sterilization

	Sterilizing Requirement	
Method	**Time (min)**	**Temperature**
Steam under pressure (autoclave)		
1. Gravity displacement	15–30	250°F (121°C)
2. Pre-vacuum	3.5–10	270°F (132°C)
Dry heat oven	120	320°F (160°C)
Unsaturated chemical vapor	20	270°F (132°C)

- Weekly testing is recommended or when changes such as repair or relocation of unit occur.[7,9]
- Equipment can be obtained for performing the testing, or commercial mail-in services are available.
- *An external chemical indicator* seals the package and changes color to show the autoclave temperature has been reached.
- *An internal chemical indicator* changes color to demonstrate the instrument was exposed to the temperature and steam for the required time.
- Biologic monitor *(spore testing)*: Tests for proper functioning of the autoclave.
  - The testing system requires use of selected test microorganisms put through a regular cycle of sterilization and then cultured. When no growth occurs, the sterilizer has performed with maximum efficiency.[9-11]
  - Microorganisms used for testing include:
    1. Steam autoclave: *Geobacillus stearothermophilus* (formerly *Bacillus stearothermophilus*) vials, ampules, or strips.
    2. Dry heat oven: *Bacillus atrophaeus* (formerly *Bacillus subtilis*) strips.
    3. Chemical vapor: *G. stearothermophilus* (formerly *B. stearothermophilus*) strips.
  - Procedures
    1. Manufacturer's directions determine the placement and location of bacterial indicators. If there are no instructions, the ampule, vial, or strip is placed in the center of a package, which in turn is placed in the middle of the load of packages to be sterilized.
    2. After the cycle has been completed at the recommended time and temperature, the ampule or strip is incubated. Ampules and vials show the color change associated with no living microorganisms, whereas the strip organisms are cultured and show no growth if the sterilizer has performed properly.
    3. **Table 7-2** lists indications for performing spore tests in dental settings. Records or logs showing dates and outcomes of each test must be maintained.
- Indications for spore testing[6,11]:
  - Once per week to verify proper use and functioning.
  - Whenever a new type of packaging material or tray is used.
  - After training new personnel to ensure proper use.
  - During initial uses of a new sterilizer to make sure the directions are being followed.

Table 7-2 Spore Testing

When	Why
Once per week	To verify proper use and functioning
Whenever a new type of packaging material or tray is used	To ensure that the sterilizing agent is getting inside to the surface of the instruments
After training of new sterilization personnel	To verify proper use of the sterilizer
New sterilizer	To make sure unfamiliar operating instructions are being followed
After repair of a sterilizer	To make sure that the sterilizer is functioning properly
With every implantable device and hold device until results of test are known	Extra precaution for sterilization of item to be implanted into tissues
After any other change in the sterilizing procedure	To make sure change does not prevent sterilization

Data from U.S. Department of Health and Human Services, Centers for Disease Control and Prevention. Guidelines for infection control in dental health-care settings—2003. *MMWR Morb Mortal Wkly Rep*. 2003;52(RR-17):27.

  - After sterilizer repair to check functioning.
  - Any load containing an implantable device should be spore tested and device should remain out of service until results are known.

Moist Heat: Steam under Pressure

Destruction of microorganisms by heat takes place because of inactivation and coagulation of essential cellular proteins or enzymes.

I. Autoclave Types

Autoclaves use steam under pressure to achieve sterilization and are available in the pre-vacuum and gravity displacement models. The two types of autoclaves differ mostly in the manner in which the evacuation of steam occurs and the process length. A time/temperature comparison of sterilization systems is provided in Table 7-1.

- Gravity displacement: Self-generation of steam forces out the air; steam enters to penetrate through the cassettes or packages.

- High-speed pre-vacuum: Pump removes the air from the chamber and allows faster penetration of the steam for sterilizing.

II. Use

- Moist heat may be used for all materials except:
  - Oils, waxes, and powders that are impervious to steam.
  - Materials that cannot be subjected to high temperatures.

III. Principles of Action

- Sterilization is achieved by action of heat; pressure serves only to attain high temperature.
- Sterilization depends on the penetrating ability of steam.
- Air must be excluded; otherwise, steam penetration and heat transfer are prevented.
- Space between objects is essential to ensure access for the steam.
- Air discharge occurs in a downward direction; load must be arranged for free passage of steam toward the bottom of autoclave.

IV. Evaluation

- Advantages
  - All microorganisms, spores, and viruses are destroyed quickly and efficiently.
  - Wide variety of materials may be treated.
  - The most economical method of sterilization.
- Disadvantages
  - If precautions are not taken, carbon steel instruments may corrode.

Dry Heat

Dry heat sterilizers achieve sterilization by oxidation of molecules, resulting in death of the organism. The most common dry sterilizers include:

- *Static air sterilizers:* Like an oven, the chamber is brought to temperature by heating coils located within the unit.
- *Forced air sterilizers:* Heated forced air is circulated at a high velocity, rapidly bringing the sterilizer to the appropriate temperature.

I. Use

- Primarily for materials that cannot be safely sterilized with steam under pressure.
- For small metal instruments enclosed in special containers or that might be corroded or rusted by moisture.

II. Principles of Action

- Sterilization is achieved by heat conducted from the exterior surface to the interior of the object; the penetration time varies among materials.
- Sterilization can result when the material is treated for a sufficient length of time at the required temperature; therefore, timing for sterilization must start when the entire contents of the sterilizer have reached the recommended temperature needed for the load.

III. Operation

- Temperature
  - A temperature of 160°C (320°F) maintained for 2 hours; 170°C (340°F) for 1 hour.[5,11] Timing starts after the desired temperature has been reached.
  - Penetration time: Heat penetration varies with different materials.
  - Nature and properties of various materials are considered.
- Care
  - Care should be taken not to overheat because certain materials can be affected. For example, temperatures over 160°C (320°F) may destroy the sharp edges of cutting instruments.

IV. Evaluation

- Advantages
  - Useful for materials that cannot be subjected to steam under pressure, such as heat-sensitive handpieces, burs, or plastics.
  - When maintained at correct temperature, this method is well suited for sharp instruments.
  - No corrosion compared with steam under pressure.
- Disadvantages
  - Long exposure time required.
  - Penetration is slow and uneven.
  - High temperature critical to certain materials.

Chemical Vapor Sterilizer

A combination of alcohols, formaldehyde, ketone, water, and acetone heated under pressure produces a gas that is effective as a sterilizing agent.

I. Use

Chemical vapor sterilization cannot be used for materials or objects that can be altered by the chemicals that make the vapor or that cannot withstand the high temperature. Examples are low-temperature melting plastics, liquids, or heat-sensitive handpieces.

II. Principles of Action

Microbial and viral destruction results from the permeation of the heated formaldehyde and alcohol. Heavy, tightly wrapped, or sealed packages would not permit the penetration of the vapors.

III. Operation

- Temperature
  - From 132°C (270°F) with 20–40 pounds' pressure in accord with the manufacturer's directions.[5,11]
- Time
  - Minimum of 20 minutes after the correct temperature and pressure have been attained. Time needs to be extended for a large load or a heavy wrap.
- Cooling at the completion of the cycle
  - Instruments should be dry. Allow instruments to cool.

IV. Care of Sterilizer

- Refilling depends on the amount of use and is needed at least every 30 cycles.
- In accord with manufacturer's instructions, the condensate tray is removed, the exhausted solution emptied, and the tray cleaned.

V. Evaluation

- Advantages
  - Corrosion- and rust-free operation for carbon steel instruments.
  - Ability to sterilize in a relatively short total cycle.
  - Ease of operation and care of the equipment.
- Disadvantages
  - Adequate ventilation is needed; cannot use in a small room.
  - Slight odor.

Intermediate-Use Steam Sterilization

Sometimes called flash sterilization, this form of rapid steam heat sterilization is a method used to sterilize unwrapped instruments for immediate use. The rapid contact with steam allows for shorter sterilization times.[11]

- Use
  - Should only be used when there is urgent need to sterilize an item.
  - Not recommended for items that require biologic spore test results before use, such as implantable items.[11]
- Care
  - Follow manufacturer's temperature and setting directions for immediate-use sterilizing.
  - Monitors and indicators should be used and checked for each cycle.
  - Items are to be used immediately after sterilizing.
  - Items are hot upon removal, so care must be used in handling.
  - Caution must be used in the transport of instruments to avoid contamination.
  - Items are meant for immediate use and should not be stored.

Chemical Liquid Sterilization

Chemical liquid sterilization is often referred to as "cold sterile." Many chemicals have been FDA approved for sterilization; however, biologic monitoring to verify sterility with this method is not possible. The CDC recommends this method of sterilization only when other methods of sterilization cannot be used.[5,11]

Care of Sterile Instruments

- Instruments stored without sealed wrappers are only momentarily sterile because of airborne contamination.
- Labeled, sterilized, and sealed packages are stored unopened in clean, dry cabinets or drawers.
  - All stored packages are dated and used in rotation.
  - Paper-wrapped packages are handled carefully to prevent tearing.
- Packages wrapped and sealed in paper may not need re-sterilizing for several months to 1 year.
- Plastic or nylon wrap with a tape or heat seal may be expected to remain sterile longer.

- The expected **shelf life** before re-sterilizing depends on the area surrounding the stored packages. A closed, protected area without exposure, such as a cabinet or drawer that can be disinfected routinely, is preferred for storage.

Chemical Disinfectants

Reducing surface contamination is beneficial in lowering the incidence of cross-contamination.[10] Healthcare facilities are expected to be kept clean and have cleaning protocol and procedures in place for all surface types.

- Chemical disinfectants are used in several forms, including:
  - Surface disinfectants.
  - Immersion disinfectants, immersion sterilants.
  - Hand rubs containing an **antimicrobial agent**.
- Each variety has specific chemicals, dilutions, and directions for application.

I. Manufacturer's Information

- All manufacturers of products should include or supply a Safety Data Sheet (SDS). An SDS provides facts about the safety and effectiveness of the product, including:
  - Effectiveness and stability expressed by:
    a. Shelf life: The expiration date indicating the termination of effectiveness of the unopened container.
    b. Use life: The life expectancy for the solution once it has been activated.
    c. Reuse life: The amount of time a solution can be used and reused while being challenged with instruments that are wet or coated with contaminants.
  - Directions for activation (mixing directions).
  - Type of container for use and storage.
  - Storage directions (light and temperature).
  - Directions for use:
    a. Precleaning and drying of items.
    b. Time/temperature ratio.
  - Instructions for disposal of used solution.
  - Warnings
    a. Toxic effects (eyes, skin).
    b. Directions for emergency care (e.g., splash in eye).

II. Categories

- Disinfectants are categorized by their biocidal activity as high level, intermediate level, or low level.
- Biocidal activity refers to the ability of the chemical disinfectant to destroy or inactivate living organisms.[11]
  - High-level disinfectants inactivate spores and all forms of bacteria, fungi, and viruses. Applied at different time schedules, the high-level chemical is either a disinfectant or a sterilant.
  - Intermediate-level disinfectants inactivate all forms of microorganisms but do not destroy spores.
  - Low-level disinfectants inactivate vegetative bacteria and certain lipid-type viruses but do not destroy spores, tubercle bacilli, or non-lipid viruses.

III. Uses

- Environmental surfaces disinfection: Following each appointment, the treatment area is cleaned and disinfected.
- Dental laboratory impressions and prostheses:
  - Impressions can be carriers of infectious material to a dental laboratory.
  - Completed prostheses must be disinfected before delivery to a patient.

IV. Principles of Action

- Disinfection is achieved by:
  - Coagulation, precipitation, or oxidation of protein of microbial cells.
  - Denaturation of the enzymes of the cells.
- Disinfection depends on the contact of the solution at the known effective concentration for the optimum period of time.
- Items are thoroughly cleaned and dried because action of the agent is altered by foreign matter and dilution.
- A solution has a specific shelf life, use life, and reuse life.
  - Some may be altered by changes in pH, or the active ingredient may decrease in potency.
  - Check manufacturer's directions.

V. Criteria for Selection of a Chemical Agent

- Objective: To select a product that is effective in the control of microorganisms and practical to use. No one product is the best choice for all dental setting. Properties of an ideal disinfectant are shown in **Box 7-1**. When choosing a product, consider the level of contamination and surface type.

Box 7-1 Properties of a Disinfectant

1	Broad spectrum	Wide antimicrobial spectrum
2	Fast acting	A rapid lethal action on all vegetative forms and spores of bacteria and fungi, protozoa, and viruses
3	Unaffected by physical factors	Active in the presence of organic matter, such as blood, sputum, and feces. Compatible with soaps, detergents, and other chemicals encountered in use
4	Nontoxic	
5	Surface compatibility	Will not corrode instruments and other metallic surfaces. Will not cause the disintegration of cloth, rubber, plastics, or other materials
6	Residual effect on treated surfaces	
7	Easy to use	
8	Odorless	Inoffensive odor to facilitate routine use
9	Economical	Reasonable cost

- Identify contamination type
  - Blood.
  - No blood.
- Clinical contact surfaces[9]
  - No blood: Use EPA-registered hospital-grade disinfectant plus hepatitis B virus (HBV) and human immunodeficiency virus (HIV) kill claim or tuberculocidal activity.
  - Blood: Use EPA-registered hospital disinfectant plus tuberculocidal activity.
- Housekeeping surfaces
  - No blood: Use EPA-registered hospital disinfectant or detergent and water.
  - Blood: Use EPA-registered hospital disinfectant plus tuberculocidal activity.

Barriers and Surface Covers

Barriers and surface covers are used to protect a surface from contaminants. They come in different sizes and shapes and are available in sheets; wraps; precut; and fitted for different items, such as hoses, light handles, keyboards, and head rests. Covers should be moisture resistant, easily removable, and disposable (**Figure 7-6**).

I. Benefits

There are many benefits to using surface barriers, not only on hard-to-clean surfaces, but also on any contact surfaces. Barriers and surface covers eliminate the contact time required by disinfectants and are chemical free, efficient, and safe. A comparison of barriers versus cleaning and disinfecting spray is shown in **Figure 7-7**.

II. Procedure

- Before treatment
  - Identify areas where barriers and covers can be used.
  - Apply the appropriate barrier prior to patient visit.
  - Be sure the barrier is secure and will not be dislodged during patient treatment.
- After treatment
  - Wear appropriate personal protective equipment (**PPE**) when removing contaminated barriers.
  - Be careful not to contaminate surfaces with gloves or unclean barriers.

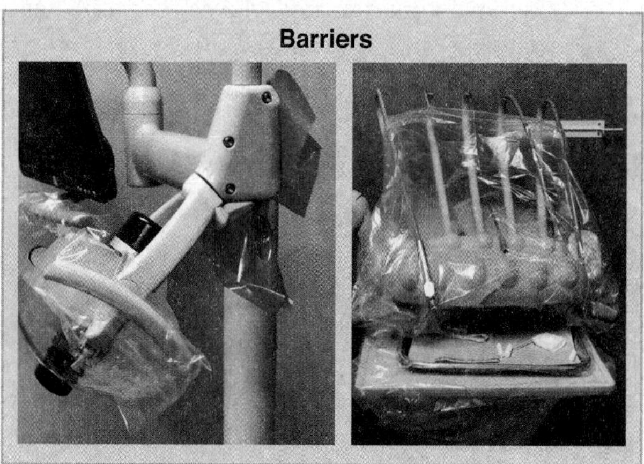

Figure 7-6 Surface Covers and Barriers

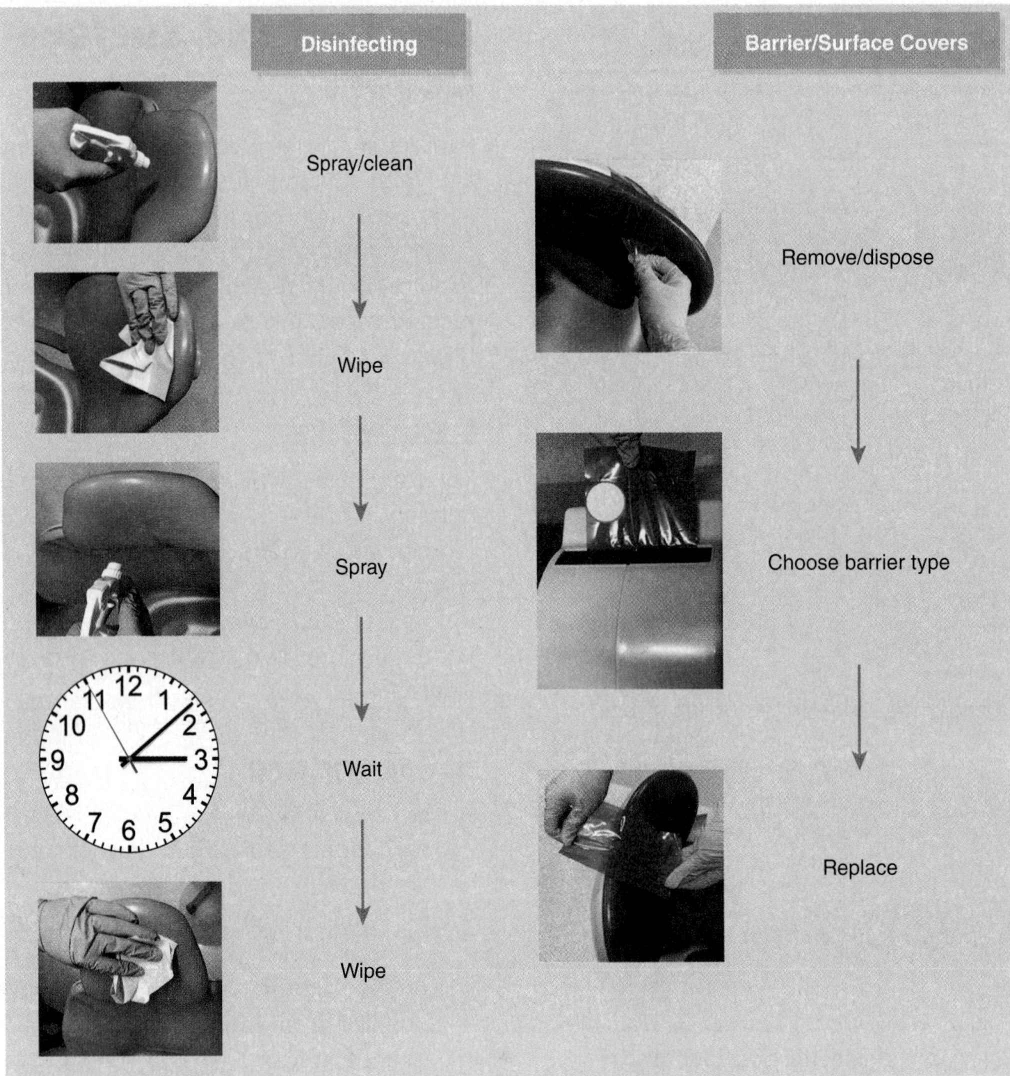

Figure 7-7 Comparison of Disinfecting versus Barriers Diagram

- If surfaces are contaminated, clean and disinfect surface.
- Discard used barriers and covers in trash according to state law.
- Remove contaminated gloves, perform hand hygiene, and apply fresh surface covers and barriers.

Preparation of the Treatment Room

- Patients may consider the cleanliness and neatness of the treatment room to reflect the conscientiousness of the dental team.
- An excellent test for effectiveness is for dental personnel to occasionally view the operatory from the patient's vantage point by becoming the patient.
- Patients may have limited knowledge of sterilization and infection control procedures and may request information.
- Appropriate infection control procedures are necessary to create an environment to minimize cross-contamination.
- If AGPs are performed, it is recommended to allow the aerosols to settle before cleaning procedures begin.[12]

I. Objective

Effective care of instruments and equipment is essential in order to control disease transmission by way of environmental surfaces and maintenance of equipment and instruments.

II. Preliminary Planning

- All surfaces and items that will be used or contacted during the appointment can be categorized as critical, semi-critical, and noncritical.
- The classification of inanimate objects (**Table 7-3**) provides a guide for analysis.

Table 7-3 Classification of Inanimate Objects

Surface Category	Definition	Sterilization/Disinfection	Examples
Critical	Penetrate soft tissue or bone	Sterilize or disposable	Needles Curets Explorers Probes
Semi-critical	Touch intact mucous membrane, oral fluids Does not penetrate	Sterilize after each use High-level disinfection when sterilization cannot be used	Radiographic bite block Ultrasonic handpiece Amalgam condenser Mirror
Noncritical	Do not touch mucous membranes (only contact unbroken epithelium)	Cleaning and tuberculocidal intermediate-level disinfection	Light handles Certain X-ray machine parts Safety eyewear
Environmental	No contact with patient surfaces (or only intact skin)	Cleaning and intermediate to low disinfection	Light handles Switches Counter tops Computers Drawer handles Faucets Equipment surfaces Housekeeping surfaces: floors, walls, and sinks

- All surfaces should be cleaned at the end of every work day.
- Preparation of treatment room when time between appointments is limited requires an efficient procedural system.

III. Surface Disinfection Procedure

- The most logical, evidence-based sequence for preparation for the appointment can then be outlined.
- Hand "touch contacts"
  - Only contact surfaces/materials essential to the procedure.
  - Plan ahead to have materials ready so cabinet knobs, drawer handles, etc. do not have to be contacted.
- Sterilizable items
  - Critical and semi-critical items must be sterilized or disposable.
- Disposable items
  - Disposable items are used wherever possible.
- Barriers
  - Barrier coverings prevent contamination from reaching surfaces.
  - Covers for light handles, counter tops, X-ray machine parts, computer keyboard, and mouse are examples.
  - Care is taken when removing the covers so as not to contaminate the object beneath.
- Items that require chemical disinfection
  - Objects and surfaces that cannot be included in one of the preceding categories are treated with a chemical disinfectant.
  - When the material is not compatible with the chemical action of the disinfectant, a disposable or coverable substitute is needed.

IV. Clean and Disinfect Environmental Surface

A. Agent

- The effectiveness of the disinfection procedure is the result of two actions[7]:
  - The physical rubbing and removal of contaminated material.
  - The chemical inactivation of the living microorganisms.
- Surface disinfectants are concentrated, premixed solutions, sprays, foams, impregnated wipes, and dissolved tablets.
  - Do not store gauze sponges in the solution because cotton fibers contained in gauze may shorten the effectiveness of disinfectants when stored in containers.[13]

B. Procedure

1. Wear your PPE as needed for the procedure, including protective eyewear, surgical mask and/or respirator, protective apparel, medical gloves, or chemical/puncture-resistant utility gloves.
2. Determine the degree of disinfection required.
3. Be sure the product has been prepared correctly and is not expired.
4. Check the label to be sure the disinfectant is compatible with the surface to be disinfected.
5. Clean blood or other potentially infectious material with a low-level or intermediate-level disinfectant effective against HBV and HIV.
6. Clean and scrub surfaces with soap and water, EPS-registered detergent, or low-level disinfectant.
7. The disinfectant must be followed by vigorous scrubbing in order to remove the film of microorganisms.
8. Scrub the disinfectant over the entire surface, with attention to irregularities where contaminated material can aggregate.
9. A disinfectant-soaked sponge or wipe in each hand can decrease the time of cleaning certain objects. Contaminated objects, such as tubing, can be held with one sponge while scrubbing with the other sponge.
10. Use a brush if surfaces do not become visibly clean from rubbing.
11. Once cleaned, spray surface again leaving the disinfectant on the surface for the recommended amount of time according to manufacturer's directions.
12. Wipe surfaces dry.

V. Unit Waterlines

- A **biofilm** of microorganisms can form on the inside of the waterline tubing during overnight standing.
- The procedure for clinical use is to flush all waterlines at least 2 minutes at the beginning of each day.
- Run water through water tubing for 30 seconds before and 30 seconds after each patient appointment.
- Tests have been conducted on tubing to hand pieces, water syringes, and ultrasonic scalers. When the lines were flushed for 2 minutes, the microbial counts were reduced.[2,5,7]
- Contaminated water cannot be used for surgical purposes or during the irrigation of pocket areas because infectious microorganisms could be introduced.
  - If contaminated water is directed forcefully into a pocket, microorganisms can enter the tissue and infection or bacteremia can result.
- Refer to the CDC Infection Prevention and Control Guidelines and Recommendations.[6]
- If dental unit is more than 20 years old, contact the manufacturer to determine if antiretraction valves are present.

Patient Preparation

- Oral procedures that penetrate tissue, such as administration of anesthesia by injection or subgingival scaling, can introduce bacteria into the tissues and hence into the bloodstream.
  - Organisms introduced into the tissue could multiply and create an abscess. Natural resistance helps the body handle and destroy invading microorganisms, provided the numbers can be kept to a minimum.
  - Though clinical research has not proven this prevents or reduces the incidence of disease transmission, it has been shown to reduce the number of microorganisms in the oral cavity, in aerosols, or introduced into the patient's bloodstream.[5,7]
- Practical procedures for the preparation of a patient include preprocedural oral hygiene measures and rinsing with an antimicrobial mouthrinse.

I. Preprocedural Oral Hygiene Measures

- Toothbrushing
  - Demonstration of biofilm removal from the teeth, tongue, and gingiva contributes to lowering the microbial count before treatment procedures.
- Rinsing
  - The numbers of bacteria on the gingival or mucosal surfaces can be reduced by the use of a preprocedural **antiseptic** mouthrinse[14,15]
  - The substantivity of 0.2% chlorhexidine provides a lowered bacterial count for more than 60 minutes.
  - Preprocedural rinsing before injections is advised.

II. Application of a Surface Antiseptic

- Before injection of anesthetic
  - As a needle is introduced into the mucosa for penetration to deeper tissues, microorganisms on the surface can be carried into the tissue.

- A topical antiseptic applied before the injection can decrease the risk of introducing microorganisms into the soft tissue.
- Before scaling and other dental hygiene instrumentation.[14,15]
  - Instrumentation in a sulcus and around the gingival margin can create breaks in the tissue where bacteria can enter.
  - Subgingival instrumentation in a pocket with broken-down sulcular epithelium contributes to the entrance of bacteria into the underlying tissues and bacteremia.[12]
  - Evidence does not currently support use of subgingival irrigation with antiseptic solutions to reduce bacteremia posttreatment, but recommend the use of a preprocedural 0.2% chlorhexidine rinse.[15,16] In the United States chlorhexidine gluconate is available in a 0.12% prescription mouthrinse.

Summary of Standard Procedures

Basic procedures for clinical management are listed here.

I. Patient Factors

- Prepare a comprehensive patient history and make necessary referrals.
- Ask the patient to rinse with an antimicrobial mouthrinse to reduce the numbers of oral microorganisms.
- Provide protective eyewear.
- Avoid elective procedures for a patient who is suffering from an infectious disease, such as a respiratory infection, or who has an open herpetic lesion on or about the lips or oral tissues.

II. Clinic Preparation

- Run water through all waterlines, including the air–water syringe, hand pieces, and ultrasonic unit, for 2 minutes at the start of the day and for at least 30 seconds before and after each use during the day.
- Disinfect all environmental surfaces that may be touch surfaces during the appointment.
  - Make an orderly sequence for surface cleaning and disinfection.
- Apply barrier covers as indicated.
- Sterilize instruments and all other equipment that can be sterilized by one of the methods for complete sterilization. Maintain closed sterilized packages until ready for use.

III. Factors for the Dental Team

- Have regular medical examinations; keep immunizations up to date; have appropriate testing on a periodic basis.
- Always use the appropriate PPE based on whether it is an AGP. (See Chapter 6.)
- Utilize thorough hand hygiene and cleansing before putting on and after removing gloves.
- Develop habits to minimize contact with switches and other parts of the dental unit, dental chair, light, and clinician's stool, and avoid all environmental contacts unrelated to the procedure at hand.

IV. Posttreatment

- Use heavy puncture-resistant utility gloves to handle contaminated, unsterile instruments.
- Follow routines to disinfect, clean, and prepare the instruments for sterilization.
- Contaminated waste is secured in a disposable plastic bag and **infectious waste** in a container with a secure lid.[1]
- Disinfect safety eyewear for patient and dental team members along with face shields, etc.

Disposal of Waste

Waste created in a dental setting can include contaminated, hazardous, or infectious/**regulated waste**.

I. Regulations

- Investigate the regulations of each town or city **sanitation** division (or health department) for rules concerning disposal of contaminated waste.
- **Figure 7-8** illustrates the universal label required by OSHA.[17] The label must be attached to containers used to store or transport **hazardous waste** materials.

II. Guidelines for Disposal of Waste

- Disposable materials, such as gloves, masks, wipes, patient bibs, or surface covers, that are contaminated with blood or body fluids but not saturated must be carefully handled and discarded in sturdy, impervious plastic bags to minimize contact.[7]
- Blood, suctioned fluids, or other liquid waste may be discharged into a sanitary sewer system in compliance with applicable local regulations.[18]

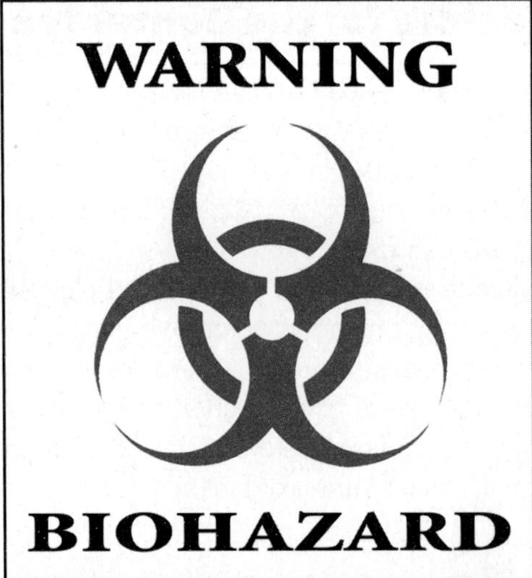

Figure 7-8 Universal Label for Hazardous Material. A hazard-warning label is fluorescent orange or orange-red with lettering or a symbol in a contrasting color. The label must be attached to containers used to store or transport waste. A label is not required for regulated waste that has been decontaminated (such as dental waste that has been autoclaved).

- Sharp items, such as needles and scalpel blades, must be placed intact into a puncture-resistant, leak-proof biohazard sharps container approved by the FDA. (See Chapter 36.)
- Human tissue, extracted teeth, and contaminated solid wastes can be disposed of according to the requirements established by local or state environmental regulatory agencies and published recommendations. Disposable bags need to be color coded or identified as biohazard.[1]
- Disposal methods for both liquid and solid chemicals vary with the type of chemical and local regulations governing waste-management practices.

Supplemental Recommendations

I. Smoking and Eating

- Smoking, drinking, and eating are banned in treatment areas.

II. Reception Area

- Should be free of toys and other reception area items that cannot be cleaned and disinfected.
- Provide hand sanitizer gel in the reception area.
- Provide face mask coverings if the patient has not brought their own.

III. Sterilization Monitoring

- Keep a written record of dates when processing tests and biologic monitor tests are performed for each sterilizer.
- Indicate advance dates for the next testing clearly on a calendar or other reference point.
- Perform tests made weekly on the same day to ensure compliance.

IV. Office Policy Manual

The clinic or office policy manual should outline procedures including the following:

- Standard precautions.
- Transmission-based precautions.
- Emergency procedures to follow when accidentally exposed are defined clearly.

Occupational Postexposure Management

Accidents happen even to the most skillful clinician. Accidental percutaneous (laceration, needlestick) or permucosal (splash to eye or mucosa) exposure to blood or other body fluids requires prompt action.

I. Significant Exposures

- Percutaneous or permucosal stick or wound with needle or sharp instrument contaminated with blood, saliva, or other body fluids.
- Contamination of any obviously open wound, nonintact skin, or mucous membrane with blood, saliva, or a combination.
- Exposure of patient's body fluids to unbroken skin is not considered a significant exposure.
- Airborne pathogen exposure such as SARS-2-CoV (coronavirus disease 2019 [COVID-19]).

II. Procedure Following Exposure

- Perform basic first aid to clean the area affected.
  - Immediately wash the wound with soap and water; rinse well.

    - Flush nose, mouth, eyes, or skin with clear water, saline, or a sterile irrigator.
- Report to designated official.
- Complete an incident report as required.
- Follow the required predetermined, posted procedures of the clinic, institution, or individual practice setting.
    - The University of California, San Francisco maintains a Clinician Consultation Center with a *PEP (postexposure prophylaxis) Quick Guide for Occupational Exposures* based on the most current U.S. Public Health Services and CDC guidelines. Consultations can be obtained by calling the Clinicians' Post-Exposure PEPline (888-448-4911).[15]
- Immediately obtain medical evaluation so if treatment is recommended, it can be initiated quickly.
- If the source (patient) is present and agrees, the patient should accompany the dental provider for medical evaluation and testing.
    - If the source is not known or unwilling to go for medical evaluation, baseline testing would be performed on the dental provider.
- If baseline testing is negative, no other follow-up may be necessary, but often 6-week follow-up testing is recommended.
- Obtain counseling services if necessary.

III. Follow-Up

- Report signs and symptoms associated with infectious disease such as COVID-19, hepatitis, or HIV.
- Obtain medical evaluation of any illness involving rash, fever or chills, dry cough and shortness of breath, feeling very tired, muscle or body aches, headache, loss of taste or smell, sore throat, congestion or runny nose, nausea or vomiting, diarrhea, or lymphadenopathy.
- Pursue counseling and further testing.

Documentation

Documentation for a patient with concerns about infection control procedures would include:

- Name, record number, address, telephone (home and cell), e-mail.
- Medical history for history of HBV, hepatitis C virus (HCV), or HIV; high-risk history associated with these diseases; patient consent to be tested for HBV, HCV, and HIV.
- HIV-positive patient: Current medications and previously taken, if they were ineffective; most recent viral load, current CD4 count if known.
- A sample progress note for a patient with concerns about infection control procedures can be reviewed in **Box 7-2**.

Box 7-2 Example Documentation: Patient with Concerns about Infection Control

- **S**—Patient presents for routine periodontal maintenance appointment. Patient asked how instruments were "cleaned" between patients.
- **O**—Health history update indicates patient has been recently diagnosed as HIV positive.
- **A**—She was concerned about an increased risk for opportunistic infections as well as the fact that her condition might increase risk for other patients seen in the office.
- **P**—Explained that standard and transmission-based precautions and infection control procedures used during all patient treatment are designed to protect all patients from cross-contamination. Explained each set of instruments is sterilized utilizing steam under pressure (autoclave). Tests for sterilization are done for each cycle of instruments, in addition to weekly and monthly tests to ensure the autoclave is functioning properly. Opened all sterilized instrument kits in her presence.

Signed: ______________________, RDH

Date: ______________________

Factors to Teach the Patient

- The meaning of "standard and transmission-based precautions" and what is included under the term; how these precautions protect the patient and the dental team members.
- The contribution of the accurately completed medical and dental personal history to the provision of the best, safest treatment possible.
- Methods for sterilization of instruments, including handpieces; how the autoclave or other sterilizer is tested daily or weekly.
- Facts about the normal oral flora and the factors that influence an increased number of bacteria on the tongue, mucosa, and in the dental biofilm on the teeth.
- Methods for personal daily control of the oral bacteria through biofilm control and tongue brushing.
- Reasons for preprocedural rinsing.
- Method for thorough rinsing.

References

1. Centers for Disease Control and Prevention. Healthcare Workers. Centers for Disease Control and Prevention. Published February 11, 2020. https://www.cdc.gov/coronavirus/2019-ncov/hcp/dental-settings.html. Accessed August 3, 2021.
2. Centers for Disease Control and Prevention. Oral health: CDC updates COVID-19 infection prevention and control guidance. Centers for Disease Control and Prevention. Published February 8, 2022. https://www.cdc.gov/oralhealth/infectioncontrol/statement-COVID.html. Accessed July 24, 2022.
3. Centers for Disease Control and Prevention, National Institute for Occupational Safety and Health. Environmental control for tuberculosis: basic upper-room ultraviolet germicidal irradiation guidelines for healthcare settings. Last reviewed June 6, 2014. https://www.cdc.gov/niosh/docs/2009-105/default.html. Accessed July 19, 2020.
4. Centers for Disease Control and Prevention. Infection prevention & control in dental settings. Published December 1, 2020. https://www.cdc.gov/oralhealth/infectioncontrol/index.html. Accessed August 16, 2021.
5. Kohn WG, Collins AS, Cleveland JL, et al. Guidelines for infection control in dental health-care settings --- 2003. *MMWR Recomm Rep*. 2003;52(RR-17):1-61. https://www.cdc.gov/mmwr/preview/mmwrhtml/rr5217a1.htm. Accessed August 18, 2021.
6. Centers for Disease Control and Prevention. Summary of Infection prevention practices in dental settings. Published October 2016. https://www.cdc.gov/oralhealth/infectioncontrol/pdf/safe-care2.pdf Accessed July 24, 2022.
7. Organization for Safety & Asepsis Procedures, Centers for Disease Control and Prevention. *From Policy to Practice: OSAP's Guide to the CDC Guidelines: A Step-by-Step Infection Prevention and Control Implementation Workbook*. 2019 ed. Organization for Safety & Asepsis Procedures: Atlanta, GA; 2019.
8. Cuny EJ. Dental infection control and technology. *Dent Assist*. 2010;6(6):24-28.
9. Centers for Disease Control and Prevention. Sterilization: Monitoring. Published February 19, 2020. https://www.cdc.gov/oralhealth/infectioncontrol/faqs/monitoring.html. Accessed August 16, 2021.
10. Schneiderman MT, Cartee DL. Surface disinfection. *Infect Control Dent Off*. 2019:169-191.
11. Center for Disease Control and Prevention. Disinfection & sterilization guidelines. Published May 24, 2019. https://www.cdc.gov/infectioncontrol/guidelines/disinfection/index.html. Accessed August 16, 2021.
12. Burger D. ADA responds to change from CDC on waiting period length. Published June 19, 2020. https://www.ada.org/en/publications/ada-news/2020-archive/june/ada-responds-to-change-from-cdc-on-waiting-period-length. Accessed August 19, 2021.
13. Molinari JA, Harte JA, Cottone JA. *Cottone's Practical Infection Control in Dentistry*. 3rd ed. Wolters Kluwer/Lippincott William & Wilkins; 2010.
14. Banakar M, Bagheri Lankarani K, Jafarpour D, Moayedi S, Banakar MH, Mohammad Sadeghi A. COVID-19 transmission risk and protective protocols in dentistry: a systematic review. *BMC Oral Health*. 2020;20(1):275.
15. Yadav S, Kumar S, Srivastava P, et al. Comparison of efficacy of three different mouthwashes in reducing aerosol contamination produced by ultrasonic scaler: a pilot study. *Indian J Dent Sci*. 2018;10(1):6-10.
16. Barbosa M, Prada-López I, Álvarez M, et al. Post-tooth extraction bacteraemia: a randomized clinical trial on the efficacy of chlorhexidine prophylaxis. *PLOS ONE*. 2015;10(5):e0124249.
17. Occupational Safety and Health Administration. Dentistry. https://www.osha.gov/dentistry/standards. Accessed August 19, 2021.
18. Sehulster LM, Chinn RYW, Arduino MJ, et al. *Guidelines for environmental Infection Control in Health-Care Facilities. Recommendations from CDC and the Healthcare Infection Control Practices Advisory Committee (HICPAC)*. Chicago, IL; American Society for Healthcare Engineering/American Hospital Association; 2004, updated July 2019.

CHAPTER 8

Patient Reception and Ergonomic Practice

Irina Smilyanski, RDH, DHS

CHAPTER OUTLINE

LEARNING OBJECTIVES

After studying this chapter, the student will be able to:

1. Describe the rules of etiquette in relationship to patient reception and care.
2. Describe the components of ergonomic practice and relationship to career longevity.
3. Identify the range of working positions for a right-handed and left-handed clinician.
4. Describe the elements of a neutral working position.
5. Recognize the causes and symptoms of the musculoskeletal disorders most often associated with the clinical practice of dental hygiene.
6. Explain the ergonomic risk factors of clinical dental hygiene practice.

The patient's presence in the office or clinic is an expression of confidence in the dentist and the dental hygienist. Confidence is inspired by the reputation for professional knowledge and skill, the appearance of the office, quality of care, and the actions of the workers in it.

- The physical arrangement and interpersonal relationships provide the setting for specific services to be performed.
- The patient's well-being is the primary consideration throughout the appointment.
- At the same time, the clinician must function effectively and efficiently in a manner that minimizes **stress** and **fatigue** to ensure personal health.
- **Musculoskeletal disorders**, **repetitive stress injuries**, and **cumulative trauma disorders** are common work-related conditions that require continuing preventive physical and mental energy by the clinical dental hygienist.
- The science of **ergonomics** has provided information for the development of standards for human performance and workplace design to maximize health, comfort, and efficiency for dental hygienists in clinical practice.

Preparation for the Patient

I. Treatment Area

The treatment area should be inviting and safe from the patient's and the clinician's perspective. It must support the best ergonomics practices, adhere to standard precautions, and be comfortable for the patient.

- Environmental surfaces: Disinfect and/or cover all clinical contact areas to control cross-contamination.
- Instruments: Maintain sterile packaged instruments sealed until the start of the actual treatment.
- Equipment: Prepare and make ready other materials that will be used, such as for the determination of blood pressure and patient instruction. Anticipate specific needs for procedures being delivered.
- Patient's dental chair: Place the patient's chair upright, chair arm adjusted for ease of access. The overhead light and other movable equipment should be moved out of the way for safe patient arrival.
- Clinician's chair: Set the clinician's chair at proper height and arrange for the proper seat and backrest angles.

II. Records

- For the patient of record, review the patient's medical and dental history for pertinent appointment information, updating, and assessment.
- Read previous appointment progress notes to focus the current treatment plan.
- Anticipate the procedures needed for a new patient.

Patient Reception

I. Introduction

- The dental assistant or the dentist may introduce the new patient to the dental hygienist, but more frequently, a self-introduction is in order.
- The patient is greeted by name, and the hygienist's name is clearly stated; for example, "Good morning, Mrs. Smith; I am Anna Jones, the dental hygienist."
- Be aware of and respect norms associated with the patient's culture. For instance, direct eye contact might be viewed differently by various cultural groups. Cultural considerations for patient communications are discussed in Chapter 3.
- Procedure for introducing the patient to others:
  - Use patient's preferred name and correct pronoun. A person's gender expression does not necessarily indicate a person's gender identity.[1]
  - An older person's name precedes the younger person's (when the difference in age is obvious).
  - In general, the patient's name precedes that of a member of the dental personnel.
  - Customarily, an older patient is not called by the first name except at the patient's request.

II. Escort Patient to Dental Chair

- Invite the patient to be seated and adjust the chair as needed. Ask the patient how you may assist them if you suspect additional assistance is needed.
- Be prepared to assist the elderly, disabled, or very small children; guide them into the chair (support the patient's arm when patient requests it).
- Assist with a wheelchair. Bring the wheelchair adjacent to the dental chair. Wheelchair procedures are described in the Wheelchair Transfer section in Chapter 51.

- Place personal items in a safe place—if possible, within the patient's view.
- Provide protective eyewear. When a patient removes personal corrective eyeglasses to put on the safety glasses provided, make sure the personal glasses are placed in their case in a safe place.
- Suggestions for helping the patient with a vision impairment may be found in Chapter 51.

Position of the Patient

I. General Positions

Four body positions for delivery of care are shown in **Figure 8-1**.

A. Upright

- This is the initial position when a patient is seated.

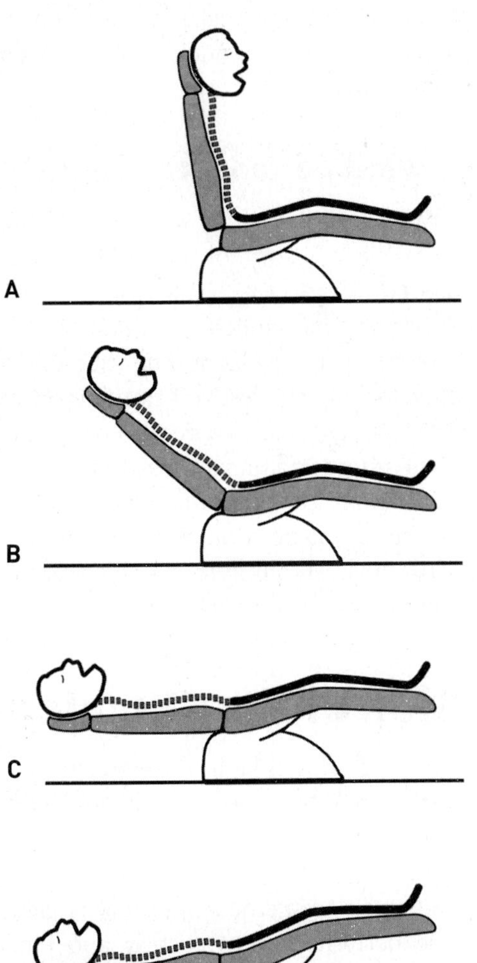

Figure 8-1 Basic Patient Positions. **A:** Upright. **B:** Semi-upright. **C:** Supine or horizontal with the brain at the same level as the heart. **D:** Trendelenburg, with the brain lower than the heart and the feet slightly elevated.

B. Semi-Upright

- The back of the chair is reclined at approximately 45° angle.
- Patients with certain types of cardiovascular, respiratory, or vertigo problems may need this position.
- **Figure 8-2** illustrates the patient and clinician using a semi-upright position during patient care.

C. Supine

- The chair is in a **supine** or flat position, the brain is at the same level as the heart.
- A patient is ideally situated for support of the circulation; rarely could a patient faint while lying in a supine position.
- The back of the chair is parallel to the floor.
- Position used most for treatment procedures.
- **Figure 8-3** illustrates the patient and clinician while using the supine position.

D. Trendelenburg

- The person is said to be placed in the **Trendelenburg position** if they are in the supine position and tipped back and down 10°–15° so that the brain is lower than the heart.
- The back of the chair is less than parallel to the floor.
- This position is utilized in management of some medical emergencies and during selected medical procedures.[2]

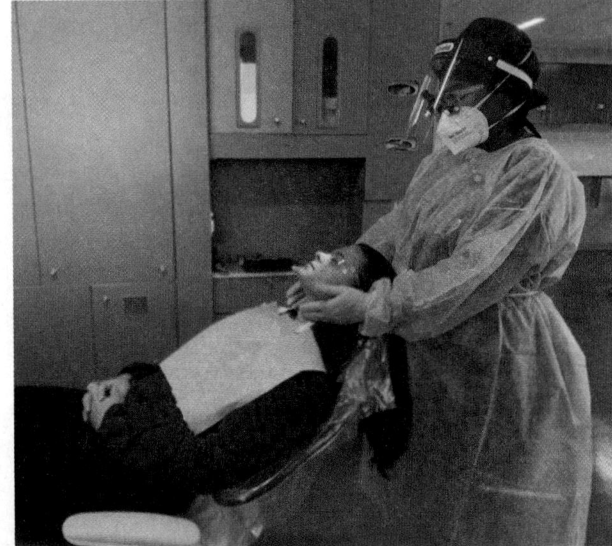

Figure 8-2 Patient in a Semi-Upright Position. This photograph illustrates ergonomic patient and clinician position for patient care in a semi-upright position when the clinician stands to provide care for the patient who cannot be moved to the supine position.

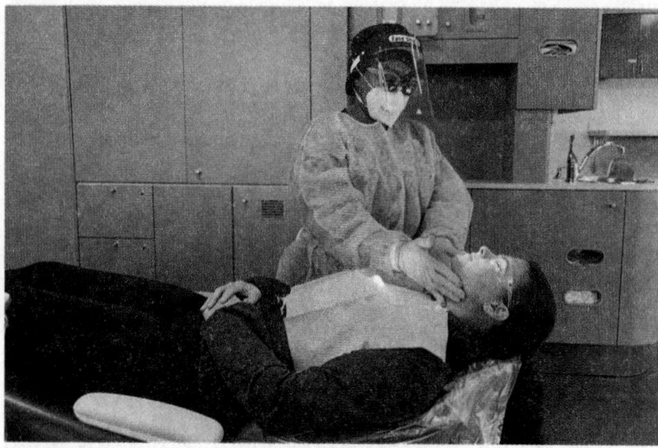

Figure 8-3 Patient in a Supine Position. This photo illustrates ergonomic patient and clinician position for patient care in a supine position. Note the neutral seating position of the clinician and the use of loupes magnifying system with attached headlight.

- Prolonged use of the Trendelenburg position can lead to adverse effects in vulnerable patients and should be avoided.

II. The Dental Chair

- A dental chair provides comfort for the patient and ergonomic access for the clinician.
- A comfortable patient is more relaxed and allows the procedure to be completed more efficiently.
- Seat and leg support move as a unit, and the back and headrest move as a unit; both are power controlled.
- A dental chair has a thin back so that the chair may be lowered close to the clinician's elbow height.
- Chair base permits the chair to be lowered as needed for appropriate treatment position.
- Chair controls need to be available from both the assistant and the clinician sides.

III. Use of Dental Chair

A. Prepositioning for Patient Reception

- Position the chair at the level comfortable for the patient when being seated; back upright.
- Move the chair arm out of patient's way on the side of approach.

B. Adjustment Steps

- The patient is seated with the chair back upright.
- Keep the chair seat and foot portion raised at first to help the patient get comfortable in the chair.
- Lower the chair back to the supine position for maxillary instrumentation and to a 20° angle with the floor for mandibular treatment.
- Adjust the headrest length/extension to accommodate for the patient's height.
- The clinician may need to ask the patient to slide up to rest the head at the upper edge of the headrest and turn head to left or right as needed for visibility and access.
- Adjust the chair height until the patient's mouth is at or slightly below the clinician's elbow height with shoulder relaxed (Figure 8-3).

C. Conclusion of Appointment

- Secure instruments on the instrument tray.
- Move the instrument tray out of the way and turn off the dental light.
- Slowly raise the back of chair to bring the patient upright.
- Bring the chair to the level comfortable for the patient when getting up.
- Request the patient remain seated in an upright position for a few seconds to avoid **postural hypotension**.

D. Contraindications for Supine Position

- Review patient history for indications of need for adaptation.
- Patient may request a position variation.
- Conditions that may contraindicate the supine position include congestive heart failure, vertigo, cervical spondylosis, and respiratory conditions such as emphysema or severe asthma.
- During the second and third trimester of pregnancy, the supine position might need to be modified.[3] Chair positioning for the pregnant patient is described in Chapter 46.

Position of the Clinician

- The clinician should be in the **neutral working position** (NWP), with good access, light, and visibility, which in turn contribute to an efficient procedure.
- The patient is positioned so dental hygiene care may be performed conveniently and efficiently within a reasonable length of time.
- The positions of the patient and the clinician are interdependent.
- When clinician and patient positioning is considered, it is realistic to remember that the patient's position will be assumed for a relatively short time compared with that of the clinician.

Neutral Working Position

I. Objectives

Objectives concern the health of the clinician, the service to be performed, and the effect on the patient. The preferred neutral position attempts to accomplish the following[4]:

- Contribute to and preserve rather than detract from clinician's health and wellness.
- Contribute to ease and efficacy of performance that encourages patient cooperation.
- Allow endurance for prolonged periods of peak efficiency.
- Reduce potential for overexertion and injury from mental and physical stress and fatigue.
- Give the patient a sense of well-being, security, and confidence.
- Accommodate a patient with special needs.

II. The Effects of NWP

- NWP needs to be developed, practiced daily, and made habitual.
- Habitual neutral position will translate to all activities outside of work as well. An internal environment can be created for ongoing physical comfort, safety, and activity.
- Without practicing the principles of neutral position on a regular daily basis, a clinician can experience discomfort, pain, and work-related stress disorders. The long-term result can be shortened or compromised career longevity with changes in daily life activities.
- Analysis and assessment of posture can give direction to corrections for treatment. Validated posture assessment instruments and evidence-based interventions are available.[5]

III. Description of Neutral Seated Position

A neutral seated position is illustrated in **Figure 8-4**. Characteristics of a neutral seated position in dentistry include[6]:

- *Back*: In neutral alignment with natural spinal curves, including cervical **lordosis**, thoracic **kyphosis**, and lumbar lordosis.
- *Head*: On top of neutral spine with forward neck flexion between 15° and 20° or less.
- *Eyes*: Directed downward to prevent neck and eye strain.
- *Shoulders*: Relaxed and parallel with the hips and floor.

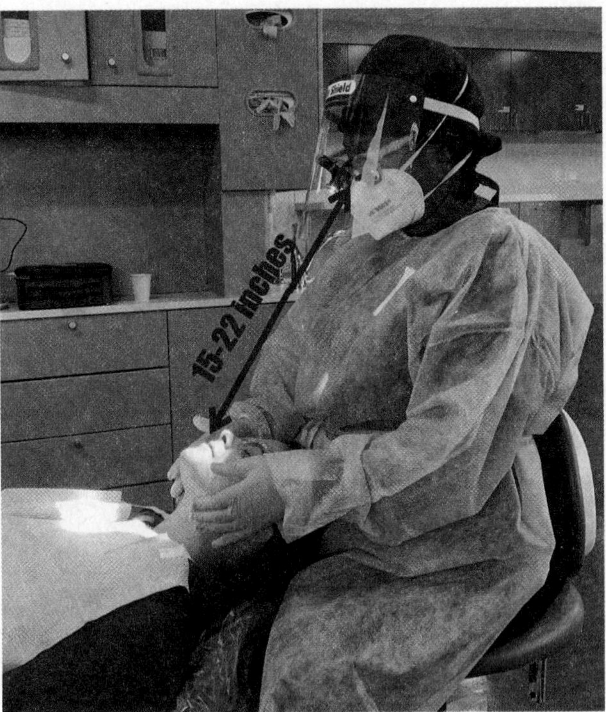

Figure 8-4 Clinician's Working Distance. Clinician in 12:00 working position, which shows the patient at the clinician's elbow level and the oral cavity of the patient between 15 and 22 inches from the clinician's eyes.

- *Elbows*: Close to the body.
- *Forearms*: Parallel with the floor.
- *Wrist*: Forearm and wrist are in a straight line.
- *Hips*: Slightly higher than knees.
- *Thighs*: Full body weight distributed evenly on seat; comfortable space (about 3 inches) between edge of seat and back of knee.
- *Knees*: Slightly apart.
- *Feet*: Flat on the floor.

IV. Clinician–Patient Positioning

A. Distance

- The position of the patient's oral cavity is adjusted to the clinician's elbow height.
- Distance from clinician's eyes to the patient's oral cavity when the clinician is seated in neutral position will be within the range of 15–22 inches.
- The distance is defined as the "working distance," which is a significant measurement when fitting magnification loupes for an individual clinician.

B. Selection

- NWP is combined with effective access to the patient for treatment procedures.

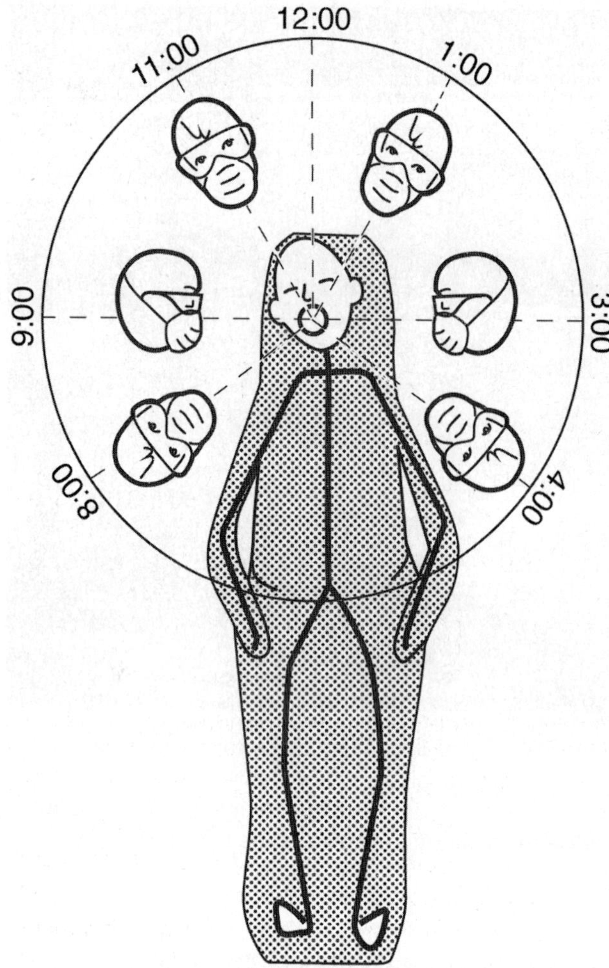

Figure 8-5 Range of Positions for Clinician. The patient's head is placed at the upper edge of the backrest or headrest for convenient access by the clinician during treatment. The range of positions is compared with the numbers on an analog clock.

- Orientation of position of the clinician to patient's oral cavity can be compared to the analog clock, with 12:00 at the top of the patient's head, as shown in **Figure 8-5**.
- Clock hours correspond with clinician–patient relation associated with instrumentation in different areas of the patient's oral cavity.

C. Flexibility

- Orientation for the right-handed clinician is associated with the 8–12 o'clock position; for the left-handed clinician, orientation is associated with the 12–4 o'clock position.
- Access and visual adjustment determine which side the clinician will select for a given procedure.
- Moving past 12 o'clock clockwise for the right-handed clinicians and counterclockwise for the left-handed clinicians improves access and visibility in certain areas.
- In treatment rooms with limited space, the dental chair may be swiveled to change the angle of the chair to allow the clinician to move past 12 o'clock position.

The Treatment Area

- The treatment area centers on the patient's oral cavity.
- The entire "work area" refers to the dental chair with patient, the unit, and the instrument tray as they are positioned for the convenience and accessibility of the clinician and clinician's assistant if available.
- For the clinician, the essentials for access and visibility for patient care are provided by the flexibility of movement of the clinician's stool and appropriate lighting, supplemented by the clinician's own visibility enhanced by wearing magnification loupes with a head light.

I. The Clinician's Chair

- The chair is a significant adjunct to the ergonomics of practice.
- Optimal chair design provides adequate support and the opportunity and means to change body posture frequently during the workday as clinicians, patients, and procedures change.
- The clinician adjusts the chair to personal specifications.

A. Characteristics of an Acceptable Chair

- *Base*: Broad and heavy with five casters; a chair with five casters provides greater stability.[4]
- *Seat design*[7]:
  - Traditional:
    - Size needs to support thighs without the back of the knees touching the edge; seamless, textured upholstery, padded firmly, with ability to tilt the seat 5°–15°; accommodates requirements for neutral seated position.
  - Saddle chair:
    - This is a relatively new type of chair modeled after a riding saddle; promotes neutral spine position and reduces muscle strain.
- *Armrests*: Adjustable at a height to support the forearm while maintaining NWP.
- *Height*: Adjustable for wide personal variability.

- *Back*: Adjustable lumbar support to accommodate different positions, procedures, and clinicians while maintaining the spinal curve.
- *Mobility*: Completely mobile; built with free-rolling casters; not connected to other dental equipment; free movement around the patient's head for instrumentation from either side.[4]
- *Adjustment*: Multiple adjustments for different positions, procedures, and clinicians; mechanisms easy to learn and use.[4]
- *Infection control friendly*: All surfaces able to withstand standard precautions regimen.

II. Vision: Lighting

- During treatment, visibility in the oral cavity is prerequisite to thoroughness without undue trauma to the tissues.
- With adequate light, efficiency increases, treatment time is decreased, and patient cooperation increases.
- Many lighting options are available. All need to be directed properly to the oral cavity for adequate visualization, optimal patient care, and clinician comfort and safety.

A. Dental Light: Suggested Features

- Is readily adjustable both vertically and horizontally.
- Beam of light is capable of being focused.
- Set within a comfortable arm's reach.

B. Dental Light: Location

- Attachment options
  - Unit attachment.
  - Ceiling-mounted light on a track.
  - Coaxial headlight can be added to improve visualization with targeted illumination.
- Dental light: adjustment principles
  - Light allows clear illumination of the entire treatment area.
  - Light is adjusted depending on the treatment area.
  - **Figure 8-6** shows position of light for maxillary and mandibular treatment.

III. Vision: Magnification

Magnification is needed to improve visualization, support NWP, and enhance treatment procedures.[8]

A. Choice of Loupe Systems

- Fixed through the lens: Customized for individuals
  - Adjusted with the clinician's prescription as needed.

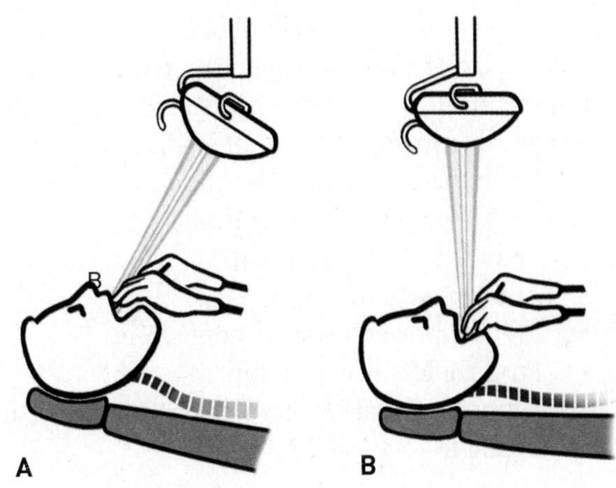

Figure 8-6 Lighting. Light does not obstruct the clinician and allows clear illumination of the treatment area. **A:** Maxillary arch; chin up position; beam of light often between 60° and 45° angle to floor. **B:** Mandibular arch; chin down position; beam of light nearly perpendicular to floor.

  - Magnifying lenses mounted directly into the lens.
  - Fixed interpupillary distance; angle of the lens not adjustable.
  - Not adjustable; enables the clinician to maintain correct posture.
- Front lens mounted without vertical adjustment
  - Prescription lenses are available.
  - Magnifying lenses mounted to a hinge on the frame; loupes can be adjusted up or down.
  - Interpupillary distance can be adjusted; angle of lens not adjustable.
- Front lens mounted with vertical adjustment
  - Prescription lenses are available.
  - Magnifying lenses mounted to a hinge on the frame; loupes can be adjusted up or down.
  - Interpupillary distance can be adjusted; angle of lens can be adjusted.

B. Features

- Proper fit is essential to successful incorporation of magnification into the clinician's treatment environment.
- Proper fit is dependent on the clinician's working distance and neutral position.
- Clinicians need to research the differences to select best option.

IV. Handpieces

- Technology has provided handpieces that are ergonomically compatible with procedures clinicians provide.

- The best designs are small, light, and well-suited for the size of a dental hygienist's hand.[9]
- Ergonomically designed handpieces are lightweight, decreasing stress on the hand and wrist.
  - Fit in the contours of the clinician's hand and allow functional light grasp.
  - Reduce fatigue and strain.
  - Allow maneuverability.
  - Provide power assist without strain.
  - Produce less heat buildup.
  - Battery operated prophy handpieces are available.

V. Cords

A. Management

- Managing cords is a significant aspect of ergonomic practice.
- Cords are part of most dental units and are an integral part of delivery of care for every patient.
- Ultrasonics, air/water syringes, slow-speed handpieces, and other power-driven equipment require cords connected to a power source.
- Improper management and inefficient design of the cords can increase drag on hand, wrist, and arm, increasing risk of repetitive injury.
- Cord design must allow for disinfection; cords should not interfere with functionality of other equipment.

B. Coiled Cords

- Can cause excessive stretching and pulling by clinician.
- Associated with bending, reaching, and awkward postures to position for treatment.
- Increase the strain on hand, wrist, arm, and shoulder of clinician.
- Provide an ergonomic risk by increasing fatigue level and creating muscle imbalances.
- Straight cords may be generally easier to manage.

Ergonomic Practice

I. Scope of Ergonomic Dental Hygiene

- Includes all practices that make work safe, decrease strain and fatigue, eliminate hazards, and improve work processes affecting the health and well-being of clinician and patient.
- **Box 8-1** lists items of the equipment, work layout, and work process organization that need attention during practice to prevent physical occupational disorders.

Box 8-1 Factors to Consider for Ergonomic Practice

Equipment

- Personal protective equipment (PPE)
- Lighting (Figure 8-6)
- Magnification, coaxial headlight
- Properly fitted gloves
- Instruments balanced, sharp, of varied diameters, with knurling on handles
- Power instruments
- Handpiece lightweight and ergonomically designed
- Cords and cord management
- Foot pedals
- Suction
- Air/water syringe

Work Layout

- Uncluttered, easy access to patient, patient records, computer, radiographs
- Counters clear with designated area for documentation
- Instrument tray within arm's reach
- Light fixture within arm's length, easy to move and adjust
- Orderly tray setup with complete armamentarium for services to be delivered
- Convenient treatment room setup and design for patient chair, air/water syringe, suction, cords, foot pedals

Work Process Organization

- Clinician NWP
- Use of magnification system supporting NWP
- Clinician–patient positioning (CPP)
- Light within easy arm's reach with clear illumination of treatment area
- Access and management of suction and air/water syringe
- Cords and cord maintenance

Instrumentation

- Instrument tray within easy reach
- Instruments are organized on tray
- Sharp instruments
- Consistent instrumentation sequence for all surfaces of sextants
- Proper grasp and fulcrum technique for dominant hand
- Proper grasp and fulcrum technique for nondominant hand
- Correct working stroke for location and type of deposit
- Inclusion of power instrumentation when indicated with appropriate management of aerosols
- Placement and access of foot pedals
- Selective polishing
- Placement and access to overgloves
- Documentation procedure

II. Related Occupational Problems

- The physical challenges inherent in dental hygiene practice place the clinicians at risk for developing work-related musculoskeletal disorders.[10]
- **Table 8-1** lists a variety of disorders that can occur among clinicians.
- Prevention of work-related musculoskeletal disorders starts at the same time as instrumentation skill development because these disorders begin in dental hygiene students.[11,12]

III. Ergonomic Risk Factors

- Prevention begins with the recognition of the **risk factors** that can point to potential body injury and more serious permanent musculoskeletal disorders.[13]
- **Table 8-2** lists and defines significant risk factors and provides examples of various practices that can lead to musculoskeletal disorders.

Self-Care for the Dental Hygienist

- Self-care and attention to the risk factors of musculoskeletal disorders are central to ergonomic practice.
- Self-care associated with **safe work practices** includes but is not limited to:
  - Wellness: Immunizations, healthy diet, adequate sleep, physical activity.

Table 8-1 Musculoskeletal Disorders Affecting Dental Hygienists

With any symptoms or any ongoing discomfort, take action to find the source of the problem and how to relieve the symptom. Prevention is the best course of action. Early intervention will decrease the risk of a more involved condition or a more costly injury. If not addressed in a timely manner, any of these conditions could lead to a limited ability to practice or total disability.

Condition	Causes	Symptoms
Carpal Tunnel Syndrome		
A symptomatic compression of the median nerve within the carpal tunnel (**Figure 8-7**)	Deviations of wrist from neutral Pinch grasp with insufficient rest	Numbness; tingling in the thumb, index, and middle fingers
Thoracic Outlet Syndrome		
Painful disorder of the fingers, hand, and/or wrist from compression of the brachial nerve plexus and vessels between the neck and shoulder	Tilting head forward Hunched and/or rounded forward shoulders Continuously reaching overhead	Numbness, tingling, and/or pain in the hand or wrist
Bursitis		
Inflammation of the bursa	Areas of friction or impingement anywhere in the body, usually the shoulder	Decreased range of motion Aching
Tendonitis		
Painful inflammation of the wrist resulting in strain	Repeated wrist extension or palmar flexion	Pain in the wrist, especially along the outer edges of the hand rather than through the center of the wrist
Disk Herniation		
Displacement of the nucleus of the disk with resultant pressure on the spinal cord or peripheral nerves	Prolonged, static postures of forward flexion, hyperextension, lateral bending, or rotation of the spine Can present on cervical, thoracic, or lumbar areas of the spine	Pain, numbness, tingling of the arm, fingers, lower back, hip, or leg

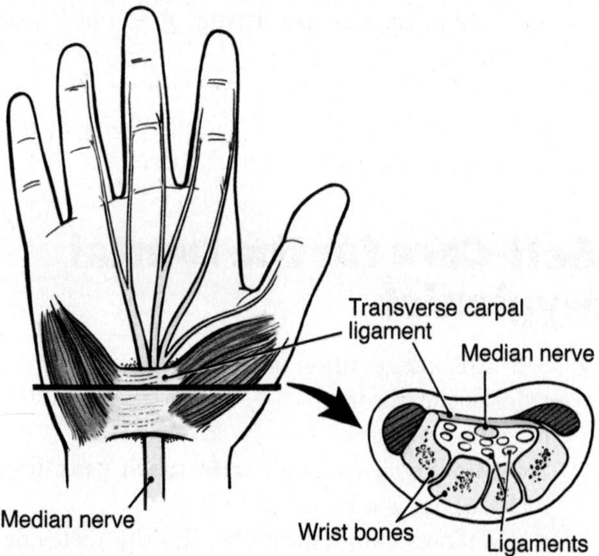

Figure 8-7 Anatomy of the Wrist (Palmar View). Left, the median nerve passes through the transverse carpal tunnel of the wrist and branches to innervate the thumb, the index and middle fingers, and the medial aspect of the ring finger. Right, cross section of wrist shows the median nerve passing through the carpal tunnel. The tunnel is formed by the concave arch of the carpal (wrist) bones and roofed over by the transverse carpal ligament.

- Standard precautions: Personal protective equipment.
- Clinical practice: Clinician–patient positioning (CPP), instrument selection and use, prevention of sharps injuries.
- NWP: In all activities, not only clinical practice.
- Stress management: Reasonable patient scheduling; adequate breaks.

I. Daily Functional Movement Exercises

- In dental hygiene practice, it is necessary to be vigilant in maintaining a healthy spine.
    - Achieving NWP throughout the work day.
    - Performing effective CPP and practicing daily functional movement exercises will support a healthy spine.
- Physical activity has a positive impact on reducing musculoskeletal symptoms; some research suggests yoga and massage have been most effective for preventing and managing symptoms.[14]
- Physical therapists can provide specific recommendations.

Table 8-2 Ergonomic Risk Factors

Intensity (strength or concentration of exposure), *frequency* (how often is the exposure), and *duration* (length of time of exposure) are related to the detrimental effects of the risk factor. A combination of risk factors intensifies risk and increases potential for injury.

Risk Factor	Definition	Example
Prolonged awkward position	Body postures that deviate from the normal resting or neutral positions	Twisting the torso during instrumentation Arm raised when scaling
Static positions (long-term static load)	Assuming and holding any position for long periods; causes muscle strain, impedes blood flow to the muscle, and leads to overuse of muscles and joints; accelerates fatigue and discomfort	Most patient treatment Bending neck for long periods Retracting cheek with nondominant hand without stable fulcrum Prolonged seated posture
Repetition	Performing the same motion or series of motions continually or frequently	Scaling and root planing Probing Exposing radiographs Using computer keyboard Writing
Force/grasp	Physical effort needed to lift, push, pull, grasp, and pinch items in the work environment Often required to handle and control equipment and tools Force increases as contact area decreases	Manual instrumentation Exposing radiographs
Environmental	Can directly influence comfort and risk of injury	Cold Heat Poor lighting Noise

Risk Factor	Definition	Example
Vibration	The physical exposure to rapidly oscillating tools or machinery	Tools such as jackhammers Additional research is needed to demonstrate the effect power scaling and handpieces have on dental personnel
Insufficient rest	Performing the same motion or series of motions continually or frequently without sufficient recovery time for muscles	Scaling procedures Probing Exposing radiographs Insufficient breaks
Stress	A physical, chemical, or emotional factor that causes bodily or mental tension and may be a factor in disease causation or fatigue Involves clinician perception of control of work environment and psychosocial factors	Poor team communication Insufficient input concerning patient workload
Poor physical fitness	Decreased capacity for body to resist the negative consequences of physical demands of dental hygiene practice	Demands of long periods of sitting Demands of repetitive movements during instrumentation

Box 8-2 Example Documentation: The Patient Who Is Unable to Tolerate the Supine Position

- **S**—Patient presents for routine 3-mo periodontal maintenance appointment; however, she came in with crutches due to a broken hip in a recent car accident. The patient provided a letter from her orthopedic surgeon clearing her for dental treatment. She is undergoing physical therapy twice a week for the next month or longer. The patient reports moderate soreness of back, arms, legs, and neck. Chief complaint is having a "dirty mouth" due to time spent in the hospital and rehab, combined with an inability to keep arms raised to clean teeth. She requests the chair remain in the upright position during treatment.
- **O**—Examination revealed limited opening of mouth, plaque index (PI) score 72%, compared with PI of 12% from last visit. Noted: moderate biofilm on maxillary and mandibular posterior teeth, supragingival calculus in the mandibular anterior region; probing mostly within 3 mm range with a few bleeding spots.
- **A**—The patient's current medical condition is preventing her from providing adequate oral self-care. Pain in arms and shoulders may be from use of crutches.
- **P**—Adjusted chair per patient's request. Limited opening and patient position caused difficulty in accessing dentition. Completed assessments only; patient requested appointment be stopped due to pain in back and legs. Advised patient to alert physician and physical therapist if there is an increase in level, duration, or frequency of pain.

Next Step: Reappoint patient in 1 month for periodontal maintenance completion pending improved physical condition.

Signed: ______________________________, RDH
Date: ______________________________

Documentation

Documentation for a patient with requirements for an alteration in dental chair positioning during instrumentation would include:

- Medical history notations indicating health history and current problem causing physical limitations or breathing difficulties.
- Notation for reference to length of appointment and time of day if needed.
- Example documentation using the SOAP format can be reviewed in **Box 8-2**.

Factors to Teach the Patient

- Discuss possible compromises to both manage the patient's concerns about positioning and the long-term impact on the dental hygienist's need to prevent musculoskeletal discomfort and pain to deliver better patient care.

References

1. Macri D, Wolfe K. My preferred pronoun is she: understanding transgender identity and oral health care needs. *Can J Dent Hyg*. 2019;53(2):110-117.
2. Rich K. Trendelenburg position in hypovolemic shock: a review. *J Vasc Nurs Off Publ Soc Peripher Vasc Nurs*. 2019;37(1):71-73.
3. Humphries A, Mirjalili SA, Tarr GP, Thompson JMD, Stone P. The effect of supine positioning on maternal hemodynamics during late pregnancy. *J Matern Fetal Neonatal Med*. 2019;32(23):3923-3930.
4. De Sio S, Traversini V, Rinaldo F, et al. Ergonomic risk and preventive measures of musculoskeletal disorders in the dentistry environment: an umbrella review. *PeerJ*. 2018;6:e4154.
5. Lietz J, Ulusoy N, Nienhaus A. Prevention of musculoskeletal diseases and pain among dental professionals through ergonomic interventions: a systematic literature review. *Int J Environ Res Public Health*. 2020;17(10):E3482.
6. Sanders MJ, Turcotte CM. Posture makes perfect. *Dimens Dent Hyg*. 2011:9(11):30-32, 35.
7. Gouvêa GR, Vieira W de A, Paranhos LR, Bernardino Í de M, Bulgareli JV, Pereira AC. Assessment of the ergonomic risk from saddle and conventional seats in dentistry: a systematic review and meta-analysis. *PloS One*. 2018;13(12):e0208900.
8. Roll SC, Tung KD, Chang H, et al. Prevention and rehabilitation of musculoskeletal disorders in oral health care professionals: a systematic review. *J Am Dent Assoc*. 2019;150(6):489-502.
9. McCombs G, Russell DM. Comparison of corded and cordless handpieces on forearm muscle activity, procedure time and ease of use during simulated tooth polishing. *J Dent Hyg*. 2014;88(6):386-393.
10. Hayes M, Cockrell D, Smith DR. A systematic review of musculoskeletal disorders among dental professionals. *Int J Dent Hyg*. 2009;7(3):159-165.
11. Netanely S, Luria S, Langer D. Musculoskeletal disorders among dental hygienists and students of dental hygiene. *Int J Dent Hyg*. 2020;18(2):210-216.
12. Hayes MJ, Smith DR, Cockrell D. Prevalence and correlates of musculoskeletal disorders among Australian dental hygiene students. *Int J Dent Hyg*. 2009;7(3):176-181.
13. Sanders MJ, Turcotte CM. Occupational stress in dental hygienists. *Work*. 2010;35(4):455-465.
14. Roll SC, Tung KD, Chang H, et al. Prevention and rehabilitation of musculoskeletal disorders in oral health care professionals: a systematic review. *J Am Dent Assoc*. 2019;150(6):489-502.

CHAPTER 9

Emergency Care

Wendy Male, MBA, BDSc, RDH

CHAPTER OUTLINE

LEARNING OBJECTIVES

After studying this chapter, the student will be able to:

1. Develop a plan to prevent and prepare for medical emergencies.
2. Identify signs and symptoms related to a possible emergency.
3. Define key words related to emergencies.
4. Describe stress minimization techniques.
5. Identify procedures for specific emergencies.
6. Incorporate documentation into the emergency plan.

Emergency Preparedness

The public expects competence in emergency situations. This chapter is designed to help prevent emergencies from escalating into more serious conditions. Emergency drills can reveal weaknesses in team responses that may identify a need for further training or education for dental office personnel.[1-3] Emergencies in the dental office were reported by more than half of those surveyed,[4-6] but the following measures may increase emergency preparedness:

- Periodic review of the literature to update drills is necessary for evidence-based responses to emergencies.
- Well-maintained emergency equipment stored in a convenient location.
- Post a *Quick Reference* with emergency equipment so it is readily available.
  - *Quick Reference* must include symptoms, equipment needed, and management of common emergencies.
- **Box 9-1** contains abbreviations.

Prevention of Emergencies

I. Attention to Prevention

Prevention of emergencies requires preparedness, alertness, and anticipation. The following patient assessment procedures may reduce the occurrence of a medical emergency:

- Thorough medical history questionnaires updated at every appointment.[7-9]
- Documentation of **baseline** vital signs, updated at each appointment.[10]
- Documentation of findings on Medical Alert Tags (wrist or ankle bracelets or necklaces that provide information on a patient's medical condition).
- Physical assessment beginning with the first interaction with a patient.[11]
- Incorporation of proper risk management and stress reduction protocols into the patient care plan.[4,9]
- Implementation of preparatory steps when a careful review and update of the patient record identifies potential risks. **Box 9-2** suggests a basic five-point plan for emergency prevention.

Box 9-1 Emergency Care Abbreviations

- **ACLS:** advanced cardiac life support
- **AED:** automated external defibrillator
- **AHA:** American Heart Association
- **ALS:** advanced life support
- **BCLS:** basic cardiac life support
- **BLS:** basic life support
- **CAD:** coronary artery disease
- **CPR:** cardiopulmonary resuscitation
- **ECC:** emergency cardiac care
- **ECG:** electrocardiogram
- **EMD:** emergency medical dispatcher
- **EMS:** emergency medical services
- **EMT:** emergency medical technician
- **EMT-P:** emergency medical technician paramedic

Box 9-2 Five-Point Plan to Prevent Emergencies

- Use systematic patient assessment procedures.
- Document and update accurate, comprehensive patient records.
- Implement stress reduction protocols.
- Recognize early signs of emergency distress.
- Organize team management plan for emergency preparedness.

II. Factors Contributing to Emergencies

- Increased number of older and medically compromised patients in society with natural teeth and dental diseases that require invasive procedures.[6,7,12-15]
- Many patients, especially older adults, are taking medications that may interact adversely with drugs used in dentistry.[6,12,14,16]
- More complex dental procedures require longer appointments.[17]
- Increased use of drugs in dentistry.[6,17]
  - Anesthesia: Local, general, conscious sedation.
  - Tranquilizers.
  - Pain medications (central nervous system depressants).
  - Antibiotics.

Patient Assessment

I. Assessment for Routine Treatment

A. First Contact

- Start with the first interaction with the patient.
- Note abnormalities of patient's voice on the telephone during appointment scheduling.

- Handwriting on dental forms can indicate steadiness, ability to communicate, and education.
- Assess overall appearance and gait when patient enters the dental office or clinic.
- Document findings in the patient's record.

B. Parts of the Assessment

- Physical assessment (signs and symptoms).
- Comprehensive patient history to include medical, dental, and psychosocial history.[4,10] See Chapter 11.
- Vital signs.
- Extraoral and intraoral examination.
- Comprehensive documentation of findings.

C. Emergency Indicators

Changes in a patient's appearance on the day of an appointment may suggest the need for preparation for emergencies.

II. The Patient's Medical History

A. Update and Document Changes

- Review the medical history at each appointment.[4,10,12]
- Discuss changes with dental team members who are providing treatment for the patient.

B. Use of Medical Alert Box

- Many dental offices utilize electronic patient records, but some continue to use paper records.
- If paper records are utilized, a chart or folder is required for confidentiality and Health Insurance Portability and Accountability Act.
- Only the patient's name and/or record number may be included on the folder or chart.
- The "Medical Alert Box" is usually located on the front page of the medical history to alert the dental team of information that may predispose a patient to a medical emergency before, during, or after dental treatment. Significant items include:
    - Physical conditions that may lead to an emergency.
    - Diseases the patient has or previously had.
    - Previous surgeries.
    - Medical emergencies the patient experienced previously.
    - Medications the patient has taken within the past 2 years.
    - Allergies and adverse drug reactions.
    - Previous adverse reactions to dental treatment.

III. Vital Signs

- Vital signs are essential to assess a patient's overall health status and to evaluate the severity of a medical emergency by comparison with baseline findings.
- A well-prepared dental team takes vital signs routinely to record baseline findings, not only during the earliest sign of emergency distress.[10]

A. The Vital Signs

Pulse, blood pressure, respirations, temperature, height, weight, and the information from the patient's personal Medical Alert Tag (bracelet, necklace, or anklet) provide essential information.

B. Baseline Vital Signs

The vital signs taken at the first appointment are considered baseline.[10] The ranges of vital signs are described in Chapter 12.

C. During Emergency

Compare vital signs to baseline findings during a medical emergency.

- Compensated shock: In most medical emergencies, patients will experience a "fight or flight" reaction to the extreme stress, during which time they are said to be compensating by trying to maintain normal bodily functions.[18]
- Hypotensive shock (compensated state): The following could indicate the patient is going into shock[18]:
    - Tachycardia.
    - Weak pulse.
    - Cold, pale skin; mottled skin; or heavy sweating.
    - Changes in consciousness (i.e. irritable, lethargic, or drowsy).
- Hypotensive shock can lead to cardiac and respiratory failure.[18]

IV. Extraoral and Intraoral Examinations

Extraoral and intraoral examinations can provide significant clues to underlying disease processes that predispose a patient to a medical emergency.

A. Extraoral

Blood disorders, cancers, and endocrine disorders may be suspected or discovered from extraoral palpation, skin color changes, abnormalities of the eyes, and asymmetry of the face or neck.

B. Intraoral

Oral manifestations and lesions can be indications of many disease states, such as diabetes, anemia, leukemia, lupus erythematosus, or human immunodeficiency virus/acquired immunodeficiency syndrome.

V. Recognition of Increased Risk Factors

The thorough and regularly updated medical and personal history, with adequate follow-up consultation with the patient's physician for integration of dental and medical care, can prevent many emergencies by alerting dental personnel to the individual patient's needs and idiosyncrasies.[4,10]

- Special needs may include[10]:
  - Specific physical conditions that may lead to an emergency (e.g., seizures and diabetes).
  - Diseases for which the patient is (or has been) under the care of a physician and the type of treatment, including medications.
  - Allergies or drug reactions or interactions.

Stress Minimization

- Stress and anxiety are the basis for many of the common emergencies that occur in a dental office or clinic.
- The clinic atmosphere and the warmth and sincerity of the personnel can help a patient feel accepted and secure.
- Develop rapport so the patient senses the clinician is empathetic, caring, and interested in alleviating the apprehension.[19]
- The apprehension and anxiety associated with dental treatment compounds the risk factors for medical emergencies.[9]

I. Recognize the Patient with Stress/Anxiety Problems

- In addition to the initial medical, dental, and psychosocial history review, use a short survey to assess dental anxiety such as the MDAS (Modified Dental Anxiety Scale).[19]
- Subjective measures of anxiety include observation of the patient for physical signs of stress such as restlessness, nervous habits, sweating, sitting on edge of chair, etc.[19]
- Objective measures might include elevated blood pressure, pulse, respirations, etc.[19]
- Elderly patients are prone to medical emergencies, as they may have cardiovascular diseases or other undiagnosed conditions.[7,12]
- Essential medications: Ensure certain medications are taken as prescribed to avoid risk of an emergency. Some medications may cause adverse reactions that can lead to a medical emergency such as **orthostatic hypotension**.

II. Stress Management

- Communicate with the patient about their fear of treatment. When a patient confides in a caregiver, trust is established, and the patient is calmer.
  - Patients who try to repress their fears are more likely to hyperventilate or experience **syncopal episodes**.
- Provide a stress reduction plan to any patient who is apprehensive or medically predisposed to emergencies.

III. Reduction of Stress

A. Appointment Scheduling

- New patient: Initial appointment for consultation and assessment provides an opportunity to build rapport and to evaluate the patient's level of anxiety. Stress reduction can be built into treatment appointments.[10,19]
- Time of appointment: Plan in accordance with personal health requirements.[9,10]
- Waiting time minimized: First appointment in the morning prevents anxiety from escalating by waiting all day for the appointment. In addition, anxiety can be decreased by taking the patient into the treatment room immediately and starting treatment promptly.[9,10,19]
- Eating requirements: Identify usual mealtime and ask about previous meal eaten to prevent **hypoglycemia**.[10]
- Length of appointment: Limited to the patient's tolerance.[10]

B. Management Strategies

- Management may be pharmacologic or psychotherapeutic (cognitive or behavioral) interventions, or a combination of both.[19]
- Pharmacologic measures include conscious sedation, inhalation sedation (e.g. nitrous oxide) or general anesthesia.[19] These require careful monitoring to prevent a medical emergency.

- Examples of psychotherapeutic interventions might include relaxation techniques, distraction, enhancing patient control, positive reinforcement, systematic desensitization, acupuncture, and guided imagery.[19]
- Adequate pain control with profound anesthesia is essential during treatment.[19]
- Patient's own prescriptions: Patients subject to emergencies are instructed to bring their own prescribed medicines (e.g., the patient with asthma or one who is subject to attacks of **angina pectoris**).

C. Posttreatment Care

- Postcare instructions for prevention and/or relief of discomfort.
- Postcare pain control as needed. **Analgesics** may be prescribed.[9]
- Consider a follow-up telephone call to an anxious patient to make certain there were no postoperative complications.

Emergency Materials and Preparation

- Organization is a key concept in emergency preparedness.[10,20]
- The first steps in preparing for managing emergencies include setting up the medical emergency equipment and a systematic action plan.[10,20-22]
- An office action plan for a medical emergency and individual acceptance of responsibility can provide the team with efficiency and composure, and minimize anxiety when the crisis occurs.[25]

I. Communication: Telephone Numbers for Medical Aid

Post emergency telephone numbers near each extension that permits outside calls.

- Rescue squads with paramedics (fire, police, or 911 in many cities in the United States and Canada).
- Ambulance service.
- Nearest hospital emergency department.
- Poison information center: 1-800-222-1222 in the United States or visit poisonhelp.org. In Canada, visit SafeMedicationUse.ca for poison center telephone listings by province.
- Primary care provider
  - List the patient's primary care provider in the permanent record in a standard, convenient place.

II. Equipment for Use in an Emergency

- Every dental office or clinic should have an emergency kit or cart,[4,10,22] and everyone in the office must be familiar with its contents. Kits can be purchased commercially (**Figure 9-1**).
- The kit must be kept in order, its contents replenished, and outdated materials replaced as needed.
- The emergency equipment should be portable, well-maintained, and kept in a place readily accessible to all treatment rooms.
  - Materials are plainly marked and kept separate from other office supplies.
  - Materials included are selected to accomplish emergency treatment by current accepted methods.
- The items included in the kit imply proper training in their use.
- Members of a team can add new items for the list in keeping with their training and abilities.
- **Table 9-1** provides a typical list of essential emergency equipment items.

III. Care of Drugs

- All dental personnel must become familiar with the emergency drugs maintained in the particular office or clinic.[17]
- Only specially trained; experienced persons will administer injectable medications.[20]
- The only drugs kept in the dental office are those the dentist or emergency team is trained to use.[17,20]

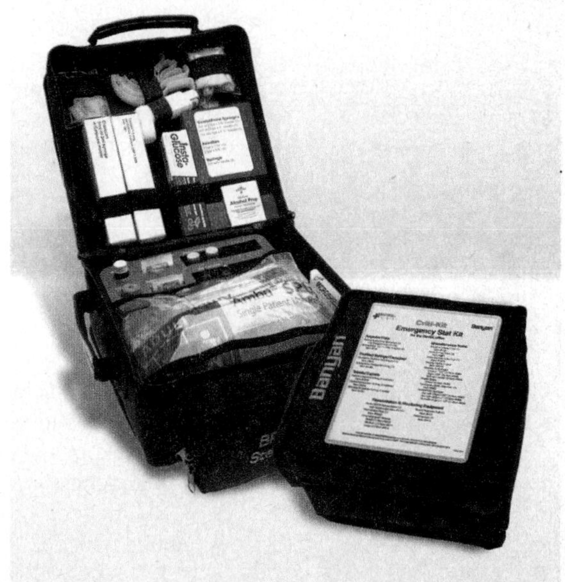

Figure 9-1 Emergency Medical Kit for the Dental Office

Table 9-1 Equipment in an Emergency Kit or Cart[a]

Category	Essential Items
Required equipment	■ Series E portable oxygen tank • Low-flow oxygen regulator • **Nasal cannula** • Simple face mask • Nonrebreather mask • Bag-valve masks (adult and pediatric) • Demand valve resuscitator ■ Automated external defibrillator (AED) ■ Oro- and nasopharyngeal airways • Sizes: Pediatric to large adult • Water-soluble lubricant ■ Sphygmomanometer • Blood pressure cuffs: Pediatric, adult regular, and large adult ■ Magill forceps ■ Disposable syringes: 2–3 mL Luer-Lok tip 21-gauge needles (assorted sizes are recommended) ■ Medical Emergency Report Forms ■ **Cricothyrotomy** equipment[b] ■ Latex-free tourniquet ■ Intravenous equipment[b]
Injectable drugs	■ Epinephrine via autoinjector (EpiPen) ■ Diphenhydramine (injectable antihistamine) ■ Cortisone[b] ■ Glucagon[b] ■ Midazolam[b] ■ Atropine[b]
Noninjectable drugs	■ Antiplatelet: Aspirin ■ Respiratory stimulant: Ammonia **vaporole** or ammonia inhalant capsule ■ Bronchodilator: Albuterol inhaler ■ Antihypoglycemic: Glucose gel, glucagon paste ■ Vasodilator: Nitroglycerin tablets, nitrolingual spray ■ Diphenhydramine tablets ■ Naloxone (Narcan): Nasal spray
Supplementary equipment	■ Thermometer ■ Blood glucose meter, lancets, and test strips ■ Pen flashlight ■ Battery operated alternative light source in case of power failure ■ Stopwatch ■ Razor (for hair removal for AED pads) ■ Scissors ■ Cotton pliers ■ Emesis basin ■ Blanket ■ Pillow ■ Inflatable splints ■ Backboard for patients who cannot be moved for cardiopulmonary resuscitation ■ Quick-activated cold packs ■ Betadine wipes (povidone-iodine antiseptic wipes) ■ Sterile packages of gauze and adhesive tape • 2 × 2 inches • 4 × 4 inches • Rolled gauze (2 × 5 inches)

[a]Check with local board of dentistry or governing body as there may be specific lists of minimum requirements for equipment and medication.
[b]Administered only by personnel with advanced medical training.

A. Identification

- The purpose and method of administration of each drug are clearly identified on the container.[17]
- A compartmentalized clear plastic cabinet or box can be useful for this purpose because the labels and instructions can be seen from the outside and efficient selection can be made.[17,22]
- The expiration date appears clearly on each item that has a limited shelf life.[17,22]
- When narcotics are included in the list of drugs available for emergencies, they are stored in a secured location other than the emergency kit, and typically purchased in pre-dosed amounts for specific emergency situations.

B. Record of Drugs

- Label each with information about shelf life and due date for replacement. Example: **Nitroglycerin** is replaced at 6 months.[17]
- Check weekly to maintain emergency kit.[17]
- A complete record of each drug must be maintained. The following are recorded:
  - Name of drug.
  - Dosage.
  - Date purchased.
  - Address of source if different from the usual local pharmacy.
  - Itemized record, signed by the staff member responsible.
  - Specific entry as each drug is used.
  - Expiration dates checked at routine intervals.
  - Instructions for disposal.

C. Disposal of Drugs

- Follow specific disposal instructions on the drug label or patient information sheet.
- Do not flush prescription drugs down the toilet.
- Take advantage of community drug take-back programs that allow the public to bring unused drugs to a central location for disposal.

IV. Medical Emergency Report Form

- **Figure 9-2** shows an example of a form that can be used to record the essential information during an emergency.
- Such a form can be filed in a patient's paper chart or scanned into the computerized chart.
- The forms can be placed on a clipboard on the emergency cart.
- A copy of the emergency report can be given to the EMS personnel to present to those in the emergency room at the hospital or other medical facility when the patient is admitted.[23]

A. Purposes

- Organize data collected during the emergency.
- Serve as a time reference during the monitoring of vital signs.
- Prepare a record from which the medical personnel can interpret the patient's condition at the time of transfer from the dental facility.[23]

B. Uses

- Evaluation for planning dental and dental hygiene appointments to avoid future emergencies for the patient.
- Provide a reference in the event legal questions arise. A well-kept record can be vital, and each emergency must be carefully recorded.[17]

V. Practice and Drill

A. Staff Instruction

- In an emergency situation, seconds count and there is no time for fumbling or discussion.
- Each member of the clinic and office staff must be thoroughly familiar with the location, purpose, effect, and application of each item of equipment and its source.[10,22]
- Each staff member also must know the order of procedures in all types of emergencies (**Figure 9-3**) and can assume any role when needed.[17,22]

B. Assignments

- Preparation: The assignment of specific responsibilities during an emergency is the result of planning by the whole team.[4,5,10]
- Substitutions: Because a staff member may be absent from the scene at the time of an emergency, each person learns and practices the duties for all positions so substitutions can be made with a minimum of discussion and no confusion.[4,5]
- **Figure 9-4** shows an example of a possible distribution of duties when three people are available to attend to the patient.
- Advantages of assignments
  - Organization efficiently uses personnel.
  - Sharing responsibility relieves pressure.
  - Duties can be carried out quietly, without excess discussion or attention from others in the clinic.
  - Necessary work gets done without duplication and without omissions.

Medical Emergency Report

Patient's Name *Smith, Joe*	Today's Date *10/27/20*

Description of incident: *Patient exhibited signs of anaphylaxis after exposure to latex gloves. Urticaria and pruritus were evident on arms, neck and chest. Signs of lip, tongue and laryngeal edema were exhibited with difficulty swallowing and breathing. Quickly explained to patient that he was having an allergic reaction. Patient was immediately given epinephrine (.3mg) via EpiPen autoinjector and EMS was summoned. 50mg of Benadryl and 100mg of Solu-Cortef were also administered IM. Oxygen was delivered by non-rebreather at 15 L/min. Within 5 minutes vital signs and symptoms improved. At 8 minutes vital signs were near baseline. Patient was released to EMS in 15 minutes and transported to the hospital.*

Time of onset		Time EMS summoned		Time EMS arrived		Time patient was released	
Stopwatch	Clock time	Stopwatch	Clock time	Stopwatch	Clock time	Stopwatch	Clock time
0:00 minutes	*10:30 am*	*0:10 minutes*	*10:30 am*	*13:00 minutes*	*10:43 am*	*15:00 minutes*	*10:45 am*

Patient released to: *EMS who transported patient to Tallahassee Memorial Regional Medical Center*

Cessation of breathing: *Ø*		Cessation of pulse: *Ø*		CPR initiated: *Ø*	
Stopwatch	Clock time	Stopwatch	Clock time	Stopwatch	Clock time
N/A	*N/A*	*N/A*	*N/A*	*N/A*	*N/A*

	Initial findings	Stopwatch times	Followup finding	Stopwatch times	Followup finding	Stopwatch times
Blood pressure	*90/60*	*2:15 minutes*	*110/80*	*5:15 minutes*	*120/80*	*8:15 minutes*
Pulse	*50 bpm*	*1:00 minutes*	*68 bpm*	*5:00 minutes*	*72 bpm*	*8:30 minutes*
Respirations	*10*	*1:30 minutes*	*12*	*5:30 minutes*	*16*	*8:00 minutes*
O_2 delivery method	*non-rebreather (15 L/min)*	*1:45 minutes*	*non-rebreather (15 L/min)*	*5:30 minutes*	*non-rebreather (15 L/min)*	*8:30 minutes*

Drugs administered	Route	Dosage	Stopwatch times
Epinephrine via EpiPen®	*I.M. (Quad)*	*.3 mg*	*0:45*
Benadryl®	*I.M. (Deltoid)*	*50 mg*	*1:15*
Solu-Cortef®	*I.M. (Deltoid)*	*100 mg*	*1:30*

Figure 9-2 Sample Medical Emergency Report. The form could be prepared in duplicate. One copy accompanies the patient to the emergency clinic, and the second copy is retained in the patient's dental record file.

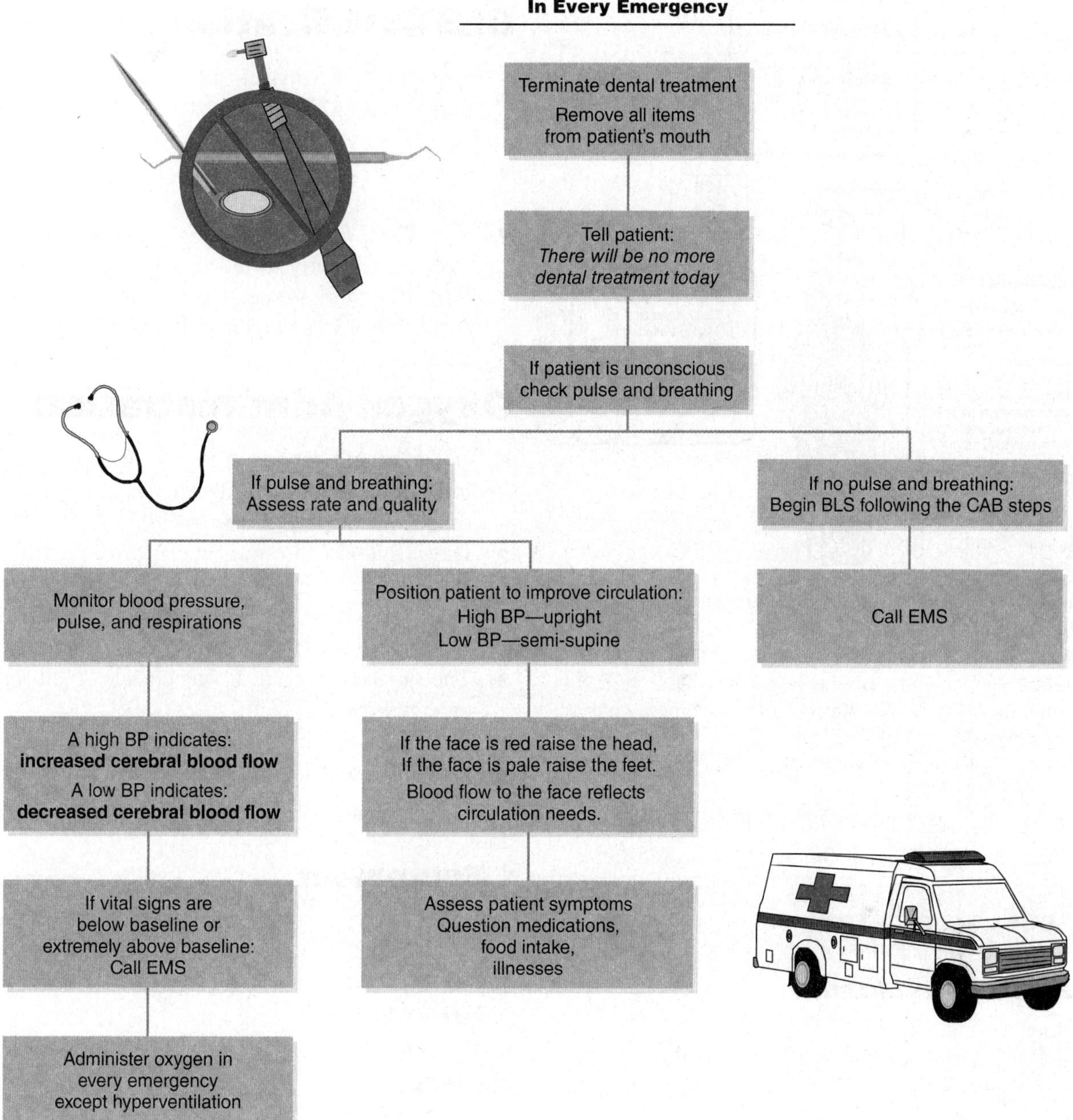

Figure 9-3 Flowchart: In Every Emergency. BLS, basic life support; BP, blood pressure; CAB, circulation–airway–breathing; EMS, emergency medical services.

C. Drills

- Check the requirements of the licensing body in your state, province, or country, as there may be a minimum requirement for the frequency of team drills. For instance, in Massachusetts, a minimum of yearly team drills is required.
- A specific emergency code call can be used when an intercom or other message system is available. Mentioning "code" in front of a number or phrase may panic the other patients; therefore, it is best to use only a number like "17."
- For each type of emergency, practice the use of procedures, including oxygen administration, resuscitation, and airway maneuvers, as well as specific positioning of a patient for all emergencies.[22]
- Equipment and materials can be checked at the time of the drill to ensure their availability and that each is in working order. One staff member should be designated to be in charge of the emergency supplies.[22]
- A record of drills must be kept with a diary of dates, procedures practiced, and names of those present.

D. New Staff Member

- Assignment of duties and practice for new members are a part of the first working day's orientation.

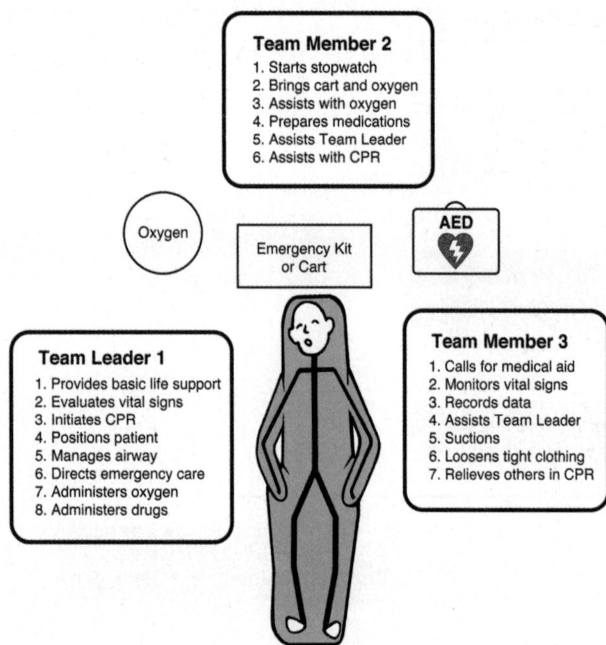

Figure 9-4 Division of Duties for Three-Person Emergency Team. Suggested distribution of responsibilities to be memorized and practiced by the dental personnel who form the emergency team. AED, automated external defibrillator; CPR, cardiopulmonary resuscitation

- Typically, BLS/CPR certification is required for licensure. However if this is not required for licensure, the new employee must identify and complete a refresher course as soon as possible.

E. Procedures Manual

A paper manual is a valuable reference, but an electronic format is a currently accepted method of storing procedure manuals. They need to be accessible from a computer or mobile device readily available in the clinic.

- Reviewed and updated three or four times each year.
- Useful during the orientation of a new member.
- Contains work assignments and checklists for equipment and resources.
- Provides reference information concerning specific emergencies organized in color-coded sections and alphabetical order to outline signs, symptoms, and initial treatment.
- Members of the team are given assignments to update the manual by conducting a critical review of the scientific literature for quality assurance and evidence-based, patient-centered care.
- All updates are referenced in the index of the manual.

BLS Certification

- Licensed dental hygienists are required to maintain a current BLS/CPR certification in most states for licensure.
- The AHA provides guidelines and training for healthcare professionals.
- The *AHA BLS for Healthcare Providers Manual* is updated regularly to reflect the most current information and procedures to follow when responding to an emergency situation.

Oxygen Administration

- Use of a high concentration of oxygen is contraindicated for chronic obstructive lung diseases, especially **emphysema**.
- Oxygen is also not indicated in the presence of hyperventilation because the patient is receiving increased amounts of oxygen in air inhaled and is in need of carbon dioxide.[17,20]
- The use of oxygen is beneficial in all other emergencies.[17]
- When the patient is not breathing, positive pressure oxygen (also known as demand valve resuscitator) delivery is needed.[20]

I. Equipment

Oxygen delivery systems with indications, flow rate, and percentage of oxygen delivered are listed in **Table 9-2**. A portable oxygen delivery system is shown in **Figure 9-5**.

A. Parts

- Oxygen resuscitation equipment consists of the following:
    - An oxygen tank.
    - A reducing valve.
    - A flow meter.
    - Tubing.
    - Mask.
    - A positive pressure bag.
- The portable E-cylinder, which can provide oxygen for 30 minutes, is the minimum size recommended. A back-up oxygen task should be kept on hand.

B. Directions

Box 9-3 outlines the steps for operation of an oxygen tank. Clear, readable directions are permanently attached to the tank's portable carriage. Practice must be a part of team drills.

Table 9-2 Oxygen Delivery Systems

Device	Indications	Flow Rate (L/min)	Oxygen Delivery (%)
Cannula	For patient who is breathing and needs low levels of oxygen	2–6	25–40
Face mask	For patient who is breathing and needs moderate levels of oxygen: ■ When cannula is not tolerated ■ When more oxygen is desired ■ Patient is in shock	8–12	60
Nonrebreather mask	For patient who is breathing and needs high levels of oxygen: ■ Patient is in shock ■ When more oxygen is desired	10–15	60–90
Bag mask	When patient has stopped breathing; bag mask is used instead of mouth-to-mouth resuscitation	10–15	90–100
Demand valve resuscitation	Positive pressure delivery of oxygen on demand	Used by emergency medical technicians or others professionally trained	100

Laminate and affix to the oxygen tank.

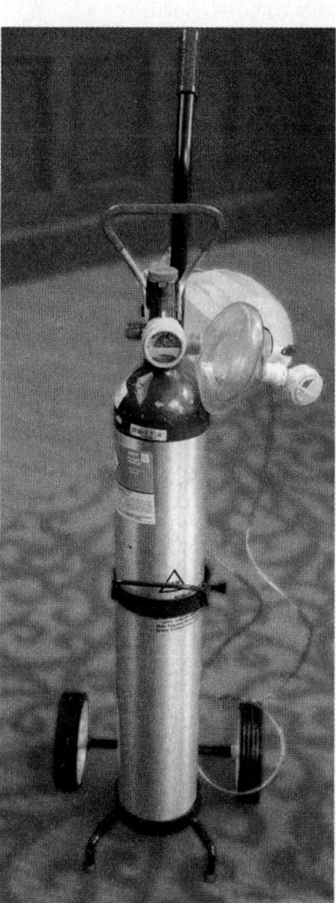

Figure 9-5 Portable Oxygen Delivery System. The portable unit is stored in an area accessible to all treatment areas in the dental clinic. If a fixed oxygen delivery system is available in the treatment area, it can be used in an emergency situation.

Box 9-3 Operation of Oxygen Tank

To turn on:

- Attach oxygen delivery system to tank.
- Turn key on top of tank in *counterclockwise direction* to open flow of oxygen.
- Adjust low-flow regulator knob and turn in the direction the arrow indicates to increase or open; many regulators are opposite of sink faucets and open clockwise instead of counterclockwise.
- Attach oxygen delivery system to patient.

To turn off:

- Remove oxygen delivery system from patient.
- Turn key on top of tank in *clockwise direction* to shut off flow of oxygen.
- Turn the low-flow regulator knob to the open position to bleed oxygen from the system.
- After bleeding, gently close the low-flow regulator knob.

Laminate and affix instructions to the oxygen tank.

II. Patient Breathing: Use Supplemental Oxygen

- Apply a full-face clear mask or a nasal cannula.
- Start supplemental oxygen at 6–10 L/min.[10]
- Monitor breathing; if breathing stops, proceed with positive pressure oxygen.

III. Patient Not Breathing: Use Positive Pressure

For persons not trained in the use of the bag-valve mask or positive pressure delivery, a mouth-to-mask procedure is used.[24]

- Apply a full-face clear mask so a tight seal is formed. One dental team member may need to apply pressure to the face mask to maintain a complete seal.
- Adjust oxygen flow so the positive pressure bag remains filled.
- Compress the bag manually, one ventilation every 5–6 seconds to provide 10–12 respirations/min for an adult. For a child, provide 1 ventilation every 3 seconds.[24]
- Watch for chest rise. When the chest does not rise, recheck airway for obstruction. Proceed with airway obstruction management.
- Call EMS.

Specific Emergencies

- Certain systemic disease conditions and physical injuries require specific treatment during an emergency.
- In **Table 9-3** and **Table 9-4**, the *Emergency Reference Charts*, several conditions are listed with their symptoms and treatment procedures.
- Some of the same conditions have been described in detail in Section IX of this text.

Table 9-3 Emergency Reference Chart: Medical Emergencies

Emergency	Signs/Symptoms	Procedure
All cases call emergency medical services (EMS) immediately if problem with: Breathing Unconsciousness **Anaphylaxis** Bleeding Poisoning Chest pain		i. Determine consciousness (tap and shout); yell for help **If patient is unconscious: Call EMS and get automated external defibrillator (AED)** i. Conduct primary assessment: • C—Circulation: check for pulse for 10 sec, if none: start compressions • A—Airway: open with head tilt-chin lift • B—Breathing: look, listen, feel; if none: give two (1-sec) breaths • D—Defibrillate: Use AED as soon as possible; provide one shock, resume cardiopulmonary resuscitation (CPR) for 2 minutes until prompted to allow the AED to check for heart rhythm. **If patient is conscious and breathing:** i. Conduct secondary assessment: a. Evaluate level of consciousness 1. Does patient know own name, location, date? 2. Use penlight to see if pupils react equally to light 3. If conscious: Check for equal hand strength by asking patient to squeeze your hands 4. Position according to signs/symptoms 5. If face is red, raise the head 6. If face is pale, raise the feet 7. Evaluate heart rate, blood pressure, respirations b. Findings in patient record or medical alert bracelet 1. Disabilities, diseases, drugs, baseline vital signs: **Call EMS**
Respiratory failure	Labored or weak respirations or cessation of breathing **Cyanosis** or ashen-white with blood loss Pupils dilated Loss of consciousness	Position: Semi-supine if not breathing; upright if breathing If visible, remove foreign material from mouth Establish airway. **Begin CPR**. If patient does not spontaneously breathe: **Call EMS** Monitor vital signs: Blood pressure, pulse, respirations Administer oxygen by nonrebreather mask if patient is already breathing

Emergency	Signs/Symptoms	Procedure
Mild airway obstruction	Good air exchange, coughing, wheezing (patient can speak)	Sit patient up Loosen tight collar, belt No treatment; let patient cough
Severe airway obstruction	Poor air exchange; noisy breathing; weak, ineffective cough; difficult respirations; gasping Unable to speak, breathe, cough Cyanosis, dilated pupils	Reassure patient Treat for complete obstruction ***Conscious patient:*** Perform Heimlich maneuver ***Patient becomes unconscious*:** **Begin CPR** ***Unconscious patient:*** **Call EMS**
Hyperventilation syndrome	Light-headedness, Anxiety, confusion Dizziness Overbreathing (25–30 respirations/min) Feelings of suffocation Deep respirations Palpitations (heart pounds) Tingling or numbness in the extremities	Terminate dental procedure Remove rubber dam and objects from mouth Position upright Loosen tight collar and/or tie Reassure patient Explain overbreathing; Request that each breath be held to a count of 10. Ask patient to breathe deeply (7–10/min) into a paper bag adapted closely over nose and mouth Never use a bag for a patient with diabetes or patients exhibiting signs of diabetic coma (e.g., fruity breath odor, **Kussmaul breathing**, lethargy, dry skin)
Heart failure	Difficult or labored breathing Pulmonary congestion with cough and difficulty breathing May cough up pink sputum Rapid, weak pulse Dilated pupils May have chest pain	Place patient in upright position. **Call EMS** Make patient comfortable: Cover with blanket Administer oxygen by nonrebreather mask Reassure patient Provide basic life support (BLS)
Cardiac arrest	Skin: Ashen gray, cold, clammy No pulse No heart sounds No respirations Eyes fixed, with dilated pupils; no constriction with light Unconscious	If conscious: ■ History of angina: Administer nitroglycerin. If no relief after a few minutes, repeat nitroglycerin. If still no relief, follow cardiac arrest protocol[4] ■ Chest pain with no history of angina, have patient chew 300–325 mg aspirin.[4,22] If unconscious: ■ **Call EMS** ■ Check oral cavity for debris or vomitus; leave dentures in place for a seal ■ **Begin CPR**[4,24]
Asthma attack	Difficulty breathing, wheezing (extreme cases—silence, indicating little to no air exchange) Cyanosis Dilated pupils Confusion due to lack of oxygen Chest pressure Sweating	Position patient upright Assist with patient's own bronchodilator (two puffs) Administer supplemental oxygen by nasal cannula Epinephrine if patient decompensates Supplemental cortisone to patients on corticosteroid therapy BLS—may need demand valve resuscitator if patient experiences respiratory depression **Call EMS**

(*continues*)

Table 9-3 Emergency Reference Chart: Medical Emergencies *(continued)*

Emergency	Signs/Symptoms	Procedure
Syncope (fainting)	Pale gray face, anxiety Dilated pupils Weakness, dizziness, faintness, nausea Profuse cold perspiration Rapid pulse at first, followed by slow pulse Shallow breathing Drop in blood pressure Loss of consciousness	Position: **Trendelenburg** Open airway Loosen tight collar, belt Place cold, damp towel on forehead Crush ammonia vaporole and place under patient's nose Keep warm (blanket) Monitor vital signs: Blood pressure, pulse, respirations Keep airway open Administer oxygen by nasal cannula Keep in supine position 10 min after recovery to prevent nausea and dizziness Reassure patient, especially during recovery
Shock	Skin: Pale, moist, clammy Rapid, shallow breathing Low blood pressure Weakness and/or restlessness Nausea, vomiting Thirst, if shock is from bleeding Eventual unconsciousness if untreated	Position: Trendelenburg Open airway Keep quiet and warm Monitor vital signs: Blood pressure, respirations, pulse Keep airway open Administer oxygen by nonrebreather bag If patient does not recover fully and/or vital signs not at baseline: **Call EMS**
Stroke (cerebrovascular accident)	**F.A.S.T**[25] **F**: Face drooping or numb on one side **A**: Arm weakness **S**: Speech difficulty (may slur words) **T**: Time to call EMS/911 Other symptoms might include confusion, vision changes, dizziness, loss of balance, or severe headache	***Conscious patient:*** ▪ **Call EMS**. Turn patient on paralyzed side; semi-upright ▪ Loosen clothing about the throat ▪ Reassure patient; keep calm, quiet ▪ Monitor vital signs: Blood pressure, pulse, respirations ▪ Administer oxygen by nasal cannula ▪ Clear airway; suction vomitus because the throat muscles may be paralyzed ***Unconscious patient:*** ▪ Position: Supine ▪ BLS ▪ CPR if indicated
Cardiovascular diseases	Symptoms vary depending on cause	***For all patients:*** ▪ **Call EMS** ▪ Be calm and reassure patient ▪ Keep patient warm and quiet; restrict effort ▪ Always administer oxygen when there is chest pain
Angina pectoris	Sudden crushing, **paroxysmal** pain in substernal area Pain may radiate to shoulder, neck, arms Pallor, faintness Shallow breathing Anxiety, fear	Position: Upright, as patient requests, for comfortable breathing If patient has been diagnosed with angina and has own nitroglycerin: Place nitroglycerin sublingually only when the blood pressure is at or above baseline Administer oxygen by nasal cannula Reassure patient Without prompt relief from nitroglycerin: **Call EMS**; treat as a **myocardial infarction**

Emergency	Signs/Symptoms	Procedure
Myocardial infarction (heart attack)	Sudden pain similar to angina pectoris, which may radiate, but of longer duration Pallor; cold, clammy skin Cyanosis Nausea Breathing difficulty Marked weakness Anxiety, fear Possible loss of consciousness	**Call EMS** Position: With head up for comfortable breathing Symptoms are not relieved with nitroglycerin Encourage to chew one adult (not enteric coated) or two low-dose "baby" aspirin if the patient has no allergy to aspirin[22] Monitor vital signs: Blood pressure, pulse, respirations Administer oxygen by nonrebreather bag Alleviate anxiety; reassure
Adrenal crisis (cortisol mental deficiency)	Anxious, stressed Confusion Pain in abdomen, back, legs Muscle weakness Extreme fatigue Nausea, vomiting Low blood pressure Elevated pulse Loss of consciousness Coma	***Conscious patient:*** ■ Terminate oral procedure ■ **Call EMS** ■ Request telephone call for medical assistance ■ Administer oxygen by nonrebreather mask ■ Monitor blood pressure and pulse ■ Place patient on stable side with legs slightly raised ***Unconscious patient:*** ■ **Call EMS** ■ BLS ■ Try ammonia vaporole when cause is undetermined ■ Administer oxygen
Insulin reaction (hyperinsulinism, hypoglycemia)	Sudden onset Skin: moist, cold, pale Confused, nervous, anxious Bounding pulse Salivation Normal to shallow respirations Convulsions (late)	***Conscious patient:*** ■ Follow the *15-15 Rule*:[26] • Administer 15 grams glucose gel (or rapidly absorbed carbohydrate) • Check blood glucose after 15 minutes • If blood glucose <70 mg/dL, administer another 15 grams glucose gel ■ Once blood glucose is >70 mg/dL, the patient should eat a source of long-acting carbohydrate like crackers and peanut butter, etc. ■ Monitor patient and only release them if blood glucose stays above 70 mg/dL to a relative, friend, etc. for transport ***Unconscious patient:*** ■ **Call EMS** ■ Administer intramuscular glucagon ■ BLS ■ Position: Supine ■ Maintain airway ■ Administer oxygen by nonrebreather bag ■ Monitor vital signs
Diabetic coma (ketoacidosis) (hyperglycemia)	Slow onset Skin: Flushed and dry Breath: Fruity odor Dry mouth, thirst Low blood pressure Weak, rapid pulse Exaggerated respirations (Kussmaul breathing)	***Conscious patient:*** ■ **Call EMS** ■ Keep patient warm ■ Administer oxygen by nasal cannula ***Unconscious patient:*** ■ BLS ■ Position: supine

(continues)

Table 9-3 Emergency Reference Chart: Medical Emergencies *(continued)*

Emergency	Signs/Symptoms	Procedure
Seizure ■ Generalized **tonic-clonic** ■ Generalized absence	Anxiety or depression Pale, may become cyanotic Muscular contractions Loss of consciousness (may be brief) Fixed posture Rhythmic twitching of eyelids, eyebrows, or head May be pale Coma	Position: Supine Create safe environment to prevent injury Do not force anything between the teeth; a soft towel or large sponges may be placed while mouth is open Do not restrain Once seizure ends, put in recovery position Monitor vital signs Administer oxygen by nasal cannula or face mask as needed Contact EMS to determine need for transport to hospital
Allergic reaction ■ Delayed (anaphylactic shock)	Skin ■ **Erythema** (rash) ■ **Urticaria** (wheals, itching) ■ **Angioedema** (localized swelling of mucous membranes, lips, larynx, pharynx) Respiratory ■ **Dyspnea** ■ Wheezing ■ Extension of angioedema to larynx: May have obstruction from swelling of vocal apparatus	Skin ■ Administer antihistamine Respiration ■ Position: Upright ■ Administer oxygen by nasal cannula ■ Epinephrine (EpiPen) may be needed if breathing difficulty ■ If airway obstruction: • Position: Supine • Airway maintenance • Determine need to **call EMS**
■ Immediate anaphylaxis	Skin ■ Urticaria (wheals, itching) ■ Flushing ■ Nausea, abdominal cramps, vomiting, diarrhea ■ Angioedema ■ Swelling of lips, membranes, eyelids ■ Laryngeal edema with difficulty swallowing Respiratory ■ Cough, wheezing ■ Dyspnea, airway obstruction ■ Cyanosis Cardiovascular collapse ■ Profound drop in blood pressure ■ Rapid, weak pulse ■ Palpitations ■ Dilation of pupils ■ Loss of consciousness (sudden) ■ Cardiac arrest	Rapid treatment needed; administer epinephrine via autoinjector (EpiPen) **Call EMS** Position: Supine (except when dyspnea predominates) Administer oxygen by nonrebreather mask BLS Monitor vital signs

Emergency	Signs/Symptoms	Procedure
Local anesthesia reactions ■ Psychogenic ■ Allergic (very rare) ■ Toxic overdose	Psychogenic: Reaction to injection, not the anesthetic ■ Syncope ■ Hyperventilation syndrome Allergic Anaphylactic shock ■ Allergic skin and mucous membrane reactions ■ Bronchial asthma attack Toxic: Effects of intravascular injection rather than increased quantity of drug (more common) ■ Stimulation phase • Anxious, restless, apprehensive, confused • Rapid pulse and respirations • Elevated blood pressure • Tremors • Convulsions ■ Depressive phase follows stimulation phase • Drowsiness, lethargy • Shock-like symptoms: Pallor, sweating • Rapid, weak pulse and respirations • Drop in blood pressure • Respiratory depression or respiratory arrest • Unconsciousness	Syncope and/or hyperventilation: See syncope procedure Mild reaction: ■ Stop injection ■ Position: Supine ■ Loosen tight clothing ■ Reassure patient ■ Monitor blood pressure, heart rate, respirations ■ Administer oxygen by nasal cannula Severe reaction: **Call EMS** ■ BLS: maintain airway ■ Administer oxygen by nonrebreather mask ■ Continue to monitor vital signs ■ CPR ■ Administration of anticonvulsant
Opioid overdose Fentanyl overdose	Trouble breathing, very slow breathing, or not breathing Unresponsive Limp, immobile Snoring, gurgling sounds Cold, clammy skin Blue lips, fingernails Drowsiness, lethargy Tiny pupils	Assess for unresponsiveness: **Call EMS** Observe breathing vs. no breathing or only gasping BLS: If unresponsive with no breathing or only gasping, begin CPR Administer naloxone 4- or 8-mg intranasal spray in one nostril (may repeat every 2 to 3 minutes in alternating nostrils until medical assistance becomes available)[27] Assess response: If patient moves purposefully, breathes regularly, moans, or otherwise responds—reassess Continue to monitor responsiveness and breathing until EMS arrives If person stops responding, begin CPR and repeat naloxone Assess response: If no response, continue CPR and use AED if available

Table 9-4 Emergency Reference Chart: Traumatic Injuries

Emergency	Signs/Symptoms	Procedure
Hemorrhage	Prolonged bleeding Spurting blood: Artery Oozing blood: Vein	Compression over bleeding area 1. Apply gauze pack with direct pressure 2. Bandage pack into place firmly where possible 3. Elevate injury above the heart if possible Severe bleeding: Digital pressure on pressure point of supplying vessel If shock symptoms: **Call EMS**
	Bleeding from tooth socket	Pack with folded gauze; do not dab Have patient bite down firmly If bleeding does not stop, instruct patient to gently bite down on a damp tea bag and hold in place for 10 min
	Nosebleed	Seat patient upright, head elevated Tell patient to breathe through mouth Apply cold application to nose Press nostril on bleeding side for a few minutes Advise patient not to blow the nose for 1 hour or more If bleeding does not stop: ■ Wet cotton rolls with water and lubricate with water-soluble lubricant ■ Pack nostril ■ Instruct patient to breathe through the mouth ■ Leave packing in place until patient sees a physician
Chemical burn	Reddened, discolored tissue	Immediate: Copious irrigation with water for 30 min Check directions on chemical container for antidote or other advice Burn caused by acid: Rinse with bicarbonate of soda; burn caused by alkali: rinse in weak acid (e.g., vinegar)
Internal poisoning	Signs of corrosive burn around or in oral cavity Evidence of empty container or information from patient Nausea, vomiting, cramps	Call Poison Control Center: 1-800-222-1222 in the United States. In Canada, visit SafeMedicationUse.ca for poison center telephone listings by province Be calm and supportive Basic life support (BLS): Airway maintenance Artificial ventilation (inhaled poison) Record vital signs Do *not* give water, milk, or Ipecac unless instructed to do so by Poison Control Center Avoid nonspecific and questionably effective antidotes, stimulants, sedatives, or other agents, which may do more harm **Call EMS**
Foreign body in eye	Tears Blinking	Wash hands Ask patient to look down Bring upper lid down over lower lid for a moment; move it upward Turn down lower lid and examine: If particle is visible, remove with moistened cotton applicator Use eye cup: Wash out eye with plain water When unsuccessful, seek medical attention: Prevent patient from rubbing eye by placing gauze pack over eye and stabilizing with adhesive tape

Emergency	Signs/Symptoms	Procedure
Chemical solution in eye	Tears Stinging	Irrigate promptly with copious amounts of water Turn head so water flows away from inner aspect of the eye; continue for 15–20 min
Dislocated jaw	Mouth is open: Patient is unable to close	Stand in front of seated patient Wrap thumbs in towels and place on occlusal surfaces of mandibular posterior teeth Curve fingers and place under body of the mandible Press down and back with thumbs, and at the same time pull up and forward with fingers (**Figure 9-6**) As joint slips into place, quickly move thumbs outward Place bandage around head under chin for support of mandible
Facial fracture	Pain, swelling **Ecchymoses** Deformity, limitation of movement **Crepitation** on manipulation Zygoma fracture: Depression of cheek Mandibular fracture: Abnormal occlusion	Place patient on side BLS Support with bandage around face, under chin, and tied on the top of the head **Call EMS**
Tooth forcibly displaced (avulsed tooth)	Swelling, bruises, or other signs of trauma depending on the type of accident	Instruct patient or parent to hold the tooth by the crown, and avoid touching the root(s) If the tooth is dirty, rinse it gently in cool water, but do not scrub it or remove tissue fragments from its root surface Keep the tooth moist by placing it in milk to transport to dentist Bring the tooth and the patient to dental office or clinic *immediately* The longer the time lapse between avulsion and replantation, the poorer the prognosis
Broken dental instrument during treatment	Instrument tip missing after use in patient's mouth	Examine carefully for broken piece A radiograph may assist in locating the broken segment of the instrument Gently sweep through the sulcus/pocket with a curet or periodontal probe to try to remove broken piece of the instrument Patient may need to be referred to an oral surgeon or periodontist for further evaluation

Documentation

All details about the patient, the treatments, reactions, healing, and comments by the patient provide crucial information in a medical emergency or posttreatment complication.

I. Comprehensive Record Keeping

- All medical findings and changes.
- Treatments provided, including types and amounts of local anesthesia, general anesthesia, nitrous oxide, or other types of sedation.[17]
- Regimens of medications prescribed for patients are crucial information should a medical emergency or a posttreatment complication occur.

II. Consultations

In the patient's record, document telephone and written responses of consultations with physicians or other healthcare providers.[17]

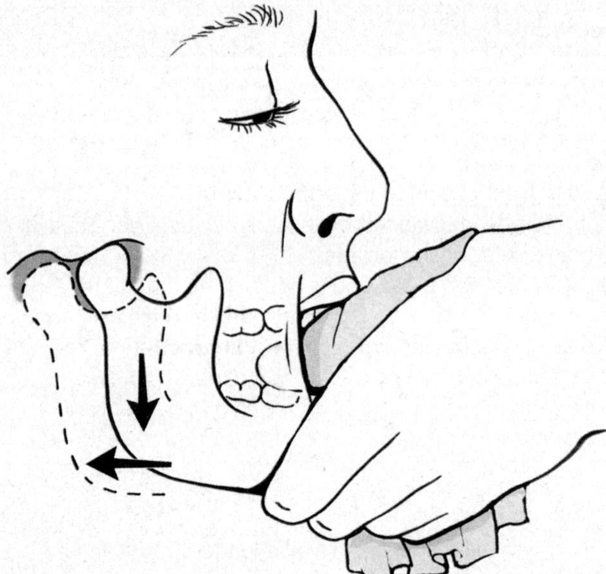

Figure 9-6 Treatment for a Dislocated Mandible. With thumbs wrapped in toweling and placed on the buccal cusps of the mandibular teeth, the fingers are curved under the body of the mandible. The jaw is pressed down and back with the thumbs while pulling up and forward with the fingers to permit the condyle to pass over the articular eminence into its normal position in the glenoid fossa. As the jaw slips into place, the thumbs are moved quickly aside.

III. New Entries

- Response to treatment: Document a patient's reactions and responses to treatments, whether they are unremarkable or remarkable.
- Previous appointment review: Complete a comprehensive review of previous appointment documentation before providing additional treatment at sequential appointments.
- Current information: Update information about the patient's health status, including vital signs as an integral part of the prevention of medical emergencies.[9]
- Emergency documentation: Include a copy of the Medical Emergency Report Form (Figure 9-2) in the patient's permanent record.
- Progress notes: **Box 9-4** contains an example progress note for an emergency that happens during an appointment.

Box 9-4 Example Documentation: Emergency during Patient Treatment

- **S**—Patient experienced blatant signs of anaphylaxis after exposure to latex gloves during a routine scaling appointment.
- **O**—Patient presented with urticaria and **pruritus** on the arms, neck, and chest. Signs of lip, tongue, and laryngeal edema were exhibited with difficulty swallowing and breathing. Quickly informed the patient that he was experiencing an allergic reaction and needed an injection of epinephrine.
- **A**—Findings indicate need for nonlatex gloves and caution during dental appointments, especially when using new materials. At 8 minutes, the patient's vital signs were near baseline. Patient was released to emergency medical services (EMS) after 15 minutes to determine the extent of anaphylaxis. Patient was in stable condition.
- **P**—Epinephrine was administered via EpiPen and EMS was summoned. About 50 mg of Benadryl and 100 mg of Solu-Cortef were also administered intramuscularly. Oxygen was delivered by nonrebreather mask at 15 L/min. A Medical Emergency Report Form was completed and given to EMS with one copy included in the patient's chart and the other sent to the patient's physician.

Signed: __________, DDS or DMD Date: __________
Signed: __________, RDH Date: __________

Factors to Teach the Patient

- Stress/anxiety minimization to prevent emergencies.
- If medications are prescribed by the dentist, review the instructions with the patient to ensure an understanding.
- Schedule appointments when there is no waiting, first appointment of the morning or afternoon.
- Eat breakfast before morning appointment, or lunch before afternoon appointment, unless instructed by the patient's physician not to eat before the appointment.
- If patient has prescription medications for emergency episodes, bring those medications to the appointment. Examples: nitroglycerin tablets for angina, asthma inhaler, glucagon for hypoglycemia.

References

1. Brooks-Buza H, Fernandez R, Stenger JP. The use of in situ simulation to evaluate teamwork and system organization during a pediatric dental clinic emergency. *Simul Healthc.* 2011;6(2):101-108.
2. Skryabina E, Reedy G, Amlot R, et al. What is the value of health emergency preparedness exercises? A scoping review study. *Int J Disaster Risk Reduct.* 2017;21:274-283.
3. Marti K, Sandhu G, Lior A, et al. Simulation-based medical emergencies education for dental students: a three-year evaluation. *J Dent Educ.* 2019;83(8):973-980.
4. Jevon P. Medical emergencies in the dental practice poster: revised and updated. *BDJ Team.* 2020;7(10):38-46.
5. Malamed SF. Medical emergencies in the dental surgery. Part 1: preparation of the office and basic management. *J Irish Dent Assoc.* 2015;61(6):302-308.
6. Vaughan M, Park A, Sholapurkar A, Esterman A. Medical emergencies in dental practice - management requirements and international practitioner proficiency. A scoping review. *Aust Dent J.* 2018;63(4):455-466.
7. Abraham-Inpijn L, Russell G, Abraham DA, et al. A patient-administered Medical Risk Related History questionnaire (EMRRH) for use in 10 European countries (multicenter trial). *Oral Surg Oral Med Oral Pathol Oral Radiol Endod.* 2008;105(5):597-605.
8. de Jong KJM, Borgmeijer-Hoelen A, Abraham-Inpign L. Validity of a risk-related patient-administered medical questionnaire for dental patients. *Oral Surg Oral Med Oral Pathol.* 1991:527-533.
9. Malamed SF. Knowing your patients. *J Am Dent Assoc.* 2010: 3S-7S.
10. Office preparedness (dental office medical emergencies). Lexicomp for Dentistry Online. https://www.wolterskluwer.com/en/solutions/lexicomp/who-we-help/dentists. Accessed September 5, 2021.
11. Reed KL. Basic management of medical emergencies: recognizing a patient's distress. *J Am Dent Assoc.* 2010;141:S20-S24.
12. Smeets EC, de Jong KJM, Abraham-Inpijn L. Detecting the medically compromised patient in dentistry by means of the medical risk-related history. *Prev Med.* 1998;27:530-535.
13. Anders PL, Comeau RL, Hatton M, et al. The nature and frequency of medical emergencies among patients in a dental school setting. *J Dent Educ.* 2010;74(4):392-396.
14. Tanzawa T, Futaki K, Kurabayashi H, et al. Medical emergency education using a robot patient in a dental setting. *Eur J Dent Educ.* 2013;17:e114-e119.
15. Smereka J, Aluchna M, Aluchna A, et al. Medical emergencies in dental hygienists' practice. *Medicine.* 2019;98(30):e16613.
16. Dawoud BE, Roberts A, Yates JM. Drug interactions in general dental practice—considerations for the dental practitioner. *Br Dent J.* 2014;216(1):15-23.
17. Malamed SF. *Medical Emergencies in the Dental Office.* 7th ed. St. Louis, MO: Mosby; 2014:3.
18. Mehra B, Gupta S. Common pediatric medical emergencies in office practice. *Indian J Pediatr.* 2018;85(1):35-43.
19. Appukuttan DP. Strategies to manage patients with dental anxiety and dental phobia: literature review. *Clin Cosmet Investig Dent.* 2016;8:35-50.
20. Rosenberg M. Preparing for medical emergencies. The essential drugs and equipment for the dental office. *J Am Dent Assoc.* 2010;141:S14-S19.
21. Haas DA. Preparing dental office staff members for emergencies. Developing a basic action plan. *J Am Dent Assoc.* 2010;141:S8-S13.
22. Dym H, Barzani G, Mohan N. Emergency drugs for the dental office. *Dent Clin N Am.* 2016;60:287-294.
23. Bost N, Crilly J, Patterson E, et al. Clinical handover of patients arriving by ambulance to a hospital emergency de partment: a qualitative study. *Int Emerg Nurs.* 2012;20: 133-141.
24. Panchal AR, Bartos JA, Cabañas JG, et al. Part 3: Adult Basic and Advanced Life Support: 2020 American Heart Association Guidelines for Cardiopulmonary Resuscitation and Emergency Cardiovascular Care. *Circulation.* 2020; 142(16_suppl_2):S366-S468.
25. American Stroke Association. Stroke symptoms. https://www.stroke.org/en/about-stroke/stroke-symptoms. Accessed September 6, 2021.
26. Centers for Disease Control and Prevention. How to treat low blood sugar. https://www.cdc.gov/diabetes/basics/low-blood-sugar-treatment.html. Accessed September 6, 2021.
27. Naloxone. Lexicomp for Dentistry Online. https://www.wolterskluwer.com/en/solutions/lexicomp/who-we-help/dentists. Accessed September 5, 2021.

SECTION III

Documentation

Introduction for Section III

Maintenance of complete records for every aspect of care provided for each patient is a key aspect of dental hygiene practice.

- Patient records may be kept in many different formats, both handwritten and electronic, in different dental settings.
- Essential factors for legal documentation of all aspects of dental hygiene care include recordkeeping that is:
    - Chronologic (each entry dated).
    - Systematic.
    - Comprehensive.
    - Accurate.
    - Unaltered.
    - Signed by the dental hygienist.

The Dental Hygiene Process of Care

- Documenting patient care is an integral component of each step in the Dental Hygiene Process of Care, as illustrated in **Figure III-1**.
- Every step in the process is documented in each patient record at the initial appointment and at every continuing care or treatment appointment.
- Comprehensive, accurate, and concise documentation of each step forms a complete and chronologic record of the patient's oral health status and treatment over time.

Ethical Applications

- A dental hygienist may be involved in a variety of moral, ethical, and legal situations related to documentation of patient information during practice.
- Understanding the patient record can be subpoenaed in the event of litigation is a basic tenet of ethical and legal risk management for professional practice.
- Knowledge of and adherence to Health Insurance Portability and Accountability Act (HIPAA) (United States) or Personal Information Protection and Electronic Documents Act (PIPEDA) (Canada) requirements for privacy and security of patient records is imperative.
- An overview of the key concepts in patient recordkeeping, with explanations and examples of ethical applications is found in **Table III-1**.

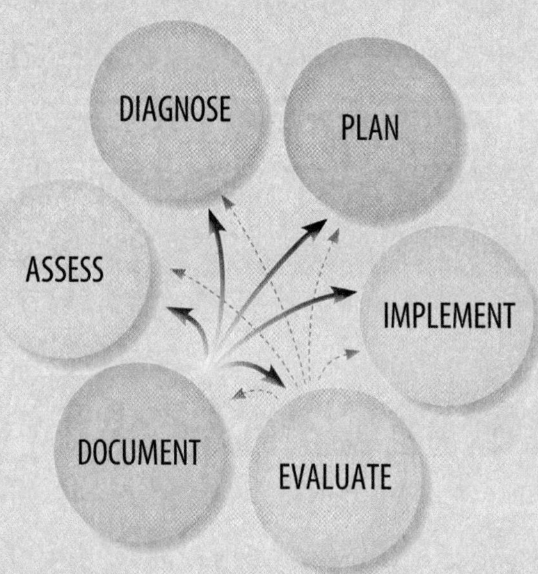

Figure III-1 The Dental Hygiene Process of Care

Table III-1 Essentials of Ethical Record-Keeping

Concept	Explanation	Ethical Application
Privacy	Patient's right to control access to identifiable personal health information.	Unless permission is given, a family member cannot receive information about the patient.
Confidentiality	The responsibility of the healthcare provider to protect patient's information.	HIPAA training is provided for new employees.
Security	Protection against unsecured patient data.	A secure computer network is used or paper records are kept in locked files.
Accuracy	Recorded information is not altered after the fact.	A new entry (dated and signed) is made in the patient's record to correct an error or omission in documentation during the patient appointment.
Authenticity	Only data actually obtained during the patient visit are recorded.	Completely document only what actually happened during a patient visit.
Impersonal/Objective	Personal opinion or negative social observations not pertinent to the patient's treatment are never placed in the patient record.	Uncooperative behavior or noncompliance are documented using subjective, factual statements.

CHAPTER 10

Documentation for Dental Hygiene Care

Linda D. Boyd, RDH, RD, EdD
Christine A. Fambely, DH, BA, MEd

CHAPTER OUTLINE

LEARNING OBJECTIVES

After studying this chapter, the student will be able to:

1. Identify and define key terms and concepts related to written and computerized dental records and charting.
2. Describe concepts related to ensuring confidentiality and privacy of patient information.
3. Compare three tooth numbering systems and apply the one used in your community.
4. Discuss the various components of a patient's comprehensive dental record.
5. Recognize and explain a systematic method for documenting patient care.

The Patient Record

I. Purposes and Characteristics

Complete and accurate documentation of patient assessment and treatment provided at each appointment facilitates communication, coordinates planning among providers, and enhances continuity of care.[1,2]

- **Patient records** serve as a basis for the evaluation of the quality of care (or standard of care) and aid when a review is made of the appropriate care for a patient.[2]
- The dental record is a legal document and is considered legal evidence in any legal or **forensic** situation.[1-3]
- Documentation in a patient record must be[1]:
  - Accurate and comprehensive.
  - Legible.
  - Objective.
- A third party should be able to read and understand what is written.
  - Avoid abbreviations unless a customized list is maintained by the practice or are documented by national dental organizations like the American Dental Association (ADA).[4]
- Patient record entries are:
  - Recorded promptly following treatment.
  - Recorded using clear, concise, objective statements.
  - Dated.
  - Signed by the clinician.

II. Components of a Patient Record

The format of a patient record will vary among private dental practices and clinics; however, essential elements remain consistent regardless of the clinical environment.

- All information collected during the initial examination and during continuing patient appointments is an official part of the permanent records.[2,4,5]
- To meet the dental hygiene standard of care, all components of the dental hygiene process of care are addressed, including the dental hygiene care plan.[6]
- Required components of a complete and regularly updated patient record include[1,5]:
  - Signed acknowledgment of information privacy and confidentiality measures (see HIPAA section in this chapter).
  - Medical history and **vital signs**.
  - Dental and psychosocial history.
  - Risk assessment (e.g. periodontal, caries, oral cancer, tobacco and/or substance use, and diabetes).
  - Clinical assessment including, but not limited to, dental charting, periodontal examination, intraoral images,[6] and radiographs.
  - Diagnosis and prognosis.
  - Treatment recommendations, record of discussion with patient about treatment options, and written treatment plan.
  - Informed consent or informed refusal for treatment.[2,7,8]
  - Treatment notes for each patient visit.
- Additional components, required when applicable, include[2]:
  - Surgery anesthesia records.
  - Study models.
  - Orthodontic records, if available.
  - Laboratory orders and test results.
  - Referral records and copies of consultation correspondence with dental specialists or medical practitioners.

III. The Handwritten Record

Historically, dental healthcare personnel have maintained handwritten documentation of patient records.

- Handwritten records must be recorded legibly in ink.
- Ideally treatment notes are completed within 24 hours[2]; however, if a late entry is necessary[1]:
  - It follows the most recent entry in the patient record.
  - It is clearly noted that it is a late entry with a cross-reference to the original chart entry.
  - It includes the date and time that the late entry was made.
- Mistakes are corrected by placing a single line through the error, writing the correct information immediately after, and signing the entry.[1,2]
- Strict infection control protocols are required to prevent contamination of paper records during patient care.
- For written records, a filing system is needed that provides accessibility to the health records only by authorized personnel.
  - Consult state and local requirements as paper records may have to be secured in a locked cabinet or room when staff is not on-site to monitor access.

IV. The Electronic Health Record

Electronic health records (EHRs) or computerized records have provided an organized mode of gathering, preserving, and sharing patient information with other healthcare professionals or providers.[9,10] The medical community was required to implement EHRs in order to receive Medicare and Medicaid reimbursement beginning in 2014.[11]

A. Benefits of an EHR

- Provides a legible longitudinal record of patient care across healthcare settings over the course of the life span accessible to authorized personnel in real time.[12]
- Has the potential to provide a standardized or structured format to gather key information with the capability for customization.[10]
  - This structured approach can provide reminders so information is not missed and it can improve efficiency of entering information into the patient record.
- Improved information sharing between providers to eliminate duplication of care.[12]
- Allows for monitoring of patient outcomes to ensure quality care and identify areas for improvement.[12]
- Interoperability of EHR systems is essential for sharing of information between medical and dental providers as well as public health entitites.[12,13]
- Allows public health entities to gather data to support decision making (i.e., during the coronavirus disease 2019 [COVID-19] pandemic).[12]
- Although not yet available in dental EHRs, many medical EHR systems allow patients access to their comprehensive health record in a timely manner.[14]
- Access to clinical decision making tools to aid in diagnosis and identification of treatment options.[10,14]

B. Challenges of an EHR

- Security of sharing protected health information (PHI) requires[9,12,14]:
  - Password-protected access to the patient record.
  - **Encryption** when PHI is transferred outside the EHR system.
  - Security measures for the server where data are backed up regularly often require external IT support.
- Creating a standardized format for gathering patient information is a challenge as it requires consensus among all healthcare providers.[5,9]
- Computerized records require computer terminals conveniently located where authorized personnel can access required information.
- Technical and computer skills of healthcare personnel.[12]
  - Support is essential so the workflow is not interrupted, impacting patient care.
  - Patient access to their records can also be impacted by computer skills as well as adequate Internet access.
- Managing safety of the EHR when entering information during patient care may require privacy screens to maintain confidentiality.
- Infection control of computer, keyboard, and mouse can be a challenge during patient care.[15,16]
  - Plastic barriers can be used for computer keyboard and mouse.[17]
  - Voice activated or speech recognition can facilitate clinical documentation and improve accuracy.[18]
  - Foot-activated entry for some patient data (e.g., periodontal probing) is also possible.

The Health Insurance Portability and Accountability Act

- The Health Insurance Portability and Accountability Act (HIPAA) of 1996 took effect for dental practices in the United States on April 14, 2003.
- The law provides federal privacy standards that protect patient records and other health-related information in an emerging electronic information environment.[19]
- The law applies to:
  - Healthcare facilities.
  - Healthcare insurance companies.
  - Healthcare providers.
- Some states may have stricter laws that take priority over the federal standards.
- The current law is divided into two separate components to address:
  - Privacy and the patient's ability to access their health information.
  - Security of patient information in healthcare settings.
- Legislation is also in place in Canada and some European countries to protect the privacy of personal information.[20,21]

- In Canada, healthcare privacy legislation is largely a provincial responsibility.[20]
  - The Personal Information Protection and Electronic Documents Act (PIPEDA) exists at the federal level.
  - There are also specific health privacy acts in most provinces.
  - Dental hygiene colleges/regulatory bodies have their own professional ethical guidelines, which reinforce the jurisdictional acts.

I. The HIPAA Privacy Rule

Establishes a national standard to protect individual's privacy and access to medical records and other health information.[22]

- Patients have the right to:
  - Receive a copy of personal health records.
  - Ask to change incorrect or incomplete information.
  - Receive reports on when, why, and with whom their health information is shared.
  - Decide, in some cases (such as marketing), whether health information can be shared.
  - Ask to be contacted regarding health information in a specific location or by a specific method such as telephone, e-mail, or mail.
  - File a complaint with the provider, health insurer, or the U.S. government regarding concerns about use of their health information.
- Healthcare facilities are responsible for:
  - Developing required privacy and confidentiality forms.
  - Adopting written privacy policies and educating staff about confidentiality of patient information.
  - Appointing staff privacy officers and privacy contact persons.
  - Providing patients with a Notice of Privacy Practices document at the beginning of their care and receiving signed acknowledgment of receipt.
  - Implementing security measures, policies, and formal protocols that protect patient information.
  - Conducting analysis of security risks and vulnerabilities.
  - Establishing sanctions for workforce members who fail to comply with policies.
- Healthcare providers are responsible for:
  - Complying with protocols and practices that protect patient information and avoiding inappropriate disclosure.

II. The HIPAA Security Rule

Updated in 2013 by establishing a national set of standards to strengthen digital security standards and enhance enforcement for protection of health information that is held or transferred in electronic form.[22]

- Comprises three separate standards[22]:
  - Administrative safeguards: Limitation of access to appropriate members in the workforce.
  - Physical safeguards: Use of storage systems and procedures that prevent access for unauthorized individuals.
  - Technical safeguards: Use of technology, such as coding and encryption, to control access to patient information.

Documenting the Extra- and Intraoral Examination

- A specific objective of the extra- and intraoral examination as a part of the total patient assessment is the recognition of deviations from normal that may be signs and **symptoms** of disease. (See Chapter 13.)
- Concentration and attention to a detailed description are necessary so each slight deviation from normal is entered on the record. An intraoral image of any lesion can be very helpful in monitoring changes.[23]

Tooth Numbering Systems

Different systems are used in the various dental offices and clinics worldwide. The three most commonly used tooth designation systems are described here.

I. Universal Numbering System

The universal numbering system (UNS) is used in the United States and it originated in 1880 with Dr. Gustav Parreidt, a German dentist.[24] The ADA adopted the numbering system in 1968. **Figure 10-1** shows the numbers corresponding to each tooth.

A. Permanent Teeth

- Start with the patient's right maxillary third molar (number 1).
- Follow around the arch to the left maxillary third molar (16).
- Descend to the left mandibular third molar (17).
- Follow around to the right mandibular third molar (32).

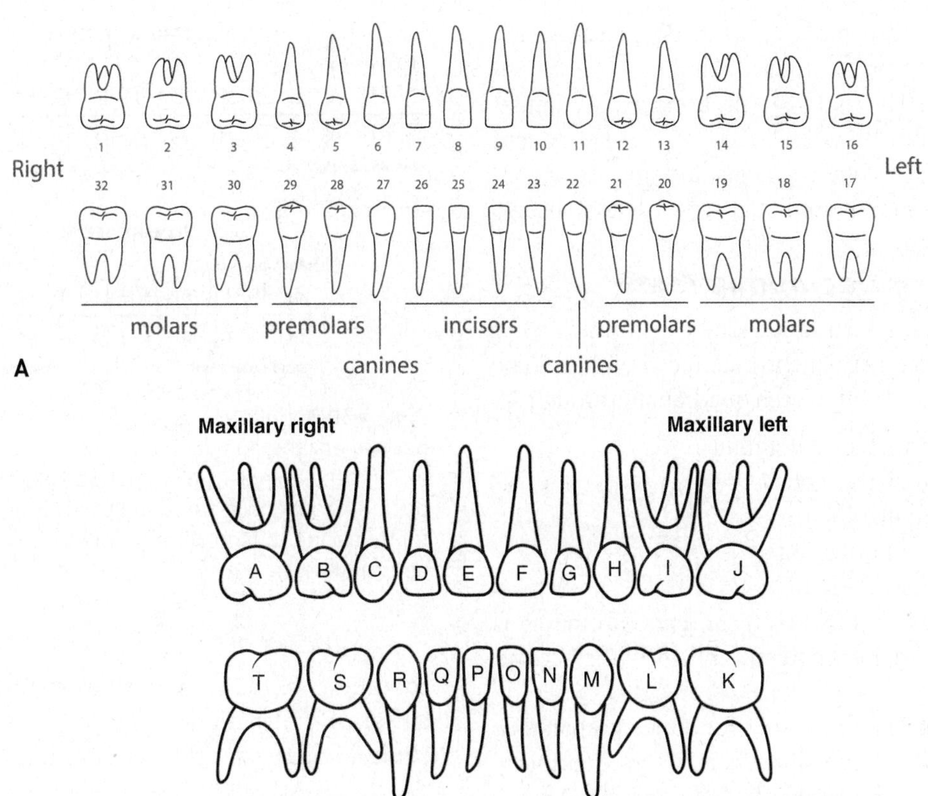

Figure 10-1 Universal Tooth Numbering. **A:** Permanent teeth are designated by numbers 1–32, starting at the maxillary right with 1 and following around to the maxillary left third molar (number 16) to the left mandibular third molar (number 17) and around to the right mandibular third molar (number 32). **B:** Primary teeth are designated by letters in the same sequence

B. Primary or Deciduous Teeth

- Use continuous upper case letters A–T in the same order as described for the permanent teeth.
- Right maxillary second molar (A) around to left maxillary second molar (J).
- Descend to left mandibular second molar (K) and around to the right mandibular second molar (T).

II. Fédération Dentaire Internationale Two Digit

The Fédération Dentaire Internationale system (**Figure 10-2**) is also called the **International** system.[25] The two-digit system uses a unique number for each tooth.

A. Permanent Teeth

Each tooth is identified by the quadrant (1 through 4) represented by the first digit. The second digit will then identify the tooth within the quadrant (1 through 8).

- Quadrant numbers: First digit
  - 1 = Patient's maxillary right
  - 2 = Maxillary left
  - 3 = Mandibular left
  - 4 = Mandibular right
- *Tooth numbers within each quadrant*: Start with number 1 at the midline (central incisor) to

PERMANENT TEETH

Q-1 Maxillary right															Q-2 Maxillary left
18	17	16	15	14	13	12	11	21	22	23	24	25	26	27	28
48	47	46	45	44	43	42	41	31	32	33	34	35	36	37	38
Mandibular right Q-4															Mandibular left Q-3

PRIMARY TEETH

Q-5 Maxillary right									Q-6 Maxillary left
55	54	53	52	51	61	62	63	64	65
85	84	83	82	81	71	72	73	74	75
Mandibular right Q-8									Mandibular left Q-7

Figure 10-2 International Tooth Numbering—Fédération Dentaire Internationale. The first digit indicates the quadrant; the second digit identifies the specific tooth. Each quadrant is numbered 1–4, with number 1 on the patient's maxillary right, number 2 on the maxillary left, number 3 on the mandibular left, and number 4 on the mandibular right. Each tooth in a quadrant is numbered 1–8 from the central incisor. Quadrants of the primary dentition are numbered from 5 through 8.

number 8, third molar. Figure 10-2 shows each tooth number in the four quadrants.

- *Designation*: The digits are pronounced separately. For example, "two-five" (25) is the permanent maxillary left second premolar, and "four-two" (42) is the permanent mandibular right lateral incisor.

B. Primary or Deciduous Teeth

Each tooth is numbered by quadrant (5 through 8) to continue with the permanent quadrant numbers. The teeth are numbered within each quadrant (1 through 5).

- Quadrant numbers: First digit
  - 5 = Maxillary right
  - 6 = Maxillary left
  - 7 = Mandibular left
  - 8 = Mandibular right
- *Tooth numbers within each quadrant:* Number 1 is the central incisor, and number 5 is the second primary molar.
- *Designation*: The digits are pronounced separately. For example, "eight-three" (83) is the primary mandibular right canine, and "six-five" (65) is the primary maxillary left second molar.

III. Palmer Notation System

Originally developed by Adolph Zsigmondy, a Viennese dentist in 1861. However, Corydon Palmer, an Ohio dentist, claimed credit for inventing the tooth numbering system and it became the Palmer System.[26]

A. Permanent Teeth

- Each tooth is designated using the numbers 1 (central incisor) through 8 (third molar) in each quadrant.
- The patient's right and left quadrants for each tooth are designated using a specific pattern of vertical and horizontal lines as shown in **Figure 10-3**.

B. Primary or Deciduous Teeth

- Upper case letters A–E are used instead of numbers to designate each tooth.

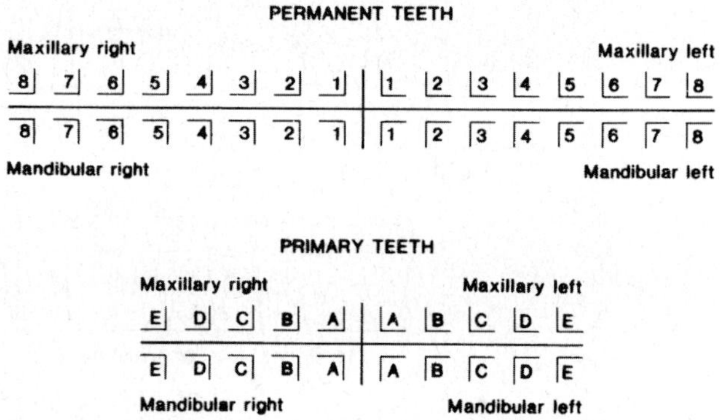

PERMANENT TEETH

Maxillary right															Maxillary left
8	7	6	5	4	3	2	1	1	2	3	4	5	6	7	8
8	7	6	5	4	3	2	1	1	2	3	4	5	6	7	8
Mandibular right															Mandibular left

PRIMARY TEETH

Maxillary right									Maxillary left
E	D	C	B	A	A	B	C	D	E
E	D	C	B	A	A	B	C	D	E
Mandibular right									Mandibular left

Figure 10-3 Palmer System Tooth Numbering. Each permanent tooth is designated by numbers 1–8, starting at the central incisor of each quadrant. Quadrants are designated by horizontal and vertical lines. Primary teeth are identified by the letters A–E, starting at the central incisor.

Charting of Hard and Soft Tissues

I. Purpose

The purpose of each type of **charting** is defined by its title. The dental **chart** (hard tissue) or **odontogram** includes diagrammatic representation of existing conditions of the teeth such as restorations and dental caries. The periodontal chart (soft tissue) includes clinical findings for the periodontium.

- Typically separate chart forms are used to record the dental and periodontal examination findings.
- Each dental and periodontal chart should include the current date to allow changes over time to be assessed.
- It is important for the symbols, drawings, and labels to be accurate representations of the oral condition.
  - In EHRs, charting symbols, etc. are standardized so separate descriptive notes may be necessary.
- An accurate, detailed, and carefully recorded charting is needed for:
  - *Care planning*: The charting is a graphic representation of the existing condition of the patient's teeth and periodontium from which needed treatment procedures can be organized into a treatment plan.
  - *Treatment*: During dental and dental hygiene appointments, the charting is useful for guiding specific procedures.
  - *Evaluation*: The outcome and degree of treatment effects are determined by comparing the findings of the initially recorded examination with periodic follow-up examinations.
  - *Protection*: In the event of a misunderstanding by a patient, or if legal questions should arise, the records and chartings are evidence.
  - *Identification*: In the event of emergency, accident, or disaster, a patient may be identified by the teeth for which a record has been maintained.[3]

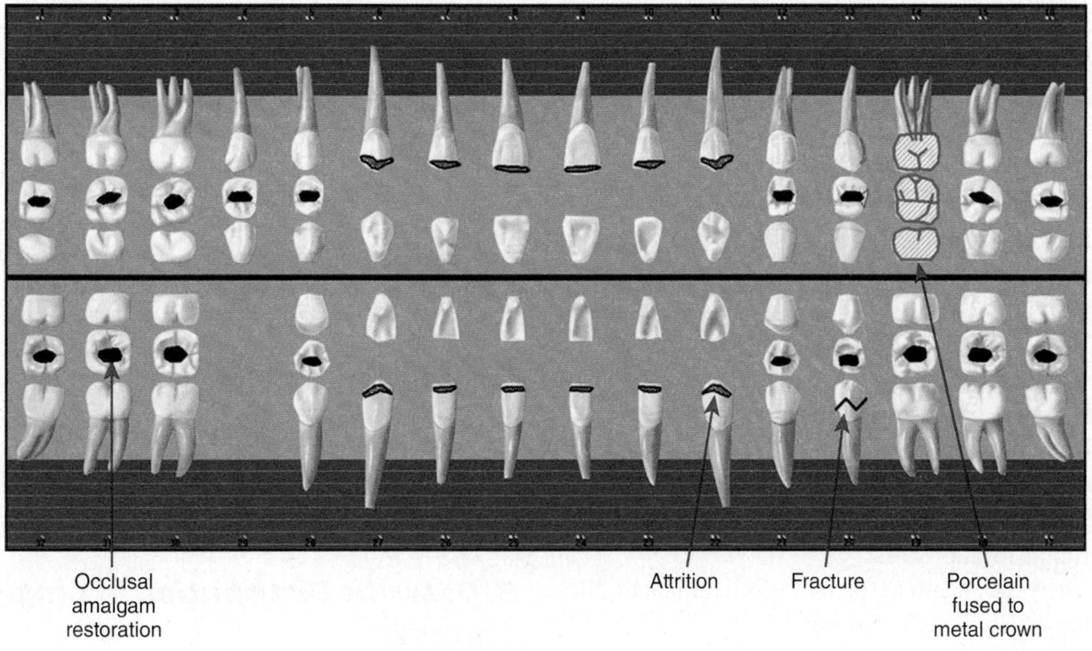

A

T#	1	2	3	4	5	6	7	8	9	10	11	12	13	14	15	16
PD	444	736	723	323	333	434	334	433	434	436	437	535	533	344	324	324
Bld	●●●					●●●	● ●	● ●	● ●	●●●	● ●	●●●		●●●	●●●	●●●
Sup																
GM	222	101	111	111	101	202	202	111	212	121	212	211	212	222	111	111
CAL	222	635	632	212	232	232	132	342	242	355	245	344	341	122	213	213
MG	545	556	656	657	657	669	659	655	337	648	859	959	645	545	545	444
FG			100											100	100	
TC														C		
PMB																
PD	546	436	635	633	324	212	212	323	333	323	324	414	325	335	335	644
Bld																
Sup																
GM	333	213	213	201	101	101	101	101	001	101	111	111	112	102	102	312
CAL	213	243	442	432	223	111	111	222	332	222	233	323	233	233	233	332
MG																
PD	545	535	533		324	423	323	323	323	323	323	323	534	436	636	645
Bld	●●●	● ●	●		●	●●●	●●●	●●●	●●●	●●●	●●●	●●●	● ●	● ●	● ●	●●●
Sup																
GM	222	111	101		111	111	111	121	111	111	111	111	112	332	222	222
CAL	323	424	432		435	532	434	444	434	434	434	232	442	104	414	423
MG																
FG														10	10	
TC				M												
PMB																
PD	535	534	533		333	334	424	533	424	335	524	433	323	436	325	535
Bld	●●●	●●●	●			●	● ●	●	● ●	●	● ●	●		● ●	●	● ●
Sup																
GM	222	212	212		111	011	101	101	111	112	111	111	111	111	111	211
CAL	313	342	321		444	343	323	432	333	243	433	344	234	347	236	346
MG	444	546	755		535	657	757	757	757	748	737	545	546	545	545	545
T#	32	31	30	29	28	27	26	25	24	23	22	21	20	19	18	17

KEY	
PD	Pocket Depth
Bld	Bleeding
Sup	Suppuration
GM	Gingival margin
CAL	Clinical attachment level
MG	Mucogingival
FG	Furcation
PMB	Mobility
TC	Missing teeth

B

Figure 10-4 Periodontal and Dental Charting. **A:** Example of dental charting notations. **B:** Example of computerized periodontal charting with key.

II. Forms Used for Charting

Many variations of chart forms are available both in paper and electronic format.

- Anatomic drawings of the teeth: **Figure 10-4** provides typical examples of EHR forms for periodontal and dental charting.
- Geometric: A diagrammatic representation that provides space to record findings for each tooth. Examples of geometric charting forms used to record a patient's disclosed biofilm for teaching personal disease control are shown in Chapter 21.

III. Sequence for Charting

A. Basic Entries

- Personal information.
- Date of appointment: Every entry must be dated.

- Missing teeth: Mark the missing teeth on the paper chart or EHR tooth chart. When radiographs are available in advance, missing teeth may be charted before the clinic appointment.

B. Systematic Procedure

- An accurate odontogram is a systematic representation of both intraoral clinical findings and radiographic findings.
- The use of a set routine is essential for a complete and accurate charting.
- Charting all of one item for the entire mouth, rather than complete charting of one tooth, helps to ensure accuracy.
  - For example, in the dental charting, record all the restorations first.
  - Then start again at the first tooth and chart all the deviations from normal.
  - Missing teeth.
  - Location of crowns, bridges, and implants.
  - Charting all restorations and deviations for each tooth separately is less efficient.
- Prepare entries that are objective, descriptive, and easily understood by other providers who read them and use them in continuing treatment.
- Additions to the records are made to show the progress of treatment and comparative observations throughout the treatment and at continuing care appointments.
- After completing treatment, a continuing care plan is outlined.

C. Radiographic Evaluation

- If the radiographs are available prior to the patient's arrival for the appointment, radiographic evaluation can be performed and the following may be noted:
  - Missing or impacted teeth.
  - Endodontic treatment.
  - Overhanging margins of existing restorations.
  - Suspicious carious lesions to evaluate further during the clinical examination.
  - Furcation radiolucency can be noted for further evaluation during the periodontal examination.
  - Radiographic bone loss (RBL) can be recorded to assist in periodontal staging.
  - Other deviations from normal evident from the radiographs.

D. Study Models

Study models are useful to record details related to occlusion. (See Chapter 16.)

Periodontal Records

I. Clinical Observations of the Gingiva

Clinical observations are recorded either on the chart form or in the patient clinic or progress notes during each patient visit. Examine gingiva and record findings before disclosing agent is used to assess the biofilm score.

A. Describe Gingiva

- Color, size, position, shape, consistency, and surface texture; extent of bleeding when probed; and areas where there is minimal attached gingiva. (See Chapter 18.)

B. Describe Distribution of Gingival Changes

- Localized or generalized; specify the areas with disease involvement as mild, moderate, or severe. Use tooth numbers to identify adjacent gingival tissue.

II. Items to Be Charted

- Gingival margin and mucogingival junction (MGJ) lines.
- Probing depths.
- Recession.
- Areas of suspected mucogingival involvement.
- Furcation involvement.
- Abnormal frenal attachments.
- Mobility and fremitus of teeth.

III. Deposits

Deposits can be recorded on dental index forms. These are illustrated in Chapter 21.

A. Stains

- Extrinsic: Record type of stain, color, and distribution; specific location by tooth number; and whether slight, moderate, or heavy.
- Intrinsic: Record separately from extrinsic and identify by type when known.

B. Soft Deposits

- Dental biofilm:
  - Record direct observations with or without disclosing agent; include distribution and degree or amount.
  - Record biofilm index or score as described in Chapter 21.

C. Calculus

- Record distribution and amount of supragingival and subgingival calculus separately for treatment planning purposes.

IV. Factors Related to Occlusion

The following list is for consideration with other records for the treatment planning. Clinical signs of trauma from occlusion are described in Chapter 16.

A. Mobility of Teeth

- Record degree of mobility for each tooth. (See Chapter 20.)

B. Fremitus

- Record the significance in relation to mobility.
- Fremitus determination is described in Chapter 20.

C. Possible Food Impaction Areas

- Ask the patient where fibrous foods usually catch between the teeth.
- Use dental floss to identify inadequate (open) contact areas that may contribute to food impaction. An example of one method for recording an open contact on a paper chart is with vertical parallel lines between teeth.

D. Occlusion-Related Habits

- Observe for evidence of, and question patient concerning, parafunctional habits, such as bruxism or clenching.
- Note wear patterns and facets.
- Note attrition.

V. Radiographic Findings

Specific notes are made to correlate the radiographic findings with the clinical observations just listed.

- If not completed prior to arrival of the patient, the following should be recorded:
    - Height of bone as related to the cemento-enamel junction (radiographic bone loss).
    - Horizontal or angular shape of remaining interdental bone.
    - Root proximity.
    - Intact, broken, or missing crestal lamina dura.
    - Furcation involvement.
    - Widening of periodontal ligament space.
    - Overhanging fillings, large carious lesions, and other dental biofilm–retention factors.
- Details of radiographic findings in periodontal disease are described in Chapter 20.

VI. Severity of Periodontal Disease

Determination of the severity of periodontal disease is based on analysis of gingival and alveolar bone changes.

- Clinical assessment procedures include periodontal probing recordings, bleeding on probing, clinical attachment level, suppuration, tooth mobility, fremitus, and the radiographic findings.[27]
- A dental or dental hygiene diagnosis statement can be developed using the disease classifications for staging and grading outlined in Chapter 19.

Dental Records

- The patient's permanent records include the clinical and radiographic findings related to the teeth, periodontal descriptors, and subjective symptoms reported by the patient.
- Occlusion and mobility of teeth may be documented during the dental or periodontal examination.
- At least annually, the dental and periodontal records should be updated to allow for comparison and monitor progress.
- Information about conditions related to the teeth as included in Chapter 16.

I. The Anatomic Tooth Chart Form

Figure 10-4 provides an example of a dental charting using anatomic tooth drawings. When charting, clinical and radiographic findings are coordinated.

II. Items to Be Charted

A list of basic items to be charted includes[27]:

- Missing teeth.
- Unerupted or supernumerary teeth.
- Existing restorations and the type of restorative materials.
- Fixed and removable prostheses.
- Dental sealants.
- Abrasion and erosion.
- Overhangs, open contacts, open margins, and other irregularities.
- Noncavitated and cavitated carious lesions.

- Inadequate contact areas and proximal surface overhangs or defects.
  - Dental floss can aid in identifying these issues.
- If indicated, pulp vitality.

Care Plan Records

- Along with a comprehensive dental treatment plan, a formal dental hygiene care plan that includes the patient's modifiable risk factors, diagnosis, preventive care plan, and nonsurgical periodontal therapy if indicated becomes part of the permanent patient record. (See Chapter 23.)

Informed Consent

- Documentation of informed consent or informed refusal prior to initiating treatment is an essential component of each patient's record.[7,27,28]
- Information about obtaining and documenting informed consent is found in Chapter 23.

Documentation of Patient Visits

I. Purpose

Documentation completed during or immediately following a patient visit, sometimes referred to as a progress note, is a chronologic history of treatment received by the patient during each appointment.[27]

II. Essentials of Good Progress Notes

- Dental hygiene progress notes document all aspects of the dental hygiene process of care and record all interactions between the patient and the practice.[4]
- In addition to documentation about treatment rendered, essential components of a patient progress note are listed in **Box 10-1**.
- Each entry in the patient record is dated and signed by the clinician.
- Only standard medical and dental abbreviations and symbols should be used, such as those recommended by the ADA.
  - If the office or clinic has preferred abbreviations or symbols, they should be documented in an office manual.[4]

Box 10-1 Essential Components of a Patient Progress Note

- Purpose of the visit
- History review
- Assessment findings
- Description of treatment provided
- Drugs (including topical or local anesthetic) administered during treatment or prescribed by the dentist
- Oral self-care and other instructions provided
- Referrals, consultations with physician or dental specialist
- Laboratory tests ordered; results of laboratory tests
- Next visit appointments scheduled or recommended; appointment cancellations
- Objective reporting of patient conversations, including telephone and e-mail
- Signature of clinician and date

- Remember to be objective in recording the accurate patient information and treatment.
  - The chart record is a legal document and could be used in a malpractice complaint.
  - HIPAA rules also allow the patient to request a copy of their records.

III. Systematic Documentation: The SOAP Approach

A systematic, standardized approach to writing patient progress notes assures that no details are missing from the patient's record.

- Many clinicians and most electronic patient record systems have developed their own systematic approach to recording patient information.
- Templates can be created in EHRs and used to make sure documentation is comprehensive.
- One approach, which uses the acronym *SOAP* as a guide, is well accepted for use in the medical and dental professions and is recommended for use by the American Pediatric Dentistry Association.[29-31]
  - S = Subjective.
  - O = Objective.
  - A = Assessment (or analysis).
  - P = Procedures (provided or planned).
- **Table 10-1** further defines the components of the SOAP acronym and provides examples of factors that are included in patient progress notes.

Table 10-1 Components of SOAP Documentation and Examples of Factors to Include in Progress Notes [29,30]

Description		Examples
S	Subjective (patient report)	■ Age and gender ■ Treatment planned for the appointment ■ Medical history provided by the patient ■ Medications and allergies ■ Patient's chief complaint ■ Patient's oral self-care regimen ■ Social history
O	Objective (observations of clinician or results of clinical examination)	■ Vital signs ■ Head and neck examination findings ■ Periodontal examination findings, bleeding, soft tissue condition ■ Hard tissue examination findings (e.g., cavitated and noncavitated lesions) ■ Radiographic findings ■ Comparison of current findings with previous findings
A	Assessment (diagnosis)	■ Risk factors for oral disease ■ Oral disease risk level, such as caries, periodontal, oral cancer ■ Dental biofilm and calculus level ■ Current periodontal diagnosis (stage and grade)
P	Plans (care or treatment provided)	■ Dental hygiene treatment provided ■ Medicaments or local anesthesia provided with details about location ■ Consult with dentist or other health providers ■ Oral self-care instructions ■ Goals for patient improvement ■ Pending/planned dental hygiene interventions

Data from American Dental Association. Templates Smart Phrases and SOAP. Accessed December 5, 2021. https://www.ada.org/resources/practice/practice-management/templates-smart-phrases-and-soap; Podder V, Lew V, Ghassemzadeh S. SOAP Notes. In: StatPearls. StatPearls Publishing; 2021. Accessed December 11, 2021. http://www.ncbi.nlm.nih.gov/books/NBK482263/

- **Box 10-2** provides an example of documentation for a patient visit written using the SOAP format.
- Additional documentation examples, each related to a clinical situation and formatted using the SOAP approach, can be reviewed near the end of each chapter of this book.

IV. Risk Reduction and Legal Considerations

- **Malpractice** allegations or complaints to the state dental board can, unfortunately, occur against even a dental hygienist who routinely meets every standard when providing dental hygiene according to the standards of care.
- Because complaints or litigation can occur years after the patient visit when the details and even the patient may have been forgotten, comprehensive documentation in each patient record entry is the best protection for the clinician against allegations of wrongdoing.

Box 10-2 Example of Patient Care Documentation: Using the SOAP Format

- **S**—Patient presents for reassessment of oral self-care 2 weeks following oral self-care instruction. Patient states that he notices a reduction in biofilm after applying what he learned at the previous appointment.
- **O**—Today's "Plaque-Free Score" = 89%; sulcus bleeding index (SBI) score = 2.
- **A**—"Plaque-Free Score" compared with previous score of 22%; SBI score compared with previous score of 5. Significant improvement in biofilm control noted in all areas except buccal surfaces of maxillary molars.
- **P**—Patient congratulated on areas of success. Additional instruction provided specifically related to biofilm removal on posterior buccal and proximal tooth surfaces. Patient observed while brushing and flossing maxillary molar areas using a mirror. Next visit: 3-month reevaluation.

Signed: ______________________, RDH
Date: ______________________

Factors to Teach the Patient

- Interpretation of all recordings; meaning of all numbers used, such as for probing depths.
- The importance of conducting a comprehensive examination of the patient before beginning treatment.
- Advantages of cooperation and patience in furnishing information to help dental personnel to interpret observations so an accurate diagnosis can be made to identify treatment options for the patient based on their individual needs.
- Assurance that all information received is confidential.

References

1. Hadden AM, FGDP(UK) Clinical Examination and Record-Keeping Working Group. Clinical examination & record-keeping: Part 1: Dental records. *Br Dent J*. 2017;223(10): 765-768.
2. American Dental Association. Writing in the dental record. https://www.ada.org/resources/practice/practice-management/writing-in-the-dental-record. Accessed December 5, 2021.
3. Forrest A. Forensic odontology in DVI: current practice and recent advances. *Forensic Sci Res*. 2019;4(4):316-330.
4. American Dental Association. Dental abbreviations, acronyms, and symbols for charting. https://www.ada.org/resources/practice/practice-management/dental-abbreviations-acronyms-and-symbols. Accessed December 5, 2021.
5. Tokede O, Ramoni RB, Patton M, Da Silva JD, Kalenderian E. Clinical documentation of dental care in an era of electronic health record use. *J Evid-Based Dent Pract*. 2016;16(3):154-160.
6. Wander P. Dental photography in record keeping and litigation. *Br Dent J*. 2014;216(4):207-208.
7. Blum IR, Hooper S. Consent to treatment in the post-Montgomery era: principles and implications for the dental team. *Prim Dent J*. 2019;8(2):40-48.
8. Ward J, Kalsi D, Chandrashekar A, et al. Shared decision making and consent post-Montgomery, UK Supreme Court judgement supporting best practice. *Patient Educ Couns*. 2020;103(12):2609-2612.
9. Hadden AM, FGDP(UK) Clinical Examination and Record-Keeping Working Group. Clinical examination & record-keeping: Part 3: Electronic records. *Br Dent J*. 2017; 223(12):873-876.
10. Joda T, Waltimo T, Probst-Hensch N, Pauli-Magnus C, Zitzmann NU. Health data in dentistry: an attempt to master the digital challenge. *Public Health Genomics*. 2019;22(1-2):1-7.
11. Agency for Healthcare Research and Quality. Module 17. Electronic Health Records and Meaningful Use. Published May 2013. https://www.ahrq.gov/ncepcr/tools/pf-handbook/mod17.html. Accessed December 9, 2021.
12. Fennelly O, Cunningham C, Grogan L, et al. Successfully implementing a national electronic health record: a rapid umbrella review. *Int J Med Inf*. 2020;144:104281.
13. Centers for Disease Control and Pevention. Public Health Data Interoperability. Published December 6, 2021. https://www.cdc.gov/datainteroperability/index.html. Accessed December 9, 2021.
14. Sulmasy LS, López AM, Horwitch CA, American College of Physicians Ethics, Professionalism and Human Rights Committee. Ethical implications of the electronic health record: in the service of the patient. *J Gen Intern Med*. 2017;32(8): 935-939.
15. Ledwoch K, Dancer SJ, Otter JA, Kerr K, Roposte D, Maillard JY. How dirty is your QWERTY? The risk of healthcare pathogen transmission from computer keyboards. *J Hosp Infect*. 2021;112:31-36.
16. Patel S, Porter K, Sammons RL. Are computer keyboards a cross-infection risk in a dental clinic? *J Infect Prev*. 2010; 11(6):206-211.
17. Porter SJ, Porter K, Sammons RL. Efficacy of cling film for barrier protection in a dental clinical environment: short communication. *J Infect Prev*. 2011;12(2):60-63.
18. Blackley SV, Huynh J, Wang L, Korach Z, Zhou L. Speech recognition for clinical documentation from 1990 to 2018: a systematic review. *J Am Med Inform Assoc JAMIA*. 2019;26(4):324-338.
19. Office for Civil Rights (OCR). HIPAA for professionals. Published September 10, 2015. https://www.hhs.gov/hipaa/for-professionals/index.html. Accessed December 5, 2021.
20. Office of the Privacy Commissioner of Canada. Summary of privacy laws in Canada. Published May 15, 2014. https://www.priv.gc.ca/en/privacy-topics/privacy-laws-in-canada/02_05_d_15/. Accessed December 5, 2021.
21. European Union. General data protection regulation (GDPR) compliance guidelines. GDPR.eu. https://gdpr.eu/. Accessed December 5, 2021.
22. Office for Civil Rights (OCR). Summary of the HIPAA security rule. Published July 26, 2013. https://www.hhs.gov/hipaa/for-professionals/security/laws-regulations/index.html. Accessed December 9, 2021.
23. Hadden AM, FGDP(UK) Clinical Examination and Record-Keeping Working Group. Clinical examination & record-keeping: Part 2: History taking. *Br Dent J*. 2017;223(11):823-825.
24. Parreidt J. *A Compendium of Dentistry for the Use of Students and Practitioners*. W.T. Keener; 1880.
25. Turp JC, Alt KW. Designating teeth: the advantages of the FDI's two-digit system. *Quintessence Int*. 1995;26(7): 501-504.
26. Harris EF. Tooth-coding systems in the clinical dental setting. *Dent Anthropol J*. 2005;18(2):43-49.
27. American Dental Hygienists' Association. *2016 Revised Standards for Clinical Dental Hygiene Practice*. Published June 2016. https://www.adha.org/resources-docs/2016-Revised

-Standards-for-Clinical-Dental-Hygiene-Practice.pdf. Accessed December 11, 2021.

28. American Dental Association. Types of consent. https://www.ada.org/resources/practice/practice-management/types-of-consent. Accessed December 11, 2021.
29. American Dental Association. Templates, smart phrases and SOAP. https://www.ada.org/resources/practice/practice-management/templates-smart-phrases-and-soap. Accessed December 5, 2021.
30. Podder V, Lew V, Ghassemzadeh S. SOAP Notes. In: *StatPearls*. StatPearls Publishing; 2021. http://www.ncbi.nlm.nih.gov/books/NBK482263/. Accessed December 11, 2021.
31. American Academy of Pediatric Dentistry. Record-keeping. In: *The Reference Manual of Pediatric Dentistry*. Chicago, IL: American Academy of Pediatric Dentistry; 2021:484-491. https://www.aapd.org/globalassets/media/policies_guidelines/bp_recordkeeping.pdf. Accessed December 11, 2021.

SECTION IV

Assessment

Introduction for Section IV

Assessment in dental hygiene practice is the collection of pertinent facts, clinical data, and dental materials, such as radiographs and study models related to the patient's oral health and overall health status.

- Initial assessment data are used:
  - In planning care.
  - As a guide during all treatment.
- After care has been provided, assessment data must be gathered again to evaluate the outcomes of the dental hygiene interventions.
- An efficiently conducted assessment and critical analysis of assessment findings:
  - Provide a permanent, continuing, accurate, and complete record of the patient's oral and general health.
  - Help formulate dental hygiene diagnostic statements from which a patient-oriented dental hygiene care plan can be prepared to include individualized preventive and treatment interventions.
  - Guide instrumentation during dental hygiene treatment.
  - Provide the basis to correlate dental hygiene care with the comprehensive dental treatment plan.

The Dental Hygiene Process of Care

- Assessment is the first step in the dental hygiene process of care, as illustrated in **Figure IV-1**.
- Critical analysis of the data identifies the patient's problems, which are used to formulate the dental hygiene diagnosis and develop an individualized care plan.
- Comprehensive and accurate assessment data aid the dental hygienist in identifying:
  - Health-related factors affecting the management of dental hygiene care.
  - Risk factors for oral or systemic disease.
  - Description of personal and culturally related habits affecting oral status.
  - Health-related attitudes of the patient and the value placed on maintenance of oral health and the prevention of disease.
  - Oral hygiene methods and communication strategies that meet the patient's needs.
- Built into the sequence of clinical procedures is the initiation of steps for arresting oral disease processes, controlling etiologic factors, and preventing episodes of recurrence of oral disease.

Ethical Applications

- An ethical theory, often based on norms or rules that ask which type of action is morally correct, offers a general approach to an ethical problem.
- A dental professional may consider the most favorable outcome of a particular situation, what guidelines to follow, or whether to rely on personal and professional virtues when making a judgment.
- A few of the many philosophical theories that apply to the delivery of dental care, with corresponding definitions, are described in **Table IV-1**.

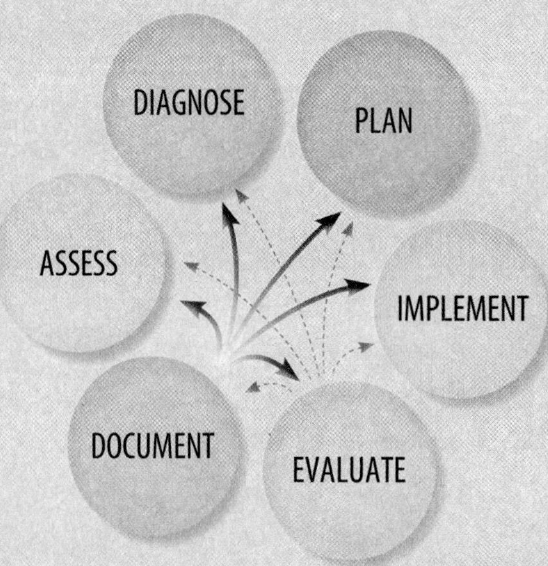

Figure IV-1 The Dental Hygiene Process of Care

Table IV-1 Some Ethical Theories

Theory	Definition	Application Examples
Deontology	A study of rules by following the proper duties or obligations pertaining to one's role.	The dental hygienist must complete accurate and detailed documentation of the services rendered for every patient.
Rights theory	Focusing on what is rightfully due to both patients and providers.	A patient has the right to be informed of what treatment the dental hygienist will perform.
Teleology	Concerned with the consequences or usefulness of one's actions; goal-driven.	A dental hygienist provides chairside education that meets the individual needs of the patient.
Utilitarianism	A form of teleology that says an action is good if it brings about the greatest pleasure for the greatest number of people.	Dental insurance companies set limits of reimbursement based on how a procedure is coded.
Virtue ethics	A moral theory that is concerned with the virtuous qualities of a professional's character (compassion, empathy, honesty, respect, wisdom, patience).	Always being honest and offering the best care to every patient.

CHAPTER 11

Medical, Dental, and Psychosocial Histories

Linda D. Boyd, RDH, RD, EdD

CHAPTER OUTLINE

LEARNING OBJECTIVES

After studying this chapter, the student will be able to:

1. Relate and define key terms and concepts utilized in the creation of patient histories.
2. Explain the significance and purpose of accurate and complete patient medical, dental, and psychosocial histories.
3. Compare and contrast the different methods available for the compilation of patient histories and the advantages and disadvantages of each.
4. Discuss how the components of patient histories relate directly to the application of patient care.

Purpose of History Taking

For safe, evidence-based dental and dental hygiene care, a thorough patient health history is an essential part of the complete assessment.[1-3] Thorough medical, dental, and psychosocial histories are used in comprehensive patient care to:

- Provide information pertinent to the etiology and diagnosis of oral conditions and the patient care plan.
- Give insight into psychosocial factors that may affect patient treatment and compliance with recommendations.
  - Identify cultural beliefs and practices that affect risk for oral disease.
  - Determine ethnic/racial influences on risk factors for oral disease.
- Reveal medical conditions that necessitate precautions, modifications, or adaptations during treatment to ensure dental and dental hygiene procedures will not harm the patient and to prevent an emergency situation.
  - In some cases, this may require a patient to seek medical care and receive clearance before treatment is performed.[2]
- Aid in the identification of possible unrecognized conditions for which the patient will be referred for further diagnosis and treatment.
- Permit appraisal of the general health and nutritional status, which, in turn, contributes to the prognosis of outcomes of patient care.
- Document records for reference and comparison over a series of appointments for periodic follow-up.
- Provide evidence in case of a legal issue.

History Preparation

The general methods in current use for obtaining a health history are the *interview*, the *questionnaire* (which may be paper or electronic), or a combination of the two. There are several methods for obtaining the history.

I. Methods

- Preappointment information
  - Basic information obtained before the initial assessment appointment can save time and facilitate the process.
  - A phone screening or teledentistry[4] interview can help determine potential medical problems, need for premedication or consultation with the patient's primary care provider (PCP), and medically compromised or physically challenged patients for whom modifications in routine care may be needed.
- History form completion
  - The history form can be provided online for the patient to download and complete, sent via e-mail, or mailed to the patient in advance of the first appointment.
  - This kind of form might include some items that can be checked or circled, with space to allow the patient to provide additional information.
- Comprehensive history
  - A comprehensive patient history must be gathered at the initial visit and is a combination of interview and questionnaire.
  - At each appointment, the history is reviewed with the patient for any changes so adjustment can be made to patient care as needed.
  - The comprehensive history should be updated annually.[1]

II. Record Forms

- Basic history forms
  - Paper forms are available commercially or from the American Dental Association (ADA) for a fee, but dental offices/clinics may prefer to develop their own.
  - ADA and other organizations have basic history forms translated into a variety of languages.
  - Electronic health (dental) systems have templates for the history and many can be customized.
- An adequate basic history form will:
  - Enable the recording of important details in a logical sequence.
  - Permit quick identification of special needs of a patient before the appointment.
  - Allow space to record the patient's own words from the interview or for notations by the patient on a questionnaire.
  - Have space for notes concerning attitudes and knowledge as stated or displayed by the patient during the history taking.
  - If a translator is not available, the form should be provided in the patient's preferred language.

III. Introduction to the Patient

- Patient education about why the information requested in the history is essential before treatment can be begin.

- Educate about the relationship between general or systemic health and oral health.
- To build rapport, allow children to participate in their history preparation, but most of the information will need to be supplied by a parent or legal guardian. The signature of the responsible adult is required on the record.

IV. Limitations of a History

Many patients cannot or will not provide complete or, in certain cases, correct information when answering medical or dental history questions. Reasons for inaccuracy or incompleteness of information can include:

- Problems related to the method of obtaining the histories, how the questions are worded, or an inadvertent lack of neutrality in the attitude of the person gathering the history.
- Difficulty in understanding because the patient cannot read or has a language barrier.
- The location in which the questionnaire is completed, such as a crowded reception area without sufficient privacy.
- The patient may withhold information, thinking there is no relationship between certain diseases or conditions and dental treatment.
- Reluctance to discuss a health condition that may be embarrassing, such as history of infectious or communicable disease. The patient may fear refusal of treatment.
- Cognitive impairment may impact the ability to understand questions or the patient may not be able to recall important information, which occurs in conditions such as traumatic brain injury or dementia.

The Questionnaire

A questionnaire by itself cannot be expected to satisfy the overall purposes of the history, but it can provide some basic personal history, dental history, and factual information in the medical history. During the interview, any positive responses on a questionnaire require further investigation with open-ended questions.[5]

I. Types of Questions

Figure 11-1 and **Figure 11-2** provide useful examples of questions necessary for a thorough patient evaluation.

- *System oriented*
  - Direct questions to determine if the patient has had a disease. Often the questions are organized as a review of body systems (e.g., the digestive system, respiratory system, or urinary system).
  - The questions may contain references to specific organs (e.g., the stomach, lungs, or kidneys).
- *Disease oriented*
  - A typical set of questions may start with "Do you have, or have you had, any of the following diseases or problems?"
  - A listing under that question contains items such as diabetes, asthma, or hypertension arranged alphabetically or grouped by systems or body organs.
  - Follow-up questions can determine dates of illness, severity, and outcome.
- *Symptom oriented*
  - In the absence of previous or current disease states, questions may lead to a suspicion of a condition, which, in turn, can provide an opportunity to recommend and refer the patient to schedule an examination with a PCP.
  - Examples of the symptom-oriented questions are "Are you thirsty much of the time?" "Have you lost weight without trying?" or "Do you have to urinate frequently during the day and/or at night?"
    - Positive answers could lead to tests for diagnosis of diabetes.
- *Culture oriented*
  - Identify ethnic or gender-related increase in risk for systemic or oral disease.
  - Determine traditional, culturally related health beliefs that may influence dental hygiene interventions or recommendations.
  - Identify herbal preparations or other traditional medications used by the patient that may affect oral care or risk for disease.

II. Advantages of a Questionnaire

- Broad in scope; useful during the interview to identify positive answers needing additional clarification.
- Time saving.
- Systematic in gathering information.
- Patient has time to think over the answers—not under pressure from the interviewer.
- Patient may write information that might not be expressed directly in an interview.
- Legal aspects of a written or an electronic record with the patient's signature.

Medical Information

Please provide the name, address, and phone number of your physician or primary care provider
None ☐

Primary care provider's first name **Primary care provider's last name**

Address **City** **State** **Zipcode**

Phone number

Date of last physical examination: ____________________
Month Year

Have you ever been hospitalized for any surgical operation or serious illness? Yes ☐ No ☐
If you answered yes, when were you hospitalized and for what? ____________________

Your height: ____________________ **Current weight:** ____________________
Feet Inches lbs

Are you wearing contact lenses? Yes ☐ No ☐

Dental Information

Please provide the name, address, and phone number of your previous dentist
None ☐

Dentist's first name **Dentist's last name**

Address/zip code **City** **State**

Phone number: ____________________

Last dental visit: ____________ Reason for the dental visit: ____________________

Name of your dental insurance co.: ____________________ Group & ID number: ____________

Mark your answer with an (X)

1. Is it important for you to keep your teeth	Yes ☐	No ☐
2. Has your medical/dental provider told you that you need to take an antibiotic prior to dental treatment?	Yes ☐	No ☐
3. Do you become anxious about having dental treatment?	Yes ☐	No ☐
4. Do you have pain or sensitivity in your mouth or teeth?	Yes ☐	No ☐
5. Have you previously or do you currently have any mouth sores?	Yes ☐	No ☐
6. Have you ever had dental x-rays taken?	Yes ☐	No ☐
7. Have you ever had periodontal surgery?	Yes ☐	No ☐
8. Do your gums bleed?	Yes ☐	No ☐
9. Do you have any dental implants?	Yes ☐	No ☐
10. Have you ever had orthodontics/braces?	Yes ☐	No ☐
11. Do you have/wear full or removable/partial dentures?	Yes ☐	No ☐

Patient Name ____________________ Record # ____________

Figure 11-1 Medical History: General Medical/Dental History

Do you have or have you ever had any of the following conditions? Mark your answer with an (x)					
Blood Disorders			**Mental Health Conditions**		
Anemia (iron/folate deficiency or sickle cell)	Yes ☐	No ☐	Anxiety disorder	Yes ☐	No ☐
Hemophilia or Von Willebrand disease	Yes ☐	No ☐	Bipolar disorder (manic depression)	Yes ☐	No ☐
Leukemia	Yes ☐	No ☐	Depression	Yes ☐	No ☐
Cardiovascular			Disordered eating or feeding	Yes ☐	No ☐
Arrhythmia or atrial fibrillation	Yes ☐	No ☐	Posttraumatic stress disorder (PTSD)	Yes ☐	No ☐
Angina	Yes ☐	No ☐	Other mental health conditions	Yes ☐	No ☐
Coronary artery disease	Yes ☐	No ☐	**Respiratory System**		
Congenital heart conditions	Yes ☐	No ☐	Asthma	Yes ☐	No ☐
Endocarditis	Yes ☐	No ☐	Emphysema	Yes ☐	No ☐
Heart attack, myocardial infarction (MI)	Yes ☐	No ☐	Chronic obstructive pulmonary disease	Yes ☐	No ☐
Heart failure	Yes ☐	No ☐	Sleep apnea	Yes ☐	No ☐
Heart murmur (mitral valve prolapse)	Yes ☐	No ☐	**Substance Use Disorders**		
Heart transplant	Yes ☐	No ☐	Alcohol use disorder	Yes ☐	No ☐
Heart valve disease, prosthetic heart valve	Yes ☐	No ☐	Prescription drug addiction	Yes ☐	No ☐
High or low blood pressure	Yes ☐	No ☐	Recreational drug addiction	Yes ☐	No ☐
Pacemaker	Yes ☐	No ☐	Tobacco addiction	Yes ☐	No ☐
Endocrine System			**Transmissible Diseases**		
Polycystic ovary syndrome	Yes ☐	No ☐	Coronavirus (COVID)	Yes ☐	No ☐
'Borderline' diabetes	Yes ☐	No ☐	Hepatitis B or C virus	Yes ☐	No ☐
Diabetes mellitus type 1	Yes ☐	No ☐	Herpes simplex virus (Type 1 or 2)	Yes ☐	No ☐
Diabetes mellitus type 2	Yes ☐	No ☐	HIV / AIDS	Yes ☐	No ☐
Pre-diabetes	Yes ☐	No ☐	Tuberculosis (TB)	Yes ☐	No ☐
Hypothyroid or hyperthyroid	Yes ☐	No ☐	Sexually transmitted disease	Yes ☐	No ☐
Gastrointestinal System			**Gender Related**		
Celiac disease	Yes ☐	No ☐	Gender affirming therapy/treatment	Yes ☐	No ☐
IBD (Crohn's disease or ulcerative colitis)	Yes ☐	No ☐	Pregnancy	Yes ☐	No ☐
Lactose intolerance	Yes ☐	No ☐	Breastfeeding/ Nursing	Yes ☐	No ☐
GERD (reflux disease, heartburn)	Yes ☐	No ☐	Menopause	Yes ☐	No ☐
Peptic ulcer disease	Yes ☐	No ☐	**Other Conditions**		
Immune System			Attention deficit disorder	Yes ☐	No ☐
Lupus	Yes ☐	No ☐	Autism spectrum	Yes ☐	No ☐
Multiple sclerosis	Yes ☐	No ☐	Cancer	Yes ☐	No ☐
Rheumatoid arthritis	Yes ☐	No ☐	Learning disability	Yes ☐	No ☐
Celiac disease	Yes ☐	No ☐	Physical limitation/disability	Yes ☐	No ☐
Other autoimmune disease	Yes ☐	No ☐	Traumatic brain injury	Yes ☐	No ☐
Liver/kidney Systems			**Additional Health Related Questions**		
Liver disease (cirrhosis, fatty liver, etc)	Yes ☐	No ☐	Have you had any of the following?		
Chronic kidney disease or kidney failure	Yes ☐	No ☐	Surgery?	Yes ☐	No ☐
Kidney transplant	Yes ☐	No ☐	Radiation therapy?	Yes ☐	No ☐
Musculoskeletal System			Chemotherapy?	Yes ☐	No ☐
Fibromyalgia	Yes ☐	No ☐	Excessive bleeding or bruising?	Yes ☐	No ☐
Osteoarthritis	Yes ☐	No ☐	Excessive thirst?	Yes ☐	No ☐
Osteoporosis	Yes ☐	No ☐	Excessive urination?	Yes ☐	No ☐
Neurological System			**Other Condition(s) Not Listed**		
Alzheimer's disease or other dementia	Yes ☐	No ☐			
Epilepsy or other seizure disorder	Yes ☐	No ☐			
Parkinson's disease or other movement disorder	Yes ☐	No ☐			
Stroke	Yes ☐	No ☐			

Patient Name ______________________________ Record # ____________

Figure 11-2 Medical History: Medical Conditions

III. Disadvantages of a Questionnaire (If Used Alone without a Follow-Up Interview)

- Impersonal; no opportunity to develop rapport.
- Inflexible; no provision for additional questioning in areas of specific importance to an individual patient.

The Interview

In long-range planning for a patient's health, much more is involved than asking questions and receiving answers. The rapport established during the interview contributes to the continued cooperation of the patient.[1,6]

I. Participants

- The interviewer is alone with the patient or parent of the child patient and, if necessary, a qualified professional translator/interpreter.

II. Setting

- A consultation room or office is preferred; if possible, move the patient away from the atmosphere of the treatment room, where thoughts may be on the services to be provided.
- The treatment room may be the only available place with privacy. If the treatment room is used for a patient interview:
  - Seat patient comfortably in upright position.
  - Turn off the dental light and close the door (if possible).
  - Sit on clinician's stool to be at eye level and face-to-face with the patient.

III. Tips and Hints for the Interview

Interviewing involves communication between individuals. Communication implies the transmission or interchange of facts, attitudes, opinions, or thoughts through words, gestures, or other means. Best practices for interviewing include the following[2,5]:

- Communication through tactful but direct questioning can elicit necessary information from the patient.
- The most effective approach for the clinician to portray is one of friendly understanding, being reassuring, nonjudgmental, and accepting to obtain accurate and complete information from the patient.
- Genuine interest and willingness to listen when a patient wishes to describe symptoms, complaints, or current health practices not only aids in establishing the rapport needed but also frequently provides insight into the patient's real attitudes and behaviors.
- By asking simple questions at first and more personal questions later after rapport has developed, the patient will be more relaxed and truthful in answering.
- The culturally sensitive dental hygienist will be aware of nonverbal communication when interviewing a patient from a different culture. (See Chapter 3.)
- Summarize what the patient has said to confirm accuracy and allow the patient to provide further explanation.

IV. Interview Form

- The history form guides the interview and notations of patient responses should be made on the form.
- Familiarity with the items on the history permits the interviewer to be comprehensive and informal without reading from a fixed list of topics, a method that may lack the personal touch necessary to gain the patient's confidence.

V. Advantages of the Interview

- Personal contact contributes to development of rapport for future appointments.
- Flexibility for individual needs; details obtained can be adapted for supplemental questions.
- Sometimes a patient has information to share that does not fit with any of the topics in the questionnaire or wants the opportunity to explain their answer to a question.

VI. Disadvantages of the Interview

- For a medically complex patient, the interview can be time consuming.
- Unless the history form is used to guide the interview, items may be omitted.
- Patient may be embarrassed to talk about personal conditions and may fail to disclose important information.

Items Included in the History

Information obtained by means of the history is directly related to the development of goals for patient care. In **Table 11-1**, **Table 11-2**, and **Table 11-3**, items are listed with possible medications and other treatments the patient may have or has had, along with suggested considerations for appointment procedures.

- In specialized practices, objectives may require increased emphasis on certain aspects of the history.
- The age group most frequently served will influence the focus of the history. For example, parental history and prenatal and postnatal information

Table 11-1 Items for the Dental History

Items to Record in the History	Possible Follow-Up Questions	Considerations for Appointment Procedures
Reason for present appointment	Tell me a little about why you are here in the office/clinic today? If experiencing pain/discomfort: ■ When did this problem start? ■ What causes pain/discomfort? ■ Has the problem gotten worse? ■ Have you done anything to relieve the pain/discomfort?	■ If the chief complaint is an emergency, it may be a priority over preventive care.
Previous dental history	■ How often do you typically get dental care? ■ Do you tend to go to the dentist only when you have a problem or toothache?	■ Understanding the patient's oral health literacy may guide patient education. ■ The patient's dental history may give insight into potential compliance with care recommendations.
Family dental history	■ Tell me about your family history of dental care, decay, gum disease. ■ Have close family members lost teeth? Do you know why they lost teeth?	■ Understanding oral health literacy will aid in educating patient about benefit for preventive care. ■ It will be important to understand the patient's oral health beliefs and practices.
Radiation history	■ What type of dental x-rays did you have? ■ When were your most recent dental x-rays? ■ Will you provide permission to request your last dental x-rays from you previous dentist? If the patient had radiotherapy for cancer: ■ Why and when did you have radiation therapy?	■ Amount of exposure for medical radiographs or radiotherapy treatment may impact the number of dental radiographs taken. ■ Educate patient about the necessity of radiographs for diagnosis. ■ Educate about the need to obtain past radiographs to monitor progression of caries/periodontal disease.
Periodontal disease	■ Have you ever been told you had periodontal disease? ■ Tell me about the treatment you have had for periodontal disease. ■ How often do you have appointments to maintain your periodontal disease?	■ Understanding the patients history of periodontal disease and treatment will provide insight into compliance with recommendations. ■ Education about the need for meticulous oral self-care and regular periodontal maintenance to prevent disease progression.
Orthodontic treatment	If the patient indicates orthodontics/braces on the dental history form: ■ What age did you start and finish treatment? ■ Do you wear a retainer or other appliance?	■ For patients receiving current treatment, a consultation with the orthodontist may be needed.

(continues)

Table 11-1 Items for the Dental History *(continued)*

Items to Record in the History	Possible Follow-Up Questions	Considerations for Appointment Procedures
Prosthodontic	If the patient reports full or removable/partial dentures: ■ When did you first get your partial/full denture? ■ Tell me how your partial/full denture fits and whether you have any issues or concerns.	■ Evaluate care of prostheses and abutment teeth and educate on best practices. ■ Consider the need for new or relined prosthesis.
Other dental treatment	■ Have you lost any teeth? Why? ■ Have you had any implants? ■ Is there any other treatment you would like to share with me?	■ Review the patient's knowledge about care of implants and refine techniques as needed. ■ Teeth lost from oral disease may indicate the need for education tailored to the patient's needs.
Injuries to head, face, or mouth	■ Have you had injuries to the head, face, and/or mouth? ■ Do you have some continuing issues from the injury? ■ Did you experience a traumatic brain injury? If yes, are there continuing effects from the injury?	■ The patient may have limitations to opening and need modifications during dental care and to preventive oral self-care techniques. ■ If the patient is healing, you may need to consult with the maxillofacial surgeon or other provider.
Temporomandibular joint (TMJ) disorder/dysfunction	■ Tell me about when the TMJ injury began and how it happened. ■ Are you experiencing pain or discomfort? ■ What treatment have you had for the condition?	■ TMJ dysfunction may limit mouth opening and the time the mouth can remain open for dental care. ■ This may require modifications of treatment and education to help the patient identify techniques for oral self-care based on their individual limitations.
Oral habits	On clinical examination, ask the following if oral signs suggest an oral habit: ■ Do you find you clench your teeth or wake with your jaw/teeth feeling sore? ■ Do you bite on objects like pens or fingernails? ■ Do you find you are unable to breathe through your nose and often breathe through your mouth? ■ Have you noticed you bite your cheek or lip, possibly when concentrating or anxious?	■ Identifying patient awareness of an oral habit may aid in determining if education or treatment is needed.
Piercing	Piercing may be visible on greeting the patient, but intraoral piercing may not be identified until the intraoral examination: ■ Do you have any piercings in your head or mouth area? ■ Where are they and when were they done? ■ Have you had any problems with infection related to the piercing?	■ Evaluate for oral health changes related to piercing. ■ Educate patient on any risks the piercings may pose.
Fluorides	■ Do you know if you lived in a community with fluoridated water when you were a child/teen? ■ Did you take fluoride supplements during childhood? ■ What fluorides have been used at past dental visits (dates/frequency)? ■ Do you (or have you) used fluorides at home (type/frequency)?	■ The fluoride history will assist in caries risk assessment. ■ Caries risk level will aid in identifying the appropriate fluoride. ■ History of compliance with fluoride use may help to identify need for education or tailoring the treatment choice to what is feasible for the patient.

Items to Record in the History	Possible Follow-Up Questions	Considerations for Appointment Procedures
Biofilm control procedures	■ Tell me what you do to clean your teeth/mouth? For toothbrushing: ■ What type of brush (manual or powered), texture of bristles, frequency of use, and frequency of having a new brush? For dentifrice: ■ What toothpaste do you use? ■ Why did you choose this toothpaste? For interdental cleaning: ■ Do you use anything to clean between your teeth? ■ What do you use and how often? For other products used: ■ Are there other things you use to clean your mouth? ■ What do you use and how often? Oral self-care instruction: ■ Has anyone provided you with education on cleaning your mouth? Did this include hands-on demonstration? ■ Are there things you have tried that worked well? Things that did not work well? Is there anything you would like to know more about while you are here today?	■ Asking a very broad question can often yield information the patient might not otherwise report. ■ Understanding the patient's oral self-care routine provides a starting point for modifications as needed for adequate biofilm control. ■ Explore challenges encountered in changing habits. ■ Adapt education to patient needs, abilities, preferences, and disease state. ■ Educate on oral biofilm being a modifiable risk factor for oral disease that the patient can control. ■ For parents/caregivers of young children, educate on need to perform and supervise oral care.

Table 11-2 Items for the Medical History

Item to Record	Possible Follow-Up Questions	Considerations for Appointment Procedures
General health and appearance	Objective observations of general health and mobility during the seating and discussion with the patient. ■ Tell me how you would describe your health.	■ Disabilities may require individualized oral self-care education. ■ Chair positioning may need adjustment for patient comfort.
Height and weight/BMI (body mass index)	■ Have you had rapid weight loss or weight gain? ■ Have you been told by your medical provider that you are either over- or underweight?	■ Marked weight change may be a symptom of undiagnosed disease, referral to PCP for evaluation. ■ Obesity is associated with periodontal disease, so nutrition counseling should support making healthy food and beverage choices. ■ Referral to a registered dietitian may be needed.
Medical examination	■ When was your most recent physical examination? ■ Have you had other medical visits? ■ Do you have any medical treatment planned? ■ Have you had recent medical tests that might affect your dental care, such as a hemoglobin A1c?	■ Consultation with PCP to clarify the patient report of medical and medication history. ■ A consultation may also be needed for clearance to ensure patient safety prior to dental care.

(continues)

Table 11-2 Items for the Medical History *(continued)*

Item to Record	Possible Follow-Up Questions	Considerations for Appointment Procedures
Major diseases/conditions, hospitalizations, surgeries	■ Have you had any major illness/condition? ■ Tell me about the type and duration of treatment/hospitalization. ■ How have you been recovering? ■ What is the status of management of the disease/condition (e.g., diabetes)?	■ Impact of illness/condition on treatment ■ Anesthetic choice/dose ■ Expected outcome from periodontal therapy based on level of control of disease
Family medical history	■ Are there certain diseases that tend to run in your family (e.g., diabetes)?	■ May need medical referral for evaluation
Medications		
Prescription medications	Based on responses to medication being taken in the medical history form: ■ What do you take this medication for? ■ When did you start taking this medication? ■ Do you follow the directions for how often to take the medication? ■ Do you take any liquid medications that might contain sugar? If yes, how often is the medication taken?	■ Consultation with PCP regarding medications and adjustments needed for dental care ■ Indications for prophylactic antibiotics ■ Adverse oral effects of medications (e.g., risk of gingival hyperplasia with phenytoin use)
Self-medication	■ Do you take any medications not prescribed by your medical provider, such as over-the-counter medications, herbals, vitamins, other supplements? ■ What do you take this for? ■ When did you start taking this medication? ■ Do you take any recreational substances? What kind and how often?	■ Information not revealed by patient could create a medical emergency. ■ Oral side effects of substance use
Blood Disorders		
Blood disorders ■ Sickle cell anemia ■ Thrombocytopenia ■ Hemophilia	■ Tell me more about your blood condition. When was it diagnosed? ■ What is being done to manage the blood disorder? ■ Have you had any unusual bleeding associated with previous dental appointments? ■ Do you have a history of coagulation disorder? ■ Do you have a history of transfusions? ■ Do you regularly use aspirin? Herbal supplements?	■ Consultation with hematologist may be necessary about providing dental care and need for prophylactic antibiotics. ■ Need for excellent oral self-care to minimize infection and bleeding ■ Avoid use of inferior alveolar and posterior superior alveolar blocks in coagulation disorders. ■ Laboratory tests for bleeding time may be needed. ■ Monitoring and application of direct pressure or hemostatic agent after scaling ■ Prevention of medical emergency
Cardiovascular System		
Angina pectoris	■ When was the last time you experienced angina? ■ How frequently does it occur? ■ What triggers your angina?	■ Have nitroglycerin tablets available within reach of the treatment area. ■ Use stress reduction protocols. ■ Morning appointments may be preferred.

Item to Record	Possible Follow-Up Questions	Considerations for Appointment Procedures
Cardiovascular diseases	■ Tell me about your heart condition. ■ Do you take medications as prescribed?	■ Consult with PCP for clearance to provide dental care. ■ Record vital signs. ■ Minimize stress.
Congenital heart disease	■ What type of congenital heart disease do you have? ■ How was the condition treated or repaired? ■ Have you ever been told by your medical or dental provider that you need to take antibiotics prior to dental care?	■ Consult with cardiologist or PCP. ■ Specific types of congenital heart disease are at risk for infective endocarditis (IE).
Endocarditis (infective endocarditis)	■ Tell me about the endocarditis you experienced. When did it happen? ■ Do you know what caused or triggered the endocarditis?	■ Consultation with PCP required to determine if antibiotic prophylaxis is necessary ■ Stress need for meticulous daily oral self-care to reduce bacterial load.
Heart failure (congestive heart failure)	■ Tell me about the history of your heart failure. ■ What symptoms (e.g. fatigue, shortness of breath, or cough) do you experience?	■ Consult with PCP to determine if any modifications are needed for dental care. ■ Short, more frequent appointments ■ Monitor vital signs. ■ May need dental chair in semi-supine position ■ There may be a bleeding tendency due to anticoagulant use.
Hypertension	■ Tell me the things you do to manage your high blood pressure. ■ Do you take the medications as prescribed by your PCP? ■ Do you experience any side effects from your medications?	■ Consult with PCP to determine type of local anesthesia and vasoconstrictor safe to use for dental care. ■ Monitor vital signs. ■ Postural hypotension (raise back of dental chair slowly). ■ Xerostomia: Manage caries risk (e.g., fluorides). ■ Gingival enlargement possible with calcium channel blockers.
Heart valve disease, prosthetic heart valve	■ Describe your heart valve disease. ■ Have you had a heart valve replacement? When was it done? ■ Did your medical provider tell you that antibiotics would be needed for dental treatment?	■ Consult with PCP about prophylactic antibiotics for dental care. ■ Stress need for meticulous daily oral self-care to reduce bacterial load.
Endocrine System		
Life cycle related ■ Puberty ■ Menstruation ■ Menopause ■ Gender affirming therapy/treatment	■ Tell me about any hormonal therapy or other treatment you are undergoing. ■ Have you noticed any changes in your oral health, such as bleeding gums?	■ Support meticulous biofilm control to prevent and manage oral disease. ■ Monitor risk for oral diseases and manage as needed. ■ There may be increased bleeding due to hormonal changes. ■ Manage symptoms reported such as xerostomia and burning mouth syndrome.

(continues)

Table 11-2 Items for the Medical History *(continued)*

Item to Record	Possible Follow-Up Questions	Considerations for Appointment Procedures
Diabetes mellitus ■ Pre-diabetes ■ Type 1 diabetes ■ Type 2 diabetes	If the patient checks yes for borderline, pre-diabetes, or type 1 or 2 diabetes: ■ When were you first told you had borderline or pre-diabetes/diabetes? ■ Describe what you do to manage your condition. ■ How well controlled is your pre-diabetes/diabetes? What was your most recent hemoglobin A1c? ■ Have you had any complications from your diabetes (vision problems, kidney failure, cardiovascular, nervous system)?	■ Assess for symptoms of undiagnosed prediabetes or diabetes (e.g., excess thirst, appetite, and urination) and refer to PCP for evaluation. ■ Prepare to manage a hypoglycemic event by having glucose and glucose monitor nearby. ■ Plan appointments around meals and medications; morning is usually best. ■ Inquire about meal consumed prior to appointment. It is ideal to have a meal balanced with fat, protein, and carbohydrate prior to appointment. ■ Frequent maintenance appointments ■ Educate the patient on the risk for more severe periodontal disease with poor diabetes control. ■ Evaluate the need for more frequent intervals for preventive care.
Pregnancy	■ When is the baby due? ■ Have you noticed any changes in your oral health, such as bleeding gums? ■ Are you experiencing heartburn or vomiting? How often does it happen?	■ May need to adjust dental chair to a semi-supine position for comfort ■ May need more frequent appointments to maintain periodontal health ■ Educate about association between periodontal disease and adverse birth outcomes and need for meticulous oral self-care. ■ Manage caries risk if vomiting or reflux is an issue with fluorides and possibly chlorhexidine.
Gastrointestinal System		
■ Crohn's disease ■ Inflammatory bowel disease ■ Celiac disease ■ Gastroesophageal reflux	■ Tell me about your condition. ■ What treatment has been done to manage the condition? ■ Tell me about diet restrictions been prescribed by your PCP/dietitian.	■ Explore side effects of condition/medications (e.g., vomiting, acid reflux) on oral cavity and esophagus. ■ If the patient has taken steroids for disease management, steroid-induced osteoporosis is possible and may impact periodontal health.
Immune System		
Allergies	■ Tell me about your allergy (e.g., latex, penicillin, pine nuts). ■ Describe the reaction you experience. ■ What treatment has been needed to manage your allergy?	■ Be prepared for a medical emergency. ■ Avoid use of substances to which the patient is allergic.
Liver/Kidney Systems		
Kidney (renal disease) ■ Hemodialysis ■ Peritoneal dialysis ■ Kidney transplant	■ Tell me about the kidney condition you reported on the medical history. ■ When was it diagnosed and what treatment has been done to manage the condition? ■ Have you ever experienced excessive bleeding following dental care?	■ Transplant protocol is for dental care to be completed prior to surgery. ■ Educate on need for meticulous biofilm removal to reduce bacterial load. ■ Consult with PCP about need for antibiotic prophylaxis. ■ Monitor and document vital signs, especially blood pressure. ■ For hemodialysis, best to treat the day after dialysis ■ Immunosuppressants for transplant may impact healing.

Item to Record	Possible Follow-Up Questions	Considerations for Appointment Procedures
Liver ■ Fatty liver ■ Cirrhosis	■ Tell me about the liver condition you noted on the medical history. ■ When were you diagnosed and how is the condition managed? ■ Have you experienced excessive bleeding after dental treatment?	■ Consult with PCP before prescribing any medication, including local anesthesia, due to impaired drug metabolism. ■ Avoid acetaminophen. ■ Monitor for oral signs of jaundice. ■ Monitoring and application of direct pressure or hemostatic agent after scaling
Mental Health Conditions		
Mental health issues	■ Tell me about the mental health condition you noted on your medical history. ■ When was it first diagnosed and how has it been treated? ■ How would you describe your compliance with the medications prescribed by your medical provider?	■ May need to consult with medical provider ■ Use a stress reduction protocol. ■ Caries risk assessment and management (e.g., xerostomia) ■ Compliance with recommendations may be an issue due to negative effects of mental health issue; may need frequent visits
Musculoskeletal System		
Arthritis Fibromyalgia Osteoporosis	■ Tell me more about the condition you checked on the medical history. ■ When were you diagnosed with the condition? How has it been treated? ■ Have you had a joint replacement? ■ What symptoms do you experience? Do they limit your ability to walk, clean your mouth, etc.? ■ Are you experiencing any issues related to your oral health or jaw (temporomandibular) joint?	■ Depending on the patient's symptoms, the dental chair may need to be in a semi-supine position. ■ Adjustments may need to be made to oral self-care recommendations to accommodate the patient's limitations. ■ Bisphosphonate use may indicate need for consultation to determine risk of osteonecrosis that may result from invasive treatment. ■ If steroids have been used long term, it may also impact bone health and healing. A consultation may be necessary prior to treatment.
Neurologic System		
Dementia Alzheimer's disease	Questions may be directed to the patient or a caregiver if indicated: ■ Tell me what you do at home to take care of your mouth. ■ Do you find reminders helpful to know when to brush, etc.?	■ A caregiver may need to be consulted for an accurate medical history. ■ The patient may not be able to provide informed consent depending on the severity of the impact of disease on cognitive functioning. ■ Providing the caregiver with oral hygiene instructions along with ways to provide the patient with reminders may aid in more effective biofilm management.
Epilepsy	■ Tell me about the seizures you experience. ■ How often do they happen? ■ What are the triggers for your seizures? ■ Have you had a seizure while in the dental office/clinic? ■ When was the last seizure?	■ Use stress management protocols. ■ Monitor medication side effects such as gingival hyperplasia (dilantin). ■ PCP consultation may be needed. ■ Prepare to manage a medical emergency for a seizure.

(continues)

Table 11-2 Items for the Medical History *(continued)*

Item to Record	Possible Follow-Up Questions	Considerations for Appointment Procedures
Cerebrovascular accident (stroke)	▪ When did the stroke occur? ▪ How has it impacted you (e.g., speech, vision, cognitive function, mobility)? ▪ Is there anything you are having difficulty with in regard to mouth care that we can help with today?	▪ Monitoring and application of direct pressure or hemostatic agent after scaling ▪ Adapt procedures and oral self-care techniques for any residual impairments.
Respiratory System		
▪ Chronic obstructive pulmonary disease ▪ Asthma ▪ Emphysema	▪ Tell me about your breathing problems. ▪ What symptoms do you experience? ▪ Are there specific triggers for an asthma attack? ▪ Do you have trouble breathing when laying down in bed (or previously in a dental chair)?	▪ May need to place patient in semi-supine position ▪ Use a stress reduction protocol. ▪ Monitor for oral candidiasis from inhalers. ▪ Nitrous oxide contraindicated ▪ Minimize aerosol-producing procedures. ▪ Keep inhaler accessible during patient care. ▪ If the patient uses tobacco, tobacco cessation should be initiated.
Transmissible Diseases		
Coronavirus disease 2019 (COVID-19)	If the patient indicates having had COVID-19 on the medical history form: ▪ When did you have COVID-19 and what treatment was involved? ▪ Do you experience any long-lasting effects from COVID-19 (long COVID)? ▪ How is this affecting your daily activities? ▪ Are you taking medications to manage the long-term effects of COVID-19? ▪ Have you been vaccinated?	▪ Ideally ask questions about exposure, current symptoms, travel, etc. prior to the patient's arrival in the office/clinic. ▪ Monitor vital signs. ▪ Monitor most recent Centers for Disease Control and Prevention and local recommendations for mitigation of community spread, as this may limit use of aerosol-producing procedures. ▪ COVID-19 can have multiorgan effects such as cardiovascular, respiratory, kidney, liver, coagulation issues, and cognitive (memory, etc.), so carefully evaluate the health history. ▪ May need consultation with PCP
Hepatitis	▪ What type of hepatitis do/did you have? ▪ Tell me about when it was diagnosed and the treatment to manage it. ▪ Do you have any long-term effects from having had hepatitis?	▪ Consultation with PCP may be needed to obtain clearance for treatment as well as any necessary modifications. ▪ Precautions against percutaneous injury ▪ Monitor for signs of oral jaundice.
Herpes simplex virus	▪ When did you first begin experiencing symptoms? ▪ What tends to trigger lesions?	▪ Postpone routine care when active oral lesions are present.
Human immunodeficiency virus (HIV) Acquired immunodeficiency syndrome (AIDS)	▪ When were you first diagnosed with HIV? ▪ What therapy/treatment has been used to manage your condition? ▪ Are you consistent with your medications? ▪ What is your current viral load and CD4 count?	▪ Consultation with PCP may be needed depending on disease management. ▪ Document oral manifestations and assist patient in management. ▪ Manage associated oral disease risk, particularly periodontal disease.

Item to Record	Possible Follow-Up Questions	Considerations for Appointment Procedures
Other Conditions		
Cancer ■ Breast cancer	■ What type of cancer did you have and what treatment did you undergo? ■ If breast cancer, when were you diagnosed? ■ What side did you have nodes removed? ■ Did you specifically have any radiation of the head and neck? ■ Were you able to get your regular dental care before cancer therapy? ■ Are you having any side effects of your treatment that are making it hard to do your daily mouth care?	■ Evaluate for neutropenia prior to dental care. ■ Patients who underwent breast cancer surgery are at increased risk of lymphedema. Determine need to take blood pressure on opposite side nodes were removed. If nodes were removed on both sides, blood pressure should be taken on the thigh with a larger cuff. ■ If patient is immunosuppressed, may be at risk of oral candidiasis and mucositis ■ Avoid tissue trauma. ■ Educate on need for meticulous biofilm removal to reduce the bacterial load. ■ Manage modifiable caries risk factors (e.g., fluorides, chlorhexidine, saliva substitutes). ■ Risk of osteonecrosis with history of bisphosphonate use
Ears ■ Deaf ■ Hard of hearing	■ Tell me how you prefer for us to communicate with you. ■ Do you wear a hearing aid?	■ Adapt patient education to meet patient needs. ■ Document degree of hearing loss and preferred method for communication.
Eyes ■ Blindness	■ How do you prefer for me to guide you to the dental chair? ■ What is the appropriate way to interact with your seeing eye dog? Where is it best for them to be located in the room with you?	■ Protective eyewear during appointment ■ Adaptations for communication with limited sight or blindness
Developmental disorder or physical disabilities Traumatic brain injury (TBI)	■ Are there any physical or learning challenges the dental team should know about in order to provide dental care? ■ What can we do here in the dental office to make you comfortable during your visit? ■ Are you having difficulty with performing your daily mouth care? For traumatic brain injury: ■ When did the injury occur and what long-term effects are you experiencing?	■ Consultation with PCP or specialist ■ Consult the *Autism Took Kit for Dental Professionals* for a specific form to use with parents prior to an appointment www.autismspeaks.org/sites/default/files/2018-08/Dental%20Professionals%20Tool%20Kit.pdf ■ Document patient needs/preferences during appointment. ■ Wheelchair accessibility and transfer ■ Techniques and patient education may need adaptation to patient needs. ■ In TBI, cognitive changes can affect memory; recommend reminders (e.g., setting calendar or cellphone reminders). ■ Schedule appointments at a time in the day when the patient is best able to be cooperative (or concentrate).

may take on particular significance for the treatment of a small child; in a pediatric dentistry practice, a special form could be developed to include all essential items.

- The American Academy of Pediatric Dentistry (www.aapd.org) has a form that can be used, which includes medical conditions, medications, dental history, supplemental questions for infants/toddlers related to dietary habits, and supplemental questions for adolescents.

- The clinician must remain current in the manifestations of systemic diseases and the medications for various conditions in order to effectively ask follow-up questions during the interview.

Table 11-3 Items for the Psychosocial History

Items to Record	Possible Follow-Up Questions	Considerations for Appointment Procedures
Personal information	■ Tell me about health beliefs or practices that relate to your oral health. ■ You noted on the medical history form that you do not have access to food each day; do you know about community resources for food in your area?	■ Try to incorporate health beliefs into education and recommendations. ■ Identify community resources as needed for support (e.g., congregate meal sites for seniors).
Daily diet	■ Tell me everything you eat and drink on a typical day. ■ Do you consume snacks in between meals? If so, what snacks do you regularly eat? ■ Do you sip on beverages or drink all at once?	■ Dependent on factors for oral disease risk, conduct a dietary assessment. ■ Provide guidance on minimizing cariogenic foods and beverages and support health food choices. ■ For medically complex patients, refer to registered dietitian nutritionist (RDN).
Alcohol consumption	■ How long have you used alcohol with your current frequency? ■ If you have felt you needed to cut down, what have you done to make changes? How successful was this? ■ Has use of alcohol affected your relationship with loved ones or your work?	■ Use of alcohol beyond guidelines may indicate a need for referral for evaluation of alcohol use disorder. ■ Resources for referral can be found at the National Institute on Alcohol Abuse and Alcoholism's Treatment Navigator (AlcoholTreatment.niaaa.nih.gov). ■ Excessive use can affect local anesthesia and healing time. ■ Diet assessment may reveal a need for referral. ■ Avoid alcohol-containing mouthrinses. ■ Patient compliance with oral health recommendations may be poor.
Tobacco/nicotine use	For patients reporting tobacco or nicotine use: ■ Have you thought about stopping use of tobacco (or nicotine)? ■ Have you tried to quit before? What did you find was most helpful? ■ Are you interested in information on quitting tobacco/nicotine use?	■ Educate patients on the association between tobacco/nicotine use and oral health (oral cancer and periodontal disease). ■ If interested in quitting, refer to resources like a national or state quitline for help (quitline.com or 1-800-QUIT-NOW).
Drug use	■ Would it be alright with you if I asked you some follow-up questions about your drug use? ■ Do you have any concerns about your use of ______________? ■ Are you interested in talking to someone about your drug use?	■ Avoid use of nitrous oxide and prescription pain medications. ■ May impact self-care, nutritional status, and healing ability ■ If interested in referral to addiction services, refer to the Substance Abuse and Mental Health Services Administation's National Helpline, 1-800-662-HELP (4357), or local resources.

I. Dental History

The dental history (Table 11-1; sample form Figure 11-1) contributes to the care provider's knowledge of:

- The immediate problem, chief complaint, cause of present pain, or discomfort in the oral cavity.
- Risk assessment forms, such as the ADA Caries Risk Assessment forms and Caries Management by Risk Assessment (CAMBRA), provide the information needed for planning individualized dental hygiene interventions based on the patient's risk factors.
- Previous dental hygiene and dental care, including preventive care, periodontal treatments, and the extent of restorative and prosthetic replacement, as well as any adverse effects.
- Personal daily oral self-care habits.

II. Medical History

Objectives of the medical history (Table 11-2) are to determine whether the patient has or has had any conditions. Sample forms for the medical conditions and medications are provided in Figure 11-2 and **Figure 11-3**. The following are categories to be assessed in a medical history:

- Personal information (Figure 11-1)
    - *Examples:* Age; address and contact information; dental insurance; physician's name and contact information; height/weight.
- Conditions that may complicate certain kinds of dental and dental hygiene treatment
    - *Examples:* Lowered resistance to infection; uncontrolled hypertension; uncontrolled diabetes; or systemic disease that requires treatment before stressful dental procedures, particularly surgery, can be carried out.
- Conditions or diseases that may require special precautions or premedication before treatment
    - *Examples:* Increased osteonecrosis risk related to previous treatment with bisphosphonates, or antibiotic coverage for the patient at risk for **infective endocarditis (IE)**.
- Conditions under treatment by a physician that require medications that may influence or contraindicate certain procedures

Please Note Any Allergies

ALLERGIES		
Antibiotics (i.e., penicillin)	Yes ☐	No ☐
Aspirin or other pain medications	Yes ☐	No ☐
Iodine	Yes ☐	No ☐
Latex products	Yes ☐	No ☐
Local anesthetic (i.e., Novocain)	Yes ☐	No ☐
Pine nuts	Yes ☐	No ☐
Other	Yes ☐	No ☐

Please list the name of any drugs you are currently taking or have previously taken in the space provided.

Place (X) in the box
If medication is current, list the dosage.

Medication	Yes	No	Dosage
Antianxiety (i.e., Xanax, benzodiazapine)	Yes ☐	No ☐	Dosage:
Antibiotics	Yes ☐	No ☐	Dosage:
Anticoagulants (i.e., warfarin, Coumadin)	Yes ☐	No ☐	Dosage:
Depression medications (i.e., Zoloft, Celexa)	Yes ☐	No ☐	Dosage:
Anti-inflammatory	Yes ☐	No ☐	Dosage:
Blood pressure medications (i.e., Norvasc, lisinopril, lopressor, hydrochlorothiazide)	Yes ☐	No ☐	Dosage:
Aspirin/pain medication	Yes ☐	No ☐	Dosage:
Anti-convulsant (i.e., Dilantin)	Yes ☐	No ☐	Dosage:
Bisphosphonates (i.e., Fosamax, Boniva)	Yes ☐	No ☐	Dosage:
Cholesterol medications (i.e., simvastatin, Lipitor)	Yes ☐	No ☐	Dosage:
Codeine	Yes ☐	No ☐	Dosage:
Diabetes medications (i.e., Metformin, Glucophage)	Yes ☐	No ☐	Dosage:
Digitalis	Yes ☐	No ☐	Dosage:
Hormone therapy (i.e., estradiol, testosterone)	Yes ☐	No ☐	Dosage:
Insulin	Yes ☐	No ☐	Dosage:
Medical marijuana	Yes ☐	No ☐	Dosage:
Nitroglycerin	Yes ☐	No ☐	Dosage:
Steroid (i.e., prednisone)	Yes ☐	No ☐	Dosage:
Thyroid medications (i.e., levothyroxine)	Yes ☐	No ☐	Dosage:
Over-the-counter medication (i.e., Zantac, Prilosec, ibuprofen)	Yes ☐	No ☐	Dosage:
Vitamin supplements	Yes ☐	No ☐	Dosage:
Herbal supplements	Yes ☐	No ☐	Dosage:
Other	Yes ☐	No ☐	Dosage:

Please explain in detail, all YES responses:

Figure 11-3 Medical History: Medications

  - *Examples:* Anticoagulant therapy such as warfarin (Coumadin) require consultation with the PCP; antihypertensive drugs may alter the amount and/or choice of local anesthetic used.
- Gender or ethnic/racial influences that increase risk for systemic and oral disease
  - *Example:* American Indian/Alaska Native, Hispanic and non-Hispanic Black populations have increased risk for diabetes.[7,8] Some racial/ethnic groups also have a higher risk for periodontal disease.[9]
- Allergic or adverse reactions
  - *Examples:* Latex hypersensitivity; previous adverse reaction to medication or anesthesia.
- Diseases and drugs with manifestations in the mouth
  - *Examples:* Phenytoin (Dilantin)-induced gingival overgrowth; infectious diseases such as herpesvirus.
- Transmissible diseases
  - *Examples:* Active tuberculosis; viral hepatitis; herpes.
- Physiologic state of the patient
  - *Examples:* Pregnancy and birth control pills.

III. Psychosocial History

- The psychosocial history (Table 11-3; **Figure 11-4**) gathers information about many aspect of the patient's life that may impact their oral and overall health[10]:
  - Health behaviors such as smoking, drug use, and dietary intake.
  - These factors may also impact dental literacy and compliance with preventive dental recommendations.
  - Social support can positively influence health behavior.
- Areas to be assessed include, but are not limited to:
  - Living situation and social support.
  - Education.
  - Employment situation.
  - Health and dental literacy levels that may influence communication.
  - Beliefs and attitudes about health, illness, and oral health.
  - Culturally related health beliefs and practices that may impact the patient's oral health.

Application of Patient Histories

- Information from the histories influences all aspects of total patient care and dental hygiene care planning.[1,2]
- Immediate evaluation of the histories is necessary before proceeding to complete the clinical assessment.[2,11,12]
- Together with information from all other parts of the diagnostic workup, the patient histories are essential for the preparation of the dental hygiene care plan.

I. Medical Consultation

Dentist and PCP need to consult relative to the patient's current therapy and medications or to elements of the patient's past health status that could influence dental treatment needs.[2,3,12]

- *Telephone or personal contact*
  - Immediate consultation for urgent treatment may be required.
  - Follow-up in writing by secure electronic communication, fax, or mail to provide a legal record of the PCP or medical provider's recommendations.
- *Written request*
  - A written request for medical consultation should be brief and include the patient's self-report of medical conditions/medication that potentially impact dental care (e.g., hemoglobin A1c to assess diabetes control), information on the oral health status, and dental/dental hygiene treatment recommended for which clearance is being requested.[11,13]
  - The PCP may be unfamiliar with dental treatments, so be specific about what you need them to approve (e.g., use of a specific amount and type of local anesthetic/vasoconstrictor).
  - A form can also be developed with space for writing the specific questions and an area for the PCP to provide the necessary recommendations.
- *Referrals*
  - Referral for medical examination when signs of a possible disease condition are present, but undiagnosed.[11,13]

II. Antibiotic Prophylaxis

- Selected patients at risk for IE receive antibiotic premedication before any oral tissue manipulation (e.g., periodontal probe or scaling) that could create a **bacteremia**.
- Review the patient medical history to identify a high-risk patient needing prophylactic antibiotics (e.g., prosthetic heart valves, history of IE, heart transplant, and some congenital heart conditions) in accordance with the recommendations of the American Heart Association (AHA) (**Box 11-1**).[14]

Please answer the following questions as accurately as possible.

Personal Information			
Do you live alone?	Yes ☐	No ☐	If not, who lives in your household?
Do you shop for food in your household?	Yes ☐	No ☐	
Do you have access to food each day?	Yes ☐	No ☐	
Do you prepare the food in your household?	Yes ☐	No ☐	How often do you prepare meals?
Do you work outside the home?	Yes ☐	No ☐	What kind of work do you do?
Do you travel for your job?	Yes ☐	No ☐	How often? On average how long are trips?
Are there any specific health beliefs or practices we should know about?	Yes ☐	No ☐	
Are you physically active daily?	Yes ☐	No ☐	
Dietary Information			
Do you eat regular meals and snacks?	Yes ☐	No ☐	What types of snacks to you typically eat? What kinds of beverages do you drink? How often?
Have you had any large weight gains or losses?	Yes ☐	No ☐	How much did you gain or lose? What was the time period?
Do you follow a specific diet?	Yes ☐	No ☐	Who prescribed the diet?
Have you eliminated any types of foods?	Yes ☐	No ☐	What types of foods? For how long? Are you being monitored by a medical provider?
Tobacco Products/Nicotine Use			
Cigarettes	Yes ☐	No ☐	Number of cigarettes per day or week:
Cigars	Yes ☐	No ☐	Number of cigars per week:
E-cigarettes/vaping	Yes ☐	No ☐	Number of cartridges per day or week:
Waterpipe/hookah	Yes ☐	No ☐	Approximate amount of time per day or week:
Smokeless	Yes ☐	No ☐	Number of cans/pouches per day/week:
Dissolvable strips, sticks, etc	Yes ☐	No ☐	Amount per day or week:
Other types of tobacco or nicotine products?	Yes ☐	No ☐	Amount per day or week:
Have you tried quitting tobacco/nicotine use in the past?	Yes ☐	No ☐	If you have tried to quit: How long did you quit last time? What did you use to help you quit? What was the longest time you have quit? What has caused you to relapse?
Alcohol Use			
Do you drink alcohol?	Yes ☐	No ☐	What kind of alcohol? How often do you have a drink containing alcohol? How many drinks containing alcohol do you have on a typical day or week?
Have you ever felt you need to cut down?	Yes ☐	No ☐	
Recreational Drugs			
Do you use any recreational drugs?	Yes ☐	No ☐	What type of drug(s)? When did you start? How often do you use drugs? In what form do you take the drug? Have you ever been in trouble because of your drug use? Have you ever tried to stop using the drug(s)? Have you ever been in rehab?

STOP

Please sign once reviewed by Forsyth School of Dental Hygiene clinician.
To the best of my knowledge, the above information is complete and correct.

Print Name: ______________________________

Signature: ______________________________ Date: ______________

Figure 11-4 Medical History: Psychosocial

Box 11-1 Cardiac Conditions That Require Antibiotic Prophylaxis before Invasive Dental and Dental Hygiene Treatment[14]

- Prosthetic heart valve.
- History of infective endocarditis.
- Congenital heart disease only in the following categories:
  - Unrepaired cyanotic congenital heart disease.
  - Completely repaired congenital heart disease with prosthetic material or device for the first 6 months after the surgery.
  - Repaired congenital heart disease with residual defects at the site or adjacent to the site of a prosthetic patch or device.
- Heart transplant recipients with heart valve disease

Data from Wilson WR, Gewitz M, Lockhart PB, et al. Prevention of viridans group streptococcal infective endocarditis: a scientific statement from the American Heart Association. *Circulation*. 2021;143(20):e963-e978.

Box 11-2 Dental and Dental Hygiene Procedures for Which Antibiotic Prophylaxis Is and Is Not Recommended for Patients at Risk of IE[14]

Dental and dental hygiene procedures that need antibiotic prophylaxis include:

- Manipulation of gingival tissue such as scaling.
- Treatment involving the apices of teeth such as root canals.
- Perforation of the oral soft tissues as in surgical procedures.

The following procedures and events do _not_ need prophylaxis:

- Local anesthetic injections in healthy tissue.
- Dental radiographs.
- Placement of adjustment of removable prostheses or orthodontic appliances.
- Placement of orthodontic brackets.
- Normal shedding of primary teeth.
- Lips or oral mucosa trauma with bleeding

Data from Wilson WR, Gewitz M, Lockhart PB, et al. Prevention of viridans group streptococcal infective endocarditis: a scientific statement from the American Heart Association. Circulation. 2021;143(20):e963-e978.

Antibiotic Prophylaxis

I. AHA Guidelines

- The AHA has made recommendations for the prevention of IE since 1955.
- Beginning with the 2007 guidelines,[15] the AHA based recommendations on review of the evidence to identify the four cardiac conditions at highest risk for IE. The guidelines were reviewed and re-affirmed in 2014 and 2021.[14]
- Maintenance of optimal oral health with daily biofilm removal and regular dental care are more important for prevention of IE from transient bacteremia created by daily activities such as toothbrushing than antibiotic prophylaxis before dental treatment.[14]

II. Recommendations Based on Principles

- The risk of adverse reactions to antibiotics outweighs the possible benefits in reducing IE.[14,16]
- It is likely only an extremely small number of cases of IE are prevented by antibiotic prophylaxis for dental procedures.[14]
- Antibiotic prophylaxis for dental procedures is recommended only for patients in the four categories at highest risk for IE.[14]
- For high-risk patients as defined by the AHA guidelines, prophylaxis is recommended for dental procedures most likely to introduce bacteria into the blood stream.[14]

III. Medical Conditions That Require Antibiotic Premedication before Invasive Dental and Dental Hygiene Procedures

- Antibiotic prophylaxis for dental procedures is recommended only in four groups at highest risk for IE (Box 11-1).
- The dental and dental hygiene procedures for which antibiotic prophylaxis for IE is and is not recommended can be found in **Box 11-2**.
- Procedures for which prophylaxis is *not* recommended include:
  - Evidence-based clinical practice guidelines developed by the ADA and American Academy of Orthopaedic Surgeons recommend against the routine use of antibiotics prior to dental procedures to prevent prosthetic joint infection.[17,18]

- However, premedication may be considered in the case of the high-risk medically complex or **immunocompromised** patient, and consultation with the patient's PCP is recommended.[19]
- Noninvasive procedures such as radiographs and placement of removable prostheses.[14]

American Society of Anesthesiologists Determination

Based on the patient's medical history, an overall estimate of medical risk of a patient can be made. American Society of Anesthesiologists (ASA) Physical Status Classification System describes six categories of physical status and provides examples of adaptations necessary for providing dental hygiene care for a patient in each category.[20]

- **ASA I:** A normal healthy patient without apparent acute or chronic disease and a normal BMI.
- **ASA II:** A patient with mild systemic disease without functional limitations that is well controlled, such as diabetes or hypertension.
- **ASA III:** A patient with one or more moderate to severe systemic diseases with significant functional limitations, such as renal failure with dialysis, unstable asthma or epilepsy, poorly controlled diabetes or hypertension, substance use disorders, history of stroke or heart attack (>3 months), or morbid obesity.
- **ASA IV:** A patient with a severe systemic disease that is a constant threat to life such as recent (<3 months) stroke or heart attack, congestive heart failure, or advanced cancer.
- **ASA V:** A moribund patient not expected to survive 24 hours with or without care such as end stage liver disease, malignant hypertension, or respiratory failure.
- **ASA VI:** A declared brain-dead patient whose organs are being removed for donor purposes.

Review and Update of History

- Updating the patient's health history at each appointment is essential to identify changes that may impact dental care.[1-3]
  - All changes in health status must be documented in the dental record with possible reassessment of the treatment or care plan.
- Following a review of the previously recorded history, questions can be directed to the patient to compare the present condition with the previous one and to determine the following:
  - Interim illnesses; changes in health.
  - Visits to physician; reasons and results.
  - Laboratory tests performed and the results; blood, urine, or other analyses.
  - Current medications.
  - Changes in the oral soft tissues and the teeth observed by the patient.

Documentation

- Date all records.
- All hard copy permanent records are written in ink.
- Electronic patient records are stored on a secure server on password-protected computers, with only office staff having access.
- All electronic charting documentation is signed electronically with safeguards in place to prevent falsification or modification of the patient records.
- The patient signature must be recorded upon completion of the health history to verify the information.[1,3]
  - The completed history for a minor or an adult unable to provide informed consent must be signed by a parent or guardian.
  - Signatures may be recorded or electronically dependent on the method in which the information is collected.
- The HIPAA guidelines should be followed to maintain confidentiality for the information obtained for a patient history.
- Alerts may be needed for patients that require antibiotic prophylaxis; coded tab systems on paper charts or pop-up alerts in electronic records should be used to notify all dental personnel to check the medical history before each appointment.
- Progress notes must document regular update of medical history and changes since last appointment.
- **Box 11-3** provides an example of a progress note related to completion of personal, dental, and medical histories.

Box 11-3 Example Documentation: Updating a Patient's Medical History

- **S**—Forty-five-year-old patient presents for routine 6-month maintenance appointment. She is new to the office and reports she has always taken penicillin prior to her "cleaning" appointments. She completed and signed a new health history form. Her medical history indicates she has a heart murmur, and she reports this is why she has been told to take penicillin before appointments. She became quite concerned about not taking antibiotics prior to the appointment.
- **O**—The recommendations for antibiotic prophylaxis were reviewed with the patient and a consult with the PCP determined she was not a candidate for premedication. A full series of radiographs was taken and the clinical examination was completed. No dental caries noted. Pocket depths in the maxillary molar area range from 5 to 6 mm with bleeding on probing. No suppuration present. No mobility. Furcation involvement Grade II on ML and DL of #2, 3, 14, and 15. Plaque score 15%, primarily in maxillary molar areas.
- **A**—Caries risk: low; periodontal risk: high; oral cancer risk: low. On the basis of the comprehensive periodontal examination and radiographic findings, she has localized Stage II, Grade A periodontitis.
- **P**—Oral self-care review of interdental brush for maxillary molar areas. Full-mouth debridement with localized scaling and periodontal debridement on #2, 3, 14, and 15. One carpule: 2% lidocaine with 1:100,000 epinephrine for a posterior superior alveolar upper right and upper left. Selective polishing: 5% sodium fluoride varnish was applied. A 3-month periodontal maintenance interval was recommended.

Signed: _______________, RDH
Date: _______________

Factors to Teach the Patient

- The need for obtaining the personal, medical, and dental history before performance of dental and dental hygiene procedures and the need for keeping the histories up to date.
- The assurance that medical histories are kept confidential.
- The relationship between oral health and general physical health.
- The interrelationship of medical and dental care.
- All patients who require antibiotic prophylaxis need special attention paid to (1) the importance of preventive dentistry, (2) the need for meticulous oral self-care and regular dental care to reduce risk for infection, and (3) the necessity for taking the prescribed prescription 1 hour before the appointment starts.

References

1. American Academy of Oral Medicine. *Clinical Practice Statement: Medical History*. https://www.aaom.com/index.php?option=com_content&view=article&id=108:medical-history&catid=24:clinical-practice-statement. Accessed December 11, 2021.
2. American Dental Association. Medical dental health history. https://www.ada.org/resources/practice/practice-management/medical-dental-health-history. Accessed December 11, 2021.
3. Greenwood M. Essentials of medical history-taking in dental patients. *Dent Update*. 2015;42(4):308-310, 313-315.
4. American Dental Association. ADA policy on teledentistry. https://www.ada.org/about/governance/current-policies/ada-policy-on-teledentistry. Accessed December 11, 2021.
5. Takemura Y, Atsumi R, Tsuda T. Identifying medical interview behaviors that best elicit information from patients in clinical practice. *Tohoku J Exp Med*. 2007;213(2):121-127.
6. American Dental Association. Writing in the dental record. https://www.ada.org/resources/practice/practice-management/writing-in-the-dental-record. Accessed December 5, 2021.
7. Poudel A, Zhou JY, Story D, Li L. Diabetes and associated cardiovascular complications in American Indians/Alaskan Natives: a review of risks and prevention strategies. *J Diabetes Res*. 2018;2018:2742565.
8. Golden SH, Yajnik C, Phatak S, Hanson RL, Knowler WC. Racial/ethnic differences in the burden of type 2 diabetes over the life course: a focus on the USA and India. *Diabetologia*. 2019;62(10):1751-1760.
9. Weatherspoon DJ, Borrell LN, Johnson CW, Mujahid MS, Neighbors HW, Adar SD. Racial and ethnic differences in self-reported periodontal disease in the multi-ethnic study of atherosclerosis (MESA). *Oral Health Prev Dent*. 2016;14(3):249-257.
10. Kye SY, Park K. Psychosocial factors and health behavior among Korean adults: a cross-sectional study. *Asian Pac J Cancer Prev*. 2012;13(1):49-56.
11. Brown RS, Farquharson AA, Pallasch TM. Medical consultations for medically complex dental patients. *J Calif Dent Assoc*. 2007;35(5):343-349.

12. American Dental Hygienists' Association. *2016 Revised Standards for Clinical Dental Hygiene Practice*. Published June 2016. https://www.adha.org/resources-docs/2016-Revised-Standards-for-Clinical-Dental-Hygiene-Practice.pdf. Accessed December 11, 2021.
13. Herrick KR, Terrio JM, Herrick C. Medical clearance for common dental procedures. *Am Fam Physician*. 2021;104(5):476-483.
14. Wilson WR, Gewitz M, Lockhart PB, et al. Prevention of viridans group streptococcal infective endocarditis: a scientific statement from the American Heart Association. *Circulation*. 2021;143(20);e963-e97.
15. Wilson W, Taubert KA, Gewitz M, et al. Prevention of infective endocarditis. *Circulation*. 2007;116(15):1736-1754.
16. American Dental Association. Antibiotic prophylaxis prior to dental procedures. Published November 8, 2021. https://www.ada.org/resources/research/science-and-research-institute/oral-health-topics/antibiotic-prophylaxis. Accessed December 24, 2021.
17. Sollecito TP, Abt E, Lockhart PB, et al. The use of prophylactic antibiotics prior to dental procedures in patients with prosthetic joints: evidence-based clinical practice guideline for dental practitioners—a report of the American Dental Association Council on Scientific Affairs. *J Am Dent Assoc*. 2015;146(1):11-16.e8.
18. Watters W, Rethman MP, Hanson NB, et al. Prevention of orthopaedic implant infection in patients undergoing dental procedures: evidence-based clinical practice guideline. *J Am Acad Orthop Surg*. 2013;21(3):180-189.
19. Abt E, Hellstein JW, Lockhart PB, et al. American Dental Association guidance for utilizing appropriate use criteria in the management of the care of patients with orthopedic implants undergoing dental procedures. *J Am Dent Assoc*. 2017;148(2):57-59.
20. American Society of Anesthesiologists. ASA Physical Status Classification System. https://www.asahq.org/standards-and-guidelines/asa-physical-status-classification-system. Accessed December 24, 2021.

CHAPTER 12

Vital Signs

Lisa B. Johnson, RDH, MPH, DHS

CHAPTER OUTLINE

LEARNING OBJECTIVES

After studying this chapter, the student will be able to:

1. List and explain the vital signs and why proper assessment is key to identifying the patient's health status.
2. Demonstrate and explain the correct procedures for assessing the vital signs: temperature, respiration, radial pulse, and blood pressure.
3. Recognize and explain factors that may affect temperature, respiration, pulse, and blood pressure.
4. Describe and evaluate equipment used for assessing temperature and blood pressure.
5. Recognize normal vital signs across varied age groups.

Introduction

Determination of four vital signs—*body temperature, pulse, respiratory rate*, and *blood pressure*—is considered standard procedure in patient care. **Table 12-1** summarizes the normal values of the four basic vital signs for infants through older adults.

I. Patient Preparation and Instruction

- Seat patient in upright position, at eye level for instruction.
- Explain the vital signs and obtain consent.
- Explain how vital signs can affect dental hygiene and dental treatment.

Table 12-1 Resting Vital Sign Ranges Infant through Older Adult[1-3]

Age (Range)	Temperature (°F)	Pulse (BPM)	Respiration (RPM)	Blood Pressure (mm Hg)	
				Systolic	Diastolic
12 mo	99.4–99.7	80–160	30–60	80–89	34–42
1–2 y	99–99.7	80–130	24–40	84–91	39–47
4–5 y	98.6–99	80–120	22–34	88–96	47–56
6–11 y	98–98.6	75–110	18–30	91–107	53–63
≥13 y	97–99	60–90	12–20	104–<120	60–<80
Adult	97–99	60–100	12–20	90–<120	60–<80
Older adult (>60)	97–99	60–100	12–20	90–<120	60–<80

- During the process, explain each step as needed by the individual patient.

II. Dental Hygiene Care Planning

- Recording vital signs contributes to the proper systemic evaluation of a patient in conjunction with the complete medical history.
- Dental hygiene care planning and appointment sequencing are directly influenced by the findings.
- When vital signs are not within normal, advise the patient consult with the primary care provider.
- Referral for medical evaluation and treatment is indicated.

Body Temperature

While preparing the patient history and making the extraoral and intraoral examinations, the need for taking the temperature may become apparent, or the dentist may have requested the procedure in conjunction with current oral disease.

I. Indications for Taking the Temperature

- For the new patient's initial permanent record along with all vital signs.
- For comprehensive examination during a continuing care appointment.
- When oral infection is known to be present.
  - Necrotizing ulcerative gingivitis or periodontitis.
  - Apical or periodontal abscess.
  - Acute pericoronitis.
- With other vital signs, prior to administration of local anesthetic.
- At any appointment when the patient reports illness or there is a suspected infection.
  - Protection of the health of the healthcare personnel and patients or families who may be exposed secondarily.
  - During epidemics when community exposure is a risk.
  - For patient's referral for medical care when indicated.

II. Maintenance of Body Temperature

- Normal
  - Adults: The normal average temperature is 98.6°F (37°C). The normal range is from 97 to 99°F (36.1 to 37.2°C).
  - Older adults: Over 70 years of age, the average temperature is slightly lower (96.8°F [36°C]).
  - Children: There is no appreciable difference between boys and girls. Average temperatures are as follows:
    - First year—99.1°F (37.3°C).
    - Fourth year—99.4°F (37.5°C).
    - Fifth year—98.6°F (37°C).
    - Twelfth year—98°F (36.7°C).
- Temperature variations
  - Fever (**pyrexia**): Values over 99.5°F (37.5°C).
  - **Hyperthermia**: Values over 104°F (40°C).
  - **Hypothermia**: Values below 96°F (35.5°C).
- Factors that alter body temperature
  - Time of day: Highest in late afternoon and early evening; lowest during sleep and early morning.
  - Temporary increase: Exercise, hot drinks, smoking, or application of external heat.
  - Pathologic states: Infection, dehydration, hyperthyroidism, myocardial infarction, or tissue injury from trauma.
  - Decrease: Starvation, hemorrhage, or physiologic shock.

III. Methods of Determining Temperature

A. Locations for Measurement

- Oral: Most common site due to ease of access.
    - Drinking hot or cold liquids just prior can affect results; wait at least 15 minutes before oral measurement is taken.
    - Not recommended for infants, young children, and unconscious or highly behavioral patients.
- Temporal artery (forehead): Measurements taken with electronic device; easily tolerated and results comparable to oral thermometers.
- Ear: With a tympanic device.
- Medical/hospital applications: Also use axilla or rectum for assessment.

B. Types of Thermometers

- Electronic oral thermometer
    - Cover with disposable protective sheath.
    - Place under tongue; short time required.
    - Read on the digital display.
- Tympanic thermometer
    - Cover with protective sheath.
    - Insert gently into ear canal.
    - Short exposure (2–5 seconds) before reading appears on digital unit.
- Temporal artery thermometer (contact and noncontact)
    - Measures the temperature of the skin over the temporal artery on the head.
    - Contact thermometer is placed on the center of the forehead, midway between the eyebrow and hairline.
    - Slide the thermometer along the forehead until the hairline is reached.
    - Read the temperature on the display.
    - Noncontact infrared thermometer (**Figure 12-1**) is held approximately 1 inch away from skin over temporal artery (the clinician should adhere to manufacturer guidelines).
    - Replace the protective cap.
    - More accurate in infants than the tympanic thermometer.

IV. Care of Patient with Temperature Elevation

- Temperature over 104°F (40°C)[4]
    - Treat as a medical emergency.
    - Transport to a hospital for medical care.

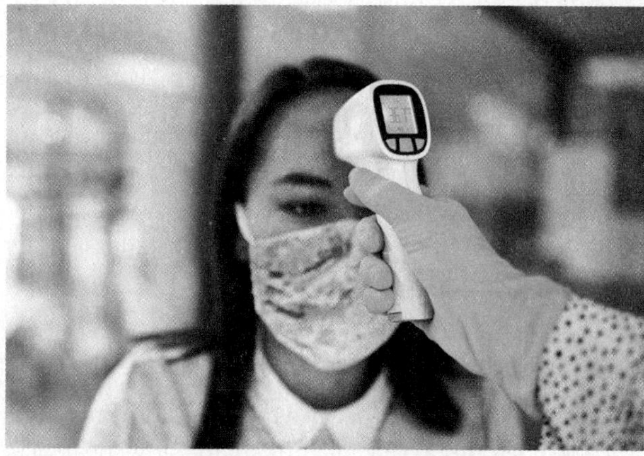

A

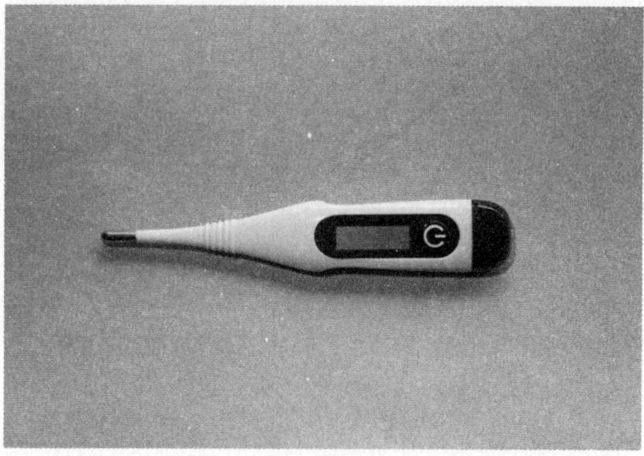

B

Figure 12-1 Types of Thermometers. **A:** Noncontact infrared thermometer. **B:** Digital thermometer.

- Temperature 99.6–104°F (37.6–40°C)[4]
    - Check possible temporary causes of pyrexia, such as hot beverage or smoking; observe patient while repeating the determination.
    - Review the dental and medical history.
    - Postpone elective oral care when there are signs of respiratory infection or other possible communicable disease.

Pulse

- The pulse is the intermittent throbbing sensation felt when the fingers are pressed against an artery.
- It is the result of the alternate expansion and contraction of an artery as a wave of blood is forced out from the heart.
- The pulse rate or heart rate is the count of the heartbeats.
- Irregularities of strength, rhythm, and quality of the pulse are noted while counting the pulse rate.

I. Maintenance of Normal Pulse

A. Normal Pulse Rates

- Adults: There is no absolute normal. The adult range is 60–100 beats per minute (BPM), slightly higher for women than for men.
- Children: The pulse or heart rate falls steadily during childhood.

B. Factors That Influence Pulse Rate

An unusually fast heartbeat (over 100 BPM in an adult) is called **tachycardia**; an unusually slow heartbeat (below 50 BPM) is **bradycardia**.

- Increased pulse: Caused by exercise, stimulants, eating, strong emotions, extremes of heat and cold, and some forms of heart disease.
- Decreased pulse: Caused by sleep, depressants, fasting, quiet emotions, and low vitality from prolonged illness.
- Emergency situations: Listed in Tables 9-3 and 9-4 in Chapter 9.

II. Procedure for Determining Pulse Rate

- Sequence
  - The pulse rate is obtained following the body temperature.
- Sites
  - Radial pulse: At the wrist (**Figure 12-2**).
  - Temporal artery: On the side of the head in front of the ear.
  - Facial artery: At the border of the mandible.
  - Carotid pulse: At the side of the upper neck near the trachea.
    - Used during cardiopulmonary resuscitation for an adult.
  - Brachial pulse: Used for an infant and is found on the inside of the upper arm between the elbow and shoulder (Figure 12-2).
- Prepare the patient
  - Explain the procedure to the patient.
  - Have the patient in a comfortable position with arm and hand supported, palm down.
  - Locate the radial pulse on the thumb side of the wrist with the tips of the first three fingers (**Figure 12-3**). Do not use the thumb because it contains a pulse that may be confused with the patient's pulse.
- Count and record
  - When the pulse is felt, exert light pressure and count for 1 minute. Use a timer, watch, or clock to monitor the time accurately. Check with a repeat count when there is a question about rate or quality of pulse.
- While taking the pulse, observe the following:
  - Rhythm: Regular, regularly irregular, irregularly irregular.
  - Volume and strength: Full, strong, poor, weak, thready.

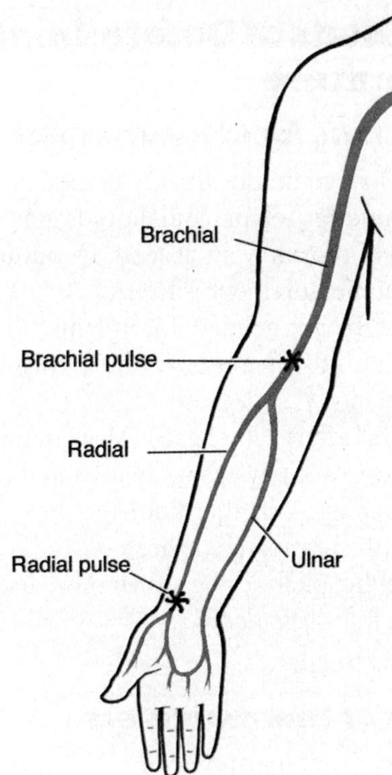

Figure 12-2 Arteries of the Arm. Note the location of the radial pulse. The brachial pulse may be felt just before the brachial artery branches into the radial and ulnar arteries.

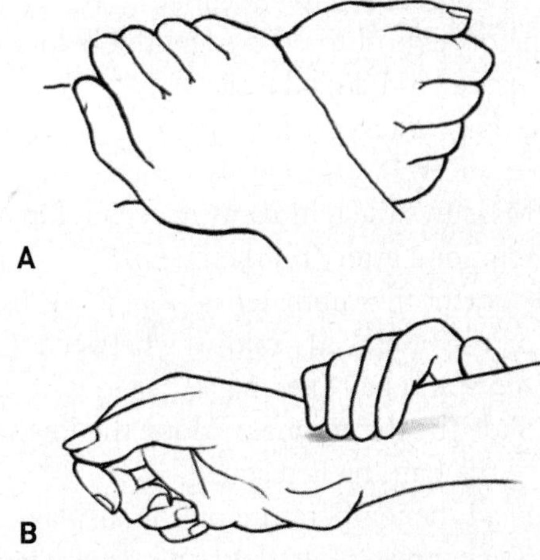

Figure 12-3 Determination of Pulse Rate. **A:** Correct position of hands. **B:** The tips of the clinician's first three fingers are placed over the radial pulse located on the thumb side of the ventral surface of the wrist.

1. Record the date and pulse rate, as BPM and with other characteristics, in patient's record. Document BPM reading prior to administering local anesthesia when included in the care plan. (See Chapter 36.)
   - A pulse rate over 100 is considered abnormal for an adult and requires further investigation before proceeding with dental treatment.

Respiration

- The function of respiration is to supply oxygen to the tissues and to eliminate carbon dioxide.
- Variations in normal respirations may be shown by such characteristics as the rate, rhythm, depth, and quality and may be symptomatic of disease or emergency states.

I. Maintenance of Normal Respirations

A respiration is one breath taken in and let out.

- Normal respiratory rate
  - Children: The respiratory rate decreases steadily during childhood.[1]
  - Adults: The adult range is from 12 to 20/min, slightly higher for women.
  - Older adults: Respiratory rate has been shown to have a higher predictive value for serious adverse events and should be considered an important component of vital sign assessment.[5]
- Factors that influence respirations: Many of the same factors that influence pulse rate also influence the number of respirations.
- A rate below 12/min (bradypnea) is considered subnormal for an adult, rate over 28 is accelerated (tachypnea), and rates over 60 are extremely rapid and dangerous.
- Increased respiration: Caused by work and exercise, excitement, anxiety, strong emotions, pain, hemorrhage, and shock.
- Decreased respiration: Caused by sleep, certain drugs, pulmonary insufficiency, and **apnea**.
- Emergency situations include **anoxia**. (See Chapter 9.)

II. Procedures for Observing Respirations

- Determine rate
  1. Make the count of respirations immediately after counting the pulse.
  2. Maintain the fingers over the radial pulse.
  3. Respirations must be counted so that the patient is not aware, as the rate may be voluntarily altered.
  4. Count the number of times the chest rises in 1 minute using a timer, watch, or clock to monitor the time. It is not necessary to count both inspirations and expirations.
- Factors to observe
  - Depth: Describe as shallow, normal, or deep.
  - Rhythm: Describe as regular (evenly spaced) or irregular (with pauses of irregular lengths between).
  - Quality: Describe as strong, easy, weak, or labored (noisy). Poor quality may have an effect on body color; for example, a bluish tinge of the face or nail beds may mean an insufficiency of oxygen.
  - Sounds: Describe deviant sounds made during inspiration, expiration, or both.
  - Position of patient: When the patient assumes an unusual position to secure comfort during breathing or prefers to remain seated upright, mark records accordingly.
- Record all findings in the patient's record.

Blood Pressure

I. Components of Blood Pressure

- Blood pressure is the force exerted by the blood on the blood vessel walls.
  - When the left ventricle of the heart contracts, blood is forced out into the aorta and travels through the large arteries to the smaller arteries, arterioles, and capillaries. The vessels of the heart are shown in Chapter 61.
  - The pulsations extend from the heart through the arteries and disappear in the arterioles.
  - During the course of the cardiac cycle, the blood pressure is changing constantly.
- Systole phase
  - The **systole phase** occurs during ventricular contraction. It is measured as systolic pressure. It is the peak, or the highest pressure exerted by the heart during contraction.
  - The normal systolic pressure for an adult is less than 120 mm Hg.
- Diastole phase
  - Diastolic pressure is the lowest pressure. The **diastole phase** is the effect of ventricular relaxation.
  - The normal diastolic pressure for an adult is less than 80 mm Hg.

- Pulse pressure
  - The **pulse pressure** is the difference between the systolic and diastolic pressures.

II. Factors That Influence Blood Pressure

- Blood pressure depends on the following:
  - Force of the heartbeat (energy of the heart).
  - Peripheral resistance; condition of the arteries; changes in elasticity of vessels, which may occur with age and disease.
  - Volume of blood in the circulatory system.
- Factors that increase blood pressure
  - Exercise, eating, stimulants, and emotional disturbance.[3]
  - Use of oral contraceptives; blood pressure increases with age and length of use.[3]
- Factors that decrease blood pressure
  - Fasting, rest, depressants, and quiet emotions.
  - Such emergencies as fainting, blood loss, shock. (See Tables 9-3 and 9-4 in Chapter 9.)

III. Equipment for Determining Blood Pressure

A sphygmomanometer is made up of a pressure-measuring device (manometer) and an inflatable cuff to wrap around the arm or, under certain circumstances, the leg.

- Mercury sphygmomanometer (analog)
  - Traditional system, but mercury is a potential health hazard because of mercury spillage and is less commonly used.[3,6]
  - Has shown to be more accurate and consistent than other types.
- Aneroid sphygmomanometer (analog)
  - Compact, portable, glass-enclosed gauge with needle for registration of blood pressure.
  - Requires regular calibration to maintain accuracy.
- Electronic sphygmomanometer (digital)
  - Automatic determination of blood pressure without use of a **stethoscope**.
  - Size: Choosing the correct size cuff (see **Figure 12-4**) is critical to accurate blood pressure results.
    - The cuff needs to be long enough to encircle 80% of the arm and wide enough to encircle 40% of the arm at its midpoint.[3]
    - A longer, wider cuff is required for obese or muscular individuals and children require pediatric-sized cuffs. Always refer to the recommended cuff sizes for accuracy of readings (**Figure 12-5**).

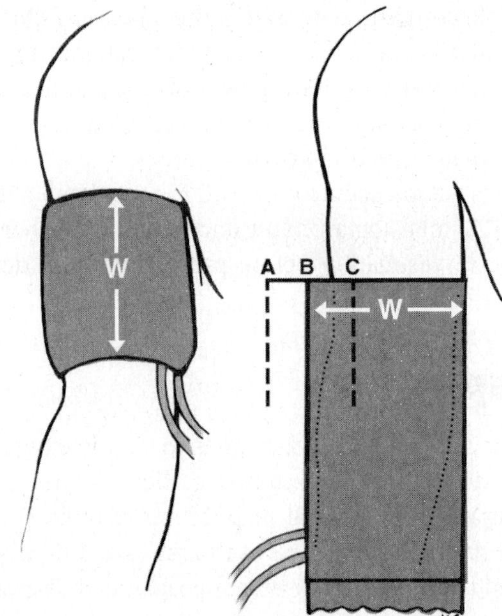

Figure 12-4 Selection of Cuff Size. The correct width (W) is 20% greater than the diameter of the arm where applied. **A:** Too wide. **B:** Correct width. **C:** Too narrow.

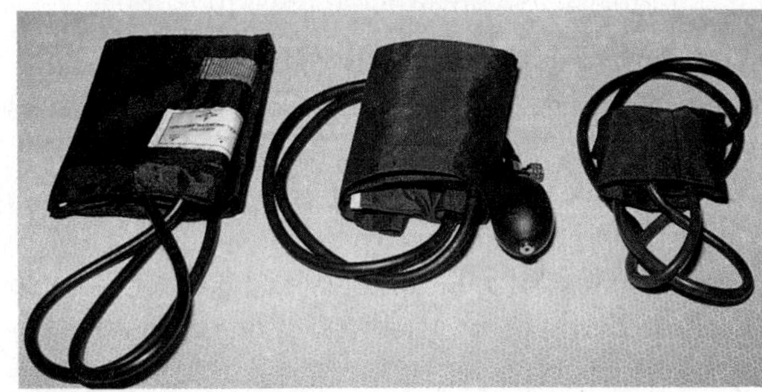

Figure 12-5 Three Sizes of Blood Pressure Cuff. Extra-large, regular, and pediatric cuffs.

- Wrist or finger devices
  - Considered to be less accurate.[3,6]
- Stethoscope
  - Consists of an endpiece with a flat diaphragm on one side and (may or may not have) a smaller, concave-shaped bell side. Both sides transmit and send sound through tubes to the earpieces.

IV. Procedure for Determining Blood Pressure

- Prepare patient.
  1. Explain the procedure briefly to the patient. Detailed explanations need to be avoided because they may excite the patient and change the blood pressure.
  2. Seat patient comfortably, with the arm slightly flexed, with palm up, and with the whole

forearm supported on a *level surface at the level of the heart*.[3]
 - Arm above heart will result in a false low reading.[6]
 - Arm below heart level will result in false high reading.[6]
 - Improper cuff selection will result in false high or low depending on size.[3,6,7]

3. Use either arm unless otherwise indicated; for example, history of vascular surgery or mastectomy would indicate the arm on opposite side should be used. Repeat blood pressure determinations need to be made on the same arm because a variation in pressure may exist between arms.[3,6,7]
4. Take pressure on bare arm, not over clothing.[6,7] Loosen a tight sleeve.
5. Select cuff size as described in Figure 12-5.

- Apply cuff.
  1. Apply the completely deflated cuff to the patient's arm, supported at the level of the heart. If the arm rests on the arm of a dental chair, lower than the heart, the diastolic pressure may show a small but significant increase.[3,6]
  2. Place the portion of the cuff that contains the inflatable bladder directly over the brachial artery. The cuff may have an arrow to show the point that is placed over the artery. The lower edge of the cuff is placed 1 inch above the antecubital fossa (**Figure 12-6**). Fasten the cuff evenly and snugly.[3,6,7]
  3. Adjust the position of the gauge/dial so it is clearly visible and facing you.
- Locate the radial pulse (Figures 12-2 and 12-3).
  1. Palpate 1 inch below the antecubital fossa to locate the brachial artery pulse (Figure 12-6).
  2. Hold the fingers on the pulse.
- Determine maximum inflation level (MIL) or estimated systolic blood pressure.
  1. Close the needle valve (air lock) attached to the hand control bulb firmly but so it may be released readily.
  2. Pump to inflate the cuff until the radial pulse stops. Monitor the gauge to note the level at which the pulse disappears. This is the estimated systolic pressure.
  3. Continue to pump until the gauge reads 30 points beyond where the radial pulse was no longer felt. This is the MIL. It means that the brachial artery is collapsed by the pressure of the cuff and no blood is flowing through. *Unless the MIL is determined, the level to which the cuff is inflated will be arbitrary. Excess pressure can be very uncomfortable for the patient.*[6]

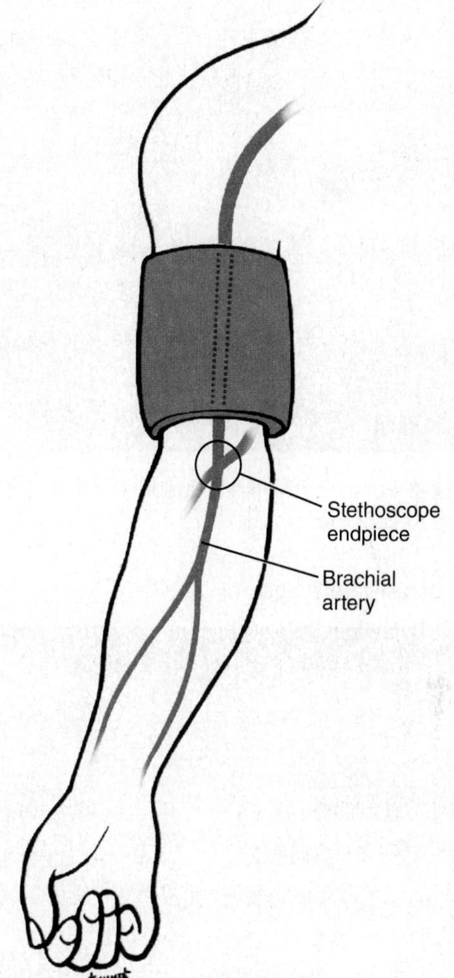

Figure 12-6 Blood Pressure Cuff in Position. The lower edge of the cuff is placed approximately 1 inch above the antecubital fossa. The stethoscope endpiece is placed over the palpated brachial artery pulse point approximately 1 inch below the antecubital fossa and slightly toward the inner side of the arm.

- Position the stethoscope.
- Place the endpiece over the palpated brachial artery, 1 inch below the antecubital fossa, and slightly toward the inner side of the arm (Figure 12-6 and **Figure 12-7**). Hold lightly in place.
  1. Earpieces should be angled forward into the ear canal for proper **auscultation** (**Figure 12-8A-B**).
  2. Manual stethoscopes can be turned on/off by rotating the endpiece. Power stethoscopes can be turned on/off by the push of a button or tap of the diaphragm.
  3. Tap gently and listen to confirm it is on (in active mode).
  4. Diaphragm or bell side of endpiece should be placed with light, steady, and complete contact with skin. Either side of the endpiece can be used for reliable measurement (Figure 12-7).[3]

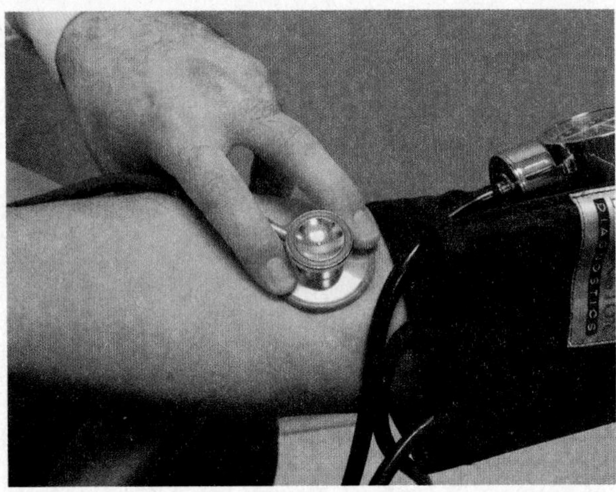

Figure 12-7 Forearm Properly Supported during Blood Pressure Assessment.

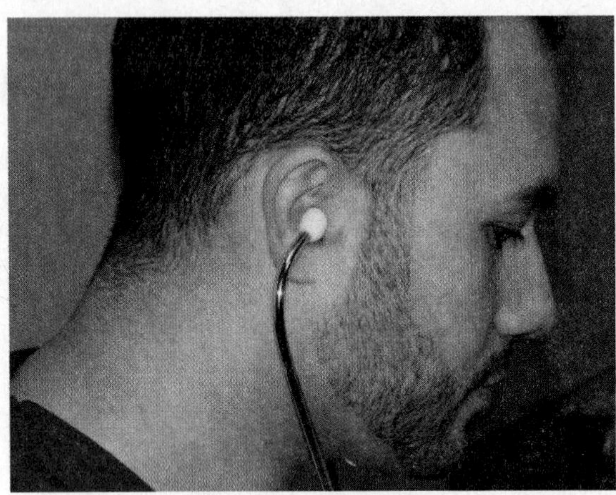

A

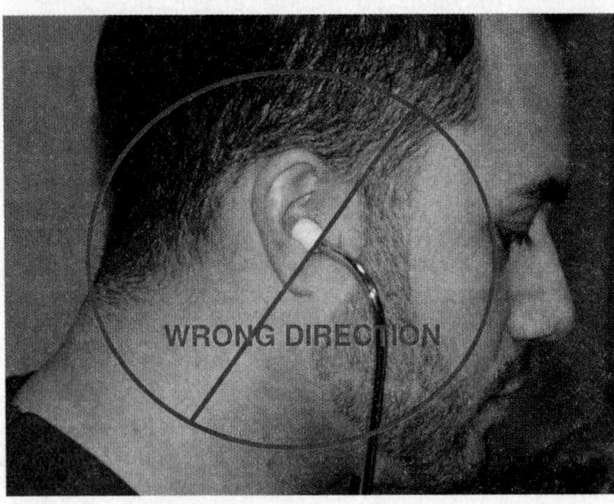

B

Figure 12-8 Placement of the Earpieces for the Stethoscope. **A:** Proper placement of the earpieces for the stethoscope. **B:** Improper placement.

5. Avoid contact with cuff to prevent extraneous sounds that may distract from **Korotkoff sounds**.

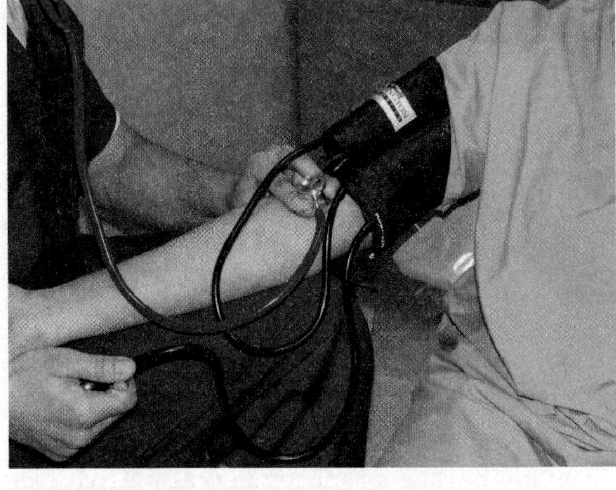

Figure 12-9 Correct Stethoscope Endpiece Placement, Away from Cuff and in Contact with Skin

6. Support patient's arm at heart level (see **Figure 12-9**). The position of the arm is critical to accuracy and can greatly influence readings. The upper arm raised above the heart can produce a false low reading and when placed below heart level will result in a false high reading.[3,6]

- Deflate the cuff gradually.
  1. Release the air lock slowly so the dial drops very gradually and steadily, approximately two to three lines.
  2. Listen for the first Korotkoff sound ("tap tap"). This is the beginning of the flow of blood past the cuff. Note the number on the dial as the *systolic pressure*.
  3. Continue to release the pressure slowly. The sound will continue, first becoming louder, then diminishing and becoming muffled, until finally disappearing. Note the number on the dial where the last distinct tap was heard. That number is the diastolic pressure.
  4. Release further (about 10 points) until all sounds cease. That is the second diastolic point. In some clinics and hospitals, the last sound is taken as the diastolic pressure.
  5. Let the rest of the air out rapidly.
- Repeat for confirmation.
  - Wait 30 seconds before inflating the cuff again.
  - More than one reading is needed within a few minutes to determine an average and ensure a correct reading.
- Record.
  - Write date, arm used, and seated or standing.
  - Record blood pressure as a fraction, for example, 110/72.

V. Hypertension (High Blood Pressure)

Hypertension (HTN) or high blood pressure (HBP) is a serious condition that affects nearly one out of every three individuals in the United States and is a leading cause of cardiovascular disease (CVD) and CVD-related deaths in the United States.[3,8]

- HTN of above 140/90 is associated with cardiovascular diseases, stroke, kidney failure, and premature death.[3,6]
- Contributing factors to hypertension include smoking, stress, obesity, alcohol and drug abuse, and lifestyle.[9]
- Information about the patient's blood pressure is essential during dental and dental hygiene appointments because special adaptations may be needed.
- Blood pressure readings are recorded with the medical history and other assessment data.
- **White-coat hypertension** is more common in older adults and reported as frequent among centenarians.[1,3,6]
  - Readings taken at the start of an appointment can be significantly higher than at the end of treatment.[7]
- To establish a baseline reading and determine the need for patient referral for medical attention, more than one reading is advised. A comparison of the reading at the beginning of the appointment with one at the end of appointment, when the patient is relaxed, may be helpful.
- Screening for blood pressure in dental practices has been shown to be an effective health service for all ages since many patients are unaware that they have hypertension (see **Table 12-2**).
- Growing evidence indicates primary hypertension is commonly asymptomatic and often unrecognized in young children and adolescents.[1]
  - Children older than 3 years who are seen in medical settings should have their blood pressure measured annually. Blood pressure should be measured at each dental encounter for children with obesity, renal disease, diabetes, or aortic arch obstruction or coarctation, or who are taking medications known to elevate blood pressure.[1]
  - Children and adolescent blood pressure should be matched to guidelines in the updated (2017) U.S. Department of Health and Human Services (USDHHS) 4th Report on Diagnosis, Evaluation, and Treatment of Blood Pressure in Children and Adolescents.[1]
  - The USDHHS guidelines use age, sex, and height percentile data to more accurately determine the presence or absence of hypertension in children and adolescents. Updated 2017 guidelines reflect normal blood pressure tables based on children with normal weight.[1]

Table 12-2 Adult Blood Pressure Classifications.[3,10,11]

Blood Pressure Classification	Systolic (mm Hg)		Diastolic (mm Hg)	Recommendations
Hypotension and **postural hypotension**	<90		<60	Observe for possible light-headedness and syncope. If persistent, referral for evaluation is indicated.
Normal/ **normotensive**	<120	and	<80	Proceed as planned.
Elevated	120–129	and	<80	Retake after 5 min. If still elevated, inform patient of elevated blood pressure. Recommend primary care provider consult and encourage lifestyle modifications.
Hypertension				
Stage 1	130–139	or	80–89	Retake after 5 min. If still elevated, inform patient of elevated blood pressure. Refer for primary care provider consult. Employ stress reduction to routine dental treatment. Modify local anesthetic to 1:100,000 vasoconstrictor.
Stage 2	≥140	or	≥90	Retake after 5 min. If still elevated, inform patient of elevated blood pressure. Refer for urgent primary care provider assessment. Delay dental treatment until hypertension is controlled.
Hypertensive crisis	>180	and/or	>120	Discontinue care and retake after 5 min to confirm findings. Refer for immediate medical care/call 911 depending on your clinic protocol.

Table 12-3 Lifestyle Modifications for Hypertension Management[1,3,9]

Modification	Recommendation	Approximate Reduction in Systolic Blood Pressure Range
Weight loss	Normal body weight maintenance based on average body mass index	5–20 mm Hg/10-kg weight loss
Dietary Approaches to Stop Hypertension (DASH)	A diet rich in fruits, vegetables, and low-fat dairy products with reduced saturated and total fat	8–14 mm Hg
Dietary sodium intake	Reduce sodium intake to ≤100 mmol/d (2.4 g sodium or 6 g sodium chloride [table salt])	2–8 mm Hg
Physical activity	Aerobic activity at least 30 min/d	4–9 mm Hg
Moderate alcohol consumption	Limit to no more than two drinks/d for most men and no more than one drink/d for women or lighter weight individuals[a]	2–4 mm Hg

[a]1 drink = 12 oz beer, 5 oz wine, or 0.5 oz distilled spirits

- Cardiovascular diseases are described in Chapter 61. That information can be a helpful introduction and is recommended for reading in conjunction with this section on the techniques for obtaining blood pressure.

VI. Blood Pressure Follow-Up Criteria

- Dental personnel have an obligation to advise and *refer for further evaluation with a medical provider.*
- Diagnosis of hypertension would never be made based on an isolated reading.
- Vital signs should be recorded for all new patients, and pre- and postoperatively if medically compromised.
- Rechecking within 1 year is recommended for persons at increased risk for hypertension, such as family history, weight gain, obesity, African American, use of oral contraceptives, smoking, and excessive alcohol consumption (see Tables 12-1 and 12-2).[1,3,9]
- Lifestyle modifications are indicated for all blood pressure classifications and HBP management should follow current evidence-based management guidelines through collaborative efforts with the patient's primary care provider.[1,3,9] Immediate consultation with a patient's primary care provider is indicated prior to dental or dental hygiene treatment when either reading is more than or equal to 180/110 (Table 12-2 and **Table 12-3**).

Documentation

Documentation in the permanent record of a patient with HBP would include the following:

- Carefully document medical history with regular updates at each maintenance appointment.
- Reminder to help patient realize the importance of regularly taking prescribed medication.
- Prepared and documented blood pressure reading at each appointment, especially when anesthesia is included in the care plan.
- **Box 12-1** contains a sample progress note.

Box 12-1 Example Documentation: Vital Signs

- **S**—Mrs. Patel apologized for arriving 5 minutes late and stated she had no concerns at the start of her dental appointment.
- **O**—Vital signs at 9:00 AM; pulse 64; respirations 12; blood pressure (right arm) 162/88 seated.
- **A**—Hypertension stage 2 range.
- **P**—Advised Mrs. Patel her blood pressure is measuring at a high and an unsafe level for treatment. Blood pressure remained elevated when reassessed 10 minutes later. Discussed hypertension range with dentist and referred patient to primary care provider for urgent follow-up. Delay maintenance appointment until hypertension under control. Follow-up later today by phone.

Signed:______________________, RDH
Date: __________

Factors to Teach the Patient

- Impact of vital signs on providing dental and dental hygiene treatment.
- The importance of having blood pressure measurements at regular intervals.
- For the patient diagnosed as hypertensive, encourage careful attention to taking medications as prescribed to control HBP.
- Encourage healthy lifestyle changes such as tobacco cessation, drug and/or alcohol counseling, modest weight loss, exercise, and healthy dietary habits (see Table 12-3).

References

1. Flynn JT, Kaelber DC, Baker-Smith CM, et al. Clinical practice guideline for screening and management of high blood pressure in children and adolescents. *Pediatrics*. 2017;140(3).
2. Fleming S, Thompson M, Stevens R, et al. Normal ranges of heart rate and respiratory rate in children from birth to 18 years of age: a systematic review of observational studies. *Lancet*. 2013;377(9770):1011.
3. Whelton PK, Carey RM, Aronow WS, et al. 2017 ACC /AHA/AAPA/ABC/ACPM/AGS/APhA/ASH/ASPC/NMA/PCNA Guideline for the prevention, detection, evaluation, and management of high blood pressure in adults: a report of the American College of Cardiology/American Heart Association Task Force on clinical practice guidelines. *J Am Coll Cardiol*. 2018;71(19):e127-e248.
4. Medline Plus. Temperature measurement. https://medlineplus.gov/ency/article/003400.htm. Accessed September 22, 2021.
5. Chester JG, Rudolph JL. Vital signs in older patients: age-related changes. *J Am Med Dir Assoc*. 2011;12(5):337-343.
6. Pickering TG, Hall JE, Appel LJ, et al. Recommendations for blood pressure measurement in humans and experimental animals: part 1: blood pressure measurement in humans: a statement for professionals from the Subcommittee of Professional and Public Education of the American Heart Association Council on High Blood Pressure Research. *Hypertension*. 2005;45(1):142.
7. Kallioinen N, Hill A, Horswill MS, Ward HE, Watson MO. Sources of inaccuracy in the measurement of adult patients' resting blood pressure in clinical settings: a systematic review. *J Hypertens*. 2017;35(3):421-441.
8. Kochanek KD, Murphy SL, Xu J, Arias E. Deaths: final data for 2017. *Natl Vital Stat Rep*. 2019;68(9):1-77.
9. Arnett DK, Blumenthal RS, Albert MA, et al. 2019 ACC/AHA guideline on the primary prevention of cardiovascular disease: executive summary: a report of the American College of Cardiology/American Heart Association Task Force on clinical practice guidelines. *Circulation*. 2019;140(11):e563-e595.
10. Bader JD, Bonito AJ, Shugars DA. A systematic review of cardiovascular effects of epinephrine on hypertensive dental patients. *Oral Surg Oral Med Oral Pathol Oral Radiol Endod*. 2013;93(6):647.
11. Guimaraes CC, Lopes LC, Bergamaschi CC, et al. Local anaesthetics combined with vasoconstrictors in patients with cardiovascular disease undergoing dental procedures: systematic review and meta-analysis. *BMJ Open*. 2021;11(7):e044357.

CHAPTER 13

Extraoral and Intraoral Examination

Lisa B. Johnson, RDH, MPH, DHS

CHAPTER OUTLINE

LEARNING OBJECTIVES

After studying this chapter, the student will be able to:

1. Explain the rationale for a comprehensive extra- and intraoral examination.
2. Explain the systematic sequence of the extra- and intraoral examination.
3. Identify normal hard and soft tissue anatomy of the head, neck, and oral cavity.
4. Describe and document physical characteristics (size, shape, color, texture, and consistency) and morphologic categories (elevated, flat, and depressed lesions) for notable findings.
5. Identify suspected conditions that require follow-up and referral for medical evaluation.

Rationale for the Extraoral and Intraoral Examination

- The extra- and intraoral examination is performed for early identification of abnormalities and pathologies, especially oral cancer.[1,2]
    - Although an essential goal of the examination is to detect cancer of the mouth at the earliest possible stage, a thorough examination may also reveal signs of thyroid disorders, eating disorders, nutritional deficiencies, sexually transmitted diseases, and a host of systemic conditions.
- Cancer prevention education for the patient is an essential component of the extra- and intraoral examination.

Components of Examination

- The standard of patient care is that the total patient is being treated, not only the oral cavity, and particularly not just the teeth and immediate surrounding tissues.
- The examination is all-inclusive to detect possible physical or psychological influences on the patient's oral health.
- Thorough examination is essential for each continuing care appointment so treatment for the control and prevention of oral diseases will be effective.
- Assessment of health-related risk factors, such as[3]:
    - History of previous cancer.
    - Family history of squamous cell carcinoma (SCC).
    - Tobacco use.
    - Alcohol use.
    - Cultural and genetic susceptibility.
    - Sun exposure and lack of use of sun protection.
    - Diet.
    - Certain surgeries such as organ or bone marrow transplant and subsequent long-term immunosuppressive medications.
    - Encounters involving orogenital contact may increase the risk of human papillomavirus (HPV) transmission.[4,5]
    - HPV vaccination status.[4,6]

I. Types of Examinations

- Comprehensive
    - A comprehensive examination includes a thorough summary of all the components of the assessment.
    - The extra- and intraoral examination is a component of a patient's complete assessment and is performed for all new patients and at each continuing care visit.
- Screening
    - Screening implies a brief, preliminary examination, usually for a particular purpose such as for initial patient assessment and triage to determine priorities for treatment.
- Limited examination
    - A type of brief examination made for an emergency situation. It may be used in the management of an acute condition.
- Follow-up
    - Brief follow-up examination to check healing following a treatment.
- Continuing care/reevaluation
    - After a specific period of time following the completion of the care plan and the anticipated restoration to health.
    - A continuing care examination is a complete reassessment from which a new dental hygiene diagnosis and care plan are derived.

II. Methods for Examination

The extra- and intraoral examination is accomplished by various visual and tactile, manual, and instrumental methods. Patient position, optimum lighting, and effective retraction for accessibility and visibility contribute to the accuracy and completeness of the examination.

- Visual examination
    - Direct observation: Visual observation is carried out in a systematic sequence to note surface appearance (color, contour, size) and to observe movement and other evidence of function.
    - Radiographic examination: The use of radiographs can reveal deviations from normal not observable by direct vision.
    - Transillumination: A strong light directed through a soft tissue or a tooth to enhance examination is useful for detecting irregularities of the teeth and locating calculus. Hold the mouth mirror to view from the lingual to see the translucency.
- Palpation
    - **Palpation** is examination using the sense of touch through tissue manipulation or pressure on an area with the gloved fingers of one hand or both.
    - Digital: The use of a single finger. Example: Index finger applied to the lingual side of

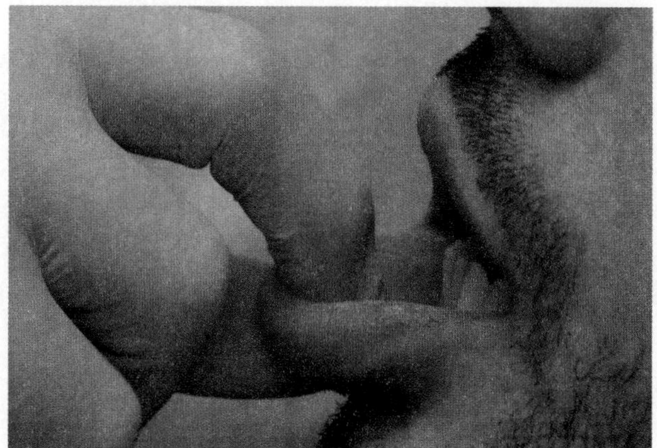

Figure 13-1 Palpation of the Lip to Illustrate the Use of a Finger and Thumb of the Same Hand

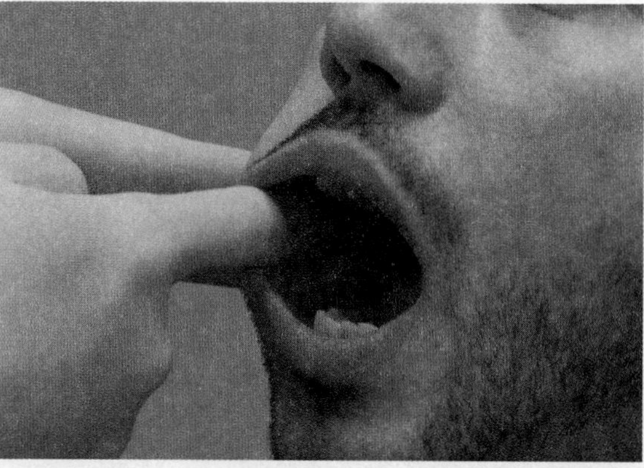

A

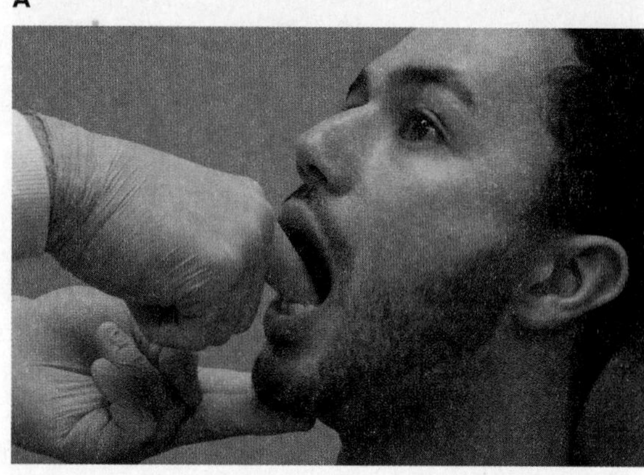

B

Figure 13-2 Bimanual Palpation. **A:** Examination of the buccal mucosa by simultaneous palpation extraorally and intraorally. **B:** Examination of the floor of the mouth by simultaneous palpation with fingers of each hand in apposition.

the mandible beneath the canine and premolar area to determine presence of a **torus** mandibularis.

- Bidigital: The use of finger and thumb of same hand. Example: Palpation of the lips (**Figure 13-1**).
- Bimanual: The use of finger or fingers and thumb from each hand applied simultaneously in coordination. Example: Index finger of one hand palpates on the floor of the mouth inside, while a finger or fingers from the other hand press on the same area from under the chin externally (**Figure 13-2A-B**).
- Bilateral: Two hands are used at the same time to examine corresponding structures on opposite sides of the body. Comparisons can be made. Example: Fingers placed beneath the chin to palpate the submandibular lymph nodes (**Figure 13-3**).

- Instrumentation
  - Examination instruments, such as a periodontal probe and an explorer, are used for specific examination of the teeth and periodontal tissues.
- Percussion
  - Percussion is the act of tapping a surface or tooth with an instrument.
  - Information about the status of health is determined either by the response of the patient or by the sound. When a tooth is known to be sensitive in any way, percussion needs to be avoided.
- Electrical test
  - An electric pulp tester may be used to detect the presence or absence of vital pulp tissue.
  - Methods for use of a pulp testing are described in Chapter 16.

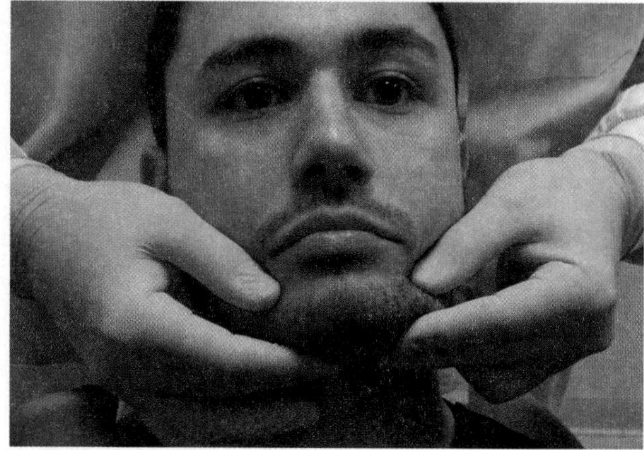

Figure 13-3 Bilateral Palpation. Bilateral palpation is used to examine corresponding structures on opposite sides of the body.

- Auscultation
  - Auscultation is the use of sound.
  - Example: The sound of clicking of the **temporomandibular joint** when the jaw is opened and closed. **Figure 13-4** shows examination of the temporomandibular joint.

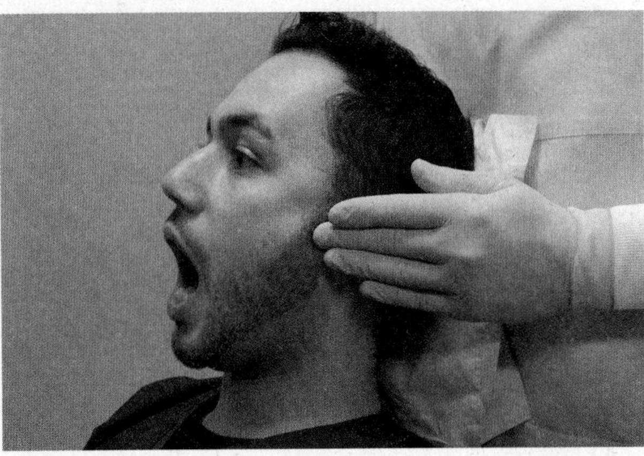

Figure 13-4 Assessment of the Temporomandibular Joint. The joint is palpated as the patient opens and closes the mouth.

III. Signs and Symptoms

- A specific objective for patient examination as a part of the complete assessment is the recognition of deviations from normal that may be signs or symptoms of disease.
- General signs and symptoms may occur in various disease conditions. Example: Fever, or increase in body temperature, accompanies most infections.
- A **pathognomonic sign or symptom** is unique to a disease and may be used to distinguish that condition from other diseases or conditions.

A. Signs

- A sign is any abnormality identified by a healthcare professional while examining a patient.
- A sign is objective information or data. Examples of signs include observable changes such as color, shape, and consistency, or abnormal findings revealed using a probe, explorer, radiograph, or other instrument for disease detection.

B. Symptoms

- A symptom is any departure from normal that may be indicative of disease.
- It is a subjective abnormality that can be observed by the patient.
- Examples are pain, tenderness, and bleeding when toothbrushing as described by the patient.

IV. Preparation for Examination

- Review the patient's health histories and dental/medical record, including risk factors, radiographs, dental caries, and periodontal and oral cancer risk assessments.
- Examine dental radiographs.
- Explain the procedures to be performed and relevance of the procedures.
    - Example: "I am going to perform an extra-/intraoral examination to look for abnormalities that can affect your oral and overall health."
    - Patient understanding the rationale for an extra- and intraoral examination is critical to acceptance and education.
    - When a patient is wearing a scarf or other head/neck covering for cultural or religious reasons, the dental hygienist uses culturally sensitive communication skills. (See Chapter 3.)

Anatomic Landmarks of the Oral Cavity

Familiarization with structures (**Figure 13-5**, **Figure 13-6**, and **Figure 13-7**) and normal anatomy is a prerequisite to understanding abnormal presentations in the head and neck region.[1,3,5]

I. Oral Mucosa

The lining of the oral cavity, the oral mucosa, is a mucous membrane composed of connective tissue covered with stratified squamous epithelium. There are three divisions or categories of oral mucosa.

A. Masticatory Mucosa

- Covers the gingiva and hard palate, the areas most used during the mastication of food.

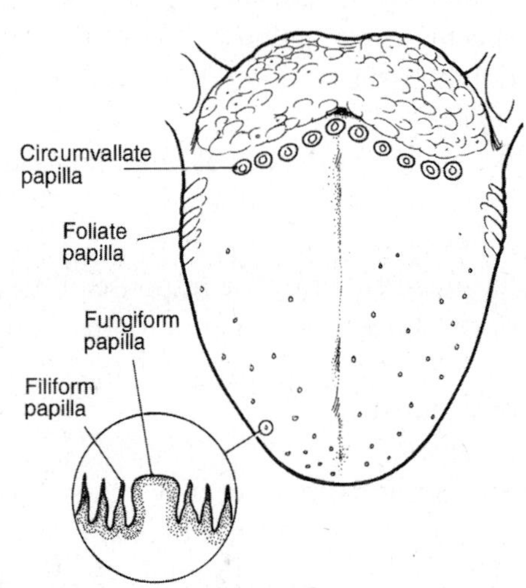

Figure 13-5 Papillae of the Tongue

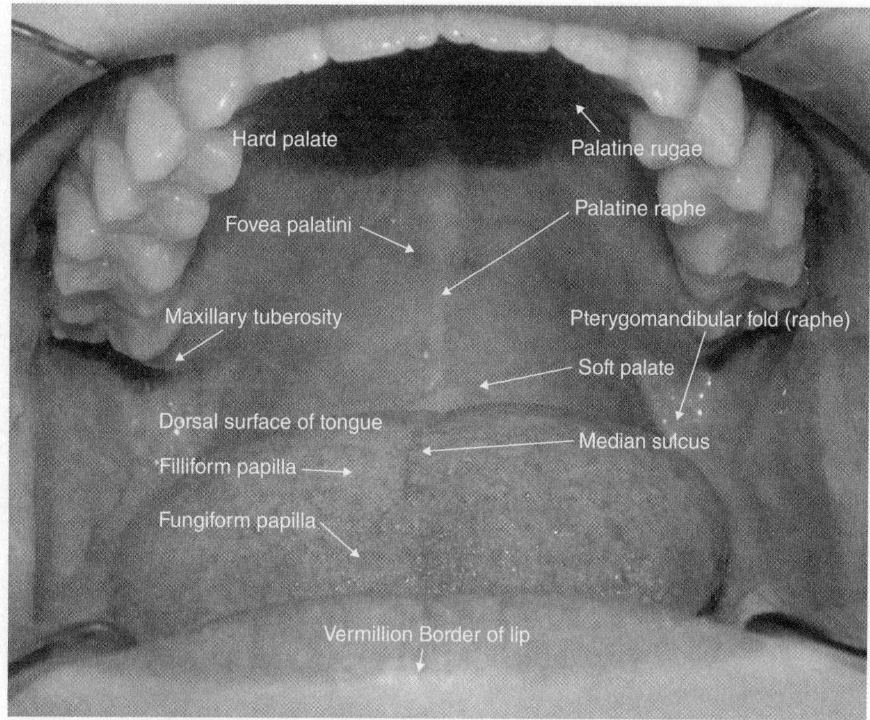

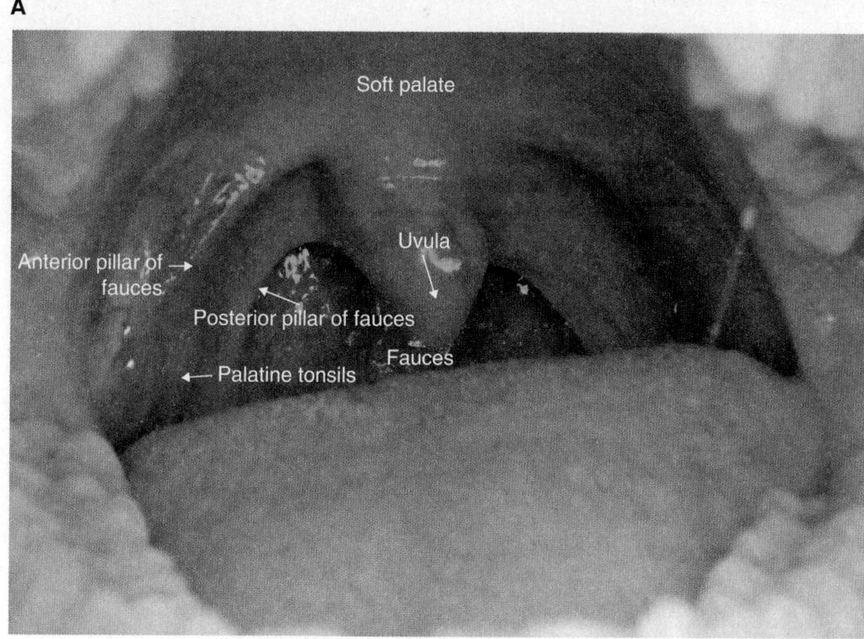

Figure 13-6 Anatomic Landmarks of the Oral Cavity—Dorsal Tongue View. **A:** View of hard and soft palate. **B:** View of uvula and oropharynx.

- Except for the free margin of the gingiva, the masticatory mucosa is firmly attached to underlying tissues.
- The normal epithelial covering is keratinized.

B. Lining Mucosa

- Covers the inner surfaces of the lips and cheeks, floor of the mouth, underside of the tongue, soft palate, and alveolar mucosa.
- These tissues are not firmly attached to underlying tissue.
- The epithelial covering is not keratinized.

C. Specialized Mucosa

- Covers the dorsum (upper surface) of the tongue.
- Composed of many **papillae**; some contain taste buds.

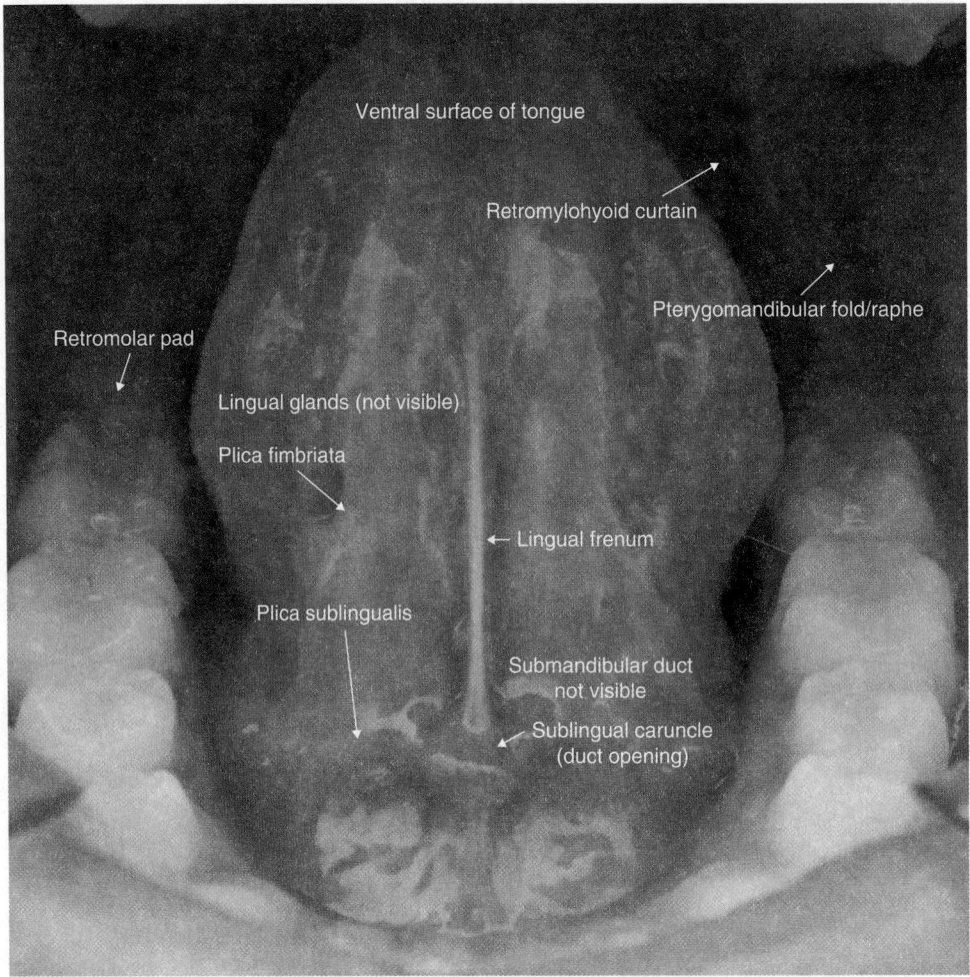

Figure 13-7 Anatomic Landmarks of the Oral Cavity—Ventral Tongue View

- The distribution of the four types of papillae is shown in Figure 13-5.
    - Filiform: Threadlike keratinized elevations that cover the **dorsal** surface of the tongue; they are the most numerous of the papillae.
    - Fungiform: Mushroom-shaped papillae interspersed among the filiform papillae on the tip and sides of the tongue; appear redder than the filiform papillae and contain variable numbers of taste buds. The inset enlargement in Figure 13-5 shows the comparative shape and size of the filiform and fungiform papillae.
    - Circumvallate (vallate): The 10–14 large round papillae arranged in a "V" between the body of the tongue and the base. Taste buds line the walls.
    - Foliate: Vertical grooves on the lateral posterior sides of the tongue; also contain taste buds.

Sequence of Examination

- Conducting an examination in a systematic sequence will minimize the possibility of excluding areas and overlooking details of importance. A systematic sequence improves efficiency, promotes professionalism, and inspires patient confidence.
- A recommended sequence for examination is outlined in **Box 13-1**, in which factors to consider during appointments are related to the actual observations made and recorded.
- This sequence is adapted from *Detecting Oral Cancer*, available from the National Institutes of Health and the National Cancer Institute.[1,2]
- In addition to proper sequence, familiarization of anatomic structures common to normal anatomy is critical to understanding abnormal findings (**Table 13-1**).

Box 13-1 Anatomic Landmarks of the Oral Cavity

- Lips
- Vermillion border
- Labial commissure
- Labial mucosa
- Buccal mucosa
- Philtrum
- Nasolabial groove
- Fauces
- Oral pharynx (includes soft palate, side and back wall of the throat, tonsils and posterior third or base of tongue)
- Vestibule
- Buccal vestibule
- Buccinator muscle
- Labial
- Buccal
- Mucobuccal fold
- Buccal frenum
- Labial frenum
- **Exostosis**
- Wharton's duct
- Lingual vein
- Sublingual fold
- Plica fimbriata
- Sublingual caruncle
- Median sulcus
- Lingual tonsils
- Lingual frenum
- Ankyloglossia
- Marginal gingiva
- Attached gingiva
- Free gingival groove
- Canine eminence
- Pterygomandibular raphe
- Parotid papilla
- Midpalatine raphe
- Palatine rugae
- Fovea palatine
- Torus palatinus
- Incisive papilla
- Uvula
- Palatine tonsils
- Pharyngeal adenoid tonsils
- Tonsillar pillars
- Tongue:
  - Dorsal
  - **Ventral**
  - Lateral border
- Filiform papilla
- Fungiform papilla
- Folate papillae
- Circumvallate papilla
- Lingual tonsils
- Stensen's duct
- Maxillary tuberosity
- Retromolar pad
- Ramus of mandible
- Zygomatic arch
- **Mandibular tori** (prevalence varies)
- Alveolar mucosa
- Mylohyoid muscle

Refer to Figures 13-6 and 13-7.

Table 13-1 Extraoral and Intraoral Examination

Sequence of Examination	Observe	Indication and Influences on Appointments
1. Overall appraisal of patient	Posture, gait General health status; size Hair; scalp Breathing; state of fatigue Voice, cough, hoarseness	Response, cooperation, attitude toward treatment Length of appointment
2. Face	Expression: Evidence of fear or apprehension Shape: Twitching; paralysis Jaw movements during speech Injuries; signs of abuse	Need for alleviation of fears Evidence of upper respiratory or other infections Enlarged masseter muscle (related to bruxism)
3. Skin	Color, texture, blemishes Traumatic lesions Eruptions, swellings Growths, **scars**, moles	Relation to possible systemic conditions Need for supplementary history Biopsy or other treatment to recommend Influences on instruction in diet

(*continues*)

Table 13-1 Extraoral and Intraoral Examination *(continued)*

Sequence of Examination	Observe	Indication and Influences on Appointments
4. Eyes	Size of pupils Color of sclera Eyeglasses (corrective) Protruding eyeballs	Dilated pupils or pinpoint may result from drugs, emergency state Eyeglasses essential during instruction Hyperthyroidism
5. Nodes (palpate) (**Figure 13-8**) a. Pre- and postauricular b. Occipital c. Submental; submandibular d. Cervical chain (Figure 13-8) e. Supraclavicular	Adenopathy; **lymphadenopathy** **Induration** or pain	Need for referral Medical consultation Ear infection Coordinate with intraoral examination
6. Glands (palpate) a. Thyroid (Figure 13-8B) b. Parotid c. Submental d. Submandibular (Figure 13-3)	Enlargement or pain Induration longer than 2 wk	Referral for medical consult
7. Temporomandibular joint (palpate) (Figure 13-4)	Limitations or deviations of movement **Trismus** Tenderness; sensitivity Noises: Clicking, popping, grating	Disorder of joint; limitation of opening Discomfort during appointment and during oral self-care
8. Lips a. Observe closed, then open b. Palpate (Figure 13-1)	Color, texture, size Cracks, angular cheilosis Blisters, ulcers Traumatic lesions Irritation from lip-biting Limitation of opening; muscle elasticity; muscle tone Evidence of mouth breathing Induration	Need for further examination: referral Immediate need for postponement of appointment when a lesion may be communicable or could interfere with procedures Care during retraction Accessibility during intraoral procedures Patient instruction: dietary, special biofilm control for mouth breather
9. Breath odor	Severity Relation to oral hygiene, gingival health	Possible relation to systemic condition Alcohol use history; special needs
10. Labial and buccal mucosa, left and right examined systematically a. Vestibule b. Mucobuccal folds c. Frena d. Opening of Stensen's duct e. Palpate cheeks (Figure 13-2A)	Color, size, texture, contour Abrasions, traumatic lesions, cheek bite Effects of tobacco use Ulcers, growths Moistness of surfaces Relation of frena to free gingiva Induration	Need for referral, biopsy, cytology Frena and other anatomic parts that need special adaptation for radiography or impression tray Avoid sensitive areas during retraction
11. Tongue a. Vestibule b. Dorsal (Figure 13-6A) c. Lateral borders d. Base of tongue (Figure 13-10) e. Deviation on extension	Shape: normal asymmetric Color, size, texture, consistency **Fissures**; papillae Coating Lesions: elevated, depressed, flat Induration	Need for referral, biopsy, cytology Need for instruction in tongue cleaning

Sequence of Examination	Observe	Indication and Influences on Appointments
12. Floor of mouth a. Ventral surface of tongue (Figure 13-7) b. Palpate (Figure 13-2B) c. Duct openings d. Mucosa, frena e. Tongue action	Varicosities Lesions: Elevated, flat, depressed, traumatic Induration Limitation or freedom of movement of tongue Frena; tongue-tie	Large muscular tongue influences retraction, gag reflex, accessibility for instrumentation Film placement problems
13. Saliva	Quantity; quality (thick, ropy) Evidence of dry mouth; lip wetting Tongue coating	Reduced in certain diseases, by certain drugs Special dental caries control program Influence on instrumentation Need for saliva substitute
14. Hard palate (Figure 13-6A)	Height, contour, color Appearance of rugae Tori, growths, ulcers	Need for referral, biopsy, cytology Signs of tongue thrust, deviate swallow Influence on radiographic film placement
15. Soft palate, uvula (Figure 13-6B)	Color, size, shape Petechiae Ulcers, growths	Referral, biopsy, cytology Large uvula influences gag reflex
16. Tonsillar region, throat (Figure 13-6B)	Tonsils: Size and shape Color, size, surface characteristics Lesions, trauma	Referral, biopsy, cytology Enlarged tonsils encourage gag reflex Throat infection, a sign for appointment postponement

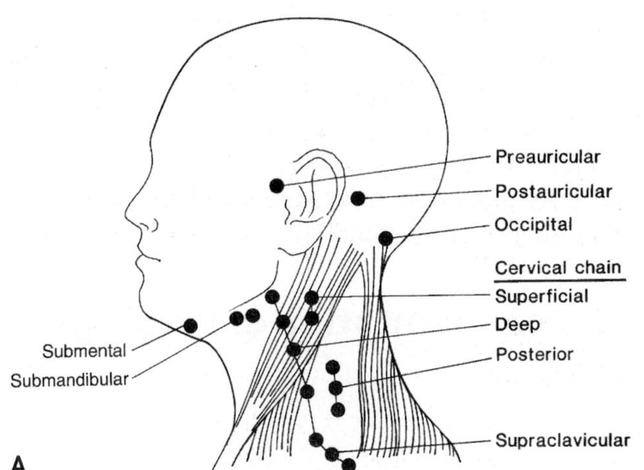

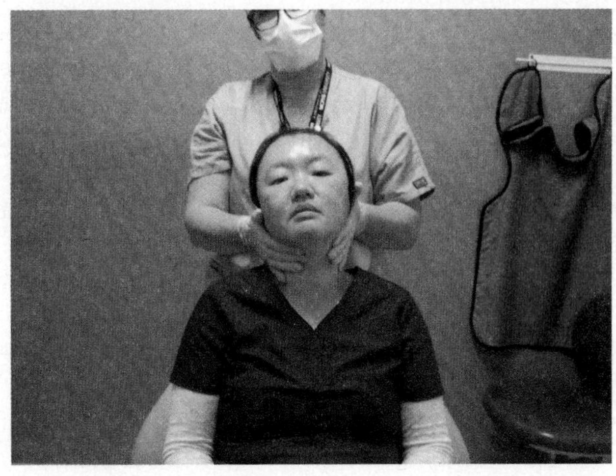

Figure 13-8 Lymph Node and Thyroid Gland Assessment. **A:** Lymph nodes. The locations of the major lymph nodes into which the vessels of the facial and oral regions drain. **B:** Examination of the thyroid gland. Identify the isthmus (center) of the thyroid gland. The butterfly-shaped gland sits below the bony protuberance or cricoid cartilage ring. Place two digits from each hand at the center of the gland and then slide digits laterally, approximately 1–2 cm from the center. Ask the patient to swallow slowly, several times and simultaneously palpate one lobe at a time while assessing for asymmetry. Observe the gland moving up and down as the patient swallows. Document any enlargement and asymmetry. Refer any aberration from normal to the patient's primary care provider for further evaluation. Note: The thyroid can be palpated from an anterior or posterior approach.[7]

I. Extraoral Examination

1. Observe patient during reception and seating to note physical characteristics and abnormalities and make an overall appraisal.
2. Observe head, face, eyes, and neck, and evaluate the skin of the face and neck.
3. Request the patient remove prosthesis prior to performing the intraoral examination. Explain how

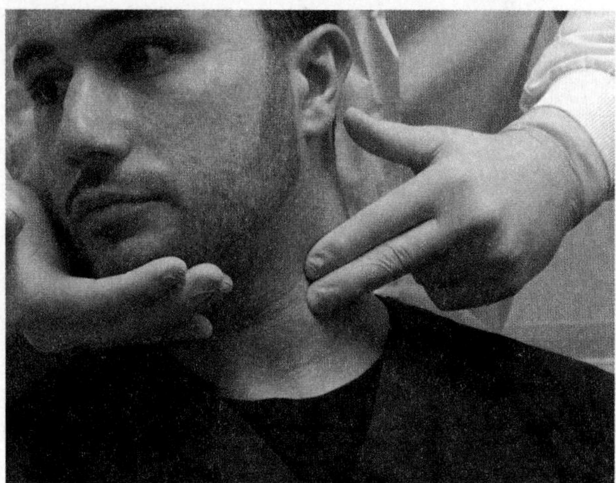

Figure 13-9 Cervical Node Palpation. Left anterior cervical lymph node chain is examined. Fingertips gently press and roll nodes along the length of the sternocleidomastoid muscle.

this will improve the ability to inspect all areas of the mouth adequately.

- If the patient is embarrassed to be seen without prosthesis, provide a tissue for them to cover their mouth when you are not examining the tissues.

4. Palpate the lymph nodes and the salivary and thyroid glands. Figure 13-8 shows the location of the major lymph nodes of the face, oral regions, and neck. Palpation is a significant component of the extra-/intraoral examination (**Figure 13-9**).
   - Note any of the following symptoms or experiences:
     - Pain or discomfort upon palpation and/or upon swallowing.
     - Persistent difficulty swallowing in the absence of pain.
     - Any recent noticeable lumps the patient may have experienced without pain.
     - Persistent earache or hoarseness of voice.[5]
5. Observe mandibular movement and palpate the temporomandibular joint (Figure 13-4). Relate to items from questions in the medical/dental history.

II. Intraoral Examination

1. Make a preliminary examination of the lips and intraoral mucosa by using a mouth mirror or a tongue depressor.
2. View and palpate lips, labial and buccal mucosa, and mucobuccal folds (Figures 13-1 and 13-2A).
3. Examine and palpate the tongue, including the dorsal and ventral surfaces, lateral borders, and

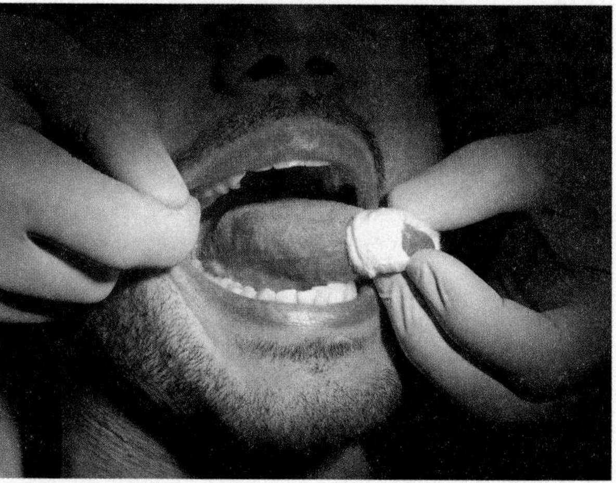

Figure 13-10 Examination of the Tongue. To observe the posterior third of the tongue and the attachment to the floor of the mouth, hold the tongue with a gauze sponge, retract the cheek, and move the tongue out, first to one side and then the other, as each section of the mucosa is carefully examined.

base. Retract to observe posterior third, first to one side and then the other (**Figure 13-10**).

4. Observe mucosa of the floor of the mouth. Palpate the floor of the mouth (Figure 13-2B).
5. Examine the hard and soft palates, tonsillar areas, and pharynx (Figure 13-6A and B). Use a mirror to observe the oropharynx, nasopharynx, and if possible, the larynx.
6. Note amount and consistency of the saliva and evidence of dry mouth (xerostomia).

III. Documentation of Findings

A. History

Question the patient to gather necessary information about the history of an oral lesion. Take care not to alarm the patient as you are just fact finding to determine the best way to proceed.

- Whether the lesion is known or not known to the patient; previous evaluation.
- If known, when first noticed; if recurrence, previous date when lesion was first noticed.
- Duration, symptoms, changes in size and appearance.

B. Location and Extent

- When a lesion is first seen, its location is noted in relation to adjacent structures.
- Document a complete description of each finding, including the location, extent, size, color,

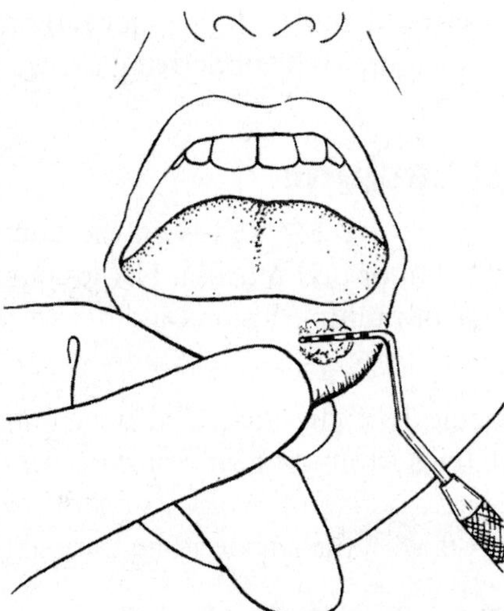

Figure 13-11 Use of a Probe to Measure a Lesion. In addition to the exact location, the width and length of a lesion are recorded. Using the probe provides a convenient method.

surface texture or configurations, consistency, **morphology**, and history.

- Intraoral photography can be of value to record images of anatomic deviations, location, and proportions.
- Descriptive words to define the location and extent include the following:
  - Localized: Lesion limited to a small focal area.
  - Generalized: Involves most of an area or segment.
  - Single lesion: One lesion of a particular type with a distinct margin.
  - Multiple lesions: More than one lesion of a particular type. Lesions may be:
    - Separate: discrete, not running together; may be arranged in clusters.
    - Coalescing: close to each other with margins that merge.

C. Physical Characteristics

- Size and shape
  - Record length and width in millimeters.
  - The height of an elevated lesion may be significant.
  - Use a probe to measure, as shown in **Figure 13-11**.
- Color
  - Red, pink, white, and red and white are the most commonly seen.
  - Other rarer lesions may be blue, purple, gray, yellow, black, or brown.
- Surface texture
  - A lesion may have a smooth or an irregular surface.
  - The texture may be papillary, verrucous or wart-like, fissured, corrugated, or crusted.
- Consistency
  - Lesions may be soft, spongy, resilient, hard, or indurated.

Morphologic Categories

- Most lesions can be classified as elevated, depressed, or flat as they relate to the normal level of the skin or mucosa.
- Flowcharts of elevated lesions (**Figure 13-12A**), depressed lesions (**Figure 13-12B**), and flat lesions (**Figure 13-12C**) break down the terms used for describing lesions in each category.

I. Elevated Lesions

An elevated lesion (Figure 13-12A) is above the plane of the skin or mucosa. Elevated lesions are considered blisterform or nonblisterform.

- Blisterform lesions contain fluid and are usually soft and translucent. They may be vesicles, pustules, or bullae.
  - Vesicle: A vesicle is a small (1 cm or less in diameter), circumscribed lesion with a thin surface covering. It may contain serum or mucin and appear white.
  - Pustule: A pustule may be more than or less than 5 mm in diameter and contain pus, giving it a yellowish color.
  - Bulla: A bulla is large (>1 cm). It is filled with fluid, usually mucin or serum, but may contain blood. The color depends on the fluid content.
- Nonblisterform lesions are solid and do not contain fluid. They may be papules, nodules, tumors, or plaques. Papules, nodules, and tumors are also characterized by the base or attachment. As shown in **Figure 13-13**, the **pedunculated** lesion is attached by a narrow stalk or pedicle, whereas the **sessile** lesion has a base as wide as the lesion itself.
  - Papule: A small (pinhead to 5 mm in diameter), solid lesion that may be pointed, rounded, or flat topped.
  - Nodule: Larger than a papule (>5 mm but <2 cm).
  - Tumor: 2 cm or greater in width. In this context, "tumor" means a general swelling or enlargement and does not refer to neoplasm, either benign or malignant.

- Plaque: Slightly raised lesion with a broad, flat top. It is usually larger than 5 mm in diameter, with a "pasted on" appearance.

II. Depressed Lesions

A depressed lesion (Figure 13-12B) is below the level of the skin or mucosa. The outline may be regular or irregular, and there may be a flat or raised border around the depression. The depth can be described as superficial or deep. A lesion greater than 3 mm is a deep lesion.

- Ulcer: Most depressed lesions are ulcers and represent a loss of continuity of the epithelium. The center is often gray to yellow, surrounded by a red border. An ulcer may result from the rupture of an elevated lesion (vesicle, pustule, or bulla).
- **Erosion**: An erosion is a shallow, depressed soft tissue lesion in which the epithelium above the basal layer is denuded. It does not extend through the epithelium to the underlying tissue.

III. Flat Lesions

A flat lesion (Figure 13-12C) is on the same level as the normal skin or oral mucosa. Flat lesions may occur as single or multiple lesions and have a regular or irregular form.

- A macule is a circumscribed area not elevated above the surrounding skin or mucosa.
  - It may be identified by its color, which contrasts with the surrounding normal tissues.

IV. Other Descriptive Terms

- **Crust**: An outer layer, covering, or scab that may have formed from coagulation or drying of blood, serum, or pus, or a combination. A crust may form after a vesicle breaks; for example, the

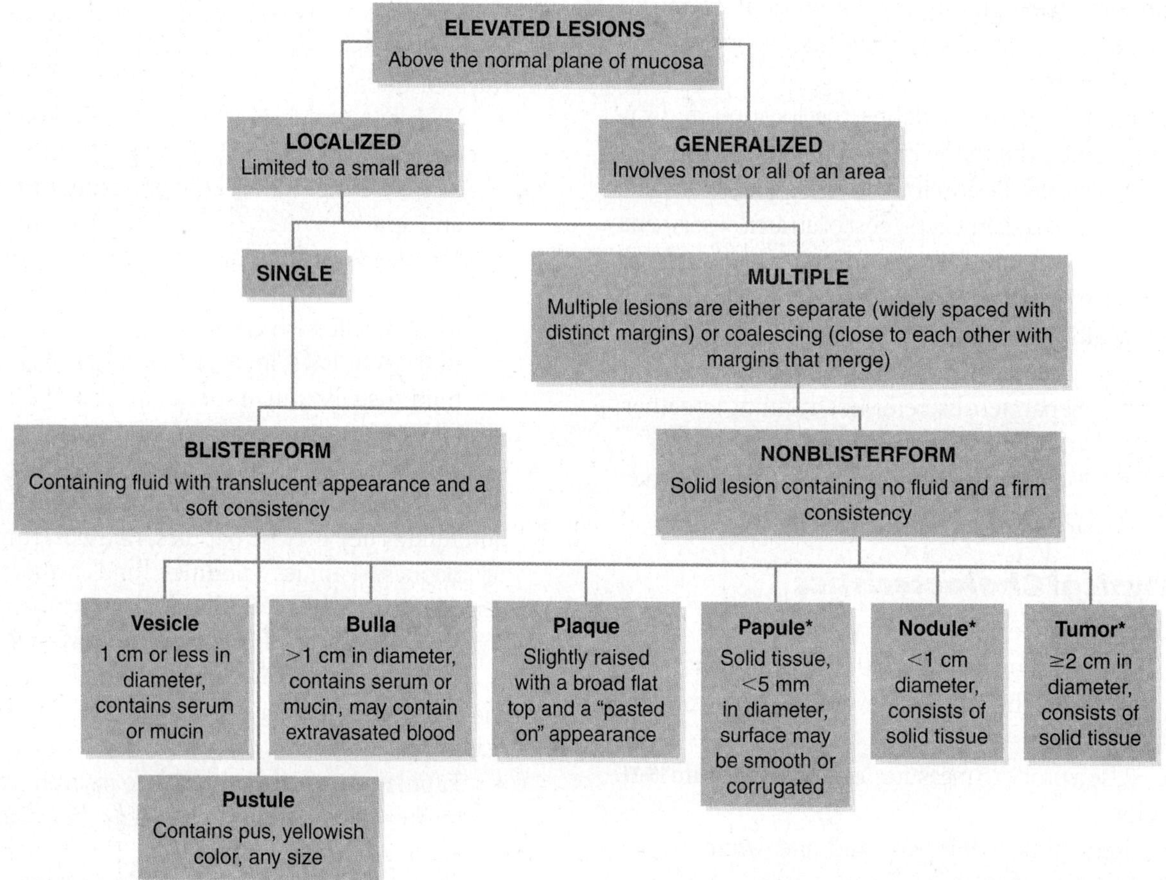

Figure 13-12 Flowcharts. **A:** Description of elevated soft tissue lesions. Elevated lesions are blisterform or nonblisterform.

A–C: Reprinted with permission from McCann AL, Wesley RK. A method for describing soft tissue lesions of the oral cavity. *Dent Hyg.* 1987;61(5):219–223.

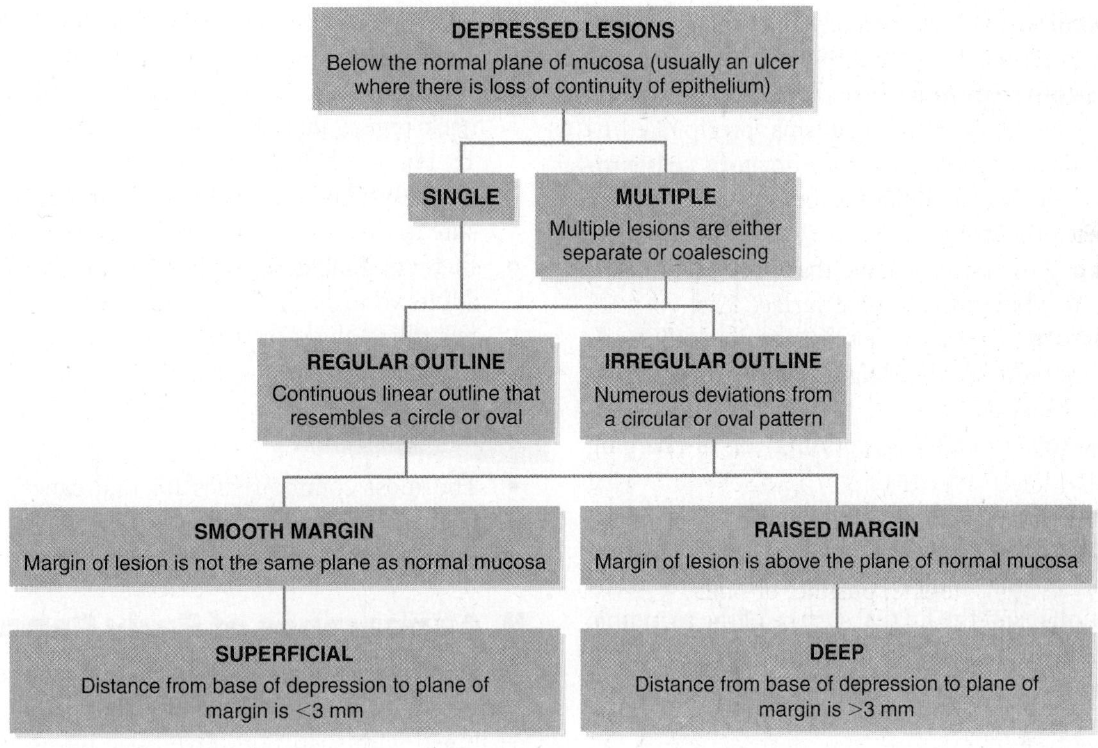

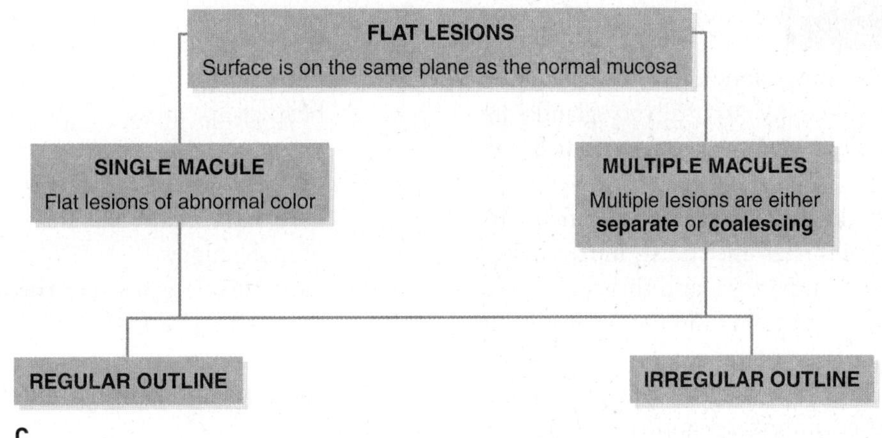

Figure 13-12 (*Continued*) **B:** Description of depressed soft tissue lesions. Depressed lesions are below the normal plane of the mucosa, usually an ulcer where there is a loss of continuity of epithelium. **C:** Description of flat soft tissue lesions. Flat lesions are level with the normal plane of the mucosa.

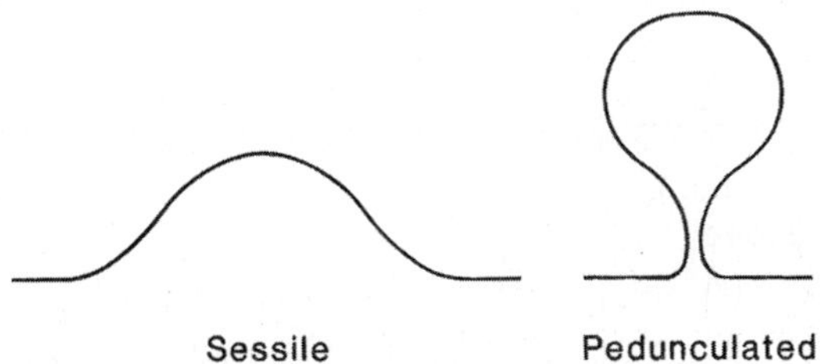

Figure 13-13 Attachment of Nonblisterform Lesions. The sessile lesion has a base as wide as the lesion itself; the pedunculated lesion is attached by a narrow stalk or pedicle.

skin lesion of chickenpox is first a macule, then a papule, then a vesicle, and then a crust.

- **Aphtha**: A small white or reddish ulcer.
- **Cyst**: A closed, epithelial-lined sac, normal or pathologic, that contains fluid or other material.
- **Erythema**: Red area of variable size and shape.
- **Exophytic**: Growing outward.
- **Idiopathic**: Of unknown etiology.
- **Indurated**: Hardened or abnormally hard.
- **Papillary**: Resembling a small, nipple-shaped projection or elevation.

- **Petechiae**: Minute hemorrhagic spots of pinhead to pinpoint size.
- **Pseudomembrane**: A loose membranous layer of exudate containing organisms, precipitated fibrin, necrotic cells, and inflammatory cells produced during an inflammatory reaction on the surface of a tissue.
- **Polyp**: Any mass of tissue that projects outward or upward from the normal surface level.
- **Punctate**: Marked with points or dots differentiated from the surrounding surface by color, elevation, or texture.
- **Purulent**: Containing, forming, or discharging pus.
- **Rubefacient**: Reddening of the skin.
- **Torus**: Bony elevation or prominence usually found on the midline of the hard palate (torus palatinus) and the lingual surface of the mandible (torus mandibularis) in the premolar area.
- **Verruca** (*verrucous* [verrucose]): A rough, wart-like growth.

Oral Cancer

- The oral cavity, oropharynx, larynx, paranasal sinuses and nasal cavity, and salivary glands are regions of the head and neck where cancer can begin.[2]
  - Cancers of the head and neck begin in the squamous cells that line moist, mucosal surfaces of the mouth, nose, and throat.[8,9]
  - Salivary glands contain different types of cells that can also become cancerous.[8,9]
- Because the early lesions are generally asymptomatic, they may go unnoticed and unreported by the patient. Observation by the dentist or dental hygienist is the principal method for the detection of oral cancer.
- The first step is to examine the entire face, neck, and oral mucous membrane of each patient at the initial examination and at each continuing care appointment (Table 13-1).
- It is necessary to know how to conduct the oral examination, most frequent sites where oral cancer occurs, characteristics of an early cancerous lesion, and procedure for referral and follow-up of when a lesion is found.
- In addition to the early lesions of oral cancers, the oral manifestations of neoplasms or abnormal growth of tissue elsewhere in the body, as well as the oral manifestations of chemotherapy, can be recognized.
- Most oral cancers are related to tobacco and/or excessive alcohol use.[5,10]
- Additional risk factors for cancer of the head and neck region include infection with HPV-16 and 18 types, multiple sex partners, weakened immune system, age 40 years and more, sun exposure to the lips, and history of cancer.[3,5,11]
- Increasing incidence of head and neck cancers in adults younger than 40 years suggests all patients, regardless of age or risk factors, must be screened for oral cancer.[10]

I. Location

- The most common sites for oral cancer are the lateral borders of the tongue, floor of the mouth, the lips, and the soft palate.

II. Appearance of Early Cancer

Early oral cancer takes many forms and may resemble a variety of common oral lesions. All types need to be examined with suspicion. Five basic forms are listed here[3,8,10]:

- White areas
  - White areas vary from a filmy, barely visible change in the mucosa to heavy, thick, heaped-up areas of dry white keratinized tissue.
  - Fissures, ulcers, or areas of induration or **sclerosis** in a white area are most indicative of malignancy.
  - Leukoplakia is a white **patch** or plaque that cannot be scraped off or characterized as any other disease. It may be associated with physical or chemical agents and the use of tobacco.
- Red areas
  - Erythroplakia is a term used to designate lesions of the oral mucosa that appear as bright red patches or plaques.
  - Lesions appear red, have a velvety consistency, and may coincide with small ulcers.
  - Erythroplakia is an oral lesion that cannot be characterized as any specific disease. It is less common than leukoplakia and more likely to manifest as dysplasia (precancerous) or malignancy.
- Ulcers
  - Ulcers may have flat or raised margins.
  - Palpation may reveal induration.
- Masses
  - Papillary masses, sometimes with ulcerated areas, occur as elevations above the surrounding tissues.

- Other masses may occur below the normal mucosa and may be found only by palpation.
- Pigmentation
  - Brown or black pigmented areas may be located on mucosa where pigmentation does not normally occur.

Clinical Recommendations for Evaluation of Oral Lesions

- Updated medical, social, and dental history along with the extra- and intraoral examination is recommended for all adult patients.[5]
- Adult patients with lesions considered to be innocuous or not suspicious for malignancy should be followed to confirm no further evaluation is needed.[5]
- Biopsy is indicated for adult patients with lesions considered to be suspicious of potential malignancy or malignant disorder or other symptoms.[5]
- Although not recommended for potential malignancy, cytologic adjuncts for minimally invasive detection of oral cancer can be performed when a patient refuses biopsy of the lesion or referral to a specialist. Cytologic adjuncts include brush cytology and toluidine blue, diffuse tissue reflectance, and laser-induced autofluorescence.[12] The rationale for performing adjunctive cytologic testing is to reinforce the need for biopsy or referral.[12]

I. Biopsy

- Biopsy is the removal and microscopic examination of a section of tissue or other material from the body for the purposes of diagnosis.
  - A biopsy is either excisional, when the entire lesion is removed, or incisional, when a representative section from the lesion is taken.
  - Considered the "gold standard" in oral cancer diagnosis.[3,8]
- Indications for biopsy
  - Any unusual oral lesion that cannot be identified with clinical certainty must be biopsied.
  - Any lesion that has not healed in 2 weeks is considered suspicious for malignancy until proven otherwise.
  - A persistent, thick, white, hyperkeratotic lesion and any mass (elevated or not) that does not break through the surface epithelium.
- Pathology report.
- Diagnostic criteria may vary, but one of the most recent guidelines for oral cytology includes the following[5]:
  - NILM (negative for intraepithelial lesion or malignancy): Normal, infection, inflammation, benign epithelial lesion, etc.
  - LSIL (low-grade squamous intraepithelial lesion): Mild to moderate dysplasia (cell changes).
  - HSIL (high-grade squamous intraepithelial lesion): Severe dysplasia.
  - SCC (squamous cell carcinoma).
  - Other malig (other malignancy).
  - IFN (indefinite for neoplasia or non-neoplasia).

Role of the Dental Hygienist in Thorough Intraoral/Extraoral Examination

- Identification of risk factors for oral cancer is an integral role in prevention of disease.
- In addition, dental hygienists play an important role educating patients about these risks, particularly as they pertain to tobacco cessation, alcohol reduction, and HPV vaccination.
- Professional continuing education and adherence to evidence-based practice guidelines can enhance the dental hygienist's confidence with current recommendations.[4,11]

Documentation

Documentation in the permanent record of a patient who had a biopsy (or smear) because of a questionable cancerous lesion is needed and must contain a minimum of the following:

- Details of the oral examination and follow-up procedures with reports from consultants, laboratories, medical follow-up, and outcomes.
- Recommendations for the frequency of a complete oral examination at future dental hygiene maintenance appointments.
- Review of lifestyle habits that may be a risk factor for an oral lesion with recommendations for specific preventive methods.
- A progress note at the patient's maintenance appointment following the biopsy with the results may be reviewed in **Box 13-2**.

Box 13-2 Example Documentation: Patient with an Oral Lesion

- **S**—50-year-old female presents for routine preventive maintenance with no current concerns at today's appointment. When questioned during intraoral examination, patient recalls accidentally biting her tongue recently.
- **O**—Patient smokes 1 pack cigarettes daily for the past 35 years and admits to drinking 1–2 beers nightly; left lateral border of tongue erythematous lesion 1 cm × 5 mm, flat.
- **A**—High risk for oral cancer, erythematous lesion requires further evaluation.
- **P**—Discuss concerns with patient regarding high-risk behaviors of tobacco use and alcohol. Recommend 2-week follow-up for reevaluation of lesion and further referral if no improvement. Recommended and offered tobacco cessation information.

Signed: ______________________, RDH
Date: ______________

Factors to Teach the Patient

- Reasons for a careful extra- and intraoral examination at each maintenance appointment.
- Guidance and support on tobacco cessation and provide appropriate referral.
- How to conduct self-examination monthly to watch for changes in oral tissues and identify lesions that last longer than 2 weeks. Examination includes the face, neck, lips, gingiva, cheeks, tongue, palate, and throat. Any changes are reported to the dentist and the dental hygienist.
- General dietary and nutritional influences on the health of the oral tissues.
  - Benefits of diet rich in fruits and vegetables.
- How the oral cavity tends to reflect the general health.
- The warning signs of oral cancer from the American Cancer Society including the following[12]:
  - A swelling, lump, or growth anywhere, with or without pain.
  - White scaly patches or red velvety areas.
  - Any sore that does not heal promptly (within 2 weeks).
  - Numbness or tingling.
  - Excessive dryness or wetness.
  - Prolonged hoarseness, sore throats, persistent coughing, or the feeling of a "lump in the throat."
  - Difficulty with swallowing.
  - Difficulty in opening the mouth.

References

1. National Institute of Health, National Institute of Dental and Craniofacial Research. *Detecting Oral Cancer: A Guide for Health Care Professionals*. Published August 2020. https://www.nidcr.nih.gov/sites/default/files/2020-10/Detecting-Oral-Cancer-Healthcare-Professionals.pdf. Accessed September 6, 2021.
2. National Cancer Institute. Oral cavity and nasopharyngeal cancer screening (PDQ®)–health Professional Version. Published August 6, 2021. https://www.cancer.gov/types/head-and-neck/hp/oral-screening-pdq. Accessed September 17, 2021.
3. Rivera C. Essentials of oral cancer. *Int J Clin Exp Pathol*. 2015;8(9):11884-11894.
4. National HPV Vaccination Roundtable. *Cancer Prevention Through HPV Vaccination: An Action Guide for Dental Health Care Providers*. Published September 2019. http://hpvroundtable.org/wp-content/uploads/2018/04/DENTAL-Action-Guide-WEB.pdf. Accessed September 6, 2021.
5. Lingen MW, Abt E, Agrawal N, et al. Evidence-based clinical practice guideline for the evaluation of potentially malignant disorders in the oral cavity: a report of the American Dental Association. *J Am Dent Assoc*. 2017;148(10):712-727.e10.
6. Patton LL, Villa A, Bedran-Russo AK, et al. Human papillomavirus vaccine: an American Dental Association clinical evaluators panel survey. *J Am Dent Assoc*. 2020;151(4):303-304.e2.
7. University of Washington Department of Medicine. Technique: thyroid exam. *Advanced Physical Diagnosis Learning and Teaching at the Bedside*. https://depts.washington.edu/physdx/thyroid/tech.html. Accessed October 27, 2021.
8. Rethman MP, Carpenter W, Cohen EEW, et al. Evidence-based clinical recommendations regarding screening for oral squamous cell carcinomas. *J Am Dent Assoc*. 2010;141(5):509-520.
9. Warnakulasuriya S. Clinical features and presentation of oral potentially malignant disorders. *Oral Surg Oral Med Oral Pathol Oral Radiol*. 2018;125(6):582-590.
10. American Cancer Society. Oral cavity and oropharyngeal cancer key statistics 2021. Published March 23, 2021. https://www.cancer.org/cancer/oral-cavity-and-oropharyngeal-cancer/about/key-statistics.html. Accessed September 17, 2021.
11. Viens LJ, Henley SJ, Watson M, et al. Human papillomavirus-associated cancers, United States, 2008-2012. *MMWR Morb Mortal Wkly Rep*. 2016;65(26):661-666.
12. Lingen MW, Tampi MP, Urquhart O, et al. Adjuncts for the evaluation of potentially malignant disorders in the oral cavity. *J Am Dent Assoc*. 2017;148(11):797-813.e52.

CHAPTER 14

Family Violence

Linda D. Boyd, RDH, RD, EdD
Lisa F. Mallonee, RDH, RD, LD, MPH

CHAPTER OUTLINE

LEARNING OBJECTIVES

After studying this chapter, the student will be able to:

1. Describe the general, extraoral, and intraoral signs of child abuse and neglect.
2. Describe the general, physical, extraoral, and intraoral signs of elder abuse and neglect.
3. Discuss the signs and attitudes of the abused in an intimate partner violence situation.
4. Discuss the role of the dental hygienist in reporting suspected abuse or neglect of children, elders, and intimate partners.
5. Discuss Munchausen syndrome by proxy and describe indicators associated with the syndrome.
6. Describe the general and behavioral indicators of human trafficking victims.

Family Violence

- **Interpersonal violence** refers to family and community violence that is a global problem with no economic, geographic, or social boundaries.[1,2]
- The entire dental team must advocate for those who experience **family violence (FV)** by identifying and reporting suspected cases to authorities.[3,4]

I. Categories of FV

- FV is abusive behavior by one individual toward another in an intimate or family relationship.[1]
    - Other terminology includes: intimate partner violence (IPV), **domestic violence** (DV), child abuse and neglect, and elder abuse and neglect.
- Those most at risk are children, the elderly, people with disabilities, Indigenous people, LGBTQ+ individuals, and women.[5-9]

II. Types of FV

- FV may include[10,11]:
    - **Physical abuse** or violence.
    - Stalking.
    - Emotional or **psychological abuse** or **neglect**.
    - **Sexual abuse** or violence.
    - **Neglect** or abandonment.
    - Medical (dental) neglect.
    - **Financial exploitation**.
- **Figure 14-1** summarizes the major types of FV.

Child Abuse and Neglect

According to the World Health Organization, "child maltreatment (including violent punishment) involves physical, sexual and psychological/emotional violence; and neglect of infants, children and adolescents by parents, caregivers and other authority figures, most often in the home but also in settings such as schools and orphanages."[6]

- In the United States, sex trafficking was added to the definition of child abuse and neglect.[11]
    - The majority of perpetrators are not the child's parents.
- Children who experience prenatal exposure to substance abuse by the mother are also considered to be victims of abuse.[11]

I. Definitions

- Child abuse: Words or actions that cause harm, potential harm, or threat to harm a child and may

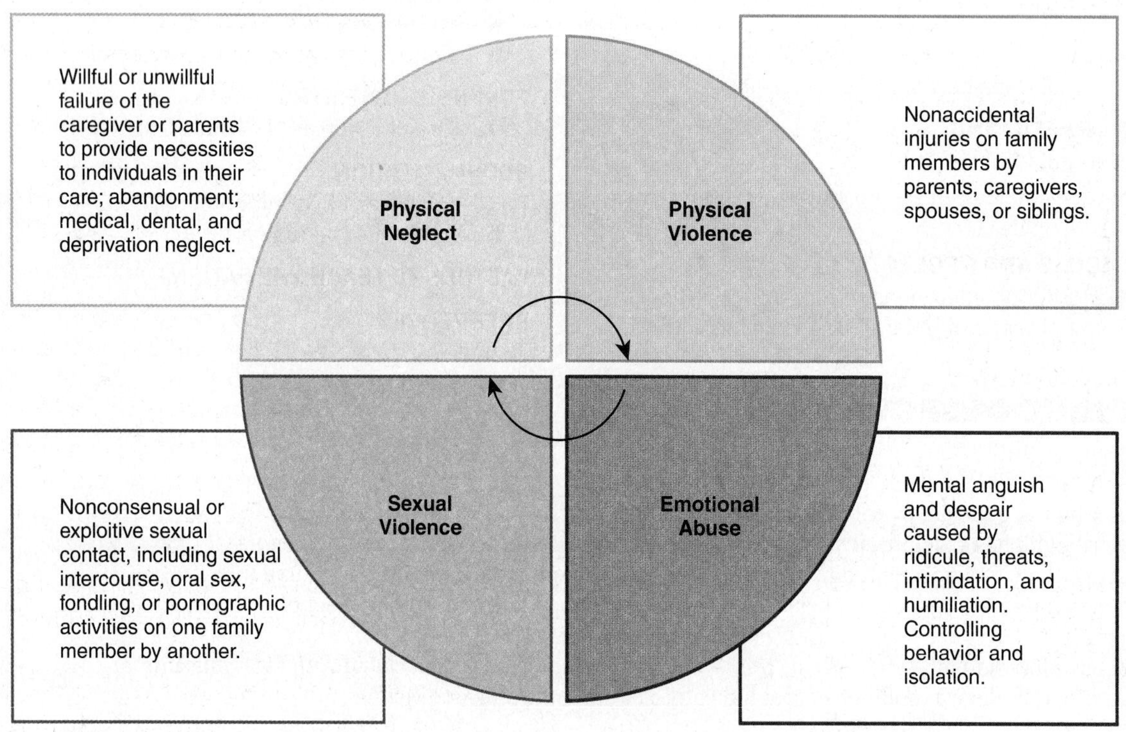

Figure 14-1 Major Types of Family Maltreatment

include physical, emotional (psychological), or sexual abuse.[12]

- Child neglect: Failure to provide for a child's basic physical, emotional, educational, and medical/dental needs. Other aspects of neglect include inadequate supervision and exposure to violent environments.[12]
- **Dental neglect**: The willful failure of a parent or guardian to seek and follow through with treatment necessary to ensure a level of oral health essential for adequate function and freedom from pain and infection.[13]

II. Risk Factors

- Risk factors for abuse or neglect are multifactorial and include individual, relational, community, and societal factors.[10]

A. Individual Risk Factors for Abuse or Neglect

- Individual risk factors for abuse include[10]:
  - Children younger than 4 years of age, with children younger than 1 year having the highest rate.[11]
  - Girls are more likely to experience child abuse or neglect.[11]
  - American Indian and Alaska Native children have the highest rate for abuse, with African-American children having the second highest rate.[11]
  - Children with special needs, particularly those with neurodevelopmental disorders like autism.[14]

B. Relational Factors for Abuse or Neglect

- Risk factors for being a perpetrator (e.g., parent or caregiver) of abuse or neglect include[11,14]:
  - Caregivers who are young, single parents or have multiple children.
  - Mental health issues such as depression are associated with neglect.
  - Those who experienced maltreatment as a child.
  - Parents or caregivers who experience family violence (IPV).
  - Drug or alcohol abuse.
  - Parents or caregivers who overreact to stress or have issues regulating emotions like anger.
  - Inadequate financial resources to meet minimum needs and high parental stress.
  - Inadequate or unsafe housing.
  - Isolation from support network.
    - The coronavirus disease 2019 (COVID-19) pandemic increased social isolation, economic challenges, unstable housing, and mental health issues, resulting in greater risk of all types of abuse and neglect.[15]
  - Caregivers in the home who are not a biological parent.

C. Community and Social Factors

- Community risk factors may include[10]:
  - Gender or social inequality.
  - Unstable or lack of adequate housing or services to support families.
  - High amounts of unemployment and/or poverty.
  - Availability of alcohol and drugs.
  - Social, economic, and health and education policies that lead to poor living standards, or to socioeconomic inequality or instability.
  - Increased stress and community isolation.

III. Consequences of Child Abuse

- Several thousand children die each year as a result of severe physical damage, and others suffer permanent brain damage or physical deformities as well as emotional trauma.[8]
- Craniofacial and head and neck injuries occur in more than one-half of child abuse cases.[10]
- Abuse should be considered in the **differential diagnosis** for any injury involving a child.

IV. General Signs of Child Abuse and Neglect

- The dental hygiene standards of practice framework promotes comprehensive patient care through thorough assessments and identifying risk factors that impede the health and wellness of the patient.[16,17]
- Recognizing signs of suspected abuse and following proper reporting protocol will promote health and safety for all individuals.
- The signs of child abuse and neglect are complex and are categorized into physical, behavioral, emotional, cognitive, and social indicators (**Table 14-1**).

Table 14-1 Indicators and Features of Child Abuse and Neglect[18-21]

Type of Child Abuse and Neglect	Physical Indicators	Behavioral Indicators	Emotional Features	Cognitive Features
Physical abuse	*Unexplained bruises and welts* ■ Face, lips, mouth ■ Torso, back, buttocks, thighs ■ Various stages of healing ■ Clustered, regular patterns ■ Reflecting shape of article used to inflict (e.g., buckle) ■ On several different areas ■ Regular appearance after absence, weekend, vacation *Unexplained burns* ■ Cigarette, cigar burns, especially on soles, palms, back, buttocks ■ Immersion burns (sock or glove-like, circular, on buttocks or genitalia) ■ Patterned: Electric burner, iron ■ Rope burns on arms, legs, or torso *Unexplained fractures* ■ Skull, nose, facial structures ■ In various stages of healing ■ Multiple or spiral fractures *Unexplained laceration or abrasion* ■ To mouth, lips, gingiva, eyes ■ To external genitalia *Malnutrition/underweight*	■ Wary of adult contacts ■ Apprehensive when others cry ■ Behavioral extremes: • Aggressive • Withdrawn ■ Frightened of parents or caregiver ■ Afraid to go home ■ Reports injury by parents ■ Risky sexual behavior	■ Higher risk for mental health issues: • Depression • Anxiety • Panic disorder • Posttraumatic stress disorder • Eating disorders • Alcohol/drug abuse • Suicide	
Physical neglect	■ Constant hunger, poor hygiene, inappropriate dress ■ Consistent lack of supervision, especially in dangerous situations or for long periods ■ Unattended physical problems or medical/dental needs ■ Abandonment	■ Begging, stealing food ■ Extended stays at school, early arrival, late departure ■ Constant fatigue, falling asleep in class ■ Impulsivity ■ Alcohol or drug abuse ■ Externalizing • Aggressive • Destructive • Antisocial/delinquency ■ Internalizing • Withdrawn • Says there is no caretaker • Difficulty making friends	■ Low self-esteem ■ Difficulty regulating emotion ■ Fewer coping strategies ■ Depression ■ Lower levels of emotional understanding of peers	■ Lower general intelligence ■ Poorer executive functioning ■ Poorer manual dexterity, auditory ■ More problems with attention ■ Better problem-solving skills

Sexual abuse	■ Difficulty in walking or sitting ■ Torn, stained, bloody underwear ■ Pain or itching in genital area ■ Bruises or bleeding on external genitalia, vaginal, or anal areas ■ Venereal disease, especially in preteen ■ Pregnancy	■ Unwilling to change for physical education class ■ Withdrawal, fantasy, or infantile behavior ■ Bizarre, sophisticated sexual knowledge or behavior ■ Poor peer relationship ■ Delinquency; runaways ■ Reports sexual assault by caretaker	■ Emotional dysregulation ■ Dissociation ■ Mental health issues (e.g., depression and compulsive behavior)	
Emotional maltreatment	■ Speech disorders ■ Lags in physical development ■ Failure to thrive	■ Habit disorders (sucking, biting, rocking, etc.) ■ Conduct disorders (antisocial, destructive) ■ Neurotic traits (sleep disorders, inhibited play) ■ Psychoneurotic behaviors (hysteria, phobia, obsession, compulsion, hypochondria) ■ Impulsivity ■ Behavioral extremes: • Compliant, passive • Aggressive, demanding ■ Overly adaptive behavior: • Inappropriately adult • Inappropriately infantile ■ Attempted suicide	■ Poor social skills ■ Difficulty making friends ■ Low self-esteem	■ Lower general intelligence ■ Poorer executive functioning

Data from Mouden LD, Lowe JW, Dixit UB. How to recognize situations that suggest abuse/neglect. *Missouri Dental J.* 1992 Nov-Dec; 26-29; Maguire SA, Williams B, Naughton AM, et al. A systematic review of the emotional, behavioural and cognitive features exhibited by school-aged children experiencing neglect or emotional abuse. *Child Care Health Dev.* 2015;41(5):641-653; Norman RE, Byambaa M de R, Butchart A, Scott J, Vos T. The long-term health consequences of child physical abuse, emotional abuse, and neglect: a systematic review and meta-analysis. *PLoS Med.* 2012;9(11):e1001349; Hébert M, Langevin R, Oussaïd E. Cumulative childhood trauma, emotion regulation, dissociation, and behavior problems in school-aged sexual abuse victims. *J Affect Disord.* 2017;225:306-312.

A. Physical Indicators

- Observe the child's nonverbal behaviors, overall appearance, alertness, responsiveness, and indicators suggestive of abuse or neglect.[22]
- Clothing is not appropriate for the weather.[23,24]
- Poor personal hygiene.[23,24]
- Failure to thrive—malnutrition.[22]
  - Body fat ratio low for child's age and height is not within normal developmental range.

B. Behavioral Features

- Externalizing is common and may include aggressive, destructive, or antisocial behavior.[19]
- Internalizing is also frequent and includes withdrawn behavior.[19]
- Impulsivity, inattention, and hyperactivity.[19]

C. Social Behavior

- Observe the parent–child relationship. Child may act differently when the parent is present than when alone, which may provide clues to the relationship.
  - The child may act withdrawn or fearful in presence of parent/caregiver.[24]
  - Observe for nonverbal cues of anxiety about answering questions about the perpetrator.[22]
- Physically neglected and/or emotionally abused children often have more difficulty with establishing and maintaining relationships.[19,24]
- A strong desire to please.[19]
- More likely to use compensation in social settings, such as being the "class clown."[19]

D. Emotional Well-Being

- Neglected children have lower self-esteem.[19]
- Difficulty regulating emotions and may fail to understand negative emotions like anger and sadness.[19,24]
- Higher levels of depressive symptoms and risk for suicide attempts are seen in children as a result of physical, sexual, and emotional abuse as well as physical neglect.[19,24,25]

E. Cognitive Features

- Neglected children may exhibit lower IQ along with less developed communication, reading, and math skills.[19]
- However, neglected children may exhibit well developed problem-solving skills.[19]

V. Extraoral Wounds and Signs of Trauma

- Common abusive injuries inflicted on children
  - Fractures and indicators of abusive injuries include[26]:
    - Infants and young toddlers rarely have accidental fractures.
    - Unexplained fractures.
    - Multiple fractures of different ages.
    - Inconsistency with the fracture and description of how it occurred.
    - Rib fractures.
    - Metaphyseal fractures.
    - Skull injuries; **edema**, combined with **ecchymosis** of varying stages.
  - Skin injuries include contusions and burns and indicators of abusive skin injuries include[26]:
    - Injuries in unusual locations (**Figure 14-2**).
    - Injuries are not consistent with the child's developmental abilities (e.g., accidental bruising in infants is rare) or with the explanation of the caregiver/parent.
    - Delays in accessing medical care.
    - A pattern is present, such as bilateral injuries or handprint.
    - Lip bruises and lacerations; angular bruising, **lichenification**, or scarring, which can be caused from gags applied to the mouth.[27]
    - Human bite marks.[26,27]
    - The number and extent of the injury are large or great in number.
  - Head injuries are responsible for most fatalities from child abuse.[26] Recognizing injuries to the head and neck from suspected child maltreatment can lead to early intervention and save lives. Abusive injuries may include[26]:
    - Bald spots (**traumatic alopecia**) caused by pulling the hair out by the roots.
    - Subdural hematomas can occur from shaking.
    - Retinal hemorrhage may occur due to head trauma.
    - **Raccoon sign**: Bilateral periorbital ecchymosis rarely occurs accidentally except when there is a broken nose.
    - Nose fractures or displacements.
- **Table 14-2** lists the possible conditions that can mimic injuries from child maltreatment.

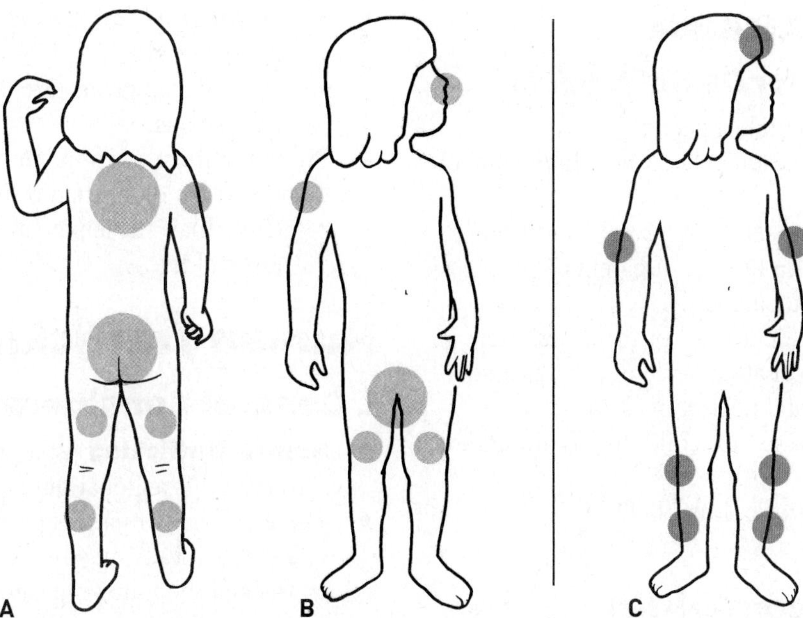

Figure 14-2 Common Sites of Children's Injuries. **A:** and **B:** Common sites of inflicted or abusive injuries. **C:** Common sites of accidental injuries.

Table 14-2 Conditions That Can Mimic Abuse

Appearance	Possible Conditions
Bruising	Accidental injuries **Idiopathic thrombocytopenia purpura** Hemophilia
Burns/red lesions	Port-wine stain Accidental burns
Skin lesions	Bullous impetigo Birthmarks

VI. Intraoral Signs of Abuse and Neglect

- A complete medical history followed by thorough intraoral/extraoral examinations are vital to assess traumatic injuries.
  - A sequential examination technique should be conducted on every patient.[16,17]
- Many injuries of the mouth in children can also be caused by accidental means. Therefore, it is important that the clinical presentation of the injuries match the explanation.
- Intraoral findings suggesting abuse may include[27]:
  - Lacerations of the tongue, buccal mucosa, or palate.
  - Lingual and labial frenal tears.
  - Discolored teeth (pulpal necrosis).
  - Burns or lacerations of the gingiva, tongue, palate, or floor of the mouth.
  - Teeth that are fractured, displaced, avulsed, or nonvital.
  - Radiographic evidence of fractures in different degrees of healing.

A. Signs of Sexual Abuse

- Bruising or petechiae of the hard or soft palate can indicate forced oral sex.[27]
- In sexually abused children, sexually transmitted diseases rarely have visible signs.[27]
- Extreme dental anxiety related to the following[28]:
  - Feelings of boundaries being invaded, feeling powerless, and feeling trapped by dental provider may cause the individual to relive the sexual abuse.
  - Sensory stimuli of taste, touch, and smell during dental care may trigger memories of the sexual abuse experience.

B. Dental Neglect

- Dental neglect is the failure of the caregiver, who is responsible for the child, to seek and complete dental care to maintain oral health with absence of pain and infection.[29]
  - Dental prevention neglect (DPN) is failure to prevent oral disease.
  - Dental treatment neglect (DTN) is failure to complete treatment of dental caries or pain.

VII. Parental Attitude

A. Risk Factors for Dental Neglect

- Risk factors for dental neglect[29]:
  - Low socioeconomic status and high cost of dental care.
  - Lower parental levels of formal education.
  - Low oral health literacy of parents.
  - Maternal dental anxiety.
  - Parental attitude toward primary dentition.
  - Irregular dental attendance of parents associated with dental neglect of children.
  - Refugee children or children of immigrant parents.
  - Religious and/or cultural beliefs.

B. Common Characteristics of Parents or Caregivers

- Characteristics of parents or caregivers who neglect their children's dental care may include[24,27,30]:
  - Disinterest or indifferent to the child.
  - Substance abuse.
  - Missed appointments and delayed treatment with repeated visits only for emergency care.
  - Lack of interest in oral hygiene education, disinterest and failure to complete treatment plan for significant oral disease.

Munchausen Syndrome by Proxy

I. General Considerations

- **Munchausen Syndrome by Proxy (MSBP)** is a type of abuse where a parent/caregiver fabricates or induces a disease in a child.[31]
  - Difficult to diagnose: Patient presents with a dramatic medical and/or dental history.
  - Disease does not follow the normal history of clinical presentation and is unsubstantiated.
  - The perpetrator may induce symptoms of disease in the child and it can lead to death.
  - Perpetrator wants to progress to more invasive diagnostic procedures for child.
- Initiated by mother of child in over 90% of cases.[32]
  - By definition, the perpetrator wants to become a sick person by way of a proxy (the child) to gain attention and sympathy from healthcare professionals.
  - Perpetrators may have a history of child maltreatment.
  - Half of caregivers are in healthcare-related professions.
- Presented most often in young children up to age 2 and seldom older than 6 years of age.[31]
  - Child may participate in the deception as they grow older.

Human Trafficking

I. General Considerations

- **Human trafficking** is a modern-day form of slavery and is a global public health issue.
- There are many nuances to the ways children and vulnerable adults may be exploited, but generally consists of the following categories[24,33,34]:
  - Sex trafficking or exploitation.
  - Labor trafficking, including exploitation in businesses such as agricultural and manufacturing, along with being forced to engage in criminal activity.
  - The majority of those trafficked for sex and labor are female and about one-half are younger than age 18 years.[35]

A. Risk Factors for Human Trafficking

- Human trafficking is multifactorial with contributing factors being individual, family, community, and societal.[35]
- Individuals most at risk include[34,35]:
  - LGBTQ.
  - Have a history of abuse and/or neglect.
  - Lack of a support system.
  - Substance abuse.
  - Homeless, currently in foster system or previous history in the system, runaways, or those in juvenile detention centers.
  - Untreated mental health issues.
  - Undocumented and migrant workers.

II. Indicators of a Patient Involved in Human Trafficking

- Dental staff must be aware of indicators of human trafficking and be able to provide resources to contact for assistance.[35]
  - 87.8% of individuals who are victims or survivors of human trafficking have seen a healthcare provider.[34]
  - The National Human Trafficking and Resource Center hotline is available to help healthcare providers and can guide the

provider in assessment and referral. There are training resources and reporting information at www.traffickingresourcecenter.org. The site also provides a way to enter your city, state, and zip code to find social and legal services for the victim or survivor.

- Indicators may include[33-35]:
  - Patient escorted by another person who seems controlling and insists on speaking for the patient.
  - Unusual behavior such as being submissive, fearful of touch, avoiding eye contact, aggressive, etc.
  - Homeless or unable to report address.
  - May have tattoos or other forms of branding of ownership (sexual exploitation).
  - May show signs of malnutrition and poor oral hygiene.
  - May show serious dental disease from neglect (infections and tooth loss).
    - Forced pulling of teeth or damage may occur as part of physical injury or torture for victims of trafficking.

Elder Abuse and Neglect

I. General Considerations

- Elder abuse and neglect occur in both institutional and community settings.[9,36]
  - Globally, one in six elders (15.7%) in community settings reports abuse/neglect.
  - In institutional settings, about one-third of residents reported psychological abuse with one in six residents reporting physical or financial abuse.
- Victims of elder abuse are more likely to die prematurely and have greater risk of morbidity and hospital admission.[9,37]

A. Risk Factors for Elder Abuse and Neglect

- Elder abuse affects all socioeconomic groups, cultures, races, and ethnicities.
- Risk factors include[36,37]:
  - Being female.
  - Cognitive impairment.
  - Functional impairment.
  - Depression.
  - Social isolation.
  - Living alone.
  - Being in an ethnic minority group.
  - Being older than age 74 years.

B. Types of Elder Abuse and Neglect

- Types of elder abuse and neglect are similar to those for family violence along with child abuse and neglect:
  - Physical abuse.
  - **Physical neglect**.
  - Psychological abuse.
  - Psychological neglect.
  - Financial exploitation.
  - Sexual abuse.
  - **Self-neglect**.
    - This may occur due to depression from loss of a loved one.

II. General Signs of Elder Abuse and Neglect

- When assessing for the possibility of abuse, it is necessary to have a working knowledge of lesions related to aging, health problems, and medications.
  - Taking a thorough history and comparing it with lesions present will help determine an appropriate differential diagnosis.
- Signs of abuse or neglect may include, but not be limited to, the following[31,32]:
  - May appear withdrawn, anxious, and shy; low self-esteem.
  - Provides an illogical explanation of how an injury occurred.
  - Depression or hostility may be exhibited.
  - May flinch at another person's movement as if expecting to be hit.
  - A sign of psychological abuse or intimidation can be deferral for response to questions to a caregiver or possible abuser.
  - May show signs of fear or apprehension if caregiver present.

III. Physical Signs of Elder Abuse and Neglect

- Physical signs of abuse and neglect may include[38]:
  - Patterned marks and bruising indicating object used to inflict injury such as belt buckle, ropes, or a hand in various stages of healing (**Figure 14-3**).
  - Open wounds, burns, cuts, or untreated injuries.
  - Broken eyeglasses.
  - Sudden behavior changes.
  - Refusal of a caregiver to allow visitors to see an older adult alone.

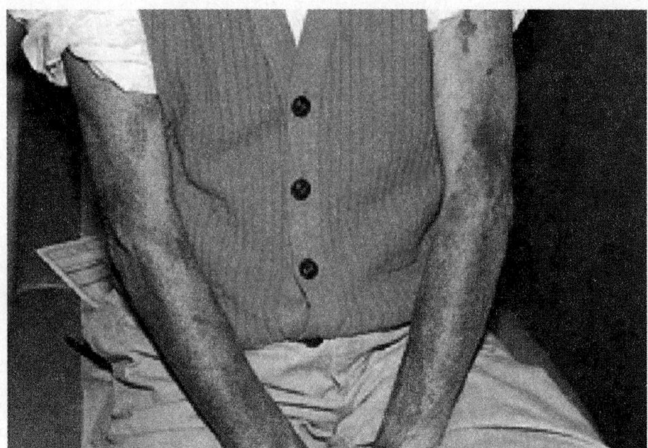

Figure 14-3 Hand- and Finger-Shaped Bruises. Large and small bruises in various stages of healing on the upper arms of this elderly patient may trigger suspicion of abuse.

Weber JR, Kelley JH. *Health Assessment in Nursing*. 2nd ed. Philadelphia, PA: Wolters Kluwer Health; 2006.

- Reports of being hit, slapped, or mistreated from an older adult.
- Broken bones, sprains, or dislocations.
- Human bite marks.
- Signs of emotional/psychological abuse may include[38]:
  - Being emotionally fragile or agitated.
  - Unresponsive and extremely withdrawn.
  - Unusual repetitive behaviors like rocking.
  - Personality changes such as being excessively apologetic and fearful of displeasing the caregiver or provider.
  - Depression or anxiety.
  - Changes in eating or sleeping habits.
- Signs of financial exploitation include[38]:
  - Changes in access to bank accounts, wills, etc.
  - The older adult reports unauthorized use or transfer of funds by a family member or someone outside the family.
- Signs of neglect and abandonment include[38]:
  - Malnutrition or **cachexia**.
  - Unsafe living conditions.
  - Unsanitary conditions, such as inadequate clothing, poor personal hygiene, etc.
  - Untreated health or dental problems.

IV. Orofacial Signs of Abuse and Neglect

- Dental team must be vigilant in discerning the indicators of elder abuse and have the proper knowledge and resources to assist elderly patients, as reporting is mandatory.[38]
- Orofacial injuries are present in over one-half of those who have experienced elder abuse.[39]
- Extraoral injuries may include[39,40]:
  - Lip trauma.
  - Bruising of facial tissues.
  - Eye injuries.
  - Fractured or bruised mandible, particularly on the left side.
  - Injuries to the cheek (zygoma), particularly on the left side.
- Intraoral injuries may include[39,40]:
  - Fractured, displaced, or avulsed teeth.
  - Lesions or sore areas in the mouth from ill-fitting dentures.
  - Deficient oral hygiene and regular dental care resulting in root caries, periodontitis, tooth loss, and denture stomatitis.
  - Fractured denture.

Intimate Partner Violence

- IPV, also known as domestic violence, has been identified as a global concern.[41,42]

I. Prevalence of IPV

- IPV may include physical violence, psychological aggression, sexual violence, and stalking.[41]
- Globally, 30% of women who had ever had a partner reported IPV.[42]
  - In the United States, 1 in 14 women and 1 in 27 men reported lifetime IPV experience.[41]
  - In Canada, 44% of women reported having ever experienced IPV.[43]
- Indigenous women had the highest prevalence of IPV in the United States (47.5%) and in Canada (61%), followed by non-Hispanic Black women (United States: 45.1%).[41,43]
- LBTQ+ women in Canada experience a high prevalence of IPV (67%).[43]
- Globally the prevalence of **intimate partner** homicide of women is 38%.[42]
  - In the United States, 70% of intimate partner homicide victims were female.[44]
  - Black and Indigenous or American Indian/Alaska Native women have the highest rate of homicide in connection with partner violence.[43]

II. Physical Injury from IPV

- Many of the same injuries listed for child and elder abuse are also evident with IPV.
- Physical injury associated with IPV may include[45]:
  - Back or neck injuries.
  - Chest injuries (e.g., broken ribs).

- Head injuries.
- Abdominal injuries.
- Upper and lower extremity injuries.
- Strangulation-related injuries such as neck bruises, voice changes, swelling, and swallowing or breathing difficulties.

- During the COVID-19 pandemic, the incidence and severity of injuries increased and healthcare providers must be vigilant to identify IPV injuries and get the individual help.[45]

III. General Health Consequences of IPV

- In addition to acute injury from IPV, there are many long-term health impacts for victims of IPV.
- The health consequences reported include[42,46,47]:
  - Chronic pain such as abdominal pain, pelvic pain, headache, and neck and low back pain.
  - Gastrointestinal disorders may include ulcers, irritable bowel syndrome, and gastroesophageal reflux.
  - Physical symptoms may include insomnia, fainting, etc.
  - Increased risk for chronic disease such as high blood pressure, strokes, and cardiovascular system.
  - Increased rates of human immunodeficiency virus (HIV) and sexually transmitted diseases.
  - Increased risk for alcohol abuse and substance abuse.
  - Mental health consequences may include depression, posttraumatic stress disorder, and suicide.
  - Unintended pregnancy, teenage pregnancy, and miscarriage.

IV. Orofacial Impact of IPV

- The most common sites for IPV injury are the head, neck, and face and may include[42]:
  - Perioral soft tissue: Contusion, laceration, and burns.
  - Teeth: Fracture, luxation, and avulsion.
  - Gingival and oral mucosa: Contusion and laceration.
  - Prosthetic device fracture.
  - Tongue: Contusion, laceration.
  - Jaw: Fracture and temporomandibular joint contusion.
  - Functional impairment:
    - Difficulty chewing.
    - Pain in face and teeth.
    - Mobility changes.
- Poor oral health behaviors due to mental health consequences of IPV, such as depression, resulting in increased risk for caries and periodontal disease.[48]
- The psychological impact of IPV may result in fear of dental treatment and avoidance of dental care.[48]

V. Role of the Dental Hygienist

- IPV may be detected in the dental setting due the frequency of orofacial injuries, so it is essential for the dental team to properly identify and make appropriate referrals to support services if IPV is suspected or reported.
- Follow dental hygiene process of care protocol to perform thorough assessments and documentation of clinical findings.[16,17]
- Practice routine inquiry, especially for women.
  - HATAH: "How are things at home?"
  - "Do you feel safe at home?"
- Perform and document detailed extraoral/intraoral findings, including photographs of injuries.[16,17]
- Provide support; encourage open communication in a nonjudgmental manner.
- Respect and maintain confidentiality; talk in a private setting.
- Offer references for counseling; telephone numbers; community services.
- Respect patient's autonomy; ask about plans for future safety.
- Prepare to share your findings with authorities when called to provide evidence.

Reporting Abuse and/or Neglect

- Dental professionals are ethically and legally mandated to report child and elder abuse and neglect.[49,50]
- Studies suggest both dentists and dental hygienists feel inadequately prepared to screen for or report abuse.[4,51] Therefore, training is critical to meet the legal obligation to report abuse.
- Despite discomfort in asking questions to screen for abuse, research shows individuals experiencing abuse want their dental provider to ask about their injuries and be given referral for assistance.[52]

I. Proper Training

- Training in the recognition and reporting of abuse and neglect needs to be implemented in every dental practice.
  - Some state governing boards require completion of continuing education courses on abuse

and neglect before licensure and re-licensure to practice dentistry and dental hygiene.

- "Prevent Abuse and Neglect through Dental Awareness" (PANDA) is a program for training dental personnel and others interested in preventing FV.[53]
  - The coalition, founded in 1992 by the Missouri Bureau of Dental Health and Delta Dental of Missouri, is a public–private partnership committed to the education of all dental professionals in the recognition and reporting of suspected cases of child abuse and neglect.
  - Since its inception, nearly all of the United States and several international coalitions have replicated the program.
- "Ask, Validate, Document, Refer (AVDR) Tutorial for Dentists" is an interactive tutorial program that utilizes a case study to demonstrate the AVDR four-step process in response to DV.[54,55]
  - *Asking* the patient about the abuse.
  - *Validating* messages that acknowledge abuse is wrong.
  - *Documenting* the signs, symptoms, and disclosures.
  - *Referring* victims to specialists and community resources.
- Project RADAR is a provider-focused initiative in healthcare settings to promote assessment and prevention of IPV.[56]
  - **R**outinely ask about IPV.
  - **A**sk directly about violence, that is, "*Has a partner hit or otherwise frightened you?*"
  - **D**ocument findings in the patient chart.
  - **A**ssess safety by asking questions such as "*Do you feel safe to return home?*"
  - **R**eview options and referrals.
- Each office should have a list of resources in the community to assist its patients.

II. Reporting Laws

- Recognizing signs of suspected abuse and following proper reporting protocol will promote health and safety for all individuals.
- It is important for all healthcare providers (including dental providers) to be observant and knowledgeable about signs and symptoms of child abuse and neglect and to know how to respond.
- Each state has laws regarding the reporting of abuse and neglect to the proper authorities.[49,50] It is imperative to research the laws for your state and have them available for reference in your office.
- Each dental practice needs a written protocol for the documentation and reporting of abuse and neglect.[17,57]

III. Required Information for Mandatory Reporting

- All states mandate healthcare workers to report suspected abuse and neglect of children, disabled individuals, and the elderly.[49,50]
- Reporting and resource hotlines are available for suspected cases of child abuse, domestic violence, human trafficking, and elder abuse and neglect (**Box 14-1**).
- When reporting suspected child maltreatment, have the following information available[49]:
  - Child's name and age.
  - Nature of the child's condition, including evidence of previous injuries.
  - Date, time, and extent of the abuse or neglect.
  - The perpetrator's (or suspected perpetrator's) identity, name, address, and relationship to the victim of abuse or neglect.

Box 14-1 Reporting and Resources Hotlines in the United States and Canada

- Child abuse national hotline:
  - United States: 800.4.A.CHILD (800.422.4453).
  - Canada: 1-800-668-6868 or text CONNECT to 686868
- Domestic violence national hotline:
  - United States: 800.799.SAFE (800.799.7233).
  - Canada: Multiple resources for family or intimate partner violence available at www.canada.ca/en/department-national-defence/campaigns/covid-19/domestic-violence.html.
- Human trafficking:
  - In the United States, victims, survivors, and witnesses can call a national 24-hour multilingual hotline: 1-888-373-7888 or text "HELP" to 233733 (BEFREE).
  - In Canada, victims, survivors, and witnesses can call a confidential 24-hour multilingual hotline: 1-833-900-1010.
- Elder abuse and neglect:
  - If it is suspected an elder is in immediate danger, call the local police or 911.
  - In the United States, the National Adult Protective Services Association website can be used to identify the number to call in your state to report a suspected case of elder abuse: www.napsa-now.org/aps-program-list/
  - In Canada, suspected elder abuse can be reported to the Seniors Safety Line at 1-866 299-1011. This number can also be given to the older adult as a source for counseling and access to support services.

- The reporter's name, affiliation, position and contact information. (In some states, the reporter's identity is confidential.)
- The information needed for reporting suspected abuse/neglect of the elderly or a disabled individual would be similar to that needed for a child.

Forensic Dentistry

Forensic dentistry is that aspect of dental science that relates and applies dental facts to legal problems.[58]

- Forensic dentistry encompasses dental identification, malpractice litigation, legislation, peer review, and dental licensure.
- Forensics is a specialty and is not within the scope of practice of any dentist or auxiliary without proper advanced training and certification or recognition.

I. Use of Forensics in Abuse Cases

- There are instances when it becomes necessary to request the aid of a forensic odontologist to determine if a particular injury, usually a bite mark, is a result of trauma caused by a particular suspect.[59]
    - Many times, the abuser will state the bite mark occurred from a sibling squabble, an animal bite, or the child self-biting.
- Two types of evidence can be obtained from a bitemark:
    - DNA from saliva.
    - Tooth impression or pattern.
- The bitemark pattern alone used as evidence in legal settings has been called into question, so the preference is for use of DNA from saliva.[59]

Documentation

I. Purposes of Documentation

- To provide authorities accurate and thorough information to support an investigation.
- To protect the abused patient from harmful circumstances or even death. A second person needs to be present to witness the examination and interview.

II. Content of the Record

- Document the date, time, and place of the examination.
- Obtain a thorough history of the injury from both the caregiver and the patient.
- Record questions and answers in the exact words of the abused patient.
- Carefully record all observations.
- Document all lesions, giving descriptive location, estimation of size, shape, and color.
    - Pay close attention to ecchymosis of varying colors and bilateral injuries.
- Use diagrams showing the location, size, and description.
- Photographs and radiographs gathered as part of comprehensive dental examination are part of the legal record and can be requested as part of a child or elder abuse investigation.
- Use the words *suspected abuse* if the patient denies abuse.
- **Box 14-2** provides a sample of documenting suspected abuse noted during a patient visit.

Box 14-2 Example Documentation: Patient Injury Related to Suspected Abuse

- **S**—A 23-year-old female presents for an emergency visit because of pain in mandibular right second premolar area. Patient complains of recent headaches and pain in right temporomandibular joint area. She states, "My boyfriend slapped me recently, but he has been under a lot of pressure lately and he didn't mean to bruise me." Patient seems nervous and agitated.
- **O**—Asked patient if this had happened before and whether she felt safe returning home. She responded that it happened once before and she felt safe returning home. Patient presents with multiple contusions on right side of face above inferior border of mandible and right buccal mucosa. Bruises are in various stages of healing; red, purple, and greenish yellow. Bruises are oval shaped about 2 to 5 cm in size. Intraoral and extraoral photographs were taken.
- **A**—Panoramic radiograph revealed a simple fracture in the body of the mandible below right second premolar area. Patient confirmed that injuries related to partner abuse.
- **P**—Reassured patient that she did not deserve to be hit even if her boyfriend was "under a lot of pressure." Given the severity of her injury, encouraged her to call the national domestic violence hotline number. Offered to initiate the call from my cell phone so the number would not be in her call history, but the patient responded that she wanted to think about it. The oral surgeon's office was called to set up an emergency appointment for evaluation of the jaw fracture.

Next step: Follow-up telephone call to patient after her scheduled appointment with the oral surgeon.
Signed: ______________________________, RDH
Date: ________________

Factors to Teach the Patient

Factors to Teach the Abused Elder or Intimate Partner

- Where help can be obtained: Emergency assistance including phone numbers and referrals.
- The tendency for the maltreatment to increase in severity and frequency over time.
- Abuse can escalate and can be life threatening.
- Maltreatment is a choice. It is used to gain power and control over another individual.

References

1. Mercy JA, Hillis SD, Butchart A, et al. Interpersonal violence: global impact and paths to prevention. In: Mock CN, Nugent R, Kobusingye O, Smith KR, eds. *Injury Prevention and Environmental Health*. 3rd ed. The International Bank for Reconstruction and Development/The World Bank; 2017. http://www.ncbi.nlm.nih.gov/books/NBK525208/. Accessed January 13, 2022.
2. Conroy S. *Family Violence in Canada: A Statistical Profile, 2019*. Canadian Centre for Justice and Community Safety Statistics; 2021:55.
3. Rodrigues JLSA, Lima APB, Nagata JY, et al. Domestic violence against children detected and managed in the routine of dentistry: a systematic review. *J Forensic Leg Med*. 2016;43:34-41.
4. de Jesus Santos Nascimento CT, de Oliveira MN, Vidigal MTC, et al. Domestic violence against women detected and managed in dental practice: a systematic review. *J Fam Violence*. Published online January 6, 2022:1-12.
5. Fiolet R, Tarzia L, Hameed M, Hegarty K. Indigenous peoples' help-seeking behaviors for family violence: a scoping review. *Trauma Violence Abuse*. 2021;22(2):370-380.
6. World Health Organization. Violence against children. Published June 8, 2020. https://www.who.int/news-room/fact-sheets/detail/violence-against-children. Accessed January 13, 2022.
7. World Health Organization. Violence against women. Published March 9, 2021. https://www.who.int/news-room/fact-sheets/detail/violence-against-women. Accessed January 13, 2022.
8. Bermea AM, Slakoff DC, Goldberg AE. Intimate partner violence in the LGBTQ+ community: experiences, outcomes, and implications for primary care. *Prim Care*. 2021;48(2):329-337.
9. Yon Y, Mikton CR, Gassoumis ZD, Wilber KH. Elder abuse prevalence in community settings: a systematic review and meta-analysis. *Lancet Glob Health*. 2017;5(2):e147-e156.
10. Centers for Disease Control and Prevention. Violence prevention. Published June 14, 2021. https://www.cdc.gov/violenceprevention/index.html. Accessed January 13, 2022.
11. US Department of Health and Human Services, Administration of Children, Youth, and Families. *Child Maltreatment 2019*. US Department of Health and Human Services; 2021:306. https://www.acf.hhs.gov/sites/default/files/documents/cb/cm2019.pdf. Accessed January 15, 2022.
12. Arias I, Leeb RT, Melanson C, Paulozzi LJ, Simon TR. *Child Maltreatment Surveillance; Uniform Definitions for Public Health and Recommended Data Elements*. Centers for Disease Control and Prevention, National Center for Injury Prevention and Control; 2008:148.
13. American Academy of Pediatric Dentistry. Oral and dental aspects of child abuse and neglect. *Pediatr Dent*. 2018;40(6):243-249.
14. van IJzendoorn MH, Bakermans-Kranenburg MJ, Coughlan B, Reijman S. Annual Research Review: umbrella synthesis of meta-analyses on child maltreatment antecedents and interventions: differential susceptibility perspective on risk and resilience. *J Child Psychol Psychiatry*. 2020;61(3):272-290.
15. Usher K, Bhullar N, Durkin J, Gyamfi N, Jackson D. Family violence and COVID-19: increased vulnerability and reduced options for support. *Int J Ment Health Nurs*. 2020;29(4):549-552.
16. American Dental Hygienists' Association. *2016 Revised Standards for Clinical Dental Hygiene Practice*. Published June 2016. https://www.adha.org/resources-docs/2016-Revised-Standards-for-Clinical-Dental-Hygiene-Practice.pdf. Accessed December 11, 2021.
17. Federation of Dental Hygiene Regulators of Canada (FDHRC). *Entry-to-Practice Canadian Competencies for Dental Hygienists*. Dental Hygiene Regulators of Canada (FDHRC); 2021:34. https://www.fdhrc.ca/wp/competency-project/. Accessed January 15, 2022.
18. Mouden LD, Lowe JW, Dixit UB. How to recognize situations that suggest abuse/neglect. *Missouri Dental J*. 1992;Nov-Dec:26-29.
19. Maguire SA, Williams B, Naughton AM, et al. A systematic review of the emotional, behavioural and cognitive features exhibited by school-aged children experiencing neglect or emotional abuse. *Child Care Health Dev*. 2015;41(5):641-653.
20. Norman RE, Byambaa M, De R, Butchart A, Scott J, Vos T. The long-term health consequences of child physical abuse, emotional abuse, and neglect: a systematic review and meta-analysis. *PLoS Med*. 2012;9(11):e1001349.
21. Hébert M, Langevin R, Oussaïd E. Cumulative childhood trauma, emotion regulation, dissociation, and behavior problems in school-aged sexual abuse victims. *J Affect Disord*. 2018;225:306-312.
22. Kellogg ND, American Academy of Pediatrics Committee on Child Abuse and Neglect. Evaluation of suspected child physical abuse. *Pediatrics*. 2007;119(6):1232-1241.
23. Stanford Medicine. Child abuse: signs & symptoms. https://childabuse.stanford.edu/screening/signs.html. Accessed January 15, 2022.
24. U.S. Department of Health and Human Services, Administration for Children and Families, Administration on Children, Youth, and Families. *Recognizing Child Abuse and Neglect: Signs and Symptoms*. Published online June 2007. https://www.childwelfare.gov/pubPDFs/signs.pdf. Accessed January 15, 2022.

25. Zatti C, Rosa V, Barros A, et al. Childhood trauma and suicide attempt: a meta-analysis of longitudinal studies from the last decade. *Psychiatry Res*. 2017;256:353-358.
26. US Department of Justice; Office of Justice Programs; Office of Juvenile Justice and Delinquency Prevention. *Recognizing When a Child's Injury or Illness Is Caused by Abuse*. Office of Justice Programs; 2014:28. http://doi.apa.org/get-pe-doi.cfm?doi=10.1037/e318182004-001. Accessed January 15, 2022.
27. Fisher-Owens SA, Lukefahr JL, Tate AR, et al. Oral and dental aspects of child abuse and neglect. *Pediatrics*. 2017;140(2).
28. Fredriksen TV, Søftestad S, Kranstad V, Willumsen T. Preparing for attack and recovering from battle: understanding child sexual abuse survivors' experiences of dental treatment. *Community Dent Oral Epidemiol*. 2020;48(4):317-327.
29. Khalid G, Metzner F, Pawils S. Prevalence of dental neglect and associated risk factors in children and adolescents: a systematic review. *Int J Paediatr Dent*. 2022;22(3):436-446.
30. Ramazani N. Child dental neglect: a short review. *Int J High Risk Behav Addict*. 2014;3(4):e21861.
31. Olczak-Kowalczyk D, Wolska-Kusnierz B, Bernatowska E. Fabricated or induced illness in the oral cavity in children: a systematic review and personal experience. *Cent Eur J Immunol*. 2015;40(1):109-114.
32. Yates G, Bass C. The perpetrators of medical child abuse (Munchausen Syndrome by Proxy): a systematic review of 796 cases. *Child Abuse Negl*. 2017;72:45-53.
33. Wood LCN. Child modern slavery, trafficking and health: a practical review of factors contributing to children's vulnerability and the potential impacts of severe exploitation on health. *BMJ Paediatr Open*. 2020;4(1):e000327. doi:10.1136/bmjpo-2018-000327
34. Toney-Butler TJ, Ladd M, Mittel O. Human trafficking. In: *StatPearls*. StatPearls Publishing; 2022. http://www.ncbi.nlm.nih.gov/books/NBK430910/. Accessed January 16, 2022.
35. Greenbaum J, Bodrick N, Committe on Child Abuse and Neglect, et al. Global human trafficking and child victimization. *Pediatrics*. 2017;140(6):e20173138.
36. Yon Y, Ramiro-Gonzalez M, Mikton CR, Huber M, Sethi D. The prevalence of elder abuse in institutional settings: a systematic review and meta-analysis. *Eur J Public Health*. 2019;29(1):58-67.
37. Dong XQ. Elder abuse: systematic review and implications for practice. *J Am Geriatr Soc*. 2015;63(6):1214-1238.
38. US Department of Justice. Red flags of elder abuse. Published June 13, 2019. https://www.justice.gov/elderjustice/red-flags-elder-abuse-0. Accessed January 16, 2022.
39. Rosen T, LoFaso VM, Bloemen EM, et al. Identifying injury patterns associated with physical elder abuse: analysis of legally adjudicated cases. *Ann Emerg Med*. 2020;76(3):266-276.
40. Petti S. Elder neglect—oral diseases and injuries. *Oral Dis*. 2018;24(6):891-899.
41. Smith SG, Chen J, Basile KC, et al. *The National Intimate Partner and Sexual Violence Survey: 2010-2012 State Report*. National Center for Injury Prevention and Control, Centers for Disease Control and Prevention; 2017:272. https://www.cdc.gov/violenceprevention/pdf/nisvs-statereportbook.pdf. Accessed August 2, 2022.
42. World Health Organization. *Global and Regional Estimates of Violence against Women: Prevalence and Health Effects of Intimate Partner Violence and Non-Partner Sexual Violence*. World Health Organization; 2013:58. https://apps.who.int/iris/handle/10665/341012. Accessed January 16, 2022.
43. Government of Canada. Fact sheet: Intimate partner violence. Published March 31, 2021. https://women-gender-equality.canada.ca/en/gender-based-violence-knowledge-centre/intimate-partner-violence.html. Accessed January 16, 2022.
44. Smith SG, Fowler KA, Niolon PH. Intimate partner homicide and corollary victims in 16 states: National Violent Death Reporting System, 2003–2009. *Am J Public Health*. 2014;104(3):461-466.
45. Gosangi B, Park H, Thomas R, et al. Exacerbation of physical intimate partner violence during COVID-19 pandemic. *Radiology*. 2021;298(1):E38-E45.
46. Rivara F, Adhia A, Lyons V, et al. The effects of violence on health. *Health Affairs*. 2019;38(10):1622-1629.
47. Campbell J, Jones AS, Dienemann J, et al. Intimate partner violence and physical health consequences. *Arch Intern Med*. 2002;162(10):1157-1163.
48. Kundu H, P B, Singla A, et al. Domestic violence and its effect on oral health behaviour and oral health status. *J Clin Diagn Res*. 2014;8(11):ZC09-ZC12.
49. U.S. Department of Health and Human Services, Children's Bureau. *Mandatory Reporters of Child Abuse and Neglect*. US Department of Health and Human Services, Children's Bureau; 2019:68. https://www.childwelfare.gov/pubPDFs/manda.pdf. Accessed August 2, 2022.
50. US Department of Justice. State elder abuse statutes. Published April 8, 2016. https://www.justice.gov/elderjustice/elder-justice-statutes-0. Accessed January 19, 2022.
51. Harris CM, Boyd L, Rainchuso L, Rothman AT. Oral health care providers' knowledge and attitudes about intimate partner violence. *J Dent Hyg*. 2016;90(5):283-296.
52. Nelms AP, Gutmann ME, Solomon ES, Dewald JP, Campbell PR. What victims of domestic violence need from the dental profession. *J Dent Educ*. 2009;73(4):490-498.
53. Northeast Delta Dental. The P.A.N.D.A. Program. https://www.nedelta.com/Providers/P-A-N-D-A-Program. Accessed January 19, 2022.
54. Futures Without Violence. The Ask, Validate, Document, Refer (AVDR) Tutorial for Dentists. Published July 1, 2014. https://www.futureswithoutviolence.org/the-ask-validate-document-refer-avdr-tutorial-for-dentists/. Accessed January 19, 2022.
55. Mythri H, Kashinath KR, Raju AS, Suresh KV, Bharateesh JV. Enhancing the dental professional's responsiveness towards domestic violence: a cross-sectional study. *J Clin Diagn Res*. 2015;9(6):ZC51-ZC53.
56. Respecting Accuracy in Domestic Abuse Reporting (RADAR). RADAR: Home Page. https://www.mediaradar.org/. Accessed January 19, 2022.
57. American Dental Association. *The ADA Principles of Ethics and Code of Professional Conduct Section on Beneficence*. https://www.ada.org/about/principles/code-of-ethics/beneficence. Accessed January 19, 2022.
58. Nagi R, Aravinda K, Rakesh N, Jain S, Kaur N, Mann AK. Digitization in forensic odontology: a paradigm shift in forensic investigations. *J Forensic Dent Sci*. 2019;11(1):5-10.
59. Bowers CM. Review of a forensic pseudoscience: Identification of criminals from bitemark patterns. *J Forensic Leg Med*. 2019;61:34-39.

CHAPTER 15

Dental Radiographic Imaging

Laura Jansen Howerton, RDH, MS

CHAPTER OUTLINE

LEARNING OBJECTIVES

After studying this chapter, the student will be able to:

1. Compare different imaging systems and describe the advantages and disadvantages of each.
2. Describe factors that influence the finished image.
3. Identify the components in the x-ray tube head and describe how images are produced.
4. Explain clinician and patient radiation protection guidelines and published recommendations for patient selection and exposure.
5. Assess need and justify radiographic exposure for each patient.

Introduction

Radiographic images are integral assessment components useful when planning comprehensive care for a patient. Images provide the clinician with valuable diagnostic information:

- Lesions, diseases, and other conditions of teeth and supporting structures.
- Localization of foreign objects.
- Assess growth and development.
- Documentation of changes in a condition over time.

The dentist is responsible for determining the need for radiographic images.

- Designation of the number and types of dental exposures is made selectively only after a review of the patient's health history and a complete clinical examination.[1]
- A history of oral and body exposures to **radiation** is recommended.
- Excessive dental exposure to low levels of ionizing radiation cannot be justified.[2]

The objective in radiography is to use procedures that expose the patient to the least possible amount of radiation to produce images of the greatest interpretive value. The first consideration is to limit the number of exposures to those that have been deemed necessary.

This chapter provides a summary of terminology and fundamentals of dental **radiology**, including:

- X-ray production.
- Procedures for image retrieval.
- Safety factors.
- Analysis of the completed images.
- The value of patient instruction.

How X-Rays Are Produced

X-ray energy is **electromagnetic ionizing radiation** of very short wavelengths, resulting from the bombardment of a target made of tungsten by highly accelerated electrons in a vacuum. Electric and magnetic fields positioned at right angles to one another produce electromagnetic energy.

The various types of energy in the electromagnetic spectrum have similar attributes. The properties of x-rays are listed in **Box 15-1**.

Essential to x-ray production are:

- A source of electrons.
- A high voltage to accelerate the electrons.
- A target to stop the electrons and convert into x-ray photons.

The parts of the tube and the circuits within the machine are designed to provide these elements.

Box 15-1 Properties of X-Rays

Characteristics
- Invisible
- No mass
- No weight

Travel
- In straight line; can be scattered
- At the speed of light

Wavelengths
- Have short wavelengths, high frequency
- Hard x-rays: Short wavelengths, high penetration
- Soft x-rays: Relatively longer wavelengths, relatively less penetrating; more likely to be absorbed into the tissue

Penetration
- Depending on atomic structure:
  - Pass through matter
  - Absorbed by matter

Causes
- Ionization
- Fluorescence of certain crystals
- Biologic changes in living cells

Produces
- A radiographic image

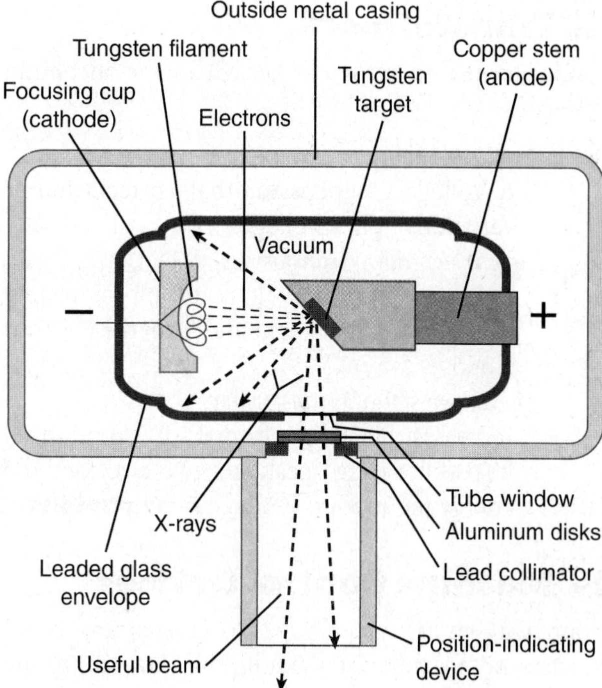

Figure 15-1 X-Ray Tube. High-speed electrons flowing from cathode to anode hit the tungsten target and create x-ray photons. X-rays exit through the tube window and position-indicating device (PID).

I. The X-Ray Tube

A. Protective Tube Housing

- A heavy metal enclosure houses the x-ray tube (**Figure 15-1**) to reduce **primary radiation** to permissible exposure levels and prevent **leakage radiation**.

B. X-Ray Tube

- A highly evacuated leaded glass tube composed of a cathode and an anode, surrounded by a refined oil with high insulating powers.

C. Cathode

- Tungsten filament, which is a coiled wire heated to generate a cloud of electrons. It is a component of the low-voltage circuit.
- Molybdenum cup around the filament helps to focus the electrons toward the anode.

D. Anode (+)

- A tungsten target embedded in a copper stem, positioned at an angle to the electron beam.

E. Aperture

- The window through which the useful beam emerges from the tube, covered with a permanent seal of glass.

F. Aluminum Disks

- Thin (0.5-mm) sheets of aluminum placed over the aperture to filter out longer-wavelength, less penetrating x-rays.

G. Lead Diaphragm

- A lead collimator with a hole to restrict the size of the x-ray beam.

H. Position-Indicating Device

- Open-ended cylinder, or rectangle, that shapes and aims the x-ray beam.

II. Circuits

A circuit is the complete path over which an electrical current may flow. Two circuits are used to produce x-rays. Two circuits used to produce x-rays are:

- Low-voltage filament circuit.
- High-voltage cathode–anode circuit.

III. Transformers

A transformer increases or decreases the incoming voltage.

- *Autotransformer*
    - A voltage compensator that corrects minor variations in line voltage.
- *Filament step-down transformer*
    - Decreases the line voltage to approximately 3 V to heat the filament and form the electron cloud.
- *High-voltage step-up transformer*
    - Increases the current from 110 V to 60 to 90 kVp (kilovoltage peak) to give electrons the energy required to produce x-ray **photons**.

IV. Machine Control Devices

Four switches are typically seen on the control panel of the x-ray machine: the on/off power switch (to the electrical outlet), the kilovoltage peak, the milliamperage, and the timer.

A. Voltage Control

Voltage is the unit of measurement used to describe the force that pushes an electric current through a circuit.

- *Circuit voltmeter*: Registers line voltage before voltage is stepped up by the transformer (with alternating current [AC], this is 110 V) or may register the kilovoltage that results after step-up.
- *kVp (selector)*: Used to change the line voltage to a selected kilovoltage peak (60–90 kVp).

B. Milliamperage Control

- *Ampere*: The unit of intensity of an electrical current produced by 1 V acting through a resistance of 1 Ω. A milliampere (mA) is 1/1,000 of an ampere.
- *Milliammeter*: Instrument used to select the actual current through the tube circuit during the time of exposure.

C. Time Control

- *X-ray timer*: A time switch mechanism used to control the length of the exposure time.
- *Time-delay switch*: Mechanism that applies power to the high-voltage circuit once the filament is heated.
- *Electronic timer*: Vacuum tube device; resets itself automatically to the last-used exposure time. The timer is calibrated in seconds or in **impulses**, with 60 impulses in each second (in a 60-cycle AC).

V. The Production of X-Rays

X-rays are produced when high-speed electrons are slowed down or stopped suddenly.

- Tungsten filament of the cathode is heated, and a cloud of electrons is produced.
- Difference in electrical potential is developed between the anode and the cathode.
- Electrons traveling at a high speed are attracted to the positively charged anode from the negatively charged cathode. When AC is used with a self-rectifying tube, the electrons are attracted back into the tungsten filament.
- Curvature of the molybdenum cup controls the direction of the electrons and causes them to be projected toward the focal spot of the anode.
- When the electron stream strikes the tungsten target, a loss of energy results.
    - Approximately 1% of the energy of electrons is converted to x-ray energy (greater percentage at higher kilovoltage peak).
    - Approximately 99% of the energy is converted to heat and is dissipated through the copper anode and oil of the protective tube housing.
- General (bremsstrahlung, or braking) radiation occurs when speeding electrons stop, "brake," or slow down near the tungsten target in the anode.
    - When an electron hits the nucleus of the tungsten atom, all of its kinetic energy is converted into a high-energy x-ray photon.
    - When an electron comes close to but misses the nucleus, an x-ray photon of lower energy is created.
    - General radiation produces x-rays of many different energies.
- Characteristic radiation results:
    - When a bombarding electron, at 70 kVp or above, displaces an electron from a shell of the target atom, ionization of the atom results.
    - Another electron in an outer shell replaces the missing electron, causing a cascading effect.

- When the displaced electron is replaced, a photon is emitted, resulting in characteristic radiation.
- Characteristic radiation contributes approximately 10% to the useful beam.

- X-rays exit the tube through the aperture to form the useful beam.
    - *Useful beam*: The part of the primary radiation that is permitted to emerge from the tube head aperture and the accessory collimating devices.
    - *Central beam* (central ray): The center of the beam of x-rays emitted from the tube.

Digital Imaging

- Traditional film-based systems to record radiographic images have been in existence in dentistry for over 100 years.
- In the late 1980s, the first direct digital imaging system was introduced and adopted by dental professionals.
- Digital imaging is a method of imaging using a **sensor**, breaking the image into small electronic pieces, and presenting and storing the image using a computer.
- Digital systems include intraoral and extraoral imaging.

I. Digital Imaging Principles

- Digital imaging requires conventional equipment to generate x-rays.
- The image is captured on sensors or plates of varying sizes, similar to conventional film.
- The information is then recorded as a digital image and displayed as **pixels** representing multiple shades of gray.
- The image is subsequently displayed on a computer monitor.
- The image can be enhanced and manipulated, by changing factors such as density and contrast. The image can be stored on the hard drive for future reference, and/or electronically sent to other professionals.[3–5]

II. Digital Imaging Equipment

A. Direct Digital Imaging

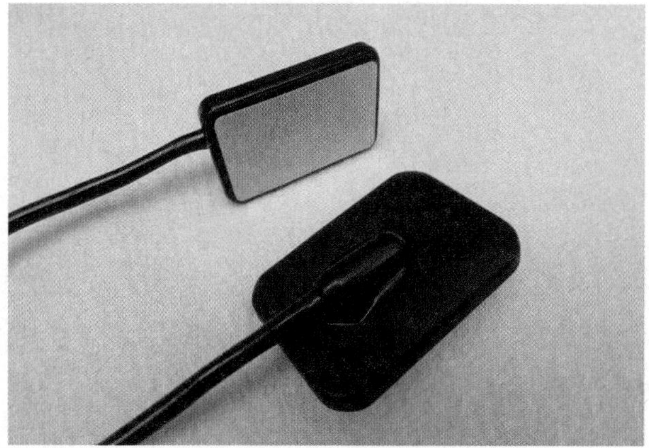

Figure 15-2 Direct Digital Sensors. Two sensor sizes are shown. Charge-coupled device or complementary metal-oxide semiconductor sensors have integrated circuits made up of a grid of small transistor elements that convert x-rays to electrons in electron wells. Each element represents one pixel in the final image. This information is passed through a cable to the computer for processing.

- A corded or cordless charge-coupled device (CCD) or complementary metal-oxide semiconductor (CMOS) sensor in a rigid case is used. Both convert x-radiation to electrons that are stored in electron wells and converted to visible images. With CMOS technology, individual pixels can be made smaller (**Figure 15-2**).
- Viewing of the image is possible on the computer screen within seconds of exposure.

B. Indirect Digital Imaging

- A cordless photostimulable phosphor (PSP) plate is used that converts x-radiation into stored energy to record the image (**Figure 15-3**).
- Information on the PSP plate is then read by a laser scanner and converted to digital data.
- The digital image is displayed on a monitor.
- Traditional films can also be scanned as **analog** images and converted to digital.

III. The Production of a Digital Image

- The sensor, direct or indirect (Figure 15-2 and Figure 15-3), is encased in a plastic sleeve (**Figure 15-4**), held in a beam alignment device, and placed in the patient's mouth.
- When exposed to radiation, an electronic charge is produced on the surface of the sensor.
- With direct digital imaging, the image is immediately converted from analog form to digital form and displayed on the monitor (**Figure 15-5**).

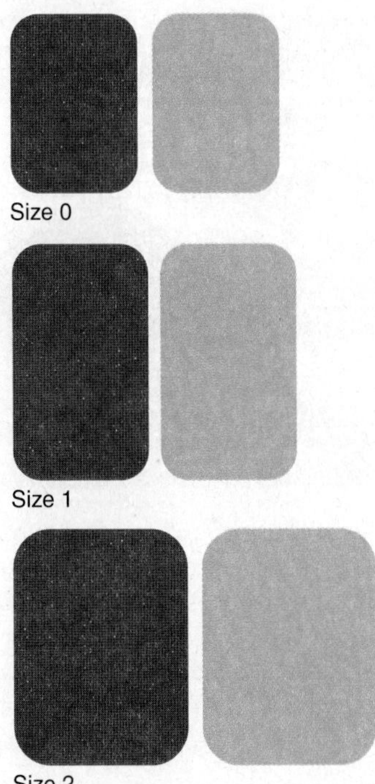

Figure 15-3 Indirect Digital Sensors. The light blue side faces the x-ray beam. The black nonexposure sides of various sizes of photostimulable phosphor (PSP) sensors are shown. Intraoral PSP sensors are available in sizes 0–4 as seen with traditional film, as well as panoramic and cephalometric sizes. The light blue side is covered with phosphor crystals that store x-ray energy when exposed. When the sensor is placed in a laser scanner, the energy is released from the phosphor layer and converted to a digital image.

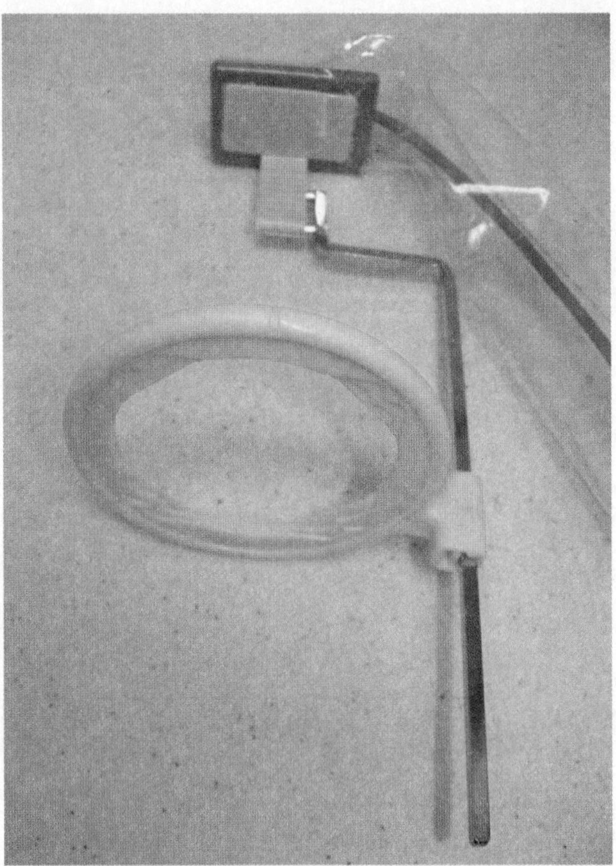

Figure 15-4 Sensor Holder in Plastic Sleeve. The sensor holder is encased in a plastic sleeve for infection control purposes.

- With indirect digital imaging, the PSP plates store the image until placed in a high-speed laser scanner, which converts the information into a **digitized** image and displays it on the monitor.
- The image can then be stored, manipulated, enhanced, retrieved, and transmitted.
- The CCD or CMOS (direct imaging) sensors can be reused immediately on the same patient or unwrapped and sanitized, according to the manufacturer's recommendations.
- The PSP (indirect imaging) plate is erased in the scanner or through being exposed to a high-intensity light box for approximately 30 seconds.
- The PSP plates resemble the shape and thickness of traditional film, which aids in receptor placement and patient tolerance.
- The CCD/CMOS sensors are thick, rigid, and bulky and are associated with patient limitations. These sensors become more user-friendly after a learning curve is achieved.
- Knowledge and experience in intraoral techniques is required for CCD/CMOS sensor exposures.[6,7]

IV. Evaluation

A. Advantages of Digital Imaging

- Less radiation exposure for the patient due to lower exposure time when compared to traditional film.
- Faster image acquisition.
- No darkroom or processing chemistry.
- Immediate feedback for diagnosis.
- Improved diagnostics through software tools.
- Effective patient education tool.
- Electronic record keeping.
- Reduced cross-contamination.
- Ability to send image electronically.

B. Disadvantages of Digital Imaging

- Initial setup expense.
- Bulky direct imaging sensors may increase receptor placement errors.
- Infection control of sensors that cannot be heat sterilized.
- Direct imaging sensors are fragile and expensive.

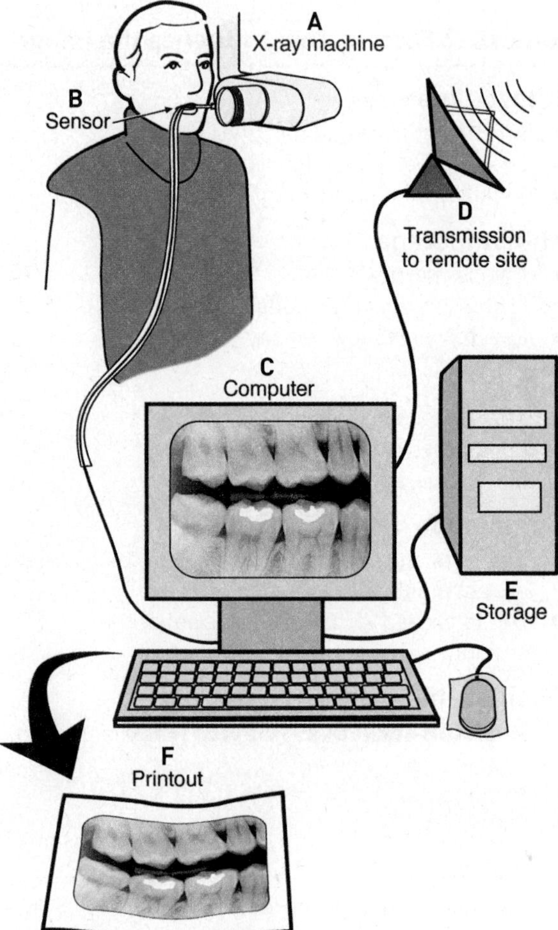

Figure 15-5 Direct Digital Imaging System. The image is exposed by an x-ray machine **(A)** and captured on a charge-coupled device or complementary metal-oxide semiconductor sensor placed intraorally **(B)**. The signal is transmitted via a cable to the computer **(C)**, where it is digitized into multiple gray levels. The image is displayed on the computer monitor, transmitted electronically to a remote site **(D)**, stored on a file server **(E)**, or printed on paper **(F)**.

Characteristics of an Acceptable Image

A *radiographic image* is the visible image on a processed film or a digitized image created by the computer.

- The image is produced after exposure to ionizing radiation that has passed through teeth or a part of the oral cavity.
- A *radiographic survey* refers to a series of radiographic images, such as four bitewing images or a complete full series.
- Before exposing a radiographic image, it is necessary to know the characteristics that are expected to result in an image of maximum diagnostic value. The basic essentials are:
    - The appearance of the image itself.
    - The region of interest is covered.
    - The quality of the processed radiograph.
- **Table 15-1** provides a list of characteristics of an acceptable image.

Table 15-1 Characteristics of an Acceptable Image

Characteristic	Appearance
Image	All portions of the region of interest mimic the actual size of the teeth, with minimal overlap and minimal distortion
Area covered	Sufficient tissue surrounding tooth for diagnostic purposes
Density	Proper density for diagnosis
Contrast	Proper contrast for diagnosis
Definition and sharpness	Clear outline of objects; minimal **penumbra**

I. Radiolucency and Radiopacity

- An image has gradations from white to black that are referred to as radiopaque or radiolucent.
- For example, a dense material, such as a metallic restoration, prevents the passage of x-rays and that area appears white or light on the processed image.
- Soft tissue does not resist passage of x-rays and appears black to gray.

II. Radiopacity

The appearance of light (white) images on an image is a result of the lesser amount of radiation that penetrates the structures and reaches the image receptor.

- A radiopaque structure inhibits the passage of x-rays.
- Examples include:
    - Enamel.
    - Dentin.
    - Metallic restorations, such as gold crowns and amalgam.
    - Implants.

III. Radiolucency

The appearance of dark images on an image is a result of the greater amount of radiation that penetrates the structures and reaches the receptor.

- A *radiolucent* structure permits the passage of radiation with relatively little attenuation by absorption.
- Examples include:
  - Pulp cavity.
  - Cysts.
  - Dental caries.
  - Periodontal ligament space.

Factors That Influence the Finished Image

As the beam leaves the x-ray tube (Figure 15-1):

- It is collimated, filtered, and allowed to travel a designated source–image receptor (or focal spot–image receptor) distance before reaching the receptor of a selected speed.
- The quality or diagnostic usefulness of the finished image, as well as the total exposure of the patient and clinician, is influenced by the *kilovoltage peak, milliampere seconds, time, collimation, filtration, target–receptor distance, object–receptor distance*, and *film speed*, as outlined in **Box 15-2**.
- Traditional film processing also directly influences the quality of the radiograph and indirectly the total exposure. Re-exposure would be necessary should the film be rendered inadequate during processing.

I. Collimation

- Collimation is the technique for controlling the size and shape of the beam of radiation emitted.
- A *collimator* is a diaphragm or system of diaphragms made of an absorbing material designed to define the dimensions and direction of a beam of radiation.

A. Purposes

- Eliminate peripheral or divergent radiation.
- Minimize exposure to patient's face.
- Minimize **secondary radiation**, which can fog the receptor and cause scatter to the patient and clinician.

B. Methods

- Lead diaphragm
  - Made of lead with a central aperture of the smallest practical diameter for making radiographic exposure.

Box 15-2 Factors That Influence the Image

Kilovoltage Peak
- Affects contrast and density
- Low kVp yields high (short-scale) contrast
- High kVp yields low (long-scale) contrast

Milliamperage
- Affects density
- High mA yields high density
- Low mA yields low density

Time
- Affects density
- Long time yields high density
- Short time yields low density

Collimation
- Restricts and shapes the beam; may be circular or rectangular
- Not to exceed 2.75 inches or 7 cm at the patient's skin

Position-Indicating Device
- **Position-indicating device (PID)** is used to direct the x-ray beam.
- Rectangular
- Cylindrical

Filtration
- Aluminum filters remove low-energy x-rays.
- Rare earth filters remove low- and high-energy x-rays.
- Methods of filtration
  - *Inherent*: Occurs when the x-ray beam passes through the internal components of the x-ray tube
    - Glass window
    - Insulating oil
    - Tube head seal
  - *Added*: Occurs when aluminum disks are added to the path of the x-ray beam
    - Aluminum disks
    - 1.5 mm for machines operating at 50–70 kVp
    - 2.5 for machines operating above 70 kVp

Total Filtration
- Combination of inherent and added filtration

Target–Receptor Distance
- Longer PID increases resolution of image
- Longer PID decreases scatter of radiation

Object–Receptor Distance
- Increased object–receptor distance achieves parallelism.
- Decreased object–receptor distance decreases penumbra.

Film Speed
- Faster speed film decreases definition; image is more grainy.

- Located between the aluminum filters in the tube head and the position-indicating device (PID).
- Recommended thickness of lead: 1/8 inch.
- Recommended maximum size of aperture: To permit a diameter of the beam of radiation equal to 2.75 inches or 7 cm at the end of the PID next to the patient's face.

- Rectangular collimation (**Figure 15-6**)
  - When used, the size of the beam is greatly reduced and patient receives approximately 66% less radiation compared to round collimation.
  - The beam of radiation's diameter is approximately 1.5 × 2 inches at the skin.
  - The collimator is rotated to accommodate receptors positioned horizontally or vertically. A rectangular PID can be used or an external collimator can be added to the open end of a cylindrical PID.
- Lead-lined cylindrical or rectangular PID
  - The PID is an open-ended cylinder, or rectangle, lined with lead, to reduce secondary radiation.

C. Relation to Techniques

- Dimensions of a #2 size receptor range in size and can be up to approximately 1.3 × 1.7 inches.
- Precise angulation techniques are required to eliminate "cone-cut" of receptor, particularly when rectangular collimation is used.
- "Cone-cut" refers to an error of technique that results when the PID is not angled with the central ray centered on the receptor being exposed.

II. Filtration

Filtration is the insertion of filters for the preferential attenuation of radiation from a primary beam of x-radiation. Two different types of filters provide filtration in the dental x-ray machine.

A. Types of Filters

- *Aluminum filters* remove low-energy x-ray photons from the x-ray beam.

B. Purpose

- To minimize exposure of the patient to unnecessary radiation.

C. Methods

- *Inherent filtration*: Includes the glass envelope encasing the x-ray tube and the glass window in the tube housing (Figure 15-1).
- *Added filtration*: Thin, aluminum disks inserted between the lead diaphragm and the x-ray tube.
- *Total filtration*: The sum of inherent and added filtration. The recommended total is the equivalent of 0.5 mm (below 50 kVp), 1.5 mm (50–70 kVp), and 2.5 mm (above 70 kVp) of aluminum.

III. Kilovoltage Peak

Kilovoltage peak is the potential difference of force that moves electrons between the negative cathode and the positive anode inside an x-ray tube.

- When the kilovoltage peak is increased, the speed of electrons is increased. The resulting x-rays have a shorter wavelength and more penetrating power.

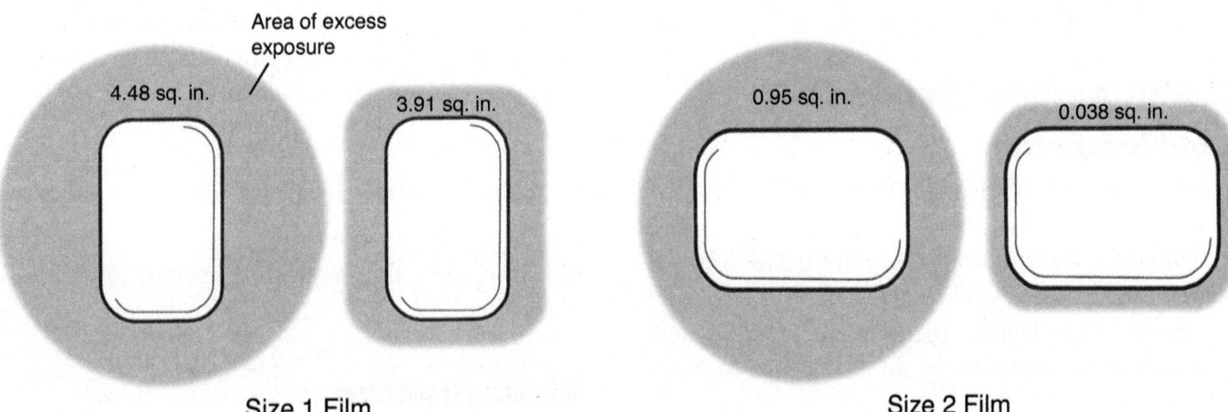

Figure 15-6 Cylindrical and Rectangular Position-Indicating Device. The useless areas of radiation seen around the edges of a receptor are greatly lessened when rectangular collimation is used, therefore sparing the patient from exposure to excessive radiation.

- kVp refers to the crest value (in kilovolts) of the potential difference of a pulsating generator. When only one-half of the wave is used, the value refers to the useful half of the cycle.

A. How kVp Affects the Image

- *Affects the contrast*
    - Low kilovoltage peak produces high contrast, with sharp black–white differences in densities between adjacent areas but a small range of distinction between subject thicknesses recorded.
    - High kilovoltage peak produces low contrast, with a wide range of subject thicknesses recorded; greater range of densities from black to white (more gray tones), which provide more interpretive details.
- *Affects the density*
    - Increased kilovoltage peak results in increased density (other factors remaining constant).
    - To maintain the same image density, the milliampere seconds is decreased as the kVp is increased.

B. Advantages of High kVp

- Permits shorter exposure time.
- Reduces exposure to tissues lying in front of the receptor.
- Facilitates the detection of bone changes.

C. Disadvantages of High kVp

- Increased radiation to tissues outside the edges of the receptor.
- More internal scattered radiation is seen at 90 kVp than at 70 kVp.

IV. Milliampere Seconds

A. Milliamperage

- The measure of the electron current passing through the x-ray tube.
- Milliamperage and time are combined to form the term milliampere seconds (mAs).
- Regulates the heat of the filament, which determines the number of electrons available to bombard the target.
- As the milliamperage is increased, the density of the image is increased.

B. Quantity of Radiation

- Quantity of radiation is expressed in milliampere seconds (mAs) or milliampere impulses (mAi).
- Definition: mAs is the milliamperes multiplied by the exposure time in seconds; mAi is the milliamperes multiplied by the exposure time in impulses.
- Example: At 10 mA for 1/2 second, the exposure of the image receptor is 5 mAs. At 10 mA for 15 impulses, the exposure of the image receptor is 150 mAi.

V. Distance

Several distances are involved in x-ray exposure. The object–receptor and the target–receptor distances are considered.

A. Object-Receptor Distance

- Refers to the distance between the object (tooth) and the receptor.
- With the paralleling technique and the use of a beam alignment device, the object–receptor distance is greater than it is for the bisecting-angle technique.
- Decreased object-receptor distance decreases image magnification.

B. Target-Receptor Distance

- The PID on the x-ray machine is designed to indicate the direction of the x-ray beam and to serve as a guide in establishing desired target–surface and target–receptor distances.
- The source is the tungsten target. The target–receptor distance is the sum total of the distance from the tungsten target to the receptor. Increased target-receptor distance decreases image magnification.

C. Advantages in the Use of a Long PID

- Decreased magnification.
- Decreased skin exposure owing to decreased scatter.

VI. Receptors

- **Receptors** refer to both traditional film and **digital sensors** used to capture a radiographic image.

- With optimum filtration, collimation, fast film, and digital sensors, the skin dose to the patient can be reduced significantly.
- Slow-speed films are no longer used in dentistry.
- Digital imaging requires a low exposure time.

A. Traditional Film Composition

A film is a thin, transparent sheet of cellulose acetate coated on both sides with an emulsion of gelatin and silver halide crystals.

- *Film base*: A flexible piece of polyester plastic that is used to provide support for the emulsion.
- *Halide crystals:* Silver bromide and silver iodide crystals are used in dental x-ray film. These crystals are sensitive to radiation and light.
- *Emulsion:* A coating of gelatinous and nongelatinous materials attached to both sides of the film base that keeps the silver halide crystals evenly dispersed in a suspension.
- *Adhesive layer:* A thin layer of adhesive material that covers both sides of the film base and keeps the emulsion on the film base.

B. Traditional Film Packet

A traditional film packet contains a sealed paper or plastic envelope that is lightproof and moisture resistant, containing an x-ray film (or two), black paper, and a thin sheet of lead foil.

- Two-film packet: Useful for sending to specialist to whom patient may be referred and for legal evidence.
- Black paper: To protect against light.
- Lead foil backing: To prevent exposure of the film by scattered radiation that could enter from back of packet and to protect the patient's tissues lying in the path of the x-ray beam.

C. Traditional Film Speed

- Film speed or film emulsion speed refers to the sensitivity of the film to radiation exposure.
- The speed is the amount of exposure required to produce a certain image density.
- The smaller the grain size, the slower the film speed and the less grainy the image.
- Classification: Films have been classified by the American National Standards Institute (ANSI) in cooperation with the American Dental Association (ADA).
- The ANSI/ADA Specification No. 22 designates six groups: A–F speed groups.
    - A, B, and C, the slowest, are associated with excess radiation exposure and are no longer used in dentistry.
    - D and E are slow speed films and not recommended.
    - F speed film is recommended for use with rectangular collimation for marked reduction in radiation exposure (if digital imaging is not available).

D. Digital Sensors

- In digital radiography, three types of receptors replace traditional film:
    - CCD.
    - CMOS.
    - PSP plates.
- CCD and CMOS detectors are known as "direct imaging sensors." When exposed to x-ray energy, an image appears on a computer monitor within seconds.
- PSP plates are known as "indirect imaging sensors." When irradiated, an image is stored on the plate until scanned by a laser. The scanner then transmits the image to the computer.
- CCD and CMOS sensors require radiation exposure times approximately 10–20% lower than "F"-speed film.
- PSP plate exposure times are similar to "F"-speed requirements.

Exposure to Radiation

I. Ionizing Radiation

Ionizing radiation is electromagnetic radiation (e.g., x-rays or **gamma** rays) or particulate radiation (e.g., electrons, neutrons, or protons) capable of ionizing air directly or indirectly.

- The phenomenon of separation of electrons from molecules to change chemical activity is called ionization.
- The organic and inorganic compounds that comprise the human body may be altered by exposure to ionizing radiation.
- The biologic effects following **irradiation** are secondary effects in that they result from physical, chemical, and biologic action set in motion by the absorption of energy from radiation.

- Factors that would influence the biologic effects of radiation are outlined in **Box 15-3**.
- Radiation to *somatic* tissues will affect only the irradiated individual, whereas radiation to *genetic* tissues will affect offspring and possibly future generations.

II. Exposure

A. Types of Exposure

Exposure is a measure of the x-radiation to which a person is exposed; this measure is based on its ability to produce ionization.

- Threshold exposure: The minimum exposure that produces a detectable degree of any given effect.
- Entrance or surface exposure: Exposure measured at the surface of an irradiated body, part, or object. It includes primary radiation and **backscatter** from the irradiated underlying tissue.
- Skin exposure: Exposure measured at the center of an irradiated skin surface area.
- Erythema exposure: The radiation necessary to produce a temporary redness of the skin.

B. Exposure Units

- The **absorbed dose** is expressed in joules/kilogram (1 rad = 0.01 J/kg).

Box 15-3 Factors That Influence the Biologic Effects of Radiation

- Quality of the radiation
- Chemical composition of the absorbing medium
- Sensitivity of tissues
- Total dose and dose rate
- Blood supply to the tissues
- Size of the area exposed
- Somatic versus genetic cells

- The units shown in **Table 15-2** are the recommendations of the International Commission on Radiation Units and Measurements.[8]
- The unit of measurement is the *gray* (Gy). An absorbed dose of 1 Gy is equal to 1 J/kg; therefore, an absorbed dose of 1 Gy is equal to 100 rad.
- The unit of biologic equivalence is the *Sievert* (Sv). 1 Sv = 100 rem.

C. Dose

- The radiation dose is the amount of energy absorbed per unit mass of tissue at a site of interest.
- A lethal dose is the amount of radiation that is or could be sufficient to cause death of an organism.

D. Permissible Dose

- The amount of radiation that may be received by an individual within a specified period without expectation of any significantly harmful result is called the permissible dose.
- Assumptions on which permissible doses are calculated include the following:
  - No irradiation is beneficial.
  - A level exists where the dose below which no somatic cellular changes can be produced.
  - Children are more susceptible than are older individuals.

E. Maximum Permissible Dose

- The maximum **dose equivalent** a person (or specified parts of that person) is allowed to receive in a stated period of time; the dose of radiation that would not be expected to produce any significant radiation effects in a lifetime.

F. Radiation Hazard

- A condition under which persons might receive radiation in excess of the maximum permissible dose is considered a hazard.

Table 15-2 Radiation Units

Definition	S.I. Unit[a]	Traditional Unit	Equivalent
Unit of radiation exposure	Coulomb per kilogram (C/kg)	Roentgen (R)	-2.58×10^{-4} C/kg = 1 R
Unit of absorbed dose	Gray (Gy)	Rad	1 Gy = 100 rad
Unit of dose equivalent	Sievert (Sv)	Rem	1 Sv = 100 rem
Unit of radioactivity	Becquerel (Bq)	Curie (Ci)	3.7×10^{10} Bq = 1 Ci

[a]S.I. (System International) is from the French Système International d'Unités.

- Exposure would be a risk in an area where x-ray equipment is being used or where radioactive materials are stored.

G. National Council on Radiation Protection and Measurements

- Maximum permissible dose limits exist for dentists and dental personnel (see **Table 15-3**).
- Limits for patients: Exposure to radiation shall be kept to the minimum level consistent with clinical requirements for accurate diagnosis based on patient need.[8]
- Radiation exposures are kept as low as reasonably achievable (ALARA). This concept is accepted and enforced by all regulatory agencies.

III. Sensitivity of Cells

A. Factors Affecting Cell Sensitivity to Radiation

- Cell differentiation: Immature cells are most sensitive.
- Mitotic activity: Rapidly reproducing cells are most sensitive when undergoing mitosis.
- Cell metabolism: Cells are more sensitive in periods of increased metabolism.

B. Radiosensitive and Radioresistant Tissues

- Radiosensitive: A cell that is sensitive to radiation.
- Radioresistant: A cell that is resistant to radiation.
- Radiation sensitivity of tissues and organs: The relative sensitivities are shown in **Box 15-4**.

C. Tissue Reaction

- Latent period
  - Lapse between the time of exposure and the time when effects are observed. (May be as long as 25 years or relatively shorter, as in the case of the production of a skin erythema.)
- Cumulative effect
  - Amount of reaction depends on dose; the reaction to radiation received in fractional doses is less than the reaction to one large dose.
  - Partial or total repair occurs as long as destruction is not complete.

Box 15-4 Radiation Sensitivity of Tissues and Organs

High Sensitivity
- Bone marrow
- Reproductive cells
- Intestines
- Lymphoid tissue

Moderately High
- Oral mucosa
- Skin

Moderate
- Growing bone
- Growing cartilage
- Small vasculature
- Connective tissue

Moderately Low
- Salivary glands
- Mature bone
- Mature cartilage
- Thyroid gland tissue

Low Sensitivity
- Liver
- Optic lens
- Kidneys
- Muscle
- Nerve

Table 15-3 Maximum Permissible Dose Equivalent Values[a] to Whole Body, Gonads, Blood-Forming Organs, Lens of Eye

Average Weekly Exposure[b]	Maximum 13-Wk Exposure	Maximum Yearly Exposure	Maximum Accumulated Exposure[c]
0.001 Sv	0.03 Sv	0.05 Sv	0.05 (*N* – 18) Sv
0.1 R	3 R	5 R	5 (*N* – 18) R[d]

[a]Exposure of persons for dental or medical purposes is not counted against their maximum permissible exposure limits.
[b]Used only for the purpose of designating radiation barriers.
[c]When the previous occupational history of an individual is not definitely known, it shall be assumed that the full dose permitted by the formula 5 (*N* – 18) has already been received.
[d]*N* = Age in years and is greater than 18. The unit for exposure is the roentgen (R) or Sievert (Sv).

- Some irreparable damage may be cumulative as more radiation is added (e.g., hair loss, skin lesions, falling blood cell count).

Risk of Injury from Radiation

- The risk of injury from dental diagnostic radiation is extremely low; however, the more radiation received, the higher the chance of cellular injuries.
- With each exposure to radiation, cellular damage is followed by repair.
- The effects of radiation exposure are cumulative, and any cellular changes not repaired result in damaged tissues.
- Most of the damage caused by dental diagnostic low-level radiation is repaired within the body cells.

I. Rules for Radiation Protection

- *Dental x-ray protection*, prepared by the National Council on Radiation Protection and Measurements,[9] provides specific information about radiation barriers, film speed group rating, personal monitoring service sources, x-ray equipment data, and operating procedure regulations.
- To protect the clinician and patient from excessive radiation, attention is paid to unnecessary radiation that may result from retakes due to inadequate clinical procedures.
- Perfecting techniques contribute to the accomplishment of minimum exposure for maximum safety.

II. Protection of Clinician

A. Protection from Primary Radiation

- Stand behind a protective barrier.
- Avoid the useful beam of radiation.
- Never hold the receptor during exposure of the patient.

B. Protection from Leakage Radiation

- Do not hold the tube housing or the PID of the machine during exposure.
- Test machine for leakage radiation.
- Wear monitoring device for testing exposure.

C. Protection from Secondary Radiation

The major sources of secondary radiation are the irradiated soft tissues of the patient. Other sources may be the leakage from the tube housing or scatter from furniture and walls contacted by the primary beam. Methods of protection are related to these sources.

Minimization of Total X-Radiation

- Use digital sensors or "F" speed film.
- Test x-ray machines periodically for radiation output and leakage.
- Replace older x-ray machines with modern equipment.

Collimation of Useful Beam

- Use diaphragms and long PIDs to collimate the useful beam to an area no larger than 2.75 inches or 7 cm in diameter at the patient. Rectangular collimation is shown to be more effective than round collimation (Figure 15-6).

Type of PID

- Use a shielded cylinder that is rectangular, long, and open ended, or use some other form of rectangular collimation.

Position of Clinician While Making Exposures

- The correct position for the clinician is behind an appropriate radiation-resistant barrier wall, preferably with a leaded window to permit a view of the patient during exposures.
- When protective barrier shielding is not available, the clinician shall stand as far as practical from the patient, at least 6 feet (2 m) in the zone between 90° and 135° to the primary central ray, as shown in **Figure 15-7**.
- Safety increases with distance.

D. Monitoring

The amount of x-radiation that reaches dental personnel can be measured economically with a personal monitoring badge. Badges can be obtained from one of several laboratories. The monitoring badge is:

- Used to measure exposure of the wearer.
- Worn at waist level for a specific period of time.
- Returned on a routine basis to the laboratory by mail and processed; its exposure is evaluated.
- Wearer is notified of the exposure totals.

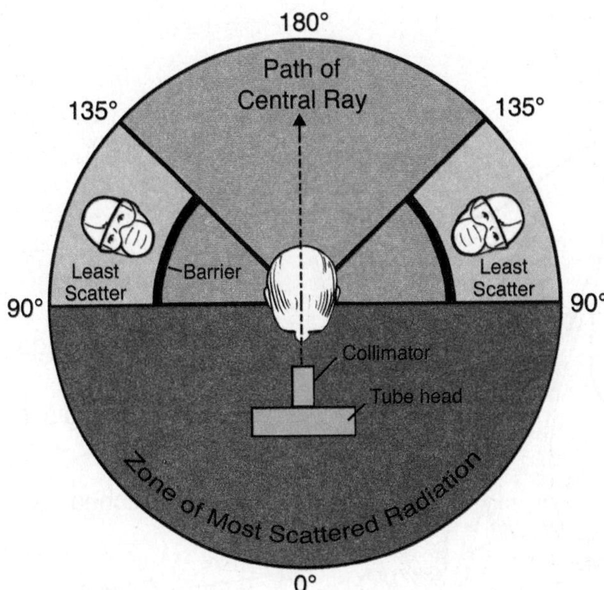

Figure 15-7 Safe Position for Clinician. While making an exposure, the clinician stands between 90° and 135° from the primary beam.

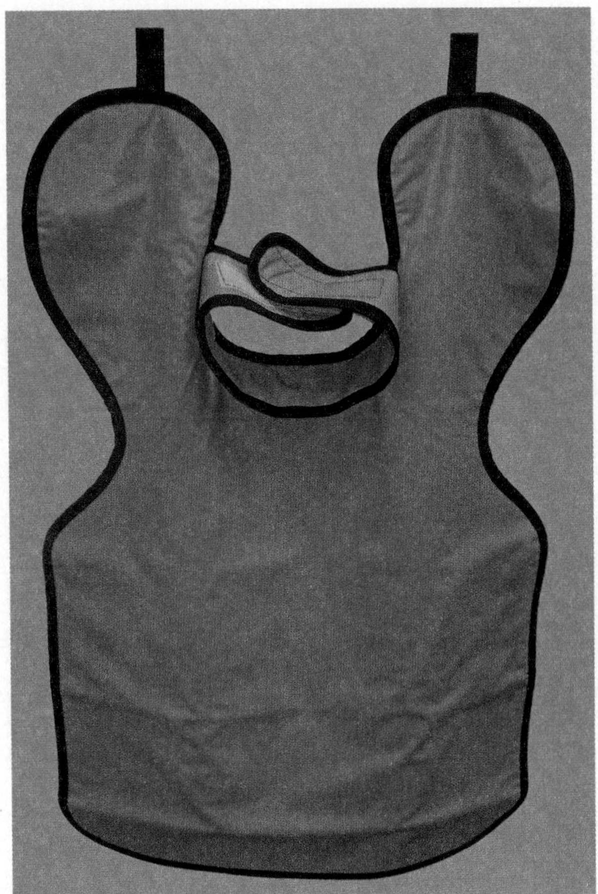

Figure 15-8 Care of Leaded Apron. The apron can be kept on a hanging device near the x-ray machine to prevent cracks and prolong the usefulness of the apron. The thyroid collar may be attached on a separate shield.

III. Protection of Patient

A. Receptors

- Use high-speed receptors.
- Use the largest intraoral receptor that can be placed skillfully in the mouth. Maximum coverage is provided in this manner with one exposure (instead of multiple).

B. Collimation

- Use diaphragms and an open-ended, shielded (lead lined), rectangular PID to collimate the useful beam.

C. Filtration

- Use filtration of the useful beam to recommended levels.

D. Processing

- Process traditional films according to the manufacturer's directions with adherence to quality assurance guidelines.

E. Total Exposure

- Do not expose the patient unnecessarily. Determine a valid reason for each exposure.

F. Patient Body Shields

- The use of leaded or lead-free alloy body shields and thyroid collars for each patient is required by law in many states and countries. The purpose of the shield is to absorb scattered rays. An acceptable lead shield contains a minimum of 0.25 mm of lead thickness.

Protective Apron

- *Types*
  - General body coverage with extensions over the shoulders and down over the gonadal area.
  - Body coverage, with cervical thyroid collar attached.
  - Body coverage, with added coverage for the back for wear during panoramic radiography.
- *Care*
  - Prevent cracks in leaded shields by hanging when not in use (**Figure 15-8**).
  - Disinfect the apron and collar before and after each use.

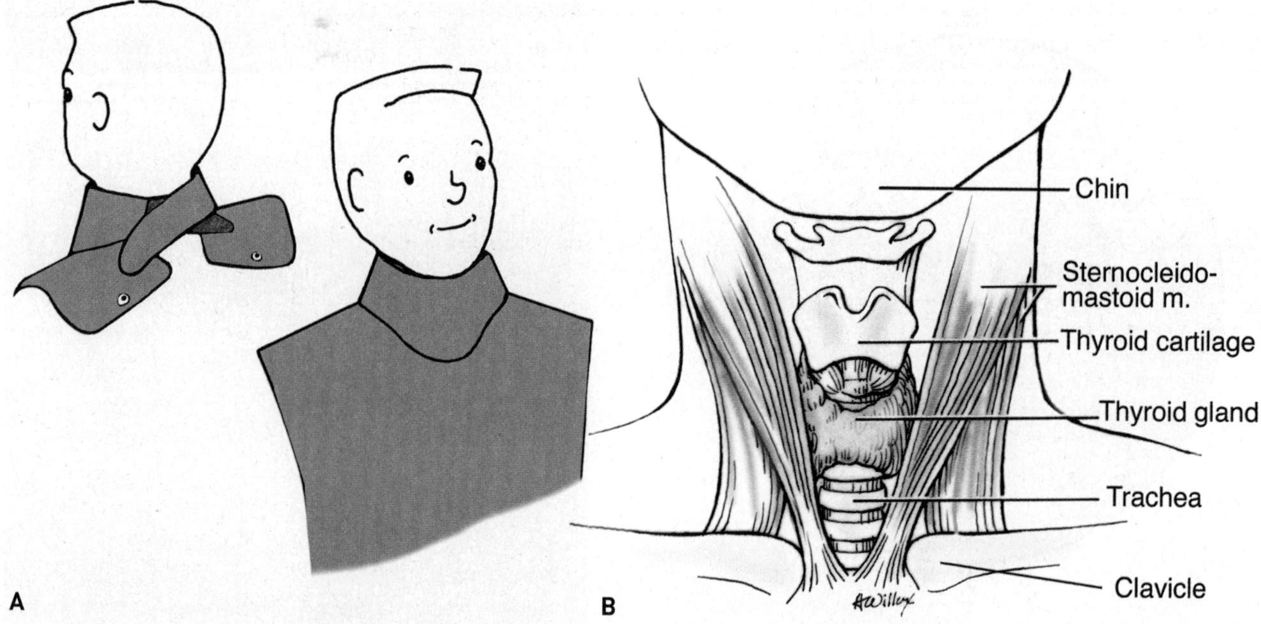

Figure 15-9 Thyroid Cervical Collar. **A:** Thyroid collar in position, covering the neck and overlapping the leaded apron used for general body coverage. Velcro tabs facilitate overlap fastening at back of neck. Collars are available in child and adult sizes. **B:** The thyroid gland is located over the trachea approximately halfway between the chin and the clavicles. The illustration shows the anatomic relationship to the sternocleidomastoid muscle.

Thyroid Cervical Collar

- Thyroid cancer can result from long-term exposure of the gland to x-rays.[10,11]
- The thyroid gland should be completely covered during exposure to x-radiation. **Figure 15-9** shows the position of a thyroid collar over the neckline of a body apron.

IV. Assessment

- An assessment regarding the need for radiographic exposure must be made for each patient based on:
  - Review of health history.
  - Preparation or review of radiation exposure history.
  - Review of medical diagnostic or therapeutic radiation.
  - Review of dates of dental surveys and availability of previous radiographs.
  - Review of clinical examination.
  - Assessment of Caries Management by Risk Assessment (CAMBRA) score.
- After assessment, consult with dentist, and obtain dentist's prescription for number and type of images needed. The ALARA concept should guide practice principles as radiation is damaging and cumulative and is to be kept to the minimum necessary to meet diagnostic requirements. Refer to the *Guidelines for Prescribing Dental Radiographs* in **Table 15-4** and **Table 15-5**.

V. Risk Reduction

A. Preparation of Clinic Facility: Infection Control Routine

- Standard infection control procedures are followed for all radiographic equipment and materials.
- Use single-use plastic barriers for all surfaces to be contacted, including x-ray machine controls.
- Use disposable materials wherever possible.
- The N95 face mask may be necessary depending on the community spread of respiratory disease.
- Wear gloves or overgloves when handling of all radiographic materials.

B. Preparation of Clinician

- Use full barrier protection that includes a cover-up gown, a mask, protective eyewear, and gloves.
- Apply standard precautions throughout the radiographic procedure.

C. Preparation of Patient

- Provide cup for holding removable dental prostheses.
- For panoramic radiographs, request patient remove oral and/or facial piercings and all other jewelry or metallic objects worn above the shoulders.
- Provide antiseptic mouth rinse to lower bacterial contamination of receptors and aerosols.

Table 15-4 Recommendations for Prescribing Dental Radiographs

	Patient Age and Dental Developmental Stage				
Type of Encounter	**Child with Primary Dentition (prior to eruption of first permanent tooth)**	**Child with Transitional Dentition (after eruption of first permanent tooth)**	**Adolescent with Permanent Dentition (prior to eruption of third molars)**	**Adult, Dentate or Partially Edentulous**	**Adult, Edentulous**
New patient being evaluated for oral diseases	Individualized radiographic examination consisting of selected periapical/occlusal views and/or posterior bitewings if proximal surfaces cannot be visualized or probed. Patients without evidence of disease and with open proximal contacts may not require a radiographic examination at this time	Individualized radiographic examination consisting of posterior bitewings with panoramic examination or posterior bitewings and selected periapical images	Individualized radiographic examination consisting of posterior bitewings with panoramic examination or posterior bitewings and selected periapical images. A full mouth intraoral radiographic examination is preferred when the patient has clinical evidence of generalized oral disease or a history of extensive dental treatment		Individualized radiographic examination, based on clinical signs and symptoms
Recall patient with clinical caries or at increased risk for caries[a]	Posterior bitewing examination at 6- to 12-mo intervals if proximal surfaces cannot be examined visually or with a probe			Posterior bitewing examination at 6- to 18-mo intervals	Not applicable
Recall patient with no clinical caries and not at increased risk for caries[a]	Posterior bitewing examination at 12- to 24-mo intervals if proximal surfaces cannot be examined visually or with a probe		Posterior bitewing examination at 18- to 36-mo intervals	Posterior bitewing examination at 24- to 36-mo intervals	Not applicable
Recall patient with periodontal disease	Clinical judgment as to the need for and type of radiographic images for the evaluation of periodontal disease. Imaging may consist of, but is not limited to, selected bitewing and/or periapical images of areas where periodontal disease (other than nonspecific gingivitis) can be demonstrated clinically				Not applicable
Patient (new and recall) for monitoring of dentofacial growth and development and/or assessment of dental/skeletal relationships	Clinical judgment as to need for and type of radiographic images for evaluation and/or monitoring of dentofacial growth and development or assessment of dental and skeletal relationships	Clinical judgment as to need for and type of radiographic images for evaluation and/or monitoring of dentofacial growth and development, or assessment of dental and skeletal relationships. Panoramic or periapical examination to assess developing third molars		Usually not indicated for monitoring of growth and development. Clinical judgment as to the need for and type of radiographic image for evaluation of dental and skeletal relationships	

(continues)

Table 15-4 Recommendations for Prescribing Dental Radiographs *(continued)*

	Patient Age and Dental Developmental Stage				
Type of Encounter	**Child with Primary Dentition (prior to eruption of first permanent tooth)**	**Child with Transitional Dentition (after eruption of first permanent tooth)**	**Adolescent with Permanent Dentition (prior to eruption of third molars)**	**Adult, Dentate or Partially Edentulous**	**Adult, Edentulous**
Patient with other circumstances including, but not limited to, proposed or existing implants, other dental and craniofacial pathoses, restorative/endodontic needs, treated periodontal disease, and caries remineralization	Clinical judgment as to need for and type of radiographic images for evaluation and/or monitoring of these conditions				

These recommendations are subject to clinical judgment and may not apply to every patient. The recommendations are to be used by dentists only after reviewing the patient's health history and completing a clinical examination. Even though radiation exposure from dental imaging is low, once a decision to obtain images is made, it is the dentist's responsibility to follow the ALARA principle to minimize patient exposure.
[a]Factors increasing risk for caries may be assessed using the ADA Caries Risk Assessment forms (0–6 years of age and over 6 years of age).
ADA, American Dental Association; ALARA, as low as reasonably achievable
American Dental Association Council on Scientific Affairs, U.S. Department of Health and Human Services, U.S. Food and Drug Administration. Dental radiographic examinations: recommendations for patient selection and limiting radiation exposure. http://www.fda.gov/Radiation-mittingProducts/RadiationEmittingProductsandProcedures/MedicalImaging/MedicalX-Rays/ucm116504.htm. Accessed March 12, 2022.

Table 15-5 Clinical Situations for Which Radiographs May Be Indicated

A. Positive Historical Findings	B. Positive Clinical Signs/Symptoms
1. Previous periodontal or endodontic treatment 2. History of pain or trauma 3. Familial history of dental anomalies 4. Postoperative evaluation of healing 5. Remineralization monitoring 6. Presence of implants, previous implant-related pathosis, or evaluation for implant placement	1. Clinical evidence of periodontal disease 2. Large or deep restorations 3. Deep carious lesions 4. Malposed or clinically impacted teeth 5. Swelling 6. Evidence of dental/facial trauma 7. Mobility of teeth 8. Sinus tract ("fistula") 9. Clinically suspected sinus pathosis 10. Growth abnormalities 11. Oral involvement in known or suspected systemic disease 12. Positive neurologic findings in the head and neck 13. Evidence of foreign objects 14. Pain and/or dysfunction of the temporomandibular joint 15. Facial asymmetry 16. Abutment teeth for fixed or removable partial prosthesis 17. Unexplained bleeding 18. Unexplained sensitivity of teeth 19. Unusual eruption, spacing, or migration of teeth 20. Unusual tooth morphology, calcification, or color 21. Unexplained absence of teeth 22. Clinical tooth erosion 23. Peri-implantitis

This list is not comprehensive.
American Dental Association Council on Scientific Affairs, U.S. Department of Health and Human Services, U.S. Food and Drug Administration. Dental radiographic examinations: recommendations for patient selection and limiting radiation exposure. http://www.fda.gov/Radiation-mittingProducts/RadiationEmittingProductsandProcedures/MedicalImaging/MedicalX-Rays/ucm116504.htm. Accessed March 12, 2022.

D. Intraoral Examination

- To determine necessary adaptations during receptor placement, there are several factors to consider. These include:
  - Accessibility, determined by height and shape of palate, flexibility of muscles of orifice, floor of the mouth, possible gag reflex, and size of tongue.
  - Position of teeth and edentulous areas.
  - Apparent size of teeth.
  - Unusual features, such as tori, crooked teeth or sensitive areas of the mucous membranes.

E. Patient Cooperation: Prevention of Gagging

- Gagging may be the result of psychological or physiologic factors.
- May present some problem in the placement of all receptors for molar imaging.
- May be initiated in the patient who ordinarily does not gag when techniques are done efficiently.

Causes of Gagging

- Hypersensitive oral tissues: Particularly common in posterior region of oral cavity.
- Techniques: Receptor moved over the oral tissues or retained in the mouth longer than is necessary.
- *Anxiety and apprehension:*
  - Fear of unknown and of the receptor touching a sensitive area.
  - Previous unpleasant experiences with radiographic techniques.
  - Failure to comprehend the clinician's instructions.
  - Lack of confidence in the clinician.

Preventive Procedures

- Inspire confidence in ability to perform the service.
- Alleviate anxiety; explain procedures carefully. Smile and display a positive attitude.
- Minimize tissue irritation.
  - Ask patient to swallow before each receptor placement.
  - Expose anterior receptors before posterior as placement is easier to tolerate.
  - Place receptor firmly and positively without sliding it over the tissue, especially the palate.
  - Rub a finger over the tissues where the receptor placement is intended to be, to help to desensitize the tissues.
  - Instruct patient to breathe through nose with quick breaths; do not suggest the patient hold their breath.
  - Use stick-on receptor cushions to make placement more comfortable.
- Use a premedicating agent prescribed by the dentist.
- Use a topical anesthetic.

Procedures for Receptor Placement and Angulation of Central Ray

- The image projected onto the receptor is a shadow of the teeth and the surrounding structures. The five principles of shadow casting should be followed during exposures, listed in **Box 15-5**.
- Two fundamental procedures are used in the production of diagnostic periapical images: the *paralleling technique* and the *bisecting angle technique*. The principles for receptor placement are shown in **Figure 15-10**.

Box 15-5 Principles of Shadow Casting

1. Place the receptor as parallel as possible to the tooth being imaged.
2. Use as small an effective focal spot as practical (dependent upon machine manufacturer).
3. Use as long a target–receptor distance as possible.
4. Use as short a object–receptor distance as possible.
5. Aim the x-ray beam perpendicular to the receptor.

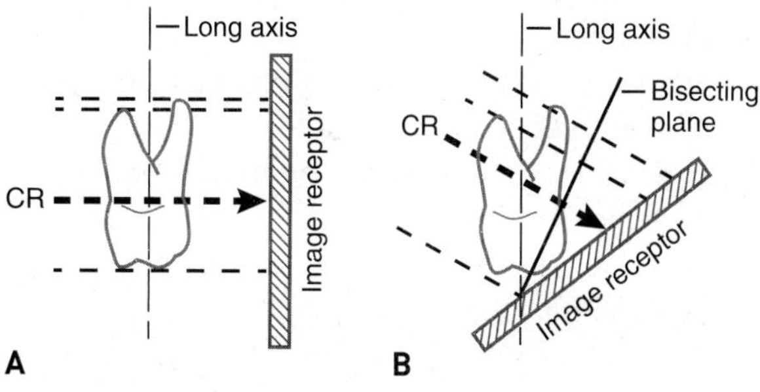

Figure 15-10 Comparison of Paralleling and Bisecting-Angle Techniques. **A:** Paralleling technique. The receptor is parallel with the long axis of the tooth and the central ray (CR) is directed perpendicular to the receptor and to the long axis of the tooth. **B:** Bisecting-angle technique. The CR is directed perpendicular to an imaginary line that bisects the angle formed by the receptor and the long axis of the tooth.

- Clinicians vary in their application of the principles of the two techniques. Basic to both the paralleling technique and the bisecting-angle technique are:
  - The primary beam passes through the teeth of interest.
  - The receptor is placed in relation to the teeth so that all parts of the region of interest are shown as close to their natural size as possible.
  - Dimensional distortion and magnification are minimized.
  - The development of a systematic, comfortable, smooth procedure saves time and energy for both patient and clinician, and the clinician is able to:
    - Increase the confidence of the patient.
    - Allow for consistency in technique.
    - Produce good-quality images.
    - Minimize the length of time the receptor remains in the patient's mouth.

Receptor Selection for Intraoral Surveys

I. Periapical Surveys

A. Area Covered

- To obtain a view of the entire tooth and its periodontal supporting structures.

B. Traditional Film Sizes

- *Child size:* No. 0 (22 × 35 mm) used for primary teeth and small mouths.
- *Anterior:* No. 1 (24 × 40 mm) used for anterior regions of adults where width of arch makes positioning of standard receptor difficult or impossible.
- *Standard:* No. 2 (31 × 41 mm) may be used for all placements.
- *Long bitewing:* No. 3 (27 × 54 mm) is not used for periapical imaging.
- *Occlusal:* No. 4 (3 x 2.25 inches) is used for occlusal imaging.

C. Digital Sensor Sizes

- No. 0 used for primary teeth and small mouths.
- No. 1 used for anterior regions of adults where width of arch makes positioning of standard receptor difficult or impossible.
- No. 2 may be used for all placements.
- No. 3 may be used to view all posterior teeth on one side of the arch; bitewing image only.

D. Number of Receptors Used in a Complete Survey

- Twelve to 18 images may compose a complete mouth survey. This is dependent upon:
  - The dentist's preferences.
  - The anatomy of the patient's mouth.
  - The size of the receptors used.

II. Bitewing (Interproximal) Surveys

A. Area Covered

- Horizontal bitewing radiographic images are exposed to view:
  - The crowns of the teeth and the alveolar crest in a dentition with normal to slight bone loss.
  - Proximal surface caries.
  - Overhanging restorations.
- Vertical bitewing radiographic images are exposed to view:
  - The crowns of the teeth and the alveolar bone level with moderate-to-severe bone loss.
  - Proximal surface caries.
  - Overhanging restorations.

B. Image Receptors

- Sizes of image receptors are shown in Figure 15-3 and Figure 15-4.
- The number and size of receptors used for bitewing surveys are determined by:
  - The size of the dental arch.
  - The number of teeth present.
  - Patient tolerance. Use largest size sensor the patient will tolerate.

III. Occlusal Surveys

A. Purpose

- To view large areas of the maxilla, mandible, or floor of the mouth.

B. Receptors

- No. 4 for use in self-contained packet or in intraoral **cassette**.
- No. 2 for child or individual areas of adult.

Periapical Survey: Paralleling Technique

The paralleling technique is based on the principles that the receptor is placed parallel to the long axis of the tooth, and the central ray is directed at a right angle to the receptor. Figure 15-10A shows the parallel relationship of the receptor with the long axis of the tooth and the right-angle direction of the central ray.

- Maxillary projections: The receptor is placed toward the midline of the palate.
- Mandibular projections: The image receptor is placed close to the teeth of interest to maintain parallelism.
- Premolar projections: The receptor is placed toward the midline, as far forward as possible to capture the distal surface of the canine.[12]

I. Patient Position

- The patient should be positioned in the dental chair with their head supported by the head rest to not only support the head, but stabilize the patient and discourage movement.
- The occlusal plane should be parallel to the floor, and the midsagittal plane perpendicular to the floor.

II. Receptor Placement and Central Ray Angulation

A. Receptor Position and Angulation of the Central Ray

The receptor is centered over the teeth to be examined.

- *Horizontal angulation* is the angle at which the central ray of the beam is directed within a horizontal plane. The central ray is directed at the center of the receptor and through the interproximal area in order to eliminate overlapping or superimposition of parts of the adjacent teeth in the image.
- *Vertical angulation* is the plane at which the central ray of the useful beam is directed within a vertical plane. Not enough vertical angulation causes elongation of the image, and too much vertical angulation causes the structures to be foreshortened.

B. Receptor Positioning Holders

- The use of a receptor holder (beam alignment device) facilitates obtaining the correct angulation of the central ray.
- Lining up the PID the guides of the beam alignment device will set the correct vertical and horizontal angulation, allowing the central ray to be perpendicular to the receptor.
- *Purposes:* The use of a beam alignment device provides:
  - Dose reduction.
  - Improved image quality.
  - Diagnostic images without frequent retakes.
  - Improved infection control.
- *Characteristics:* An effective beam alignment device has characteristics such as the following:
  - Simple and adaptable to all intraoral placements.
  - Aids in reducing radiation exposure to patient.
  - Aids in alignment of x-ray beam.
  - Comfortable for the patient.
  - Minimal complexity for learning.
  - Disposable or conveniently sterilized.
- Types of beam alignment devices
  - Several types of common beam alignment devices are listed in **Box 15-6**.
- Examples of widely used types include the following:
  - Rinn X-C-P film and sensor holders. A plastic and stainless steel beam alignment device is used with the paralleling technique.
  - Bite blocks vary depending on the receptor selected.
  - Styrofoam disposable bite block for use with a traditional film or digital PSP plate when utilizing the paralleling or bisecting-angle techniques (**Figure 15-11**).

III. Paralleling Technique Basics

A. Accuracy

- The paralleling technique gives a more accurate size and shape of dental structures with less distortion and superimposition of other anatomic structures when compared to the bisecting-angle technique.

Box 15-6 Beam Alignment Devices

Bite blocks, plastic or foam
Stabe (Styrofoam disposable film/photostimulable phosphor plate holder)
Snap-a-ray
X-C-P (extension cone paralleling)
B-A-I (bisecting-angle instrument)
V.I.P. (versatile intraoral positioner)
Hemostat with rubber bite block

Supplements

Removable denture may be left in place when imaging the opposite arch; the denture may help to stabilize the receptor.
Cotton rolls may stabilize edentulous areas to achieve parallelism.

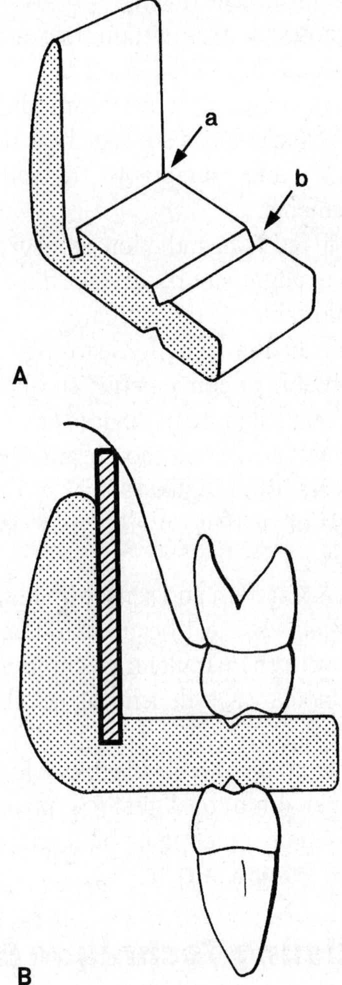

Figure 15-11 Styrofoam Disposable Bite Block. **A:** Empty bite block to show: a, slot for insertion of the receptor, and b, break-off point to shorten the bite surface for use in the mandibular posterior positions. **B:** Receptor placement for maxillary molar projection for patient with a high palatal vault.

B. Horizontal Ray Direction

- No x-radiation is directed toward the thyroid gland, whereas with the bisecting-angle technique, several maxillary radiographs require a relatively steep vertical angulation. The thyroid protective collar is recommended.

Bitewing Survey

Figure 15-12 shows in diagram form:

- The position of the horizontal molar bitewing receptor in relation to the teeth.
- The correct horizontal and vertical angulation.
- An example of a premolar and molar bitewing image.

I. Patient Position

A. Patient Position

- Patient in upright position:
  - Midsagittal plane is perpendicular to the floor.
  - Occlusal plane is parallel with the floor.

B. Vertical Angulation of Central Ray

- Set at +10° for horizontal or vertical bitewing projection (Figure 15-12B) if using a bitewing tab.

C. Horizontal Angulation of Central Ray

- The horizontal angulation is adjusted to direct the central ray perpendicular to the center of the receptor.

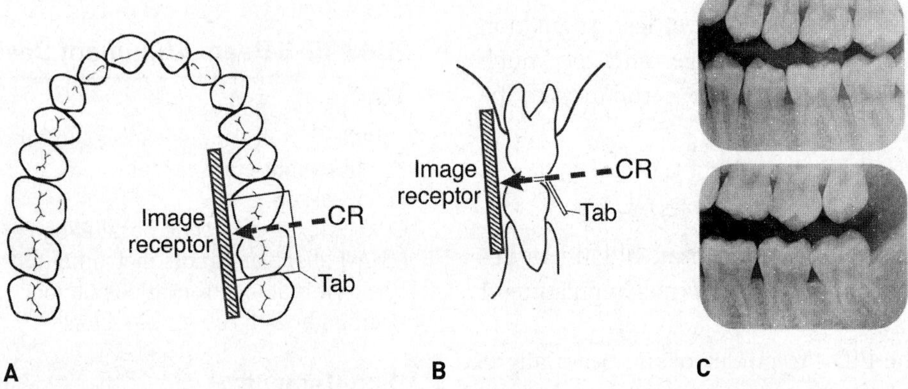

Figure 15-12 Horizontal Bitewing Radiograph. **A:** Receptor position showing horizontal angulation for molar projection, with central ray (CR) directed through the interproximal space to the center of the receptor. Receptor is centered over the second molar. **B:** Vertical angulation set at +10° if using a bitewing tab. **C:** Example bitewing images for premolar placement (above) and molar placement (below).

- The central ray passes through the interproximal space or parallel to a line through the interproximal spaces of the teeth of interest (Figure 15-12A).

II. Receptor Placement: Horizontal Bitewing Survey

- Molar
  - Standard receptor in horizontal position.
  - Center the receptor on the second molar (see Figure 15-12).
- Premolar
  - Standard receptor in horizontal position.
  - Center the receptor over the second premolar to include the distal surfaces of maxillary and mandibular canines.

III. Receptor Placement: Vertical Bitewing Survey

- Molar
  - Standard receptor in vertical position.
  - Center the receptor on the second molar (see **Figure 15-13**).
- Premolar
  - Standard receptor in vertical position.
  - Center the receptor over the second premolar to include the distal surfaces of the maxillary and mandibular canines.
- Anterior
  - Although not often used, vertical bitewing images may be exposed in the anterior region of the mouth to reveal interproximal levels of bone between the incisors and canines.
  - Center receptor at proximal space between the lateral incisor and canine.

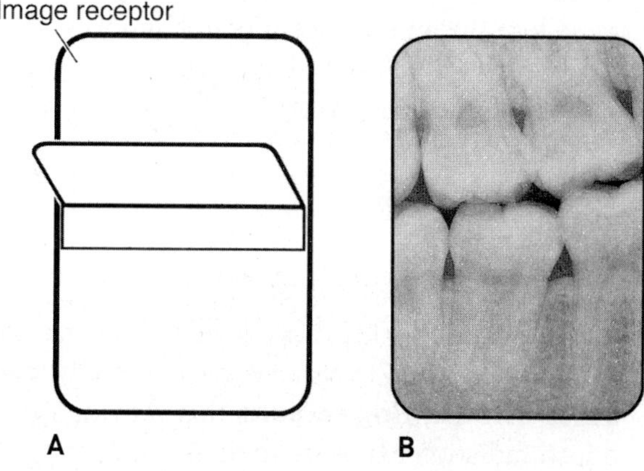

Figure 15-13 Vertical Bitewing Image. **A:** Vertical bitewing receptor with the tab positioned over the center of the receptor. **B:** Image of maxillary and mandibular molar regions. Receptor is placed centered over the mandibular second molar.

  - Center receptor at midline of the arch for the central bitewing image.

Periapical Survey: Bisecting-Angle Technique

The bisecting-angle technique is based on the geometric principle that the central ray is directed perpendicular to an imaginary line that bisects the angle formed by the long axis of the tooth and the plane of the receptor.

- Figure 15-10B illustrates the relationship of the long axis of the tooth, the receptor, and the bisected angle formed by these two planes.
- Types of receptor holders:
  - *Rinn snap-a-ray:* A rigid plastic receptor holder without a backing plate to prevent bending, used in both posterior and anterior regions. Useful in patients who cannot tolerate the receptor backing devices of a bite block.
  - *Rinn B-A-I film and sensor holders:* A plastic and stainless steel receptor holder with an aiming device used with the bisecting-angle technique.
  - *Styrofoam disposable holder:* A disposable bite block used with the bisecting-angle or paralleling technique.

Occlusal Survey

The occlusal technique is used to examine larger areas of the jaws and is a supplemental technique usually used in conjunction with the periapical and/or bitewing image.

I. Purpose of the Occlusal Technique

- To observe areas not shown on intraoral projections.
- To locate the extent and size of larger lesions.
- To supplement the angulation provided by other image receptors for such conditions as fractures, impacted teeth, or salivary duct calculi.

II. Maxillary Midline Topographic Projection

A. Position of Patient Head

- The line from the tragus of the ear to the ala of the nose is parallel with the floor.

B. Position of Receptor

- The exposure side of the receptor is toward the palate.
- Posterior border of receptor is brought back as close to the third molar region as possible. Receptor is held between the teeth with a soft edge-to-edge closure.

C. Angulation

- The PID is directed toward the bridge of the nose at a +65° angle.

III. Mandibular Topographic and Cross-Sectional Projection

A. Position of Patient's Head

- The head is tilted directly back at approximately –55 degrees. For the cross-sectional projection, the central ray is directed perpendicular to the receptor (90 degrees).

B. Position of Image Receptor

- The exposure side of the receptor is toward the floor of the mouth.
- The posterior border of the receptor is in contact with the soft tissues of the retromolar area.
- The receptor is held between the teeth with a soft edge-to-edge bite.

C. Angulation

- Topographical: Point PID at chin for incisal region: −55° angle.
- Cross-sectional: Direct PID under the chin for the floor of the mouth, perpendicular to the receptor.

Panoramic Images

- Panoramic imaging is an extraoral technique that produces an image with a wide view of the structures of the oral cavity on a single image.
- The panoramic image demonstrates a loss of sharpness and detail and should not be compared to the diagnostic information found on periapical images. The principal advantages of panoramic images are:
  - Broad coverage of facial bones and teeth.
  - Low patient radiation dose.
  - Convenience of the examination for the patient.
  - Short time required for exposure of a panoramic image.
  - Useful for patients who cannot open their mouths very wide.
  - Useful patient education tool.

I. Technique Basics

A panoramic image is an extraoral radiographic projection used to examine the maxillary and mandibular jaws on a single image.

- The movement of the receptor and tube head produces an image through the process known as tomography.
- The prefix *tomo* means section; tomography is a radiographic technique that depicts one layer or section of the body in focus while surrounding structures in other planes are blurred.
- In a panoramic tomograph, the attempt is to image the maxillary and mandibular arches in focus on one receptor.
- The receptor and tube head rotate around the patient's head in opposite directions.
- The focal trough refers to the area where structures are most clearly in focus during the exposure.

A. Patient Position

- Patient positioning depends on the manufacturer's instruction of the panoramic unit and the height of the patient, whether seated or standing.
  - Stabilize the head with a chin support or one of several types of head positioner characteristic of each machine.
  - Position the patient to ensure that the Frankfort plane (floor of the orbit and the external auditory meatus) is parallel to the floor and the midsagittal plane is perpendicular to the floor.
  - Close the anterior teeth on the grooves of the bite block to ensure that the arches are placed within the focal trough.

B. Cassette

- Curved or flat.
- Rigid or flexible.
- Marked to denote left or right side of the patient.
- Contains calcium tungstate or preferably **rare earth intensifying screens** that provide for reduced radiation exposure to the patient.

II. Uses of Panoramic Imaging

- The numerous applications for panoramic images are outlined in **Box 15-7**.

Box 15-7 Uses for Panoramic Images

- Detection and diagnosis of oral pathologic lesions
- Evaluation of impacted teeth
- Examination of the extent of large lesions
- Survey for edentulous patients
- Detection of calcified carotid arteries: Potential stroke victims
- Evaluation of growth and development for pedodontic patients
- Evaluation of teeth and jaw position for orthodontic patients
- Detection of fractured jaws and traumatic injuries
- When intraoral projections are impossible, such as patients with the following conditions:
  - Trismus
  - Parkinson's disease
  - Cerebral palsy
  - Hyperactive gag reflex

- Not for routine use for patients seeking general oral care. Panoramic imaging should not be used as a substitute for a periapical survey due to magnification and overlap of anatomy.

III. Limitations

- Loss of definition and detail compared with periapical images.
- Distortion of structures and findings.
- Inadequate for examination of detailed periodontal structures and interproximal dental caries.

A. *Inferiority of Definition and Detail*

Causes of poor definition include:

- Use of intensifying screens.
- Increased object–receptor distance.
- Movement of x-ray tube and receptor.

B. *Distortion*

- Magnified images are produced because of increased distance between the receptor and object.
- Overlapping
- With the panoramic technique, the head and teeth remain in a fixed position. The angulation of the x-ray beam and position of the receptor are manufactured for the "average" size of patient. Altered positions may be required for children or large individuals.

IV. Procedures

Learning to use panoramic equipment is usually straightforward and uncomplicated. Each machine has its own step-by-step directions that can be learned readily from the manufacturer's instructions.

A. *Patient Preparation*

- Thyroid shield
  - Cannot be used because it blocks the x-ray beam.
  - A special leaded shield for panoramic imaging is available with coverage over the shoulders and down the back.

B. *Receptor*

- Receptor sizes are typically either 5 × 12 or 6 × 12 inches. Fast-speed film or digital sensors are recommended to minimize radiation exposure to the patient.

C. *Processing*

- Regular processing solutions for intraoral films are used for traditional panoramic film.

Infection Control

I. Practice Policy

- Personnel of each office or clinic can determine a specific protocol appropriate to their facility and the type of processing used.
- A written policy is necessary for infection control during receptor exposure, processing, and mounting and during management of the completed images throughout clinical treatment appointments.[13]

II. Basic Procedures

Basic procedures are followed to prevent cross-contamination during transport to the digital laser scanner or darkroom and during use of manual and automatic processing equipment.[13] Steps are outlined in **Box 15-8**.

III. No Touch Method for Receptors

- With gloved hands and under appropriate safelight, pull open packets by the tab or from the barrier envelopes (**Figure 15-14**).

Box 15-8 Basic Infection Control Procedures

- Digital photostimulable phosphor (PSP) plates and traditional films covered with contaminated saliva are confined to a disposable cup after exposure.
- Gloved hands do not come in contact with walls, doors, light switches, and other environmental surfaces when transporting a cup of contaminated exposed PSP plates to the scanner or traditional films to the dark room.
- The darkroom or computer monitor/keyboard work area is prepared by the disinfection of all touch surfaces, and the counter is covered with clean paper.
- Traditional processing procedures may reduce the bacterial counts, but the potential for cross-contamination still exists.
- Dispose of PSP plate and traditional film wrappers, cups, and contaminated gloves with contaminated waste. Lead foil is disposed of according to environmental waste guidelines.

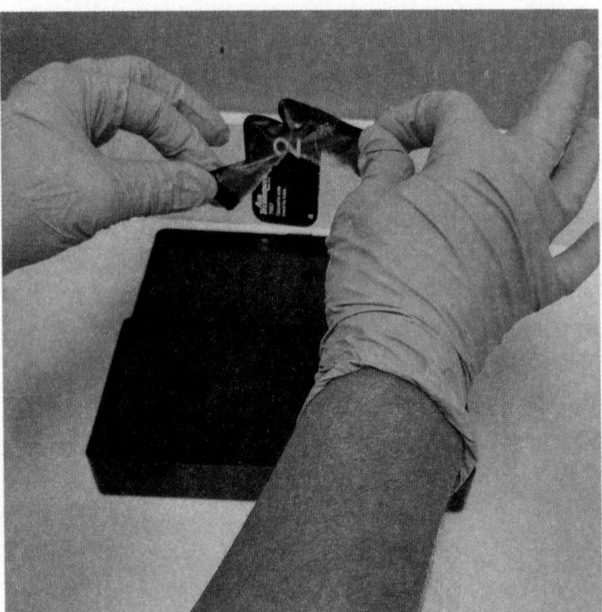

Figure 15-14 Photostimulable Phosphor (PSP) Plate Barrier. Opening PSP plate barrier over a transport box using the no-touch method. Plastic barriers placed over intraoral receptors are used to protect receptors from salivary contamination.

- Allow films/PSP plates to drop out into a cup, transport box, or the clean barrier-covered surface.
- Do not touch the films/PSP plates. Remove gloves, wash hands, and place films on hangers or into the automatic processor, being careful to touch the films by the edges only. Place PSP plates into the laser scanner.
- Dispose of waste properly.
- Alternative no-touch method.
  - Wear overgloves over powder-free treatment gloves and remove them after dropping film/PSP plates into the cup.
  - Films/PSP plates are then processed while wearing powder-free treatment gloves.

Traditional Film Processing

Film processing is the chemical transformation of the **latent image**, produced in a traditional film emulsion by exposure to radiation, into a stable image visible by transmitted light.

I. Image Production

- Film emulsion contains crystals of silver halides (bromide and iodide).
- Development consists of selective reduction of affected silver halide salts to metallic silver grains.
- X-ray exposure changes the silver halides to silver and halide ions.
- Developer reacts with the halide ions, leaving only the metallic silver in an arrangement corresponding with the radiolucency and radiopacity of the tissues being exposed.
- Fixation consists of selective removal of unaffected silver halide crystals.
- Fixer removes only those crystals of silver halide that were not exposed to radiation.
- Washing removes processing chemicals.
- End result is a *negative*, showing various degrees of lightness and darkness (microscopic grains of black metallic silver).

II. Darkroom and Lighting Fundamentals

- Find and eliminate all possible light leaks while standing inside a darkroom.
- Safelighting:
  - Fifteen-watt bulb or less.
  - Light-emitting diode safelight can be used.
  - Positioned a minimum of 4 feet above the working surface.
  - Filter is selected according to film type.

III. Automated Processing

Automatic film processing refers to the use of equipment designed to transport film mechanically through a series of solutions under controlled conditions. The film is transported from the entry slot to the developer, fixer, water bath, dryer, and exit slot.

A. Advantages of Automated Processing

- Consistency of results.
- Conservation of time by dental personnel.
- Dried radiographs in 4–6 minutes.

B. Principles of Operation

- Rollers or tracks are used to carry traditional film through developing, fixing, washing, and drying. Some machines may process only standard intraoral films, whereas others may also accommodate extraoral sizes.
- Increased temperature decreases processing time.

IV. Manual Processing

The darkroom has tanks of chemicals and water for processing traditional films by hand: the developing tank, fixing tank, and water bath. In most darkrooms, the developer solution is in the left tank, the water bath is in between both tanks with circulating water, and the fixer solution is in the right tank.

A. Processing Temperature and Times

- The quality of the radiographic image depends greatly on the processing time and temperature. Optimal developing condition for manual processing is 68°F for 5 minutes.
- Higher temperatures would produce films with excessive density; cooler temperatures, too little density. Follow manufacturer's directions for proper time and temperature settings.

B. Equipment and Steps for Manual Processing

- Check level and temperature of solutions with processing thermometer; stir solutions with stirring rods.
- Turn on safelights and turn off overhead white lights.
- Unwrap films with gloved hands and drop onto a paper towel. Once all films have been unwrapped, discard gloves.
- Load films onto metal hangers.
- Immerse film in the developer; activate timer according to the temperature of the developer solution.
- When timer buzzes, place film rack in circulating water for a 30-second rinse.
- Immerse the films in the fixer solution for twice the development time; activate timer.
- When timer buzzes, place the film rack in circulating water for 10 minutes.
- Dry films thoroughly before handling. This may take up to 1 hour.

C. Disposal of Liquid Chemicals

Fixer and developer solutions are considered environmentally hazardous waste material and are disposed of according to governmental regulations.

Handheld X-Ray Devices

X-ray devices held by the operator are now used in dentistry. Lightweight, handheld x-ray units provide a way to bring radiographic diagnostic examinations into such places as nursing homes, outreach, temporary, and emergency clinics (**Figure 15-15**).

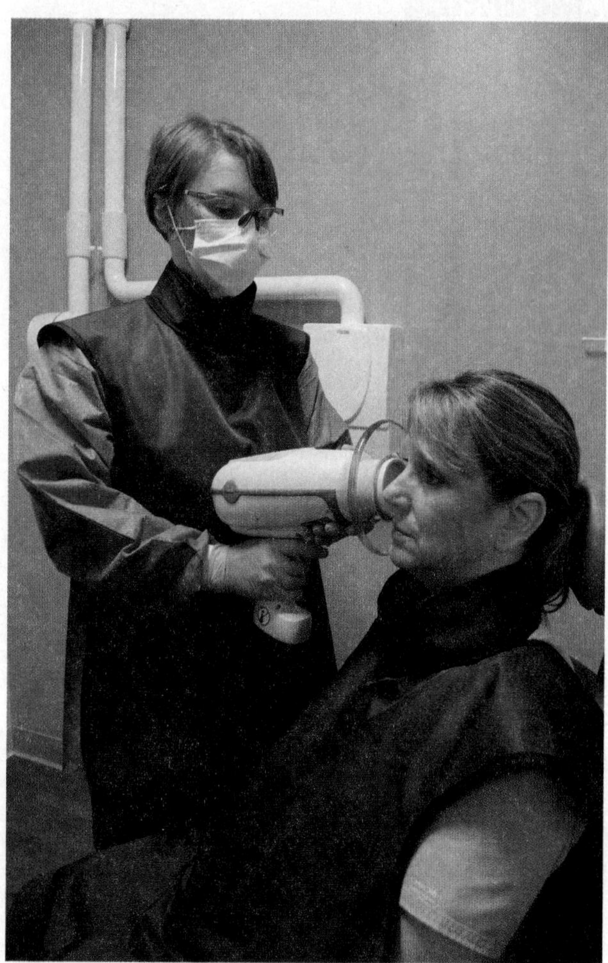

Figure 15-15 Handheld X-Ray Device. The position of the operator in relation to the handheld x-ray device affects the radiation exposure received by the operator.

- Use only Food and Drug Administration–approved devices.
- Units are safe if tube head shielding and backscatter ring shield are in place.
- Institute proper position of the handheld unit relative to the operator to keep operator exposure levels low.
- Use of personal monitoring is recommended when using handheld x-ray units.
- Training and usage protocols must be in place to ensure compliance.[14]

Analysis of Completed Images

The images are mounted and examined on a computer monitor or at a viewbox. Interpretation of images may be difficult, and the determination of a pathologic condition requires keen evaluation. The dentist is responsible for the diagnosis of the information found on dental images.

I. Mounting

- If using traditional film, legibly mark the mount with the name of patient, age, date, and name of dentist; printing is preferred.
- Handle radiographs only by the edges with clean, dry hands.
- Arrange radiographs in front of the viewbox on clean, dry paper.
- The embossed dot near the edge of the radiograph is the guide to mounting; the raised side of the dot is on the facial side.
- Identify individual radiographs by teeth and other anatomic landmarks.
- Approved mounting system is as follows: Looking at the teeth from outside the mouth, the teeth are viewed and mounted in the same manner as the approved tooth numbering system.

II. Anatomic Landmarks

A. Definition

An anatomic landmark is an anatomic structure that may serve as an aid in the localization and identification of the regions portrayed by an image. The teeth are the primary landmarks.

B. Landmarks That May Be Seen in Individual Images

- *Maxillary molar:* Maxillary sinus, zygomatic process, zygomatic (malar) bone, hamular process, coronoid process of the mandible, maxillary tuberosity, lateral pterygoid plate.
- *Maxillary premolar:* Maxillary sinus.
- *Maxillary canine:* Maxillary sinus, junction of the maxillary sinus and nasal fossa (Y-shaped).
- *Maxillary incisors:* Incisive foramen, nasal septum and fossae, anterior nasal spine (V-shaped), median palatine suture, symphysis of the maxillae.
- *Mandibular molar:* Mandibular canal, internal oblique ridge, external oblique ridge, mylohyoid ridge, submandibular gland fossa.
- *Mandibular premolar:* Mental foramen.
- *Mandibular incisors:* Lingual foramen, mental ridge, genial tubercles, symphysis of the mandible. Nutrient canals are also easily viewed.

III. Identification of Errors

Table 15-6 outlines the more common errors, their causes, and the keys to correction.

A. Causes

Errors may be related to any step in the entire procedure, including receptor placement, angulation, exposure, processing if using traditional film, and care and handling of the receptors.

B. Error Types

- Distortion: An inaccuracy in the size or shape of an object in the image. Distortion is brought about by misalignment of the PID relative to the object. Vertical distortion produces elongation or foreshortening of the object.
- Fog: A darkening of the whole or part of an image by sources other than the radiation of the primary beam to which the receptor was exposed. Types of fog include chemical, light, and radiation.
- Artifact: A blemish or an unintended image that can result from faulty manufacture, manipulation, exposure, or processing of a receptor.

IV. Interpretation

- Images are used in conjunction with clinical assessment for a complete treatment care program for the patient.
- As part of the permanent record, images help to document the oral condition at a specific point in time, for comparison, or for legal and forensic purposes.
- The quality of the images determines their value for diagnostic interpretation.

Table 15-6 Analysis of Images: Causes of Errors

	Error	Cause: Factors in Correction
Image	Elongation	Insufficient vertical angulation
	Foreshortening	Excessive vertical angulation
	Superimposition (overlapping)	Incorrect horizontal angulation (central ray not directed through interproximal space)
	Partial image	Cone-cut (incorrect direction of central ray or incorrect image receptor placement) Incompletely immersed in processing tank Traditional film touched other film or side of tank during processing
	Blurred or double image	Patient, tube, or image receptor movement during exposure Image receptor exposed twice
	Stretched appearance of trabeculae or apices	Bent traditional film or PSP plate
	No image	Machine malfunction from time switch to wall plug Failure to turn on the machine Traditional film placed in fixer before developer
Density	Too dark	Excessive exposure for all receptors For traditional film: Excessive developing Developer too warm Unsafe safelight Accidental exposure to white light
	Too light	Insufficient exposure for all image receptors For traditional film: Insufficient development or excessive fixation Solutions too cool Use of old, contaminated, or poorly mixed solutions Film placement: tube side not placed toward teeth Film used beyond expiration date
Fog	Chemical fog	For traditional film: An imbalance or deterioration of processing solutions
	Light fog	For traditional film: An unintentional exposure to light to which the emulsion is sensitive, either before or during processing Unsafe safelight Darkroom leak Holding unprocessed films too close to the safelight too long Improper storage of unused traditional film
	Radiation fog	Traditional film exposed to scatter radiation before processing
Reticulation	Puckered or pebbly surface	For traditional film: Sudden temperature changes during traditional film processing, particularly from warm solutions to very cold water

(continues)

Table 15-6 Analysis of Images: Causes of Errors (continued)

	Error	Cause: Factors in Correction
Artifacts	Dark lines	Bent or creased film or PSP plate Fingernail used to grasp traditional film or PSP plate For traditional film: Static electricity when removed from wrapper with excessive force
	Herringbone pattern (light film)	Traditional film packet placed in mouth backward and exposed
Discoloration	Stains and spots	For traditional film: Unclean film hanger Spattering of developer, fixer, dust Insufficient rinsing after developing before fixing Splashing dry negatives with water or solutions Air bubbles adhering to surface during processing (insufficient agitation) Overlap of film on film in tanks or while drying Paper wrapper stuck to film (film not dried when removed from patient's mouth)
	Stains at later date after storage of completed radiographs	For traditional film: Incomplete processing or rinsing Storage in too warm a place Storage near chemicals

PSP, photostimulable phosphor

- Procedures for the preparation of images are perfected so that the images have maximum interpretability with minimum radiation exposure of the patient.

A. Prerequisites for Interpretation

- Mounting: Mount traditional radiographs in an opaque mount to prevent light between each radiograph from creating glare.
- Viewbox: Use an adequately lighted viewbox for traditional films. Holding the radiographs up to view by window, room, or unit light is inadequate and not recommended.
- Digital software tools: Use magnifiers or a magnifying glass to examine images, manipulate brightness and contrast, invert image densities, etc., to enhance diagnostic capabilities.

B. Systematic Examination

- Observe one radiographic feature at a time. It is important to note comparisons for each change over the entire survey, and comparisons to past surveys if available.
- When examining a particular tooth, compare the appearance of that tooth in each image in which it appears, including bitewings. At different angulations, different findings may become apparent.

C. Correlation with Clinical Examination

- Correlation of radiographic findings with the clinical examination, using probe and explorer, is basic to an understanding of the true oral condition of the patient.
- A description of examination of the teeth is found in Chapter 16 and of the periodontal tissues in Chapter 20.

Ownership

- Radiographic images belong to the dental practice, even though the patient paid to have the images exposed.
- Patient has a right to a copy of their records and their images.
- If using traditional films, originals are kept by the dental practice and a duplicate series is given to the patient.

Documentation

I. Radiation Exposure History

- Inquire whether the patient is receiving or has recently received radiation therapy. It may be necessary to minimize the number of exposures.

A consultation with the patient's physician is recommended.

- Maintain an exposure log for each patient that indicates the date and number of exposures, and document the findings.

II. Patient Care Progress Notes

Patient care progress notes include the following components:

- Patient complaint, if applicable, including:
  - Location of symptomatic area.
  - Duration and severity of symptoms.
- Clinical findings.
- Recommended diagnostic procedures.
  - Explain to patient necessity of images for accurate diagnosis and treatment.
  - Patient has the right to refuse dental imaging.
  - Obtain the patient's signature to a statement of refusal in the event a legal issue should arise. The patient's signature does not protect providers if an improper diagnosis is made due to a lack of dental radiographs. It is the responsibility of the dental provider to follow the standard of care.
- Type of images (periapical or bitewing), number of exposures, and area(s) exposed.
- **Box 15-9** provides example documentation for the patient who has received dental images.

Box 15-9 Example Documentation: Assessment for Dental Radiographic Examination

- **S**—Patient presents for routine maintenance appointment and complains about heat sensitivity related to tooth #10. The patient stated that he was hit in the mouth with a soccer ball approximately a year ago.
- **O**—Last images consisted of four bitewings exposed 2 years ago. The most recent periapical radiograph of tooth #10, dated 3 years ago, reveals a healthy lamina dura and periodontal ligament space. The patient has several porcelain-fused-to-metal crowns and large amalgam restorations in the posterior sextants. Teeth in the anterior sextants are natural and contain no restorative materials.
- **A**—Discussed with the patient that #10 may have been traumatized and that periapical pathology may exist. He has recently undergone numerous medical imaging procedures and requests minimal radiation exposure today.
- **P**—After a complete clinical examination, two premolar and two molar bitewing images, along with one periapical image of #10 were exposed.

Next steps: Tooth #10 revealed periapical pathology. The patient was referred to an endodontist for care.

Signed: ______________________________, RDH
Date: ________________

Factors to Teach the Patient

When the Patient Asks about the Safety of Radiation

- Patients ask questions about safety factors, and occasionally a patient may refuse to have any images exposed. The patient can be reassured with confidence, instructed as to why images are necessary at this time, and informed about how modern equipment and techniques are in accord with radiation standards.
- Adapt the answer to the patient. Certain patients have more fear; others have more knowledge about x-radiation. The clinician who expresses confidence aids in allaying fears. Hesitation increases the patient's doubt.
- Radiographic examinations are essential to diagnosis and treatment. Without the information provided, the clinician can only guess at conditions not visible clinically.
- The benefits resulting from the intelligent use of dental images outweigh any possible negative effects.
- Modern x-ray machines are equipped for safety. Simple details about filtration, collimation, film speed, use of protective shields, and short exposure times can be explained.

Educational Features in Dental Images

- Position of unerupted permanent teeth in relation to primary teeth.
- Detection of early cavitated carious lesions not visible by clinical examination.
- Effects of loss of teeth and the importance of having replacement options.
- Periodontal changes and other pathologic conditions appropriate to an individual patient.

References

1. American Dental Association Council on Scientific Affairs, U.S. Department of Health and Human Services, U.S. Food and Drug Administration. The selection of patients for dental radiographic examinations. https://www.fda.gov/radiation-emitting-products/medical-x-ray-imaging/selection-patients-dental-radiographic-examinations. Accessed March 12, 2022.
2. National Research Council, (BEIR-VII Phase 2). *Health Risks of Exposure to Low Levels of Ionizing Radiation*. Washington, DC: National Academies Press; 2006. https://www.nap.edu/catalog/11340/health-risks-from-exposure-to-low-levels-of-ionizing-radiation. Accessed March 12, 2022.
3. Parks ET. Digital radiographic imaging: is the dental practice ready? *JADA*. 2008;139(4):477-481.
4. van der Stelt, PF. Better imaging: the advances of digital radiography. *JADA*. 2008;139(suppl 3):7S-13S.
5. Gart C, Zamanian K. Global trends in dental imaging: the rise of digital. *Dental Tribune*. July 27, 2010. https://us.dental-tribune.com/news/global-trends-in-dental-imaging-the-rise-of-digital/. Accessed March 12, 2022.
6. Matzen LH, Christensen J, Wenzel A. Patient discomfort and retakes in periapical examination of mandibular third molars using digital receptors. *Oral Surg Oral Med Oral Pathol Oral Radiol Endod*. 2009;107(4):566-572.
7. Williamson GF. Intraoral imaging: basic principles, techniques and error correction, March 2018. *Dentalcare.com Professional Education*. https://www.dentalcare.com/en-us/professional-education/ce-courses/ce559. Accessed March 12, 2022.
8. International Commission on Radiation Units and Measurements. Radiation quantities and units. *ICRU Report No. 33*. Washington, DC: ICRU; 1980.
9. National Council on Radiation Protection and Measurements. Radiation protection in dentistry. *NCRP Report No. 145*. Washington, DC: NCRP; 2003. https://ncrponline.org/publications/reports/ncrp-reports-145/. Accessed March 12, 2022.
10. White SC, Mallya SM. Update on the biological effects of ionizing radiation, relative dose factors and radiation hygiene. *Aust Dent J*. 2012;57(suppl 1):2-8.
11. Anjum M, Godward S, Williams D, et al. Dental x-rays and the risk of thyroid cancer: a case-control study. *Acta Oncol*. 2010;49(4):447-453.
12. Thomson EM. Reduce retakes. *Dimens Dent Hyg*. 2011;9(10):58-61.
13. Frommer HH, Stabulas-Savage JJ. *Radiology for the Dental Professional*. 9th ed. St. Louis, MO: Mosby; 2011.
14. Makdissi J, Pawar RR, Johnson B, Chong BS. The effects of device position on the operator's radiation dose when using a handheld portable x-ray device. *Dentomaxillofac Radiol*. 2016;45(3):20150245.

CHAPTER 16

Hard Tissue Examination of the Dentition

Linda D. Boyd, RDH, RD, EdD
Lorie Speer, RDH, MSDH

CHAPTER OUTLINE

LEARNING OBJECTIVES

After studying this chapter, the student will be able to:

1. Identify the three divisions of the human dentition: primary teeth, mixed (transitional) dentition, and permanent teeth.
2. Recognize and explain the various developmental and noncarious dental lesions.
3. Describe types of dental injuries and tooth fractures that may occur.
4. List the G.V. Black classification, American Dental Association Caries Classification, and International Caries Detection and Assessment System classification of dental carious lesions used for diagnosis, treatment planning, management, cavity preparations, and finished restorations.
5. Explain the initiation and development of early childhood caries.
6. Compare methods for determining the vitality of the pulp of a tooth.
7. Provide a list of the factors to be observed and recorded during a complete dental charting with a new patient.
8. Explain the basic principles of occlusion.
9. Classify occlusion on a patient or case study according to Angle's classification and describe facial profile associated with each classification.
10. Describe functional and parafunctional contacts.
11. Give examples of parafunctional habits.
12. Discuss types of occlusal trauma and explain the effects on the oral structures.
13. List the purposes and uses of study models.
14. Identify and explain the purposes and uses of study models in the clinical practice of dental hygiene.

Clinical examination and assessment of the teeth are essential before treatment to provide guidelines for treatment planning, instrumentation, instruction, and follow-up evaluation.

- Background study of dental anatomy, oral histology, and oral pathology is essential to the examination of the hard tissues of the oral cavity.

The Dentitions

The three divisions are the **primary (deciduous) dentition**, **mixed (transitional) dentition**, and **permanent dentition**.

I. Primary (Deciduous) Dentition

- Formation of the primary teeth begins in utero.
- The weeks in utero when each primary tooth begins to mineralize and the average age after birth when the enamel is completely formed before the date of eruption is found in Chapter 47.

II. Mixed or Transitional Dentition

- Mixed or transitional **dentition** occurs between the ages of 6 and 12 years when primary teeth are being exfoliated and permanent teeth erupt.
- **Succedaneous** teeth are permanent teeth that erupt into the positions of exfoliated primary teeth.
- **Figure 16-1** illustrates the mixed dentition of a child approximately 6 years of age just as the first permanent molars are erupting.

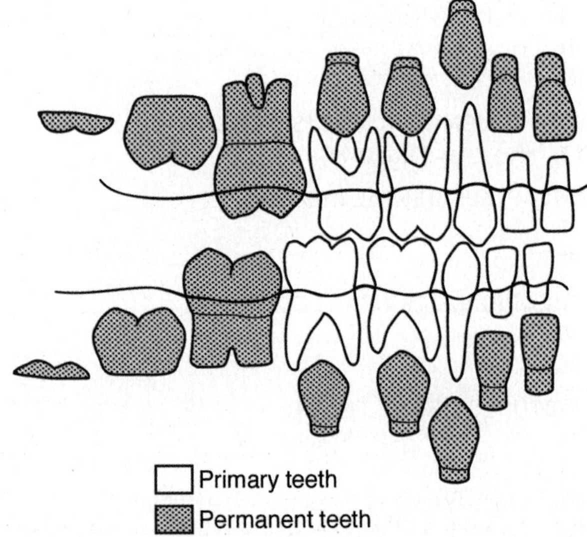

Figure 16-1 Mixed Dentition at Approximately Age 6 Years. The average child has 20 primary teeth in place, and root resorption of the incisors has started as the developing permanent incisors move into position. The first permanent molars are partially erupted.

Table 16-1 Tooth Development and Eruption: Permanent Teeth[1-3]

		Crown Formation Begins	Crown Completed (Years)	Eruption (Years)	Root Completed (Years)
Maxillary	Central incisor	3–4 mo	4–5	7–8	10
	Lateral incisor	10-12 mo	4–5	8–9	11
	Canine	4–5 mo	6–7	11–12	13–15
	First premolar	1.5–2 y	5–6	10–11	12–13
	Second premolar	2–2.5 y	6–7	10–12	12–14
	First molar	At birth	2.5–3	6–7	9–10
	Second molar	2.5–3 y	7–8	12–13	14–16
	Third molar	7–9 y	12–16	17–21	19–21
Mandibular	Central incisor	3–4 mo	4–5	6–7	7.5-8
	Lateral incisor	3–4 mo	4–5	7–8	8-9
	Canine	4–5 mo	6–7	9–10	11–13
	First premolar	1.5–2 y	5–6	10–12	12–13.5
	Second premolar	2.5–3 y	6-7	11–12	13.5–14
	First molar	At birth	2.5–3	6–7	8.5–10
	Second molar	2.5–3 y	7–8	11–13	14–15
	Third molar	8–10 y	12–16	17–21	19–21

Data from Logan WH, Kronfield R. Development of the human jaws and surrounding structures from birth to age fifteen. *JADA*. 1933;35(20):379-424; Orban B. *Oral Histology and Embryology*. St. Louis, MO: Mosby; 1944. Schour I, McCall JO. Chronology of the human dentition. In: Orban B, ed. *Oral Histology and Embryology*. St Louis, MO: Mosby; 1944:240.

III. Permanent Dentition

- Consists of 32 teeth that replace the primary teeth and serve throughout life.
- Mineralization of the permanent teeth starts at birth and continues into adolescence. The chronology of development and eruption of the permanent teeth is listed in **Table 16-1**.
- There may be variations in development and eruption based on factors such as genetics and gender.
- Roots are completely formed about 3 years after eruption into the oral cavity.

IV. The Teeth

- Clinical crown is the part of the tooth above the attached periodontal tissues. It can be considered the part of the tooth that is visible (not covered with gingiva) when in the mouth and where restorative treatment procedures are performed (**Figure 16-2**).
- Clinical root is the part of the tooth not visible because it is below the base of the gingival sulcus or periodontal pocket (is not visible when in the mouth). It is the part of the root to which periodontal fibers are attached.
- Anatomic crown is the part of the tooth covered by enamel.
- Anatomic root is the part of the tooth covered by cementum.

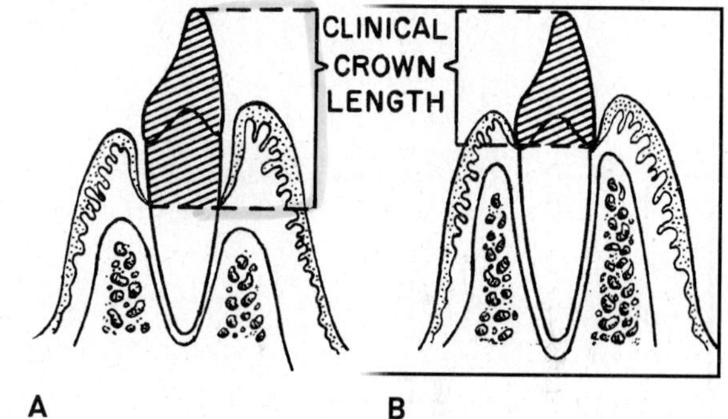

Figure 16-2 Clinical Crown. The part of the tooth that is above the attached periodontal tissue. **A:** When the periodontal pocket depth is increased, the clinical crown extends to a position at which the clinical crown length is greater than the clinical root length. The clinical root is the part of the tooth with attached periodontal tissues. **B:** When the clinical attachment level is at the cementoenamel junction, the clinical crown and the anatomic crown are the same.

Hard Tissue Examination Procedure

The hard tissue examination includes dental charting of the existing restorations along with carious lesions and noncarious lesions. Radiographs are utilized to aid in identification of carious lesions and other pathologies. Documentation of occlusion and preparation of study models to aid with treatment planning are also part of the hard tissue examination. **Table 16-2** lists factors to observe during the hard tissue examination.

Table 16-2 Examination of the Teeth

Feature	To Observe	Dental Hygiene Implication
Morphology	Number of teeth (missing teeth verified by radiographic examination) Size, shape Arch form Position of individual teeth (**diastema**) Injuries: fractures of the crown (root fractures observed in radiographs)	Selection and adaptation of instruments Areas prone to dental caries initiation, particularly difficult-to-reach areas during biofilm control Pulp test for vitality may be indicated
Development	Anomalies and developmental defects Pits and white spots	Distinguish **hypoplasia** and dental fluorosis from demineralization Identify pits for sealants
Eruption (**Table 16-1**)	Sequence of eruption: Normal, irregular Unerupted teeth observed in radiographs	Care in using floss in the col area where the epithelium is usually less mature in young children Orthodontic needs Procedures for preservation of primary teeth
Deposits (**Table 17-1**) Food debris Biofilm Calculus Supragingival Subgingival	Overall evaluation of oral self-care and biofilm control measures Relation of appearance of teeth to gingival health Extent and location of biofilm, debris, and calculus Calculus and the tooth surface pocket wall	Need for instruction and guidance Frequency of follow-up and maintenance appointments
Stains (see Chapter 17) Extrinsic Intrinsic	Extrinsic: Colors relate to causes Intrinsic: Dark, grayish Tobacco stain	Need to test pulp vitality Stain removal procedures; selection of polishing agent Dentifrice recommendation Biofilm control emphasis for biofilm-related stains Provide information concerning oral effects of tobacco use Tobacco cessation program (see Chapter 32)
Noncarious lesions	Attrition: Primary and permanent Abrasion: Physical agents that may be a cause Erosion	Evaluate modifiable risk factors and initiate appropriate prevention Dietary analysis Habit evaluation
Exposed cementum	Relation to gingival recession, pocket formation Areas of narrow attached gingiva Hypersensitivity	Special care areas such as narrow attached gingiva Nonabrasive dentifrice advised Prevention of root surface caries Care during instrumentation Indication for application of desensitizing agent

Dental caries	Areas of demineralization Stages of carious lesions Proximal lesions observed in radiographs **Arrested caries** Root caries	Charting Treatment plan Cavitated vs. noncavitated Preventive program for caries management based on modifiable factors for caries risk (i.e., fluoride, dietary factors) Follow-up and frequency of maintenance
Restorations	Contour of restorations, overhangs Proximal contact Surface smoothness Staining	Chart inadequate margins Selection of instruments and polishing agents Dentifrice selection to prevent discoloration
Factors related to occlusion	Health of supporting structures; observation of radiographs for signs of trauma from occlusion	Need for study of bruxism and other parafunctional habits
Tooth wear	Facets; worn-down cusp tips	Chart inadequate contacts for corrective measures
Proximal contacts	Assess difficulty in flossing Areas of food retention	Evaluate appropriate interdental cleaning aid
Mobility	Degree; comparison of chartings Assess for fremitus Possible causes	Need for reduction of related inflammatory factors Dentist will identify and treat factors related to occlusal trauma
Classification	Position of teeth Angle's classification	Relationship to orthodontic treatment needs
Habits	Nail or object biting; lip or cheek biting Observe effects on lip, cheek, teeth **Tongue thrust**; reverse swallow	Guidance for habit correction when indicated
Edentulous areas	Radiographic evaluation for impacted, unerupted teeth; supernumerary teeth; retained root tips; other deviations from normal	Alternative fulcrum selection during instrumentation Applied biofilm control procedures for abutment teeth
Replacement for missing teeth Dentures Partial dentures Implants	Teeth and tissue that support a prosthesis Cleanliness of a prosthesis Factors that contribute to food and debris retention	Instruction in care of fixed and removable dentures Identify cleaning aid for under fixed partial denture
Saliva	Amount and consistency Dryness of mouth	Identify appropriate caries management for xerostomia (i.e., fluorides, saliva substitute) Avoid alcohol-containing mouth rinse

I. Dental Charting of Existing Restorations

- Missing, **supernumerary**, or unerupted teeth are recorded.
- A systematic approach to charting restorations should be utilized to avoid errors, for example, start with tooth #1.

II. Assessment of Noncarious and Carious Lesions

A. Visual Examination Procedure

- Carefully visually inspect each surface, use air to clean and dry tooth surface, and utilize adequate lighting.[4,5]
- Observe changes in the color and translucency of tooth structure.
- Changes noted can then be studied in the radiograph or documented for future review.
- Variations in color and translucency include the following:
  - Chalky white areas of demineralization.
  - Grayish-white discoloration of marginal ridges caused by dental caries of the proximal surface underneath.
  - Grayish-white color spreading from margins of restorations.
- Transillumination is especially useful for anterior teeth and unrestored posterior teeth.

B. Radiographic Examination

- Carefully review and interpret radiographic findings to identify areas to investigate during the clinical examination. Neither radiographic nor clinical examination is complete without the other.
- In addition to possible caries lesions, other important areas to investigate in the radiographic examination include anomalies, impactions, fractures, internal and root **resorption**, and periapical radiolucencies.
- Panoramic, extraoral, or occlusal radiographs are needed for detecting or defining anomalies and pathologic lesions outside the scope of periapical radiographs.

C. Clinical Examination Procedure

- If caries cannot be confirmed visually or radiographically, gently use a rounded or ball-end explorer to confirm visual findings.[4,5]
  - It is essential not to break through a remineralizing tooth surface with a sharp explorer.

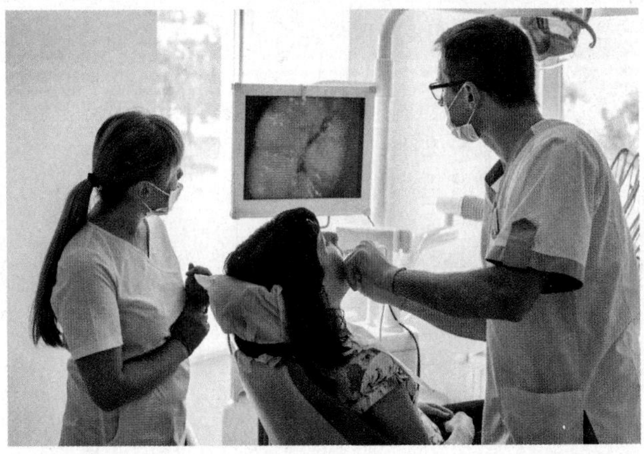

Figure 16-3 Clinical Assessment Tools. Intraoral camera used during dental examination to record oral conditions and to educate patient about their oral health.

- Intraoral images can also document the existing oral condition and provide visual representation of treatment needs both for documentation in the patient record and to educate the patient (**Figure 16-3**).

D. Document the Following

- Existing restorations.
- Developmental enamel lesions.
- Noncarious cervical lesions (NCCLs).
- Carious lesions using a recognized classification system described later in the chapter.
- Any other pathology noted during the radiographic or clinical examination.

III. Occlusion

Assessment of occlusion will include:

- Normal occlusion.
- Malocclusion.
- Malrelations of groups of teeth.
- Malpositions of individual teeth.
- Dynamic (or functional) occlusion.
- Traumatic occlusion.

IV. Study Models

Study models may be taken to assess and document occlusal relationships.

Developmental Enamel Lesions

I. Enamel Hypoplasia

Enamel hypoplasia is a defect that occurs as a result of a disturbance during formation of the enamel matrix.

A. Types and Etiology

- Genetic[6]:
  - **Amelogenesis imperfecta** is a hereditary enamel defect in which the enamel is either thin or absent. The enamel may also have surface pitting or vertical grooves.
  - Other inherited syndromes associated with enamel defects may be associated with dermatologic conditions or defects in mineralization such as hypoparathyroidism.
- Systemic conditions contributing to enamel hypoplasia during tooth development may include[6]:
  - Metabolic disturbances such as celiac disease and chronic renal or liver disease.
  - Infections causing fever such as chicken pox, rubella, measles, or congenital syphilis.
  - Chemicals and drugs such as fluoride and tetracycline.
  - Nutritional deficiencies like rickets.
  - Preterm birth.
- Local insults to developing tooth may include:
  - Trauma.
  - Periapical inflammation of a primary tooth may injure the developing permanent tooth.

B. Appearance

- The teeth may appear yellow or brown.
- Systemic
  - Also called "chronologic hypoplasia" because the lesions are found in areas of the teeth where the enamel was forming during the systemic disturbance.
  - Single narrow zone (smooth or pitted): Disturbance lasted a short period of time.
  - Multiple (may appear as furrows or horizontal rows of dimples in the enamel)[7]: Disturbance to the ameloblast occurred over a period of time or several times (**Figure 16-4**).
  - Teeth most frequently affected are the first molars, incisors, and canines because the disturbances generally occur during the first year when those teeth are mineralizing.
- Hypoplasia of congenital syphilis
  - Transmission of syphilis from mother to fetus after the 16th week of pregnancy may alter the development of the tooth germs.
  - **Figure 16-5** illustrates tooth forms that may result, including the mulberry molar. The mesiodistal width may be reduced, and incisors are frequently narrowed at the incisal third, as shown by the Hutchinson's incisors and the peg lateral incisor.
- Local enamel hypoplasia
  - A single tooth with a yellow or brown intrinsic stain.

II. Hypomineralization

- **Hypomineralization** occurs during the maturation stage of enamel mineralization.[6,8,9]
- Hypomineralization may result in a higher risk for hypersensitivity, tooth wear, and dental caries.[6,8]

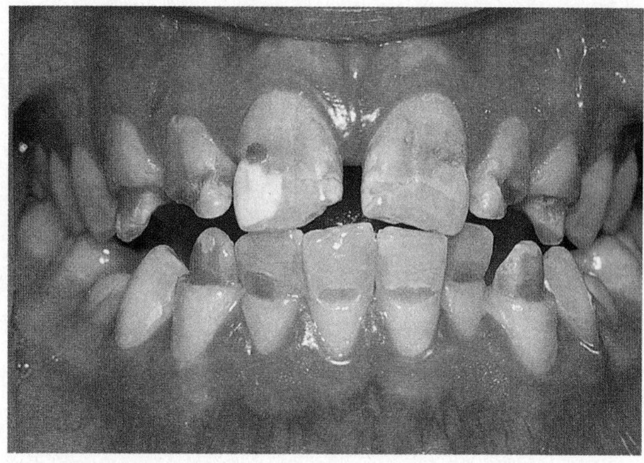

Figure 16-4 Enamel Hypoplasia. Enamel hypoplasia, usually in the form of white or brown grooves or pits, at a level corresponding with the stage of development of the teeth.

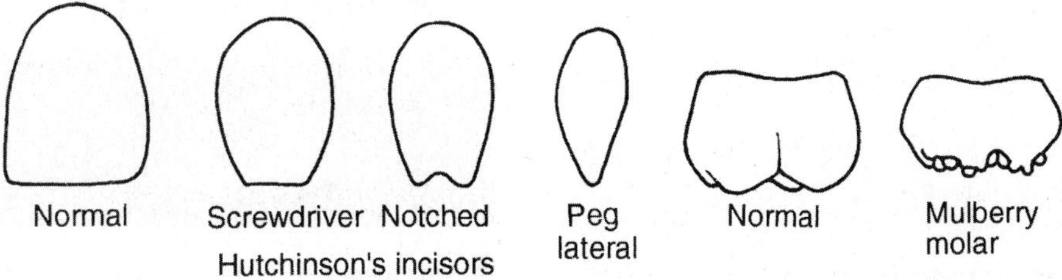

Figure 16-5 Crown Forms of Enamel Hypoplasia. Hutchinson's incisors and mulberry molars are typical crown forms that result from congenital syphilis. The central incisors are narrowed at the incisal third, and the lateral incisors may be conical or peg shaped.

A. Etiology

- Children with celiac disease are at risk for hypomineralization because of malabsorption and potential for mineral deficiencies.[6]
- Chronic liver or kidney disease may impact mineralization during tooth development.[6]
- Early childhood illness associated with a high fever such as chicken pox, respiratory, and urinary tract infections.[6,9]
- Chemicals and drugs such as fluoride and tetracycline.[6]

B. Types

- Molar incisor hypomineralization (MIH) appears as yellow or brownish demarcated areas on one or more permanent molars and incisors.[6,8]
    - Prevalence tends to be highest in Australia, some areas of Europe, Brazil, and Iraq.
    - Occasionally the defects may involve the primary second molars along with the permanent canines and premolars.[8,9]
- Amelogenesis imperfecta
    - In the hypomineralized type, enamel is a normal thickness, but opaque and brittle.[8]
- Dental fluorosis[8]
    - Exposure of the **enamel organ** to excessive fluoride during development.
    - Severe forms appear yellow/brown and the enamel is prone to breakdown.

III. Hypomaturation

- **Hypomaturation** occurs during the last stages of mineralization from a decrease in deposition of mineral.[6]
- The enamel may appear opaque or discolored and fracture easily.[6]

Developmental Defects of Dentin

I. Types and Etiology

A. Genetic[3]

- Current genetic evidence suggests there is just one gene responsible for disturbances in dentin development with a range of severity.[10]
- **Dentinogenesis imperfecta** (DI) characteristics vary from mild to severe. Milder forms were previously named dentin dysplasia.
    - Mild-severity DI characteristics[10]:
        - Normal to light gray discoloration of the crown.
        - Pulp chamber may be thistle-shaped.
- In moderate to severe DI characteristics[10]:
    - Crowns may be blue, gray, or brown opalescent in color.
    - Shortened, bulbous tooth crowns.
    - Alterations in the pulp from complete obliteration to an enlarged pulp.
    - Thin and shortened roots.
    - Increased incidence of periapical pathology.
    - More severe DI may be associated with more fragile bones (osteogenesis imperfecta).[6,10]

Noncarious Dental Lesions

I. Attrition

Attrition is the wearing away of a tooth as a result of tooth-to-tooth contact (**Figure 16-6**).

A. Occurrence

- Location
    - May be found on occlusal, incisal, and proximal surfaces.
- Impact of age and gender
    - Effects of attrition are cumulative over time, so an increase in attrition is often associated with increasing age.[11]

B. Etiology

- Bruxism
    - There are two main types of **bruxism**: Sleep (nocturnal) and awake bruxism (tooth clenching).[11]

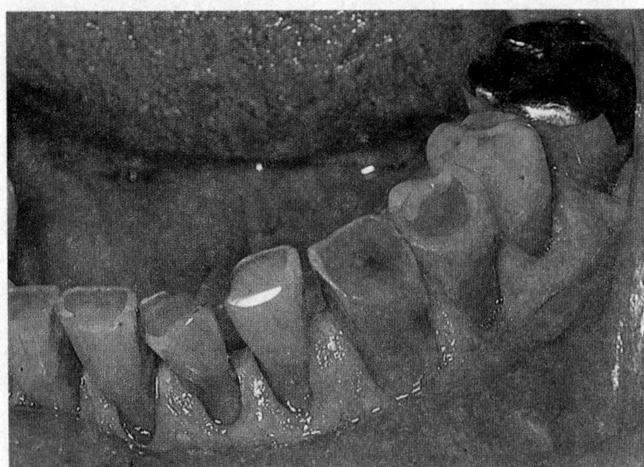

Figure 16-6 Attrition. The incisal surfaces of mandibular anterior teeth have been worn to expose the dentin. Dentin usually appears as a yellow-brown line or ring.

Reproduced from Langlais RP, Miller CS. *Color Atlas of Common Oral Diseases*. Philadelphia, PA: Lea & Febiger; 1992. Used with permission.

- Sleep bruxism (SB) in children is associated with many factors including, but not limited to, male gender, secondhand smoke exposure, restless sleep, loud snoring, and headache.[12]
- Sleep bruxism in adults has been strongly associated with childhood SB, chronic migraine, and gastroesophageal reflux disease (GERD).[13]

- Occlusal interferences may also be a risk factor for attrition.
- Modifying factors for attrition include[11]:
  - Ecstasy (MDMA, or 3, 4-methylenedioxymeth amphetamine) use includes bruxism as a side effect.
  - Habit of chewing on hard foods like bones.
  - SSRIs (selective serotonin uptake inhibitors) used as an antidepressant may cause bruxism.

C. Appearance

- Initial lesion
  - Small shiny, flat, worn spot on the surface of a tooth known as a **facet** is found on a cusp tip or ridge, or slight flattening of an incisal edge.
- Advanced
  - Gradual reduction in cusp height; flattening of incisal or **occlusal plane** as shown in Figure 16-6.
  - Staining of exposed dentin.
  - Radiographically the pulp chamber and canals may be narrowed and sometimes obliterated as a result of formation of secondary dentin.

II. Erosion

Erosion is the loss of tooth substance by a chemical process that does not involve known bacterial action.

A. Occurrence

- Location
  - Facial or lingual surfaces are mostly commonly affected (**Figure 16-7**).
  - Erosion can result from **endogenous** and **exogenous** acid sources.[14]
- Usually involves multiple teeth.

B. Etiology

- Exogenous (extrinsic) acid sources may include[14]:
  - Occupational acid exposure: Battery, ammunition, or galvanizing factory workers; wine tasters; and professional swimmers.

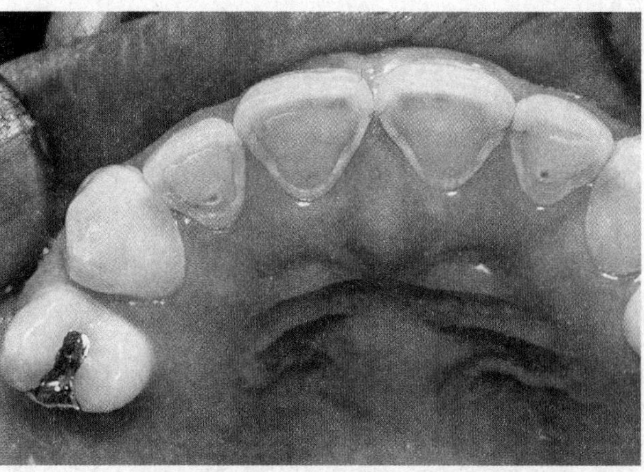

Figure 16-7 Erosion. Enamel erosion on the lingual of mandibular anterior teeth caused by chronic vomiting in bulimia.

  - Acidic food: Acidic soft drinks, sports drinks, citrus fruits or drinks, vinegar, and wine.
  - Acidic drugs: Aspirin, iron tablets, and vitamin C supplements.
  - Substance use disorders: Alcohol and Ecstasy (MDMA).
- Endogenous (intrinsic) acid sources include[14]:
  - Eating disorders: Bulimia.
  - Gastroesophageal reflux disease. GERD

C. Erosion Process

- Exposure to acid causes loss of the outermost enamel and dentin and softening (demineralization) of the tooth surface.[15]
- This softened surface is easily removed by mechanical forces, such as toothbrushing.[15]

D. Appearance

- Smooth, shallow, hard, shiny (in contrast to **dental caries**, in which appearance is soft and discolored).
- Shape varies from shallow saucer-like depressions of the cusps to deep wedge-shaped grooves; margins are not sharply demarcated.
- May progress to involve the dentin and stimulate secondary dentin.

Noncarious Cervical Lesions

- NCCLs are lesions resulting from loss of tooth structure near the cementoenamel junction not related to dental caries.[16]

- The lesions typically are wedge-shaped and at least 1 mm deep.
- NCCLs impact the structural integrity of the tooth and esthetics, may retain dental biofilm, and exhibit dentin hypersensitivity.
- Typically NCCLs are multifactorial and more than one type of lesion may be present (e.g., erosion and abrasion).[17]

I. Abrasion

Abrasion is the mechanical wearing away of tooth substance by forces other than mastication.

A. Occurrence

- Exposed root surfaces.
- Cervical areas are the most commonly affected tooth surface (Figure 16-7).[18]

B. Etiology

- The action of microorganisms is not implicated in the development of abrasion. However, dental caries may occur in the abraded area as a secondary lesion.
- Primary factors impacting development of cervical abrasion include the abrasiveness of the dentifrice, stiffness of the toothbrush bristles, and the area where the patient first begins brushing.[18,19] **Figure 16-8** shows the effect on the root surface.
- *Occupational causes*: Cement factories and granite workers along with iron miners.[18]

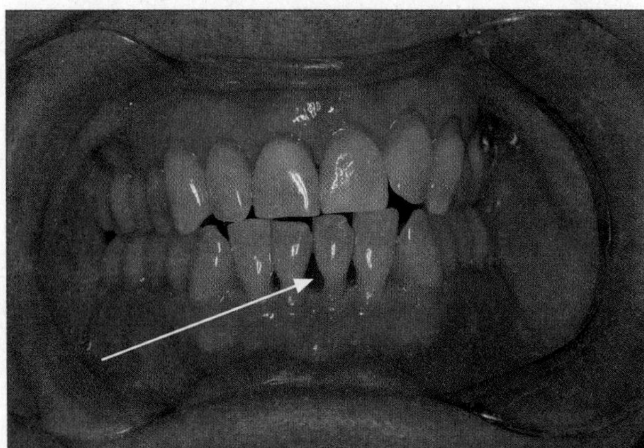

Figure 16-8 Abrasion. The lower anterior teeth exhibit areas of abrasion. Note that the area of abrasion on the root surface undermines the enamel.

Photograph courtesy of Dr. Paul Epstein, DMD.

- Habits putting the patient at risk for abrasion include pipe smoking, chewing pens, betel nut chewing, and pica (eating nonfood items).[18]

C. Appearance

- V or wedge shaped with hard, smooth, shiny surface and clearly defined margins.
- Lesions typically occur on exposed cementum, then extend into the dentin.

II. Abfraction

Abfraction means to break away and results from microfractures in the hydroxyapatite crystals of enamel and dentin.[17]

A. Occurrence

- Primarily occurs on buccal surfaces.
- Wedge- or V-shaped lesions with relatively sharp angles.

B. Etiology

- Multifactorial.
- Research has not confirmed that occlusal factors are the cause.[17]
- Dentin demineralization may increase the risk of abfraction, and occlusal forces may increase progression of the lesion.[17]

C. Appearance

- V or wedge shaped with hard, smooth, shiny surface and clearly defined margins.
- Except for incisal biting habits, the lesions occur initially on exposed cementum, then extend into the dentin.

Fractures of the Teeth

- Trauma to the face may involve fractured bones and teeth in addition to soft tissue injuries. Fractured jaw and methods of treatment are described in Chapter 56.
- Emergency care for a forcibly displaced tooth is found in Chapter 9.

I. Causes of Tooth Fractures

- Automobile, bicycle, and diving accidents.
- Contact sports when mouth protectors are not worn.
- Blows to the face.
- Falls.

II. Description

A. Line of Fracture

- May be horizontal, diagonal, or vertical.
- **Figure 16-9** illustrates fractures of a central incisor.

B. Radiographic Signs of Trauma

- Widened periodontal ligament (PDL) space.
- Radiolucent fracture line.
- Radiopaque areas where fracture segments overlap.
- Tooth displacement.

III. Classification of Traumatic Dental Injuries

Both primary and permanent dentitions are included. The *International Association of Dental Traumatology* guidelines for management of traumatic dental injuries include[20,21]:

- Fracture
  - Incomplete fracture of enamel of tooth (cracks) without loss of tooth structure.
  - Coronal fracture of enamel only.
  - Fracture of enamel and dentin with or without pulpal involvement.
  - Fracture of enamel, dentin, and cementum with or without pulpal involvement.
  - Fracture of root of tooth.
  - Fracture involves alveolar bone.
- **Luxation** (dislocation) of the tooth
  - Concussion: Normal mobility with sensitivity to percussion and touch.
  - Subluxation: Injury to supporting tooth structures with loosening, but no displacement of the tooth.
  - Extrusive luxation is displacement of the tooth from the socket so it appears elongated with increased mobility.
  - Lateral luxation is when the tooth is displaced laterally (in a palatal/lingual or facial direction) and usually associated with alveolar bone fracture.
  - Intrusive luxation is a tooth displaced apically into the alveolar bone.
- **Avulsion** is the complete displacement of the tooth out of its socket due to forcible trauma.

IV. Recommendations for Treatment

- Diagnosis and planning are necessary for satisfactory healing.
- Guidelines for treatment planning have been prepared by the *International Association of Dental Traumatology* and include[20,21]:
  - Clinical diagnosis and immediate emergency treatment.
  - Radiographs to detect root fracture.
  - Location of tooth fragments.
  - Pulp testing.
  - Mobility; tenderness.
  - Follow-up for additional requirements.

Dental Caries

The international consensus definition of dental caries:

> Dental caries is a biofilm-mediated, diet modulated, multifactorial, non-communicable, dynamic disease resulting in net mineral loss of dental hard tissues. It is determined by biological, behavioral, psychosocial, and environmental factors (p. 8).[22]

I. Development of Dental Caries

Requirements for the development of a **carious** lesion are microorganisms, fermentable carbohydrate,

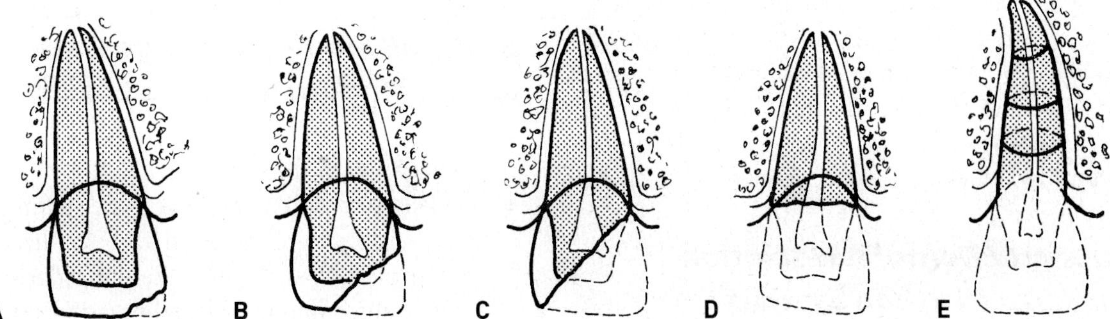

Figure 16-9 Fractures of Teeth. **A:** Enamel fracture. **B:** Crown fracture without pulpal involvement. **C:** Crown fracture with pulpal involvement. **D:** Fracture of crown and root near neck of tooth. **E:** Root fractures involving cementum, dentin, and the pulp may occur in the apical, middle, or coronal third of the root.

and a susceptible tooth surface. Chapter 33 shows four overlapping circles to illustrate the essential factors in dental caries initiation.

- Dental biofilm contains many types of bacteria. Classic theory is that *Streptococcus mutans* and *Lactobacillus* are primarily responsible for dental caries; however, research suggests the **oral microbiome** is much more complex than originally thought and caries results from an imbalance in the oral microbes.[23] The role of oral microbiome, dental biofilm, and other factors involved in dental caries development is described in Chapter 17.

II. Classification of Carious Lesions

A. G.V. Black's Classification[24]

- The standard method for classifying dental caries/restorations was developed by Dr. G.V. Black,[24] a noted dental educator who divided the categories into classes according to surfaces of the teeth.
- The G.V. Black classification was associated with a surgical approach where diseased portions of the tooth were removed with placement of restorations. **Figure 16-10** defines and illustrates the classifications.
- This classification system applies when completing the dental charting of existing restorations.

B. International Caries Classification and Management System

- The International Caries Classification and Management System (ICCMS) approach classifies the tooth surface from healthy to severe decay and allows for early detection of enamel changes that will benefit from remineralization.[4]
- The goal of this standardized system is for early detection in order to make informed decisions about caries management. **Figure 16-11** describes and illustrates the International Caries Detection and Assessment System (ICDAS). More information can be found at www.iccms-web.com/.

C. American Dental Association Caries Classification System

- The Caries Classification System (CCS) ranges from a healthy or sound tooth to noncavitated lesions to advanced carious lesions.[5]
- Each tooth surface is scored according to the presence or absence of a carious lesion, severity of the change, and estimation of activity or progression.[5] This information is then used to determine management or treatment options.

Enamel Caries

I. Stages in the Formation of a Carious Lesion

A. ICCMS Initial Stage Caries or CCS Initial Caries Lesion

In this stage, there is demineralization of the enamel. This may also be called early caries or an incipient lesion.[4,5,25]

- Subsurface demineralization: Acid products from **cariogenic** dental biofilm pass through microchannels (pores) from the surface of the enamel to the subsurface area in the dentin.
- First clinical evidence: First visual changes in enamel may appear whitish/yellowish (white spot lesion); when dried, the surface may be opaque or dull rather than shiny as in health.
  - There is no breakthrough or **cavitation** of the enamel surface.
  - Surface may become brownish over time or in pits and fissures.
- Remineralization: At this stage, the dental hygienist and patient are central to preventing progression of the lesion with meticulous daily oral biofilm removal and remineralization. Approaches to control and management of caries are discussed in more detail in Chapter 25.
- Chapter 34 shows examples of levels of concentration of fluoride in surface enamel and in a white demineralized area.

B. ICCMS Moderate Stage Caries or CCS Moderate Caries Lesion

- In this stage, the lesion has progressed to localized breakdown of the enamel.[4,5,25]
- Breakdown of enamel over the demineralized area: Visible to observation with localized breakdown of enamel or an underlying dark shadow with transillumination. Radiographically, the radiolucency extends into the dentin.
- Progression of carious lesion: Follows general direction of enamel rods.

CLASSIFICATION: LOCATION	APPEARANCE	METHOD OF EXAMINATION
Class I. Cavities in pits or fissures a. Occlusal surfaces of premolars and molars b. Facial and lingual surfaces of molars c. Lingual surfaces of maxillary incisors	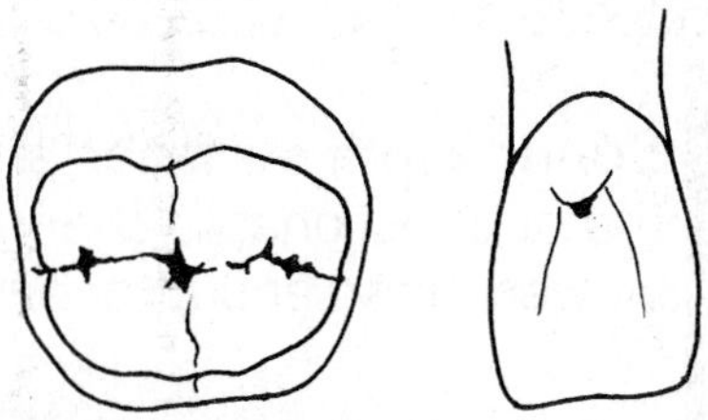	Direct or indirect visual Radiographs not useful
Class II. Cavities in proximal surfaces of premolars and molars	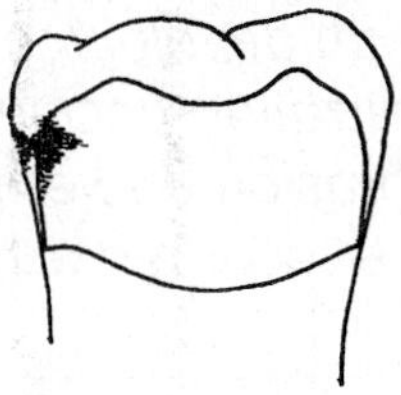	Early caries: by radiographs only Moderate caries not broken through from proximal to occlusal: 1. Visual by color changes in tooth and loss of translucency. 2. Radiograph Extensive caries involving occlusal: direct visual
Class III. Cavities in proximal surfaces of incisors and canines that do not involve the incisal angle	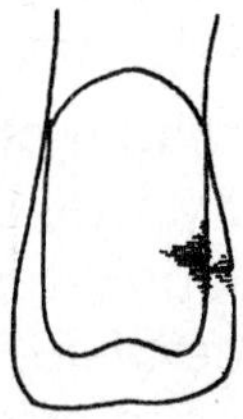	Early caries: by radiographs or transillumination Moderate caries not broken through to lingual or facial: 1. Visual by tooth color change 2. Radiograph Extensive caries; direct visual
Class IV. Cavities in proximal surfaces of incisors or canines that involve the incisal angle	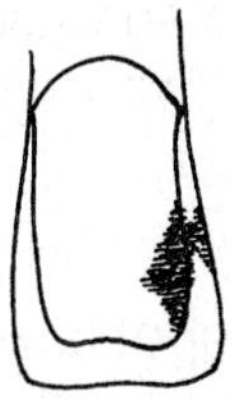	Visual Transillumination
Class V. Cavities in the cervical 1/3 of facial or lingual surfaces (not pit or fissure)	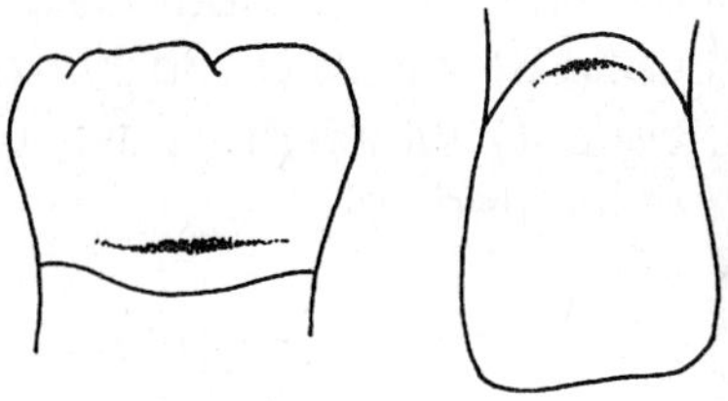	Direct visual: dry surface for vision Dull probe to distinguish demineralization: whether rough or hard and unbroken Areas may be sensitive to touch
Class VI. Cavities on incisal edges of anterior teeth and cusp tips of posterior teeth	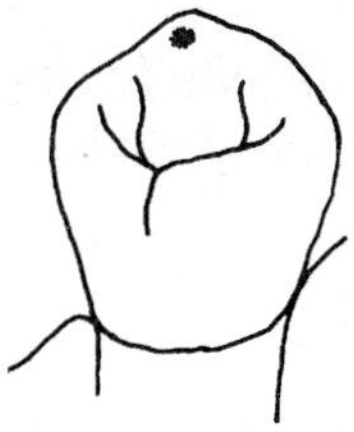	Direct visual May be discolored

Figure 16-10 G.V. Black's Classification of Carious Lesions

- Spread of carious lesion: Spreads at dentinoenamel junction; continues along the dentinal tubules (**Figure 16-12**).

C. ICCMS Extensive Stage Caries or CCS Advanced Caries Lesion

- Cavitation exposing dentin.[4,5,25]
- Radiographically, the radiolucency extends into the inner half of dentin or into the pulp.[5,25]

II. Nomenclature by Surfaces

- Simple cavity: Involves one tooth surface. Example: Occlusal cavity.
- Compound cavity: Involves two tooth surfaces. Example: Mesio-occlusal cavity, referred to as an "M-O" cavity.
- Complex cavity: Involves more than two tooth surfaces. Example: Mesio-occlusal-distal, referred to as an "M-O-D" cavity.

Definition of ICCMS™ Caries Merged categories

Caries categories		
Sound surfaces (ICDAS™ code 0)	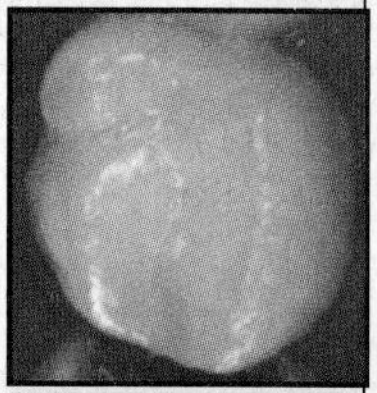 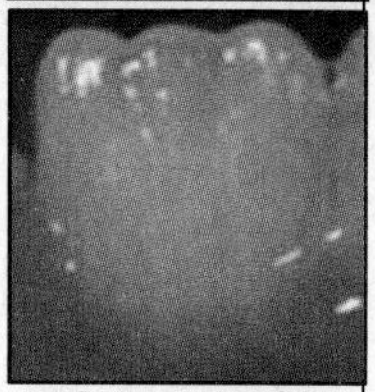	**Sound tooth surfaces** show no evidence of visible caries (no or questionable change in enamel translucency) when viewed clean and after prolonged air-drying (5 seconds). 8-9 *(Surfaces with developmental defects such as enamel hypomineralization (including fluorosis), tooth wear (attrition, abrasion and erosion), and extrinsic or intrinsic stains will be recorded as sound).*
Initial stage caries (ICDAS™ codes 1 and 2)	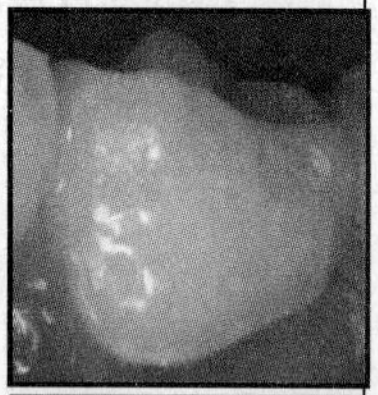 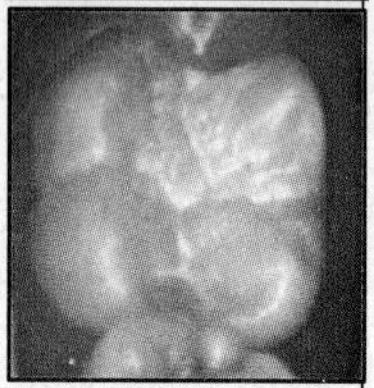	**First or distinct visual changes in enamel** seen as a carious opacity or visible discoloration (white spot lesion and/or brown carious discoloration) not consistent with clinical appearance of sound enamel (ICDAS™ code 1 or 2) and which show no evidence of surface breakdown or underlying dentine shadowing.
Moderate stage caries (ICDAS™ codes 3 and 4)	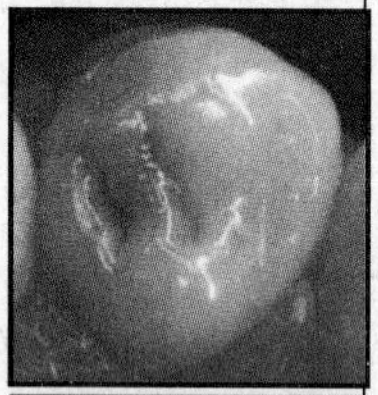 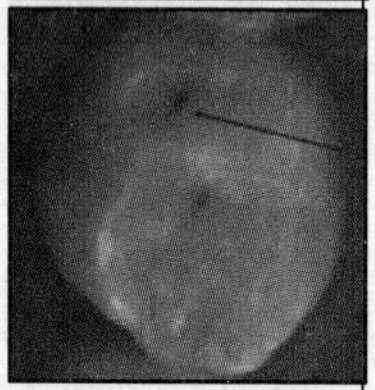	A white or brown spot lesion with **Localized enamel breakdown,** without visible dentine exposure (ICDAS™ code 3), **or an Underlying dentine shadow** (ICDAS™ code 4), which obviously originated on the surface being evaluated. *(To confirm enamel breakdown, a WHO/CPI/PSR ball-end probe can be used gently across the tooth area—a limited discontinuity is detected if the ball drops into the enamel micro-cavity/discontinuity).*
Extensive stage caries (ICDAS™ codes 5 and 6)	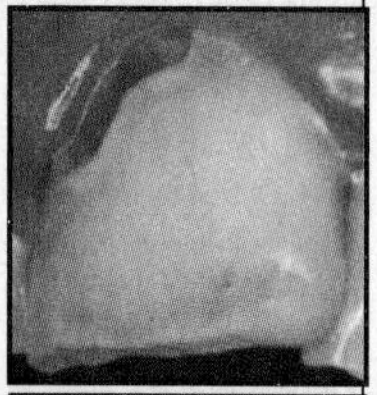 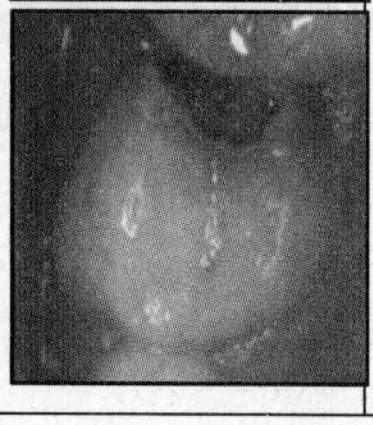	A **distinct cavity** in opaque or discolored enamel **with visible dentine** (ICDAS™ code 5 or 6). *(A WHO/CPI/PSR probe can confirm the cavity extends into dentine).*

Figure 16-11 Definition of International Caries Classification and Management System (ICCMS) Caries Categories

Reproduced from Pitts NB, Ismail AI, Martignon S, Ekstrand K, Douglas GVA, Longbottom C; ICDAS Foundation. ICCMS International Caries Classification and Management System (ICCMS) Guide for Practitioners and Educators. 2014; https://iccms-web.com/uploads/asset/592845add7ac8756944059.pdf. Accessed July 2, 2019.

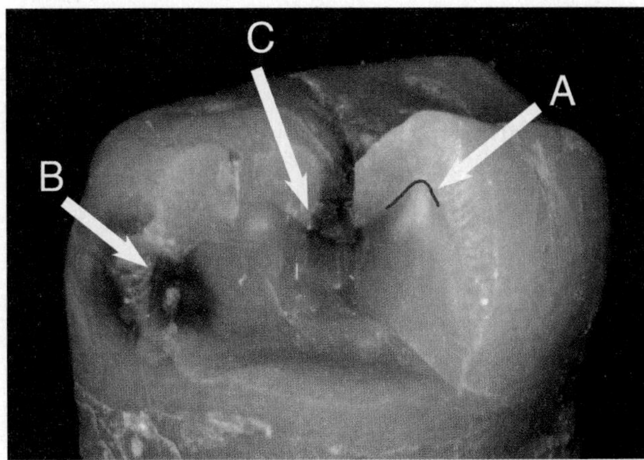

Figure 16-12 Dental Caries. The red line labeled **(A)** follows the dentinoenamel junction (DEJ) of one cusp. The arrow labeled **(B)** points to caries that began on the smooth proximal surface of the tooth enamel, showing that when it reaches dentin, it spreads out along the DEJ. The arrow labeled **(C)** points to pit and fissure caries, which began in the occlusal pit (almost hidden from view clinically) showing that once it reaches dentin, it also spreads out at the DEJ.

Reproduced from Weiss G, Scheid R. *Woelfel's Dental Anatomy*. 8th ed. Philadelphia, PA: Lippincott Williams & Wilkins; 2012.

III. Types of Dental Caries

A. Pit and Fissure

- Caries begins in a minute fault in the enamel.
- Pit or fissure irregularity occurs where three or more lobes of the developing tooth join; closure of the enamel plates is imperfect. Examples: occlusal pits of molars and premolars.

B. Smooth Surface

- Caries begins in smooth surfaces where there is no pit, groove, or other defect.
- It occurs in areas where dental biofilm is protected from removal, such as proximal tooth surfaces, protected areas near a contact, cervical thirds of teeth, and other difficult-to-clean areas.

C. Primary

- Occurs on a surface not previously affected.
- Also called initial caries.
- Early lesions may be referred to as **incipient caries**.

D. Recurrent

- Occurs on a surface adjacent to a restoration.
- **Recurrent caries** may become very involved because it can be difficult to detect radiographically and clinically.

E. Arrested

- Carious lesion that has not changed and does not show a tendency to progress further.
- Frequently has a hard surface and takes on a dark brown or reddish-brown color.

F. Rampant Caries

- Sudden, rapidly spreading caries resulting in early pulp involvement in which typically 10 or more new lesions occur each year on tooth surfaces not typically affected.
- The three types include early childhood, adolescent, and xerostomia-induced **rampant caries**.
- Restoration is often challenging due to the deep, burrowing nature of the decay.

Early Childhood Caries

- Early childhood caries (ECC) is one or more decayed, missing, or filled primary tooth surface in a child younger than the age of 6 years.[22,26]
    - Other names for the condition include nursing bottle mouth, baby bottle syndrome, baby bottle tooth decay, and prolonged nursing habit.
- Common risk factors are enamel defects, increased consumption of fermentable carbohydrates (e.g., sugary snacks/beverages, bottle at bedtime, prolonged at-will breastfeeding at night), low parental education/oral health literacy, and low socioeconomic status.[26,27] ECC is discussed in more detail in Chapter 47.

I. Microbiology

- High levels of *S. mutans* is a strong risk indicator for the initiation of ECC.[27]
- *Candida* may also be a risk factor.[27]

II. Clinical Appearance

- Demineralization begins along the cervical third of the maxillary anterior teeth as white spot lesions which then become cavitated (**Figure 16-13**).
- As the lesions progress, the caries spread to the maxillary and mandibular molars.
- Eventually, the crown of the tooth may be destroyed to the gingival margin, abscesses may develop, and the child may suffer severe pain and discomfort.

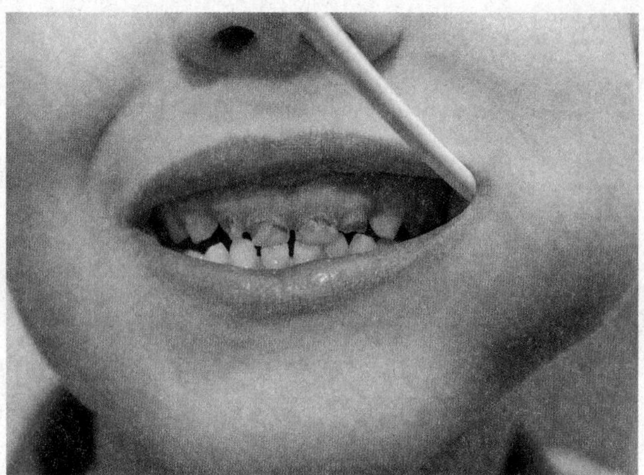

Figure 16-13 Early Childhood Caries. The lesions begin on the maxillary anterior teeth along the cervical areas and progress quickly from white spot lesions to cavitated lesions.

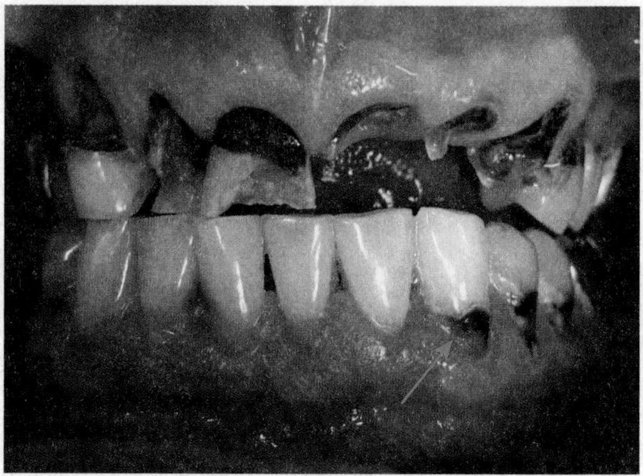

Figure 16-14 Root Caries. A root surface lesion starts near the cementoenamel junction after gingival recession has exposed the root surface. The lesion is progressive, undermining the enamel.

Courtesy of Dr. Richard J. Foster, Guilford Technical Community College, Jamestown, NC.

Root Caries

- **Root caries** is a soft, progressive lesion of cementum and dentin that involves bacterial infection, tends to be shallow, and may spread laterally below the CEJ (**Figure 16-14**).
  - It is also called cemental caries, cervical caries, or radicular caries.
- Multifactorial disease increasing in prevalence in older adults as they age and retain more natural teeth.[28]

I. Stages in the Formation of a Root Surface Lesion

The ICCMS provides criteria for the stages and activity of root caries.[4,25] The American Dental Association CCS uses the same criteria for root caries as for other caries.

A. Initial Lesion

- A clearly demarcated discoloration (light/dark brown or black) below the cementoenamel junction with no cavitation.

B. Moderate/Extensive Lesion

- Discolored (light/dark brown or black) area on the root surface with cavitation. May have a leathery texture.

II. Factors Associated with Root Caries

- A systematic review identified the following risk factors for root caries[28]:
  - Age: People are retaining their teeth longer and root surfaces become physiologically (aging) or pathologically exposed due to periodontal disease, providing a susceptible root surface.
  - Lower socioeconomic status.
  - Tobacco users.
  - History of root caries.
  - Gingival recession.
  - Poor oral biofilm removal.
  - Higher levels of *S. mutans* or lactobacilli.

Testing for Pulp Vitality

- Diagnosis of pulp vitality is made with the patient history, clinical and radiographic examinations, and diagnostic testing.
- **Pulp vitality testing** (**Figure 16-15**) may or may not be in the scope of practice for the dental hygienist within your state.
- Any tooth suspected of being nonvital needs to be tested for pulpal vitality or degree of vitality.
- The two basic types of pulp testing are thermal and electric.

I. Causes of Loss of Vitality

- A tooth may become nonvital from bacterial causes, particularly invasion of the pulp from dental caries or periodontal diseases.

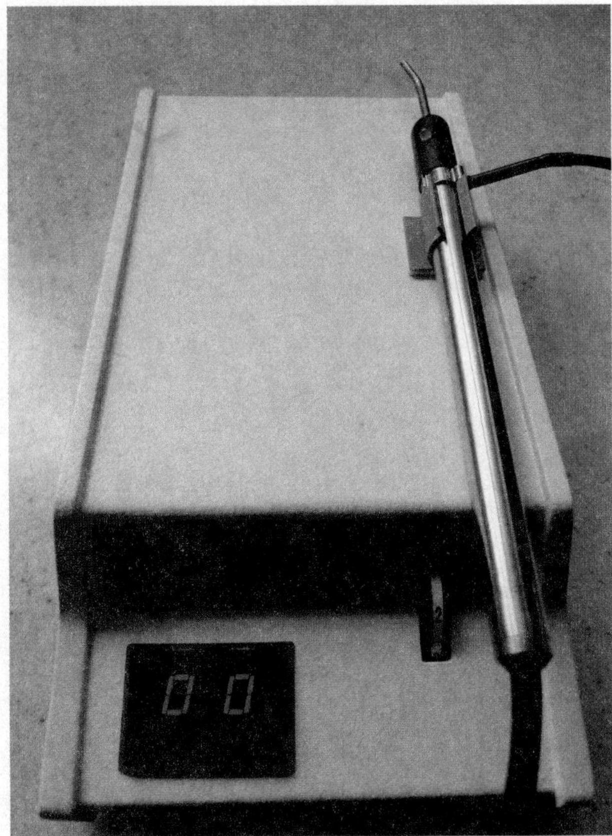

A

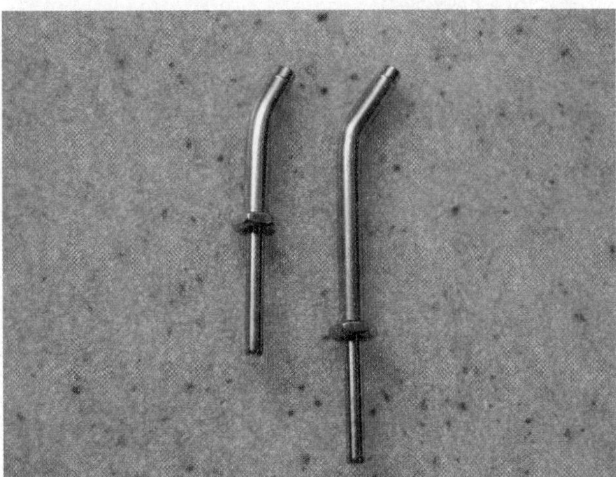

B

Figure 16-15 Pulp Testing Equipment. **A:** This is a sample electrical pulp vitality testing machine. **B:** The tips used for the vitality testing.

Courtesy of Susan Jenkins, MCPHS University Forsyth School of Dental Hygiene.

- Physical causes may be mechanical or thermal injuries. Examples of mechanical injuries are trauma, such as a blow, or iatrogenic dental procedures, such as cavity preparation or orthodontic movement done too rapidly.

II. Indications for Pulp Vitality Testing

- Pulp vitality testing may be used for the following[29]:
  - Diagnosis to assess origin of oral pain.
  - Evaluation of apical radiolucency.
  - Prior to dental procedures when pulp health may be questionable, that is, advanced dental caries.
  - Assessment following trauma or orthognathic surgery.
  - Monitoring of orthodontic procedures.

III. Response to Pulp Testing

- Pulp testing is based on the knowledge that a stimulus can create pain to which a patient will react. The pulp tester, therefore, determines the conduction of stimuli to the sensory receptors.
  - Pulp sensibility to thermal or electric stimuli is the most common method used, although there is ongoing research with other pulp vitality tests to also assess blood flow.[30]
- The vitality of the pulp depends on the density of the nerve fibers; however, recent research suggests a determination of the blood flow may be more accurate in identifying vital and necrotic pulp tissue.
- Outcomes for pulp testing:
  - Pulp is normal in response to stimuli of pulp testing.
  - Pulpitis is present as indicated by an exaggerated response to pain. Pulpitis can be reversible or irreversible.
  - There is no response because the pulp is necrotic.

IV. Thermal Pulp Testing

Cold or hot stimuli may be used. For all methods, a control test is performed on a healthy tooth on the opposite side of the arch. A positive response indicates pulpal health.[30]

- Cold testing may be accomplished with an ice, ethyl chloride on a cotton pellet, carbon dioxide, or dry ice. Isolate the test teeth and dry with gauze.
- Heat testing is done with gutta-percha or compound material heated to melting and applied directly to the tooth. This is technique sensitive and may result in overheating the pulp.

V. Electrical Pulp Tester

Electric stimuli are used to stimulate intact nerves in the pulp (Figure 16-15A and B) and are reliable in identifying healthy pulp tissue.[30] This will feel like a tingling sensation to the patient.

- The pulp tester probe is applied to the tooth in question and the intensity of the electric stimuli is gradually increased to a preselected value.
- The tooth in question is isolated (e.g., with a rubber dam) to prevent spread of the stimuli to nearby teeth.
- A digital display provides values for when the patient first feels the stimuli.
- *Note:* Studies show the use of electrical devices (e.g., ultrasonic scalers, pulp testers) in patients with cardiac implantable devices such as pacemakers produced only slight interference, but did not interfere with overall function.[31]

Occlusion

Static occlusal relationships are seen when the jaws are closed in **centric occlusion**, that is, the maximum intercuspation or contact of the teeth of the opposing arches. There are a number of occlusion classification systems, but Dr. Edward Hartley Angle is credited with first describing an occlusal classification system in 1900.[32] Dr. Angle based his classification on the relationship of the first molars.

I. Normal Occlusion

Normal occlusion is the ideal mechanical relationship between the teeth of the maxillary arch and teeth of the mandibular arch with an even bilateral distribution of occlusal forces between maxillary and mandibular arches that is symmetrical (**Figure 16-16**).[32]

A. Facial Profile

- Mesognathic: Slightly protruded jaws, which give the facial outline a relatively flat appearance (straight profile) (**Figure 16-17**).

B. Molar Relation

- The mesiobuccal cusp of the maxillary first permanent molar occludes with the buccal groove of the mandibular first permanent molar.[32]
- Occlusal force is greater on the posterior teeth than on the anterior teeth.

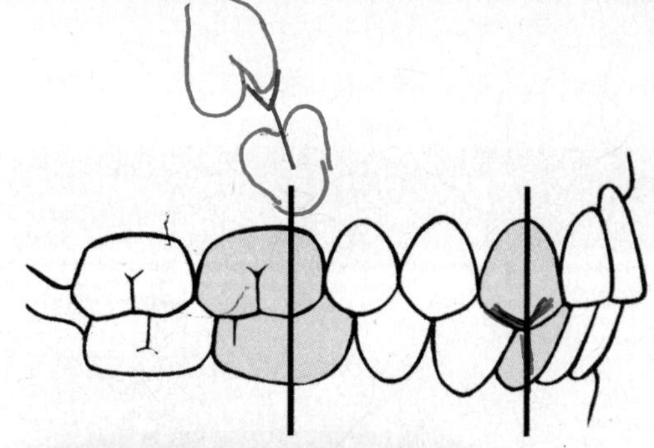

Normal (Ideal) Occlusion
Molar relationship: mesiobuccal cusp of maxillary first permanent molar occludes with the buccal groove of the mandibular first permanent molar.

Malocclusion
Class I: Neutrocclusion
Molar relationship: same as Normal, with malposition of individual teeth or groups of teeth.

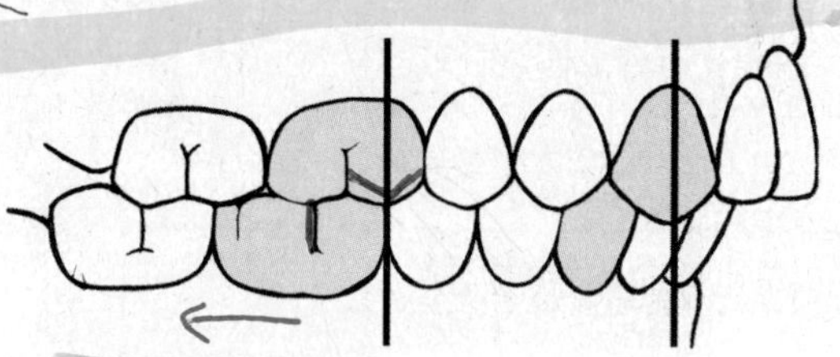

Class II: Distocclusion
Molar relationship: buccal groove of the mandibular first permanent molar is distal to the mesiobuccal cusp of the maxillary first permanent molar by at least the width of a premolar.
Division 1: mandible is retruded and all maxillary incisors are protruded.

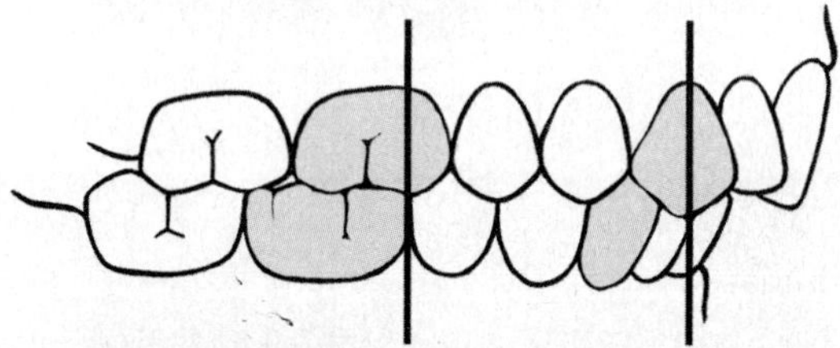

Class II: Distocclusion
Division 2: mandible is retruded and one or more maxillary incisors are retruded.

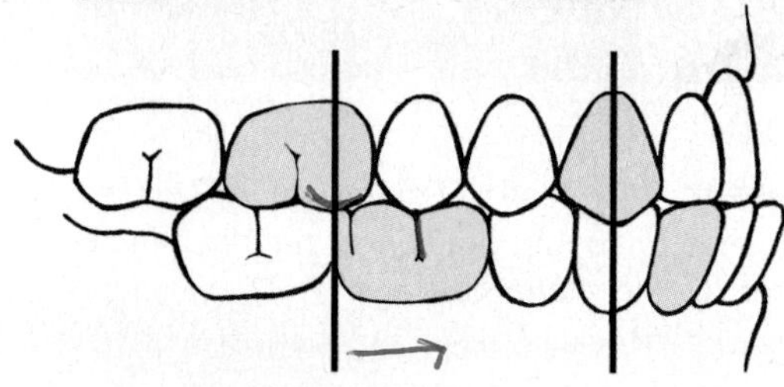

Class III: Mesiocclusion
Molar relationship: buccal groove of the mandibular first permanent molar is mesial to the mesiobuccal cusp of the maxillary first permanent molar by at least the width of a premolar.

Figure 16-16 Normal Occlusion and Classification of Malocclusion

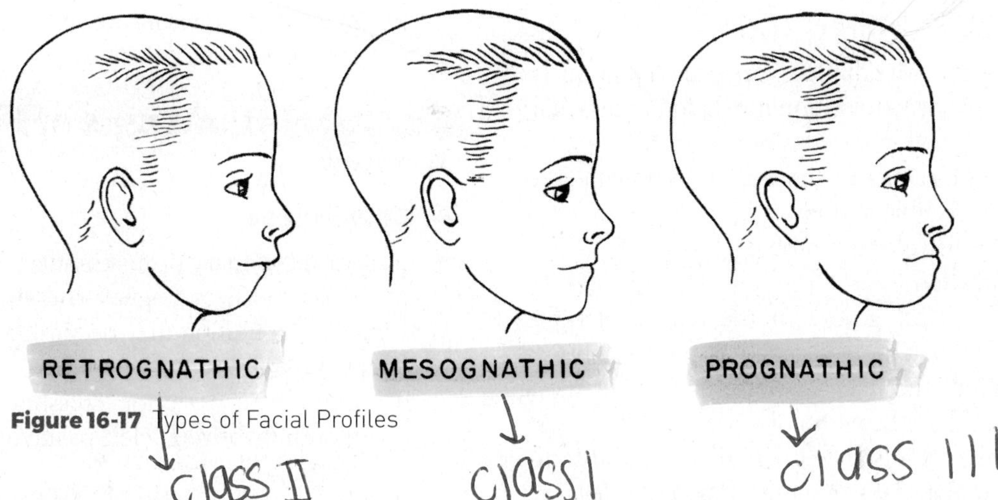

Figure 16-17 Types of Facial Profiles

C. Canine Relation

- The maxillary permanent canine occludes with the distal half of the mandibular canine and the mesial half of the mandibular first premolar.[32]

II. Malocclusion

Malocclusion is any deviation from the physiologically acceptable relationship of the maxillary arch and/or teeth to the mandibular arch and/or teeth. Because the mandible is movable and the maxilla is stationary, the classes describe the relationship of the mandible to the maxilla. Three general classes of malocclusion are described in the following sections. These classes are designated by Roman numerals (Figure 16-16).

A. Class I

- Facial profile: Mesognathic.
- Molar relation: First molars are usually in normal occlusion, but one or more may be in lingual or buccal occlusion.[32]
- Canine relation: Same as normal occlusion.
- Malposition of individual teeth or groups of teeth[32]:
  - Crowded maxillary or mandibular anterior teeth.
  - Protruded or retruded maxillary incisors.
  - Anterior or posterior crossbite.
  - Mesial drift of molars resulting from premature loss of teeth.

B. Class II

- Description: Mandibular teeth posterior (or distal) to normal position in their relation to the maxillary teeth. This class has two divisions.[32]
- Facial profile: Retrognathic with a prominent maxilla and a mandible posterior to its normal relationship (convex profile). Lower lip is full and often rests between the maxillary and mandibular incisors and the mandible appears retruded (Figure 16-17).
- Molar relation
  - The buccal groove of the mandibular first permanent molar is distal to the mesiobuccal cusp of the maxillary first permanent molar by at least the width of a premolar.[32]
  - When the distance is less than the width of a premolar, the relation is classified as *tendency toward Class II*.
- Canine relation
  - The distal surface of the mandibular canine is distal to the mesial surface of the maxillary canine by at least the width of a premolar.[32]
  - When the distance is less than the width of a premolar, the relation is classified as *tendency toward Class II*.
- *Class II, Division 1*
  - Description: The maxillary arch is narrow and lengthened with protruding maxillary incisors.[32]
  - General types of conditions that frequently occur in Class II, Division 1 malocclusion: Deep overbite, excessive overjet, abnormal muscle function (lips), short mandible, or short upper lip.
- *Class II, Division 2*
  - Description: Less narrowing of the maxillary arch, and the mandible is retruded with one or more maxillary incisors are retruded or lingually inclined.[32]
  - General types of conditions that frequently occur in Class II, Division 2 malocclusion: Maxillary lateral incisors protrude while both central incisors retrude, crowded maxillary anterior teeth, or deep overbite.[32]

C. Class III

- Description: Mandibular teeth are anterior (or mesial) to normal position in relation to maxillary teeth.[32]
- Facial profile: Prognathic with a prominent, protruded mandible and lower lip and normal (usually) maxilla (concave profile) (Figure 16-17).
- Molar relation
  - The buccal groove of the mandibular first permanent molar is mesial to the mesiobuccal cusp of the maxillary first permanent molar by at least the width of a premolar.[32]
  - When the distance is less than the width of a premolar, the relation is classified as *tendency toward Class III*.
- Canine relation
  - The distal surface of the mandibular canine is mesial to the mesial surface of the maxillary canine by at least the width of a premolar.[32]
  - When the distance is less than the width of a premolar, the relation is classified as *tendency toward Class III*.
- General types of conditions that occur in Class III malocclusion
  - True Class III: Maxillary incisors are lingual to mandibular incisors in an anterior crossbite (**Figure 16-18**).
  - Maxillary and mandibular incisors are in edge-to-edge occlusion.
  - Mandibular incisors are very crowded but lingual to maxillary incisors.

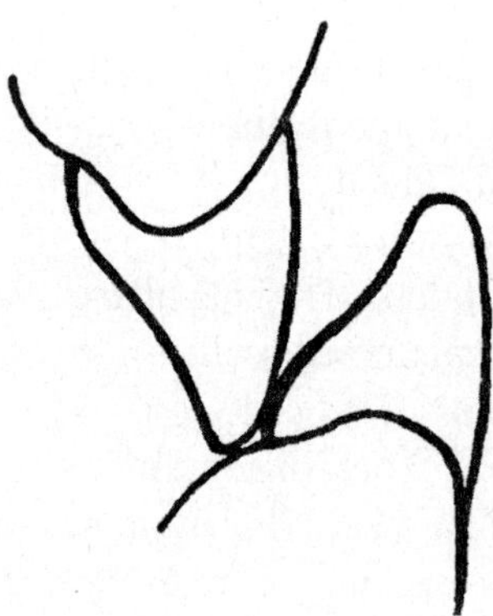

Figure 16-18 Anterior Crossbite. Maxillary anterior teeth are lingual to mandibular anterior teeth. Anterior crossbite occurs in Angle's Class III malocclusion.

III. Malrelationships of Dental Arches

A. Crossbites

- *Posterior:* Maxillary or mandibular posterior teeth are either facial or lingual to their normal position. This condition may occur bilaterally or unilaterally (**Figure 16-19**).
  - Causes of posterior crossbite can include mouth breathing, cleft palate/lip, and thumb sucking.[33]
- *Anterior:* Maxillary incisors are lingual to the mandibular incisors (Figure 16-18).

B. Edge-to-Edge Bite

Incisal surfaces of maxillary anterior teeth occlude with incisal surfaces of mandibular teeth instead of overlapping as in normal occlusion (**Figure 16-20**).

C. End-to-End Bite

Molars and premolars occlude cusp-to-cusp as viewed mesiodistally (**Figure 16-21**).

D. Open Bite

Lack of occlusal or incisal contact between certain maxillary and mandibular teeth because either or both have failed to reach the line of occlusion. The teeth will not come together, and a space remains as a result of the arching of the line of occlusion (**Figure 16-22**).

E. Overjet

The horizontal distance between the labioincisal surfaces of the mandibular incisors and the linguoincisal surfaces of the maxillary incisors (**Figure 16-23**).

- One way to measure the amount of overjet is to place the tip of a periodontal probe on the labial surface of the mandibular incisor and, holding it horizontally against the incisal edge of the maxillary tooth, read the distance in millimeters.

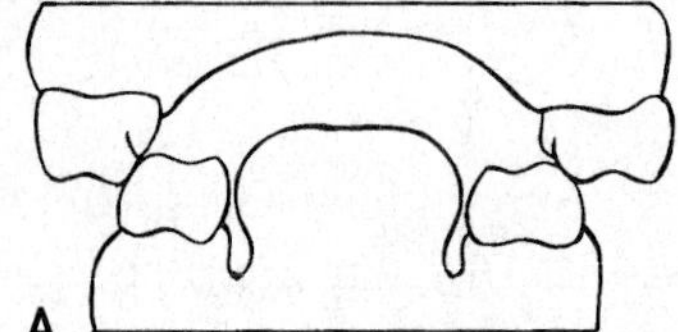

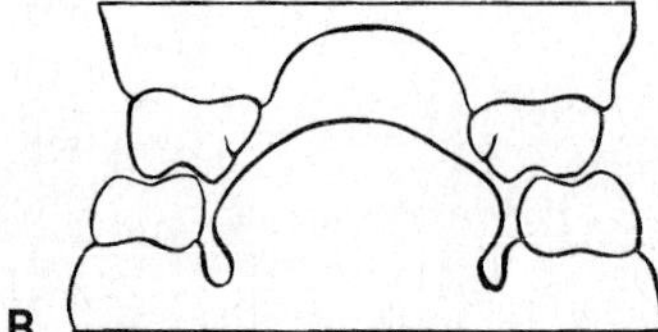

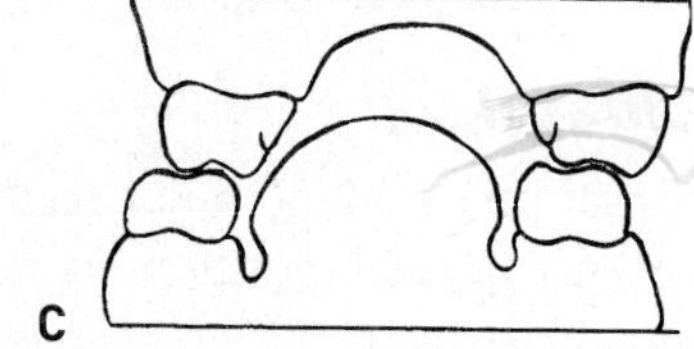

Figure 16-19 Posterior Crossbite. **A:** Mandibular teeth lingual to normal position. **B:** Mandibular teeth facial to normal position. **C:** Unilateral crossbite: Right side, normal; left side, mandibular teeth facial to normal position.

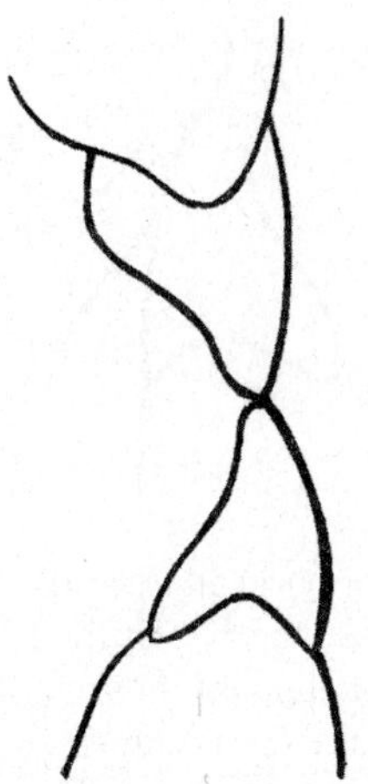

Figure 16-20 Edge-to-Edge Bite. Incisal surfaces occlude.

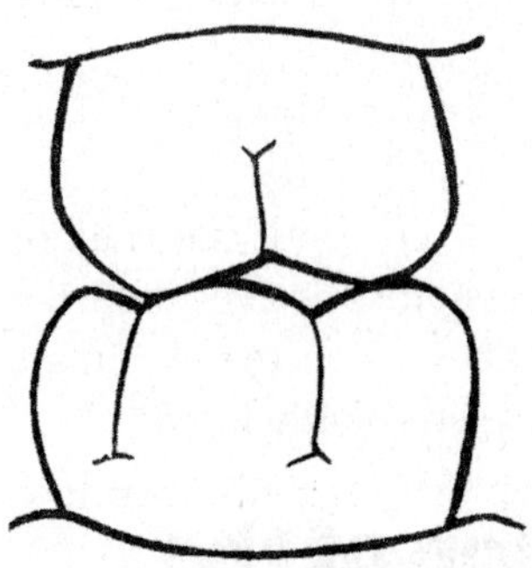

Figure 16-21 End-to-End Bite. Molars in cusp-to-cusp occlusion as viewed from the facial.

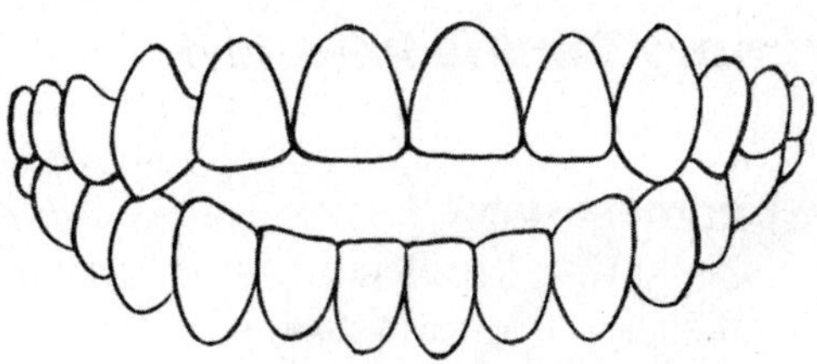

Figure 16-22 Open Bite. Lack of incisal contact. Posterior teeth in normal occlusion.

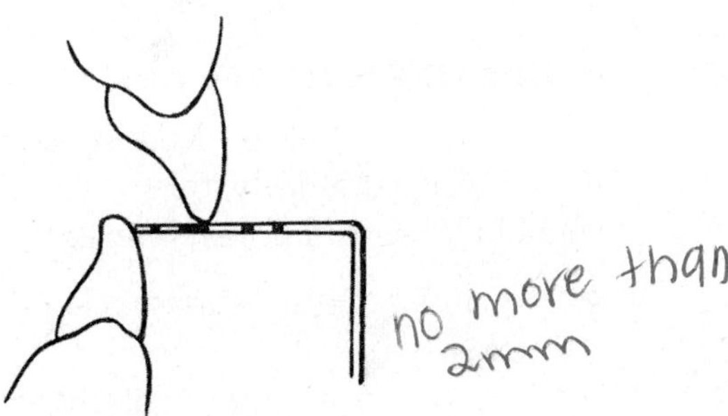

Figure 16-23 Overjet. Maxillary incisors are labial to the mandibular incisors. Measurable horizontal distance is evident between the incisal edge of the maxillary incisors and the incisal edge of the mandibular incisors. A periodontal probe can be used to measure the distance.

F. Underjet

Maxillary teeth are lingual to mandibular teeth. Measurable horizontal distance between the labioincisal surfaces of the maxillary incisors and the linguoincisal surfaces of the mandibular incisors (**Figure 16-24**).

G. Overbite

Overbite, or vertical overlap, is the vertical distance by which the maxillary incisors overlap the mandibular incisors.

- Normal overbite: An overbite is considered normal when the incisal edges of the maxillary teeth are within the incisal third of the mandibular teeth,[32] as shown in **Figure 16-25** in side view and in **Figure 16-26A** in anterior view.
- Moderate overbite: An overbite is considered moderate when the incisal edges of the maxillary teeth appear within the middle third of the mandibular teeth (**Figure 16-26B**).
- Deep (severe) overbite
  - Deep (severe): When the incisal edges of the maxillary teeth are within the cervical third of the mandibular teeth (**Figure 16-26C**).

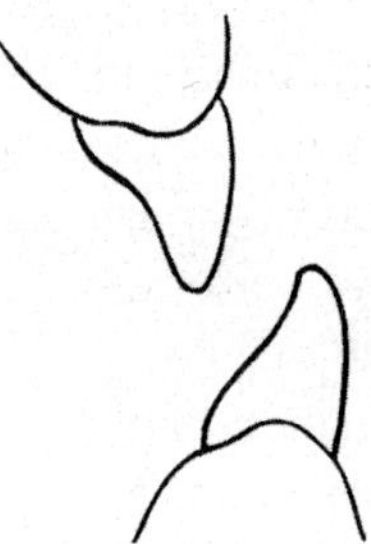

Figure 16-24 Underjet. Maxillary incisors are lingual to the mandibular incisors. Measurable horizontal distance is evident between the incisal edges of the maxillary incisors and the incisal edges of the mandibular incisors.

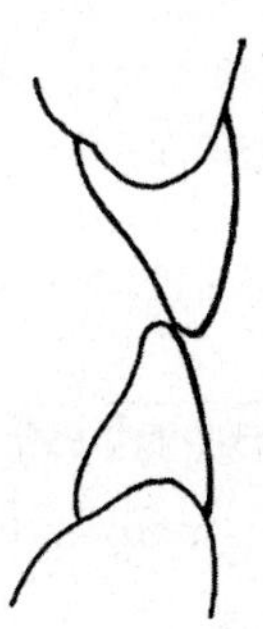

Figure 16-25 Normal Overbite. Profile view to show the position of the incisal edge of the maxillary tooth within the incisal third of the facial surface of the mandibular incisor.

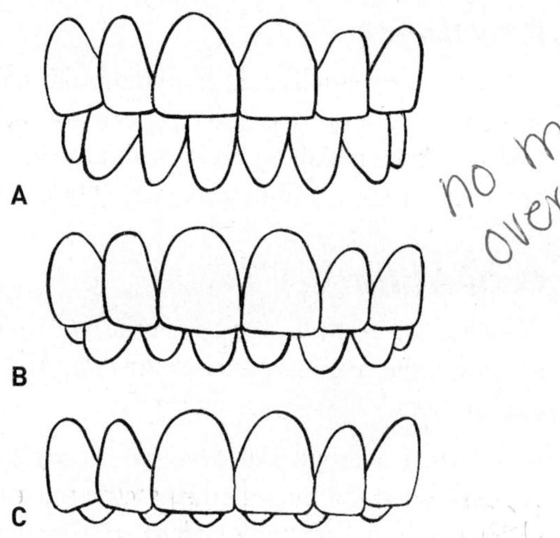

Figure 16-26 Overbite, Anterior View. **A:** Normal overbite: Incisal edges of the maxillary teeth are within the incisal third of the facial surfaces of the mandibular teeth. **B:** Moderate overbite: Incisal edges of maxillary teeth are within the middle third of the facial surfaces of the mandibular teeth. **C:** Severe overbite: The incisal edges of the maxillary teeth are within the cervical third of the facial of the mandibular teeth. When the incisal edges of the mandibular teeth are in contact with the maxillary lingual gingival tissue, the overbite is considered very severe.

- Very deep: When, in addition, the incisal edges of the mandibular teeth are in contact with the maxillary lingual gingival tissue. A side view of very deep overbite is shown in **Figure 16-27**.

- Clinical examination of overbite
    - Direct observation: With the posterior teeth closed together, the lips can be retracted and the teeth observed, as in Figure 16-27. The degree of anterior overbite is judged by the position of the incisal edge of the maxillary teeth:
    - Mirror view: By placing a mouth mirror under the incisal edge of the maxillary teeth, one can sometimes see the mandibular teeth in contact with the maxillary palatal gingiva. When contact is not visible, an examination of the lingual gingiva may reveal teeth prints or at least enlargement and redness from the contact.

IV. Malalignment of Teeth

- Malalignment or malposition refers to one or more teeth in an altered position in an otherwise normal occlusion.
- Terminology for the malalignment include:
    - Labioversion: A tooth that has assumed a position labial to normal.

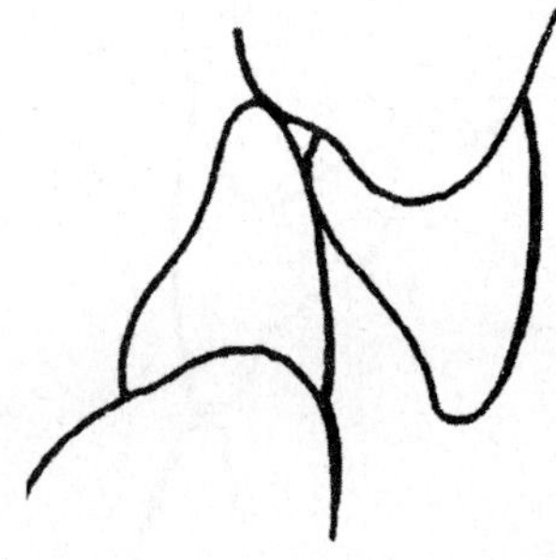

Figure 16-27 Deep (Severe) Anterior Overbite. Incisal edge of the maxillary tooth is at the level of the cervical third of the facial surface of the mandibular anterior tooth. See the facial view in Figure 16-26C.

    - Linguoversion: Tooth position is lingual to normal.
    - Buccoversion: Tooth position is buccal to normal.
    - Supraversion: Elongated above the line of occlusion.
    - Torsiversion: Tooth is turned or rotated.
    - Infraversion: Tooth is depressed below the line of occlusion (e.g., primary tooth that is submerged or ankylosed).

Occlusion of the Primary Teeth

I. Normal Occlusion

A. Primary Canine Relation

Same as permanent dentition.

- *With* **primate space**[34]:
    - Mandibular: Between mandibular canine and first molar (**Figure 16-28A**).
    - Maxillary: Between maxillary lateral incisor and canine (**Figure 16-28B**).
- *Without primate spaces:* Closed arches put the child at risk for crowding of the permanent dentition.

B. Second Primary Molar Relation

The mesiobuccal cusp of the maxillary second primary molar occludes with the buccal groove of the mandibular second primary molar.

- Variations in distal surface relationships: Terminal step.
    - The distal surface of the mandibular primary molar is mesial to that of the maxillary, thereby forming a mesial step (**Figure 16-29A**).
    - Morphologic variation in molar size; maxillary and mandibular primary molars have approximately the same mesiodistal width.

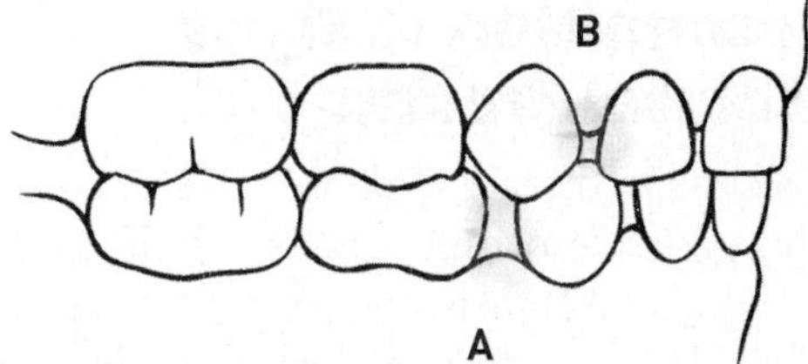

Figure 16-28 Primary Teeth with Primate Spaces. **A:** Mandibular primate space between the canine and the first molar. **B:** Maxillary primate space between the lateral incisor and the canine.

- Variation: Terminal plane.
  - The distal surfaces of the maxillary and mandibular primary molars are on the same vertical plane (**Figure 16-29B**).
  - The maxillary molar is narrower mesiodistally than the mandibular molar (occurs in many patients).
- Effects on occlusion of first permanent molars
  - Terminal step: First permanent molar erupts directly into proper occlusion (Figure 16-29A).
  - Terminal plane: First permanent molars erupt end to end. With mandibular primate space, early mesial shift of primary molars into the primate space occurs, and the permanent mandibular molar shifts into proper occlusion. Without primate spaces, late mesial shift of permanent mandibular molar into proper occlusion occurs, following **exfoliation** of second primary molar (Figure 16-29B).

II. Malocclusion of the Primary Teeth

Same as permanent dentition.

Dynamic or Functional Occlusion

In contrast to static occlusion, which pertains to the relationship of the teeth when the jaws are closed, dynamic (or functional) occlusion consists of all contacts during chewing, swallowing, or other normal action.

- Dynamic occlusion has two guidance systems[35]:
  - The posterior guidance system of the mandible is the temporomandibular joint.
  - The anterior guidance is provided by the canines during lateral excursion of the mandible.
- Masticatory (chewing) performance or efficiency depends on the type and severity of malocclusion as well as the number and location of teeth.[36]

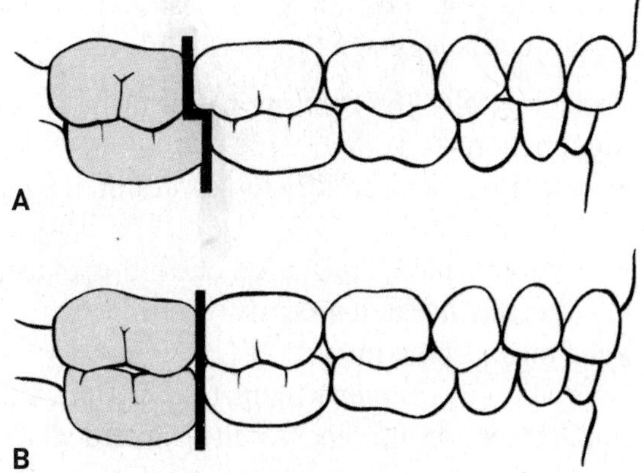

Figure 16-29 Eruption Patterns of the First Permanent Molars. **A:** Terminal step. The distal surface of the mandibular second primary molar is mesial to the distal surface of the maxillary primary molar. **B:** Terminal plane. The distal surfaces of the mandibular and maxillary second primary molars are on the same vertical plane; permanent molars erupt in end-to-end occlusion.

I. Types of Occlusal Contacts

A. Functional Contacts

Functional contacts are the normal contacts that are made between the maxillary teeth and the mandibular teeth during chewing and swallowing.

B. Parafunctional Activity

Parafunctional describes abnormal or deviated function.

- Pathologic wear occurs as a result of parafunctional activity and may result in[37]:
  - Accelerated tooth wear creating facets and attrition.
  - Pulpal involvement.
  - Tooth movement changing interocclusal relationships.
- Etiology may include:
  - Tooth-to-tooth contact: Clenching and bruxism.
  - Tooth-to-hard-object contacts: Nail biting; occupational use of such objects as tacks or pins; use of smoking equipment, such as a pipe stem or hard cigarette holder.
  - Tooth-to-oral-tissues contacts: Lip or cheek biting.

II. Proximal Contacts

Proximal contacts or interproximal interface is the common boundary of two adjacent teeth. It is dynamic and varies with age, crowding, masticatory (chewing) force, and tooth alignment.

- Physiologically, the contacts perform the following functions[38]:
  - Dissipates masticatory forces around the dental arch.
  - Prevents mesial migration or drifting of teeth.
  - Protects the arch integrity.
  - Prevents food impaction.
- Aberration in proximal contacts can ultimately impact bone health and result in interdental crestal bone loss and periodontal breakdown in the col area.[38]

Trauma from Occlusion

Trauma to the periodontium by dynamic (or functional) or parafunctional forces that exceed the adaptive and reparative capacities is called **occlusal trauma**.[39]

I. Types of Occlusal Trauma

- Historically, occlusal trauma has been classified as follows[39]:
  - *Primary occlusal trauma* results from excessive occlusal force on a tooth with normal bone support.
  - *Secondary occlusal trauma* results when normal or abnormal occlusal forces are placed on a tooth with bone loss and inadequate alveolar bone support.
- There has been controversy that the effects on the periodontium are similar with primary and secondary occlusal trauma and the following types are more descriptive:
  - Acute trauma from occlusion happens unexpectedly as a result of biting on a hard object.
  - Chronic trauma from occlusion is an ongoing, long-term pathology.

II. Effects of Trauma from Occlusion

The main purpose of the oral attachment apparatus (PDL, cementum, and alveolar bone) is to keep the tooth in the socket in a functional state. In a healthy situation, occlusal pressures and forces during chewing and swallowing are readily dispersed or absorbed and no unusual effects are produced.

- However, secondary occlusal trauma may be a factor in the rate of progression of existing periodontal disease.[39]

III. Recognition of Signs of Occlusal Trauma

No one clinical or radiographic finding clearly defines the presence of trauma from occlusion. Diagnosis of the condition is complex. Clinical findings listed here are recorded for evaluation and correlation with the patient history and all other clinical determinations.

A. Clinical Findings Associated with Occlusal Trauma

- Clinical signs of occlusal trauma[39]:
  - Progressive change in tooth mobility.
  - **Fremitus** is movement of the teeth subjected to dynamic or functional occlusion. It can be assessed by gently palpating the buccal aspect of the teeth as the patient taps up and down.
  - Discomfort or sensitivity of teeth to pressure, chewing, and/or percussion.
  - Tooth drifting or **pathologic migration**.
  - Fractured teeth.
- Radiographic signs of occlusal trauma[39]:
  - Thickening of the lamina dura. Note: Thickened lamina dura is frequently associated with teeth that have undergone orthodontic treatment and may not be associated with occlusal trauma.
  - Widening of PDL space, particularly angular thickening (triangulation).
  - Root resorption.

Study Models

A **study model** provides a life-size reproduction of the teeth, gingiva, and adjacent structures, which can be used in the assessment and care of a patient (**Figure 16-30**).

- The study models, radiographs, and clinical examination with recordings and chartings, together with the medical and dental histories, are utilized in the diagnosis, comprehensive care planning, and treatment.

I. Purposes and Uses

- Serve as a permanent record of the patient's present condition, including:
  - Existing and missing teeth.
  - Tooth position and tooth anatomy.

- Position, size, and shape of the gingiva and interdental papillae.
- Position of frena.

- During examination of the occlusion, to observe the static relations (Angle's classification, malrelationship of dental arches, and malalignment of individual teeth) and other features, such as wear patterns and the effects of premature loss of teeth.

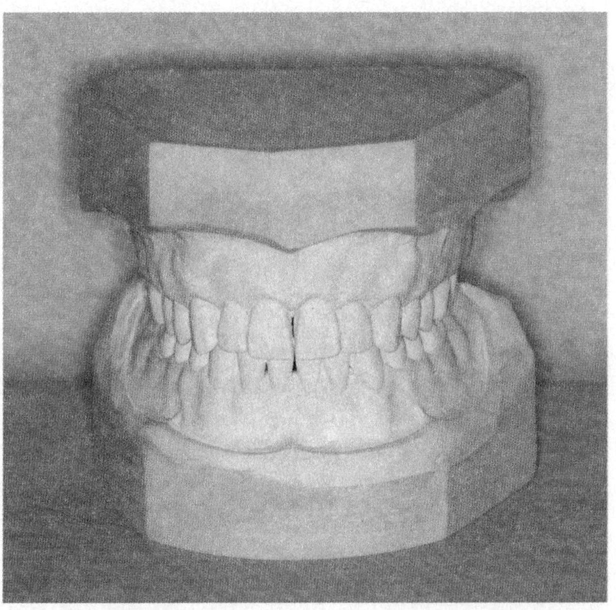

Figure 16-30 Trimmed and Finished Study Models

- An effective visual aid to use when the oral conditions are explained and the dental and dental hygiene care plans are presented; to enable the patient to visualize and understand the need for the specific care outlined.
- Provide assistance during forensic examination along with dental charting and radiographs.

The Interocclusal Record

I. Purposes

- **Interocclusal record** or *bite registration* relates the maxillary and mandibular models correctly.
- Many, if not most, models orient to each other readily in only one position.
- When such problems as open bite, crossbite, **edentulous** areas, or end-to-end (or edge-to-edge) relations interfere with direct occlusion of the models, a bite registration is needed.
- Placed between the models during trimming and storage to prevent breakage of the model teeth.

Documentation

Documentation of the findings from the hard tissue examination includes existing and missing teeth, existing restorations, white spot and cavitated carious lesions, noncarious lesions, NCCLs, and fractures (see **Figure 16-31**). In addition, occlusal findings are also

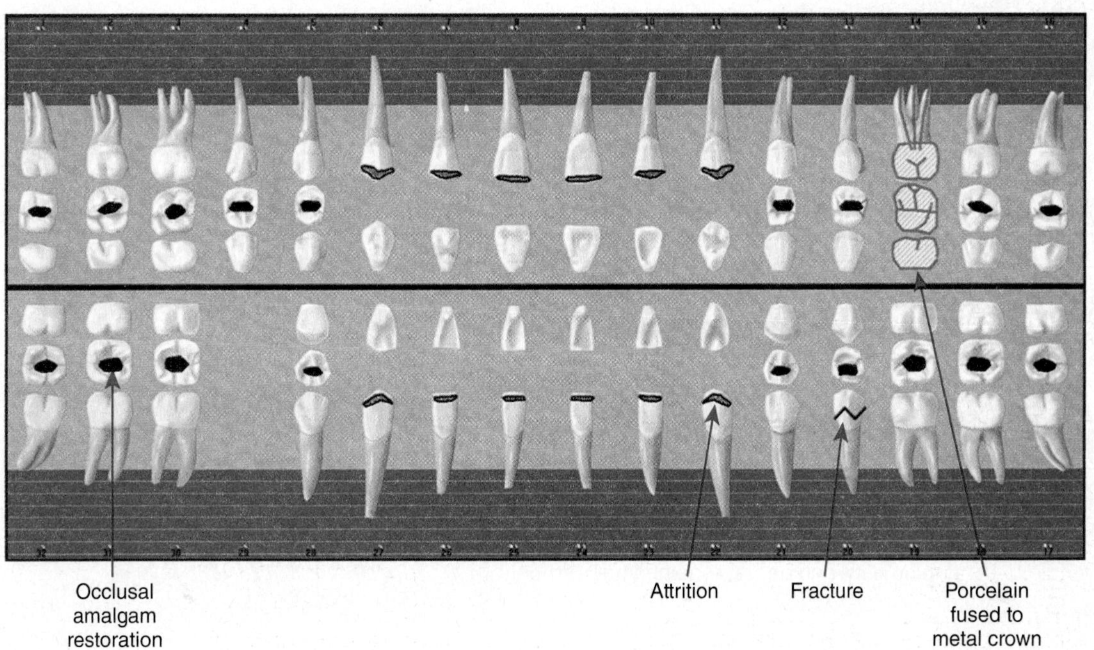

Figure 16-31 Sample Dental Charting. This is an example of dental charting. Symbols and colors used for various conditions will vary between offices/clinics.

recorded in the patient dental chart. In addition to charting conditions, the following should be documented in the clinical notes:

- If study models and interocclusal record are indicated, this should also be documented in the chart notes.
- Record occlusal habits including bruxism, clenching, or other parafunctional habits along with any patient reports of discomfort associated with these habits.
- Previous orthodontic treatment; dates, patient report of satisfaction.
- Sample progress notes are included in **Box 16-1** and **Box 16-2**.

Factors to Teach the Patient

- Education on the benefits (function and esthetics) of orthodontic care to patients referred by the dentist to an orthodontist.
- Impact of chewing (masticatory) efficiency on food selection in the diet, which impact nutritional status and health.
- Education on the need to correct oral habits with negative impacts on oral health.
- The space-maintaining function of the primary teeth in prevention of malocclusion of the emerging permanent teeth in children.
- The role of malocclusion as a predisposing factor for dental biofilm retention increasing the risk of dental caries and periodontal infections.
- Dental biofilm removal methods for reducing dental calculus and soft deposit retention in areas where teeth are crowded, displaced, or otherwise not in normal occlusion.
- The relation of the occlusion and the position of the teeth to the patient's selection of oral self-care products such as interdental aids.
- Need for continuing care appointments related to malocclusion and while in the process of having orthodontic therapy.

Box 16-1 Example Documentation: The Patient with Noncarious Tooth Lesions

- **S**—An 87-year-old male patient presents for new patient examination. He states, "My lower front teeth seem to be wearing away. About a month or so ago, I noticed some pieces chipped off my upper front tooth. In fact two of them are feeling kind of sharp." Further questioning revealed his wife reported he grinds his teeth at night and he states he often chews on a pencil while working on his daily crossword puzzle.
- **O**—Generalized advanced attrition and enamel fractures on 7, 8, and 9.
- **A**—Patient needs referral for comprehensive dental diagnosis and treatment plan.
- **P**—Discussed risk to oral health status related to oral habits such as grinding and biting on hard objects. Answered patient questions about potential treatment options. Provided assurance that the dentist would thoroughly discuss the specific options best for the patient's particular circumstances. Referred to attending dentist for diagnosis and treatment planning.

Signed: ____________________, RDH
Date: ____________________

Box 16-2 Example Documentation: Patient Needing Orthodontic Referral

- **S**—A 9-year-old female patient, accompanied by her mother, presents for routine continuing care and oral examination. Chief complaint: Mother states, "Since the last time we saw you, I notice her teeth are all coming in crooked and her smile seems lopsided to me. Does she need to see an orthodontist?"
- **O**—No changes in health history; no significant extraoral, intraoral, or radiographic findings. Good tissue health and low caries risk. Occlusion classification: Class II, Division 2 with retruded maxillary incisors, maxillary left lateral incisor, and canine in buccoversion and rotated. Facial profile is normal.
- **A**—Referral for orthodontic assessment is indicated.
- **P**—Prophylaxis completed. Panoramic radiograph taken and a copy provided to the mother along with contact information for two local orthodontists who have treated our patients in the past. Discussed why her child's caries risk may be increased during orthodontic procedures and stressed the importance of maintaining the regular schedule of continuing care and dental hygiene appointments.

Signed: ____________________, RDH
Date: ____________________

References

1. Logan WHG, Kronfeld R. Development of the human jaws and surrounding structures from birth to the age of fifteen years. *J Am Dent Assoc*. 1933;20(3):379-428.
2. Schour I, McCall JO. Chronology of the human dentition. In: *Oral Histology and Embryology*. St. Louis, MO: Mosby; 1944:240.
3. Smith BH. Standards of human tooth formation and dental age assessment. In: *Advances in Dental Anthropology*. New York: Wiley-Liss Inc.; 1991:143-148.
4. Ismail AI, Pitts NB, Tellez M, et al. The International Caries Classification and Management System (ICCMS): an example of a caries management pathway. *BMC Oral Health*. 2015;15(Suppl 1):S9:9
5. Young DA, Nový BB, Zeller GG, et al. The American Dental Association Caries Classification System for clinical practice: a report of the American Dental Association Council on Scientific Affairs. *J Am Dent Assoc 1939*. 2015;146(2):79-86.
6. Seow WK. Developmental defects of enamel and dentine: challenges for basic science research and clinical management. *Aust Dent J*. 2014;59(Suppl 1):143-154.
7. Caruso S, Bernardi S, Pasini M, et al. The process of mineralisation in the development of human tooth. *Eur J Paediatr Dent*. 2016;17(4):322-326.
8. da Cunha Coelho ASE, Mata PCM, Lino CA, et al. Dental hypomineralization treatment: a systematic review. *J Esthet Restor Dent*. 2019;31(1):26-39.
9. Silva MJ, Scurrah KJ, Craig JM, Manton DJ, Kilpatrick N. Etiology of molar incisor hypomineralization: a systematic review. *Community Dent Oral Epidemiol*. 2016;44(4):342-353.
10. de La Dure-Molla M, Philippe Fournier B, Berdal A. Isolated dentinogenesis imperfecta and dentin dysplasia: revision of the classification. *Eur J Hum Genet EJHG*. 2015;23(4):445-451.
11. Rees JS, Somi S. A guide to the clinical management of attrition. *Br Dent J*. 2018;224(5):319-323.
12. Guo H, Wang T, Niu X, et al. The risk factors related to bruxism in children: a systematic review and meta-analysis. *Arch Oral Biol*. 2018;86:18-34.
13. Castroflorio T, Bargellini A, Rossini G, Cugliari G, Deregibus A. Sleep bruxism and related risk factors in adults: a systematic literature review. *Arch Oral Biol*. 2017;83:25-32. 2
14. Schlueter N, Luka B. Erosive tooth wear–a review on global prevalence and on its prevalence in risk groups. *Br Dent J*. 2018;224(5):364-370.
15. Attin T, Wegehaupt FJ. Methods for assessment of dental erosion. *Monogr Oral Sci*. 2014;25:123-142.
16. Teixeira DNR, Thomas RZ, Soares PV, Cune MS, Gresnigt MMM, Slot DE. Prevalence of noncarious cervical lesions among adults: a systematic review. *J Dent*. 2020;95:103285. 5
17. Nascimento MM, Dilbone DA, Pereira PN, Duarte WR, Geraldeli S, Delgado AJ. Abfraction lesions: etiology, diagnosis, and treatment options. *Clin Cosmet Investig Dent*. 2016;8:79-87.
18. Milosevic A. Abrasion: a common dental problem revisited. *Prim Dent J*. 2017;6(1):32-36.
19. Wiegand A, Kuhn M, Sener B, Roos M, Attin T. Abrasion of eroded dentin caused by toothpaste slurries of different abrasivity and toothbrushes of different filament diameter. *J Dent*. 2009;37(6):480-484.
20. Bourguignon C, Cohenca N, Lauridsen E, et al. International Association of Dental Traumatology guidelines for the management of traumatic dental injuries: 1. Fractures and luxations. *Dent Traumatol*. 2020;36(4):314-330.
21. Fouad AF, Abbott PV, Tsilingaridis G, et al. International Association of Dental Traumatology guidelines for the management of traumatic dental injuries: 2. Avulsion of permanent teeth. *Dent Traumatol*. 2020;36(4):331-342.
22. Machiulskiene V, Campus G, Carvalho JC, et al. Terminology of dental caries and dental caries management: consensus report of a workshop organized by ORCA and Cariology Research Group of IADR. *Caries Res*. 2020;54(1):7-14.
23. Tanner ACR, Kressirer CA, Rothmiller S, Johansson I, Chalmers NI. The caries microbiome: implications for reversing dysbiosis. *Adv Dent Res*. 2018;29(1):78-85.
24. Black GV. *A Work on Operative Dentistry*. Vol 1. 3rd ed. Chicago, IL: Medico-Dental Publishing Company; 1908.
25. Pitts NB, Ismail AI, Martignon S, Ekstrand K, Douglas GVA, Longbottom C. *ICCMS Guide for Practitioners and Educators*. King's College London Dental Institute; 2014:84.
26. Tinanoff N, Baez RJ, Diaz Guillory C, et al. Early childhood caries epidemiology, aetiology, risk assessment, societal burden, management, education, and policy: global perspective. *Int J Paediatr Dent*. 2019;29(3):238-248.
27. Thang Le VN, Kim JG, Yang YM, Lee DW. Risk factors for early childhood caries: an umbrella review. *Pediatr Dent*. 2021;43(3):176-194.
28. Zhang J, Sardana D, Wong MCM, Leung KCM, Lo ECM. Factors associated with dental root caries: a systematic review. *JDR Clin Transl Res*. 2020;5(1):13-29.
29. Tomer AK, Raina AA, Ayub F, Bhatt M. Recent advances in pulp vitality testing: a review. *Int J Appl Dent Sci*. 2019; 5:8-12.
30. Alghaithy RA, Qualtrough AJE. Pulp sensibility and vitality tests for diagnosing pulpal health in permanent teeth: a critical review. *Int Endod J*. 2017;50(2):135-142.
31. Niu Y, Chen Y, Li W, Xie R, Deng X. Electromagnetic interference effect of dental equipment on cardiac implantable electrical devices: a systematic review. *Pacing Clin Electrophysiol*. 2020;43(12):1588-1598.
32. Angle EH. *Treatment of Malocclusion of the Teeth and Fractures of the Maxillae; Angle's System*. 6th ed. Philadelphia, PA: White Dental Manufacturing Co.; 1900. //catalog.hathitrust.org /Record/007651376
33. Saghiri MA, Eid J, Tang CK, Freag P. Factors influencing different types of malocclusion and arch form: a review. *J Stomatol Oral Maxillofac Surg*. 2021;122(2):185-191.
34. Vegesna M, Chandrasekhar R, Chandrappa V. Occlusal characteristics and spacing in primary dentition: a gender comparative cross-sectional study. *Int Sch Res Not*. 2014;2014:Article ID 512680.
35. Davies S, Gray RMJ. What is occlusion? *Br Dent J*. 2001;191(5):235-245.
36. Magalhães IB, Pereira LJ, Marques LS, Gameiro GH. The influence of malocclusion on masticatory performance: a systematic review. *Angle Orthod*. 2010;80(5):981-987.
37. Alani A, Patel M. Clinical issues in occlusion–Part I. *Singapore Dent J*. 2014;35:31-38.
38. Sarig R, Lianopoulos NV, Hershkovitz I, Vardimon AD. The arrangement of the interproximal interfaces in the human permanent dentition. *Clin Oral Investig*. 2013;17(3): 731-738.
39. Fan J, Caton JG. Occlusal trauma and excessive occlusal forces: narrative review, case definitions, and diagnostic considerations. *J Periodontol*. 2018;89(Suppl 1):S214-S222.

CHAPTER 17

Dental Soft Deposits, Biofilm, Calculus, and Stain

Catherine A. McConnell, RDH, BDSc, MEd, GCCT
Linda D. Boyd, RDH, RD, EdD

CHAPTER OUTLINE

EXTRINSIC STAINS
- **I.** Yellow Stain
- **II.** Green Stain
- **III.** Black-Line Stain
- **IV.** Tobacco Stain
- **V.** Brown Stains
- **VI.** Orange and Red Stains
- **VII.** Metallic Stains

ENDOGENOUS INTRINSIC STAINS
- **I.** Pulpless or Traumatized Teeth
- **II.** Disturbances in Tooth Development
- **III.** Drug-Induced Stains and Discolorations

EXOGENOUS INTRINSIC STAINS
- **I.** Restorative Materials
- **II.** Stain in Dentin
- **III.** Other Local Causes

DOCUMENTATION

FACTORS TO TEACH THE PATIENT

REFERENCES

LEARNING OBJECTIVES

After studying this chapter, the student will be able to:

1. Define acquired pellicle and discuss the significance and role of the pellicle in the maintenance of oral health.
2. Describe the different stages in biofilm formation and identify the changes in biofilm microorganisms as biofilm matures.
3. Differentiate between the types of soft and hard deposits.
4. Recognize the factors that influence the accumulation of biofilm, calculus, and stain.
5. Explain the location, composition, and properties of dental biofilm, calculus, and stain.
6. Identify the modes of attachment of supra- and subgingival calculus to dental structure.
7. Describe the clinical and radiographic characteristics of supra- and subgingival calculus and its detection.
8. Educate patients regarding the etiology and prevention of dental biofilm, calculus, and stain.
9. Differentiate between exogenous and endogenous stains and identify extrinsic and intrinsic dental stains and discolorations.
10. Determine the appropriate clinical approaches for stain removal and maintenance.
11. Design biofilm, calculus, and stain management strategies to meet each patient's individual needs.

Dental Biofilm and Other Soft Deposits

During clinical examination of the teeth and surrounding soft tissues, soft and hard deposits are assessed. The presence of **dental biofilm** is a primary risk factor for gingivitis, inflammatory periodontal diseases, and dental caries.[1]

- The soft deposits are referred to as acquired pellicle, dental biofilm, **materia alba**, and food debris.
- A comparison of the types of dental deposits with descriptions is found in **Table 17-1**.

Acquired Pellicle

- The acquired pellicle is a thin, **acellular** tenacious film formed of proteins, carbohydrates, and lipids.[2,3]
- Pellicle is uniquely positioned at the interface between the tooth surfaces and the oral environment. It forms over exposed enamel, dentin, mucosa, and restorative materials.
- The thickness of the enamel pellicle varies from 100 to 1,300 nm and thickness of the dentin pellicle varies from 300 to 1,200 nm.[2,4]
  - Thickness is dependent on its intra-oral location, time of formation, variations between individuals, and permanent versus primary dentition.[2]
  - The pellicle is thickest near the buccal gingival margin and thinner palatally where it is exposed to the forces of the tongue.[2]

I. Pellicle Formation

- Immediately upon exposure to saliva after eruption or after all soft and hard deposits have been removed from the tooth surfaces (such as by rubber cup or air polishing), the pellicle begins to form and is fully formed within 30 to 90 minutes.[3,4]
- Composition: Primarily glycoproteins, selectively **adsorbed** by the hydroxyapatite of the tooth surface.
  - Protein components are derived from the saliva, oral mucosal cells, gingival crevicular fluid (GCF), and **microorganisms**.[3]

Table 17-1 Tooth Deposits

Tooth Deposit	Description	Derivation	Removal Method
Acquired enamel pellicle	Translucent, homogeneous, thin, structured film covering and adherent to the surfaces of the teeth, restorations, calculus, and other surfaces	Supragingival: Saliva, oral mucosa, microorganism Subgingival: Gingival crevicular fluid	Toothbrush and appropriate interdental aid such as floss
Acquired dentin pellicle[2]	Translucent, two-layer structure, adheres to exposed dentin and restorative materials	Saliva, gingival crevicular fluid, and dentinal fluid	Toothbrush and appropriate interdental aid
Microbial (bacterial) biofilm Nonmineralized	Dense, organized bacterial communities embedded in EPS matrix adheres tenaciously to the teeth, calculus, prostheses, and other surfaces in the oral cavity	Colonization of oral microorganisms	Toothbrush and appropriate interdental aid such as floss
Materia alba Nonmineralized	Loosely adherent, unstructured, white or grayish-white mass of oral debris and bacteria that lies over dental biofilm	Incidental accumulation	Vigorous rinsing and water irrigation can remove materia alba
Food debris Nonmineralized	Unstructured, loosely attached particulate matter	Food retention following eating	Self-cleansing activity of tongue and saliva Rinsing vigorously removes debris Toothbrushing, flossing, and other aids
Calculus Mineralized	Calcified dental biofilm; Hard, tenacious mass that forms on the clinical crowns of the natural teeth and on dentures and other oral appliances	Biofilm **mineralization**	
a. Supragingival	Occurs coronal to the margin of the gingiva; is covered with dental biofilm	Source of minerals is saliva	Manual instrumentation Ultrasonic instrumentation
b. Subgingival	Occurs apical to the margin of the gingiva; is covered with dental biofilm	Source of minerals is gingival crevicular fluid	Manual instrumentation Ultrasonic instrumentation

- Initial attachment of bacteria to the pellicle is by selective adherence of microorganisms and occurs about 30 minutes after pellicle formation begins.[2,3]
  - Salivary proteins have a high affinity for the hydroxyapatite tooth surface and contribute to pellicle adherence and formation.[2]

II. Types of Acquired Pellicle

A. Acquired Enamel Pellicle

- Acquired enamel pellicle (AEP) is translucent and not readily visible until application of a disclosing agent.
  - Pellicle can take on extrinsic stain and become gradations of brown, gray, or other colors.
  - When stained with a disclosing agent, pellicle appears thin, with a pale staining that contrasts with the thicker, darker staining of dental biofilm.

B. Acquired Dentin Pellicle

- Acquired dentin pellicle (ADP) occurs on dentin exposed by recession.[2]

III. Functions of Pellicle

The pellicle plays an important role in the maintenance of oral health.[2,3] The various functions of the pellicle include[2,3]:

- Regulation of mineral homeostasis
  - Protects against acid-induced enamel demineralization (this role is more limited on dentin surfaces).
  - The pellicle structure may serve as a scaffold for remineralization.
  - May protect against erosion.
- Host defense and microbial colonization
  - About 8% of the proteins in the pellicle have antimicrobial functions.

- The bacterial colonization depends on specific protein binders in the pellicle. Some protein components inhibit binding and others promote adherence.
- Bacterial adherence and aggregation begin the process of biofilm formation.

- Lubrication
    - Pellicle keeps surfaces moist and prevents drying, which in turn enhances the efficiency of speech and mastication.
    - The AEP lubricating properties may also protect against abrasive damage.

IV. Removal of Pellicle

- Pellicle is not resilient enough to withstand oral self-care.
- Extrinsic factors that may interfere with pellicle formation and **maturation** include[5]:
    - Abrasive toothpastes.
    - Whitening products.
    - Intake of acidic foods and beverages.

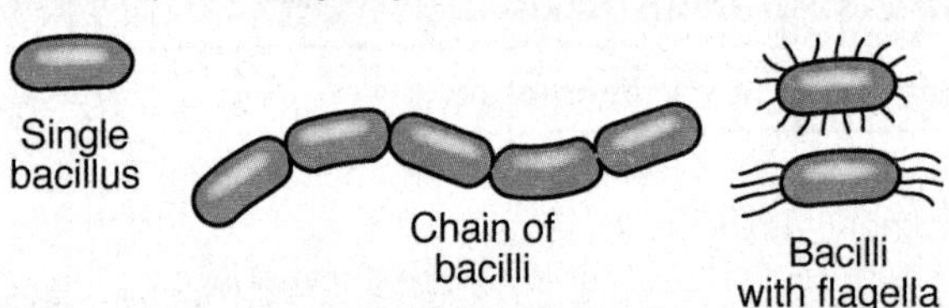

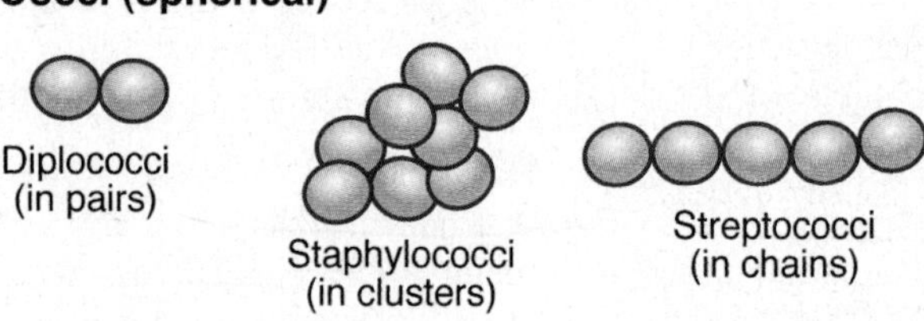

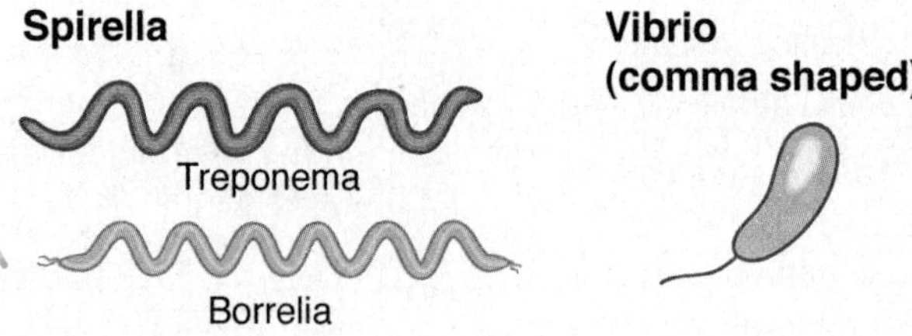

Figure 17-1 Bacilli, Cocci, Spirella, and Vibrio

Reproduced from Sakai J. *Practical Pharmacology for the Pharmacy Technician*. Baltimore, MD: Lippincott Williams & Wilkins; 2008.

Dental Biofilm

The **oral microbiome** is composed of microorganisms, their genetic makeup, and the environments found in the oral cavity.[6]

- The mouth has a number of environments, including the teeth, gingival sulcus, attached gingiva, tongue, oral mucosa, lips, and hard and soft palates, with their own microbial inhabitants.[6]
- The permanent teeth, as the only nonshedding surface in the body, serve as a unique environment for biofilm formation and maturation.[6]
- The microorganisms in the oral cavity perform both pro- and anti-inflammatory activities, which maintain homeostasis in health.[6]
- Dental biofilm is a dynamic, structured community of microorganisms, encapsulated in a self-produced **extracellular polymeric substance (EPS)** forming a **matrix** around microcolonies.
    - The matrix is composed of polysaccharides, proteins, and other compounds; it acts to protect the biofilm from the host's immune system and antimicrobial agents.
    - The microcolonies are separated by a network of open water channels that supply nutrients deep within the biofilm community.
- The three-dimensional structure of biofilms enhances their ability to communicate with each other, adapt, and respond to their environment.
- Adheres to the pellicle coating on all hard and soft oral structures, including teeth, existing calculus, and fixed and removable restorations.
- There are over 700 distinct microorganisms in the oral cavity, including bacteria, viruses, protozoa, and yeast.[6] Morphologic forms of bacteria found within biofilms are shown in **Figure 17-1**.

I. Steps in the Formation of Oral Biofilm

Biofilm formation involves a series of complex microbial interactions (**Figure 17-2**).

- The close proximity of microbial species allows for changes in gene expression, which impact the growth and capabilities of the biofilm community to cause disease.[1]

A. Step 1—Pellicle Formation

- The acquired pellicle provides the glycoproteins for microorganism adhesion.

B. Step 2—Initial Adhesion

- Biofilm formation begins with initial attachment of **planktonic** bacterial cells to the pellicle on the tooth surface.[7]

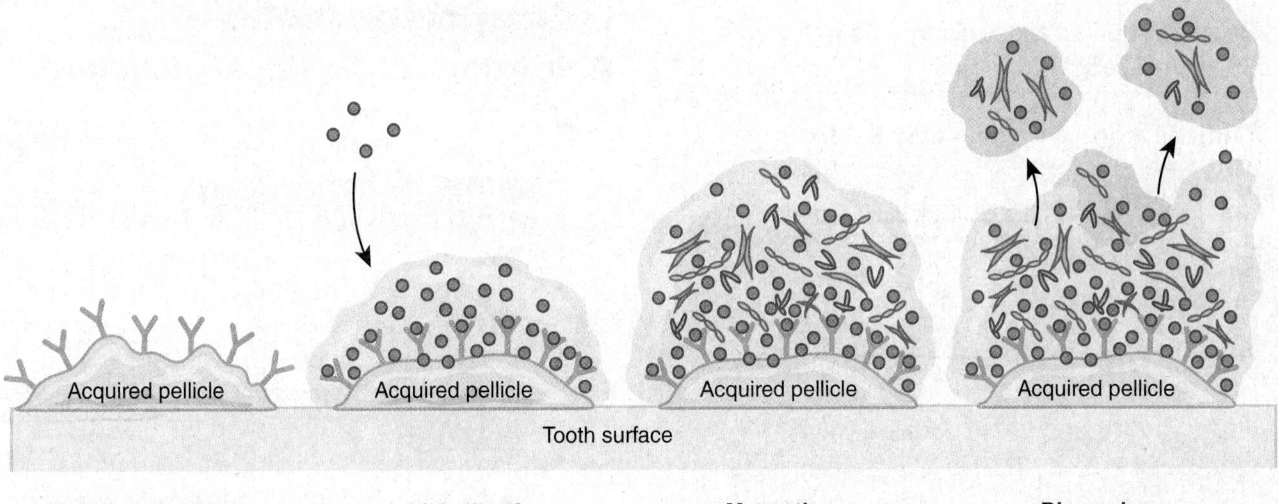

Figure 17-2 Biofilm Microorganisms

Data from Huang R, Li M, Gregory RL. Bacterial interactions in dental biofilm. Virulence. 2011 Sep 1;2(5):435-44

- Microbes attach to the pellicle by means of fimbriae and pilli along with electrostatic interactions.[8]
- Initially, the adherent cells are not "committed" to this process and it is reversible. When cells are disrupted (with oral self-care activities), they may dislodged from the surface.[7]
- The early colonizers attached to the pellicle begin to excrete extracellular polymeric substance (EPS) to help bacteria bind together (co-adhesion) and to the pellicle.[7]
  Components of the EPS include:
  - Polysaccharides, glucans, and fructans, or levans produced by certain bacteria within the community and from dietary sucrose.
  - EPS provides a scaffold to anchor the bacteria together, increasing adherence to dental and other structures and providing protection as the bacterial community continues to grow.[6]
  - EPS contains components such as antimicrobial enzymes to protect the biofilm.[6]
- At this stage, the cocci adhere to filamentous bacteria, creating structural components of biofilm such as *corn cob* or *bristle brush* forms.[6,7]

C. Step 3—Maturation

- Later colonizing bacteria attach to the early colonizers to form microcolonies.[7] The metabolism of one species of bacteria may be a source of nutrients to another species, resulting in food chains or webs within the biofilm.[1,7]
- This stage is also characterized by further development of the biofilm architecture to enhance the cell-to-cell communication process, also known as **quorum sensing**.[6]
- Quorum sensing controls the growth of the microbial community and signals microorganisms when to leave the biofilm to find new sites.[7]
- Maturation occurs by 72 hours.[6]

D. Step 4—Detachment and Dispersion

- Bacterial colonies mature and release planktonic cells to spread and colonize other areas within the oral cavity.
- Bacteria convert to motile forms in order to disperse.[7]
- Bacteria can disperse as single cells or in clumps.[7]

II. Changes in Biofilm Microorganisms

- Dental biofilm consists of a complex mixture of microorganisms in microcolonies. The microbial density is very high and increases as biofilm ages and matures.
- The potential for the development of dental caries and/or gingivitis increases with more microorganisms, especially as the numbers of **pathogenic** microorganisms outnumber the nonpathogenic microorganisms.[6,9]
- With undisrupted biofilm for approximately 7 days, gram-negative anaerobic bacteria growth is favored, which increases risk for dental caries and gingivitis, and eventually other inflammatory periodontal diseases increase.[6]

Box 17-1 Loe's Classic Gingivitis in Man Study in 1965[10]

Time Frame	Microbiologic Findings
Day 1–2	Early biofilm consists primarily of gram-positive cocci with small accumulations of **leukocytes**
Day 2–4	The cocci still dominate while increasing numbers of gram-positive filamentous form and slender rods join the surface of the cocci colonies, along with more leukocytes
Day 5–10 (on average)	Filaments increase in numbers, and a mixed **flora** appears comprising rods, filamentous forms, and fusobacteria with heavy accumulations of leukocytes
Day 10–21	Gingivitis is clinically evident in 10 to 21 days

- Although there is significant variability between individuals in the pattern of dental biofilm development, the changes in **oral flora** follow a general pattern (Figure 17-2).
- The formation of dental biofilm may vary by days of accumulation (**Box 17-1**).

Supragingival and Subgingival Dental Biofilm

Recent technology innovations in DNA sequencing and fluorescent in situ hybridization (FISH) have allowed for a more in-depth understanding of the science of biofilms.[11,12]

I. Supragingival Biofilm

- Supragingival biofilm has greater variability in architecture than subgingival biofilm and typically consists of two layers of predominantly gram-positive **aerobic** bacteria[12]:
    - The first layer (basal layer) adheres to the tooth surface and is composed of streptococci, *Actinomyces*, filamentous bacteria, yeast, and *Lactobacillus*.
    - The second layer forms on top of the basal layer and includes streptococci and *Lactobacillus*.

II. Subgingival Biofilm

A. Subgingival Biofilm Architecture

- Subgingival biofilm is made up of four layers, which includes predominantly gram-negative **anaerobic** and motile organisms. The organisms present will vary in health and disease, but may contain the following[11]:
    - The first layer (basal layer) contains bacteria such as *Actinomyces*.
    - Intermediate layers contain bacteria such as *Tannerella forsythia* and *Fusobacterium nucleatum*.
    - Top layers contain spirochetes and this is typically where the periodontal pathogens such as *Porphyromonas gingivalis and P. endodontalis* may be located.

B. Subgingival Biofilm

The subgingival microbiome is very complex, and the bacteria present in health versus disease shift to a disease-associated community.[13] There are core species of bacteria that do not change from health to disease, such as Campylobacter gracilis and Fusobacterium nucleatum ss. Vincentii.[13]

- Subgingival microbiome in health[11]
    - Primarily gram-positive cocci and rods with a few gram-negative species.
    - *Corynebacterium* aid in forming the structure of early biofilm.
    - *Rothia* are involved with cell-cell aggregation in early biofilm formation.
- Subgingival microbiome associated with gingivitis[11,13]
    - There is a greater biofilm mass with more diversity and a higher number of bacterial species in gingivitis.
    - There is a shift from gram-positive species to gram-negative aerobic organisms in gingivitis.
    - Bacteria most associated with clinical signs of gingivitis and inflammation are *Prevotella* and *Selenomonas*.
- Periodontal-associated subgingival microbiome[11,13]
    - Significant shifts in the composition of the biofilm communities occur with more bacterial species in periodontitis as compared to health. Increased diversity in the microbiome is a unique feature of periodontitis.
    - Bacteria seen in health are still present, but **dysbiosis** results in shifts to periodontitis-associated species. Periodontal

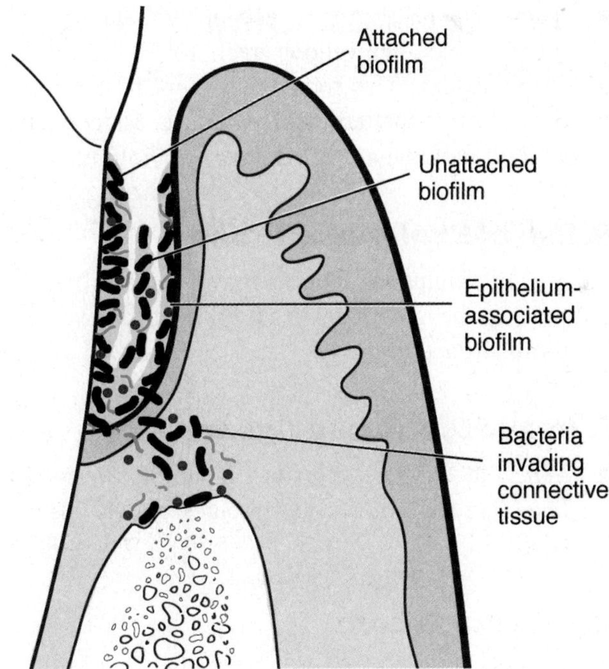

Figure 17-3 Bacterial Invasion. Diagram of a periodontal pocket shows attached and unattached biofilm (planktonic) bacteria within the pocket epithelium, in the connective tissue, and on the surface of the bone.

pathogens have been found to be present in the adjacent epithelial cells and underlying connective tissue (**Figure 17-3**).[14]

Composition of Dental Biofilm

- Microorganisms and EPS comprise 20% of the biofilm that are organic and inorganic solids. The other 80% is water.
- Composition differs among individuals and among tooth surfaces.

I. Inorganic Elements

A. Calcium and Phosphorus

- Calcium, phosphorus, and magnesium are more concentrated in biofilm than in saliva.[15]
- Saliva transports the minerals during the mineralization and demineralization processes.

B. Fluoride

- Fluoride concentration in biofilm is higher in the presence of fluoridated water, following professional topical fluoride applications, and with the use of fluoride-containing dentifrices and oral rinses for 3 to 6 hours before returning to baseline.[16]

II. Organic Elements

The organic EPS forms a scaffold for biofilm development and contains primarily polysaccharides and proteins, with small amounts of lipids.[17]

A. Polysaccharides (Carbohydrates)

- In addition to dietary sucrose and starch, polysaccharides are metabolized by bacteria such as *S. mutans* to produce glucans and fructans.[17]
- The glucans provide binding sites for microorganisms, especially *S. mutans,* which facilitates clustering and adherence of the bacteria to the tooth.[17]

B. Proteins

- The proteins of supragingival biofilm bind with glucans supporting further growth of biofilm.[17]

Clinical Aspects of Dental Biofilm

I. Distribution of Biofilm

A. Location

- *Supragingival biofilm*: Coronal to the gingival margin.
- *Gingival biofilm*: Forms on the external surfaces of the oral epithelium and attached gingiva.
- *Subgingival biofilm*: Located between the epithelial attachment and the gingival margin, within the sulcus or pocket.
- *Fissure biofilm*: Develops in pits and fissures of the teeth.

B. By Surfaces

- *During formation*
  - Supragingival biofilm formation begins at the gingival margin, particularly on proximal surfaces, and extends coronally when left undisturbed.
  - It spreads over the gingival third and on toward the middle third of the crown.
- *Tooth surfaces involved*
  - Biofilm is heaviest on lingual, posterior, and proximal surfaces.[18]
  - Anterior surfaces have the least biofilm.[18]

C. Factors Influencing Biofilm Accumulation

- Dental biofilm accumulates readily around crowded teeth as shown in **Figure 17-4**. With effective biofilm control, biofilm accumulation around crowded teeth is not greater than that around well aligned teeth.
  - Special accommodations such as using a toothbrush placed in a vertical position can remove thick biofilm on the lingual surface of the crowded mandibular anterior.
- Rough surfaces: Biofilm develops more rapidly on rough tooth surfaces, existing calculus, poorly contoured restorations, and removable appliances; thick, dense deposits can be difficult to remove.
- Occlusion: Deposits may extend over an entire crown of a tooth that is unopposed, out of occlusion, or not actively used during mastication.

D. Removal of Biofilm

- Toothbrushing and interdental cleaning are the most universal daily mechanical disruption methods.

II. Detection of Biofilm

A. Direct Vision

- *Thin biofilm:* May be translucent and therefore not visible without a disclosing agent.

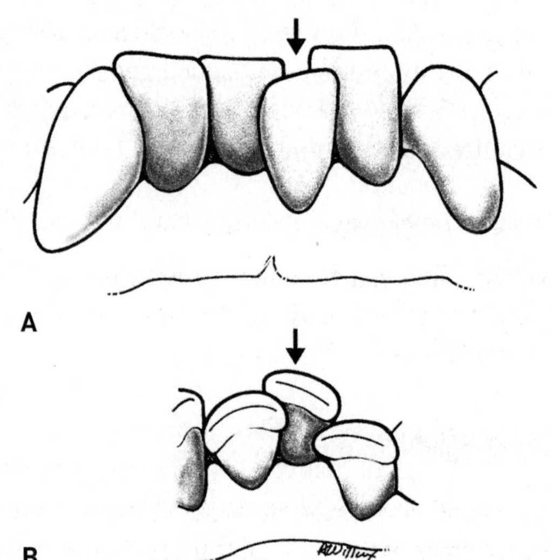

Figure 17-4 Biofilm Accumulation in Protected Areas. **A:** Crowded mandibular anterior teeth demonstrate dental biofilm after use of a disclosing agent. Thickest biofilm is on proximal surfaces and at cervical thirds of teeth. **B:** Note central incisors with thick extensive biofilm on the less accessible protected surfaces.

- *Stained biofilm:* Extrinsic stains may make biofilm more visible (e.g., yellow, green, tobacco stains).
- *Thick biofilm:* The tooth may appear dull and dingy, with a matted fur-like surface. Materia alba or food debris may collect over the biofilm.

B. Use of Explorer or Probe

- *Biofilm disruption:* Biofilm may be disturbed by passing the side of an explorer or probe over the tooth surface.

C. Use of Disclosing Agent

- When a disclosing agent is applied, biofilm takes on the color and becomes readily visible (Figure 17-4).

D. Clinical Record

- A Biofilm Control record should be used to document initial biofilm accumulation, followed by continuing changes over the treatment and follow-up appointments.
- Record biofilm by location and thickness (slight, moderate, or heavy). For objective evaluations, use of an index or a biofilm score is recommended. (See Chapter 21.)

Significance of Dental Biofilm

- Biofilm plays a major role in the initiation and progression of dental caries and periodontal diseases, caused by pathogenic microorganisms found in oral biofilms.[1]
- Biofilm is significant in the formation of **dental calculus**, which is essentially mineralized dental biofilm.

I. Dental Caries

- Dental caries is a disease of the dental calcified structures (enamel, dentin, and cementum) characterized by demineralization of the mineral components and dissolution of the organic matrix. (See Chapter 16.)
- The sequence of events leading to demineralization and dental caries is shown in **Figure 17-5**.

A. The Caries Microbiome

- Dysbiosis of the microbiome results in changes in the microbiome communities with reduced

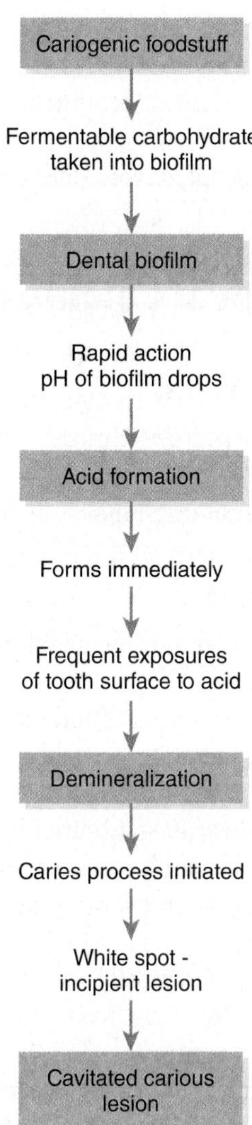

Figure 17-5 Development of Dental Caries. Flowchart shows the step-by-step action within the microbial biofilm on the tooth surface.

diversity to favor caries initiation. This dysbiosis may occur due to decreased salivary flow resulting in a reduced buffering capacity and/or frequent fermentable carbohydrate exposure.[19,20]

- Acid tolerant *S. mutans* and *S. sobrinus*, predominantly, and lactobacilli are thought to be the major bacteria associated with caries, particularly in those with poor biofilm removal without access to regular dental care.[19,21]
- For populations with lower caries rates, *S. mutans* may be lower and other acidogenic bacteria such as *Actinomyces* may be predominant.[19,21]

B. The pH of Biofilm

- Acid formation begins *immediately* once a **cariogenic** substance is taken into the biofilm, resulting in a rapid drop in the pH of the biofilm.[22]
- Critical pH for enamel demineralization averages 5.5, although other factors impact decalcification.[23]
- The critical pH for root surface demineralization may be higher because of the lower mineral content of dentin and cementum.[23]
  - The critical pH for demineralization of dentin is approximately 6.7, which is particularly relevant for patients with multiple areas of recession and xerostomia.[24]
- The extent of demineralization depends on the length of time and frequency the pH is below critical level; biofilm composition, pH-lowering ability of the microorganisms, and action of saliva are additional factors that affect the caries process.[22]

C. Effect of Diet on Biofilm

- Cariogenic foods
  - In a diet high in fermentable carbohydrates, biofilm communities shift to bacteria with higher pH-lowering ability.[22]

Materia Alba

I. Clinical Appearance and Content

- Materia alba is a soft, whitish tooth deposit that is clinically visible without application of a disclosing agent. It may have a cottage cheese–like texture and appearance.
- Materia alba is an unorganized accumulation of living and dead bacteria, desquamated epithelial cells, disintegrating **leukocytes**, salivary proteins, and food debris. This differentiates it from organized oral biofilms.

II. Prevention

- Materia alba can be removed with the basic mechanical oral self-care procedures. (See Chapters 26 and 27.)

Food Debris

- After food consumption, food remnants may collect in areas of the cervical third and proximal embrasures of the teeth.
- Vertical **food impaction** results during mastication as food is forced into open contact areas (loss of proximal contact), dental diastemas, poorly contoured restorations, or occlusal irregularities such as plunger cusps.[25]

- Left unattended, the accumulation of food debris adds to a general unsanitary condition of the mouth and may contribute to the initiation of dental caries and oral malodor.[26]

Calculus

Dental calculus is dental biofilm mineralized by crystals of calcium phosphate mineral salts between previously living microorganisms.[27]

- The calculus is covered with a layer of nonmineralized dental biofilm containing live bacteria.[27]
- The hard, tenacious mass forms on the clinical crowns of natural teeth, dental implants, dentures, and other dental prostheses.
- Dental calculus is classified by its location on a tooth surface as related to the adjacent free gingival margin, that is, *supragingival* and *subgingival* calculus as shown in **Figure 17-6**.

I. Supragingival Calculus

A. Location

- Forms on clinical crowns coronal to the margin of the gingiva.
- Forms on implants, complete and partial dentures.

B. Distribution: Most Frequent Sites

- On the lingual surfaces of mandibular anterior teeth and the facial surfaces of maxillary first and second molars, opposite the openings of the ducts of the submandibular and parotid salivary glands.
  - **Figure 17-7** shows heavy supragingival calculus forming a continuous "bridge" across several teeth.
- On the crowns of teeth out of occlusion, nonfunctioning teeth, or teeth that are neglected during daily biofilm removal (toothbrushing or interdental care).
- On surfaces of dentures, dental prostheses, and oral piercings.

II. Subgingival Calculus

A. Location

- Forms apical to the margin of the gingiva and extending toward the clinical attachment on the root surface.
- Forms on dental implants.

B. Distribution

- May be generalized or localized on single teeth or a group of teeth.
- Heaviest deposits are related to areas most difficult for the patient to access during personal oral biofilm removal procedures.
- **Figure 17-8** illustrates subgingival calculus on an extracted molar and premolar. In **Figure 17-9A** and **B**, ledges of interproximal calculus can be seen radiographically.
  - The calculus typically will form at the cementoenamel junction as recession and pocket formation continue.
  - The color of subgingival calculus comes from exposure to the products of blood and blood breakdown products.

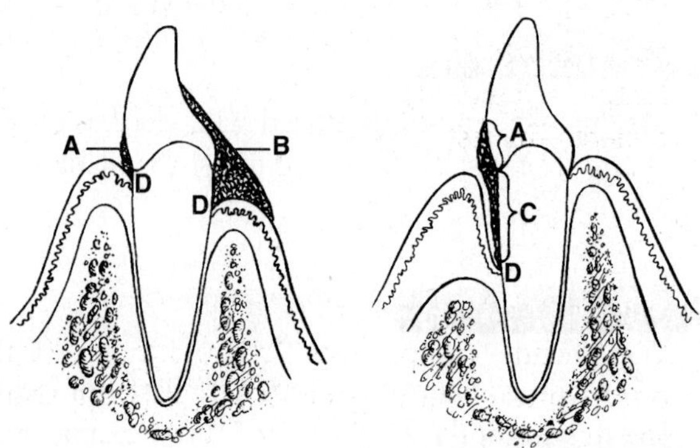

Figure 17-6 Dental Calculus. **A:** Supragingival calculus on the cervical third of a mandibular anterior tooth extends slightly subgingivally. **B:** Supragingival calculus over crown, exposed root surface, and the margin of the gingiva. **C:** Subgingival calculus along root to the base of a periodontal pocket. **D:** Base of pocket.

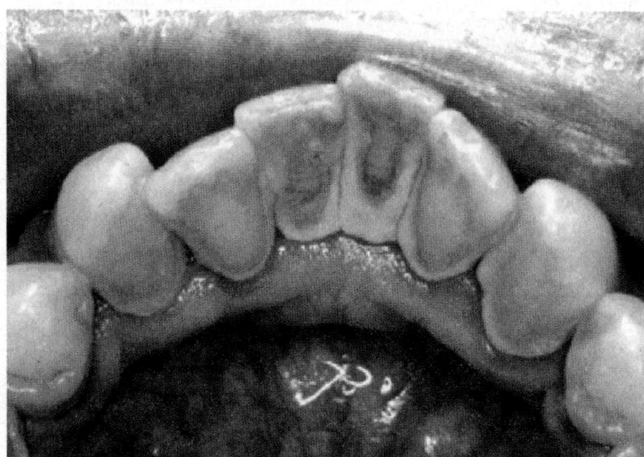

Figure 17-7 Supragingival Calculus. Heavy calculus deposits on the lingual surfaces of the mandibular anterior teeth. These deposits are so large that they interfere with the patient's oral self-care efforts. In addition, calculus deposits harbor living bacteria that are in constant contact with the gingival tissue.

Reproduced from Nield-Gehrig J, Willmann D. *Foundations of Periodontics for the Dental Hygienist.* 3rd ed. Philadelphia, PA: Lippincott Williams & Wilkins; 2011.

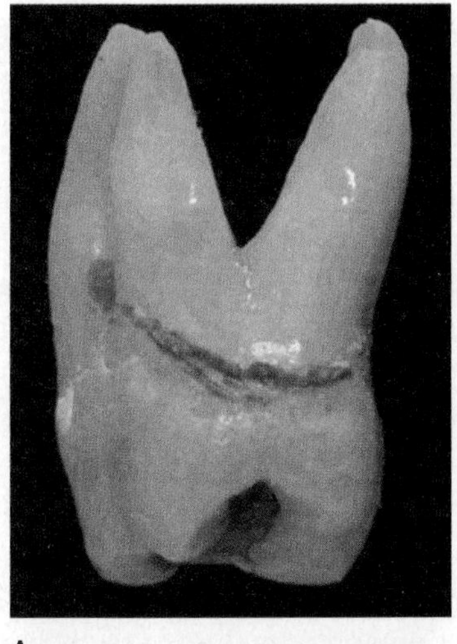

A

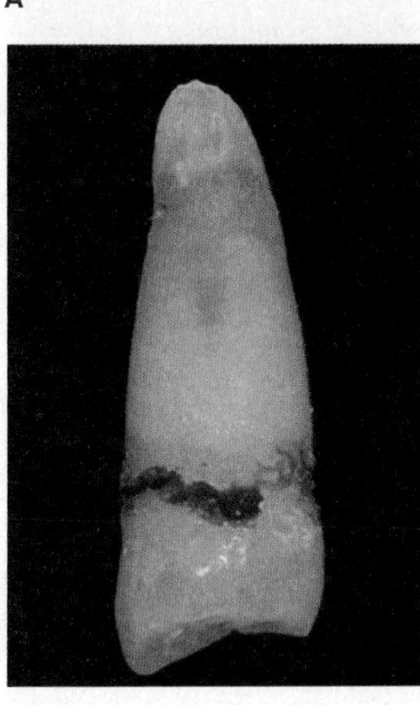

B

Figure 17-8 Subgingival Calculus on Extracted Teeth. **A:** On a maxillary first molar, calculus that formed in the subgingival environment is dark brown because elements of blood were incorporated during calcification. Additionally, some of the bacteria that are formed in calculus produce pigment. It can be seen here on surfaces where it most commonly forms and is often missed during periodontal instrumentation: near the cementoenamel junction (CEJ), at line angles, in grooves (the concavity just coronal to the buccal furcation), and furcations. **B:** Calculus at and apical to the CEJ on a premolar.

Reproduced from Weiss G, Scheid R. *Woelfel's Dental Anatomy.* 8th ed. Philadelphia, PA: Lippincott Williams & Wilkins; 2012.

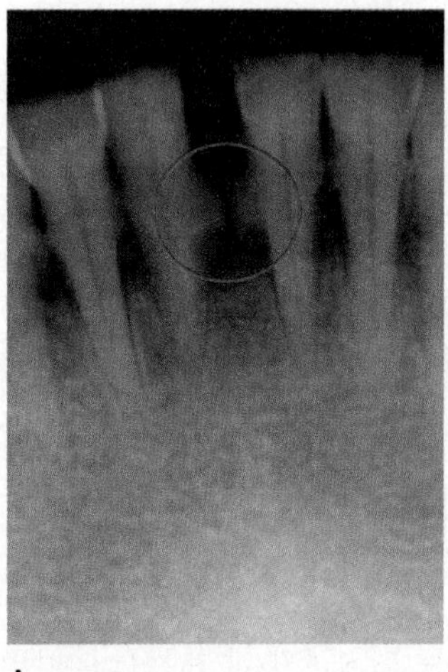

A

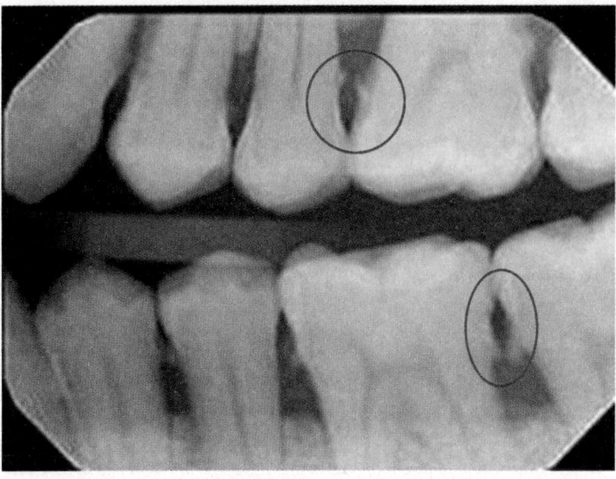

B

Figure 17-9 Subgingival Calculus in Radiographs. **A:** Heavy supra- and subgingival proximal calculus is shown on the mandibular anterior teeth (#24–25). **B:** The bitewing radiographs show heavy ledges or spines of subgingival calculus in the proximal areas of premolar and molar areas.

Calculus Composition

- Calculus is composed of inorganic and organic components and water.
- The percentages vary depending on the age, hardness of a deposit, and location of the calculus (supragingival calculus in maxillary molar areas tends to be higher in calcium, phosphorus, and ash content than on the lingual of mandibular anterior teeth).[24]
- Mature calculus usually contains inorganic components; the rest is organic components and water.

I. Inorganic Content

A. Major Inorganic Components

- The main components are calcium (Ca), phosphorus (P), carbonate (CO_3), sodium (Na), and magnesium (Mg).[28]

B. Trace Elements

- Trace elements include copper (Cu), zinc (Zn), strontium (Sr), manganese (Mn), silicon (Si), fluorine (F), iron (Fe), and potassium (K).[28]

C. Fluoride in Calculus

- Fluoride is present primarily as part of hydroxyapatite in supragingival dental calculus.[28]
- The concentration of fluoride in calculus varies depending on the patient's exposure to fluoridated drinking water, topical applications, dentifrices, or any form in contact with the external surface of the calculus.

D. Crystals

- Dental calculus contains four types of calcium phosphate crystals:
  - Brushite
  - Octocalcium phosphate
  - Hydroxyapatitie
  - Whitlockite[27]

E. Composition of Calculus

- Dental enamel is the most highly mineralized tissue in the body and contains 95% to 97% inorganic salts; dentin contains 65% and cementum and bone contain 45% to 70%.[28]
- Supragingival calculus has an average mineral content of 37% with amounts as high as 80%.[27]
  - The predominant inorganic component in exterior layers of supragingival calculus is octacalcium phosphate, with hydroxyapatite being more dominant in older calculus.[27]
- Subgingival calculus has an average mineral content of 58% with maximum content of 60–80%.[27]
  - The predominant inorganic component of subgingival calculus is whitlockite.[27]

II. Organic Content

- The organic proportion of calculus consists of various types of microorganisms, desquamated epithelial cells, leukocytes, and mucin from the saliva.
- Substances identified in the organic matrix include lipids such as free fatty acids and phospholipids and a protein portion.[29]

Calculus Formation

- Calculus results from the deposition of minerals into a biofilm organic matrix.
- Mineralization of supragingival and subgingival calculus is essentially the same, although the source of the elements for mineralization is not the same.

I. Factors in Rate of Calculus Formation

- Genetic and individual variation in saliva composition and flow.[27]
  - In heavy calculus formers, saliva contains higher levels of calcium and three times greater levels for phosphorus than light calculus formers.[27]
- Diet, especially alkaline food, foods high in silicon like rice, and refined carbohydrates.[27,29]
- Individual variations in bacterial load.[27]
- Age, race, and gender.[27]
- More severe periodontal disease.[30]
- Malposition and crowding of teeth.[30]
- Lower levels of S. *mutans*.[30]
- Inhibitors of calculus formation (i.e., urea, zinc, and pyrophosphates).[28,29]

II. Precursor to Calculus Mineralization

- Nonmineralized biofilm is necessary for initiation of calculus formation.
- In supragingival biofilm, filamentous microorganisms are oriented at a right angle to the tooth and provide the matrix for the deposition of minerals.[27]
- In subgingival biofilm, cocci, rods, and filamentous bacteria do not form a distinct pattern in relation to the tooth.[27]

III. Mechanism of Calculus Mineralization

- **Supersaturation** of saliva is the driving force for mineralization.[29,31]
- Dead microorganisms degrade and mineral deposition begins using the cell walls of the bacteria.[29]
- The initial calcium phosphate crystals form by binding with phospholipids in the cell membranes of the bacteria.[29]
- These early crystals are typically brushite, which progress through transformation stages of maturation as mineralization continues to octacalcium phosphate, whitlockite, and finally to a stable hydroxyapatite phase.[28]
- The final stable phase occurs around 8 months.[28]
- Calculus forms in layers.
  - In supragingival calculus, the layers are heterogeneous and each may have a different mineral content.[27]

- In subgingival calculus, the layers are more similar or homogeneous with equal mineral density.[27]
- The layers of calculus are called *incremental lines*.[29] The lines are evidence calculus grows or increases by apposition of new layers.

IV. Types of Calculus Deposits

The surface of the calculus is typically rough and can be detected with an explorer. The exception is veneer-type calculus, which is smooth and difficult to detect with an explorer.

- Crusty, spiny, or nodular deposits.
- Ledge or ring formation.
- Thin, smooth veneers.
- Finger- and fern-like formations.
- Individual calculus islands or spots.

V. Formation Time

- The average time required for the primary soft deposit to change to the mature mineralized stage is about 12 days.[27]
  - Half of mineralization can begin in the first two days when a patient's daily oral self-care is inadequate.[27]
- Formation time depends on individual factors previously mentioned.

Attachment of Calculus

- The ease or difficulty of calculus removal is related to the manner of attachment of the calculus to the tooth surface.

I. Attachment by Means of an Acquired Pellicle

- In early calculus formation, the attachment is superficial because no interlocking with the tooth surface occurs and calculus can be easily removed.

II. Attachment to Minute Irregularities in the Tooth Surface

- Dentin irregularities include cracks, resorption, and carious defects.[32]
  - Cemental irregularities include tiny spaces left at previous locations of **Sharpey's fibers**, resorption lacunae, root gouging from improper scaling, and cemental tears.
- Calculus is difficult to remove when it is attached by this method because it becomes locked into the irregularities.

III. Attachment by Direct Contact with the Tooth Surface

- Interlocking of inorganic apatite crystals of the enamel and cementum with the calcium phosphate crystals of the calculus.[33]
- Research suggests this mode of attachment results in a portion of the calculus that is prone to fracture during removal, but it may leave calculus crystals attached to the tooth surface.[33]

Clinical Implications of Dental Calculus

- There has been a long-standing debate over whether subgingival calculus has a role in periodontal disease.[27]
- Given calculus is always covered by a layer of unmineralized viable biofilm, it is likely the biofilm is responsible for the initiation of the immune response in gingivitis and periodontitis.[27]
  - Calculus is a *secondary* etiologic factor in periodontitis because it acts as a reservoir for bacteria and endotoxins.[27]
  - The progression of calculus apically is responsible for the deepening of the pocket and loss of attachment due to the layer of biofilm covering it.
  - Research has shown that removal of the biofilm on subgingival calculus results in healing of periodontal tissues.[27]
- The cornerstone of nonsurgical periodontal therapy is the daily control of biofilm by the patient, supplemented by definitive professional supra- and subgingival instrumentation to reduce or eliminate gingival inflammation and bleeding on probing and regular periodontal maintenance or supportive care.[27,34]
  - However, understanding the mode of attachment is important to recognize that calculus is prone to fracture during removal and may leave calculus crystals attached to the tooth surface.[33]
  - These remaining calcium phosphate crystals may then serve as a nidus for continued biofilm formation.[33]
  - It is important to meticulously debride subgingival biofilm given complete removal of calculus is not feasible.[27]

Clinical Characteristics

- Identification of calculus prior to removal depends on knowledge of its appearance, consistency, and distribution.
- Appointment planning, selection of instruments, and techniques depend on understanding the texture, morphology, and mode of attachment of calculus. **Table 17-2** lists a summary of clinical characteristics.

I. Supragingival Examination

A. Direct Examination

- Supragingival deposits may be seen directly or indirectly, using a mouth mirror.

Table 17-2 Clinical Characteristics of Dental Calculus[27,29,30,33]

Characteristic	Supragingival Calculus	Subgingival Calculus
Color	White, creamy yellow, or gray May be stained by tobacco, food, tea, or coffee Slight deposits may be invisible until dried with compressed air	Light to dark brown, dark green, or black due to gingival crevicular fluid, blood and blood breakdown products
Shape	**Amorphous**, bulky Gross deposits may: ▪ Form interproximal bridge between adjacent teeth (Figure 17-7) ▪ Extend over the margin of the gingiva ▪ Form based on the anatomy of the teeth; contour of gingival margin; and pressure of the tongue, lips, cheeks	Conforms to the root surface due to constraints of the pocket wall Calculus formations occur in the following forms: ▪ Crusty, spiny, or nodular ▪ Ledge or ringlike ▪ Thin, smooth veneers ▪ Finger- and fern-like ▪ Individual calculus islands
Consistency and texture	Moderately hard Newer deposits less mineralized (37%) Porous surface covered with nonmineralized biofilm	Harder and more mineralized (58%) than supragingival calculus Surface covered with dental biofilm
Size and quantity	Quantity has direct relationship to: ▪ Personal oral self-care ▪ Diet ▪ Individual characteristics, such as diet and salivary flow ▪ Position of the teeth ▪ Use of tobacco products	Quantity is related to: ▪ Personal oral self-care ▪ Individual characteristics, such as age ▪ Bacterial load ▪ Disease severity
Distribution on individual tooth	Coronal to margin of gingiva	Apical to margin of gingiva Extends to bottom of the pocket and follows contour of soft-tissue attachment
Distribution on teeth	Symmetrical arrangement on teeth, except when influenced by: ▪ Malpositioned teeth ▪ Unilateral hypofunction ▪ Inconsistent personal oral self-care Location related to openings of the salivary gland ducts: ▪ Facial surface of maxillary molars ▪ Lingual surface of mandibular anterior teeth	Heaviest on proximal surfaces, lightest on facial surfaces Occurs with or without associated supragingival deposits

Data from Akcalı A, Lang NP. Dental calculus: the calcified biofilm and its role in disease development. *Periodontol 2000*. 2018;76(1):109-115. doi:10.1111/prd.12151; Jin Y, Yip H-K. Supragingival calculus: formation and control. *Crit Rev Oral Biol Med*. Published online 2002:16; Fons-Badal C, Fons-Font A, Labaig-Rueda C, Fernanda Solá-Ruiz M, Selva-Otaolaurruchi E, Agustín-Panadero R. Analysis of predisposing factors for rapid dental calculus formation. *J Clin Med*. 2020;9(3):E858. doi:10.3390/jcm9030858; Rohanizadeh R, LeGeros RZ. Ultrastructural study of calculus–enamel and calculus–root interfaces. *Arch Oral Biol*. 2005;50(1):89-96. doi:10.1016/j.archoralbio.2004.07.001

B. Use of Compressed Air

- Small amounts of calculus may be invisible when they are wet with saliva.
- With adequate light and drying with air, small deposits usually become visible.

II. Subgingival Examination

A. Visual Examination

- Dark edges of calculus may be seen at or just beneath the gingival margin.
- Gentle air blast can deflect the gingival margin from the tooth to gain some visibility into the coronal portion of the pocket.

B. Gingival Tissue Color Change

- Dark calculus may be visible as a dark shadow along the gingiva and suggest the presence of subgingival calculus.

C. Tactile Examination

- *Probe*: While probing for sulcus/pocket characteristics, a rough subgingival tooth surface may be felt when calculus is present.
- *Explorer*: With a subgingival explorer like an ODU 11/12, each tooth is explored carefully to the base of the pocket to detect any calculus deposits.

D. Radiographic Examination

- Radiographic examination may detect large calculus deposits on proximal surfaces (see Figure 17-9A and B).

E. Dental Endoscopy

- The use of the dental endoscope in deep pockets and furcations can detect otherwise undetectable calculus, especially burnished or veneer-type calculus.[35]

Prevention of Calculus

- Risk factors related to calculus formation are similar to those for dental biofilm formation and relate to the patient's daily biofilm removal regime.

I. Personal Dental Biofilm Control

A. Objective

- Regular removal of dental biofilm by appropriately selected brushing, interdental care, and supplementary methods is a major factor in the control of dental calculus reformation.

B. Oral Self-Care Education

- Patient education includes[34]:
  - Identification and hands-on demonstration of the oral hygiene aids appropriate for the patient's needs.
  - Follow-up at continuing care appointments to commend the patient's successes and review and refine techniques as necessary to overcome barriers.
  - Identification of dietary behaviors that may be enhancing biofilm growth, such as sugar-sweetened beverages and sugary snacks between meals.

II. Regular Professional Continuing Care

- Professional maintenance or supportive periodontal care appointments on a regular basis supplement daily oral self-care.[34]
- With emphasis on good oral hygiene and routine professional removal, low levels of supragingival and subgingival calculus can be maintained.[27]

III. Anticalculus Dentifrice

A. Objective

- Calculus-control dentifrices aim to inhibit calculus crystal growth, which may lessen the amount of calculus formation.[29] (See Chapter 28.)
- Dentifrices do not have an effect on existing calculus deposits; however, they may prevent formation of new supragingival calculus.
- For a patient who cannot control supragingival calculus, and hence cannot achieve optimum gingival tissue health, an anticalculus dentifrice may provide motivation, as well as be a supplement to mechanical biofilm removal efforts.

B. Chemotherapeutic Anticalculus Agents

- Agents used in "tartar-control" mouth rinses or dentifrices are mineralization inhibitors.
  - Examples include pyrophosphates and zinc citrate.[29]

Dental Stains and Discolorations

- Discolorations of the teeth and restorations occur in three general ways[36]:
  - Adhered directly to the tooth surfaces.
  - Contained within calculus or pellicle.
  - Incorporated within the tooth structure or the restorative material.

Significance of Dental Stains

- The significance of stain is primarily the appearance or cosmetic (esthetic) effect.[37]
- In general, any detrimental effect on the teeth or gingival tissues is related to the dental calculus in which the stain occurs.
- Certain stains provide a means of evaluating adequate oral self-care for management of dental biofilm.

I. Classification of Stains

A. Classified by Location

- **Extrinsic** stain: Occurs on the external surface of the tooth and may be removed by procedures of toothbrushing, scaling, and/or polishing.
  - Origins are metallic and nonmetallic.[36]
- **Intrinsic** stain: Occurs due to changes in structural composition or thickness of the enamel.
  - Internalized discoloration: Extrinsic stain is internalized into the tooth structure following development.[36]
  - Occurs in development defects and acquired defects like restorative materials.

B. Classified by Source

- **Exogenous** stain: Develops or originates from sources outside the tooth.
  - Exogenous stains may be extrinsic and stay on the outer surface of the tooth or intrinsic and become incorporated within the tooth structure.
- **Endogenous** stain: Develops or originates from within the tooth.
  - Endogenous stains are always intrinsic and usually are discolorations of the dentin reflected through the enamel.

II. Recognition and Identification

More than one type of stain may occur and more than one etiologic factor may cause the stains and discolorations of an individual's dentition. A differential diagnosis may be needed in order to plan whether an appropriate intervention is indicated.

A. Medical and Dental History

- Developmental delays; medications; use of tobacco, marijuana, or betel or areca nut; and fluoride histories all contribute necessary information.
- Thorough medical, dental, and social histories and cultural practices can provide information to supplement clinical observations.

B. Food Diary

- Assessment of a patient's food diary may aid in identifying certain contributing factors.
  - Examples of staining from beverages include tea, coffee, dark-colored juices, and wine.

C. Oral Hygiene Habits

- The history of oral self-care routines may help explain the presence of certain stains.

III. Application of Procedures for Stain Removal

A. Stains Occurring Directly on the Tooth Surface

- Stains directly associated with the pellicle on the surface of the enamel or exposed cementum are removed as much as possible during toothbrushing or interdental cleaning.
- Certain stains can be removed with debridement and/or polishing. (See Chapter 42.)
- When stains are tenacious, avoid excessive polishing. Use the most conservative approach with the least abrasive polishing agent to prevent the following:
  - Excess tooth structure or abrasion of the gingival margin.
  - Removal of a layer of fluoride-rich tooth surface.
  - Overheating of the dental structure with a power-driven polisher.

B. Stains Incorporated within Acquired Pellicle

- When stain is included within the acquired pellicle, it can be removed with a toothbrush and interdental aid(s).

C. Stains Incorporated within the Tooth

- When stain is intrinsic, whether exogenous or endogenous, it cannot be removed by scaling or polishing. Evaluation for possible whitening procedures may be considered. (See Chapter 43.)
- If stain removal is inadequate, microabrasion is another noninvasive approach that can be used.[37]
- For more extensive deep staining, porcelain veneers or crowns may be necessary to restore esthetics.[37]

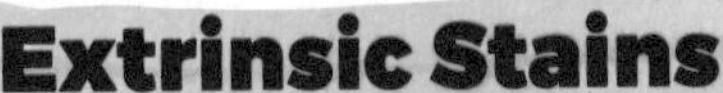

Extrinsic Stains

There are two broad categories for extrinsic stains[36]:

- Directed extrinsic stains caused by compounds, organic chromogens, attached to the pellicle producing a stain.
- Indirect extrinsic stains result from chemical interaction with the tooth surface that creates a colored stain.

The most frequently observed stains—yellow, green, black line, and tobacco—are described first; descriptions of the less common orange, red, and metallic stains follow.

I. Yellow Stain

A. Clinical Features

- Dull, yellowish discoloration of dental biofilm is illustrated in **Figure 17-10**.

B. Distribution on Tooth Surfaces

- Yellow stain can be generalized or localized.

C. Occurrence

- More common in older adults.
- More evident when oral self-care is inadequate.

D. Etiology

- Dietary sources.
- Tobacco use.

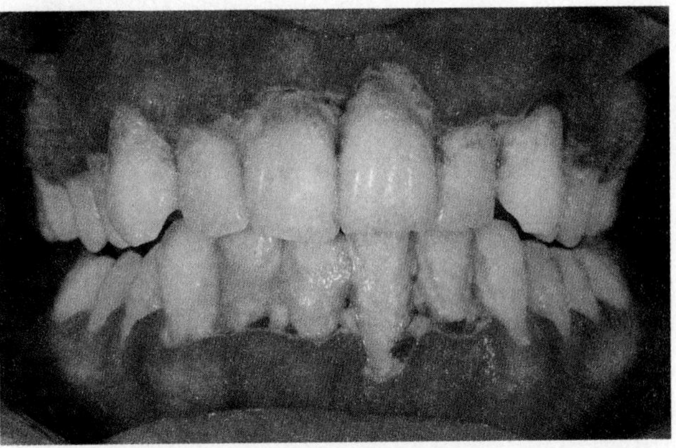

Figure 17-10 Yellow Stain. Generalized, dull, yellowish discoloration of dental biofilm.

II. Green Stain

A. Clinical Features

- Light or yellowish green to very dark green.[38]
- Occurs in three general forms:
  - Small curved line following contour of facial gingival margin.
  - Irregular coverage of flat tooth surfaces.
  - Streaked, following grooves or lines in enamel.

B. Distribution on Tooth Surfaces

- Most frequently facial gingival third of maxillary anterior teeth.[38]

C. Composition

- **Chromogenic** bacteria.
- Decomposed hemoglobin.
- Inorganic elements include copper, nickel, and other elements in small amounts.[38]

D. Occurrence

- May occur at any age; primarily found in childhood.
- Collects on both permanent and primary teeth.

E. Recurrence

- Recurrence depends on thoroughness of oral self-care.

F. Etiology

- Green stain results from poor oral hygiene, dental biofilm retention, chromogenic bacteria, and gingival hemorrhage.[38]

- Chromogenic bacteria are nourished in dental biofilm where the green stain is produced.[38]
- Blood pigments from hemoglobin are decomposed by bacteria.[38]

G. Clinical Approach

- The patient may be able to remove the soft deposits with a toothbrush during oral self-care education.
- Choose the least abrasive polishing agent for stain removal.

H. Other Green Stains

- In addition to the clinical entity known as "green stain" that was just described, dental biofilm and acquired pellicle may become stained a green color by a variety of substances.
- Differential distinction may be determined by questioning the patient or from items in the medical or dental histories. Green discoloration may result from the following:
  - **Chlorophyll** preparations.
  - Metallic dust produced by some industries.
  - Green tea.
  - Certain drugs, such as smoking marijuana.

III. Black-Line Stain

- Black-line stain is a highly retentive black or dark-brown calculus-like stain that forms along the gingival third near the gingival margin. It may occur on primary or permanent teeth.

A. Other Names

- Pigmented dental biofilm, brown stain, black stain.

B. Clinical Features

- Continuous or interrupted fine line formed by pigmented spots, 1-mm wide (average), no appreciable thickness.
  - May be a wider band or even occupy entire gingival third in severe cases (rare).
- Appears black at bases of pits and fissures.
- Lower numbers of cariogenic microorganisms compared to dental biofilm that is not discolored.[39]
  - Although more research is needed, some studies have found a lower prevalence of caries in children with black-line stain.[39,40]

C. Distribution on Tooth Surfaces

- Facial and lingual surfaces; follows contour of gingival margin onto proximal surfaces.
- Rarely on facial surfaces of maxillary anterior teeth.
- Most frequently: Lingual and proximal surfaces of maxillary posterior teeth and occlusal pits.

D. Composition and Formation

- Black-line stain is composed of chromogenic microorganisms embedded in a ferric matrix with a higher phosphorus–calcium content.[39]
- Attachment of black-line stain to the tooth is by a pellicle-like structure.

E. Occurrence

- Occurrence increases with age, although most research has been done with children.[39]

F. Recurrence

- Black-line stain tends to form again despite regular personal care.
- Quantity may be less when biofilm control procedures are meticulous.

G. Predisposing Factors

- No definitive etiology, but several have been proposed, including[39]:
  - *Actinomyces* may be involved in growth of the black pigmentation.
  - Dietary habits.
  - Conflicting data exist about a connection between black-line stain and poor oral hygiene.
  - Iron supplements may promote development.

IV. Tobacco Stain

A. Clinical Features

- Light brown to dark leathery brown or black (**Figure 17-11**).
- Incorporated in calculus deposit.
- Heavy deposits (particularly from smokeless tobacco) may penetrate irregularities in the enamel and become exogenous intrinsic.

B. Distribution on Tooth Surface

- Diffuse staining of dental biofilm.
- Narrow band that follows contour of gingival crest, slightly above the crest.
- Wide, firm, tar-like band may cover the cervical third and extend to the central third of the crown, primarily on lingual surfaces.

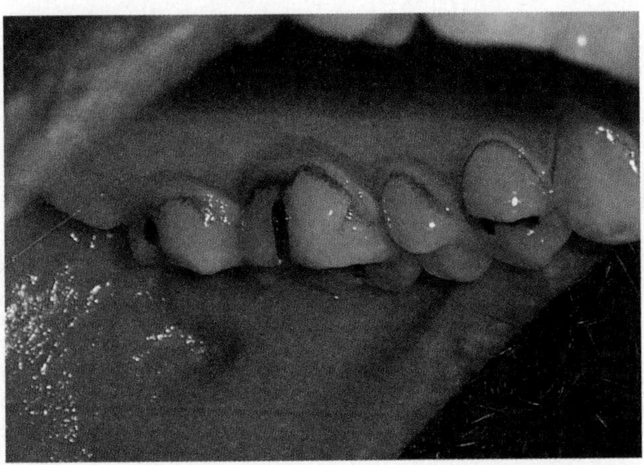

Figure 17-11 Tobacco Stain. Dark brown band following contour of gingival crest.

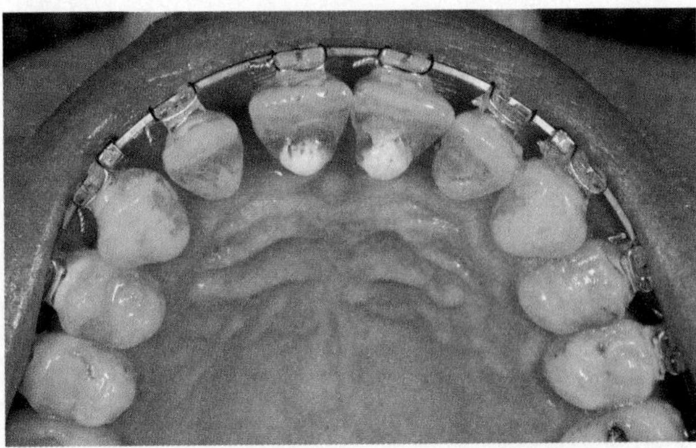

Figure 17-12 Brown Stain. Most likely caused by pigmented foods or drinks.

C. Composition

- Tar and products of combustion.[38]
- Brown pigment from smokeless tobacco.

D. Predisposing Factors

- Smoking or chewing tobacco or use of hookah to inhale tobacco. The quantity of stain is not necessarily proportional to the amount of tobacco used.
- Inadequate oral self-care.
- Extent of dental biofilm and calculus available for adherence.

V. Brown Stains

A. Clinical Features

- The pellicle can take on stains of various colors that result from chemical alterations.
- Found primarily on buccal of maxillary molars and lingual of mandibular anterior surfaces.

B. Predisposing Factors

- Poor oral hygiene may be associated with it.
- Tannins in tea, coffee, soy sauce, and other foods may also deposit in the pellicle, resulting in brown stain (**Figure 17-12**).

C. Stannous Fluoride

- Light brown, sometimes yellowish, stain forms on the teeth in the pellicle.
  - Studies suggest minimal stain accumulation after 6 months with twice daily use, so it is important to weigh the risk of stain with the benefits of use in reducing gingivitis and as an antiplaque agent.[41]
- The brown stain results from the formation of stannous sulfide or brown tin oxide from the reaction of the tin ion in the fluoride compound.[41]

D. Antimicrobial Agents

- Chlorhexidine and essential oil/phenol are used in mouth rinses and are effective against biofilm formation.[42]
- Chromogenic polyphenols in the diet such as coffee, tea, and wine may interact with chlorhexidine and worsen the staining.[36]
- A brownish stain on the tongue and tooth surfaces may result, usually more pronounced on proximal and other surfaces less accessible to routine biofilm control procedures.[36]
- The stain also tends to form more rapidly on exposed roots than on enamel. Tooth staining is considered a significant side effect.
- Clinical implications
  - Stain may not be removable from enamel defects, anterior composite, and crown- or veneer-type restorations.
  - Careful consideration of risk versus benefit of use as an antimicrobial agent is needed by the patient and clinician.

E. Betel/Areca

- The betel nut is a seed of the *Areca catechu*, a type of palm tree.
  - The nut is ground and other ingredients such as flavoring and tobacco may be added to create a "chew" or "**quid**." Betel chewing is common among people of all ages in Micronesian islands, such as Guam, and Asian countries, particularly China.[43] In the Polynesian islands,

the use has cultural connections and is used in religious ceremonies.
- The discoloration imparted to the teeth is a dark mahogany brown, sometimes almost black. It may become thick and hard, with partly smooth and partly rough surfaces.
- Microscopically, the black deposit consists of microorganisms and mineralized material with a laminated pattern characteristic of subgingival calculus.[44]

F. Swimmer Stain

- Frequent exposure to pools disinfected with chlorine or bromine can cause yellowish or dark brown stains on the facial surfaces of maxillary and mandibular incisor teeth.[45]

VI. Orange and Red Stains

A. Clinical Appearance

- Orange or red stains appear at the cervical third.

B. Distribution on Tooth Surfaces

- More frequently on anterior than on posterior teeth.

C. Occurrence

- Rare (red rarer than orange).

D. Etiology

- Possibly chromogenic bacteria.
- Poor oral hygiene.[36]

VII. Metallic Stains

A. Metals or Metallic Salts from Metal-Containing Dust of Industry

- Clinical appearance/examples of colors on teeth[36]:
  - Copper or brass: Green or bluish-green.
  - Iron: Brown to greenish-brown.
  - Nickel: Green.
  - Cadmium: Yellow or golden brown.
- Distribution on tooth surfaces
  - Primarily anterior; may occur on any teeth.
  - Cervical third more commonly affected.
- Manner of formation
  - Industrial workers inhale dust through the mouth, bringing aerosolized metallic particles in contact with teeth.
  - Metal imparts color to pellicle.
  - Occasionally, stain may penetrate tooth surface and become exogenous intrinsic stain.
- Prevention
  - Workers need to be advised to wear a mask while working.

Endogenous Intrinsic Stains

I. Pulpless or Traumatized Teeth

Not all pulpless teeth discolor. However, traumatized teeth that have not been treated endodontically often discolor.

A. Clinical Appearance

- A wide range of colors exists; stains may be light yellow-brown, slate gray, reddish-brown, dark brown, bluish-black, or black. Others have an orange or greenish tinge.

B. Etiology

- Blood and other pulp tissue elements may be available for breakdown as a result of hemorrhages in the pulp chamber, root canal treatment, or necrosis and decomposition of the pulp tissue.[36]
- Pigments from the decomposed hemoglobin and pulp tissue penetrate and discolor the dentinal tubules.

II. Disturbances in Tooth Development

- Stains incorporated within the tooth structure may be related to the period of tooth development.[36,46]
- Defective tooth development may result from factors of genetic abnormality or environmental influences during tooth development.

A. Hereditary: Genetic

- **Amelogenesis imperfecta**: The enamel is partially or completely missing due to a generalized disturbance of the ameloblasts. Teeth are yellow to yellowish-brown.
- **Dentinogenesis imperfecta** (*opalescent dentin*): The dentin is abnormal as a result of disturbances in the odontoblastic layer during development. The teeth appear translucent or opalescent and vary in color from yellow-brown to blue-gray.[46]

B. Developmental Enamel Defects

- Development enamel defects (DDE) include enamel hypoplasia, enamel opacity, and molar-incisor hypomineralization (MIH) and result from damage to the tooth germ during development; the location of the defect(s) is typically related to the timing of the injury during development.[47]

- *Generalized* **hypoplasia** (**chronologic** hypoplasia resulting from ameloblastic disturbance of short duration) may extend across multiple teeth and color may vary from chalky white to yellow or brown.[48]
- *Local hypoplasia* affects a single tooth (e.g., individual white spots, caused by trauma to a primary tooth).

- Clinical appearance[48]:
  - Teeth erupt with white spots, pits, or grooves depending on the severity of the injury to the tooth germ.
  - Over time, the enamel hypoplasia defects are prone to extrinsic stain.
- Etiology[47,48]
  - Trauma or **infection** of an individual tooth.
  - Rubella infection or disease causing a high fever.
  - Drug intake during pregnancy.
  - Preterm birth.
  - Hypocalcemia (low calcium) levels such as in premature infants.

C. Dental Fluorosis

- Dental fluorosis was originally called "brown stain." Later, Dr. Frederick S. McKay studied the condition and described it in the dental literature as "mottled enamel."
- Etiology
  - Enamel hypomineralization results from ingestion of excessive fluoride ion from any source during the period of mineralization. The enamel alterations are a result of toxic damage to the ameloblasts.
  - Severity is related to the age and dose of fluoride exposure.[49,50]
- Fluorosis classification
  - There are several indices for classifying fluorosis.[50] (See Chapter 34.)
- Clinical appearance
  - When the teeth erupt, the color of the enamel ranges from chalky white spots to brown. Depending on the severity of the enamel defect(s), discoloration may occur over time.[49]
  - Severe effects of excess fluoride during development may produce cracks or pitting. This condition and appearance led to the name *mottled enamel*.

III. Drug-Induced Stains and Discolorations

A. Tetracycline

- Tetracycline antibiotics have an affinity for calcium and form complexes with hydroxyapatite crystals in mineralized tissues (**Figure 17-13**).[51]
- Discoloration of a child's teeth may result when the drug is administered to the mother during the fourth month of pregnancy or to the child in infancy and early childhood.[51]
- Etiology
  - The discoloration depends on the dosage, length of time used, and type of tetracycline prescribed.[51]
- Clinical appearance[51]
  - Discoloration may be generalized or localized to individual teeth that were developing at the time of administration of the antibiotic.
  - Color of teeth may be light green to dark yellow, or a gray-brown, with or without banding and approximate age when the antibiotic was taken.
  - The patient's medical history may reveal the illness for which the antibiotic was prescribed.

B. Minocycline

- Unlike tetracycline, minocycline has been reported to cause generalized intrinsic staining posteruption.[52]
- Clinical appearance
  - Use of minocycline can result in a generalized intrinsic blue-gray to gray staining of the permanent teeth.[52]

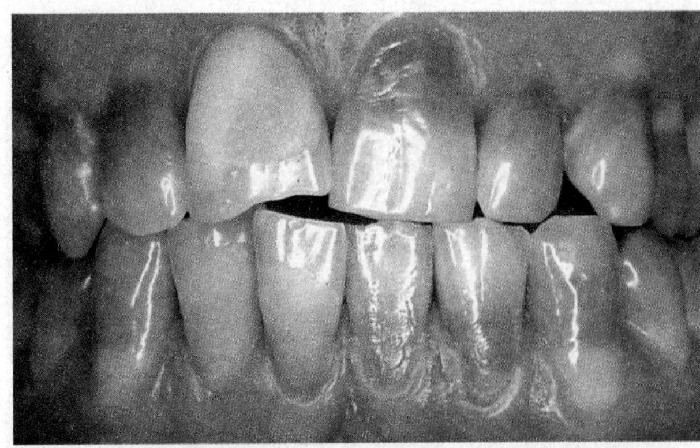

Figure 17-13 Tetracycline Stain. Tetracycline staining in this permanent dentition resulted from the administration of tetracycline antibiotic during the time that crowns formed. Teeth have the appearance of yellow to gray-brown horizontal bands across the crowns. (The staining on tooth no. 8 has been covered with a tooth-colored restorative material such as composite resin.)

Courtesy of Carl Allen, DDS, MSD.

- Etiology
  - Several theories exist about the mechanism related to intrinsic and extrinsic mechanisms for the stain.[52]

Exogenous Intrinsic Stains

- When intrinsic stains come from an outside source, not from within the tooth, the stain is called exogenous intrinsic.
- Extrinsic stains result from stain in the tooth following development and may occur when the stain penetrates enamel defects and exposed dentin to become intrinsic (**Figure 17-14**). These may also be called internalized discoloration.[36]
- The sources of these stains may include:[36]
  - Developmental defects.
  - Acquired defects such as tooth wear and gingival recession.
  - Dental caries.
  - Restorative materials.

I. Restorative Materials

A. Silver Amalgam

- Silver amalgam can impart a gray to black discoloration to the tooth structure around a restoration.
- Tin migrates from the amalgam restoration into the enamel and dentin.[36]

B. Endodontic Therapy

- Discoloration tends to be most evident on the cervical third of the crown and root surface.[53]
- Materials used during endodontic therapy can cause intrinsic staining.[53]
  - Endodontic sealers may cause stain ranging in color from orange-red to gray.
  - Endodontic medicaments, which may include tetracycline, may cause a dark brown intrinsic stain.
  - Portland cement–based materials may cause a gray intrinsic stain.
  - Antibiotic pastes used in regenerative endodontic procedures may also contain tetracycline, but also ciprofloxacin, metronidazole, or minocycline, and result in a green-brown staining.

II. Stain in Dentin

- Discoloration resulting from a carious lesion is an example.
- Arrested decay or secondary dentin can present as black stain on severely decayed teeth. The surface is hard and glossy, and stain cannot be removed.

III. Other Local Causes

- Enamel erosion is the loss of hard tissue by chemical means such as acidic foods (including carbonated drinks), eating disorders (bulimia), and gastroesophageal reflux disease.[54,55]
  - Resulting thinner enamel allows the yellow color of the underlying dentin to show through and cause the teeth to appear duller gray or yellow (**Figure 17-15**).
- Attrition of occlusal surfaces can result in loss of enamel, allowing a yellow or brown outline of dentin to show through (**Figure 17-16**).

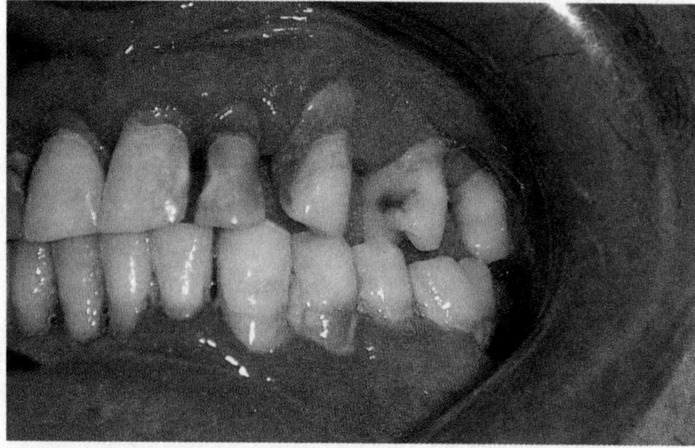

Figure 17-14 Exogenous Intrinsic Stain. Most likely from an outside source such as tobacco or food and becomes intrinsic over time. Areas of attrition allow yellow color of underlying dentin to be exposed and become further stained.

Photograph used by permission of Dr. Julius Manz, San Juan College, NM.

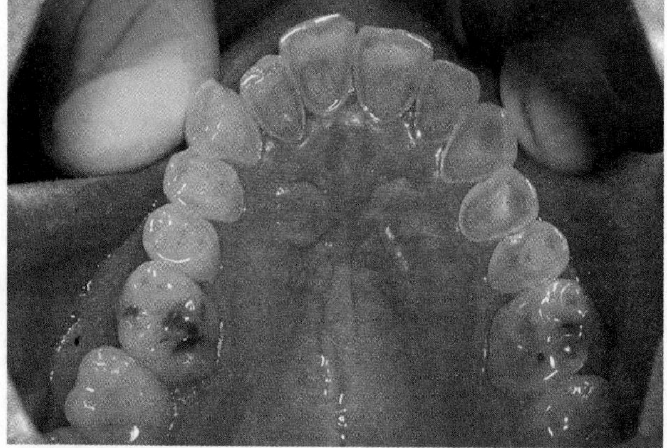

Figure 17-15 Enamel Erosion. The extensive enamel erosion reveals the yellow color of the dentin on the lingual surfaces of anterior teeth and premolars. This individual had chronic severe gastroesophageal reflux disease (GERD) of more than 10 years' duration.

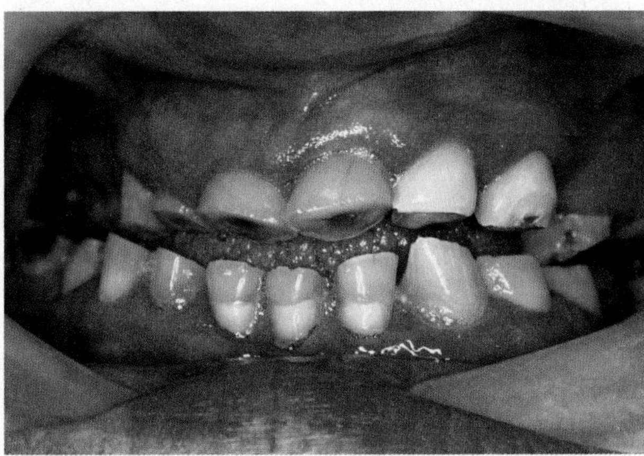

Figure 17-16 Attrition. Attrition of the maxillary teeth exposing the yellow dentin and brown of the pulp chamber.

Courtesy of Dr. Richard Foster, Guilford Technical Community College, Jamestown, NC.

Documentation

The permanent records for each patient should include information relating to the soft deposits, calculus, and stain, including:

- Clinical description of appearance of the teeth relative to the biofilm, materia alba, or food debris as indications of the personal oral care on a daily basis.
- The extent of supragingival and subgingival deposits (slight, moderate, or heavy) should be described in the initial examination record and charted to show location for reference during the clinical removal and during teaching personal care for prevention.
- Record color, type, extent, and location of stains with the patient's examination and assessment.
- Personal patient care procedures demonstrated, preventive measures discussed, and frequency of continuing care appointments recommended.

See **Box 17-2** for a sample documentation note.

Box 17-2 Example Documentation: Patient with Calculus and Stain

- **S**—Male patient, aged 35 years, medical history indicates no medication, no health compromise. Cigarette smoker, 1/2 pack per day. Patient presents for new patient exam. His last dental cleaning was 2 years ago. Chief complaint: Oral malodor, bleeding gums when brushing, and he would like whiter teeth.
- **O**—Generalized pocket depths of 3 mm or less with bleeding on probing. Light, localized subgingival calculus. Light generalized supragingival calculus with generalized moderate tobacco stain.
- **A**—Poor oral self-care with generalized moderate gingivitis and coated tongue. Discuss and demonstrate proper oral self-care instruction. Bass method brushing, daily flossing, oral rinsing, and tongue cleaning. Evaluate patient's readiness for smoking cessation.
- **P**—Medical/dental history, intra-extraoral examination performed, completed new patient periodontal chart-odontogram, full mouth radiographic series, caries assessment, and consultation with dentist. Oral self-care instruction along with smoking cessation counseling. Prophylaxis completed with subgingival debridement mandible only. Educated patient regarding the etiology and significance of dental biofilm, calculus, tongue coating, and stain accumulation. Patient advised to return for debridement of maxillary arch followed by a 3-month preventive maintenance appointment to monitor patient's oral self-care and offer smoking cessation support.

Next step: Reappoint in 1 week to complete debridement and follow-up soft-tissue evaluation. Reappoint in 3 months for preventive maintenance appointment.

Signed: ______________________________, RDH

Date: ______________________________

Factors to Teach the Patient

- Location, composition, and properties of dental biofilm and calculus with emphasis on its role in dental caries and periodontal infections.
- Effects of personal oral care procedures in the prevention of dental biofilm, calculus, and stain.
- Biofilm control procedures with special adaptations for individual needs.
- Sources of cariogenic foodstuff in the diet and frequency of consumption in relation to dental caries formation.
- What calculus is and how it forms from dental biofilm.
- Etiology of individual's dental stains and discolorations with suggestions for modification of sources of extrinsic stain.
- Advantages of a smoking cessation program.
- Effect of tetracyclines on developing teeth. Need to avoid use during pregnancy and by children to age 12 years.
- Select products with an American Dental Association or Canadian Dental Association Seal of Acceptance.

References

1. Marsh PD, Zaura E. Dental biofilm: ecological interactions in health and disease. *J Clin Periodontol*. 2017;44(S18):S12-S22.
2. Rasputnis W, Schestakow A, Hannig M. The dentin pellicle: a neglected topic in dental research. *Arch Oral Biol*. 2021;129:105212.
3. Siqueira WL, Custodio W, McDonald EE. New insights into the composition and functions of the acquired enamel pellicle. *J Dent Res*. 2012;91(12):1110-1118.
4. Hannig M. Ultrastructural investigation of pellicle morphogenesis at two different intraoral sites during a 24-h period. *Clin Oral Investig*. 1999;3(2):88-95.
5. Hara AT, Zero DT. The caries environment: saliva, pellicle, diet, and hard tissue ultrastructure. *Dent Clin North Am*. 2010;54(3):455-467.
6. Seneviratne C, Zhang C, Samaranayake L. Bacterial biofilm and associated infections. Chin J Dent Res. 2011;14(2):87-94.
7. Huang R, Li M, Gregory RL. Bacterial interactions in dental biofilm. Virulence. 2011;2(5):435-444.
8. Jamal M, Ahmad W, Andleeb S, et al. Bacterial biofilm and associated infections. J Chin Med Assoc. 2018;81(1):7-11.
9. Kilian M, Chapple ILC, Hannig M, et al. The oral microbiome - an update for oral healthcare professionals. *Br Dent J*. 2016;221(10):657-666.
10. Loe H, Theilade E, Jensen SB. Experimental gingivitis in man. *J Periodontol*. 1965;36:177-187.
11. Abusleme L, Hoare A, Hong B-Y, Diaz PI. Microbial signatures of health, gingivitis, and periodontitis. *Periodontol 2000*. 2021;86(1):57-78.
12. Zijnge V, van Leeuwen MBM, Degener JE, et al. Oral biofilm architecture on natural teeth. *PLoS One*. 2010;5(2):e9321.
13. Curtis MA, Diaz PI, Van Dyke TE. The role of the microbiota in periodontal disease. *Periodontol 2000*. 2020;83(1):14-25.
14. Tribble GD, Lamont RJ. Bacterial invasion of epithelial cells and spreading in periodontal tissue. *Periodontol 2000*. 2010;52(1):68-83.
15. Tanaka M, Matsunaga K, Kadoma Y. Correlation in inorganic ion concentration between saliva and plaque fluid. *J Med Dent Sci*. 2000;47(1):55-59.
16. Naumova EA, Kuehnl P, Hertenstein P, et al. Fluoride bioavailability in saliva and plaque. *BMC Oral Health*. 2012;12:3.
17. Koo H, Allan RN, Howlin RP, Stoodley P, Hall-Stoodley L. Targeting microbial biofilms: current and prospective therapeutic strategies. *Nat Rev Microbiol*. 2017;15(12):740-755.
18. Sreenivasan PK, Prasad KVV. Distribution of dental plaque and gingivitis within the dental arches. *J Int Med Res*. 2017;45(5):1585-1596.
19. Tanner ACR, Kressirer CA, Rothmiller S, Johansson I, Chalmers NI. The caries microbiome: implications for reversing dysbiosis. *Adv Dent Res*. 2018;29(1):78-85.
20. Ribeiro AA, Azcarate-Peril MA, Cadenas MB, et al. The oral bacterial microbiome of occlusal surfaces in children and its association with diet and caries. *PLoS One*. 2017;12(7):e0180621.
21. Johansson I, Witkowska E, Kaveh B, Lif Holgerson P, Tanner ACR. The microbiome in populations with a low and high prevalence of caries. *J Dent Res*. 2016;95(1):80-86.
22. Lingström P, van Ruyven FO, van Houte J, Kent R. The pH of dental plaque in its relation to early enamel caries and dental plaque flora in humans. *J Dent Res*. 2000;79(2):770-777.
23. Bowen WH. The Stephan Curve revisited. *Odontology*. 2013;101(1):2-8.
24. Hoppenbrouwers PM, Driessens FC, Borggreven JM. The mineral solubility of human tooth roots. *Arch Oral Biol*. 1987;32(5):319-322.
25. Khairnar M. Classification of food impaction - revisited and its management. *Indian J Dent Res*. 5(1):1113-1119.
26. Aylıkcı BU, Çolak H. Halitosis: from diagnosis to management. *J Nat Sci Biol Med*. 2013;4(1):14-23.
27. Akcalı A, Lang NP. Dental calculus: the calcified biofilm and its role in disease development. *Periodontol 2000*. 2018;76(1):109-115.
28. Abraham J, Grenón M, Sánchez HJ, Pérez C, Barrea R. A case study of elemental and structural composition of dental calculus during several stages of maturation using SRXRF. *J Biomed Mater Res Part A*. 2005;75A(3):623-628.
29. Jin Y, Yip H-K. Supragingival calculus: formation and control. *Crit Rev Oral Biol Med*. 2002;13(5):426-441.
30. Fons-Badal C, Fons-Font A, Labaig-Rueda C, Fernanda Solá-Ruiz M, Selva-Otaolaurruchi E, Agustín-Panadero R. Analysis of predisposing factors for rapid dental calculus formation. *J Clin Med*. 2020;9(3):E858.
31. Carino A, Ludwig C, Cervellino A, Müller E, Testino A. Formation and transformation of calcium phosphate phases under biologically relevant conditions: experiments and modelling. *Acta Biomater*. 2018;74:478-488.
32. Selvig KA. Attachment of plaque and calculus to tooth surfaces. *J Periodontal Res*. 1970;5(1):8-18.
33. Rohanizadeh R, LeGeros RZ. Ultrastructural study of calculus–enamel and calculus–root interfaces. *Arch Oral Biol*. 2005;50(1):89-96.
34. Sanz M, Herrera D, Kebschull M, et al. Treatment of stage I-III periodontitis-the EFP S3 level clinical practice guideline. *J Clin Periodontol*. 2020;47(Suppl 22):4-60.
35. Osborn JB, Lenton PA, Lunos SA, Blue CM. Endoscopic vs. tactile evaluation of subgingival calculus. *J Dent Hyg*. 2014;88(4):229-236.
36. Watts A, Addy M. Tooth discolouration and staining: a review of the literature. *Br Dent J*. 2001;190(6):309-316.
37. Kapadia Y, Jain V. Tooth staining: a review of etiology and treatment modalities. *Acta Sci Dent Sci*. 2018;2(6):67-70.
38. Prathap S, Rajesh H, Boloor VA, Rao AS. Extrinsic stains and management: a new insight. *J Acad Indus Res*. 2013;1(8):435-442.
39. Elelmi Y, Mabrouk R, Masmoudi F, Baaziz A, Maatouk F, Ghedira H. Black stain and dental caries in primary teeth of Tunisian preschool children. *Eur Arch Paediatr Dent*. 2021;22(2):235-240.
40. Asokan S, Varshini KR, Geetha Priya PR, Vijayasankari V. Association between black stains and early childhood caries: a systematic review. *Indian J Dent Res*. 2020;31(6):957-962.
41. Milleman KR, Patil A, Ling MR, Mason S, Milleman JL. An exploratory study to investigate stain build-up with long term use of a stannous fluoride dentifrice. *Am J Dent*. 2018;31(2):71-75.
42. Figuero E, Herrera D, Tobías A, et al. Efficacy of adjunctive anti-plaque chemical agents in managing gingivitis: a systematic review and network meta-analyses. *J Clin Periodontol*. 2019;46(7):723-739.
43. Saraswat N, Pillay R, Everett B, George A. Knowledge, attitudes and practices of South Asian immigrants in developed countries regarding oral cancer: an integrative review. *BMC Cancer*. 2020;20(1):477.

44. Reichart PA, Lenz H, König H, Becker J, Mohr U. The black layer on the teeth of betel chewers: a light microscopic, microradiographic and electronmicroscopic study. *J Oral Pathol*. 1985;14(6):466-475.
45. Escartin JL, Arnedo A, Pinto V, Vela MJ. A study of dental staining among competitive swimmers. *Community Dent Oral Epidemiol*. 2000;28(1):10-17.
46. American Academy of Pediatric Dentistry, Council on Clinical Affairs. Guideline on dental management of heritable dental developmental anomalies. *Pediatr Dent*. 2016;38(6):302-307.
47. Bensi C, Costacurta M, Belli S, Paradiso D, Docimo R. Relationship between preterm birth and developmental defects of enamel: a systematic review and meta-analysis. *Int J Paediatr Dent*. 2020;30(6):676-686.
48. Rodd HD, Graham A, Tajmehr N, Timms L, Hasmun N. Molar incisor hypomineralisation: current knowledge and practice. *Int Dent J*. 2021;71(4):285-291.
49. Fejerskov O, Manji F, Baelum V. The nature and mechanisms of dental fluorosis in man. *J Dent Res*. 1990;69 Spec No:692-700; discussion 721.
50. Rozier RG. Epidemiologic indices for measuring the clinical manifestations of dental fluorosis: overview and critique. *Adv Dent Res*. 1994;8(1):39-55.
51. Thomas MS, Denny C. Medication-related tooth discoloration: a review. *Dent Update*. 2014;41(5):440-447.
52. Good M, Hussey D. Minocycline: stain devil?: your access options. *Br J Dermatol*. 2003;149(2):237-239.
53. Krastl G, Allgayer N, Lenherr P, Filippi A, Taneja P, Weiger R. Tooth discoloration induced by endodontic materials: a literature review. *Dent Traumatol*. 2013;29(1):2-7.
54. Ortiz ADC, Fideles SOM, Pomini KT, Buchaim RL. Updates in association of gastroesophageal reflux disease and dental erosion: systematic review. *Expert Rev Gastroenterol Hepatol*. 2021;15(9):1037-1046.
55. Chan AS, Tran TTK, Hsu YH, Liu SYS, Kroon J. A systematic review of dietary acids and habits on dental erosion in adolescents. *Int J Paediatr Dent*. 2020;30(6):713-733.

CHAPTER 18

The Periodontium

Linda D. Boyd, RDH, RD, EdD
Esther M. Wilkins, BS, RDH, DMD

CHAPTER OUTLINE

LEARNING OBJECTIVES

After studying this chapter, the student will be able to:

1. Recognize normal tissues of the periodontium.
2. Identify and describe the clinical features of the periodontium.
3. Describe the characteristics of healthy gingiva.
4. Compare and contrast the characteristics of gingiva in health and disease.
5. Describe the characteristics of healthy gingiva following periodontal surgery.

The Normal Periodontium

The **periodontium** is the functional unit of tissues surrounding and supporting the tooth. It is made up of two parts: the gingiva, which protects the underlying tissues, and the **attachment apparatus**, which consists of the periodontal ligament (PDL), cementum, and alveolar bone.[1] Recognizing normal, healthy periodontium by clinical observation and periodontal assessment is an essential component of accurate diagnosis and treatment planning.

I. Gingiva

The gingiva surrounds the roots of the teeth, alveolar bone, and underlying connective tissue.

Anatomically the gingiva is made up of the free gingiva, interdental gingiva (interdental papilla), and attached gingiva.[2]

A. Free Gingiva (Marginal Gingiva)

In health, the **free gingiva** surrounds the tooth, but is not attached to the tooth or alveolar bone. It connects with the attached gingiva at the free gingival groove and attaches to the tooth at the coronal portion of the **junctional epithelium (JE)** as shown in **Figure 18-1** and **Figure 18-2** to form the **gingival sulcus**.

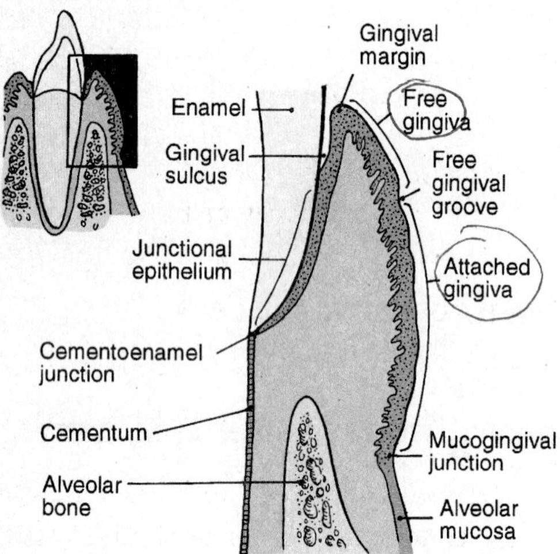

Figure 18-1 Parts of the Gingiva. Cross-sectional diagram shows the parts of the gingiva and adjacent tissues of a partially erupted tooth. Note that the junctional epithelium is on the enamel.

- Gingival margin (gingival crest, margin of the gingiva, or free margin, Figures 18-1 and 18-2)
  - Location: This is the edge of the gingiva, nearest to the incisal or occlusal surface.
  - The gingival margin is 0.08–2.1 mm coronal to the cementoenamel junction (CEJ) in health.[3]
  - Marks the opening of the gingival sulcus.
- Free gingival groove
  - Location: The **free gingival groove** is a shallow, linear groove demarcating the free from the attached gingiva. In health, there may be a free gingival groove visible in about one-third of adults.[4]
  - In the absence of inflammation and pocket formation, the gingival groove runs parallel with and about 0.5–1.5 mm from the gingival margin.[5]
  - The gingival groove is approximately at the level of the bottom of the gingival sulcus.
- Oral epithelium (outer gingival epithelium, **Figure 18-3**)
  - Location: Covers the free gingiva from the gingival groove over the gingival margin.
  - Composed of keratinized stratified squamous epithelium.
  - Cells turn over every 9–12 days.[4]

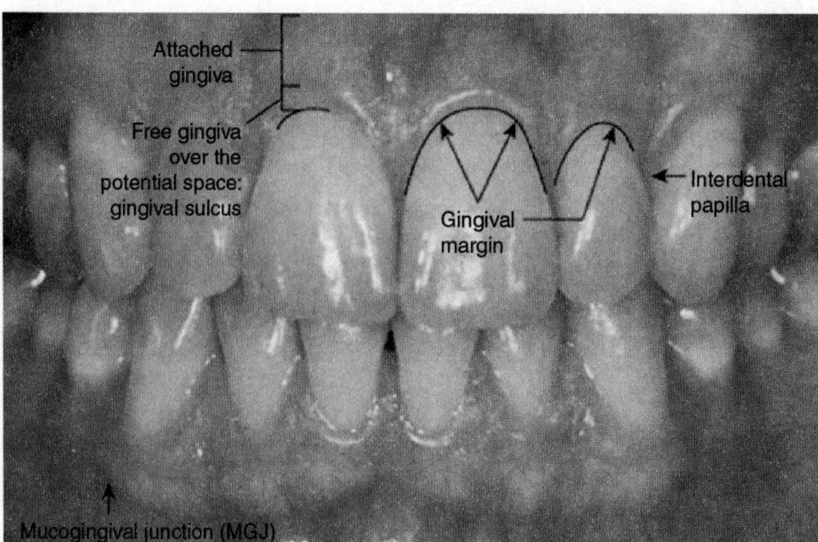

Figure 18-2 Picture of Gingival Tissues. Gingiva surrounds each tooth, forming a characteristic scalloped shape gingival margin. Interproximal papillae fill the spaces between most teeth. The potential space between the free gingiva and the tooth can be accessed with a periodontal probe. The attached gingiva is firmly attached to the underlying bone. The mucogingival junction (MGJ) is where the attached gingiva and alveolar mucosa meet.

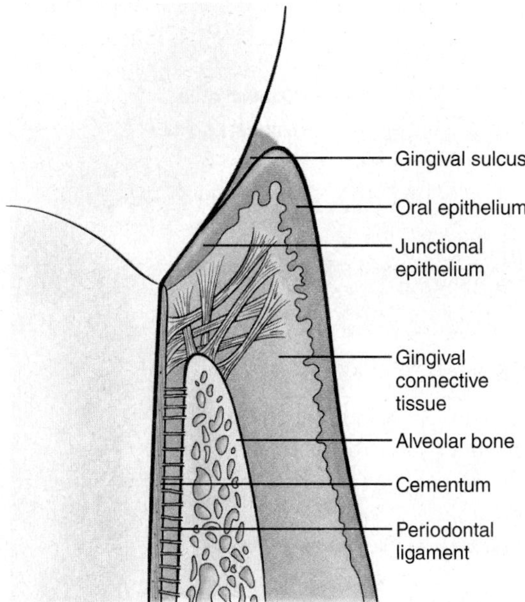

Figure 18-3 The Gingival Tissues. Cross-sectional diagram shows the relationships of the oral, sulcular, and junctional epithelium and the connective tissue.

B. Gingival Sulcus

- Location: The gingival sulcus is the crevice or space between the free gingiva and the tooth extending from the free gingival margin to the JE (Figure 18-1 and Figure 18-3).
- Sulcular epithelium
  - The continuation of the oral epithelium from the free gingiva.
  - Nonkeratinized.[1]
  - Plays a crucial role in sealing off the oral environment from the periodontal tissues.
- Depth of sulcus
  - Average histologic depth of the healthy sulcus is about 0.8–2.1 mm with no bleeding on probing.[3]
  - Average clinical **probing depth** of the normal gingival sulcus is 1.3–2.7 mm.[3]
- Gingival crevicular fluid or sulcular fluid
  - The **gingival crevicular fluid (GCF)** is a serum-like fluid that seeps from the connective tissue through the epithelial lining of the sulcus or pocket.
  - Flow rate is slight to none in a normal sulcus; GCF flow rate reflects changes in permeability of the tissue due to inflammation.[6]
  - It is part of the local defense mechanism and is able to transport many substances, including endotoxins, enzymes, antibodies, and certain systemically administered drugs.
  - Possible use as a diagnostic aid for periodontal disease activity because the composition changes in the presence of inflammation.[6,7]

C. Interdental Gingiva (Interdental Papilla)

- Location
  - In health, the **interdental gingiva** or **interdental papilla** occupies the interproximal area between two adjacent teeth that are in contact (see Figure 18-2).
  - The tip and lateral borders are continuous with the free gingiva, whereas other parts of the papilla are attached gingiva.
  - An interproximal area is also called an **embrasure**.
- Shape
  - Varies with spacing or overlapping of the teeth: The interdental gingiva may be flat or saddle shaped when there are wide spaces between teeth, or it may be tapered and narrow when teeth are crowded or overlapped.
  - Between anterior teeth: Pointed, pyramidal.
  - Between posterior teeth
    - Flatter than anterior papillae because of wider teeth, wider contact areas, and flattened interdental bone.
    - Two papillae, one facial and one lingual, connected by a col, are found when teeth are in contact.
- Col — nonkeratinized
  - A **col** is the depression under the contact area between a lingual or palatal and facial papilla that conforms to the proximal contact area, as shown in **Figure 18-4A** and **B**.
  - The width of the col from buccal to lingual ranges from 2 to 6 mm and the depth ranges from 0.3 to 1.5 mm.[8]
  - The center of the col area is not usually keratinized and thus is more susceptible to infection.[8]
- Papillary height
  - A classification system for papillary height[9] is as follows (**Figure 18-5A-D**):
    - Normal: The interdental papilla fills the space between teeth.
    - Class I embrasure: The tip of the interdental papilla is apical to the contact point of adjacent teeth, but the interproximal CEJ is not visible.
    - Class II embrasure: The tip of the interdental papilla is at or apical to the interproximal CEJ, but coronal to the height of the facial CEJ.
    - Class III embrasure: Complete loss of the interdental papilla due to extensive gingival recession.

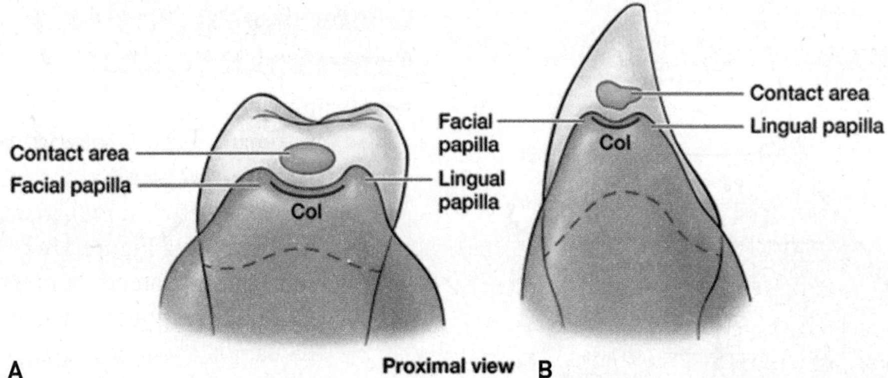

Figure 18-4 Col. A col is the depression between the lingual or palatal and the facial papillae under the contact area. **A:** Mesial of mandibular molar to show wide col area. **B:** Mesial of mandibular incisor to show a narrow col. The col deepens when gingival enlargement occurs.

Reproduced from Nield-Gehrig J, Weiss G. *Fundamentals of Periodontal Instrumentation and Advanced Root Instrumentation*. 7th ed. Philadelphia, PA: Lippincott Williams & Wilkins; 2012.

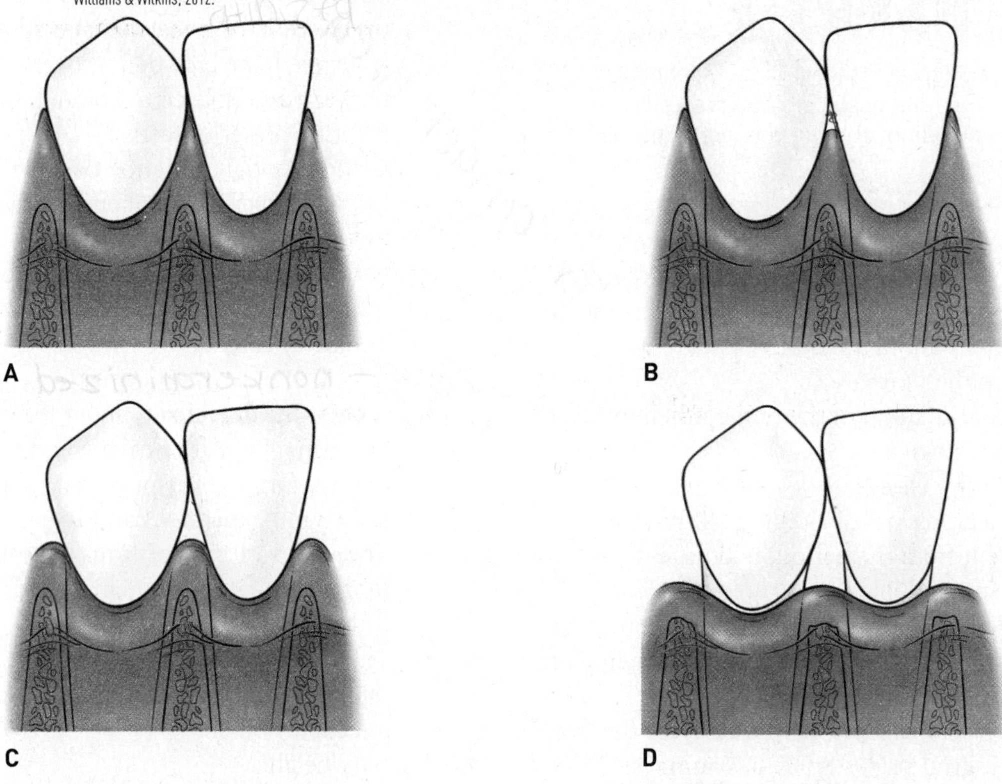

Figure 18-5 Interdental Embrasure Classifications. **A:** Normal papilla—fills the space between teeth. **B:** Class I embrasure—tip of interdental papilla is apical to the contact point, but the interproximal cementoenamel junction (CEJ) is not visible. **C:** Class II embrasure—tip of interdental papilla is at or apical to the interproximal CEJ, but coronal to the facial CEJ. **D:** Class III embrasure—the interdental papilla is at or apical to the level of the facial CEJ.

D. Junctional Epithelium

- Description
  - The junctional epithelium (JE) is a stratified squamous **nonkeratinized mucosa** made up of two strata (layers), one adjacent to the connective tissue and the other facing the tooth surface.
  - The JE is continuous with the sulcular epithelium and completely encircles the tooth to form a tight seal.
  - JE cells have wider fluid-filled intercellular spaces that contain polymorphonuclear leukocytes and monocytes that pass into the gingival sulcus to manage the constant microbial challenge.[10]
  - JE cells turn over rapidly in about 5 days.[8]
- Size
  - The JE may be 15 to 30 cells in thickness where it joins the sulcular epithelium and

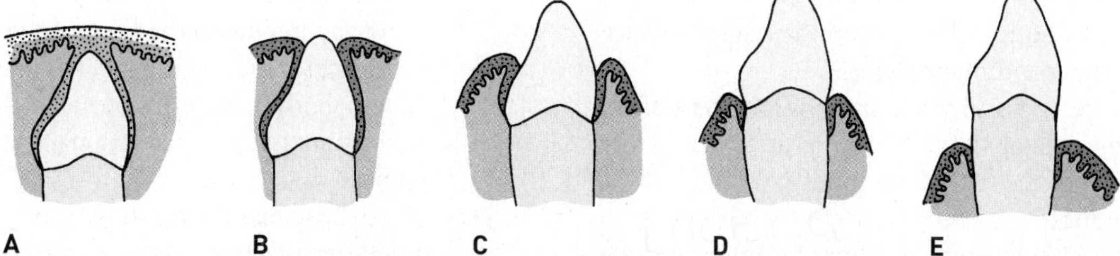

Figure 18-6 Tooth Eruption and the Gingiva. **A:** Before eruption, the oral epithelium covers the tooth. **B:** As the tooth emerges, the reduced epithelium joins the oral epithelium as the gingival sulcus is formed. **C:** Partial eruption with the junctional epithelium (JE) along the enamel. **D:** Eruption complete, with JE at the cementoenamel junction. **E:** From disease or other cause, the attachment migrates along the root surface, exposing the cementum.

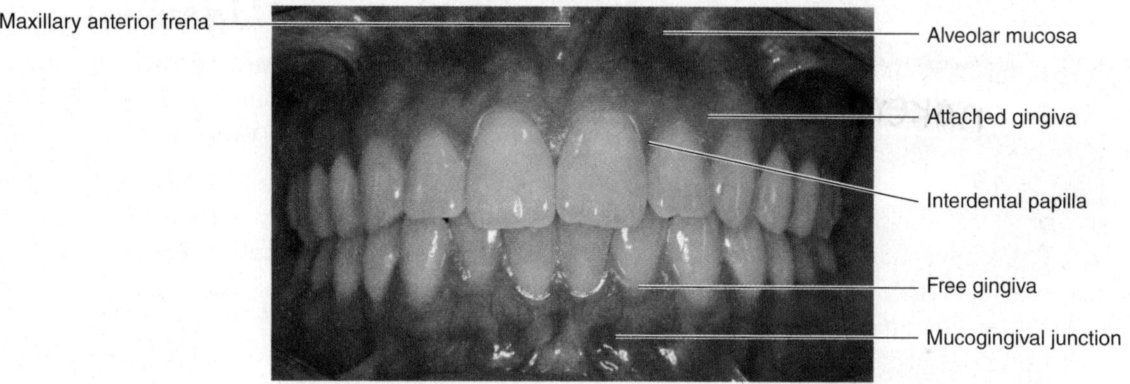

Figure 18-7 Parts of the Gingiva

tapers down to 1 to 3 cells in thickness at the apical end.[10]
  - The length ranges from 0.25 to 1.35 mm.[10]
- Position
  - As the tooth erupts, the attachment is on the enamel; during eruption, the **epithelium** migrates toward the CEJ (**Figure 18-6A–C**).
  - At full eruption, the attachment is usually on the cementum, where it becomes firmly attached (**Figure 18-6D**).
  - With wear of the tooth on the incisal or occlusal surface and with periodontal infections, the attachment migrates along the root surface (**Figure 18-6E**).
- Relation of crest of alveolar bone to the attached gingival tissue
  - The distance between the epithelial attachment and the crest of the alveolar bone is approximately 2.15 to 2.30 mm.[11] This is also referred to as the **biologic width**.
  - This distance is maintained in disease when the epithelium moves along the root surface and bone loss occurs.
- Epithelial attachment to the tooth surface
  - The JE attaches gingiva to the tooth and tissue by a basal lamina and **hemidesmosomes**.[8]

E. Attached Gingiva

- Extent
  - The **attached gingiva** is continuous with the **oral epithelium** of the free gingiva and is covered with keratinized stratified **squamous epithelium**.
  - Maxillary palatal gingiva is continuous with the palatal mucosa.
  - Attached gingiva of the mandibular facial and lingual gingiva and maxillary facial gingiva are demarcated from the alveolar mucosa by the **mucogingival junction (MGJ)** (Figure 18-1, Figure 18-2, and **Figure 18-7**).
- Attachment
  - Firmly bound to the underlying alveolar bone.
- Shape
  - Follows the depressions between the eminences of the roots of the teeth.

F. Mucogingival Junction

- Location
  - The MGJ is where the attached gingiva and the alveolar mucosa meet (Figure 18-1, Figure 18-2, and Figure 18-7).

- A mucogingival line is found on the facial surface of both arches and on the lingual surface of the mandibular arch.
- There is no alveolar mucosa on the palate. The palatal tissue is firmly attached to the bone of the roof of the mouth.

- Appearance
  - The MGJ appears as a line, a contrast can be seen between the pink of the **keratinized**, stippled, attached gingiva, and more vascular alveolar mucosa that is a deeper reddish-pink.
  - In the anterior area the MGJ is scalloped, but it is fairly straight in posterior areas.

G. Alveolar Mucosa

- Description nokeratinized
  - Movable tissue loosely attached to the underlying bone.
  - It has a smooth, shiny surface with nonkeratinized, thin epithelium. Underlying capillaries may often be visible through the epithelium.
- Frena (singular: Frenum or frenulum)
  - Description: A **frenum** is a narrow fold of mucous membrane connecting more fixed tissue to movable mucosa, for example, from the attached gingiva at the MGJ to the lip, cheek, or undersurface of the tongue. A frenum serves to restrict movement.
  - Locations
    - Maxillary and mandibular anterior frena: At midlines between central incisors. Figure 18-7 shows the location of the maxillary anterior frena.
    - Lingual frenum: Connects undersurface of the tongue to the floor of the mouth.
    - Buccal frena: In the canine–premolar areas, both maxillary and mandibular.
  - Attachment of frena in relation to the attached gingiva
  - Closely associated with the MGJ.
  - When the attached gingiva is narrow or missing, the frena may pull on the free gingiva and displace it laterally. A "tension test" can be used to locate frenal attachments and check the adequacy of the attached gingiva. (See Chapter 20.)

II. Periodontal Ligament

The **periodontal ligament (PDL)** is the fibrous connective tissue that surrounds and attaches the alveolar bone to the cementum (**Figure 18-8**).

- The PDL acts as an interface between bone and tooth and allows for movement to distribute the chewing or **masticatory forces**.[12]
- It is composed of cells and an extracellular compartment.[1]
  - Cells include osteoblasts, osteoclasts, fibroblasts, epithelial cells, and cementoblasts.
  - The extracellular compartment contains collagen fiber bundles in a ground substance.
- The fibers inserted into the cementum on one side and the alveolar bone on the other are called **Sharpey's fibers**.
- The two general groups of fibers are the gingival groups (**Figure 18-9**) (around the cervical area within the gingival tissues) and the principal fiber groups (surrounding the root).[1]

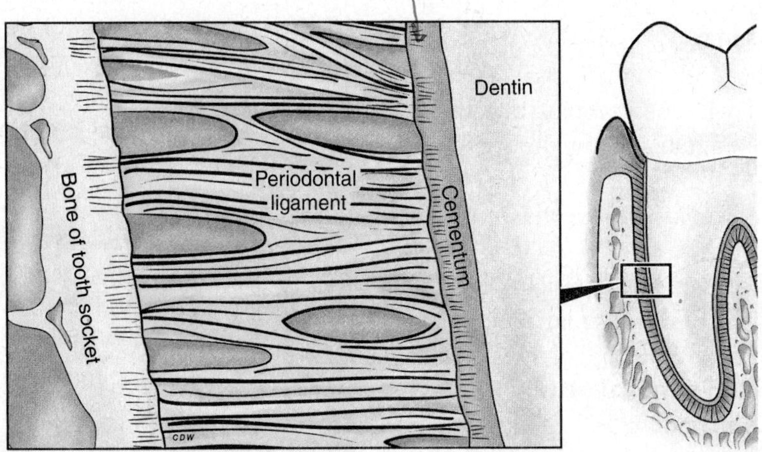

Figure 18-8 Periodontal Ligament. On the tooth side, the ends of the periodontal ligament fibers are anchored in the cementum of the root. On the bone side, the ends of the periodontal ligament fibers are anchored in the alveolar bone of the tooth socket.

A. Gingival Fiber Groups

- Dentogingival fibers (free gingiva): From the cementum in the cervical region into the free gingiva to give support to the gingiva.
- Alveologingival fibers (attached gingiva): From the alveolar crest into the free and attached gingiva to provide support.
- Circumferential fibers (circular): Continuous around the neck of the tooth to help to maintain the tooth in position.

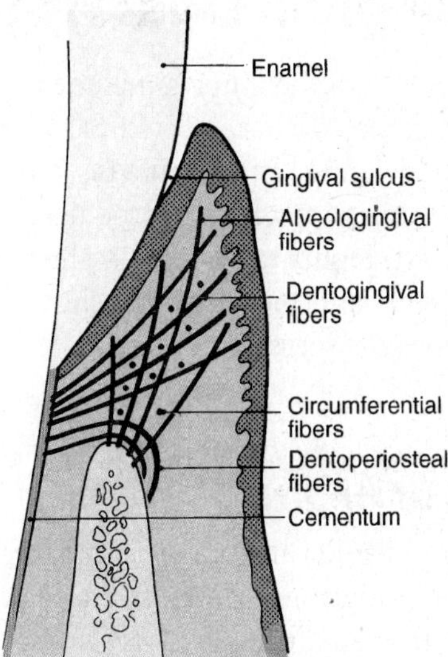

Figure 18-9 Gingival Fiber Groups. Cross section of the gingiva shows the relation of the gingival fiber groups to the gingival sulcus, free gingiva, cementum, and alveolar bone.

- Dentoperiosteal fibers (alveolar crest): From the cervical cementum over the alveolar crest to blend with fibers of the periosteum of the bone.
- Transseptal fibers: From the cervical area of one tooth across to an adjacent tooth (on the mesial or distal only) to provide resistance to separation of teeth.

B. Principal Fiber Groups

The five principal groups of collagen fibers (**Figure 18-10**) are named for their location on the root and for their direction. They are also called the dentoalveolar fiber groups.

- Apical fibers: Extend from the root apex to adjacent surrounding bone to resist vertical forces.
- Oblique fibers: Extend obliquely from the cementum to bone in a coronal direction and are the majority of the principal fibers. They help the tooth to resist vertical and unexpected strong forces.[13]
- Horizontal fibers: From the cementum in the middle of each root to adjacent alveolar bone to resist tipping of the tooth.
- Alveolar crest fibers: From the alveolar crest to the cementum just below the CEJ to resist intrusive forces.
- Interradicular fibers: From cementum between the roots of multi-rooted teeth to the adjacent bone to resist vertical and lateral forces.

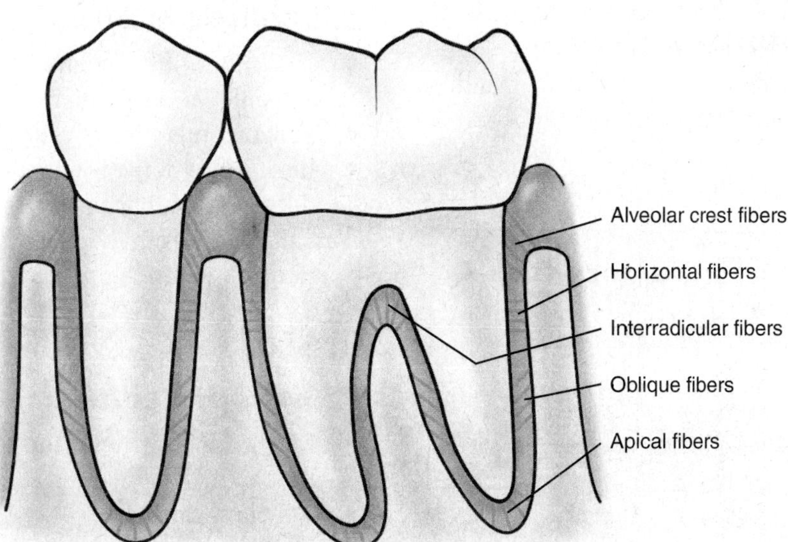

Figure 18-10 Principal Fiber Groups of the Periodontium. The five principal groups (apical, oblique, horizontal, alveolar crest, and interradicular) are shown. The transseptal fibers of the gingival fiber groups are also shown as they span across from the cervical area of one tooth to the neighboring tooth.

III. Cementum

The cementum is a thin layer of calcified connective tissue that covers the tooth from the CEJ to, and around, the apical foramen.

A. Functions

- Supports the tooth along with the alveolar bone by serving as the attachment for periodontal fiber groups of the PDL.[14]
- Seals the tubules of the root dentin.

B. Characteristics

- Thickness is 50–200 μm.[14]
- Thickness of cementum increases with age.
- Two types of cementum:[14]
    - Acellular cementum is on the cervical half to two-thirds of the root and serves as a place for attachment of the PDL fibers.
    - Cellular cementum is found primarily on the apical half or third of the root and serves as a repair tissue to fill defects.
- Relationship of enamel and cementum at the cervical area is shown in **Figure 18-11**. Estimates for the relationship of enamel to cementum are as follows:
    - A gap between cementum and enamel exposing dentin in 10–40% of teeth.
    - Enamel and cementum meet edge-to-edge in 50–70% of the teeth.
    - The cementum overlaps the enamel in approximately 7–14%.[15]

IV. Alveolar Bone

The alveolar bone is a specialized part of the mandibular and maxillary bones with a primary function to support the teeth.

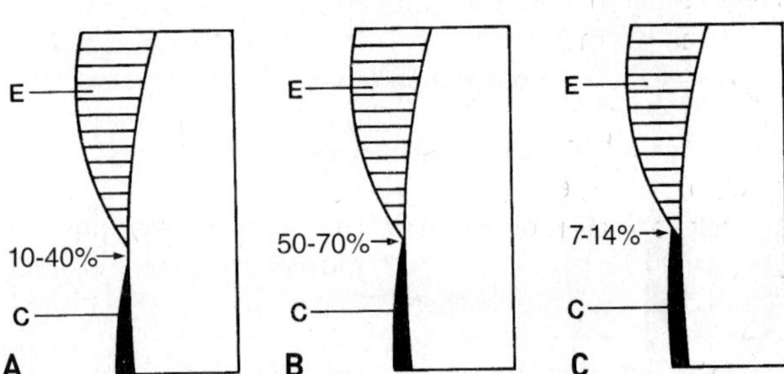

Figure 18-11 Relationship of Enamel and Cementum. The possible relationships of the enamel and the cementum of the cementoenamel junction. **A:** The cementum and the enamel do not meet, and there is a small zone of dentin exposed in 10–40% of teeth. **B:** The cementum meets the enamel in approximately 50–70% of teeth. **C:** The cementum overlaps the enamel in 7–14% of teeth.

- Description
    - Alveolar bone undergoes rapid and continual remodeling due to the demands of tooth eruption, orthodontic tooth movement, and occlusal forces.[16]
    - The architecture is similar to other bone tissues, but the rate of bone remodeling is unique to alveolar bone.[16]
    - When teeth are lost, the alveolar bone is progressively resorbed.

The Gingival Description

The examination of the gingiva includes evaluation of color, size, shape, consistency, surface texture, position, MGJs, bleeding, and **exudate**. These are summarized in **Table 18-1**, which can be used as a clinical reference chart. **Figure 18-12A** and **B** show an image of healthy gingiva, and **Figure 18-12C** shows gingiva exhibiting signs of disease (gingivitis).

I. Color

A. Signs of Health

- Pale pink: Darker in people with darker complexions due to melanin pigmentation (Figure 18-12B).
- Factors influencing color
    - Vascular supply.
    - Thickness of epithelium.
    - Degree of keratinization.
    - Physiologic pigmentation

B. Changes in Disease

- In chronic inflammation: Dark red, bluish red, magenta, or deep blue.
- In acute inflammation: Bright red.
- Extent: Deep involvement can be expected when diffuse color changes extend into the attached gingiva, or from the marginal gingiva to the MGJ, or through into alveolar mucosa.

II. Size

A. Signs of Health

- Free gingiva: Flat, not enlarged; fits snugly around the tooth.
- Attached gingiva
    - Width of attached gingiva varies among patients and among teeth for an individual from 1–9 mm.[17]
    - Wider in maxilla than mandible; broadest zone related to incisors, narrowest at the canine and premolar regions.

Table 18-1 Examination of the Gingival Clinical Markers

	Appearance in Health	Changes in Disease Clinical Appearance	Causes for Changes
Color	Uniformly pale pink or coral pink Variations in pigmentation related to complexion, race	Acute: Bright red Chronic: Bluish pink, bluish red, magenta Attached gingiva: Color change may extend to the mucogingival line	Inflammation Capillary dilation Increased blood flow Vessels engorged Blood flow sluggish Venous return impaired **Anoxemia** Increased fibrosis Deepening of pocket, mucogingival involvement
Size	Not enlarged Fits snugly around the tooth	Enlarged	**Edematous**: Inflammatory fluid, cellular exudate, vascular engorgement, hemorrhage Fibrotic: New collagen fibers
Shape (contour)	Marginal gingiva: Flat, knife-edged, follows a curved line about the tooth Papillae: Normal contact: papilla is pointed and pyramidal; fills the interproximal area space (diastema) between teeth; gingiva is flat or saddle shaped	Marginal gingiva: Rounded, rolled Papillae: Bulbous, flattened, blunted, cratered	Inflammatory changes: Edematous or fibrous **Bulbous** with gingival enlargement Cratered in necrotizing ulcerative gingivitis
Consistency	Firm Attached gingiva firmly bound to underlying bone	Soft, spongy: Dents readily when pressed with probe Associated with red color, smooth shiny surface, loss of stippling, bleeding on probing	Edematous: Fluid between cells in connective tissue Fibrotic: Collagen fibers
Surface texture	Free gingiva: Smooth Attached gingiva: Stippled	Acute condition: Smooth, shiny gingiva Chronic: Hard, firm, with stippling, sometimes heavier than normal	Inflammatory changes in the connective tissue; Edema, cellular infiltration Fibrosis
Position of gingival margin	Fully erupted tooth: Margin is 1–2 mm above CEJ, at or slightly below the enamel contour	Enlarged gingiva: Margin is higher on the tooth, above normal, pocket deepened Recession: Margin is more apical; root surface is exposed	Edematous or fibrotic JE has migrated along the root; gingival margin follows
Position of JE	During eruption along the enamel surface (Figure 18-6) Fully erupted tooth: the JE is at the CEJ	Position determined by the use of probe, is on the root surface	Apical migration of the epithelium along the root

(continues)

Table 18-1 Examination of the Gingival Clinical Markers *(continued)*

	Appearance in Health	Changes in Disease Clinical Appearance	Causes for Changes
Mucogingival junctions	Make clear demarcation between the pink, stippled, attached gingiva and the darker alveolar mucosa with smooth shiny surface	No attached gingiva: Color changes may extend full height of the gingiva; mucogingival line obliterated Probing reveals that the bottom of the pocket extends into the alveolar mucosa Frenal pull may displace the gingival margin from the tooth	Apical migration of the JE Attached gingiva decreases with pocket deepening Inflammation extends into alveolar mucosa
Bleeding	No spontaneous bleeding or upon probing	Spontaneous bleeding Bleeding on probing: Bleeding near margin in acute condition; bleeding deep in pocket in chronic condition	Degeneration of the sulcular epithelium with the formation of pocket epithelium Blood vessels engorged Tissue edematous
Exudate	No exudate expressed on pressure or during probing	White, yellow, or green suppuration, visible on digital pressure or during probing Amount not related to pocket depth	Inflammation in the connective tissue Excessive accumulation of white blood cells with serum and tissue makes up the exudate (suppuration or pus)

CEJ, cementoenamel junction; JE, junctional epithelium

B. Changes in Disease

- Free gingiva and papillae
    - Become enlarged.
    - May be localized or limited to specific areas or generalized throughout the gingiva.
    - The col deepens as the papillae increase in size.
- Attached gingiva: Decreases in amount as the pocket deepens.

C. Enlargement from Drug Therapy

- Certain drugs used for specific systemic therapy cause gingival enlargement as a side effect such as phenytoin, cyclosporine, and nifedipine (calcium channel blocker).[18]

III. Shape (Form or Contour)

A. Signs of Health

- Free gingiva
    - Follows a curved line around each tooth; may be straighter along wide molar surfaces.
    - The margin is knife-edged or slightly rounded on facial and lingual gingiva; closely adapted to the tooth surface.
- Papillae
    - Facial and lingual gingiva are pointed or pyramidal papillae with a col area under the contact between adjacent teeth.
    - Spaced teeth (with diastemata). Interdental gingiva is flat or saddle shaped.

B. Changes in Disease

- Free gingiva: Rounded or rolled.
- Papillae: Blunted, flattened, bulbous, cratered (**Figure 18-13A–C**).
- "McCall's festoon": An enlargement of the marginal gingiva with the formation of a lifesaver-like gingival prominence. Frequently, the total gingiva is very narrow, with associated apparent recession, as shown in **Figure 18-13D**.
- "Stillman's cleft" (**Figure 18-14A** and **B**).
    - A localized recession may be V shaped, apostrophe shaped, or form a slit-like indentation. It may extend several millimeters toward the MGJ or even to or through the junction.
- Floss cleft: A cleft created by incorrect floss positioning appears as a vertical linear or V-shaped fissure in the marginal gingiva and can result in bone loss if not corrected.[19]

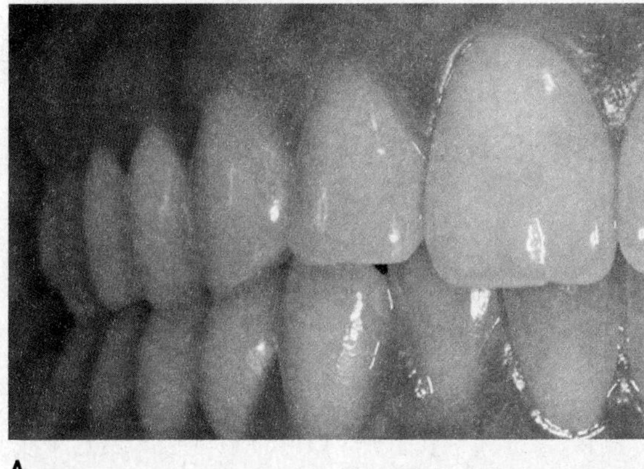

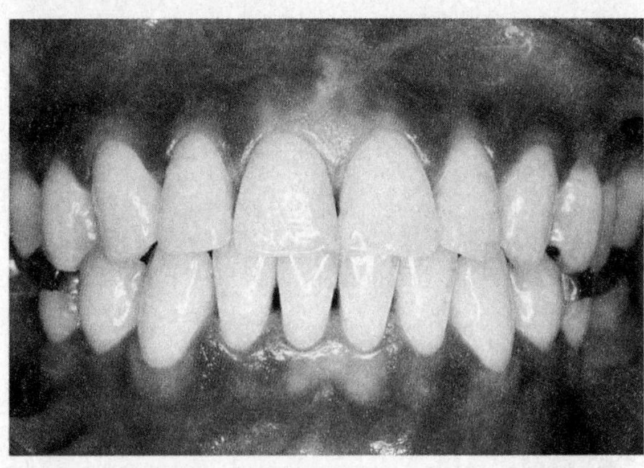

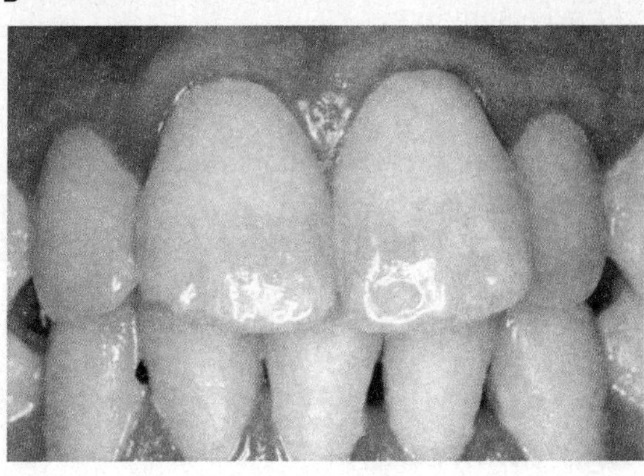

Figure 18-12 Signs of Health. **A:** Health: Coral pink color, stippling is evident, gingival margins are knife-edged, and interdental papilla are pointed. **B:** Pigmentation of the gingiva showing how the gingiva can vary in color in some patients. Signs of disease. **C:** Pinkish-red color, loss of stippling, redness and enlargement of gingival margin, and interdental papilla are slightly bulbous in maxillary areas.

A and **C:** Reproduced from Nield-Gehrig J, Weiss G. *Fundamentals of Periodontal Instrumentation and Advanced Root Instrumentation*. 7th ed. Philadelphia, PA: Lippincott Williams & Wilkins; 2012.

- Usually occurs at one side of an interdental papilla.
- The injury can develop when dental floss is curved repeatedly in an incomplete "C" around the line angle so the floss is pressed across the gingiva.

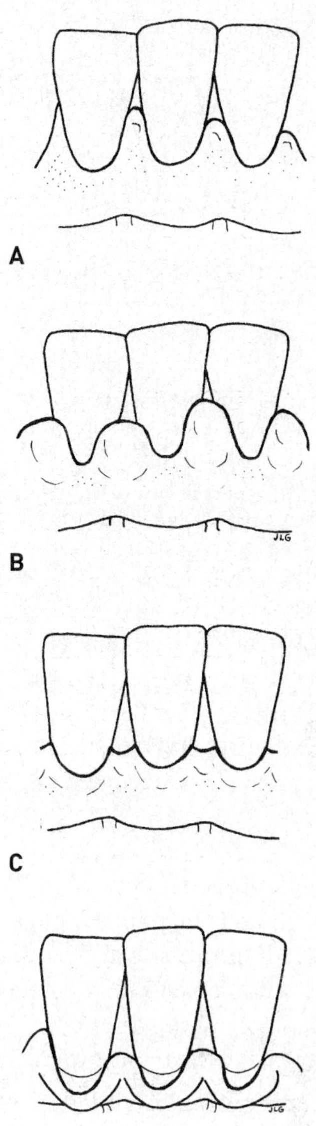

Figure 18-13 Gingival Shape or Contour. **A:** Blunted papillae. **B:** Bulbous papillae. **C:** Cratered papillae. **D:** Rolled, lifesaver-shaped "McCall's festoons."

IV. Consistency

A. Signs of Health

- Attached gingiva is bound firmly to the underlying bone.

B. Changes in Disease

- To determine consistency: Gently press side of probe on free gingiva. Soft, spongy gingiva dents readily; firm, hard tissue resists.
- Soft, spongy gingiva: Related to acute stages of inflammation with increased infiltration of fluid and inflammatory elements.
  - The tissue appears red, may be smooth and shiny with loss of stippling.

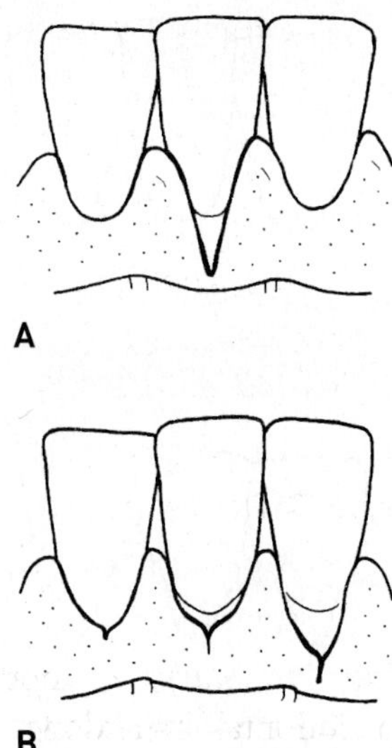

Figure 18-14 Gingival Clefts. **A:** V-shaped Stillman's cleft. **B:** Slit-like Stillman's clefts of varying degrees of severity in relation to the mucogingival junction.

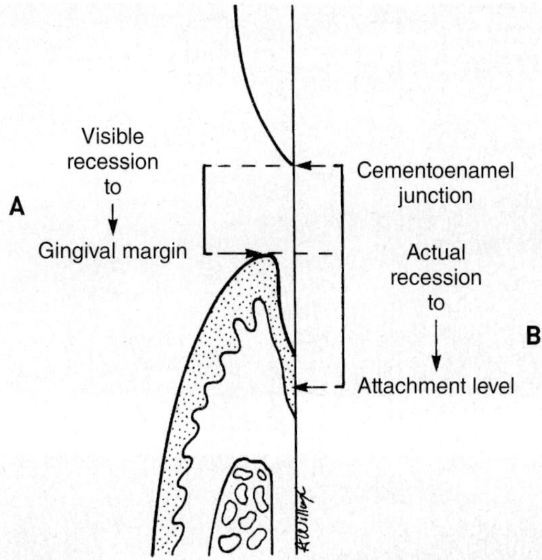

Figure 18-15 Gingival Recession. **A:** Clinically visible recession of the gingival margin with root surface apparent to the eye. **B:** The actual recession exposes the root surface as the periodontal attachment migrates along the root surface.

    - Tissue may be **friable** or thin and fragile.
    - Has marginal enlargement and bleeds readily on probing.
- Firm, hard gingiva: Related to chronic inflammation with increased fibrosis.
    - Fibrotic tissue may appear pink and firm with no bleed on probing even in the presence of inflammation, particularly in individuals who smoke.[20]
- Retraction of the margin away from the tooth: Normally, the free gingiva fits snugly about the tooth.
    - When the margin tends to hang slightly away or is readily displaced with a light air blast, it suggests the gingival fibers that support the margin have been destroyed (**Figure 18-15**).

V. Surface Texture

A. Signs of Health

- Free gingiva: Smooth.
    - Attached gingiva: **Stippled** (minutely "pebbled" or "orange peel" surface).
    - Interdental gingiva: The free gingiva is smooth; the center portion of each papilla is stippled.

B. Changes in Disease

- Inflammatory changes: May be loss of stippling, with smooth, shiny surface.
- **Hyperkeratosis**: May result in a leathery, hard, or nodular surface.
- Chronic disease: Tissue may be hard and **fibrotic**, with a normal pink color and normal or deep stippling.

VI. Position

- The actual position of the gingiva is the level of the epithelial attachment. It is not directly visible but can be determined through periodontal probing.
- The apparent position of the gingiva is the level of the gingival margin or crest of the free gingiva that is seen by direct observation.

A. Signs of Health

For the fully erupted tooth in an adult, the apparent position of the gingival margin is at the level of, or slightly below, the enamel contour or prominence of the cervical third of a tooth.

B. Changes in Disease

- Effect of gingival enlargement: When the gingiva is enlarged, the gingival margin is coronal to the CEJ, partially or nearly covering the anatomic crown as seen in Dilantin hyperplasia.
- Effect of gingival recession
    - Definition: Recession is the exposure of root surface resulting from the apical migration of the JE exposing the CEJ (Figure 18-15).
    - Actual recession: The recession is measured from the CEJ to the gingival margin.

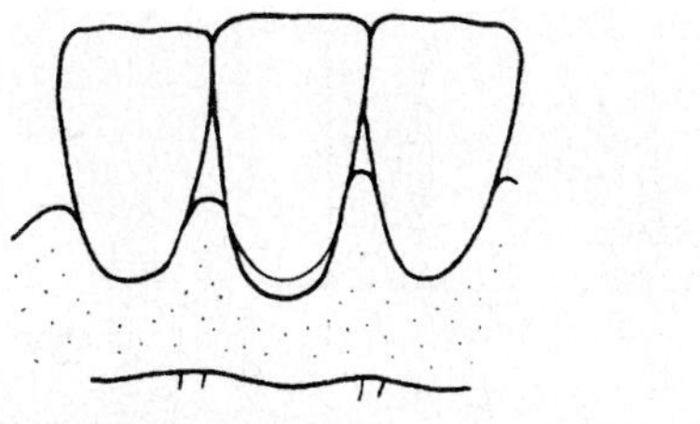
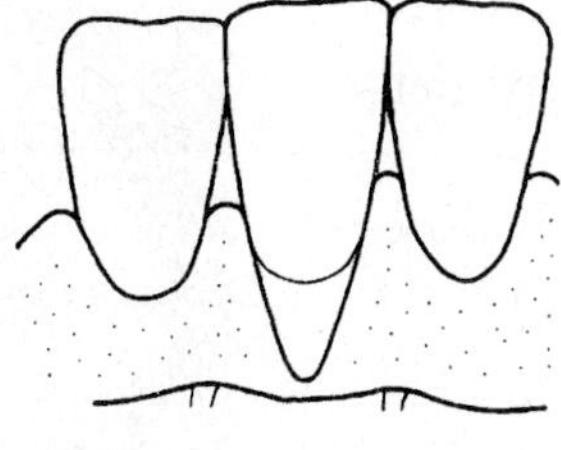
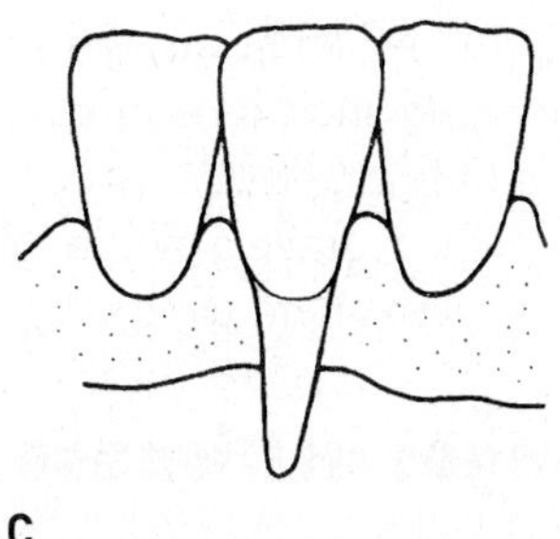

Figure 18-16 Localized Recession. A single tooth may show narrow or wide, deep or shallow recession. **A:** Wide, shallow. **B:** Wide, deep, with narrow attached gingiva. **C:** Narrow, deep, with missing attached gingiva.

- Visible recession: Exposed root surface visible on clinical examination from the gingival margin to the CEJ.
- Localized recession (**Figure 18-16**): A localized recession may be narrow or wide and deep or shallow. The root surface is denuded, and the visible recession may extend to or through the MGJ.
- Measurement: Both actual and visible recession can be measured with a periodontal probe from the CEJ. Total recession is the distance from the CEJ to the bottom of the sulcus.

VII. Bleeding

A. Signs of Health

- Traditionally the definition of gingival health has been no bleeding on periodontal probing[20]; however, the 2017 World Workshop on the Classification of Periodontal and Peri-Implant Disease and Condition defines gingival health as one or two sites of gingival inflammation.[21] The case definition for gingivitis is $<$10% of sites bleed on probing.[21]

B. Changes in Disease

- Sulcular epithelium becomes a diseased pocket epithelium.
- The ulcerated pocket wall bleeds spontaneously or during periodontal probing.

VIII. Exudate

A. Signs of Health

There is no exudate in health.[7]

B. Changes in Disease

- Increased GCF in presence of inflammation with flow rate increasing as periodontal disease progresses.[7,22]
- **Suppuration (or pus)** is another indicator of active periodontal breakdown and may be seen in about 25% of patients with chronic periodontitis.[23]

The Gingiva of Young Children

I. Signs of Health

A. Primary Dentition

- Color: Pink.
- Shape: Thick, rounded, or rolled.
- Consistency: Less fibrous than adult gingiva; not as tightly adapted to the teeth.
- Surface texture: May or may not have stippling; in children with healthy gingiva, stippling may be present in less than 50%.[24]
- Attached gingiva: Width of attached gingiva in children is typically between 4 and 5 mm.[25]
- Interdental gingiva
  - Anterior: The maxillary midline **diastema** is present in the primary dentition in 97% of cases[26] and is considered normal; the papillae in areas of diastemas are flat or saddle shaped.
  - Posterior: Col between facial and lingual papillae when teeth are in contact (Figure 18-4A).

B. Mixed Dentition

- Constant state of change with periods of inflammation related to exfoliation and eruption.[27]
- Free gingiva may appear rolled or rounded, slightly reddened, shiny, and with a lack of firmness.
- The gingiva covers a varying portion of the anatomic crown, depending on the stage of eruption (Figure 18-6).

- Alveolar bone height varies during exfoliation and eruption and should be monitored until the dentition is fully erupted.[27]
- The attached gingiva width gradually increases once the permanent teeth erupt completely.[25,28]

II. Changes in Disease

- Gingivitis occurs frequently in children but is usually reversible with improved oral self-care without leaving permanent damage.
- Mucogingival problems can occur in children. The recognition of deficiencies of attached gingiva has particular significance for the child who will need orthodontic treatment.[23]
    - However, managing gingival inflammation and thickness of the gingiva are more important than the width of the gingiva.[28]
- A periodontal examination is conducted at dental visits for early diagnosis of periodontal disease according to the Academy of Periodontology and American Academy of Pediatric Dentistry.[29–31]
- The British Society of Periodontology and the British Society of Paediatric Dentistry recommend the use of the Simplified Basic Periodontal Examination for screening of children and adolescents.[31]

The Gingiva after Periodontal Surgery

I. Pocket Reduction Surgery

- The characteristics of "normal healthy gingiva" take on different dimensions for the patient who has completed treatment for pockets, bone loss, and other signs of a periodontal infection.
- The JE may be apical to the CEJ (see **Figure 18-17**).
- After healing, in health the stable patient should have sulcus depths ≤4 mm with <10% bleeding on probing. Any remaining sites ≥4 mm should have no bleeding on probing according to the 2017 World Workshop on the Classification of Periodontal and Peri-Implant Diseases and Conditions.[21]
- With each periodontal maintenance appointment, a careful examination is necessary to control factors that may permit recurrence of disease.

II. Gingival Grafting Surgery

- Depending on the exact type of gingival or connective tissue grafting surgery performed, examination shows changes from the initial evaluation.

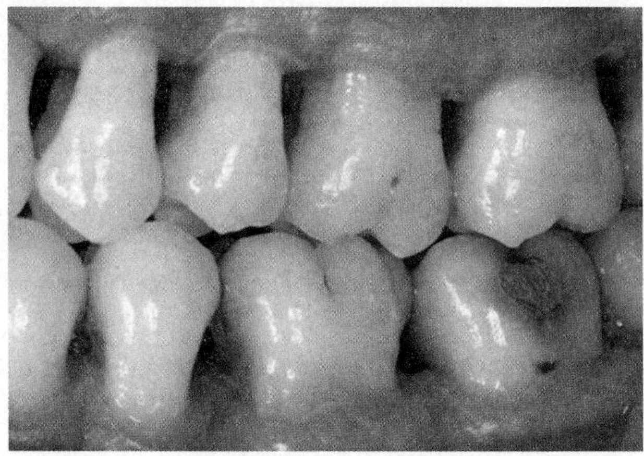

Figure 18-17 Gingiva after Pocket Reduction Periodontal Surgery. The gingival margin is significantly apical to cementoenamel junction leading to exposure of the root surface and root concavities. The embrasures (space) between teeth is no longer filled by the papillae.

Reproduced from Nield-Gehrig J, Weiss G. *Fundamentals of Periodontal Instrumentation and Advanced Root Instrumentation*. 7th ed. Philadelphia, PA: Lippincott Williams & Wilkins; 2012.

    - For example, where the initial examination showed a deficiency of attached gingiva with frenal pull, mucogingival surgery may have created new attached gingiva.

III. Implant Surgery

- Gingiva around the implant should have the same color and consistency as gingiva surrounding a natural tooth. (See Chapter 31.)
- Contour of the gingiva will depend on the placement of the implant, but may result in open embrasures interproximally like those seen after pocket reduction surgery.

Documentation

The permanent records of a patient who received treatment for a gingival or periodontal condition would have a minimum of the following:

- Health history with routine follow-up recorded for each visit.
- Initial charting and descriptive material to show disease symptoms with information to show need for and actual treatment carried out by a series of progress notes at each appointment with changes identified resulting from specific treatment.
- Individual oral self-care instruction with biofilm scores to monitor progress. Any personal care products recommended, their demonstration, and report of use by the patient. Record of

improvements in gingival health noted over the series of appointments.

- Patient's own comments related to oral health change, habit changes, dietary changes, all successes, along with an agreement to a recommended plan for a periodontal maintenance program.
- A progress note for an individual patient appointment may be read in **Box 18-1**.

Factors to Teach the Patient

- Role and responsibility for self-management of periodontal disease.
- Characteristics of normal healthy gingiva.
- The significance of bleeding; healthy tissue does not bleed.
- Relationship of findings during a gingival examination to the daily oral self-care procedures for infection control.
- The special attention needed for an area of gingival recession to prevent abrasion, inflammation, and further involvement.
- How the brushing method, stiffness of toothbrush filaments, abrasiveness of a dentifrice, and pressure applied during brushing can be factors in gingival recession.

Box 18-1 Example Documentation: Description of the Periodontium

- **S**—55-year-old Hispanic female presents for continuing care appointment with chief complaint of bleeding when she brushes her teeth.
- **O**—Gingival description: Color: Normal pigmentation, generalized dark reddish inflammation of free gingival margin. Size: General slight enlargement of interdental papilla. Shape: Bulbous areas in maxillary anterior. Consistency: Generally soft and spongy, shiny surface, generalized bleeding on probing. Probing depths generally 3–4 mm. Biofilm score: 50%.
- **A**—Diagnosis is plaque-induced gingivitis.
- **P**—Oral biofilm was disclosed and patient demonstrated toothbrushing and flossing technique. Review of modified Bass technique was provided to assist in accessing biofilm along gingival margins. Floss technique was good, but the patient needs to be more consistent flossing daily. Treatment goals: (1) brush 2×/day, (2) flossing daily, and (3) reduce bleeding on probing by 20%. Subgingival debridement and prophylaxis completed. Five percent sodium fluoride varnish applied because of moderate caries risk. Next visit: 6-month continuing care.

Signed: ______________________________, RDH
Date: ______________________________

References

1. Nanci A, Bosshardt DD. Structure of periodontal tissues in health and disease. *Periodontol 2000*. 2006;40:11-28.
2. Bartold PM, Walsh LJ, Narayanan AS. Molecular and cell biology of the gingiva. *Periodontol 2000*. 2000;24(1):28-55.
3. Ainamo J, Loe H. Anatomical characteristics of gingiva. A clinical and microscopic study of the free and attached gingiva. *J Periodontol*. 1966;37(1):5-13.
4. Leblebicioglu B, Claman L. Periodontal anatomy. In: RC Scheid, G Weiss, eds. *Dental Anatomy*. 9th ed. Philadelphia, PA: Wolters Kluwer; 2016:215-248.
5. Orban B. Clinical and histologic study of the surface characteristics of the gingiva. *Oral Surg Oral Med Oral Pathol*. 1948;1(9):827-841.
6. Gupta G. Gingival crevicular fluid as a periodontal diagnostic indicator. II: Inflammatory mediators, host-response modifiers and chair side diagnostic aids. *J Med Life*. 2013;6(1):7-13.
7. Fatima T, Khurshid Z, Rehman A, Imran E, Srivastava KC, Shrivastava D. Gingival crevicular fluid (GCF): a diagnostic tool for the detection of periodontal health and diseases. *Molecules*. 2021;26(5):12088.
8. Schroeder HE, Listgarten MA. The gingival tissues: the architecture of periodontal protection. *Periodontol 2000*. 1997;13(1):91-120.
9. Nordland WP, Tarnow DP. A classification system for loss of papillary height. *J Periodontol*. 1998;69(10):1124-1126.
10. Bosshardt DD, Lang NP. The junctional epithelium: from health to disease. *J Dent Res*. 2005;84(1):9-20.
11. Schmidt JC, Sahrmann P, Weiger R, Schmidlin PR, Walter C. Biologic width dimensions: a systematic review. *J Clin Periodontol*. 2013;40(5):493-504.
12. Ho SP, Kurylo MP, Fong T, et al. The biomechanical characteristics of the bone-periodontal ligament-cementum complex. *Biomaterials*. 2010;31(25):6635-6646.
13. Cho MI, Garant PR. Development and general structure of the periodontium. *Periodontol 2000*. 2000;24:9-27.
14. YamamotoT, Hasegawa T, Yamamoto T, Hongo H, Amizuka N. Histology of human cementum: its structure, function, and development. *Jpn Dent Sci Rev*. 2016;52(3):63-74.
15. Astekar M, Kaur P, Dhakar N, Singh J. Comparison of hard tissue interrelationships at the cervical region of teeth based on tooth type and gender difference. *J Forensic Dent Sci*. 2014;6(2):86-91.
16. Sodek J, McKee MD. Molecular and cellular biology of alveolar bone. *Periodontol 2000*. 2000;24(1):99-126.
17. Lang NP, Loe H. The relationship between the width of keratinized gingiva and gingival health. *J Periodontol*. 1972;43(10):623-627.
18. Trackman PC, Kantarci A. Molecular and clinical aspects of drug-induced gingival overgrowth. *J Dent Res*. 2015;94(4):540-546.

19. Hallmon WW, Waldrop TC, Houston GD, Hawkins BF. Flossing clefts. Clinical and histologic observations. *J Periodontol.* 1986;57(8):501-504.
20. Meitner SW, Zander HA, Iker HP, Polson AM. Identification of inflamed gingival surfaces. *J Clin Periodontol.* 1979;6(2):93-97.
21. Chapple ILC, Mealey BL, Van Dyke TE, et al. Periodontal health and gingival diseases and conditions on an intact and a reduced periodontium: consensus report of workgroup 1 of the 2017 World Workshop on the Classification of Periodontal and Peri-Implant Diseases and Conditions. *J Clin Periodontol.* 2018;45(Suppl 20):S68-S77.
22. Goodson JM. Gingival crevice fluid flow. *Periodontol 2000.* 2003;31:43-54.
23. Silva-Boghossian CM, Neves AB, Resende FA, Colombo AP. Suppuration-associated bacteria in patients with chronic and aggressive periodontitis. *J Periodontol.* 2013;84(9):e9-e16.
24. Bimstein E, Peretz B, Holan G. Prevalence of gingival stippling in children. *J Clin Pediatr Dent.* 2003;27(2):163-165.
25. Maynard JG, Ochsenbein C. Mucogingival problems, prevalence and therapy in children. *J Periodontol.* 1975;46(9):543-552.
26. Gkantidis N, Kolokitha OE, Topouzelis N. Management of maxillary midline diastema with emphasis on etiology. *J Clin Pediatr Dent.* 2008;32(4):265-272.
27. Drummond BK, Brosnan MG, Leichter JW. Management of periodontal health in children: pediatric dentistry and periodontology interface. *Periodontol 2000.* 2017;74(1):158-167.
28. Wyrębek B, Orzechowska A, Cudziło D, Plakwicz P. Evaluation of changes in the width of gingiva in children and youth. Review of literature. *Dev Period Med.* 2015;19(2):212-216.
29. Califano JV; Research, Science and Therapy Committee American Academy of Periodontology. Position paper: periodontal diseases of children and adolescents. *J Periodontol.* 2003;74(11):1696-1704.
30. American Academy of Pediatric Dentistry. Classification of periodontal diseases in infants, children, adolescents, and individuals with special health care needs. In: *The Reference Manual of Pediatric Dentistry*. Chicago, IL: American Academy of Pediatric Dentistry; 2021:435-449.
31. Cole E, Ray-Chaudhuri A, Vaidyanathan M, Johnson J, Sood S. Simplified basic periodontal examination (BPE) in children and adolescents: a guide for general dental practitioners. *Dental Update.* 2014;41(4):328-337.

CHAPTER 19

Periodontal Disease Development

Linda D. Boyd, RDH, RD, EdD
Esther M. Wilkins, BS, RDH, DMD

CHAPTER OUTLINE

LEARNING OBJECTIVES

After studying this chapter, the student will be able to:

1. List and describe the modifiable and nonmodifiable risk factors for periodontal disease.
2. Explain the signs and symptoms of periodontal disease.
3. Define the stages of development for periodontal lesions.
4. Apply the staging and grading of periodontal disease in the current classification system.
5. Describe the dental hygienist's role in educating the patient about management of modifiable risk factors for periodontal disease.

The periodontium gives the support needed to maintain the teeth in function (**Figure 19-1**).

- Periodontal diseases are chronic diseases initiated by microorganisms in the dental biofilm, which collects on the teeth when oral self-care is inadequate.

Periodontal-Systemic Disease Connection

- There has been significant research on the association between periodontal infections and a number of systemic diseases and conditions, including[1,2]:
    - Cardiovascular disease.
    - Adverse pregnancy outcomes, including premature low birth weight babies.
    - Respiratory disease.
    - Chronic kidney disease.
    - Rheumatoid arthritis.
    - Obesity.
    - Cognitive impairment.
    - Osteoporosis.
    - Inflammatory bowel disease.
    - Some cancers.
- Despite the association, periodontal disease has not been shown to *cause* systemic disease.
- The mechanism for the association is not yet clear, but infection and inflammation are common elements of all the diseases and conditions.[3]
- The association between periodontal infection and various systemic diseases/conditions makes it critical for early identification, treatment, and management of periodontal disease (infection) by dental and dental hygiene professionals as part of the interprofessional healthcare team.

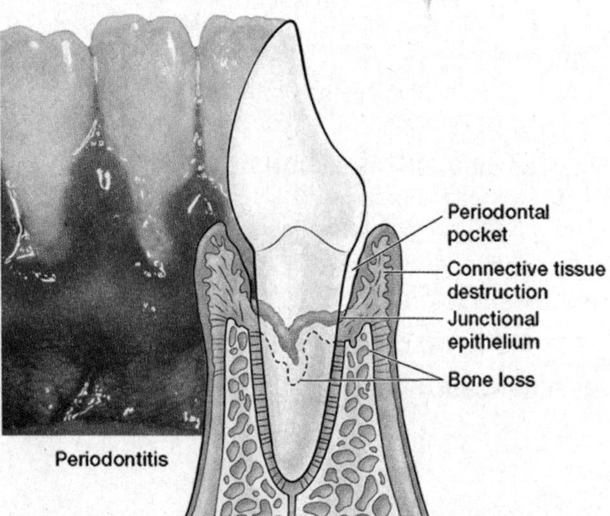

Figure 19-1 Clinical Changes in Periodontitis. Periodontitis is characterized by inflammation within the supporting tissues of the teeth, progressive destruction of the periodontal ligament, and loss of supporting alveolar bone.

Risk Assessment

I. Types of Factors Involved

Complicating and risk factors for disease development may be etiologic, predisposing, or contributing. They are delineated as follows:

- Etiologic factor: The actual cause of a disease or condition.
- Predisposing factor: Renders a person susceptible to a disease or condition.
- Contributing factor: Lends assistance to, supplements, or adds to a condition or disease.
- Risk factor: Increases the probability that disease will occur.
- Etiologic, predisposing, and contributing factors may be local or systemic, defined as follows:
    - Local factor: A factor in the immediate environment of the oral cavity or specifically in the environment of the teeth and periodontium.
    - Systemic factor: A factor that results from or is influenced by a general physical or mental disease or condition.

II. Risk Assessment Tools

- Risk assessment identifies the level of likelihood for developing and progression of periodontal disease and is an integral part of individualizing preventive strategies and periodontal treatment.[4,5]
- Risk assessment may reduce the need for more advanced periodontal therapy and improve patient outcomes to reduce oral healthcare costs.[4]
- Examples of periodontal risk assessment (PRA) tools:
  - **Periodontal risk calculator (PRC)** is a web-based risk assessment tool that uses known factors such as smoking history, diagnosis of diabetes, and periodontal history and status to predict risk for periodontal disease and has shown a high level of accuracy in a 15-year study.[4,6,7]
  - A **periodontal risk assessment (PRA)** tool based on tooth loss, genetic, and systemic conditions and periodontal status can also be located on the Internet at www.perio-tools.com/pra/en/ and has been shown to predict the progression of periodontal disease.[4,8]
- In the 2017 World Workshop on the Classification of Periodontal and Peri-Implant Diseases and Conditions, risk factors were incorporated into the grading of periodontal disease as part of estimating response to therapy and future risk for progression of disease.[9]
  - In the periodontal classification system, these are called *grade modifiers* and include diabetes and smoking.
- Risk assessment can be used to educate the patient about the level of risk and the factors that can be modified. The patient can use the tools to manage their personal disease risk.
- The clinician uses the risk assessment information to identify the modifiable risk factors to be addressed in the treatment plan.

Etiology of Periodontal Disease

- Microorganisms, in the form of subgingival biofilms forming communities called microbiomes, are the primary etiologic agents of periodontal disease/infection.[4,10]
  - The microbiome complexity and diversity increase in **periodontitis** when compared to health.[10]
  - The microbiome of **gingivitis** is not the same as in periodontitis.[10]
  - The type of organisms shifts to gram-negative anaerobic species including *Porphyromonas gingivalis*, *Tannerella forsythia* (previously known as *Bacteroides forsythus*), *Treponema denticola*, and *Fretibacterium* species.[10]

Risk Factors for Periodontal Diseases

- Identification of risk factors for periodontal diseases can provide significant insight into assessment and care planning for an individual patient.
- The various periodontal pathogenic microorganisms do not affect all people with the same degree of severity suggesting host factors play a significant role.[2]

I. Modifiable Risk Factors

- The common risk factors for periodontal disease and systemic disease include tobacco exposure, diabetes, metabolic syndrome (MetS), obesity, diet, and excess alcohol intake.[3]
  - These are all modifiable risk factors; however, most require an interprofessional collaboration with medical providers.

A. Tobacco Use

- The evidence provides strong support that smoking is an independent risk factor for periodontal disease (see **Figure 19-2**).[3,9]
- Smoking increases risk of periodontal disease by 85%.[11]
- Periodontal treatment may be less effective in smokers than in those who do not smoke.

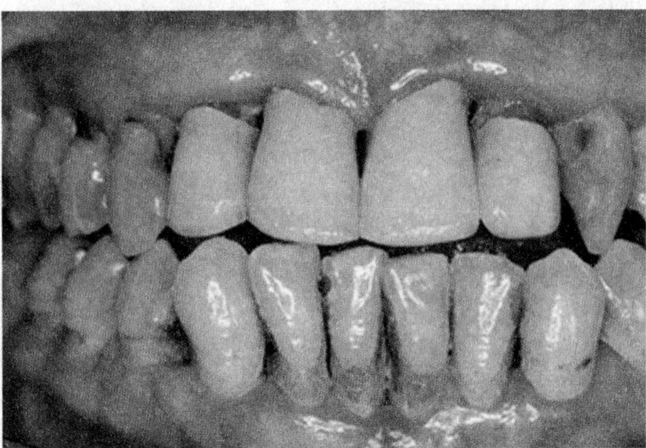

Figure 19-2 Attachment (Bone Loss) in Smoker.
A 58-year-old female, cigarette smoker of 20 pack years with advanced periodontitis. Note that clinical signs of inflammation, such as marginal redness, are minimal. The teeth are discolored due to nicotine deposits.

- Users of smokeless tobacco products experience oral effects, including predisposition to oral cancer. Periodontal **lesions** with severe recession and clinical attachment loss (CAL) occur where the quid of smokeless tobacco is held.[12]
- Evidence is emerging to show that cannabis or marijuana use is an independent risk factor for periodontitis with odds almost double in those who were frequent cannabis users.[13–14]

B. Diabetes Mellitus

- Periodontal disease and diabetes mellitus have a bidirectional relationship, meaning a patient who does not control blood glucose is more likely to have more severe periodontal disease.[15]
- Poor control of blood glucose (glycemic control) increases the risk of developing periodontal disease and results in poor outcomes to treatment.[3,9,15]
- As a result of the increase in diabetes in the U.S. population, there is an increase in prevalence of periodontitis in children and adolescents with type 1 diabetes mellitus.[16]
- Although diabetes is a chronic disease, research suggests management of periodontal infection results in improvement in control of blood glucose.[3,17]

C. Metabolic Syndrome

- MetS is a group of risk factors for heart disease and diabetes that includes hypertension, hyperglycemia, excess abdominal fat, and high cholesterol/triglycerides.
- MetS increases risk of periodontal disease.[3,18]
- A systematic review and meta-analysis found individuals with MetS are 38% more likely to have periodontitis.[3,18]

D. Obesity

- Obesity prevalence is about 42.4% in the United States and continues to increase, resulting in a major public health problem.[19]
- Obesity, overweight, weight gain, and increased waist circumference are emerging as risk factors for periodontal disease in adults, adolescents, and children.[3, 20,21]
- The odds of having periodontal disease in obese and overweight individuals is doubled.[3]

E. Alcohol Consumption

- Alcohol intake is associated with an increased risk for periodontal disease.[22]
- The risk in women was doubled and for men, the risk was 25% greater for periodontal disease with heavy alcohol (>30 grams/day or >2 standard drinks) consumption.[23]

F. Diet

- Macronutrient and micronutrient intake may be modifying factors in periodontal disease.[3,24]
    - Macronutrient intake such as high carbohydrate intake impacts glycemic control and may be involved in initiation of the inflammatory state in periodontal disease.[24]
    - Micronutrient deficiencies, such as vitamin C, vitamin D, or vitamin B_{12}, may impact onset, healing, and progression of periodontal disease.[24]

G. Psychosocial Factors

- Some research suggests individuals under psychological stress, anxiety, or depression may be more susceptible to periodontal disease.[3,25]

H. Medications

- Medications for specific systemic conditions can lead to gingival enlargement.[26] The enlarged tissue encourages dental biofilm retention and complicates removal, thus increasing the potential for periodontal infections. These medications may or may not be modifiable and consultation with the medical provider is required.
    - *Phenytoin-induced gingival enlargement:* Phenytoin is a drug used to control seizures (see **Figure 19-3**).

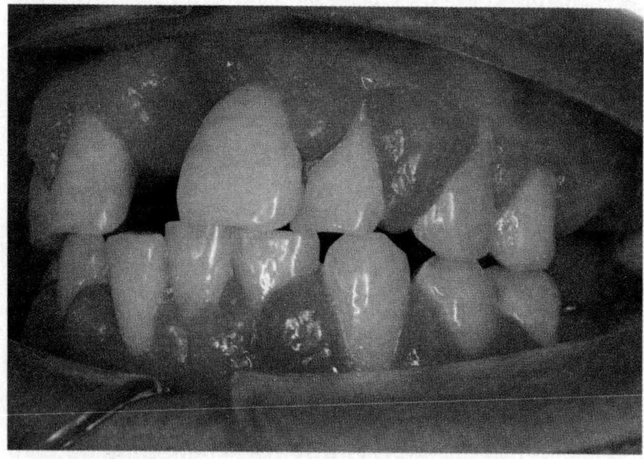

Figure 19-3 Hypertension Drug–Induced Gingival Hyperplasia

- *Cyclosporine-induced gingival enlargement:* Cyclosporine is an immunosuppressant drug used for patients with organ transplants to prevent rejection.
- *Nifedipine-induced gingival enlargement:* Nifedipine is a calcium-channel blocker used in the treatment of angina and ventricular arrhythmias.
- Oral contraceptives with high doses of estrogen, progestin, or both.[26]

II. Nonmodifiable Risk Factors

A. Genetic Predisposition

- Approximately one-third of the risks for periodontal disease are related to genetic factors.[27]
- Genetic testing is likely to become more cost effective and will benefit patients and dental providers in targeting those at risk to provide enhanced prevention.

B. Host Response

- Host response refers to the way an individual's immune response interacts with bacteria to resolve inflammation.
- Bacteria initiates an inflammatory response in periodontal disease; in susceptible individuals, the body's immune response becomes chronic, resulting in tissue destruction.[28]
- In addition to chronic diseases that impair the immune response, such as diabetes, genetic disorders associated with deficiencies in the immune system, such as Down syndrome, also result in a higher prevalence and severity of periodontal disease.[2,9]

C. Osteoporosis

- Research suggests an association between osteoporosis and periodontal disease with three times the risk of greater than 4 mm of CAL.[2,29]
- There was a five times greater risk of CAL greater than or equal to 6 mm.[29]
- In osteopenia, there was nearly a two times greater risk of more than 4 mm of CAL.[29]

D. Age

- Age also is factored into the 2017 periodontal grading system to take into consideration more severe periodontal disease at an earlier age.[9]
  - The grading of periodontitis is related to the potential for disease progression and will be described later in this chapter.

III. Local Factors

- Although dental biofilm is the primary etiologic factor in the development of inflammatory gingival and periodontal diseases, a variety of other factors predispose some patients to the retention of bacterial deposits and to the development of periodontal disease.[30]
  - Retentive areas may be associated with rough surfaces of teeth and restorations; tooth contour and position; and gingival size, shape, and position.
  - **Iatrogenic** causes (factors created by professionals during patient treatment) or neglect of proper treatment can impact development and progression of periodontal disease.
  - Factors such as mastication (chewing), saliva, the tongue, cheeks, lips, oral habits, and personal biofilm control procedures contribute to retention.

A. Dental Factors

- Tooth surface irregularities: Pellicle and biofilm microorganisms attach to defective or rough surfaces, include the following:
  - Pits, grooves, cracks.
  - Calculus.
  - Exposed altered cementum with irregularities.
  - Demineralization and cavitated dental caries.
  - Iatrogenic factors such as rough or grooved surfaces left after scaling or inadequately contoured dental restorations (**Figure 19-4B**).
- Tooth contour: Altered shape may interfere with oral self-cleansing mechanisms. (See Chapters 16 and 27.)
  - Congenital abnormalities: Extra or missing cusps or a bell-shaped crown with prominent facial and lingual contours that tend to provide deeper retentive areas in the cervical third.
  - Teeth with flattened proximal surfaces have faulty contact with adjacent teeth, thus permitting debris to wedge between the teeth.
  - Occlusal and incisal surfaces altered by attrition interrupt normal excursion of food during chewing. Marginal ridges have worn down.
  - Areas of erosion and abrasion.
  - Carious lesions.
  - Heavy calculus deposits; biofilm retained on rough surface.
  - Overcontoured, undercontoured, or overhanging restorations (see **Figure 19-5**).

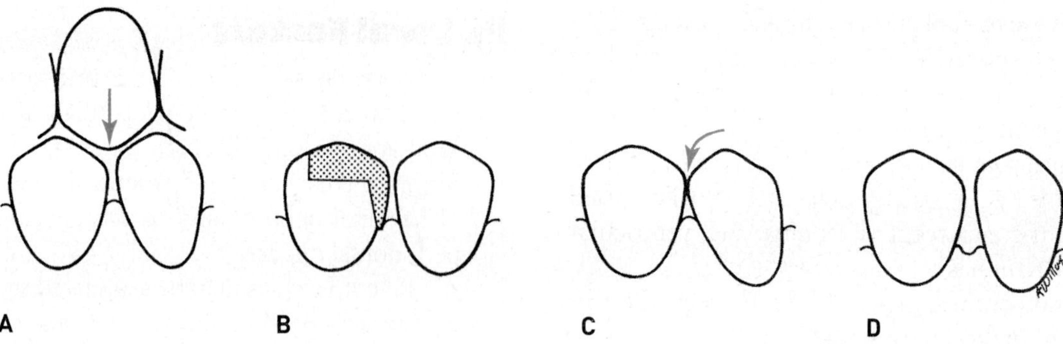

Figure 19-4 Effect of Tooth Position. **A:** Food impaction area, shown by plunger cusp (with arrow) directing pressure between lower teeth with open contact area. **B:** Inadequate restoration without proximal contact and with overhang. **C:** Tipped tooth leaving irregular marginal ridge relation. **D:** Natural open contact (diastema) with saddle-shaped gingival margin.

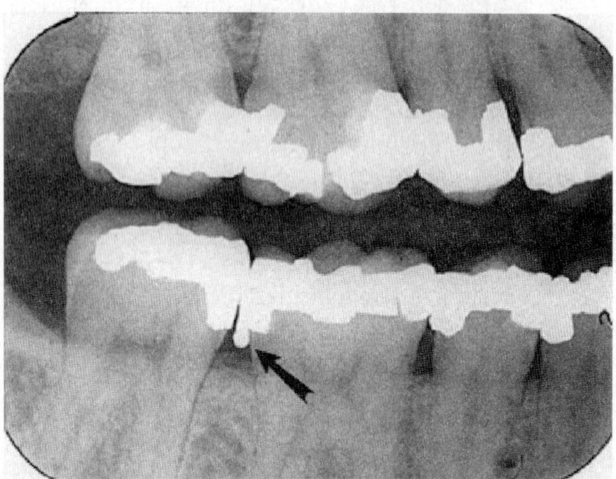

Figure 19-5 Restoration with an Overhang. The distal surface of the mandibular first molar in this radiograph has a faulty restoration that creates a food trap and harbors biofilm.

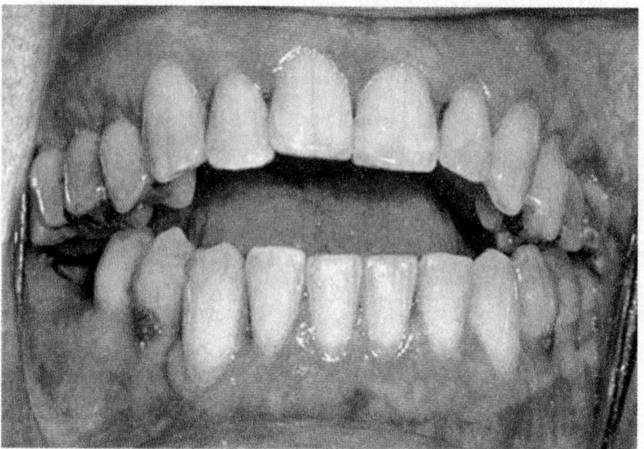

Figure 19-6 Anterior Open Bite

- Tooth position
  - Malocclusion: Irregular alignment of a single tooth or groups of teeth leaves areas prone to collection of biofilm formation.
    - Crowded or overlapped.
    - Rotated.
    - Deep anterior overbite. (See Chapter 16.)
    - Mandibular teeth force food particles against maxillary lingual surface.
    - Lingual inclination of mandibular teeth allows maxillary teeth to force food particles against mandibular facial gingiva.
  - Tooth adjacent to edentulous area may be inclined or migrated; contact missing.
  - When an opposing tooth is missing, the tooth may extrude beyond the line of occlusion.
  - Related to eruption
    - Incomplete eruption: The teeth do not erupt into the line of occlusion.
    - Partially erupted impacted third molar.
  - Lack of function or the use of teeth eliminates or decreases effectiveness of natural cleansing:
    - Lack of opposing teeth.
    - Open bite (**Figure 19-6**).
    - Marked maxillary anterior protrusion.
    - Crossbite with limited lateral excursion.
    - Unilateral chewing.
  - Food **impaction**
    - Created by the combined effect of tooth contour, missing proximal contact, proximal carious lesions, and irregular marginal ridge relationship.
    - Inclination related to loss of adjacent tooth and a plunger cusp from the opposite arch (**Figure 19-4A**).
  - Defective contact area
    - Restoration margin is faulty, and the contact area is missing, improperly located, or unnaturally wide (Figure 19-4B).
    - Inclined tooth with irregular marginal ridge relation (**Figure 19-4C**).
  - Dental appliances and prostheses
    - Orthodontic appliances provide retentive areas (see **Figure 19-7**).

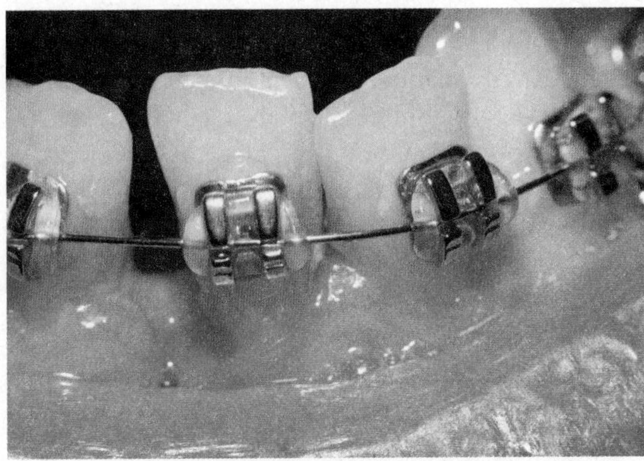

Figure 19-7 Orthodontic Appliances as a Predisposing Factor for Periodontal Disease. Infrequent oral self-care and biofilm accumulation contribute to inflammation and heightened periodontal risk.

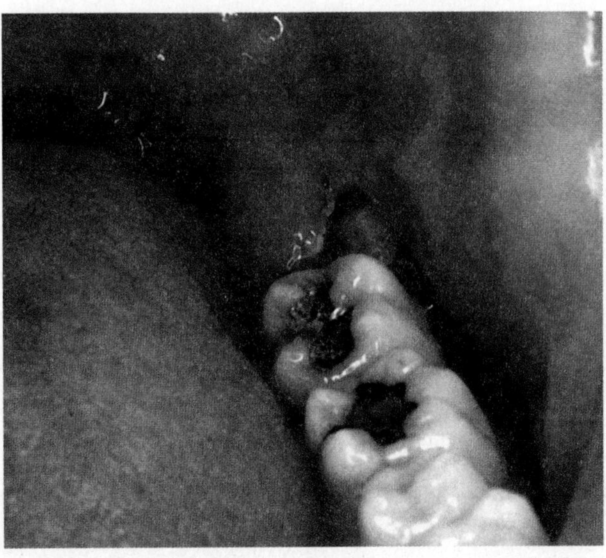

Figure 19-8 Operculum Is a Flap of Tissue over a Partially Erupted Third Mandibular Molar. This flap makes removal of biofilm difficult and may lead to inflammation and infection.

  - Fixed partial denture with deficient margin on an abutment tooth or an unusually shaped pontic.
  - Removable partial denture with poorly fitting clasps.

B. Gingival Factors

- *Position*
  - Deviations from normal provide retentive areas for biofilm.
  - Gingival recession: May expose root irregularities that serve as areas for biofilm retention.
  - Enlarged gingival margin or papillae: Extended to or over the height of contour.
  - Reduced height of interdental papilla creating an open interdental area.
  - Operculum: Tissue flap over occlusal surface of an erupting tooth (**Figure 19-8**).
  - Periodontal pocket: Depth and shape can make biofilm removal difficult.
  - Calculus creating a rough retentive surface.
- *Size and contour*
  - Deviation of shape of enlarged gingiva: Rolled, bulbous, and cratered.
  - Combination with presence of irregular restorations or dental prosthesis can result in marked biofilm retention.
- *Effect of mouth breathing*
  - Dehydration of oral tissues in the anterior region leads to changes in size, shape, surface texture, and consistency.

C. Other Factors

A variety of factors may predispose or contribute to the progression of periodontal infections. Some of the items listed here may have an indirect effect, whereas others have a direct effect on the oral tissues.

- Personal oral self-care is the first step in preventing and managing periodontal disease[15] and is affected by the following factors:
  - Neglect: This can lead to generalized dental biofilm accumulation and disease promotion.
  - Inadequate biofilm control techniques: Incorrect use of brush and/or interdental cleaning aids.
  - Lack of access to the oral health aids needed for adequate dental biofilm removal.
  - Lack of awareness of need for biofilm removal: Cleansing habits, including both self-cleansing mechanisms and mechanical biofilm removal, depend in part on an individual's perception and feeling of debris through taste and tongue activity. This can become impaired in individuals with some conditions like poststroke.
- Diet and eating habits.
  - Soft foods tend to be less nutrient dense and more retentive than fibrous, firm foods.
  - Masticatory deficiencies limit diet selection. Missing teeth, ill-fitting partial dentures, and various occlusal deficiencies alter diet selection and eating habits.[31]

Pathogenesis of Periodontal Diseases

Pathogenesis refers to the process by which a disease develops and progresses. The primary etiology of periodontal disease is bacteria that initiate an inflammatory process.

- The inflammatory process is very complex and influenced by patient and environmental factors; progression of disease is impacted by the individual's response to the bacterial challenge.[32]

I. Acute Inflammatory Response

- When the immune response is working effectively with no disease modifiers (e.g., diabetes or smoking), the presence of biofilm results in gingival inflammation with no breakdown of tissue.[32]
- Activation of the local acute inflammatory response begins the process of lesion development.

II. Development of Gingival and Periodontal Infection

- The stages of development of gingivitis and periodontitis are a complex, nonlinear process.[33]
- With an accumulation of dental biofilm on the cervical tooth surface adjacent to the gingival margin, an inflammatory reaction is initiated, and the immune system responds.
- Progression of periodontal lesions has traditionally been divided into the *initial lesion, early lesion, established lesion*, and *advanced lesion*.

A. The Initial Lesion

- Inflammatory response to dental biofilm[34]
  - Occurs within 2–4 days in response to bacterial accumulation.
  - Migration and **infiltration** of white blood cells (neutrophils) into the junctional epithelium and gingival sulcus result from the natural body response to infectious agents.
  - Increased flow of gingival crevicular fluid.
  - Early breakdown of **collagen** of the supporting gingival fiber groups. (See Chapter 18.)
  - Fluid fills the spaces in the connective tissue.
- Clinical appearance
  - No clinical evidence of change may appear in the earliest phases.
  - Marginal redness with enlargement due to the fluid collection follows as the infection develops.

B. The Early Lesion

- Increased inflammatory response[34]
  - Dental biofilm becomes older and thicker (4–10 days; time reflects individual differences).
  - Infiltration of fluid, macrophages, T-cells, and neutrophils with a few plasma cells migrating into the connective tissue.
  - Breakdown of collagen fiber support to the gingival margin.
  - Epithelium proliferation: Epithelial extensions and rete ridges are formed.
- Clinical appearance
  - Early signs of gingivitis become apparent with slight gingival enlargement; will become an established lesion if undisturbed.
  - Early gingivitis is reversible when biofilm is controlled and inflammation is reduced. Healthy tissue may be restored.
  - Susceptibility of individuals varies; time before lesion becomes established varies.

C. The Established Lesion

- Progression from the early lesion to the established lesion occurs in approximately 2–3 weeks.[34]
  - Migration of B-lymphocytes and plasma cells within connective tissue are characteristics of the established lesion.
  - Formation of pocket epithelium.
    1. Proliferation of the junctional and sulcular epithelium continues in an attempt to wall out the inflammation.
    2. Pocket epithelium is more **permeable**; areas of ulceration of the lining epithelium develop.
    3. Early pocket formation with bleeding on probing.
  - Collagen destruction continues; connective tissue fiber support is lost.
  - Progression to the early periodontal lesion may occur or the established lesion may remain stable for extended periods of time.
- Clinical appearance
  - Clear evidence of inflammation is present with marginal redness, bleeding on probing, and spongy marginal gingiva.
  - This is followed by chronic fibrosis development.

D. The Advanced Lesion

- Extension of inflammation
  - The two hallmarks of the advanced lesion, which is when the lesion progresses to

periodontitis, are alveolar bone resorption and collagen breakdown.[33] B-lymphocytes and plasma cells are thought to influence both these processes due to the cytokines released.[33]

- Progressive destruction of connective tissue
  - Connective tissue fibers below the junctional epithelium are destroyed; the epithelium migrates along the root surface.
  - Coronal portion of junctional epithelium becomes detached.
  - Exposed cementum where Sharpey's fibers were attached becomes altered by the host response to the bacterial challenge.
  - Diseased cementum contains a thin superficial layer of endotoxins from the bacterial breakdown.
  - Without treatment, loss of attachment results in increased pocket depth.
- Characteristics of the advanced lesion
  - Pocket formation, bleeding, inflammation, and bone loss are all signs of periodontitis.
  - Persistence of the chronic inflammatory process; plasma cells predominate.
  - Junctional epithelium continues to migrate; lesion extends through connective tissue.
  - Periods of disease inactivity alternate with periods of activity.

Gingival and Periodontal Pockets

- The presence or absence of infection distinguishes a pocket from a sulcus and the level of attachment on the tooth distinguishes a gingival pocket from a periodontal pocket.
- A pocket has an inner wall (the tooth surface) and an outer wall (the sulcular epithelium or pocket epithelium) of the free gingiva. The two walls meet at the base of the pocket.
  - The base of the pocket is the coronal margin of the attached periodontal tissues.
  - Histologically, the base of a healthy sulcus is the coronal border of the junctional epithelium, whereas the base of a pocket (diseased sulcus) may be at the coronal border of the connective tissue attachment.
- Substances found in a pocket
  - Communication of the gingival sulcus to the oral cavity provides an opportunity for dental biofilm microbial communities to develop and progress in complexity from organisms found in health to those present in gingivitis and periodontitis.[10]
  - Microorganisms and their products: Enzymes, endotoxins, and other metabolic products.
  - Gingival crevicular fluid.
  - **Desquamated** epithelial cells.
  - Leukocytes, the numbers of which increase with increased inflammation in the tissues.
  - Purulent exudate made up of living and broken-down leukocytes, living and dead microorganisms, and serum.
- Pockets are divided into gingival and periodontal types to clarify the degree of anatomic involvement.
- Periodontal pockets are further categorized by their position in relation to the alveolar bone, that is, whether their pocket base is suprabony or intrabony (**Figure 19-9**).

I. Gingival Pocket or Pseudopocket

- Definition: A pocket formed by gingival enlargement without apical migration of the junctional epithelium (Figure 19-9B).[35]
- The margin of the gingiva has moved toward the incisal or occlusal without the deeper periodontal structures becoming involved.
- The tooth wall of the pocket is enamel.
- During eruption, the base of the sulcus is at various levels along the enamel. The base of the sulcus of a fully erupted tooth is near the cementoenamel junction.
- All gingival pockets are suprabony (the base of the pocket is coronal to the crest of the alveolar bone).

II. Periodontal Pocket

- Definition: A pocket formed as a result of disease or degeneration causing apical migration of the junctional epithelium along the cementum.[35]
- The periodontal deeper structures (attachment apparatus) are involved (i.e., the cementum, periodontal ligament, and bone).[35]
  - The tooth wall of the pocket is cementum or partly cementum and partly enamel.
  - Detachment of junctional epithelium leads to the pocket formation.
  - Pocket epithelium permeability increases with migration of neutrophils, lymphocytes, and plasma cells.
  - An active phase of destruction of connective tissue then occurs and fibroblasts and collagen fibers are replaced by inflammatory and immune cells.

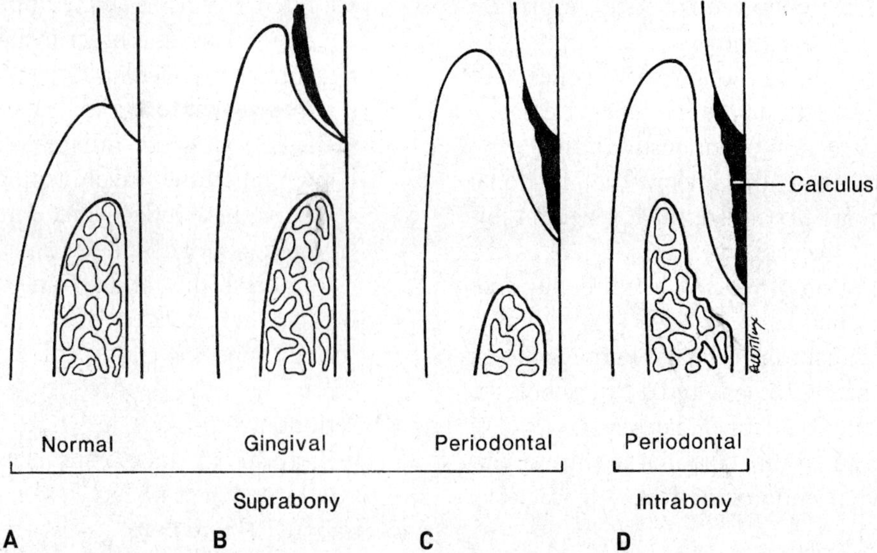

Figure 19-9 Types of Periodontal Pockets. **A:** Normal relationship of the gingival tissue and the cementoenamel junction in a fully erupted tooth. **B:** Gingival pocket showing attachment at the cementoenamel junction and the pocket formed by enlarged gingival tissue. There is no bone loss. **C:** Periodontal pocket showing attachment on cementum with root surface exposed. Gingival tissue has enlarged. **D:** Periodontal intrabony pocket with the bottom of the pocket within the bone. See the text for further description of each type of pocket.

- Periodontal pockets may be suprabony or intrabony.
  - Suprabony: Pocket in which the base of the pocket is coronal to the crest of the alveolar bone (Figure 19-9A–C).
  - Intrabony: Pocket in which the base of the pocket is below or apical to the crest of the alveolar bone (Figure 19-9D). "Intra" means located within the bone. The term "infrabony" is used in some texts. "Infra" means under or beneath.

III. Tooth Surface Irregularities

- Supragingival tooth surface irregularities are detected by drying the surface and observing under adequate direct or indirect light; limited use of the sharp tip of an explorer is recommended.
- Subgingival examination is dependent, for the most part, on tactile and auditory sensitivity transmitted by a probe or an explorer.
- Causes of surface roughness on the enamel surface include the following:
  - Structural defects: Cracks and grooves.
  - Demineralization; cavitated dental caries.
  - Calculus deposits and heavy stain deposits.
  - Erosion, abrasion.
  - Pits and irregularities from hypoplasia.
- Root surface irregularities
  - Diseased cementum.
  - Cemental resorption.
  - Root caries.
  - Abrasion.
  - Calculus.
  - Deficient or overhanging filling (see Figure 19-5).
  - Grooves from improper instrumentation.
- Irregularities at the cementoenamel junction
  - The relationships of enamel and cementum at the cementoenamel junction are shown in Chapter 18.

Complications Resulting from Periodontal Disease Progression

I. Furcation Involvement

Furcation involvement means the clinical attachment level and bone loss have extended into the furcation area between the roots of a multirooted tooth (see the Glickman furcation grades in **Figure 19-10**). Glickman furcation grades are also discussed in Chapter 20.

- Presence of furcation involvement increases the risk of tooth loss.[36]
  - It is difficult to adequately remove biofilm and calculus from the furcation area (see

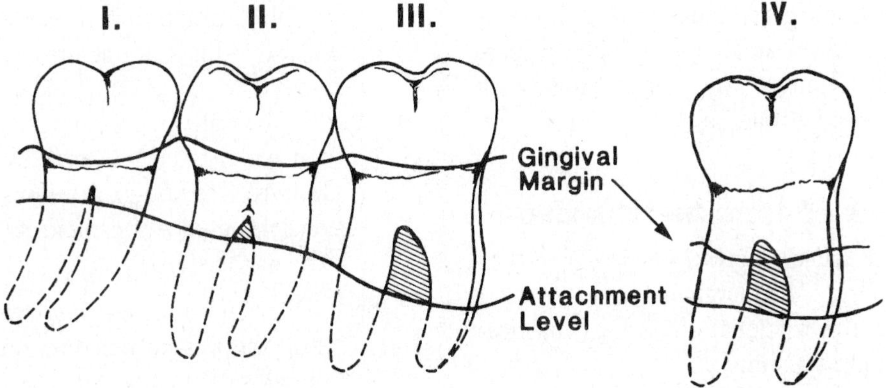

Figure 19-10 Classification of Furcations. **I:** Early, beginning involvement. **II:** Moderate involvement, in which the furcation can be probed but not through and through. **III:** Severe involvement, when the bone between the roots is destroyed and a probe can be passed through. **IV:** Same as III, with clinical exposure resulting from gingival recession.

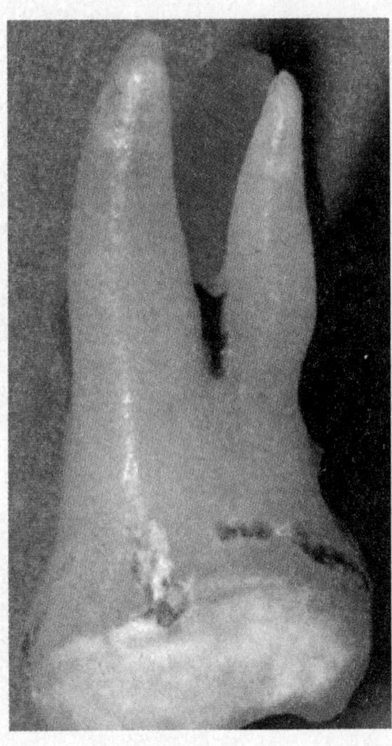

Figure 19-11 Calculus in the Furcation Area and Root Depressions. This extracted molar has mineralized deposits (calculus) in the furcation. Once disease progresses into the furcation area, access for removal becomes difficult.

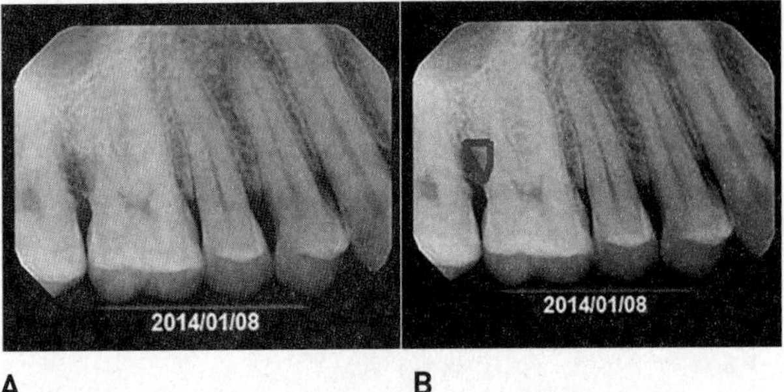

Figure 19-12 Furcation Involvement. **A:** Note radiolucency in the furcation area on the distolingual of the maxillary first molar. **B:** The red triangle outlines the radiolucency in the furcation area.

Figure 19-11) for both the dental hygienist and the patient, making it challenging to manage the inflammation and infection in this area.

A. Clinical Observations

- When the gingiva over the furcation has not receded, the following may be seen:
  - The furcation is covered by the periodontal pocket wall.
  - No differences in color, size, or other tissue changes may exist to differentiate the area from adjacent gingiva, but when color changes do exist, they provide clues to guide further examination.
  - A radiolucency in the furcation area (sometimes called a furcation arrow) may be noted on the radiographs (**Figure 19-12**).
- When the gingiva over a molar furcation recedes, the root division may be seen directly (Figure 19-10).

B. Detection

A suggested procedure for probing furcation areas is described in Chapter 20.

II. Mucogingival Involvement

A pocket that extends to or beyond the mucogingival junction and into the alveolar mucosa is described as *mucogingival involvement* (**Figure 19-13**). There is no attached gingiva in the area, and a probe can pass through the pocket and beyond the mucogingival junction into the alveolar mucosa.

A. Significance of Attached Gingiva

- Functions of attached gingiva
  - Give support to the marginal gingiva.
  - Withstand the frictional stresses of mastication and toothbrushing.
  - Provide attachment or a solid base for the movable alveolar mucosa for the action of the cheeks, lips, and tongue.
- Barrier to passage of inflammation
  - The junctional epithelium (epithelial attachment) acts as a barrier to keep infection outside the body.
  - With destruction of the connective tissue and periodontal ligament fibers under the junctional epithelium, the epithelium migrates along the root.
  - The thickness of the gingiva and managing gingival inflammation are more important than the width of the gingiva, so biofilm removal is essential.[37,38]

B. Clinical Observations

- Color changes, tension test, and probe measurements are used during assessment of the mucogingival areas. (See Chapter 20.)
- Thickness of attached gingiva: In patients with a thin type of gingiva, the periodontal probe will be visible through the gingiva when probing and these individuals are at greater risk for gingival recession.[38]
- Width of keratinized or attached gingiva: Current evidence suggests 1–2 mm of attached gingiva is desirable, although a minimal amount is not needed if the patient can execute optimal biofilm control at the site(s).[38]
  - When the attached gingiva measures 1–2 mm and there is no bleeding on probing or marginal inflammation, it is recorded and reevaluated at each continuing care or periodontal maintenance appointment (see **Figure 19-14A** and **B**).

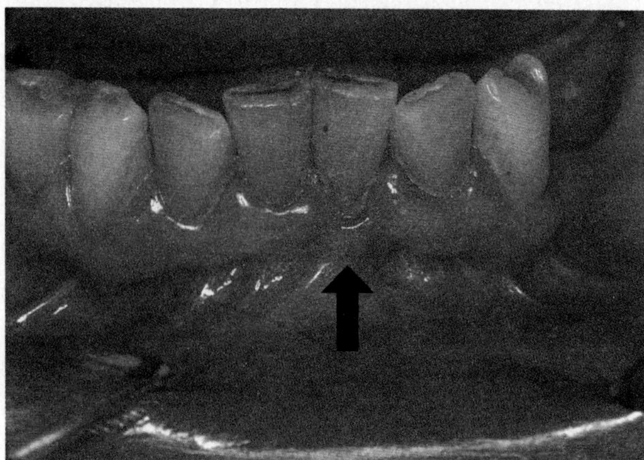

Figure 19-13 Mucogingival Defect. A mucogingival defect is suspected at tooth #24, which has a very narrow zone of keratinized gingiva.

Reproduced from Weiss G, Scheid R. *Woelfel's Dental Anatomy*. 8th ed. Philadelphia, PA: Lippincott Williams & Wilkins; 2012.

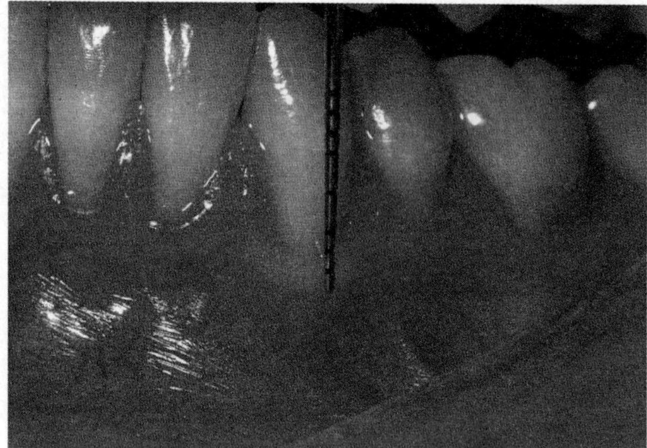

A

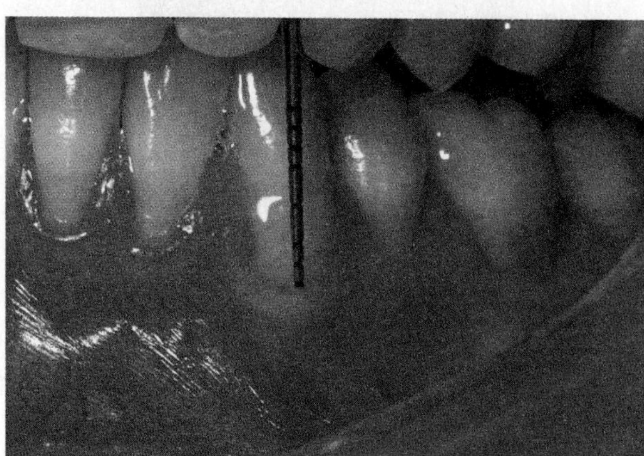

B

Figure 19-14 Measuring for a Mucogingival Defect.
A: The width of keratinized gingiva is measured at 2 mm.
B: The probe depth is measured at less than 2 mm (only 1 mm), indicating no mucogingival defect. If the probe depth reached or exceeded the mucogingival junction (exceeded the width of keratinized gingiva), there would be no attached gingiva, and a mucogingival defect would be present.

Reproduced from Weiss G, Scheid R. *Woelfel's Dental Anatomy*. 8th ed. Philadelphia, PA: Lippincott Williams & Wilkins; 2012.

- Long-term, longitudinal studies have shown that in the absence of inflammation and good biofilm control, areas with a narrow band of attached gingiva can be maintained for long periods.[38]
- A patient with such an area needs specific instruction in biofilm control procedures for preventive maintenance.

C. Mucogingival Deformities and Conditions Classification

- The 2017 World Workshop on the Classification of Periodontal and Peri-Implant Diseases and Conditions proposed a new classification for mucogingival conditions based more on treatment and potential for root coverage. It is quite complex and includes the following components[38]:
  - Periodontal biotype related to the thickness of the gingiva, width of keratinized tissue, tooth dimension, and bone thickness.
  - Gingival recession related to interdental CAL, facial/lingual attachment loss, severity, gingival thickness and width, cervical carious or noncarious lesions, hypersensitivity, and esthetic concerns.
  - Lack of keratinized gingiva.
  - Frenum position.
  - Gingival excess.
  - Abnormal color.

The Recognition of Gingival and Periodontal Infections

I. The Clinical Examination

The recognition of normal gingiva, gingival infections, and deeper periodontal involvement depends on a systematic, step-by-step examination.

- It is necessary to know the *extent* of the disease:
  - *Gingival infections* are confined to the gingiva.
  - *Periodontal infections* include all parts of the periodontium, namely, the gingiva, periodontal ligament, bone, and cementum.
- A comprehensive periodontal examination to gather assessment information and identify the signs of inflammation includes the following:
  - Gingival tissue changes (color, size, shape, surface texture, position).
  - Mucogingival involvement (width of attached gingiva).
  - Probing depths.
  - Clinical attachment levels.
  - Bleeding on probing.
  - Exudate or suppuration.
  - Furcation involvement.
  - Dental biofilm and calculus distribution.
  - Tooth mobility.
  - Fremitus.
  - Radiographic evaluation.

II. Signs and Symptoms

- Patients may or may not have specific symptoms to report because periodontal infections may be painless.
- Symptoms the patient reports may include:
  - Bleeding gingiva while brushing or flossing.
  - On occasion, spontaneous bleeding of the gingiva.
- Other possible symptoms the patient may notice include[39]:
  - Sensitivity to hot and cold.
  - Tenderness or discomfort while eating or pain after eating.
  - Food retained between the teeth.
  - Bad breath.
  - Chronic bad taste.
  - A feeling the teeth are loose.

III. Causes of Tissue Changes

- Disease changes produce alterations in color, size, position, shape, consistency, surface texture, bleeding tendency, and exudate production.
- To understand the changes that take place in the gingival tissues during the transition from health to disease, the clinician must understand:
  - The role of the bacterial biofilm in the development of disease.
  - The inflammatory response initiated by the body.
- When the products of the biofilm microorganisms cause breakdown of the intercellular substances of the sulcular epithelium, injurious agents can pass into the connective tissue, where an inflammatory response is initiated.
- An inflammatory response means there is increased blood flow, increased permeability of capillaries, and increased collection of defense cells and tissue fluid.
- The changes produce tissue alterations, such as in color, size, shape, and consistency.

Classification of Periodontal Health

- Before reviewing the classification of gingival and periodontal conditions, it is important to first define the classifications of periodontal health.[28]
- Signs associated with periodontal health on an intact periodontium, as well as a reduced periodontium that is stable, include[39]:
  - <10% of sites exhibit bleeding on probing.
  - Probing depths ≤3 mm.
- Additional signs of health for a stable patient with a reduced periodontium include:
  - Control of modifying factors, such as optimal control of diabetes and reduction or cessation of smoking.
  - No probing depths >4mm that bleed on probing.

Classification of Gingivitis

Gingivitis continues to be designated as plaque-induced and nonplaque-induced gingivitis classifications. An overview is shared here, but there are many complexities to the classifications, so the original 2017 World Workshop articles or a current periodontology text should be reviewed.

I. Dental Plaque Biofilm-Induced Gingivitis

- Dental biofilm is the primary etiology, but the extent and severity may be impacted by local and systemic factors.
- No loss of attachment for an intact periodontium; however, gingivitis can also occur on a reduced periodontium and appears as inflammation of the gingival margin with no progression of attachment loss.
- The inflammation is reversible with thorough biofilm removal.

A. Dental Plaque Biofilm-Induced Gingivitis Clinical Description

- Clinical signs include[39]:
  - Swelling and blunting of papilla.
  - ≥10% of sites exhibit bleeding on probing.
  - Redness.
  - Probing depths ≤3 mm.

B. Factors for Dental Plaque Biofilm-Induced Gingivitis

- Systemic conditions may also modify plaque-induced gingivitis and include[39]:
  - Metabolic factors, such as hyperglycemia in poorly controlled diabetes.
  - Hematologic factors include blood malignancies like leukemia. Gingival signs of leukemia include enlarged, glazed, spongy gingiva that is red to deep purple in color.
  - Smoking.
  - Nutritional factors, such as malnutrition.
  - Pharmacologic factors (i.e. drug-induced xerostomia).
  - Elevated sex steroid hormones can exacerbate gingivitis and include:
    - Puberty.
    - Menstruation.
    - Pregnancy.
    - Oral contraceptives.
- Local risk factors (predisposing factors) include[39]:
  - Dental biofilm retention such as poorly contoured restorations and crowded or malposed teeth.
  - Hyposalivation or **xerostomia**: Sjogren's syndrome, medication, anxiety, etc. may result in xerostomia.

C. Drug-Induced Gingival Enlargement

- A number of drugs, such as antiepileptic drugs (e.g., Dilantin and valproate), calcium-channel blockers (e.g., nifedipine, verapamil, diltiazem), immunosuppressants (e.g., cyclosporine), and high-dose oral contraceptives.[26]
- Occurs most commonly in the anterior areas and usually seen earliest in the papilla.

II. Nondental Plaque-Induced Gingivitis

For nonplaque-induced gingivitis, management of the biofilm will not resolve the inflammation.[39]

A. Genetic/Developmental Disorders

- Genetic causes of gingivitis are rare; an example is hereditary gingival fibromatosis.[40]

B. Specific Infections

- Bacterial origin[40]
  - Necrotizing gingivitis and stomatitis are due to underlying risk factors such as poor oral hygiene, stress, and compromised immunity with no loss of attachment.
  - Sexually transmitted disease such as gonorrhea and syphilis.
  - Tuberculosis.
- Viral origin[40]
  - Herpes simplex: Primary herpetic infection or gingivostomatitis resulting in many vesicles that rupture, leaving irregular mucosal ulcers.
  - Human papilloma virus.
  - Varicella-zoster virus.
- Fungal infections such as candidosis.[40]

C. Inflammatory and Immune Conditions

- Autoimmune diseases (e.g., lupus erythematosus, lichen planus).
- Hypersensitivity reactions (contact allergies).
- Granulomatous inflammatory conditions (e.g., Crohn's disease).

D. Reactive Processes

- Lesions are thought to be due to a response to local irritation or trauma and may include pyogenic granuloma (pregnancy), fibrous epulis, etc.[40]

E. Neoplasms

- Premalignant lesions such as leukoplakia and erythroplakia.
- Malignant conditions such as leukemia and lymphoma.

F. Endocrine, Nutritional, and Metabolic Diseases

- Vitamin deficiencies like scurvy (vitamin C).[40]

G. Traumatic Lesions

- Physical/mechanical insults (e.g., toothbrush abrasion, habits causing self-injury).[40]
- Chemical insults (e.g., etching, cocaine, dentifrice ingredients).[40]
- Thermal insults (e.g., mucosal burns).[40]

H. Gingival Pigmentation

- Gingival pigmentation may be the result of smoker's melanosis, amalgam tattoo, or drug induced (minocycline).[40]

Classification of Periodontitis

The classification of periodontitis focuses on detectable interdental CAL.[9]

I. Periodontitis Classifications

A. Necrotizing Periodontitis

- Necrotizing periodontal disease (NPD) begins as an acute condition with rapid tissue destruction, but NPD may also become chronic.
- Characterized by a history of pain, ulceration of the gingival margin, and punched out papillae.[9]
- A major predisposing factor is a compromised host immune response. Factors associated with host response include[41]:
  - Human immunodeficiency virus/acquired immunodeficiency syndrome (HIV/AIDS): CD4 counts less than 200 and detectable viral load.
  - Immunosuppression.
  - Severe malnutrition.
  - Psychological stress and insufficient sleep.
  - History of NPD and poor oral self-care.

B. Periodontitis as a Manifestation of Systemic Disease

- Genetic disorders are rare, but may be significantly impact periodontal status. These include immunologic, metabolic, and endocrine disorders, and connective tissue, oral mucosa, and gingival tissue diseases.[37]
- Systemic diseases have a variable effect on the course of periodontitis, but can influence the occurrence and severity. These include[37]:
  - Diabetes mellitus.
  - Obesity.
  - Osteoporosis.
  - Arthritis (rheumatoid and osteoarthritis).
  - Emotional stress and depression.
  - Smoking.
  - Medications.

- Systemic disorders associated with loss of periodontal tissue independent of periodontitis include[37]:
  - Neoplasms (odontogenic tumors and squamous cell carcinoma).
  - Other disorders such as hyperparathyroidism and scleroderma.

C. Periodontitis

The periodontitis case definition or classification system aids in identification of disease, risk factors for progression of disease, and individualized approaches to management and treatment of the disease. The 2017 World Workshop on the Classification of Periodontal and Peri-Implant Diseases and Conditions system for classification of periodontitis takes into account the following elements[9]:

- *Severity* relates to the periodontal attachment loss at diagnosis and affects the complexity of management and treatment.
- *Complexity of management* includes factors such as probing depths, type of bone loss (vertical vs. horizontal), furcation involvement, occlusal issues.
- *Extent* refers to the number of teeth and distribution of the periodontitis and uses the terminology *localized* (<30% of teeth affected), *generalized* (>30% of teeth affected), and *molar–incisor involvement only*.
- *Rate of progression* is primarily dependent on radiographic evidence over time of attachment loss, but other methods to assess progression are under investigation.
- *Risk factors.*

II. Terminology for Staging Periodontitis

As previously noted, the staging of periodontitis includes severity, complexity, and extent and distribution (**Figure 19-15**).[9]

- Stage I is mild periodontitis.
- Stage II is moderate periodontitis.
- Stage III is severe periodontitis.
- Stage IV is very severe or advanced periodontitis.

A. Severity

- Interdental CAL at site of greatest loss[9]:
  - Slight or mild: 1–2 mm CAL.
  - Moderate: 3–4 mm CAL.
  - Severe or advanced: >5 mm CAL.
- Radiographic bone loss (RBL)[9]
  - Coronal third (<15%).

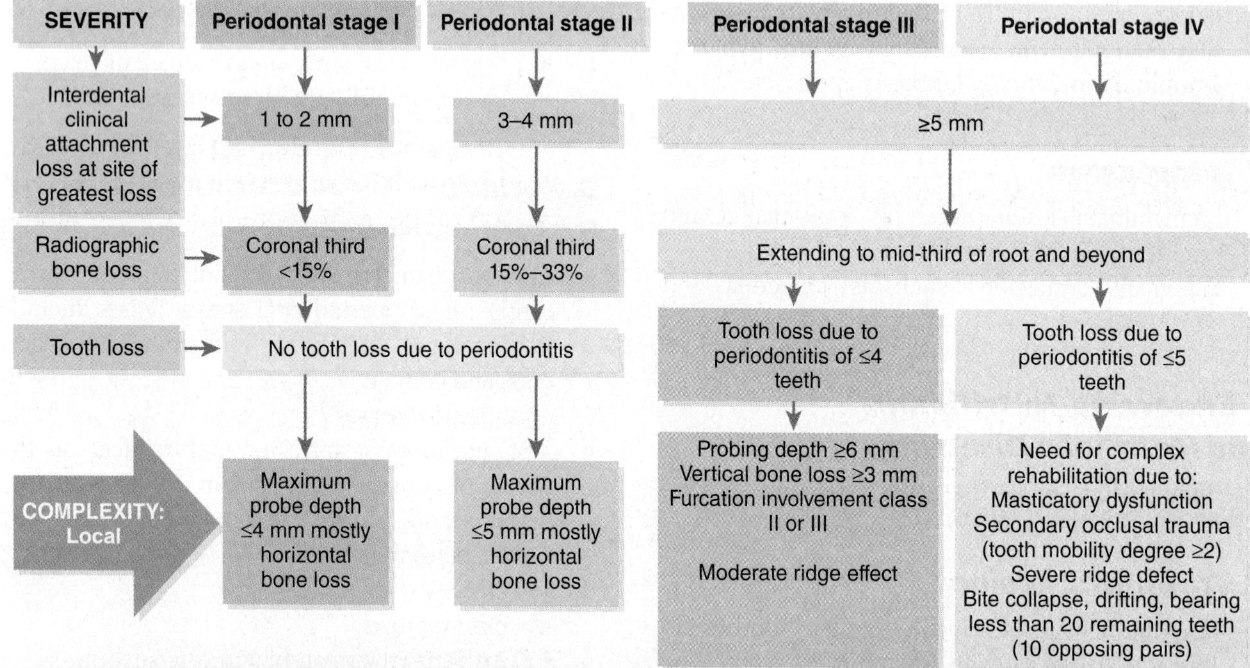

Figure 19-15 Periodontitis Stage Flow Chart

Lori J. Giblin-Scanlon, RDH, DHSc, Forsyth School of Dental Hygiene.

  - Coronal third (15–33%).
  - Extends beyond mid-third of root apically.
- Tooth loss
  - No tooth loss due to periodontitis.
  - Loss of four or fewer teeth due to periodontitis.
  - Loss of five or more teeth due to periodontitis.

B. Complexity

- Pocket depth
  - Maximum pocket depth less than 4 mm.
  - Pocket depths greater than 5 mm.
  - Pocket depths greater than 6 mm.
- Type of bone loss
  - Horizontal bone loss.
  - Vertical bone loss greater than or equal to 3 mm.
- Furcation involvement.
- Occlusal issues.

C. Extent and Distribution

- *Localized*: The gingiva is involved on a single tooth or a specific group of teeth (<30% of teeth involved).
- *Generalized*: The gingiva is involved on all or nearly all of the teeth throughout the mouth (>30% of teeth involved).
- *Molar/incisor pattern*: Bone loss limited to molar and incisor areas may suggest a more aggressive or rapid progression of disease (formerly called juvenile periodontitis).

Although not included in the staging of periodontitis, the following terminology may also be used when describing the extent and distribution of gingival inflammation.

- *Marginal*: A change confined to the free or marginal gingiva. This is specified as either localized or generalized.
- *Papillary*: A change involving a papilla but not the rest of the free gingiva around a tooth. A papillary change may be localized or generalized.
- *Diffuse*: Spread out, dispersed; affects gingival margin, attached gingiva, and interdental papillae; may extend into alveolar mucosa.

III. Terminology for Grading Periodontitis

Grading of periodontitis allows for recognition of factors that may impact the progression and management of the disease and includes primary criteria, grade modifiers, risk of systemic impact of periodontitis, and biomarkers (**Figure 19-16**).[9]

- Grade A denotes a slow rate of progression.
- Grade B is potential for a moderate rate of progression.
- Grade C is suggestive of a rapid rate of progression.

A. Primary Criteria

- Direct evidence of progression[9]
  - No evidence of bone loss over 5 years (radiographic or CAL).
  - Less than 2 mm over 5 years.
  - Greater than or equal to 2 mm over 5 years.
- Percentage bone loss divided by age.[9] For example: RBL is 30% and age is 60 = 0.5. If the RBL is 30% and the age is 25, then the result is 1.2. This accounts for more severe bone loss at an early age.
  - Less than 0.25.
  - 0.25–1.0.
  - Greater than 1.0.
- Case phenotype[9]
  - Heavy biofilm with low levels of destruction.
  - Destruction consistent with biofilm.
  - Destruction in excess of expectations given biofilm present and evidence of rapid progression.

B. Grade Modifiers (Risk Factors)

- Smoking
  - Nonsmoker.
  - Smokes fewer than 10 cigarettes/day.
  - Smokes more than 10 cigarettes/day.
- Diabetes
  - No diabetes.
  - Hemoglobin A1c (HbA1c) less than 7.0 in patients with diabetes.
  - HbA1c greater than or equal to 7.0 in patients with diabetes.

C. Risk of Systemic Impact of Periodontitis

- If laboratory values are available, a measure of inflammation is C-reactive protein. This can also be used as part of the grading.
  - Less than 1 mg/L.
  - 1–3 mg/L.
  - Greater than 3 mg/L.

D. Biomarkers

- Biomarkers that serve as indicators of bone loss or CAL have not been definitively identified, but the grading system allows for these to be added as more evidence emerges.

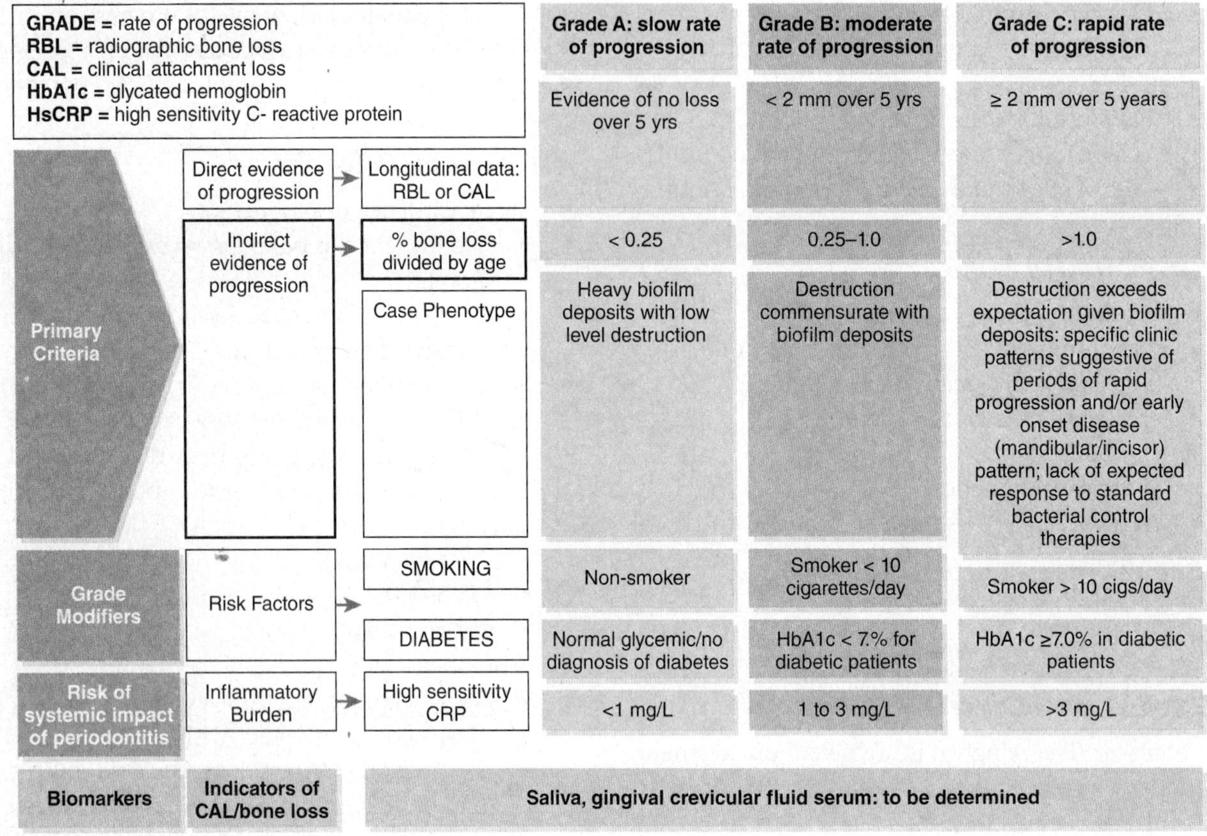

Figure 19-16 Periodontitis Grade Flow Chart

Lori J. Giblin-Scanlon, RDH, DHSc, Forsyth School of Dental Hygiene.

IV. Steps to Staging and Grading the Periodontal Classification

- *Step 1*: Initial assessment
  - The patient history, risk assessment, clinical examination, radiographs, and periodontal examinations are completed.
- *Step 2*: Establish stage
  - Identify areas of interdental CAL.
  - Rule out nonperiodontal causes for loss of attachment.
  - Evaluate extent of RBL and maximum CAL.
  - Identify type of bone loss (horizontal or vertical).
  - Determine number of teeth missing due to periodontitis.
  - Confirm presence or absence of furcation involvement.
  - Identify occlusal issues (e.g., occlusal trauma).
  - Evaluate the extent and distribution of disease and factors impacting complexity.
- *Step 3*: Establish grade
  - Identify the rate of bone loss, either CAL or RBL, over time based on past records.
  - From medical and psychosocial history, assess risk factors such as smoking and diabetes control. It may be necessary to consult with the medical provider to obtain the HbA1c to assess diabetes control.
  - Evaluate attachment loss in relationship to the amount of biofilm present.
  - Assess rate of progress by dividing RBL (% bone loss) by age.
- A simplified diagram of the classifications for periodontal health, gingival, and periodontal diseases is provided in **Figure 19-17**.

Acute Periodontal Lesions

The acute periodontal lesions are classified according to the etiology.[41]

I. Periodontal Abscess

- Periodontal abscess in periodontitis patient (in a preexisting periodontal pocket) subcategories include[41]:

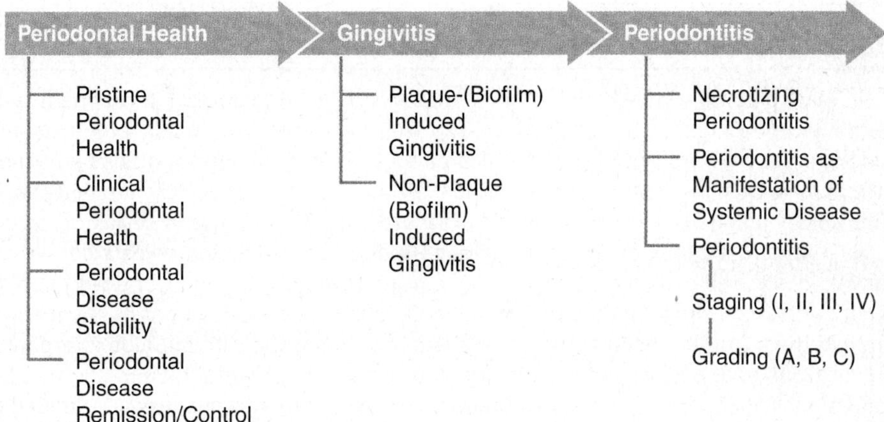

Figure 19-17 Classifications of Periodontal Health, Gingivitis, and Periodontitis

    - Acute exacerbation may occur in untreated periodontitis or during periodontal maintenance.
    - After treatment, abscesses may occur postscaling, postsurgery, and postmedication.
- Periodontal abscess in nonperiodontitis patient subcategories include[41]:
    - Impaction such as popcorn hull, dental floss.
    - Harmful habits such as nail biting.
    - Orthodontic treatment with changes in occlusion.
    - Gingival overgrowth.
    - Alteration of the root surface such as a root fracture or enamel pearl.

II. Necrotizing Periodontal Diseases

NPD typically is acute, which would fall into the acute periodontal condition, but may become chronic and then classified as periodontitis as previously described.[41]

- NPD in chronically, severely compromised patients subcategories include[41]:
    - HIV/AIDS and conditions causing immunosuppression in adults.
    - In children, NPD may occur in severe malnutrition, severe viral infections, or extreme living conditions (such as lack of stable living situations).
- NPD in temporarily and/or moderately compromised patients subcategories include[41]:
    - Gingivitis or periodontal patients with predisposing factors such as stress, nutrition, smoking; and previous NPD.

III. Endo-Periodontal Lesions

This classification was updated from the 1999 classifications to focus on the current clinical condition and lesions in those with and without periodontitis to cover a broader range of situations.[41]

- Endo-periodontal lesion with root damage[41]
    - This subclassification includes root fracture or crack, root canal perforation, and external root resorption.
- Endo-periodontal lesions without root damage[41]
    - This includes lesions in patients with and without periodontitis and uses a grading system (1–3) which is beyond the scope of dental hygiene care.

Documentation

Documentation for a patient to determine periodontal classification includes:

- Initially, a complete history and assessment is documented, to include:
    - Medical, dental, and psychosocial history.
    - Chief complaint or problem.
    - Consultation with primary care providers for additional information (e.g., history and current HbA1c for a patient with diabetes).
    - Risk assessment and identification of modifiable risk factors for oral disease.
    - Comprehensive periodontal examination.
    - Periodontal classification.
- A sample progress note may be reviewed in **Box 19-1**.

Box 19-1 Example Documentation: Patient with Periodontal Disease

- **S**—A 58-year-old male presents with chief complaint of painful, bleeding gums. On the medical history the patient reports having type 2 diabetes and hypertension. He reports his A1c was 8.2 at his last appointment. The patient takes Metformin and Cardizem. Patient indicates he smokes 1 pack/day and has smoked since he was 13 years old. He reports both his mother and father lost all their teeth because of gum disease.
- **O**—Extraoral/intraoral findings were normal. Blood pressure: 120/80. Full mouth series of radiographs taken and reviewed. No new dental caries. A comprehensive periodontal examination reveals generalized 5- to 6-mm pocket depths with localized bleeding on probing. Radiograph reveals 4–5 mm of CAL with approximately 20–33% bone horizontal loss. No mobility was noted. Grade I furcation involvement on the meso-lingual and disto-lingual of the maxillary molars. The gingiva is pink and fibrotic with bulbous interdental papillae throughout. Generalized heavy supragingival and subgingival calculus. Dental biofilm score 40%.
- **A**—The periodontal classification is generalized Stage III, Grade C periodontitis. Recommended patient return for four appointments of NSPT using local anesthesia followed by a reevaluation in 4–6 weeks.
- **P**—Patient education about the risk factors for periodontal disease present including biofilm, genetic history of periodontal disease, lack of diabetes control, and tobacco use. The patient is interested in tobacco cessation and was referred to the state quit line and his primary care provider. Oral self-care was reviewed with a soft toothbrush and interdental brush and the patient demonstrated good technique. Patient referred to his primary care provider for follow-up on his diabetes control prior to beginning NSPT to facilitate healing. Next visit: Begin NSPT maxillary right quadrant and review oral self-care. Follow-up about progress on tobacco cessation and diabetes management.

Signed: ______________________________, RDH
Date: ________________________________

Factors to Teach the Patient

- Educate the patient about the connections between periodontal disease and systemic disease related to the patient's medical history.
- Describe the risk factors that put the patient at risk for periodontal disease and assist the patient in identifying ways to manage the modifiable risk factors.
- Explain a normal sulcus versus a diseased periodontal pocket.
- Explain the need for a comprehensive periodontal examination to assess the extent and severity of disease.
- Clarify the need for adequate oral self-care and continuing care to prevent or manage periodontal disease (infection).

References

1. Linden GJ, Lyons A, Scannapieco FA. Periodontal systemic associations: review of the evidence. *J Periodontol*. 2013; 84(suppl 4):S8-S19.
2. Albandar JM, Susin C, Hughes FJ. Manifestations of systemic diseases and conditions that affect the periodontal attachment apparatus: case definitions and diagnostic considerations. *J Periodontol*. 2018;89(suppl 1):S183-S203.
3. Genco RJ, Genco FD. Common risk factors in the management of periodontal and associated systemic diseases: the dental setting and interprofessional collaboration. *J Evid Based Dent Pract*. 2014;14(suppl):4-16.
4. Lang NP, Suvan JE, Tonetti MS. Risk factor assessment tools for the prevention of periodontitis progression a systematic review. *J Clin Periodontol*. 2015;42(suppl 16):S59-S70.
5. Ferraiolo DM. Predicting periodontitis progression? *Evid Based Dent*. 2016;17(1):19-20.
6. Page RC, Krall EA, Martin J, Mancl L, Garcia RI. Validity and accuracy of a risk calculator in predicting periodontal disease. *J Am Dent Assoc*. 2002;133(5):569-576.
7. Page RC, Martin J, Krall EA, Mancl L, Garcia R. Longitudinal validation of a risk calculator for periodontal disease. *J Clin Periodontol*. 2003;30(9):819-827.
8. Lang NP, Tonetti MS. Periodontal risk assessment (PRA) for patients in supportive periodontal therapy (SPT). *Oral Health Prev Dent*. 2003;1(1):7-16.
9. Tonetti MS, Greenwell H, Kornman KS. Staging and grading of periodontitis: Framework and proposal of a new classification and case definition. *J Periodontol*. 2018;89(Suppl 1):S159-S172.
10. Abusleme L, Hoare A, Hong BY, Diaz PI. Microbial signatures of health, gingivitis, and periodontitis. *Periodontol 2000*. 2021;86(1):57-78.

11. Leite FRM, Nascimento GG, Scheutz F, López R. Effect of smoking on periodontitis: a systematic review and meta-regression. *Am J Prev Med*. 2018;54(6):831-841.
12. Kamath KP, Mishra S, Anand PS. Smokeless tobacco use as a risk factor for periodontal disease. *Front Public Health*. 2014;2:195.
13. Chaffee BW. Cannabis use and oral health in a national cohort of adults. *J Calif Dent Assoc*. 2021;49(8):493-501.
14. Shariff JA, Ahluwalia KP, Papapanou PN. Relationship between frequent recreational cannabis (marijuana and hashish) use and periodontitis in adults in the United States: National Health and Nutrition Examination Survey 2011 to 2012. *J Periodontol*. 2017;88(3):273-280.
15. Sanz M, Ceriello A, Buysschaert M, et al. Scientific evidence on the links between periodontal diseases and diabetes: consensus report and guidelines of the joint workshop on periodontal diseases and diabetes by the International Diabetes Federation and the European Federation of Periodontology. *Diabetes Res Clin Pract*. 2018;137:231-241.
16. Ismail AF, McGrath CP, Yiu CK. Oral health of children with type 1 diabetes mellitus: a systematic review. *Diabetes Res Clin Pract*. 2015;108(3):369-381.
17. Teshome A, Yitayeh A. The effect of periodontal therapy on glycemic control and fasting plasma glucose level in type 2 diabetic patients: systematic review and meta-analysis. *BMC Oral Health*. 2016;17(1):31.
18. Daudt LD, Musskopf ML, Mendez M, et al. Association between metabolic syndrome and periodontitis: a systematic review and meta-analysis. *Braz Oral Res*. 2018;32:e35.
19. Hales CM, Carroll MD, Fryar CD, Ogden CL. *Prevalence of obesity and severe obesity among adults: United States, 2017–2018*. NCHS Data Brief, no 360. Hyattsville, MD: National Center for Health Statistics; 2020.
20. Keller A, Rohde JF, Raymond K, Heitmann BL. Association between periodontal disease and overweight and obesity: a systematic review. *J Periodontol*. 2015;86(6):766-776.
21. Martens L, De Smet S, Yusof MY, Rajasekharan S. Association between overweight/obesity and periodontal disease in children and adolescents: a systematic review and meta-analysis. *Eur Arch Paediatr Dent*. 2017;18(2):69-82.
22. Pulikkotil SJ, Nath S, Muthukumaraswamy, Dharamarajan L, Jing KT, Vaithilingam RD. Alcohol consumption is associated with periodontitis. A systematic review and meta-analysis of observational studies. *Community Dent Health*. 2020;37(1):12-21.
23. Alsharief M, Kaye EK. Alcohol consumption may increase the risk for periodontal disease in some adult populations. *J Evid Based Dent Pract*. 2017;17(1):59-61.
24. Chapple IL, Bouchard P, Cagetti MG, et al. Interaction of lifestyle, behaviour or systemic diseases with dental caries and periodontal diseases: consensus report of group 2 of the joint EFP/ORCA workshop on the boundaries between caries and periodontal diseases. *J Clin Periodontol*. 2017; 44(suppl 18):S39-S51.
25. Decker A, Askar H, Tattan M, Taichman R, Wang HL. The assessment of stress, depression, and inflammation as a collective risk factor for periodontal diseases: a systematic review. *Clin Oral Investig*. 2020;24(1):1-12.
26. Hughes FJ, Bartold PM. Periodontal complications of prescription and recreational drugs. *Periodontol 2000*. 2018; 78(1):47-58.
27. Nibali L, Bayliss-Chapman J, Almofareh SA, Zhou Y, Divaris K, Vieira AR. What is the heritability of periodontitis? A systematic review. *J Dent Res*. 2019;98(6):632-641.
28. Cekici A, Kantarci A, Hasturk H, Van Dyke TE. Inflammatory and immune pathways in the pathogenesis of periodontal disease. *Periodontol 2000*. 2014;64(1):57-80.
29. Penoni V, Fidalgo TK, Torres SR, et al. Bone density and clinical periodontal attachment in postmenopausal women: a systematic review and meta-analysis. *J Dent Res*. 2017;96(3): 261-269.
30. Murakami S, Mealey BL, Mariotti A, Chapple ILC. Dental plaque-induced gingival conditions. *J Periodontol*. 2018; 89(suppl 1):S17-S27.
31. Iwasaki M, Hirano H, Ohara Y, Motokawa K. The association of oral function with dietary intake and nutritional status among older adults: latest evidence from epidemiological studies. *Jpn Dent Sci Rev*. 2021;57:128-137.
32. Loos BG, Van Dyke TE. The role of inflammation and genetics in periodontal disease. *Periodontol 2000*. 2020;83(1):26-39.
33. Kornman KS. Mapping the pathogenesis of periodontitis: a new look. *J Periodontol*. 2008; 79(suppl 8):1560-1568.
34. Page RC, Schroeder HE. Pathogenesis of inflammatory periodontal disease. A summary of current work. *Lab Invest*. 1976;34(3):235-249.
35. Bosshardt DD. The periodontal pocket: pathogenesis, histopathology and consequences. *Periodontol 2000*. 2018;76(1): 43-50.
36. Huynh-Ba G, Kuonen P, Hofer D, et al. The effect of periodontal therapy on the survival rate and incidence of complications of multirooted teeth with furcation involvement after an observation period of at least 5 years: a systematic review. *J Clin Periodontol*. 2009;36(2):164-176.
37. Jepsen S, Caton JG, Albandar JM, et al. Periodontal manifestations of systemic diseases and developmental and acquired conditions: Consensus report of workgroup 3 of the 2017 World Workshop on the Classification of Periodontal and Peri-Implant Diseases and Conditions. *J Periodontol*. 2018;89 (suppl 1):S237-S248.
38. Cortellini P, Bissada NF. Mucogingival conditions in the natural dentition: narrative review, case definitions, and diagnostic considerations. *J Periodontol*. 2018;89(suppl 1):S204-S213.
39. Chapple ILC, Mealey BL, Van Dyke TE, et al. Periodontal health and gingival diseases and conditions on an intact and a reduced periodontium: consensus report of workgroup 1 of the 2017 World Workshop on the Classification of Periodontal and Peri-Implant Diseases and Conditions. *J Clin Periodontol*. 2018;45(suppl 20):S68-S77.
40. Holmstrup P, Plemons J, Meyle J. Non-plaque-induced gingival diseases. *J Clin Periodontol*. 2018;45(suppl 20):S28-S43.
41. Herrera D, Retamal-Valdes B, Alonso B, Feres M. Acute periodontal lesions (periodontal abscesses and necrotizing periodontal diseases) and endo-periodontal lesions. *J Periodontol*. 2018;89(suppl 1):S85-S102.

CHAPTER 20

Periodontal Examination

Linda D. Boyd, RDH, RD, EdD
Esther M. Wilkins, BS, RDH, DMD

CHAPTER OUTLINE

LEARNING OBJECTIVES

After studying this chapter, the student will be able to:

1. Describe the components of a comprehensive periodontal examination.
2. List the instruments used for a periodontal examination.
3. Explain the technique for use of the periodontal probe and explorers.
4. Explain how procedure for the comprehensive examination will be described to the patient.

Basic Instruments for Examination

- Parts of the dental and periodontal clinical examinations are made by direct visual observation, whereas other parts require **tactile** examination using a **periodontal probe** and/or an **explorer**.
- Basic instrument setups for all patients with permanent teeth should include at least a mouth mirror, periodontal probe, furcation probe, and a subgingival explorer such as an ODU (Old Dominion University) EXD11/12.
- The general principles of instrumentation are described in Chapter 37.

The Mouth Mirror

I. Purposes and Uses

A. Indirect Vision

- Indirect vision is used for all surfaces where direct vision is not possible.
- Examples are the distal surfaces of posterior teeth and lingual surfaces of anterior teeth.

B. Indirect Illumination

- The mirror is used to reflect the light from the dental overhead light or headlamp worn by the clinician to any area of the oral cavity.

C. Transillumination

- Transillumination refers to reflection of light through the teeth.
  - Mirror is used to reflect light from the lingual aspect of the teeth while examined from the facial.
  - Mirror is used for indirect vision on the lingual while light from the overhead dental light passes through the teeth. Dental caries or calculus deposits appear opaque.

D. Retraction

- The mirror is used to protect or prevent interference by the cheeks, tongue, or lips.

II. Procedure for Use

A. Grasp and Rest

- Use modified pen grasp with finger rest on a tooth surface near the working area.
- Provides stability and control.
- Assists in retraction of lips and cheek.
- Exercises for gaining skill in control of instruments are described in Chapter 37.

B. Retraction

- Adjust the mirror position so the angles of the mouth are protected from undue pressure by the shank of the mirror.
- If needed, use a thin layer of water-based lubricant on dry or cracked lips and corners of mouth.

C. Maintain Clear Vision

- Rub the surface of the mirror along the buccal mucosa to coat mirror with thin transparent film of saliva or use warm water to prevent the mirror from fogging.
- Request that the patient breathe through the nose to prevent condensation of moisture on the mirror.

Air-Water Syringe

I. Purposes and Uses

A. Procedure for Use

- Use with caution because the air-water syringe creates aerosols and leads to potential airborne contamination.
  - See Chapter 7 for guidance on managing aerosols. In particular, having adequate air filtration, barriers between patient chairs, using appropriate PPE, and use of high speed evacuation (HVE) suction.[1]

- Grasp the handle of the air–water syringe; place thumb on button to activate air.
- Test the air flow before using in the mouth so the strength of flow can be controlled.
- Apply a controlled, steady stream of air directly to the area being assessed. The clinician needs to thoroughly dry the area to increase visibility.
- Supplement air drying with use of the HVE and folded gauze sponge placed in vestibule to maintain a dry field.

B. To Improve and Facilitate Examination Procedures

- Make a thorough and more accurate examination.
- Dry supragingival calculus to facilitate identification.
  - Small deposits may be light in color and not visible until they are dried.
  - Dried calculus appears chalky and presents a contrast to tooth color.
- Deflect the free gingival margin (GM) for observation into the subgingival area. Subgingival calculus usually appears darker than supragingival calculus.
- Identify areas of demineralization and carious lesions.
- Recognize location and condition of restorations, particularly composite or tooth-colored restorations.

C. To Improve Visibility of the Treatment Area during Instrumentation

- Provide dry area for finger rest for stability during instrumentation.
- Facilitate effective scaling techniques.
- Minimize appointment time.
- Evaluate complete removal of supragingival calculus.

D. To Prepare Teeth and/or Gingiva for Certain Procedures

- Examples are to dry surfaces for:
  - Application of caries-preventive agents when indicated.
  - Preparation to make impression for study model.

E. Precautions

- Avoid sharp blasts of air on cervical areas of teeth or open carious lesions due to possible sensitivity of these areas. Such areas may be dried by blotting with a gauze sponge or cotton roll to avoid patient discomfort.
- As previously noted, the use of the air–water syringe is considered an aerosol-generating procedure (AGP) and care must be taken to follow appropriate infection control protocols to minimize risk for spread of infectious disease.[1]
- Avoid directing air toward the posterior region of the patient's mouth as it may cause coughing.
- Avoid startling the patient; give a warning when air is to be applied.

Explorers

I. General Purposes and Uses

- To detect, by tactile sense, the texture and character of the tooth surfaces.
  - For calculus detection, irregularities in the tooth surface, defects in margins of restorations, and other irregularities not apparent to direct visual observation.
  - An explorer is used to confirm direct observation. Avoid use of a sharp explorer on white spot lesions (demineralized tooth surfaces with potential to be remineralized).[2-3]
- To define the extent of instrumentation needed and guide techniques.
  - For nonsurgical periodontal instrumentation (scaling and root instrumentation).
  - Removing an overhanging filling.
- To evaluate when calculus has been adequately removed or restoration overhang removed.

II. Specific Explorers and Their Uses

- A variety of explorers are available, as shown by the examples in **Figure 20-1**.
- Explorer design impacts accessibility to proximal and root surfaces along with flexibility and tactile sensitivity.

A. Subgingival Explorers

- Use:
  - Subgingival use of explorers such as the ODU 11/12 is facilitated by an angled shank with a short tip (Figure 20-1C).
  - Supragingival use of TU-17 (Figure 20-1D): It may be adapted to all surfaces of anterior teeth, but is especially useful for proximal surface examination.

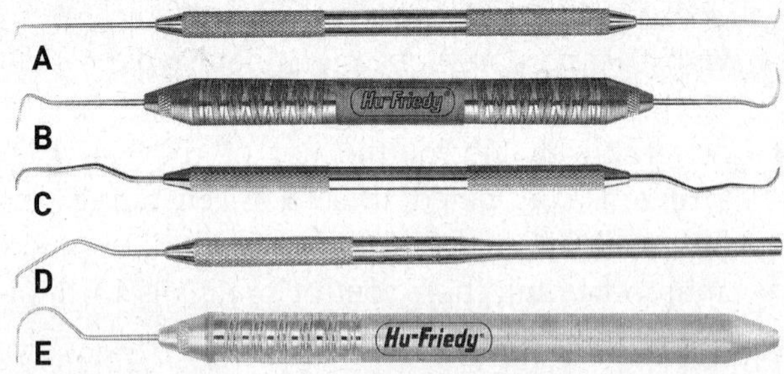

Figure 20-1 Explorers. **A:** Pigtail. **B:** Cowhorn. **C:** ODU 11/12. **D:** TU 17. **E:** Shepherd hook/No. 23.

- Features for subgingival examination:
  - Back of tip can be applied directly to the base of the pocket without trauma or laceration.
  - The short tip can be adapted to rounded tooth surfaces and line angles.
  - Narrow short tip can be adapted at the base where the pocket narrows without undue displacement of the pocket soft tissue wall.

B. Supragingival Explorers

- A sharp explorer should not be used to examine pits and fissures and supragingival smooth surface white spot lesions.[2-4]
- Shepherd hook explorer (Figure 20-1E):
  - Use: Examining surfaces and margins of restorations and sealants.
- Pigtail or cowhorn (Figure 20-1A and B):
  - Use: Proximal surfaces for calculus or margins of restorations.
  - Adaptability: As paired, curved tips, they are applied to opposite tooth surfaces.

Basic Procedures for Use of Explorers

- Development of ability to use an explorer and a probe is achieved first by learning the anatomic features of each tooth and root surface and the types of irregularities that may be encountered.
- The second step is repeated practice of techniques for application of the instruments to develop fine motor skills.[5]
- The objective is to adapt the instruments in a routine manner that relays consistent comparative information about the nature of the tooth surface.
- Concentration, patience, attention to detail, and being alert to irregularities, however small they may seem, are necessary.

I. Use of Sensory Stimuli

- A slender, wirelike explorer such as the ODU 11/12 has a greater degree of flexibility that contributes to increased tactile sensitivity for the clinician when a light grasp is used.

II. Tooth Surface Irregularities

- Three basic tactile sensations can be distinguished when probing or exploring.
  - Normal tooth surface.
    - Tooth structure: The smooth surface of enamel and root surface; anatomic configurations, such as cingula or furcations.
    - Restored surfaces: Smooth surfaces of metal (gold, amalgam) versus the feeling of composite; smooth margin of a restoration.
  - Irregularities created by excess or elevations in the surface.
    - Deposits: Calculus.
    - Anomalies: Enamel pearl.
    - Restorations: Overcontoured, irregular margins (overhangs).
  - Irregularities caused by depressions in the tooth surface.
    - Tooth surface: Demineralized or carious lesion, abrasion, erosion, or pits such as those caused by enamel hypoplasia.
    - Restorations: Deficient margin, rough surface.

III. Types of Stimuli

During exploring and probing, recognition of irregularities can be made through auditory and tactile means.

A. Tactile

- Tactile sensitivity is a very complex neurologic process with interaction among cognitive, sensory, and neuromuscular systems going on simultaneously.[5]
  - For calculus detection, tactile sensitivity consists of stimuli from vibrations created from the instrument passing over the tooth surface to the fingers and ultimately to the brain that interprets what we are feeling.
- Tactile sensations, for example, may be the result of the explorer catching on an overcontoured restoration, encountering an elevated calculus deposit, or simply passing over a rough tooth surface.

B. Auditory

- As an explorer or a probe moves over the surface of enamel, cementum, a metallic restoration, a composite restoration, or any irregularity of tooth structure or restoration, a difference in texture is apparent. With each contact, sound may be created.

- The rough cementum or calculus is scratchy or may present as a distinctive click. Sometimes, a metallic restoration may "squeak" or have a metallic "ring." With experience, differentiations can be detected.

Explorers: Supragingival Procedures

I. Use of Vision

- Visual examination of coronal tooth surfaces is most effective in combination with tactile examination with an explorer.[5]
- Visual examination with adequate light and air, proper retraction, and use of a mouth mirror can minimize unnecessary exploration.
- Visual examination can be effective for identification of supragingival calculus because when the tooth is dried, it can generally be seen as either chalky white or brownish-yellow in contrast to tooth color.

II. Facial and Lingual Surfaces

- Adapt 1–2 mm of the working end to the tooth surface, keeping the explorer continuously adapted to the tooth.
- Move the instrument in short walking strokes over the surface being examined.
- Careful noninvasive examination can be made by gently using the side of the explorer to feel for roughness, which may indicate demineralization. Applying pressure to puncture or scratch the surface can result in cavitation that requires restoration and is to be avoided.[2,3]

III. Proximal Surfaces

- Lead with the tip onto a proximal surface, rolling the handle between the fingers to ensure adaptation around the line angle. Keep the side of the point of the explorer in contact with the tooth surface at all times to avoid tissue trauma.
- Explore under the proximal contact area when there is recession of the papilla and the area is exposed. Overlap strokes from facial and lingual surfaces to ensure full coverage.

Explorers: Subgingival Procedures

I. Essentials for Detection of Tooth Surface Irregularities

- Light grasp to improve tactile sensitivity.
- Consistent finger rest with light pressure.
- Keep the last 1–2 mm of working end of the explorer tip in contact with the tooth to prevent tissue trauma. Do not remove from the pocket for each stroke.
- Use a "walking" stroke (**Figure 20-2**) with a light grasp.

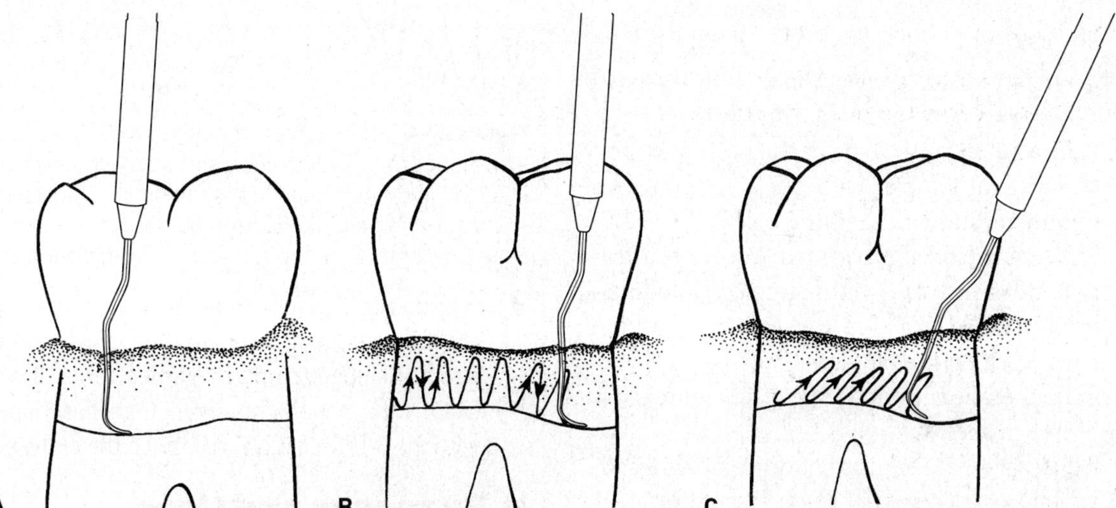

Figure 20-2 Use of Subgingival Explorer. **A:** The lower shank (next to tip) is held parallel with the long axis of the tooth. The explorer is passed into the pocket and lowered until the back of the working tip meets resistance from the attached periodontal tissue at the base of the pocket. **B:** Vertical walking stroke. With the side of the tip in contact with the tooth surface at all times, the explorer is moved over the surface. **C:** Diagonal walking stroke. Complete exploration of the surface is needed; therefore, groups of strokes are overlapped.

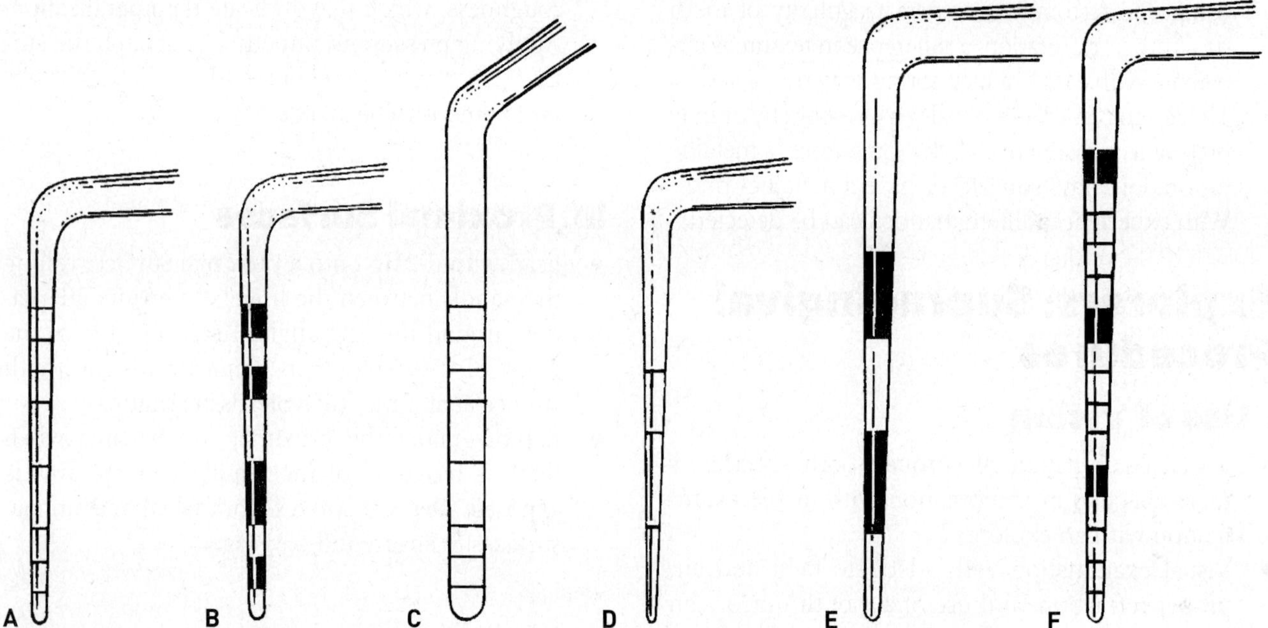

Figure 20-3 Examples of Probes. Names and calibrated markings shown are **A:** Williams (1-1-1-2-2-1-1-1), **B:** Williams, color-coded, **C:** Goldman-Fox (1-1-1-2-2-1-1-1), **D:** Michigan O (3-3-2), **E:** Hu-Friedy or Marquis color-coded (3-3-3-3 or 3-3-2-3), and **F:** Hu-Friedy UNC 15 (each millimeter to 15), color-coded at 5-10-15.

- Use short, controlled strokes to allow adaptation of the instrument to the tooth/root surface and depth of the sulcus/pocket.

Periodontal Probe

- The periodontal probe is an essential component of assessment and diagnosis of the patient's periodontal disease status.[6]

I. Types of Probes

Four generations of periodontal probes include[6]:

- First-generation or conventional manual periodontal probes remain the gold standard.
  - **Figure 20-3** shows some of the most common periodontal probes with their markings in millimeter increments from 1 to 3.
  - Probes specifically designed to assess furcation areas with and without colored millimeter markings, such as the Nabers furcation probe (see **Figure 20-4**).
- Second-generation periodontal probes are constant force probes.
  - Advantages are consistent force, but disadvantages are cost and patient discomfort.
- Third-generation periodontal probes are automated constant force probes with the same advantages and disadvantages of the second-generation probes. They are used primarily in clinical research.

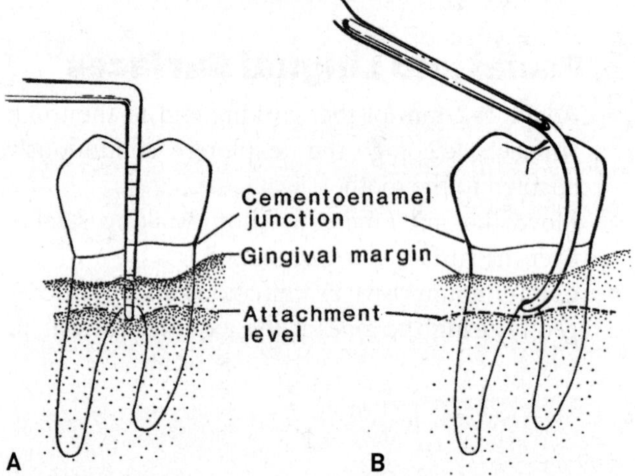

Figure 20-4 Furcation Examination. **A:** Limited access of a straight probe to examine a furcation. Williams probe inserted into bifurcation in area of gingival recession shows probing depth of 3 mm. **B:** Nabers furcation probe used to examine the topography of the furcation area.

- Fourth-generation periodontal probes use ultrasonographic technology to map the periodontal probing depth in an attempt to gather three-dimensional (3-D) information; however, high costs and issues with the 3-D imaging have limited their advancement.

II. Purposes and Uses

A probe is used for the following purposes.

A. Measure the Probing Depth (PD)

- Measure distance from the gingival margin to the base of the sulcus.

B. Measure Location of Gingival Margin (GM) in Relation to Cementoenamel Junction (CEJ)

- The distance from the GM to the CEJ determines the recession.
- The distance from the GM to CEJ is used along with the PD measurement to calculate the **clinical attachment level (CAL)**. This is described in more detail later in the chapter.
- The CAL is used as part of diagnosing the periodontal classification.
- Care is needed in measuring the location of the GM when it is coronal to the CEJ or the CAL will be inaccurate.

C. Measure Mucogingival Junction (MGJ) Location

- The distance from the GM to the mucogingival junction (MGJ) and subtract the PD to determine the amount of attached gingiva.
- Also check the pull of the frena to assess the pull on the attached gingiva

D. Make Other Gingival Determinations

- Evaluate bleeding on probing (BOP).
  - In the Classification of Periodontal Disease case definitions of health and disease, bleeding on probing is a key indicator.[7]
- Calculate a gingival bleeding index.
- Evaluate exudate or suppuration.
- Determine the consistency of the gingival tissue.

E. Provides Assessment Data for Diagnosis and Treatment Planning

- The assessment data gathered with the periodontal probe allow for calculation of the CAL that is used as part of classification of periodontal disease. The diagnosis (classification) and prognosis are used to guide the best options for treatment.
- The PD and state of inflammation determine the choice of instrument(s) for subgingival scaling and maintenance debridement.
- The periodontal probe, in conjunction with the explorer, is used to detect anatomic configuration of roots, subgingival deposits, and root irregularities that may complicate instrumentation.

F. Evaluate Treatment Outcomes

- Evaluate posttreatment tissue response to nonsurgical periodontal treatment as well as at periodic maintenance examinations.
- Evaluate patient's oral self-care.
- Identify signs of health when probing, including the following:
  - Less than 10% of sites exhibit BOP with no exudate.
  - Reduced PD; comparison of pretreatment and posttreatment PD.
  - Tissue is firm.

G. Evaluation at Continuing Care and Periodontal Maintenance Appointments

- At each continuing care appointment, a reevaluation is needed.
- To identify early disease changes that require additional professional treatment.

III. Description of Manual Periodontal Probes

- A probe is a slender instrument with a smooth, rounded tip designed for examination of the depth and topography of a gingival sulcus or periodontal pocket.
- A probe has three parts: the handle, angled shank, and working end, which is the probe itself.

A. Materials

- Stainless steel.
- Plastic.

B. Characteristics

- *Straight working end:*
  - Tapered, round, flat, or rectangular in cross section with a smooth, rounded end.
  - Calibrated in millimeters at intervals specific for each kind of probe; some have color coding. Figure 20-3 shows a comparison of a few typical markings; **Table 20-1** lists probe markings with examples.
- *Curved working end*: Paired furcation probes have a smooth, rounded end for investigation of the topography and anatomy around roots in a furcation. Examples are the Nabers 1N and 2N probes (Figure 20-4B).

Table 20-1 Types of Probes

Probe Markings (mm)	Examples	Description
Marks at 1-2-3-5-7-8-9-10	Williams	Round, tapered (available with color code)
	Glickman	Round, narrow diameter, fine
	Merritt B	Round, with longer lower shank Round, single bend to shank
Marks at 3-3-2	Michigan O Marquis M-1	Round, fine, tapered, narrow diameter
Marks at 3-6-9-12 3-6-8-11 (and other variations)	Michigan O Marquis Nordent	Round, tapered, fine Color-coded
Marks at each mm to 15	UNC 12 or 15	Round Color-coded at 5-10-15
Marks at 3-5-7-10	Perioscreen®	Round Color-coded with green and red to indicate the absence and presence of periodontal disease
Marks at 3.5-5.5-8.5-11.5	World Health Organization (WHO) probe (Figure 21-7)	Round, tapered, fine, with ball end Color-coded
Marks at 3-5-9-12 No marks	Nabers 1N, 2N	Curved, with curved shank for furcation examination

C. Selection

- Regular use of the same type of periodontal probe results in greater consistency of readings.[8]
- Following are the important features to be considered in probe selection:
  - Adaptability: The probe needs to be adaptable around the complete circumference of each tooth, both posterior and anterior, so that no millimeter area of the sulcus can be neglected. Flat probes require more attention to adaptation and are useful primarily on facial and lingual surfaces.
  - Markings: Research suggests the UNC15 with markings in 1-mm increments may provide more accurate PD measurement.[8] This minimizes inaccuracies of rounding up PDs when between probe markings.

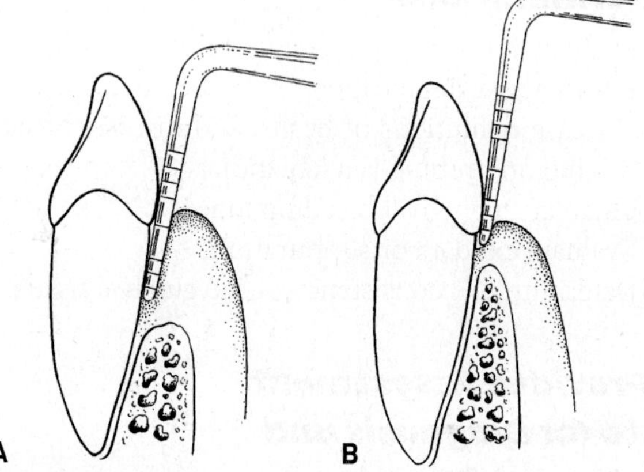

Figure 20-5 Probing Depth (PD). A pocket is measured from the gingival margin (GM) to the attached periodontal tissue. Shown is the contrast of probe measurements with GMs at the same level. **A:** Deep periodontal pocket (7 mm) with apical migration of attachment. **B:** Shallow sulcus (2 mm) with the attachment near the cementoenamel junction.

Guide to Periodontal Probing

I. Pocket Characteristics

- A pocket is measured from the base of the pocket to the GM. **Figure 20-5** shows GMs at the same level on two teeth with measurement of probing depths.
- The pocket (or sulcus) is continuous around the tooth and the entire sulcus needs to be measured. "Spot" probing is inadequate for a thorough assessment for periodontal classification and treatment planning.

- The depth tends to vary around an individual tooth; PD rarely measures the same all around a tooth or even around one surface of a tooth.
  - The GM varies in its position on the tooth.
- Proximal surfaces are approached by entering from both the facial and lingual aspects of a tooth.
  - Gingival and periodontal infections begin in the col area more frequently than in other areas. (See Chapter 19.)
  - PD may be deepest directly under the contact area because of crater formation in the alveolar bone (**Figure 20-6**).
- Anatomic features of the tooth surface wall of the pocket influence the direction of probing. Examples are concave surfaces, anomalies, shape of cervical third, and position of furcations.

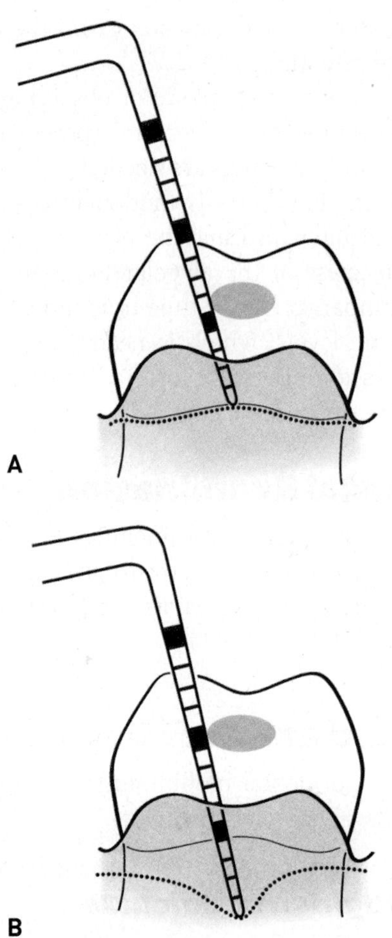

Figure 20-6 Proximal Surface Probing. **A:** Probe must be applied more than halfway across from facial to overlap with probing from the lingual. **B:** Probe in area of crater formation. Probing is often deeper on the proximal surface under the contact area than on the facial or lingual surfaces.

II. Evaluation of Tooth Surface

- During the movement of the probe, calculus and tooth surface irregularities can be felt and evaluated.
- The information obtained is used to plan the appointments for subgingival debridement.

III. Factors Affecting Probe Accuracy

- The general objectives of probing are accuracy and consistency so recordings can be used for comparison with future periodontal examinations, as well as with colleagues in practice together.
- At the same time, patient discomfort and trauma to the tissues must be minimized.
- Probing is influenced by many factors, such as those described in the following topics.

A. Stage and Extent of Periodontal Disease

- Diseased tissue offers less resistance, so that with increased severity of inflammation, the probe inserts to a deeper level.[6]
  - In gingivitis and periodontitis: The probe tip passes through the junctional epithelium to reach attached connective tissue fibers and may overestimate the attachment loss.[6]

B. The Periodontal Probe

- **Calibration**: Must be accurately marked.
- Thickness: The recommended probe tip diameter is 0.6 mm.[9]
- Readability: Markings and color coding are easy to read.

C. Placement Problems

- Anatomic variations: Tooth contours, furcations, contact areas, and crowding.
- Interferences: Calculus, irregular margins of restorations, and fixed dental prostheses.
- Accessibility and visibility: Obstructed by tissue bleeding, biofilm, limited opening by patient, and macroglossia.

Preliminary Assessment Prior to Periodontal Examination

The American Academy of Periodontology's Parameter on the Comprehensive Periodontal Examination includes the following.[2,10]

I. Medical History

- A thorough medical history is taken and reviewed to identify issues that may affect treatment and outcomes.
- Patients at risk of bacteremia may need antibiotic prophylaxis before examination or instrumentation. (See Chapter 11.)

II. Dental and Psychosocial History

- Document the dental history, including oral self-care habits, previous dental history, and chief complaint. (See Chapter 11.)
- Psychosocial history may include information such as marital status, living situation, financial situation, work habits, diet, substance use, stress, and oral health literacy. (See Chapter 11.)
    - Psychosocial factors are taken into consideration when planning treatment and setting treatment goals.

III. Vital Signs

- Vital signs are taken at each new patient appointment, at follow-up appointments for those with hypertension, and prior to treatment requiring local anesthesia. (See Chapter 12.)

IV. Extraoral/Intraoral Examination

- An extraoral/intraoral examination should be done at each examination appointment. (See Chapter 13.)

V. Risk Assessment

- The American Academy of Periodontology suggests risk assessment is an important aspect of treatment planning to identify patient modifiable risks that need to be addressed.[11]
- Risk assessment for dental caries, periodontal disease, and oral cancer are conducted. (See Chapters 19 and 25 for information on risk assessment tools.)
- Additional risk assessment for factors such as diabetes, tobacco use, or substance use may be performed based on individual needs of the patient. (See Chapter 54 for information on diabetes, Chapter 32 for information on tobacco use, and Chapter 59 for information on substance use.)

VI. Radiographic Examination

- Radiographs provide essential information to aid and supplement clinical findings to develop the periodontal classification (diagnosis), prognosis, and treatment plan.[12-13]
    - In the 2017 Classification of Periodontal Diseases, radiographic bone level (RBL) is used to assess severity of periodontitis.[13]
- The need for radiographs is based on the radiographic history of the patient and current guidelines. (See Chapter 15.)
- During the examination, and especially during the periodontal examination, the radiographs must be available for viewing.
    - When the radiographs are not available at the time of the initial examination, a definitive diagnosis (periodontal classification) and treatment plan cannot be completed.
    - Radiographs free from errors in technique and viewed with magnification on an adequately lighted viewbox or on the computer are essential.
- Selection of radiographs: For observing evidence of periodontal involvement, periapical radiographs and bitewings are needed.
    - When bone loss is moderate to severe, vertical bitewings may be necessary to evaluate the crest of the alveolar bone and to allow comparisons over time to identify changes in bone levels, which is needed to assess progression of disease for grading of periodontal disease.[13] (See Chapter 15.)

VII. Dental Examination

- The dental examination includes documentation of missing teeth, caries, restorations, tooth position, parafunctional habits, and occlusion. (See Chapter 16.)

VIII. Hard and Soft Deposits

The location of dental biofilm and calculus is documented. (See Chapter 17.)

A. *Supragingival Calculus*

- Distribution
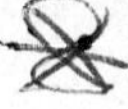
    - Supragingival calculus is generally localized on the lingual surfaces of the mandibular anterior teeth and the facial surfaces of the maxillary first and second molars, opposite the openings to the salivary ducts.

- Amount
  - Indicate a subjective description of the amount using terms such as slight, moderate, and heavy.

B. Subgingival Calculus

- Distribution
  - Subgingival calculus can be either localized or generalized. Record in relation to PD on a chart or form to show exact locations.
- Amount
  - Indicate a subjective description of the amount using terms such as slight, moderate, and heavy.
- Type
  - Include descriptive terminology for the type of calculus deposits. (See Chapter 17.)

Parameters of Care for the Periodontal Examination

I. Periodontal Probing Procedure

A. Periodontal Probe Insertion

- Grasp probe with modified pen grasp.
- Establish finger rest on a neighboring tooth, preferably in the same dental arch.
- Keep probe against the tooth near the GM. The cervical third of a primary tooth is more convex (**Figure 20-7**).
- Gently slide the tip under the GM.
  - Healthy or firm fibrotic tissue: Insertion is more difficult because of the close adaptation of the tissue to the tooth surface; underlying gingival fibers are strong and tight.
  - Spongy, soft tissue: GM is loose and flabby because of the destruction of underlying gingival fibers. Probe inserts readily, and bleeding can be expected on gentle probing.

B. Advance Probe to Base of Pocket

- Hold the probe tip against the tooth surface; probe should be kept parallel with long axis of the tooth for vertical insertion. The shape of the crown can make it difficult to maintain this angulation (Figure 20-7).
- Slide the probe along the tooth surface vertically down to the base of the sulcus or pocket.
  - Maintain the tip of the probe in contact with the tooth.

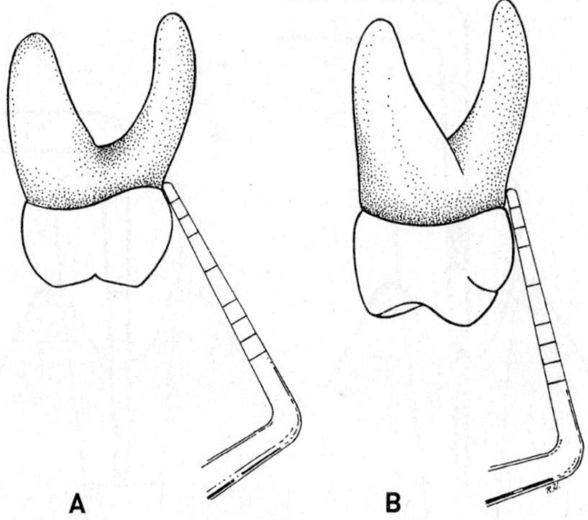

Figure 20-7 Primary and Permanent Maxillary Molars. **A:** Accentuated convexity of the cervical third and widespread roots of the primary molar complicate probe placement. Probe may encounter the root. **B:** Permanent tooth with less convexity of the cervical third and roots that are less widely spread.

  - As the probe is moved down the side of the tooth, roughness may be felt, which may be calculus.
  - When obstruction by a hard bulky calculus deposit is encountered, lift the probe away from the tooth and follow over the edge of the calculus until the probe can move vertically into the pocket again.
  - The base of the sulcus or pocket feels soft and elastic (compared with the hard tooth surface and calculus deposits).
  - The force used is approximately 0.20 g (50 N/cm^2) once the tension of the attached periodontal tissue at the base of the pocket is felt.[9,15]
- Position the probe so measurement can be read.[15]
  - Bring the probe to position as nearly parallel with the long axis of the tooth as possible for reading the depth.
  - Interference of the contact area does not permit placing the probe parallel for the measurement directly beneath the contact area. Hold the side of the shank of the probe against the contact to minimize the angle (Figure 20-6).

C. Reading the Probe Measurement

- Measurement for a PD is made from the GM to the attached periodontal tissue or base of the sulcus or pocket.
- A comparison of pocket measurement using probes with different markings is shown in **Figure 20-8**.

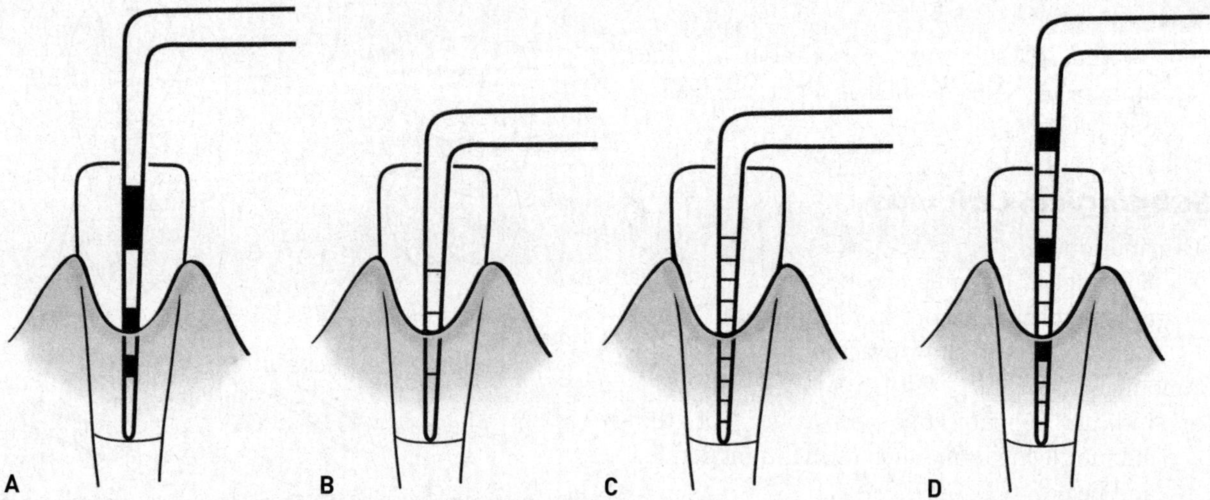

Figure 20-8 Comparison of Probe Readings. Measurement of the same 5-mm pocket with four different probes. **A:** Color-coded. **B:** Michigan O. **C:** Williams. **D:** Hu-Friedy UNC 15.

- When the GM appears at a level between probe marks, round up to the higher marking on the probe for the final measurement.

D. Circumferential Probing

- Probe stroke
  Maintain the probe in the sulcus or pocket of each tooth as the probe is moved in a walking stroke in the direction of the blue arrow in **Figure 20-9**.
  - It is not necessary to remove the probe and reinsert it to make individual readings. Use a continuous walking stroke to avoid missing a deep pocket area.
  - Repeated withdrawal and reinsertion cause unnecessary trauma to the GM and increases posttreatment discomfort.
- Walking stroke
  - Keep the side of the tip of the probe in contact with the tooth at the base of the pocket.
  - Slide the probe up (coronally) about 1–2 mm and back to the attachment in a "touch ... touch ... touch ..." rhythm (Figure 20-9).
  - Observe and record probe measurement at the GM at each location as noted in **Figure 20-10**.
  - Advance millimeter-by-millimeter along the facial and lingual surfaces into the proximal areas of each tooth.

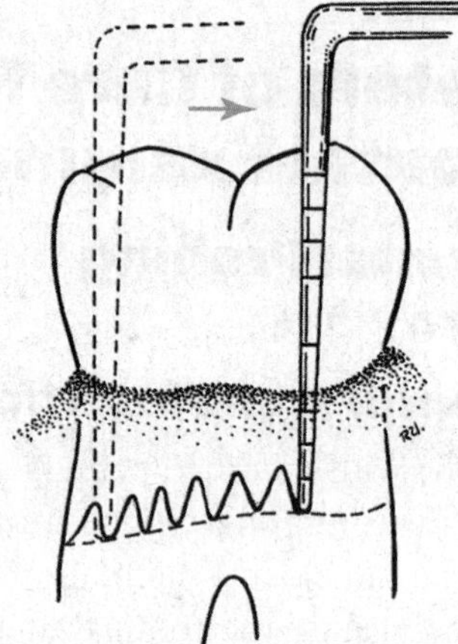

Figure 20-9 Probe Walking Stroke. The side of the tip of the probe is held in contact with the tooth. From the base of the pocket, the probe is moved up and down in 1-to 2-mm strokes as it is advanced in the direction indicated by the blue arrow in 1-mm steps. The attached periodontal tissue at the base of the pocket is contacted on each downward stroke to identify probing depth in each area.

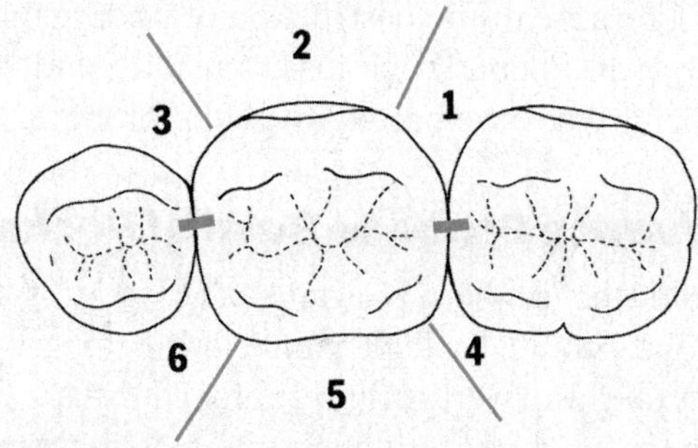

Figure 20-10 Recording Periodontal Probing Depths. The pocket/sulcus is measured completely around each tooth. Record the deepest measurement for each of the six areas around the tooth. Areas 1, 3, 4, and 6 extend from the line angle to under the contact area.

E. Adaptation of Probe for Individual Teeth

- Molars and premolars
  - Orient the probe at the distal line angle for both facial and lingual application.

- Insert the probe at the distal line angle and probe in a distal direction.
- As the distal proximal area is probed, the probe should touch the contact area and be slanted toward the midline of the proximal surface in the col area (Figure 20-6).
- Note the PD and slide the probe back to the distal line angle. Proceed in the mesial direction around the mesial line angle and across the mesial surface.
- The probing depth on the mesial is measured in the same manner as the distal proximal surface, and the probe should touch the contact area and be slanted to the midline of the col area where the proximal measurement is read.
- Overlap strokes from facial surface with strokes from lingual surface to ensure full coverage of the proximal area.

- Anterior teeth
  - Initial insertion may be at the distal line angle or from the midline of the facial or lingual surfaces.
  - Proceed around the distal line angle and across the distal surface; reinsert and probe the other half of the tooth.

F. Recording of Probing Measurements

- Six measurements are recorded for each tooth: Three from the facial and three from the lingual or palatal, as shown in Figure 20-10.
- For each of the six areas, the deepest probing measurement is recorded.
- Two recordings each are made for proximal areas: Numbers 3 and 6 for the mesial and numbers 1 and 4 for the distal in Figure 20-10. Frequently the deepest probing will be in the col, directly under the contact area.
- Recordings of PDs are part of the total periodontal charting.
- **Figure 20-11** illustrates a typical chart form in which boxes are provided for recording PD, furcations, and mobility for each tooth (this chart form is missing the MGJ measurements). Many electronic charts also provide an area to calculate the CAL.

G. Sources of Error in Periodontal Probing

- Sources of error in periodontal probing include[15]:
  - Resistance of tissues that is affected by the level of inflammation in the tissues.
  - Calculus.
  - Diameter and/or variations in standardization of the probe marks.
  - Clinician errors in angulation and/or insertion.
  - Probing pressure or force.

II. Clinical Attachment Level

- Attachment level refers to the position of the periodontal attached tissues at the base of a sulcus or pocket.
- CAL is measured from a fixed point to the attachment, whereas the PD is measured from a changeable point (the crest of the free gingiva) to the attachment (**Figure 20-12A**).

A. Rationale

- Stability of attachment is a characteristic of health.
- A loss of clinical attachment is a primary clinical feature of periodontitis as the junctional epithelium migrates toward the apex.[16]
- When periodontal disease is active, pocket formation and migration of the attachment along the cemental surface continue.
- Evaluation can be made of the outcome of periodontal treatment and the stability of the attachment during maintenance examinations.

B. Procedure

- Selecting a fixed point
  - CEJ is used unless it cannot be detected because of abrasion or a restoration.
  - Margin of a permanent restoration.
- Measuring in the presence of visible recession
  - CEJ is visible.
  - Measure from the CEJ to the GM (**Figure 20-12B**).
  - The CAL is calculated by *addition* of the probing depth to the GM to CEJ distance (PD + GM = CAL).
- Measuring when the CEJ is covered by the gingiva margin
  - Slide the probe along the tooth surface into the pocket until the CEJ is felt (**Figure 20-12C**). This is the CEJ to GM measurement.
  - *Subtract* the distance from the CEJ to GM from the total PD to the attachment (PD − GM = CAL).
- Measuring when the GM is level with the CEJ
  - With the GM at the CEJ, that measurement is the same as the PD.
  - The PD *equals* the CAL when the GM is level with the CEJ (**Figure 20-12D**).

PERIODONTAL CHART

Date 3/4/2019

Patient Last Name Does   First Name Jane   Date Of Birth

✓ **Initial Exam**   **Reevaluation**   Clinician Wilkins

	1	2	3	4	5	6	7	8	9	10	11	12	13	14	15	16
Mobility		0	0	0	0	0	0	0	0	0	0	0	0	0	0	
Implant																
Furcation																
Bleeding on Probing																
Plaque																
Gingival Margin		2 0 1	1 0 0	1 -2 0	0 -2 0	1 -3 1	1 0 1	1 0 1	0 0 0	0 0 0	0 -2 0	0 0 0	0 0 0	1 0 1	1 0 2	
Probing Depth		5 6 7	6 4 6	5 2 5	4 3 4	3 2 3	2 2 2	2 2 2	3 2 2	2 1 2	2 1 2	3 2 3	3 3 4	4 2 7	5 5 6	

Buccal

Lingual

	1	2	3	4	5	6	7	8	9	10	11	12	13	14	15	16
Gingival Margin		2 1 1	1 0 0	1 0 1	1 0 1	0 0 0	0 0 0	0 0 0	0 0 0	0 0 0	0 0 0	0 0 0	0 0 0	0 0 0	1 0 1	
Probing Depth		6 4 6	6 3 6	4 3 4	3 2 3	2 1 1	2 1 1	2 1 2	2 1 2	2 1 1	2 1 1	3 2 2	3 2 3	4 4 6	6 3 6	
Plaque																
Bleeding on Probing																
Furcation																
Note																

Mean Probing Depth = **3** mm   Mean Attachment Level = **-2.7** mm   48% Plaque   42% Bleeding on Probing

	32	31	30	29	28	27	26	25	24	23	22	21	20	19	18	17
Note																
Furcation																
Bleeding on Probing																
Plaque																
Gingival Margin		2 1 1	1 1 1	1 1 1	1 1 1	0 0 0	0 0 0	0 0 0	0 0 0	0 0 0	0 0 1	1 0 1	1 1 1	2 3 2	2 2 3	
Probing Depth		6 5 5	4 5 5	3 2 3	3 2 3	3 2 2	2 1 2	2 1 2	2 1 2	2 1 2	2 2 3	3 2 2	3 2 3	5 4 6	7 6 8	

Lingual

Buccal

	32	31	30	29	28	27	26	25	24	23	22	21	20	19	18	17
Gingival Margin		2 1 1	1 -1 1	0 -2 0	0 -2 0	0 0 0	0 -1 0	0 -1 0	0 -1 0	0 -1 0	0 0 0	1 -2 1	1 -2 1	1 0 1	1 0 2	
Probing Depth		6 4 5	4 3 4	4 2 3	3 1 2	3 1 2	2 2 2	2 1 2	2 1 2	2 1 2	2 2 3	3 2 3	3 2 3	3 2 2	3 2 4	
Plaque																
Bleeding on Probing																
Furcation																
Implant																
Mobility		0	0	0	0	0	0	0	0	0	0	0	0	0	0	

Figure 20-11 Sample Periodontal Chart Form. There are boxes to record the gingival margin, probing depth, plaque, bleeding on probing, furcations, and mobility. The form is missing boxes to record the mucogingival junction and boxes to calculate the clinical attachment level (CAL). The CAL is however graphically displayed by the blue band. (The blank form is available on perio-tools.com.)

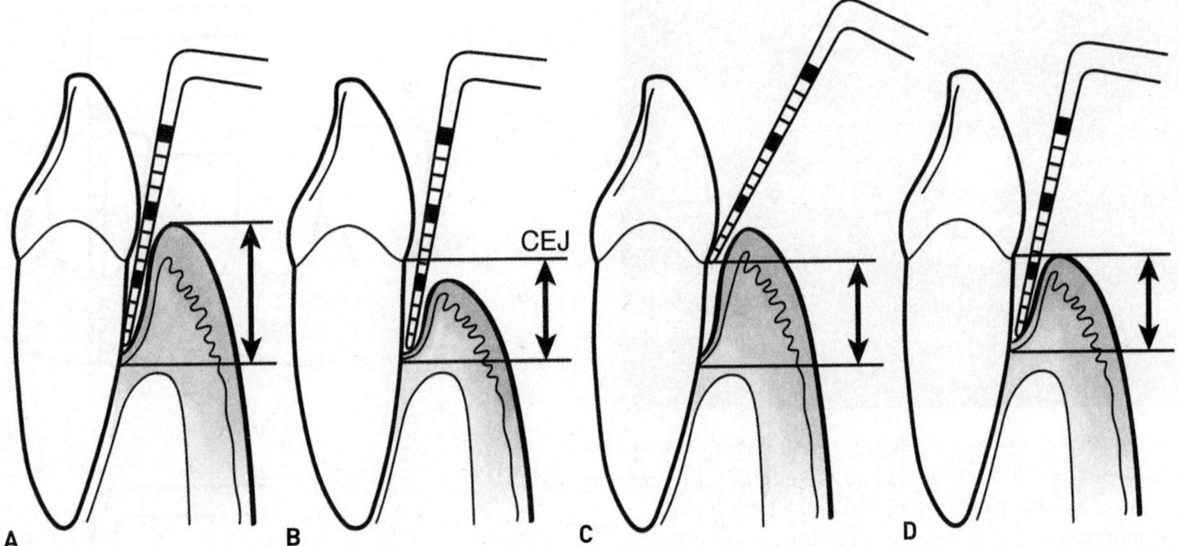

Figure 20-12 Clinical Attachment Level (CAL). **A:** Probing depth is measured from the gingival margin (GM) to the attached periodontal tissue. **B:** CAL in the presence of gingival recession is measured directly from the cementoenamel junction (CEJ) to the attached tissue. **C:** CAL when the GM covers the CEJ: First the CEJ is located as shown, and then the distance to the CEJ is measured and subtracted from the probing depth (PD). **D:** The CAL is equal to the PD when the GM is at the level of the CEJ.

III. Mucogingival Examination

A. Methods for Identifying MGJ

- Purposes
  - To detect adequacy of the width of the attached gingiva.
  - To locate frenal attachments and their proximity to the free gingiva.
- **Tension test procedure**
  - Retract cheeks and lips laterally by grasping the lips with the thumbs and index fingers.
  - Move the lips and cheeks up and down and back and forth, creating tension between the attached gingiva and mucosa to make the MGJ visible (**Figure 20-13**).
  - Follow around from the molar areas on the right to molar areas on the left, both maxillary and mandibular. Observe frenal attachments.
- Lingual (mandible)
  - Hold a mouth mirror to tense the mucosa of the floor of the mouth, gently retracting the side of the tongue, so that the MGJ is clearly visible.
  - Request patient move the tongue to the left, to the right, and up to touch the palate.
- Fold (or wrinkle) test procedure
  - Retract the lip gently, but not to the point of tension between the attached gingiva and buccal mucosa.
  - The periodontal probe is oriented horizontal to the MGJ and very gentle pressure is used to fold or wrinkle the mucosa toward the GM (see **Figure 20-14**).[17]
  - This procedure can be used if the MGJ cannot be easily visualized with the tension test method.

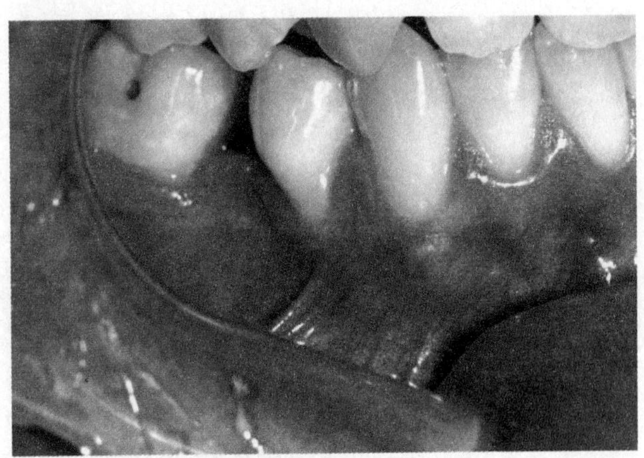

Figure 20-13 Tension test. The tension test can be used to differentiate unattached mucosa and attached gingiva to aid in identifying the location of the MGJ to more accurately calculate the quantity of attached gingiva.

Courtesy of Dr. Ralph Arnold.

B. Measurement of Width of Attached Gingiva

- Place the probe (no pressure) on the external surface of the gingiva and measure from the MGJ to the GM to determine the total width of the gingiva (**Figure 20-15A**).
- Measure PD (**Figure 20-15B**).

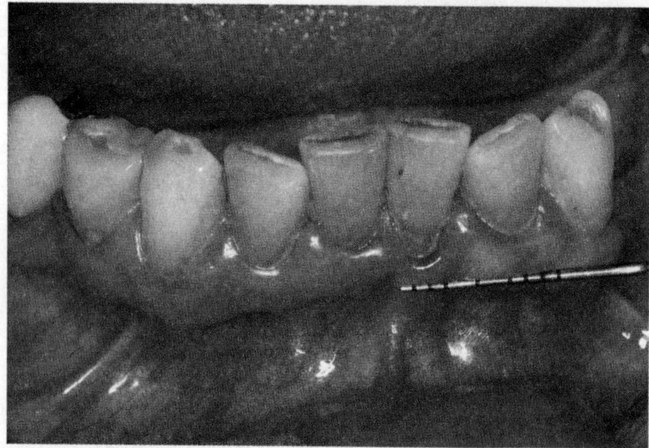

Figure 20-14 Wrinkle or Fold Test for a Mucogingival Defect. A mucogingival defect is suspected at tooth #24, which has a very narrow zone of keratinized gingiva. The periodontal probe is positioned at the mucogingival junction and very gently moved coronally against the mucosa. Blanching or wrinkling of the mucosa at the gingival margin indicates no attached gingiva.

Reproduced from Weiss G, Scheid R. *Woelfel's Dental Anatomy*. 8th ed. Philadelphia, PA: Lippincott Williams & Wilkins; 2012.

- Calculate the width of attached gingiva by *subtracting* the PD from the total width of the gingiva.
- Record findings.

C. Areas at Risk for Mucogingival Conditions

- Primary factors putting an area at risk for a recession[18]:
  - Absence of attached gingiva.
    - When a pocket extends to or beyond the MGJ, the probe may pass through into the alveolar mucosa when probing the pocket.
  - Reduced alveolar bone thickness due to abnormal tooth positioning in the arch.
- Inconsistent findings in research suggest the following may also be risk factors for recession, but more research is needed[18]:
  - Improper toothbrushing.
  - Cervical restoration margins.
  - Orthodonture, but it is more likely a result of the direction of tooth movement and thickness of the alveolar bone and gingiva.

IV. Mobility Examination

- Because of the nature and function of the periodontal ligament, teeth have a slight normal mobility.
- Mobility can be considered abnormal or pathologic when it exceeds normal.

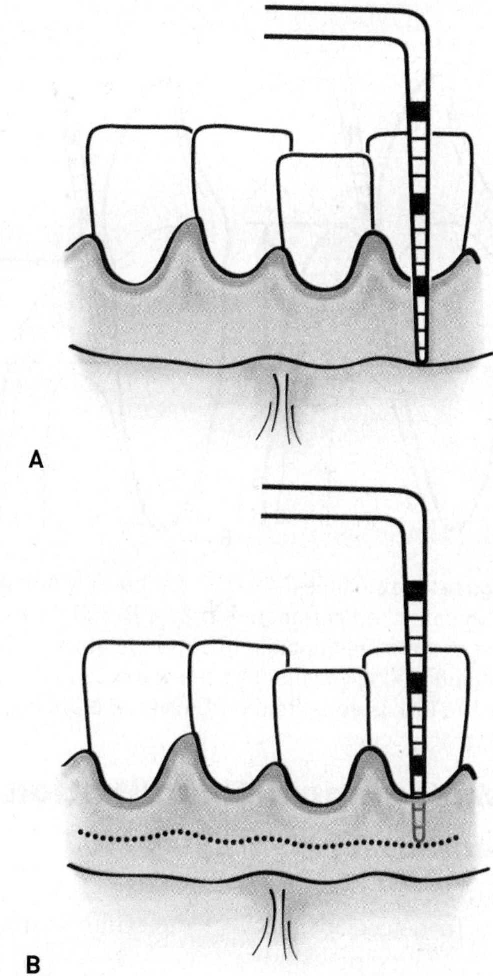

Figure 20-15 Measuring Attached Gingiva. **A:** Measure the total gingiva by laying the probe over the surface of the gingiva and measuring from the free margin to the mucogingival junction. **B:** Measure the probing depth (PD). Dotted line represents the base of the pocket. Subtract the PD (B) from the total gingiva (A) to obtain the width of attached gingiva. The area illustrated shows 2 mm of attached gingiva.

- Increased mobility can be a clinical sign of trauma from occlusion.

A. Procedure for Determination of Mobility

1. Position the patient for clear visibility with good light.
2. Stabilize the head: Motion of the head, lips, or cheek can interfere with an accurate evaluation of tooth movement.
3. Use two single-ended metal instruments with wide blunt ends, held with a modified pen grasp (**Figure 20-16**).
   - The use of wooden tongue depressors or plastic mirror handles is not recommended because of their flexibility.

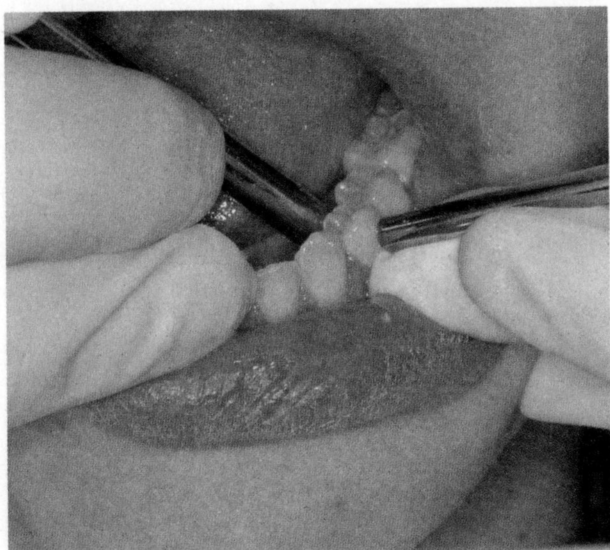

Figure 20-16 Method for Determining Tooth Mobility. **A:** Two rigid instrument handles are applied to the tooth to see if it can be displaced either buccolingually or mesiodistally. For teeth with severe mobility, the tooth can be depressed or rotated (which is category 3 mobility). **B:** Technique for determining buccolingual mobility. Light, alternating (reciprocating) buccolingual forces are applied and movement observed relative to adjacent teeth.

- Testing with the fingers without the metal instruments can be misleading because the soft tissue of the fingertips can move and give an illusion of tooth movement.

1. Apply specific, firm finger rests (fulcrums): A standardized finger rest pressure contributes increased consistency to the determinations. The teeth may be dried with air or gauze to prevent slipping of the instruments or the finger on the finger rest.
2. Apply the blunt ends of the instruments to opposite sides of a tooth, and rock the tooth to test horizontal mobility. Keep both instrument ends on the tooth as pressure is applied first from one side and then the other.
3. Test vertical mobility (depression of the tooth into its socket) by applying pressure with one of the mirror handles to the occlusal or incisal surface.
4. Move from tooth to tooth in a systematic order.

B. Record Degree of Movement

The most widely used method to assess tooth mobility is the Miller Index, first described in 1938.[19]

- *Scale*
  - The N, 1, 2, 3 or I, II, III are frequently used, sometimes with a plus sign (+) to indicate mobility between numbers.
- *Recording*
  - Although subjective, interpretation may be considered as follows[10]:
    - N: Normal, physiologic.
    - 1: Slight mobility, greater than normal.
    - 2: Moderate mobility, greater than 1 mm displacement.
    - 3: Severe mobility, moves vertically and is depressible in the tooth socket.
- *The letter N means normal mobility.*
  - All teeth that have a periodontal ligament have normal mobility. No tooth has zero mobility, except in a condition such as ankylosis in which there is no periodontal ligament.
- *Chart form*
  - A chart form such as Figure 20-11 provides for a place to record mobility. Preferably more than one space is available, so comparative readings can be recorded at successive maintenance appointments.

V. Fremitus

A. Definition

- **Fremitus** means palpable vibration or movement.
- In dentistry, fremitus refers to the vibratory patterns of the teeth. A tooth with fremitus has excess contact, possibly related to a premature contact. Usually, the tooth also demonstrates some degree of mobility because the excess contact forces the tooth to move.
- The test is used in conjunction with occlusal analysis and adjustment.
- Because fremitus depends on tooth contact, determination is made only on the maxillary teeth.

B. Procedure for Determination of Fremitus

1. Seat the patient upright with the head stabilized against the headrest; the occlusal biting plane is parallel with the floor.
2. Gently place the index finger on the facial surface of each maxillary tooth at about the cervical third (**Figure 20-17**).
3. Request the patient close the back teeth together in a functional occlusion and tap up and down repeatedly.[20]
4. Start with the most posterior maxillary tooth on one side and move the index finger tooth by tooth around the arch.
5. Record by tooth number the teeth where vibration is felt and the teeth where actual movement

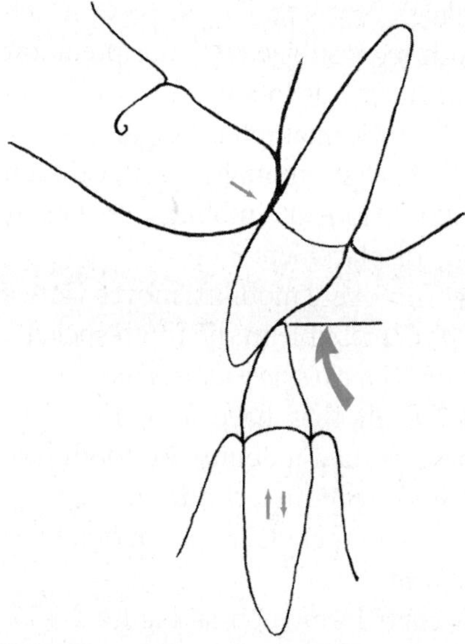

Figure 20-17 Fremitus. With the patient seated upright and the head stabilized against the headrest, an index finger is placed firmly over the cervical third of each maxillary tooth in succession starting with the most posterior tooth on one side and moving around the arch. The patient is asked to click the posterior teeth.

is noted. The degree recorded may be subjective, but the following range has been suggested:

- N: Normal (without vibration or movement).
- +: One-degree fremitus; only slight vibration can be felt.
- ++: Two-degree fremitus; the tooth is clearly palpable but movement is barely visible.
- +++: Three-degree fremitus; movement is clearly observed visually.

VI. Furcation Examination

When a pocket extends into a furcation area, special adaptation of the probe must be made to determine the extent and topography of the furcation involvement.

A. Anatomic Features

- Bifurcation (teeth with two roots)
  1. Mandibular molars: The furcation area is accessible for probing from the facial and lingual surfaces (Figure 20-4).
  2. Maxillary first premolars: The furcation area is accessible from the mesial and distal aspects, under the contact area.
  3. Primary mandibular molar: Widespread roots.
- Trifurcation (teeth with three roots)
  1. Maxillary molars: A palatal root and two buccal roots, the mesiobuccal and the distobuccal roots. Access for probing is from the buccal (**Figure 20-18A**), mesiolingual, buccal (**Figure 20-18B**), and distolingual surfaces (**Figure 20-18C**).
  2. Maxillary primary molars: Widespread roots (Figure 20-7).

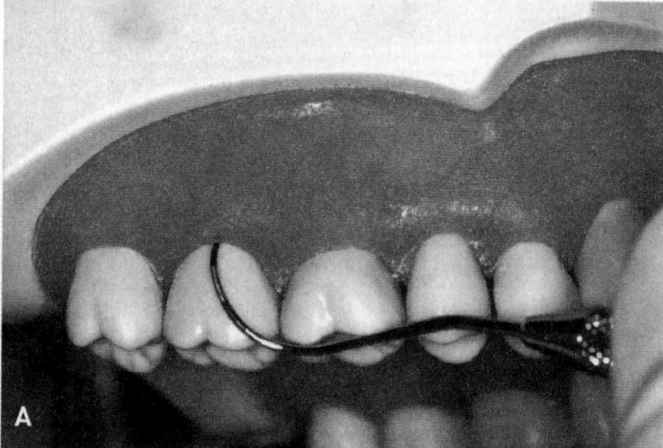

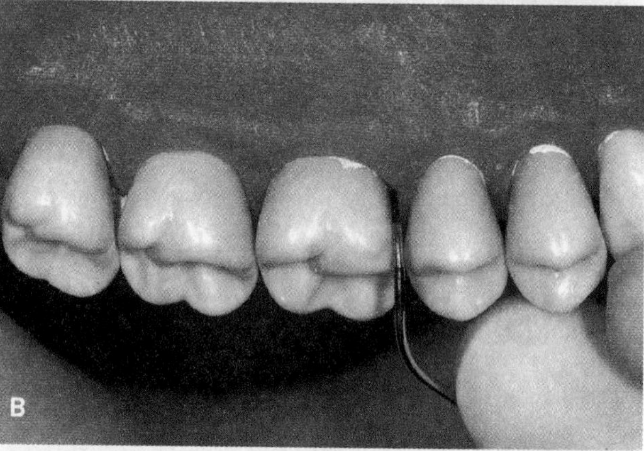

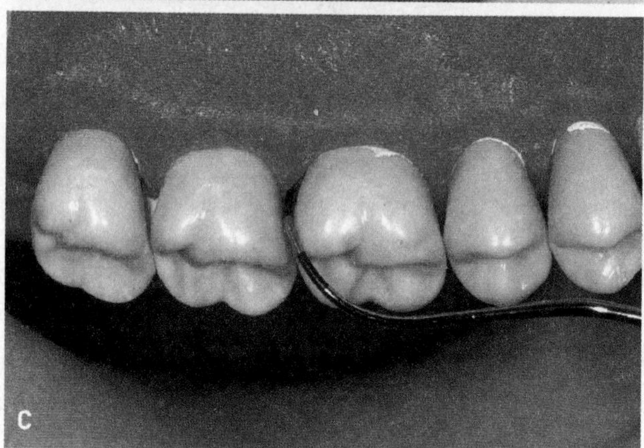

Figure 20-18 Three Locations Used to Confirm Maxillary Molar Furcation Involvement. **A:** Buccal view: Buccal furcation is probed midbuccal. The furcation probe is shown as it enters the potential furcation near the middle of the facial surface of this maxillary molar. **B:** Palatal view: The mesial furcation on a maxillary molar is accessed through the palatal embrasure since the mesiobuccal root is wider than the palatal root. **C:** Palatal view: The distal furcation on a maxillary molar is probed through the palatal embrasure here, although the distobuccal root is about as wide as the palatal root.

B. Examination Methods

- Furcation measurement procedure[21]:
  - Review the radiograph for signs of furcation involvement or radiolucency (**Figure 20-19**).
  - Using knowledge of the anatomy of the multirooted teeth, use a furcation probe, such as the Nabers 1N or 2N probe, to walk around the area sulcus to identify the entrance to the furcation (Figure 20-4).[22]
  - If the Nabers probe enters the furcation, note the distance from the entrance to the furcation until resistance is felt, which provides the vertical depth of the furcation.
- Furcation grades
  - Furcation involvement is usually classified by the amount of bone destroyed in the furcation area. The most common classification is the Glickman furcation grades[23,24]:
    - Grade I: Early, beginning involvement. A probe can enter the concavity of the furcation but the bone between the roots (interradicular) is intact.
    - Grade II: Moderate involvement. Bone has been destroyed to an extent that permits Nabers probe to enter the furcation area between the roots but not extend all the way through to the opposite side.
    - Grade III: Severe involvement. A probe can be passed between the roots through the entire furcation.
    - Grade IV: Same as grade III, with exposure resulting from gingival recession, especially after periodontal therapy.
- Difficulties encountered in measurement of the furcation[21]
  - Anatomic variations that complicate furcation examination are fused roots, anomalies such as extra roots, or low or high furcations.
  - Force, tip diameter, angulation, and type of probe used.
  - Tissue quality variation.
  - Interference by calculus, crown contour, or overhanging restorations.

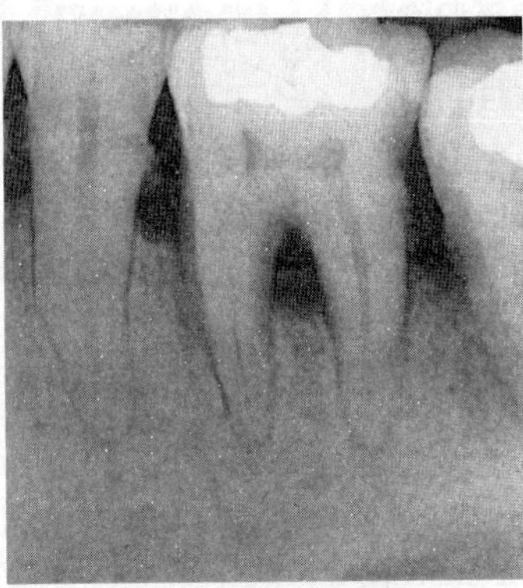

Figure 20-19 Furcation Involvement. The furcation involvement (radiolucency) is easily visible on the mandibular first molar in this radiograph.

Radiographic Changes in Periodontal Disease

I. Bone Level

A. Normal Bone Level

The crest of the interdental bone appears from 1.0 to 1.5 mm from the CEJ and is horizontal from the CEJ of one tooth to the adjacent tooth (**Figure 20-20**).

B. Bone Level in Periodontal Disease

The height of the bone is lowered progressively as the inflammation is extended and bone is destroyed.

II. Shape of Remaining Bone

A. Horizontal Bone Loss

- When the crest of the bone is parallel with a line between the CEJs of two adjacent teeth, the term horizontal bone loss is used (**Figure 20-21**).
- When inflammation is the sole destructive factor, the bone loss usually appears horizontal.
- Extent of disease is considered to be generalized if >30% of areas involved and localized if <30% of sites are involved.[16]

B. Angular or Vertical Bone Loss

- Reduction in height of crestal bone that is irregular; the bone level is not parallel with a line joining the adjacent CEJs (**Figure 20-22**).

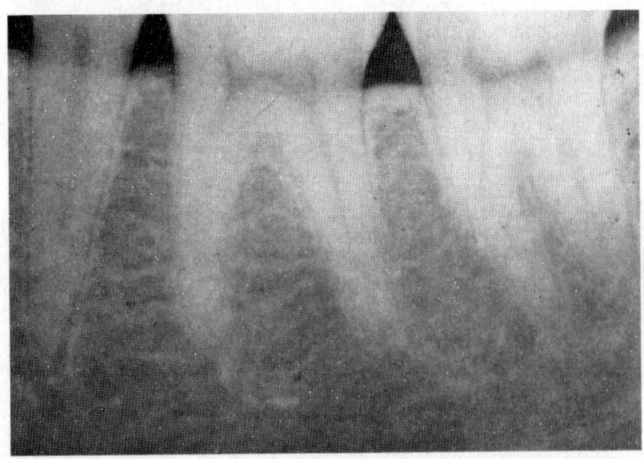

Figure 20-20 Normal Bone Level. Radiograph showing normal bone level, 1–1.5 mm from the cementoenamel junction.

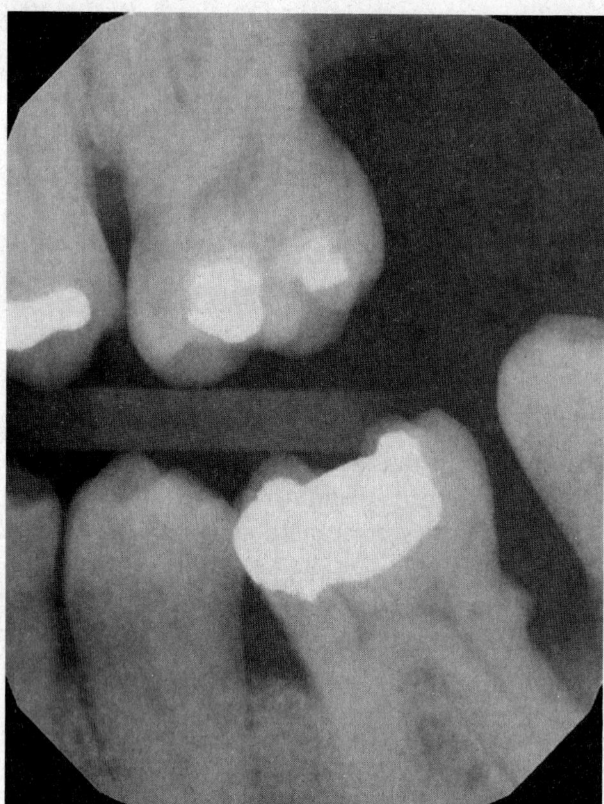

Figure 20-21 Horizontal Bone Loss. Note that the level of the crestal bone is parallel with a line between the cementoenamel junctions of the mandibular second premolar and the mesially tipped first molar (also note calculus on the distal surface of the mandibular first molar).

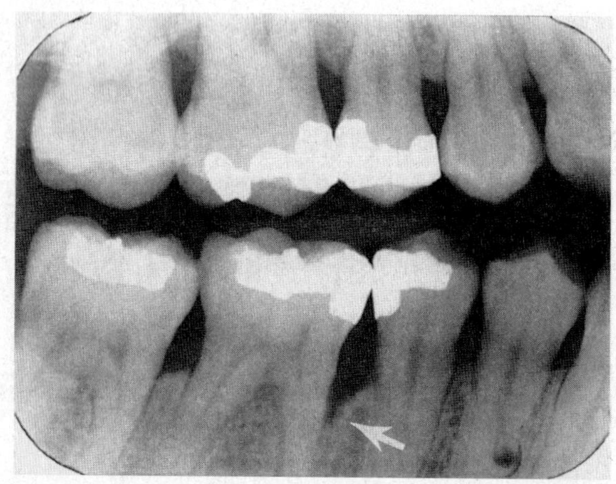

Figure 20-22 Vertical Bone Loss. The arrow points to vertical bone loss on the mesial surface of the mandibular first molar.

- Angular bone loss is more commonly localized; rarely generalized.
- When inflammation and trauma from occlusion are combined in causing the destruction and irregular shape of the bone, the bone may appear with "angular defects" or with "vertical bone loss."

III. Crestal Lamina Dura

A. Normal

- White, radiopaque; continuous with and connects the lamina dura about the roots of two adjacent teeth; covers the interdental bone of the two molars in Figure 20-20.

B. Evidence of Disease

- The crestal lamina dura is indistinct, irregular, radiolucent, and fuzzy (Figures 20-21 and 20-22).

IV. Furcation Involvement

A. Normal

- Bone fills the area between the roots (Figure 20-20).

B. Evidence of Disease

- Radiolucent area in the furcation (Figure 20-19).
- Early furcation involvement shown in the mandibular second molar in Figure 20-22 may appear as a small radiolucent black area or as a slight thickening of the periodontal ligament space. It can be confirmed by clinical assessment with a Nabers probe.
- Furcation involvement of maxillary molars may become more advanced before radiographic evidence is seen. Superimposition of the palatal root may mask a small area of involvement.
- When the height of the interdental bone in the radiograph is at the level of the furcation, it can be used as an approximate guide to possible furcation involvement.[25]
- Maxillary first premolar furcation involvement cannot be seen in a radiograph with correct vertical and horizontal angulation because the roots are superimposed.

V. Periodontal Ligament Space

A. Normal

- The periodontal ligament is connective tissue and, hence, appears as a fine black radiolucent line next to the root surface.
- On its outer side is the lamina dura—the bone that lines the tooth socket and appears radiopaque.

B. Evidence of Disease

- Widening or thickening.
- Angular thickening or triangulation: Widened only near the coronal third, near the crest of the interdental bone.

- Periodontal ligament space widening may occur along an entire side of a root to the apex or around the root (Figure 20-19): When viewed at different angulations (in the various radiographs of a complete survey), the ligament space may reveal varying thicknesses, thus showing the disease involvement is not consistent around the entire root or that other structures are superimposed.

Other Radiographic Findings

- Any other radiographic findings related directly or indirectly to periodontal involvement and contributing factors are noted in the record.
- Certain findings have a direct relation to dental hygiene care and instruction, particularly local factors that contribute to food impaction or biofilm retention.

I. Calculus

- Gross deposits, primarily those on proximal surfaces, may be seen in radiographs (Figure 20-21).
- Radiographs have very limited value for calculus detection, so clinical assessment with an explorer is needed to determine the location and extent of the deposit.
- Radiographs should *not* be taken after nonsurgical periodontal therapy to evaluate calculus removal to minimize patient exposure to radiation.

II. Overhanging Restorations

- Some proximal overhanging margins may be seen on radiographs.
- The use of an explorer is necessary to detect irregular margins and to examine all proximal margins that do not reveal irregularities in the radiographs.

III. Dental Caries

- See Chapter 16.

Documentation

Documentation in the permanent record for a patient with a gingival or periodontal condition needs to include a minimum of the following:

- Findings by clinical observation and comprehensive periodontal examination leading to the dental hygiene diagnosis (periodontal classification).
- Outcomes of risk assessment, particularly the modifiable risk factors, are important to document so they can be considered in planning treatment.
- A sample progress note documenting a dental hygiene appointment can be found in **Box 20-1**.

Box 20-1 Example Documentation: Periodontal Examination Findings

- **S**—Mr. Jones presents to the dental office for his first visit. He just moved to Boston a few months ago and needs a routine examination and "cleaning." He does not report any concerns about his mouth at this time. Mr. Jones reports he just had a physical examination with his new physician and was diagnosed with prediabetes and was put on metformin. His A1c was 6.5. He lives alone and eats out once or twice a day. He reports brushing daily, but he says he will not floss so don't lecture him about it.
- **O**—His vital signs are normal, with a BP of 120/79. Extraoral examination/intraoral examination were normal. No full mouth series of radiographs in 5 years and his risk assessment indicated he was at high caries and periodontal risk. Comprehensive examination findings included a broken filling DO-#30 and a broken mesiolingual (ML) cusp on #31. He has generalized 5- to 6-mm probing depths (4-5 mm CAL) with BOP in all posterior areas with marginal inflammation. Grade I furcations noted ML and DL of #2, 3, 14, and 15. No mobility. Adequate attached gingiva in all areas.
- **A**—The periodontal diagnosis is Stage 2 Grade B periodontitis. High caries and periodontal risk. Slight-to-moderate localized subgingival calculus. Plaque score 60%.
- **P**—Patient education for oral self-care included refinement of modified Bass brushing technique in posterior areas along with introduction of floss picks for interdental care. Patient demonstrated both home care aids and liked the floss picks. Education about periodontal disease and association with diabetes was discussed along with his diagnosis and need for nonsurgical periodontal therapy (NSPT) by quadrant with local anesthesia in posterior areas. The patient was shocked by the findings because he has been having "cleanings" every 6 months at his previous dental office, but he indicated he had never had all the "measuring" done before. He was very thankful to learn about the association between diabetes and periodontal disease. He seemed highly motivated to improve his oral health. The dentist also discussed the need for a crown on #31 and replacement of the filling on #30 once the NSPT was complete. Next visit: NSPT maxillary right quadrant with local anesthesia and review of oral self-care.

Signed: ______________________, RDH
Date: ________________

Factors to Teach the Patient

- The need for a comprehensive examination to ensure treatment is planned to meet all of the patient's needs.
- The value of the various components of the comprehensive examination in assessing the patient's oral health. Examples are the complete radiographic survey and comprehensive periodontal examination.
- Why bleeding can occur when probing. More bleeding is a sign of periodontal disease.
- Relation of probing depth measurements to normal sulci.
- Significance of the periodontal findings such as mobility, furcation involvement, or inadequate attached gingiva.

References

1. Centers for Disease Control and Prevention. Guidance for Dental Settings. Updated September 10, 2021. https://www.cdc.gov/coronavirus/2019-ncov/hcp/dental-settings.html. Accessed December 29, 2021.
2. Ismail AI, Pitts NB, Tellez M, et al. The International Caries Classification and Management System (ICCMSTM): An example of a caries management pathway. *BMC Oral Health.* 2015;15(Suppl 1):S9.
3. Young DA, Nový BB, Zeller GG, et al. The American Dental Association Caries Classification System for clinical practice: a report of the American Dental Association Council on Scientific Affairs. *J Am Dent Assoc.* 2015;146(2):79-86.
4. Mattos-Silveira J, Oliveira MM, Matos R, Moura-Netto C, Mendes FM, Braga MM. Do the ball-ended probe cause less damage than sharp explorers?-An ultrastructural analysis. *BMC Oral Health.* 2016;16:39.
5. El-Kishawi M, Khalaf K, Winning T. How to improve fine motor skill learning in dentistry. *Int J Dent.* 2021;2021:6674213.
6. Elashiry M, Meghil MM, Arce RM, Cutler CW. From manual periodontal probing to digital 3-D imaging to endoscopic capillaroscopy: recent advances in periodontal disease diagnosis. *J Periodontal Res.* 2019;54(1):1-9.
7. Chapple ILC, Mealey BL, Van Dyke TE, et al. Periodontal health and gingival diseases and conditions on an intact and a reduced periodontium: consensus report of workgroup 1 of the 2017 World Workshop on the Classification of Periodontal and Peri-Implant Diseases and Conditions. *J Clin Periodontol.* 2018;45(Suppl 20):S68-S77.
8. Holtfreter B, Alte D, Schwahn C, Desvarieux M, Kocher T. Effects of different manual periodontal probes on periodontal measurements. *J Clin Periodontol.* 2012;39(11):1032-1041.
9. Garnick JJ, Silverstein L. Periodontal probing: probe tip diameter. *J Periodontol.* 2000;71(1):96–103.
10. American Academy of Periodontology. Parameter on comprehensive periodontal examination. *J Periodontol.* 2000;71(5)(suppl):847–848.
11. American Academy of Periodontology. American Academy of Periodontology statement on risk assessment. *J Periodontol.* 2008;79(2):202.
12. Corbet EF, Ho DK, Lai SM. Radiographs in periodontal disease diagnosis and management. *Aust Dent J.* 2009;(54)(suppl 1):S27-S43.
13. Tonetti MS, Greenwell H, Kornman KS. Staging and grading of periodontitis: framework and proposal of a new classification and case definition. *J Periodontol.* 2018;89(Suppl 1):S159-S172.
14. Larsen C, Barendregt DS, Slot DE, Van der Velden U, Van der Weijden F. Probing pressure, a highly undervalued unit of measure in periodontal probing: a systematic review on its effect on probing pocket depth. *J Clin Periodontol.* 2009;36(4):315-322.
15. Andrade R, Espinoza M, Gómez EM, Espinoza JR, Cruz E. Intra- and inter-examiner reproducibility of manual probing depth. *Braz Oral Res.* 2012;26(1):57-63.
16. Papapanou PN, Sanz M, Buduneli N, et al. Periodontitis: consensus report of workgroup 2 of the 2017 World Workshop on the Classification of Periodontal and Peri-Implant Diseases and Conditions. *J Periodontol.* 2018;89(Suppl 1) 1:S173-S182.
17. Guglielmoni P, Promsudthi A, Tatakis DN, Trombelli L. Intra- and inter-examiner reproducibility in keratinized tissue width assessment with 3 methods for mucogingival junction determination. *J Periodontol.* 2001;72(2):134-139.
18. Cortellini P, Bissada NF. Mucogingival conditions in the natural dentition: narrative review, case definitions, and diagnostic considerations. *J Clin Periodontol.* 2018;45(Suppl 20):S190-S198.
19. American Academy of Periodontology. Parameters of mucogingival conditions. *J Periodontol.* 2000;71(suppl):861-862.
20. Laster L, Laudenbach KW, Stoller NH. An evaluation of clinical tooth mobility measurements. *J Periodontol.* 1975; 46(10):603–607.
21. Davies SJ, Gray RJ, Linden GJ, James.JA Occlusal considerations in periodontics. *Br Dent J.* 2001;191(11):597–604.
22. Karthikeyan BV, Sujatha V, Prabhuji ML. Furcation measurements: realities and limitations. *J Int Acad Periodontol.* 2015;17(4):103–115.
23. Eickholz P, Kim TS. Reproducibility and validity of the assessment of clinical furcation parameters as related to different probes. *J Periodontol.* 1998;69(3):328-336.
24. Al-Shammari KF, Kazor CE, Wang HL. Molar root anatomy and management of furcation defects. *J Clin Periodontol.* 2001;28(8):730-740.
25. Grover V, Malhotra R, Kapoor A, et al. Correlation of the interdental and the interradicular bone loss: a radiovisuographic analysis. *J Indian Soc Periodontol.* 2014;18(4):482-487.

CHAPTER 21

Indices and Scoring Methods

Lisa F. Mallonee, RDH, RD, LD, MPH
Charlotte J. Wyche, RDH, MS

CHAPTER OUTLINE

LEARNING OBJECTIVES

After studying this chapter, the student will be able to:

1. Identify and define key terms and concepts related to dental indices and scoring methods.
2. Identify the purpose, criteria for measurement, scoring methods, range of scores, and reference or interpretation scales for a variety of dental indices.
3. Select and calculate dental indices for a use in a specific patient or community situation.

This chapter provides an introduction to scoring methods used by clinicians, researchers, and community practitioners to evaluate **indicators** of oral health **status**. It is not possible to explain all of the many dental indices that have been used in a variety of settings, but the most notable, current, and widely used indices and scoring methods are described in this chapter.

Types of Scoring Methods

Indices and scoring methods are used in clinical practice and by community programs to determine and record the oral health status of individuals and groups.

I. Individual Assessment Score

A. Purpose

In clinical practice, an **index**, or a scoring system, for an individual patient can be used to measure the amount or condition of oral disease or related condition in individuals or a population for purposes of evaluation, education or motivation.[1]

- An index is based on a graduated scale with defined upper and lower limits.
- Used for data collection and comparisons of individuals or population groups using established criteria.
- Frequently used in clinical trials.

B. Uses

- To provide individual assessment to help a patient recognize an oral problem.
- To reveal the degree of effectiveness of oral hygiene practices.
- To motivate the patient during preventive and professional care for the elimination and control of oral disease.
- To evaluate the success of individual oral self-care, professional treatment, and status of oral disease over a period of time by comparing index scores.

II. Clinical Trial

A. Purpose

A clinical trial is planned to determine the effect of an agent or a procedure on the prevention, progression, or control of a disease.

- The trial is conducted by comparing an experimental group with a control group that is similar to the experimental group in every way, except for the variable being studied.
- Examiners who collect dental index data for research are **calibrated** or trained to measure the index in exactly the same way each time.
- Examples of indices used for clinical trials are the biofilm index (BI)[2,3] and the patient hygiene performance (PHP).[4]

B. Uses

- To determine baseline **data** before experimental factors are introduced.
- To measure the effectiveness of specific agents for the prevention, control, or treatment of oral conditions.
- To measure the effectiveness of mechanical devices for personal care, such as toothbrushes, interdental cleaning devices, or irrigators.

III. Epidemiologic Survey

A. Purpose

The word **epidemiology** denotes the study of disease characteristics of populations rather than individuals. Epidemiologic surveys provide information on the trends and patterns of oral health and disease in populations.

B. Uses

- To determine the **prevalence** and **incidence** of a particular condition occurring within a given population.
- To provide baseline data on indicators that show existing dental health status in populations.

- The *Surgeon General's Report(s) on Oral Health in America* used epidemiologic data to identify oral health disparities in certain populations.[5,6]
- To provide data to support recommendations for public health interventions to improve the health status of populations, such as those provided in the U.S. *Healthy People 2030* document.[7]

IV. Community Surveillance

A. Purpose

Community oral health assessment is a multifaceted process of identifying factors that affect the oral health status of a selected population. Community **surveillance** of oral health indicators and **determinants** can be accomplished at many levels.

- Government agencies, local community-based service-providing agencies, and professional associations are examples of groups that collect data to determine oral health status by conducting oral health **screenings**.
- Information from community-wide oral screenings can be used when planning local community-based oral health services or education.
- An example of a system designed to be used by a community-based group is the Association of State and Territorial Dental Directors' (ASTDD) Basic Screening Survey.[8]

B. Uses

- To assess the needs of a community.
- To help plan community-based health promotion/disease prevention programs.
- To compare the effects or evaluate the results of community-based programs.

Indices

An index is a way of expressing clinical observations by using numbers. The use of numbers can provide standardized information to make observations of a health condition consistent and less subjective than a word description of that condition.

I. Descriptive Categories of Indices

A. General Categories

- Simple index: Measures the presence or absence of a condition. An example is the biofilm index that measures the presence of dental biofilm without evaluating its effect on the gingiva.
- Cumulative index: Measures all the evidence of a condition, past and present. An example is the DMFT index for dental caries.

B. Types of Simple and Cumulative Indices

- Irreversible index: Measures conditions that will not change. An example is an index that measures dental caries experience.
- Reversible index: Measures conditions that can be changed. Examples are indices that measure dental biofilm.

II. Selection Criteria

A useful and effective index:

- Is simple to use and calculate.
- Requires minimal equipment, expense, and time to complete.
- Is acceptable to the individuals being measured; does not cause discomfort.
- Has clear-cut criteria that are readily understandable.
- Is objective—free from subjective interpretation.
- Has **validity**—measures what it is intended to measure
- Has **reliability**—is reproducible by the same examiner or different examiners.
- Is quantifiable—statistics can be applied to data collected.

Oral Hygiene Status (Biofilm, Debris, and Calculus)

Indices that measure oral hygiene status can be used in a clinical setting to educate and motivate an individual patient. When data are collected in a community setting, such as a nursing home, the findings can help determine how daily oral care is being provided and monitor the results of oral hygiene education programs.

I. Biofilm Index (BI)

This index was historically known as plaque index (PI).[2,3]

A. Purpose

- To assess the thickness of biofilm at the gingival area.

B. Selection of Teeth

- The entire dentition or selected teeth can be evaluated.
- *Areas examined:* Examine four gingival areas (distal, facial, mesial, and lingual) systematically for each tooth.
- *Modified procedures:* Examine only the facial, mesial, and lingual areas. Assign double score to the mesial reading and divide the total by 4.

C. Procedure

- Dry the teeth and examine visually using adequate light, mouth mirror, and probe or explorer.
- Evaluate dental biofilm on the cervical third; pay no attention to biofilm that has extended to the middle or incisal thirds of the tooth.
- Use probe to test the surface when no biofilm is visible. Pass the probe or explorer across the tooth surface in the cervical third and near the entrance to the sulcus. When no biofilm adheres to the probe tip, the area is scored 0. When biofilm adheres, a score of 1 is assigned.
- Use a disclosing agent, if necessary, to assist evaluation for the 0–1 scores. When the Pl I is used in conjunction with the gingival index (GI), the GI is completed first because the disclosing agent masks the gingival characteristics.
- Include biofilm on the surface of calculus and on dental restorations in the cervical third in the evaluation.
- Criteria

Biofilm Index

Score	Criteria
0	No biofilm.
1	A film of biofilm adhering to the free gingival margin and adjacent area of the tooth. The biofilm may be recognized only after application of disclosing agent or by running the explorer across the tooth surface.
2	Moderate accumulation of soft deposits within the gingival pocket that can be seen with the naked eye or on the tooth and gingival margin.
3	Abundance of soft matter within the gingival pocket and/or on the tooth and gingival margin.

D. Scoring

- BI for area
  - Each area of a tooth (distal, facial, mesial, lingual, or palatal) is assigned a score from 0 to 3.
- BI for a tooth
  - Scores for each area are totaled and divided by 4.
- BI for groups of teeth
  - Scores for individual teeth may be grouped and totaled and divided by the number of teeth. For instance, a BI may be determined for specific teeth or groups of teeth. The right side of the dentition may be compared with the left.
- BI for the individual
  - Add the scores for each tooth and divide by the number of teeth examined. The BI score ranges from 0 to 3.
- Suggested range of scores for patient reference

Rating	Scores
Excellent	0
Good	0.1–0.9
Fair	1.0–1.9
Poor	2.0–3.0

- BI for a group
  - Add the scores for each member of a group and divide by the number of individuals.

II. Biofilm Control Record (BCR)

This index was previously known as the plaque control record.[9]

A. Purpose

- To record the presence of dental biofilm on individual tooth surfaces to permit the patient to visualize progress while learning biofilm control.

B. Selection of Teeth and Surfaces

- All teeth are included. Missing teeth are identified on the record form by a single, thick horizontal line.
- Four surfaces are recorded: Facial, lingual, mesial, and distal.
- Six areas may be recorded. The mesial and distal segments of the diagram may be divided to

provide space to record proximal surfaces from the facial separately from the lingual or palatal surfaces (**Figure 21-1**).[10]

C. Procedure

- Apply disclosing agent or give a chewable tablet. Instruct patient to swish and rub the solution over the tooth surfaces with the tongue before rinsing.
- Examine each tooth surface for dental biofilm at the gingival margin. No attempt is made to differentiate the quantity of biofilm.
- Record by making a dash or color in the appropriate spaces on the diagram (Figure 21-1) to indicate biofilm on facial, lingual, palatal, mesial, and/or distal surfaces.

D. Scoring

- Total the number of teeth present and multiply by 4 to obtain the number of available surfaces. Count the number of surfaces with biofilm.
- Multiply the number of biofilm-stained surfaces by 100 and divide by the total number of available surfaces to derive the percentage of surfaces with biofilm.
- Compare scores over subsequent appointments as the patient learns and practices biofilm control. Ten percent or less biofilm-stained surfaces can be considered a good goal, but if the biofilm is regularly left in the same areas, special instruction is indicated.
- Calculation: Example for biofilm control record
  - Individual findings: 26 teeth scored; 8 surfaces with biofilm.
  - Multiply the number of teeth by 4: $26 \times 4 = 104$ surfaces.
  - Percentage with biofilm =

$$\frac{\textit{Number of surfaces with biofilm} \times 100}{\textit{Number of available tooth surfaces}} = \frac{8 \times 100}{104}$$

$$= \frac{800}{104}$$

$$= 7.7\%$$

- Interpretation
  - Although 0% is ideal, less than 10% biofilm-stained surfaces has been suggested as a guideline in periodontal therapy. After initial therapy and when the patient has reached a 10% level of biofilm control or better, necessary additional periodontal and restorative procedures may be initiated.[9] In comparison, a similar evaluation using a biofilm-free score would mean that a goal of 90% or better biofilm-free surfaces would have to be reached before the surgical phase of treatment could be undertaken.

III. Biofilm-Free Score (BFS)

This index was historically called the plaque-free score.[11]

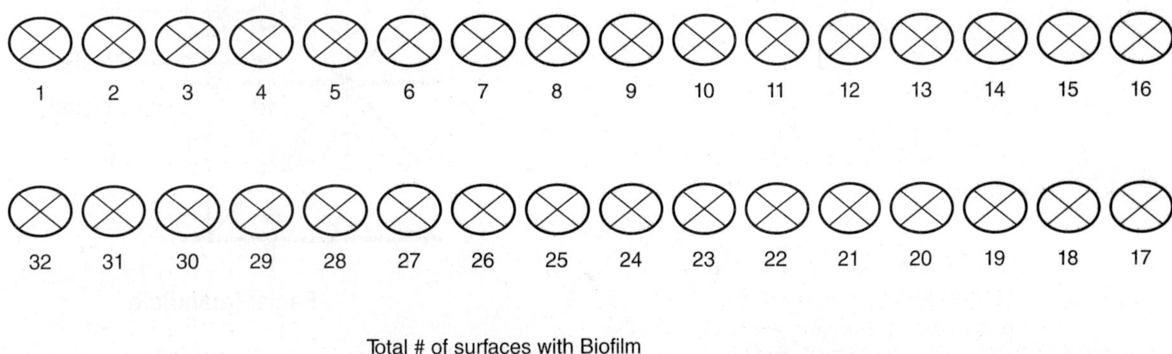

Figure 21-1 Biofilm Control Record. Diagrammatic representation of the teeth includes spaces to record biofilm on six areas of each tooth. The facial surfaces are on the outer portion and the lingual and palatal surfaces are on the inner portion of the arches. Teeth are numbered by the American Dental Association system on the inside and by the Fédération Dentaire Internationale system on the outside.

A. Purpose

- To determine the location, number, and percentage of biofilm-free surfaces for individual motivation and instruction. Interdental bleeding can also be documented.

B. Selection of Teeth and Surfaces

- All erupted teeth are included. Missing teeth are identified on the record form by a single, thick horizontal line through the box in the chart form.
- Four surfaces are recorded for each tooth: Facial, lingual or palatal, mesial, and distal.

C. Procedure

- Biofilm-free score
  - Apply disclosing agent or give chewable tablet. Instruct patient to swish and rub the solution over the tooth surfaces with the tongue before rinsing.
  - Examine each tooth surface for evidence of biofilm using adequate light and a mouth mirror.
  - The patient needs a hand mirror to see the location of the biofilm missed during personal hygiene procedures.
  - Use an appropriate tooth chart form or a diagrammatic form, such as that shown in **Figure 21-2**. Red ink for recording the biofilm is suggested when a red disclosing agent is used to help the patient associate the location of the biofilm in the mouth with the recording.
- Papillary bleeding on probing
  - The small circles between the diagrammatic tooth blocks in Figure 21-2 are used to record proximal bleeding on probing.
  - Improvement in the gingival tissue health will be demonstrated over a period of time as fewer bleeding areas are noted.

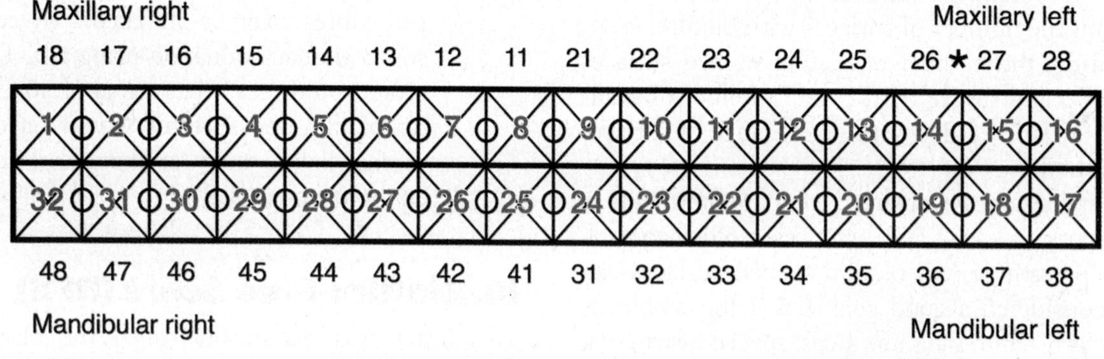

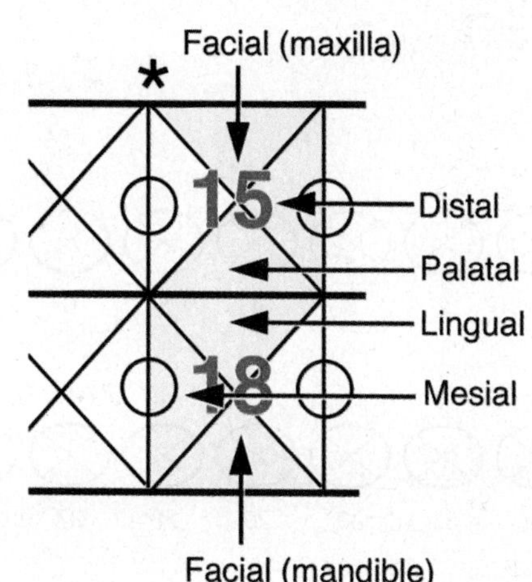

Figure 21-2 Biofilm-Free Score. **A:** Diagrammatic representation of the teeth used to record biofilm and papillary bleeding. **B:** Enlargement of one section of the diagram shows tooth surfaces. Teeth are numbered by the American Dental Association system inside each block and by the Fédération Dentaire Internationale system outside each block.

Reproduced from Grant DA, Stern IB, Listgarten MA. *Periodontics*. 6th ed. St. Louis, MO: Mosby; 1988:613.

D. Scoring: Biofilm-Free Score

- Total the number of teeth present.
- Total the number of surfaces with biofilm that appear in red on the tooth diagram.
- To calculate the biofilm-free score:
  - Multiply the number of teeth by 4 to determine the number of available surfaces.
  - Subtract the number of surfaces with biofilm from the total available surfaces to find the number of biofilm-free surfaces.
  - Biofilm-free score

$$\frac{\textit{Number of Biofilm-free surface} \times 100}{\textit{Number of available surfaces}}$$

$$= \textit{Percentage of biofilm-free surfaces}$$

- Evaluate biofilm-free score: Ideally, 100% is the goal. When a patient maintains a percentage under 85%, check individual surfaces to determine whether biofilm is usually left in the same areas. To prevent the development of specific areas of periodontal infection, remedial instruction in the areas usually missed is indicated.
- Calculation: Example for biofilm-free score
  - Individual findings: 24 teeth scored and 37 surfaces with biofilm.
  - Multiply the number of teeth by 4: $24 \times 4 = 96$ available surfaces.
  - Subtract the number of surfaces with biofilm from total available surfaces: $96 - 37 = 59$ biofilm-free surfaces.
  - Percentage of biofilm-free surfaces

$$\frac{59 \times 100}{96} = 61.5\%$$

- Interpretation
  - On the basis of the ideal 100%, 61.5% is poor. More personal daily oral care instruction is indicated.

E. Scoring: Papillary Bleeding on Probing

- Total the number of small circles marked for bleeding. A patient with 32 teeth has 30 interdental areas. The mesial or distal surface of a tooth adjacent to an edentulous area is probed and counted.
- Evaluate total interdental bleeding. In health, bleeding on probing does not occur.

IV. Patient Hygiene Performance (PHP)[4]

A. Purpose

- To assess the extent of biofilm and debris over a tooth surface. Debris is defined for the PHP as a soft foreign material consisting of dental biofilm, materia alba, and food debris loosely attached to tooth surfaces.

B. Selection of Teeth and Surfaces

- Teeth examined:

Maxillary	Mandibular
No. 3 (16)[a]	No. 19 (36)
Right first molar	Left first molar
No. 8 (11)	No. 24 (31)
Right central incisor	Left central incisor
No. 14 (26)	No. 30 (46)
Left first molar	Right first molar

[a]Fédération Dentaire Internationale system tooth numbers are in parentheses.

- Substitutions
  - When a first molar is missing, is less than three-fourths erupted, has a full crown, or is broken down, the second molar is used.
  - The third molar is used when the second is missing.
  - The adjacent central incisor is used for a missing incisor.
- Surfaces
  - The facial surfaces of incisors and maxillary molars and the lingual surfaces of mandibular molars are examined.

C. Procedure

- Apply disclosing agent. Instruct the patient to swish for 30 seconds and expectorate, but not rinse.
- Examination is made using a mouth mirror.

- Each tooth surface to be evaluated is subdivided (mentally) into five sections (**Figure 21-3A**) as follows:
  - Vertically: Three divisions—mesial, middle, and distal.
  - Horizontally: The middle third is subdivided into gingival, middle, and occlusal or incisal thirds.
- Each of the five subdivisions is scored for the presence of stained debris as follows:

Patient Hygiene Performance

Score	Criteria
0	No debris (or questionable).
1	Debris definitely present.
M	When all three molars or both incisors are missing.
S	When a substitute tooth is used.

D. Scoring

- Debris score for individual tooth
  - Add the scores for each of the five subdivisions. The scores range from 0 to 5. Examples are shown in **Figure 21-3B** and **Figure 21-3C**.
- PHP for the individual
  - Total the scores for the individual teeth and divide by the number of teeth examined. The PHP ranges from 0 to 5.
- Suggested range of scores for evaluation

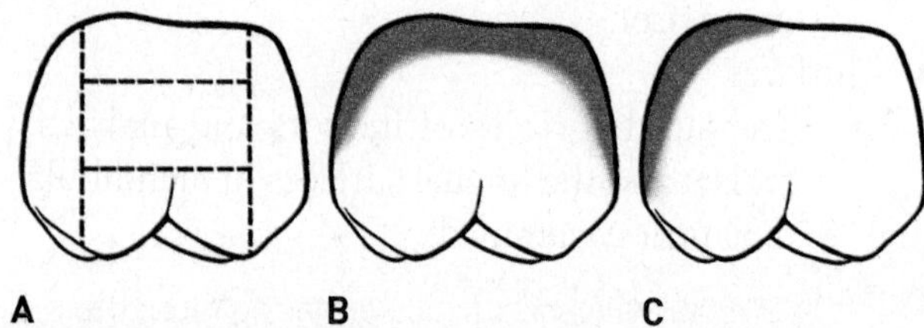

Figure 21-3 Patient Hygiene Performance. **A:** Oral debris is assessed by dividing a tooth into five subdivisions, each of which is scored 1 when debris is shown to be present after use of a disclosing agent. **B:** Example of debris score of 3. Shaded portion represents debris stained by disclosing agent. **C:** Example of debris score of 1.

Data from Podshadley AG, Haley JV. A method for evaluating oral hygiene performance. *Public Health Rep.* 1968;83(3):259-264.

Rating	Scores
Excellent	0 (no debris)
Good	0.1–1.7
Fair	1.8–3.4
Poor	3.5–5.0

- Calculation: Example for an individual

Tooth	Debris Score
No. 3 (16)	5
No. 8 (11)	3
No. 14 (26)	4
No. 19 (36)	5
No. 24 (31)	2
No. 30 (46)	3
Total	22

$$\frac{\textit{Total debris score}}{\textit{Number of teeth scored}} = \frac{22}{6} = 3.67$$

- Interpretation
  - According to the suggested range of scores, this patient with a PHP of 3.67 would be classified as exhibiting poor hygiene performance.
- PHP for a group
  - To obtain the average PHP score for a group or population, total the individual scores and divide by the number of people examined.

V. Simplified Oral Hygiene Index (OHI-S)[12,13]

A. Purpose

- To assess oral cleanliness by estimating the tooth surfaces covered with debris and/or calculus.

B. Components

- The simplified oral hygiene index (OHI-S) has two components: the simplified debris index (DI-S) and the simplified calculus index (CI-S). The two scores may be used separately or may be combined for the OHI-S.

C. Selection of Teeth and Surfaces

- Identify the six specific teeth (see **Figure 21-4**)
  - Posterior: The facial surfaces of the maxillary molars and the lingual surfaces of the

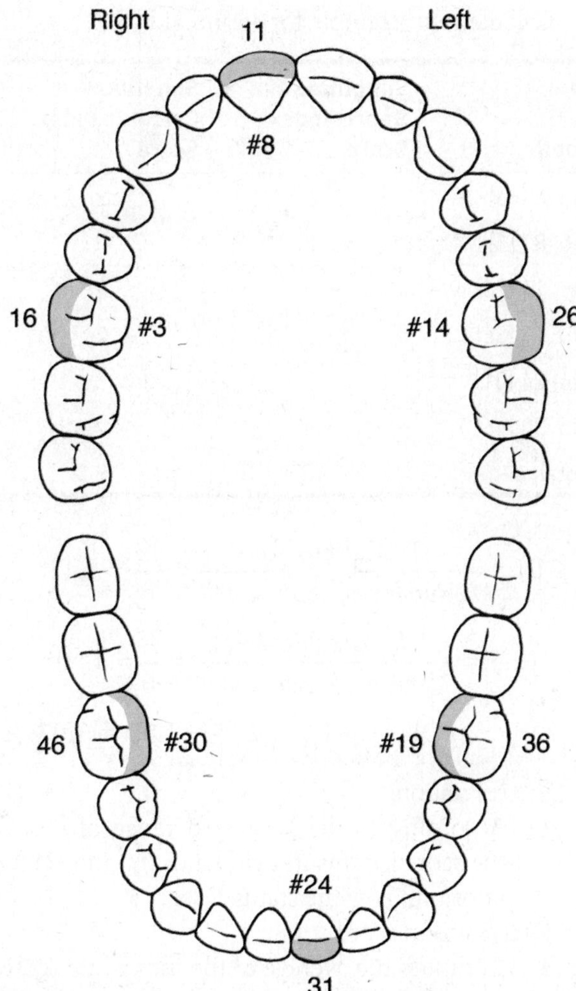

Figure 21-4 Simplified Oral Hygiene Index. Six tooth surfaces are scored as follows: facial surfaces of maxillary molars and of the maxillary right and mandibular left central incisors, and the lingual surfaces of mandibular molars. Teeth are numbered by the American Dental Association system on the lingual surface and by the Fédération Dentaire Internationale system on the facial surface.

mandibular molars are scored. Although usually the first molars are examined, the first fully erupted molar distal to each second premolar is used if the first molar is missing.

- Anterior: The facial surfaces of the maxillary right and the mandibular left central incisors are scored. When either is missing, the adjacent central incisor is scored.

- Extent
  - Either the facial or lingual surfaces of the selected teeth are scored, including the proximal surfaces to the contact areas.

D. Procedure

- Qualification: At least two of the six possible surfaces are examined to calculate an individual score.
- Record six debris scores
  - Definition of oral debris: Oral debris is a soft foreign matter, such as dental biofilm, material alba, and food debris on the surfaces of the teeth.
- Examination: Move the side of the tip of a probe or an explorer across the tooth surface to estimate the surface area covered by debris.
- Criteria (see **Figure 21-5** and the Debris Index table next).

Simplified Debris Index (DI-S)

Score	Criteria
0	No debris or stain present.
1	Soft debris covering not more than one-third of the tooth surface being examined, or presence of extrinsic stains without debris, regardless of surface area covered.
2	Soft debris covering more than one-third but not more than two-thirds of the exposed tooth surface.
3	Soft debris covering more than two-thirds of the exposed tooth surface.

- Record six calculus scores
- Examination: Use an explorer to estimate surface area covered by supragingival calculus deposits. Identify subgingival deposits by exploring and/or probing. Record only definite deposits of hard calculus.
  - Criteria: Location and tooth surface areas scored are illustrated in **Figure 21-6**.

Simplified Calculus Index (CI-S)

Score	Criteria
0	No calculus present.
1	Supragingival calculus covering not more than one-third of the exposed tooth surface being examined.
2	Supragingival calculus covering more than one-third but not more than two-thirds of the exposed tooth surface, or the presence of individual flecks of subgingival calculus around the cervical portion of the tooth.
3	Supragingival calculus covering more than two-thirds of the exposed tooth surface or a continuous heavy band of subgingival calculus around the cervical portion of the tooth.

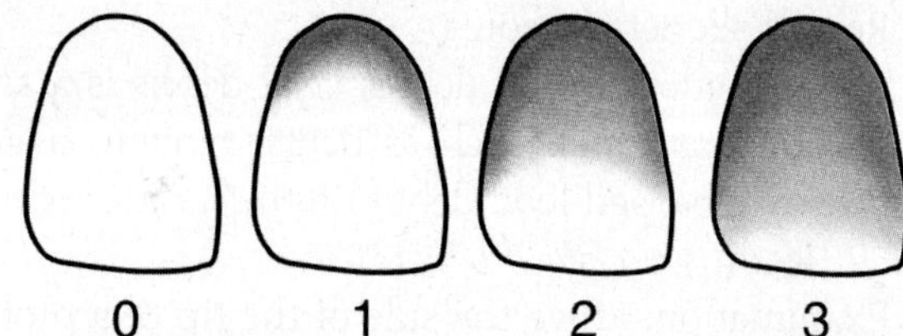

Figure 21-5 Simplified Oral Hygiene Index. For the debris index, six teeth (Figure 21-3) are scored. Scoring of 0–3 is based on tooth surfaces covered by debris as shown.

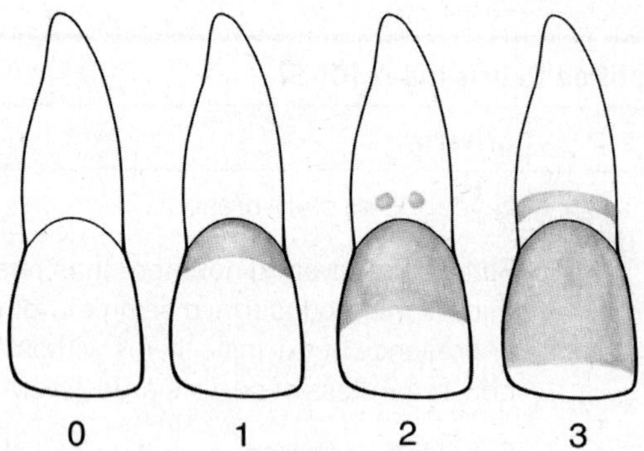

Figure 21-6 Simplified Oral Hygiene Index. For the calculus index, six teeth (Figure 21-3) are scored. Scoring of 0–3 is based on location and tooth surface area with calculus as shown. Note slight subgingival calculus recorded as 2 and more extensive subgingival calculus as 3.

E. Scoring

- *OHI-S individual score.*
- Determine separate DI-S and CI-S.
  - Divide each total score by the number of teeth scored (6).
  - DI-S and CI-S values range from 0 to 3.
- Calculate the OHI-S.
  - Combine the DI-S and CI-S.
  - OHI-S value ranges from 0 to 6.
- Suggested range of scores for evaluation[13]

Rating	Scores
Individual simplified debris index (DI-S) and the simplified calculus index (CI-S)	
Excellent	0
Good	0.1–0.6
Fair	0.7–1.8
Poor	1.9–3.0
OHI-S (combined DI-S and CI-S)	
Excellent	0
Good	0.1–1.2
Fair	1.3–3.0
Poor	3.1–6.0

- Calculation: Example for an individual

Tooth	Simplified Debris Index Score	Simplified Calculus Index Score
No. 3 (16)	2	2
No. 8 (11)	1	0
No. 14 (26)	3	2
No. 19 (36)	3	2
No. 24 (31)	2	1
No. 30 (46)	2	2
Total	13	9

$$DI\text{-}S = \frac{\textit{Total debris score}}{\textit{Number of teeth scored}} = \frac{13}{6} = 2.17$$

$$CI\text{-}S = \frac{\textit{Total calculus scores}}{\textit{Number of teeth scored}} = \frac{9}{6} = 1.50$$

$$\text{OHI-S} = \text{DI-S} + \text{CI-S} = 2.17 + 1.50 = 3.67$$

- Interpretation
  - According to the suggested range of scores, the score for this individual (3.67) indicates a poor oral hygiene status.
- OHI-S group score
  - Compute the average of the individual scores by totaling the scores and dividing by the number of individuals.

Gingival and Periodontal Health

Measurements for gingival and periodontal indices have varied over the years. Two indices, not completely described here, are of historic interest.

- The papillary-marginal-attached index, attributed to Schour and Massler[14] and later revised by Massler,[15] was used to assess the extent of gingival changes in large groups for epidemiologic studies.
- The periodontal index of Russell,[16] another acclaimed contribution to the study of disease incidence, was a complex index that accounted for both gingival and periodontal changes. Its aim was to survey large populations.
- For patient instruction and motivation, several bleeding indices and scoring methods have been developed.
- Bleeding on gentle probing or flossing is an early sign of gingival inflammation and precedes color changes and enlargement of gingival tissues.[17,18]

- Bleeding on probing is an indicator of the progression of periodontal disease, so testing for bleeding has become a significant procedure for assessment prior to treatment planning, after therapy to show the effects of treatment, and at maintenance appointments to determine continued control of gingival inflammation.

I. Periodontal Screening and Recording (PSR)[19,20,21]

A. Purpose

To assess the state of periodontal health of an individual patient.

- A modified form of the original community periodontal index of treatment needs (CPITN) index.[22]
- Designed to indicate periodontal status in a rapid and effective manner and motivate the patient to seek necessary complete periodontal assessment and treatment.
- Used as a screening procedure to determine the need for comprehensive periodontal evaluation.

B. Selection of Teeth

- The dentition is divided into sextants. Each tooth is examined. Posterior sextants begin distal to the canines.

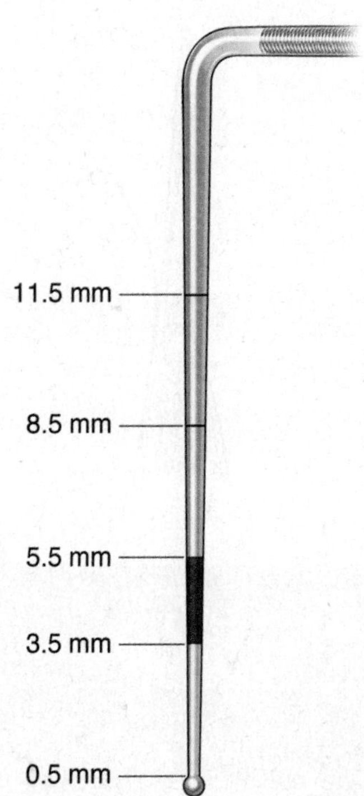

Figure 21-7 World Health Organization (WHO) Periodontal Probe. The specially designed WHO probe measures 3.5-, 5.5-, 8.5-, and 11.5-mm intervals. This probe is used to make determinations for the periodontal screening and recording and the community periodontal index.

Data from Fédération Dentaire Internationale. A simplified periodontal examination for dental practices. Based on the Community Periodontal Index of Treatment Needs—CPITN. *Aust Dent J.* 1985;30(5):368-370.

C. Procedure

- Instrument: Probe originally designed for World Health Organization (WHO) surveys (**Figure 21-7**), with markings at intervals from tip: 3.5, 5.5, 8.5, and 11.5 mm.
- Color coded between 3.5 and 5.5 mm.
- Working tip: A ball 0.5 mm in diameter. The functions of the ball are to aid in the detection of calculus, rough overhanging margins of restorations, and other tooth surface irregularities, and also to facilitate assessment at the probing depth and reduce risk of overmeasurement.
- Probe application
  - Insert probe gently into a sulcus until resistance is felt.
  - Apply a circumferential walking step to probe systematically about each tooth through each sextant.
  - Observe color-coded area of the probe for prompt identification of probing depths.
  - Each sextant receives one code number corresponding to the deepest position of the color-coded portion of the probe.
- Criteria
  - Five codes and an asterisk are used. **Figure 21-8** shows the clinical findings, code significance, and patient management guidelines.
  - Each code may include conditions identified with the preceding codes; for example, Code 3 with probing depth from 3.5 to 5.5 mm may also include calculus, an overhanging restoration, and bleeding on probing.
  - One need not probe the remaining teeth in a sextant when a Code 4 is found. For Codes 0, 1, 2, and 3, the sextant is completely probed.
- Recording
  - Use a simple six-box form to provide a space for each sextant. The form can be made into peel-off stickers or a rubber stamp to facilitate recording in the patient's permanent record.
  - One score is marked for each sextant; the highest code observed is recorded. When indicated, an asterisk is added to the score in the individual space with the sextant code number.

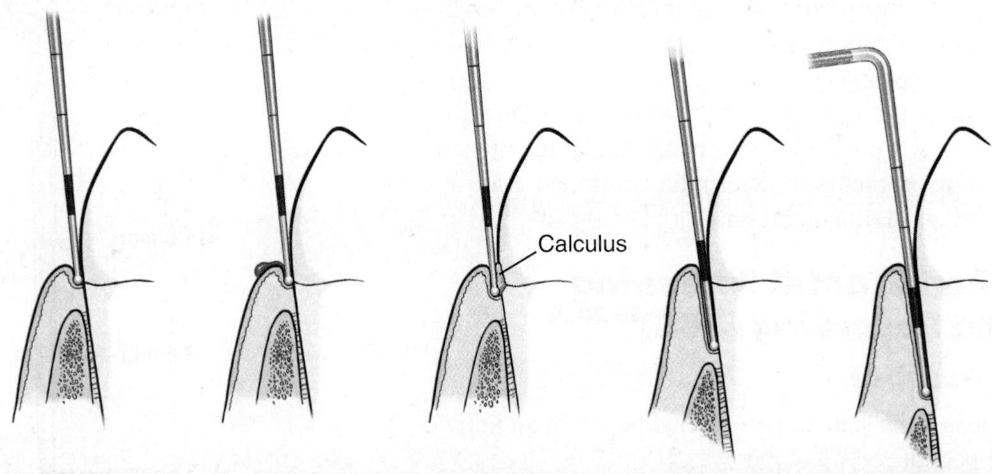

PSR and CPI sextant scores	Code 0	Code 1	Code 2	Code 3	Code 4
CPI description	• Entire black band of the probe is visible.	• Entire black band of the probe is visible, but bleeding is present after gentle probing.	• Entire black band is visible, but calculus is present. • Bleeding may or may not be present.	• 4 to 5 mm pocket depth. • Black band on probe partially hidden by gingival margin.	• 6 mm or greater pocket depth. • Black band of probe completely hidden by gingival margin.
PSR sextant code description	• Colored area of probe completely visible. • No calculus, defective restoration margins, or bleeding.	• Colored area of probe completely visible. • No calculus or defective restoration margins. • Bleeding after gentle probing.	• Colored area of probe completely visible. • Supra- or subgingival rough surface or calculus. • Defective restoration margins.	• Colored area of probe only partially visible. • Calculus, defective restorations, and bleeding may or may not be present.	• Colored area of probe completely disappears (probing depth of 5.5 mm or greater).
PSR management guidelines	• Biofilm control instruction. • Preventive care.	• Biofilm control instruction. • Preventive care.	• Biofilm control instruction. • Complete preventive care. • Calculus removal. • Correction of defective restoration margins.	• Comprehensive periodontal assessment and treatment plan is indicated.	• Comprehensive periodontal assessment and treatment plan is indicated.

Figure 21-8 Community Periodontal Index (CPI) and Periodontal Screening and Recording (PSR) Codes

Data from Petersen PE, Baez RJ. *Oral Health Surveys: Basic Methods*. 5th ed. Geneva: World Health Organization; 2013. https://apps.who.int/iris/bitstream/handle/10665/97035/9789241548649_eng.pdf. Accessed April 25, 2022; American Academy of Periodontology. Parameter on comprehensive periodontal examination. *J Periodontol*. 2000;71(5 suppl):847-848.

D. Scoring

- Follow-up patient management
  - Patients are classified into assessment and treatment planning needs by the highest coded score of their periodontal screening and recording (PSR).
- Calculation: Example 1: PSR Sextant Score

4*	2	3
3	2*	4*

- Interpretation
  - With Codes 3 and 4, a comprehensive periodontal examination is indicated. The asterisks indicate furcation involvement in two sextants and a mucogingival involvement in the mandibular anterior sextant. When the patient is not aware of the periodontal involvement, counseling is important if cooperation and compliance are to be obtained.
- Calculation: Example 2: PSR Sextant Score

2	1	2
2	1*	2*

- Interpretation
  - An overall Code 2 can indicate calculus and overhanging restorations that can be removed. All restorations are checked for recurrent dental caries. Appointments for instruction in dental biofilm control are of primary concern.
    - In this example, the asterisks in two sextants indicate a notable clinical feature such as minimal attached gingiva.

II. Community Periodontal Index (CPI)[1,22]

A. Purpose

To screen and monitor the periodontal status of populations.

- Originally developed as the CPITN index that included a code to indicate an individual and group-summary recording of treatment needs. However, because of changes in management of periodontal disease, the treatment needs portion of the index has been eliminated.
- One component of a complete oral health survey[1] designed by the WHO that includes the assessment of many oral health indicators, including mucosal lesions, dental caries, fluorosis, prosthetic status, and dentofacial anomalies.
- Later modified to form the PSR index for scoring individual patients.

B. Selection of Teeth

- The dentition is divided into sextants for recording on the assessment form.
- Posterior sextants begin distal to canines.

Adults (20 Years and Older)

- A sextant is examined only if there are two or more teeth present that are not indicated for extraction.
- Ten index teeth are examined.
- The first and second molars in each posterior sextant. If one is missing, no replacement is selected and the score for the remaining molar is recorded.
- The maxillary right central incisor and mandibular left central incisor.
- If no index teeth or tooth is present in the sextant, then all remaining teeth in the sextant are examined and the highest score is recorded.

Children and Adolescents (7–19 Years of Age)

- Six index teeth are examined; the first molar in each posterior quadrant and the maxillary right and the mandibular left incisors.
- For children younger than age 15 years, periodontal pocket depth is not recorded to avoid the deepened sulci associated with erupting teeth. Only bleeding and calculus are considered.

C. Procedure

- Instrument: A specially designed probe is used to record both the community periodontal index (CPI) and PSR. The probe is described in Figure 21-7.
- Criteria: CPI score.
- Five codes are used to record bleeding, calculus, and periodontal pocket depth. Criteria for the CPI codes are similar to the criteria for the PSR, as illustrated in Figure 21-8 and the Community Periodontal Index table next.

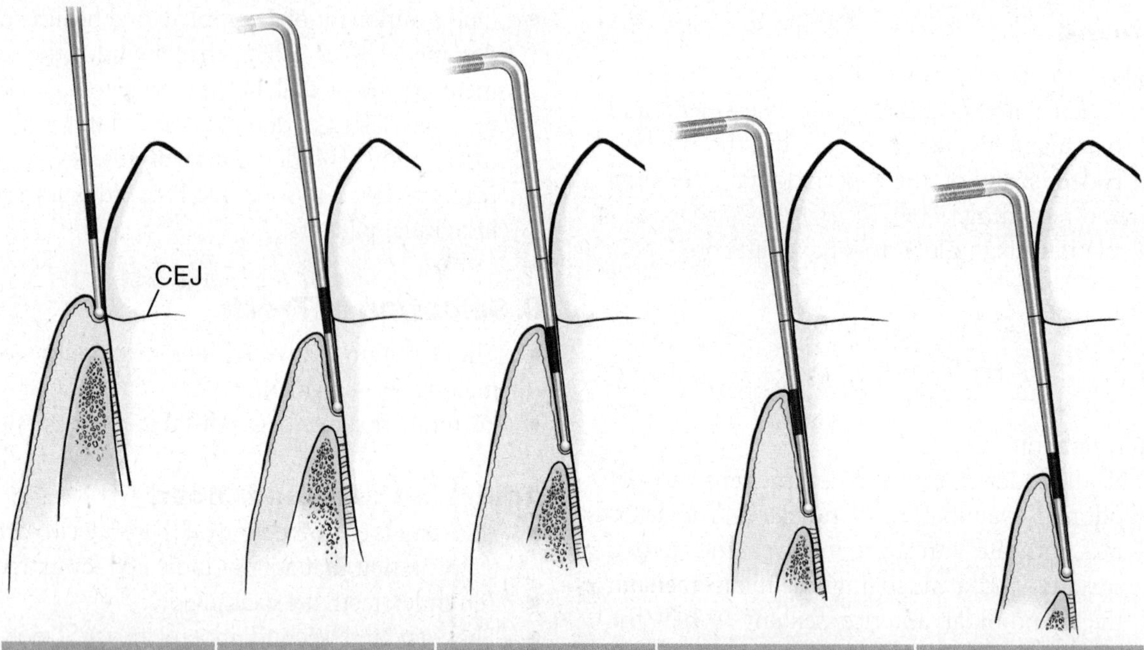

Code 0	Code 1	Code 2	Code 3	Code 4
• 0 to 3 mm loss of attachment. • Cementoenamel junction (CEJ) is covered by gingival margin and CPI score is 0 to 3. If CEJ is visible, or if CPI score is 4, LOA codes 1 to 4 are used.	• 3.5 to 5.5 mm loss of attachment. • CEJ is within the black band on the probe.	• 6 to 8 mm loss of attachment. • CEJ is between the top of the black band and the 8.5 mm mark on the probe.	• 9 to 11 mm loss of attachment. • CEJ is between the 8.5 mm and 11.5 mm marks on the probe.	• 12 mm or greater loss of attachment. • CEJ is beyond the highest (11.5 mm) marks on the probe.

Figure 21-9 Loss of Attachment (LOA) Codes

Data from Petersen PE, Baez RJ. *Oral Health Surveys: Basic Methods*. 5th ed. Geneva: World Health Organization; 2013. https://apps.who.int/iris/bitstream/handle/10665/97035/9789241548649_eng.pdf. Accessed April 25, 2022; American Academy of Periodontology. Parameter on comprehensive periodontal examination. *J Periodontol*. 2000;71(5 suppl):847-848.

Community Periodontal Index

Code	Criteria
0	Healthy periodontal tissues.
1	Bleeding after gentle probing; entire colored band of probe is visible.
2	Supragingival or subgingival calculus present; entire colored band of probe is visible.
3	4- to 5-mm pocket; colored band of probe is partially obscured.
4	6 mm or deeper; colored band on the probe is not visible.

- Criteria: Loss of attachment (LOA) code.
  - In conjunction with the CPI, the WHO probe is also used to record LOA. The five LOA codes used are illustrated in **Figure 21-9**. LOA is not recorded for individuals younger than 15 years of age.

Loss of Attachment (LOA) Code	Criteria
0	0–3 mm LOA
1	4–5 mm LOA
2	6–8 mm LOA
3	9–11 mm LOA
4	12 mm or greater LOA

III. Sulcus Bleeding Index (SBI)[17]

A. Purpose

- To locate areas of gingival sulcus bleeding and color changes in order to recognize and record the presence of early (initial) inflammatory gingival disease.

B. Areas Examined

- Four gingival units are scored systematically for each tooth: the labial and lingual marginal gingiva (M units) and the mesial and distal papillary gingiva (P units).

C. Procedure

- Use standardized lighting while probing each of the four areas.
- Walk the probe to the base of the sulcus, holding it parallel with the long axis of the tooth for M units, and directed toward the col area for P units.
- Wait 30 seconds after probing before scoring apparently healthy gingival units.
- Dry the gingiva gently if necessary to observe color changes clearly.
- Criteria

Sulcular Bleeding Index

Code	Criteria
0	Healthy appearance of P and M, no bleeding on sulcus probing.
1	Apparently healthy P and M showing no change in color and no swelling, but bleeding from sulcus on probing.
2	Bleeding on probing and change of color caused by inflammation. No swelling or macroscopic edema.
3	Bleeding on probing and change in color and slight edematous swelling.
4	Bleeding on probing and change in color and obvious swelling or bleeding on probing and obvious swelling.
5	Bleeding on probing and spontaneous bleeding and change in color, marked swelling with or without ulceration.

D. Scoring

- Sulcus bleeding index (SBI) for area
  - Score each of the four gingival units (M and P) from 0 to 5.
- SBI for tooth
  - Total scores for the four units and divide by 4.
- SBI for individual
  - Total the scores for individual teeth and divide by the number of teeth. SBI scores range from 0 to 5.

IV. Gingival Bleeding Index (GBI)[23]

A. Purpose

- To record the presence or absence of gingival inflammation as determined by bleeding from interproximal gingival sulci.

B. Areas Examined

Each interproximal area has two sulci, which can be scored as one interdental unit or scored separately.

- Certain areas may be excluded from scoring because of accessibility, tooth position, diastemata, or other factors, and if exclusions are made, a consistent procedure is followed for an individual and for a group if a study is to be conducted.
- A full complement of teeth has 30 proximal areas. In the original studies, third molars were excluded, and 26 interdental units were recorded.[23]

C. Procedure

- Instrument
  - Unwaxed dental floss is used.
- Steps
  - Pass the floss interproximally first on one side of the papilla and then on the other.
  - Curve the floss around the adjacent tooth and bring the floss below the gingival margin.
  - Move the floss up and down for one stroke, with care not to lacerate the gingiva. Adapt finger rests to provide controlled, consistent pressure.
  - Use a new length of clean floss for each area.
  - Retract for visibility of bleeding from both facial and lingual aspects.
  - Allow 30 seconds for reinspection of an area that does not show blood immediately either in the area or on the floss.
- Criteria
  - Bleeding indicates the presence of disease. No attempt is made to quantify the severity of bleeding.

D. Scoring

- The numbers of bleeding areas and scorable units are recorded. Patient participation in observing and recording over a series of appointments can increase motivation.

V. Eastman Interdental Bleeding Index (EIBI)[24,25]

A. Purpose

- To assess the presence of inflammation in the interdental area as indicated by the presence or absence of bleeding.

B. Areas Examined

- Each interdental area around the entire dentition.

C. Procedure

- Instrument
  - Triangular wooden interdental cleaner.
- Steps
  4. Gently insert a wooden cleaner into each interdental area in such a way as to depress the papilla 1–2 mm (**Figure 21-10**), then immediately remove.
  5. Make the path of insertion horizontal (parallel to the occlusal surface), taking care not to angle the point in an apical direction.
  6. Insert and remove four times; move to next interproximal area.
  7. Record the presence or absence of bleeding within 15 seconds for each area.

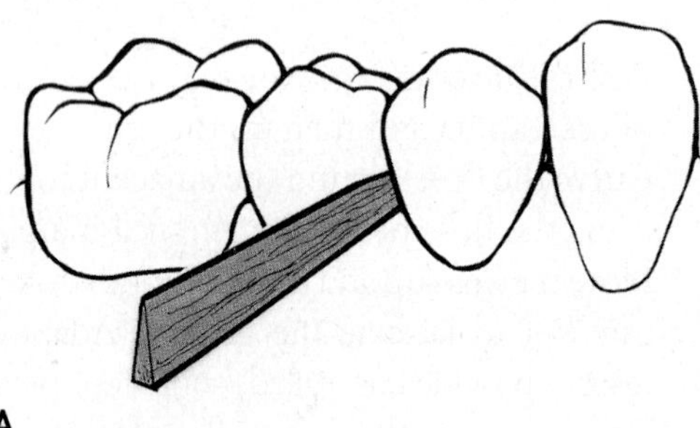

A

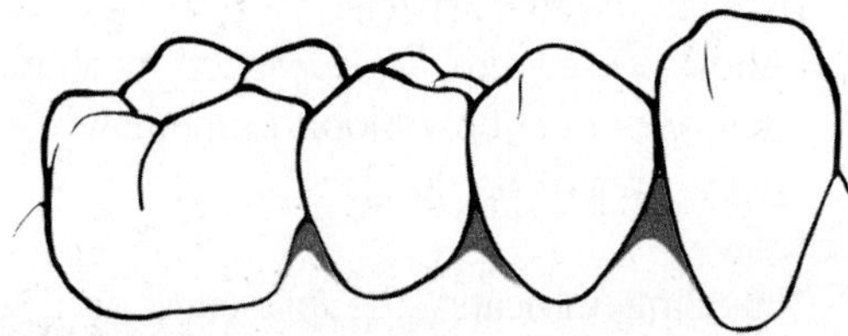

B

Figure 21-10 Eastman Interdental Bleeding Index. The test for interdental bleeding is made by inserting a wooden interdental cleaner into each interdental space. **A:** Wooden interdental cleaner inserted in a horizontal path, parallel with the occlusal surfaces. **B:** The presence or absence of bleeding is noted within a quadrant 15 seconds after final insertion. Bleeding indicates the presence of inflammation.

D. Scoring

- Number of bleeding sites
  - The number may be totaled for an individual score for comparison with scores over a series of appointments.
- Percentage scores
  - Index is expressed as a percentage of the total number of sites evaluated. Calculations can be made for total mouth, quadrants, or maxillary versus mandibular arches.
- Calculation example
  - An adult with a complete dentition has 15 maxillary and 15 mandibular interproximal areas. The Eastman interdental bleeding index revealed 13 areas of bleeding. To calculate percentage:

$$\frac{\textit{Number of bleeding areas}}{\textit{Total number of areas}} \times 100 = \textit{Percent bleeding area}$$

$$\frac{13}{30} \times 100 = 43\%$$

VI. Gingival Index (GI)[3]

A. Purpose

- To assess the severity of gingivitis based on color, consistency, and bleeding on probing.

B. Selection of Teeth and Gingival Areas

A GI may be determined for selected teeth or for the entire dentition.

- Areas examined
  - Four gingival areas (distal, facial, mesial, and lingual) are examined systematically for each tooth.
- Modified procedure
  - The distal examination for each tooth can be omitted. The score for the mesial area is doubled and the total score for each tooth is divided by 4.

C. Procedure

- Dry the teeth and gingiva; under adequate light, use a mouth mirror and probe.
- Use the probe to press on the gingiva to determine the degree of firmness.
- Slide the probe along the soft-tissue wall near the entrance to the gingival sulcus to evaluate bleeding (**Figure 21-11**).
- Criteria

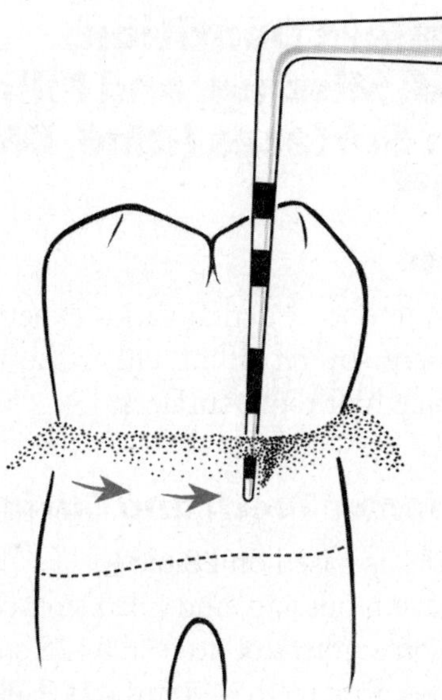

Figure 21-11 Gingival Index. Probe stroke for bleeding evaluation. The broken line represents the level of attachment of the periodontal tissues. The probe is inserted a few millimeters and moved along the soft-tissue pocket wall with light pressure in a circumferential direction. The stroke shown here is in contrast with the walking stroke used for probing depth evaluation and measurement.

Gingival Index Code	Criteria
0	Normal gingiva.
1	Mild inflammation—slight change in color, slight edema. *No bleeding* on probing.
2	Moderate inflammation—redness, edema, and glazing. *Bleeding* on probing.
3	Severe inflammation—marked redness and edema. Ulceration. Tendency to *spontaneous bleeding*.

D. Scoring

- GI for area
  - Each of the four gingival surfaces (distal, facial, mesial, and lingual) is given a score of 0–3.
- GI for a tooth
  - Scores for each area are totaled and divided by 4.
- GI for groups of teeth
  - Scores for individual teeth may be grouped and totaled and divided by the number of teeth. A GI may be determined for specific teeth, group of teeth, quadrant, or side of mouth.
- GI for the individual
  - Scores for each tooth are added up and divided by the number of teeth examined. Scores range from 0 to 3.
- Suggested range of scores for patient reference

Rating	Scores
Excellent (healthy tissue)	0
Good	0.1–1.0
Fair	1.1–2.0
Poor	2.1–3.0

- Calculation: Example for an Individual
  - Using six teeth for an example of screening; teeth selected are known as the **Ramfjord index teeth**.[26]

Tooth No.	M	F	D	L	
3 (16)	3	1	3	1	
9 (21)	1	0	1	1	
12 (24)	2	1	2	0	
19 (36)	3	1	3	3	
25 (41)	1	1	1	1	
28 (44)	2	1	2	0	
Total	12	5	12	6	= 35

$$\textit{Gingival index} = \frac{\textit{Total score}}{\textit{Number of surfaces}} = \frac{35}{24} = 1.46$$

- Interpretation
  - According to the suggested range of scores, the score for this individual (1.46) indicates only fair gingival health (moderate inflammation).
  - The ratings for each gingival area or surface can be used to help the patient compare gingival changes and improve oral hygiene procedures.
- GI for a group
  - Add the individual GI scores and divide by the number of individuals examined.

VII. Modified Gingival Index (MGI)[27,28]

A. Purpose

- Adaptation of the original GI that eliminates probing in the sulcus; less sensitive measure of gingivitis since it relies only on visual observation.
- Probing requirement was removed to reduce disruption of plaque biofilm disruption, avoid potential gingival trauma, and eliminate need for multiple probing assessments to increase reliability.

B. Areas Examined

- Assesses full mouth or gingiva of selected teeth.
- Gingiva is divided into marginal and papillary units.

C. Scoring

- Scores the extent and severity of gingival inflammation using five ordinal numbers.
- Scoring of mild and moderate inflammation differs from original GI.
- Calculates mean scores for individuals and population groups.
- Criteria:

Modified Gingival Index Code	Criteria
0	Normal, healthy tissue.
1	Mild inflammation; involves any part of the gingiva *not entire* marginal or papillary gingival unit.
2	Mild inflammation involved the *entire* marginal or papillary gingival unit.
3	Moderate inflammation.
4	Severe inflammation.

Dental Caries Experience

Dental caries experience data are most useful when measuring the prevalence of dental disease in groups rather than individuals. The population scores can document such information as the number of persons in any age group who are affected by dental caries, the number of teeth that need treatment, or the proportion of teeth that have been treated.

I. Permanent Dentition: Decayed, Missing, and Filled Teeth or Surfaces (DMF, DMFT, or DMS)[29]

A. Purpose

- To determine total dental caries experience, past and present, by recording either the number of affected teeth or tooth surfaces.

B. Selection of Teeth and Surfaces

- The DMFT is based on 28 teeth.
- The decayed, missing, and filled surfaces (DMFS) is based on surfaces of 28 teeth; 128 surfaces.
  - 16 posterior teeth × 5 surfaces (facial, lingual, mesial, distal, and occlusal) = 80 surfaces.
  - 12 anterior teeth × 4 surfaces (facial, lingual, mesial, and distal) = 48 surfaces.
  - Teeth missing due to dental caries are recorded using five surfaces for posterior and four surfaces for anterior teeth.
- Teeth not counted.
  - Third molars.
  - Unerupted teeth. A tooth is considered erupted when any part projects through the gingiva. Certain types of research may require differentiation between clinical emergence, partial eruption, and full eruption.
  - Congenitally missing and supernumerary teeth.
  - Teeth removed for reasons other than dental caries, such as an impaction or during orthodontic treatment.
  - Teeth restored for reasons other than dental caries, such as trauma (fracture), cosmetic purposes, or use as a bridge abutment.
  - Primary tooth retained with the permanent successor erupted. The permanent tooth is evaluated because a primary tooth is never included in this index.

C. Procedures

- Examination
  - Examine each tooth in a systematic sequence.
  - Observe teeth by visual means as much as possible.
  - Use adequate light.
  - Review the stages of dental caries in Chapter 25.
- Criteria for recording[29]
  - Each tooth is recorded once when using the DMFT index.

- Five surfaces for posterior teeth and four surfaces for anterior teeth are recorded when using the DMFS index.
- DMF indices use a dichotomous scale (present or absent) to record decay.

DMF Rating	Criteria
Decayed (D)	Visible dental caries is present or both dental caries and a restoration are present.
Missing (M)	A tooth extracted because of dental caries or when it is carious, nonrestorable, and indicated for extraction.
Filled (F)	Any permanent or temporary restoration is present or a defective restoration without evidence of dental caries is present.

D. Scoring

- Individual DMF
  - Total each component separately.
    - *Total D + M + F = DMF*
  - *Example:* An individual presents with dental caries on the mesial and occlusal surfaces of a posterior tooth and caries on the mesial surface of an anterior tooth. A molar tooth and an anterior tooth are missing because of dental caries and there is an amalgam restoration on the mesial–distal–occlusal surfaces of a posterior tooth.
    - *DMFT = 2 + 2 + 1 = 5*
    - *DMFS = 3 + 9 + 3 = 15*
- A DMF score may have different interpretations. For example, an individual with a DMF score of 15 who has experienced regular dental care may have a distribution such as D = 0, M = 0, F = 15.
- Group DMF
  - Total the DMFs for each individual examined.
  - Divide the total DMFs by the number of individuals in the group.
- Calculation:
  - *Example:* A population of 20 individuals with individual DMF scores of 0, 0, 0, 0, 2, 2, 3, 3, 3, 4, 9, 9, 9, 10, 10, 10, 11, 11, 12, and 16 equals a group total DMF of 124.

$$\frac{124}{20} = 6.2 = \textit{the average DMF for the group}$$

  - This DMF average represents accumulated dental caries experience for the group.

- The differences in caries experience between two groups of individuals within this population are notable and influence interpretation of the results. For the first 10 individuals, the group average is 17/10 = 1.7 and for the second 10 individuals the average DMF is 107/10 = 10.7.
- Scores for these two groups can be presented separately because of the wide difference.
- Average DMF scores can also be presented by age group.
- Specific treatment needs of a group
  - To calculate the percentage of DMF teeth that need to be restored, divide the total D component by the total DMF.
- Calculation:
  - *Example 1:* To calculate the *percentage of DMF teeth* that need to be restored, divide the total D component by the total number of DMF teeth.
    - *D = 175, M = 55, F = 18*
    - *Total DMFT = 248*

$$\frac{D}{DMF} = \frac{175}{248} = 0.71 \textit{ or}$$

71% of the teeth need restorations

  - *Example 2:* The same type of calculations can be used to determine the *percentage of all teeth* missing in a group of individuals.
    - *20 individuals have 28 × 20 = 560 permanent teeth.*
    - *D = 175, M = 55, F = 18 or nearly 10% of all their teeth lost because of dental caries.*

$$\frac{M}{\textit{Total \# of teeth}} = \frac{55}{560} = 0.098$$

II. Primary Dentition: Decayed, Indicated for Extraction, and Filled (df and def)[30,31]

A. Purpose

- To determine the dental caries experience for the primary teeth present in the oral cavity by evaluating teeth or surfaces.

B. Selection of Teeth or Surfaces

- deft or dft: 20 teeth evaluated.
- defs or dfs: 88 surfaces evaluated.
  - Posterior teeth: Each has five surfaces: facial, lingual or palatal, mesial, distal, and occlusal. (8 teeth × 5 surfaces = 40 surfaces.)
  - Anterior teeth: Each has four surfaces: facial, lingual or palatal, mesial, and distal (12 teeth × 4 surfaces = 48 surfaces).

- Teeth not counted
  - Missing teeth, including unerupted and congenitally missing.
  - Supernumerary teeth.
  - Teeth restored for reasons other than dental caries are not counted as f.

C. Procedure

- Instruments and examination
  - Same as for DMF.
- Criteria

Decayed, Indicated for Extraction, Filled (df and def)

Rating	Criteria
d	Primary teeth (or surfaces) with dental caries but not restored.
e	Primary teeth (or number of surfaces) that are *indicated for extraction* because of dental caries.
f	Primary teeth (or surfaces) restored with an amalgam, composite, or temporary filling. Each tooth (or surface) is scored only once. A tooth with recurrent caries around a restoration receives a "d" score.

- Difference between deft/defs and dft/dfs
  - In the deft and defs, both "d" and "e" are used to describe teeth with dental caries. Thus, d and e are sometimes combined, and the index becomes the dft or dfs.

D. Scoring

- Calculation:
  - *Example 1:* Individual def: A 2½-year-old child has 18 teeth. Teeth A (55) and J (65) are unerupted. There is no sign of dental caries in teeth M (73), N (72), O (71), P (81), Q (82), and R (83). All other teeth have two carious surfaces each, except tooth B (54), which is broken down to the gum line.

  Summary:

  Total number of teeth = 18
  Number of "d" teeth = 11
  Number of "e" teeth = 1
  Number of "f" teeth = 0
  def = d + e + f = 11 + 1 + 0 = 12
- Interpretation
  - Twelve of 18 teeth (67%) with carious lesions indicates a serious need for dental treatment and a caries management program for the child.
- Calculation: Example 2: Individual dfs
  - Using the same 2½-year-old child to calculate dfs: Eleven teeth each have two carious surfaces: 11 × 2 = 22 carious surfaces

  Tooth B has 1 × 5 = 5 carious surfaces

  Total dfs: d + f = 27 + 0 = 27
- Interpretation
  - The child has 48 total anterior surfaces (12 teeth × 4 surfaces) and 30 total posterior surfaces (6 teeth × 5 surfaces) to total 78 surfaces.

$$\frac{dfs}{Number\ of\ surfaces} = \frac{27}{78}$$

= 0.35 or 35% of the surfaces in need of dental treatment

E. Mixed Dentition

- A DMFT or DMFS and a deft or defs are never combined or added together.

III. Primary Dentition: Decayed, Missing, and Filled (dmf)[30,31]

A. Purpose

- To determine dental caries experience for children. Only primary teeth are evaluated.

B. Selection of Teeth or Surfaces

- dmft: 12 teeth evaluated (8 primary molars; 4 primary canines).
- dmfs: 56 surfaces evaluated.
  - Primary molars: 8 × 5 surfaces each = 40
  - Primary canines: 4 × 4 surfaces each = 16
- Each tooth is counted only once. When both dental caries and a restoration are present, the tooth or surface is scored as "d."

C. Procedure

- Instruments and examination are the same as for DMF.
- Criteria for dmft or dmfs:

dmf Rating	Criteria
d	Primary molars and canines (or surfaces) that are carious.
m	Primary molars and canines (or surfaces) that are missing. A primary molar or canine is presumed missing because of dental caries when it has been lost before normal exfoliation.
f	Primary molars and canines (or surfaces) that have a restoration but are without caries.

Table 21-1 ECC and S-ECC Case Definition

Age	Birth to 3 Years (0–35 Months)	3–4 Years (36–47 Months)	4–5 Years (48–59 Months)	5–6 Years (60–71 Months)
ECC	One or more teeth with decayed (either cavitated or noncavitated), missing, or filled surfaces			
S-ECC	▪ Any sign of smooth surface caries	▪ One or more cavitated or filled smooth surfaces in primary maxillary anterior teeth ▪ One or more missing teeth due to caries OR dmfs score ≥4	▪ One or more cavitated or filled smooth surfaces in primary maxillary anterior teeth ▪ One or more missing teeth due to caries OR dmfs score ≥5	▪ One or more cavitated or filled smooth surfaces in primary maxillary anterior teeth ▪ One or more missing teeth due to caries OR dmfs score ≥6

Data from: Drury TF, Horowitz AM, Ismail AI, et al. Diagnosing and reporting early childhood caries for research purposes. *J Public Health Dent.* 1999;59(3):192-197.

D. Scoring

- Calculation: Example 1: Individual dmf
  - A 7-year-old boy has all primary molars and canines present. Examination reveals two carious surfaces on one molar tooth, one missing canine tooth, and one two-surface amalgam filling on a molar tooth:
    - *dmft* = 1 + 1 + 1 = 3
    - *dmfs* = 2 + 4 + 2 = 8

E. Mixed Dentition

- Permanent and primary teeth are evaluated separately. A DMFT or DMFS and a dmft or dmfs are never added together.

IV. Early Childhood Caries (ECC)[32]

A. Purpose

- To provide case definitions that determine dental caries experience and severity in children 5–6 years of age or younger.

B. Selection of Teeth or Surfaces

- Each surface (mesial, distal, facial, lingual, and occlusal) of each tooth visible in the child's mouth is evaluated. Only primary teeth are scored.

C. Procedure

- Visual examination of all surfaces of each erupted tooth.
- Categorized according to age and severity.
  - Early childhood caries (ECC) applies to children 6 years of age and younger.
  - Severe early childhood caries (S-ECC) applies to children 5 years of age and younger.
- Criteria for case definitions are included in **Table 21-1**.

D. Scoring

- A designation of early childhood caries (ECC) or severe early childhood caries (S-ECC) for a particular individual relates the age of the child with the status of DMFT surfaces observed.
- Community-based surveys identify the percentage of a population with ECC and/or S-ECC.

V. Root Caries Index (RCI)[33]

A. Purpose

- To determine total root caries experience for individuals and groups and provide a direct, simple method for recording and making comparisons.

B. Selection of Teeth

- Up to four surfaces (mesial, distal, facial, and lingual/palatal) are counted for each tooth.
- Only surfaces with visible gingival recession are counted.
- Teeth with multiple roots and extreme recession, though rare, could present with two or three lesions on the same surface. In this case, the most severe lesion is selected for recording and each surface is counted only once.

C. Procedure

- Examination
  - Use adequate retraction and light to examine each tooth.
  - Apply current knowledge of the stages of dental caries to prevent damage to remineralizing areas during examination. Only cavitated lesions are recorded.
- Record a rating for each root surface.

Root Caries Index Rating	Criteria
NoR	Root surface with a covered cementoenamel junction and no visible recession (R = recession).
R-D	Root surface with recession present and root caries present (D = decay).
R-F	Root surface with recession present and the surface is restored (F = filled).
R-N	Root surface with recession, but no caries or restoration is present.
M	The tooth is missing.

D. Scoring

- Calculation: Formula

$$\frac{[R-D]+[R-F]}{[R-D]+[R-F]+[R-N]} \times 100 = RCI$$

- Calculation: Example individual root caries index (RCI)
  - A man, aged 70, presents with 23 natural teeth (23 × 4 = 92 surfaces). Clinical examination reveals:
    R − D = 26
    R − F = 8
    R − N = 58

$$RCI = \frac{26+8}{26+8+58} = \frac{34}{92} \times 100 = 36.9\%$$

- Interpretation
  - A score of 36.9% means that of all tooth surfaces with visible gingival recession, 36.9% have a history of root caries (cavitated or restored) carious lesions.
- Group or community RCI
  - The R − D, R − F, and R − N scores for all individuals in the group are added together and the RCI formula is calculated using the total scores.

Dental Fluorosis

Dental indices such as the Thylstrup–Fejerskov index,[34] the fluorosis risk index,[35] and the developmental defects of dental enamel index[36,37] have been used to investigate the effects of fluoride concentration on dental enamel. The two indices described here are the most commonly used for community-based assessment.

I. Dean's Fluorosis Index[38]

A. Purpose

- To measure the prevalence and severity of dental fluorosis.
- Originally developed in the 1930s and refined in 1942 to relate the severity of hypomineralization of dental enamel to concentration of fluoride in the water supply.
- Considered less sensitive than some other measures of fluorosis, but still recommended for use in community studies.

B. Selection of Teeth

- The smooth surface enamel of all teeth is examined.

C. Procedure

- Each tooth is visually examined for signs of fluorosis and assigned a numerical score using the descriptive categories listed in **Table 21-2**.

D. Scoring

- An individual fluorosis score is assigned using the highest numerical score recorded for two or more teeth.
- Community levels of fluorosis are indicated by the percentage of individuals in the **sample** or population that receives scores in each category.

II. Tooth Surface Index of Fluorosis (TSIF)[39]

A. Purpose

- To measure the prevalence and severity of dental fluorosis.
- More sensitive than Dean's index in identifying the mildest signs of fluorosis.

B. Selection of Teeth

- The smooth surface enamel, cusp tips, and incisal edges of all teeth are examined.

C. Procedure

- Each tooth is examined visually and assigned a numerical score using the criteria in **Table 21-3**.

Table 21-2 Scoring System for Dean's Fluorosis Index

Category	Description	Numerical Score
Normal	Smooth, creamy white tooth surface	0
Questionable	Slight changes from normal transparency	1
Very mild	Small, scattered opaque areas; less than 25% of tooth surface	2
Mild	Opaque areas; less than 50% of tooth surface	3
Moderate	Significant opaque and/or worn areas; may have brown stains	4
Severe	Widespread, significant hypoplasia, pitting, brown staining, worn areas, and/or a corroded appearance	5

Data from Dean HT. The investigation of physiological effect by the epidemiological method. In: Moulton FR, ed. *Fluorine and Dental Health*. Washington, DC: American Association for the Advancement of Science; 1942:23-71.

Table 21-3 Scoring System for Tooth Surface Index of Fluorosis

Description	Numerical Score
No evidence of fluorosis	0
Areas with parchment-white color; less than one-third of visible tooth surface; includes fluorosis confined to anterior incisal edges and posterior cusp tips	1
Parchment-white color on at least one-third but less than two-thirds of visible tooth surface	2
Parchment-white color on at least two-thirds of visible tooth surface	3
Staining (from light to very dark brown) in conjunction with parchment-white areas as described above in levels 1, 2, or 3	4
Discrete stained and rough pitted areas, but no staining on intact enamel surfaces	5
Discrete pitting plus staining of intact enamel surfaces	6
Confluent pitting over large areas of tooth surface; anatomy of tooth may be altered; dark-brown stain usually present	7

Reproduced from Horowitz HS, Driscoll WS, Meyers RJ, et al. A new method for assessing the prevalence of dental fluorosis—the tooth surface index of fluorosis. *J Am Dent Assoc.* 1984;109(1):37-41.

D. Scoring

- Tooth surface index of fluorosis (TSIF) data are presented as a distribution citing the percentage of the population with each numerical score, rather than as mean scores for the entire group.

Community-Based Oral Health Surveillance

Community oral health screenings can be performed at every level: local, national, and worldwide. Data collected by such screenings are useful for monitoring health status and determining population access to or need for oral health services.

I. WHO Basic Screening Survey

The WHO screening survey includes the CPI and the LOA indices described earlier.[1]

A. Purpose

- To collect comprehensive data on oral health status and dental treatment needs of a population.

This system is suitable for surveying both adults and children.

B. Tissues/Areas Examined

Survey categories include the following:

- Orofacial (intraoral and extraoral) lesions and anomalies.
- Temporomandibular joint status.
- Periodontal status.
- Dentition status and treatment needs.
- Prosthetic status and need.
- Need for immediate care/referral.

C. Procedures

- Standardized assessment form with boxes for data entry identifies the codes and descriptive criteria for each **data collection** category.

- Standardized codes facilitate computerized data entry and analysis.
- Photographs in the training manual provide examples of criteria for each code.

D. Scoring

- Data can be analyzed by survey team or arrangements can be made for data entry forms to be analyzed by the WHO.

II. Association of State and Territorial Dental Directors' (ASTDD) Basic Screening Survey[8]

A. Purpose

- Developed by the ASTDD to provide oral screening for adult, school age, and/or preschool populations.
    - Data levels are consistent with monitoring the U.S. Public Health Service national health objectives.
    - Data collected can easily be compared with data collected by other communities and states using the data collection techniques.
- The system was designed to be used by screeners with or without dental background because:
    - Sometimes nondental personnel have better access to some population groups.
    - Some communities have little access to dental public health professionals.

B. Selection of Teeth

- All teeth are examined, but each individual patient receives one score for each category.

C. Procedure

- Oral screening can be combined with an optional questionnaire that collects additional data on demographics and access to dental care.
- Screeners are trained and calibrated. They record oral findings using photographs and detailed descriptions of associated criteria.

D. Scoring

- **Table 21-4** outlines the scoring criteria and categories recorded for preschool and school children.
- **Table 21-5** lists the scoring criteria and categories recorded for older adults.
- Data from each indicator can be compiled and expressed in frequency graphs or tables as a percentage of the population that exhibits a specific category trait.

Table 21-4 Association of State and Territorial Dental Directors' Basic Screening Survey Scoring Criteria: Preschool and School Children

Criteria	Score	Preschoolers	School Children
Untreated caries (≥0.5 mm discontinuity in tooth surface)	0 = No untreated caries 1 = Untreated caries	✓	✓
Treated decay (amalgam, composite, or temporary filling)	0 = No treated decay 1 = Treated decay	✓	✓
Sealants on permanent molars	0 = No sealants 1 = Sealants		✓
Treatment urgency	0 = No obvious problem (routine dental care indicated) 1 = Early dental care (within 2 wk) 2 = Urgent care (as soon as possible—presents with pain, swelling, etc.)	✓	✓

A ✓ mark indicates that the oral condition category is scored in that particular age group. Some categories (i.e., sealants) are not scored in all age groups.
Data from ASTDD Basic Screening Surveys. Association of State and Territorial Dental Director website. http://www.astdd.org/basic-screening-survey-tool. Updated January 2022. Accessed April 25, 2022.

Table 21-5 Association of State and Territorial Dental Directors' Basic Screening Survey Scoring Criteria: Older Adults

Criteria	Score
Removable upper denture	0 = No 1 = Yes
If yes: Do you wear upper denture when eating?	0 = No 1 = Yes
Removable lower denture	0 = No 1 = Yes
If yes: Do you wear lower denture when eating?	0 = No 1 = Yes
Number of upper natural teeth (include root fragments)	Range 0–16
Number of lower natural teeth (include root fragments)	Range 0–16
Root fragments	0 = No 1 = Yes 9 = Edentulous
Untreated decay	0 = No 1 = Yes 9 = Edentulous
Need for periodontal care	0 = No 1 = Yes 9 = Edentulous
Suspicious soft-tissue lesions	0 = No 1 = Yes 9 = Edentulous
Treatment urgency	0 = No obvious problem—next scheduled visit 1 = Early care—within next several weeks 2 = Urgent care—within next week—pain or infection
Obvious tooth mobility (optional indicator)	0 = No 1 = Yes 0 = Edentulous
Severe dry mouth (optional indicator)	0 = No 1 = Yes

Data from ASTDD Basic Screening Surveys. Association of State and Territorial Dental Director website. http://www.astdd.org/basic-screening-survey-tool. Updated January 2022. Accessed April 29, 2022.

Box 21-1 Example Documentation: Use of a Dental Index during Patient Assessment

- **S**—Patient presents for reassessment of biofilm and bleeding levels 14 days following oral hygiene instructions that were provided during the previous appointment.
- **O**—Biofilm-free score = 89% compared with previous score of 22%; SBI score = 2 compared to previous score of 5.
- **A**—Significant improvement noted in scores except on maxillary facial surfaces.
- **P**—Patient congratulated on areas of success. Additional instruction provided specifically related to biofilm removal on posterior facial and proximal tooth surfaces. Patient observed while brushing and flossing maxillary molar areas using a mirror.

Next Step: 3 months re-evaluation.
Signed: ____________________, RDH
Date: ______________

Documentation

Factors related to dental indices to document in the patient records include:

- Name of the index or indices used.
- Score calculated for the index.
- Objective statement that provides an interpretation of the index score.
- Follow-up instructions provided to the patient.
- An example of documentation for use of a dental index appears in **Box 21-1**.

Factors to Teach Patient or Members of the Community

- How an index is used and calculated, and what the scores mean.
- Purpose for the selection of the particular index being used.
- Correlation of index scores with current oral health practices and procedures.
- Procedures to follow to improve index scores and bring the oral tissues to health.

References

NOTE: Many of the citations below may seem not to be current or even seem completely out-of-date; however, the reader will note that most are "classic" references, which refer to the development and first use of the index.

1. Petersen PE, Baez, RJ. *Oral Health Surveys: Basic Methods*. 5th ed. Geneva, Switzerland: World Health Organization; 2013. https://apps.who.int/iris/bitstream/handle/10665/97035/9789241548649_eng.pdf. Accessed April 25, 2022.
2. Silness J, Loe H. Periodontal disease in pregnancy. II. correlation between oral hygiene and periodontal condition. *Acta Odontol Scand*. 1964;22:121-135.
3. Löe H. The gingival index, the plaque index and the retention index systems. *J Periodontol*. 1967;38(6 suppl):610-616.
4. Podshadley AG, Haley JV. A method for evaluating oral hygiene performance. *Public Health Rep*. 1968;83(3):259-264.
5. U.S. Department of Health and Human Services. *Oral Health in America: A Report of the Surgeon General*. Rockville, MD: U.S. Department of Health and Human Services, National Institute of Dental and Craniofacial Research, National Institutes of Health; 2000:63-89.
6. National Institutes of Health. *Oral Health in America: Advances and Challenges*. Bethesda, MD: US Department of Health and Human Services, National Institutes of Health, National Institute of Dental and Craniofacial Research; 2021. https://www.nidcr.nih.gov/sites/default/files/2021-12/Oral-Health-in-America-Advances-and-Challenges.pdf. Accessed April 28, 2022.
7. Healthy People 2030. Objectives and data: oral conditions. https://health.gov/healthypeople/objectives-and-data/browse-objectives/oral-conditions. Accessed April 25, 2022.
8. Association of State and Territorial Dental Directors. *Basic Screening Surveys*. Reno, NV: ASTDD; 2022. http://www.astdd.org/basic-screening-survey-tool/. Accessed April 25, 2022.
9. O'Leary TJ, Drake RB, Naylor JE. The plaque control record. *J Periodontol*. 1972;43(1):38.
10. Ramfjord SP, Ash MM. *Periodontology and Periodontics*. Philadelphia, PA: WB Saunders Co; 1979:273.
11. Grant DA, Stern IB, Everett FG. *Periodontics*. 5th ed. St. Louis, MO: Mosby; 1979:529-531.
12. Greene JC, Vermillion JR. The simplified oral hygiene index. *J Am Dent Assoc*. 1964;68:7-13.
13. Greene JC. The Oral Hygiene Index—development and uses. *J Periodontol*. 1967;38(6 suppl):625-637.
14. Schour I, Massler M. Prevalence of gingivitis in young adults. *J Dent Res*. 1948;27(6):733.
15. Massler M. The P-M-A index for the assessment of gingivitis. *J Periodontol*. 1967;38(6 suppl):592-601.
16. Russell AL. A system of classification and scoring for prevalence surveys of periodontal disease. *J Dent Res*. 1956;35(3):350-359.
17. Mühlemann HR, Son S. Gingival sulcus bleeding—a leading symptom in initial gingivitis. *Helv Odontol Acta*. 1971;15(2):107-113.
18. Meitner SW, Zander HA, Iker HP, et al. Identification of inflamed gingival surfaces. *J Clin Periodontol*. 1979;6(2):93-97.
19. American Academy of Periodontology. Parameter on comprehensive periodontal examination. *J Periodontol*. 2000;71(5 suppl):847-848.
20. Khocht A, Zohn H, Deasy M, et al. Assessment of periodontal status with PSR and traditional clinical periodontal examination. *J Am Dent Assoc*. 1995;126(12):1658-1665.
21. Periodontal screening and recording training program kit. Chicago, IL: American Dental Association and American Academy of Periodontics; 1992.
22. Ainamo J, Barmes D, Beagrie G, et al. Development of the World Health Organization (WHO) community periodontal index of treatment needs (CPITN). *Int Dent J*. 1982;32(3):281-291.
23. Carter HG, Barnes GP. The gingival bleeding index. *J Periodontol*. 1974;45(11):801-805.
24. Abrams K, Caton J, Polson A. Histologic comparisons of interproximal gingival tissues related to the presence or absence of bleeding. *J Periodontol*. 1984;55(11):629-632.
25. Caton JG, Polson AM. The interdental bleeding index: a simplified procedure for monitoring gingival health. *Compend Contin Educ Dent*. 1985;6(2):88, 90-92.
26. Ramfjord SP. Indices for prevalence and incidence of periodontal disease. *J Periodontol*. 1959;30:51-59.
27. Chattopadhyay A. *Oral Health Epidemiology: Principals and Practice*. Sudbury, MA: Jones and Bartlett; 2011.
28. Lobene RR, Weatherford T, Ross NM, Lamm RA, Menaker L. A modified gingival index for use in clinical trials. *Clin Prev Dent*. 1986;8(1):3-6.
29. U.S. Department of Health and Human Services, Public Health Service, National Institutes of Health. *Oral Health Surveys of the National Institute of Dental Research, Diagnostic Criteria and Procedures*. Bethesda, MD: National Institute of Dental Research; 1991.
30. Klein H, Palmer CE, Knutson JW. Studies on dental caries. I. dental status and dental needs of elementary school children. *Public Health Rep*. 1938;53(19):751-765.
31. Gruebbel AO. A measurement of dental caries prevalence and treatment service for deciduous teeth. *J Dent Res*. 1944;23:163-168.
32. Drury TF, Horowitz AM, Ismail AI, et al. Diagnosing and reporting early childhood caries for research purposes. *J Public Health Dent*. 1999;59(3):192-197.
33. Katz RV. Assessing root caries in populations: the evolution of the root caries index. *J Public Health Dent*. 1980;40(1):7-16.
34. Thylstrup A, Fejerskov O. Clinical appearance of dental fluorosis in permanent teeth in relation to histologic changes. *Community Dent Oral Epidemiol*. 1978;6(6):315-328.
35. Pendrys DG. The fluorosis risk index: a method for investigating risk factors. *J Public Health Dent*. 1990;50(5):291-298.
36. Fédération Dentaire Internationale. An epidemiological index of developmental defects of dental enamel (DDE Index). Commission on Oral Health, Research and Epidemiology. *Int Dent J*. 1982;32(2):159-167.
37. Clarkson J, O'Mullane D. A modified DDE index for use in epidemiological studies of enamel defects. *J Dent Res*. 1989;68(3):445-450.
38. Dean HT. The investigation of physiological effect by the epidemiological method. In: FR Moulton, ed. *Fluorine and Dental Health*. Washington, DC: American Association for the Advancement of Science; 1942:23-71.
39. Horowitz HS, Driscoll WS, Meyers RJ, et al. A new method for assessing the prevalence of dental fluorosis—the tooth surface index of fluorosis. *J Am Dent Assoc*. 1984;109(1):37-41.

SECTION V

Dental Hygiene Diagnosis and Care Planning

Introduction for Section V

After the initial assessment is completed, as described in Section IV, the data are assembled, sequenced, and analyzed in preparation for planning dental hygiene treatment and education interventions that help the patient acquire and maintain optimum oral health.

The Dental Hygiene Process of Care

Figure V-1 shows the position of diagnosis and care planning in the total Dental Hygiene Process of Care.

- Dental hygiene diagnosis:
  - Identification of an existing oral health problem that a dental hygienist is qualified and licensed to treat within the scope of dental hygiene practice.[1]
  - Development of evidence-based diagnostic statements based on patient assessment data about the patient's condition.[2]
- The formal, written dental hygiene care plan, integrated with the total treatment plan for the patient, is used to:
  - Identify evidence-based dental hygiene interventions based on diagnostic statements that define patient needs.
  - Educate the patient.
  - Secure informed consent for treatment.
  - Communicate planned dental hygiene interventions with other oral care team members.

Ethical Applications

- Basic concepts of healthcare law apply to all dental hygiene professionals.
- The dental hygiene practice acts of each state or province govern the scope of dental hygiene functions and the criteria for licensure.
- The potential for an ethical situation arises anytime a dental hygienist interacts with:
  - A patient.
  - Members of the dental or interprofessional healthcare team.
  - Other individuals involved in the special needs of the patient, such as family and caregivers.
- A dental hygienist who provides ethical patient care:
  - Is cognizant of the respect each patient deserves.
  - Maintains communication among all parties responsible for dental and dental hygiene treatment.
  - Attains knowledge of current standards of care and legal scope of practice.
  - Possesses the ability to assess and justify the reporting of unacceptable practices.
- Selected legal concepts and suggestions for application are described in **Table V-1**.

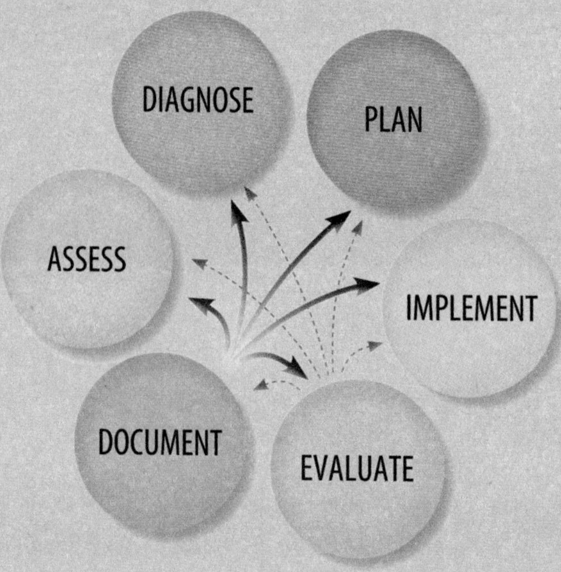

Figure V-1 The Dental Hygiene Process of Care

Table V-1 Legal and Ethical Concepts

Legal Concept	Explanation	Application Examples
Professional liability	A licensed professional is legally accountable for all actions; bound by the law.	Responsibility for actions and decisions made during patient care.
Scope of practice	A dental hygienist is legally bound to provide care within the dental hygiene scope of practice.	Adherence to dental hygiene licensure requirements and performance of functions defined as legal within each state's Dental Hygiene Practice Act.
Standard of care	A professional uses: ■ Ordinary and reasonable skill commonly used by other dental professionals. ■ Prudent judgment. ■ All available resources to determine standards of practice.	Analyzing the patient's assessment data before selecting dental hygiene interventions.
Informed consent	Voluntary affirmation by a patient to allow examination or treatment by authorized dental hygienist or other member of the dental team.	An ongoing process of communication and education about oral health treatment options, not merely a printed form to sign.
Negligence/malpractice	Failure to perform professional duties according to the accepted standard of care.	Failure to inform and refer a patient when concerns outside the scope of dental hygiene practice exist.

References

1. American Dental Hygienists' Association. *Diagnosis-Position Paper*. Published online September 2015. https://www.adha.org/resources-docs/Diagnosis-Position-Paper.pdf. Accessed January 20, 2022.
2. Federation of Dental Hygiene Regulators of Canada (FDHRC). *Entry-to-Practice Canadian Competencies for Dental Hygienists*. Published 2021. https://www.fdhrc.ca/wp/competency-project/. Accessed January 15, 2022.

CHAPTER 22

Dental Hygiene Diagnosis

Linda D. Boyd, RDH, RD, EdD
Catherine G. Ranson, RDH, MET

CHAPTER OUTLINE

LEARNING OBJECTIVES

After studying this chapter, the student will be able to:

1. Explain the significance of developing a dental hygiene diagnosis as a component of the dental hygiene process of care.
2. Formulate a dental hygiene diagnosis based on the assessment findings.
3. Identify and define key terms and concepts related to planning dental hygiene care.
4. Identify and explain assessment findings and individual patient factors that affect patient care.
5. Identify additional factors that influence planning for dental hygiene care.

Introduction

- Four basic steps to be considered when planning patient care are as follows[1]:
  1. Collect and analyze **assessment** information.
  2. Establish the **diagnosis**.
  3. Select treatment and education interventions based on the diagnostic findings.
  4. Develop a formal plan for care.
- In the dental hygiene process of care, the **dental hygiene diagnosis** is the result of analysis and synthesis of assessment data and the application

of clinical judgment and critical thinking skills.[2,3] (See Chapter 1.)
- Then, using an **evidence-based approach**, a dental hygiene care plan and appointment sequence are formalized.[2,3]

Assessment Findings

Clinical assessment findings play a key role in the development of the dental hygiene diagnosis and dental hygiene care plan.

I. Chief Complaint

- The **chief complaint** (concern) is the patient's statement regarding the reason for seeking dental and dental hygiene care.[2]
- A significant concern expressed by the patient, such as pain, must be addressed before initiating dental hygiene treatment to alleviate pain.

II. Risk Factors

- **Risk factors** increase the patient's potential for diminished oral health status.
    - **Modifiable risks factors** are determinants that can be modified by intervention, thereby reducing the probability or progression of disease.
- **Anticipatory guidance** through preventive education and counseling is an essential component of the care plan for a patient exhibiting one or more risk factors.

A. Individual Risk Factors for Periodontal Diseases

- Risk factors recognized based on the evidence for the 2017 World Workshop on the Classification of Periodontal and Peri-Implant Diseases and Conditions include[4]:
    - Diabetes (poorly controlled).
    - Cigarette smoking.
    - Age as related to radiographic bone loss (RBL).
    - Inflammatory burden (measured by high sensitivity C-reactive protein [CRP]).
        - Associated with systemic diseases like cardiovascular disease.
- Emerging risk factors include[4]:
    - Obesity.
    - Specific genetic factors.
    - Nutrition.
    - Physical activity.

B. Periodontal Disease Association with Systemic Conditions

Current research suggests periodontal disease is associated with a variety of systemic conditions, including:
- Cardiovascular disease.[5]
- Diabetes mellitus.[6]
- Metabolic syndrome (a cluster of health conditions that increase risk for heart disease and diabetes).[7]
- Obesity.[6]
- Respiratory disease including asthma, pneumonia, and chronic obstructive pulmonary disease (COPD).[8]
- Adverse pregnancy outcome.[9]
- Osteoporosis.[6]

C. Risk Factors for Dental Caries

- The current **best practice**, evidence-based approach for management of dental caries is by identifying and managing risk factors.[10,11]
- Risk factors for dental caries include[11]:
    - Heavy plaque biofilm.
    - Dietary factors (frequent use of cariogenic foods/beverages).
    - Low fluoride exposure.
    - Visible caries or white spot lesions.
    - Recent restorative treatment (last 2 years for children <6 years old and last 3 years for those >6 years old).
    - Tooth morphology and position (deep occlusal pits and fissures, exposed root surfaces, rotated positioning).
    - Xerostomia.
    - Recreational drug use.
    - Orthodontic appliances.
    - Low health literacy and/or low socioeconomic status
    - For children: Primary caregiver with current or recent history of dental caries.

D. Risk Factors for Oral Cancer

- Risk factors for oral and oropharyngeal cancer include[12]:
    - Tobacco use of any kind.
    - Betel quid and gutka.
    - Heavy alcohol use.
    - Excessive sun exposure (lips and face).
    - Exposure to the human papillomavirus.
    - Male gender.
    - Older than 55 years of age.
    - **Genetic susceptibility**.

III. Patient's Overall Health Status

A. Physical Status

- The extent of the patient's medical, physical, and psychological risk determines modifications necessary during treatment.
- Examples of systematic approaches used to assess physical status include:
  - The **American Society of Anesthesiologists' (ASA)** classification system (**Table 22-1**).[13]
  - The Oral, Systemic, Capability, Autonomy, and Reality (OSCAR) Planning Guide (**Table 22-2**).[14]

B. Tobacco Use

- Tobacco in all forms affects oral status and dental hygiene treatment outcomes.

Information on planning dental hygiene interventions for the patient who uses tobacco is discussed in Chapter 32.

IV. Oral Healthcare Literacy Level of the Patient

- Before planning individualized patient care, the patient's oral **health literacy** is assessed.[15]

Table 22-1 ASA Physical Status Classification System[13]

	ASA Classification	Examples of Physical or Psychosocial Manifestations	Dental Hygiene Treatment Considerations
ASA I	No systemic disease; a normal, healthy patient with little or no dental anxiety	Non smoker Healthy body weight ADL/IADL level = 0	No modifications necessary
ASA II	Mild systemic disease or extreme dental anxiety	Well-controlled mild chronic conditions (e.g., diabetes, epilepsy) Mild lung disease Mild obstructive sleep apnea Smoker Social drinking Overweight or obese Healthy pregnant woman ADL/IADL level = 1	Minimal risk; minor modifications to treatment and/or patient education may be necessary
ASA III	Systemic disease that limits activity but is not incapacitating	Functional limitations with 1 or more chronic conditions Poorly controlled disease (e.g., diabetes) Substance abuse Morbid obesity Severe obstructive sleep apnea ESRD with dialysis Autism at the severe end of the spectrum ADL/IADL level = 2 or 3	Elective treatment is not contraindicated, but serious consideration of treatment and/or patient/caregiver education modifications may be necessary
ASA IV	Incapacitating disease that is a constant threat to life	Unstable cardiovascular conditions Severe respiratory distress Ventilator dependent	Conservative, noninvasive management of emergency dental conditions only; more complex dental intervention may require hospitalization during treatment; caregiver training for daily oral care may be necessary
ASA V	Patient is not expected to survive	Multiple organ system failure Respiratory failure	Only palliative treatment is provided to keep the patient comfortable and out of pain

ADL, activities of daily living; ASA, American Society of Anesthesiologists; IADL, instrumental activities of daily living
Data from American Society of Anesthesiologists. ASA physical status classification system. http://www.asahq.org/resources/clinical-information/asa-physical-status -classification-system.

- From that baseline, education can build on current knowledge rather than provide information too far above or below the patient's current literacy.

V. Oral Self-Care Ability

- The patient's ability to manipulate a toothbrush and interdental aid in order to comply with suggested oral care regimens will determine the success of planned interventions.
- Patients with disabilities or physical limitations will require modification to ensure adequate daily oral biofilm removal.
- An **activities of daily living (ADL/IADL)** classification level provides a simple means of summarizing a person's ability to carry out the basic tasks needed for self-care (**Table 22-3**).
  - The ADL/IADL classification will aid in determining whether adaptive or assistive aids or caregiver training for personal oral care procedures are necessary.

Table 22-2 The Oral, Systemic, Capability, Autonomy, and Reality Planning Guide

Issue	Factors of Concern
A systematic approach to identifying factors to evaluate when planning dental hygiene care	
Oral	Teeth, restorations, prostheses, periodontium, pulpal status, oral mucosa, occlusion, saliva, tongue, alveolar bone
Systemic	Normative age changes, medical diagnoses, pharmacologic agents, interdisciplinary communication
Capability	Functional ability, self-care, caregivers, oral hygiene, transportation to appointments, mobility within the dental office
Autonomy	Decision-making ability, dependence on alternative or supplemental decision makers
Reality	Prioritization of oral health, financial ability or limitations, significance of anticipated life span

Reprinted with permission from Ship JA, Mohammad AR, eds. *Clinician's Guide to Oral Health in Geriatric Patients*. Baltimore, MD: American Academy of Oral Medicine; 1999:21.

Periodontal Risk and Diagnosis

Planning for the number and length of appointments in a treatment sequence is influenced by[2,3,16]:

- Patient's modifiable risk factors (see Risk Factors section).
- Periodontal diagnosis.

I. Current Periodontal Status

A description of past and current periodontal conditions, as well as risk factors affecting the progress of disease, determine a patient's current periodontal status. (See Chapter 19.)

II. Classification of Periodontal Disease

- The extent, severity, and risk for progression of disease can be characterized using the 2017 World Workshop Periodontal Classification Staging and Grading.[4]
- The periodontal staging and grading will aid in determining the sequences and number of appointments required for initial nonsurgical periodontal therapy.[4,16]

Table 22-3 Measures of Patient Functioning

Examples of ADL	Examples of IADL	Levels
Brushing Flossing Applying interdental aids Feeding Ambulation (walking) Bathing Continence Communication Dressing Toileting Transfer (from bed to toilet) Grooming	Maintaining self-care regimens Ability to make and keep dental appointments Writing Cooking Shopping Climbing stairs Managing medication Reading Cleaning Using telephone	*Level 0:* Ability to perform the task without assistance *Level 1:* Ability to perform the task with some human assistance; may need a device or mechanical aid but or still independent *Level 2:* Ability to perform the task with partial assistance *Level 3:* Requires full assistance to perform the task; totally dependent

ADL, activities of daily living; IADL, instrumental activities of daily living

A. Gingivitis

- Inflammation of the gingiva is characterized by changes in color, form, size, position of margin, with bleeding on probing, and no attachment loss.

B. Stage I Periodontitis

- Mild periodontitis with progression of inflammation into the deeper periodontal structures with slight bone loss and connective tissue attachment; subgingival calculus and measurable pocket depth with bleeding on probing.

C. Stage II Periodontitis

- Moderate periodontitis, with increased destruction of the periodontal structures, increased probing depths with bleeding, and noticeable loss of interdental bony support with early to moderate furcation invasions; mobility and fremitus.

D. Stage III or Stage IV Periodontitis

- Further progression of periodontal inflammation with increased probing depths with bleeding, major loss of bony support, furcation invasions, possible evidence of trauma from occlusion with increased tooth mobility and fremitus, and other signs and symptoms.

III. Parameters of Care

- Clinical diagnosis, therapeutic goals, treatment considerations, and outcomes assessment for periodontal disease are outlined in the following documents[4,16,17]:
  - American Academy of Periodontology Parameters of Care
  - 2017 World Workshop periodontal classification
  - European Federation of Periodontology (EFP) clinical practice guidelines for treatment of Stage 1-III periodontitis.
- Planning considerations are determined by the severity of infection.

Dental Caries Risk Level

- Restorative treatment for dental caries is provided by the dentist or dental therapist; however, the plan for dental hygiene care includes interventions aimed at managing risk factors for dental caries.[11]
- Protocols and treatment guidelines for caries management based on risk factors are found in Chapter 25 for adults and Chapter 47 for children ages 0–5 years.

The Dental Hygiene Diagnosis

The diagnosis is a fundamental component of medical and dental care.

- The dental hygiene diagnosis is part of the process of care, involving the use of evidence-based analysis of the assessment findings to determine the patient's or community's dental hygiene needs.[2,3,18]
- The dental hygiene diagnosis provides a basis for the dental hygiene care plan (therapeutic and preventive).[2,3,18]

I. Basis for Diagnosis

- The basis for the diagnosis includes the following[1-3,17,18]:
  - Patient interview data (chief complaint, identification of oral problems, and comprehensive personal/social, medical, and dental health histories).
  - Physical assessment data (vital signs, extraoral and intraoral tissue examination, and dental and periodontal chartings).
  - Radiographic series.

II. Diagnostic Statements

- Provide the basis for development of the care plan that focuses on education, oral self-care, prevention, dental hygiene treatment within the scope of dental hygiene practice and referral.[3,17]
- Diagnostic statements include the diagnosis and the risk factors contributing to the condition diagnosed.
- Examples of dental hygiene diagnostic statements are listed in **Table 22-4**.

The Dental Hygiene Prognosis

The **dental hygiene prognosis** is a component of medical and dental care. Prognosis is a forecast of the outcome of a disease or condition. In the dental hygiene process of care, prognosis refers to the following[3,19]:

- A look ahead to an anticipated outcome or end point expected from the dental hygiene intervention selected for an individual patient.
- Expressed in general terms for either an individual tooth or the overall prognosis for the patient's

Table 22-4 Examples of Dental Hygiene Diagnostic Statements

Problem	Risk Factors and Etiology
Hypersensitivity	Related to gingival recession resulting in exposed root surfaces
Gingivitis	Related to biofilm accumulation causing inflammation
Increased caries risk (Caries Management By Risk Assessment [CAMBRA] level = extreme)	Related to previous history of dental caries and consumption of sugar-sweetened beverages frequently throughout each day
Biofilm control record score = fair to poor score	Related to limited ability to perform oral self-care tasks (activities of daily living Level 3)
Decreased saliva flow/xerostomia	Related to side effect of medication
Red patchy tissue on palate appears to be nicotine stomatitis	Related to regular tobacco use
Generalized Stage II, Grade C periodontitis	Related to inadequate biofilm control, lack of regular professional dental care, radiographic evidence of interdental clinical attachment loss, and HbA1c of 9.

teeth. Typically, the overall prognosis will be determined in consultation with the dentist.

- Based on treatment and self-care behavior goals agreed upon by the patient and clinician during the planning phase of care.

I. Criteria for Various Prognoses

The criteria for various prognoses are listed in **Box 22-1**.

II. Factors in Assigning a Prognosis

- Individual tooth prognosis[4,19,20]:
  - Percentage of bone loss.
  - Clinical attachment loss.
  - Extent and type of bone loss (vertical versus horizontal).
  - Presence and severity of furcation involvement.
  - Mobility.
  - Caries.
  - Tooth position.
  - Occlusal trauma.

Box 22-1 Criteria for Various Prognoses[4,16,19,21]

Prognosis following periodontal therapy is determined by the following factors:

Good

- Control of etiologic factors
- Adequate biofilm management
- No clinical attachment loss
- Bleeding on probing <10%
- Regular professional preventive care
- Non smoker
- Good control of diabetes

Fair

- Control of etiologic factors
- Adequate patient oral biofilm management
- Bleeding on probing >10%
- Interdental clinical attachment loss 1–4 mm
- Radiographic bones loss less than 15–33%
- Probing depths <5mm
- Class I furcation involvement
- No molar mobility

Poor

- Inadequate patient oral biofilm management due to challenges with exposed root morphology and/or dexterity issues
- Greater than 33% radiographic attachment loss
- Interdental attachment loss >5 mm
- Pocket depths >6mm
- Areas of vertical bone loss
- Furcation involvement Class II
- Molar mobility Class II
- Inadequate management of diabetes
- Tobacco use

Questionable

- Inadequate patient oral biofilm management due to challenges with exposed root morphology and/or dexterity issues
- Inadequate ongoing diabetes control
- Greater than 50% attachment loss with poor crown-to-root ratio
- Class II furcation or Class III furcation
- Greater than Class II mobility
- Root proximity
- Tobacco use
- Tooth loss due to periodontal disease

Hopeless

- Inadequate attachment to maintain the tooth

Data from McGuire, MK. Prognosis vs outcome: predicting tooth survival. *Compend Contin Educ Dent*. 2000;21:217-220, 222, 224.

- Crown-to-root ratio.
- Root form such as fused roots.

- Overall prognosis
  - Age.
  - Medical status.
  - Rate of disease progression.
  - Patient cooperation and compliance with recommendations.
  - Compliance with recommendations.
  - Oral habits and behaviors.
  - Oral health literacy

Putting It All Together

The dental hygiene student is often challenged to put together all the assessment information they have gathered to develop the diagnosis and prognosis in preparation for development of the care plan (also referred to as a treatment plan).

I. Evaluation of Assessment Data

All the assessment information provided is analyzed and interpreted in order to determine interventions for the care plan.

- The Comprehensive Patient Assessment and Diagnosis Worksheet (see **Figure 22-1**) provides an approach to gather information together in one document to assist in the development of the diagnosis, prognosis, and care or treatment plan. The form includes the following components:
  - Summary of significant medical and dental history.

Comprehensive Patient Assessment and Diagnosis Worksheet

Student Name ____________ **Patient Name** ____________ **Patient Record#** ________ **Date** ________

Medical History (significant findings):		*Relevant Dental History (dental knowledge and behaviors):* *History of NSPT: Yes/No If yes, when and what?*		
Chief Complaint (reason for visit)	Plaque Score _____%	*Gingival Description:*		Periodontal Diagnosis: Caries Diagnosis:
Local Risk Factors: ☐ Poor OH ☐ Calculus level (1, 2, 3, 4) ☐ Defective Restoration/Caries ☐ Orthodontics ☐ Malocclusion/Trauma ☐ Open Contact/Foot Retention ☐ Root Morphology/concavities ☐ Toothbrush Trauma ☐ Missing Teeth ☐ Previous HS of Perio/Reduced peridontium	**Acquired Risk Factors:** ☐ Genetics ☐ Cardio Disease ☐ Stress ☐ Obesity ☐ Endocrine Disorder ☐ Prediabetes/Diabetes ☐ Cancer ☐ Hormones ☐ Osteoporosis ☐ Hematologic Disorder ☐ Immuno-Compromised Host ☐ Nutritional Status ☐ Smoking ☐ Xerostomia ☐ Medication	**Risk Factors/Indicators:** ☐ Age, Ethnicity Gender ☐ Infrequent maintenance ☐ Knowledge level ☐ Psychological Factors ☐ Cultural Influence ☐ History of periodontal disease	**Periodontal Assessment** # of teeth/#of sites **Total Teeth** ___ ___ Bleeding ___ ___ Furcation ___ ___ Mobility ___ ___ **Probe depth** 1–3mm ___ ___ 4–5mm ___ ___ 6 or more ___ ___ **CAL:** 1–3mm ___ ___ 4–5mm ___ ___ 6 or more ___ ___	**RADIOGRAPHIC INTERPRETATION/EVALUATION** **Alveolar Bone Loss/crestal irregularities: List Tooth #s** Slight (10–20%) ______ Moderate (20–40%) ______ Severe (>40%) ______ Horizontal ______ Vertical ______ Increased PDL Width ______ Periapical Pathology ______ Close Root Proximity ______ Furcation Radiolucency's ______ Caries ______

PROGNOSIS: ***Prognosis following periodontal therapy is determined by the present of one or more of the following factors.***

GOOD = Adequate control of etiologic factors, patient self-care ability, and periodontal support.

FAIR = Adequate control of etiologic factors and patient self-care ability & less than 25% attachment loss, class I or less furcation involvement.

POOR = Greater than 50% attachment loss with class II furcation & patient self-care difficult due to location and depth of furcation.

QUESTIONABLE = Greater than 50% attachment loss with poor crown to root ration; poor root form: instrumentation access; inaccessible Class II/II furcation; > than 2+ mobility; significant root proximity.

HOPELESS = Inadequate attachment to maintain the tooth.

Source: McGuire, MK. Prognosis vs outcome: predicting tooth survival. *Compend Contin Educ* Dent. 2000; 21:217-220,222,224

PERIODONTAL CLASSIFICATION: EXTENT, SEVERITY AND STAGING/TREATMENT

	Gen. >30%	Local <30%	Grade A	Grade B	Grade C	Pro	Scaling in presence of mod-sev. inflamm.	Perio. Main.	NSPT	NSPT
HEALTH										
Gingivitis Plaque Induced										
Gingivitis Non-Plaque Induced										
Stage I Periodontitis										
Stage II Periodontitis										
Stage III Periodontitis										
Stage IV Periodontitis										
Acute Periodontal Lesions (Periodontal Abscess/ Necrotizing Periodontal Disease)										
Periodontal-Endo Lesions										
Mucogingival Conditions										
Other										

Date/Faculty/What was reviewed? ____/____/____________
____/____/____________

Figure 22-1 Comprehensive Patient Assessment and Diagnosis Worksheet. The comprehensive assessment form includes a summary of significant medical and dental history findings, client's chief complaint, periodontal and caries diagnosis, local and acquired risk factors, radiographic findings, and treatment prognosis. The form can be utilized as a worksheet for the clinician to develop the dental hygiene care plan.

Data from American Academy of Periodontics. All Parameters of Care. 2022. http://www.joponline.org/toc/jop/71/5-s; Tonetti MS, Greenwell H, Kornman KS. Staging and grading of periodontitis: Framework and proposal of a new classification and case definition. *J Periodontol.* 2018;89 Suppl 1:S159-S172; Genco RJ, Borgnakke WS. Risk factors for periodontal disease. *Periodontol 2000.* 2013;62(1):59-94; Genco RJ. Genco FD. Common risk factors in the management of periodontal and associated systemic diseases: the dental setting and interprofessional collaboration. *J Evid Based Dent Pract.* 2014;14(Suppl):4-16.

- Chief complaint.
- Risk factors.
- Summary of periodontal examination findings.
- Summary of radiographic interpretation.
- Periodontal classification.
- Diagnosis.
- Prognosis.

II. Selection of Dental Hygiene Interventions

Dental hygiene interventions are planned based on the following[2,3]:

- Evaluation of individual patients' needs to develop personal goals and the interventions to aid the patient in achieving optimal oral health.
- Clinical findings.
- Evidence-based interventions to prevent or manage oral disease.
    - Selecting interventions based on evidence from the professional literature can improve opportunities for achieving successful outcomes from dental hygiene treatment.
    - The patient can benefit when the dental hygienist has developed skills in accessing and evaluating the scientific literature.

III. Dental Hygiene Care Plan

- Chapter 23 outlines specific procedures for preparation and documentation of a formal written dental hygiene care (treatment) plan.

Documentation

- All assessment findings are documented in preparation for development of a dental hygiene care plan.
- When patient treatment records are not computerized, all entries are recorded in ink.
- All entries are dated and signed by the dental hygiene clinician.
- Standardized abbreviations are used to document all information; misunderstandings can lead to legal involvement.
- Example documentation for an assessment appointment prior to development of a dental hygiene care plan is found in **Box 22-2**.
- A suggested format for documenting a dental hygiene care plan is found in Chapter 23.

Box 22-2 Example Documentation: Assessment before Developing a Dental Hygiene Care Plan

- **S**—A 35-year-old Asian female patient presents for initial new patient visit. Patient states no dental concerns.
- **O**—Completed assessment data collected and documented, including vital signs, medical, social and dental histories, intraoral and extraoral examination findings, and dental radiographs, in preparation for developing a formal written dental hygiene care plan. All findings documented on the appropriate assessment forms.
- **A**—Analysis of assessment findings and risk factors will be reviewed prior to development of a final care plan.
- **P**—Briefly discussed assessment findings and their relevance to the care plan that will be prepared. Informed patient the dentist and dental hygienist together would complete both a comprehensive dental hygiene care plan and dental treatment plan. Explained that the plan would take into consideration all of the examination findings and assessment of risk factors for oral disease identified during this assessment appointment. Patient had no questions at this point. Appointment scheduled in 2 weeks.

Next steps: Completed plan for both dental and dental hygiene treatment will be presented to patient at next appointment, scheduled in 2 weeks.
Signed: ____________________, RDH
Date: ________________

Factors to Teach the Patient

- A clear explanation of how assessment data are used in planning dental hygiene care.
- The importance of using scientific evidence of success in the selection of patient-specific therapeutic and preventive interventions.
- Why disease control measures are learned before and monitored throughout dental hygiene care.
- Facts of oral disease prevention and oral health promotion relevant to the patient's current level of healthcare literacy and individual risk factors.
- The long-term positive effects of comprehensive continuing care.

References

1. Newsome P, Smales R, Yip K. Oral diagnosis and treatment planning: part 1. introduction. *Br Dent J*. 2012;213(1): 15-19.
2. Federation of Dental Hygiene Regulators of Canada (FDHRC). *Entry-to-Practice Canadian Competencies for Dental Hygienists*. Published2021.https://www.fdhrc.ca/wp/competency-project/. Accessed January 15, 2022.
3. American Dental Hygienists' Association. *2016 Revised Standards for Clinical Dental Hygiene Practice*. Published June 2016. https://www.adha.org/resources-docs/2016-Revised-Standards-for-Clinical-Dental-Hygiene-Practice.pdf. Accessed December 11, 2021.
4. Tonetti MS, Greenwell H, Kornman KS. Staging and grading of periodontitis: framework and proposal of a new classification and case definition. *J Periodontol*. 2018;89(Suppl 1):S159-S172.
5. Sanz M, Marco Del Castillo A, Jepsen S, et al. Periodontitis and cardiovascular diseases: consensus report. *J Clin Periodontol*. 2020;47(3):268-288.
6. Jepsen S, Caton JG, Albandar JM, et al. Periodontal manifestations of systemic diseases and developmental and acquired conditions: consensus report of workgroup 3 of the 2017 World Workshop on the Classification of Periodontal and Peri-Implant Diseases and Conditions. *J Periodontol*. 2018;89 (Suppl 1):S237-S248.
7. Gobin R, Tian D, Liu Q, Wang J. Periodontal diseases and the risk of metabolic syndrome: an updated systematic review and meta-analysis. *Front Endocrinol*. 2020;11:336.
8. Gomes-Filho IS, daCruz SS, Trindade SC, et al. Periodontitis and respiratory diseases: a systematic review with meta-analysis. *Oral Dis*. 2020;26(2):439-446.
9. Bi WG, Emami E, Luo ZC, Santamaria C, Wei SQ. Effect of periodontal treatment in pregnancy on perinatal outcomes: a systematic review and meta-analysis. *J Matern Fetal Neonatal Med*. 2021;34(19):3259-3268.
10. Featherstone JDB, Chaffee BW. The evidence for Caries Management by Risk Assessment (CAMBRA®). *Adv Dent Res*. 2018;29(1):9-14.
11. Featherstone JDB, Crystal YO, Alston P, et al. Evidence-based caries management for all ages-practical guidelines. *Front Oral Health*. 2021;2:14.
12. American Cancer Society. Risk factors for oral cavity and oropharyngeal cancers. https://www.cancer.org/cancer/oral-cavity-and-oropharyngeal-cancer/causes-risks-prevention/risk-factors.html. Accessed October 23, 2021.
13. American Society of Anethesiologists. ASA Physical Status Classification System. https://www.asahq.org/standards-and-guidelines/asa-physical-status-classification-system. Accessed December 24, 2021.
14. Ship JA, Mohammed AR. *The Clinician's Guide to Oral Health in Geriatric Patients*. American Academy of Oral Medicine; 1999.
15. Baskaradoss JK. Relationship between oral health literacy and oral health status. *BMC Oral Health*. 2018;18(1):172.
16. Sanz M, Herrera D, Kebschull M, et al. Treatment of stage I-III periodontitis: the EFP S3 level clinical practice guideline. *J Clin Periodontol*. 2020;47(Suppl 22):4-60.
17. American Academy of Pediatric Dentistry. Parameters of Care. *J Periodontol*. 2000;71(5 Suppl):847-883.
18. American Dental Hygienists' Association. *Diagnosis-Position Paper*. Published online September 2015. https://www.adha.org/resources-docs/Diagnosis-Position-Paper.pdf. Accessed January 20, 2022.
19. Nunn ME, Carney WG, McNally SJ. The Miller-McEntire score for molars provides an evidence-based approach to assigning periodontal prognosis for molar teeth. *J Evid Based Dent Pract*. 2015;15(2):73-76.
20. Muzzi L, Nieri M, Cattabriga M, Rotundo R, Cairo F, Pini Prato GP. The potential prognostic value of some periodontal factors for tooth loss: a retrospective multilevel analysis on periodontal patients treated and maintained over 10 years. *J Periodontol*. 2006;77(12):2084-2089.
21. McGowan T, McGowan K, Ivanovski S. A novel evidence-based periodontal prognosis model. *J Evid Based Dent Pract*. 2017;17(4):350-360.

CHAPTER 23

The Dental Hygiene Care Plan

Linda D. Boyd, RDH, RD, EdD
Catherine G. Ranson, RDH, MET

CHAPTER OUTLINE

LEARNING OBJECTIVES

After studying this chapter, the student will be able to:

1. Discuss objectives for developing a dental hygiene care plan and how it fits within the comprehensive treatment plan.
2. Identify the components of a dental hygiene care plan.
3. Prepare a written dental hygiene care plan from a dental hygiene diagnosis.
4. Apply procedures for discussing a care plan with the dentist and the patient.
5. Identify and apply measures for obtaining informed consent and informed refusal.

Preparation of a Dental Hygiene Care Plan

A formal, written, evidence-based **dental hygiene care plan** is an essential component of the comprehensive dental treatment plan.[1,2]

I. Objectives

Objectives of the dental hygiene care plan include the following:

- Address patient needs identified from assessment data.
- Reassess previous treatment goals and identify barriers to success.
- Develop treatment goals in collaboration with the patient to address problems and modifiable risk factors.
- Identify treatment option interventions and recommendations based on current scientific evidence including the need for referral.
- **Prioritize** the sequence of education, preventive services, and treatment in the care plan.
- Collaborate with the dentist to integrate the dental hygiene care plan into the comprehensive dental treatment plan (**Table 23-1**).

Components of a Written Care Plan

- A dental hygiene care plan may be written using a variety of formats.
- Software for electronic patient records include a treatment plan template that can be used to develop a dental hygiene care plan.
- **Figure 23-1** is a suggested template for a patient-specific care plan that follows the dental hygiene process of care.
- The recommended components of a written care plan are described in this section.

Table 23-1 Components of a Comprehensive Dental Treatment Plan

Phase	Procedures	Included in the Dental Hygiene Care Plan
Phase 1 Urgent/Diagnostic	▪ Emergency care (pain, biopsy)	
	▪ Consultation with medical providers and provide referrals as needed	
	▪ Summary of information from assessment	✓
	▪ Develop dental hygiene diagnosis	✓
	▪ Establish patient-centered oral health goals	✓
Phase 2 Disease Control	▪ Dental biofilm control by patient	✓
	▪ Additional preventive measures (e.g., diet changes, fluorides, mouthguard) to address modifiable risk factors	✓
	▪ Professional supra- and subgingival biofilm and calculus removal	✓
	▪ Restore cavitated lesions and correct conditions impairing biofilm removal (e.g., overhangs)	
Outcomes Evaluation of Phase 2	▪ Evaluation of oral health goals and revise as needed	✓
	▪ Periodontal assessment data	✓
	▪ Adequacy of dental biofilm control by patient	✓
	▪ Patient compliance with treatment recommendations	✓
Phase III Rehabilitation or Corrective Therapy	▪ Periodontal surgery if healing was inadequate from nonsurgical periodontal therapy	
	▪ Endodontic	
	▪ Orthodontics	
	▪ Fixed/removable prostheses	
	▪ Implant placement	
Maintenance or Supportive Therapy	▪ Appointments for continuing care and re-evaluation	✓
	▪ Refining patient biofilm control techniques and management of modifiable risk facts	✓

PATIENT SPECIFIC DENTAL HYGIENE CARE PLAN

Patient Name: Age: Gender: Record #: Date:

Initial Therapy Maintenance Re-evaluation

Health /Social History Findings Impacting Treatment:

ASA Classification: ____________

Systemic Disease: ____________

Medications: ____________

Health Behaviors/Cultural Factors: ____________

Modifiable Risk Factors:

Related to Dental Hygiene Diagnosis: ____________

____

Related to Periodontal Diagnosis: ____________

____

Dental Hygiene Diagnosis (Related to Risk Factors and Etiology):

Periodontal Diagnosis and Status (Active or Stable, Classification, Extent, Stage, Grade):

Caries Management Risk Assessment (CAMBRA) level: ☐ Low ☐ Moderate ☐ High ☐ Extreme

Medical and Dental Referrals Required:

Radiographic Exposures Completed/Interpreted: (identify film or digital)

☐ PAN ☐ FMX ☐ 2 BWX ☐ 4/6 BWX

Initial Biofilm Score:

Planned Interventions (to arrest or control disease and regenerate, restore, or maintain health)		
Clinical/Addresses DH Diagnosis and Periodontal Diagnosis	**Education/Counseling**	**Oral Hygiene Instruction/ Oral Self - Care (evidence-based & patient centered rationale)**
1)		
2)		

Recommended Oral Self-Care Aids:

Recommended Preventive Agents and Chemotherapeutics (include type and percentage) (home use)

☐ Dentifrices: ☐ Mouthrinses: ☐ Fluoride:

Expected Outcomes		
Patient - Centered Goals	**Evaluation Methods**	**Time Frame**
1)		
2)		

Figure 23-1 Patient-Specific Dental Hygiene Care Plan. The written care plan includes a summary of assessment findings and modifiable risk factors, the dental hygiene diagnosis, planned dental hygiene interventions, expected outcomes based on patient-centered goals, an appointment plan that sequences treatment procedures and education interventions for each appointment, and a section for patient signature indicating informed consent for the planned care.

Previous Treatment Goals Met/Not Met:

Recommended Dental Hygiene Treatment

- ☐ Prophylaxis
- ☐ Periodontal Maintenance
- ☐ Non-Surgical Periodontal Therapy: Quadrant(s): ________
- ☐ Non-Surgical Periodontal Therapy 1-3 Teeth ________________
- ☐ Scaling in the Presence of Inflammation
- ☐ Local Anesthesia:
- ☐ Power Scaling
- ☐ Selective Polish Agent:
- ☐ Topical Fluoride: Agent:
- ☐ Sealants: Tooth #(s)
- ☐ Custom Tray: Type
- ☐ Education
- ☐ Nutritional Analysis
- ☐ Other:

Estimated Number of Treatment Appointments:

Recommended Maintenance or Continuing Care Interval with Rationale:

Appointment Plan (sequence of planned interventions)	
Appt#	**Plan for Treatment, Services** **Plan for Education, Counseling, and Oral Hygiene Instruction**

Figure 23-1 (*Continued*)

I. Individual Patient Considerations

- Basic demographic information, such as age, gender identity, etc.
- Patient chief complaint or concerns.
- Social determinants of health including transportation, oral health literacy, access to healthy food, financial situation, etc.[2,3]
  - In Canada, this includes Jordan's Principle to ensure First Nations children have access to care.[2]
- Health and oral health beliefs/cultural beliefs.[4,5]
  - Cultural sensitivity is an important aspect of working with a patient to determine what options for care best meet their needs and fit within their belief system.

II. Assessment Findings and Risk Factors

This section of the plan contains a summarized description of significant findings.

A. Medical, Social, and Dental History

- American Society of Anesthesiologists (ASA) classification.
- Systemic diseases and conditions: Current and past.
- Medications.
- Health behaviors.
- Dental anxiety.
- Cultural factors.
- Functional assessment.

B. Health Risk Factors

- Increased risk of systemic disease due to oral infection.
- Potential for compromised treatment outcomes.

III. Periodontal Classification

- Periodontal classification (stage and grade). (See Chapter 19.)

IV. Caries Risk

- Utilize patient's caries risk level and modifiable risk factors for dental caries to guide the preventive aspects of the dental hygiene care plan. (See Chapter 25.)
- For instance:
  - Selection of treatment interventions, such as oral self-care, dental sealants, fluoride, chlorhexidine, etc.

V. Diagnosis

- There may be multiple diagnoses based on analysis of the assessment data.
- Provides the basis for the treatment or care plan.
- Examples of dental hygiene diagnostic statements can be found in Chapter 22.

VI. Patient-Centered Oral Health Goals

- Based on the diagnosis, the clinician will collaborate with the patient to create goals for the outcomes of treatment linked to the dental hygiene disease status and modifiable risk factors.
- The establishment of patient-centered goals is designed to accomplish the following:
  - Prioritize the modifiable risk factors for oral health disease.
  - Reflect priorities for the patient.
  - Address cognitive, psychomotor, and affective aspects of the patient-specific oral health needs.
  - Describe observable behaviors with measurable outcomes.
  - Define the time frame to achieve the goal.

VII. Planned Interventions

Dental hygiene interventions are measures applied to prevent, regenerate, restore, or maintain oral health and are specific to the individual patient's assessment findings and patient-centered goals. The interventions may include[1,2,6]:

- Education and counseling in topics such as etiology and progression of oral disease and elimination of risk factors.
- Individualized oral hygiene instructions and personal daily oral self-care regimens based on patient needs and abilities.
- Preventive measures, such as dental sealants, to maintain tooth integrity.
- Clinical treatments, such as nonsurgical periodontal therapy (subgingival instrumentation) and debridement, to arrest or control existing disease.
  - **Table 23-2** provides some considerations for care or treatment planning for periodontal therapy.

VIII. Expected Outcomes

A plan for treatment outcomes or goals, created in consultation with the patient:

- Identify short-term goals to move the patient toward the long-term goal to enhance success. (See Chapter 24.)
- Clearly define how progress toward each goal will be measured.
- Identify a realistic time frame for measuring success of treatment goal outcomes.

XI. Re-evaluation

- Re-evaluation is an essential component of assessing treatment outcomes. (See Chapter 44.)
- At the re-evaluation appointment[1,2]:
  - New assessment data are collected and analyzed. For instance:
    - Following initial treatment, such as nonsurgical periodontal therapy assessment, data should be collected at a subsequent appointment for comparison to assess resolution in pocket depths, bleeding, and improved management of oral biofilm.
  - Determine if the treatment goals have been met, partially met, or not met and revise treatment goals as needed.
  - Determine the continuing care or maintenance appointment interval.

X. Appointment Sequence

- Prioritize interventions.
- Outline a sequence of interventions.

Table 23-2 Periodontal Treatment Planning Considerations[4]

Clinical Diagnosis	Therapeutic Goals	Treatment Considerations
Biofilm-induced gingivitis	■ To establish gingival health through elimination of etiologic factors	■ Individualized patient education based on modifiable risk factors ■ Attainment of adequate biofilm control ■ Supra- and subgingival debridement ■ Restorative correction of biofilm-retentive factors
Stage I–III Periodontitis ■ Slight to moderate loss of periodontal support	■ To arrest progression of disease and prevent recurrence ■ To preserve health and function	■ Individualized patient education based on modifiable risk factors (e.g., tobacco cessation) ■ Management of chronic disease (e.g., diabetes) ■ Attainment of adequate biofilm control ■ Supra- and subgingival debridement • Often divided into quadrant or half mouth subgingival instrumentation appointments depending on severity of disease ■ Restorative correction of biofilm-retentive factors ■ Adjunctive antimicrobial agents ■ If resolution of the condition does not occur, consider periodontal surgery in pocket depths > 6 mm
Stage IV Periodontitis ■ Advanced loss of periodontal support	■ To alter or eliminate microbial etiology and infrabony defects ■ To arrest progression of disease	■ Initial therapy as described for Stages I–III ■ If resolution of the condition does not occur, consider periodontal surgery ■ In a compromised patient unable to tolerate survey, provide additional localized subgingival debridement along with ongoing maintenance care
Periodontal maintenance or supportive periodontal care	■ To minimize the recurrence and progression of the disease ■ To reduce the incidence of tooth loss	■ Comparison of clinical data to previous baseline measurements ■ Assessment of biofilm management and refinement of oral self-care ■ Counseling on control of modifiable risk factors ■ Thorough subgingival removal of biofilm

- Can be modified at each appointment to respond to new information or an immediate need of the patient.

Additional Considerations

I. Role of the Patient

A. Purpose

- The willingness and/or ability of the patient to participate in reducing risk factors and changing oral health behaviors will be the key to reaching goals set during planning.

B. Procedure

- Determine the patient's level of understanding of dental diseases, risk factors, and oral health behaviors.
- Determine the patient's physical ability to manipulate recommended oral care aids.
- Determine **lifestyle factors** and oral health beliefs that impact the patient's ability to comply with oral health recommendations.
- Educate patients regarding the importance of their role in eliminating modifiable risk factors, setting oral health goals, and complying with recommendations.

II. Pain and Anxiety Control

A. Purpose

- Control of discomfort during treatment procedures will enhance patient compliance with completion of the dental hygiene care plan.

B. Procedures

- When there is a patient complaint of pain or discomfort, treat those areas first.

- For a patient with dental anxiety, the clinician may choose to treat either the quadrant with the fewest teeth or the least severe periodontal infection first to ensure the following:
    - Make the first scaling less complicated.
    - Help orient an anxious patient to clinical procedures.
- If there is no dental anxiety, treat the quadrant with more severe disease first so that healing can be monitored at the following appointments.
- When two quadrants are to be treated at the same appointment, selecting a maxillary and mandibular quadrant on the same side minimizes the patient's posttreatment discomfort.
- The need for local anesthesia is determined by:
    - Depth, bleeding, and severity of inflammation of periodontal pockets and furcation involvement.
    - The patient's previous pain control experiences.
    - Consistency and distribution of calculus.
    - Potential patient discomfort during scaling.
    - Sensitivity of the patient's tissues during instrumentation.

Sequencing and Prioritizing Patient Care

I. Objectives

Reasons for preparing a well-sequenced dental hygiene care plan are:

A. To Provide Evidence-Based, Individualized Patient Care

- Determined by analysis of assessment data.
- Based on evidence-based approaches to care.
- Enhanced by the clinician's clinical judgment in applying evidence-based care.

B. To Eliminate or Control Etiologic and Predisposing Disease Factors and Prevent Recurrence of Disease

- Educate patient on etiologic agents in both dental caries and periodontal diseases.
- Dental hygiene interventions should address modifiable risk factors to minimize or prevent progression of oral disease.
    - Counseling on prevention measures and elimination of modifiable risk factors.
    - Instruction in daily oral self-care techniques.
    - Encouragement of regularly scheduled maintenance follow-up for dental hygiene care.

C. To Eliminate the Signs and Symptoms of Disease

- Measures to eliminate signs of infection such as gingival bleeding and probing depths are included in the care plan.

II. Factors Affecting Sequence of Care

Treatment sequence defines the order in which the parts of an individual dental hygiene care plan are to be carried out. Sequence planning involves:

- Identification of overall treatment and education patterns appropriate for an individual patient's needs.
- Outline of a series of appointments, with specific services, treatment procedures, and educational interventions included.
- The sequence should be flexible to adjust to meet the patient needs.
    - For instance, the dental hygiene care plan may be for nonsurgical periodontal therapy on the maxillary and mandibular right. When the patient arrives, they have an unexpected meeting and can only stay to complete one quadrant so another appointment is added to the plan.

A. Urgency

Discomfort or pain that requires urgent care could apply to:

- An area with an abscess.
- Severe carious lesion(s).
- Mucositis or other mucosal lesions.

B. Existing Etiologic Factors

- In patients with periodontal disease or risk for dental caries, success of the treatment depends on thorough, daily biofilm removal.
    - Biofilm control measures are introduced, and success is evaluated before additional oral hygiene aids are presented so the patient does not become overwhelmed.

C. Severity and Extent of the Condition

- The number and length of appointments and the sequencing of procedures planned are affected by the severity of the condition.

- Findings that indicate the severity of gingival or periodontal infection include:
  - Changes in color, size, shape, or consistency of the gingiva.
  - Probing depths.
  - Bleeding on probing.
  - Suppuration or exudate.
  - Mobility of the teeth.
  - Furcation involvement.
  - Clinical and radiographic signs of attachment or bone loss.

D. Individual Patient Requirements

Items from a patient's history that may require adaptation in appointment length, spacing, or sequencing when planning dental hygiene care include:

- Antibiotic premedication
  - Current recommended standard prophylactic regimens and a list of conditions that require antibiotic premedication are found in Chapter 11.
  - Efficient use of appointment time and/or spacing of appointment dates will avoid unnecessary extra antibiotic coverage.
- Systemic diseases
  - Chronic disease may influence the complexity of the procedure(s) and length of appointments.
  - The patient should be educated on the associations between periodontitis and systemic conditions that may influence oral disease. For instance, poorly controlled diabetes may result in progression and more severe periodontitis. This may in turn, worsen diabetes control.[7]
- Disability
  - Physical limitations will require adaptation of the appointment plan. (See Chapter 51.)
  - Intellectual disabilities, Alzheimer's disease, and dementia may require adjustments to the dental hygiene care plan and require more engagement of a caregiver to assist the patient.

Presenting the Dental Hygiene Care Plan

Before treatment begins, the dental hygiene care plan must be coordinated with a comprehensive treatment plan.

I. Presenting the Plan to the Collaborating Dentist

A. Purpose

- To integrate the dental hygiene care plan into the patient's comprehensive treatment plan.
- To provide a coordinated dental and dental hygiene statement to the patient regarding oral health needs.

B. Procedure

- Follow sequence on the patient's written care plan.
- Summarize demographic data.
- Summarize major systemic and dental health assessment findings.
- Summarize risk factors.
- Summarize periodontal assessment findings.
- Provide the preliminary periodontal classification for confirmation by the dentist (if required in your scope of practice).
- Indicate suggested intervention strategies, goals, expected outcomes, and referrals to other health-care providers.
- Outline suggested appointment sequence and services to be provided.
- Be prepared to give detail and answer questions.

II. Explaining the Plan to the Patient

- Good communication skills are essential to build a trusting relationship with the patient.
- Use of radiographs and an intraoral camera during presentation of the plan for care provides visual documentation of need for oral health interventions.
- Using a motivational interviewing approach while discussing the plan can help determine and respond to the patient's readiness to change health behaviors that increase risk for oral disease. (See Chapter 24.)

A. Purpose

- To provide the patient with information needed to give **informed consent** for treatment.
- To reinforce the patient's role in setting and reaching oral health goals outlined in the plan.

B. Procedure

- Position the patient in an upright position, face-to-face with clinician.
- Use terminology appropriate to the patient's level of oral health literacy.
- If appropriate, educate the patient regarding link between systemic and their oral disease.
- Present information using visual aids such as the patient's own radiographs, dental models,

drawings or pictures, videotapes, brochures, or an intraoral camera.

- Educate the patient regarding recommended dental hygiene services, appointment sequence, expected outcomes, and referrals to other healthcare providers.
- Engage the patient in planning and setting goals.
- Be prepared to give detail and answer questions.
- Obtained signed informed consent.

Informed Consent

- Obtaining **consent** is about providing relevant information so that an educated decision about treatment can be made by the patient.[2,8,9]
- It is every patient's right to possess knowledge that will[8,9]:
  - Aid the patient in making optimal decisions for their oral health.
  - Allow shared decision making with the oral care provider while treatment is being planned.
- Adequate documentation of informed consent in the patient's record includes evidence that the patient has received the information listed in **Box 23-1**.[2,3]
- Informed consent is a legal concept that can exist even without a written document.
- Informed consent can be lacking even when a document has been signed if the patient has not had the opportunity to comprehend and evaluate the risks and benefits of the suggested treatment.[8,9]
- **Implied consent**, granted by the patient's presence in the dental chair, only applies to nontreatment procedures, such as data collection, and treatment planning.

Box 23-1 Criteria for Adequate Content in Informed Consent[10,11]

- Complete description of the procedure including:
  - The patient's diagnosis
  - Nature and purpose of proposed treatment
  - Rationale for treatment
  - Duration of treatment
  - Effects of patient's current medical status on treatment.
- Risks and limitations of the proposed treatment, including probability of risk occurring.
- Benefits of the treatment including prognosis.
- Alternative evidence-based treatment options available, including no treatment and the consequences of no treatment.
- Purpose of treatment.
- Demonstration the patient understands the information and has had all questions answered.
  - Invite the patient to tell the clinician what they understand about the information provided to ensure understanding.
  - For those with limited English language skills, a translator may be needed (and required in some states).
  - For the visually impaired, the document may need to be provided in an alternative format.
  - For minors and individuals with cognitive impairment, the legal guardian must be included in discussion of treatment options in order to provide informed consent.[10,12]
- Demonstration of informed consent or informed refusal must be signed by the patient or guardian.

Data from American Academy of Pediatric Dentistry. Guideline on informed consent. Revised 2015. https://www.aapd.org/globalassets/media/policies_guidelines/bp_informedconsent.pdf. Accessed July 4, 2019; Glick A, Taylor D, Valenza JA, Walji MF. Assessing the content, presentation, and readability of dental informed consents. *J Dent Educ.* 2010;74(8):849-861.

I. Informed Consent Procedures

- **Box 23-2** provides information for obtaining informed consent.
- The patient must be informed of all evidence-based treatment options available, choose the treatment option, and provide informed consent or informed refusal to follow the recommendations in the agreed-upon care plan.
- It may be necessary to provide forms written in simpler terms, larger print, or the patient's primary language.
- Patients do not always remember the information they received during informed consent; therefore, written documentation of all information provided for the patient is essential.[13]
- Review your state's, province's, or country's laws related to informed consent, as often a signature of the patient (or guardian), dental provider, and a witness may be required prior to beginning treatment.

II. Informed Refusal

- The patient's right to autonomy in making decisions regarding oral treatment requires that practitioners respect a patient's decision to refuse treatment.[10,11]
- **Informed refusal of care** as well as any recommended treatment options must be documented in the patient's permanent record.

Box 23-2 Informed Consent[10,11]

Information to Disclose

- *Diagnosis*: Description of patient's problem(s).
- *Treatment*: Description and purpose of the proposed treatment(s).
- *Alternatives*: Evidence-based alternatives to the proposed treatment(s).
- *Consequences*: Risks and benefits of all proposed treatment alternatives, including physical and psychological effects and costs.
- *Prognosis*: Expected outcome with treatment(s), with alternative treatment(s), and without treatment.

Principles of Informing

- Assess the patient's ability to give informed consent.
- Oral health literacy and cognitive ability may require adjusting the terminology so the patient can understand.
- Encourage the patient (or legal guardian) to ask questions.
- Continue to assess the patient's understanding and answer questions as often as necessary.
- Document all relevant factors and include the signed form in patient record.

- Depending on the state or province practice act, this may or may not protect clinicians who provide treatment that does not meet the standard of care from legal action.
  - According to the American Academy of Pediatric Dentistry, an informed refusal typically does not release the provider from the standard of care and the patient can be asked to get a second opinion or be dismissed from the practice.[10]

Documentation

- A written dental hygiene care plan documents all information related to each component of the formal plan as described in this chapter and illustrated in Figure 23-1.
- Example documentation for a patient appointment to explain the dental hygiene care plan and obtain informed consent is found in **Box 23-3**.

Box 23-3 Example Documentation: Presentation of Care Plan and Informed Consent for Dental Hygiene Care

- **S**—A 35-year-old female patient presents 2 weeks following assessment data collection appointment. Patient expects to discuss the formal written dental hygiene care plan related to periodontal treatment.
- **O**—No changes in patient's health history or other relevant assessment findings since previous appointment for data collection. Written dental hygiene care and comprehensive treatment plan completed and available.
- **A**—Patient appeared engaged in the discussion and eager to begin treatment.
- **P**—Explained all assessment findings and risk factors; discussed dental hygiene diagnosis, patient-centered oral health goals, planned interventions, expected outcomes of treatment, and referrals to other healthcare providers. Responded to numerous questions related to the rationale for scheduling multiple treatment appointments. Patient stated that all questions had been answered, then signed/dated the informed consent form. Copy of signed care plan was given to patient and a copy was placed in the patient record.

Next step: Begin treatment as described for appointment #1 on the care plan form.

Signed: ______________________, RDH

Date: ____________

Factors to Teach the Patient

- The purpose of the dental hygiene care plan.
- The importance of collaboration of the dental team with the patient to develop treatment goals to guide the care plan.
- The responsibility of the patient to improve the success of the treatment planned to attain optimal oral health.
- The patient's rights and responsibilities regarding informed consent and refusal.

References

1. American Dental Hygienists' Association. 2016 Revised Standards for Clinical Dental Hygiene Practice. Published June 2016. https://www.adha.org/resources-docs/2016-Revised-Standards-for-Clinical-Dental-Hygiene-Practice.pdf. Accessed December 11, 2021.
2. Federation of Dental Hygiene Regulators of Canada (FDHRC). *Entry-to-Practice Canadian Competencies for Dental Hygienists*. Published 2021. https://www.fdhrc.ca/wp/competency-project/. Accessed January 15, 2022.
3. Healthy People 2030, US Department of Health and Human Services, Office of Disease Prevention and Health Promotion. Social determinants of health. https://health.gov/healthypeople/objectives-and-data/social-determinants-health. Accessed January 22, 2022.
4. Smith A, MacEntee MI, Beattie BL, et al. The influence of culture on the oral health-related beliefs and behaviours of elderly Chinese immigrants: a meta-synthesis of the literature. *J Cross Cult Gerontol*. 2013;28(1):27-47.
5. Butani Y, Weintraub JA, Barker JC. Oral health-related cultural beliefs for four racial/ethnic groups: assessment of the literature. *BMC Oral Health*. 2008;8(1):26.
6. Sanz M, Herrera D, Kebschull M, et al. Treatment of stage I-III periodontitis: the EFP S3 level clinical practice guideline. *J Clin Periodontol*. 2020;47(Suppl 22):4-60.
7. Cao R, Li Q, Wu Q, Yao M, Chen Y, Zhou H. Effect of non-surgical periodontal therapy on glycemic control of type 2 diabetes mellitus: a systematic review and Bayesian network meta-analysis. *BMC Oral Health*. 2019;19(1):176.
8. Moreira NCF, Pachêco-Pereira C, Keenan L, Cummings G, Flores-Mir C. Informed consent comprehension and recollection in adult dental patients: a systematic review. *J Am Dent Assoc*. 2016;147(8):605-619.e7.
9. Pietrzykowski T, Smilowska K. The reality of informed consent: empirical studies on patient comprehension-systematic review. *Trials*. 2021;22(1):57.
10. American Academy of Pediatric Dentistry. Informed consent. Published online 2019. https://www.aapd.org/globalassets/media/policies_guidelines/bp_informedconsent.pdf. Accessed January 22, 2022.
11. Glick A, Taylor D, Valenza JA, Walji MF. Assessing the content, presentation, and readability of dental informed consents. *J Dent Ed*. 2010;74(8):849-861.
12. Conti A, Delbon P, Laffranchi L, Paganelli C. Consent in dentistry: ethical and deontological issues. *J Med Ethics*. 2013;39(1):59-61.
13. Ferrús-Torres E, Valmaseda-Castellón E, Berini-Aytés L, Gay-Escoda C. Informed consent in oral surgery: the value of written information. *J Oral Maxillofac Surg*. 2011;69(1):54-58.

SECTION VI

Implementation: Prevention

Introduction for Section VI

The aim of health promotion and disease prevention is to help each patient accept responsibility for lifelong health practices and daily oral self-care regimens that prevent oral disease.

- Implementation of the prevention care plan is a significant component of both the dental hygiene care plan and the total treatment plan.
- The influence of oral health on total body health may be a new concept for many patients.
- In the sequence of patient treatment, introduction to preventive measures occurs first, before treatment interventions are implemented.

The Dental Hygiene Process of Care

- The implementation phase of the Dental Hygiene Process of Care, illustrated in **Figure VI-1**, provides the dental hygiene interventions identified in a patient's dental hygiene care plan.
- Dental hygiene patient education and counseling interventions are:
  - The basis for oral health promotion and disease prevention.
  - Selected using individualized patient assessment data.
  - Designed to meet oral health goals developed in concert with the patient.
- The patient's commitment to daily self-care before and after treatment is essential to keep the teeth and gingival tissues free from new or recurrent disease caused by the microorganisms of dental biofilm.
- The dental hygienist has the responsibility to:
  - Consider each patient's current oral health practices, cultural factors, physical abilities, and life circumstances when implementing the preventive care plan.
  - Implement dental hygiene interventions for each patient that attain and maintain oral health and contribute to systemic health.
  - Educate about oral disease and prevention modalities based on individualized patient needs.
  - Identify an approach that will motivate each patient to accept and adhere to recommended preventive procedures and self-care protocols.

Ethical Applications

- When complex ethical issues and dilemmas arise in the dental setting, the ethically competent dental hygienist can:
  - Understand the patient perspective.
  - View a concern from various perspectives.
  - Determine who is responsible.
  - Document and share clear, concise, and objective evidence.
  - Communicate clearly with all parties involved in the situation.
  - Act within acceptable moral standards to determine an acceptable decision.

- To resolve an ethical dilemma, the dental hygienist can use professional judgment, reflection about dental hygiene core values, and the components of moral reasoning.
- Solving an ethical dilemma often leads to the examination of issues using questions, as listed in **Table VI-1**.

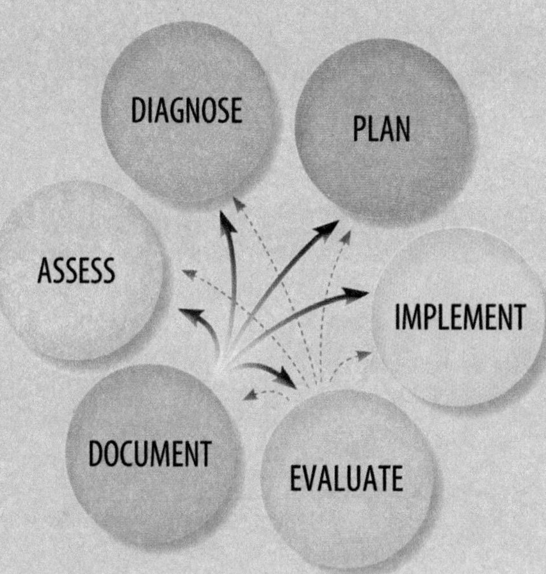

Figure VI-1 The Dental Hygiene Process of Care

Table VI-1 Decision Alternatives through Questioning

Ethical Decision Concept	Questions to Ask	Application Examples
Recognize conflict	What are the specific details of the case? Are there issues of rights or moral character involved? At what level does the conflict exist?	Consider the role of the dental hygienist for each of the ethical principles outlined in the code of ethics.
Accumulate possible options	What alternative actions are available? Whose interests are at stake? What resources would other professionals use?	Review the Dental Practice Act to determine limitations of actions that can be taken by the dental hygienist, the dentist, and other healthcare providers.
Evaluate the alternatives	Which decision would lead to the best consequences overall? Are all individuals involved being respected and treated fairly? Which alternative(s) could be developed into a general rule to follow?	Review the entries in a patient's record to determine if all points of view from the case have been included.
Reflect on the decision	Can the action taken be justified as the best choice? What alternative actions could be selected?	Discuss a similar situation at the next office/staff meeting to enhance responsiveness to ethical protocols and evaluate the course of action.

CHAPTER 24

Preventive Counseling and Behavior Change

Marsha A. Voelker, CDA, RDH, MS

CHAPTER OUTLINE

LEARNING OBJECTIVES

After studying this chapter, the student will be able to:

1. Explain the steps in a preventive program, identify the need to conduct preventive counseling, and describe the proper setting.
2. Describe the importance of partnering with the patient to come up with a plan for change.
3. Describe and explain the methods of motivational interviewing.
4. Describe how to recognize and explore the patient's ambivalence and describe techniques to elicit and recognize change talk.
5. Understand and explain various plans to strengthen the patient's commitment for change.

The dental hygienist is a primary care provider of preventive services. A specialist in oral health care, the dental hygienist is involved at all levels of prevention.

- Within the process of dental hygiene care, the needs of a patient are assessed from the histories and clinical findings. Then a dental hygiene diagnosis is made, and the care plan is outlined.
- When planning the sequence of treatment for the patient, initiation of preventive measures precedes clinical services except in an emergency.
- Oral health can only be attained and maintained if the patient learns and practices proper daily self-care.

Steps in a Preventive Program

Each patient needs a preventive care plan. To plan and carry out a program takes a collaborative effort by the patient and members of the dental team.

I. Assess the Patient's Needs

- Review all information from the histories, radiographic data, clinical examinations, and chartings.
- Identify the presence and severity of infection and the risk factors for systemic and oral disease.
- Utilize indices to evaluate the extent of the need and provide a baseline for continuing comparisons.
- For most patients, a dental biofilm score can be helpful to show the patient the extent of bacterial accumulation.
- A discussion of caries and periodontal risk factors illustrates the dental concerns to the patient.
- The patient's use of oral aids (toothbrushing, flossing, interproximal aids) is assessed for proper technique.
- Factors to consider during assessment:
    - Explore what will work for the patient to make the needed changes.
    - Determine the patient's **motivation** and confidence to make changes.
    - Consider what the patient values. The cultural values and beliefs can either promote or block the patient's efforts to make an oral health change.

II. Plan for Interventions

- Apply information about the patient, such as educational level, occupation, socioeconomic background, cultural influences, and attitudes regarding oral care.
- Determine the current personal oral care procedures carried out by the patient and their frequency.
- Note factors that may affect the patient's dexterity when using oral cleaning devices. This information is helpful when the clinician is determining the appropriate oral health aid options to provide the patient.
- Recognize the influence of age, physical limitations, and cognitive disabilities. Determine whether another person (parent or other caregiver) is needed to carry out the necessary procedures.
- Discuss procedures needed and develop goals, both short- and long-term, with the patient.
- Discuss with the patient the expected oral health clinical outcomes.

III. Implement the Plan

- Initiate **preventive counseling** to help the patient become aware of oral health problems. This includes **learning** and practicing more effective health **behaviors**.
- Explore what oral aids and preventive measures the patient utilizes daily and motivation for oral self-care.
- Show methods for self-**evaluation**.
- Explore the patient's diet in relation to caries risk or periodontal conditions. (See Chapter 33).
- Introduce tobacco cessation when indicated. (See Chapter 32.)
- Change takes time and preventive counseling needs to be revisited at each appointment.

IV. Perform Clinical Preventive Services

- Scaling for complete calculus and biofilm removal.
- Application of caries-preventive agents: such as fluoride and/or dental sealants. (See Chapters 34 and 35.)

V. Evaluate Progressive Changes

- Have the patient demonstrate procedures for oral self-care to determine a need for modifications in technique.
- Record a dental biofilm score at each appointment and compare previous recordings with the patient.
- At appropriate intervals, perform periodontal probing to note improvement or changes in tissue quality, bleeding on probing, and probing depths.
- For goals that have not been met, collaborate with the patient to revise them.

VI. Plan Short- and Long-Term Continuing Care

- Determine appropriate maintenance intervals.
- Re-evaluate to monitor continuance of preventive practices.
- Provide supplemental care for the patient who does not respond to initial therapy.

Patient Counseling

- Personalized preventive counseling contributes to the knowledge, values, and practices of the individual. Then, through the individual, these ideas can be passed on to the family and the community.
- Periodontal infections and dental caries can be prevented or controlled and, therefore, teeth preserved throughout the lifetime of the individual.
- An intra- and extraoral examination is done to recognize possible pathology requiring exfoliative cytology and/or biopsy.
- For most patients, focus is placed on prevention and control of dental caries and/or periodontal infection.
- Other preventive measures involving oral trauma need to be brought to the patient's attention, such as mouth protectors for contact sports and accidents that lead to fractured anterior teeth in children.
- Knowledge and belief in health facts are not enough. Benefits result only when a partnership between the clinician and patient is established and patient **autonomy** is taken into consideration.

I. When to Conduct

- Preventive counseling is conducted after the clinician has completed the patient assessment.
- When having a conversation regarding preventive strategies, clinicians need to remember the patient is the decision maker and is key to making a sustainable **behavior change**.
- Preventive counseling is provided at each appointment to follow-up on the goals, both short- and long-term, established at the previous appointment.
- By revisiting goals at each appointment, the clinician is aware of how the patient is progressing toward the established oral health change. An example is provided in **Box 24-1**.
- Clinicians need to recognize that health behavior changes do not happen after one preventive counseling session.

Box 24-1 Example of Revisiting Patient Progress at Subsequent Appointments

- The patient's long-term goal is to floss 7 days a week and short-term goal is to begin flossing at least 3 days a week. The patient comes for the 3-month continuing care appointment and has only been flossing two times a week.
- Clinician provides affirmation about the progress the patient has made by flossing twice a week.
  - The clinician elicits from the patient obstacles encountered and ideas to overcome those obstacles.
  - The clinician may find out the floss is breaking a lot when flossing or not getting into the embrasure space well.
- Therefore, the clinician will need to explore and elicit from the patient what other options may work to be successful.

- Patient education may take multiple sessions before progress is made toward change. An example would be patients who are smokers who may require multiple quit attempts due to the addictive nature of nicotine.

II. The Setting for Preventive Counseling

- Usually, preventive counseling will take place in the dental hygiene treatment room with the patient placed in an upright position in the dental chair.
- The most effective counseling approach is with the clinician sitting face-to-face with the patient in a neutral position and maintaining eye contact.
- Face-to-face positioning style allows the patient to recognize the clinician is attentive, focused, and **listening** as well as builds a trusting relationship.
- Providing the appropriate setting for the clinician to explore the patient's ideas and thoughts toward an oral health behavior change is needed to maintain patient autonomy.

Patient Motivation and Behavior Change

- Control and management of oral health conditions are dependent upon the oral self-care and **compliance** of the patient.[1]
- Traditionally, behavior change in the dental field has been approached in a prescriptive, authoritative manner where the clinician provides the information and shows the patient what to do.[2]

Table 24-1 Key Concepts of the Health Belief Model

Perceived susceptibility	Chances of getting a condition
Perceived severity	Seriousness of the disease and the effects
Perceived benefits	Effectiveness of the recommended action to reduce risk
Perceived barriers	Tangible and psychological costs of the recommended action
Cues to action	Strategies to motivate readiness
Self-efficacy	Confidence in the ability to take action

Table 24-2 Transtheoretical Model—The Six Stages of Change

Precontemplation	Patient not intending to take action in future
Contemplation	Patient intends to change in next 6 months
Preparation	Patient intends to take action in immediate future
Action	Patient made modifications to life style within the past 6 months
Maintenance	Patient working to prevent relapse
Termination	Patient has no temptation and 100% self-efficacy

- However, research has concluded changes needed to prevent further disease do not happen only by providing knowledge or information to a patient.[2–7]
- Many health behavior change theories (Health Belief Model and Transtheoretical Model) have provided important perspectives on the factors to promote change and maintenance.

I. Health Belief Model

- Developed in 1950s in an effort to explain unsuccessful attempts to engage patients in programs to prevent or detect disease.[8,9]
- Later, the model expanded to include patients' responses to symptoms, behavioral response to diagnosis of illness, and compliance with medical regimens.[8,9]
- The model is utilized to explain change and maintenance of health behavior and provide a guiding framework for health behavior interventions.
- **Table 24-1** provides the key concepts of the Health Belief Model.

II. Transtheoretical Model

- The Transtheoretical Model suggests health behavior change involves progress through six stages of change.[9–12]
- **Table 24-2** provides the six stages of change.

III. Motivation for Health Behavior Change

- Different theories have identified the following as important for clinicians to understand regarding behavioral change: various signs to change, six stages of change, self-efficacy, social support, and decisional processes.[9,10]
- All the various theories focus attention on the need to enhance a patient's motivation toward change. Therefore, the development of an effective approach for overcoming resistance to change was established, which is **motivational interviewing** (MI).[11]

Motivational Interviewing[13]

- MI and brief motivational interviewing are person-centered, goal-directed methods of **communication** for eliciting and strengthening intrinsic motivation for positive change.
- MI has been applied successfully within many health professions. This includes tobacco cessation, diabetes management and eating behavior which all impact oral health.[2,14-21]
- Brief motivational interviewing[13,22-24] during a dental hygiene appointment assists the clinician to:
  - Effectively **elicit** the patient's own understanding of current oral health status and ideas about needed behavior change.
  - Avoid imposing the clinician's own ideals for behavior change onto the patient.
- Brief motivational interviewing is utilized in a healthcare or dental setting when MI is conducted in a brief amount of time, such as 5–10 minutes.[2,14,15,19,22-24]
- **Table 24-3** lists the basic components of the MI approach to changing a patient's health behaviors.

Table 24-3 Basic Components of Motivational Interview (MI)

Spirit of MI Elements (PACE)	Guiding Principles (RULE)	Implementation Process
■ **P**artnership **A**cceptance • Absolute worth • Accurate empathy • Autonomy support • Affirmation ■ **C**ompassion **E**vocation	■ Resist righting reflex ■ Understand the patient's motivation ■ Listen to the patient ■ Empower the patient	■ Engaging ■ Focusing ■ Evoking ■ Planning

I. Elements of the "Spirit of MI"

- The "spirit of MI" is how a clinician relates to the patient through communication and interactions.
- Four interrelated elements of the spirit of MI can be easily remembered using the acronym PACE: partnership, acceptance, compassion, and **evocation**.

A. Partnership[25]

- Establish a positive interpersonal environment that encourages change but is not intimidating.
- Avoid the trap of communicating based entirely on professional expertise.
- Understand patients as individuals and attempt to see the world from their perspective.
- Patients are experts on themselves; it is more effective to elicit the patient's own ideas for change than to impose personal ideals or push expertise and knowledge.

B. Acceptance[25]

- The **spirit of MI** is an attitude of acceptance of what the patient brings.
- However, to accept a person does not mean to approve of the patient's actions and maintaining the status quo.
- There are four patient-centered conditions that convey acceptance.
  1. Absolute worth[25]
     - Honor the patient's worth and potential as a human being.
     - Respect the patient as an individual who has worth in their own right.
  2. Accurate empathy[25]
     - Empathy is not sympathy. The empathetic clinician demonstrates an active interest in understanding the patient's perspective.
  3. Autonomy support[13,25]
     - Autonomy is the patient's irrevocable right to choose and make an educated decision without being coerced, persuaded, or pressured.
     - The "spirit" of MI honors, respects, and provides support for a patient's autonomy.
     - Allows for patients to have complete independence to choose for themselves.
  4. Affirmation[13,25]
     - **Affirmation** instills hope and belief that the patient can indeed change and the recognition provides support and encouragement to the patient.

C. Compassion[25]

- Compassion is commitment to promoting the welfare and prioritizing the needs of the patient.
- The clinician is addressing the patient's best interests and needs and not the clinician's agenda.
- A compassionate manner can assist with establishing trust with the patient.

D. Evocation[13,25]

- Commitment to elicit patients' assessment of their own strengths, thoughts, ideas, and resources is necessary for successful preventive counseling and behavior change.
- Patients provide a lot of information to the clinician about what will work for them in order to achieve their oral health goals through evocation.
- The overall spirit of MI begins with the premise that patients already have within them much of what is needed.
- The task of the clinician is to elicit and draw the motivation for change out of the patient.

II. Guiding Principles[13]

- MI has four guiding principles that assist the clinician in maintaining a rapport with the patient.
- The four principles can be remembered with the acronym RULE: resist–understand–listen–empower.

A. Resist Righting Reflex[13]

- Clinicians often have a desire to help and fix what is wrong and take the "expert role."

- This approach is not patient centered.
- This communication technique overshadows the patient's ability to share their ideas, experiences, and obstacles for goal setting.
- The urge to correct the patient's problem is often an automatic or reflexive habit.
- The reflexive nature of the clinician response can negatively effect the clinician-patient relationship because patients tend to resist persuasion, especially when they are ambivalent about change.
- Instead, to establish and maintain the collaborative spirit of MI, it is necessary to explore by eliciting the patient's own motivation and ideas for change.

B. Understand the Patient's Motivation[13]

- Determine the patient's reasons for change rather than focusing on the clinician's perspective about why the patient needs to make the change.
- Be interested in the patient's concerns, values, and motivations.
- Utilize MI to evoke and explore the patient's perception about their current situation and motivations for change.
- Help the patient voice their own arguments for behavior change.

C. Listen to the Patient[13]

- Patients appreciate a good listener, and a truly good listener will forgo their own agenda in the interest of giving full attention to understanding the patient.
- The expectation of a clinician typically has been to know all the answers and give them to the patient.
- Patients have ideas about how to make the change.
- **Active listening** requires more than the clinician asking questions.
- Listening involves the clinician demonstrating an empathetic interest in understanding the patient.
- A good listener does not direct or instruct, agree or disagree, persuade or advise, or warn or analyze what a patient says. There is no agenda to achieve other than understanding the world of the patient.

D. Empower the Patient[13]

- Patient empowerment is about supporting the patient's right to autonomy.
- Outcomes of behavior change increase when patients take an active interest and role in their own health care.
- Encourage patients by exploring how they can make a difference in their oral health by listening and understanding the patient's own ideas for change.
- Patients are more likely to take steps toward change when they are included in the discussion and take an active role in the decision making.

III. Processes of MI[25]

- The four processes of MI form the flow of how clinicians use MI to direct patient behavior change.
- The flow of the four processes throughout a conversation with a patient will overlap and repeat. These processes are like the stair steps illustrated in **Figure 24-1**, in which each process builds upon the other yet continues as the foundation.
- **Box 24-2** provides a checklist of questions to help the clinician gauge the success of their MI approach at each step.

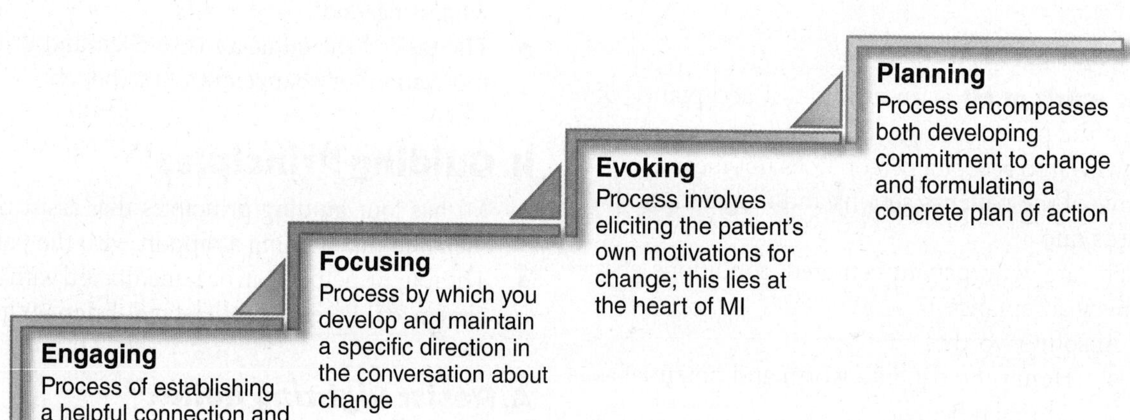

Figure 24-1 Four Processes of Motivational Interviewing

Box 24-2 Clinician Checklist of the Four Processes of Motivational Interviewing[25]

Engaging

- How comfortable is the patient in talking to me (clinician)?
- Do I understand the patient's perspective and concerns?
- Does this feel like a collaborative partnership?

Focusing

- Are we (clinician and patient) working together for a common purpose?
- What are the patients goals for change?
- Does this conversation feel more like dancing or a wrestling match?

Evoking

- What are the patient's reasons for change?
- Is the reluctance to change about confidence or importance?
- What change talk am I hearing?
- Is the righting reflex causing me (the clinician) to be the one arguing for change, instead of the patient?

Planning

- What would be a reasonable next step toward change?
- Am I remembering to evoke rather than prescribe a plan for the patient?
- Am I offering needed information or advice with permission when appropriate?
- Am I eliciting the patient's ideas for making the change?

Box 24-3 Motivational Interview: Information Exchange

Clinician: Mrs. Poe, do you mind if I discuss your oral assessment findings? (Ask permission)

Patient: Sure, that is fine.

Clinician: Great, we can discuss three areas of the assessment: Extra/intraoral findings, dental evaluation, or periodontal evaluation. Which would you like to begin with first? (Agenda setting)

Patient: Since I have a family history of gum disease, let's begin with the periodontal evaluation.

Clinician: Since you have a family history of gum disease, tell me what you know about gum disease. (Elicit)

Patient: My grandparents both wear dentures and my father has a couple of missing teeth due to bone loss. Gum disease involves the loss of bone.

Clinician: Yes, that is correct. Gum disease, also known as periodontal disease, involves the loss of bone. What do you know about the various types of periodontal disease? (Elicit)

Patient: Nothing, I didn't realize there were different types. Can you tell me more about the kinds and how they relate to my current oral health?

Clinician: Sure, I will be happy to elaborate (pulls out a chart illustrating the various stages). Gingivitis is reversible and inflammation of the gums, slight periodontitis includes slight bone loss and recession, moderate periodontitis is the beginning of bone loss between the roots of the teeth and mobility, and severe periodontitis is more advanced bone loss around the teeth and teeth may feel loose. Currently you have slight periodontitis due to the recession and slight bone loss revealed in the radiographs in conjunction with the probe readings taken today. (Provide) What are your thoughts about the information i have shared? (Elicit)

MI Implementation

I. Information Exchange[13]

- To provide information to a patient, begin by asking permission.
- Asking permission to provide information indicates respect and increases the willingness of the patient to hear what the clinician has to say.

A. Ask Permission[13,25]

- There are two approaches a clinician utilizes to ask the patient's permission to provide further detail or additional information.
- The clinician can:
  - Relay information when a patient asks the clinician for that information.
  - Directly ask permission to provide information even when the patient has not directly requested the information.
- For example, "I would like to discuss with you the assessment pertaining to your oral health; do you mind if I take a few minutes to go over my findings and address any concerns you may have?"
- **Box 24-3** provides an example of information exchange utilizing asking permission.

B. Elicit Provide Elicit[13]

A strategy for easy exchange of information that maintains patient autonomy is the elicit-provide-elicit (EPE) approach.

- Three general functions of eliciting are:
  - Asking permission.
  - Exploring the patient's prior knowledge.

- Determining the patient's interest in the information that may be provided by the clinician.
- An exploration of the patient's prior knowledge is necessary.
    - This avoids the "expert trap" so patients are not told things they already know.
    - It also allows the clinician to fill in any variances or gaps in the patient's knowledge.
- Querying interest allows the clinician to:
    - Determine what the patient would like to know most.
    - Provide the information that increases attention and receptiveness.
    - Increase patient compliance.[10]
- Box 24-3 also provides an example utilizing the EPE strategy of information change.

II. Agenda Setting[13,25]

- Agenda setting (agenda mapping) is a brief discussion in which the patient is given as much decision-making freedom as possible to set the agenda for what information and recommendations the clinician provides and for when the information is provided.
- An agenda setting approach provides the patient with a list of topics regarding oral health and allows them to choose which topic to discuss first.
- For example, "Mrs. Smith, there are three areas we can discuss regarding the assessment findings, which are extraoral/intraoral evaluation, dental evaluation, and periodontal evaluation. Which area would you like to discuss first?"
- There may be areas the dental hygienist is concerned about; however, if the clinician decides the topic of conversation without consulting the patient, an opportunity to learn what behavior change the patient may be most ready to discuss is lost.
- Respect for the patient's autonomy to choose what topics to discuss will increase the patient's willingness to listen.

III. Core Skills[13,24-25]

- The core skills for MI are better known by the acronym OARS:
    - **O**pen-ended questions.
    - **A**ffirmations.
    - **R**eflective listening.
    - **S**ummary.
- **Box 24-4** provides an example of a brief patient conversation that illustrates MI core skills.

A. Open-Ended versus Closed-Ended Questions[13,25]

- A skillful blend of open-ended questions and **reflective listening** is essential in the MI approach to patient counseling.
- Open-ended questions permit the patient to think about the response. This may yield information and insight about topics the clinician may have missed.
- This style of questioning invites conversation focused in a particular direction and provides insight into the patient's values, understanding of the oral health status, as well as the ability to change.
- Examples of open-ended questions include:
    - "What brings you here today?"
    - "How do you hope your life might be like in 5 years?"
    - "What do you know about cavities?"

Box 24-4 Motivational Interview: Core Skills

Clinician: Mr. Brooks, I notice you are a smoker from your chart. Tell me what you know about smoking cessation. (Open-ended question)

Patient: Yes, I do smoke and have for several years. I have been lectured in the past about smoking by previous healthcare providers and they mentioned something regarding smoking cessation. I think smoking cessation is guidance to quit smoking.

Clinician: I am not here to lecture you at all about smoking Mr. Brooks, but I am here to assist you with ways to quit when you are ready. Seems you have tried to quit before since you are familiar with the smoking cessation program to guide smokers on alternatives ways to quit. (Reflection) What further information have you received regarding smoking cessation? (Open-ended question)

Patient: Well, they told me there are medications and patches that could be used to assist with quitting. I have tried going cold turkey in the past. I need something to assist me with decreasing the number of cigarettes per day. Cold turkey does not work because it was just too much to handle with all the stress and I need something that will help me quit but slowly.

Clinician: I commend you on your efforts in the past to quit smoking and it seems you have really given thought to quitting based on what you are telling me your past experience. (Affirmation) You realize going cold turkey was not the best route and you need a way to decrease the amount of nicotine daily—more of a gradual way to quit smoking. (Summary)

- Box 24-4 provides an example of a patient conversation that begins with an open-ended question.
- Closed-ended questions, while good for gathering specific types of information, tend to limit the person's options for responding. An example: "Do you smoke?"
- Closed-ended questions can disguise themselves as an open-ended question.
  - An example would be "So what are you hoping to do: quit or cut down?"
  - This type is termed a "leading" question and does not allow the patient the option to elaborate nor provide patient autonomy.

B. Affirmations[24-25]

- Affirmations emphasize the positive attributes, particularly concerning strengths the patient has expressed in regard to making a behavior change.
- Affirmations help encourage and support a patient.
- Affirmations are genuine and contain a reflection of what is true regarding the patient.
- Patients are more likely to spend time with, trust, listen to, and be open with a healthcare provider who they perceive recognizes and affirms their strengths.
- Affirmations decrease or reduce defensiveness.
- Encourage self-affirmation by asking the patient to describe strengths and past successes. This type of self-affirming has been shown to facilitate openness.[26-27]
- Good affirmations center on the word "you." Using statements beginning with "I" will focus more on the clinician than on the patient.
- Example of an affirmation statement: "Your intention was good even though it didn't turn out as you would like."
- An example of a patient conversation that includes affirmation is found in Box 24-4.

C. Reflective Listening[13,24-25]

- Reflective listening (reflection) is a response to what the patient is conveying with a statement or summary that is more than repeating verbatim what the patient has said.
- This allows the patient to know the clinician is hearing and understanding.
- Two categories for reflections are simple reflection and complex reflection.
- Simple reflection is slightly rephrasing the content that was relayed to you by the patient.
- **Box 24-5** provides an example of a simple reflection.
- Complex reflection:
  - Adds meaning or emphasis to what the patient said.
  - Makes a guess about the unspoken content or what might come next.
  - Tends to move the conversation forward.
  - **Box 24-6** provides an example of a complex reflection.

Box 24-5 Motivational Interview: Reflective Listening—Simple Reflection

Patient: I know what you're trying to do is help me, but I'm just not going to do that!

Clinician: On the one hand, you know there are some real problems here, and on the other, what I suggested is just not acceptable to you.

Box 24-6 Motivational Interview: Reflective Listening—Complex Reflection

Patient: You're probably going to give me a laundry list of ways to take care of my mouth that I need to stick to, and tell me I have to get some of those interproximal brushes, superfloss, power toothbrush, and a bunch of other products. I don't have time for all that!

Clinician: If I were to tell you a whole lot of things you have to do, it would immobilize you even further. It's ironic, isn't it? When you feel like you are being forced to do something, it actually prevents you from doing what you want to do.

D. Summarizing

Summarizing information provided by the patient:

- Pulls together several items or ideas that a patient has provided.[13,24-25]
- Is affirming because it implies the clinician remembers what the patient said and wants to understand.
- Assists the patient to reflect and think about the various experiences they communicated.

Exploring Ambivalence[13,25]

- Patients often experience conflicting feelings about changing health behaviors.
- On one hand, they may appreciate and value knowledge and recommendations the dental

hygienist provides about how to attain and maintain their oral health.

- On the other hand, they often have very mixed feelings about how successful they could be at implementing the recommendations the care provider has suggested.
- The most effective way to explore and respond to a patient's **ambivalence** is by using the OARS core skills discussed in the previous section of this chapter.

I. Sustain Talk versus Change Talk[13,24-25]

- Listening carefully to the patient and responding appropriately is an important MI skill.
- Conversations with a patient may balance between **sustain talk** and **change talk**.
- A patient who is happy about current health-related behaviors will exhibit more discussion about maintaining the status quo (sustain talk) than someone who is ready to change.
- The skillful clinician who hears only sustain talk can use MI techniques to determine what information the patient is interested in receiving about oral health status and explore ambivalence.
- During patient conversations, the clinician may hear change talk, through patient statements that seem preparatory or mobilizing toward changing behaviors.
- When this occurs, the clinician can move to reflecting the change talk and eliciting a plan for change.
- Responding to both sustain talk and change talk, a clinician can use the MI process (OARS) to explore the patient's ambivalence toward change and to understand the issues that may be inhibiting their desire, motivation, or ability to change behaviors.

II. Decisional Balance[25]

A. The Balancing Act

- Decisional balance is the point at which a patient is determining whether the benefits outweigh the risks of the current behavior.
- The clinician can use this as an opportunity to explore and elicit more information from the patient about the pros and cons for making or not making the change.
- The key to success in this process is for the clinician to take a neutral position and provide a balanced way for the patient to explore the pros and cons of a behavior change.[27]
- The clinician's role is to elicit the patient's perception of:
    - Advantages of maintaining current behavior.
    - Disadvantages of maintaining the current behavior.
    - Advantages of making the change.
    - Disadvantages of making the change.
- The approach is very helpful when a patient seems to be uncertain about making a change.

B. Pro–Con Matrix

- Use of a pro–con matrix, illustrated in **Figure 24-2**, can also be beneficial in exploring decisional balance.
- The clinician can reflect and ask "What else?" at each interval during the patient's listing of pros and cons of making the change.
- When the decisional balance matrix has been completed, the clinician will focus on key items regarding the change of the behavior and provide a summary.
- **Box 24-7** provides an example of the pro–con matrix in a conversation with a patient.

III. Readiness Ruler[25]

- A readiness ruler, illustrated in **Figure 24-3**, provides a visual aid during a discussion and is useful if the clinician is not sure how important, confident, or motivated the patient is toward making the behavior change.
- Example questions to ask when using the ruler are:
    - "How important is it to make this change?"
    - "On a scale of 1–10, where 1 means not motivated and 10 means extremely motivated, how motivated are you in making this change?"
- Use of a ruler can not only tell the clinician about the patient's motivation, confidence, or

Pro–Con Matrix	*Pros*	*Cons*
If I don't change	A	B
If I do change	D	C

Figure 24-2 Decisional Balance: Pro and Con Matrix

Box 24-7 Motivational Interview: Pro–Con Matrix

Clinician: What are the pros for not preventing cavities?
Patient: There are none really, but I really do like my soda and it provides me with the caffeine needed to stay alert after being up all night studying.
Clinician: So, soda is your caffeine supply. (Reflection) What are the cons if you don't change?
Patient: I will continue to spend money on cavities. I want to keep my teeth and have them for a long time. Maintaining good oral health is important, but I don't know if I can quit my soda habit completely. I could make modifications with my snacks.
Clinician: You value your oral health and are willing to make modifications in your diet to prevent cavities. However, you are not willing to give up soda. (Reflection)
Patient: Yes, I would lose my caffeine source, so I would fall asleep during my classes and not be able to study the hours I need for my classes.
Clinician: I see, you feel your performance in school would decrease due to lack of caffeine source. What are the cons for making the change? (Reflection, Open-ended Question)
Patient: None really except if I give up soda, maybe lack of sleep. But maybe I could manage my time better and go to sleep at an earlier time.
Clinician: It is obvious you have no desire to quit drinking soda at this time. What are the pros if you do make the change? (Reflection, Open-ended Question)
Patient: I would not have to spend money on repairing my teeth. I really would like to keep my teeth. I could substitute fruit or vegetable for a candy bar when craving a snack. Maybe reduce the amount of soda and replace with caffeinated cold or hot tea without sugar.
Clinician: It seems that you have a good understanding regarding how you can prevent cavities and know it is important to maintain good oral health. You want to have your teeth for a long time, but you feel it will be hard for you to give up soda completely. However, you mentioned substituting fruit or vegetables for snacks instead of candy or try to reduce your soda intake with a sugar-free, less acidic caffeinated choice or hot tea without sugar. (Affirmation, Summary)

importance for the change, but also the readiness ruler can elicit change talk.

- For example: A patient states they are a 5 on the scale from 1 to 10, the clinician responds, "So you are a 5? Why not a 3 or 4?"

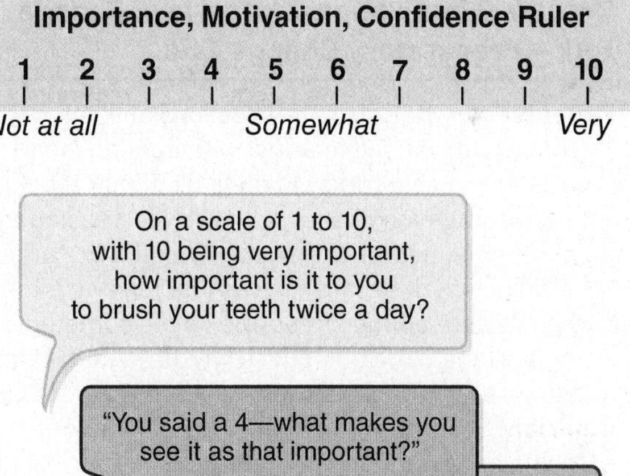

Figure 24-3 Readiness for Change Ruler. The utilization of this ruler will assist the clinician with eliciting the patient's importance, motivation, or confidence in making the change.

Box 24-8 Motivational Interview: Readiness Ruler

Clinician: On a scale of 1–10, where 1 means not confident and 10 means extremely confident, how confident are you in quitting smoking?
Patient: I'd say a 5.
Clinician: You are a 5, why not a 3 or 4?
Patient: Because I have tried in the past and have been successful, but at the same time I have some obstacles to overcome.
Clinician: You have learned from your past what works for you and you know the obstacles you have to overcome. What are some ways for you to get to a 6 or 7?

- This approach can encourage the patient to explain why the behavior being discussed is important enough to designate it a 5 on the scale.
- Then the clinician can ask, "What are some ways for you to get to a 6 or 7?" to elicit the patient's ideas and potential strategies for making the change. **Box 24-8** provides an example of the use of the readiness ruler.

Eliciting and Recognizing Change Talk[13,24,25]

- During a conversation with a patient, the clinician needs to be able to elicit and recognize when change talk is exhibited.

Box 24-9 Motivational Interview: Change Talk—Preparatory Change Talk

Patient: I know there are medications and patches that could be used to assist with quitting. I have tried going cold turkey in the past. (Desire) I need something to assist me with decreasing the number of cigarettes per day. (Need) Cold turkey does not work because it was just too much to handle with all the stress and I need something that will help me quit but slowly. I can quit if I go slowly and have the support. (Ability)

Clinician: Seems you have really given thought to being successful in quitting based on your past experience. You realize going cold turkey was not the best route and you need a way to decrease the amount of nicotine daily. More of a gradual way to quit smoking.

Patient: Yes, I can quit with assistance and guidance. I really want to quit because I would like to be around for my wife and kids. (Reason) Plus I need to get in better health. (Need)

Box 24-10 Motivational Interview: Change Talk—Mobilizing Change Talk

Clinician: You value your health and family. You know you can quit smoking if you have something to assist with quitting. You mentioned using patches or medications in assisting.

Patient: Yes, I have already researched the cost and the effectiveness of the patches and medications, plus chewing gums for quitting smoking. I intend to begin with the patches (Commitment), which I have already purchased (Action toward). I have scheduled an appointment with my physician to discuss which medication will not interfere with my heart medications. (Taking steps)

- When change talk is heard in a conversation with the patient, the clinician provides reflection statements that incorporate and summarize the change talk.
- **Box 24-9** and **Box 24-10** provide examples of a conversation between a patient who is making change talk and a clinician who reflects and summarizes the patient's change talk.

I. Preparatory Change Talk[13,25]

- Skillful application of MI can allow the clinician to elicit further information about the patient's desire, ability, reasons, and needs for making the behavior change.
- It is important for the clinician to be actively listening for the themes present in preparatory change talk and reflect those statements back to the patient when they occur in conversation.
- Some examples of change talk during a patient/clinician conversation are found in Box 24-9.
- The DARN acronym (desire, ability, reasons, need) is useful for remembering the four components of preparatory change talk that initiate the behavior change process.

A. Desire[13,25]

- During patient conversations, listen for words associated with desire for change.
- Examples of patient statements that the clinician may hear are "I want to…," "I would like…," or "I wish…"
- When eliciting change talk, the clinician can pose questions that encourage the patient to express a desire for change.
- An example question for eliciting desire is, "How would you like for things to change?"

B. Ability[13,25]

- The theme of ability in change talk displays what a patient is thinking about regarding their capability or potential to make a change.
- Statements may be expressed during a conversation to demonstrate ability would include words like "can" or "could."
- Statements the clinician can use to elicit ability change talk are:
  - "What would you be willing to do?"
  - "What are some ideas you have for how to change?"

C. Reasons[13,25]

- This form of change talk expresses the patient's specific rationale or personal reasons for making a certain change.
- Examples of statements a clinician can use to elicit the patient's reasons for making a change are:
  - "What might be the good things about making this change?"
  - "What would be the downside of changing how things are now?"

D. Need[13,25]

- Need is expressed by patients when they recognize the urgency or begin to understand that they must make a change.

- Words associated with need change talk are "must," "have to," "got to," "should," "ought," or "need to."
- Example questions for eliciting the need to change are:
  - "What needs to happen?"
  - "How important is it for you to make this change?"[1]

II. Mobilizing Change Talk[13]

- The acronym CAT can be used for remembering the three key components (commitment, activation, and taking steps) of mobilizing change talk.
- The clinician responds to the patient's mobilizing change talk with reflection, affirmation, and encouragement.
- Box 24-10 provides an example of mobilizing change talk expressed in a conversation.

A. Commitment[13]

- Clinicians can gauge a patient's commitment to change during a conversation either by listening for commitment statements or eliciting the patient's commitment for change.
- **Table 24-4** provides patient statements that indicate high or low level of commitment to change.

B. Activation[13]

- Clinicians may encounter change talk that indicates action toward change, and these types of statements mean the patient has taken some step toward change.
- For example, the patient might say: "I have bought dental floss" or "I have purchased a power toothbrush."

C. Taking Steps[13]

- Patients express steps they have already taken in making the change.

Table 24-4 Patient Statements Indicating Commitment

Low-Level Commitment	High-Level Commitment
I will think about it I'll consider it I plan to, I hope to, I will try to	I will, I promise, I guarantee, I am ready to I intend to

- For example, "I just began flossing twice a week" or "I have just started eating healthy snacks between meals instead of a candy bar."
- An example eliciting question is, "What have you done to make this change?"

Strengthening Commitment (The Plan)[13,24,25]

- The goal when having a conversation with a patient about making health behavior change is to have the patient come up with a plan to make the change.
- The signs a patient may be ready to proceed to a plan are:
  - An increase in change talk.
  - Talk about taking steps toward the change.
  - Diminished sustain talk.
  - Questions about making the change.
- It is important that the patient provide the solutions for change and the clinician allow the patient to develop the solutions that will work best for them.
- Patients are more successful and committed to a plan if their own ideas and needs are incorporated.
- The clinician utilizes the same MI techniques (OARS) when having a conversation regarding the patient's plan.
- After the patient articulates the plan, the clinician can summarize the patient's plan and follow-up with a commitment question.
- **Box 24-11** provides a conversation with a patient that leads to a plan.
- There are three scenarios when it comes to planning.

I. Clear Plan[25]

- The first planning scenario is when the patient knows what they want or need to do.
- If the patient has decided on a clear plan for change and they know how they will accomplish it, there is no need to explore other paths.
- Even when there is a clear plan, elicit the patient's thoughts about obstacles or unanticipated difficulties that may arise with the plan. In addition, discuss ideas the patient has about how to overcome these obstacles in order to be successful.

II. Several Clear Options[25]

- The second planning scenario is when the patient has determined there is more than one clear plan for working toward the goal.

Box 24-11 Motivational Interview: The Plan

Clinician: Mrs. Poe, you have quit in the past and now you have some options to assist you with quitting. You know cold turkey did not work well in the past attempt to quit, but you seem to be highly interested in using the nicotine patch and gum for your next quit attempt. (Summary)

Patient: Yes, after discussing the various options, I am going to get the nicotine patches and gum to assist me with quitting. I really think this option will be more successful for me.

Clinician: Any thoughts on when you will begin the process of quitting? (Eliciting)

Patient: Well, I am under a bit of stress right now and the holidays are coming up. Maybe January 1st.

Clinician: Seems smoking is a stress reliever for you and you would like to wait 4 months before beginning the smoking cessation program. (Reflection)

Patient: Yes, smoking is a stress reliever and really all I am doing is trying to go slowly with quitting, so I am going to go out and get the patches and gum and begin on Monday with decreasing the amount I smoke a day. (Change talk) I can do other things to relieve my stress by walking or jogging, which I already do daily. I just will increase it when I feel more stressed. (Change talk)

Clinician: You have some alternative ways to relieve your stress that are not different from your daily routine now. Your plan is to begin with the patches and gum on Monday and slowly decrease the number of cigarettes you smoke. Seems you want to be completely off of cigarettes by January 1. When you feel more stress you will extend your exercise time. (Summary—the plan)

Patient: Yes, that is the plan.

Clinician: Great, I will make a note in your chart and follow-up with you at your next periodontal maintenance appointment.

- Through agenda setting, the clinician can help the patient prioritize and choose among the various plans.

III. Brainstorming[25]

- The last category of planning is when a patient has neither a clear plan nor an obvious set of options to choose from for making the desired behavior change.
- The conversation with the patient is a brainstorming-type session from which the clinician elicits ideas the patient has about making the change.
- The clinician utilizes agenda setting to determine what the patient would like to pursue initially from the ideas established.

MI with Pediatric Patients and Caregivers[28-31]

- MI can be utilized with pediatric patients and parents or other caregivers.
- The same core skills are utilized to explore ambivalence or elicit change talk.
- The age and self-care ability of the child determines whether the conversation regarding preventive behavior change is directed toward the child or the caregiver.
- **Box 24-12** provides an example conversation utilizing MI with a pediatric patient and caregiver.

Motivational Training and Coaching

- MI workshops alone are unlikely to provide the skills needed to develop competency in application of MI in patient care.[15,22]
- In order to become proficient with MI, introductory and advanced MI courses or workshops where feedback is provided through MI practice and coaching is recommended.[25,32-33]
- Therefore, skill development is an ongoing process and MI must coincide with classroom, practice, and coaching in order to be properly trained.[25,32-33]
- There is additional information located on the MI Network of Trainers website (www.motivationalinterviewing.org), with additional information regarding trainings clinicians may attend as well as many other resources pertaining to MI.[34]

Documentation

Routine documentation for a MI session includes a minimum of the following information:

- Assessment findings and areas of concern (disease status and risk).
- Patient's stage of readiness for making a change.
- Patient's motivation for change.

Box 24-12 Motivational Interview: The Pediatric Patient and Caregiver

Background: Jimmy is 8 years old and has been seeing the dentist since age 1 year. Mom is with Jimmy today for his 6-month visit. No past history of cavities. It is time for Jimmy to have some bitewings today, which mom has approved. The radiographs reveal Jimmy has proximal lesions on teeth #3, 14, 19, and 30 and incipient lesions present on several other teeth. Use of disclosing solution reveals a biofilm score of 80%.

Clinician: Jimmy, what do you know about cavities? (Eliciting)

Patient: All I know about cavities is there are bugs that eat away at your tooth if you don't brush and eat too much sugar.

Clinician: Yes, if you don't take care of teeth and eat properly, teeth can become decayed. (Affirmation, reflective listening) Remember when the dentist was doing his examination and he mentioned there were a few areas where there were cavities? (Closed-ended question)

Patient: Yes, does that mean I have teeth that have decayed?

Clinician: Yes, Jimmy you do have areas of decay. May I bring your mom back to discuss what was found today when the dentist did his exam? (Asking permission)

Patient: Sure.

Clinician: (Brings mom back to discuss findings) Mrs. Jones, the dentist found cavities during Jimmy's examination today that were not there 6 months ago. Are you aware of any changes in Jimmy's diet? (Eliciting)

Mrs. Jones (Mom): Well, I have noticed he does consume a lot of sports drinks and soft drinks between meals. He has a candy bar at least once a week, but he brushes twice a day for 2 minutes.

Clinician: Seems he enjoys sports drinks and soft drinks, and Jimmy, I commend you on your brushing habits. (Affirmation) Jimmy and I reviewed his brushing technique today to ensure he was effectively getting all the plaque off when he brushes. What do you think may be contributing to his recent decay? (Eliciting, Open-ended Question)

Box 24-13 Example Documentation: Motivational Interview (MI) Session during a Patient Appointment

- **S**—A 30-year-old White male presents for 3-month continuing care visit. Previous assessment indicates high intake of sugar-sweetened beverages. Previous entries in patient record indicate ongoing recommendations for limiting intake of sugar-sweetened beverages. Patient states today that he sips three to five cans of cola-type beverage during the day and evening. He indicates he knows the beverages are what "cause my cavities" and that he would like to change his behavior so he wouldn't "get any more cavities," but that his motivation for behavior change on the readiness ruler is "about a 2."
- **O**—Previous history of significant smooth surface decay, and today's examination indicates two new cavitated lesions on anterior facial surfaces, which were documented on the patient's dental chart.
- **A**—Patient has knowledge of the cause of dental decay but expresses ambivalence to change that can correct the problem.
- **P**—Used MI approach and the pro–con matrix to help the patient explore his ambivalence to behavior change and to explore factors that might affect his ability to change behavior and stop continually drinking sugar-sweetened beverages. He will continue to explore other ways he can cut down and might begin drinking bottle water with sugar-free flavoring.

Next Steps: Continue to use MI approach to provide follow-up discussion and encouragement during patient's visit for restorative treatment in 2 weeks and at his next dental hygiene appointment in 3 months.

Signed: ______________________________, RDH
Date: ______________________________

- The outcome of the conversation with the patient regarding the area(s) of concern, such as:
  - Knowledge and understanding of their disease status and risk.
  - What the patient would like to address first.
  - What has worked in the past or what has not worked in the past.
  - How they plan to make the change.
  - Short- and long-term goals for making the change.
  - When they plan to begin to make the change.
- A documentation example is found in **Box 24-13**.

Factors to Teach the Patient

- Discuss preventive measures and suggested care plan options pertaining to the clinical assessment findings.
- Elicit what the patient knows about periodontal disease or their risk for caries and have a discussion utilizing the MI methods regarding possible changes the patient can pursue.
- Discuss self-assessment and alternative methods (disclosing agent) for determining the health of gingiva.
- Determine the patient's self-care technique (e.g., toothbrushing power or manual, flossing) and provide suggestions if need to modified technique to be effective.
- Provide the patient with various options regarding preventive measures for the disease status to choose those that will be effective.
- Elicit from the patient's short- and long-term goals pertaining to what the patient would like to achieve regarding disease status and overall self-care.

References

1. Gao X, Lo EC, Kot SC, Chan KC. Motivational interviewing in improving oral health: a systemic review of randomized controlled trials. *J Periodontol*. 2014;85(3):426-437.
2. Bray KK, Catley D, Voelker MA, Liston R, Williams KB. Motivational interviewing in dental hygiene education: curriculum modification and evaluation. *J Dent Educ*. 2013;77(12): 1662-1669.
3. Croffoot C, Krust Bray K, Black MA, Koerber A. Evaluating the effects of coaching to improve motivational interviewing skills of dental hygiene students. *J Dent Hyg*. 2010;84(2):57-64.
4. Kalsbeek H, Truin GJ, Poorterman JH, van Rossum GM, van Rijkom HM, Verrips GH. Trends in periodontal status and oral hygiene habits in Dutch adults between 1983 and 1995. *Community Dent Oral Epidemiol*. 2000;28(2):112-118.
5. Ronis DL, Lang WP, Farghaly MM, Passow E. Tooth brushing, flossing, and preventive dental visits by Detroit-area residents in relation to demographic and socioeconomic factors. *J Public Health Dent*. 1993;53(3):138-145.
6. Smedslund G, Berg RC, Hammerstrøm KT, et al. Motivational interviewing for substance abuse. *Cochrane Database Syst Rev*. 2011;(5):CD008063.
7. Yevlahova D, Satur J. Models for individual oral health promotion and their effectiveness: a systematic review. *Aust Dent J*. 2009;54(3):190-197.
8. Glanz K, Lewis FM, Rimer BK. *Health Behavior and Health Education*. 2nd ed. San Francisco, CA: Jossey-Bass; 1997:41-59.
9. Emmons KM, Rollnick D. Motivational interviewing in health care settings: opportunities and limitations. *Am J Prev Med*. 2001;20(1):68-74.
10. Prochaska JO, Velicer WF. The transtheoretical model of health behavior change. *Am J Health Promot*. 1997;12(1):38-48.
11. Wilson GT, Schlam TR. The transtheoretical model and motivational interviewing in the treatment of eating and weight disorders. *Clin Psychol Rev*. 2004;24(3):361-378.
12. Bundy C. Changing behaviour: using motivational interviewing techniques. *J R Soc Med*. 2004;97(suppl 44):43-47.
13. Rollnick S, Miller WR, Butler CC. *Motivational Interviewing in Health Care: Helping Patients Change Behavior*. New York, NY: The Guilford Press; 2008:3-107.
14. Rubak S, Sandbaek A, Lauritzen T, Christensen B. Motivational interviewing: a systematic review and meta-analysis. *Br J Gen Pract*. 2005;55(513):305-312.
15. Lundahl BW, Kunz C, Brownell C, Tollefson D, Burke BL. A meta-analysis of motivational interviewing: twenty-five years of empirical studies. *Res Social Work Prac*. 2010;20(2): 137-159.
16. Lundahl B, Moleni T, Burke BL, et al. Motivational interviewing in medical care settings: a systematic review and meta-analysis of randomized controlled trials. *Patient Educ Couns*. 2013;93(2):157-168.
17. Hettema J, Steele J, Miller WR. Motivational interviewing. *Annu Rev Clin Psychol*. 2005;1:91-111.
18. Soria R, Legido A, Escolano C, Yeste AL, Montoya J. A randomised controlled trial of motivational interviewing for smoking cessation. *Br J Gen Pract*. 2006;56(531):768-774.
19. Koeber A, Crawford J, O'Connell K. The effects of teaching dental students brief motivational interviewing for smoking cessation counseling: a pilot study. *J Dent Educ*. 2003;67(4):439-447.
20. Hettema JE, Hendricks PS. Motivational interviewing for smoking cessation: a meta-analytic review. *J Consult Clin Psychol*. 2010;78(6):868-884.
21. Martins RL, McNeil DW. Review of motivational interviewing in promoting health behaviors. *Clin Psychol Rev*. 2009; 29:283-293.
22. Rollnick S, Heather N. Negotiating behavior change in medical settings: the development of brief motivational interviewing. *J Mental Health*. 1992;1(1):25-38.
23. Gilliam DG, Yusuf H. Brief motivational interviewing in dental practice. *Dent J*. 2019;7(51):1-9.
24. Bhat A, Rajesh G, Mohanty VR, Shenoy R, Pai M. Motivational interviewing as tool for behavior change: implications for public health dentistry. *World J Dentist*. 2020;11(3):241-246.
25. Miller WR, Rollnick S. *Motivational Interviewing: Helping People Change*. 3rd ed. New York, NY: The Guilford Press; 2013:3-292.
26. Critcher CR, Dunning D, Armor DA. When self-affirmations reduce defensiveness: timing is key. *Pers Soc Psychol Bull*. 2010;36(7):947-959.
27. Janis IL, Mann L. *Decision Making: A Psychological Analysis of Conflict, Choice and Commitment*. New York, NY: Free Press; 1977.
28. Skaret E, Weinstein P, Kvale G, Raadal M. An intervention program to reduce dental avoidance behavior among adolescents: a pilot study. *Eur J Paediatr Dent*. 2003;4:191-196.

29. Wu L, Gao X, Lo ECM, et al. Motivational interviewing to promote oral health in adolescents. *J Adolescent Health*. 2017;61:378-384.
30. Weinstein P, Harrison R, Benton T. Motivating parents to prevent caries in their young children: one-year findings. *J Am Dent Assoc*. 2004;135(6):731-738.
31. Weinstein P, Harrison R, Benton T. Motivating mothers to prevent caries: confirming the beneficial effect of counseling. *J Am Dent Assoc*. 2006;137:789-793.
32. Miller WR, Yahne CE, Moyers TB, Martinez J, Pirritano M. A randomized trial of methods to help clinicians learn motivational interviewing. *J Consult Clin Psychol*. 2004;72:1050-1062.
33. Fuhrmann S, Kitzmann J, Isailor-Schochlin M, et al. Can motivational interviewing for dental settings be taught online? Results of an uncontrolled interventional trial. *Eur J Dent Educ*. 2022;26(2):254-262.
34. Motivational Interviewing Network of Trainers. MINT excellence in motivational interviewing: MI Training and Resources. http://www.motivationalinterviewing.org/. Accessed September 1, 2021.

CHAPTER 25

Protocols for Prevention and Control of Dental Caries

Michelle Hurlbutt, RDH, MSDH, DHSc
Linda D. Boyd, RDH, RD, EdD

CHAPTER OUTLINE

LEARNING OBJECTIVES

After studying this chapter, the student will be able to:

1. Describe the dental caries disease process.
2. Identify factors contributing to demineralization and remineralization.
3. Distinguish each step in caries management.
4. Evaluate each patient for individual risk for caries disease.
5. Apply caries risk status in developing individualized caries management protocols and carefully document.

History of Dental Caries Management

- In the early half of the 20th century, the history of **dental caries** management included placing restorations, removing diseased teeth, and providing prosthetic replacements.
- Reductions in caries incidence of 40% to 60% since 1945 in the United States were observed for those fortunate enough to live in communities with community water fluoridation.[1]
- As the 20th century progressed, a decrease in dental caries prevalence was generally related to the widespread home use of fluoride dentifrices and mouthrinses as well as professional topical applications of solutions, gels, and varnishes.
- In the early 21st century, studies revealed dental caries prevalence has remained the same and even increased in some populations in the United States as a result of lack of access to care.[2]
- Evidence suggests the prevalence of untreated dental caries decreased among preschoolers during 2011–2014 but the prevalence of having no dental caries in permanent teeth in children and adolescents has remained unchanged.[3]
- Dental caries remains a major public health problem in adults, adolescents, and children.

The Dental Caries Process

- Dental caries is a biofilm-mediated, diet-modulated, multifactorial, noncommunicable, dynamic disease[4] resulting in a net mineral loss of the hard tissues.
- This disease affects a majority of the world's population across the life span.
- The type of cariogenic bacteria associated with this disease is not present at birth and is most commonly transmitted from mother to child through vertical transmission.[5,6]
- When a caries lesion occurs in the oral cavity, strategies exist to control the disease, reverse it in its early stages, and prevent further progression.
- Dental hygienists have current evidence-based research to educate their patients to increase their understanding of the dental caries process and prevent oral disease.
  - The extended ecological plaque hypothesis proposes that dental caries is the result of a shift in the ecological balance of dental plaque toward a more cariogenic flora.[7]
  - The basic caries process starts with certain **acidogenic bacteria** and **aciduric bacteria** in dental biofilm acting to metabolize the fermentable carbohydrates ingested by the patient.[8]
  - The acids formed demineralize the enamel, cementum, and/or dentin and lead to mineral loss and cavity formation.
  - On the tooth surface, a continuous process of **demineralization** and **remineralization** is occurring.
  - This process is ongoing and takes place throughout the life of the tooth.
  - Protocols exist to address caries disease prevention and management at the various stages of lesion development; the goal being to halt and control the disease process.
  - The interrelationship of the microorganisms, tooth, salivary factors, and cariogenic foods in the caries process is discussed in Chapter 33.

I. Acidogenic and Aciduric Bacteria

- Acidogenic and aciduric bacteria produce acid as a result of metabolizing fermentable carbohydrates consumed by the individual.
- When acidogenic and aciduric bacteria predominate the oral flora, the risk for dental caries increases.
- Although there are many acid-forming and acid-tolerant bacteria present, two groups of bacteria predominate in the caries process: the mutans streptococci (*Streptococcus mutans* and *Streptococcus sobrinus* are two most prevalent bacteria in the group) as well as *Lactobacillus* and *Actinomyces* and non-*Actinomyces* species.[4,7] *Bifidobacteria* are also associated with early childhood caries.[9]
- Mutans streptococci are infectious organisms that colonize the teeth and help to form the dental biofilm because they create a sticky environment for survival and multiplication.
- Mutans streptococci and *Bifidobacteria* are most active during the initial stages of demineralization and caries formation, whereas the lactobacilli are more active during the progression of the caries.
- Permanent colonization of a child's teeth with the mutans streptococci group can take place soon after tooth eruption. Transmission of the acid-forming organisms is usually from close family members, particularly the mother.[10]

- *Candida albicans* is also detected in association with the caries pathogen *S. mutans* in plaque samples from children with early childhood caries.[11]

II. Role of Fermentable Carbohydrates

- Commonly consumed fermentable carbohydrates include sugars (sucrose, glucose, fructose) and processed starches.[12]
- Acids produced during the metabolic processes include acetic, lactic, formic, and propionic.
- Frequency and form of fermentable carbohydrates enhance the amount of biofilm and acid produced and results in increased demineralization.[12-14]

III. Acid Production

- The acid formed passes freely into the tiny diffusion channels between the enamel rods or into the exposed root surfaces.
- Acids can dissolve the enamel crystals into calcium and phosphate ions.
- The subsurface initial carious lesion is formed and appears clinically as a **white spot lesion**. (See Chapter 16.)

IV. Demineralization

- Demineralization and remineralization are natural processes as the fluids in the oral cavity constantly strive to maintain equilibrium.[15]
  - Demineralization is the process by which the minerals of the tooth structure are dissolved into solution by organic acids produced from acidogenic bacteria that metabolize fermentable carbohydrates.
  - With repeated bathing of the tooth surface with the acids, the tooth demineralization can outpace the remineralization process. The end product of this activity is the cavitated carious lesion.
  - Smooth surface and pit and fissure carious lesions can result when cariogenic nutrients are available.

V. Remineralization

Remineralization is the natural repair process of moving minerals back into the subsurface of the intact enamel. Saliva provides protective factors to promote remineralization.[15]

A. Saliva

- Protective factors of healthy saliva can balance or reverse the destruction of the tooth structure.
- The functions of saliva related to caries management include[16]:
  - **Buffering** of acids and clearance of bacteria and food debris.
  - Supplying minerals to replace calcium and phosphate ions dissolved from the tooth during demineralization.
- Low saliva flow (**hyposalivation** or **xerostomia**) reduces buffering capacity and aids in the demineralization process.
- Maintaining a neutral or basic saliva pH of 7 is necessary to maximize remineralization. After an exposure to fermentable carbohydrate, the pH drops to the critical pH of 5.5, at which point demineralization occurs.[7]
- Exposure to topical fluoride can increase available salivary levels of fluoride.
  - Saliva is a reservoir for fluoride to aid in remineralization.
  - Fluoride accumulation in saliva comes from many sources, including water, dentifrice, mouthrinse, and professionally applied therapies.[17]

B. Fluoride Mechanisms of Action

- Inhibits demineralization: Fluoride available in biofilm and saliva can flow into the enamel diffusion channels and root surface and attach in the form of hydrogen fluoride (HF) as the oral environment attempts to achieve equilibrium.[18]
- Enhances remineralization: Sufficient saliva is integral in this process.
  - The buffering properties of saliva can neutralize acid pH.
  - This change in pH can reverse the equilibrium, driving calcium, phosphate, and fluoride ions into the tooth surface.[18]
  - The resulting fluorapatite bond is stronger and less acid soluble than the hydroxyapatite bond, resulting in a stronger tooth surface than the original bond.
- Inhibits bacterial growth:
  - In the biofilm, the HF diffuses through the cell membrane of acidogenic bacteria.
  - Fluoride ions interfere with the essential enzyme activity within the bacterial cell wall.[17]

Dental Caries Classifications

- There are several stages of caries development from noncavitated to **cavitated carious lesion** using either the American Dental Association (ADA) Caries Classification System (CCS) or **International Caries Classification and Management System (ICCMS)**.
- Early diagnosis and detection of carious lesions still in the subsurface, incipient, or noncavitated state allows the clinician to educate the patient, provide strategies to manage risk of further progression of the lesion, and provide preventive treatments to reverse the lesion.
- Examination for caries detection clinically and radiographically are reviewed in Chapter 16.

I. Reversible Stages of Dental Carious Lesion

Chapter 16 reviews the stages of caries lesion development.

- The stages when caries development is still reversible include the following[19,20]:
  - ICCMS Initial Stage Caries or CCS Initial Caries Lesion when there is no **cavitation** of the lesion (see **Figure 25-1**).
- The stages when caries development is irreversible include the following[19,20]:
  - ICCMS Moderate Stage Caries or CCS Moderate Caries Lesion where there is cavitation of the enamel.
  - ICCMS Extensive Stage Caries or CCS Advanced Caries Lesion where the lesion extends into the dentin.

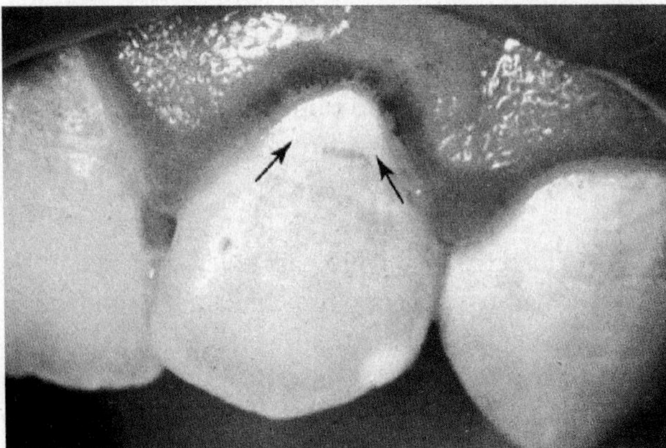

Figure 25-1 Initial Caries Lesion (White Spot Lesion). Smooth surface demineralization appearing as chalky white area (at arrows) seen in the cervical third of a maxillary lateral incisor is evidence of the first stages of dental caries. If this demineralization continues, this area could develop a cavitation that would need to be restored

Caries Risk Assessment Systems

Risk assessment is commonly used to assess the risk factors for disease so that individualized prevention and management plans can be developed and implemented.

- **Caries risk assessment (CRA)** is an essential component in the decision-making process for patient-centered caries management.[21] CRA can be defined as the clinical process of establishing the probability of a patient to develop new caries lesions or the likelihood of a change to the size or activity of lesions already present over a certain period of time.
  - The most powerful single factor in caries prediction for all age groups is previous caries experience.
  - The ideal CRA will be evidence based, inexpensive, and easy to use in the process of patient care.
  - Identifying the validity of a CRA system long term in prevention of caries and stopping progression of early lesions is still undergoing further research.
- Risk factors fall into two categories:
  - Modifiable risk factors.
  - Nonmodifiable risk factors.

I. ADA Caries Risk Assessment

- This tool was developed based on expert opinion and available evidence.
- This CRA has assessment forms for age 0–6 years and those older than age 6 years.
- The assessment includes the following factors[22]:
  - Contributing conditions such as fluoride exposure, consumption of sugary foods/drinks, eligibility for government programs, dental home, and family caries experience (ages 0–6 years).
  - General health conditions such as special healthcare needs, eating disorders, medication-induced xerostomia, drug/alcohol abuse, and chemo/radiation therapy.

- Clinical conditions such as radiographic caries lesions, missing teeth due to caries, noncavitated lesions, visible plaque biofilm, interproximal restorations, exposed root surfaces, fixed or removable prosthetic/orthodontic appliances, and salivary flow.
- Risk levels include low, moderate, and high risk.

II. American Academy of Pediatric Dentistry (AAPD) Caries-Risk Assessment Tool (CAT)

- The AAPD used a systematic review process to update the CAT tool in 2014.[23]
- The CAT is for infants, children, and adolescents.
  - 0–3-year-olds for nondental providers such as physicians.
  - 0–5-year-olds for dental providers.
  - Older than 6-year-olds for dental providers.
- The assessment includes the following factors:
  - Biologic factors such as sugar-containing snacks or beverages, special healthcare needs, recent immigrant, low socioeconomic status, and active caries in primary caregiver.
  - Protective factors such as fluoride exposure, brushing daily, professional topical fluoride, and regular dental care.
  - Clinical findings such as decayed/missing/filled surfaces or defective restorations, white spot lesions, elevated streptococci levels, and plaque.
- Risk levels include:
  - Low and high for the nondental providers.
  - Low, moderate, and high for dental providers.

III. Cariogram

- The Cariogram is a visual representation of the interaction of caries with various etiologic factors to predict future risk. Originally developed in 1976, decades of trials were conducted to validate it before it was launched online in 1997.[24]
- The assessment includes the following factors:
  - Bacteria, including dental plaque amount and mutans streptococci count.
  - Diet, including fermentable carbohydrates and frequency.
  - Susceptibility, such as fluoride exposure and use, saliva secretion, and buffering capacity.
  - Circumstances, such as past caries experience and related diseases.
- Risk is displayed as a pie chart and the percentage of chance to avoid new caries is displayed, as well as the contribution of each of the factors on the risk of new caries.

IV. Caries Management by Risk Assessment (CAMBRA)

- **CAMBRA** was developed following two consensus conferences beginning in 2003 in California. Large-scale pilot tests were conducted and the assessment form was modified and disseminated in 2007 and 2021.[8,25]
- CAMBRA has assessment forms for age 0–5 years and those age 6 years through adult. (See Chapter 47 for risk factors.)
- The assessment includes the following categories of factors for ages 6 years through adult[25]:
  - Disease indicators (clinical examination) such as visible or radiographic caries, white spot lesions, new radiographic noncavitated lesions, and restorations in last 3 years.
  - Biologic risk factors such as heavy plaque, deep pits and fissures, reduced saliva flow, exposed roots, and orthodontic appliances.
  - Biologic or environmental risk factors include frequent snacking, medications causing xerostomia, and recreational drug use.
  - Protective factors include normal salivary flow, fluoridated water, fluoride toothpaste, fluoride varnish twice/year, 0.05% sodium fluoride mouthrinse, prescription fluoride toothpaste, and chlorhexidine use 7 days/month.
- Risk levels are low, moderate, high, or extreme.

V. International Caries Classification and Management System (ICCMS)

- ICCMS was developed through a consensus process by an international group of experts after review of the evidence.[21]
- The assessment includes the following factors:
  - Medical history, such as prescribed and recreational drugs and conditions resulting in hyposalivation.
  - Head and neck radiation.
  - Sugary foods and beverages.
  - Low fluoride exposure.
  - Primary caregiver caries experience.
  - Oral hygiene behaviors and heavy plaque biofilm.
  - Socioeconomic status.
  - Caries experience and presence of active carious lesions.

    - Exposed root surfaces.
    - Oral appliances such as orthodontic retainers and partial dentures.
- The risk levels utilized by this system include low-, medium-, or high-risk categories.

Implementation of CRA in the Process of Care

- The clinic or office must first identify which risk assessment system will be implemented.
- During review of the medical, dental, and psychosocial history, identify risk factors for caries such as medical conditions or medications that cause xerostomia. (See Chapter 11.)
    - Complete the portion of the risk assessment related to the medical, dental, and psychosocial history, which should include diet assessment.
- The radiographic and clinical examination are used to assess some of the risk factors. (See Chapters 13, 15–17, and 20.)
    - Some risk assessment systems require assessment of saliva and bacteria, so this needs to be implemented at this point in the care process.
- Once the risk assessment is complete, using clinical judgment and the results of the risk assessment, the clinician needs to identify risk level and which risk factors are modifiable.
    - The modifiable risk factors are the ones to target for management when developing the care (treatment) plan to reduce the risk of caries progression or development.

Caries Risk Management Systems

Just as there are a number of CRA systems available, there are several caries risk management systems and a brief overview will be provided.

I. AAPD Caries Risk Management Protocol

- The AAPD protocol is based on evidence-based literature and judgment of an expert panel.[23]
- The protocol is based on risk and takes into account the level of patient/parent cooperation.
- The protocols are based on the age category of the child/adolescent and include the following:
    - Diagnostics: Recommended frequency for radiographs and professional dental care.
    - Interventions: Brushing frequency with fluoridated toothpaste, frequency of professional application of fluoride, use of fluoride supplements when appropriate, diet counseling, use of xylitol-containing products, and sealants.
    - Restorative: Active surveillance for progression of incipient lesions, restoration of cavitated lesions, and interim therapeutic restorations (when possible for very young children 1–3 years old).

II. Caries Management by Risk Assessment (CAMBRA)

- The CAMBRA recommendations are based on available evidence and were developed by consensus of the Western CAMBRA Coalition.[22]
- The management protocol is based on risk level and clinical judgment of the clinician.
- The protocols vary based on risk level and may include the following[22]:
    - Diagnostics: Frequency of radiographs, examinations, and preventive care.
    - Interventions: Diet counseling; oral hygiene instruction; and use of fluoride rinses, sealants, bacterial testing, antimicrobial treatments such as chlorhexidine rinse, calcium phosphate paste, prescription fluorides, baking soda rinses, and xylitol products.
    - Restorative: Glass ionomer resins, early minimally invasive for those at high risk to delay invasive restorative treatment.
- Research suggests patients who are compliant with recommendations based on their level of risk show a statistically significant reduction in caries.[20]

III. International Caries Classification and Management System (ICCMS)

- The **International Caries Detection and Assessment System (ICDAS)** and ICCMS systems are based on extensive critical analyses of the literature and consensus from a global group of experts.[19]
- The ICCMS is a systematic guide for the critical decisions clinicians need to make to develop a management plan based on caries risk.
- The protocols vary by risk level and may include the following[19]:
    - Diagnostics: Frequency of exams and professional preventive care.

- Interventions: Oral self-care, dietary counseling to reduce frequency of intake of fermentable carbohydrates, fluoridated toothpaste, fluoride varnish, high-dose fluoride pastes (5,000 ppm F), and sealants.
- Restorative: POP (tooth-preserving operative procedures).

Planning Care for the Patient's Caries Risk Level

- The dental hygienist is challenged to select a caries management strategy to meet the needs of each individual patient.
- The care plan will not only need to provide for treatment of existing nonreversible carious lesions, but also provide a framework for changes in personal care previously unrecognized by the patient to prevent development of new lesions.
  - Dental carious lesions contain large numbers of acidogenic and aciduric bacteria, especially mutans streptococci and lactobacilli. Cavitated carious lesions need to be restored or bacteria from within the lesion will remain a source of infection.
  - Restorative materials containing fluoride are recommended wherever possible.
  - Family members can continue to harbor cariogenic microorganisms, so having close family members address carious lesions will further reduce individual exposure to these pathogens.[5,6,10]
- A plan for care is individualized depending on the disease risk level, physical and cognitive abilities, and patient or parent desire to change.
- It is essential to partner with the patient in setting goals and planning care in order to work with the patient for a successful caries management plan. (See Chapter 24 for additional information.)
- What follows are general recommendations for management of caries risk levels, but see **Table 25-1** for more detail.

Table 25-1 Comparison of Caries Management Systems/Guidelines[23,25,26]

	Caries Risk Level			
Caries Management System/ Guideline	Low	Moderate	High	Extreme
ICCMS	■ Brushing: 2X/day with fluoride toothpaste ■ Oral health education ■ Diet counseling: Reduce sugar intake ■ Regular dental visits	■ Brushing: 2X/day with higher concentration fluoride (>1,450 ppm) or prescription toothpaste ■ Prescription fluoride mouthrinse ■ Sealants ■ Fluoride varnish 2X/year ■ 2% NaF fluoride gel ■ Dental visits every 3 months, including topical fluoride ■ Dietary counseling ■ Reduce use of recreational drugs ■ Change medications causing xerostomia when possible	■ Brushing: 2X/day with higher concentration fluoride (>1,450 ppm) or prescription toothpaste ■ Prescription fluoride mouthrinse ■ Sealants ■ Fluoride varnish 4X/year ■ 2% NaF fluoride gel ■ Dental visits every 3 months, including topical fluoride ■ Dietary counseling (reduce added sugars and frequency) ■ Reduce use of recreational drugs ■ Change medications causing xerostomia when possible	

(continues)

Table 25-1 Comparison of Caries Management Systems/Guidelines[23,25,26] *(continued)*

	Caries Risk Level			
Caries Management System/ Guideline	**Low**	**Moderate**	**High**	**Extreme**
CAMBRA	▪ Brushing 2X/day with fluoride toothpaste ▪ Radiographs: 12–24 months ▪ Dental visits: 6–12 months	▪ Brushing 2X/ day with fluoride toothpaste ▪ Prescription fluoride (5,000 ppm) toothpaste 2X/ day or 0.05% NaF mouthrinse daily ▪ Fluoride varnish every 6 months ▪ Diet counseling ▪ Sealants on at-risk pits and fissures ▪ Radiographs: 6–12 months ▪ Dental visits every 6 months	▪ Brushing 2X/day with fluoride toothpaste ▪ Prescription (5,000 ppm) fluoride toothpaste 2X/day ▪ Fluoride varnish every 3 months ▪ Chlorhexidine mouthrinse (0.12%) 1X/day for 1 week each month ▪ Diet counseling: reduce between meal snacking ▪ Sealants on at-risk pits and fissures ▪ Radiographs: 6–12 months ▪ Dental visits every 6 months	▪ Brushing 3X/day with fluoride toothpaste ▪ Prescription (5,000 ppm) fluoride toothpaste ▪ Fluoride varnish every 1–3 months ▪ Chlorhexidine mouth rinse (0.12%) 1X/day for 1 week each month ▪ Diet counseling: Reduce between meal snacking ▪ Rinse multiple times/day with baking soda solution ▪ Home fluoride trays may be need to manage caries risk ▪ For early lesions, silver diamine fluoride or ITR (interim therapeutic restoration) may be considered ▪ Radiographs: 6–12 months ▪ Dental visits every 6 months
American Academy of Pediatric Dentistry (AAPD)	▪ Brushing 2X/day with fluoride toothpaste ▪ Drink fluoridated water ▪ Diet counseling ▪ Sealants ▪ Radiographs every 12–24 months ▪ Dental visits every 6–12 months	▪ Brushing 2X/ day with fluoride toothpaste ▪ Drink fluoridated water ▪ Fluoride supplements (for nonfluoridated community water supply) ▪ Diet counseling ▪ Sealants ▪ Professional topical fluoride every 6 months ▪ Radiographs every 6–12 months ▪ Dental visits every 6 months	▪ (<6 years old) Brushing 2X/day fluoride toothpaste ▪ (>6 years old) Brushing with 5% prescription fluoride toothpaste ▪ Drink fluoridated water ▪ Fluoride supplements (for nonfluoridated community water supply) ▪ Professional topical ▪ Diet counseling ▪ Sealants ▪ Professional topical fluoride every 3 months ▪ Silver diamine fluoride on cavitated lesions ▪ Radiographs every 6 months ▪ Dental visits every 3 months	

I. The Patient with Low Caries Risk

- Primary prevention remains a top priority, as changes in habits may increase caries risk.
- Provide the patient with positive feedback and education so oral, periodontal, and dental health can be maintained.
- Review with the patient the existing habits that categorize them at low caries risk, such as good oral daily biofilm removal, healthy snacking habits, normal salivary flow, and daily exposure to fluoridated toothpaste and/or fluoridated water supply.
- Recommend routine continuing care appointments.

II. The Patient with Moderate Caries Risk

- This patient exhibits factors increasing their risk for developing dental carious lesions.
- Provide the patient with positive feedback and support for the protective factors they currently exhibit, such as fluoride use, healthy snacking habits, or sugar-free chewing gum use.[25,27]
- Motivational interviewing engages the patient in choosing behavior changes to increase compliance and success in reducing caries.[20, 21]
- Work with the patient to plan strategies to reduce risk factors, such as acidic beverages, frequent fermentable carbohydrate snacks, and improved daily biofilm removal.
- Increase protective factors such as use of prescription fluoride toothpaste, fluoride varnish, and sealants.[17,28,29]
- Discuss addition of caries-preventive foods to diet, such as nuts, sugar-free yogurt, and cheese.[30]
- Increasing protective factors can be accomplished by the dental hygienist, especially application of fluoride varnish and sealant placement.
- Recommend appropriate continuing care schedule.

III. The Patient with High and Extreme Caries Risk

The patient at high risk for caries displays active carious lesions, has a recent history of restoration to repair carious lesions, or may have medications or systemic factors that cause severe dry mouth (patients who are at high risk and also suffer from dry mouth are categorized as extreme risk).

- Improved biofilm removal.
- Dietary counseling to reduce intake of fermentable carbohydrates.
- Initial one to three fluoride varnish application followed by application once every 3 months.[26]
- Diamine fluoride application may also be indicated for early lesions to prevent progression.[23]

Continuing Care

- Continuing care appointments include the following:
    - Biofilm control assessment: Use disclosing agent and record the biofilm score. Address oral self-care issues.
    - Reassess caries risk.
    - Clinical detection for demineralization areas, need for sealants, and poor margins on restorations.
    - Radiographs prescribed as indicated by level of risk and clinical findings.
    - Assess patient compliance with caries management recommendations.
    - Determine changes needed in caries management protocol.

Documentation

- CRA, risk level, and compliance with management protocols are documented at each continuing care visit.
- Thorough documentation includes assessment results, collaboration with the patient, health promotion education, and evaluation of patient attainment of goals at each appointment.
    - Initial planning: Record all instructions and survey report from the analysis of risk factors.
    - Note specific oral self-care and dietary changes recommended and progress in meeting goals.
    - Note any phone or e-mail follow-up messages.
    - At continuing care, note patient comments on individual efforts, likes and dislikes, successes, and changes that can be made to improve success.
    - Set new goals.
    - A sample of documentation can be found in **Box 25-1**.

Box 25-1 Example Documentation: Patient with High Caries Risk

- **S**—Admits drinking soda in the afternoon while studying. Chews lots of gum containing sugar. Brushes twice daily, but admits to flossing only a couple of times a week. Snacks frequently.
- **O**—Resting pH—7.2; CRA—moderate. Moderate generalized biofilm in embrasures on disclosing with plaque-free score of 50%.
- **A**—Increased risk for dental caries.
- **P**—Recommend patient drink soda only during meals and sip fluoridated water while studying, chew sugar-free or xylitol gum, and use 1.1% sodium fluoride gel or paste daily. Discussed alternatives to flossing. Demonstrated interdental brushes. Pt. liked interdental brushes and said he would try to use them daily while studying. Reassess at 6-month continuing care visit.

Signed: ____________________, RDH
Date: ____________________

Factors to Teach the Patient

- The causes and process of caries development.
- Explain to the patient what demineralization means and how they can prevent it from progressing to a cavity that needs restoration.
- How remineralization can be helped by using fluoride toothpaste and drinking fluoridated water daily.
- Use of appropriate fluoride based on risk for dental caries is necessary throughout life.

References

1. Chankanka O, Cavanaugh JE, Levy SM, et al. Longitudinal associations between children's dental caries and risk factors. *J Public Health Dent*. 2011;71(4):289-300.
2. Beltrán-Aguilar ED, Barker L, Dye BA. Prevalence and severity of dental fluorosis in the United States, 1999-2004. *NCHS Data Brief*. 2010;(53):1-8.
3. Dye BA, Mitnik GL, Iafolla TJ, Vargas CM. Trends in dental caries in children and adolescents according to poverty status in the United States from 1999 through 2004 and from 2011 through 2014. *J Am Dent Assoc* 2017;148(8):550-565.e7.
4. Machiulskiene V, Campus G, Carvalho JC, et al. Terminology of dental caries and dental caries management: consensus report of a workshop organized by orca and Cariology Research Group of IADR. *Caries Res*. 2020;54(1):7-14.
5. Childers NK, Momeni SS, Whiddon J, et al. Association between early childhood caries and colonization with *Streptococcus mutans* genotypes from mothers. *Pediatr Dent*. 2017;39(2):130-135.
6. Caufield PW, Dasanayake AP, Li Y, Pan Y, Hsu J, Hardin JM. Natural history of *Streptococcus sanguinis* in the oral cavity of infants: evidence for a discrete window of infectivity. *Infect Immun*. 2000;68(7):4018-4023.
7. Takahashi N, Nyvad B. The role of bacteria in the caries process: ecological perspectives. *J Dent Res*. 2011;90(3):294-303.
8. Featherstone JDB, Chaffee BW. The evidence for Caries Management by Risk Assessment (CAMBRA®). *Adv Dent Res*. 2018;29(1):9-14.
9. Palmer CA, Kent R, Loo CY, et al. Diet and caries-associated bacteria in severe early childhood caries. *J Dent Res*. 2010; 89(11):1224-1229.
10. Kaan AMM, Kahharova D, Zaura E. Acquisition and establishment of the oral microbiota. *Periodontol 2000*. 2021; 86(1):123-141.
11. Garcia BA, Acosta NC, Tomar SL, et al. Association of *Candida albicans* and Cbp+ *Streptococcus mutans* with early childhood caries recurrence. *Sci Rep*. 2021;11(1):10802.
12. Hancock S, Zinn C, Schofield G. The consumption of processed sugar- and starch-containing foods, and dental caries: a systematic review. *Eur J Oral Sci*. 2020;128(6):467-475.
13. Pitchika V, Standl M, Harris C, et al. Association of sugar-sweetened drinks with caries in 10- and 15-year-olds. *BMC Oral Health*. 2020;20(1):81.
14. Marshall TA, Broffitt B, Eichenberger-Gilmore J, Warren JJ, Cunningham MA, Levy SM. The roles of meal, snack, and daily total food and beverage exposures on caries experience in young children. *J Public Health Dent*. 2005;65(3):166-173.
15. González-Cabezas C. The chemistry of caries: remineralization and demineralization events with direct clinical relevance. *Dent Clin North Am*. 2010;54(3):469-478.
16. Pedersen AML, Sørensen CE, Proctor GB, Carpenter GH, Ekström J. Salivary secretion in health and disease. *J Oral Rehabil*. 2018;45(9):730-746.
17. Featherstone JD. Prevention and reversal of dental caries: role of low level fluoride. *Community Dent Oral Epidemiol*. 1999;27(1):31-40.
18. Rošin-Grget K, Peroš K, Sutej I, Bašić K. The cariostatic mechanisms of fluoride. *Acta Medica Acad*. 2013;42(2):179-188.
19. ICCMS Caries Management. ICDAS. ICCMS. Published 2020. https://www.iccms-web.com/content/icdas. Accessed November 6, 2021.

20. Young DA, Nový BB, Zeller GG, et al. The American Dental Association Caries Classification System for clinical practice: a report of the American Dental Association Council on Scientific Affairs. *J Am Dent Assoc* 2015;146(2): 79-86.
21. Cagetti MG, Bontà G, Cocco F, Lingstrom P, Strohmenger L, Campus G. Are standardized caries risk assessment models effective in assessing actual caries status and future caries increment? A systematic review. *BMC Oral Health*. 2018;18(1):123.
22. American Dental Association. Caries Risk Assessment and Management. Published June 9, 2021. https://www.ada.org/en/member-center/oral-health-topics/caries-risk-assessment-and-management. Accessed November 6, 2021.
23. American Academy of Pediatric Dentistry. Guideline on caries-risk assessment and management for infants, children, and adolescents. *Pediatr Dent*. 2016;38(6):142-149.
24. Bratthall D, Hänsel Petersson G. Cariogram—a multifactorial risk assessment model for a multifactorial disease. *Community Dent Oral Epidemiol*. 2005;33(4):256-264.
25. Featherstone JDB, Crystal YO, Alston P, et al. Evidence-based caries management for all ages-practical guidelines. *Front Oral Health*. 2021;2:14.
26. ICCMS Caries Management. Education. Published 2020. https://www.iccms-web.com/content/iccms-usage/education. Accessed November 6, 2021.
27. Ismail AI, Pitts NB, Tellez M, et al. The International Caries Classification and Management System (ICCMSTM) an example of a caries management pathway. *BMC Oral Health*. 2015;15(Suppl 1):S9.
28. Janakiram C, Deepan Kumar CV, Joseph J. Xylitol in preventing dental caries: A systematic review and meta-analyses. *J Nat Sci Biol Med*. 2017;8(1):16-21.
29. Kashbour W, Gupta P, Worthington HV, Boyers D. Pit and fissure sealants versus fluoride varnishes for preventing dental decay in the permanent teeth of children and adolescents. *Cochrane Database Syst Rev*. 2020;11:CD003067.
30. Gul P, Akgul N, Seven N. Anticariogenic potential of white cheese, xylitol chewing gum, and black tea. *Eur J Dent*. 2018;12(2):199-203.

CHAPTER 26

Oral Infection Control: Toothbrushes and Toothbrushing

Heather L. Reid, RDH, MS
Linda D. Boyd, RDH, RD, EdD

CHAPTER OUTLINE

DEVELOPMENT OF TOOTHBRUSHES
- **I.** Origins of the Toothbrush
- **II.** Early Toothbrushes

MANUAL TOOTHBRUSHES
- **I.** Characteristics of an Effective Manual Toothbrush
- **II.** General Description
- **III.** Handle
- **IV.** Brush Head
- **V.** Filaments (or Bristles)

POWER TOOTHBRUSHES
- **I.** Effectiveness
- **II.** Purposes and Indications
- **III.** Description

TOOTHBRUSH SELECTION FOR THE PATIENT
- **I.** Influencing Factors
- **II.** Toothbrush Characteristics
- **III.** Stiffness of Filaments or Bristles

METHODS FOR MANUAL TOOTHBRUSHING

THE BASS AND MODIFIED BASS METHODS
- **I.** Purposes and Indications
- **II.** Procedure
- **III.** Limitations

THE STILLMAN AND MODIFIED STILLMAN METHODS
- **I.** Purposes and Indications
- **II.** Procedure
- **III.** Limitations

THE ROLL OR ROLLING STROKE METHOD
- **I.** Purposes and Indications
- **II.** Procedure
- **III.** Limitations

CHARTERS METHOD
- **I.** Purposes and Indications
- **II.** Procedure
- **III.** Limitations

THE HORIZONTAL (OR SCRUB) METHOD
- **I.** Purposes and Indications
- **II.** Procedure
- **III.** Limitations

THE FONES (OR CIRCULAR) METHOD
- **I.** Purposes and Indications
- **II.** Procedure
- **III.** Limitations

LEONARD'S (OR VERTICAL) METHOD
- **I.** Purposes and Indications
- **II.** Procedure
- **III.** Limitations

METHOD FOR POWER TOOTHBRUSHING
- **I.** Procedure
- **II.** Limitations

SUPPLEMENTAL BRUSHING METHODS
- **I.** Occlusal Brushing
- **II.** Brushing Difficult-to-Reach Areas
- **III.** Tongue Cleaning

LEARNING OBJECTIVES

After studying this chapter, the student will be able to:

1. Identify the characteristics of effective manual and power toothbrushes.
2. Differentiate among manual toothbrushing methods, including limitations and benefits of each.
3. Describe the different modes of action of power toothbrushes.
4. Identify the basis for power toothbrush selection.
5. Describe tongue cleaning and its effect on reducing dental biofilm.
6. Identify adverse effects of improper toothbrushing on hard and soft tissues.

Development of Toothbrushes

The toothbrush has been the principal instrument in general use for oral care and is a necessary part of oral disease control.[1-4] There is a long history of development of toothbrushes since ancient times.

I. Origins of the Toothbrush

- Evidence of toothbrushes has its origins in the Babylonian chew sticks in early 3500 BC.[5]
- The "chew stick," which has been considered the primitive toothbrush, appears in the Chinese literature around 1600 BC.[5]
    - Care of the mouth was associated with religious training and ritual: the Buddhists had a "toothstick," and the Mohammedans used the "miswak" or "siwak."
    - Chew sticks are made from various types of wood by crushing the end of a twig or root and spreading the fibers in a brush-like manner.
    - Miswaks are used in many African and Middle Eastern countries and evidence suggests[4] they have antimicrobial properties.[6]

II. Early Toothbrushes

- It is believed the first toothbrush made of horsehair **bristles** was mentioned in the early Chinese literature around 1000 AD.[5]
- Pierre Fauchard in 1728 in *Le Chirurgien Dentiste* described many aspects of oral health. He was critical of the toothbrush made of horse's hair because it was too soft and advised the use of sponges to vigorously rub the teeth.[7]
- One of the earlier toothbrushes made in England was produced by William Addis around 1780.[8]
    - By the early 19th century, craftsmen in various European countries constructed handles of gold, ivory, or ebony in which replaceable brush heads could be fitted.
    - The first patent for a toothbrush in the United States was issued to HN Wadsworth in 1860.[9]
- In the early 1900s, celluloid began to replace bone handles.
- Nylon bristles were introduced by Dupont De Nemours in 1938.[10]
    - World War II prevented Chinese export of wild boar bristles, so synthetic materials were substituted for natural bristles.
    - Since then, synthetic materials have improved and manufacturers' specifications standardized.

- Most toothbrushes are made exclusively of synthetic materials.
- The first **power toothbrush** to appear in the American market was a Broxodent in 1960.[10]

Manual Toothbrushes

Little evidence exists related to the most effective characteristics of a toothbrush and other aspects of toothbrushing, so clinical experience and individual patient needs will guide recommendations.[11]

I. Characteristics of an Effective Manual Toothbrush

- Conforms to individual patient requirements in size, shape, and texture.
- Easily and efficiently manipulated.
- Readily cleaned and aerated; impervious to moisture.
- Durable and inexpensive.
- Soft bristles.[12]
- Multilevel or angled bristles.[12,13]
- **End-rounded** filaments free of sharp or jagged edges.[12]
- Designed for utility, efficiency, and cleanliness.
- In the United States, look for the ADA (American Dental Association) Seal of Acceptance, and in Canada, look for the CDA (Canadian Dental Association) Seal.

II. General Description

A. Parts (Figure 26-1)

- Handle: The part grasped in the hand during toothbrushing.
- Head: The working end; consists of **tufts** of **bristles** or **filaments**.
- Shank: The section that connects the head and the handle.

B. Dimensions

- Recommendations in the literature and in different countries seem to vary.

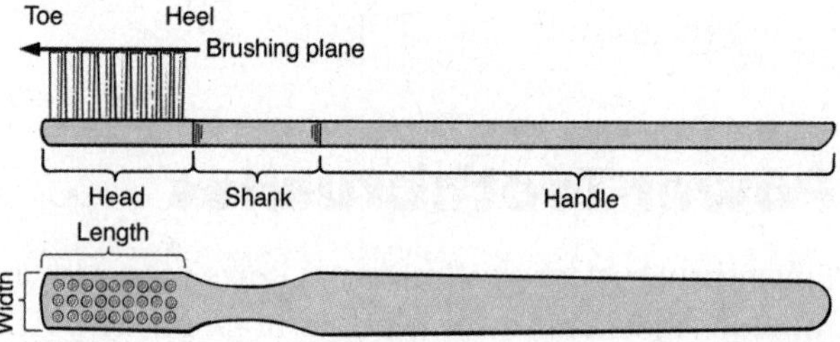

Figure 26-1 Parts of a Toothbrush

- Generally, the following should be considered in recommending a toothbrush to a patient[13]:
  - Length of the toothbrush head should cover two to three posterior teeth.
  - Width of the **toothbrush head** should cover the intercuspal distance of the first molar.
- General recommendations from the ADA for dimensions include:
  - Total brush length: About 15–19 cm (6–7.5 inches); junior and child sizes are shorter.
  - Head: Length of brushing plane, 25.4–31.8 mm (1–1.25 inches); width, 7.9–9.5 mm (5/16–3/8 inch).
  - Bristle or filament height: 11 mm (7/16 inch).

III. Handle

A. Composition

- Manufacturing specifications: Most often a single type of plastic, or a combination of polymers.
- Properties: Combines durability, imperviousness to moisture, pleasing appearance, low cost, and sufficient maneuverability.

B. Shape

- Preferred characteristics
  - Easy to grasp.
  - Does not slip or rotate during use.
  - No sharp corners or projections.
  - Lightweight, consistent with strength.
- Variations
  - A twist, curve, offset, or angle in the shank with or without thumb rests may assist the patient in adaptation of the brush to difficult-to-reach areas.
  - A handle of larger diameter may be useful for patients with limited dexterity, such as children, aging patients, and those with a disability.

IV. Brush Head

A. Design

- Length: May be 5–12 tufts long and 3–4 rows wide.
- Shape and size: A variety of brush head shapes and sizes from rounded to tapered to angled are available.
- Arrangement of bristle tufts varies in configuration and angulation as shown in **Figure 26-2**.

B. Brushing Plane (Lateral Profile)

- Length: Range from filaments of equal lengths (flat planes) to those with variable lengths, such as rippled, scalloped, tapered, bi-level, multilevel, and angled (Figure 26-2).

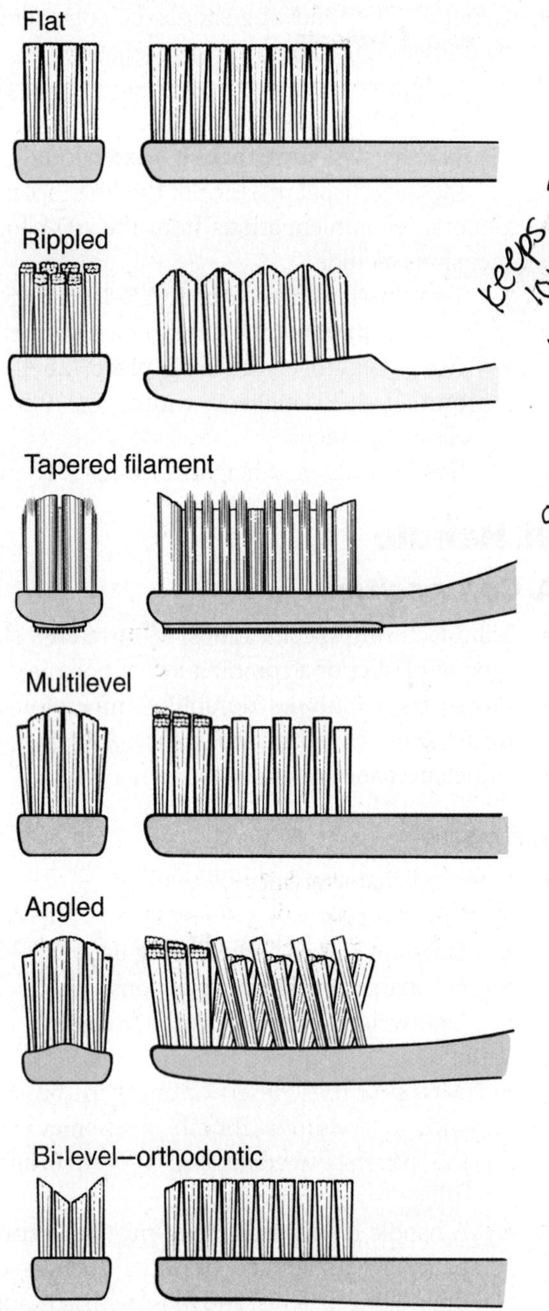

Figure 26-2 Manual Brush Trim Profiles. A variety of filament profiles are available. In addition to the classic flat planed brush, other trims include the rippled, tapered filaments, bi-level, multilevel, and angled brushes. Brushes for use over orthodontic appliances are made with various bi-level shapes.

- Efficiency in biofilm removal:
  - Research results have demonstrated plaque and gingivitis are better reduced through use of modern bristle technology (i.e., angled, tapered, criss-cross designs versus traditional flat trim designs).[14,15]
  - Ultimately, efficiency in cleaning the hard-to-reach areas, such as extension onto proximal surfaces, malpositioned teeth, or exposed root surfaces, depends on individual patient abilities and understanding.

V. Filaments (or Bristles)

- Most current toothbrushes have nylon filaments.
  - The physical properties of natural bristles cannot be standardized.
  - A comparison of natural bristles and synthetic filaments is reviewed in **Table 26-1**.
- Many manufacturers of synthetic filaments refer to filaments as "bristles" when communicating with consumers on the toothbrush package and in advertising.
  - Dental professionals need to be aware that most manufacturers of toothbrushes today produce brushes using "synthetic filaments" but still refer to these as "bristles."
- Companies that produce a toothbrush with "natural bristles" may distinguish themselves by using the word "natural" in the product description.
- The **bristle stiffness** depends on the diameter and length of the filament.[4] Brushes designated as soft, medium, or hard may not be consistent among manufacturers.

A. Filament or Bristle Design

- A variety of filament designs are available and may include, but are not limited to, end-rounded, feathered, microfine, and conical shaped.
- Another factor to keep in mind is that the quality of end-rounding varies in both adult and children's toothbrushes depending on the manufacturer.[16] Natural bristles cannot be end-rounded.
- Some evidence suggests end-rounded bristles are less abrasive to gingival damage than bristles that are non-end-rounded (**Figure 26-3** for examples); however, the overall conclusion by a systematic review found the association of rounding of filaments (or bristles) to gingival recession to be inconclusive.[17]

Power Toothbrushes

Power brushes are also known as power-assisted, automatic, mechanical, or electric brushes. The ADA Council on Scientific Affairs evaluates power brushes for the reduction of dental biofilm and gingivitis.[18]

Table 26-1 Comparison of Natural Bristles and Synthetic Bristles or Filaments

	Natural Bristles	Bristles/Filaments
Source	Historically made from hog or wild boar hair	Synthetic, plastic materials, primarily nylon
Uniformity	No uniformity of texture. Diameter or wearing properties depending upon the breed of the animal, geographic location, and season in which the bristles were gathered	Uniformity controlled during manufacturing
Diameter	Varies depending on portion of the bristle taken, age, and life of animal	Ranges from extra soft at 0.075 mm (0.003 inch) to hard at 0.3 mm (0.012 inch)
End shape	Deficient, irregular, frequently open ended	End-rounded
Advantages and disadvantages	Cannot be standardized Wear rapidly and irregularly Hollow ends allow microorganisms and debris to collect inside	Rinse clean, dry rapidly Durable and maintained longer End-rounded and closed, repel debris and water More resistant to accumulation of microorganisms

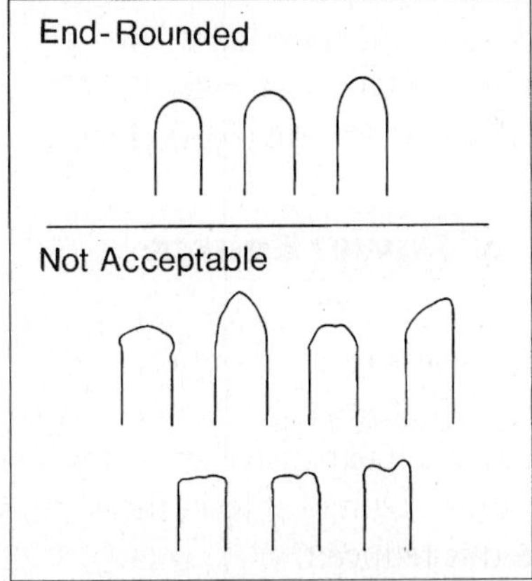

Figure 26-3 End-Rounded Filaments. Examples of the shape of acceptable end-rounding and of those that are not acceptable are shown.

Data from Silverstone LM, Featherstone MJ. A scanning electron microscope study of the end rounding of bristles in eight toothbrush types. *Quintessence Int.* 1988;19(2):87-107; and Checchi L, Minguzzi S, Franchi M, et al. Toothbrush filaments end-rounding: stereomicroscope analysis. *J Clin Periodontol.* 2001;28(4):360-364.

I. Effectiveness

A. Evolution

- Power toothbrushes have evolved over time due to improved designs and features.
- Power toothbrushes of the 1960–1980 era mimicked the motions of manual brushing.
- Current power brushes move at speeds and motions that often cannot be duplicated by manual brushes.

B. Power Toothbrushes versus Manual Toothbrushes

- There is moderate evidence that power toothbrushes result in a 10% to 20% reduction in plaque and about a 10% reduction in gingivitis when compared to manual toothbrushes.[19]
- Rotating oscillating action power toothbrushes have been shown to be more effective than side-to-side power brushes for reducing plaque and gingivitis.[1]
- Sonic power toothbrushes have not been shown to be more effective than other types of power toothbrushes.[20-25]
- Power toothbrushes, as compared to their manual counterparts, do not damage gingival tissues as much; they may be less damaging because they have mechanisms to alert the patient when they apply excessive force.[4,11] However, when not used properly, power toothbrushes may be more abrasive.[26,27]
- Ultimately, recommendations are based on patient needs and preference.

II. Purposes and Indications

A. Purpose

- Recommended for physically able patients with ineffective manual biofilm removal techniques.
- Facilitate **mechanical dental biofilm control** or removal of food debris from the teeth and the gingiva.
- Reduce calculus and extrinsic dental stain buildup.[28]

B. Indications for Use of Power Toothbrush

Power brushes can be useful for many patients, including:

- Those with a history of failed attempts at more traditional biofilm removal methods.
- Those undergoing orthodontic treatment.

- Those undergoing complex restorative and prosthodontic treatment.
- Aggressive brushers
    - Many models of power toothbrushes will shut off automatically if too much pressure is applied during brushing, which can be a benefit for those who have a tendency to apply too much pressure.[4,11]
- Patients with disabilities or limited dexterity.
    - The large handle of a power brush can be of benefit.
    - Handle weight needs to be considered for these patients.
- When a parent or caregiver must brush for the patient.

III. Description

A. Motion

- The motion of the head of power toothbrushes varies between models and may include one or more of the following (**Table 26-2**)[12]:
    - Rotation oscillation.
    - Counter oscillation.
    - Sonic or ultrasonic motion.
    - Side to side.
    - Circular.

B. Speeds

- Vary from low to high.
- Generally, power brushes with replaceable batteries move more slowly than those with rechargeable batteries and have been shown to be less effective in plaque biofilm removal.[25,29]
- Movement per minute varies from 3,800 to over 48,000 depending on the manufacturer and type (battery, sonic, or ultrasonic).

C. Brush Head Design

- Adult: The variety of shapes continues to evolve, but a few examples are illustrated in **Figure 26-4**. They may be small and round, or like traditional manual heads. Trim profiles include flat, bi-level, rippled, or angled.
- Child: A child's power brush head should be specially designed to accommodate a smaller mouth, as shown in **Figure 26-5**.

D. Filaments or Bristles

- Made of soft, end-rounded nylon.
- Diameters: From extra soft, 0.075 mm (0.003 inch), to soft, 0.15 mm (0.006 inch).

E. Types of Power Source

- Direct
    - Utilizes an electrical outlet.
- Replaceable batteries
    - Relatively inexpensive and convenient.
    - As most batteries lose their power, brush speed is reduced.
    - Advise patients to select a brush that has a water tight handle to avoid corrosion of batteries.

Table 26-2 Power Toothbrush Motions

Motion	Description
Rotational	Moves in a 360° circular motion.
Counterrotational	Each tuft of filaments moves in rotational motion; each tuft moves counter-directional to the adjacent tuft.
Oscillating	Rotates from center to the left, then to the right; degree of rotation varies from 25° to 55°.
Pulsating	When brush head is on the tooth, pulsations are directed toward the interproximal areas.
Cradle or twist	Side to side with an arc.
Side to side	Side to side perpendicular to the long axis of the brush handle.
Translating	Up and down parallel to the long axis of the brush handle.
Combination	Combination of simultaneous yet different types of movement.
Ultrasonic	Brush head vibrates at ultrasonic frequency (>250 kHz).

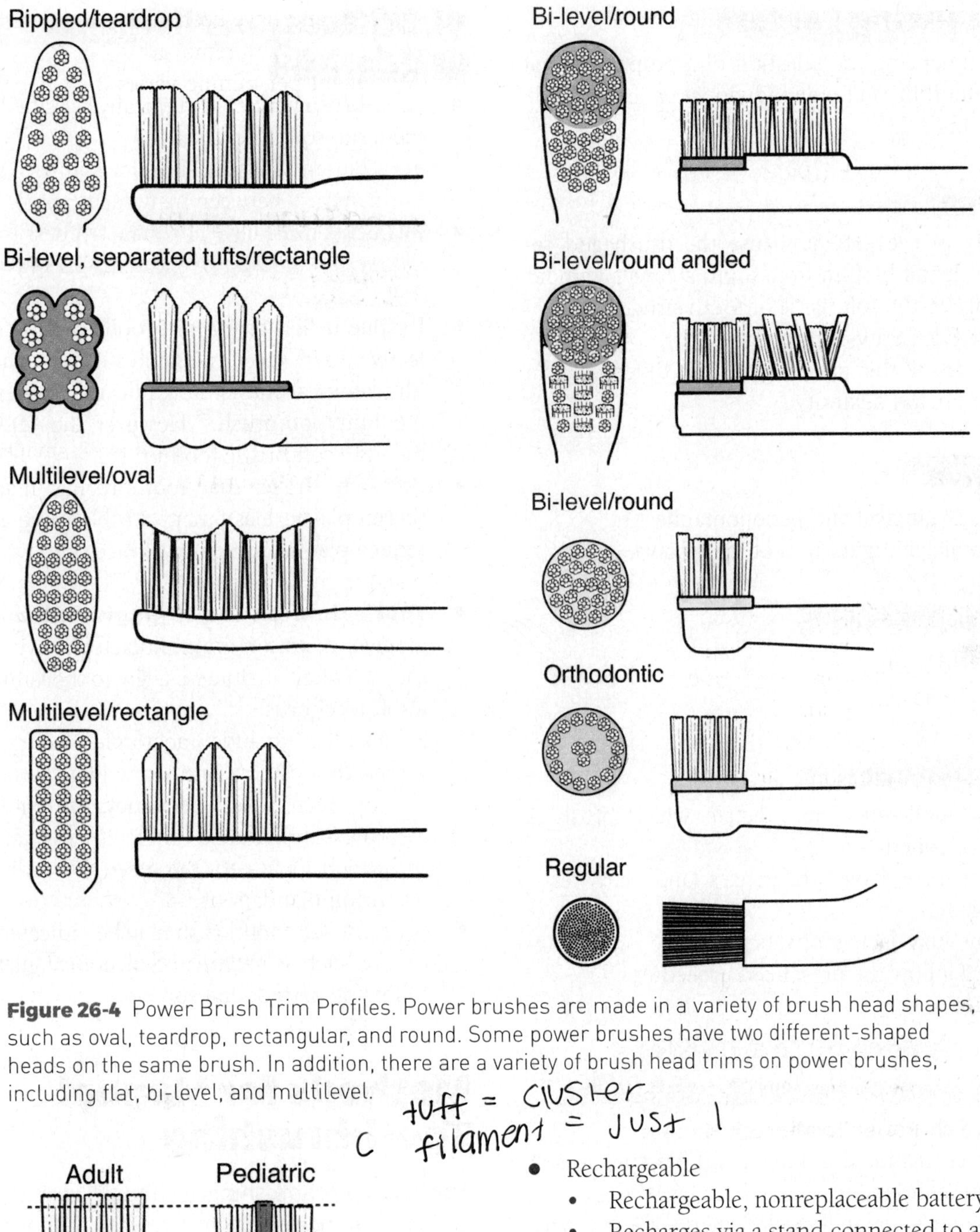

Rippled/teardrop

Bi-level, separated tufts/rectangle

Multilevel/oval

Multilevel/rectangle

Bi-level/round

Bi-level/round angled

Bi-level/round

Orthodontic

Regular

Figure 26-4 Power Brush Trim Profiles. Power brushes are made in a variety of brush head shapes, such as oval, teardrop, rectangular, and round. Some power brushes have two different-shaped heads on the same brush. In addition, there are a variety of brush head trims on power brushes, including flat, bi-level, and multilevel.

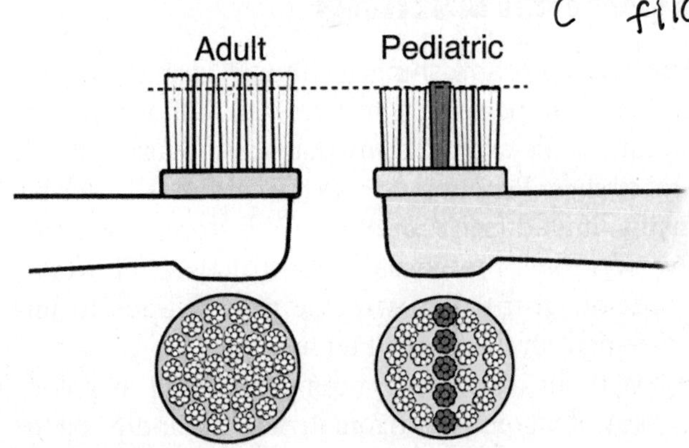

Figure 26-5 Child Power Brush Profile. Power brushes for children could necessitate smaller head sizes and shorter filaments to allow for access to tight posterior areas. Raised blue filaments allow for better access to occlusal pits and fissures.

- Rechargeable
  - Rechargeable, nonreplaceable battery.
  - Recharges via a stand connected to an electrical outlet.
- Disposable
  - Batteries cannot be replaced or recharged.

Toothbrush Selection for the Patient

Overarching factors in toothbrush selection include the quality of clinical research supporting the efficacy and safety of the brush and the ADA or CDA Seal of Approval, along with the clinical decision making of the clinician regarding what is best for an individual patient.

I. Influencing Factors

Factors influencing the selection of a proper manual or power toothbrush for an individual patient include the following:

A. Patient

- Ability of the patient to use the brush and remove dental biofilm from tooth surfaces without damage to the soft tissue or tooth structure.
- Manual dexterity of the patient.
- The age of the patient and the differences in dentition and dexterity.

B. Gingiva

- Status of gingival and periodontal health.
- Anatomic configurations of the gingiva.

C. Position of Teeth

- Crowded teeth.
- Open contacts.

D. Compliance

- Patient preference may dictate which brush is recommended.
- Patient may have preferences and may resist change.
- Patient may lack motivation, ability, or willingness to follow the prescribed procedure.

E. Specific Factors to Consider for Selection of Power Toothbrush

- Replaceable brush head.
- Features that include a timer and pressure sensor.
- Patient affordability.
  - Battery-operated models are often less expensive and may be a good way for the patient to try out a power toothbrush before investing in a more expensive rechargeable model.

II. Toothbrush Characteristics

- Brush head selection is dependent on the patient's ability to maneuver and adapt the brush correctly to all facial, lingual, palatal, and occlusal surfaces for dental biofilm removal.
- Some research suggests angled tufted designs of manual toothbrush heads and rotating, oscillating round power brush heads are most effective.[14,20,30]

III. Stiffness of Filaments or Bristles

- Toothbrush bristles are typically classified as hard, medium, soft, or extra soft.
  - The same classification for stiffness (i.e., soft) may vary between manufacturers.[31]
- Filaments must have adequate stiffness to remove plaque biofilm and do no harm to oral soft and hard tissues.
- Despite beliefs that a soft toothbrush is more effective, more recent research suggests plaque biofilm removal may be significantly better with a medium toothbrush.[32] However, the ADA recommends a soft bristle toothbrush.[12]
- Research shows that toothbrushes made from thermoplastic elastomer, a rubber-like material, reduce plaque and gingival bleeding, when compared to nylon bristles.[32]
- **Tooth abrasion** and/or **gingival abrasion** and gingival recession are multifactorial even though they are often attributed solely to the failure to use a soft toothbrush.[11]
  - Factors include anatomic features (e.g., tooth position and crowding), toothbrushing technique, frequency, duration, force (pressure), and self-inflicted gingival trauma, which point to the need to individualize recommendations.[33]
- An extra-soft toothbrush may be indicated in conditions such as necrotizing ulcerative gingivitis or following periodontal surgery.

Methods for Manual Toothbrushing

The ideal toothbrushing technique is one that the patient can perform effectively to remove plaque biofilm while avoiding any damage to hard and soft oral tissues. Research on which method is better remains limited (see **Box 26-1** for a historical perspective on proper toothbrushing instruction). However, hands-on instruction with the patient leads to improvement in their brushing methods.[34,35]

- Without instruction, normal brushing may consist of vigorous horizontal, vertical, and/or circular strokes.[35]
- Manual toothbrushing methods include the following:
  - Sulcular: Modified Bass.
  - Roll: Rolling stroke, modified Stillman.

Box 26-1 Historical Perspective on Proper Toothbrushing Instruction

Koecker, in 1842, wrote that after the dentist has scaled off the tartar, the patient will clean the teeth every morning and after every meal with a hard brush and an astringent powder. For the inner surfaces, he recommended a conical-shaped brush of fine hog's bristles. For the outer surfaces, he believed in an oblong brush made of the "best white horse-hair." He instructed the patient to press hard against the gums so the bristles go between the teeth and "between the edges of the gums and the roots of the teeth. The pressure of the brush is to be applied in the direction from the crowns of the teeth toward the roots, so that the mucus, which adheres to the roots under the edges of the gums, may be completely detached, and after that removed by friction in a direction toward the grinding surfaces."

Koecker L. Exhibiting a new method of treating the diseases of the teeth and gums. In: *Principles of Dental Surgery.* Baltimore, MD: American Society of Dental Surgeons; 1842:155-156.

- Vibratory: Stillman, Charters, Bass.
- Horizontal (or scrub).
- Circular: Fones.
- Vertical: Leonard.

The Bass and Modified Bass Methods

The Bass and modified Bass methods are widely accepted as effective methods for dental biofilm removal adjacent to and directly beneath the gingival margin (sulcus) despite conflicting evidence.[11,35,36] They are considered to be types of **sulcular brushing**, which may be more effective than other methods, and generally are recommended by the ADA.[12,37] The areas at the gingival margin and in the col are the most significant in the control of gingival and periodontal infections.

I. Purposes and Indications

- Dental biofilm removal adjacent to and directly beneath the gingival margin.
- Open embrasures, cervical areas beneath the height of contour of the enamel, and exposed root surfaces.
- Adaptation to abutment teeth or implants, under the gingival border of a fixed partial denture.

II. Procedure

A. Position the Brush[38]

- Direct the filaments apically (up for maxillary, down for mandibular teeth).
- First, position the sides of the filaments parallel with the long axis of the tooth (**Figure 26-6A**).
- From that position, turn the brush head toward the gingival margin to make approximately a 45° angle to the long axis of the tooth (**Figure 26-6B**).
- Direct the filament tips into the gingival sulcus (Figure 26-6A and B).

B. Strokes[31,38]

- Press lightly so the filament tips enter the gingival sulci and embrasures and cover the gingival margin. Do not bend the filaments with excess pressure.
- Vibrate the brush back and forth with very short strokes without disengaging the tips of the filaments from the sulci (Figure 26-6C).

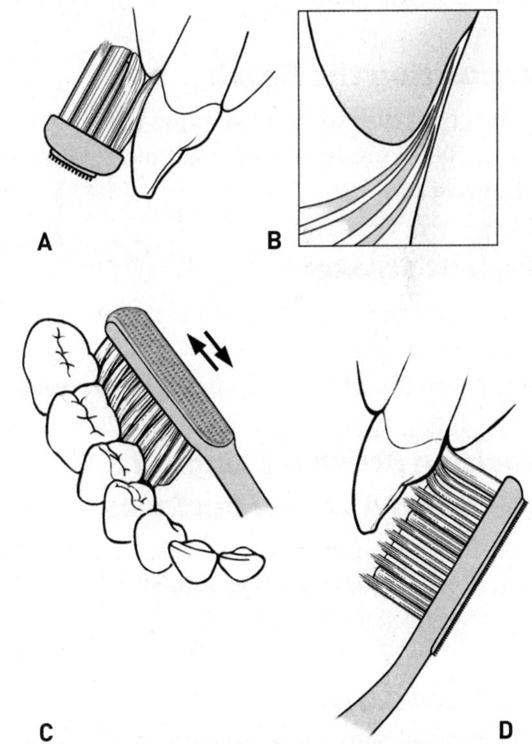

Figure 26-6 Bass/Modified Bass Method of Brushing. **A:** Filament tips are directed into the gingival sulcus at approximately 45° to the long axis of the tooth. **B:** Brushes designed with tapered filaments reach below the gingival margin with ease. **C:** Brush in position for lingual surfaces of mandibular posterior teeth. **D:** Position for palatal surface of maxillary anterior teeth.

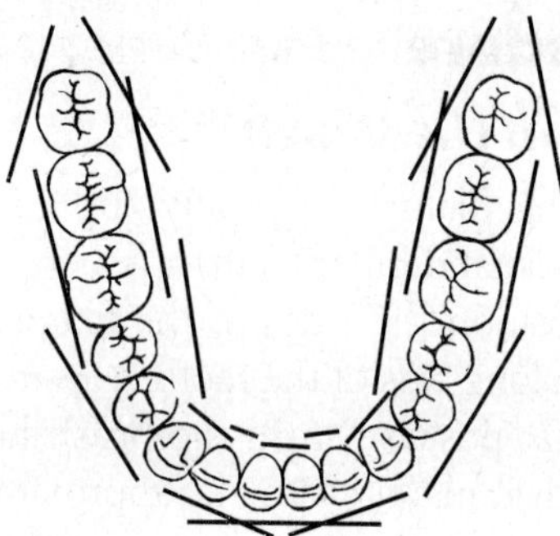

Figure 26-7 Brushing Positions. Each brush position, as represented by a black line, will overlap the previous position. Note placement at canines, where the distal aspect of the canine is brushed with the premolars and the mesial aspect is brushed with the incisors. Short lines on the lingual anterior aspect indicate a brush placed vertically. The maxillary teeth require a similar number of brushing positions.

- Count at least 10 vibrations.
- In the modified Bass method, the vibratory, sulcular brush stroke is followed by rolling the toothbrush down over the crown of the tooth to clean the rest of the tooth surface.

C. Reposition the Brush

- Apply the brush to the next group of two or three teeth. Take care to overlap placement, as shown in **Figure 26-7**.

D. Repeat Stroke

- The entire stroke (steps A–C) is repeated at each position around the maxillary and mandibular arches, on both facial and lingual tooth surfaces.

E. Position Brush for Lingual and Palatal Anterior Surfaces

- Tilt the brush handle somewhat vertically for the anterior components (**Figure 26-6D**).[12] The bristles are directed into the sulci.

III. Limitations

- The toothbrush bristles extend only 0.9 mm below the gingival margin, so plaque removal in the sulcus is limited.[39]
- An individual who is an aggressive brusher may interpret "very short strokes" into a vigorous horizontal scrubbing motion, causing injury to the gingival margin.
- Dexterity requirement for the vibratory stroke may be difficult for certain patients.

The Stillman and Modified Stillman Methods

The modified Stillman method is considered a sulcular brushing technique along with the modified Bass method.

I. Purposes and Indications

- As originally described by Stillman,[40] the method is designed for massage and stimulation, as well as for cleaning the cervical areas. The modified Stillman method adds a rolling stroke to the vibratory stroke to clean the crown of the tooth.[41]
- Dental biofilm removal from cervical areas below the height of contour of the crown and from exposed proximal surfaces.
- General application for cleaning tooth surfaces and massage of the gingiva.

II. Procedure[40]

A. Position the Brush

- Place side of brush on the attached gingiva: The filaments are directed apically (up for maxillary, down for mandibular teeth) in **Figure 26-8A**. When the plastic portion of the brush head is level with the occlusal or incisal plane, generally the brush is at the proper height, as shown in Figure 26-7A.
- The brush ends are placed partly on the gingiva and partly on the cervical areas of the tooth and directed slightly apically.

B. Strokes

- Press to flex the filaments: The sides of the filaments are pressed lightly against the gingiva, and blanching of the tissue occurs (**Figure 26-8B**).
- Angle the filaments: Turn the handle by rotating the wrist so that the filaments are directed at an angle of approximately 45° with the long axis of the tooth.
- Activate the brush: Use a slight rotary motion. Maintain light pressure on the filaments, and keep the tips of the filaments in position on the tooth surface. Count to 10 slowly as the brush is vibrated by a rotary motion of the handle.
- Roll and vibrate the brush: Turn the wrist and work the vibrating brush slowly down over the gingiva and tooth. Make some of the filaments reach interdentally (**Figure 26-8C**).

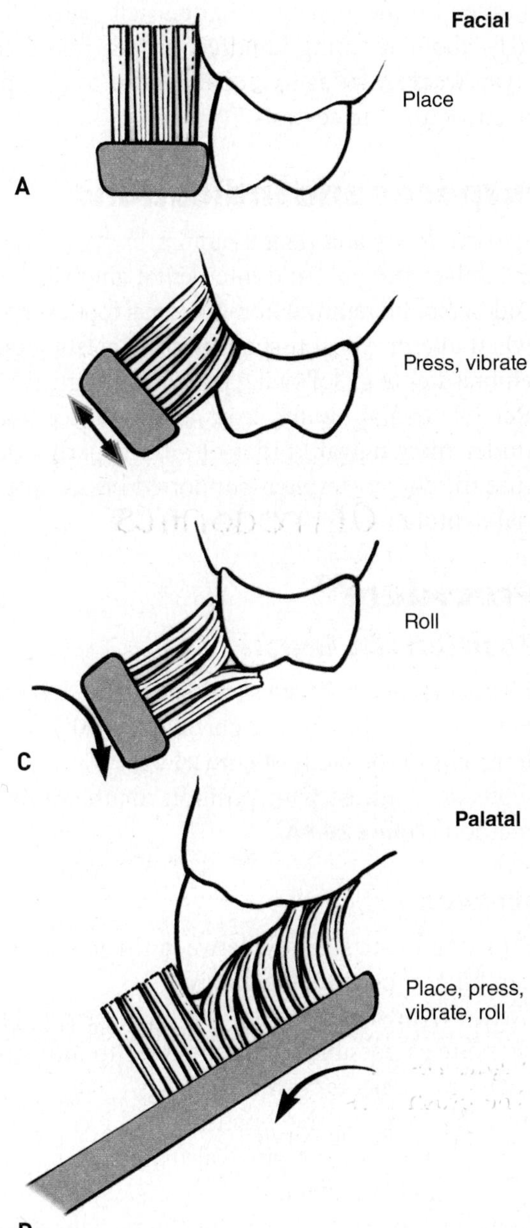

Figure 26-8 Modified Stillman Method of Brushing. **A:** Initial brush placement with sides of bristles or filaments against the attached gingiva. **B:** The brush is pressed and angled, then vibrated. **C:** Vibrating is continued as the brush is rolled slowly over the crown. **D:** Using the toe of the brush, place the bristles into the gingival sulcus of the maxillary anterior teeth, press lightly, vibrate the bristles, and use a rolling stroke to clean the remainder of the lingual surface. Repeat for each anterior tooth and for the mandibular teeth.

C. Replace Brush for Repeat Stroke

- Reposition the brush by rotating the wrist. Avoid dragging the filaments back over the free gingival margin by holding the brush slightly away from the tooth.

D. Repeat Stroke Five Times or More

- The entire stroke (steps A–C) is repeated at least five times for each tooth or group of teeth. When moving the brush to an adjacent position, overlap the brush position.

E. Position Brush for Anterior Lingual and Palatal Surfaces

- Position the brush somewhat vertically using the toe of the brush head for the anterior components (**Figure 26-8D**).
- Press and vibrate, roll, and repeat.

III. Limitations

- Careful placement of a brush with end-rounded filaments is necessary to prevent tissue laceration. Light pressure is needed.
- Patient may try to move the brush into the rolling stroke too quickly, and the vibratory aspect may be ineffective for biofilm removal at the gingival margin.

The Roll or Rolling Stroke Method

I. Purposes and Indications

- Removing biofilm, materia alba, and food debris from the teeth without emphasis on gingival sulcus.
  - Used in conjunction with a vibratory technique such as modified Bass, Charters, and Stillman methods.
- Can be particularly helpful when there is a question about the patient's ability to master and practice a more complex method.

II. Procedure[42]

A. Position the Brush

- Filaments: Direct filaments apically (up for maxillary, down for mandibular teeth).
- Place side of brush parallel to and against the attached gingiva: The filaments are directed apically. When the plastic portion of the brush head is in level with the occlusal or incisal plane, generally the brush is at the proper height, as shown in Figure 26-8A.

B. Strokes

- Press to flex the filaments: The sides of the filaments are pressed lightly against the gingiva. The gingiva will blanch.

- Roll the brush slowly over the teeth: As the brush is rolled, the wrist is turned slightly. The filaments remain flexed and follow the contours of the teeth, thereby permitting cleaning of the cervical areas. Some filaments may reach interdentally.

C. Replace and Repeat Five Times or More

- Repeat the entire stroke: The entire stroke (steps A and B) is repeated at least five times for each tooth or group of teeth.
- Rotate the wrist: When the brush is removed and repositioned, the wrist is rotated.
- Stretch the cheek: The brush is moved away from the teeth, and the cheek is stretched facially with the back of the brush head. Be careful not to drag the filament tips over the gingival margin when the brush is returned to the initial position.

D. Overlap Strokes

- When moving the brush to an adjacent position, overlap the brush position, as shown in Figure 26-7.

E. Position Brush for Anterior Lingual or Palatal Surfaces

- Tilt the brush slightly vertically and use the toe of the brush head to access the lingual surfaces of the anterior teeth.
- Press (down for maxillary, up for mandibular) until the filaments lie flat against the teeth and gingiva.
- Press and roll (curve up for mandibular, down for maxillary teeth).
- Replace and repeat five times for each brush width.

III. Limitations

- Brushing too high during initial placement can lacerate the alveolar mucosa.
- Minimal plaque removal interproximally or in sulcular areas.
- Tendency to use quick, sweeping strokes results in failure to adequately remove plaque biofilm from the cervical third of the tooth because the brush tips pass over rather than into the area, likewise for the interproximal areas.

Charters Method

Charters strongly believed in prevention and felt dentists were not doing their "full duty" if they were not taking the time to teach patients a system of home care.[43] He advocated for personal demonstration of techniques by the patient. Charters felt particularly strongly about teaching children proper home care and even went so far as to recommend it to be a part of the curriculum in schools.[43]

I. Purposes and Indications

- Loosen debris and dental biofilm.[43]
- Stimulate marginal and interdental gingiva.[43]
- Aid in biofilm removal from proximal tooth surfaces when interproximal tissue is missing creating open embrasures (e.g., following periodontal surgery).[43]
- Remove dental biofilm from abutment teeth and under the gingival border of a fixed partial denture (bridge) or implant-supported bridge or partial denture.

II. Procedure[43]

A. Position the Brush

- Filaments: Direct bristles at 90° angle to the teeth.
- Place side of brush at right angles (90°) to the long axis of the teeth (**Figure 26-9B**).
- Note the contrast with position for the Stillman method (**Figure 26-9A**).

B. Strokes

- Press the bristles gently between the teeth, being careful not to injure the gingiva.
- With the bristles between the teeth, use as little pressure as possible and make three to four small rotary movements with the bristles.
  - The sides of the bristles should come into contact with the gingival margin to massage or stimulate them.
- Remove the brush from the interproximal area and move to the next area.

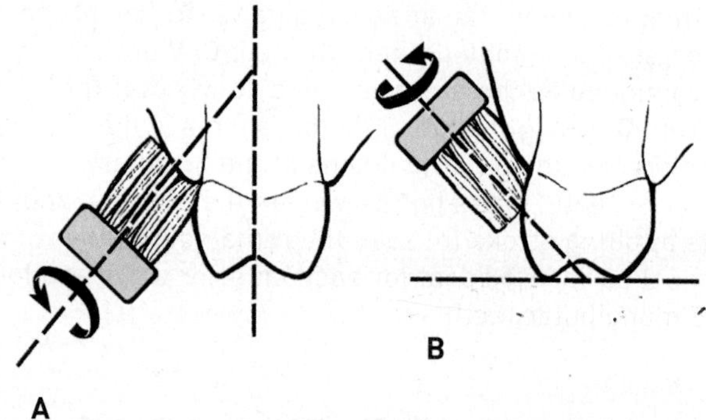

Figure 26-9 Stillman and Charters Methods Compared. **A:** Stillman: The brush is angled at approximately 45° to the long axis of the tooth. **B:** Charters: The brush is angled at approximately 45° to the occlusal plane, with brush tips directed toward the occlusal or incisal surfaces.

C. Reposition the Brush and Repeat

- Repeat steps for strokes described previously three to four times in each area on the maxillary and mandibular arches.

D. Overlap Strokes

- Move the distance of one embrasure and repeat the process *to overlap strokes.*

III. Limitations

- Brush ends do not engage the gingival sulcus to disturb subgingival bacterial accumulations.
- In some areas, the correct brush placement is limited or impossible; modifications become necessary, consequently adding to the complexity of the procedure.

The Horizontal (or Scrub) Method

I. Purposes and Indications

- Research suggests the horizontal toothbrushing method is appropriate for children younger than 6 years for use on occlusal and lingual surfaces; however, the method should be combined with other techniques.[44]
- Once the child reaches the late mixed dentition stage, modification to another technique can be initiated as the horizontal method has limitations in terms of thorough plaque biofilm removal.

II. Procedure

A. Position the Toothbrush

- Filaments: Direct bristles at right angle to the tooth.
- Place toothbrush head at a 90° angle to the long axis of the teeth on both buccal and lingual posterior surfaces.
- For anterior teeth, the head of the toothbrush is held parallel to the long axis of the tooth and the toe of the brush is used.

B. Stroke

- Bristles are moved in a gentle back and forth motion on the posterior surfaces, buccal, lingual, and occlusal.
- Bristles are moved in an up and down motion on the anterior teeth using the toe of the toothbrush.

III. Limitations

- Although this method can remove plaque biofilm on buccal and lingual surfaces, it does not reach interproximal areas.[33]
- There are also concerns about this method resulting in cervical abrasion if excessive pressure along with an abrasive toothpaste is used in adults.[11]

The Fones (or Circular) Method

I. Purpose and Indications

- This method is easy for children to learn and may be easier than the horizontal method to switch to more appropriate techniques as the child ages.[44]

II. Procedure

- Place toothbrush at 90° to the long axis of the teeth, buccal and lingual, and press bristles gently against the teeth.

A. Stroke

- Bristles are moved in a circular motion several times in each area and then the brush is moved to a new area (**Figure 26-10**).

III. Limitations

- Efficiency of plaque removal was the lowest as compared to sulcular and horizontal brushing methods.[45,46]

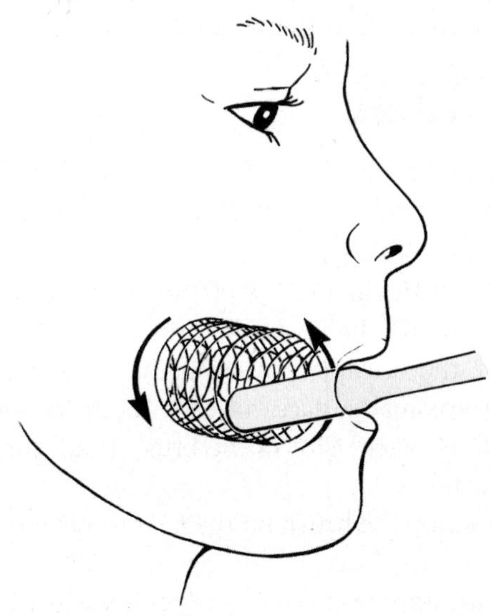

Figure 26-10 Fones Method of Brushing. With the teeth closed, a circular motion extends from the maxillary gingiva to the mandibular gingiva using light pressure.

Leonard's (or Vertical) Method

I. Purpose and Indication

- May work well for small children.

II. Procedure

- Place toothbrush at 90° to the long axis of the teeth, buccal and lingual, and press bristles gently against the teeth.
- The teeth are edge to edge.

A. Stroke

- Bristles move in an up and down motion with light pressure on the tooth surfaces. Move systematically from area to area around the mouth.

III. Limitations

- Much like the rolling stroke, there is minimal plaque removal interproximally and in the sulcular areas.[47]

Method for Power Toothbrushing

As previously noted, a systematic review found powered toothbrushes reduced plaque biofilm and gingivitis better than a manual toothbrush and may be of benefit for some individuals.[19] However, the type of power supply, mode of action of the powered toothbrush, brushing duration, and method of instruction are factors impacting the effectiveness of biofilm removal.[25]

I. Procedure

Although no clearly defined brushing method has been evaluated, the following was developed by the Swiss Dental Society[31]:

- Place bristles at a 45° to 90° angle to the long axis of the tooth, then turn the brush on.
- Move the brush over the buccal (or lingual) and interproximal surfaces of each tooth (or area depending on the size of the brush head) for about 5 seconds.
- Reposition the brush on the next tooth and repeat both on the buccal and lingual surfaces in a systematic approach.
- Many powered toothbrushes have a built-in 2 minute timer which can signal to the patient the minimum brushing time.

II. Limitations

- Cost for the rechargeable models can be an economic hardship for some patients.
- Some people may not like the sound or vibration of the powered toothbrushes, especially those with oral hyposensitivity. However, desensitization may allow for power toothbrushes to be used and they have been shown to be effective in those with autism.[48]

Supplemental Brushing Methods

I. Occlusal Brushing

A. Purpose

- Loosen food debris and biofilm microorganisms in pits and fissures.
- Remove biofilm from the margins of occlusal restorations.
- Clean pits and fissures to prepare for sealants.

B. Procedure

- Place brush head on the occlusal surfaces of molar teeth with filament tips pointed into the occlusal pits at a right angle.
- Position the handle parallel with the occlusal surface.
- Extend the toe of the brush to cover the distal grooves of the most posterior tooth (**Figure 26-11**).
- Strokes: The two acceptable strokes include:
    - Vibrate the brush in a slight circular movement while maintaining the filament tips on the occlusal surface throughout a count of 10. Press moderately so filaments do not bend but go straight into the pits and fissures.

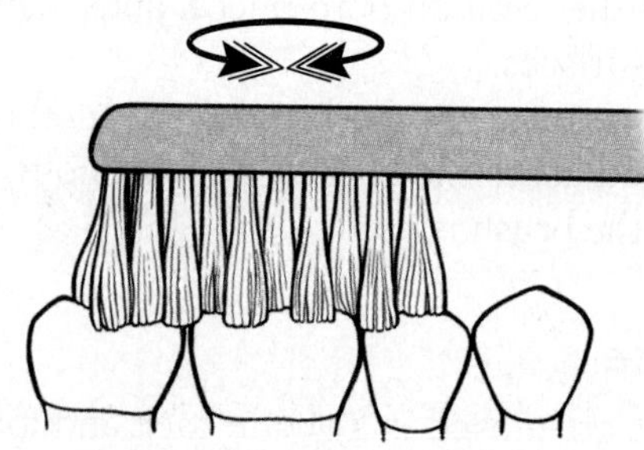

Figure 26-11 Occlusal Brushing. Small circular or vibrating strokes with light pressure while maintaining filament tips on the occlusal surface permit tips to work their way into pits and fissures.

    • Force the filaments against the occlusal surface with sharp, quick strokes; lift the brush off each time to dislodge debris; repeat 10 times.
- Overlap previous stroke by moving the brush to the premolar area. Gradually progress around each maxillary and mandibular arch until all occlusal surfaces have been thoroughly debrided.

II. Brushing Difficult-to-Reach Areas

A. Adaptations

- Hands-on demonstration by the patient is essential so the clinician can assess dexterity and ability of the patient to reach difficult areas. This also allows the clinician to determine if a different oral hygiene aid may be more effective.
- Use of disclosing solution to make biofilm visible to the patient and clinician in difficult-to-reach areas may be useful in order to work with the patient to modify the technique for effective plaque biofilm removal.
- At successive appointments, the difficult-to-reach areas should be monitored with continued refinement of oral self-care techniques.

B. Areas for Special Attention

- Distal surfaces of most posterior teeth (**Figure 26-12**). At best, the brush may reach only the distal line angles and a single- or end-tufted brush may be necessary. (See Chapter 27.)
- Facially displaced teeth, especially canines and premolars, where the zone of attached gingiva and buccal alveolar bone on the facial surface may be minimal. These areas are at risk for gingival recession and toothbrush abrasion.
- Lingually inclined teeth such as the maxillary anterior teeth.
- Exposed root surfaces: Cemental and dentinal surfaces.
- Overlapped teeth or wide embrasures, which may require use of vertical brush position (**Figure 26-13**).
- Surfaces of teeth next to edentulous areas.

III. Tongue Cleaning

The dorsum of the tongue is an ideal environment for harboring bacteria and is a key component of the overall oral self-care process.[49]

A. Anatomic Features of the Tongue Conducive to Debris Retention[49]

- Surface papillae: Numerous filiform papillae extend as minute projections, whereas fungiform papillae are not as high and create elevations and depressions that entrap debris and microorganisms. These papillae provide a large surface area for the microflora of the tongue.
- Fissures may be several millimeters deep and also provide a surface for bacterial growth.

B. Microorganisms of the Tongue

- Anaerobic bacteria involved in the production of volatile sulfur compounds related to oral malodor (bad breath) or **halitosis** reside on the tongue.[49]

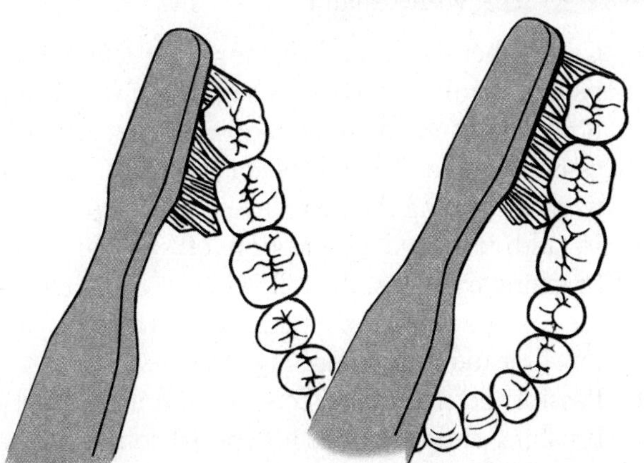

Figure 26-12 Brushing Problems. Brush placement to remove biofilm from the distal surfaces of the most posterior teeth. The distobuccal surface is approached by stretching the cheek; the distolingual surface is approached by directing the brush across from the canine of the opposite side.

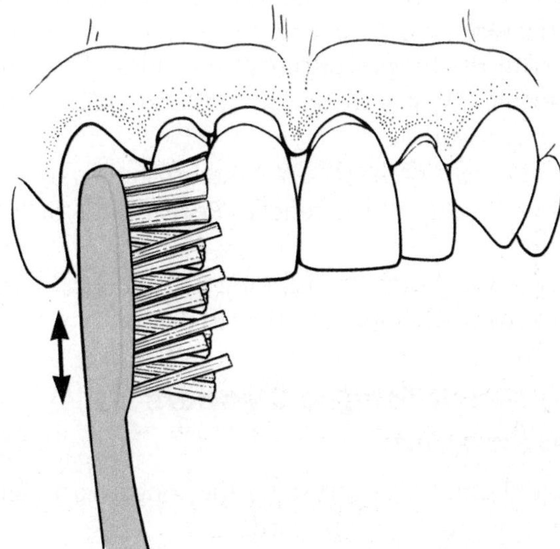

Figure 26-13 Brush in Vertical Position. For overlapped teeth, open embrasures, and selected areas of recession, the dental biofilm on proximal tooth surfaces can be removed with the brush held in a vertical position.

- Periodontal pathogens such as *Porphyromonas gingivalis, Prevotella intermedia*, and *Aggregatibacter actinomycetemcomitans* are also found on the dorsum of the tongue.[49,50]
- Microorganisms in saliva are typically the same as those found on the tongue.

C. Purposes and Indications

- Remove or reduce tongue coating.
  - Tongue coating is a white-brownish layer on the dorsum of the tongue and is made up of desquamated epithelial cells, blood cells and metabolites, food debris, and bacteria.[49]
  - The composition of the coating is affected by factors including periodontal status, salivary flow, age, tobacco use, and oral hygiene.[49]
  - The tongue coating is implicated in halitosis.
- Reduces bacterial load. However, research has not indicated that this reduces the periodontal pathogens on the dorsum of the tongue or in the saliva, so the effect may be primarily on the bacteria producing halitosis.[50]
- Reduces potential for halitosis.[51] Tongue brushing and scraping can be effective in reducing halitosis. According to some research findings, the effect is unclear or may only provide short-term benefit.[3,49]
- Improves taste sensation in smokers and nonsmokers.[52]

D. Brushing Procedure

- Hold the brush handle at a right angle to the midline of the tongue and direct the brush tips toward the throat.
- With the tongue extruded, the sides of the filaments are placed on the posterior part of the tongue surface.
- With light pressure, draw the brush forward and over the tip of the tongue. Repeat three or four times.
- A power brush should only be used for tongue cleaning when the switch is in the "off" position.

E. Types of Tongue Cleaners and Scrapers

As an alternative to brushing the tongue, a tongue cleaner or scraper can be used.

- Tongue cleaners or scrapers are typically made of plastic or a flexible metal strip. A variety of tongue cleaners and scrapers are available and may include the following:

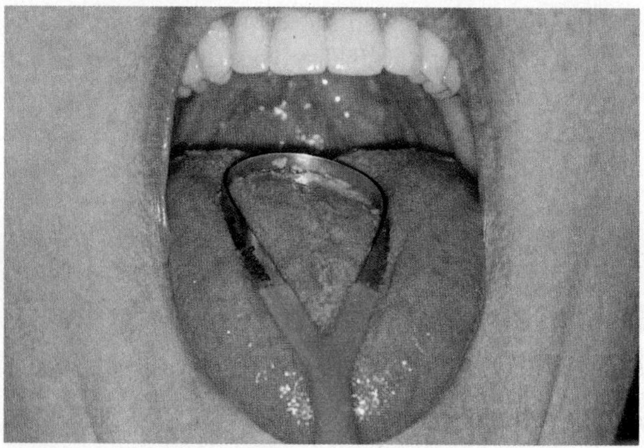

Figure 26-14 Tongue Cleaners or Scrapers. A variety of plastic or flexible metal cleaners are available to clean the dorsal surface of the tongue.

  - Loop with a single handle (**Figure 26-14**).
  - Curved with two ends to hold.
  - Raised, textured rubber pad on the back side of the toothbrush head.
- Procedure
  - Place the cleaner toward the most posterior area of the dorsal surface (Figure 26-14).
  - Press with a light but firm stroke, and pull forward.
  - Repeat several times, covering the entire surface of the tongue.
  - Wash the tongue cleaner under running water to remove debris.

Guidelines for Toothbrushing Instructions

- Comprehensive toothbrushing instruction for a patient involves teaching what, when, where, and how. Hands-on demonstration by the patient is essential. (See Chapter 24 for guidance on effectively educating the patient.)
- In addition to a description of specific toothbrushing methods, the following sections address the grasp, sequence, frequency, duration, and force for toothbrushing.
- Possible detrimental effects from improper toothbrushing and variations for special conditions are described.

I. Toothbrush Grasp

A. Objectives of Instruction on Grasp

- Ability to manipulate the brush for successful removal of dental biofilm.

- A light, controlled grasp accomplishes the following:
  - Control of the brush during all movements.
  - Effective positioning at the beginning of each brushing stroke, follow-through during the complete stroke, and repositioning for the next stroke.
  - Sensitivity to the amount of pressure applied.

B. Procedure

- Grasp the toothbrush handle in the palm of the hand with the thumb against the shank.
  - Grasp the brush near the head so it can be controlled effectively.
  - Do not grasp so close to the head of the brush that manipulation of the brush is hindered or fingers touch the anterior teeth when moving the brush head to molar regions.
- Position according to the brushing method to be used.
- Adapt grasp for the various positions of the brush head on the teeth throughout the procedure; adjust to permit unrestricted movement of the wrist and arm.
- Apply appropriate pressure for removal of the dental biofilm avoiding excessive pressure that results in soft-tissue trauma.

II. Brushing Sequence

- There is no one recommended sequence for brushing. Research suggests similar results irrespective of whether patients begin on the buccal or lingual surfaces.[53]
- The brushing process should be approached in a systematic way to ensure complete coverage for each tooth surface. Technique based on sequence creates habit, which may increase effectiveness.[54]
- Divide the mouth into sextants or quadrants.
- Start brushing from a molar region of one arch around to the midline facial then lingual followed by brushing the occlusal surfaces.
- Repeat in the opposing arch.
- Each brush placement should overlap the previous one for thorough coverage as shown in Figure 26-7.
- Approaches to address areas where patients may have more difficulty removing plaque biofilm may include:
  - Changing the sequence and starting with areas where the patient misses plaque biofilm, such as the lingual of the mandibular right for a right-handed patient and mandibular left for a left-handed patient.
  - Specific areas with active periodontal disease.

III. Frequency of Brushing

- Brushing a minimum of two times/day has been shown to reduce caries incidence and severity of periodontal disease.[55,56] Research indicates low frequency of toothbrushing as a risk factor for diabetes, dyslipidemia, and cardiovascular disease.[57]
- Regular daily oral self-care is most effective at reducing risk and severity of oral disease. Infrequent brushing results in higher odds for dental caries and more severe periodontal disease.[55,56]
- Failure to adequately disturb plaque biofilm allows for continued maturation, which increases the pathogenic potential of the biofilm. (See Chapter 17.)
- Quality of brushing technique for plaque biofilm removal is equally important as the frequency.

IV. Duration of Brushing

- The average times for brushing range from 60 to 80 seconds in the literature.[58]
- Several factors impact the time required for each individual, including tendency to accumulate plaque, psychomotor skills, position of the teeth, orthodontics, etc.
- Research suggests an increase in plaque biofilm removal with increased brushing time.[59] However, more recent research with power toothbrushes suggests that there is no additional benefit beyond 120 seconds or 2 minutes for brushing duration.[60]

A. The Count System

To ensure thorough coverage with an even distribution of effort in all areas, a system of counting can be useful.

- Count the number of strokes in each area (or 5 or 10, whichever is most appropriate for the particular patient) for modified Stillman or other methods in which a stroke is used.
- Count slowly to 10 for each brush position while the brush is vibrated and filament ends are held in position for the Bass, Charters, or other vibratory method.

B. The Clock System

- For some patients, watching a clock or an egg timer can be helpful to gauge the time they spend brushing.

- However, using a timer does not guarantee thorough biofilm removal, because the easily accessible areas may get more brushing time.

C. Combination

- For many patients, the use of the "count" system in combination with the "clock" system may be most effective.

D. Built-in Timers

- Many power toothbrushes have built-in timers.
- Signals may be set for 30 seconds, 1 or 2 minutes.
- Timers can motivate patients to increase the total time spent brushing.

E. Oral Hygiene Mobile Applications

There are a variety of mobile toothbrushing applications (also known as apps) available for download on a variety of electronic devices, including cell phones and tablets, which provide an interactive brushing experience and reminders, thus enhancing patient oral hygiene.[61-63]

- These applications may include the following features[63]:
  - Educational videos and texts.
  - Goal setting with reminders such as "Time to brush!" set to times designated by the patient.
  - Monitoring of oral hygiene behaviors through reports and graphs of how often a patient brushes or flosses and the duration.
  - Feedback on progress toward goals such as badges for children.
  - Peer support through sharing of progress with friends.
- Research suggests these mobile applications hold promise in terms of improving oral hygiene.
  - In adolescents, use of a mobile app resulted in reductions in gingivitis and plaque compared to verbal oral hygiene instructions.[62] The use of apps also helps to establish good oral health habits.[64]
  - In another study, the majority (>90%) of participants said the app motivated them to brush their teeth longer.[61]

V. Toothbrushing Force

- Toothbrushing force has been evaluated in terms of the impact on gingival recession and tooth abrasion as well as on effectiveness of plaque biofilm removal.[60,65,66]
  - Most research suggests plaque removal is improved with force up to a point, beyond which there is no benefit and potential harm.[66]
- Suggested optimal brushing force for plaque removal:
  - Manual toothbrushing: 400 g.[66]
  - Power toothbrushing: 150 g.[60]
- Although force alone does not cause soft- and hard-tissue injury (i.e., gingival recession and tooth abrasion), it is important to provide patient education to avoid aggressive brushing techniques while effectively removing plaque biofilm.[67]
  - Many power toothbrushes have a mechanism to alert the user to excessive force, which may help them to adjust the force applied.[68,69]

VI. General Toothbrushing Instruction

A. Preparation for Instructing Patient

- The dental hygienist must become familiar with an oral self-care product before providing patient education.
- For power toothbrushes, review manufacturer instructions and practice with a toothbrush model, if available, prior to instructing the patient on using it effectively.

B. Patient Education

- Research suggests the most effective teaching strategies for patient education include computer technology, audio and videotapes, written materials, and demonstrations.[70]
  - Verbal instructions alone had only a small effect on patient outcomes (i.e., plaque biofilm removal) and should not be used as a stand-alone educational strategy.
  - Demonstrations had the largest effect on patient outcomes and are an essential component of educating the patient.
  - Multiple educational strategies lead to further improvement in patient outcomes.
- When initially introducing a new power toothbrush or oral self-care aid, a demonstration model and/or video can be helpful to introduce the new product to the patient.
  - Adult learning theory suggests patients come to us with experience, so it is important to understand what the patient already knows prior to beginning patient education.[71]

- Like motivational interviewing, adult learning theory stresses the importance of the adult patient establishing the learning goals. (See Chapter 24.)
- If a patient is familiar with an oral self-care tool such as a toothbrush, allow the patient to demonstrate their technique and help refine it as needed to be effective.

- Disclosing the plaque biofilm in the patient's mouth can be very useful to provide the patient with a way to visualize the biofilm and its removal when practicing brushing and other oral self-care aid techniques. Do not forget to provide the patient with a hand mirror.
  - Disclosing plaque biofilm makes it easy for the patient and clinician to assess whether the techniques have been effective in biofilm removal.
  - In subsequent follow-up appointments, disclosing the plaque biofilm is also a way for the patient and clinical to assess progress toward plaque biofilm removal goals and to identify problem areas requiring further modification of techniques or a different oral self-care aid.
- Observe the patient's technique and refine as needed to show the patient how to adapt the brush head to reach difficult areas.

C. *Toothbrushing Procedure*

- Select a brush size and shape appropriate for the individual patient.
- Select a dentifrice with minimum abrasiveness.
- Place a small amount of fluoride dentifrice on the brush and spread the dentifrice over the teeth.
- For a manual toothbrush:
  - Place the brush on the most posterior maxillary molar and begin moving around each arch on the buccal and then lingual surfaces using the chosen toothbrushing method until all surfaces are completed.
  - Move the brush to the mandibular teeth and repeat. This sequence may vary depending on the preferences of the patient.
  - Brush the occlusal surfaces of first the maxillary and then the mandibular teeth.
- For a power toothbrush, place the brush in the mouth before turning the power on to prevent splatter.
  - Place the brush on the most posterior maxillary molar and move the brush around all surfaces, including angling into interproximal areas of each tooth if using a small circular brush.
  - If using a more typical rectangular brush head, start in the posterior and work on each area individually before moving to the next.
  - Carefully angle the brush head to access rotated, crowded, or otherwise displaced teeth.

Toothbrushing for Special Conditions

Prolonged failure to remove plaque biofilm is not indicated because of the association between oral infection and inflammation and many systemic diseases/conditions.[72] Examples of conditions that may require a temporary modification of oral self-care routines may include, but are not limited, to the following conditions.

I. Acute Oral Inflammatory or Traumatic Lesions

When an acute oral condition precludes normal oral self-care, instruct the patient to:

- Brush all areas of the mouth not affected and if tolerable clean the affected area with an extra-soft toothbrush. Reducing the bacterial load is essential to aid in healing.
- Rinse with a warm saline solution to encourage healing and debris removal.
- Consider prescribing an antimicrobial rinse like chlorhexidine to aid in the reduction of bacterial load until normal oral self-care can resume.
- Resume regular biofilm control measures on the affected area as soon as possible.

II. Following Periodontal Surgery

Provide specific instructions concerning brushing while sutures and/or a dressing are in place.

- Perform oral self-care in the areas not involved in the surgery as usual.
- Follow directions provided by the periodontal office for care of the surgical area.
- Rinsing and brushing the surgical area may not be recommended until at least 24 hours after surgery, at which time care should be taken to avoid the gingival areas when brushing.
  - If gingival grafting was done, no brushing may be allowed until the postoperative follow-up appointment.
- An antimicrobial rinse like chlorhexidine may be prescribed to aid with reducing the bacterial load and to aid in healing while the oral self-care process is modified.

III. Following Dental Extraction

- Clean the teeth adjacent to the extraction site the day following surgery.
- Brush areas not involved in the surgery as usual to reduce biofilm and promote healing.
- Beginning 24 hours after surgery, rinse the mouth with a warm, mild saline solution after each meal or snack to help remove food debris from the extraction site.
- Detailed instructions for pre- and post-surgery are found in Chapter 56.

IV. Oral Self-Care of the Neutropenic Patient

Neutropenia or a low white blood cell count (<500 absolute neutrophil count) occurs during treatment such as chemotherapy, radiotherapy, and bone marrow transplant associated with many cancers. Neutropenia puts the patient at increased risk for life-threatening infection. Oral complications can significantly impact the patient's quality of life and ability to recover primarily due to the impact on adequate nutrient intake.[73] (See Chapter 62.)

A. Oral Complications[73]

- **Mucositis** (inflammation and ulceration of the mucous membranes of the mouth and throat).
- Xerostomia (dry mouth).
- **Dysgeusia** (changes in taste).
- Fungal and viral infections such as *Candida* and herpetic lesions.
- **Trismus** (reduce opening of the mouth).
- Diffuse pain.
- Aggravation of existing periodontal diseases.

B. Oral Care Recommendations

- The Joint Task Force of the Multinational Association of Supportive Cancer Care in Cancer/International Society of Oral Oncology (MASCC/ISSOO) and European Society for Blood and Marrow Transplantation developed a protocol for basic oral care for before, during, and after treatment.[73]
- Ongoing interprofessional collaboration with the oncology team by the dental team is essential to maintain the patient's oral health.
- Prevention of infection in the oral cavity is needed to minimize the risk of systemic infection during this immune-compromised state. The following recommendations have been made by the MASCC/ISSOO guidelines:
    - Brush a minimum of two times/day with an extra-soft or soft toothbrush with the bristles softened in hot water.
    - If mucositis is present, a topical anesthetic mouthrinse, such as morphine 0.2%, may be necessary for brushing to help minimize oral pain.[74]
    - Replace the toothbrush regularly. It is suggested to replace the brush prior to each neutropenic cycle, meaning it should be replaced prior to the beginning of each chemotherapy or radiotherapy treatment cycle.
    - Use a fluoride toothpaste; non-mint flavored may be more comfortable if the patient is experiencing mucositis. A prescription fluoride gel, toothpaste, or rinse may also be recommended depending on the patient's caries risk and ability to be compliant with oral self-care.
    - The use of chlorhexidine for preventive measures of oral mucositis is not recommended.[74]
    - Interproximal cleaning should be done regularly using aids the patient is familiar with to avoid self-injury. (See Chapter 27.)
    - Clean the tongue by either brushing or using a tongue cleaner/scraper.
    - Any dental prostheses should be cleaned according to instructions found in Chapter 30.

Adverse Effects of Toothbrushing

I. Soft-Tissue Lesions

- Gingival abrasion
    - Evidence of toothbrushing alone resulting in gingival recession is unclear.[17] However, frequency, duration, force, abrasiveness of the dentifrice, and technique may be implicated in recession.[11]
    - Localized gingival abrasion or trauma may occur with vigorous toothbrushing and is most common on the mid-facial aspect on canines, first premolars, or teeth in labioversion or buccoversion.
    - The appearance may be a distinct surface wound where the epithelial tissue has been denuded or it may be punctate lesions that appear as red pinpoint spots.

- To prevent further gingival abrasion, recommend use of a soft toothbrush with end-rounded filaments and observe the patient's toothbrushing technique and modify it as needed.

II. Hard-Tissue Lesions

- Dental abrasion
  - These lesions result from mechanical abrasion and typically appear as wedge-shaped indentations in cervical areas with a smooth, shiny surface. (See Chapter 16.)
  - These lesions are multifactorial and include use of an abrasive dentifrice, stiff toothbrush bristles, occupational causes, and habits such as chewing on pens.[75]
  - Primarily on facial surfaces, especially of canines, premolars, and sometimes first molars, or on any tooth in buccoversion or labioversion, because typically more force is applied to these areas during toothbrushing.
  - When adjacent teeth are involved, the lesions appear in a linear pattern across the quadrant or sextant.
  - Educate the patient about the presence of the abrasion and advise use of a soft toothbrush with end-rounded bristles along with use of a less abrasive dentifrice. The patient should then demonstrate their brushing technique to determine what modifications are necessary.
  - A power toothbrush that alerts the user when too much pressure is applied may be helpful to train the patient not to use excessive force when brushing.

III. Bacteremia

- Evidence suggests daily oral activities including chewing, toothbrushing, and flossing can produce transient bacteremia.[76]
  - The incidence and magnitude of bacteremia are significantly higher in patients with more dental biofilm accumulation and gingival inflammation following toothbrushing.
  - Power toothbrushes cause more bacteremia than manual toothbrushes.[77,78]
- Despite these findings, there is no clear association of transient bacteremia and infective endocarditis.
- However, it suggests the need for patients, especially those who are medically compromised, to maintain meticulous removal of dental biofilm on a daily basis to minimize the magnitude of bacteremia.

Care of Toothbrushes

When discussing the type and features of the toothbrush selected for an individual patient, the number of brushes needed and the frequency of replacement should be included.

I. Supply of Brushes

- Recommend at least two brushes for home use so they can be rotated to ensure they dry thoroughly between brushings. Most people will also want a third toothbrush in a portable container for use at work, school, or travel.
- Purchase of brushes needs to be staggered so that all brushes are not new at the same time and, more importantly, so that they are not old at the same time, thereby resulting in less than optimum biofilm removal.

II. Brush Replacement

Evidence shows toothbrushes with heavy wear are less effective at plaque removal than those with less wear.[12,79]

- There is no ideal timeframe for toothbrush replacement, but a general recommendation is at least every 2–3 months.
- Brushes need to be replaced before filaments become splayed or frayed or lose resiliency.
- The point at which a toothbrush needs replacement is influenced by many factors, including frequency and method of use.

III. Cleaning Toothbrushes

- Clean the toothbrush thoroughly after each use.
- Rinse the brush head with tap water until completely clean of visible debris, dentifrice, and bacteria from between the filaments.[80]
- Allow to dry thoroughly.

A. Toothbrush Contamination

- Toothbrush contamination has been explored in the literature.[81,82] Transmission of bacteria to others in the household has also been suggested, but little evidence exists to support it at this time.

- Toothbrushes become contaminated with pathogenic microorganisms during use as well as the way in which they are stored.[81-83]

B. Toothbrush Disinfection

- Though there is no evidence of harmful effects from the bacteria harbored in toothbrushes, the ADA recognizes individuals may opt for further disinfection.[12]
- Evidence shows toothbrushes soaked in 3% hydrogen peroxide or Listerine mouthwash have 85% less bacterial load.[12,84]
- Individuals with a higher risk for systemic infection, such as those with compromised immune systems, may benefit from the following:[80]
  - Rinse with an antimicrobial mouthrinse prior to brushing to reduce bacterial load.
  - Use of a toothpaste may also reduce bacterial load.[85]
  - Soak the toothbrush in an antimicrobial rinse such as essential oil mouthwash, cetylpyridinium chloride, or chlorhexidine after brushing.[81]
- Toothbrush sanitization using microwaves or ultra violet rays shows a significant reduction in bacteria.[86]

IV. Brush Storage

- Brushes need to be kept in open air with the head in an upright position, apart from contact with other brushes, particularly those of another person to avoid cross contamination.[80]
- Do not store in closed containers. If a portable brush container is used, try to dry the toothbrush prior to putting it in the container. A closed container encourages bacterial growth.[80,81]

Documentation

In the dental chart or record, the documentation for initial toothbrush instruction will include the following:

- Type of toothbrush patient has used to date: manual versus power.
- Recommended changes in type of brush or method of use.
- Description of soft tissue health and/or plaque score with goal(s) for improvement.
- Description of toothbrush education and areas patient has difficulty reaching.
- Tongue cleaning method education provided.
- **Box 26-2** shows a sample documentation for toothbrush selection and toothbrushing method.

Box 26-2 Example Documentation: Toothbrush Selection and Toothbrushing Method

- **S**—A 30-year-old male presents for his 6-month preventive appointment with a chief complaint of gums bleeding during toothbrushing. Patient has a negative medical history and reports taking no medications. Patient reports brushing once per day with a hard manual toothbrush and uses a back and forth "scrubbing" method.
- **O**—Intraoral assessment reveals generalized moderate edema, marginal erythema, and moderate bleeding on probing. Moderate plaque is noted along the gingival margin of posterior teeth. Ulcerations and denuded gingiva noted, particularly on the left side maxillary facial and mandibular molar lingual surfaces. Biofilm-free score 63%.
- **A**—Acute tissue trauma related to the use of hard toothbrush and scrubbing method.
- **P**—Oral self-care instructions given using a soft toothbrush, recommended twice daily using the modified Stillman method. Flossers were introduced to the patient for removal of interdental plaque biofilm. Patient demonstrated modified Stillman method intraorally with some challenges on the lingual of mandibular molars. Patient demonstrated successfully the use of flossers. Patient committed to try the following behavior modifications: increase frequency of brushing from 1 to 2× a day, and floss at least 4× a week. Increase biofilm-free score to 85% at re-evaluation appointment.

Next visit—6–8 weeks re-evaluation of gingival condition, plaque-free score, evaluate biofilm removal, and assess patient's toothbrushing and flossing technique. Modify as needed. Determine appropriate continuing care visit for the patient.

Signed: ____________________, RDH
Date: ______________

Factors to Teach the Patient

- The effect of dental biofilm formation on the teeth and gingiva.
- Rationale for thorough daily removal of dental biofilm from the teeth, especially before going to sleep.
- The type of brush: manual, power, or both, recommended to maintain optimal oral health for a particular patient.
- Individualized hands-on instruction using an appropriate manual or power brushing method.
- Proper care and maintenance of manual and power brushes.
- Indications for and use of a tongue cleaner.

References

1. Arweiler NB, Auschill TM, Sculean A. Patient self-care of periodontal pocket infections. *Periodontol 2000*. 2018;76(1):164-179.
2. Berchier CE, Slot DE, Haps S, Van der Weijden GA. The efficacy of dental floss in addition to a toothbrush on plaque and parameters of gingival inflammation: a systematic review. *Int J Dent Hyg*. 2008;6(4):265-279.
3. Slot DE, De Geest S, van der Weijden FA, Quirynen M. Treatment of oral malodour. Medium-term efficacy of mechanical and/or chemical agents: a systematic review. *J Clin Periodontol*. 2015;42(suppl 16):S303-S316.
4. Van der Weijden FA, Slot DE. Efficacy of homecare regimens for mechanical plaque removal in managing gingivitis a meta review. *J Clin Periodontol*. 2015;42(suppl 16):S77-S91.
5. Gurudath G, Vijayakumar K, Arun R. Oral hygiene practices: ancient historical review. *J Orofac Res*. 2012;2:225-227.
6. Aumeeruddy MZ, Zengin G, Mahomoodally MF. A review of the traditional and modern uses of *Salvadora persica* L. (Miswak): toothbrush tree of Prophet Muhammad. *J Ethnopharmacol*. 2018;213:409-444.
7. Guerini V. *A History of Dentistry from the Most Ancient Times Until the End of the Eighteenth Century*. Philadelphia, PA: Lea & Febiger; 1909.
8. McCauley HB. Toothbrushes, toothbrush materials and design. *J Am Dent Assoc*. 1946;33(5):283-293.
9. Wadsworth HN. Toothbrush. U.S. Patent US 28,794 A. 1860.
10. Library of Congress. Everyday mysteries: who invented the toothbrush and when was it invented? Published 2019. https://www.loc.gov/rr/scitech/mysteries/tooth.html. Accessed August 8, 2021.
11. Asadoorian J. Canadian Dental Hygienists Association position paper: tooth brushing. *CJDH*. 2006;40(5):232-248.
12. American Dental Association. Oral health topics: toothbrushes. Published 2019. https://www.ada.org/en/member-center/oral-health-topics/toothbrushes. Accessed August 5, 2021.
13. Chun JA, Cho MJ. The standardization of toothbrush form in Korean adult. *Int J Clin Prev Dent*. 2014;10(4):227-236.
14. Slot DE, Wiggelinkhuizen L, Rosema NA, Van der Weijden GA. The efficacy of manual toothbrushes following a brushing exercise: a systematic review. *Int J Dent Hyg*. 2012;10(3):187-197.
15. Xu Z, Cheng X, Conde E, Zou Y, Grender J, Ccahuana-Vasquez RA. Clinical assessment of a manual toothbrush with CrissCross and tapered bristle technology on gingivitis and plaque reduction. *Am J Dent*. 2019;32(3):107-112.
16. Turgut MD, Keceli TI, Tezel B, Cehreli ZC, Dolgun A, Tekcicek M. Number, length and end-rounding quality of bristles in manual child and adult toothbrushes. *Int J Paediatr Dent*. 2011;21(3):232-239.
17. Rajapakse PS, McCracken GI, Gwynnett E, Steen ND, Guentsch A, Heasman PA. Does tooth brushing influence the development and progression of non-inflammatory gingival recession? A systematic review. *J Periodontol*. 2007;34:1046-1061.
18. American Dental Association. Acceptance program: guidelines for toothbrushes. Published 1996. http://www.ada.org/en/science-research/ada-seal-of-acceptance/how-to-earn-the-ada-seal/guidelines-for-product-acceptance. Accessed December 21, 2017.
19. Yaacob M, Worthington HV, Deacon SA, et al. Powered versus manual toothbrushing for oral health. *Cochrane Database Syst Rev*. 2014(6):Cd002281.
20. Deacon SA, Glenny AM, Deery C, et al. Different powered toothbrushes for plaque control and gingival health. *Cochrane Database Syst Rev*. 2010;8:CD004971.
21. Nash DA, Friedman JW, Mathu-Muju KR, et al. A review of the global literature on dental therapists. Community Dent Oral Epidemiol. 2014;42(1):1-10.
22. Grender J, Adam R, Zou Y. The effects of oscillating-rotating electric toothbrushes on plaque and gingival health: A meta-analysis. Am J Dent. 2020;33(1):3-11.
23. van der Sluijs E, Slot DE, Hennequin-Hoenderdos NL, Valkenburg C, van der Weijden F. Dental plaque score reduction with an oscillating-rotating power toothbrush and a high-frequency sonic power toothbrush: a systematic review and meta-analysis of single-brushing exercises. *Int J Dent Hyg*. 2021;19(1):78-92.
24. Grender J, Adam R, Zou Y. The effects of oscillating-rotating electric toothbrushes on plaque and gingival health: a meta-analysis. *Am J Dent*. 2020;33(1):3-11.
25. Erbe C, Jacobs C, Klukowska M, Timm H, Grender J, Wehrbein H. A randomized clinical trial to evaluate the plaque removal efficacy of an oscillating-rotating toothbrush versus a sonic toothbrush in orthodontic patients using digital imaging analysis of the anterior dentition. *Angle Orthod*. 2019;89(3):385-390.
26. Schmickler J, Wurbs S, Wurbs S, et al. The influence of the utilization time of brush heads from different types of power toothbrushes on oral hygiene assessed over a 6-month observation period: a randomized clinical trial. *Am J Dent*. 2016;29(6):307-314.
27. Rosema N, Slot DE, van Palenstein Helderman WH, Wiggelinkhuizen L, Van der Weijden GA. The efficacy of powered toothbrushes following a brushing exercise: a systematic review. *Int J Dent Hyg*. 2016;14(1):29-41.
28. Bizhang M, Schmidt I, Chun YP, Arnold WH, Zimmer S. Toothbrush abrasivity in a long-term simulation on human dentin depends on brushing mode and bristle arrangement. *PLoS One*. 2017;12(2):e0172060.
29. Hamza B, Uka E, Körner P, Attin T, Wegehaupt FJ. Effect of a sonic toothbrush on the abrasive dentine wear using toothpastes with different abrasivity values. *Int J Dent Hyg*. 2021;19(4):407-412.
30. Sharma NC, Galustians HJ, Qaqish J, Cugini M, Warren PR. The effect of two power toothbrushes on calculus and stain formation. *Am J Dent*. 2002;15(2):71-76.
31. van der Sluijs E, Slot DE, Hennequin-Hoenderdos NL, Valkenburg C, van der Weijden F. Dental plaque score reduction with an oscillating-rotating power toothbrush and a high-frequency sonic power toothbrush: a systematic review and meta-analysis of single brushing exercises. *Int J Dent Hyg*. 2021;19(1):78-92.
32. Davidovich E, Ccahuana-Vasquez RA, Timm H, Grender J, Cunningham P, Zini A. Randomised clinical study of plaque removal efficacy of a power toothbrush in a paediatric population. *Int J Paediatr Dent*. 2017;27(6):558-567.
33. Baruah K, Thumpala VK, Khetani P, Baruah Q, Tiwari RV, Dixit H. A review of toothbrushes and toothbrushing methods. *Int J Pharm Sci Invention*. 2017;6(5):29-38.
34. Versteeg PA, Rosema NA, Timmerman MF, Van der Velden U, Van der Weijden GA. Evaluation of two soft manual toothbrushes with different filament designs in relation to gingival abrasion and plaque removing efficacy. *Int J Dent Hyg*. 2008;6:166-173.
35. Litonjua LA, Andreana S, Bush PJ, Cohen RE. Toothbrushing and gingival recession. *Int Dent J*. 2003;53(2):67-72.

36. Brothwell DJ, Jutai DKG, Hawkins RJ. An update of mechanical oral hygiene practices: evidence-based recommendations for disease prevention. *J Can Dent Assoc*. 1998;64(4):295-306.
37. Poyato-Ferrera M, Segura-Egea JJ, Bullon-Fernandez P. Comparison of modified Bass technique with normal toothbrushing practices for efficacy in supragingival plaque removal. *Int J Dent Hyg*. 2003;1(2):110-114.
38. Smutkeeree A, Rojlakkanawong N, Yimcharoen V. A 6-month comparison of toothbrushing efficacy between the horizontal scrub and modified Bass methods in visually impaired students. *Int J Paediatr Dent*. 2011;21(4):278-283.
39. Ausenda F, Jeong N, Aresenault P, et al. The effect of the Bass intrasulcular toothbrushing technique on the reduction of gingival inflammation: a randomized clinical trial. *J Evid Based Dent Pract.* 2019;19(2):106-114.
40. Bass CC. An effective method of personal oral hygiene, Part II. *J Louisiana State Med Soc*. 1854;106:100-102.
41. Waerhaug J. Effect of toothbrushing on subgingival plaque formation. *J Periodontol*. 1981;52(1):30-34.
42. Stillman PR. A philosophy of the treatment of periodontal disease. *Dent Digest*. 1932;38(9):314.
43. Hirschfeld I. *The Toothbrush: Its Use and Abuse*. Brooklyn, NY: Dental Items of Interest Pubs; 1939.
44. Gibson JA, Wade AB. Plaque removal by the Bass and roll brushing techniques. *J Periodontol*. 1977;48:456-459.
45. Charters W. Home care of the mouth. I. proper home care of the mouth. *J Periodontol*. 1948;19(4):136-137.
46. Bok HJ, Lee CH. Proper tooth-brushing technique according to patient's age and oral status. *Int J Clin Prev Dent*. 2020, 16(4):149-153.
47. Patil SP, Patil PB, Kashetty MV. Effectiveness of different tooth brushing techniques on the removal of dental plaque in 6-8 year old children of Gulbarga. *J Int Soc Prev Community Dent*. 2014;4(2):113-116.
48. Janakiram C, Varghese N, Venkitachalam R, Joseph J, Vineetha K. Comparison of modified Bass, Fones and normal tooth brushing technique for the efficacy of plaque control in young adults: a randomized clinical trial. *J Clin Exp Dent*. 2020;12(2):e123-e129.
49. Shick RA, Ash MM. Evaluation of the vertical method of toothbrushing. *J Periodontol*. 1961;32(4):346-353.
50. Vajawat M, Deepika PC, Kumar V, Rajeshwari P. A clinicomicrobiological study to evaluate the efficacy of manual and powered toothbrushes among autistic patients. *Contemp Clin Dent*. 2015;6(4):500-504.
51. Roldan S, Herrera D, Sanz M. Biofilms and the tongue: therapeutical approaches for the control of halitosis. *Clin Oral Investig*. 2003;7(4):189-197.
52. Laleman I, Koop R, Teughels W, Dekeyser C, Quirynen M. Influence of tongue brushing and scraping on the oral microflora of periodontitis patients. *J Periodontal Res*.2018;53(1): 73-79.
53. Van der Sleen MI, Slot DE, Van Trijffel E, Winkel EG, Van der Weijden GA. Effectiveness of mechanical tongue cleaning on breath odour and tongue coating: a systematic review. *Int J Dent Hyg*. 2010;8(4):258-268.
54. Timmesfeld N, Kunst M, Fondel F, Guildner C, Steinbach S. Mechanical tongue cleaning is a worthwhile procedure to improve the taste sensation. *J Oral Rehabil*. 2021, 48:45-54.
55. Van der Sluijs E, Slot DE, Hennequin-Hoenderdos NL, Van der Weijden GA. A specific brushing sequence and plaque removal efficacy: a randomized split-mouth design. *Int J Dent Hyg*. 2018;16(1):85-91.
56. Nandlal B, Shanbhog, R, Godhi B, Sunila BS. Evaluating the change in skills observed with a novel brushing technique based on sequence learning using video bio-feedback system in children. *Highl Med Medical Sciences*. 2021;14:31-36.
57. Kumar S, Tadakamadla J, Johnson NW. Effect of toothbrushing frequency on incidence and increment of dental caries: a systematic review and meta-analysis. *J Dent Res*. 2016;95(11):1230-1236.
58. Zimmermann H, Zimmermann N, Hagenfeld D, Veile A, Kim TS, Becher H. Is frequency of tooth brushing a risk factor for periodontitis? A systematic review and meta-analysis. *Community Dent Oral Epidemiol*. 2015;43(2):116-127.
59. Zoraya SI, Azhar AAB. Association between toothbrushing and cardiovascular disease risk factors: a systematic review. *Adv Health Sci Res*. 2019;25:23-29.
60. Gunjalli G, Kumar KN, Jain SK, Reddy SK, Shavi GR, Ajagannavar SL. Total salivary anti-oxidant levels, dental development and oral health status in childhood obesity. *J Int Oral Health*. 2014;6(4):63-67.
61. Van der Weijden G, Timmerman M, Nijboer A, Lie M, Van der Velden U. A comparative study of electric toothbrushes for the effectiveness of plaque removal in relation to toothbrushing duration. Timerstudy. *J Clin Periodontol*. 1993;20(7):476-481.
62. McCracken GI, Janssen J, Swan M, Steen N, de Jager M, Heasman PA. Effect of brushing force and time on plaque removal using a powered toothbrush. *J Clin Periodontol*. 2003;30(5):409-413.
63. Underwood B, Birdsall J, Kay E. The use of a mobile app to motivate evidence-based oral hygiene behaviour. *Br Dent J*. 2015;219(4):E2.
64. Alkadhi OH, Zahid MN, Almanea RS, Althaqeb HK, Alharbi TH, Ajwa NM. The effect of using mobile applications for improving oral hygiene in patients with orthodontic fixed appliances: a randomised controlled trial. *J Orthod*. 2017;44(3):157-163.
65. Nolan SL, Giblin-Scanlon LJ, Boyd LD, Rainchuso L. Theory based development and beta testing of a smartphone prototype developed as an oral health promotion tool to influence ECC. *J Dent Hyg*. 2018;92(2):6-14.
66. Lozoya CJS, Giblin-Scanlon L, Boyd LD, Nolen S, Vineyard J. Influence of a smartphone application on the oral health practices and behaviors of parents of preschool children. *J Dent Hyg*. 2019;93(5):6-14.
67. Van der Weijden GA, Timmerman MF, Reijerse E, Snoek CM, van der Velden U. Toothbrushing force in relation to plaque removal. *J Clin Periodontol*. 1996;23(8):724-729.
68. Van der Weijden GA, Timmerman MF, Danser MM, Van der Velden U. Relationship between the plaque removal efficacy of a manual toothbrush and brushing force. *J Clin Periodontol*. 1998;25(5):413-416.
69. Wiegand A, Schlueter N. The role of oral hygiene: does toothbrushing harm? *Monogr Oral Sci*. 2014;25:215-219.
70. Janusz K, Nelson B, Bartizek RD, Walters PA, Biesbrock AR. Impact of a novel power toothbrush with SmartGuide technology on brushing pressure and thoroughness. *J Contemp Dent Pract*. 2008;9(7):1-8.
71. Van der Weijden FA, Campbell SL, Dorfer CE, Gonzalez-Cabezas C, Slot DE. Safety of oscillating-rotating powered brushes compared to manual toothbrushes: a systematic review. *J Periodontol*. 2011;82(1):5-24.
72. Friedman AJ, Cosby R, Boyko S, Hatton-Bauer J, Turnbull G. Effective teaching strategies and methods of delivery for

patient education: a systematic review and practice guideline recommendations. *J Cancer Educ*. 2011;26(1):12-21.

73. Papadakos CT, Papadakos J, Catton P, Houston P, McKernan P, Jusko Friedman A. From theory to pamphlet: the 3Ws and an H process for the development of meaningful patient education resources. *J Cancer Educ*. 2014;29(2):304-310.
74. Linden GJ, Herzberg MC. Periodontitis and systemic diseases: a record of discussions of working group 4 of the Joint EFP/AAP Workshop on Periodontitis and Systemic Diseases. *J Periodontol*. 2013;84(4 suppl):S20-S23.
75. Elad S, Raber-Durlacher JE, Brennan MT, et al. Basic oral care for hematology-oncology patients and hematopoietic stem cell transplantation recipients: a position paper from the joint task force of the Multinational Association of Supportive Care in Cancer/International Society of Oral Oncology (MASCC/ISOO) and the European Society for Blood and Marrow Transplantation (EBMT). *Support Care Cancer*. 2015;23(1):223-236.
76. Elad S, Kin Fon Cheng K, Lall RV, et al. MASCC/ISOO clinical practice guidelines for the management of mucositis secondary to cancer therapy. *Cancer*. 2020;126(19):4423-4431.
77. Milosevic A. Abrasion: a common dental problem revisited. *Prim Dent J*. 2017;6(1):32-36.
78. Tomas I, Diz P, Tobias A, Scully C, Donos N. Periodontal health status and bacteraemia from daily oral activities: systematic review/meta-analysis. *J Clin Periodontol*. 2012;39(3):213-228.
79. Misra S, Percival R, Devine D, Duggal M. A pilot study to assess bacteraemia associated with tooth brushing using conventional, electric or ultrasonic toothbrushes. *Eur Arch Paediatr Dent*. 2007;8(1):42-45.
80. Bhanji S, Williams B, Sheller B, Elwood T, Mancl L. Transient bacteremia induced by toothbrushing a comparison of the Sonicare toothbrush with a conventional toothbrush. *Pediatr Dent*. 2002;24(4):295-299.
81. Van Leeuwen MPC, Van der Weijden FA, Slot DE, Rosema MAM. Toothbrush wear in relation to toothbrushing effectiveness. *Int J Dent Hyg*. 2019;17(1):77-84.
82. American Dental Association, Council on Scientific Affairs. Toothbrush care: cleaning, storing and replacement. Updated February 26, 2019. https://www.ada.org/resources/research/science-and-research-institute/oral-health-topics/toothbrushes. Accessed November 11, 2021.
83. Frazelle MR, Munro CL. Toothbrush contamination: a review of the literature. *Nurs Res Pract*. 2012;2012:420630.
84. Ankola AV, Hebbal M, Eshwar S. How clean is the toothbrush that cleans your tooth? *Int J Dent Hyg*. 2009;7(4):237-240.
85. Wetzel WE, Schaumburg C, Ansari F, Kroeger T, Sziegoleit A. Microbial contamination of toothbrushes with different principles of filament anchoring. *J Am Dent Assoc*. 2005;136(6):758-765; quiz 806.
86. Beneduce C, Baxter KA, Bowman J, Haines M, Andreana S. Germicidal activity of antimicrobials and VIOlight Personal Travel Toothbrush sanitizer: an in vitro study. *J Dent 2010*;38(8):621-625.
87. Warren DP, Goldschmidt MC, Thompson MB, Adler-Storthz K, Keene HJ. The effects of toothpastes on the residual microbial contamination of toothbrushes. *J Am Dent Assoc*. 2001;132(9):1241-1245.
88. Agrawal SK, Dahal S, Bhumika TV, Nair NS. Evaluating sanitization of toothbrushes using various decontamination methods: a meta-analysis. *J Nepal Health Res Counc*. 2019;16(41):364-371.

CHAPTER 27

Oral Infection Control: Interdental Care

Lisa J. Moravec, RDH, MSDH

CHAPTER OUTLINE

LEARNING OBJECTIVES

After studying this chapter, the student will be able to:

1. Review the anatomy of the interdental area and explain why toothbrushing alone cannot remove biofilm adequately for prevention of periodontal infection.
2. Describe embrasure size and patient status of health or disease as factors for evidence-based clinical decision making regarding which interdental device to recommend.
3. Describe the types of interdental brushes and explain why they may be more effective than floss for some patients.
4. Describe the types of dental floss and outline the steps for use of floss or floss loops for biofilm removal from proximal tooth surfaces.
5. Develop a list of the types and purposes of various floss aids, including floss holders and power flossing devices, and provide a rationale for the choice of the best ones to meet a specific patient's needs.
6. Demonstrate and recommend other interdental devices for biofilm removal, including an interdental rubber tip, a toothpick holder, a wooden interdental cleaner, and oral irrigation.

Overview of Interdental Care

Toothbrushing alone cannot accomplish biofilm removal from proximal tooth surfaces and adjacent gingiva to the same degree that it does for the facial, lingual, and palatal aspects. Therefore, interdental biofilm control is essential to complete the patient's oral self-care program.

Interdental cleaning devices ideally should be user-friendly, be effective with plaque removal, and have no deleterious effects on the soft or hard tissues.[1] When the preventive treatment plan is outlined for an individual, assessment is made of the oral condition, the problem areas, and the overall prognosis for improvement or maintenance of gingival health.

- Measures for interdental biofilm control are selected to complement biofilm control by toothbrushing.[2]
- The addition of floss or interdental brushes used with toothbrushing may reduce gingivitis and dental biofilm.[3]
- Daily interdental cleaning is necessary for dental biofilm removal and to reduce gingival inflammation.[2]

The Interdental Area

- In health, the interdental gingiva fills the **interproximal space** and under the contact of the adjacent teeth.
- When the interdental papilla is missing or reduced in height, the shape of the interdental gingiva changes.
- Factors impacting the papilla height include[4]:
  - Shape of the tooth.
  - Interproximal bone height.
  - Thickness of the gingiva.
- **Figure 27-1** shows a Class II embrasure from the proximal surface with the **col** and from the facial surface.
- The classification system on papillary height is illustrated in Chapter 18.

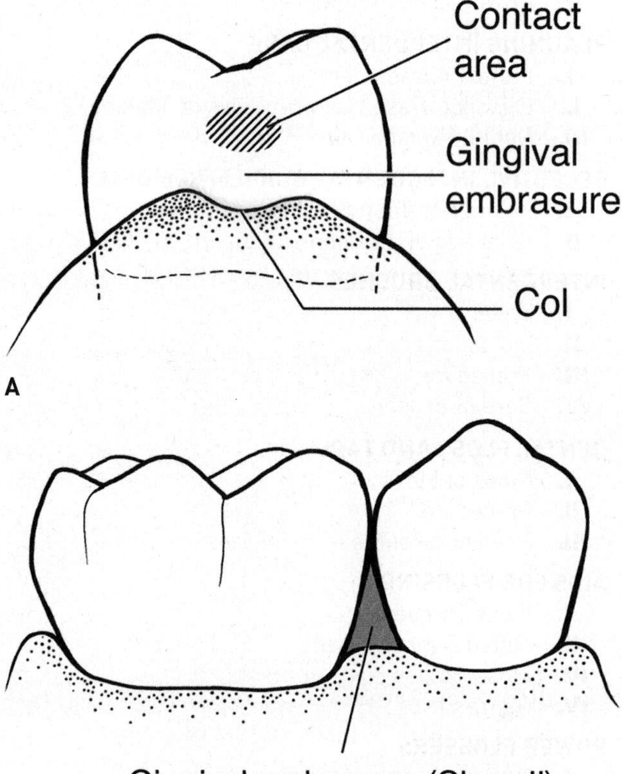

Figure 27-1 Class II Gingival Embrasure. **A:** Embrasure shown from the proximal surface with the col. **B:** Facial view, with gingival embrasure shown in blue.

I. Anatomy of the Interdental Area

A review of the gingival and dental anatomy of the interdental area can give meaning to and clarify the role and purpose of the various devices available for interdental care.

A. Posterior Teeth

- Between adjacent posterior teeth are two papillae, one facial and one lingual or palatal.
- The papillae are connected by a col, a depressed concave area that follows the shape of the apical border of the contact area (Figure 27-1).

B. Anterior Teeth

- Between anterior teeth in contact is a single papilla with a pyramidal shape.
- Tip of the papilla may form a small col under the contact area.

C. Epithelium

- The epithelium covering a col is usually thin and not **keratinized epithelium**.
- Col epithelium is less resistant to infection than keratinized surfaces.
- Inflammation in the papilla leads to enlargement; with increased inflammatory cells and edema, the col becomes deeper.
- The col area is inaccessible for ordinary toothbrushing and microorganisms may be harbored in the concave center.
- The incidence of gingivitis is greatest in the interdental tissues.[5]
- Bacteria accumulate in a biofilm on the tooth surface and affect the adjacent periodontal tissue which can lead to periodontal disease.[6]

II. Proximal Tooth Surfaces

- With bacterial infection and loss of attachment, the interdental papillae height is reduced, exposing the proximal tooth surfaces.
- Root concavities, grooves, and furcation areas provide areas for biofilm accumulation and contribute to causation of periodontal disease.[7]
- Irregularities of tooth position, such as rotation or overlapping, and deviations related to malocclusion or tooth loss may also be present.
- The increased root surface and complexity of the root morphology may make removal of bacterial deposits more difficult.

Planning Interdental Care

I. Patient Assessment

A. History of Personal Oral Care

- Self-care history includes type of toothbrush, dentifrice, and adjunct interdental aids currently used (i.e., dental floss, interdental brush, oral irrigation device).[8]
- Frequency and time spent.
- Assess barriers to effective interdental care, including patient preference and compliance.

B. Dental and Gingival Anatomy

- Position of teeth.
- Types and shapes of embrasures: Variation throughout the dentition (i.e., may recommend floss for anterior teeth with tight embrasures and interdental brush for posterior teeth with larger spaces).
- Clinical attachment level: Classification of the periodontal condition.
- Prostheses present: Special interdental care required for fixed and removable prostheses.
- Areas where toothbrush cannot reach.

C. Extent and Location of Dental Biofilm

- Preparation of a biofilm score or biofilm-free score to show the patient the extent of biofilm needing removal on a daily basis. (See Chapter 21.)
- Use of a disclosing agent to show specific sites where biofilm accumulates.
- Evidence of the patient's ability to care for difficult-to-access areas.

D. Personal Factors

- Disability that limits one's ability to carry out needed personal oral hygiene as well as patient compliance with interdental care.
- Oral health literacy about and appreciation for interdental oral care. Clinician should educate patient about the cause of disease, explain biofilm, and teach how to effectively remove biofilm from interdental space.[9]

II. Evidence-Based Clinical Decision Making

- Before selecting an interdental aid, the clinician must clinically assess and make a determination of periodontal health, gingivitis, or periodontitis. Periodontal health is defined by absence of clinically detectable inflammation (no bleeding on probing, erythema, edema, patient symptoms, clinical attachment loss or bone loss).[10]
- Embrasure size and patient status of health or disease are key factors in selection of interdental device.[9]
- Type I Embrasure: Dental floss is indicated for individuals with healthy tissues with high levels of patient compliance. Due to low compliance and/or gingival inflammation, other interdental cleaning devices should be considered.[11,12]
- For individuals with closed embrasures who lack motivation and/or dexterity, the use of easy flossers/floss holders, rubber interdental cleaners/soft picks, oral irrigation, or small interdental brushes are alternatives to traditional dental floss.
- Type II and Type III Embrasure: High quality evidence indicates use of interdental brushes are the most effective interproximal cleaning device for open embrasure spaces[9] and for periodontal maintenance patients.[11,12]

III. Dental Hygiene Care Plan

A. Objectives

- Utilize motivational interviewing to select appropriate interdental aids to help the patient reach optimum oral health. (See Chapter 24.)
- Determine if challenges with compliance exist, including lack of motivation to adhere or patient not remembering instructions for oral self-care.[7]
- Educate the patient on the oral care aids selected.
- The patient must accept responsibility for daily personal care and work as a partner with the oral health team.

B. Initial Care Plan

- Assess oral health behavior to create an individualized care plan that is sustainable and requires minimal reinforcement.[13]
- At first, the simplest procedures are selected for convenience and ease of learning based on the patient's current knowledge, preferences, and oral self-care habits.
- Minimum frequency: Twice daily.
- Keep the daily oral self-care regimen at a realistic level with respect to the time the patient is able or willing to spend.

Selective Interdental Biofilm Removal

I. Relation to Toothbrushing

- Vibratory and sulcular toothbrushing, such as that performed with the Charters, Stillman, and Bass methods, can be successful to some degree in removing dental biofilm near the line angles of the facial and lingual or palatal embrasures.
- Brushing in a vertical position is effective for additional access around line angles onto the proximal surfaces. (See Chapter 26.)

II. Selection of Interdental Aids

- The ideal interdental cleaning aid needs to be user-friendly, remove biofilm effectively, and cause no damage to soft tissues or hard tissues.[1]
- Choices are dependent on oral self-care abilities, embrasure size, disease status, and the risk for future recurrence.
- Flossing is typically recommended for patients with healthy gingiva and normal gingival contour, but is technique sensitive and requires instruction and reinforcement by a dental professional.
- High-quality flossing is a difficult skill for most patients; therefore, other interdental devices may be more effective with higher patient compliance.
- A patient working to control or arrest disease may need more frequent oral self-care than a patient in the maintenance phase.
- With the judicious selection and use of the various methods for interdental care, the dedicated patient can accomplish disease control.
- When gingival inflammation is present, interdental brushes are the preferred interdental cleaning aid.[11,12]
- Periodontal patients who have experienced gingival recession or attachment loss have concave surfaces in the interdental space and furcation areas that require special consideration.
- Stable periodontitis patients remain at higher risk for recurrent disease; therefore, ongoing risk assessment is necessary as part of optimal patient management.[10]

Interdental Brushes

I. Types

A. Small Insert Brushes with Reusable Handle

- Soft nylon filaments are twisted into a fine stainless steel plastic-coated wire. This brush is disposable and inserted into a plastic handle with an angulated shank (**Figure 27-2A**).
- The small tapered or cylindrical brush heads are of varying sizes, approximately 12–15 mm (1/2 inch) in length and 3–5 mm (1/8–1/4 inch) in diameter.

B. Travel Interdental Brush

- Reuseable travel interdental brushes are also available and may be more convenient for patients when away from home
    - Soft nylon filaments are twisted into a fine stainless steel plastic-coated wire.
    - The wire is continuous with the handle, which is approximately 35–45 mm (1½–1¾ inches) in length (**Figure 27-2B**).

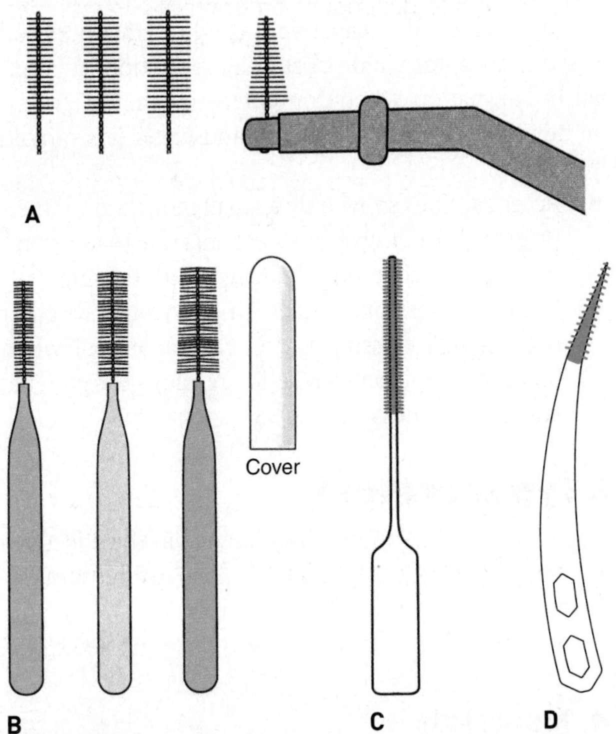

Figure 27-2 Interdental Brushes and Cleaners. **A:** Insert brushes for a reusable handle with an angulated shank. **B:** Reusable travel interdental brush with filaments twisted onto a fine plastic-coated wire that ends in a handle and cover. **C:** Disposable interdental cleaner. **D:** Disposable curved interdental cleaner.

- The very short, soft filaments form a narrow brush approximately 30–35 mm (1¼–1½ inches) in length and 5–8 mm (1/4–5/16 inches) in diameter (Figure 27-2B).

C. Rubber Interdental Cleaners

- Similar to an interdental brush, but do not have a wire. The rubber interdental cleaner or "soft-pick" has small elastomeric fingers that are perpendicular to a plastic core (**Figure 27-2C** and **D**).[14]
- The soft-pick is effective at biofilm removal and reducing gingival bleeding.[15,16]
- Rubber interdental picks are becoming increasingly popular with patients due to ease of use; patients may find them to be more comfortable than wire interdental brushes during insertion.[17]
- Rubber interdental picks may not remove as much biofilm due to fewer bristles[17] so selection of interdental device to best fit the patients' needs is important.

II. Indications for Use

- It is suggested that interdental brushes should be the first choice for interproximal cleaning.[2]
- Patient preference and anatomy need to be considered when selecting size and style.
    - Interdental brushes have been shown to be easier to use and preferred by patients.[18]
    - Size of the interdental embrasure also determines the choice of interdental brush or cleaner.
- Interdental brushes are more effective in biofilm removal than floss when the brush fills the embrasure.[2,3]

A. For Removal of Dental Biofilm and Debris

- Proximal tooth surfaces adjacent to open embrasures, orthodontic appliances, fixed prostheses, dental implants, periodontal splints, and space maintainers are well suited to interdental brushes and cleaners.
- Concave proximal surfaces are used where dental floss and other interdental aids cannot reach (**Figure 27-3A**). Floss will not access a concave surface, whereas the interproximal brush can reach and cleanse (**Figure 27-3B**).[1,8,14,19,20]
    - In patients with open embrasures and moderate to severe attachment loss, the interdental brush is often more effective than floss. However, it is important to choose an interdental

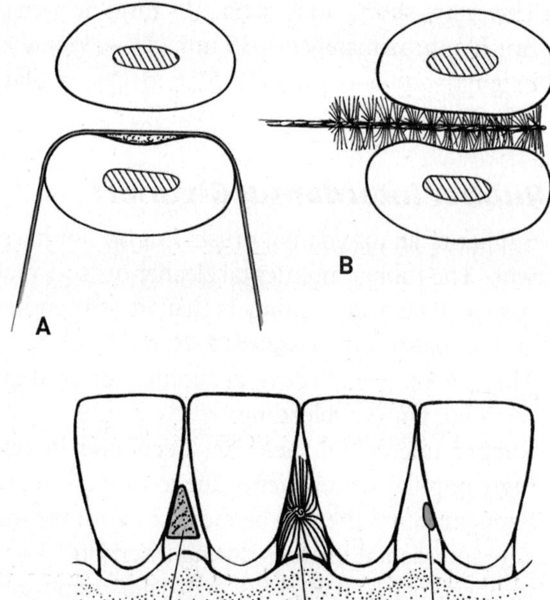

Figure 27-3 Interdental Care. **A:** Floss positioned on the mesial surface of a maxillary first premolar shows the inability of the floss to remove dental biofilm on a concave proximal tooth surface. **B:** The use of an interdental brush in the same interproximal area to show how dental biofilm can be removed from the proximal surfaces. **C:** Comparison of the access of a wooden tip, an interdental brush, and a piece of dental floss to an open interdental area.

brush that fills the embrasure to effectively clean concavities (**Figure 27-3C**).
  - Interdental brushes are a great choice for periodontal patients with larger interdental spaces with recession or root exposure.[2]
- Exposed Class IV furcation areas (see Chapter 20).

B. For Application of Chemotherapeutic Agents

- Fluoride dentifrice, gel, and/or mouthrinse for prevention of dental caries, particularly root surface caries, and for surfaces adjacent to any prosthesis.
- Antimicrobial agents for control of dental biofilm and the prevention of gingivitis.
- Desensitizing agents.

III. Procedure

- Select brush of appropriate diameter to fill the embrasure.
- Insert at an angle in keeping with gingival form; brush in and out.
- For wide embrasures, it is important to remember to apply pressure against the proximal root surfaces to remove the biofilm thoroughly.
  - Insert the interdental brush as shown in Figure 27-3B–C.
  - Apply pressure toward the mesial proximal surface to remove biofilm.
- Then apply pressure toward the distal proximal surface and remove the biofilm.

IV. Care of Brushes

- Clean the brush during use to remove debris and biofilm by holding under running water.
- Clean thoroughly after use and dry in open air.
- Discard before the filaments become deformed or loosened.

Dental Floss and Tape

Despite daily dental floss along with toothbrushing being recommended to a majority of patients, effectiveness, compliance, and patient dexterity are limitations. High-quality flossing is difficult to achieve and may not confer significant oral health benefits over brushing alone if ineffectively used.[17] Unsupervised flossing does not yield substantial reduction in gingival inflammation when compared to other interdental devices (interdental brushes and water-jets ranked higher).[21]

- Recent studies show only a small reduction in interproximal bleeding in most patients due to low compliance and technique challenges with flossing.[1,2]
- Dental professionals need to determine whether high-quality flossing is an achievable goal when making individualized self-care plans for patients and effectiveness of plaque removal.

I. Types of Floss

- Research has shown no difference in the effectiveness of waxed or unwaxed floss for biofilm removal[22]; however, the effectiveness of flossing for biofilm removal is not supported by evidence.[18,19]

A. Materials

- *Silk*: Historically, floss was made of silk fibers loosely twisted together to form a strand and waxed for proximal surface cleaning.
- *Nylon*: Nylon multifilaments, waxed or unwaxed, have been widely used in circular (floss) or flat (tape) form for biofilm removal from proximal tooth surfaces.

- *Polytetrafluoroethylene (PTFE)*: Monofilament PTFE is used for biofilm removal from proximal tooth surfaces.

B. Features of Waxed Floss

- Smooth surface provided by the wax coating helps the floss slide through the contact area.
- Easing the floss between the teeth may minimize tissue trauma.
- Wax gives strength and durability during application to minimize breakage.

C. Features of Unwaxed Floss

- Thinner floss may be helpful when contact areas are tight.
- Care must be taken to avoid injury when guiding floss through a tight contact area or when moving floss on the tooth surface in an apical direction.
- Unwaxed floss may become frayed due to irregular tooth surface, rough surface of a restoration, or calculus deposit and cause the patient to become frustrated, thereby resulting in lost motivation to floss regularly.

D. Features of PTFE

- Monofilament type resists breakage or shredding when passed over irregular tooth surface, restoration, or calculus deposit.
- Reduces the force required to pass the floss through the contact, which may improve patient compliance with regular flossing and reduce tissue injury or trauma.[23]

E. Enhancements

- Color and flavor have been added to dental floss.
- Therapeutic agents added include fluoride and whitening agents; however, limited research has been published relative to their effectiveness.
- Dental floss that expands in contact with moisture to fill interproximal spaces better.

II. Procedure

- When dental floss is applied with good technique to a flat or convex proximal tooth surface, biofilm can be removed.
- Older biofilm is tenacious and may require more strokes for removal.
- When floss is placed over a concave surface, contact is not possible (Figure 27-3A), and supplementary devices are needed to remove biofilm completely.

A. Sequence of Flossing

- There is no ideal time to floss, but it may be helpful to floss before brushing to help dislodge food debris and plaque biofilm.

B. Floss Preparation

- **Figure 27-4** outlines the flossing steps described in detail here in this section.
- Hold a 12- to 15-inch length of floss with the thumb and index finger of each hand; grasp firmly with only 1/2-inch of floss between the fingertips. The ends of the floss may be tucked into the palm and held by the ring and little finger, or the floss may be wrapped around the middle fingers (**Figure 27-4A** and **B**).
- A circle of floss or "floss loop" may be made by tying the ends together; the circle may be rotated as the floss is used (**Figure 27-5**).
  - Advantages of creating a floss circle include improved user compliance and easier handling, less waste, and increased floss hygiene and biofilm removal efficacy.[24]

C. Application

- Maxillary teeth: Direct the floss upward by holding the floss over two thumbs or a thumb and an index finger as shown in **Figure 27-4C**. Rest a side of a finger on the teeth of the opposite side of the maxillary arch to provide balance and a fulcrum.
- Mandibular teeth: Direct the floss down by holding the two index fingers on top of the strand. One index finger holds the floss on the lingual aspect and the other on the facial aspect. The side of the finger on the lingual side is held on the teeth of the opposite side of the mouth to serve as a fulcrum or rest.

D. Insertion

- Hold floss firmly in a diagonal or oblique position.
- Guide the floss past each contact area with a gentle back and forth or sawing motion (**Figure 27-4D**).
- Control floss to prevent snapping through the contact area into the gingival tissue.

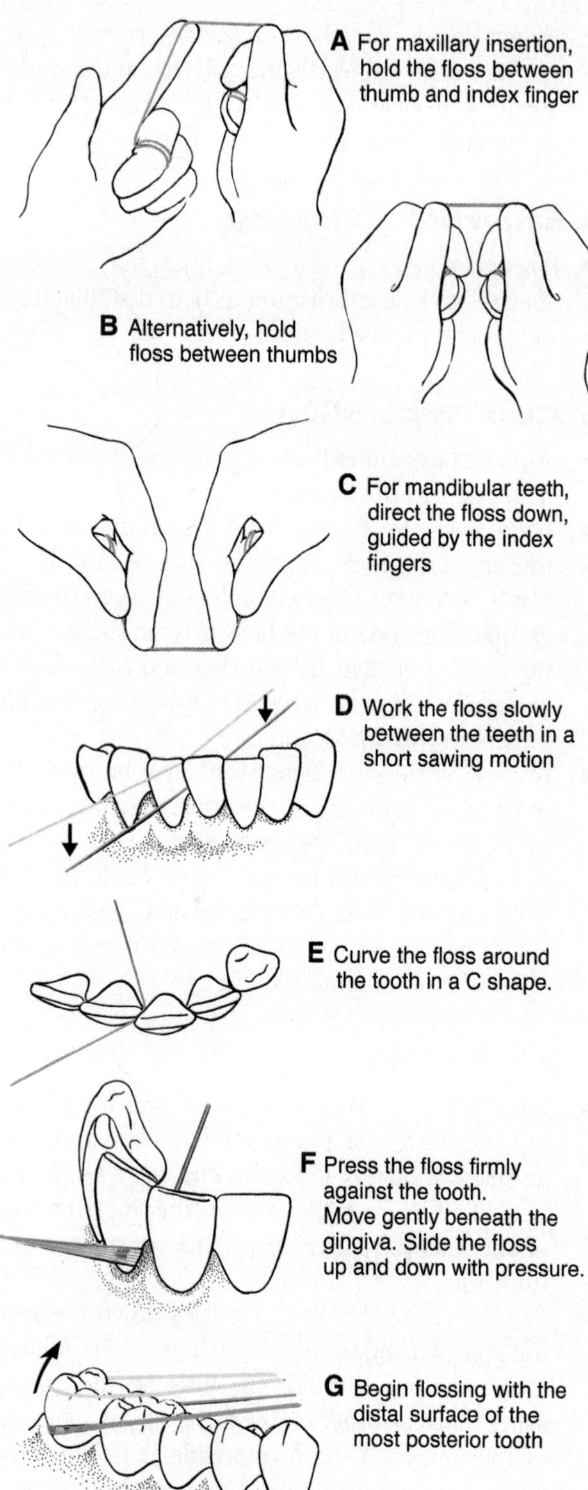

Figure 27-4 Use of Dental Floss.

E. Cleaning Stroke

- Clean proximal tooth surface separately; for the distal aspect, curve the floss mesially, and for the mesial aspect, curve the floss distally, around the tooth (**Figure 27-4E–F**).

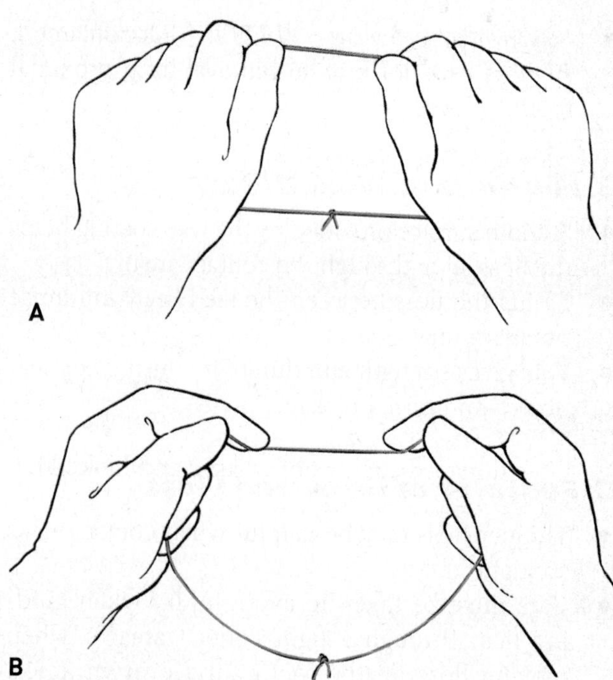

Figure 27-5 Circle of Floss. The ends of the floss can be tied together for convenient holding. A child may be able to manage floss better with this technique. **A:** Floss held for maxillary teeth. **B:** Floss held for mandibular teeth.

- Pass the floss below the gingival margin, curve to adapt the floss around the tooth, press against the tooth, and slide up and down over the tooth surface several times.
- Move the floss to a new, unused portion for each proximal tooth surfaces.
- Loop the floss over the distal surfaces of the most posterior teeth in each quadrant and the teeth next to edentulous areas (**Figure 27-4G**). Hold firmly against the tooth and move the floss in an up-and-down motion.

III. Prevention of Flossing Injuries

- Location: **Floss cuts** or **clefts** occur primarily on facial and lingual or palatal surfaces directly beside or in the middle of an interdental papilla. They appear as straight-line cuts beginning at the gingival margin and may result in a floss cleft if the tissue is repeatedly injured.[25]
- Causes
  - Using a piece of floss that is too long between the fingers when held for insertion.
  - Snapping the floss forcefully through the contact area.

- Not curving the floss about the tooth adequately and cutting into the gingival margin.

Aids for Flossing

I. Floss Threader

A floss threader is used for biofilm and debris removal around orthodontic appliances or under fixed partial dentures (**Figure 27-6**).

A. Description

- Floss threaders are flexible plastic and look like a needle with a very large loop at the end through which regular floss is placed.

B. Indication for Use

- Biofilm removal from mesial and distal abutments and under pontic of a fixed partial denture, implant, orthodontic arch wire, or other fixed prosthesis.

C. Procedure

- Individual surface of tooth or implant
  - Take a 12- to 18-inch piece of floss and thread it through the loop on the threader.
  - Put the floss threader under the appliance and pull the floss under the fixed appliance (**Figure 27-6A**).
  - Then curve the floss in a "C" shape around the proximal surface to remove dental biofilm (**Figure 27-6B** and **D**).
- Fixed partial denture
  - Thread floss under pontic and apply to distal surface of the mesial abutment and mesial surface of the distal abutment (Figure 27-6B–D).

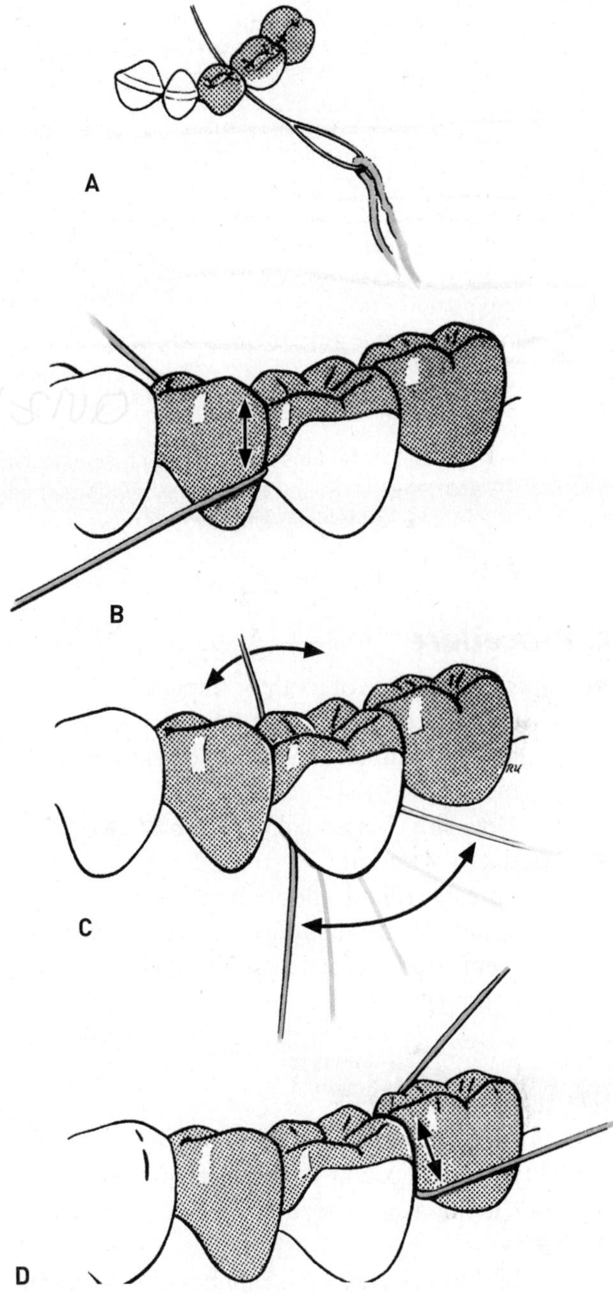

Figure 27-6 Use of Floss Threader. **A:** Use floss threader to draw the floss between abutment and pontic. **B:** Apply floss to the distal surface of the mesial abutment; pull through 1 or 2 inches. **C:** Slide floss under pontic. Move back and forth several times, as shown by the arrows, to remove dental biofilm from the gingival surface of the pontic. **D:** Apply new section of floss to the mesial surface of the distal abutment.

II. Tufted Dental Floss

A. Description

Tufted dental floss is regular dental floss alternated with a thickened tufted (spongy) portion. This type of floss is commercially available.

- *Single, precut lengths*
  - Available in pre-cut 2-foot lengths composed of a 5-inch tufted portion adjacent to a 3-inch stiffened end for inserting under a fixed appliance or orthodontic attachment (**Figure 27-7A**).
- Example: Super Floss.

B. Indication for Use

- Biofilm removal from mesial and distal abutments and under the pontic of a fixed partial denture, implant, or orthodontic appliance. The stiff end of the tufted floss is inserted like a floss threader.

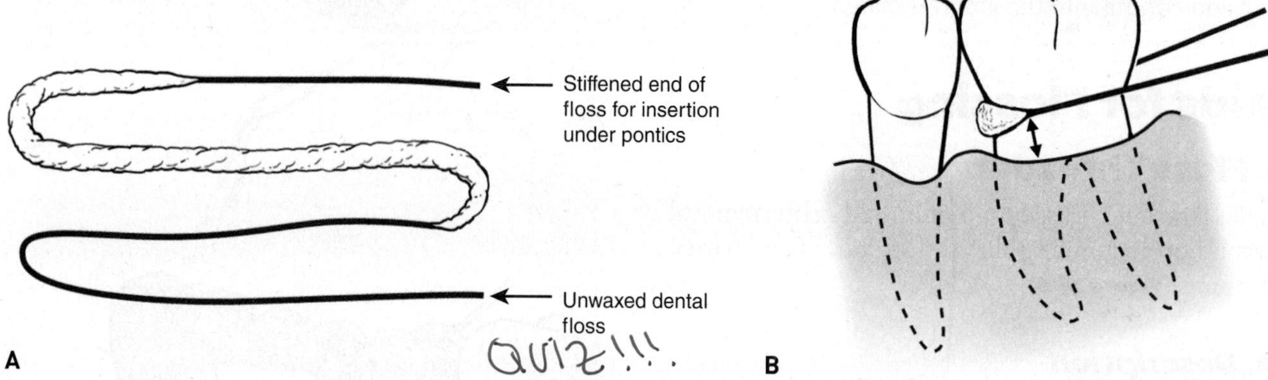

Figure 27-7 Tufted Dental Floss. A common brand available is called Super Floss, which is available **(A)** in a precut length with a tufted portion and a 3-inch stiffened end for insertion under a fixed prosthesis. **B:** How the tufted part of the floss might be used interproximally to remove biofilm is shown.

C. Procedure

- Individual surface of tooth or implant
  - Curve floss and/or tufted portion around the tooth or implant in a "C" to remove dental biofilm.
  - Move floss horizontally (**Figure 27-7B**).
- Fixed partial denture
  - Thread tufted floss under pontic and apply to distal surface of the mesial abutment and mesial surface of the distal abutment.

III. Floss Holder

A floss holder can be helpful for a person with a disability or for a parent or caregiver providing oral hygiene care for a child or adult.

- Types
  - Multiuse: Using 12–15 inches of floss, wrapping end around button and threading up across slot on prongs and back down toward button on the other side to keep floss taut (**Figure 27-8**).
  - Single-use: Disposable floss holder for single use (**Figure 27-9A-D**). These disposable flossers go by many names, which include, but are not limited to, sword floss, floss picks, or easy flossers.
- Indications for use
  - The mechanical properties, including floss tension and angle, are important considerations when selecting a floss holder.[26]
  - The effectiveness of holders maintaining adequate tension of floss through proximal contacts while not displacing the tissue is crucial for proper use.[26]
  - A novel two-handle flossing system (Gumchucks) increases control and dexterity, allowing young children to make the "C" shape while flossing,[27] and is an effective alternative to string floss that allows children to floss with greater speed and efficacy (**Figure 27-10**).[28]
- Procedure
  - Use the same insertion and application procedure as previously described for flossing for use of the floss holder (Figure 27-9A-D) and single-use flossers such as the dual handle flosser (Figure 27-10).

IV. Gauze Strip

- Uses
  - For proximal surfaces of widely spaced teeth.
  - For surfaces of teeth next to edentulous areas.
  - For outer mesial and distal surfaces of abutment teeth of a fixed partial denture.
  - For areas under posterior cantilevered section of a fixed appliance, such as the distal portion of a denture supported by implants.
- Procedure
  - Cut 1-inch gauze bandage into a 6- to 8-inch length, and fold in thirds or down the center.
  - Position the fold of the gauze on the cervical area next to the gingival crest and work back and forth several times; hold ends in a distal direction to clean a mesial surface, and in a mesial direction to clean a distal surface (**Figure 27-11**).

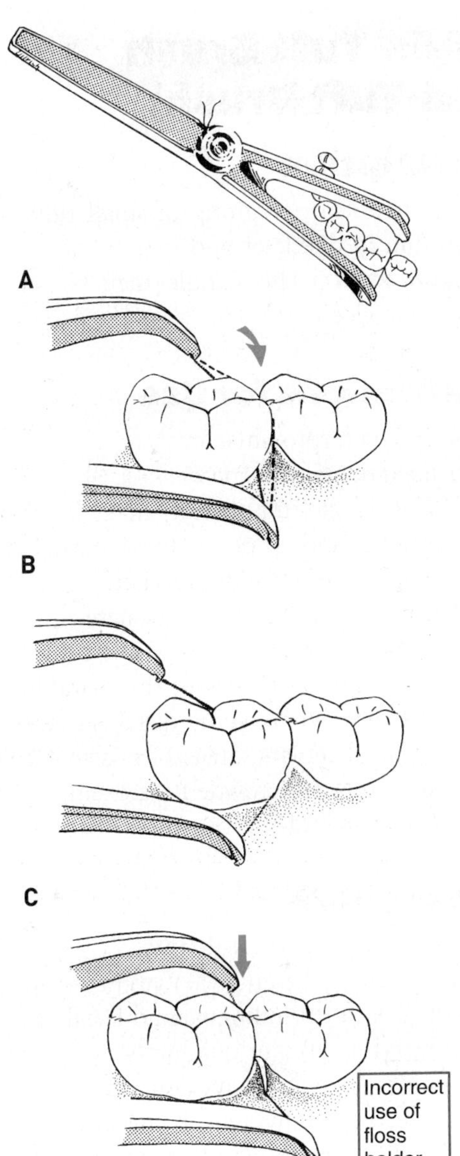

Figure 27-8 Use of a Floss Holder. **A:** The floss is held over the proximal contact for insertion. A hand rest is maintained on the chin to prevent excess pressure. **B:** As the floss is lowered gently and drawn through the contact area, the holder is pulled mesially when the floss is applied to the distal surface and pushed distally when the floss is applied to the mesial surface. **C:** Floss is lowered slightly below the gingival margin. **D:** Floss cut in the papilla when used incorrectly.

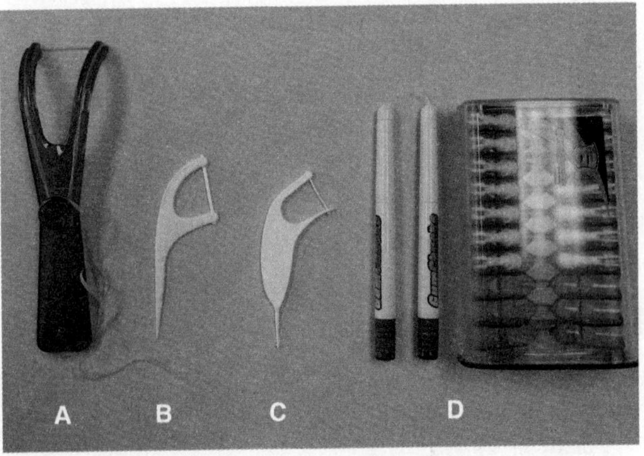

Figure 27-9 Disposable Single-Use Floss Holders. **A:** Reusable floss holder device. **B:** Disposable floss holder. **C:** Ortho floss holder. **D:** Flossing aid with two handles and disposable tips.

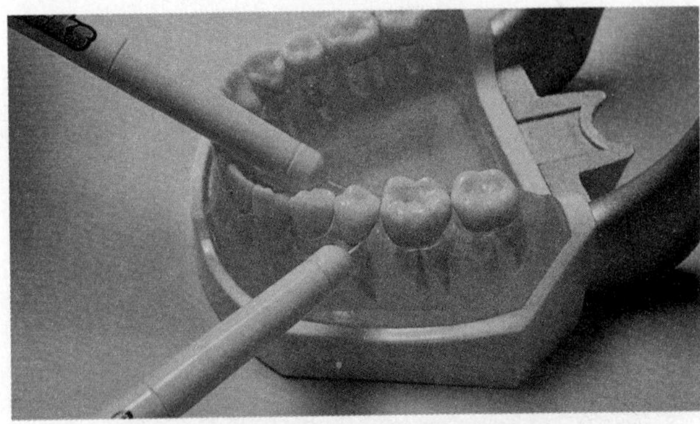

Figure 27-10 Use of a flossing aid with two handles. The procedure is the same as described for Figure 27-9.

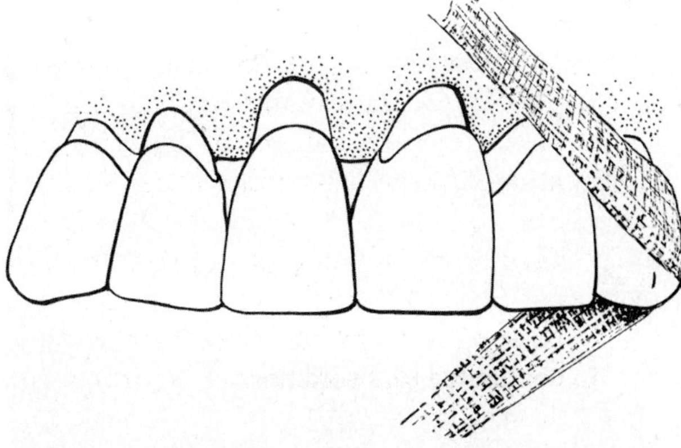

Figure 27-11 Gauze Strip. A 6- or 8-inch length of 1-inch bandage is folded in thirds and placed around a tooth adjacent to an edentulous area, a tooth with interdental spacing, or the distal surface of the most posterior tooth. A back-and-forth motion is used to clean the dental biofilm from the surface.

Power Flossers

I. Description

- Several types of power flossers are available.
  - One type of power flosser is battery operated and uses a disposable flexible nylon tip for interproximal care (**Figure 27-12A**).

- Another type of power flosser is an air flosser, which uses bursts of air and water droplets to disrupt dental biofilm (**Figure 27-12B**).
- Patient acceptance regarding comfort when compared to dental floss was higher, with the microdroplet device being more effective at reducing biofilm.[29]

II. Indications for Use

- May be helpful for patients who are unable to use regular floss or those with manual dexterity issues.
- A power flosser can also be helpful for those who do not clean interproximally regularly and want to try this tool.

III. Procedure

- If the device has a reservoir, fill it with water.
- Standing near the sink, point the flosser interproximally and activate the device.
- Move systematically through the mouth on the facial and lingual interproximal areas.

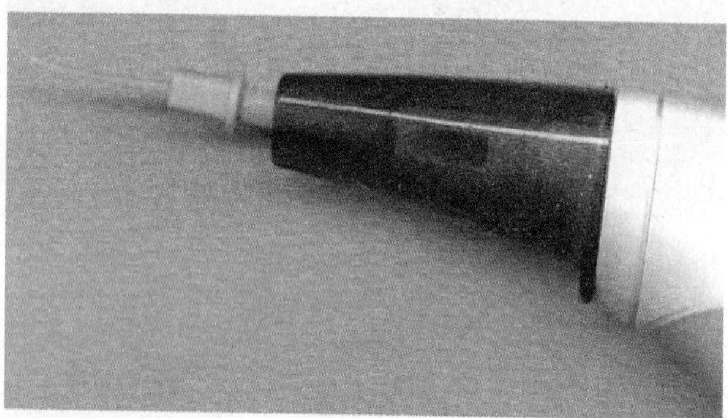

A

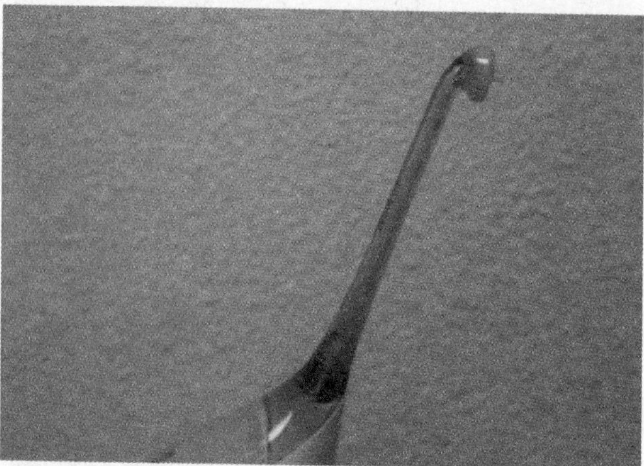

B

Figure 27-12 Power Dental Flossing Devices. **A.** An example of a powered dental flossing device. **B.** Air flosser.

Single-Tuft Brush (End-Tuft Brush)

I. Description

- The single tuft, or group of small tufts, may be 3–6 mm in diameter and may be flat or tapered (**Figure 27-13**). The handle may be straight or contra-angled.

II. Indications for Use

- For open interproximal areas
- For fixed dental prostheses
  - The single-tuft brush may be adaptable around and under a fixed partial denture, pontic, orthodontic appliance, precision attachment, or implant abutment.
- For difficult-to-reach areas
  - The lingual surfaces of the mandibular molars, abutment teeth, distal surfaces of the terminal molars, areas of missing teeth, and teeth that are crowded are examples of areas where an end-tuft brush may be of value.

III. Procedure

- Direct the tip of the tuft into the interproximal area and along the gingival margin; go around the distal surfaces from lingual and facial of the most distal teeth in all four quadrants.
- Combine a rotating motion with intermittent pressure, especially in the interproximal areas, to reach as much of the proximal surfaces as possible.
- Use a sulcular brushing stroke.

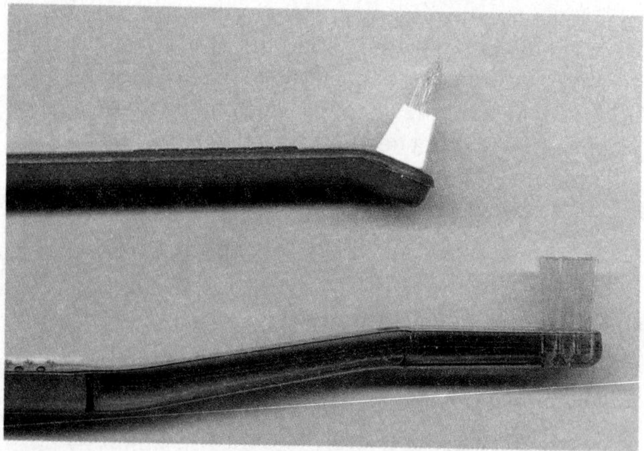

Figure 27-13 End-Tuft Brushes. End-tuft brushes come in flat and tapered shapes and can be used to clean areas that are difficult to access with a standard toothbrush.

Interdental Tip

The interdental tip may be called a rubber tip or rubber tip stimulator.

I. Composition and Design

- Conical or pyramidal flexible rubber tip may be attached to the end of the handle of a toothbrush or is on a single plastic handle (**Figure 27-14**).

II. Indications for Use

- For cleaning debris from the interdental area.
- For biofilm removal at and just below the gingival margin.
- The rubber tip is sometimes recommended for stimulation of gingival blood flow, although literature to support this is absent.
- After periodontal surgery, the rubber tip may also be used to shape the interproximal area during healing.

III. Procedure

- Trace along the gingival margin with the tip positioned just beneath the margin (1–2 mm). The adaptation is similar to the toothpick in holder (**Figure 27-15**).
- Rinse the tip as indicated during use to remove debris, and wash thoroughly at the finish.

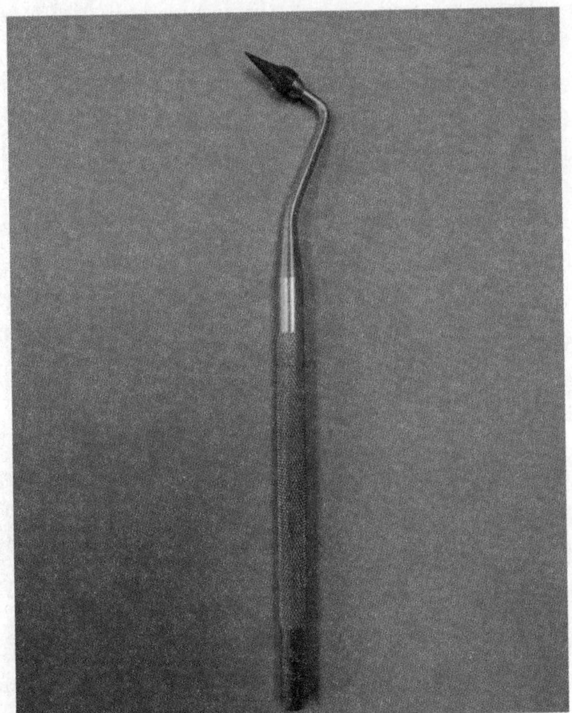

Figure 27-14 Rubber Tip (Also Called a Rubber Tip Stimulator) with Handle.

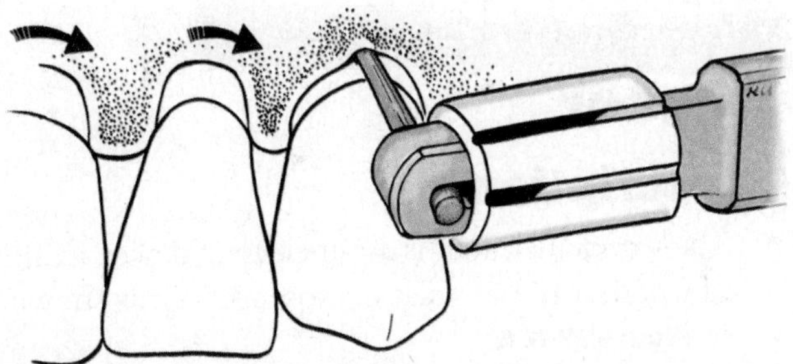

Figure 27-15 Toothpick in Holder for Dental Biofilm at Gingival Margin. The tip is placed at or just below the gingival margin. Gently trace the gingival margin of each tooth.

Toothpick in Holder

I. Description

A round toothpick is inserted into a plastic handle with contra-angled ends for adaptation to the tooth surface at the gingival margin for biofilm removal. The device is also called a Perio-Aid.

II. Indications for Use

- Patient with periodontitis
  - For biofilm removal at and just under the gingival margin; for interdental cleaning, particularly for concave proximal tooth surfaces; and for exposed furcation area.[30]
- Orthodontic patient
  - For biofilm removal at gingival margin above bands.

III. Procedure

A. Prepare Instrument

- Insert round, tapered toothpick into the end of the holder. One type of holder has angulated ends for use in various positions.
- Twist the toothpick firmly into place. Break off the long end so that sharp edges do not scratch the inner cheek or the tongue during use.

B. Application

- Apply toothpick at the gingival margin.
  - To remove biofilm just below the gingival margin, position the toothpick tip to a 70° angle to the long axis of the tooth and gently trace slightly subgingivally along the gingival margin from one interproximal space to the next[30] (Figure 27-15).
- For hypersensitive spots, usually at the cervical third of a tooth, the patient can use the tip daily to massage dentifrice for desensitization on the sensitive area.

Wooden Interdental Cleaner

I. Description

- The wooden cleaner is a 2-inch-long device made of wood. It is triangular in cross section, as shown in **Figure 27-16A**.
- A common brand is Stimudent.

II. Indications for Use

- Application
  - For cleaning proximal tooth surfaces where the tooth surfaces are exposed and interdental gingivae are missing. Space must be adequate, otherwise the gingival tissue can be traumatized.[31]
- Advantages
  - Ease of use.
  - Transported easily and can be used throughout the day.
  - Patients use woodsticks more frequently than dental floss.[31]
  - Although woodsticks do not remove biofilm as effectively as dental floss, research suggests they significantly reduce bleeding and interdental inflammation.[31]
- Limitations
  - As with most interdental devices, the wooden cleaner is advised only for patients who follow instructions carefully.
  - The wooden interdental cleaner cannot access root concavities and irregularities in proximal areas to adequately remove dental biofilm.
  - Difficult to use in posterior areas and from the lingual aspect of the teeth.[31]

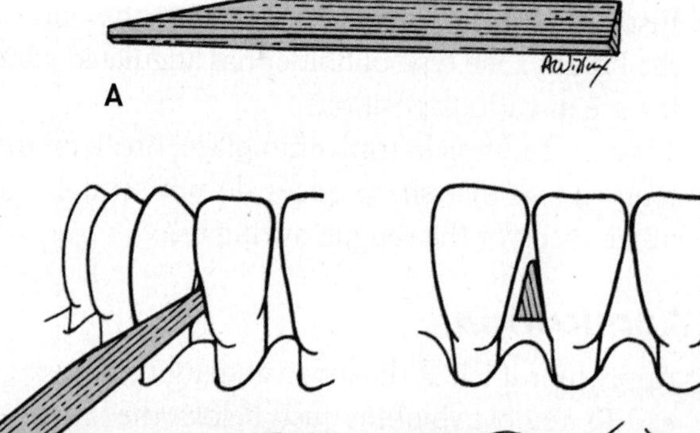

Figure 27-16 Wooden Interdental Cleaner. **A:** The 2-inch wooden triangular cleaner. **B:** Application on the proximal surface of a tooth with a type III embrasure. The base of the triangle is on the gingival side. **C:** The side of the triangle is rubbed in and out against the proximal surface to remove dental biofilm.

III. Procedure

- Fulcrum
  - Teach the patient to use a fulcrum by placing the hand on the cheek or chin or by placing a finger on the gingiva convenient to the place where the tip will be applied.
- Preparation
  - Soften the wood by placing the pointed end in the mouth and moistening with saliva.
- Patient instructions
  - Hold the base of the triangular wedge toward the gingival border of the interdental area and insert with the tip pointed slightly toward the occlusal or incisal surfaces to follow the contour of the embrasure (**Figure 27-16B-C**).
  - Clean the tooth surfaces by moving the wedge in and out while applying a burnishing stroke with moderate pressure first to one side of the embrasure and then to the other side, about four strokes each.
  - Discard the wooden cleaner as soon as the first signs of splaying are evident.

Oral Irrigation

I. Description

- The oral irrigator was introduced in 1962 and may also be called a water flosser.[32]
- Studies have shown oral irrigators lower bleeding and gingivitis indices, even if plaque levels are not affected.[3, 21,32,33]
- Oral irrigators and interdental brushes are recommended over dental floss for implant maintenance[17] and subjects undergoing orthodontic treatment.[34]
- **Irrigation** is the targeted application of a pulsated or steady stream of water or other **irrigant** for preventive or therapeutic purposes.
  - The purpose of irrigation is to reduce the bacteria and inflammatory mediators that lead to the initiation or progression of periodontal infections.
  - For the patient, irrigation can be a part of routine oral self-care.
- Water flossers use a pulsated stream of water under pressure.[35]
  - The water flossers have been shown to remove supragingival interproximal biofilm and reduce gingival inflammation.[35-40] However, the research has been funded by a single manufacturer, so there is a risk of bias and more

research is needed. Thus, the benefit of oral irrigation is reduction of gingivitis and this effect may not be related to biofilm removal.[18]

- The research on the benefits of **subgingival irrigation** with or without antimicrobial agents in managing microbial and clinical signs of periodontal disease remains inconsistent and more study is needed.[32,41]
  - The oral irrigator does not appear to reduce visible dental biofilm; however, it may have positive effects on gingival health over toothbrushing alone.[18,32]
  - In addition, some research suggests reduced counts of periodontal pathogens.[42]

II. Types of Devices

- Countertop power-driven model has a large reservoir for liquid (**Figure 27-17A**).
- Cordless model has a large base to serve as a reservoir for liquid and is good for travel (**Figure 27-17B**).
  - The handle is bulky because of the reservoir and may be too heavy for some patients.
- The shower model attaches to the showerhead or faucet and uses the pressure of the shower water, which may be somewhat lower than the irrigation delivered by the countertop model.

III. Delivery Tips

- A tongue cleaner to remove bacteria and debris (**Figure 27-18A**).
- A regular brush head is used like a manual toothbrush with water. It has no rotational or vibratory action (**Figure 27-18B**).
- A filament-type tip can be used in hard to reach areas and around dental implants or bridges (**Figure 27-18C**).
- An orthodontic tip is available to remove debris and loose dental biofilm from brackets, wires, and bands (**Figure 27-18D**).
- The subgingival tip is designed for subgingival irrigation with a soft rubber tip (**Figure 27-18E**) to be placed below the gingival margin.
- Standard jet tip delivers a steady flow of irrigant (**Figure 27-18F**)

IV. Procedure

These are general instructions for use of an oral irrigator:

- Fill the reservoir with water or other irrigant.
- Choose the appropriate tip.
- Direct the jet tip toward the interdental area until almost touching the tooth surface.
- Hold the tip at a right angle (90°) to the long axis of the tooth for **supragingival irrigation** to remove food debris and loose dental biofilm.
- Lean over the sink to minimize splatter and splashing water on the mirror, countertop, and floor.
- Turn the unit on using low power and increase the water pressure to a rate that is comfortable.
- Use a systematic approach for moving through the mouth such as, maxillary arch first, then the mandibular, facial, palatal, and lingual.
- When done, empty the reservoir to prevent bacterial growth.

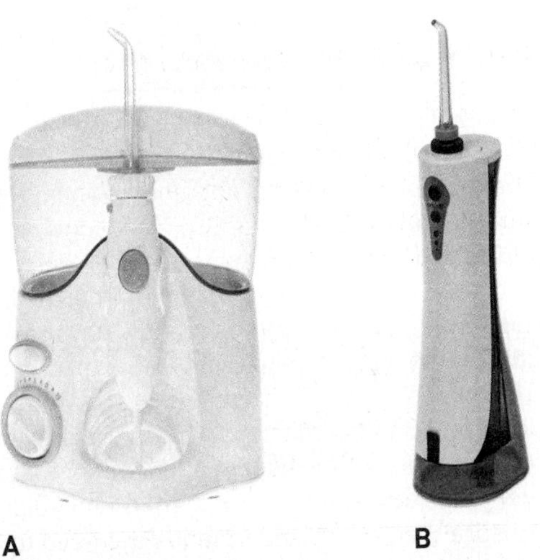

Figure 27-17 Water and Air Flossers. **A:** A countertop dental water jet with rechargeable power toothbrush. **B:** A countertop dental water jet.

A: © olegganko/Shutterstock; B: © ai_stock/Shutterstock

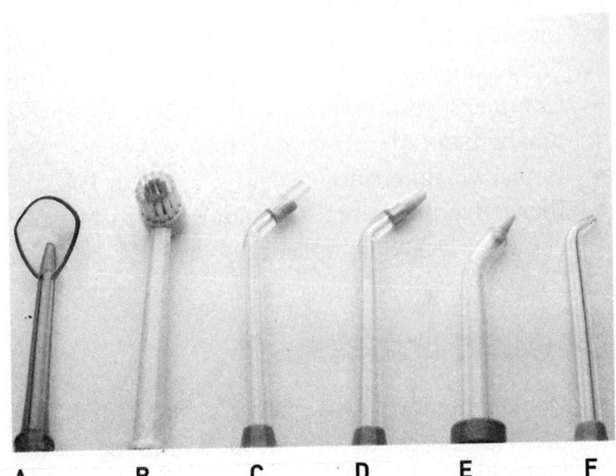

Figure 27-18 Tips for Water Irrigator. **A.** Tongue cleaner **B.** Toothbrush tip. **C.** Plaque Seeker tip. **D.** Orthodontic tip. E. Pik Pocket tip. **F.** Classic jet tip.

© aon168/Shutterstock

V. Applications for Practice

Regular use of daily personal oral irrigation is beneficial.[32] Use a patient-centered approach to evaluate each patient's needs individually to determine which techniques, products, or devices are appropriate.

A. Reduction of Gingival Inflammation

- The evidence is inconsistent on improving parameters of periodontal health, but there was a positive trend toward improving gingival health.[32]
  - A recent orthodontic study found the powered oral hygiene regimen (electric toothbrush and AirFloss Pro) was significantly more effective than a manual regimen (manual toothbrush and string floss) in reducing plaque on bracketed and nonbracketed teeth, and in reducing gingival bleeding and gingival inflammation in orthodontic subjects.[34]

B. Problem Areas

- Areas that are difficult to access with traditional mechanical methods:
  - Open interdental areas.
  - Malpositioned teeth.
  - Exposed furcations.

C. Special Needs Areas

- Prosthetic replacements such as a bridge with a pontic for a missing tooth and fixed partial dentures.
- Orthodontic appliances.
- Intermaxillary fixation appliances for orthognathic surgery and fractured jaw.
- Complex restorations and other extensive rehabilitation.
- Implant maintenance.
- Ineffective interdental technique due to physical ability or lack of compliance.

Documentation

- Documentation for a patient's interdental care progress needs to include a minimum of the following:
  - All interdental aid recommendations and demonstrations with the patient.
- A sample documentation can be found in **Box 27-1**.

Box 27-1 Example Documentation: Recommendations for Daily Interdental Care

- **S**—A 54-year-old male patient presents for routine 3-month continuing care appointment. Patient states, "I do not floss regularly as it is difficult for me, even with the floss holder you gave me last time. Is there another way to clean that area?"
- **O**—Generalized recession and extensive loss of interdental papilla on most posteriors. Observed patient has large hands and limited dexterity when trying to floss. Due to the open embrasure spaces, floss will not be effective in cleaning all surfaces of his teeth.
- **A**—Interdental brush may be a better choice than tufted floss for more thorough cleaning of the wide embrasure spaces in that area of his mouth.
- **P**—Provided instructions for use of two different sizes of interdental brushes with a tapered or cone shape as well as an interdental brush handle with replaceable inserts. The larger size will be used for the patient's posterior teeth with wider embrasures and the smaller size for the anterior areas. Observed patient use of the interdental brushes and worked with him to refine his technique. The patient felt these would do a better job of removing the debris and biofilm and will use these in every space where they fit and is easier for him to use. Samples of the types of interdental brushes were provided and suggestions where he can purchase replacements.

Signed: ______________________________, RDH
Date: ______________

Factors to Teach the Patient

- Use of disclosing solution will provide the patient with a visual understanding of the limitation of the toothbrush in accessing and cleaning the interdental area thoroughly.
- Discuss dental biofilm and how it collects on the proximal tooth surfaces when left undisturbed.
- Educate the patient on the reason why the interdental area is more vulnerable to infection.
- Use hands-on demonstrations to show how interdental aids are used to clean the proximal tooth surfaces. It is essential the patient also demonstrates the use of the interdental aids.
- Ensure the patient understands the need to ask the dental professional about new products they see advertised and whether the product meets the patient's individual oral self-care needs.

References

1. Salzer S, Slot DE, Van der FA Weijden, CE. Dorfer efficacy of inter-dental mechanical plaque control in managing gingivitis—a meta-review. *J Clin Periodontol*. 2015;42(suppl 16):S92-S105.
2. Chapple IL, Van der Weijden F, Doerfer C, et al. Primary prevention of periodontitis: managing gingivitis. *J Clin Periodontol*. 2015;42(suppl 16):S71-S76.
3. Worthington HW, MacDonald L, Pericic TP, et al. Home use of interdental cleaning devices, in addition to toothbrushing, for preventing and controlling periodontal diseases and dental caries. *Cochrane Database Syst Rev*. 2019;4(4): CD012018.
4. Joshi K, Baiju CS, Khashu H, Bansal S, Maheswari IB. Clinical assessment of interdental papilla competency parameters in the esthetic zone. *J Esthetic Rest Dent*. 2017;29(4):270-275.
5. Smukler H, Nager MC, Tolmie PC. Interproximal tooth morphology and its effect on plaque removal. *Quintessence Int*. 1989;20(4):249-255.
6. Graves DT, Corrêa JD, Silva TA. The oral microbiota is modified by systemic diseases. *J Dent Res*. 2019;98(2):148-156.
7. Kaur S, Gupta R, Dahiya P, Kumar M. Morphological study of proximal root grooves and their influence on periodontal attachment loss. *J Indian Soc Periodontol*. 2016;20(3):315-319.
8. Drisko CL. Periodontal self-care: evidence-based support. *Periodontol 2000*. 2013;62(1):243-255.
9. Liang P, Ye S, McComas M, Kwon T, Wang CW. Evidence-based strategies for interdental cleaning: a practical decision tree and review of the literature. *Quintessence Int*. 2021;52(1):84-95.
10. Chapple ILC, Mealey BL, Van Dyke TE, et al. Periodontal health and gingival diseases and conditions on an intact and a reduced periodontium: Consensus report of workgroup 1 of the 2017 World Workshop on the Classification of Periodontal and Peri-Implant Diseases and Conditions. *J Periodontol*. 2018;89(Suppl 1):S74-S84.
11. Slot DE, Valkenburg C, Van der Weijden GAF. Mechanical plaque removal of periodontal maintenance patients: a systematic review and network meta-analysis. *J Clin Periodontol*. 2020;47(Suppl 22):107-124.
12. Sanz M, Herrera D, Kebschull M, et al. Treatment of stage I-III periodontitis-the EFP S3 level clinical practice guideline. *J Clin Periodontol*. 2020;47(Suppl 22):4-60.
13. Wilder RS, Bray KS. Improving periodontal outcomes: merging clinical and behavioral science. *Periodontol 2000*. 2016; 71(1):65-81.
14. Graziani F, Palazzolo A, Gennai S, et al. Interdental plaque reduction after use of different devices in young subjects with intact papilla: a randomized clinical trial. *Int J Dent Hyg*. 2018;16(3):389-396.
15. Abouassi T, Woelber JP, Holst K, et al. Clinical efficacy and patients' acceptance of a rubber interdental bristle. A randomized controlled trial. *Clin Oral Investig*. 2014;18(7):1873-1880.
16. Hennequin-Hoenderdos NL, van der Sluijs E, van der Weijden GA, Slot DE. Efficacy of a rubber bristles interdental cleaner compared to an interdental brush on dental plaque, gingival bleeding and gingival abrasion: a randomized clinical trial. *Int J Dent Hyg*. 2018;16(3):380-388.
17. Graetz C, Schoepke K, Rabe J, et al. In vitro comparison of cleaning efficacy and force of cylindric interdental brush versus an interdental rubber pick. *BMC Oral Health*. 2021;21(1):194.
18. Ng E, Lim LP. An overview of different interdental cleaning aids and their effectiveness. *Dent J*. 2019;7(2):56.
19. Berchier CE, Slot DE, Haps S, Van der Weijden GA. The efficacy of dental floss in addition to a toothbrush on plaque and parameters of gingival inflammation: a systematic review. *Int J Dent Hyg*. 2008;6(4):265-279.
20. Larsen HC, Slot DE, Van Zoelen C, Barendregt DS, Van der Weijden GA. The effectiveness of conically shaped compared with cylindrically shaped interdental brushes - a randomized controlled clinical trial. *Int J Dent Hyg*. 2017;15(3):211-218.
21. Kotsakis GA, Lian Q, Ioannou AL, Michalowicz BS, John MT, Chu H. A network meta-analysis of interproximal oral hygiene methods in the reduction of clinical indices of inflammation. *J Periodontol*. 2018;89(5):558-570.
22. Ciancio SG, Shibly O, Farber GA. Clinical evaluation of the effect of two types of dental floss on plaque and gingival health. *Clin Prev Dent*. 1992;14(3):14-18.
23. Dörfer CE, Wündrich D, Staehle HJ, Pioch T. Gliding capacity of different dental flosses. *J Periodontol*. 2001;72(5):672-678.
24. Azcarate-Velázquez F, Garrido-Serrano R, Castillo-Dalí G, Serrera-Figallo MA, Gañán-Calvo A, Torres-Lagares D. Effectiveness of flossing loops in the control of the gingival health. *J Clin Exp Dent*. 2017;9(6):e756-e761.
25. Hallmon WW, Waldrop TC, Houston GD, Hawkins BF. Flossing clefts. Clinical and histologic observations. *J Periodontol*. 1986;57(8):501-504.
26. Wolff A, Staehle HJ. Improving the mechanical properties of multiuse dental floss holders. *Int J Dent Hyg*. 2014;12(4):245-250.
27. Kiran SD, Ghiya K, Makwani D, Bhatt R, Patel M, Srivastava M. Comparison of plaque removal efficacy of a novel flossing agent with the conventional floss: a clinical study. *Int J Clin Pediatr Dent*. 2018;11(6):474-478.
28. Lin J, Dinis M, Tseng CH, et al. Effectiveness of the GumChucks flossing system compared to string floss for interdental plaque removal in children: a randomized clinical trial. *Sci Rep*. 2020;10(1):3052.
29. Stauff I, Derman S, Barbe AG, et al. Efficacy and acceptance of a high-velocity microdroplet device for interdental cleaning in gingivitis patients: a monitored, randomized controlled trial. *Int J Dent Hyg*. 2018;16(2):e31-e37.
30. Lewis MW, Holder-Ballard C, Selders RJ Jr, Scarbecz M, Johnson HG, Turner EW. Comparison of the use of a toothpick holder to dental floss in improvement of gingival health in humans. *J Periodontol*. 2004;75(4):551-556.
31. Hoenderdos NL, Slot DE, Paraskevas S, Van der Weijden GA. The efficacy of woodsticks on plaque and gingival inflammation: a systematic review. *Int J Dent Hyg*. 2008;6(4):280-289.
32. Husseini A, Slot DE, Van der Weijden GA. The efficacy of oral irrigation in addition to a toothbrush on plaque and the clinical parameters of periodontal inflammation: a systematic review. *Int J Dent Hyg*. 2008;6(4):304-314.
33. Bertl K, Edlund Johansson P, Stavropoulos A. Patients' opinion on the use of 2 generations of power-driven water flossers and their impact on gingival inflammation *Clin Exp Dent Res*. 2021;7(6):1089-1095.
34. Nammi K, Starke EM, Ou SS, et al. The effects of use of a powered and a manual home oral hygiene regimen on plaque and gum health in an orthodontic population. *J Clin Dent*. 2019;30(Spec No A):A1-A8.
35. Goyal CR, Lyle DM, Qaqish JG, Schuller R. Efficacy of two interdental cleaning devices on clinical signs of inflammation:

a four-week randomized controlled trial. *J Clin Dent*. 2015;26(2):55-60.

36. Barnes CM, Russell CM, Reinhardt RA, Payne JB, Lyle DM. Comparison of irrigation to floss as an adjunct to tooth brushing: effect on bleeding, gingivitis, and supragingival plaque. *J Clin Dent*. 2005;16(3):71-77.
37. Goyal CR, Lyle DM, Qaqish JG, Schuller R. Evaluation of the plaque removal efficacy of a water flosser compared to string floss in adults after a single use. *J Clin Dent*. 2013;24(2):37-42.
38. Goyal CR, Lyle DM, Qaqish JG, Schuller R. Comparison of water flosser and interdental brush on reduction of gingival bleeding and plaque: a randomized controlled pilot study. *J Clin Dent*. 2016;27(2):61-65.
39. Goyal CR, Lyle DM, Qaqish JG, Schuller R. The addition of a water flosser to power tooth brushing: effect on bleeding, gingivitis, and plaque. *J Clin Dent*. 2012;23(2):57-63.
40. Lyle DM, Goyal CR, Qaqish JG, Schuller R. Comparison of water flosser and interdental brush on plaque removal: a single-use pilot study. *J Clin Dent*. 2016;27(1):23-26.
41. Nagarakanti S, Gunupati S, Chava VK, Reddy BV. Effectiveness of subgingival irrigation as an adjunct to scaling and root planing in the treatment of chronic periodontitis: a systematic review. *J Clin Diagn Res*. 2015;9(7):ZE06-ZE9.
42. Pandya DJ, Manohar B, Mathur LK, Shankarapillai R. Comparative evaluation of two subgingival irrigating solutions in the management of periodontal disease: a clinicomicrobial study. *J Indian Soc Periodontol*. 2016;20(6):597-602.

CHAPTER 28

Dentifrices and Mouthrinses

Amy N. Smith, RDH, MPH, PhD
Kristeen Perry, RDH, MS

CHAPTER OUTLINE

CANADIAN DENTAL ASSOCIATION SEAL PROGRAM

- **I.** Purpose of Seal Program
- **II.** Product Submission and Acceptance Process
- **III.** Use of Seal

DOCUMENTATION

FACTORS TO TEACH THE PATIENT

REFERENCES

LEARNING OBJECTIVES

After studying this chapter, the student will be able to:

1. Identify and define the active and inactive components in dentifrices and mouthrinses.
2. Explain the mechanism of action for preventive and therapeutic agents in dentifrices and mouthrinses.
3. Explain the purpose and use of dentifrices and mouthrinses.
4. Discuss regulatory agencies for medicines and healthcare products and their purpose.
5. Explain the American Dental Association Seal of Acceptance program or Canadian Dental Association Seal Program and their purpose.

Chemotherapeutics

Recent advances in understanding the pathogenesis of periodontitis have led to alternative therapies that focus on reduction of inflammation in the oral cavity using both mechanical devices and chemotherapeutics.

- Inflammation of periodontal tissues has an impact on the human body beyond the oral cavity.
- Oral inflammation has been linked to several conditions, including diabetes and heart disease.[1,2]
- Increased inflammation associated with diabetes can make a patient more susceptible to periodontal disease.[2,3]
- Oral pathogens can travel to the lungs, causing healthcare-associated pneumonia.[4]
- Either the clinician or the patient can administer chemotherapeutics.

Dentifrices

The benefits of using dentifrices may be preventive, therapeutic, or cosmetic. A dentifrice is a substance applied with a toothbrush or other applicator for:

- Removal of biofilm, stain, and other soft deposits from the gingiva and tooth surfaces.
- Application of therapeutic agents.
- Superficial cosmetic effects.

Preventive and Therapeutic Benefits of Dentifrices

I. Prevention of Dental Caries

- Although fluoride has long been recognized as an anticariogenic agent, the addition of stannous fluoride to a dentifrice was problematic because of lack of compatibility with abrasive agents.[5]
- The first caries-preventive dentifrice contained stannous fluoride (0.4%). It became available commercially in 1955.[6]
- Xylitol, a flavoring agent in some dentifrices, has been shown to provide anticaries benefits.[7]
- Additional information about fluoride dentifrices is described in Chapter 34.

II. Remineralization of Early Noncavitated Dental Caries

- Fluoride enhances remineralization as described in Chapters 25 and 34.

III. Reduction of Biofilm Formation

- Agents used:
  - Zinc citrate.
  - Stannous fluoride.

IV. Reduction of Gingivitis/Inflammation

- An antigingivitis dentifrice can contribute to the improved health of gingival tissue.
- Stannous fluoride has been shown to decrease bleeding sites and reduce the severity of gingivitis.[8,9]
- Dentifrice containing 0.454% stannous fluoride was shown to improve patients' scores on bleeding and gingival indices.[9]
  - Note: Research on the efficacy of this stannous fluoride toothpaste was sponsored by the product manufacturer, which has the potential to introduce bias.

V. Reduction of Dentinal Hypersensitivity

- For in-home treatment of dentinal hypersensitivity, chemical occlusion (potassium nitrate and sodium fluoride) of the dentinal tubules and nerve desensitization are most effective.[10]
- In-home treatment is the first intervention for dentinal hypersensitivity, but if it is not effective, in-office treatments are recommended.[10]
- More information on reducing dentinal hypersensitivity is discussed in Chapter 41.

VI. Reduction of Supragingival Calculus Formation

- "Tartar-control" dentifrices shown to help inhibit supragingival calculus may contain:
  - Pyrophosphate salts.[11]
  - Zinc salts (zinc chloride and zinc citrate).[11]
  - Sodium hexametaphosphate.[12]

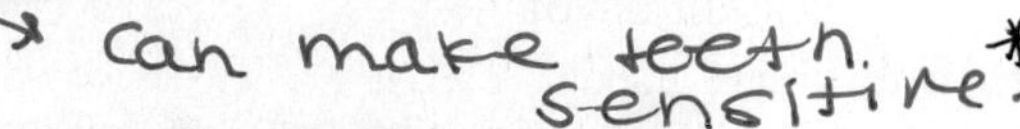

Cosmetic Effects of Dentifrices

I. Removal of Extrinsic Stain

- The pigments from foods, tobacco, or chemical agents may become imbedded in the acquired pellicle and dental biofilm.
- Cosmetic results from dentifrice are based on:
  - Mechanical removal of the stained biofilm.
  - Delivery of a bleaching agent.
- Each commercially available product needs to be evaluated individually for efficacy and patient acceptance.
- More information on tooth stains is provided in Chapters 17 and 42.

II. Reduction of Oral Malodor (Halitosis)

- Certain ingredients added to a dentifrice can reduce oral malodor on a temporary basis by inhibiting the production of volatile sulfur compounds (VSCs).
- Chlorhexidine (CHX), cetylpyridinium chloride (CPC), and zinc formulations have a beneficial effect on reducing oral malodor via reduction of VSCs.[13,14]
- Stannous fluoride combined with sodium hexametaphosphate can reduce VSC production.[15]

Basic Components of Dentifrices: Inactives

- Most dentifrices share a common composition of ingredients needed for a stable formulation.
- Dentifrices are sold primarily as pastes and gels. The common ingredients and their function are listed in **Table 28-1**.
- In addition to the inactive ingredients described in Table 28-1, a therapeutic dentifrice will have a drug or chemical agent stated as an active ingredient for a specific preventive or therapeutic action.
- The active ingredient represents approximately 1.5% to 2% of the dentifrice's formulation.
- Therapeutic agents are described in **Table 28-2**.

I. Detergents (Foaming Agents or Surfactants)

- Purposes
  - Lower surface tension.
  - Penetrate and loosen surface deposits.
  - Suspend debris for easy removal by toothbrush.
  - Emulsify/disperse the flavor oils.
  - Contribute to foaming action.

Table 28-1 Ingredients and Function of Commercially Available Dentifrices

Ingredient	Function	Average Formulation Percentage (%)
Surfactant/ detergent	Foaming and cleansing	1–2
Abrasive	Cleaning and polishing	20–40
Binder	Thickening agent and stabilizes formula	1–2
Humectant	Prevents water loss/ hardening of dentifrice	20–40
Preservative	Prevents microorganisms from destroying the dentifrice in storage	2–3
Flavoring	Sweetener	1–1.5
Water	Maintains the ingredient in formulation	20–40

Table 28-2 Therapeutic Active Ingredients in Dentifrices

Benefit	Active Ingredients
Antibiofilm/ antigingivitis	Stannous fluoride, zinc citrate
Anticalculus	Tetrapotassium pyrophosphate, tetrasodium pyrophosphate, sodium hexametaphosphate, zinc compounds
Desensitizer	Potassium nitrate, potassium citrate, potassium chloride, stannous fluoride, strontium chloride
Oral malodor	Essential oils, chlorine dioxide, stannous fluoride/sodium hexametaphosphate

- Substances used
  - Sodium lauryl sulfate USP.
  - Sodium N-lauroyl sarcosinate.

II. Cleaning and Polishing Agents (Abrasives)

- Purposes
  - Cleans well with no damage to tooth surface.
  - A polishing agent is used to produce a smooth tooth surface.
  - A smooth surface can prevent or delay the accumulation of stains and deposits.
- Primary abrasives used[16]:
  - Silica, silicates, and hydrated silica gels.
  - Calcium carbonate.
  - Dicalcium phosphate.
  - Sodium bicarbonate.

III. Binders (Thickeners)

- Purposes
  - Stabilize the formulation.
  - Prevent separation of the solid and liquid ingredients during storage.
- Types used
  - Mineral colloids.
  - Natural gums.
  - Seaweed colloids.
  - Synthetic celluloses.

IV. Humectants (Moisture Stabilizers)

- Purposes
  - Retain moisture.
  - Prevent hardening on exposure to air.
- Substances used
  - Xylitol.
  - Glycerol.
  - Sorbitol.

V. Preservatives

- Purposes
  - Prevent bacterial growth.
  - Prolong shelf life.
- Substances used
  - Alcohol.
  - Benzoates.
  - Dichlorinated phenols.

VI. Flavoring Agents (Sweeteners)

- Purposes
  - Impart a pleasant flavor for increased patient acceptance.
  - Mask other ingredients that may have a less pleasant flavor.
- Substances used
  - Essential oils (peppermint, cinnamon, wintergreen, clove).
  - Artificial noncariogenic sweeteners (xylitol, glycerol, sorbitol).

Active Components of Dentifrices

Dentifrice selections offer a variety of active ingredients that may help prevent caries, dentin hypersensitivity, biofilm formation, gingivitis, calculus formation, and oral malodor.

- The first active ingredient introduced in a dentifrice was fluoride. Major developments in active ingredients have been made since then.
  - Specific active ingredients are summarized in Table 28-2.

Selection of Dentifrices

I. Prevention or Reduction of Oral Disease

- Dental caries.
- Fluoride-containing dentifrice during remineralization program. (See Chapters 25 and 34.)
- Dentinal hypersensitivity.
- Gingivitis.
- Calculus formation.
- Oral malodor/reduction of VSCs.

II. Considerations for the Pediatric Patient

- Birth to first tooth eruption
  - Caregivers can clean the child's gingiva with a soft infant toothbrush or cloth and water.
- Eruption of first tooth
  - Caregivers can begin to start brushing twice daily using fluoridated toothpaste and a soft, appropriately sized toothbrush.
  - Use a very small "smear" or rice-sized amount of toothpaste to brush the teeth of a child younger than 3 years of age.[17] The small smear of fluoride paste is shown in Chapter 47.
- 2–5 years old
  - The caregiver can dispense a "pea-sized" amount of toothpaste for children over 3 years of age and perform or assist child's tooth brushing.[17] (See Chapter 47 for an illustration of "pea-sized.")
  - Caregivers need to recognize that young children do not have the ability to brush their teeth effectively without help and supervision.
  - Caregivers brushing their own teeth at the same time as the child can provide the child with a role model for brushing habits.
  - Children should be supervised until they are able to adequate remove plaque biofilm, spit out toothpaste, and not swallow excess toothpaste during brushing.

III. Patient-Specific Dentifrice Recommendations

- Dentifrice recommendations are a key part of personal daily care planning and are patient specific.
- Considerations include:
  - Patient's current oral condition.
  - Any patient complaint/concern.
  - Sensitivities or allergies to a specific ingredient.
  - Propensity of staining (stannous fluoride–containing dentifrice).
  - Patient's nontherapeutic/cosmetic choices.
  - Expectation of compliance. When a dentifrice does not appeal in either taste or texture, it will not be used regardless of therapeutic benefits.
  - Personal trial is needed before a recommendation is made. Dental hygienists need firsthand experience with each product they recommend.

Mouthrinses

- Mechanical aids may not be sufficient to maintain optimum oral health for certain patients and may be supplemented with the use of a chemotherapeutic mouthrinse.
- The benefits of using a mouthrinse may be one or more of the following: preventive, cosmetic, and therapeutic.
- Chemotherapeutic rinses may have active ingredients to reduce inflammation.
- Cosmetic rinses can provide some extrinsic stain removal when it is superficial in unattached biofilm.
- **Therapeutic rinses** have healing properties that are delivered by rinsing or irrigation device.
- Delivery: Rinsing can deliver an agent less than 2 mm into the sulcus or pocket and is not a delivery of choice for patients with moderate or deep pockets.[18]
- Functions: A list of general functions of **chemotherapeutic agents** is provided in **Box 28-1**.

Purposes and Uses of Mouthrinses

I. Before Professional Treatment

- To reduce the numbers of intraoral microorganisms to lower the bacterial load.
- To reduce contamination during aerosol generating procedures such as use of a handpiece or ultrasonic scaler.

II. Self-Care

- As part of personal oral self-care for specific needs.
- Biofilm control.

Box 28-1 Functions of Chemotherapeutic Agents

- Remineralization: Restore mineral elements.
- Antimicrobial: Bactericidal or bacteriostatic.
  - Biofilm control.
  - Gingival health: Reduction/prevention of gingivitis.
- **Astringent**: Shrink tissues.
- Anodyne: Alleviate pain.
- Buffering: Reduce oral acidity.
- Deodorizing: Neutralize odor.
- Oxygenating: Cleanse.

- Dental caries prevention through remineralization of noncavitated early dental caries.
- Prevention of gingivitis.
- Contribute to malodor control.
- Posttreatment therapy following nonsurgical periodontal therapy:
  - Periodontal surgery.
  - Removal of teeth.

Preventive and Therapeutic Agents of Mouthrinses

I. Fluoride

A. Mechanism of Action

- Stannous fluoride
  - Deposit of fluoride ion on enamel.
  - Tin ion from stannous fluoride interferes with cell metabolism for antimicrobial effect.
- Sodium fluoride:
  - Deposit of fluoride ion on enamel.
  - Cariostatic: Inhibits demineralization and enhances remineralization.

B. Availability and Use

- Available in varying concentrations.
- Uses:
  - Prevention of demineralization.
  - Reduction of hypersensitivity.
  - Reduction of gingivitis.

C. Efficacy

- Reduction in biofilm or dental caries when rinse is used topically by the patient.

D. Considerations

- Stannous: Tooth staining; flavor.
- Instruct patient to expectorate/not to swallow.

II. Chlorhexidine

A. Mechanism of Action

- The mechanisms of action of chlorhexidine (**CHX**) include the following:
  - A cationic bisbiguanide with broad antibacterial activity.
  - Binds to oral hard and soft tissues.
  - Attaches to bacterial cell membrane, thereby damaging the cytoplasm and causing lysis.
  - Binds to pellicle and salivary mucins to prevent biofilm accumulation.
  - Bactericidal and bacteriostatic depending on concentration.
  - Bactericidal concentrations cause cell lysis.
  - Bacteriostatic concentrations interfere with cell wall transport system.
  - The substantivity of CHX: 8–12 hours.
  - Antimicrobial and antigingivitis agent.

B. Availability and Uses

- CHX is the most effective antimicrobial and antigingivitis agent available for clinical use.[19,20]
  - Mouthrinse available by prescription in a 0.12% solution in the United States (higher concentrations are available in other countries); postsurgery for enhanced wound healing (**Figure 28-1**).
- Recommended uses:
  - Preprocedural rinse to reduce bacterial load before aerosol-producing procedures.
  - Before, during, and after periodontal debridement.
  - Patients who are at a high risk for dental caries.
  - Immunocompromised individuals who are more susceptible to infection.
  - Postsurgery for enhanced wound healing.

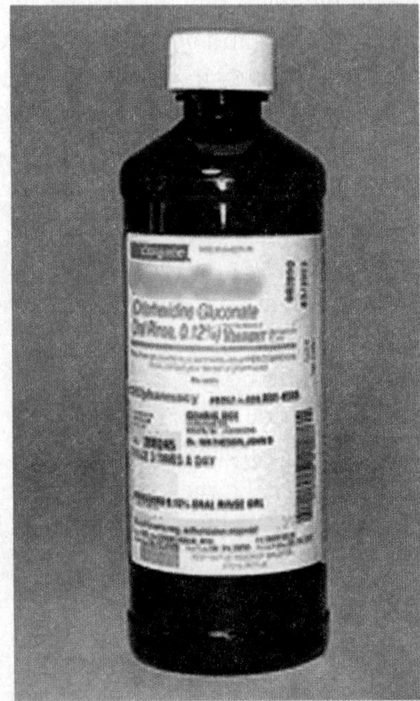

Figure 28-1 Therapeutic Mouthrinse. Chlorhexidine gluconate mouthrinse aids in plaque biofilm control and requires a prescription for purchase.

Reproduced from Nield-Gehrig J, Willmann D. Foundations of Periodontics for the Dental Hygienist. 3rd ed. Philadelphia, PA: Lippincott Williams & Wilkins; 2011.

C. Efficacy

- CHX is safe and effective in:
  - Preventing and controlling biofilm formation.
  - Reducing viability of existing biofilm.
  - Inhibiting and reducing the development of gingivitis.[20]
  - Reducing mutans streptococci.[20]

D. Considerations

- Low level of toxicity due to poor absorption through mucous membranes.
- Staining of teeth, including smooth surfaces, pits and fissures, restorations, and soft tissues (**Figure 28-2**).
- Increase in supragingival calculus formation.
- Altered taste perception.
- Minor irritation to soft tissues, lips, and tongue.

Some research suggests CHX interacts with and is inactivated by sodium lauryl sulfate (a surfactant used in dentifrices) when rinsing is performed immediately after brushing. However, a recent systematic review and meta-analysis indicates that sodium lauryl sulfate does not interfere with the antiplaque effect of CHX.[21]

III. Phenolic-Related Essential Oils

A. Mechanism of Action

- Disrupt cell walls and inhibit bacterial enzymes.
- Decrease pathogenicity of biofilm.
- Antimicrobial and antigingivitis agent.

B. Availability and Uses

- A combination of thymol, eucalyptol, menthol, and methyl salicylate is available as a brand name product and generic product.
- Recommended uses:
  - Individuals unable to perform adequate brushing and flossing.
  - Initially or periodically to help improve management of dental biofilm.
  - Adjunct for mechanical self-care routines that are not sufficient in reducing biofilm, bleeding, and gingivitis.
  - Preprocedural rinse to reduce bacterial load before instrumentation-producing aerosols.

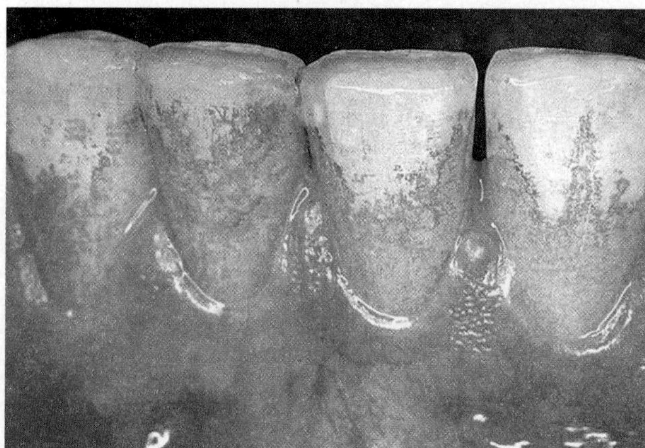

Figure 28-2 Chlorhexidine Stain

Reproduced from Nield-Gehrig J. *Fundamentals of Periodontal Instrumentation and Advanced Root Instrumentation.* Philadelphia, PA: Lippincott Williams & Wilkins; 2011.

C. Efficacy

- Significant reduction in the levels of biofilm and gingivitis.[20,22]

D. Considerations

- Burning sensation.
- Bitter taste.
- Poor substantivity.
- Efficacy of individual rinses based on following the manufacturer's instructions and not casual use of the rinse.
- Contraindicated for current or recovering alcoholics due to alcohol content.

IV. Quaternary Ammonium Compounds

A. Mechanism of Action

- The mechanisms of action of quaternary ammonium compounds include[23]:
  - Cationic agents that bind to oral tissues.
  - Rupture the cell wall and alter the cytoplasm.
  - Initial attachment to oral tissue is very strong, but released rapidly.
  - Decreases the ability of bacteria to attach to the pellicle.
  - Low substantivity.

B. Availability and Uses

- The most commonly used agent is CPC, at 0.05% to 0.07%.
- Recommended uses:
  - Reduction in biofilm accumulation.
  - Adjunct for mechanical self-care routines.

C. Efficacy

- Weak evidence for reductions in biofilm and gingivitis and more research is recommended.[24]

- Possible inhibition of calculus formation.[24]
- Preliminary research has shown that CPC inactivated SARS-CoV-2, but the clinical efficacy has not been investigated.[25]

D. Considerations

- Staining of teeth and tongue.[26]
- A burning sensation and occasional desquamation.[26]

V. Oxygenating Agents

A. Mechanism of Action[27]

- Alters bacterial cell membrane, increasing permeability.
- Poor substantivity.

B. Availability and Uses

- The common agents available in commercial rinses are 10% carbamide peroxide and 1.5% hydrogen peroxide.
- Recommended for short-term use to reduce the symptoms of pericoronitis and necrotizing ulcerative gingivitis.[27]

C. Efficacy

- Negligible antimicrobial effect.
- Debriding agent.
- Despite early suggestions of efficacy, hydrogen peroxide has not been proven to inactivate or reduce the viral load of SARS-CoV-2 when used as a mouthrinse.[25]

D. Considerations

- Does not consistently prevent plaque biofilm accumulation short term, but when used long term, some reduction in gingival redness has been noted.[27]
- Occasional reports of erosive changes to oral mucosa.[27]

VI. Oxidizing Agents

A. Mechanism of Action

- Neutralization of VSCs that contribute to oral malodor.

B. Availability and Uses

- Common agents available in commercial rinses are chlorine dioxide (ClO_2) and chlorine dioxide/zinc combination.

C. Efficacy

- Mainly used for management of halitosis.[28]

D. Consideration

- Diluted 0.25% to 0.5% sodium hypochlorite used as a mouthrinse twice per week showed significant reductions in bleeding on probing (BOP), dental biofilm, and gingival inflammation.[29,30]

Commercial Mouthrinse Ingredients

Ingredients and their functions are listed in **Table 28-3**.

I. Active Ingredients

- Commercial mouthrinses generally contain more than one active ingredient and, therefore, may advertise multiple claims for use.
- Factors that influence how effective an agent may be:
  - Dilution by the saliva.

Table 28-3 Typical Commercial Mouthrinse Formulation

Ingredient	Function
Alcohol	Enhances flavor impact and contributes to cleansing
Flavor	Used to enhance taste and makes breath temporarily fresh
Humectant	Adds "body" and inhibits crystallization around closure
Surfactant	Solubilizes the flavor and provides foaming action
Water	Major vehicle to carry other ingredients
Preservative	Preserves aqueous formulation
Dyes	Add color
Sweeteners	Contribute to overall flavor perception
Flavor	Makes mouthrinse pleasant to use
Active or functional ingredients	Provide therapeutic and/or benefits

- Length of time the agent is in contact with the tissue or bacteria.
- Evidence supporting the particular product.
- General characteristics of an effective chemotherapeutic agent are shown in **Box 28-2**.

II. Inactive Ingredients

A. Water

- Makes up the largest percentage by volume.

B. Alcohol

- Use of alcohol in mouthrinses[31]:
  - Increases the solubility of some active ingredients.
  - Acts as a preservative.
  - Percentage varies from 18% to 27%.
  - Enhances flavor.
- No link to oral cancer has been found with regular use of an alcohol-containing mouthrinse.[32]

C. Flavoring

- Essential oils and derivatives (eucalyptus oil, oil of wintergreen).
- Aromatic waters (peppermint, spearmint, wintergreen, or others).
- Artificial noncariogenic sweetener.

III. Patient-Specific Mouthrinse Recommendations

Mouthrinses are formulated for a variety of oral benefits, including mouth freshening, prevention of caries, biofilm control, and control of oral malodor. Several factors are considered when making a mouthrinse recommendation, including:

- Is the patient currently able to control biofilm through other methods?
- Does the patient consider rinsing a substitute for other mechanical procedures such as brushing and interproximal biofilm removal?
- Does the patient's substance abuse history contraindicate recommending an alcohol-containing mouthrinse?
- Could the patient's xerostomia be worsened by the drying effect of an alcohol-containing mouthrinse?

IV. Contraindications

- The use of a mouthrinse can enhance a patient's oral self-care regimen. The patient needs to understand why rinsing is not a substitute for brushing or use of interproximal aids.
- Some agents are contraindicated for children younger than 6 years of age who have a tendency to swallow instead of expectorate.
- Review manufacturer's instructions for age limits as they vary by product.
- Contraindicated in patients with physical or cognitive challenges who cannot follow rinsing instructions.

Procedure for Rinsing

- Many patients, particularly children, must be shown specifically how to rinse. The method can be practiced under supervision.
- **Box 28-3** suggests steps for teaching a patient to rinse.

Box 28-2 Characteristics of an Effective Chemotherapeutic Agent

- Nontoxic: The agent does not damage oral tissues or create systemic problems.
- No or limited absorption: The action is confined to the oral cavity.
- Substantivity: The ability of an agent to be bound to the pellicle and tooth surface and be released over a period of time with retention of potency.
- Bacterial specificity: May be broad-spectrum, but with an affinity for the pathogenic organisms of the oral cavity.
- Low-induced drug resistance: Low or no development of resistant organisms to agent.

Box 28-3 Steps: How to Rinse

- Take a small amount of the fluid into the mouth.
- Close lips; hold teeth slightly apart.
- Force the fluid through the interdental areas with pressure.
- Use the lips, cheeks, and tongue action to force the fluid back and forth between the teeth.
- Balloon the cheeks, then suck them in, alternately several times.
- Divide the mouth into three parts—front, right, and left.
- Concentrate the rinsing first on the front, then on the right, and then on the left side.
- Expectorate.
- Follow manufacturer's directions on amount, length, and frequency of rinsing.

Emerging Alternative Practices

I. Oil Pulling

- The ancient practice of swishing with 10 mL (one tablespoon) of sesame or coconut oil.[33,34]
- Reduction of biofilm.[33,34]
- Reduction of bacteria causing caries, gingivitis, halitosis, and oral thrush.[33,34]

Agencies Regulating Medicine and Healthcare Products

The purpose of the U.S. Food and Drug Administration (FDA) is to ensure the safety and efficacy of medical and dental drugs, equipment, and devices that affect living tissue. All drugs require FDA approval. Rinses and dentifrices are classified by the FDA as cosmetic, **therapeutic**, or a combination of cosmetic and therapeutic.[35]

I. Regulatory Agencies Overview

- Regulatory agencies for oversight of medicine and healthcare products globally include some of the following:
    - United States: Food and Drug Association (FDA)
    - Canada: Health Canada (HC)
    - United Kingdom: Medicines and Healthcare Products Regulatory Agency (MHRA)
    - European Union: European Medicines Agency (EMA)
    - South Africa: South African Health Products Regulatory Authority (SAHPRA)

II. Role of the Regulatory Agencies for Medicines and Healthcare Products

- Regulate safety, quality, and efficacy of drugs, equipment, and devices.
    - Some devices and equipment may be exempt from (dental water jets, power and manual toothbrushes, dental floss) if they have existing or reasonably similar characteristics as previously approved devices of the same type.

III. Dental Product Regulation

- Dental products regulated will vary from agency to agency, but may include:
    - Infection control products.
    - Dental equipment such as ultrasonic instruments.
    - Diagnostic test kits (i.e., dental caries detection devices).
    - Prosthetic and restorative materials such as implants.
    - Surgical and periodontal materials such as guided tissue regeneration membranes, bone-filling material, and growth factors.
    - Prescription drugs, controlled and sustained-release devices, and chemotherapeutics.
    - In the case of dentifrice and mouthrinses, the FDA has reviewed active ingredients under over-the-counter (OTC) monographs, which are regulations that specify the active ingredients and permissible levels of those ingredients, as well as statements required on product labels.[36]

IV. Research Requirements and Documentation

- **Table 28-4** outlines the documentation process for a product to receive FDA approval.[37]
    - Regulatory agencies in other countries may have a different process, but rigor in the evidence needed for approval is always a part of this process.

Seal of Acceptance Program

I. American Dental Association Seal of Acceptance

- The American Dental Association (ADA) has promoted safety and effectiveness of dental products for over 92 years.[38]
- The ADA Seal of Acceptance Program, which evaluates OTC products offered to consumers, has been in place since 1931, and is internationally recognized.[38]
- Unlike the FDA, the ADA Seal Program is voluntary, and a company must apply to obtain it by making a product submission.[38]
- Products are awarded the ADA Seal only after the ADA Council on Scientific Affairs has thoroughly

Table 28-4 Food and Drug Administration Clearance Documentation Process for Oral Care Products

Phase	Study Type	Purpose
Preclinical	Animal studies	Safety/toxicity
I.	Clinical trial with small sample population (20–80)	Determine dosing/safety, how drug is metabolized and excreted, and side effects
II.	Clinical trial with a larger sample population (100–200) who have disease or condition that the product is designed to treat. The test drug is compared to a standard treatment or placebo known as a control	Provides further safety data and preliminary evidence of efficacy
III.	Clinical trial with a large sample population (1,000–3,000) who have a disease or condition to test efficacy, monitor side effects, and identify treatment parameters. The test drug is compared to a standard treatment or placebo known as a control	Identify possible less obvious side effects
IV.	Clinical trials on products that are already approved and on the market	Continue to measure long-term benefits, risks, and optimal protocol

evaluated clinical and laboratory studies on a product and determined that it meets the ADA criteria for safety and effectiveness, when used as directed.[38]

II. Purposes of the Seal Program

The ADA Seal of Acceptance Program is designed to[38]:

- Help the public and dental professionals make informed decisions about consumer dental products.
- Study and evaluate products for safety and efficacy, when used as directed.
- Inform members of the dental team and the public about the safety and efficacy of each product that is accepted.
- Maintain liaisons with regulatory agencies and research and professional organizations.

III. Product Submission and Acceptance Process

A. Information Required from the Company

- A company submitting an application for the ADA Seal must submit the following[38]:
  - Complete ingredient listing.
  - Objective data from clinical and laboratory studies that support the product's safety, and claimed effectiveness, when used as directed.
  - Compliance with specific product category; acceptance guidelines if applicable.
  - Evidence of good manufacturing processes.

B. Evaluation

- Involves members of the ADA Council on Scientific Affairs, comprising of member dentists from various dental specialities and research scientists.
- Acceptance is for a 5-year period, after which the company can reapply for a new 5-year acceptance.
- Any changes in the product pertaining to composition, manufacturer, claims, etc. need to be communicated to the seal program.

IV. Acceptance and Use of the Seal

- The requirements for use of the seal include the following[38]:
  - Claims of product effectiveness on labeling and in advertising and promotional materials must first be approved by the Council on Scientific Affairs.
  - The use of the ADA Seal (**Figure 28-3**) on labeling and in promotional materials must be accompanied by an ADA-approved Seal Statement.
  - The Seal Statement tells the consumer what specific claims have been reviewed and approved and indicates why the particular product was accepted.

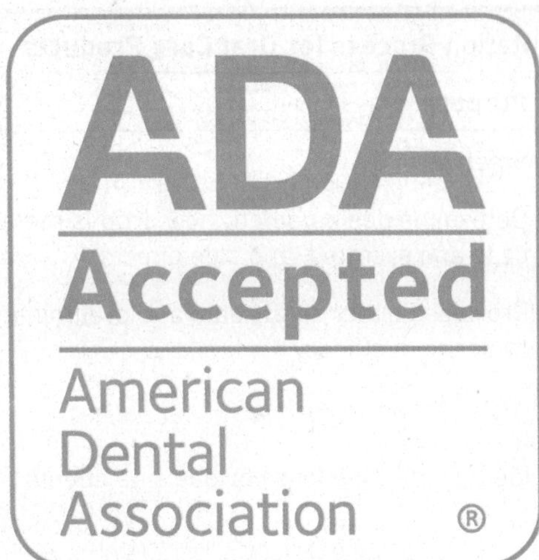

Figure 28-3 ADA Seal of Acceptance, the American Dental Association, Council on Scientific Affairs. The Seal is awarded to consumer products that meet ADA guidelines for safety and effectiveness.

Reprinted with permission of the ADA Council on Scientific Affairs.

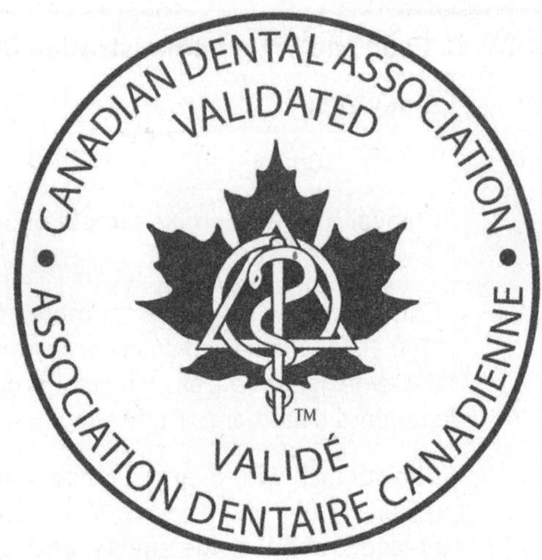

Figure 28-4 CDA Seal of Acceptance, the Canadian Dental Association. The Seal is awarded to consumer products that will deliver oral health benefits validated by CDA and claimed by the manufacturer.

Reproduced from Canadian Dental Association. www.cda-adc.ca/seal.

- A product search can be done on the www.ada.org website to obtain detailed information on each of the accepted products to help consumers and dental professionals select OTC oral care products.[38]
  - Information is included for each product on the basis for acceptance (i.e., the data on which acceptance is based), indications, directions for use, ingredients, label warnings, and company contact information.
  - The Seal website also allows comparisons of the attributes of two to six products in a given product category.
  - This information is printable and can be used to help consumers make informed decisions about the oral care products they use.
  - It can also be useful to dental professionals in recommending OTC oral care products to their patients.
  - Visit www.mouthhealthy.org for preventive oral health resources and ADA Seal product information for patients.
  - Visit www.ada.org/seal for more information on the ADA Seal Program and for access to product information on ADA-accepted products.

Canadian Dental Association Seal Program

- The Canadian Dental Association (CDA) seal (**Figure 28-4**) validates the claims made by the manufacturer about a specific oral health benefit of a product.[39]

I. Purpose of Seal Program

- Provides assurance a product will improve oral health as claimed.
- For the manufacturer, the seal differentiates the product from others on the market by supporting the oral health benefits of using the product.[39]

II. Product Submission and Acceptance Process

- Participation of manufacturers in applying for the seal is voluntary.
- A completed CDA Seal application is required from the manufacturer and reviewed by a panel of experts.
- Research conducted to support the product is reviewed and the experts may identify additional research needed.
- The oral health benefit claimed must be measurable and clinically significant as it relates to therapeutic, cosmetic, or preventive effects of using the product.

III. Use of the Seal

- Once a CDA Seal is approved, the CDA Seal Statement for the product must specify the oral health benefit(s) verified by the CDA.[39]
- A product search can be done to obtain detailed information on each of the accepted products to help consumers and dental professionals select OTC oral care products.[39]
  - Visit www.cda-adc.ca/en/oral_health/seal/products/seal for more information on the CDA Seal Program and for access to product information on CDA-accepted products.

Documentation

- Information to be documented in the patient's permanent record will include a minimum of the following:
    - Recommended dentifrice and mouthrinse for daily oral self- care: nonalcohol-containing mouthrinse and antibacterial dentifrice.
    - Patient instructed on proper usage, including amount and frequency of use.
- Summary of current oral findings indicating need for recommendations provided.
- Example documentation is provided in **Box 28-4**.

Box 28-4 Example Documentation: Choosing a Mouthrinse for a Patient with Xerostomia

- **S**—A 76-year-old male presented for a routine maintenance appointment. His chief complaint is a dry mouth. He reports no medication and although he has a history of smoking, he quit 40 years ago. Patient states he eats a lot of apples and other fruits. Patient stated he has been using a "great mouthwash" for the past 25 years. Patient believes it is helping "toughen up his gums" because his mouth is so dry.
- **O**—Extraoral: No significant findings. The intraoral examination reveals decreased salivary flow. The periodontal examination reveals generalized 3- to 4-mm pocket depths with no bleeding on probing present.
- **A**—Patient presents with xerostomia and a history of smoking that increases his risk for caries, oral cancer, and periodontal disease.
- **P**—Discussed xerostomia and probable causes. Discussed the effects of alcohol on the oral cavity and recommended mouthwash that does not contain alcohol to reduce the incidence of dry mouth.

Signed: ______________________, RDH
Date: ______________

Factors to Teach the Patient

- Significance of American Dental Association or Canadian Dental Association Seal, especially that it is a voluntary program and lack of a seal on a product does not signify it is unsafe.
- To ask the dental hygienist and dentist about new dentifrices and mouthrinses, best way to use, and appropriateness for personal needs.
- How to avoid impulse buying with regard to dentifrices, mouthrinses, and other chemical agents. To seek professional advice to avoid contraindications with oral condition and restorations.
- To understand compliance with recommended chemical agent is directly related to expected outcomes (results or improvements).
- Why the use of chemotherapeutics is not a substitute for proper and daily mechanical biofilm removal.
- To check the ingredients of mouthrinses to prevent the purchase of high-alcohol content if xerostomia is a problem.

References

1. Holmlund A, Lampa E, Lind L.Poor response to periodontal treatment may predict future cardiovascular disease. *J Dent Res*. 2017;96(7):768-773.
2. Oberoi SS, Harish Y, Hiremath S, Puranik M. A cross-sectional survey to study the relationship of periodontal disease with cardiovascular disease, respiratory disease, and diabetes mellitus. *J Indian Soc Periodontol*. 2016;20(4):446-452.
3. D'Aiuto F, Gable D, Syed Z, et al. Evidence summary: the relationship between oral diseases and diabetes. *Br Dent J*. 2017;222(12):944-948.
4. Manger D, Walshaw M, Fitzgerald R, et al. Evidence summary: the relationship between oral health and pulmonary disease. *Br Dent J*. 2017;222(7): 527-533.
5. Mellburg JR. Fluoride dentifrices: current status and prospects. *Int Dent J*. 1991;41(1):9-16.
6. Fischman SL. The history of oral hygiene products: how far have we come in 6000 years? *Periodontol 2000*. 1997;15:7-14.
7. Janakiram C, Deepan Kumar CV, Joseph J. Xylitol in preventing dental caries: a systematic review and meta-analyses. *J Natural Sci Biol Med*. 2017;8(1):16-21.
8. Biesbrock A, He T, DiGennaro J, et al. The effects of bioavailable gluconate chelated stannous fluoride dentifrice on gingival bleeding: meta-analysis of eighteen randomized controlled trials. *J Clin Periodontol*. 2019;46(12):1205-1216.
9. Parkinson C, Milleman K, Milleman J. Gingivitis efficacy of a 0.454% w/w stannous fluoride dentifrice: a 24-week randomized controlled trial. *BMC Oral Health*. 2020;20(1):89.
10. Moraschini V, da Costa LS, Dos Santos GO. Effectiveness for dentin hypersensitivity treatment of non-carious cervical lesions: a meta-analysis. *Clin Oral Investig*. 2018;22(2):617-631.

11. Netuveli GS, Sheiham A. A systematic review of the effectiveness of anticalculus dentifrices. *Oral Health Prev Dent.* 2004;2(1):49-58.
12. Winston JL, Fiedler SK, Schiff T, Baker R. An anticalculus dentifrice with sodium hexametaphosphate and stannous fluoride: a six-month study of efficacy. *J Contemp Dent Pract.* 2007;8(5):1-8.
13. Seemann R, Conceicao MD, Filippi A, et al. Halitosis management by the general dental practitioner—results of an international consensus workshop. *J Breath Res.* 2014;8(1):017101.
14. Mendes L, Coimbra J, Pereira A, Resende M, Pinto M. Comparative effect of a new mouthrinse containing chlorhexidine, triclosan and zinc on volatile sulphur compounds: a randomized, crossover, double-blind study. *Int J Dent Hyg.* 2016;14(3):202-208.
15. Farrell S, Barker ML, Gerlach RW. Overnight malodor effect with a 0.454% stabilized stannous fluoride sodium hexametaphosphate dentifrice. *Compend Contin Educ Dent.* 2007;28(12):658-661.
16. Schemehorn BR, Moore MH, Putt MS. Abrasion, polishing, and stain removal characteristics of various commercial dentifrices in vitro. *J Clin Dent.* 2011;22(1):11-18.
17. AAPD Council on Clinical Affairs. Fluoride therapy. *Oral Health Pol Recomm.* 2018;40(6):251-252.
18. Wunderlich RC, Singelton M, O'Brien WJ, Caffesse RG. Subgingival penetration of an applied solution. *Int J Periodontics Restorative Dent.* 1984;4(5):64-71.
19. Van Strydonck DA, Slot DE, Van der Velden U, et al. Effect of a chlorhexidine mouthrinse on plaque, gingival inflammation and staining in gingivitis patients: a systematic review. *J Clin Periodontol.* 2012;39(11):1042-1055.
20. Neely AL. Essential oil mouthwash (EOMW) may be equivalent to chlorhexidine (CHX) for long-term control of gingival inflammation but CHX appears to perform better than EOMW in plaque control. *J Evid Based Dent Pract.* 2012;12(suppl 3):69-72.
21. Elkerbout TA, Slot DE, Bakker EW, Van der Weijden GA. Chlorhexidine mouthwash and sodium lauryl sulphate dentifrice: do they mix effectively or interfere? *Int J Dent Hyg.* 2016;14(1):42-52.
22. Araujo MWB, Charles CA, Weinstein RB, et al. Meta-analysis of the effect of an essential oil-containing mouthrinse on gingivitis and plaque. *J Am Dent Assoc.* 2015;146(8):610-622.
23. Sanz M, Serrano J, Iniesta M, Santa Cruz I, Herrera D. Antiplaque and antigingivitis toothpastes. *Monogr Oral Sci.* 2013;23:27-44.
24. Gunsolley JC. Clinical efficacy of antimicrobial mouthrinses. *J Dent.* 2010;38(suppl 1):S6-S10.
25. Haps S, Slot DE, Berchier CE, Van der Weijden GA. The effect of cetylpyridinium chloride-containing mouth rinses as adjuncts to toothbrushing on plaque and parameters of gingival inflammation: a systematic review. *Int J Dent Hyg.* 2008;6(4):290-303.
26. Carrouel F, Gonçalves L, Conte M, et al. Antiviral activity of reagents in mouth rinses against SARS-CoV-2. *J Dent Res.* 2021;100(2):124-132.
27. Hossainian N, Slot DE, Afennich F, Van der Weijden GA. The effects of hydrogen peroxide mouthwashes on the prevention of plaque and gingival inflammation: a systematic review. *Int J Dent Hyg.* 2011;9(3):171-181.
28. Shinada K, Ueno M, Konishi C, et al. Effects of a mouthwash with chlorine dioxide on oral malodor and salivary bacteria: a randomized placebo-controlled 7-day trial. *Trials.* 2010;11:14.
29. Gonzalez S, Cohen CL, Galván M, Alonaizan FA, Rich SK, Slots J. Gingival bleeding on probing: relationship to change in periodontal pocket depth and effect of sodium hypochlorite oral rinse. *J Periodontal Res.* 2015;50(3):397-402.
30. De Nardo R, Chiappe V, Gómez M, Romanelli H, Slots J. Effects of 0.05% sodium hypochlorite oral rinse on supragingival biofilm and gingival inflammation. *Int Dent J.* 2012;62(4):208-212.
31. Gandini S, Negri E, Boffetta P, La Vecchia C, Boyle P. Mouthwash and oral cancer risk quantitative meta-analysis of epidemiologic studies. *Ann Agric Environ Med.* 2012;19(2):173-180.
32. Naseem M, Khiyani M, Nauman H, et al. Oil pulling and importance of traditional medicine in oral health maintenance. *Int J Health Sci.* 2017;11(4):65-70.
33. Aceves Argemí R, González Navarro B, Ochoa García-Seisdedos P, Estrugo Devesa A, López-López J. Mouthwash with alcohol and oral carcinogenesis: systematic review and meta-analysis. *J Evid Based Dent Pract.* 2020;20(2):101407.
34. Shanbhag VK. Oil pulling for maintaining oral hygiene—a review. *J Tradit Complement Med.* 2017;7(1):106-109.
35. Woolley J, Gibbons T, Patel K, Sacco R. The effect of oil pulling with coconut oil to improve dental hygiene and oral health: a systematic review. *Heliyon.* 2020;6(8):e04789.
36. U.S. Food and Drug Administration. Division of Dermatology and Dental Products (DDDP). https://www.fda.gov/about-fda/center-drug-evaluation-and-research/division-dermatology-and-dental-products-dddp. Accessed August 29, 2021.
37. U.S. Food and Drug Administration. Drug Application Process for Nonprescription Drugs. https://www.fda.gov/drugs/types-applications/drug-applications-over-counter-otc-drugs. Accessed August 29, 2021.
38. American Dental Association. ADA Seal and Acceptance Program and Products. https://www.ada.org/en/science-research/ada-seal-of-acceptance. Accessed August 29, 2021.
39. Canadian Dental Association. CDA Seal Program. https://www.cda-adc.ca/en/oral_health/seal/. Accessed October 11, 2021.

CHAPTER 29

The Patient with Orthodontic Appliances

Jessica August, MS, RDH

CHAPTER OUTLINE

LEARNING OBJECTIVES

After studying this chapter, the student will be able to:

1. Recognize the key words and terminology used in orthodontic therapy.
2. Explain the advantages and disadvantages of bonded brackets.
3. Summarize the clinical procedures for bonding and debonding.
4. Develop oral self-care recommendations for the orthodontic patient to address effective biofilm removal and reduce risk for dental caries and periodontal disease.

An individualized preventive program that includes a specific plan of instruction, motivation, and supervision is essential for the patient with orthodontic **appliances**.

Cemented Bands and Bonded Brackets

- Resin-bonded **brackets** have been used widely in orthodontic treatment.
  - Brackets are usually placed on the facial surfaces of the teeth; however, occasionally brackets are **bonded** to the lingual surfaces.
  - Brackets aid in the application and control of applied forces necessary to accomplish tooth movement and bone remodeling for orthodontic therapy.
  - The function is to retain the **arch wire**.
  - The two types of brackets are illustrated in **Figure 29-1** and **Figure 29-2**.
- In some cases, circumferential molar **bands** are used.
  - For example, for jaw stabilization following orthognathic surgery or when additional strength is needed to hold palatal bars, elastics, or other special devices.

I. Advantages of Bonded Brackets[1]

- Improved aesthetics.
- Improved gingival condition due to better access for control of dental biofilm at the cervical third of the teeth.

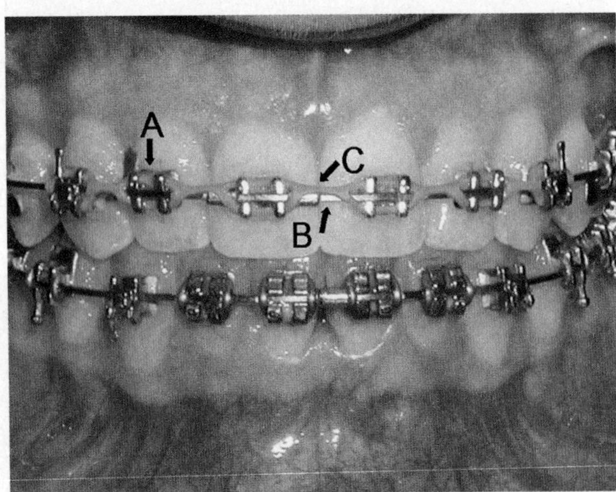

Figure 29-1 Fixed Appliance System. **A:** Bonded brackets. **B:** With arch wire. **C:** Held in place by elastomers.

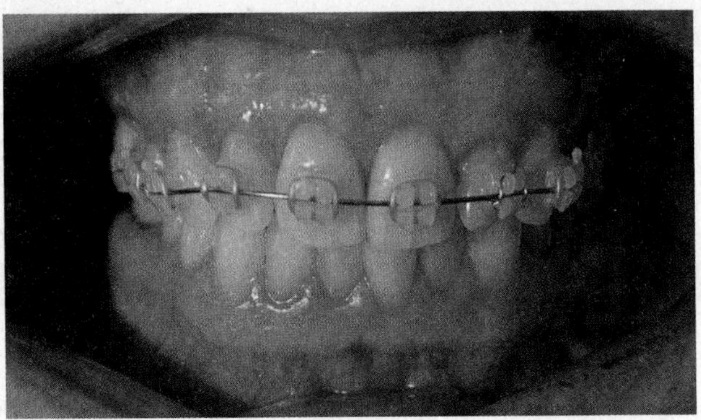

Figure 29-2 Fixed Appliance System. Bonded clear brackets with arch wire.

- Dental caries on proximal surfaces can be detected and treated without bracket removal.
- Patient will immediately be aware when a bracket loosens, whereas an unsecured band may go undetected.
- Placement factors include:
  - No need for tooth separation (as required for band placement); results in less patient discomfort and no band spaces to close at the end of treatment.
  - Lingual brackets ("invisible braces") may be used for specially selected cases.
  - Placement of brackets is faster and easier than placement of bands.

II. Disadvantages of Bonded Brackets[1]

- **Shear bond strength** of the various materials differs, but all the generally available adhesives had higher than recommended bond strength.[2]
- Brackets may detach more readily than a band because attachment may be weaker with less surface area in contact with tooth.
- Rebonding a loose bracket is more time-consuming and requires more tooth preparation than recementing a loose band.
- **Debonding** at the end of treatment is more time-consuming than debanding, with more potential for damage to the tooth surface because of surface area covered by the adhesive.

III. Fixed Appliance System

A. Brackets

- Materials
  - Metal (stainless steel) (Figure 29-1).
  - Plastic (polycarbonate).
  - Plastic with metal reinforcements.
  - **Ceramic** (Figure 29-2).

- Forms: Brackets are made in many styles, shapes, and sizes for different teeth, each designed to accomplish a specific objective of treatment. The basic forms are single or twin, as illustrated in **Figure 29-3**.
- Base: The base of the bracket is prepared with a mesh backing to assist in retaining the resin **bonding** agent.
  - The mesh backing, or bonding pad, is made to the exact size of the bracket to minimize the gaps between the composite–enamel junction, which can harbor bacteria that cause demineralization.

B. Arch Wire

- The arch wire attaches to the bracket to generate and distribute forces that guide orthodontic tooth movement.
- Arch wires are made of stainless steel or an alloy of chromium or titanium, and they may be round, rectangular, or multi-strand. The arch wire is illustrated in Figures 29-1 and 29-2.

C. Elastomers

- **Elastomers** are available in latex and nonlatex materials and come in a wide variety of colors.
- Elastomers are used as chains and on individual teeth for the following purposes:
  - Hold wires in the brackets (Figure 29-1).
  - Apply light continuous force to close spaces between teeth.[3]

IV. Removable Aligner System

Clear **aligner systems** are an increasingly popular orthodontic technique for aligning teeth and correcting malocclusions.

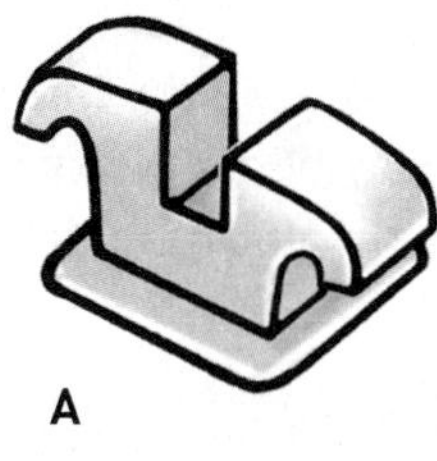

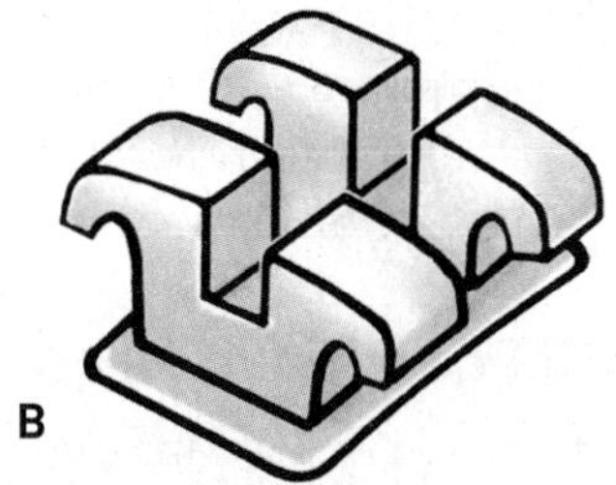

Figure 29-3 Orthodontic Brackets. **A:** Single bracket with an incisal and a cervical wing. **B:** Twin, or Siamese, bracket with two wings on each side of the central groove where the arch wire is held. The shape and style of each bracket vary with the tooth on which the bracket will be located.

A. Overview of Removable Aligner System[4]

- An individual treatment plan is developed and a series of custom, clear thermoplastic aligners are fabricated.
- With each set of aligners, the misaligned teeth are progressively moved.

B. Clinical Procedure

- A consultation with the orthodontist will determine the need for orthodontic treatment.
  - Fixed and removable orthodontic options are evaluated to meet the individual patient needs.
  - Not every patient is a candidate for removable aligner systems.
- Upper and lower impressions are taken, and the aligners are fabricated.
- The study models are scanned into a computer to make a three-dimensional model of the step-by-step process for movement of the teeth.
- Retention attachments are bonded on the teeth, so the aligner has an area to clip into place.
- A series of aligners are given to the patient to wear per instructions.
  - Each tray is worn for approximately 2 weeks.
- The patient will visit the orthodontist on a regular basis for adjustments and monitoring of progress.
- Impressions are taken to fabricate **retainers** to stabilize the tooth position after active treatment.

Clinical Procedures for Bonding

I. Assessment Examination

Before bonding, documentation of any irregularities of the patient's teeth, such as white spots or cracks, is required to prevent misunderstanding by the patient after debonding.[5]

II. Procedural Steps

- The principles for pit and fissure sealants apply for bonding orthodontic brackets. (See Chapter 35.)
  - After bonding, the area around the bracket is carefully cleaned of excess material. Excess material around the bracket serves as a site for biofilm accumulation.[6]

III. Characteristics of Bonding Relating to Debonding

A. Nature of the Bond

- The acid etch exposes the prism structure of enamel and creates microclefts. (See Chapter 35.)
- On the bracket side, the resin becomes locked into the mesh base.

B. Effect of Filler Particles

- Adding fillers to the resin increases bond strength, hardness, and wear resistance.[7]
  - Heavily filled resins (composites) perform better for the posterior teeth because posterior attachments are subject to high forces of mastication.
- Ease of debonding is related to the type of resin and length of etching time.
  - Heavily filled composites are thicker and less viscous; they may be more difficult to remove.
  - Etching time of 30 seconds significantly improved bond strength for orthodontic brackets.[8]
- The bond is stronger when a thinner layer of resin is placed between the tooth surface and the bracket.
- Anterior brackets can be bonded with a lightly filled resin, whereas posterior teeth need a resin with more filler to prevent detachment.

IV. Use of Fluoride-Releasing Bonding System

- Demineralization around brackets can result in an increased risk of dental caries for even the most conscientious patient.[9]
- Use of fluoride-releasing bonding systems such as glass ionomers have been shown to have positive preventive results.[10]

Dental Hygiene Care

- The patient may be under orthodontic care with regular appointments for a long period, frequently years.
- Periodic communication between the orthodontist and the patient's referring dentist and dental hygienist is required to coordinate oral self-care instruction along with other essential dental and dental hygiene care.
- Regular dental hygiene preventive care and motivation for oral self-care are essential during orthodontic treatment.[11]

I. Complicating Factors: Risk Factors

A. Age Groups

- Many orthodontic patients are in the preteen and teenage years, periods when the incidence of gingivitis is high.
  - The incidence of periodontal infection increases from early childhood to late teenage years.
- There is a significant increase in the number of adult patients seeking orthodontic treatment.
  - As with younger patients, the risk factors for caries and periodontal diseases increase.
  - The adult orthodontic patient may be taking medications or have a systemic condition that can complicate therapy.
  - The adult patient may present with various classifications of periodontal disease, which can complicate orthodontic treatment as well as management of the periodontal status.[12,13]

B. Periodontal Health[14]

- Evidence suggests an increase in the quantity and quality of oral microorganisms with orthodonture, but this is short term if the patient maintains good oral self-care.[6]
- Regular periodontal assessment is essential, including periodontal probing in adolescents and young adults during orthodontic treatment, since this is an age group when periodontal disease may develop.
- Dental biofilm retention around orthodontic appliances may lead to gingivitis.
- The degree can vary from slight to severe with gingival enlargement, particularly of the interdental papillae.
- The tissue may greatly enlarge and cover the **fixed appliance**. In some cases, it may be necessary to remove the bracket until the patient can improve oral hygiene and resolve the inflammation.

C. Position of Teeth

- Teeth that are malpositioned are more susceptible to the retention of dental biofilm and are more difficult to clean.
- With the severe malocclusions presented by orthodontic patients at the outset, this factor becomes even more significant.

D. Problems with Appliances

- **Orthodontic appliances** retain biofilm and debris.
- Accidents may cause a bracket to become detached.

E. Self-Care Is Difficult

- The appliances interfere with the application of the toothbrush, interdental aids, and other devices used for dental biofilm control.
- Instruction needs to be very specific and reviewed at each appointment.

II. Oral Disease Control

A meticulous program for dental caries and periodontal disease control is needed.

- The selection of biofilm control procedures for an individual patient is determined by the periodontal status, anatomic features of the gingiva, position of the teeth, and type and position of the orthodontic appliance.

A. General Oral Self-Care Instructions[11,14]

- Give oral self-care instructions before appliances are placed, with the goal of having the oral tissues healthy and the patient motivated to perform thorough daily biofilm removal.
- Encourage the patient to perform brushing and interdental care in front of a mirror so the technique is accurate and thorough.
  - Place emphasis on sulcular brushing and cleaning the area between the orthodontic bands and brackets and the gingiva.
- Disclosing solution is useful to help the patient self-evaluate biofilm removal; however, it may be difficult to remove from the bonding resin.
- Interdental aids
  - A floss threader may be helpful to provide access to interproximal areas around arch wires for biofilm removal.
  - Tufted dental floss used in the floss threader can remove the biofilm more efficiently than regular dental floss.
  - A single-tuft brush or end tuft brush can be particularly beneficial around individual teeth that are hard to access with a regular toothbrush.
  - Travel interdental brushes can provide access to areas around and under the arch wires and come in a container that is easy for patients to use away from home.
  - Review Chapter 27 for interdental aids, such as tufted floss, interdental brushes, floss threaders, and irrigation options, that may be effective for each patient.
- Caries prevention is a necessary part of minimizing and preventing white spot lesions.
  - Recommend an approved fluoride dentifrice, professionally applied fluoride varnish, and prescribed home fluoride gel or paste to aid in dental caries control.[15] (Review Chapter 34 for recommendations for fluoride dentifrices, gels, and mouthrinses.)
  - Sugar-free mints containing xylitol may be used between meals.
  - Dietary counseling is needed to ensure a patient understands the foods and beverages most likely to impact future dental caries.
  - For patients with xerostomia, saliva substitutes and dry mouth products may help reduce caries risk.
- Recommend an approved mouthrinse to aid in dental caries control and periodontal inflammation control.

B. Toothbrush Selection

Research found manual and power toothbrushes were not significantly different in terms of effectiveness.[16]

- Power brush
  - Sonic toothbrushes performed slightly better than other power or manual toothbrushes in reducing gingivitis, plaque, and interdental bleeding.[16]
  - See Chapter 26 for more information on power brushes.
- Manual brush
  - Soft brush: A soft brush with end-rounded filaments is recommended.
  - Bilevel: A special bilevel orthodontic brush designed with spaced rows of soft nylon filaments and a shorter middle row that can be applied directly over the appliance is shown in **Figure 29-4**. It is used with a short horizontal stroke.

C. Toothbrushing Procedure

- Sulcular brushing (**Figure 29-5A** and **B**): A sulcular method is needed by most patients for cleaning the appliances and maintaining the gingiva.

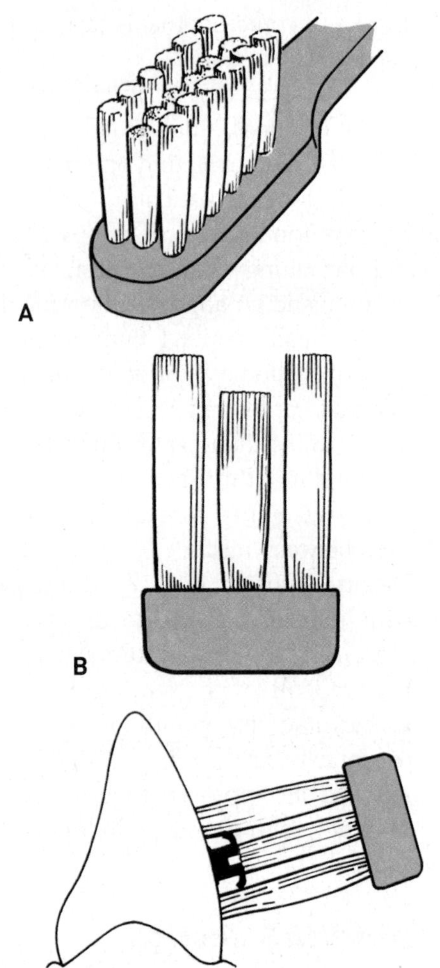

Figure 29-4 Orthodontic Bilevel Toothbrush. **A:** Middle row of filaments trimmed shorter to fit over a fixed appliance. **B:** Cross section. **C:** Brush held over a bracket.

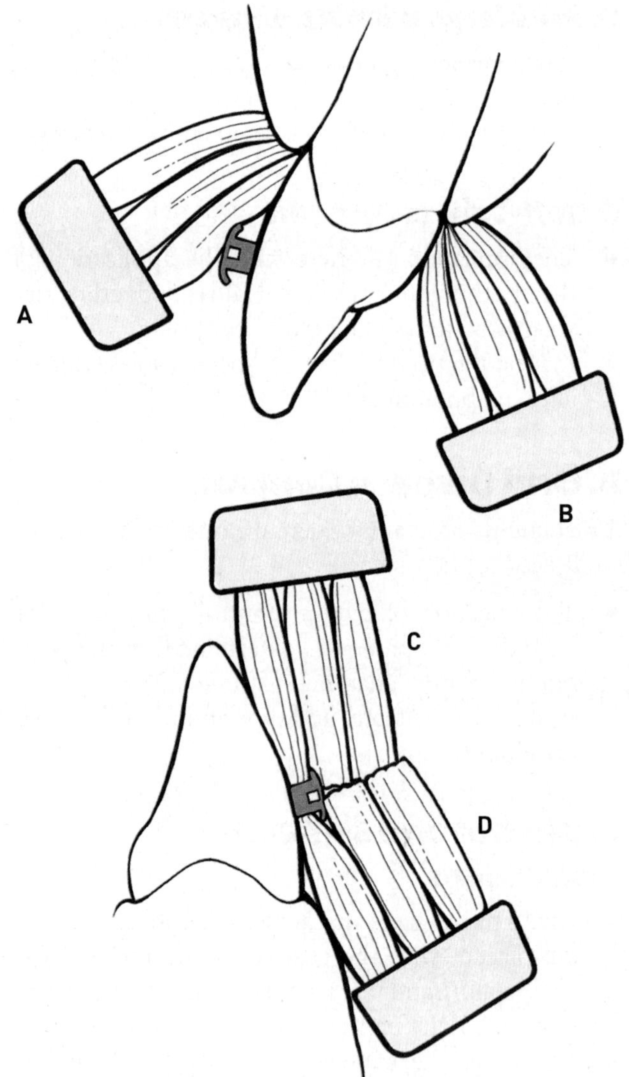

Figure 29-5 Toothbrushing for Orthodontic Appliance. **A** and **B:** Sulcular brushing for periodontal tissues. **C:** Brush in Stillman position for occlusal side of bracket and arch wire. **D:** Cleaning the gingival side of bracket using brush in Charters brushing position.

- Lingual and palatal: Approach to brushing is similar to the basic strokes used on the facial surfaces. (Figures 29-5A and 5B)
- Adapt toothbrush for appliance
  - Place the brush with filament ends directed toward the occlusal surface (Charters position, **Figure 29-5D**) to clean under the wire and bracket for mandibular arch, place in Stillman position for the opposite side (**Figure 29-5C**).
- Clean all surfaces of biofilm and food debris
  - Insert the brush from below, over, and above the arch wire; rotate and vibrate to remove biofilm and debris.

D. Additional Measures

- Keep the oral self-care routine as simple as possible; it can be a challenge to find the most effective therapeutic aids for the individual needs of the patient.
  - When suggesting a new aid, be sure to eliminate one that did not work well for the patient, so the patient does not become overwhelmed.
- Document changes to the oral care plan in the patient's chart.
- Oral irrigation:
  - Most patients who wear orthodontic appliances can benefit from the regular use of water irrigation for removal of loose dental biofilm and food debris.[17]
  - Oral irrigation, particularly with an orthodontic tip, before brushing is recommended so debris is removed to provide access to enamel surfaces for the fluoride dentifrice. (See Chapter 27.)

E. Dental Hygiene Instrumentation

- Manual instrumentation around orthodontic bands and brackets is challenging. The use of an ultrasonic or piezoelectric scaler may be helpful for debridement.
- The use of an air-powder polisher may be indicated to remove debris since the bands and brackets can tear polishing cups and the agent is less abrasive than polishing paste.[18,19]
- Use appropriate precautions for managing aerosols produced. (See Chapter 42.)

Clinical Procedures for Band Removal and Debonding

Following completion of active orthodontic therapy, bands and brackets are removed mechanically followed by removal of residual adhesive (cement) and bonding material.

- Two types of iatrogenic damage to enamel occur during adhesive and bonding removal[20]:
  - Loss of enamel from etching, grinding, and polishing.
  - Increased enamel roughness by scratching or creating wear facets.
- Objectives for adhesive (cement) and debonding procedure[20]:
  - Remove resin bulk.
  - Minimize damage to pulpal tissue.
  - Leave enamel surface smooth.
  - Prevent excess enamel loss.

I. Band Removal

- Bands are generally removed with orthodontic band-removing pliers.
- The remaining dental adhesive (cement) is removed primarily by rotary burs.
- Complete removal is critical to prevent biofilm retention and support periodontal health.

II. Clinical Procedures for Debonding

Dental hygienists and dental assistants may be involved in removal of orthodontic appliances, which may include use of slow- and/or high-speed handpieces depending on the scope of practice; as such, it is important clinicians know the scope of practice in their state, province, or county.

A. Method Types

- Mechanical, electrothermal, laser, and ultrasonic methods have been studied in an attempt to determine which debonding method is the most efficient and effective, provides the least discomfort for the patient, and causes the least damage to enamel.[20]
  - Tungsten-carbide burs are the fastest and most effective but require a multistep process to polish the enamel for finishing.
  - The most destructive tools for resin removal include Arkansas stones, green stones, diamond burs, steel burs, and lasers.[20]

B. Steps in Removal of Residual Resin Bonding

1. Examination
   - Varying amounts of resin remain after the bracket is removed, particularly in normal anatomic grooves, as shown in **Figure 29-6**.
   - During debonding, frequent examination is necessary using visual and tactile methods.
   - **Box 29-1** contains a summary of the steps necessary for complete removal of the orthodontic adhesive resin.
2. Identification of residual resin
   - Visual: When dry, the resin appears dull and opaque compared to the shiny enamel.
   - Tactile: Application of an explorer reveals a rough surface, sometimes with catches along the margin of a resin tag. Filler particles from the resin may abrade the metal explorer tip, leaving a gray line on the resin surface.
   - Use of loupes for magnification to evaluate the tooth surface.

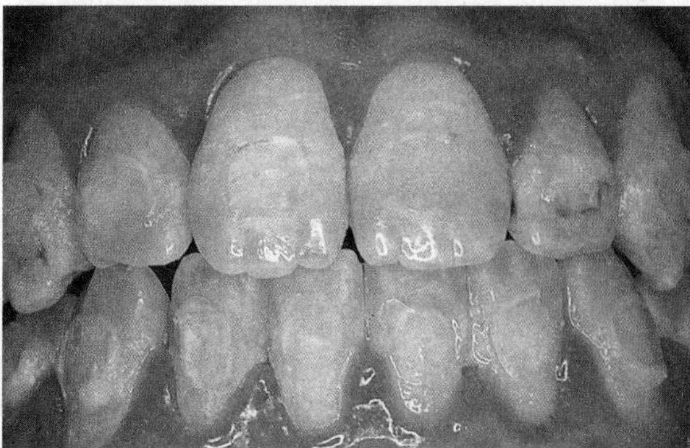

Figure 29-6 Facial View of Anterior Teeth with Adhesive Resin Remaining Following Removal of Orthodontic Brackets

Box 29-1 Steps for Orthodontic Adhesive Resin Removal Using Burs and Polishing Instruments

1. Identify the location and extent of the resin with an explorer, disclosing solution, and patient feedback.
2. Using a tapered, tungsten-carbide finishing bur in a low-speed handpiece, move the bur from the cervical to incisal/occlusal portion of the resin in a light, brush-like stroke.
3. Evaluate progress frequently by rinsing and drying the tooth surfaces.
4. Polish each surface with aluminum oxide polishing points, followed by aluminum oxide polishing cups.
5. Use a rubber cup in a slow-speed handpiece to polish each surface with a fine pumice slurry. Use intermittent strokes.
6. Use a brown polishing cup in a slow-speed handpiece to polish the enamel surfaces.
7. Use a green polishing cup in a slow-speed handpiece to provide the final finish to the enamel surfaces.

3. Removal of resin from tooth surface[20]
   - Bur selection: Use a tapered, plain-cut, tungsten-carbide finishing bur with a low-speed handpiece, as illustrated in **Figure 29-7**.
   - Speed: Use low speed to control production of heat that may cause damage to the pulp.
   - Stroke: Use a smooth, evenly applied, light brush stroke in one direction to prevent faceting of the tooth surface.
   - Direction: Work systematically from the cervical portion of the resin; move toward incisal or occlusal third. When removed, the resin resembles fine white shavings, as seen in **Figure 29-8**.
   - Evaluate frequently to prevent excessive removal of enamel. Rinse frequently, dry, and evaluate the surface. The resin will appear opaque in contrast to the glossy enamel.
4. Final finish[20]
   - Objective: Restore pretreatment enamel surface finish.
   - Examination: Perform visual and tactile examination to distinguish areas of normal enamel from irregularities.
   - Application of aluminum oxide finishing points and cups
     - Use the finishing points first to remove any fine scarring resulting from the burs (**Figure 29-9**).
     - Use a low-speed handpiece.

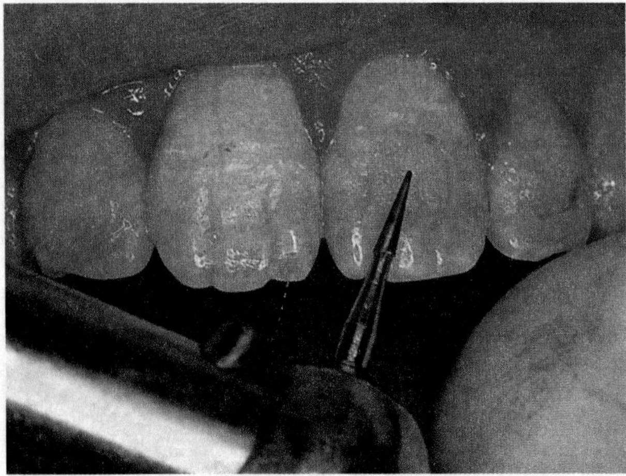

Figure 29-7 Use of Tapered, Tungsten-Carbide Finishing Bur on Low-Speed Handpiece to Remove Bulk of Adhesive Resin

Reprinted with permission from Gutmann ME. Composite adhesive resin removal following orthodontic treatment. *J Pract Hyg*. 1996;5:16.

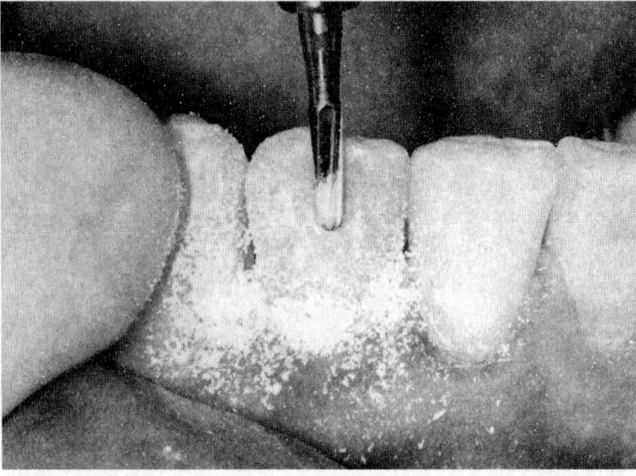

Figure 29-8 Adhesive Shavings Following Use of Bur

Reprinted with permission from Gutmann ME. Debonding orthodontic adhesives. *J Dent Hyg*. 1985;59:369.

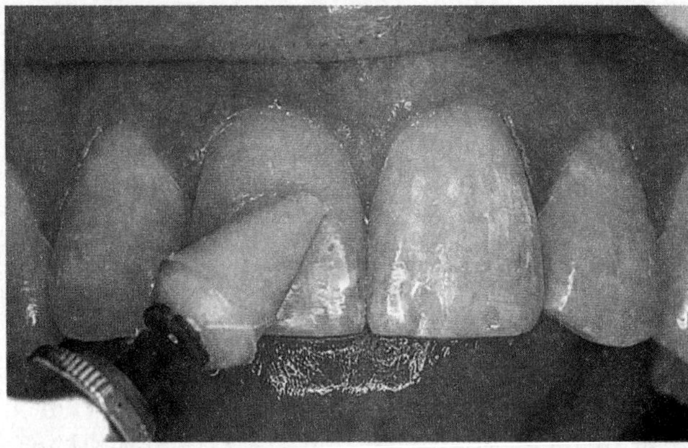

Figure 29-9 Aluminum Oxide Finishing Point to Remove Any Enamel Scarring Resulting from Bur

Reprinted with permission from Gutmann ME. Composite adhesive resin removal following orthodontic treatment. *J Pract Hyg*. 1996;5:16.

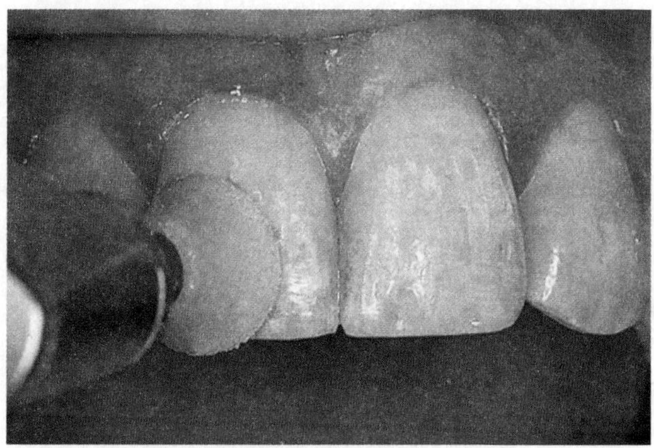

Figure 29-10 Aluminum Oxide Finishing Cup to Remove Any Enamel Scarring Resulting from Bur

Reprinted with permission from Gutmann ME. Composite adhesive resin removal following orthodontic treatment. *J Pract Hyg*. 1996;5:16.

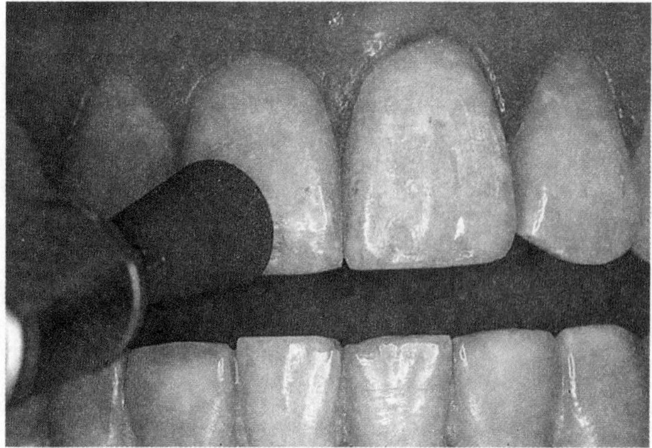

Figure 29-12 Brown Polishing Cup Provides Maximum Gloss to Enamel Surface

Reprinted with permission from Gutmann ME. Composite adhesive resin removal following orthodontic treatment. *J Pract Hyg*. 1996;5:16.

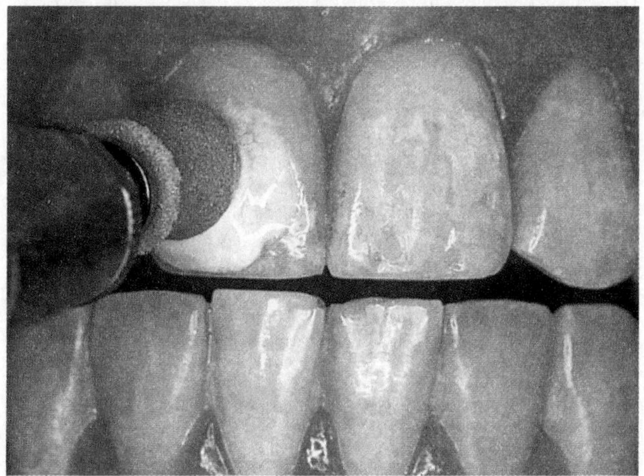

Figure 29-11 Polishing with Fine Pumice Slurry and Rubber Cup

Reprinted with permission from Gutmann ME. Composite adhesive resin removal following orthodontic treatment. *J Pract Hyg*. 1996;5:16.

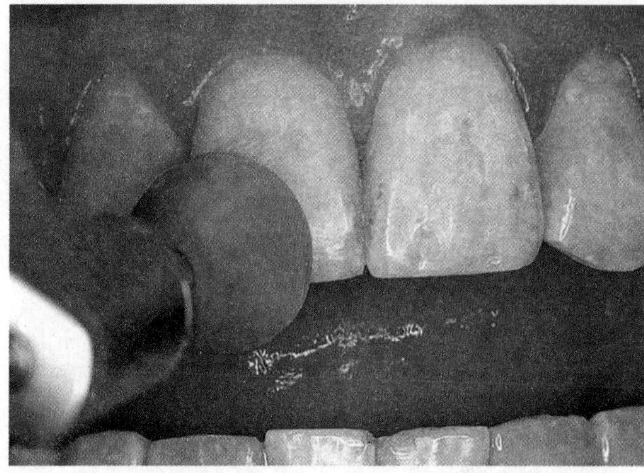

Figure 29-13 Final Polishing with Green Polishing Cup

Reprinted with permission from Gutmann ME. Composite adhesive resin removal following orthodontic treatment. *J Pract Hyg*. 1996;5:16.

    - Follow with aluminum oxide cups and move from area to area in a cervical-to-incisal/occlusal direction (**Figure 29-10**).
- Application of the rubber cup
    - Use a fine pumice water slurry, as shown in **Figure 29-11**.
    - Polish in a wet field to prevent overheating.
    - Use intermittent strokes to avoid overheating and move from tooth to tooth.
- Final polish: Use brown followed by green polishing cups to produce a natural-appearing, glossy enamel surface (**Figures 29-12** and **29-13**).

After debonding, topical fluoride varnish application is recommended for caries prevention and to reverse white spot lesions.[21]

Postdebonding Evaluation

- Each step of bonding and debonding has a damaging effect on the enamel surface.
- The clinician must avoid unnecessary trauma during the various procedures.

I. Enamel Loss

- Total enamel loss from etching, bracket removal, residual resin removal, surface finishing, and application of pumice averages approximately 55 μm.[20]
    - Use of a tungsten-carbide finishing bur results in enamel loss from 22.8 to 50.5 μm.[20]
- Enamel loss is greater when filled resins (composites) are used for bonding than when unfilled resins are used.

- The loss is also greater when a rotating bristle brush rather than a rubber cup is used with the abrasive for finishing.
- The external layer of enamel is the most fluoride-rich enamel.[20]
    - Without care during debonding, the entire protective layer can be removed.
- When multiple bonding and debonding procedures are performed, such as when a bracket becomes detached, the enamel loss is compounded.
- Careful selection of instruments and abrasives, along with minimal instrumentation, is necessary to minimize enamel loss.

II. Demineralization (White Spot Lesions)

- White demineralization areas or dental caries are relatively common findings after orthodontic treatment.[22]
- Dental biofilm retention on appliances and the resin, along with the difficulty of biofilm removal by the patient, contribute to demineralization and dental caries.

III. Etched Enamel Not Covered by Adhesive

- Surface areas etched but not covered with adhesive resin may be remineralized when the fluoride contact is increased through regular patient and professional applications.
- Etched enamel has a high fluoride uptake.

Orthodontic Retention

- After fixed appliances have been removed, a retainer is worn to prevent movement of the teeth while the bone and other supporting tissues are stabilizing.
    - One type of removable retainer is the **Hawley retainer**, as shown in **Figure 29-14**.
- The use of a fixed retainer appliance provides another source for retention of dental biofilm.
- General care and cleaning procedures for a removable retainers include:
    - Clean the appliance after each meal and before bedtime.
    - Instructions for cleaning procedures and agents for removable appliances are similar to the care of the removable denture. (See Chapter 30.)
    - Brush and rinse teeth and gingival tissue under the appliance each time the appliance is removed.
    - Keep appliance in a container with water when it is out of the mouth.

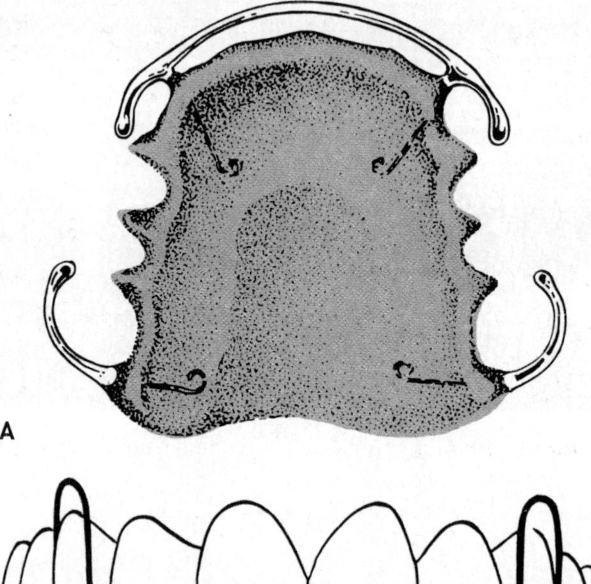

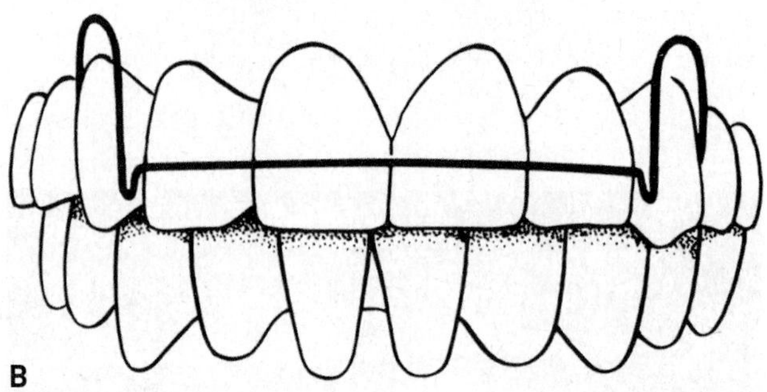

Figure 29-14 Hawley Retainer. **A:** Removable acrylic retainer with facial retaining wire and clasps to be worn after removal of a fixed orthodontic appliance. **B:** Anterior view shows a Hawley appliance in position. The method for cleaning the appliance is similar to that for cleaning a removable denture.

Postdebonding Preventive Care

I. Periodontal Evaluation

- A complete examination with a careful periodontal assessment is necessary because many changes take place during treatment.
- Thorough periodontal debridement.
- Intraoral images assist the patient in comparing gingival tissue changes and teeth before and after treatment.
- Apply disclosing agent for documentation of biofilm and patient instruction.

II. Dental Examination

- Examination for demineralization (white spots) and dental caries is essential.
- Dental biofilm retention by orthodontic appliances can be problematic for the patient.
    - The configurations of the appliances make biofilm control extremely difficulty for the patient.

    - Biofilm collects on brackets and some resins even when the patient's oral hygiene is generally good.[6]
- Composite resin may remain on the tooth surface where the bracket was removed leading to biofilm retention.

III. Fluoride Therapy

- A complete program of fluoride therapy, professionally applied at frequent maintenance appointments and used by the patient daily, is essential both during and following orthodontic therapy.[15]
- Application of a fluoride varnish immediately following bonding can help to reduce demineralization by up to 38% to 44%.[21,23,24] Varnish applications need to become a part of every maintenance appointment.

Documentation

- Document treatment goals and progress toward goals with any changes at each appointment.
- Assess the patient's oral health along with changes in risk for oral disease, and record in the dental chart.
- Evaluate effectiveness of the patient's oral self-care and adjustments needed for continued improvement.
- Monitor patient compliance with use of home fluorides.
- A sample progress note may be found in **Box 29-2**.

Box 29-2 Example Documentation: Patient Following Completion of Orthodontic Treatment

- **S**—A 16-year-old female patient presents for 6-month maintenance appointment. Patient has recently completed orthodontic treatment. Patient reports the soreness she had following band removal has subsided.
- **O**—Assessment data collected include marginal redness with bleeding on probing on the mandibular anterior teeth. Hard-tissue examination findings include areas of demineralization on the maxillary anterior teeth. Calculus localized to the mandibular anterior teeth.
- **A**—Patient is at a high caries risk level. Caries prevention and remineralization of enamel are essential.
- **P**—Assessment data collected and documented. Health history update, extra- and intraoral examination, full-mouth periodontal assessment, and biofilm score using disclosing solution. Manually scaled to completion and applied fluoride varnish. Oral self-care instructions reviewed. Demonstrated flossing and positioning of the toothbrush for more effective biofilm removal. Patient observed while brushing and flossing mandibular anterior teeth. Recommended prescription 1.1% sodium fluoride toothpaste.

Next steps: Schedule continuing care appointment in 3 months to reevaluate demineralized areas.

Signed: ______________________________, RDH

Date: ________________

Factors to Teach the Patient

- The significance of dental biofilm around orthodontic appliances and the teeth.
- How to apply the toothbrush (power or manual) and adjunctive aids to remove dental biofilm from the bracket, the arch wire, and the teeth.
- How, when, and why to use fluoride rinses, toothpaste, and prescription gels/pastes.
- The frequency for professional follow-up during and after orthodontic therapy.

References

1. Zachrisson BU, Usumez S, Buyukyilmaz T. Bonding in orthodontics. In: Graber LW, Vanarsdall RL, Vig KWL, Huang GJ, eds. *Orthodontics: Current Principles and Techniques*. 6th ed. St. Louis, MO: Elsevier; 2017:813-867.
2. Sharma S, Tandon P, Nagar A, et al. A comparison of shear bond strength of orthodontic brackets bonded with four different orthodontic adhesives. *J Orthod Sci*. 2014;3(2):29-33.
3. Baratieri C, Mattos CT, Alves Jr M, et al. In situ evaluation of orthodontic elastomeric chains. *Braz Dent J*. 2012; 23(4):394-398.
4. Rossini G, Parrini S, Castroflorio T, Deregibus A, Debernardi CL. Efficacy of clear aligners in controlling orthodontic tooth movement: a systematic review. *Angle Orthod*. 2015;85(5): 881-889.

5. Heravi F, Rashed R, Raziee L. The effects of bracket removal on enamel. *Aust Orthod J*. 2008;24(2):110-115.
6. Freitas AO, Marquezan M, Nojima Mda C, DS Alviano DS, LC, Maia LC. The influence of orthodontic fixed appliances on the oral microbiota: a systematic review. *Dental Press J Orthod*. 2014;19(2):46-55.
7. Najafi-Abrandabadi A, Najafi-Abrandabadi S, Ghasemi A, Kotick PG. Microshear bond strength of composite resins to enamel and porcelain substrates utilizing unfilled versus filled resins. *Dent Res J*. 2014;11(6):636-644.
8. Firoozmand LM, Brandão JV, Fialho MP. Influence of microhybrid resin and etching times on bleached enamel for the bonding of ceramic brackets. *Braz Oral Res*. 2013;27(2):142-148.
9. Farronato G, Giannini L, Galbiati G, et al. Oral tissues and orthodontic treatment: common side effects. *Minerva Stomatol*. 2013;62(11-12):431-446.
10. Prabhakar AR, Dhanraj K, Sugandhan S. Comparative evaluation in vitro of caries inhibition potential and microtensile bond strength of two fluoride releasing adhesive systems. *Eur Arch Paediatr Dent*. 2014;15(6):385-391.
11. Migliorati M, Isaia L, Cassaro A, et al. Efficacy of professional hygiene and prophylaxis on preventing plaque increase in orthodontic patients with multibracket appliances: a systematic review. *Eur J Orthod*. 2015;37(3):297-307.
12. Gkantidis N, Christou P, Topouzelis N. The orthodontic-periodontic interrelationship in integrated treatment challenges: a systematic review. *J Oral Rehabil*. 2010;37(5): 377-390.
13. Christensen L, Luther F. Adults seeking orthodontic treatment: expectations, periodontal and TMD issues. *Br Dent J*. 2015;218(3):111-117.
14. Levin L, Einy S, Zigdon H, Aizenbud D, Machtei EE. Guidelines for periodontal care and follow-up during orthodontic treatment in adolescents and young adults. *J Appl Oral Sci*. 2012;20(4):399-403.
15. Benson PE, Parkin N, Dyer F, et al. Fluorides for the prevention of early tooth decay (demineralised white lesions) during fixed brace treatment. *Cochrane Database Syst Rev*. 2013;12:CD003809.
16. Sharma R, Trehan M, Sharma S, Jharwal V, Rathore N. Comparison of effectiveness of manual orthodontic, powered and sonic toothbrushes on oral hygiene of fixed orthodontic patients. *Int J Clin Pediatr Dent*. 2015;8(3):181-189.
17. Barnes CM, Russell CM, Reinhardt RA, Payne JB, Lyle DM. Comparison of irrigation to floss as an adjunct to tooth brushing: effect on bleeding, gingivitis, and supragingival plaque. *J Clin Dent*. 2005;16(3):71-77.
18. Leite Bdos S, Fagundes NC, Aragón ML, Dias CG, Normando D. Cleansing orthodontic brackets with air-powder polishing: effects on frictional force and degree of debris. *Dental Press J Orthod*. 2016;21(4):60-65.
19. Camboni S, Donnet M. Tooth surface comparison after air polishing and rubber cup: a scanning electron microscopy study. *J Clin Dent*. 2016;27(1):13-18.
20. Janiszewska-Olszowska J, Szatkiewicz T, Tomkowski R, Tandecka K, Grocholewicz K. Effect of orthodontic debonding and adhesive removal on the enamel—current knowledge and future perspectives—a systematic review. *Med Sci Monit*. 2014;20:1991-2001.
21. Vicente A, Ortiz Ruiz AJ, García López M, Martínez Beneyto Y, Bravo-González LA. Enamel resistance to demineralization after bracket debonding using fluoride varnish. *Sci Rep*. 2017;7(1):15183.
22. Heymann GC, Grauer D. A contemporary review of white spot lesions in orthodontics. *J Esthet Restor Dent*. 2013;25(2):85-95.
23. Vivaldi-Rodrigues G, Demito CF, Bowman SJ, Ramos AL. The effectiveness of a fluoride varnish in preventing the development of white spot lesions. *World J Orthod*. 2006;7(2):138-144.
24. Demito CF, Vivaldi-Rodrigues G, Ramos AL, Bowman SJ. The efficacy of a fluoride varnish in reducing enamel demineralization adjacent to orthodontic brackets: an in vitro study. *Orthod Craniofac Res*. 2004;7(4):205-210.

CHAPTER 30

Care of Dental Prosthesis

Kristeen Perry, RDH, MS
Linda D. Boyd, RDH, RD, EdD

CHAPTER OUTLINE

LEARNING OBJECTIVES

After studying this chapter, the student will be able to:

1. Identify the causes and prevention of tooth loss.
2. Describe the anatomic features of an edentulous oral cavity.
3. Describe the types and components of fixed and removable oral prostheses.
4. Describe the methods for marking a denture for permanent identification.
5. Develop an individualized patient oral self-care regimen for fixed and removable prostheses.
6. Provide a careful evaluation of an oral prosthesis to include clinical examination of the prosthesis, related soft tissue, and patient concerns.
7. Explain the causes and prevention of denture-induced oral lesions.
8. List the steps to provide professional cleaning of fixed and removable prostheses.

Missing Teeth

- A patient may have one or more missing teeth or may have a treatment plan for tooth extractions.
- A patient should be informed of the various options to replace missing teeth as well as the risk factors associated with not replacing the missing teeth.
  - Providing objective information on treatment alternatives and acting as a patient advocate allows the patient to make informed, autonomous decisions about personal oral health.
- A long history of poor oral self-care, neglecting professional dental and dental hygiene care, carious lesions, and periodontal infections may have led to tooth loss; trauma is another common cause of tooth loss.
- A fully **edentulous** patient has no teeth.
  - Absence of teeth may be congenital or due to loss from a variety of causes such as a traumatic accident or lack of knowledge about oral disease prevention.
  - An edentulous patient may have dental implants to improve the function and stability of an **overdenture** dental **prosthesis**.[1]
- A partially edentulous patient has one or more, but less than all, of their natural teeth.
- A partially edentulous patient may have a **complete denture** opposing an arch with all natural teeth or various kinds of fixed or removable partial prostheses.

The Edentulous Mouth

I. Bone

- Residual ridges[2]
  - After the teeth are removed, the **residual ridges** enter into a continuing bone remodeling process.
  - The alveolar bone, which had supported the teeth, undergoes resorption. The rate and amount of bony resorption vary with each individual.
  - Major bony changes occur during the first year after the teeth are removed, but changes continue throughout life.
  - Mandibular bone loss is generally greater than maxillary bone loss.
  - Bone remodeling and soft-tissue healing may make it necessary to have dentures rebased, relined, or remade at intervals.
- Tori and exostoses
  - Benign bony outgrowths may interfere with the fabrication and wearing of dentures.
  - Because of the size, shape, or location, excess bone often needs to be removed surgically before a **denture** can be constructed.
  - Torus palatinus: Bony enlargement located over the midline of the palate.
  - Torus mandibularis: Bony mass generally located on the lingual in the region of the premolars.
  - Exostosis: A bony protuberance generally located on the buccal aspects of maxilla and/or mandible.

II. Mucous Membrane

- Composition: Oral mucosa is composed of masticatory, lining, and specialized mucosa.
  - Masticatory mucosa covers the edentulous ridges and the hard palate. The mucous membrane covering the bony ridges is made up of two layers—the lamina propria and the surface-stratified squamous epithelium—which is keratinized in the healthy mouth.
  - Lining mucosa covers the floor of the mouth, vestibules, and cheeks.

- Specialized mucosa covers the dorsal surface of the tongue and contains filiform, fungiform, and circumvallate papillae. (See Chapter 13.)
- Composition: Submucosa
  - Underneath the mucous membrane is the submucosa, which is attached to the underlying bone.
  - The submucosa is composed of connective tissue with vessels, nerves, adipose tissue, and glands.
  - The support or cushioning effect for the denture depends on the makeup of the submucosa, which varies throughout the mouth.
- Tension test
  - Examine the edentulous mouth by retracting the lips and cheeks using a tension test technique. (The tension test is described in Chapter 20.)
  - A line of demarcation similar to the mucogingival junction is apparent, separating the attached tissue over the bony ridge and the loose lining mucosa of the vestibule.
  - Frenal attachments can be observed.

Purposes for Wearing a Fixed or Removable Prosthesis

The benefits of replacing missing teeth with a fixed or removable prosthesis include the following[3]:

- Replace missing teeth and adjacent structures.
- Presence of teeth has an esthetic role.
- Restore facial contour, including lip support and temporomandibular joint position.
- Provide function.
- Enhance ability to eat a variety of healthy foods such as chewy meat and fresh vegetables/fruit.
- Promote proper speech and enunciation.

I. Replacement Options

- Replacement options include the following (see **Box 30-1**):
  - Fixed prosthesis.
  - Removable prosthesis.
  - Dental implants. (See Chapter 31.)
- Dental hygienist's role.
  - Explain each choice for the patient.
  - Answer questions from the patient.
  - Prepare notes from the patient's medical and dental histories, risk factors, intraoral/extraoral examination, and other pertinent observations to assist the dentist.

Box 30-1 Types of Oral Prostheses

Fixed

Fixed partial denture
Implant-supported complete denture

Removable

Removable partial denture
Natural tooth supported
Implant supported
Complete denture
Overdenture
Obturator

II. Consequences of Not Replacing Missing Teeth

- Replacement for a missing tooth may not be indicated for a patient who has sufficient remaining teeth for function; for example, the following are generally not replaced after extraction:
  - Third molars.
  - Second molars that are extracted and have no opposing teeth.
  - Teeth extracted for orthodontic purposes.
- Consequences of not replacing missing teeth include:
  - Migration of adjacent teeth: Tilting and rotation of teeth may complicate future replacement options or lead to periodontal problems due to difficulty in biofilm control and misdirected occlusal forces when chewing.
  - Migration of opposing teeth: An unopposed tooth may **supererupt**.
  - Remaining teeth may suffer from the added function and stress: May lead to fractures and tooth loss.
  - Loss of **occlusal vertical dimension**: Missing teeth may result in **overclosure** of the occlusion or bite and can lead to temporomandibular joint disorders.
  - Loss of vertical dimension may promote pooling of saliva which may promote fungal or yeast growth resulting in **angular cheilitis** at the corners of the mouth.

Fixed Partial Denture Prostheses

I. Description

- **Fixed partial dentures**, commonly called bridges, are composed of the following, as shown in **Figure 30-1**:
  - **Abutments.**

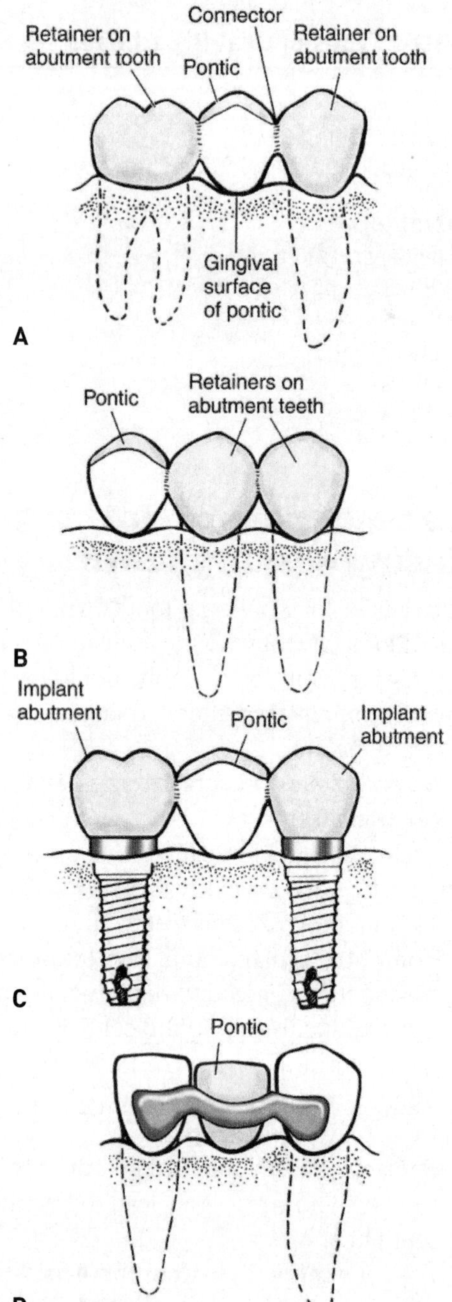

Figure 30-1 Fixed Partial Dentures. **A:** Characteristic parts of a mandibular three-unit fixed partial denture. Cast gold crowns on the abutment teeth serve as the retainers for the bridge. **B:** Cantilever bridge supported by a double abutment. **C:** Fixed partial denture with implant abutments. **D:** Fixed resin-retained partial prosthesis.

- Connectors.
- **Pontics**.
- Bridges can be fabricated from various materials, including:
  - Metals.
  - Ceramics: Porcelain is used most often.
  - Combination of both.
- A fixed partial denture is affixed to the teeth or implants with special cement and is not removable.

II. Types of Fixed Partial Dentures

- Natural tooth supported
  - Traditional/bilateral: Supported by one or more natural teeth at each end, as shown in Figure 30-1A.
  - Cantilever: Pontic supported by one or more teeth at one end only, as shown in Figure 30-1B.
  - Resin retained: Wing-like extensions are bonded with resin cement to etched enamel. Requires minimal or no preparation for tooth structure. Also called a Maryland Bridge and shown in Figure 30-1D.
- Implant supported
  - For implant supported fixed partial dentures and overdentures, the endosseous (endosteal) implant is used most often for support (Figure 30-1C).

III. Criteria for Fixed Partial Dentures

- Biologically and esthetically harmonious with the teeth and surrounding periodontium.
- All parts accessible for cleaning by the patient and the dental professional.
- Does not interfere with the cleaning regimen for the remaining natural dentition.
- Does not traumatize oral tissues.
- Restores function of the missing tooth or teeth.

Removable Partial Denture Prostheses

I. Description

- A removable partial denture (RPD) replaces one or more, but less than all, of the natural teeth and associated structures.
- The partial denture can be removed from the mouth.
- The denture base rests on the oral mucosa and houses the artificial teeth.

II. Types of Removable Partial Dentures

- A typical partial denture consists of a metal framework made of chrome cobalt.
- The framework engages abutment teeth or an abutment implant with a wide variety of clasp assemblies and **rest** seats or **precision attachments**.

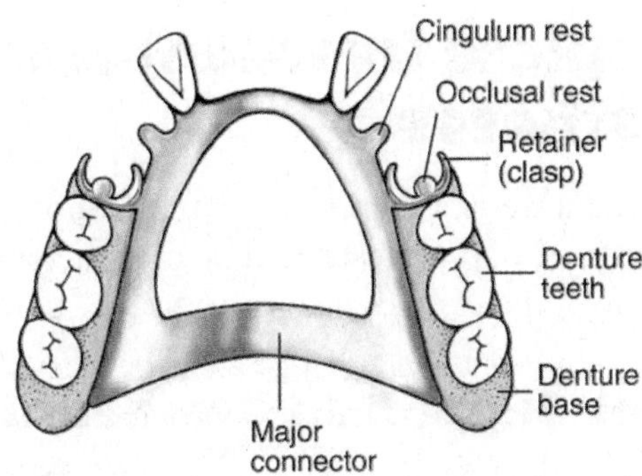

Figure 30-2 Removable Partial Denture (RPD). Components of a RPD shown for a maxillary prosthesis.

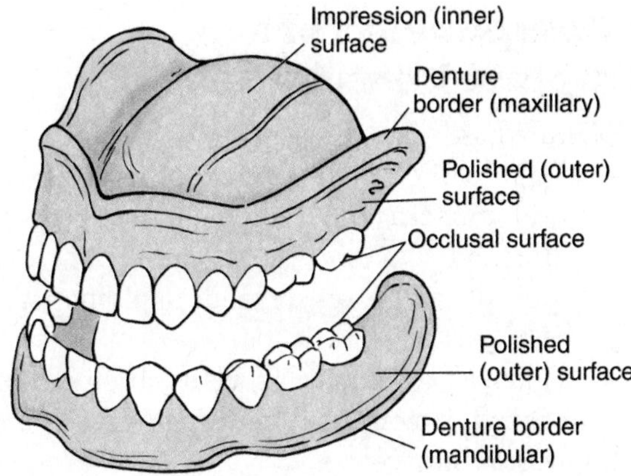

Figure 30-3 Complete Denture. The surfaces and borders of maxillary and mandibular dentures.

- Depending on the location and number of remaining natural teeth, a partial denture may receive all its support from the teeth or it may be partially tooth-borne, partially implant-borne, or partially tissue-borne.
- The base is made of plastic acrylic resin.
- The teeth are made of porcelain, plastic resin, or metal.
- The basic parts of an RPD are shown in **Figure 30-2**.

Complete Denture Prosthesis

I. Description

- Complete denture replaces a full arch, maxillary and/or mandibular, missing teeth.
- A new prosthesis requires several adjustment visits with the dentist.
- The entire dental team needs to work together to assist the patient through the process of losing teeth and adjusting to a new prosthesis.
- Components of a complete denture are shown in **Figure 30-3**.

II. Types of Complete Dentures[4]

- Tissue-supported complete denture: A removable dental prosthesis that replaces the entire dentition and associated structures of the maxilla or the mandible and rests on the **denture foundation area**, the mucosal-covered alveolar ridge.
- Implant denture: A complete dental prosthesis supported in part or whole by one or more dental implants. The denture itself is not an implantable device.
- Overdenture: A removable prosthesis that rests on one or more remaining natural teeth and/or dental implants. It is also called an overlay prosthesis. (See Chapter 31 for more on dental implants.)
- **Interim denture** or provisional prosthesis: A removable dental prosthesis is designed to enhance esthetics, stabilization, and/or function for a limited period, after which it is to be replaced by a definitive prosthesis.
  - Often such prostheses are used to assist in determining the therapeutic effectiveness of a specific treatment plan or the form and function of the planned definitive prosthesis.
- **Immediate denture**: A denture fabricated for placement immediately following the removal of a natural tooth or teeth.
  - An immediate or interim denture tends to loosen after the significant remodeling of bone and soft tissue that follows surgery.
  - The denture may be relined temporarily with a soft liner or a tissue conditioning material.
  - The patient may use a **denture adhesive** until the majority of healing occurs.
  - After approximately 6 months, dentures are remade, relined, or rebased.
- Denture for primary teeth
  - Dentures occasionally must be constructed to replace primary teeth.
  - The teeth may be congenitally missing (**anodontia**) or may have been extracted due to rampant caries or trauma.
  - Early childhood dental caries can break down the teeth severely soon after eruption.
  - To provide esthetics and function, dentures can be constructed for the cooperative child.
  - As the permanent teeth begin to erupt, the denture is adjusted to allow for eruption.
  - A caries management program based on caries risk is essential to prevent caries. (See Chapter 25.)

III. Components of a Complete Denture

- Denture base
  - The part of a denture that rests on the oral mucosa and to which the teeth are attached.
  - Most denture bases are made of plastic acrylic resin.
  - Others may be metal, such as chrome cobalt or gold, in combination with a plastic resin.
- Impression surface[4]
  - The tissue or inner surface of the denture that is not polished.
  - Lies directly on the residual ridges and adjacent tissues.
  - The denture's impression (inner) surface may be lined with a long-term material for removal to be removed by the patient, such as a temporary soft liner, a tissue conditioner, or a permanent soft silicone liner.
  - A patient may place a denture-adhesive material on the impression surface of the denture before inserting the denture.
    - A denture adhesive is a commercially available paste or powder preparation.
    - The adhesive is used to improve denture retention, stabilization, and comfort, as recommended by the dentist.
    - The denture adhesive should be removed from the denture during daily cleaning and from soft tissues to enable visual examination.
    - The patient should be discouraged from using an adhesive indefinitely in the attempt to cope with ill-fitting dentures that need to be adjusted or remade.
- Polished surface: The external or outer surface is polished.
- Occlusal surface: The surface of a denture that makes contact or near-contact with the corresponding surface of the opposing denture or natural teeth.
- Teeth
  - The denture teeth may be made of plastic acrylic resin, composite resin, porcelain, or polymethyl methacrylate.
  - A patient may request to have decorative facings incorporated into certain teeth.
  - Metal occlusal surfaces may be present, for example, to maintain a stable vertical dimension of occlusion when opposing teeth may cause excessive wear.

Complete Overdenture Prostheses

An overdenture is a complete denture supported by both retained natural teeth and/or implants and the soft tissue of the residual alveolar ridge.

I. Root-Supported Overdenture

- An overdenture may be possible for any patient when the clinical crowns are not restorable and the root is caries-free and periodontally healthy.
  - Tooth crowns are reduced to short, rounded preparations or to the level and contour of the gingival margin and require endodontic therapy.
- The advantages of maintaining tooth roots as abutments to support an overdenture include[5,6]:
  - Significantly less alveolar bone resorption in the maxilla and mandible when compared with edentulous patients with complete dentures.
  - Better stability and retention of a mandibular prosthesis.
  - Improved masticatory (chewing) ability and efficiency.
  - Retain some tactile and proprioceptive senses for the patient because the periodontal ligament is present.
  - Increase the patient's psychological acceptance of the denture. The patient does not feel that all natural teeth have been lost.
  - Invasive surgery is not needed when compared with implant placement, which may not be advisable in an individual who is medically complex and/or has special needs.
- Teeth frequently selected for overdenture abutments are the mandibular and maxillary canines.
- Regular preventive care and meticulous daily self-care are essential because the most common causes of abutment tooth loss in overdenture patients include[7]:
  - Periodontal disease.
  - Caries.

II. Implant-Supported Overdenture

- Implants can be placed to help stabilize dentures and are becoming more widely used than root-supported overdentures.
  - A mandibular overdenture supported by two implants had been shown to be cost-effective with good long-term survival.[8]

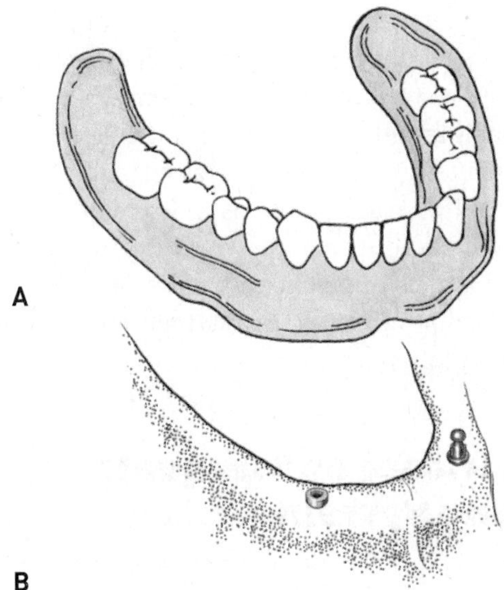

Figure 30-4 Overdenture. **A:** Mandibular complete denture. **B:** Examples of two different types of implant abutments. Generally, the same type of abutments is used in a denture.

    - However, for maxillary overdentures, four or more implants are necessary for the best long-term success, making them less cost-effective.[9]
- Mandibular implants are generally placed in the position of the mandibular canine, as shown in **Figure 30-4**.
- The advantages of an implant-supported overdenture include[10]:
    - No risk for dental caries as seen with the abutment roots used in a root-supported overdenture.
    - Less alveolar bone loss when compared with complete dentures.
    - Improved stability and retention when compared with a complete denture.
    - Better chewing ability and quality of life.
- Peri-implant hygiene is described in Chapter 31.

Obturator

I. Description

- An **obturator** is a prosthesis designed to close a congenital or acquired opening, such as a cleft of the hard palate.
- Made with a resin base and retainer clasps that provide stability for the appliance.
- Depending on the exact location of the palatal defect, an obturator may extend to include anterior prosthetic teeth.
- See **Figure 30-5A–B** for an example of a palatal defect and corresponding obturator.

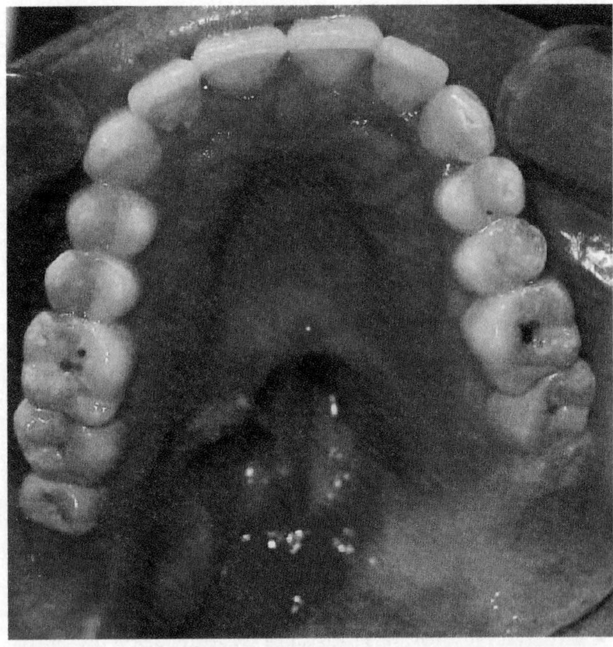

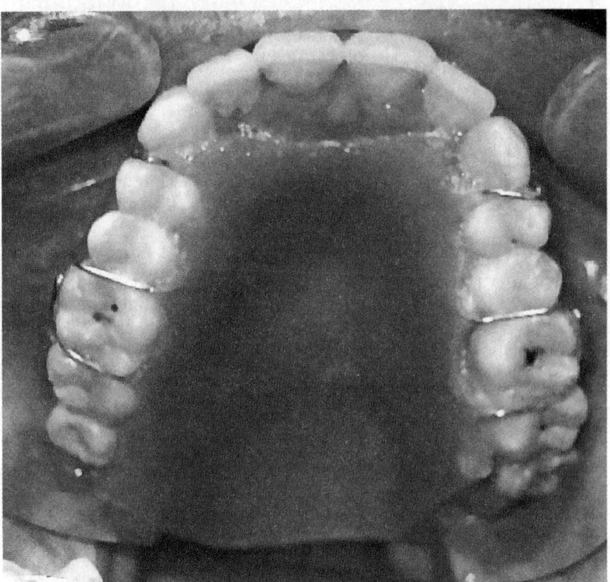

Figure 30-5 **A:** Palatal defect. **B:** Corresponding obturator.

Ahmed B (2015) Rehabilitation of Surgically Resected Soft Palate with Interim Velopharyngeal Obturator. *Int J Oral Craniofac Sci 1*(2): 031-033. DOI: 10.17352/2455-4634.000006

II. Purposes and Uses

- A variety of medical and physical conditions benefit from use of an obturator, including:
    - Loss or perforation of the palate due to chronic cocaine abuse.[11]
    - Patient with a loss of the palate due to trauma.
    - Patients with previous cancers involving the maxilla.
    - Patients with cleft palate. (See Chapter 49.)

III. Clinical Applications

- Depending on the size of the palatal defect, the obturator may need to stay in place in the mouth during parts of the intraoral and extraoral examination and treatment procedures to prevent choking or aspiration of water or other materials used in the oral cavity.
- Obturators need to be removed during exposure of radiographic images. An appliance with metal clasps will interfere with the radiolucency of the teeth and surrounding tissues.
- Removal of an obturator during dental hygiene therapy may be necessary to ensure access for complete calculus and biofilm removal and treatment of natural tooth surfaces.
- Professional care of an obturator follows procedures for cleaning an RPD.
- Instruction for patient's daily cleaning and care of the obturator is the same as the care given to an RPD.
- Patients may need to sleep with the obturator in place when the defect is severe, which may cause the underlying mucosa to become desiccated and the tissue may spontaneously begin to bleed.
- Sleeping with an obturator in place increases the risk for demineralization and dental caries in the abutment teeth as well as the incidence of **denture stomatitis**.
- When the patient must sleep with the obturator in place, it is advisable the obturator be removed for short periods during the day to allow the tissue to rest.

IV. Professional Continuing Care

- A minimum of three visits each year to the dentist and dental hygienist is recommended for continuing care, depending on patient compliance and risk factors for oral disease.
- The palatal defect will change over time and the dentist will need to adjust the obturator along with providing routine preventive dental care.

Denture Marking for Identification

Marking is required by law in some countries and in most states of the United States. However, there is no universal denture marking system. The need for denture marking is apparent in a variety of situations, including[11]:

- In forensic dentistry, or for identification of victims of war, disasters such as flood or fire, or transportation catastrophes, the dentition has been used increasingly as a means of identification.
- Prompt identification can be urgent when an individual is found unconscious from illness or injury or is suffering from amnesia as a result of psychiatric or traumatic causes, as well as suffering from Alzheimer's disease.
- The dentures of people in long-term residence or care facilities must be marked with identification information.

I. Criteria for an Adequate Marking System

Information on the denture must be specific so that rapid identification is possible. Criteria for the marking system include[12]:

- For the denture
  - No adverse effects on denture material.
  - No change to the strength, surface texture, or fit of the denture.
  - Placed in an unobtrusive position for esthetic reasons.
- The marking system must be:
  - Easy to learn and simple to carry out.
  - Inexpensive.
  - Durable. When the information is incorporated during denture processing, it is permanent. A surface marker for a denture already in use needs to be able to withstand denture-cleaning methods for a reasonable period of time.
- Characteristics of the material used
  - Fire and humidity resistant: When the label is placed inside the posterior section of a denture, the surrounding tongue and maxillofacial parts offer protection.
  - Radiopaque: A metal marker can be of use as a means of identification by radiographic examination in the event the radiolucent acrylic denture is accidentally swallowed.

II. Inclusion Methods for Marking

Inclusion methods are more permanent, but tend to be more expensive, require special equipment, and require trained personnel.[12,13]

- ID-Band
  - A shallow indentation is made on the denture for a stainless-steel metal band containing the

patient identification and covered with clear acrylic resin.
  - The Swedish ID-Band is the international standard.
- ID-Strip
  - Identification information can be placed on the surface of the impression to be incorporated when the denture is fabricated.
- Electronic microchip
  - A microchip can be incorporated in the denture because of the small size and esthetic acceptability.
  - A disadvantage is higher cost.
- Laser etching
  - Copper vapor laser has been used to mark dentures with metal frameworks, **removable partial dentures**, and other metallic restorations.
  - This method is expensive and requires specialized equipment and personnel.
- Radio-frequency identification (RFID) tags
  - RFID tags are small and can be incorporated into the denture resin.
  - They permit rapid identification and can store large amounts of data.
  - Not widely used due to the high cost.
- Bar codes
  - Bar codes can be printed on silk and incorporated into a denture with clear acrylic resin.
  - A disadvantage is that it requires expensive special equipment.

III. Surface Markers

Surface markers are not as durable, but instruction can be provided for persons not trained in dental laboratory methods. In a skilled nursing facility or other long-term care institution that has no resident dentist or dental hygienist, it may be possible to teach a nurse or other staff member to mark dentures of residents as they are admitted. The methods described as follows have been used for this purpose[12,13]:

- Permanent marker or pen
  - After cleaning and drying the denture, a small area near the posterior of the outer or polished denture surface is rubbed with an emery board until it is rough.
  - Name, initials, or other identification is printed on the roughened area with an indelible pen and dried.
  - Two or three coats of a fingernail acrylic (heavy nail protector) are painted over the area; each layer is dried before applying the next.
  - Surface markings have been found to last up to 6 months.
  - Light-cured materials may also be used.
- Engraving tool or dental bur
  - An engraving tool or round dental bur may be used to enter the name on the denture.
  - The engraving should be covered with a denture acrylic and processed to provide a smooth surface that will not retain food debris.

IV. Information to Include on a Surface Marker

- For residents of a home or institution, using only the person's name and initials can suffice for temporary surface marking.
- In a community, country, or international situation, the name alone would not provide enough identification, and the Social Security number, armed services serial number, or the equivalent in other countries has been included.
- Other identification, such as blood type and vital drug or disease condition, has been suggested.
- In certain countries, the dentist's registration or hospital number has been used. In Sweden, the patient's date of birth and national registration number have been marked on the dentures.
- Markings that can provide *immediate* identification are preferred.

Professional Care Procedures for Patients with Fixed Prostheses

Guidelines for professional care for patients with fixed dental prostheses include the following[14]:

- Medical, dental, psychosocial history, and vital signs. (See Chapters 11 and 12.)
- Extraoral/intraoral examination. (See Chapter 13.)
- Risk assessments for oral disease.
- Radiographs according to recognized guidelines. (See Chapter 15.)
- Comprehensive dental and periodontal examination. The following should be carefully evaluated[15]:
  - Margins of fixed prostheses for possible dental caries and other irregularities.
  - Monitoring of periodontal health and changes in mobility or loss of attachment.
  - One or more bridge abutments can become loose or fracture.

- Abutment teeth may also fracture.
- Monitor for radiographic or clinical signs of loss of pulp vitality. (See Chapters 16 and 20 for more on dental and periodontal examinations.)

- Dental and dental hygiene diagnosis and care planning.
- Oral hygiene education for existing natural dentition along with fixed prostheses. (See Chapters 26 and 27.)
- Prophylaxis or periodontal treatment as indicated by the examination findings.
  - See Chapter 31 for care of implant-supported fixed prostheses.
- Preventive services to address modifiable risk factors such as fluoride varnish, prescription fluorides, chlorhexidine mouthrinse, tobacco intervention, and nutrition counseling. (See Chapters 32, 33, and 34.)
- Continuing care at a minimum of a 6-month interval, with more frequent intervals needed for those who are at higher risk or unable to perform adequate oral self-care.

Patient Self-Care Procedures for Fixed Prostheses

I. Debris Removal

- Use an oral irrigator for loose debris removal throughout the dentition for a first step.
  - Facilitates next step: Biofilm removal with a toothbrush and other aids.
  - Procedure for use of an oral irrigator is described in Chapter 27.

II. Biofilm Removal from Abutment Teeth

- Nearly all the methods proposed for dental biofilm control are applicable to abutment teeth. (See Chapters 26 and 27.)
- The proximal surface of an abutment tooth and the gingiva adjacent to a pontic require special attention.
- Toothbrushing
  - Sulcular brushing is generally indicated.
- Dentifrice selection
  - A nonabrasive dentifrice is indicated to prevent the abrasion of the prosthesis surfaces and areas of exposed root on abutment teeth.
  - Fluoride-containing dentifrice is recommended for protection of remaining natural tooth surfaces, particularly exposed cementum.
- Additional interdental care
  - The method of interdental care is selected based on the manual dexterity of each patient and the type of prosthesis.
  - An interdental cleaning device is adapted specifically to the proximal surfaces of the abutments.
- Interdental cleaning methods and devices are described in Chapter 27.

III. Preventive Agents

- Those at risk for caries or periodontal disease may also benefit from prescription fluoride (5000 ppm fluoride).[14]
- Short-term 0.12% chlorhexidine mouthrinse as needed.[14]

IV. Care of the Fixed Prosthesis

- Areas requiring emphasis
  - The area beneath the pontics and the connectors is particularly prone to biofilm retention.
- Toothbrushing
  - A toothbrush in the Charters position may be helpful for cleaning the gingival surface of the pontic from the facial aspect. (See Chapter 26.)
  - The filaments can be directed under the pontic to clean the gingival surface.
- Dental floss for threader
  - Tufted dental floss is most efficient for cleaning a fixed partial denture as it can be passed under the pontic(s). (See Chapter 27.)
  - Thread a 12- to 15-inch length into a floss threader. Several types are available and are shown in **Figure 30-6**.
  - Apply threader between abutment, pontic, and gingiva (Figure 30-6).
  - Draw the floss through and use a single or double thickness for oral self-care (**Figure 30-7**).
- Other interdental devices
  - A single-tuft brush can be recommended and demonstrated as needed for individual prosthesis. (See Chapter 26.)
  - Small interdental brushes may be used mesial and distal to the pontic and natural teeth when space allows access. (See Chapter 27.)
- Additional factors
  - Instruct the patient to inform the dental team when any problem or change with the fixed prosthesis becomes apparent.

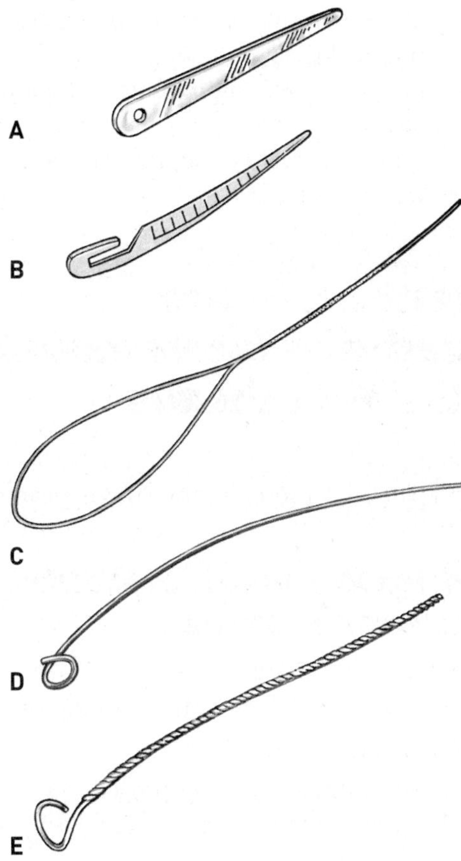

Figure 30-6 Floss Threaders. **A:** Clear plastic with closed eye. **B:** Tinted plastic with open eye. **C:** Soft plastic loop. **D:** Flexible wire. **E:** Twisted wire.

Professional Care Procedures for Patients with Removable Partial Prosthesis

The guidelines for the care of patients with removable partial prostheses are similar to those for fixed prostheses in regard to the examination and care of the natural dentition present.[14]

- Medical, dental, psychosocial history, and vital signs. (See Chapters 11 and 12.)
- Remove prosthesis for evaluation and cleaning (described in next section).
  - It is typically easiest to have the patient remove the prosthesis because the patient is familiar with the path of insertion and removal.
  - When a patient is unable to remove the appliance, the dental hygienist proceeds as follows:
    - Exert an even pressure on both sides of the denture simultaneously as the clasps slide up over their abutment teeth.

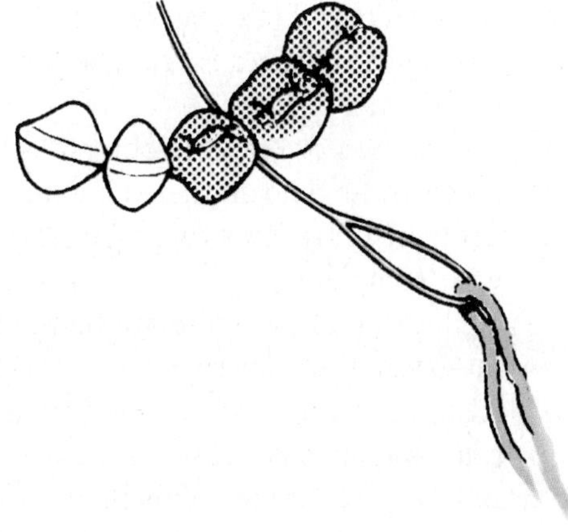

Figure 30-7 Use of Floss Threader to Draw the Floss or Tufted Floss between Abutment and Pontic

    - The line of insertion and removal of a partial denture is designed and constructed for an even, vertical movement.
    - Avoid grasping the clasp assemblies of the prostheses, which may damage or bend a clasp.
  - Prevent cross-contamination when receiving a removable prosthesis from a patient by wearing personal protective equipment and offering a disposable cup or resealable plastic bag to place the prosthesis in; rinse the prosthesis to remove any loose debris.
- Extraoral/intraoral examination. (See Chapter 13.)
  - Careful monitoring of the palatal tissue and edentulous ridges for signs of oral mucosal lesions (OMLs) is essential, as about one-third of removable prosthesis wearers exhibit stomatitis.[16,17]
  - Risk assessments for oral disease
  - Radiographs according to recognized guidelines (see Chapter 15)
  - Comprehensive dental and periodontal examination. The following should be carefully evaluated[14]:
    - Check the condition of the removable prostheses by looking for fractures, cracks, chipped and worn teeth, and broken clasps.
    - Evaluate the fit and function of the prostheses. (See Chapters 16 and 20 for more on dental and periodontal examinations.)
  - Dental and dental hygiene diagnosis and care planning
  - Oral hygiene education for existing natural dentition along with prostheses (see Chapters 26 and 27)

- Biofilm control is a major factor in maintaining the long-term health of abutment teeth for an RPD.[16]
- The biofilm or oral microbiome is different in those who are dentate with partial dentures versus those who are edentulous with complete dentures.[17] When natural teeth are present, there are higher levels of *Actinomyces*, *Haemophilus*, *Corynebacterium*, and *Veillonella*, with fewer *Lactobacillus* and *Streptococcus*.[17]

- Prophylaxis or periodontal treatment as indicated by the examination findings
  - See Chapter 31 for care of implant-supported fixed prostheses.
- Clean removable prosthesis.
  - Place in a cleaning solution in a resealable plastic bag in an **ultrasonic cleaner** as shown in **Figure 30-8**.
  - After removal from the cleaning solution, carefully brush the prosthesis with a denture brush and wrap in a wet paper towel or put in a new resealable plastic bag with water to keep it moist until patient care is complete.
- Preventive services to address modifiable risk factors such as fluoride varnish, prescription fluorides, chlorhexidine mouthrinse, tobacco intervention, and nutrition counseling. (See Chapters 28, 32, 33, and 34).
- Continuing care at a minimum of a 6-month interval, with more frequent intervals needed for those who are at higher risk or unable to perform adequate oral self-care.

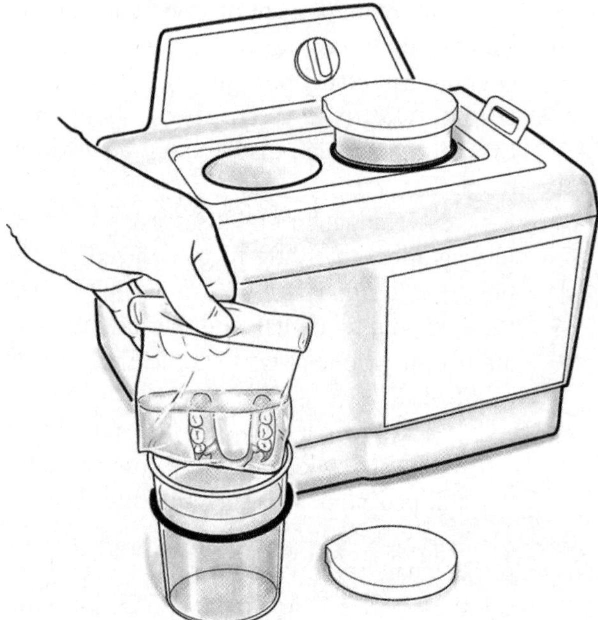

Figure 30-8 Ultrasonic Denture Cleaner. First, the removable prosthesis is placed in a sealed bag with cleaning solution and placed in a container filled with water. The container is then placed in an ultrasonic unit and the time is set according to manufacturer directions.

Patient Self-Care Procedures for Removable Partial Prostheses

Poor oral hygiene increases risk of OMLs like stomatitis in both partial and complete prosthesis wearers.[17,18]

I. Biofilm Removal for Abutment Teeth and Implants

See Chapters 26, 27, and 31 for oral self-care procedures for the abutment teeth and implants.

- Biofilm control
  - Prior to oral hygiene procedures, remove the RPD to access the natural teeth and/or implants.
  - Oral hygiene aids should be chosen according to patient's risk assessment, specific oral health needs, abilities, and preferences.
  - Meticulous biofilm removal must be emphasized to prevent dental caries and/or periodontal infection involving abutment tooth, which can lead to additional tooth loss. Tooth loss impacts the longevity of the RPD and may impact options for replacement.
- Dental caries and periodontal disease prevention
  - Abutment teeth are at increased risk for dental caries and periodontal disease.[7,8]
  - Daily oral self-care, topical fluoride use (e.g., fluoridated toothpaste, 5000-ppm prescription fluoride paste or gel), and diet changes may be necessary to reduce caries risk.[14] (See Chapter 25.)

II. Patient Education on Proper Use of Removable Prosthesis

- Partial dentures should be removed at night or for a 6- to 8-hour-period daily.[14,16,18,19]
  - Not removing the RPD overnight may result in inflammation from exposure to microorganisms.
- Clean the prosthesis as recommended at least twice a day.[14,18,19]

- Proper storage at night in a recommended cleaning solution.[14]
- Regular dental examinations are needed to identify when the RPD needs to be replaced.[14]

III. Cleaning the Prosthesis

A. Rinsing

- Rinsing is used to remove food debris when complete cleaning of the prosthesis is not possible.
  - Remove the partial denture, rinse under running water.
  - Rinsing does not remove biofilm, which is attached firmly, so it is not a substitute for complete biofilm removal and disinfection.

B. Mechanical Denture Cleansing

- Guidelines recommend brushing the RPD twice a day.[14]
  - Brushing is primarily for biofilm removal but is considered the least effective method to disinfect a partial or complete prosthesis.[18]
- Precautions to take when brushing an RPD include:
  - Partially fill the sink with water and line the sink with a washcloth or towel to prevent breakage if the prosthesis is dropped.
  - Carefully hold the RPD in the palm of the hand as described in **Box 30-2**.

Box 30-2 Procedure for Cleaning Denture by Brushing

1. Spread a towel, washcloth, or rubber mat over the bottom of the sink to serve as a cushion should the denture be dropped; partially fill the sink with water.
2. Grasp denture in palm of hand securely, but without squeezing because dentures can be broken.
3. Apply warm water, nonabrasive cleanser, and brush all areas of the denture. Pay particular attention to the impression surfaces where configurations of the surface correspond with those of the oral topography. The anterior areas of the inner surfaces of both the maxillary and mandibular dentures require special adaptations of the brush.
4. Rinse denture and brush under running water. Use the brush to remove denture cleanser that may be retained in the grooves.
5. Visually check each area carefully for biofilm.

- Denture brush: A good-quality soft denture brush with end-rounded filaments is recommended.[14,20] The styles of denture brushes vary.
  - One type shown in **Figure 30-9** is designed with two arrangements of filaments:
    - Round arrangement to access the inner, curved impression surface.
    - Rectangular portion for convenient adaptation to the polished and occlusal denture surfaces.
- Clasp brush
  - A specially designed, narrow, tapered brush about 2–3 inches long that can be adapted to the inner surfaces of clasps or **precision attachments** is recommended and shown in **Figure 30-10**.
  - Difficult-to-clean clasp assemblies have internal surfaces prone to biofilm accumulation that can be removed carefully with a clasp brush.
- Brushing the RPD with denture-cleaning creams and pastes
  - *Precaution*: All denture creams and pastes are to be used extraorally and may cause adverse effects such as damage to the esophagus, seizures, vomiting, etc., if misused.[21]
  - The American College of Prosthodontists does not recommend use of traditional toothpastes

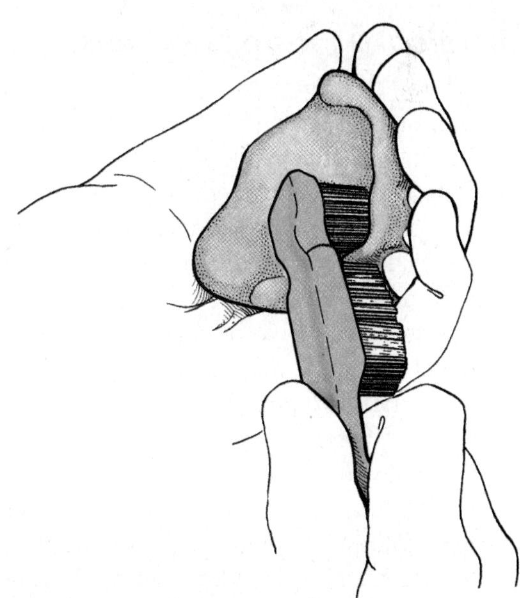

Figure 30-9 Denture Brush. The denture is held securely, but without squeezing, in the palm of the nonworking hand. Place a washcloth in the bottom of the sink and partially fill with water. The specially designed brush is preferred because one group of tufts is arranged to provide access to the inner impression surface of the denture, as shown.

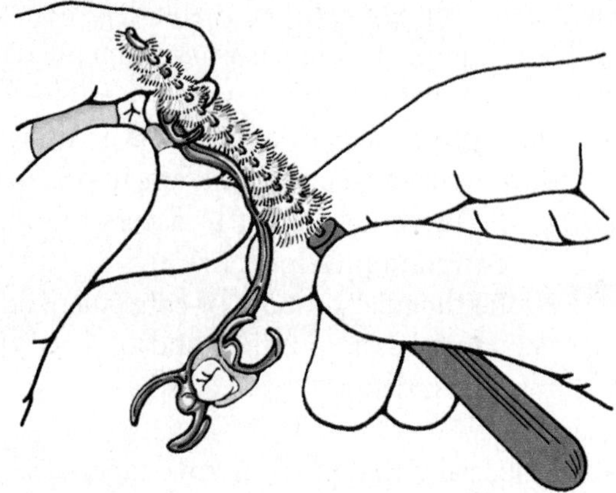

Figure 30-10 Clasp Brush. A brush specially designed to remove dental biofilm from the inside surfaces of clasps is available. The denture must be held carefully to avoid accidents.

on RPDs because they may be too abrasive for the acrylic resin and may scratch it, leading to a nidus for biofilm attachment.[16,20,22]

- Choose a cream or paste specifically designed for RPDs or dentures. Choices may also include a dishwashing liquid.[22] However, it should be noted that brushing alone has not been shown to eliminate *Candida*, so immersion in a denture cleanser is recommended in addition to brushing.[21]

C. Chemical Denture Cleansers

- Procedure
  - Denture cleansers should be used with the RPD outside the mouth to prevent adverse effects as previously noted.[21]
  - The procedure for soaking an RPD in a commercially available denture cleanser is discussed in **Box 30-3**.
  - The solution should be changed and the container should be cleaned daily to prevent contamination and growth of microorganisms.
- Types of denture cleansers
  - Generally available in powder or tablet form and include a variety of active agents such as hypochlorite, peroxide, and enzymes.[21]
    - Research has shown denture cleansers with sodium hypochlorite are most effective at killing pathogens such as *Candida* and methicillin-resistant *Staphylococcus aureus*.
    - However, soaking for longer than 10 minutes in a sodium hypochlorite solution may damage the RPD.
  - Manufacturer instructions vary and should be carefully followed.
    - The dental hygienist should ask the patient what kind of cleaning products are being used and review the instructions with them.
  - Carefully rinse after using denture-cleaning solutions prior to reinserting them in the oral cavity.
  - Immerse the RPD in water or cleansing solution when not in the mouth to avoid warping.

Box 30-3 Procedure for Cleaning a Denture by Immersion

- Place denture in a plastic container with a fitted cover specifically for this purpose.
- Use only warm water, which promotes the action of the cleanser, for rinsing and mixing the solution. Hot water is never used because it can distort plastic resin.
- Follow manufacturer's specifications to ensure correct dilution of cleanser and time length for immersion.
- Check that the denture is completely submerged in the solution; cover the container.
- When the denture is removed, rinse under running water and remove loosened debris and chemicals before proceeding to clean by brushing.
- Empty and clean container daily. Mix fresh solution to prevent contamination and growth of microorganisms.

Professional Care Procedures for Complete Dentures

At the continuing care appointments, the dental hygienist and the dentist will evaluate the health of the oral mucosa, the prosthesis, the patient's compliance with personal care, prosthesis retention, and any issues the patient has with the appliance.

- A professional denture cleaning in a dental office or clinic is suggested annually to minimize calculus and biofilm accumulation over time.[21]
  - Ultrasonic cleaning can be done in the dental office with an approved denture-cleaning solution such as Biosonic Enzymatic and Ultra-Kleen (Sterilex) and has been shown to improve bacterial kill rates.[21]

    - An example of dentures placed in sealed bag filled with denture cleaner to be placed in an ultrasonic cleaner is shown in Figure 30-7.
- Avoid scaling the prosthesis with a sharp instrument to remove calculus deposits, as it may scratch the resin or denture teeth, resulting in a nidus for biofilm and calculus accumulation.

I. Denture Deposits

- Accumulation of stains and deposits on dentures varies among individuals in a manner similar to that on natural teeth. The phases of deposit formation may be divided as follows:
- Mucin and food debris on the denture surfaces
    - Readily removed by rinsing, brushing, and irrigation.
- Denture pellicle and denture biofilm
    - Denture pellicle forms readily after a denture is cleaned.
    - Denture biofilm or the oral microbiome is different in those who are edentulous with complete dentures versus those who are dentate with partial dentures.[13]
    - For edentulous denture wearers, the biofilm is much less diverse and consists primarily of *Actinobacteria* and *Bacilli* with over 70% of dentures showing colonization by *Candida*.[17]
    - In stomatitis, denture biofilm contains *C. albicans* along with higher levels of *Prevotella* and *Veillonella*.[17]
- *Denture calculus*
    - When biofilm is not thoroughly removed on a regular basis, calcification occurs within 3 days and is completely calcified by 2 weeks.[23]
- *Stains*
    - Dentures can become stained similarly to natural teeth.
    - Frequent causes of stain include tobacco, marijuana, betel nut, red wine, coffee, and tea.

II. Removal of Denture

- It is usually most comfortable for the patient to remove the denture.
- The clinician may remove dentures for certain patients, particularly those with a physical limitation or in an emergency situation.
- Although denture removal may be complicated by anatomic features of an individual mouth, a general procedure is outlined in **Box 30-4**.

Box 30-4 Method for Removal of a Complete Denture

The clinician follows standard procedures for infection control while removing and handling the denture from the patient's mouth.

The Complete Maxillary Denture

1. Right-handed clinician is positioned at 11–12 o'clock; left-handed clinician is at 12–1 o'clock.
2. Grasp the anterior portion of the denture firmly with the thumb on the facial surface at the height of the border of the denture under the lip and the index finger on the palatal surface.
3. With the other hand, elevate the lip to expose the border of the denture to break the seal.
4. Remove the denture gently in a downward and forward direction.

The Complete Mandibular Denture

1. Right-handed clinician is positioned at 8–9 o'clock; left-handed clinician is at 3–4 o'clock.
2. Grasp the denture firmly on the facial surface with the thumb and on the lingual surface with the index finger.
3. With the other hand, retract the lower lip forward and remove the denture gently.

III. Care of Dentures during Intraoral Procedures

- Provide a disposable cup and tissue for the patient's use when requesting the patient remove or insert the denture.
- Rinse in running water being careful to avoid splashing to remove any unattached debris.
- Professionally clean the denture in an ultrasonic denture cleaner, following manufacturer's instructions, with appropriate cleaning solution.
- Follow strict procedures to protect the denture from exposure to unclean areas during transportation and when in the ultrasonic cleaner.
- Provide a clean disposable cup or sterile container with a fitted cover to hold the prosthesis after rinsing.
- Immerse denture in water after cleaning to prevent drying, which can cause distortion of the denture.[21]
- Place container in a safe place away from treatment area to prevent spilling or inadvertently discarding it.

- At the end of the appointment, remember to rinse and return the denture before dismissing the patient from the dental chair.

Patient Self-Care Procedures for Complete Dentures

I. General Education Prior to Denture Placement

- The preparation for **denture insertion** has to begin well in advance of delivery.
- Be sensitive to the patient's emotional state about becoming edentulous[24] and be prepared to help them adapt to the new prosthesis.
- Patient expectations about esthetics and function may impact satisfaction, so this must be carefully assessed prior to beginning treatment.[24]
- Develop an individualized plan appropriate for educating the patient on the self-care for the new prosthesis.

II. Education for the New Denture Wearer

The dental hygienist plays a valuable role in educating the new prosthesis wearer on its use, limitations, and functions. Education should include the following[25]:

- Each patient is different and progress in adjusting to new dentures cannot be compared with someone else.
- Patients may have to adapt to their appearance with new dentures. Many people may have had missing or broken teeth, so the change in vertical dimension and appearance require time for adjustment.
- Chewing or mastication with new dentures is a challenge for some and may take 6–8 weeks.
  - It may take time for the facial and masticatory muscles to learn to keep the denture in place and to go through the motion of chewing.
  - Hypersalivation may occur for the first few days; however, in individuals with xerostomia, the lack of saliva can affect the comfort of the denture as well as swallowing ability.
  - Initially, the patient may want to eat a softer diet, eat more slowly, and cut fibrous foods into small pieces.
  - Avoid biting with the front teeth and bite into food such as a sandwich more toward the corners of the mouth, distributing food on both sides of the mouth to avoid dislodging the denture.
- Cover the mouth when coughing and sneezing as dentures may loosen and come out.
- An upper denture can affect taste and swallowing.
- New dentures can affect speech, so patients may need to practice.
- Choosing a high-protein, healthy diet is important as those with dentures typically eat a less nutrient-dense diet with higher levels of sucrose and refined carbohydrates.
  - Patients may choose to lightly steam fresh vegetables or cut them into small pieces to make them easier to chew.
  - Cooked whole-grain cereals and grains are also a good source of fiber and B vitamins.
  - Cutting fresh fruit will also make it easier for new denture wearers to eat a healthy diet.
  - Those who are edentulous tend to be at risk of malnutrition, so including good sources of protein (dairy, fish, meat, chicken, and eggs) will be important for new denture wearers.
- Denture care will be discussed in more detail in the next section.

III. Denture Cleaning

A. Purpose

- Prevent prosthesis-related OMLs such as traumatic ulcers, hyperplasia, angular cheilitis, and denture stomatitis.[18,21]
- Reduce levels of dental biofilm, bacteria, and fungi.[21]
- Prevent halitosis (oral malodor).
- Maintain appearance of the denture.

B. Denture Care Recommendations[1]

The recommendations for the patient self-care of the complete denture are essentially the same as for RPDs[21], so refer back to that section for additional detail.

- Thoroughly remove dental biofilm on the oral tissues with a soft toothbrush and complete denture with a denture brush daily.
  - Ideally the patient should clean (or at least rinse) the denture after meals to remove loose food debris.
  - At least once a day, a soft toothbrush with end-rounded filaments should be applied lightly over the ridges and in the vestibules using long, straight strokes from posterior to anterior to remove debris and biofilm.
  - Clean the tongue daily.

- A nonabrasive denture cleanser is used only when the denture is not in the mouth.
- Thoroughly rinse to remove denture cleanser prior to reinsertion in the mouth.
    - Residual chemical agents, such as essential oils, may cause inflammatory or allergic reactions of the oral mucosa, and phenolic agents can have deleterious effects on plastic resin.
- Soaking the denture in a denture cleanser when not in the mouth may reduce bacterial levels and dental biofilm.
    - Denture cleansers have a variety of active ingredients, for example, peroxide, enzymes, and hypochlorite.
    - Recommend products shown to be safe and effective for denture use by looking for the American Dental Association Seal of Acceptance or the Canadian Dental Association Seal.
    - The patient should follow manufacturer's instructions.
- Recommend the patient remove the denture and leave it out overnight or for another extended period during the day as those who wear them continually have a greater risk of *Candida*-related denture stomatitis.[18,21]
- When the denture is not in the mouth, it should be stored in water.
- Those wearing upper and lower dentures need an annual dental examination to assess the oral tissues and the prosthesis.[21]

C. Denture Adhesives

- Benefits of denture adhesives[26]:
    - Research shows dental adhesives significantly improve denture retention.
    - Dental adhesive may improve chewing by enhancing retention and stability.
    - An adhesive may be necessary for the new denture patient as the immediate, interim denture begins to loosen with healing of the underlying tissues.
        - However, the patient needs regular evaluation to determine the need for possible reline or rebase of the denture. In some cases, a new denture may be indicated.[21]
- The practitioner needs to provide education on the use of a denture adhesive and include the following[21]:
    - Dental adhesive choice is personal, but research suggests the most effective are creams, followed by powder, with the strips being least effective.[26]
    - Clean and dry the surface where the denture adhesive will be applied.
    - Use only three or four pea-sized dollops of denture-adhesive cream on each denture.
    - For powder denture adhesives, dampen denture surface and apply a thin film to the entire surface and shake off the excess.
    - If using pad adhesives, adapt the size to the surface to be placed against the tissue.
    - Avoid zinc-containing adhesives due to adverse side effects.
    - Once the adhesive is applied, seat the denture and hold firmly in place for 5–10 seconds.
    - Bite firmly to spread the adhesive.
    - It is not recommended dentures be worn continuously (24 hours/day) because of risk for denture stomatitis.
    - Denture adhesives need to be thoroughly removed from the prosthesis and oral tissues daily.

D. Reline or Rebase of Denture

- A reline of a denture is used to resurface the base material of the tissue side of the denture to provide an improved fit and retention.[4]
- A rebase of the denture is done by a dental laboratory and is replacement of the entire denture resin base material and resetting of the denture teeth.

Denture-Induced Oral Mucosal Lesions (OMLs)

Regular intraoral examination of the oral cavity and evaluation of the denture will help to identify and manage denture-induced oral lesions.[27]

- Education of the patient is essential, as a majority of those with dentures think they no longer need to have regular dental visits.

I. Contributing Factors for Denture-Induced OMLs

The factors causing OMLs under dentures are complex. The literature suggests the following:

- Ill-fitting dentures[27]
    - Food particles become lodged under an ill-fitting denture and may irritate the soft tissues and provide an environment for growth of microorganisms.
    - Because tissue changes under dentures can occur gradually over a long period, the patient may not be aware of developing disease.

- Improper storage of denture[18]
    - Storage of the denture in water when not in the mouth increased risk of OMLs by eight times.
    - Leaving the denture dry also resulted in a six times higher risk of OMLs.
- Inadequate or improper oral hygiene[18,27]
- Continuous wearing of dentures
    - Nocturnal wearing of dentures more than doubles the risk of oral lesions, such as denture stomatitis.[18,21]
- Chemotoxic effect from residual cleansing paste or solution not thoroughly rinsed from the denture
- Allergy to the denture base (rare)
- Patient self-treatment with over-the-counter products for relining
- Xerostomia due to medications or medical conditions[27]

II. Types of Denture-Induced OMLs

A. Denture-Induced Irritation (Also Called Traumatic Ulcers or Sore Spots)

- Appearance: Isolated, red, inflamed area, sometimes ulcerated (**Figure 30-11**).
- Contributing factors: New denture wearer, trauma from an ill-fitting denture, an overextended denture flanges, unbalanced occlusion, a rough spot on a denture surface, a tongue bite, or a foreign object caught under the denture.[27]
- The ulcer may resemble a cancerous lesion and need to be biopsied when it persists longer than 7–14 days after denture adjustment.

B. Denture Stomatitis

- Inflammatory condition of high prevalence among denture wearers and may be characterized by the following[27,28]:
    - Generalized inflammation and erythema of mucosa covered by the denture (**Figure 30-12**).
    - May be asymptomatic, but some patients may experience pain, itching, or a burning sensation.
    - Denture stomatitis is often associated with *C. albicans*.[21,29]
    - More common in the maxilla.
    - More frequently diagnosed in females than males.
- Etiologic factors include the following[21,28]:
    - Poor denture hygiene.
    - Continuous denture wearing, particularly nocturnal use of dentures.

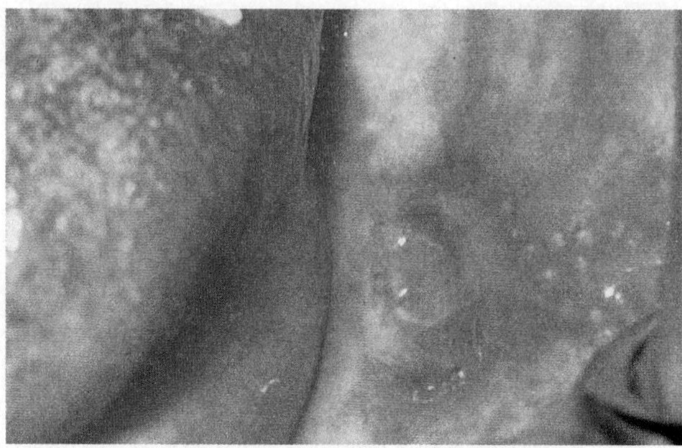

Figure 30-11 Traumatic Ulcer: Molar Area, Under Denture

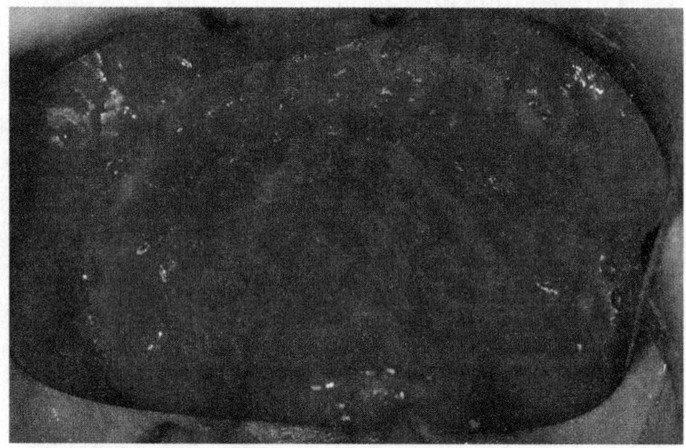

Figure 30-12 Erythema and Papillary Hyperplasia Seen with Denture Stomatitis

    - Cigarette smoking.
    - Wearing dentures longer than 5 years.
    - Elderly denture wearer.
    - Trauma from ill-fitting denture.
- Treatment may include[21]:
    - Denture adjustments or fabrication of new denture.
    - Testing for *Candida* and prescription of appropriate antifungal medication.
    - Attention to daily denture care to manage dental biofilm with regular removal of food debris from under the denture.

C. Angular Cheilitis

- Appearance
    - Deep fissuring at the angles of the mouth, with cracks, ulcerations, and erythema (**Figure 30-13**).
    - Moist with saliva or sometimes dry with a crust.
- Contributing factors
    - Local factors including infection by *C. albicans*.
    - Poor oral hygiene.

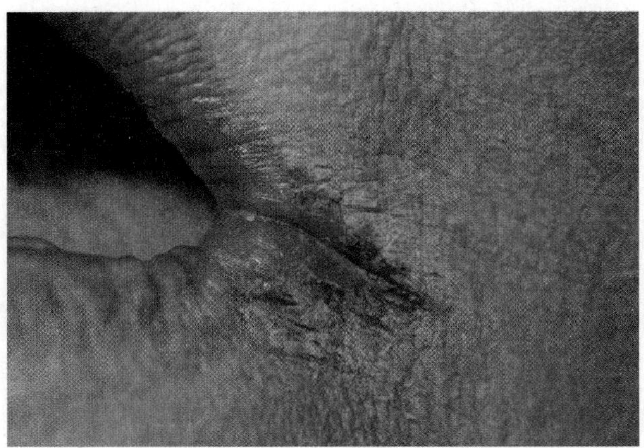

Figure 30-13 Angular Cheilitis

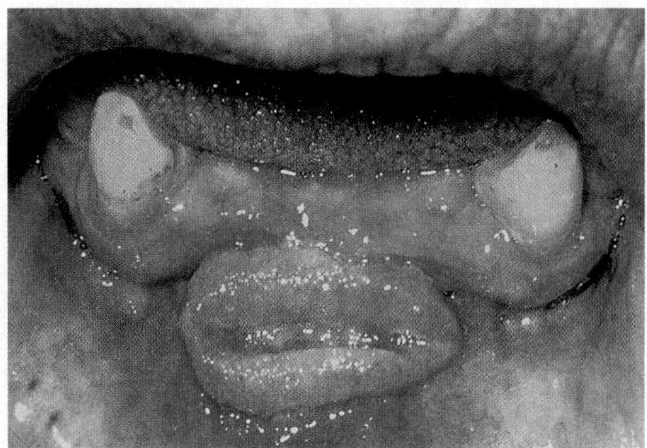

Figure 30-14 Epulis Fissuratum at Partial Denture Flange

- Irritation from saliva is associated with anatomic changes that make the folds at the corners of the mouth deeper and more pronounced.
- B-vitamin deficiency can further complicate angular cheilitis, particularly in debilitated and dependent elder patients, so encouraging adequate nutrition is important.
- Prevalence is higher in females than in men; associated with use of removable denture and not closely associated with being edentulous.

- Prescription antifungal medication may be indicated depending on the etiology.

D. Tissue Hyperplasia

There are several types of tissue hyperplasia seen in those who wear dentures.

- Epulis fissuratum[27]
  - Long-standing chronic inflammatory tissue appears as tissue growth over the alveolar ridges (**Figure 30-14**).
  - The etiology is often multifactorial and may include poor oral self-care, smoking, and ill-fitting dentures.
  - It may be treated by surgical removal by scalpel or laser.
  - Management: closely related to inflammatory hyperplasia.
- Inflammatory hyperplasia[27]
  - Inflammatory hyperplasia is located on the palate, rarely outside the confines of the bony ridges.
  - The lesion appears as a group of closely arranged, pebble-shaped, red, edematous projections.
  - Associated primarily with chronic injury from poor-fitting dentures.
  - Management: Replacement or adjustment of denture will often resolve the inflammation.
- Flabby ridge[27]
  - Mobile soft tissue on the superficial aspect of the alveolar ridge due to a replacement by fibrous tissue.
  - Typically located on the anterior aspect of the maxilla.
  - Management
    - Surgical excision prior to construction of the denture.
    - Construction of fixed or removable implant retained denture.
    - Construction of denture without surgical excision.
    - When treatment planning for a denture, it is better to have a poor ridge than no ridge for retention purposes.

Documentation

The following items need to be included in the permanent record of a patient with a fixed or removable prosthesis:

- Review medical history; make necessary additions to the record.
- Chief complaint will reveal any discomfort the patient is experiencing.
- Description of the prostheses and stability.
- Intraoral findings describing soft tissue and any pathologic changes of the mucosa or attached gingiva, health of abutment teeth to identify mobility, dental caries, or wear facets.
- Evaluation of abutment implants.
- Individualized regimen for oral self-care, including prevention recommendations for those with remaining teeth to address modifiable caries risk factors.
- An example progress note can be found in **Box 30-5**.

Box 30-5 Example Documentation: Partial Denture

- **S**—A 63-year-old female presents for an adult prophylaxis appointment with chief complaint, "My partial feels loose and lifts off the top of my mouth when I chew meats."
- **O**—Intraoral examination: Slight edematous tissue mesial to #6 and #11, with redness noted on palate where removable partial denture (RPD) rests, probing depths 3 mm or less except the mesial facial #6 and #11; where 4-mm probing measurements are noted, tissue has slight generalized marginal erythema with generalized, moderate biofilm. Light generalized stain and calculus on natural dentition, the RPD teeth, and the tissue-supported surface of the RPD.
- **A**—Ill-fitting, unstable RPD with retained calculus is contributing to gingival inflammation and increased risk for oral trauma.
- **P**—RPD placed in sealed bag with cleaning solution and placed in a container filled in the ultrasonic unit to remove calculus; upon subsequent visual inspection, all calculus was removed and there were no fractures or roughness noted. Advised patient to clean RPD daily and remove nightly to rest the underlying mucosa. Reminded her to keep the denture soaking in water when it is out of her mouth during the night. Proper technique for denture cleaning was demonstrated and practiced by the patient. Dispensed new denture toothbrush and clasp brush and advised patient to purchase American Dental Association–recommended denture cleanser.

Next steps: Schedule with dentist for RPD evaluation to determine possible reline or replacement.

Signed: ____________________________, RDH
Date: : _______________

Factors to Teach the Patient

- How to perform self-examination of the oral tissues.
- Dentures may need to be replaced periodically as the bone and tissue under the denture change.
- The importance of careful removal of dental biofilm from the prosthesis on a regular basis to prevent tissue inflammation and possible *Candida* infection.
- The need for careful oral self-care of abutment teeth whether natural tooth or implant.
- How tongue cleaning contributes to complete oral health.
- The significance of regular maintenance appointments: intraoral/extraoral screening for pathology, especially oral cancer screening; professional cleaning of remaining teeth and prostheses; and prosthesis evaluation and adjustments as needed.
- The importance of seeking professional evaluation if any problems arise with existing prostheses; never attempt to repair or adjust a prosthesis.

References

1. Tealdo T, Menini M, Bevilacqua M, et al. Immediate versus delayed loading of dental implants in edentulous patients' maxillae: a 6-year prospective study. *Int J Prosthodont*. 2014;27(3):207-214.
2. Mosnegutu A, Wismeijer D, Geraets W. Implant-supported mandibular overdentures can minimize mandibular bone resorption in edentulous patients: results of a long-term radiologic evaluation. *Int J Oral Maxillofac Implants*. 2015;30(6):1378-1386.
3. Yunus N, Masood M, Saub R, Al-Hashedi AA, Taiyeb Ali TB, Thomason JM. Impact of mandibular implant prostheses on the oral health-related quality of life in partially and completely edentulous patients. *Clin Oral Implants Res*. 2016;27(7):904-909.
4. Academy of Prosthodontics Foundation. The glossary of prosthodontic terms: ninth edition. *J Prosthet Dent*. 2017;117(5S):e1-e105.
5. Van Waas MA, Jonkman RE, Kalk W, Van 't Hof MA, Plooij J, Van Os JH. Differences two years after tooth extraction in mandibular bone reduction in patients treated with immediate overdentures or with immediate complete dentures. *J Dent Res*. 1993;72(6):1001-1004.
6. Ettinger RL, Qian F. Longitudinal assessment of denture maintenance needs in an overdenture population. *J Prosthodont*. 2019;28(1):22-29.
7. Ettinger RL. Tooth loss in an overdenture population. *J Prosthet Dent*. 1988;60(4):459-462.
8. Zhang Q, Jin X, Yu M, et al. Economic evaluation of implant-supported overdentures in edentulous patients: a systematic review. *Int J Prosthodont*. 2017;30(4):321-326.
9. Di Francesco F, De Marco G, Capcha EB, et al. Patient satisfaction and survival of maxillary overdentures supported by four or six splinted implants: a systematic review with meta-analysis. *BMC Oral Health*. 2021;21(1):247.

10. Carlsson GE. Implant and root supported overdentures—a literature review and some data on bone loss in edentulous jaws. *J Adv Prosthodontics*. 2014;6(4):245-252.
11. Blanco GF, Madeo MC, Vázquez ME, Martínez M. Case for diagnosis. Palate perforation due to cocaine use. *An Bras Dermatol*. 2017;92(6):877-878.
12. Datta P, Sood S. The various methods and benefits of denture labeling. *J Forensic Dent Sci*. 2010;2(2):53-58.
13. Bathala LR, Rachuri NK, Rayapati SR, Kondaka S. Prosthodontics an "arsenal" in forensic dentistry. *J Forensic Dent Sci*. 2016;8(3):173.
14. Bidra AS, Daubert DM, Garcia LT, et al. Clinical practice guidelines for recall and maintenance of patients with tooth-borne and implant-borne dental restorations. *J Prosthodont*. 2016;25(suppl 1):S32-S40.
15. Tan K, Pjetursson BE, Lang NP, Chan ES. A systematic review of the survival and complication rates of fixed partial dentures (FPDs) after an observation period of at least 5 years. *Clin Oral Implants Res*. 2004;15(6):654-666.
16. Szalewski L, Pietryka-Michalowska E, Szymansky J. Oral hygiene in patients using removable dentures. *Polish J Public Health*. 2017;127(1):28-31.
17. O'Donnell LE, Robertson D, Nile CJ, et al. The oral microbiome of denture wearers is influenced by levels of natural dentition. *PLoS One*. 2015;10(9):e0137717.
18. Ercalik-Yalcinkaya S, Ozcan M. Association between oral mucosal lesions and hygiene habits in a population of removable prosthesis wearers. *J Prosthodont*. 2015;24(4):271-278.
19. Cakan U, Yuzbasioglu E, Kurt H, et al. Assessment of hygiene habits and attitudes among removable partial denture wearers in a university hospital. *Niger J Clin Pract*. 2015;18(4):511-515.
20. American Dental Association. *Healthy Mouth: removable partial dentures*. https://www.mouthhealthy.org/en/az-topics/d/dentures-partial. Accessed September 1, 2021.
21. American College of Prosthodontists. Dentures FAQs. https://www.gotoapro.org/dentures-faq/#445. Accessed September 1, 2021.
22. Felton D, Cooper L, Duqum I, et al. Evidence-based guidelines for the care and maintenance of complete dentures: a publication of the American College of Prosthodontists. *J Prosthodont*. 2011;20(suppl 1):S1-S12.
23. Matsumura K, Sato Y, Kitagawa N, Shichita V, Kawata D, Ishikawa M. Influence of denture surface roughness and host factors on dental calculi formation on dentures: a cross-sectional study. *BMC Oral Health*. 2018;18(1):78.
24. Kudsi Z, Fenlon MR, Johal A, Baysan A. Assessment of psychological disturbance in patients with tooth loss: a systematic review of assessment tools. *J Prosthodont*. 2020;29(3):193-200.
25. Goiato MC, Filho HG, Dos Santos DM, Barão VA, Júnior AC. Insertion and follow-up of complete dentures: a literature review. *Gerodontology*. 2011;28(3):197-204.
26. Shu X, Fan Y, Lo ECM, Leung KCM. A systematic review and meta-analysis to evaluate the efficacy of denture adhesives. *J Dent*. 2021;108:103638.
27. Mubarak S, Hmud A, Chandrasekharan S, Ali AA. Prevalence of denture-related oral lesions among patients attending College of Dentistry, University of Dammam: a clinico-pathological study. *J Int Soc Prev Community Dent*. 2015;5(6):506-512.
28. Gendreau L, Loewy ZG. Epidemiology and etiology of denture stomatitis. *J Prosthodont*. 2011;20(4):251-260.
29. Gleiznys A, Zdanavičienė E, Žilinskas J. *Candida albicans* importance to denture wearers: a literature review. *Stomatologija*. 2015;17(2):54-66.

CHAPTER 31

The Patient with Dental Implants

Carol Tran, BOH, PhD
Linda D. Boyd, RDH, RD, EdD

CHAPTER OUTLINE

LEARNING OBJECTIVES

After studying this chapter, the student will be able to:

1. Describe the concepts, technology, and terminology relevant to implant dentistry.
2. Develop a knowledge base related to osseointegration and ancillary procedures in oral implantology.
3. Describe patient selection factors and education essentials.
4. Explain maintenance of dental implants in the clinical setting.
5. Recognize and manage dental implant problems, complications, and failures.

Dental implants offer a means of tooth replacement to preserve surrounding oral tissues normally compromised by a missing tooth.

- Dental implants simulate natural tooth roots.
  - Dental implants may replace one tooth or multiple teeth for a partially or completely edentulous patient.
- Knowledge of dental implants is essential for all dental hygienists who are responsible for professional maintenance and monitoring of peri-implant health.
- Patients often have questions and/or concerns for the dental hygienist regarding their treatment options, which presents an opportune time for education to dispel confusion, alleviate fears, or reinforce a decision to proceed with needed treatment.
- The success of a dental implant can depend on many factors, including patient compliance and skills for daily care of the prosthesis and the surrounding soft tissues.
- Frequent maintenance appointments (supportive periodontal and implant therapy) for careful supervision and patient motivation are essential components of implant success.

Bone Physiology

Alveolar bone is of critical importance to the planning and execution of dental implants. A careful assessment of the quantity and quality of bone provides a foundation for proper treatment planning and a more predictable surgical outcome.

- Bone is a dynamic tissue that is cellular and vascular.
  - Osteocytes: Mediate activity.
  - Osteoblasts: Repair and regeneration.
  - Osteoclasts: Remodeling and homeostasis.
- Key function: To provide structural support to various loads or stresses.

I. Bone Classification

- Bone is classified according to its density as follows[1]:
  - D1: Dense cortical bone.
  - D2: Thick, dense to porous cortical bone on crest and coarse trabecular bone within.
  - D3: Thin, porous cortical bone on crest and fine trabecular bone within.
  - D4: Fine trabecular bone.
  - D5: Immature, nonmineralized bone.
- The density of bone in a potential implant site determines factors such as:
  - Time frame for integration of the implant.
  - Window of time for prosthetic loading.

II. Biomechanical Force

- Wolff's law (1892) states bone is laid down in areas of greatest stress and is resorbed in areas where it is not stressed.[2]
- The patient needs to understand the implication of biomechanical force on the alveolar process.[2]
  - Bone will resorb when teeth are removed and mechanical stress is no longer applied to the bone.
  - Dental implants preserve surrounding bone through function, which supplies the needed load and stress.

III. Grafting and Regeneration

- Areas of insufficient bone due to previous resorption or tooth loss can be grafted to create a suitable recipient site for dental implant placement.
- Site preparation measures for implant therapy include:
  - Atraumatic extraction with ridge and/or socket preservation.
  - Ridge augmentation.[3]
  - Maxillary **sinus augmentation**, also called a "sinus lift."[4]
- Options for grafting and regeneration of recipient sites include[3]:
  - Autograft: Bone obtained from the patient, harvested from a donor site.
  - Allograft: Bone obtained from another human (cadaver bone).
  - Xenograft: Bone obtained from another species (cow/bovine; horse/equine).
  - **Alloplast**: Synthetic derivative of bone (e.g., beta-tricalcium phosphate).

Osseointegration

Successful tooth replacement is accomplished by **osseointegration**, which means direct bone anchorage to an implant body. When viewed at a light microscopic level, osseointegration reveals direct contact between bone and implant with no intervening connective tissue. The process of osseointegration is a dynamic process and includes the following stages[5]:

- Initial healing stage takes place up to 1 year.
- Second stage when bone actively remodels and may take up to 5 years.
- Third stage includes fewer osteocytes and less bone remodeling.

Implant Interfaces

An implant has an inner interface with the *bone* and a *soft-tissue* interface where the **abutment**, post, or other protruding portion of the implant is surrounded by the mucosal or gingival tissue.

I. Implant–Bone Interface

A. Osseointegration

- Refers to direct structural and functional union between the implant and healthy living bone.
- Indicates successful placement of the implant.
- No mobility evident.

B. Fibrous Encapsulation

- Fibrous encapsulation refers to the infusion of connective tissue cells between the implant body and surrounding bone.
- Indicates failure of osseointegration.
- Mobility of the implant is evident.

II. Implant–Soft-Tissue Interface

- The external environment of an implant is the oral cavity, with saliva, dental biofilm, and debris.
- **Biologic seal (perimucosal seal)**: Between the implant and the soft tissue, a biologic seal exists to prevent microorganisms and inflammation-producing agents from entering the tissues.
  - The peri-implant junction is similar to the junctional epithelium (JE) in a natural tooth.[6]
- The biologic width around an implant is 3–4 mm, which is slightly longer than in a natural tooth (~2 mm).[6]
- Soft-tissue connection: Peri-implant sulcular epithelium is in contact with the implant surface.[6]
  - The peri-implant epithelium (PIE) performs a similar function to the JE of a natural tooth.
  - Hemidesmosomes and basal lamina connect the PIE cells to the titanium of the implant much like JE cells connect to natural teeth.

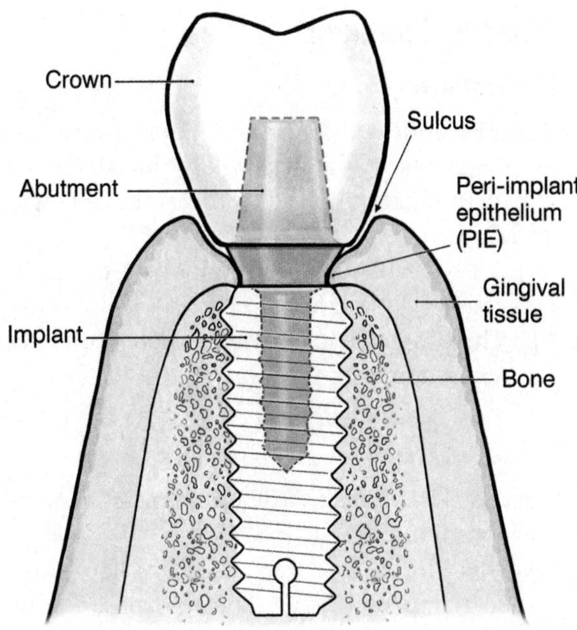

Figure 31-1 The Implant–Soft-Tissue Interface. At the implant–soft-tissue interface, there can be no connective tissue fiber attachment as when bone is present. The peri-implant epithelium (PIE) attachment resembles a long junctional epithelial attachment.

- The PIE attachment is weaker than the JE–tooth interface.
- The long JE of an implant is parallel to the implant, surrounding it, but with no attachment creating a cuff of tissue.
- No connective tissue fibers (Sharpey's fibers) exist to hold the attachment as with a natural tooth.
- Normal periodontal tissue has a blood supply from both alveolar bone and the periodontal ligament (PDL); however, the peri-implant tissue has no PDL, resulting in a reduced blood supply.
- The reduced blood supply and weaker PIE–titanium interface reduces resistance to bacterial invasion and to penetration of the periodontal probe during probing.[7,8]
- **Figure 31-1** illustrates the implant–soft-tissue interface at the peri-implant epithelium.

Types of Dental Implants

Over the years, a variety of dental implant systems have been tried clinically and studied with research.[9] They are **subperiosteal**, **transosseous**, and **endosseous**. Currently, endosseous or "root form" implants are the most widely used.

I. Subperiosteal

A. Definition

- Custom-fabricated framework of metal that rests over the bone of the mandible or maxilla, under the periosteum. Indicated under the following conditions[10]:
  - A removable denture cannot be retained because of lack of bone.
  - There is inadequate alveolar bone for endosseous implants.

B. Description[10]

- Material: **Titanium** or Vitallium (cobalt–chromium–molybdenum).
- Two step: In the first step, a surgical flap is used to reflect mucosal tissues and to expose the underlying bone. An impression is made of the bony ridge. The metallic unit is cast and then placed in a second surgical step. Usually, four posts protrude into the oral cavity to hold the complete denture.
- One step: Computer-assisted **tomography** design and manufacturing have been applied, using a reformatted computed tomography scan from which approximate casts of the maxilla or mandible can be made. The implant is designed on this replica and is placed in one surgical procedure (**Figure 31-2**).

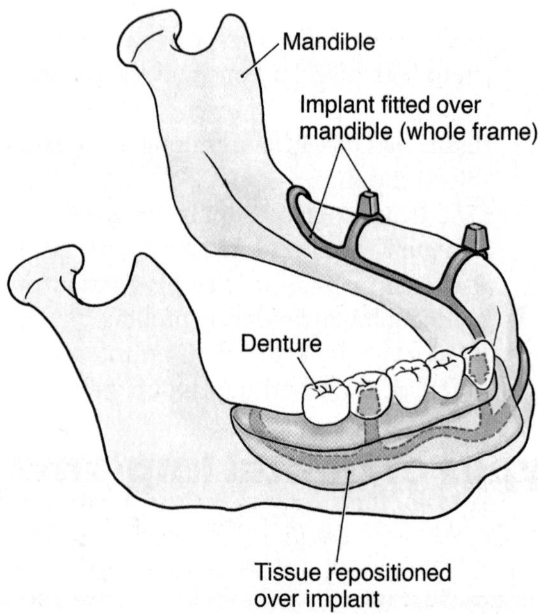

Figure 31-2 Subperiosteal Implant. The custom-fabricated framework is shown on the left-hand side of the mandible; on the right-hand side, the framework is shown by dotted lines under the denture.

II. Transosseous (Transosteal)

A. Definition

- A dental implant that penetrates both cortical plates and passes through the full thickness of the alveolar bone.
- Also known as a mandibular staple implant or staple bone implant.

B. Description[11]

- Materials: Stainless steel, ceramic-coated materials, and **titanium alloy**.
- A metal plate, fitted to the inferior border of the mandible, has five to seven pins extending toward the occlusal surface.
- Usually, two terminal pins protrude into the oral cavity to hold the overdenture. The pins are connected by a crossbar (**Figure 31-3**).
- The transosteal implant can be used when the patient has an edentulous mandible with little mandibular bone.

III. Endosseous (Endosteal) Implant

A. Definition

- An implant placed within the bone to replace a single tooth or provide support for the replacement of complete or partial loss of teeth.
- Early forms (endosteal): Blade or plate form.
- Current forms (endosseous): "**Root form**" or cylindrical; can be threaded, smooth, perforated, or solid (**Figure 31-4**).[12]

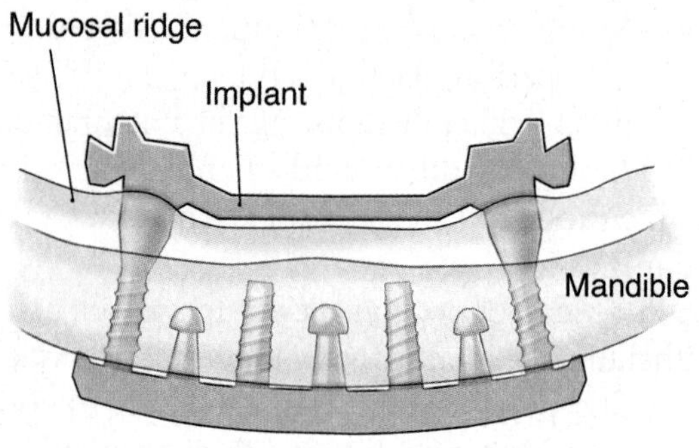

Figure 31-3 Transosteal Implant. Mandibular staple bone plate in the anterior region shows metal plate at the lower border of the mandible, with pins extending toward the occlusal surface. Terminal pins protrude into the oral cavity to hold the overdenture. This is not common.

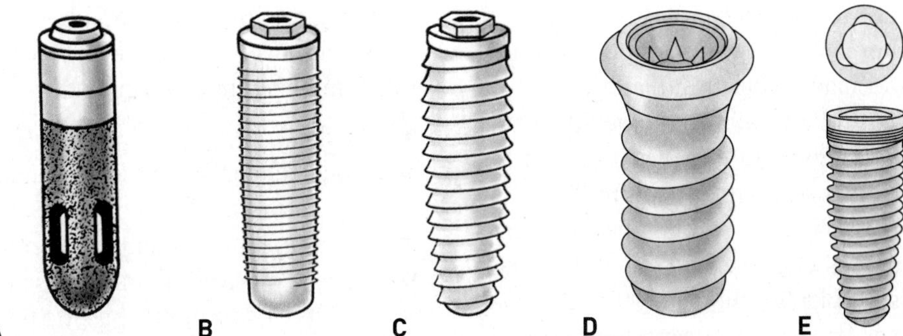

Figure 31-4 Endosseous Root Form Implants. **A:** Cylinder type. **B** and **C:** Screw types (external hex). **D:** Screw type, tissue level, internal hex. **E:** Screw type, bone level, internal hex.

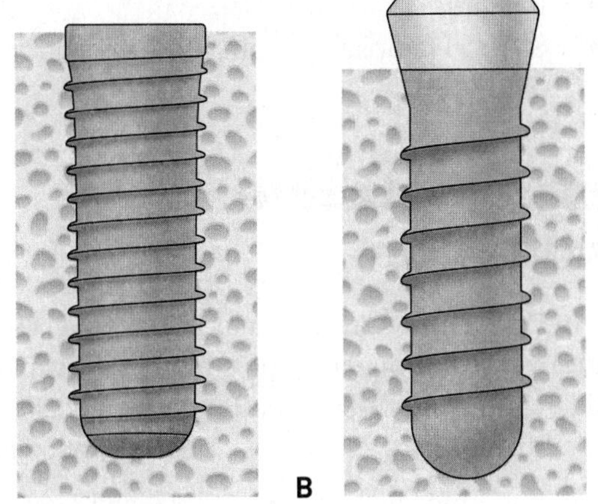

Figure 31-5 Endosseous Implant Types. **A:** Bone level. **B:** Tissue level.

- The endosseous implant may be placed so it emerges into the oral cavity at the bone level or tissue level (see **Figure 31-5**).

B. Description

- Material: Primarily sandblasted and acid-etched titanium or titanium alloy (Ti-6Al-4V).
- May be placed in one or two phases[13]:
  - Immediate implant placement: The implant is placed immediately following extraction of the tooth. This approach has a lower survival rate versus a two-phase delayed implant approach.
  - Two-phase implant placement: After tooth extraction, the site is allowed to heal prior to placement of the implant fixture and left covered by a periodontal flap for several months while the implant integrates with the bone. In a second stage of the surgical procedure, the abutment post is exposed. Placement of the crown or prosthesis follows.
- **Figure 31-6** illustrates the parts of an endosseous implant and the surrounding biologic tissues.

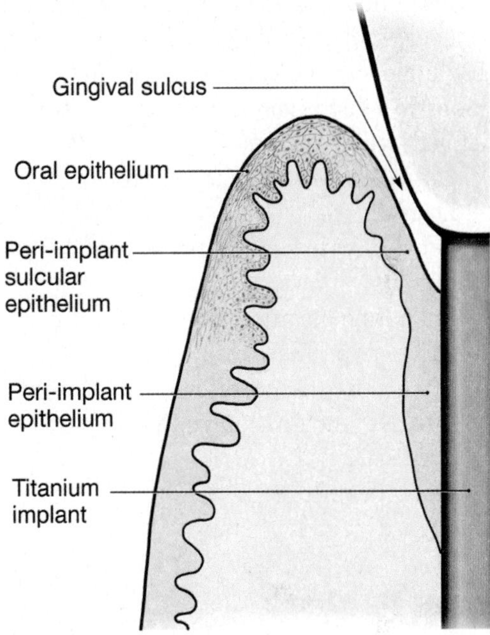

Figure 31-6 Parts of an Endosseous Implant. The crown, abutment, and implant are shown in relation to the surrounding bone and soft tissues.

Patient Selection

Patient selection depends on key factors that may impact osseointegration of the dental implant and success of treatment. These factors include primarily systemic health, condition of the jaws, and other local factors.[14]

I. Systemic Health

- Medical history: Careful review of the medical history and conditions is crucial to implant survival. Conditions that impact dental implant success include[14]:
  - Tobacco may adversely affect wound healing, and jeopardize the success of dental implants and bone health.[15] Tobacco cessation should be addressed (see Chapter 32).

- Alcohol abuse use may cause changes in alveolar bone healing impacting osseointegration and may result in implant failure.
- Poorly controlled diabetes mellitus impacts osseointegration and increases risk for peri-implantitis and implant failure.[16]
- Osteoporosis may have some impact on bone healing and osseointegration, but of greater concern is the bisphosphonate medication that patients may be taking to treat osteoporosis.
- Patients using anticoagulant medications require consultation with the primary care provider to evaluate suitability for a dental implant.
- Immunosuppressant therapy may also negatively impact healing.

- Absolute contraindications: There are a few conditions in which dental implants are not recommended, which include[14]:
  - Untreated periodontal disease
  - Liver disease.
  - Renal disease such as renal insufficiency and uremia.
  - Endocrine disorders such as hyperthyroidism and hypopituitarism.
  - Connective tissue disease and autoimmune diseases, such as lupus, that impact connective tissue.
  - Blood disorders.
  - High-dose radiotherapy.

II. Local Factors

Local factors include history and presence of oral disease along with status of oral soft and hard tissue in the area for the dental implant.[14]

- Periodontal disease
  - Presence of periodontal pathogens is a risk factor for development of peri-implantitis.
  - Previous untreated or uncontrolled periodontitis.
- Patient's compliance and ability to maintain a high level of oral self-care.
- Soft-tissue architecture, including tissue height and adequate attached gingiva.
- Architecture of the implant site, including bone volume, soft tissue, and root proximity of surrounding teeth.

Evaluation for Implant Placement

Implant therapy typically requires collaboration of a team, which may include the dentist or specialist placing the implant, general dentist or prosthodontist restoring the implant, dental hygienist, dental laboratory technician, and patient. Prior to placement, the following need to be evaluated[17]:

- Medical and psychological evaluation.
- Comprehensive dental examination.
  - Periodontal and restorative status of all teeth.
- Assessment of patient expectations of outcomes.
- Patient motivation and oral self-care abilities.
- Habits or conditions placing the patient at risk for implant failure, such as alcohol abuse, periodontal disease.
- Preparation of diagnostic aids:
  - Diagnostic models or casts.
  - Imaging.
  - Surgical template or computer-guided implant placement.

Postrestorative Evaluation

Once the implant is fully integrated in the bone and restorative work is complete, a postrestorative evaluation is made to establish a baseline for maintenance. Periodic evaluation of the implant includes the following[17]:

- Radiographic appearance of implant and surrounding alveolar bone.
- Occlusal evaluation including assessment of implant and/or crown mobility.
- Peri-implant tissue health: No inflammation, no calculus or biofilm, and no suppuration or bleeding.
- Peri-implant probing: Initial data serve as baseline for comparison during the maintenance phase.[18]
  - The seventh European Workshop of Periodontology consensus report and 2017 World Workshop on the Classification of Periodontal and Peri-Implant Diseases and Conditions indicates probing of implants is necessary to assess and monitor peri-implant health.[18,19]
  - Use very light pressure or force to gently probe (approximately 0.25 N) the implant. Remember the PIE–titanium interface is weaker and less resistant to bacterial invasion and penetration of the periodontal probe.[7]
  - Peri-implant pocket depths should be less than 5 mm and may not indicate pathology in the absence of bleeding or suppuration.[8,19]
  - Record presence of bleeding on probing, suppuration, and pocket depth.
- Sufficiency of patient's oral self-care.
- Patient comfort.

Peri-Implant Preventive Care

A key requirement for implant success is the disease control program for the tissue surrounding the implant. Failure of dental implants is associated with increased biofilm accumulation, so meticulous daily oral self-care is essential for implant success.[20,21]

I. Care of the Natural Teeth

- Periodontal disease is a risk factor for peri-implantitis and implant failure and must be controlled prior to implant placement.[22,23]
- After the placement of the implants, the maintenance program emphasizes care of the natural teeth and tissues as well as the peri-implant tissues.[21]

II. Implant Biofilm

- Although the biofilm formation process on implant surfaces is similar to that of teeth, the characteristics of the implant surface may also impact the amount and composition of the biofilm.[23]
- The oral microbiome of an implant may be more diverse when compared to natural teeth and continues to be studied.[24]
- The development of peri-implant disease is closely related to the host response to the microbiome composition and if the implant prosthesis is cleansable.
    - Host response is impacted by smoking, environmental factors, and the patient's general status.[23]

III. Planning the Oral Disease Control Program

A. Relation to Treatment

Supervision of a patient's oral hygiene and oral self-care regimen begins before the surgical phase for implant placement and carries on throughout the treatment phases.

B. Types of Prostheses

- Implant-supported **prostheses** may be partial, complete, fixed, removable, or single-tooth replacements. (See Chapter 30 for care instructions.)
- Prostheses may be removable or fixed (screwed or cemented into place).

C. Monitoring Prostheses Fit

- Regular dental examinations are recommended to monitor implant-supported restorations and prostheses and adjust or repair as needed.[21]
- Instruct and demonstrate to the patient how to monitor the fit of the implant prosthesis.

IV. Maintenance of Implant-Supported Restorations

- Regular professional maintenance is required. Guidelines suggest at least a 6-month interval, but this may need to be more frequent dependent upon the patient's needs.[21]
- Each patient needs an individualized plan to effectively manage dental biofilm.
- Choose instruments and oral self-care aids compatible with the material and type of implant.
- Toothbrushes
    - Select either a manual or a powered toothbrush with smooth, soft, and end-rounded filaments to prevent damage to the titanium and peri-implant tissue.
- Interdental care
    - Interdental brushes with nylon-coated wires work well to clean embrasure spaces and areas around implant-supported restorations. (See Chapter 27.)
    - A floss threader can be used to position dental floss around an abutment and under a fixed prosthesis. (See Chapter 30.)
    - Clinical practice guidelines from the American College of Prosthodontists also suggest the option of a water flosser or air flosser.[20] However, the research on use of the water flosser is industry-supported, which introduces the chance of bias, so further independent research is needed.[25]
    - The end tufted brush with soft filaments is used on distal surfaces of terminal teeth or in lingual and palatal embrasure spaces. (See Chapter 27.)

V. Antimicrobial Use

A. Toothpaste

- To prevent caries in natural teeth, a fluoride toothpaste is recommended.

B. Mouthrinse

- Use of chlorhexidine gluconate is recommended short term to manage inflammation of soft tissues around implants.[20,21]
- However, irrigation with chlorhexidine was more effective at reducing biofilm and reducing bleeding than use as a mouthrinse.[26]

- Essential oil mouthrinse such as Listerine as an adjunct to mechanical biofilm removal resulted in reductions in plaque and marginal peri-implant bleeding.[26]

VI. Fluoride Measures for Dental Caries Control

- Patients with natural teeth and multiple or complex restorations should be advised to use a prescription fluoride such as a 5000-ppm sodium fluoride gel or toothpaste.[21]
- Avoid acidulated fluoride preparations due to possible etching effects on the implant surface.

Continuing Care

Periodic care for professional maintenance and monitoring is scheduled according to the complexity of the restoration or prosthetic superstructure and the patient's ability to perform adequate oral self-care.[21]

I. Basic Criteria for Implant Success

- The long-term success of an implant is assessed during dental examinations at least every 6 months.[21]
- A successful implant meets the following criteria[27]:
  - No visible inflammation, pink as opposed to red, no tissue swelling, tissues appear to be firm compared to soft and loose.[19]
  - No pain or tenderness reported by the patient.
  - No mobility of the implant(s).
  - Radiograph: Less than 2-mm radiographic bone loss from initial surgery.[19]
  - No bleeding, suppuration, or increased depths beyond baseline on gentle probing with a plastic probe (**Figure 31-7**).
  - No movement or loose components in the prosthesis; check for cracks, fractures, and missing or unsecured screws by close visual inspection while applying coronally directed force to superstructure using a rigid single-ended instrument such as a mirror handle.

II. Frequency of Appointments

- When the original teeth were lost due to inadequate daily biofilm control by the patient, a more intense program of education and monitoring may be needed.

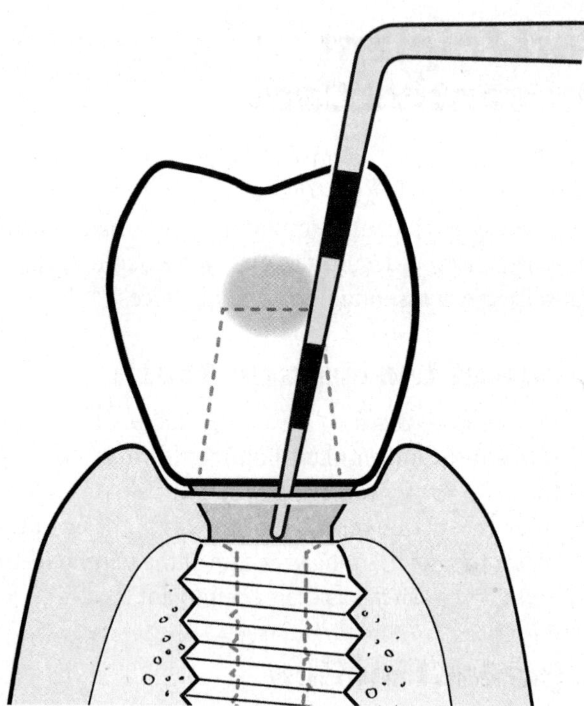

Figure 31-7 Probing an Implant. Using a probe, probe with gentle pressure to assess pocket depth and bleeding on probing.

- Professional maintenance at least every 6 months based on individual needs is recommended.[21]

III. The Continuing Care Appointment

Once osseointegration has been achieved, maintenance of the soft tissues to prevent peri-implantitis is essential to minimize risk for implant failure.[17,20,21,26,28]

A. Health History Review, Vital Signs, and Intraoral/Extraoral Examination

- Basic review questions can reveal the present state of health, recent illnesses, changes in medications, and other current information.
- Comparisons with previous records permit assessment of vital signs and extraoral/intraoral observations.

B. Selective Radiographs

- A standardized procedure using a film placement device and a paralleling technique is recommended to allow comparison of marginal bone level changes from the original level.
- Remodeling of bone of up to 1.5 mm typically occurs in the first year and 0.2 mm annually thereafter.[8,27]

- Cone-beam computed tomography is used to aid evaluation of the alveolar bone and other surrounding structures for implant placement.

C. Periodontal Assessment

- Peri-implant tissue: Visual examination to assess changes in color, size, shape, and consistency.
- Dental biofilm
  - Use a disclosing solution to identify biofilm and to aid in patient education.
  - Utilize a plaque index to monitor biofilm to allow for comparison between maintenance appointments.[29]
  - Assess biofilm accumulation patterns to aid in patient education.
- Probing
  - A plastic probe is suggested.[29]
  - Light pressure of 0.15–0.25 N is recommended.[7,18]
  - Pressure-sensitive probes are available to guard against excess insertion pressure.
  - Pocket depths should be compared with baseline measurements.[17] Probing depths more than 6 mm with bleeding on probing are indicators of peri-implantitis.[18-20,28]
  - Bleeding on probing is recorded as it is an indication of peri-implantitis.[17-19,29]
  - Suppuration or exudate is also an indicator of implant disease.[17-19,29]
- Mobility determination
  - Mobility is assessed.[29]
  - Inform the dentist and/or implant surgeon immediately of noticeable mobility.
- Recession
  - Measure and document changes in location of the gingival margin in relation to the restoration margins.[29]
- Calculus
  - Mineralized deposits usually are not extensive, hard, or firmly attached to implant abutments or other protruding parts.
  - Semisoft, partially mineralized deposits can be effectively removed with floss or instruments designed for use on implants.
- Residual cement
  - When the implant crown is permanently cemented to the abutment, residual cement is a significant risk factor for iatrogenic peri-implant disease.[28,30,31]
  - Cement residue goes largely undetected on postrestorative radiographs.
  - Be alert to clinical signs of inflammation, especially idiopathic change in an otherwise stable implant, since cement-associated peri-implantitis may not appear for many years following implant restoration.
  - Typically cement cannot be removed with nonsurgical treatment, so these patients need to be referred back to the surgeon who placed the implant for further evaluation and treatment.[29]

D. Dental Biofilm Control

- Biofilm control is essential for long-term implant success, so this must be continuously reinforced with the patient.[18,29]
- Review the patient's current oral self-care regimens and identify areas needing improvement based on biofilm, pocket depth increases, and bleeding points.
- The patient should demonstrate oral self-care techniques and work with the clinician to refine techniques to improve effective biofilm removal.

E. Instrumentation

- Biofilm removal: Soft deposits are removed from the implant abutment with dental floss or implant instrument.
  - Air polishing with subgingival powder (glycine or erythritol) has been shown to be safe and effective in debriding the implant surface of dental biofilm and is effective in treating sites of mucositis.[32,33]
- Calculus removal: Specialized implant-specific instruments, typically made of plastic, are indicated for hard deposits remaining after soft deposit removal.[29]
  - Current implant-specific instruments mimic traditional universal curettes and sickle scalers in design.
  - Implant-specific plastic-covered ultrasonic tips and inserts are available for peri-implant debridement. Use low power when instrumenting implant abutments with an ultrasonic device with tips designed to be safe around abutments.[29]
- Stain removal: Unless it is necessary for esthetics, stain removal is not included routinely.
  - When selective stain removal with a rubber cup is indicated, only a nonabrasive agent is used and applied gently to avoid damaging the surface.

    - Tin oxide or nonabrasive toothpaste may be suitable for polishing agents.
- Professional subgingival irrigation: The use of 0.12% chlorhexidine after professional instrumentation may be an alternative treatment when peri-implantitis has been identified. Irrigation with chlorhexidine gluconate has been shown to be a safe procedure around implants.[20,21,26]

Classification of Peri-Implant Disease

There are two basic peri-implant diseases: **peri-implant mucositis** and **peri-implantitis**.[19]

I. Peri-Implant Mucositis

Peri-implant mucositis is reversible. A recent meta-analysis found the prevalence of peri-implant mucositis to be approximately 30%.[34]

A. Diagnostic Criteria

The diagnostic criteria for peri-implant mucositis have not been universally agreed upon, but the most common signs include the following[18,35]:

- An inflammatory lesion in the mucosa similar to gingivitis.
- Bleeding and/or suppuration on gentle probing.
- An increase in probing depth (due to tissue inflammation and not bone loss).
- No bone loss has occurred.

B. Treatment

- Prevention and management of peri-implant mucositis includes patient compliance with meticulous biofilm removal daily with either a manual toothbrush or a powered toothbrush and appropriate interdental aids. Regular reinforcement for oral self-care is an important part of managing peri-implant disease.
- Use of antimicrobial toothpaste.[21]
- Short-term daily 0.12% chlorhexidine gluconate mouthrinse for home use and chlorhexidine gel application in the dental office (available in some countries).[21]
- Professional peri-implant debridement with appropriate hand instruments (implant-safe scalers) and/or powered instruments such as a subgingival air-polishing system.[20,32]
- Regular professional care may be required at short intervals such as 3–4 months to resolve the mucositis.[35]

II. Peri-Implantitis

The prevalence of peri-implantitis at the implant level varies in the literature from approximately 9% to 13%.[36]

A. Diagnostic Criteria[18,19]

- Evidence of gingival inflammation in peri-implant tissues.
- Bleeding on gentle probing and exudate or suppuration is common.
- Increase in probing depths beyond baseline after implant healing, but probing depths more than 6 mm with bleeding on probing are at greater risk for progression of the peri-implantitis.
- Crestal bone loss on radiographs, and/or increasing probing depths compared to baseline.
- If no initial radiographs, or initial probing depths are available, greater than or equal to 6 mm and/or probing depths with bleeding.

B. Treatment

- Nonsurgical treatment[37]:
    - Biofilm control daily by the patient is critical.
    - Professional debridement of biofilm and calculus from the implant surface.
    - Adjunctive antimicrobials such as chlorhexidine may be used in conjunction with debridement.
- Surgical treatment[37]:
    - Guided bone regeneration.
- New treatment approaches include[37]:
    - Laser-assisted nonsurgical treatment using carbon dioxide and diode lasers to decontaminate the implant surface have shown some positive outcomes, but more research is recommended.
    - Photodynamic therapy has also shown positive results, but more research is needed.

Documentation

The implant therapy team must collaborate when planning, treating, and maintaining an implant. For documenting appointments for a patient with a dental implant, the following factors are recorded in the progress note:

- Consultation before implant treatment plan:
    - Patient advised of all options to replace missing tooth/teeth.
    - Patient understands surgical, prosthetic, and maintenance phases of dental implant therapy.
    - Expected benefits, principal risks, and potential complications of dental implant therapy have been fully explained.

- Alternatives to suggested dental implant treatment have been outlined.
- The patient is ready to take responsibility for thorough daily oral self-care to manage biofilm.
- The need for ongoing professional maintenance appointments has been fully explained to patient.

- Examination as follows includes:
  - Verify dental implant locations with chart and current radiographs.
  - Peri-implant tissue tone, color, and texture.
  - Presence of inflammation: note erythema, edema, and/or exudate.
  - Probe implant with gentle pressure.
  - Assess implant mobility.
  - Take a radiograph if signs of peri-implant disease are present, and/or every 12 months to look for changes in bone level.
  - Prosthesis integrity and stability.
  - Note quantity and location of biofilm and calculus accumulations.
- Carefully document continuing care procedures.
- An example of a progress note appears in **Box 31-1**.

Box 31-1 Example Documentation: Patient with Implants

- **S**—Patient presents for continuing care 3 months following final seating of implant prosthesis for tooth #3. No chief complaint or concerns.
- **O**—Intraoral/extraoral examination within normal limits. Peri-implant soft tissue appears healthy with no bleeding. Biofilm score of less than 10%. One periapical radiograph within normal limits; no mobility evident of implant fixture or prosthesis; no biofilm or calculus accumulation on tooth #3.
- **A**—Periapical implant appears healthy and well-integrated.
- **P**—Treatment: Reinforce implant cleaning procedures with floss, periodontal debridement with implant safe instruments. Next: Three-month continuing care. Copy report to surgeon and general dentist.

Signed: ______________________, RDH
Date: ______________

Factors to Teach the Patient

- How dental implants preserve and maintain surrounding bone.
- How to care for implants; special needs related to the titanium surfaces.
- How the health of the periodontal tissues and the duration of the implants and prostheses depend on meticulous daily self-care by the patient.
- The role of biofilm in peri-implant diseases.
- How a history of periodontitis may place a patient at increased risk for peri-implantitis.
- The complexity and dedication needed to maintain thorough daily oral self-care of complex restorations often associated with implant therapy.
- Why frequent, ongoing professional maintenance care and annual radiographs to document bone height around implants are necessary.
- When to call the office to address potential or suspected problems around an implant, for example, peri-implant bleeding, soreness, or pain.

References

1. Misch DE.*Contemporary Implant Dentistry*. 3rd ed. St. Louis, MO: Mosby; 2008.
2. Huiskes R, Ruimerman R, Van Lenthe GH, Janssen JD. Effects of mechanical forces on maintenance and adaptation of form in trabecular bone. *Nature*. 2000;405(6787):704-706.
3. Milinkovic I, Cordaro L. Are there specific indications for the different alveolar bone augmentation procedures for implant placement? A systematic review. *Int J Oral Maxillofac Surg*. 2014;43(5):606-625.
4. Stern A, Green J. Sinus lift procedures: an overview of current techniques. *Dent Clin North Am*. 2012;56(1):219-233.
5. Insua A, Monje A, Wang HL, Miron RJ. Basis of bone metabolism around dental implants during osseointegration and peri-implant bone loss. *J Biomed Mater Res A*. 2017;105(7): 2075-2089.
6. Atsuta I, Ayukawa Y, Kondo R, et al. Soft tissue sealing around dental implants based on histological interpretation. *J Prosthodont Res*. 2016;60(1):3-11.
7. Gerber JA, Tan WC, Balmer TE, Salvi GE, Lang NP. Bleeding on probing and pocket probing depth in relation to probing pressure and mucosal health around oral implants. *Clin Oral Implants Res*. 2009;20(1):75-78.

8. Coli P, Christiaens V, Sennerby L, Bruyn H. Reliability of periodontal diagnostic tools for monitoring peri-implant health and disease. *Periodontol 2000*. 2017;73(1):203-217.
9. Esposito M, Ardebili Y, Worthington HV. Interventions for replacing missing teeth: different types of dental implants. *Cochrane Database Syst Rev*. 2014;(7):CD003815.
10. Homoly PA. The restorative and surgical technique for the full maxillary subperiosteal implant. *J Am Dent Assoc*. 1990;121(3):404-407.
11. Cranin AN, Sher J, Schilb TP. The transosteal implant: a 17-year review and report. *J Prosthet Dent*. 1986;55(6):709-718.
12. Niznick GA. Endosseous dental implant. *Google Patents*; 2006.
13. Mello CC, Lemos CAA, Verri FR, et al. Immediate implant placement into fresh extraction sockets versus delayed implants into healed sockets: a systematic review and meta-analysis. *Int J Oral Maxillofac Surg*. 2017;46(9):1162-1177.
14. Bryington M, De Kok IJ, Thalji G, Cooper LF. Patient selection and treatment planning for implant restorations. *Dent Clin North Am*. 2014;58(1):193-206.
15. Strietzel FP, Reichart PA, Kale A, et al. Smoking interferes with the prognosis of dental implant treatment: a systematic review and meta-analysis. *J Clin Periodontol*. 2007;34(6):523-544.
16. Naujokat H, Kunzendorf B, Wiltfang J. Dental implants and diabetes mellitus: a systematic review. *Int J Implant Dent*. 2016;2(1):5.
17. American Academy of Pediatrics. Periodontology Parameter on placement and management of the dental implant. *J Periodontol*. 2000;71(5 suppl):870-872.
18. Lang NP, Berglundh T. Peri-implant diseases: where are we now?—Consensus of the Seventh European Workshop on Periodontology. *J Clin Periodontol*. 2011;38(suppl 11): 178-181.
19. Renvert S, Persson GR, Pirih FQ, Camargo PM. Peri-implant health, peri-implant mucositis, and peri-implantitis: case definitions and diagnostic considerations. *J Periodontol*. 2018;89(suppl 1):S304-S312.
20. Bidra AS, Daubert DM, Garcia LT, et al. A systematic review of recall regimen and maintenance regimen of patients with dental restorations. Part 2: implant-borne restorations. *J Prosthodont*. 2016;25(suppl 1):S16-S31.
21. Bidra AS, Daubert DM, Garcia LT, et al. Clinical practice guidelines for recall and maintenance of patients with tooth-borne and implant-borne dental restorations. *J Am Dent Assoc*. 2016;147(1):67-74.
22. Sgolastra F, Petrucci A, Severino M, Gatto R, Monaco A. Periodontitis, implant loss and peri-implantitis. A meta-analysis. *Clin Oral Implants Res*. 2015;26(4):e8-16.
23. Stacchi C, Berton F, Perinetti G, et al. Risk factors for peri-implantitis: effect of history of periodontal disease and smoking habits. A systematic review and meta-analysis. *J Oral Maxillofac Res*. 2016;7(3):e3.
24. Pokrowiecki R, Mielczarek A, Zaręba T, Tyski S. Oral microbiome and peri-implant diseases: where are we now? *Ther Clin Risk Manag*. 2017;13:1529-1542.
25. Qaqish JG, Schuller R. Efficacy of two interdental cleaning devices on clinical signs of inflammation: a four-week randomized controlled trial. *J Clin Dent*. 2015;26:55-60.
26. Grusovin MG, Coulthard P, Worthington HV, George P, Esposito M. Interventions for replacing missing teeth: maintaining and recovering soft tissue health around dental implants. *Cochrane Database Syst Rev*. 2010(8):CD003069.
27. Misch CE, Perel ML, Wang HL, et al. Implant success, survival, and failure: the International Congress of Oral Implantologists (ICOI) Pisa Consensus Conference. *Implant Dent*. 2008;17(1):5-15.
28. Schwarz F, Derks J, Monje A, Wang HL. Peri-implantitis. *J Clin Periodontol*. 2018;45(suppl 20):S246-S266.
29. Todescan S, Lavigne S, Kelekis-Cholakis A. Guidance for the maintenance care of dental implants: clinical review. *J Can Dent Assoc*. 2012;78:c107.
30. Quaranta A, Lim ZW, Tang J, Perrotti V, Leichter J. The impact of residual subgingival cement on biological complications around dental implants: a systematic review. *Implant Dent*. 2017;26(3):465-474.
31. Staubli N, Walter C, Schmidt JC, Weiger R, Zitzmann NU. Excess cement and the risk of peri-implant disease—a systematic review. *Clin Oral Implants Res*. 2017;28(10):1278-1290.
32. Schwarz F, Becker K, Renvert S. Efficacy of air polishing for the non-surgical treatment of peri-implant diseases: a systematic review. *J Clin Periodontol*. 2015;42(10):951-959.
33. Shrivastava D, Natoli V, Srivastava KC, et al. Novel approach to dental biofilm management through Guided Biofilm Therapy (GBT): a review. *Microorganisms*. 2021;9(9):1966.
34. Lee C-T, Huang Y-W, Zhu L, Weltman R. Prevalences of peri-implantitis and peri-implant mucositis: systematic review and meta-analysis. *J Dent*. 2017;62:1-12.
35. Jepsen S, Berglundh T, Genco R, et al. Primary prevention of peri-implantitis: managing peri-implant mucositis. *J Clin Periodontol*. 2015;42(suppl 16):S152-S157.
36. Rakic M, Galindo-Moreno P, Monje A, et al. How frequent does peri-implantitis occur? A systematic review and meta-analysis. *Clin Oral Investig*. 2018;22(4):1805-1816.
37. Romanos GE, Javed F, Delgado-Ruiz RA, Calvo-Guirado JL. Peri-implant diseases: a review of treatment interventions. *Dent Clin North Am*. 2015;59(1):157-178.

CHAPTER 32

The Patient with Nicotine Use Disorders

Kelley Martell, RDH, BSDH, MSDH

CHAPTER OUTLINE

HEALTH HAZARDS AND CURRENT TRENDS

COMPONENTS OF NICOTINE PRODUCTS AND TOBACCO SMOKE

METABOLISM OF NICOTINE

I. Nicotine from Smoking

ALTERNATIVE TOBACCO PRODUCTS

I. Electronic Nicotine Delivery Systems (ENDS)
II. Smokeless Tobacco
III. Waterpipe/Tobacco Smoking

SYSTEMIC EFFECTS

I. Cardiovascular Diseases
II. Pulmonary Conditions
III. Cancer
IV. Tobacco and Use of Other Drugs

ENVIRONMENTAL TOBACCO SMOKE

I. Cardiovascular Effects
II. Toxicity
III. Cardiovascular Effects

PRENATAL AND CHILDREN

I. In Utero
II. Infancy
III. Young Children

ORAL MANIFESTATIONS OF TOBACCO AND NICOTINE USE

TOBACCO AND PERIODONTAL INFECTIONS

I. Effects on the Periodontal Tissues
II. Mechanisms of Periodontal Destruction
III. Response to Treatment

NICOTINE ADDICTION

I. Tolerance
II. Dependence
III. Addiction
IV. Withdrawal

TREATMENT

I. Reasons for Quitting
II. Self-Help Interventions
III. Assisted Strategies

PHARMACOTHERAPIES USED FOR TREATMENT OF NICOTINE ADDICTION

I. Objectives and Rationale
II. Considerations
III. Contraindications
IV. Nicotine Replacement Therapy

NICOTINE-FREE THERAPY

I. Bupropion SR
II. Varenicline Tartrate
III. Combination Therapies
IV. Second-Line Medications
V. Alternative Cessation Therapies

DENTAL HYGIENE CARE FOR THE PATIENT WHO USES NICOTINE

ASSESSMENT

I. Patient History
II. Extraoral Examination
III. Intraoral Examination

LEARNING OBJECTIVES

After studying this chapter, the student will be able to:

1. Recognize the health hazards associated with nicotine use.
2. Identify components of conventional tobacco and alternative nicotine products.
3. Explain various mechanisms for nicotine delivery.
4. Describe the metabolism of nicotine.
5. Recognize the oral manifestations of nicotine use.
6. Recognize the effects of environmental tobacco smoke (ETS).
7. Assess and develop a dental hygiene care plan for the patient who uses nicotine.
8. Recognize protocols for developing a nicotine cessation program.
9. Identify the pharmacotherapies and behavioral therapies used for treatment of nicotine addiction.

The oral effects associated with nicotine use are well documented and show there is no safe form that to consume.[1-3] Information provided by oral health professionals has been shown to have a powerful influence on patients' intentions to stop or not begin using nicotine products.[4,5] Dental and dental hygiene professionals are in an ideal position and have a responsibility to provide patients who use nicotine products with the most up-to-date information regarding cessation. Engagement in this important dialogue with patients in the clinical dental setting can help to ensure better oral and overall health outcomes for individuals struggling with nicotine addiction.[6]

Health Hazards and Current Trends

Nicotine is toxic to humans. Nicotine use is the single greatest preventable cause of disease and premature death in the world.[1]

- Approximately 50 million Americans engage in some form of tobacco usage.[7-10] This includes combustible tobacco products, electronic nicotine delivery systems (ENDS), cigars, cigarillos, regular pipes, waterpipes (hookahs), and smokeless tobacco.[7-10]
- Although cigarette smoking has declined in the past few years, it remains the most commonly used nicotine product, followed closely by ENDS.[8,9,11] The use of multiple forms of tobacco products is another growing trend, especially among noncigarette users, known as polytobacco use.[11-14]
- ENDS products are most frequently used in combination with conventional cigarettes.[11]
- As years of use accumulate, so do the systemic and oral health effects of all forms of nicotine.[1,15]
- Life expectancy of nicotine users is shortened by an average of 10–14 years.[1]
- Offspring of smokers are more likely to become smokers.[1] Approximately 4.9 million middle- and high school–aged youth use tobacco products.[16]
- Approximately 40% of high school students have reported electronic cigarette use by the senior year.[17]
- Approximately 16 million Americans suffer from a disease caused by smoking.[1,10]
- Ninety percent of deaths from lung cancer are attributed to smoking.[10]
- Annual U.S. healthcare costs to treat nicotine-related illness exceed $170 billion.[18]

- The majority of cigarette smokers (68%) desire to quit smoking but do not receive consistent cessation support from their healthcare provider.[19]

Components of Nicotine Products and Tobacco Smoke

- **Nicotine** is the chief psychoactive ingredient in tobacco that causes addiction.[20,21]
- Nicotine is considered toxic and 60 mg can cause fatality.[20]
- Cigarette smoke is a complex mixture containing an estimated 7,357 chemical compounds.[15]
- Over 90 of the chemicals and chemical compounds in nicotine products and tobacco smoke are identified by the Food and Drug Administration (FDA) as being unsafe or having unsafe potential.[21]
- These chemicals or chemical compounds can be categorized as a **carcinogen** (cancer-causing), respiratory toxicant, cardiovascular toxicant, reproductive or developmental intoxicant, addictive, or combination of these agents.[21,22]
- The following chemical components in tobacco products have the greatest potential for harmful systemic effects: 1,3-butadiene (cancer); acrolein and acetaldehyde (respiratory); and cyanide, arsenic, and cresols (cardiovascular).[1,22]
- **Table 32-1** lists differences in the quantity of nicotine delivered by tobacco products: the amount and rate at which a nicotine-containing product delivers nicotine to the bloodstream is a determinant of its addiction potential.[21,23]

Table 32-1 Nicotine Levels of Various Tobacco Products[21,23,24]

Products	Amount of Nicotine Delivery
Cigarette	0.7–2.0 mg
Electronic Cigarette (ENDS)	40 mg per pod (JUUL)
Box Mod Vape Device	3–36 mg/mL
Cigars	13–15 mg
Bidi	1.5–4.1 mg
Moist snuff	0.01–7.8 mg/g
Hookah smoking (45 min–1 hr)	Equivalent to inhaling 100–200 times the volume of smoke from one cigarette

Metabolism of Nicotine

- Absorption of nicotine occurs through most of the body's membranes. It is most readily absorbed through lung tissues, but also well absorbed through skin, oral and buccal mucosa; nasal membranes; and the gastrointestinal tract.[20,25]
- Delivery method affects the way nicotine is absorbed into the body. For example, inhaled tobacco is efficiently absorbed via the membranes in the lung.[20]
- Another factor affecting absorption is the pH level of the product. The more basic the medium, the easier the absorption.[15]
- Several factors influence absorption from smoked tobacco (cigarettes, pipes, and cigars), as identified in **Figure 32-1**. Regardless of the type of tobacco used, nicotine is primarily metabolized by the liver and excreted in the urine.[20,25]

I. Nicotine from Smoking

A. Absorption: Lungs

- Nicotine enters the lungs and quickly passes into arterial circulation by way of blood vessels lining the sacs of the bronchi.[25]

B. Distribution

- To the brain: Nicotine is delivered efficiently to the brain by the bloodstream in 20 seconds or less.[25]
- Following the onset of nicotine use, peak plasma concentration of nicotine in the brain occurs in approximately 5 minutes.[20]
- Dissemination: Nicotine is spread to nearly all body tissues.[20]
- Changes in the liver: Nicotine is metabolized in the liver primarily as **cotinine**.[25]
    - Cotinine concentrations in the blood, urine, hair, and saliva are used to assess[25]:
        - Whether a person uses nicotine products.
        - The extent of use.
        - The level of exposure of nonsmokers to passive or environmental smoke.

Alternative Nicotine-Containing Products

Alternative tobacco products (**ATPs**) are products that deliver nicotine via alternative methods other than cigarettes, such as ENDS (e-cigarettes, vape pens),

CENTER FOR TOBACCO PRODUCTS

How a Cigarette Is Engineered

The design and content of cigarettes continue to make them attractive, addictive, and deadly.[1] Every day, more than 1,300 people in the United States die because of cigarette use.[2]

Filter [3,4,5]

- Typically made from bundles of thin, hair-like fibers.
- Designed to trap smoke, but only stops a small portion of the smoke from being inhaled.
- The filter (and ventilation holes) in most cigarettes may lead smokers to inhale more deeply, pulling dangerous chemicals farther into their lungs.

Tipping paper [6]

- Wraps around the filter, connecting it to the rest of the cigarette.
- **Ventilation holes**, if unblocked, dilute inhaled smoke with air.
- Manufacturers have chosen to place the ventilation holes where they are. The holes are largely ineffective. Because of their location, most smokers unknowingly block them with their fingers or lips.

Cigarette paper [3]

- Holds the tobacco filler.
- Manufacturers add chemicals to the paper to control how fast the cigarette burns.
- Smokers inhale everything that is burned—the tobacco filler, the paper... everything.

Additives [10,11,12]

Manufacturers can **add hundreds of ingredients** to a cigarette to make smoking more appealing and to mask the harshness of smoke.

Certain **additives**, like sugars, can form cancer-causing chemicals when they are burned.

Sugar and flavor* additives can change the taste of smoke and make it easier to inhale, but no less harmful.

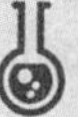

Ammonia and other **chemicals** added to tobacco may increase the absorption of nicotine, which is addictive.

Some additives are **bronchodilators** that could increase the amount of dangerous chemicals absorbed by the lungs.

Tobacco filler [7,8,9]

- Made up of chopped tobacco leaves, stems, reprocessed pieces, and scraps.
- Dangerous chemicals can form in and be deposited on tobacco during the processing of the tobacco leaves.
- Other dangerous chemicals are created when the tobacco filler is burned.

**In 2009, The Family Smoking Prevention and Tobacco Control Act banned characterizing flavors in cigarettes, except for tobacco and menthol flavors.*

FDA'S REGULATORY AUTHORITY: The FDA Center for Tobacco Products (CTP) has broad authority, via the Tobacco Control Act, to regulate the manufacturing, distribution, and marketing of tobacco products. To protect public health, CTP has the authority to regulate what ingredients tobacco manufacturers can put into their products.

(1) U.S. Department of Health and Human Services. *A Report of the Surgeon General: How Tobacco Smoke Causes Disease* (Fact Sheet). Atlanta, GA: U.S. Department of Health and Human Services, Centers for Disease Control and Prevention, National Center for Chronic Disease Prevention and Health Promotion, Office on Smoking and Health; 2010. **(2)** U.S. Department of Health and Human Services. *The Health Consequences of Smoking—50 Years of Progress: A Report of the Surgeon General.* Atlanta, GA: U.S. Department of Health and Human Services, Centers for Disease Control and Prevention, National Center for Chronic Disease Prevention and Health Promotion, Office on Smoking and Health; 2014. **(3)** Taylor MJ. The role of filter technology in reduced yield cigarettes. Filtrona. World Tobacco Exhibition Kunming. **(4)** Kiefer JE, Mumpower RC II. *Parameters That Affect the Pressure Drop and Efficiency of Cellulose Acetate Cigarette Filters.* Research Laboratories, Tennessee Eastman Company; 2004; Bates number: 81052204/2269. **(5)** U.S. Department of Health and Human Services. *Let's Make the Next Generation Tobacco-Free: Your Guide to the 50th Anniversary Surgeon General's Report on Smoking and Health* (Consumer Booklet). Atlanta, GA: U.S. Department of Health and Human Services, Centers for Disease Control and Prevention, National Center for Chronic Disease Prevention and Health Promotion, Office on Smoking and Health; 2014. **(6)** Browne CL. *The Design of Cigarettes.* 3rd ed. Charlotte, NC: C Filter Products Division, Hoechst Celanese Corporation; 1990. **(7)** Spears AW. Effect of manufacturing variables on cigarette smoke composition. *CORESTA Bulletin d'Information.* 1974;6:65-78. **(8)** Geiss O, Kotzias D. *Tobacco, Cigarettes, and Cigarette Smoke: An Overview.* European Commission, Directorate-General, Joint Research Centre; 2007. **(9)** Baker R. A review of pyrolysis studies to unravel reaction steps in burning tobacco. *Journal of Analytical and Applied Pyrolysis.* 1987;11:555-573. **(10)** U.S. Department of Health and Human Services. *How Tobacco Smoke Causes Disease: The Biology and Behavioral Basis for Smoking-Attributable Disease: A Report of the Surgeon General.* Atlanta, GA: U.S. Department of Health and Human Services, Centers for Disease Control and Prevention, National Center for Chronic Disease Prevention and Health Promotion, Office on Smoking and Health; 2010. **(11)** Rabinoff M, Caskey N, Rissling A, Park, C. Pharmacological and chemical effects of cigarette additives. *American Journal of Public Health.* 2007;97(11):1981-1991. **(12)** Talhout R, Opperhuizen A, Amsterdam J. Sugars as tobacco ingredient: Effects on mainstream smoke composition. *Food and Chemical Toxicology.* 2006;44(11):1789-1798.

Last Updated October 2016
CTP-62-P

www.fda.gov/tobacco  @FDATobacco 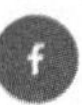 facebook.com/fda

Figure 32-1 Components of Mainstream Smoke and Factors Influencing Absorption by the Lungs

U.S. Food and Drug Administration. https://www.fda.gov/tobacco-products/products-ingredients-components/how-cigarette-engineered.

smokeless tobacco, waterpipes, cigars, and dissolvable and gel tobacco forms.

- ATPs contain nicotine and other harmful or potentially harmful constituents.[13]
- ATPs are not considered safe or a safe alternative to cigarette smoking and should not be utilized for nicotine cessation.[13,26]
- Evidence shows individuals who use an ATP are at higher risk of using other forms of tobacco.[13,14,26,]
- All ATP packages and advertisements require a warning statement regarding nicotine and addiction.[13,18]
- The FDA regulates the manufacturing, importing, packaging, labeling, advertising, and distribution of ATP-associated components, excluding accessories.[27]

I. Electronic Nicotine Delivery Systems (ENDS)

- Use of Electronic Nicotine Delivery Systems (ENDS) is also known as vaping.[28]
- ENDS are the second most popular nicotine product behind conventional tobacco cigarettes.[8,27,28]
- ENDS are battery-operated devices designed to heat and deliver aerosolized nicotine to its user.[28]
- ENDS do not contain tobacco but are composed of nicotine, propylene glycol, glycerin, flavoring agents (diacetyl), heavy metals (nickel and lead), and carbonyl compounds (formaldehyde and acrolein).[14,15,28]
- Using ENDS may lead youth and young adults to try conventional tobacco products, which are known to increase morbidity and mortality rates.[1,13,26,29]
- ENDS devices consist of a battery, heater, cartridge, and other parts (**Figure 32-2**). Variations in product design including resembling a cigarette, small fluid tank, or USB drive.[28,29]
- Puffing on the device activates the heating element, and the solution is then vaporized and inhaled through a mouthpiece.[28,29]
- Ingestion of the flavorant diacetyl has been linked to a condition known as "popcorn lung" or bronchiolitis obliterans.[30]
- Other adverse health effects from components such as solvents, flavorants, and toxicants when heated and aerosolized are unknown.[29]
- To date, the FDA has not approved the safety of ENDS, its use in NRT, or its use as an effective method of smoking cessation.[29,31,32]

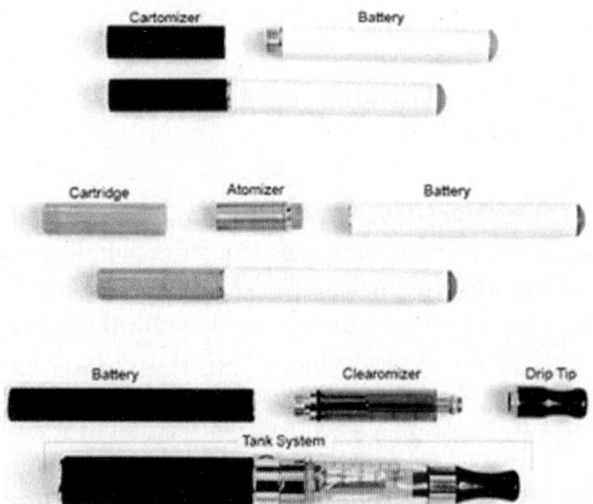

Figure 32-2 There Are a Number of Parts and Components in ENDS Products

U.S. Food and Drug Administration. https://www.fda.gov/tobacco-products/products-ingredients-components/e-cigarettes-vapes-and-other-electronic-nicotine-delivery-systems-ends.

- To understand health effects of the long-term use of ENDS, additional well-designed research is necessary.[15,21,25,28]

II. Smokeless Tobacco

Smokeless tobacco is the term applied to noncombustible tobacco products that are not smoked but placed in the mouth, typically between the cheek and gingiva or lower lip, gingiva, and mucosa.[33,34] Depending on the product, smokeless tobacco can be moist or dry and can be chewed, spit, or swallowed.[33]

- Snuff is a fire-cured, finely ground, or powdered tobacco sold in both dry and moist forms or bag-like pouches; not chewed, but a small amount ("pinch" or "quid") is placed and held between check and "gums."[33,34]
- Snuff can also be sniffed or inhaled into the nose.[33,34]
- Snus is moist snuff distributed in a prepackaged pouch and does not require spitting.[33,34]
- Similar to snuff, chewing (spit) tobacco is available in loose-leaf, twist/roll, and plug forms manufactured by air-drying tobacco leaves; it is held inside the cheek or lower lip and gingiva, and/or chewed.[33,34]
- The most harmful carcinogen found in smokeless tobacco is the tobacco-specific **nitrosamines** (TSNAs). These chemical compounds are usually formed during the growing, curing, fermenting, and aging of tobacco process.[34]

- Other cancer-causing substances found in smokeless tobacco include benzo(a)pyrene, formaldehyde, acetaldehyde, arsenic, nickel, cadmium, and polonium-210.[34]

A. Absorption: Oral Cavity

- Nicotine is directly absorbed through the oral mucous membranes.[25]
- Once smokeless tobacco is placed in the mouth, the amount of nicotine absorbed is three to four times the amount delivered by a cigarette.[15] Per day, a user may keep snuff in the mouth for approximately 11–14 hours.
- Nicotine concentration steadily increases with use and slowly declines over 2 hours and is at a negligible level within 24 hours.[25]
- Smokeless tobacco users experience nicotine blood plasma levels similar to the nicotine blood levels of smokers.[25]

B. Absorption: Intestinal

- Most tobacco juice produced by smokeless tobacco is spit out.[34]
- Juice that is intentionally and/or accidentally swallowed by the user is absorbed through the blood vessels lining the small intestine.[34]

III. Waterpipe Tobacco Smoking

A **waterpipe** is a device used to smoke tobacco, also known as hookah, shisha, and hubble-bubble (**Figure 32-3**).[35,36]

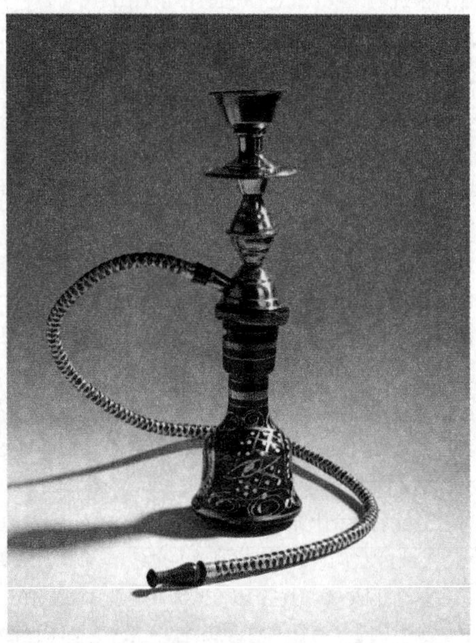

Figure 32-3 An Example of a Waterpipe or Hookah

- Tobacco used in the waterpipe is available in a variety of flavors.[36]
- Waterpipe smoking can lead to nicotine dependence and has similar health risks as smoking of cigarettes.[36,37]
- A waterpipe commonly has a head, body, water bowl, and a hose with a mouthpiece and is indirectly heated by charcoal.[37]
- Significant association with respiratory diseases, oral cancer, cardiovascular disease, lung cancer, delivering a low-birth-weight baby, metabolic syndrome, and mental health disorders.[38]

Systemic Effects of Nicotine

- The use of nicotine products influences every system of the body.[1] **Table 32-2** lists smoking-related conditions.
- The diseases that affect each system have consequences ranging from mild to deadly.[1]

I. Cardiovascular Diseases

- Smoking tobacco and consuming other nicotine-containing products contribute to 32% of all coronary heart disease deaths.[1] Nicotine products aggravate and accelerate the development of atherosclerosis and are a major risk factor for coronary heart disease, the leading cause of death for Americans.[1]

II. Pulmonary Conditions

- Smoking is the major cause of chronic obstructive pulmonary disease (COPD), including emphysema and chronic bronchitis.[1] More information on COPD is provided in Chapter 60.
- Emphysema slowly diminishes a person's ability to breathe due to the destruction of bronchial alveoli.[1,39]
- Chronic bronchitis is a condition in which the airways produce excess mucus, which forces the smoker to cough frequently.[40]
- In addition to contributing to COPD, use of ENDS products has been strongly associated with the pulmonary disease called electronic-cigarette, or vaping, product use–associated lung injury (EVALI).[41] To date, over 2,800 cases, including 68 deaths, have been reported.[28]
    - Vitamin E acetate, a component of all ENDS products, was found in all EVALI patient samples.[41,42]

Table 32-2 Disease Consequences of Nicotine and Tobacco Use[1]

Cancer	Respiratory Diseases	Cardiovascular Diseases	Pregnancy Infant Health	Other Conditions
Oral cavity Lung Larynx Trachea Oropharynx Esophagus Stomach Bladder Cervix Bronchus Kidney and ureter Pancreas Acute myeloid leukemia Liver Breast Colorectal	Chronic obstructive pulmonary disease Emphysema Asthma Pneumonia Tuberculosis Pulmonary infections EVALI	Atherosclerosis Coronary heart disease Aortic aneurysm Early abdominal aortic atherosclerosis in young adults Stroke	Ectopic pregnancy Fetal neonatal death/stillbirth Preterm delivery Congenital defects Orofacial clefts Reduced fertility Growth delay Sudden infant death syndrome Low birth weight	Immune function Diabetes Rheumatoid arthritis Male sex function (erectile dysfunction) Blindness Cataracts Age-related macular degeneration

EVALI, electronic-cigarette, or vaping, product use–associated lung injury

III. Cancer

- Smoking is responsible for 80% of lung cancers in the United States. Lung cancer is the leading cause of death among cancers, for both men and women.[43]
- Smoking causes 30% to 40% of all U.S. deaths annually.[43] Smoking can cause many different types of cancers, including lung, larynx/throat, oropharynx, esophagus, trachea, stomach, liver, pancreas, kidney, bladder, cervix, and colorectal.[1,43]
- Tobacco is one of the strongest risk factors for head and neck cancers.[44] The increased use of tobacco products increases the risk of developing oral cancer.

IV. Tobacco and Use of Other Drugs

- Smokers are more likely to consume alcohol. The combined use of alcohol and tobacco places the patient at higher risk for neoplasms and other oral problems.[1,45]

Environmental Tobacco Smoke

- Environmental tobacco smoke (ETS) is a passive or involuntary smoke nonusers are exposed to secondhand in room air when burning tobacco products are present.[1]
- The principal contributor is **sidestream smoke**, the material emitted from burning tobacco products between puffs.[46]
- Other components include exhaled mainstream smoke directly from the user and vaporized compounds diffused through a cigarette wrapper.[46]
- In indoor areas, environmental smoke can last for many hours, depending on ventilation. Exposure for certain workers and family members can be extensive.[46]
- Secondhand smoke at any level is deemed unsafe and harms anyone that is exposed to it.[1,19,43,44]
- Approximately 58 million Americans are exposed to passive smoke.[45,46]
- Exposure to secondhand smoke is most prevalent among children, African Americans, those living below the poverty level, and those living in multi-unit rental housing.[45,46]
- The aerosol emissions from ENDS is another toxic secondhand and thirdhand exposure for nonusers.[29,47]

I. Toxicity

- Many chemicals are contained in passive smoke, including the same carcinogenic compounds as those in mainstream smoke. Some toxic components are actually in higher concentrations in sidestream smoke than in mainstream smoke.[15,46]

- Chemicals present in ETS include irritants and systemic toxicants (hydrogen cyanide and sulfur dioxide), mutagens and carcinogens (benzo[a]pyrene and formaldehyde), and reproductive toxicants (nicotine, cadmium, and carbon monoxide).[46,48]
- Of the 250 toxic chemicals in ETS, there are at least 50 associated with cancer.[46]

II. Cardiovascular Effects

- Both active and passive exposure to smoke have similar effects on the cardiovascular system.[1,19,43]
- Coronary heart disease and death.[1,15,46]
- A causal relationship exists between secondhand smoke exposure and increased risk of stroke.[1,15]

Prenatal and Children

The fetus, infant, and growing child are exposed to ETS through the following ways[1,46,47]:

- Homes and cars where smoking is permitted.
- Public environments in which smoking is permitted.
- Other enclosed environments that allow smoking, such as restaurants and sporting events.
- Nonsmoking mothers who are exposed to ETS expose their unborn child to tobacco smoke constituents, such as carbon monoxide, nicotine, and cotinine.
- Parental smoking is a strong determinant of smoking uptake among children and adolescents.[49]
- Data on developmental defects due to parental ENDS usage are currently inconclusive but all efforts should be made to avoid usage or exposure to aerosols during pregnancy.[50]

I. In Utero

- Nicotine crosses the placenta and concentrates in the fetus at slightly higher levels than the mother.[1,49]
- Adverse pregnancy risks include miscarriage, low birth weight, placenta previa, preterm delivery, spontaneous abortion, and stillbirth.[1,51,52]
- Evidence shows maternal smoking in early pregnancy can cause orofacial clefts.[1]
- Evidence shows a causal relationship between maternal smoking and ectopic pregnancy.[1]

II. Infancy[1,43,51]

- Chemicals are passed to the baby in the breast milk of mothers who smoke.
- Acute effects include increased incidence of upper respiratory tract illness.
- ETS increases risk of an infant developing a lower respiratory illness.
- Nicotine can increase the risk of sudden infant death syndrome in infants of smokers.

III. Young Children[1,27,46]

- ETS affects lung development with symptoms of coughing, phlegm, and wheezing.
- Children who are exposed to passive smoking, particularly prenatal and postnatal maternal smoking, are at significant risk for onset of wheezing illness and asthma.
- Children have an increased incidence of middle ear infections.

Oral Manifestations of Tobacco and Nicotine Use

- The numerous oral conditions attributed to nicotine use vary with the type of (smoke or smokeless tobacco) and the form in which it is used (cigarettes, pipes, cigars, chewing tobacco, moist and dry snuff, ENDS, waterpipe, hookah).[1]
- Pattern and severity of clinical presentation vary with frequency and duration of nicotine use.[53]
- Research indicates ENDS have shown oxidative stress, increased risk of infection, and cell death to the epithelium tissue.[54-56]
- Cracked and broken teeth, as well as gingival and cheek mucosa pain, have been reported with ENDS usage.[57]
- Increased pocket depth, vasoconstriction, and radiographic bone loss have all been shown with ENDS use.[58-60]
- **Table 32-3** lists examples of the wide variety of oral consequences of nicotine use; periodontal diseases and oral cancers provide the most serious destructive effects.
- A comprehensive extraoral/intraoral examination is the most efficient and effective method for detecting nicotine-related conditions in and around the mouth.
  - The extraoral/intraoral examination gives visual examples to use in encouraging the patient to begin a nicotine cessation program.

Tobacco and Periodontal Infections

- Tobacco use is a major risk factor for the development and progression of periodontitis.[1,35,60-62]
- Users are at a high risk for developing more severe periodontitis than nonusers.[61]

Table 32-3 Oral Consequences of Nicotine Use

Cancer and Precancer	Periodontal Factors	Soft-Tissue Problems	Hard-Tissue Problems	Esthetic Factors	Excerbation—Oral Signs in Systemic Diseases
Squamous cell leukoplakia (ST) Homogeneous Nonhomogeneous Verrucous	Acute necrotizing ulcerative gingivitis (ANUG) and acute necrotizing ulcerative periodontitis (ANUP) Relapse during maintenance Increased risk for peri-implantitis and peri-implant bone loss Localized recession and clinical attachment loss	Nicotine stomatitis (P) Smoker's melanosis Black hairy tongue Median rhomboid glossitis Leukodema (P) Hyperkeratosis (ST) Dry socket Delayed wound healing Cheek mucosa pain	Cracked or broken teeth Occlusal or incisal abrasion (P, ST) Cervical abrasion (ST) Dehiscence of bone (ST) Tooth loss	Halitosis Dental stains Prosthesis stains Orthodontic appliance stains Discoloration of restorations Impaired taste and smell	HIV/AIDS Type 1 and type 2 diabetes

AIDS, acquired immunodeficiency syndrome; HIV, human immunodeficiency syndrome; P, pipe; ST, smokeless tobacco; no notation, smoked tobacco.

I. Effects on the Periodontal Tissues

- Gingivitis[35,54,56,59,63,64]
    - The degree of inflammatory response to dental biofilm accumulation is reduced compared with nonsmokers.
    - Nicotine use may affect treatment and therapeutic outcomes for plaque-induced gingivitis.
- Periodontitis in tobacco and e-cigarette users[62,65,66]
    - Increased rate and severity of periodontal destruction.
    - Increased bone loss, attachment loss, and pocket depths.
    - Diminished gingival blood flow and gingival crevicular flow.
    - Increased tooth loss from periodontal causes.[67]
    - Prevalence and severity may lessen with cessation.

II. Mechanisms of Periodontal Destruction

- Host response: Lowered immune response.[54,56,68]
- Impaired neutrophils: Decreased chemotaxis, phagocytosis, and adherence.[15,68]
- Impairment of revascularization; disruption of immune response; impact on healing; increased risk of periodontal disease.[1,66]
- Peri-implant bone loss in ENDS users.[58,60]
- Increased levels of inflammatory mediators and greater localized tissue destruction.[60]
- Negative effect on bone metabolism; after menopause, women smokers have a deficit in bone density; smoking can also influence osteoporosis.[1]

III. Response to Treatment

- People who use tobacco and nicotine products have a weakened response to conventional therapy.[69]
- Smoking has a negative impact on bone regeneration after periodontal therapy[70]
- Implants have higher risk for failure due to implantitis and peri-implant bone loss.[71]
- Delayed healing after surgical and nonsurgical procedures.[72]
- Therapeutic effects of nonsurgical procedures may improve with cessation.[73]

Nicotine Addiction

- Nicotine is tobacco's psychoactive agent (one that produces feelings of pleasure and well-being), and its use leads to tolerance, dependence, and addiction.
- No one starts using nicotine to become addicted to it.

I. Tolerance

- *Physiologic adaptation*
    - Tolerance refers to the user's need to increase the amount of the product used over time as it becomes less and less effective in creating the desired feeling of well-being.[74]
- *Amount of use*
    - To sustain the positive feelings associated with tobacco use, more and more has to be used.[74]

II. Dependence

- Characteristics
    - As increased amounts are needed over time, the loss of control over the amount and frequency of nicotine use show evidence of dependence.[74]
    - Facts about nicotine dependency are included in **Box 32-1**.
- Reinforcing effect[74]
    - Nicotine intensifies the release of dopamine by the brain, thereby increasing a feeling of pleasure and the compulsion to use tobacco.
    - Positive reinforcement is produced with nicotine use, and abrupt stopping produces withdrawal symptoms.

Box 32-1 Facts about Nicotine Dependency[53,75,76]

- Nicotine is the most addictive drug in the United States.
- Nicotine addiction is similar to that produced by other substances such as alcohol, cocaine, and heroin.
- Those who have a high tolerance to nicotine experience less nausea and dizziness following initial use.
- Nicotine abuse: Any use of nicotine products is considered a health hazard. Therefore, the use of any amount is considered abuse.
- Nicotine addiction may be the most challenging of all addictions for complete recovery.
- Many nicotine users make many unsuccessful quit attempts before stopping use for indefinite or extended periods of time.
- Successfully quitting smokeless tobacco use may be equally or more difficult than stopping smoking.

Data from National Institute on Drug Abuse. Research Report Series: Is Nicotine Addictive? Bethesda, MD: National Institutes of Health, National Institute on Drug Abuse; 2012; American Psychiatric Association. Diagnostic and Statistical Manual of Mental Disorders (DSM-IV). 5th ed. Washington, DC: American Psychiatric Association; 013:571-589

III. Addiction

- Under federal law, tobacco companies are required to make the following statements regarding nicotine addiction and nicotine manipulation[31]:
    - Here is the truth: Smoking is highly addictive. Nicotine is the addictive drug in tobacco.
    - Conventional tobacco and e-cigarette companies intentionally designed products with enough nicotine to create and sustain addiction.
    - Quitting is extremely difficult once addicted.
    - When you ingest nicotine, chemical changes occur in the brain—that is why quitting is so hard.
    - Defendant tobacco companies intentionally designed cigarettes to make them more addictive.
    - Cigarette companies control the impact and delivery of nicotine in many ways, including designing filters and selecting cigarette paper to maximize the ingestion of nicotine, adding ammonia to make the cigarette taste less harsh, and controlling the physical and chemical makeup of the tobacco blend.
- ENDS products, such as JUUL, contain nicotine salt up to a content of 5%, potentially creating nicotine dependence in as little as one pod.[77]
- To date, there is no regulation of the concentration of nicotine in an ENDS device in the United States.[77]
- **Addiction** is a chronic, progressive, relapsing disease characterized by compulsive use of a substance.[74]
- The effects result in physical, psychological, and/or social harm to the user, but use continues despite that harm.[77]
- Nicotine is more addictive than alcohol and other drugs of abuse in terms of the proportion of those who are exposed and subsequently become dependent.
- The pattern of relapse is identical for nicotine, alcohol, and heroin.
- Factors affecting the development of addiction include:
    - Properties of psychoactive drug (dose).
    - Genetic predisposition to dependence.[78]
    - Family, peer influences, and social acceptance.
    - Neuropsychiatric disorders.[79]
    - Cost and availability of the drug.
    - Influence of advertising.

Box 32-2 Criteria for Nicotine Withdrawal Syndrome[74,80,81]

- Dysphoric or depressed mood
- Insomnia
- Irritability, frustration, and anger
- Anxiety
- Difficulty concentrating
- Restlessness
- Decreased heart rate
- Increased appetite or weight gain
- Cravings for tobacco
- Impulsivity
- **Anticipatory anhedonia**

IV. Withdrawal

- Withdrawal refers to the effects of cessation of nicotine use by an individual in whom dependence is established.[74]
- When users of nicotine products stop abruptly, within 24 hours, they can experience maximal physical and/or psychological (e.g., anxiety, irritability, depressed mood) withdrawal symptoms.[80]
- **Box 32-2** identifies typical nicotine withdrawal symptoms.
- Duration[4,80]
    - Patients may experience withdrawal symptoms in as little as 3 hours, and relapse within a week is common.
    - Most symptoms diminish over a few weeks when relapse does not occur.
- Cravings for nicotine, increased appetite, and weight gain are greatest in the first 3 months after cessation.[82]
    - Nicotine replacement is associated with less weight gain.[82]
- Alleviation of symptoms
    - **Table 32-4** lists activities to help overcome withdrawal symptoms.
    - The goal is to prevent relapse.[78]

Treatment

Cessation from nicotine has increased over the past years, with two-thirds of smokers reporting an interest in quitting.[18,19,83] Nicotine cessation methods or treatment for nicotine addiction fall into two categories: *self-help* (unassisted) and *assisted strategies*.[83]

- Nonpharmacologic cessation strategies, such as behavioral counseling, should be attempted prior to introduction of pharmacologic treatment such as NRT, varenicline, and bupropion.[83,84]

Table 32-4 Alleviating Nicotine Withdrawal Symptoms[76,85]

Symptoms	Activities
Mood changes, anxiety, nervousness, irritability	Breathe deeply or other relaxation techniques. Take a walk or other physical activity. Remind yourself the feeling is temporary and will pass. Make a list of things you enjoy doing instead of smoking. Reduce or avoid caffeine intake from coffee, soda, tea, and energy drinks. Avoid places and situations where you most commonly used tobacco.
Sleep disturbances	Avoid caffeine; drink a glass of warm milk instead. Avoid alcohol. Consider relaxation techniques. Avoid naps; take a warm bath or meditate. Read a book, listen to soothing music. Avoid use of electronic devices before bedtime.
Appetite increase	Eat only when you are hungry. Eat low-fat, low-calorie snacks. Chew sugarless gum or eat sugarless hard candy. Drink additional glasses of water. Physical activity.
Cravings	*Delay smoking or dipping*: Use tactics such as waiting 1 more minute; often cravings pass in 5 or 10 minutes. *Distract yourself*: Be physically active; take a walk; call a friend. *Drink water*: To fight off cravings. *Deep breaths*: Relax! Close your eyes and take 10 deep breaths; exhale through pursed lips. *Discuss your feelings*: With someone close to you or a support group. Consult with your medical or dental provider about options for nicotine replacement.

I. Reasons for Quitting

Success cannot be expected unless the individual takes responsibility and believes in the significance of the effort. Typical reasons include the following[15,18,84]:

- General health awareness.
- Specific health problems directly or indirectly related to nicotine use.

- Coughing and lack of breath while exercising.
- Halitosis and yellow-stained teeth.
- Effect on family
  - Need to act as a role model.
  - Awareness of effects of ETS.
- Effect of smoking and/or ETS on fetus during pregnancy.
- Cost.
- Social pressure and restrictions on smoking in many settings.
- Personal recognition of the dangers of nicotine addiction and the desire to regain control of one's life.

II. Self-Help Interventions

When attempting to quit, fewer than one-third of nicotine users currently use an evidence-based cessation treatment. As a result, fewer than 1 in 10 reported success in cessation.[19]

- The following methods are used either singularly or, most commonly, in conjunction with one another[86]:
  - Go "cold turkey" all at once.
  - Reduce number of daily nicotine exposures.
  - Join a family member or friend in the nicotine cessation effort.
  - Select over-the-counter (OTC) nicotine replacement patches, gum, or lozenges.
  - Transitioned to a "light" version of cigarettes.
- Neither the FDA nor current clinical guidelines recommend ENDS for tobacco cessation.
- Recent evidence supports the reduction of smoking as a short-term harm reduction strategy and the cessation of smoking using NRTs as a long-term strategy[18]
- Dental practitioners are in an ideal position to advise nicotine users on cessation techniques by providing effective counseling and highlighting the various nicotine-induced oral diseases.[6,87,88]

III. Assisted Strategies

- Counseling
  - Interventions provided by oral health professionals can help patients in tobacco cessation.[88]
  - Provide a brief intervention for cessation to all nicotine users at every appointment.[4,87,88]
  - Tailor cessation discussion to the individual user's specific needs.[64]
  - Provision of practical counseling, including problem-solving and skills training.[4]
  - Provision of in-office social support: "Our office staff and I are willing to assist you."[4]
  - Customized Internet-based interventions with and without behavioral support can be an effective method for cessation.[89,90]
- Pharmacotherapies
  - **Table 32-5** provides an overview of FDA-approved first-line pharmacotherapies.
- Combination
  - Counseling combined with pharmacotherapy has been shown to be effective in helping patients to quit nicotine use.[18,91]

Pharmacotherapies Used for Treatment of Nicotine Addiction

I. Objectives and Rationale

- Make it easier to abstain from cigarettes or other ATP by partial replacement of nicotine or by counteracting nicotine's action.[4]
- Reduce withdrawal symptoms.[4,92]
- Fulfill, in part, the craving for nicotine by sustaining tolerance.[93]
- Provide some effects (mood, cognitive changes) previously delivered from nicotine-containing products.[93]

II. Considerations

- NRT and pharmacotherapy have been shown to be safe and effective in assisting in nicotine cessation.[18,91,94]
- Discourage casual use of pharmacotherapies. Failure as a result of improper use can discourage future quit attempts.
- Inform patient of potential adverse effects: nausea and vomiting.[93]
- Consult primary care provider before use if younger than 18 years or has a medical contraindication.[18]
- Should be used cautiously with pregnant patients and only under direct supervision from a maternal healthcare provider.[95]

III. Contraindications

- Self-medication without professional examination and advice is strongly discouraged.
- Nicotine gum, lozenge, and inhaler: Avoid eating or drinking acidic beverages for 15 minutes before and during use due to decreased nicotine absorption.[4]
- Patients with history of seizures and history of eating disorders are cautioned in using bupropion SR.[4]

Table 32-5 Suggestions for the Clinical Use of Pharmacotherapies for Smoking Cessation[4]

Pharmacotherapy	Precautions/ Contraindications	Side Effects	Dosage	Duration	Availability
Bupropion SR	History of seizure History of eating disorder Using monoamine oxidase inhibitor	Insomnia, dry mouth	Days 1–3: 150 mg each morning Day 4–end: twice daily; take evening dose 8 hr before sleep	Start 1–2 wk before quit date Use 2–6 mo	Zyban Wellbutrin SR Generic (prescription only)
Varenicline[a]	Kidney problems or on dialysis Has not been studied in pregnant or nursing women; FDA warning re: potential for agitation, depressed mood, atypical behavior, or suicidal thoughts	Nausea; insomnia; abnormal, vivid, or strange dreams Constipation, gas, and/or vomiting	Days 1–3: 0–5 mg once in morning Days 4–7: 0.5 mg twice daily Day 8 though end of treatment: 1 mg twice daily	Use 3–6 mo Start 1 wk before quit date	Chantix (prescription only)
Nicotine gum	Temporomandibular disorder Caution for denture wearers	Mouth soreness Dyspepsia Headaches	1–24 cigs/day: 2 mg gum (up to 24 psc/day) 20+ cigs/day or smokeless tobacco: 4 mg gum (up to 24 psc/day)[b]	Up to 12 wk or as needed	Nicorette gum (OTC only) Generic available
Nicotine inhaler	Asthma COPD	Local irritation of mouth and throat	6–16 cartridges/ day[b]	Up to 6 mo; taper at end	Nicotrol inhaler (prescription only)
Nicotine nasal spray	Nasal polyps Rhinitis Sinusitis Asthma	Nasal and throat irritation Dependence potential	8–40 doses/day (no more than 48 sprays in 24 hr)	3–6 mo; taper at end	Nicotrol NS (prescription only)
Nicotine transdermal patch	Allergy to patch adhesive Do not use if have severe eczema or psoriasis Do not cut patches	Local skin reaction Insomnia Changes in dreams Headache	One patch per day If 10 cigs/day: 21 mg 4 wk 14 mg 2–4 wk 7 mg 2–4 wk If <10/day: 14 mg 4 wk, then 7 mg 4 wk One patch per day	8–12 wk	Nicoderm CQ (OTC only) Generic patches (prescription and OTC) Nicotrol (OTC only)

(continues)

Table 32-5 Suggestions for the Clinical Use of Pharmacotherapies for Smoking Cessation[4] *(continued)*

Pharmacotherapy	Precautions/ Contraindications	Side Effects	Dosage	Duration	Availability
Nicotine lozenge	One lozenge at a time	Mouth soreness Dyspepsia Nausea Headache Cough Hiccups Heartburn Flatulence	2 mg if smoke/ chew after 30 min of waking; 4 mg if smoke/chew within 30 min of waking Maximum 20 lozenges in 24 hr[b]	3–6 mo Wks 1–6:1 every 1–2 hr Wks 7–9:1 every 2–4 hr; Wks 10–12:1 every 4–8 hr	Commit ■ Mint ■ Cherry ■ Original (OTC only) Generic available
Nicotine mini lozenge	Same as above	Same as above	2 mg if smoke/ chew after 30 min of waking; 4 mg if smoke/chew within 30 min of waking Maximum 24 mini lozenges/day[b]	Same as above	Nicorette mini ■ Mint (OTC only)

[a]Varenicline (Chantix) information. March 17, 2014. https://www.chantix.com/index.aspx.
[b]Nothing to eat or drink 15 min prior to or during use.
COPD, chronic obstructive pulmonary disease; FDA, Food and Drug Administration; OTC, over-the-counter.
Data from Fiore MC, Jaén CR, Baker TB, et al. Treating tobacco use and dependence: 2008 update. In: *Quick Reference Guide for Clinicians*. Rockville, MD: U.S. Department of Health and Human Services, Public Health Service; 2009.

IV. Nicotine Replacement Therapy

- The objective of NRTs is to help prevent withdrawal symptoms and to promote nicotine cessation.[84]
- NRT lasts typically 12 weeks but may be longer for those more strongly addicted.[84]
  - Longer term NRT has not been associated with an increased risk of harm.
- NRTs are less likely to cause dependence compared to tobacco products.[84]
- Dental hygienists are in an ideal position to discuss the immediate delivery of nicotine to the brain during consumption of nicotine-containing products. Furthermore, they are poised to educate patients about the differences in nicotine delivery of various NRTs, particularly those that are available OTC.
- Research is still inconclusive regarding the effectiveness of NRTs for individuals aged 20 years and younger.[84]
- Nicotine gum[4]
  - Available in 2-mg and 4-mg dosages.
  - More highly dependent patients are more successful with cessation with a 4-mg dosage.[94]
  - Considered a short-acting NRT to reduce acute nicotine cravings faster than patches.[93]
  - Transmucosal delivery: Nicotine is released in the mouth during "chewing."
  - Description: Nicotine gum is sweetened with xylitol and has either a mild mint, cinnamon, or orange flavor.
  - Directions: Chew one piece slowly until tingling or peppery taste is achieved; "park" gum in buccal vestibule; resume chewing when peppery taste or tingle fades; and repeat chew/park activity for approximately 30 minutes.
- Nicotine patch[4,94]
  - Releases nicotine at a steady rate and is considered a "controlled" NRT.[93]
  - Designed to release between 5 mg and 22 mg of nicotine over a 24-hour period, similar to plasma nicotine levels of a moderate-to-heavy cigarette smoker.[94]
  - **Transdermal** delivery: Nicotine is released through skin.
  - Directions: Place a new patch on a hairless location upon rising; if sleep disruption occurs, remove 24-hour patch before bedtime or use 16-hour patch.

    - Patches should be moved to different locations daily to avoid skin irritation.[94]
- Nicotine inhaler[4,93,94]
    - **Transmucosal** delivery: Primarily used to satisfy the *hand-to-mouth*-ritual while delivering nicotine to the oral cavity in a concentration similar to nicotine gum.[94]
    - Nicotine is released in the mouth during inhalation or puffing; hold vapor in oral cavity for absorption, but do not inhale.
    - Requirements: Store inhaler and cartridges in a warm place when temperatures drop below 40°F to prevent a decline in delivery of nicotine from the inhaler to the oral cavity.
- Nicotine nasal spray[4]
    - Nasal mucous membrane delivery: Nicotine is released through lining of nose in a dose of 0.5 mg per 50-uL squirt.[94]
    - Dose delivery: Avoid sniffing, swallowing, or inhaling while administering doses, as these increase irritating effects.
    - Directions: Tilt head slightly back while delivering spray.
    - Precaution for heavy smoker: Increased dose.
- Nicotine lozenge[2]
    - Transmucosal delivery: Nicotine is released in the mouth as lozenge dissolves.
    - Description: The lozenge is sweetened with mannitol and aspartame and flavored with a mild mint or cherry.
    - Dose delivery: See Table 32-5.
    - Directions: Do not bite or chew lozenge as it dissolves in the mouth; this can cause more nicotine to be swallowed quickly and may result in indigestion and/or heartburn.

Nicotine-Free Therapy

I. Bupropion SR[4,93]

- The first non-nicotine medication shown to be effective for tobacco cessation and approved by the FDA for that use.
- Can control both craving and withdrawal symptoms.[93]
- Mechanism of action: Blocks neural uptake of dopamine and/or norepinephrine.
- Additional dosing information is listed in Table 32-5.
- Use should begin 1–2 weeks prior to "quit date."[93]
- Take second dose 8 hours after first dose with an evening meal to reduce sleep disturbances.
- Bupropion SR can be used in combination with NRTs.
- Bupropion has not been shown to be an effective cessation method for adolescents, 20 years and younger.[4,93]

II. Varenicline Tartrate[4]

- The second non-nicotine medication shown to be effective for smoking cessation and approved by the FDA for that use.
- Has shown superior reductions in nicotine cravings and withdrawal symptoms to both NRT and bupropion for greater than 6 months.[87]
- *Mechanism of action*: A partial nicotine agonist (blocks nicotine receptors in brain). It also causes reduction in dopamine release.
    - Always take after meals with full glass of water, to reduce nausea.
    - Take second dose 8 hours after first dose with evening meal to reduce sleep disturbances.
    - Can be started 1–2 weeks before "quit date."[92]
    - Additional dosing information is listed in Table 32-5.
- Not currently recommended for use in combination with NRTs.

III. Combination Therapies

- Certain combinations of first-line medications have been shown to be effective smoking cessation treatments.
- Clinical trials suggest combining the slow delivery of a NRT medication with the faster delivery of a nicotine patch or gum can help to control acute cravings and nicotine withdrawal symptoms.[96]
- Nicotine users are 5% to 36% more likely to successfully quit if employing combination therapy.[92]
- Effective combination medications are[85]
    - Long-term (>14 weeks) combined NRT (e.g. nicotine patch + nicotine gum or spray).
    - NRT + varenicline.
    - NRT + bupropion SR.
    - Varenicline + bupropion SR.

IV. Second-Line Medications

- Second-line medications are pharmacotherapies for which there is evidence of efficacy for treating tobacco dependence, but they have a more limited role because of the following reasons[4]:
    - The FDA has not approved them for tobacco dependence treatment.
    - Second-line treatments, clonidine and nortriptyline, can be considered for use on a case-by-case basis after first-line treatments have been used or considered and while under a primary care provider's supervision.[4]

V. Alternative Cessation Therapies

- Research suggests alternative aids such as acupuncture and hypnotherapy may help with smoking cessation.[84]
  - It is unclear whether these alternative nicotine-cessation aids are as effective as pharmocotherapies.

Dental Hygiene Care for the Patient Who Uses Nicotine

- The majority of people who smoke state they would like to quit, and almost half say they have tried to quit in the past 12 months.[18]
- The nicotine-using patient presents a unique challenge to the oral health team. Specific treatment modifications are indicated and should highlight prevention of the oral implications of nicotine usage.
- Helping the patient to quit using nicotine becomes an integral part of the dental hygiene care plan as it supports improvement in oral and overall health outcomes.[87,88]

Assessment

I. Patient History

- Nicotine use status is assessed at each appointment.
- The basic history form used by all patients includes questions to determine whether the patient currently uses nicotine and, if so, what type (cigarette, ENDS, other ATPs, and/or smokeless). A sample of a tobacco use assessment form is shown in **Figure 32-4**. (See Chapter 11 for an example of a history form.)
- Concomitant use of alcohol and other **psychoactive drugs** (substances that can alter mood, behavior, or cognitive processes) with tobacco may necessitate modifications of approaches to tobacco/nicotine cessation.
- Healthcare providers should record nicotine use status as a *vital sign* along with temperature, pulse, respiratory rate, and blood pressure.

II. Extraoral Examination

- Breath and body odor
  - Halitosis.
  - Smoke from tobacco products clings to skin, hair, and clothes and results in body odor.[48]

Tobacco Products			
Cigarettes	YES ( )	NO ( )	Number of cigarettes per day or week:
Cigars	YES ( )	NO ( )	Number of cigars per week:
E-cigarettes	YES ( )	NO ( )	Number of cartridge per day or week:
Waterpipe/hookah	YES ( )	NO ( )	Approximate amount of time per day or week:
Smokeless	YES ( )	NO ( )	Number of cans/pouches per day/week:
Dissolvable strips, sticks, orbs, etc.	YES ( )	NO ( )	Amount per day or week:
Other types of tobacco products?	YES ( )	NO ( )	Amount per day or week:
Have you tried quitting tobacco use in the past?	YES ( )	NO ( )	If you have tried to quit: How long did you quit last time? What did you use to help you quit? What was the longest time you have quit? What has caused you to relapse?

Figure 32-4 Sample Tobacco Use Assessment Form

- Fingers
  - Smokers of nonfiltered cigarettes may have a yellowish-brown discoloration of the fingers and fingernails.
- Skin
  - Smokers experience premature and more extensive facial wrinkling.[1]
- Lips
  - Cigar smokers are at risk for development of precancerous and cancerous lip lesions.[12]

III. Intraoral Examination

Oral consequences of tobacco use are listed in Table 32-3. An outline for conducting a thorough intraoral examination for the patient who uses tobacco is provided in Chapter 13.

Clinical Treatment Procedures

- Patients who use tobacco or nicotine-containing products may require longer and/or more frequent appointments due to the presence of increased risk for the following[69,87]:
  - Dental stain.
  - Calculus.
  - Dental caries.
  - Periodontal disease.

I. Dental Biofilm Control/Caries Control

- Self-care for daily dental biofilm control is the first priority in the care plan.
- Meticulous oral self-care is required by this group of high-risk patients owing to their susceptibility to dental caries, periodontal infections, and other soft-tissue alterations.

II. Nonsurgical Periodontal Therapy

- Inform the patient healing will be jeopardized by continued nicotine use, and users should not anticipate similar treatment outcomes as nonusers.[56,69]
- Inform the patient nicotine cessation would improve the results of treatment.[69,73]
- When using power-driven instruments:
  - Take precautions to protect the patient from aerosol-containing bacteria and debris (smokers often have pulmonary and cardiovascular complications).[1]

III. Other Patient Instruction

- Diet and nutrition
  - Tobacco users may be poorly nourished because nicotine use suppresses appetite.[97]
  - Conversely, the desire to avoid weight gain through tobacco use may impede a patient's willingness to quit.[4]
  - Suggestions about diet and exercise are included as a part of the cessation program.[4]

Tobacco Cessation Program

- A program for tobacco cessation is an essential component of the oral healthcare plan for all tobacco-using patients.[87,98]
- The treatment of tobacco use and dependence will often require multiple appointments, repeated interventions, and multiple attempts to quit.[4,87,98]
- The dental setting provides an excellent opportunity to assist tobacco users in tobacco cessation.[87,99,100]
- Interventions and their outcomes will vary depending on the motivation and experience of the clinician and the patient's acceptance of, and adherence to, the regimen
- Even a minimal intervention conducted by a clinician may help a patient become nicotine free.[98]

Motivational Interviewing

The use of brief motivational interviewing is an effective method of tobacco cessation.

- Motivation and improving self-confidence increase likelihood of tobacco cessation.[101]
- Motivational interviewing techniques are described in Chapter 24, which can be useful in encouraging behavior change for patients.

The "5 A's"

The "5 A's"—ask, advise, assess, assist, arrange—provide the basis for a brief, simple, but effective tobacco dependence intervention for clinicians.[4,102] A tobacco/nicotine cessation flowchart is presented in **Figure 32-5** to aid in decision making.

I. Ask

- Health history
  - Ask all patients about nicotine use.[4,98,102]

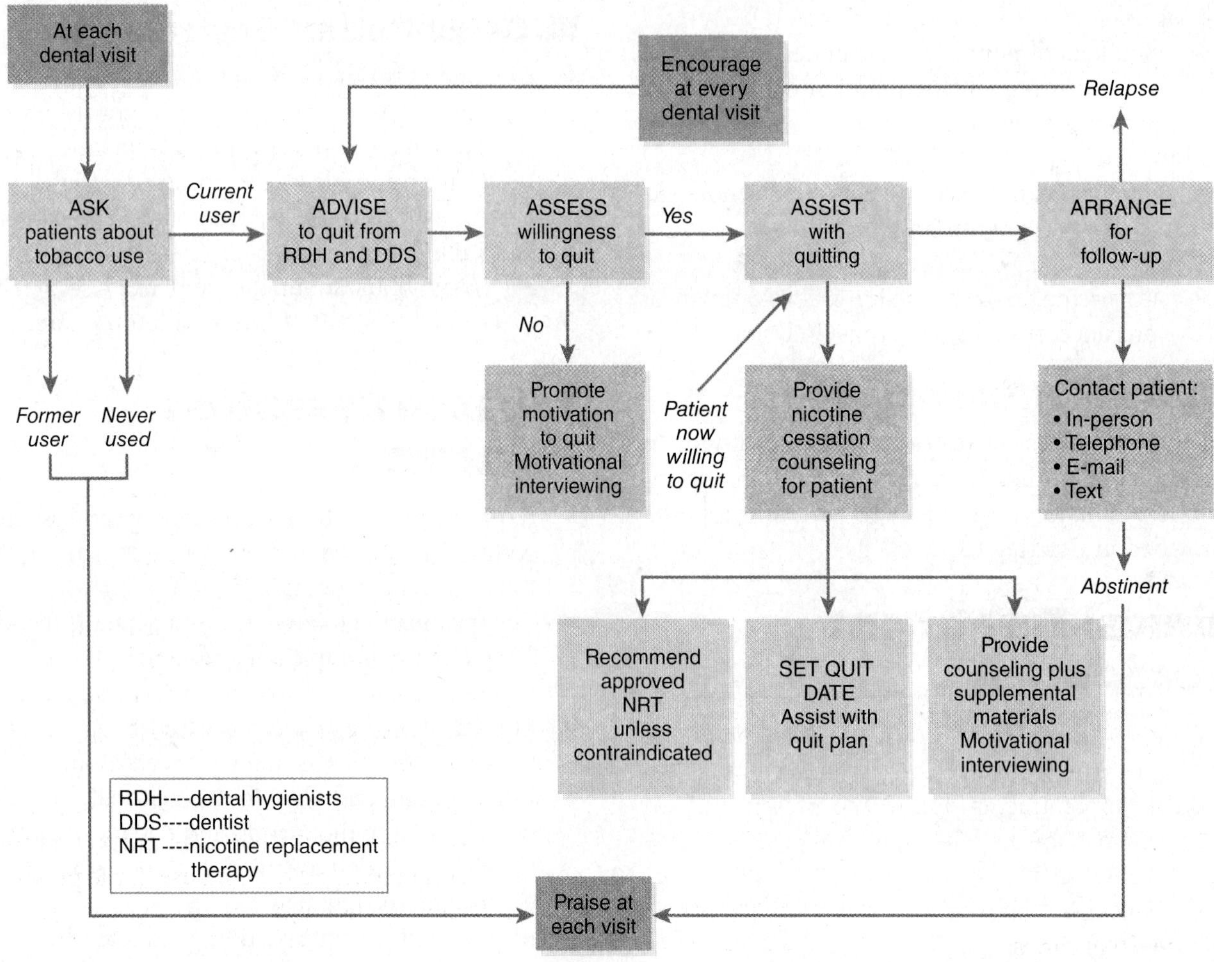

Figure 32-5 Tobacco/Nicotine Cessation Flowchart. Flowchart to show how the 5 A's can be incorporated into the clinical setting.

Data from Fiore MC, Jaén CR, Baker TB, et al. Treating tobacco use and dependence: 2008 update. In: *Quick Reference Guide for Clinicians*. Rockville, MD: U.S. Department of Health and Human Services, Public Health Service; 2009.

    - Include questions about nicotine use on the health history form and document nicotine use at every appointment. (See Chapter 11.)
- Nonjudgmental follow up questions
    - During review of the health history, present questions related to nicotine use nonjudgmentally.
    - Address nicotine use as a health issue, not as a moral and/or social issue.
    - Obtain facts without placing the patient on the defensive.
- Gain patient's trust and confidence[4]
    - Express empathy and support patient's decision to choose or reject change.
    - Social disapproval of nicotine use is increasing, and patients may hesitate to disclose their habit.
- Children and adolescents
    - E-cigarettes are the most common tobacco product used among adolescents.[8,29]
    - Risk factors affecting a child or adolescent initiating tobacco use include being male, White, and from a rural area; having parents with lower education levels; having friends and parents who use tobacco; feeling tobacco/nicotine is low risk; and having experienced highly stressful events.[103]
    - Brief counseling, including risk assessment, needs to be implemented to prevent initiation of nicotine use. Assessment should include parent history of nicotine use, product access, smoking among peers, and nicotine advertisement exposure.[4]
    - For children and adolescents who have not tried tobacco or nicotine products, it is critical to provide a prevention message.[103]
    - For parents of younger children, discuss the effects of secondhand smoke on health, developmental risks, and how tobacco or nicotine use places the child at risk for use.[103]
    - Group-based behavioral interventions may be helpful in adolescent nicotine cessation.[104]

II. Advise

A. Never Users/Former Users

- Advise every patient about nicotine use.
- Praise "never users" and "former users" for their nicotine-free behavior.
- Reinforcement counters the nicotine industry's message and other enticements to begin nicotine use and can help prevent relapse.

B. Current Users

1. Stop now: Clearly advise the patient about the importance of *stopping* now. Present the advice in a caring, compassionate manner so patients realize clinicians are interested in their health and well-being.
2. Show: Have patients *look* in their mouths during the initial oral examination to observe the clinical effects of nicotine use.
   - Advice needs to be relevant to existing conditions.
   - Existing oral conditions may serve as strong motivators to quit.
3. Listen:
   - Ask patients whether they want to quit and their reasons. Most users want to quit. Their reasons may have little to do with health, but verbalizing the reasons forces patients to focus and strengthen their reasons.
   - *Listening* to the patient allows the clinician to support the patient's thoughts and provide appropriate reinforcement.

III. Assess

1. Assess the patient's readiness to quit.
   - Ask the patient: "Are you ready to quit?"
2. If the patient is ready:
   - Determine whether the patient could best be treated in your practice. (A patient may have multiple problems necessitating referral.)
   - If treatment is provided in your office, go to the *assist* step.
3. If the patient is not ready to quit, use the "5 R's"[69]:
   - *Relevance*: Patient indicates personal importance of quitting.
   - *Risks*: Patient identifies negative consequences of continued use.
   - *Rewards*: Patient identifies personal benefits of quitting.
   - *Roadblocks*: Patient identifies barriers to quitting, and clinician helps address barriers.
   - *Repetition*: Reinforce the motivational message at every visit.

IV. Assist

A. Establish a Quit Plan

- Set a quit date, preferably within 2–4 weeks.[69]
- Have the patient tell family, friends, and coworkers about quitting and request their understanding and support.[69]
- Warn the patient to anticipate challenges to the planned quit attempt, particularly during the first few weeks. This includes nicotine withdrawal symptoms.
- Ask the patient to remove all nicotine-related products from home, car/truck, and work sites.[69]

B. Provide Practical Counseling

- Total abstinence is *essential:* "not even a single puff or dip after the quit date."
- Review past quit attempts and identify what helped and challenges or triggers that contributed to relapse.[69]
  - Because alcohol can cause relapse, the patient needs to limit/abstain from alcohol use.
- Quitting is more difficult when there is another user in the household. Nicotine-using housemates are encouraged to avoid use in the presence of the patient attempting to quit.
- Provide the local or state quitline number, as quitline counseling has been shown to be very helpful in supporting cessation.[18]

C. Pharmacotherapy

- The combination of nicotine cessation counseling and medication is more effective than either counseling or medication alone.[18,85]
- Suggest the use of approved OTC or prescription pharmacotherapy. Refer to Table 32-5.
- Evidence supports combining short- and long-term NRT to assist in cessation and relapse prevention.[18]

D. Provide Educational Information

- Agencies publishing motivational materials are listed in **Table 32-6**.
- The *2020 Surgeon General's Report on Smoking Cessation* indicates the following supplemental interventions for smoking cessation have evidence for being effective[18]:
  - Smartphone apps for cessation.
  - Short text message cessation programs.
  - Web or Internet-based interventions for smoking cessation.[105]

Table 32-6 Sources for Tobacco Cessation Patient Educational Materials

Name of Source	Telephone Numbers	Links
American Lung Association		www.lung.org/quit-smoking
National Cancer Institute		https://smokefree.gov/
Centers for Disease Control and Prevention (CDC) Tobacco Information and Prevention Tips		www.cdc.gov/tobacco/quit_smoking
The Truth Initiative		https://truthinitiative.org/what-we-do/quit-smoking-tools
Nicotine Anonymous		www.nicotine-anonymous.org
National Alliance for Tobacco Cessation		www.becomeanex.org
Substance Abuse and Mental Health Services Administration (SAMHSA)		https://store.samhsa.gov/product/You-Can-Quit-Tobacco/SMA18-5069YCQ
You Can Quit Smoking—Agency for Healthcare Research and Quality		www.ahrq.gov/prevention/guidelines/tobacco/clinicians/index.html
CDC	National Quit Line 1-800—Quit-Now (1-800-784-8669)	www.smokefree.gov Can access state quitlines through National Quit Line number
CDC smokefree.gov		quitSTART App (Find the app in Google Play or Apple Store)

- Specific educational materials are available for the following groups and can be made available in the office or clinic:
  - Various cultures and ethnic groups.
  - Different levels of education and literacy.
  - Readers of all ages.

V. Arrange

A. Follow-up

- Essential for successful quit rates.[4,98]
- Provide written documentation as a reminder, listing their quit date.
- Suggest posting quit-date reminders in visible locations, such as refrigerator door or bathroom mirror or placing a laminated post-it note with the quit date between cellophane and paper of the cigarette package.[4,98]

B. Contact the Patient before the Quit Date

- Assure patient of care provider's sincere interest in their nicotine cessation attempt via telephone call, email, or text message.
- Inquire:
  - If information provided at initial contact has been helpful.
  - If the patient has any questions regarding the information received.
- Follow-up contact[4,69,98]
  - Follow up, either in person or via telephone or e-mail.
  - Timely intervals would be once within the first week after the quit date, when the patient's physical withdrawal symptoms are most intense, and again at the end of the first, second, and third months of their cessation.
  - More than four contacts with patient help to increase long-term abstinence.
  - Follow-up at regularly scheduled continuing care appointments.
- Actions during follow-up contact[4,69]
  - Congratulate and praise patients who have remained nicotine free.
  - Provide the opportunity for patients to ask questions. If they have none, encourage the patient to contact you if questions arise.

- If relapse has occurred, ask the patient to reflect on and record the circumstances that led to use.
- Encourage the patient to set another quit date, reminding the patient that a lapse can be a learning experience.
- Review the use of NRT.
- Provide agencies and local contact numbers for the patient who requests a more intensive cessation program.

The Team Approach

Evidence concludes that oral health professionals provide and support tobacco cessation interventions.[100,106]

I. Organize the Clinic Team

- Select a team coordinator.
- The coordinator does not do everything, but sees that everything is done.
- Responsibilities
  - Identify nicotine use status at patient's first visit.
  - Record appropriate documentation in patient's records.
  - Ensure all nicotine-using patients are offered the opportunity to enter a cessation program.
  - Contact patients for follow-up.
  - Act as a coach for patients who relapse.
  - Maintain a supply of literature for patients.

II. Organize a Nicotine-Free Environment

- Display nicotine use prevention and cessation materials in the office or clinic.

III. Organize a Tobacco User Tracking System

- Nicotine use assessment form: Figure 32-3.
- Patient chart: Records should include documentation of advice provided to quit, patient response, interest in quitting, and progress in cessation.
- Nicotine status on records: Clearly mark records (paper or electronic) so status can be immediately seen by all providers.

Advocacy

I. Public Health Policy

- *The Surgeon General's Report on Oral Health* in 2000 was the first report of a Surgeon General focused on oral health, and the report specifically identified tobacco use as a risk factor for oral cavity and pharyngeal cancer.[107]
- Healthcare providers can help nicotine users quit and can become partners with one another and with community programs to prevent diseases and promote good health habits.
- The Centers for Disease Control and Prevention has been supporting state-based nicotine control coalitions in all 50 states. Many local communities and municipalities are considering or have adopted smoke-free workplace ordinances.[108]
- Oral health professionals can be valuable and collaborative partners in these programs.[87,98,106]

II. Community Oral Health Educational Programs

No community oral health program can be considered complete without inclusion of nicotine prevention, control, and cessation education. Excellent materials are available from many nonprofit and professional organizations.

Documentation

Careful and complete documentation of nicotine use is a component of each patient assessment. It is part of the health history for new patients and part of the clinical (progress) notes for maintenance patients.

- Include nicotine history and/or current use, type of nicotine, and amount typically used.
- Age, ethnicity, gender, and periodontal and overall dental status, as well as oral cancer screening findings.
- Patient interest/confidence motivation/readiness to quit and previous quit attempts and techniques used.
- Options for cessation presented to patient and referrals to primary care provider for examination/treatment.
- **Box 32-3** contains an example for nicotine use assessment and cessation treatment.

Box 32-3 Example Documentation: Tobacco Use Assessment and Cessation Treatment

- **S**—A 45-year-old African American male presents for second quadrant scaling, upper left (UL) with local anesthesia, and postscaling evaluation of first quadrant, upper right (UR). Cigarette smoker for 15 years; 1–2 packs a day. Patient states his oral self-care has improved since the initial quadrant scaling. Patient's chief complaint: Gums still sore from previous scaling appointment.
- **O**—Intraoral assessment reveals slow healing for first quadrant scaling with localized inflammation and erythematous areas, evidence of nicotine stomatitis, other oral cancer finding negative, and no cavitated carious lesions. Periodontal examination findings: UL quadrant with generalized 5–6 mm pocket depths, and 7 mm pocket on #15 MB, bleeding on probing #14 and 15 buccal.
- **A**—Patient presents with a high risk for oral and systemic disease due to tobacco dependence. Provided patient with smoking cessation basics, and explanation of oral and systemic effects of tobacco use. Brief discussion indicated patient is motivated to quit because he and his wife are expecting their first baby but reports previous attempts to quit "cold turkey" were unsuccessful due to weight gain, mood swings, and increased stress.
- **P**—Patient congratulated on wanting to quit and reminded previous attempts at quitting should not be looked upon as failures. Introduced various options for cessation support. Patient agreed to Internet option www .smokefree.gov, with quitting apps; walked patient through the website. Additionally, patient agreed to 21 mg nicotine transdermal patch, transitioning to 14 mg, then 7 mg patch over 8–10 weeks, combining patch therapy with nicotine gum to help prevent weight gain and provide relief for additional withdrawal symptoms and cravings. Follow-up by telephone in 1 week and re-evaluate at next visit scheduled in 2 weeks.

Next visit: Scale lower right quadrant with local anesthesia, reassess UL quadrant, and continue tobacco cessation counseling.

Signed: ______________________, RDH
Date: ________________

Factors to Teach the Patient

- The most effective method to stop nicotine use is never to start.
- How to perform a regular self-examination of the oral cavity.
- Pregnant women who use nicotine products can harm the developing fetus and the newborn infant.
- Young children may experiment with or use nicotine products. Parents can be educated so that they are prepared to provide guidance.
- *All* forms of social nicotine use can lead to addiction.
- Nonsmokers who breathe ETS can incur the same serious health problems as primary nicotine users; children are especially susceptible.
- Smokeless tobacco use is *not* a safe alternative to smoking.
- Oral health team members can help patients become nicotine free.
- Learn about local or state nicotine legislation and public health policy to make informed choices related to a nicotine-free society.

References

1. United States Department of Health and Human Services. *The Health Consequences of Smoking—50 Years of Progress: A Report of the Surgeon General*. US Department of Health and Human Services, Centers for Disease Control and Prevention (US); 2014:943. http://www.ncbi.nlm.nih.gov/books/NBK179276/. Accessed August 31, 2021.
2. Tomar SL, Asma S. Smoking-attributable periodontitis in the United States: findings from NHANES III. National Health and Nutrition Examination Survey. *J Periodontol*. 2000;71(5):743-751.
3. Wendell KJ, Stein SH. Regulation of cytokine production in human gingival fibroblasts following treatment with nicotine and lipopolysaccharide. *J Periodontol*. 2001;72(8):1038-1044.
4. Fiore MC, Jaen CR, Baker TB. *Treating Tobacco Use and Dependence: 2008 Update*. U.S. Department of Health and Human Services; 2008.

5. Chaffee BW. Electronic cigarettes: trends, health effects and advising patients amid uncertainty. *J Calif Dent Assoc.* 2019;47(2):85-92.
6. Martell KM, Boyd LD, Giblin-Scanlon LJ, Vineyard J. Knowledge, attitudes, and practices of young adults regarding the impact of electronic cigarette use on oral health. *J Am Dent Assoc.* 2020;151(12):903-911.
7. Creamer MR, Wang TW, Babb S, et al. Tobacco product use and cessation indicators among adults — United States, 2018. *MMWR Morb Mortal Wkly Rep.* 2019;68(45):1013-1019.
8. Villarroel M, Cha A, Vahratian A. Electroninc cigarette use among adults, 2018. Published April 28, 2020. https://www.cdc.gov/nchs/products/databriefs/db365.htm. Accessed August 4, 2021.
9. Hu SS, Neff L, Agaku IT, et al. Tobacco product use among adults - United States, 2013-2014. *MMWR Morb Mortal Wkly Rep.* 2016;65(27):685-691.
10. Centers for Disease Control and Prevention. Fact sheets on smoking and tobacco use. Centers for Disease Control and Prevention. Published December 14, 2020. https://www.cdc.gov/tobacco/data_statistics/fact_sheets/index.htm. Accessed August 6, 2021.
11. Kypriotakis G, Robinson JD, Green CE, Cinciripini PM. Patterns of tobacco product use and correlates among adults in the population assessment of tobacco and health (PATH) study: a latent class analysis. *Nicotine Tob Res.* 2018;20(Suppl 1):S81-S87.
12. Sung H-Y, Wang Y, Yao T, Lightwood J, Max W. Polytobacco use of cigarettes, cigars, chewing tobacco, and snuff among US adults. *Nicotine Tob Res.* 2016;18(5):817-826.
13. McMillen R, Maduka J, Winickoff J. Use of emerging tobacco products in the United States. *J Environ Pub Health.* 2012;2012:e989474.
14. Harrell PT, Naqvi SMH, Plunk AD, Ji M, Martins SS. Patterns of youth tobacco and polytobacco usage: the shift to alternative tobacco products. *Am J Drug Alcohol Abuse.* 2017;43(6):694-702.
15. Centers for Disease Control and Prevention (US), National Center for Chronic Disease Prevention and Health Promotion (US), Office on Smoking and Health (US). *How Tobacco Smoke Causes Disease: The Biology and Behavioral Basis for Smoking-Attributable Disease: A Report of the Surgeon General.* Centers for Disease Control and Prevention; 2010. http://www.ncbi.nlm.nih.gov/books/NBK53017/. Accessed July 31, 2021.
16. Centers for Disease Control and Prevention. Vital signs: Youth tobacco use surged from 2017-2018. Centers for Disease Control and Prevention. Published February 21, 2019. https://www.cdc.gov/vitalsigns/youth-tobacco-use/index.html. Accessed August 31, 2021.
17. Overbeek DL, Kass AP, Chiel LE, Boyer EW, Casey AMH. A review of toxic effects of electronic cigarettes/vaping in adolescents and young adults. *Crit Rev Toxicol.* 2020;50(6):531-538.
18. United States Public Health Service Office of the Surgeon General, National Center for Chronic Disease Prevention and Health Promotion (US) Office on Smoking and Health. *Smoking Cessation: A Report of the Surgeon General.* US Department of Health and Human Services; 2020. http://www.ncbi.nlm.nih.gov/books/NBK555591/. Accessed August 31, 2021.
19. Babb S. Quitting smoking among adults — United States, 2000–2015. *MMWR Morb Mortal Wkly Rep.* 2017;65.
20. Maisto SA, Galizio M, Connors GJ. *Drug Use and Abuse.* Cengage Learning; 2018.
21. Food and Drug Administration. Harmful and potentially harmful constituents in tobacco products and tobacco smoke: established list. Published online October 7, 2019. https://www.fda.gov/tobacco-products/rules-regulations-and-guidance/harmful-and-potentially-harmful-constituents-tobacco-products-and-tobacco-smoke-established-list. Accessed August 31, 2021.
22. Centers for Disease Control and Prevention. Biomonitoring summary. Published May 24, 2019. https://www.cdc.gov/biomonitoring/Cotinine_BiomonitoringSummary.html. Accessed August 6, 2021.
23. Djordjevic MV, Doran KA. Nicotine content and delivery across tobacco products. *Handb Exp Pharmacol.* 2009;(192):61-82.
24. Lawler TS, Stanfill SB, deCastro BR, et al. Surveillance of nicotine and pH in cigarette and cigar filler. *Tob Regul Sci.* 2017;3(Suppl 1):101-116.
25. Benowitz NL, Hukkanen J, Jacob P. Nicotine chemistry, metabolism, kinetics and biomarkers. *Handb Exp Pharmacol.* 2009;(192):29-60.
26. Popova L, Ling PM. Alternative tobacco product use and smoking cessation: a national study. *Am J Public Health.* 2013;103(5):923-930.
27. USPHS, Office of the Surgeon General. *Preventing Tobacco Use among Youth and Young Adults: A Report of the Surgeon General.* U.S. Department of Health and Human Services, Public Health Service, Office of the Surgeon General; 2012.
28. Centers for Disease Control and Prevention. Smoking and tobacco use; electronic cigarettes. Centers for Disease Control and Prevention. Published May 12, 2021. https://www.cdc.gov/tobacco/basic_information/e-cigarettes/about-e-cigarettes.html. Accessed July 31, 2021.
29. US Department of Health and Human Services. *E-Cigarette Use among Youth and Young Adults: A Report of the Surgeon General-Executive Summary.* US Department of Health and Human Services, Centers for Disease Control and Prevention, National Center for Chronic Disease Prevention and Health Promotion, Office of Smoking and Health; 2016. https://www.dupagepediatrics.com/storage/app/media/e-cigarette20use20among20youth20and20young20adults-20a20report20of20the20surgeon20general.pdf. Accessed July 31, 2021.
30. Gaur R, Ram G. Popcorn lung: the e-disease. *Int J Pharmaceut Chem Biol Sci.* 2021;11(1):16-18.
31. Food and Drug Administration. Deeming tobacco products to be subject to the federal food, drug, and cosmetic act, as amended by the family smoking prevention and tobacco control act; restrictions on the sale and distribution of tobacco products and required warning statements for tobacco products; final rule. *Federal Register.* 2015;81(90):134.
32. Food and Drug Administration. Vaporizers, e-cigarettes, and other electronic nicotine delivery systems (ENDS). *FDA.* Published online August 18, 2021. https://www.fda.gov/tobacco-products/products-ingredients-components/vaporizers-e-cigarettes-and-other-electronic-nicotine-delivery-systems-ends. Accessed August 31, 2021.
33. Centers for Disease Control and Prevention. Smokeless tobacco: products and marketing. Smoking and tobacco use. Published May 14, 2021. https://www.cdc.gov/tobacco/data_statistics/fact_sheets/smokeless/products_marketing/index.htm. Accessed August 23, 2021.
34. World Health Organization. *Smokeless Tobacco and Some Tobacco-Specific n-Nitrosamines.* International Agency for Research on Cancer; 2007.

35. Munshi T, Heckman CJ, Darlow S. Association between tobacco waterpipe smoking and head and neck conditions: a systematic review. *J Am Dent Assoc*. 2015;146(10):760-766.
36. Maziak W. Consensus statement on assessment of waterpipe smoking in epidemiological studies. *Tob Control*. 2017;26(3): 338-343.
37. Food and Drug Administration. Hookah tobacco (shisha or waterpipe tobacco). *FDA*. Published online January 3, 2020. https://www.fda.gov/tobacco-products/products-ingredients-components/hookah-tobacco-shisha-or-waterpipe-tobacco. Accessed August 23, 2021.
38. Waziry R, Jawad M, Ballout RA, Al Akel M, Akl EA. The effects of waterpipe tobacco smoking on health outcomes: an updated systematic review and meta-analysis. *Int J Epidemiol*. 2017;46(1):32-43.
39. American Lung Association. Emphysema. Published August 31, 2021. https://www.lung.org/lung-health-diseases/lung-disease-lookup/emphysema. Accessed August 31, 2021.
40. American Lung Association. Chronic bronchitis. Published August 31, 2021. https://www.lung.org/lung-health-diseases/lung-disease-lookup/chronic-bronchitis. Accessed August 31, 2021.
41. Blount BC, Karwowski MP, Shields PG, et al. Vitamin E acetate in bronchoalveolar-lavage fluid associated with EVALI. *N Eng J Med*. 2020;382(8):697-705.
42. Centers for Disease Control and Prevention. Outbreak of lung injury associated with the use of e-cigarette, or vaping, products. Centers for Disease Control and Prevention. Published August 3, 2021. https://www.cdc.gov/tobacco/basic_information/e-cigarettes/severe-lung-disease.html. Accessed October 23, 2021.
43. American Cancer Society. Cancer facts & figures 2020. Published August 31, 2021. https://www.cancer.org/research/cancer-facts-statistics/all-cancer-facts-figures/cancer-facts-figures-2020.html. Accessed August 31, 2021.
44. American Cancer Society. Risk factors for oral cavity and oropharyngeal cancers. https://www.cancer.org/cancer/oral-cavity-and-oropharyngeal-cancer/causes-risks-prevention/risk-factors.html. Accessed October 23, 2021.
45. Centers for Disease Control and Prevention. Health effects of secondhand smoke. Smoking and Tobacco Use. Published February 27, 2020. https://www.cdc.gov/tobacco/data_statistics/fact_sheets/secondhand_smoke/health_effects/index.htm. Accessed August 31, 2021.
46. Centers for Disease Control and Prevention, Office on Smoking and Health. *The Health Consequences of Involuntary Exposure to Tobacco Smoke: A Report of the Surgeon General*. Centers for Disease Control and Prevention; 2006:709. https://www.ncbi.nlm.nih.gov/books/NBK44328/. Accessed October 23, 2021.
47. Wills TA, Soneji SS, Choi K, Jaspers I, Tam EK. E-cigarette use and respiratory disorders: an integrative review of converging evidence from epidemiological and laboratory studies. *Eur Respir J*. 2021;57(1):1901815.
48. National Cancer Institute, Division of Cancer Control & Population Sciences. *Health Effect of Exposure to Environmental Tobacco Smoke. Tobacco Control Monograph No. 10*. US Department of Health and Human Services, National Institutes of Health, National Cancer Institute; 1999:430. https://cancercontrol.cancer.gov/brp/tcrb/monographs. Accessed August 31, 2021.
49. Leonardi-Bee J, Jere ML, Britton J. Exposure to parental and sibling smoking and the risk of smoking uptake in childhood and adolescence: a systematic review and meta-analysis. *Thorax*. 2011;66(10):847-855.
50. Orzabal M, Ramadoss J. Impact of electronic cigarette aerosols on pregnancy and early development. *Curr Opin Toxicol*. 2019;14:14-20.
51. Ko T-J, Tsai L-Y, Chu L-C, et al. Parental smoking during pregnancy and its association with low birth weight, small for gestational age, and preterm birth offspring: a birth cohort study. *Pediatr Neonatal*. 2014;55(1):20-27.
52. Hackshaw A, Rodeck C, Boniface S. Maternal smoking in pregnancy and birth defects: a systematic review based on 173 687 malformed cases and 11.7 million controls. *Hum Reprod Update*. 2011;17(5):589-604.
53. National Institute of Dental and Craniofacial Research. Oral cancer. Published July 2018. https://www.nidcr.nih.gov/health-info/oral-cancer/more-info. Accessed August 31, 2021.
54. Pushalkar S, Paul B, Li Q, et al. Electronic cigarette aerosol modulates the oral microbiome and increases risk of infection. *iScience*. 2020;23(3):100884.
55. Ji EH, Sun B, Zhao T, et al. Characterization of electronic cigarette aerosol and its induction of oxidative stress response in oral keratinocytes. *PLoS One*. 2016;11(5):e0154447.
56. Karaaslan F, Dikilitaş A, Yiğit U. The effects of vaping electronic cigarettes on periodontitis. *Aust Dent J*. 2020;65(2):143-149.
57. Cho JH. The association between electronic-cigarette use and self-reported oral symptoms including cracked or broken teeth and tongue and/or inside-cheek pain among adolescents: a cross-sectional study. *PLoS One*. 2017;12(7):e0180506.
58. Al-Aali KA, Alrabiah M, ArRejaie AS, Abduljabbar T, Vohra F, Akram Z. Peri-implant parameters, tumor necrosis factor-alpha, and interleukin-1 beta levels in vaping individuals. *Clin Implant Dent Relat Res*. 2018;20(3):410-415.
59. Yang I, Sandeep S, Rodriguez J. The oral health impact of electronic cigarette use: a systematic review. *Crit Rev Toxicol*. 2020;50(2):97-127.
60. Sinha DK, Vishal, Kumar A, Khan M, Kumari R, Kesari M. Evaluation of tumor necrosis factor-alpha (TNF-α) and interleukin (IL)-1β levels among subjects vaping e-cigarettes and nonsmokers. *J Family Med Prim Care*. 2020;9(2): 1072-1075.
61. Eke PI, Wei L, Thornton-Evans GO, et al. Risk indicators for periodontitis in US adults: NHANES 2009 to 2012. *J Periodontol*. 2016;87(10):1174-1185.
62. Baumeister S-E, Freuer D, Nolde M, et al. Testing the association between tobacco smoking, alcohol consumption, and risk of periodontitis: a Mendelian randomization study. *J Clin Periodontol*. 2021;48(11):1414-1420.
63. Silva H. Tobacco use and periodontal disease—the role of microvascular dysfunction. *Biology*. 2021;10(5):441.
64. Hanioka T, Ojima M, Tanaka K, Matsuo K, Sato F, Tanaka H. Causal assessment of smoking and tooth loss: a systematic review of observational studies. *BMC Public Health*. 2011;11:221.
65. Akram Z, Aati S, Alrahlah A, Vohra F, Fawzy A. Longitudinal evaluation of clinical, spectral and tissue degradation biomarkers in progression of periodontitis among cigarette and electronic cigarette smokers. *J Dent*. 2021;109:103678.
66. Figueredo CA, Abdelhay N, Figueredo CM, Catunda R, Gibson MP. The impact of vaping on periodontitis: a systematic review. *Clin Exp Dent Res*. 2021;7(3):376-384.

67. Souto MLS, Rovai ES, Villar CC, Braga MM, Pannuti CM. Effect of smoking cessation on tooth loss: a systematic review with meta-analysis. *BMC Oral Health*. 2019;19(1):245.
68. Sundar IK, Javed F, Romanos GE, Rahman I. E-cigarettes and flavorings induce inflammatory and pro-senescence responses in oral epithelial cells and periodontal fibroblasts. *Oncotarget*. 2016;7(47):77196-77204.
69. Chaffee BW, Couch ET, Vora MV, Holliday RS. Oral and periodontal implications of tobacco and nicotine products. *Periodontol 2000*. 2021;87(1):241-253.
70. Patel RA, Wilson RF, Palmer RM. The effect of smoking on periodontal bone regeneration: a systematic review and meta-analysis. *J Periodontol*. 2012;83(2):143-155.
71. Naseri R, Yaghini J, Feizi A. Levels of smoking and dental implants failure: a systematic review and meta-analysis. *J Clin Periodontol*. 2020;47(4):518-528.
72. Kotsakis GA, Javed F, Hinrichs JE, Karoussis IK, Romanos GE. Impact of cigarette smoking on clinical outcomes of periodontal flap surgical procedures: a systematic review and meta-analysis. *J Periodontol*. 2015;86(2):254-263.
73. Fiorini T, Musskopf ML, Oppermann RV, Susin C. Is there a positive effect of smoking cessation on periodontal health? A systematic review. *J Periodontol*. 2014;85(1):83-91.
74. Baker TB, Breslau N, Covey L, Shiffman S. DSM criteria for tobacco use disorder and tobacco withdrawal: a critique and proposed revisions for DSM-5. *Addiction*. 2012;107(2):263-275.
75. National Institutes of Health, National Institute on Drug Abuse. Is nicotine addictive? National Institute on Drug Abuse. Published January 2020. https://www.drugabuse.gov/publications/research-reports/tobacco-nicotine-e-cigarettes/nicotine-addictive. Accessed October 21, 2021.
76. Smokefree.gov. Managing withdrawal. https://smokefree.gov/challenges-when-quitting/withdrawal/managing-withdrawal. Accessed October 21, 2021.
77. The Truth Initiative. E-cigarettes: Facts, stats and regulations. https://truthinitiative.org/research-resources/emerging-tobacco-products/e-cigarettes-facts-stats-and-regulations. Accessed August 29, 2021.
78. Benowitz NL. Nicotine addiction. *N Engl J Med*. 2010; 362(24):2295-2303.
79. Hahad O, Daiber A, Michal M, et al. Smoking and neuropsychiatric disease-associations and underlying mechanisms. *Int J Mol Sci*. 2021;22(14):7272.
80. Conti AA, Tolomeo S, Steele JD, Baldacchino AM. Severity of negative mood and anxiety symptoms occurring during acute abstinence from tobacco: a systematic review and meta-analysis. *Neurosci Biobehav Rev*. 2020;115:48-63.
81. Hughes JR, Klemperer EM, Peasley-Miklus C. Possible new symptoms of tobacco withdawal II: anhedonia-a systematic review. *Nicotine Tob Res*. 2020;22(1):11-17.
82. Pankova A, Kralikova E, Zvolska K, et al. Early weight gain after stopping smoking: a predictor of overall large weight gain? A single-site retrospective cohort study. *BMJ Open*. 2018;8(12):e023987.
83. Giulietti F, Filipponi A, Rosettani G, et al. Pharmacological approach to smoking cessation: an updated review for daily clinical practice. *High Blood Press Cardiovasc Prev*. 2020;27(5):349-362.
84. Patnode CD, Henderson JT, Thompson JH, Senger CA, Fortmann SP, Whitlock EP. Behavioral counseling and pharmacotherapy interventions for tobacco cessation in adults, including pregnant women: a review of reviews for the U.S. preventive services task force. *Ann Intern Med*. 2015;163(8):608-621.
85. National Cancer Institute, National Institute of Medicine. Handling withdrawal symptoms & triggers when you decide to quit. Published June 16, 2020. https://www.cancer.gov/about-cancer/causes-prevention/risk/tobacco/withdrawal-fact-sheet. Accessed October 21, 2021.
86. Rodu B, Plurphanswat N. Quit methods used by American smokers, 2013–2014. *Int J Environ Res Public Health*. 2017;14(11):1403
87. Chaffee BW, Urata J, Couch ET, Silverstein S. Dental professionals' engagement in tobacco, electronic cigarette, and cannabis patient counseling. *JDR Clin Translat Res*. 2020; 5(2):133-145.
88. Gonseth S, Abarca M, Madrid C, Cornuz J. A pilot study combining individual-based smoking cessation counseling, pharmacotherapy, and dental hygiene intervention. *BMC Public Health*. 2010;10:348.
89. Berg CJ, Krishnan N, Graham AL, Abroms LC. A synthesis of the literature to inform vaping cessation interventions for young adults. *Addict Behav*. 2021;119:106898.
90. Prutzman YM, Wiseman KP, Grady MA, et al. Using digital technologies to reach tobacco users who want to quit: evidence from the National Cancer Institute's smokefree.gov initiative. *Am J Prevent Med*. 2021;60(3):S172-S184.
91. Stead LF, Lancaster T. Combined pharmacotherapy and behavioural interventions for smoking cessation. *Cochrane Database Syst Rev*. 2012;(10).
92. Lindson N, Chepkin SC, Ye W, Fanshawe TR, Bullen C, Hartmann-Boyce J. Different doses, durations and modes of delivery of nicotine replacement therapy for smoking cessation. *Cochrane Database Syst Rev*. 2019;2019(4): CD013308.
93. Lindson-Hawley N, Hartmann-Boyce J, Fanshawe TR, Begh R, Farley A, Lancaster T. Interventions to reduce harm from continued tobacco use. *Cochrane Database Syst Rev*. 2016;2016(10):CD005231.
94. Agency for Healthcare Research and Quality. Clinical guidelines for prescribing pharmacotherapy for smoking cessation. Published August 28, 2021. http://www.ahrq.gov/prevention/guidelines/tobacco/prescrib.html. Accessed August 28, 2021.
95. American College of Obstetricians and Gynecologists. *Tobacco and Nicotine Cessation during Pregnancy*. ACOG; 2020. https://www.acog.org/en/clinical/clinical-guidance/committee-opinion/articles/2020/05/tobacco-and-nicotine-cessation-during-pregnancy. Accessed October 24, 2021.
96. Shah SD, Wilken LA, Winkler SR, Lin S-J. Systematic review and meta-analysis of combination therapy for smoking cessation. *J Am Pharm Assoc*. 2008;48(5):659-665.
97. Pengpid S, Peltzer K. Tobacco use and associated health risk behaviours among university students in 27 countries. *Int J Adolesc Med Health*. 2020;34(2):131-137.
98. Moafa I, Hoving C, van den Borne B, Jafer M. Identifying behavior change techniques used in tobacco cessation interventions by oral health professionals and their relation to intervention effects—a review of the scientific literature. *Int J Environ Res Public Health*. 2021;18(14):7481.
99. Centers for Disease Control and Prevention. Smoking cessation—the role of healthcare professionals and health systems. Published February 24, 2020. https://www.cdc.gov/tobacco/data_statistics/sgr/2020-smoking-cessation/fact-sheets/healthcare-professionals-health-systems/index.html. Accessed August 26, 2021.

100. Holliday R, Hong B, McColl E, Livingstone-Banks J, Preshaw PM. Interventions for tobacco cessation delivered by dental professionals. *Cochrane Database Syst Rev*. 2021;2:CD005084.
101. Lindson-Hawley N, Thompson TP, Begh R. Motivational interviewing for smoking cessation. *Cochrane Database Syst Rev*. 2015;(3):CD006936.
102. Chaffee BW, Couch ET, Ryder MI. The tobacco-using periodontal patient: the role of the dental practitioner in tobacco cessation and periodontal diseases management. *Periodontol 2000*. 2016;71(1):52-64.
103. US Preventive Services Task Force, Owens DK, Davidson KW, et al. Primary care interventions for prevention and cessation of tobacco use in children and adolescents: US Preventive Services Task Force Recommendation Statement. *JAMA*. 2020;323(16):1590-1598.
104. Fanshawe TR, Halliwell W, Lindson N, Aveyard P, Livingstone-Banks J, Hartmann-Boyce J. Tobacco cessation interventions for young people. *Cochrane Database Syst Rev*. 2017;2017(11):CD003289.
105. Cutrona SL, Sadasivam RS, DeLaughter K, et al. Online tobacco websites and online communities—who uses them and do users quit smoking? The quit-primo and national dental practice-based research network Hi-Quit studies. *Transl Behav Med*. 2016;6(4):546-557.
106. Carr AB, Ebbert J. Interventions for tobacco cessation in the dental setting. *Cochrane Database Syst Rev*. 2012;(6):CD005084.
107. U.S. Department of Health and Human Services. *Oral Health in America: Surgeon General's Report*. U.S. Department of Health and Human Services, National Institute of Dental and Craniofacial Research, National Institutes of Health; 2000:308. https://www.cdc.gov/oralhealth/publications/sgr2000_05.htm. Accessed October 24, 2021.
108. Centers for Disease Control and Prevention. Best practices for comprehensive tobacco control programs—2014. Smoking and Tobacco Use. Published May 19, 2021. https://www.cdc.gov/tobacco/stateandcommunity/best_practices/index.htm. Accessed August 31, 2021.

CHAPTER 33

Diet and Dietary Analysis

Lisa F. Mallonee, RDH, RD, LD, MPH

CHAPTER OUTLINE

NUTRIENT STANDARDS FOR DIET ADEQUACY IN HEALTH PROMOTION
- **I.** Government Standards
- **II.** Dietary Standards
- **III.** Dietary Guidelines for Americans
- **IV.** MyPlate Food Guidelines
- **V.** Recommended Food Intake Patterns

ORAL HEALTH RELATIONSHIPS
- **I.** Skin and Mucous Membrane
- **II.** Periodontal Tissues
- **III.** Tooth Structure and Integrity
- **IV.** Dental Caries

COUNSELING FOR DENTAL CARIES CONTROL

THE DIETARY ASSESSMENT
- **I.** Purposes of a Dietary Assessment
- **II.** Preliminary Preparation for Dietary Assessment
- **III.** Forms Used for Assessment
- **IV.** Presentation of the Food Record to the Patient
- **V.** Receiving the Completed Food Record
- **VI.** Analysis of Dietary Intake

PREPARATION FOR ADDITIONAL COUNSELING
- **I.** Define Objectives
- **II.** Planning Factors
- **III.** Appropriate Teaching Materials

COUNSELING PROCEDURES
- **I.** Setting
- **II.** Setting the Stage for a Successful Counseling Session
- **III.** Presentation of Findings
- **IV.** Specific Dietary Recommendations

EVALUATION OF PROGRESS
- **I.** Immediate Evaluation
- **II.** Three-Month Follow-Up
- **III.** Six-Month Follow-Up
- **IV.** Overall Evaluation

DOCUMENTATION

FACTORS TO TEACH THE PATIENT

REFERENCES

LEARNING OBJECTIVES

After studying this chapter, the student will be able to:

1. Recognize oral manifestations of vitamin and mineral deficiencies.
2. Explain the function of nutrients in maintaining oral and overall health.
3. Identify good food sources for each micronutrient relevant to oral health.
4. Determine the caries risk potential of a patient's food record.
5. Access and utilize the MyPlate website for diet analysis and as a tool for patient education.

Nutrition is an integral part of an individual's general health as well as the health status of the oral cavity. The health of oral tissues can be affected by nutrition, diet, and food habits.

- The interrelationship among nutritional status, systemic diseases, and oral conditions supports the need for timely and effective diet intervention.
- Within the scope of practice, the dental hygienist has a responsibility to assess, screen, and deliver nutritional information and instruction as part of comprehensive education in health promotion and disease prevention and intervention.
- Dietary and nutritional counseling, as part of a dental caries risk assessment and management program and periodontal health maintenance, is an essential part of the dental hygiene care plan.

Nutrient Standards for Diet Adequacy in Health Promotion

- Patient education should center on helping patients learn about selection of foods that make up a balanced **diet** for maintenance of optimum health and reduced oral disease risk.

I. Government Standards

A. Purposes of Standards

- Facilitate education for individuals about dietary needs and goals to achieve and maintain health.
- Prevent deficiency diseases and help achieve diet adequacy for the public.
- Make recommendations relative to poor food habits, such as missed meals, omission of essential foods and **nutrients**, and fad dieting.
- Make specific recommendations for oral health.
- Motivate for behavioral modification.

B. Guidelines

- Provided through printed and web-based educational materials.
- Reflect public health concerns as they relate to nutrition.

II. Dietary Standards

A. Dietary Reference Intakes (DRI)

- **Dietary Reference Intakes (DRIs)** is a comprehensive term for categories of reference values to meet the general nutrient needs for the healthy population to prevent deficiencies, toxicities, and chronic disease.
- Encompasses the current nutrient recommendations made by the Institute of Medicine (IOM), National Academy of Sciences, and Food and Nutrition Board.[1]
- The categories include:
  - **Recommended Dietary Allowance (RDA)**.
  - **Estimated Average Requirement (EAR)**.
  - **Adequate Intake (AI)**.
  - **Tolerable Upper Intake Level (UL)**.
- Established for vitamins and minerals.

B. Recommended Dietary Allowances (RDAs)

- Recommended amounts of **macronutrients** and **micronutrients** needed to consume daily to maintain good health and prevent deficiency.[2]
- Categorized by age and sex; do not include special needs such as illness.

C. Estimated Average Requirements (EARs)

- Estimates the nutritional requirements of the average individual.[1]
- Categorized by age and sex.
- Provide the foundation for the RDAs.

D. Adequate Intakes (AIs)

- Recommended nutrient intake utilized when there is not enough information to establish an EAR.[2,3]
- AIs have been established for calcium, vitamin D, and fluoride for all age groups.

E. Tolerable Upper Intake Levels (ULs)

- Maximum intake by an individual that is unlikely to create risks of adverse health effects in almost all healthy individuals.
- ULs were established to avoid toxicity due to excess intake of specific nutrients from food, fortified food, water, and nutrient supplements.[2,3]

III. Dietary Guidelines for Americans

- Established by U.S. Department of Agriculture (**USDA**) and U.S. Department of Health and Human Services as the basis for a federal nutrition

Box 33-1 Key Recommendations: Dietary Guidelines for Americans, 2020–2025

- Follow a healthy pattern of eating at every life stage.
- Consume nutrient-dense food and beverage choices based on personal preferences, cultural norms, and budgetary considerations.
- Limit consumption of alcohol and foods/beverages with added sugars, saturated fats, and sodium.
- Consume a diet rich in nutrient-dense foods and monitor intake of calories.

Data from U.S. Department of Agriculture and U.S. Department of Health and Human Services. *Dietary Guidelines for Americans, 2020–2025*. 9th ed. December 2020. www.DietaryGuidelines.gov. Accessed April 23, 2022.

policy based on the most recent scientific evidence review.
- Provides information and advice for choosing healthy eating patterns that focus on consuming **nutrient-dense** foods to promote a healthy weight and reduce risk of chronic disease.
- Used as the basis for developing nutrition-related programs, educational materials, and consumer health messages to promote healthy eating patterns at home, school, work, community, and retail food establishments.
- **Box 33-1** lists key recommendations in the 2015–2020 Dietary Guidelines for Americans.

IV. MyPlate Food Guidelines

- Originally developed as a "Food Pyramid" by the USDA in 1991.[4]
- Newest version established in June 2011 using the graphic representation of a "dinner-plate" icon as illustrated in **Figure 33-1**.
- Colorful graphic provides a visual reminder of the approximate proportions of five food groups necessary for a healthy diet.
- Educational materials accompanying the MyPlate food guidance system encourage consumers to build a healthy plate:
    - Make half the plate vegetables and fruits.
    - Switch to fat-free or low-fat milk.
    - Choose whole grains.
    - Vary protein choices to include seafood and legumes and keep meat portions small.
    - Cut back on foods high in solid fat, added sugars, and salt.
    - Eat the right amount of calories to maintain a healthy weight.
    - Enjoy food, but eat less and keep track of what is consumed.

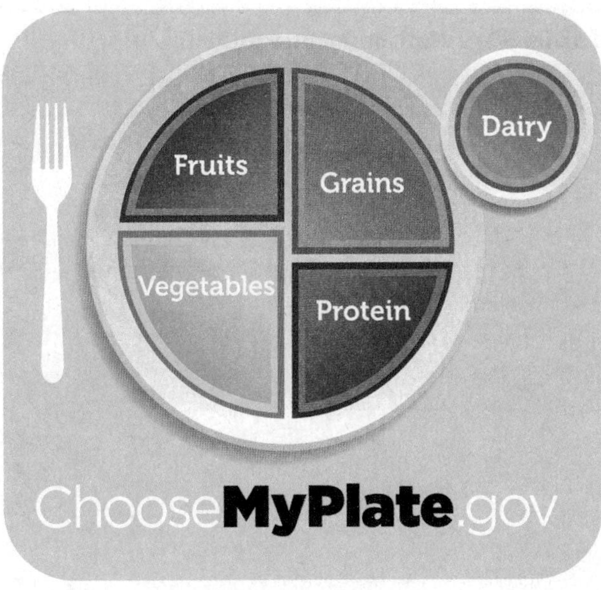

Figure 33-1 ChooseMyPlate Guidelines Icon

U.S. Department of Agriculture, Center for Nutrition Policy and Promotion. ChooseMyPlate guidelines. 2011. https://www.myplate.gov/. Accessed April 23, 2022.

    - Cook more often at home and choose lower calorie options when eating out.
    - Limit alcoholic beverages.
    - Be physically active.

V. Recommended Food Intake Patterns

- Estimated calorie needs and recommended amounts of food from each food group accompany the MyPlate food guidelines.
- Individual dietary plans that estimate calorie needs based on age, sex, weight, height, and activity levels can be created.
- Provides option to create a dietary plan to maintain current weight or achieve a healthier weight.

Oral Health Relationships

- Nutrition, diet, and oral and systemic health are closely interrelated:
    - Healthy masticatory function of the dentition contributes to proper dietary selection for maintenance of the nutritional status of the entire body.
    - Healthy diet selection provides essential nutrients for optimum health of oral tissues and prevention of **nutrient deficiency**. **Table 33-1** outlines micronutrients relevant to oral health, their function, associated deficiency state(s), toxicity states that can occur if consumed in excess, and food sources.

Table 33-1 Nutrients Relevant to Oral Health

Nutrient	Function	Oral Implications of Deficiency	Food Source
Vitamin A (retinol, provitamin A carotene)	▪ **Antioxidant** ▪ Bone and tooth development ▪ Skin and mucous membrane integrity ▪ Cell differentiation; essential for reproduction ▪ Vision in dim light	▪ Enamel hypoplasia ▪ Defective dentin formation ▪ Poor growth ▪ Keratinization of epithelium ▪ Toxic in large doses: headache, vomiting, double vision, dry mucous membranes, joint pain, liver damage	Retinol: found only in animal foods such as egg yolk, liver, fortified milk, cream, cheeses Provitamin A (beta carotene): green leafy vegetables; orange-, red-, and yellow-pigmented fruits and vegetables
Vitamin D (calciferol)	▪ Aids in the absorption of calcium and phosphorus ▪ Mineralization of bone	▪ Enamel hypoplasia ▪ Loss of lamina dura ▪ Toxic in large doses: hypercalcemia	Exposure to sunlight, fortified milk, fish oils
Vitamin E (tocopherol)	▪ Antioxidant	▪ Low incidence of deficiency or toxicity	Whole grains, wheat germ, vegetable oils, legumes, seeds, nuts
Vitamin K (quinone)	▪ Synthesis of prothrombin in blood clotting and bone proteins	▪ Prolonged clotting time ▪ Hemorrhage ▪ Toxic in large doses: patients on blood thinners need to limit dietary intake	Synthesized by intestinal bacterial flora; dark green leafy vegetables, liver
Thiamin (vitamin B_1)	▪ Acts as coenzyme in carbohydrate and amino acid metabolism	▪ Glossitis ▪ Discoloration of gingival tissues ▪ Beriberi: weight loss, fatigue, edema, depression	Enriched whole grains and cereals, pork, nuts, seeds, legumes
Riboflavin (vitamin B_2)	▪ Coenzyme in energy metabolism of fat, carbohydrate, and protein	▪ **Ariboflavinosis** ▪ Angular cheilosis ▪ Glossitis ▪ Edema of pharyngeal and oral mucous membranes ▪ Angular stomatitis	Dairy, enriched whole grains and cereals, rice, mushrooms, liver
Niacin (vitamin B_3)	▪ Coenzyme in energy metabolism of fat, carbohydrate, and protein	▪ Pellagra: diarrhea, dermatitis, dementia, and death ▪ Toxicity not seen in food sources	Eggs, meat, poultry, fish, grains, peanuts, legumes, green leafy vegetables
Pyridoxine (vitamin B_6)	▪ Coenzyme in amino acid and lipid metabolism ▪ Hemoglobin synthesis ▪ Homocysteine metabolism	▪ Glossitis	Potatoes, beef liver, salmon, bananas
Cobalamin (vitamin B_{12})	▪ Maturation of red blood cells (RBCs) ▪ Requires intrinsic factor from parietal cells for absorption ▪ Cofactor in folate and homocysteine metabolism	▪ Pernicious anemia secondary to lack of intrinsic factor and total **vegan diet**	Found only in animal foods or fortified cereals/grains
Folate (folic acid)	▪ Maturation of RBCs ▪ DNA synthesis ▪ Homocysteine metabolism	▪ Glossitis ▪ Chronic periodontitis ▪ Megaloblastic anemia ▪ Cleft lip and palate ▪ May promote *Candida* infection	Green leafy vegetables, brewer's yeast, spinach, melons, lemons, bananas, legumes, fortified grains

Nutrient	Function	Oral Implications of Deficiency	Food Source
Ascorbic acid (vitamin C)	▪ Antioxidant ▪ Collagen synthesis ▪ Wound healing ▪ Aids in absorption of iron	▪ Weakened collagen formation ▪ Poor wound healing ▪ Gingivitis ▪ Petechial hemorrhages	Citrus fruits, broccoli, strawberries, peppers, tomatoes, cantaloupe
Calcium	▪ Muscle contraction ▪ Blood clotting ▪ Nerve impulse transmission ▪ Calcification of bones and teeth	▪ Incomplete calcification of bones and teeth ▪ Tooth mobility or premature loss of teeth	Dairy products, tofu, fortified foods, soy milk, green leafy vegetables, canned salmon and sardines
Phosphorus	▪ Important for bone and teeth formation ▪ Acid–base balance ▪ Muscle contraction	▪ Incomplete calcification of teeth ▪ Compromised alveolar integrity may result	Dairy products, meat, poultry, nuts, legumes, whole-grain cereals
Magnesium	▪ Bone strength and rigidity ▪ Hydroxyapatite crystal formation ▪ Nerve impulse ▪ Muscle contraction	▪ Gingival hypertrophy ▪ Alveolar bone fragility	Wheat bran, whole grains, green leafy vegetables, legumes, nuts, chocolate
Fluoride	▪ Prevention of dental caries ▪ Remineralization	▪ Increased incidence of caries ▪ Toxicity: mottled enamel ▪ Can alter amelogenesis ▪ Decreased resistance to caries	Fluoridated water, tea, seaweed, toothpaste

Data from Palmer CA, Boyd L. The minerals and mineralization. In Palmer CA, Boyd LD, eds. *Diet and Nutrition in Oral Health*. 3rd ed. Upper Saddle River, NJ: Pearson Prentice Hall; 2017; Palmer CA. Vitamins today. In Palmer CA, Boyd LD, eds. *Diet and Nutrition in Oral Health*. 3rd ed. Upper Saddle River, NJ: Pearson Prentice Hall; 2017; U.S. Department of Agriculture and U.S. Department of Health and Human Services. Dietary Guidelines for Americans, 2020–2025. 9th ed. December 2020. www.DietaryGuidelines.gov. Accessed April 27, 2022; National Institutes of Health, Office of Dietary Supplements. *Dietary supplement fact sheets*. https://ods.od.nih.gov/factsheets/list-all. Accessed April 27, 2022.

I. Skin and Mucous Membrane

- Relevant vitamins: vitamin A, vitamin B complex, and ascorbic acid (vitamin C).
- Relevant minerals: zinc and iron.

II. Periodontal Tissues

Periodontal diseases are not caused by nutritional deficiencies, but **malnutrition** may contribute to the progression of periodontal disease symptoms and influence healing following treatment.

- Nutritional deficiencies do not cause periodontal diseases. Without local factors, including the periodontal pathogens in biofilm, biofilm-retentive factors (such as calculus and defective restorations), and lack of the oral self-care to remove biofilm, periodontal infections cannot occur.
- Severe deficiencies are rare in developed countries. Symptoms of deficiencies such as those listed in **Table 33-2** may be seen in cases of severe deprivation, starvation, and patients with long-term alcoholism or other drug addictions.
- RDAs are essential to the health of the periodontal tissues. As part of total body health, the daily diet nourishes the oral tissues.
- The physical characteristic of the diet contributes. A soft, sticky diet that stays on the tooth surfaces, especially cervical third and proximal areas, encourages biofilm buildup and proliferation of bacteria, including the periodontal pathogens.
- Malnutrition suppresses the immune system and impairs the host's reaction to infections. Increased activity of pathogenic microorganisms may result in increased periodontal disease.
- Nutrients contribute to healing and tissue repair.[5] The elements strongly associated with wound healing include vitamin B complex, vitamin C (ascorbic acid), and dietary calcium.
  - *B complex* refers to all the water-soluble vitamins, except vitamin C. They are thiamin (vitamin B_1), riboflavin (vitamin B_2), niacin (vitamin B_3), pyridoxine (vitamin B_6), cobalamin (vitamin B_{12}), biotin, folic acid, and pantothenic acid. Each member of the B complex has individual functions.

Table 33-2 Oral Manifestations of Nutrient Deficiencies

Oral Symptoms Associated with the Tongue	Nutrient Deficiency
Altered taste sensations	Riboflavin, thiamin, zinc, vitamin A, vitamin B_{12}
Glossitis	Folate, niacin, riboflavin, vitamin B_6, vitamin B_{12}
Glossodynia	Niacin, vitamin B_6, vitamin B_{12}
Sore or burning tongue	Iron, niacin, riboflavin, thiamin, vitamin B_6, vitamin B_{12}
Oral Symptoms Associated with Mucosal Tissue	
Angular cheilosis	Folate, iron, riboflavin, vitamin B_6, vitamin B_{12}
Candidiasis	Folate, iron, zinc, vitamin A, vitamin C
Delayed wound healing	Riboflavin, zinc, vitamin A, vitamin C
Mucositis/ stomatitis	Folate, niacin, thiamin, vitamin B_{12}

Data from Palmer CA, Boyd LD. Principals of diet screening, risk assessment and guideance. In Palmer CA, Boyd LD, eds. *Diet and Nutrition in Oral Health*. Upper Saddle River, NJ: Pearson Prentice Hall; 2017; National Institutes of Health. Office of Dietary Supplements. *Dietary supplement fact sheets*. https://ods.od.nih.gov/factsheets/list-all. Accessed April 27, 2022.

- Vitamin C is needed for collagen formation and intercellular material, and healing tissues after procedures including periodontal debridement.
- Dietary calcium. About 99% of the calcium in the body is in the bones and teeth, 1% is in the body tissues and fluids; essential for cell metabolism, muscle contraction, and nerve impulse transmission. Vitamin D is necessary for the continuous exchange of calcium between the blood, skeletal bones, and other cells.
- Low dietary intake of calcium and vitamin D can negatively impact alveolar bone integrity in periodontal disease. Loss of alveolar bone and soft-tissue attachment are typical of periodontal disease progression. Supplementation of these nutrients has been shown to reduce alveolar bone loss.[6,7]
- Current and former smokers with low dietary vitamin C intake are at risk for more severe periodontal disease.[8,9] The IOM suggests smokers need 35 mg more vitamin C per day than nonsmokers.[10]

- Obesity and oral disease
  - Obesity and periodontal disease have an association with each other, and inflammation is the proposed mechanism for this relationship.[11,12]
  - Higher **body mass index** and waist circumference have been correlated with increased incidence of dental caries and periodontal disease.[11-13]
  - As with all chronic diseases, it is the dental professional's role to promote healthy lifestyle choices, including, but not limited to, oral self-care, tobacco cessation, healthy food choices adequate physical exercise, and weight control to manage and/or prevent progression of disease.
  - Referral to a primary care provider or registered dietitian nutritionist is indicated if dietary guidance is indicated for weight control.
- Dietary considerations post-periodontal surgery
  - Following periodontal surgical intervention, patients may need to alter diet consistency during the healing period.
  - A soft diet of high-quality protein is indicated for adequate wound healing. Puddings, scrambled eggs, milkshakes, yogurt, and cottage cheese have high-quality protein to promote healing.
  - Chewing firm foods increases salivary flow. Saliva acts as a buffer, and increased saliva aids in oral clearance.

III. Tooth Structure and Integrity

- Nutrients and health of tooth structure
  - Adequate nutrition during tooth development is essential for mineralization.
  - Relevant minerals: calcium, phosphorus, magnesium, and fluoride.
  - Relevant vitamin: vitamin A.
- Dietary assessment
  - Diet assessment during early tooth development is essential to assist parents in caries prevention.
  - Anticipatory guidance for the parents of infants, children, and adolescents can be found in Chapters 46 and 47.

IV. Dental Caries

- Prevention[14]
  - Fluoride is an essential mineral for dental caries prevention.
  - Contributing factors in dental caries formation are illustrated in **Figure 33-2**.

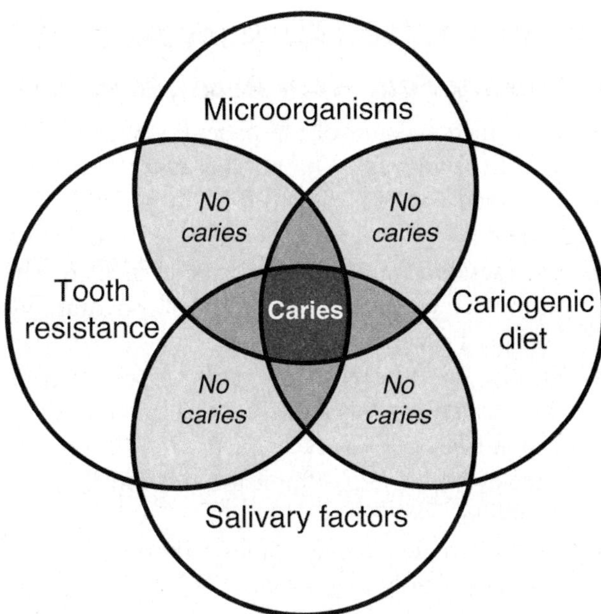

Figure 33-2 Dental Caries Process. Four overlapping circles illustrate the factors involved in the development of dental caries. All four act together, and as shown by the center, dental caries results.

Data from U.S. Department of Health and Human Services, Public Health Service, National Institute of Dental Research. Broadening the Scope. Long-Range Research Plan for the 1990s. Washington, DC: U.S. Government Printing Office; 1990. NIH Publication No. 90-1188.

- Role of cariogenic foods[15]
  - Dental caries is a result of biofilm and excess **cariogenic** foods, not a nutrient deficiency.
  - *Streptococcus mutans*, lactobacilli, and other acid-forming organisms use fermentable carbohydrates from the diet to produce acids.
- Consistency of food
  - Soft, sticky foods cling to the teeth and gingiva and encourage biofilm accumulation.[15]
  - Microorganisms are protected and nourished in dental biofilm on the tooth, leading to increased acid formation.
- Dietary assessment and counseling
  - Use of **dietary assessment** and patient instruction relative to dental caries control.
  - Personal recommendations foster behavioral modification in disease prevention.

Counseling for Dental Caries Control

- Risk factors (see Chapter 25)
  - Inadequate biofilm removal.
  - Dexterity issues that may affect oral self-care and ability to effectively remove biofilm.
  - Inadequately mineralized tooth enamel, such as in enamel hypoplasia or demineralization.
  - Did not live in an area with fluoridated water or consume fluoride during formative years of tooth development.
  - Frequent snacks with fermentable carbohydrates, consumption of slow-dissolving foods and acidic beverages between meals.
  - Altered salivary flow such as in drug-induced xerostomia.
  - Figure 33-2 illustrates the relationship of all four factors involved in the development of dental caries.
- Preventive measures that support dietary control
  - Adequate plaque biofilm removal.
  - Modification of intake of cariogenic foods and acidogenic beverages.
  - Strengthening the tooth surface to resist caries activity with appropriate office and home fluorides.
  - Pit-and-fissure sealants.
  - Restoration of existing carious lesions.
  - Routine preventive care at intervals specific to patient need (3, 4, or 6 months)

The Dietary Assessment

- Dietary assessment is an integral part of disease prevention and health promotion in the scope of dental hygiene care.[16]
- The patient and dental hygienist have the opportunity to collaborate in the evaluation of diet adequacy and in diet intervention.

I. Purposes of a Dietary Assessment

- Identify patients who may be at nutritional and oral health risk based on reported dietary habits.
- Review nutritional status of an individual with regard to overall dietary requirements based on height, weight, sex, and activity level.
- Identify cariogenic eating patterns and/or food groups not regularly consumed, which may result in nutrient-related oral manifestations.
- Refer to a **registered dietitian (RD)** or **registered dietitian nutritionist (RDN)** when intervention beyond the scope of dental hygiene practice is indicated.
- Provide an opportunity for a patient to be more consciously aware of personal dietary habits and the potential impact on oral and systemic health by:
  - Recording frequency of consumption of cariogenic food and acidogenic beverages.

- Obtaining an overall picture of the types of food in the patient's diet, food preferences, and quantity of food eaten.
- Focused observation and discussion of food/beverage habits and snacking patterns.
- Determine the overall adequacy and consistency of the diet.
  - Identify food groups that are not regularly consumed or lacking in the diet.
  - Identify fibrous foods regularly consumed.
  - Identify soft, sticky foods frequently consumed.
- Collaborate with the patient to make suggestions for modification in nutritional adequacy of the diet in health promotion.
- Plan with the patient for necessary changes to improve the health of the oral mucosa and periodontium and to prevent dental caries.

II. Preliminary Preparation for Dietary Assessment

A. Patient History

- Information obtained from medical, dental, and social histories is essential in assessing oral health and nutritional status:
  - Disease states
  - Disabilities
  - Dexterity issues
  - Medications
  - Avoidance of foods due to mouth pain or missing teeth
  - Learning limitations
  - Significant unintentional change in body weight
  - Factors influencing food use and food intake.
  - Dietary influences can be identified by intraoral and extraoral examination, which may reveal oral tissue changes suggestive of nutritional deficiencies.

B. Clinical Evaluation

- High-risk patients can be identified by noting factors suggestive of a dietary problem.
- Clinical examination and charting of cavitated carious lesions and demineralizing areas.
- Identification of any abnormalities in the patient's overall appearance: weight, skin, nails, and hair.
- Table 33-2 lists oral manifestations of severe deficiencies.

III. Forms Used for Assessment

*A. Twenty-Four Hour Recall (**Table 33-3**).*

- A detailed account of the patient's dietary intake over the previous 24 hours (**Box 33-2**)
- Obtained during face-to-face discussion with patient.
- Assesses food groups; nutrients; diet adequacy; form, frequency, and timing of carbohydrate intake; and snacking patterns.
- Results are reviewed and appropriate instruction given at appointment or a follow-up appointment.
- Quick and easy to administer and can be done chairside.
- Is limited to 1-day intake; therefore, it is not necessarily representative of a patient's normal diet.

B. Dietary Food Record: 3, 5, or 7 Days

- A more accurate account of a patient's intake.
- Food record can be modified to include 3, 5, or 7 days (**Figure 33-3**).
- Patient completes food record for 3, 5, or 7 days, inclusive of 1 weekend day.

Table 33-3 **Twenty-Four Hour Recall Dietary Intake Form**

NAME______________________________
AGE______SEX______Height______Weight______
Activity Level:

- Physically active less than 30 minutes daily
- Physically active 30–60 minutes daily
- Physically active more than 60 minutes daily

Foods/Beverages Consumed (Include Time)	Quantity Eaten (cup, oz, tbsp, tsp, etc.)	Location Consumed/ Preparation Method
BREAKFAST		
SNACK		
LUNCH		
SNACK		
DINNER		
SNACK		

Box 33-2 Example 24-Hour Recall Dietary Intake

7:30 AM Breakfast Orange juice Bagel Cream cheese Coffee Milk Sugar Brushed teeth 2 minutes	 1/2 cup Whole 2 tablespoons 2 cups 1/2 cup 2 packets	 Bagel shop
10:00 AM Snack Chocolate chip cookies Orange soda	 2 cookies 12 oz can	 Prepared at home
1:00 PM Lunch Mushroom pizza Orange soda Cheese cake Used floss picks	 2 slices 12 oz can 1 slice	 School cafeteria
4:00 PM Snack Whole-wheat pretzels	 1 bag	 Vending machine
7:00 PM Dinner Turkey Potato Sour cream Broccoli Olive oil Gravy	 6 oz 1 medium 2 tablespoons 1 cup 2 tablespoons ½ cup	 Prepared at home Roasted Baked Steamed Packet mix
9:30 PM Snack Popcorn Brushed teeth 2 minutes, flossed, and used antibacterial rinse prior to bedtime	 3 cups	 Home/ microwave

- Affords the patient a more active role in the dietary assessment and a chance to observe areas that require modification.
- Request patient return the completed food record at follow-up visit.
- At follow-up visit, the patient's food record is evaluated for:
  - Eating patterns.
  - Consumption and frequency of fermentable carbohydrates.
  - Nutritional adequacy.
- Noncompliance may occur due to the following reasons:
  - Time consuming for the patient and the person assessing the diet.
  - Reliance on patient to accurately report intake.
  - Foods not written down immediately may be forgotten.

IV. Presentation of the Food Record to the Patient

- Explain the purpose
  - Identify oral disease risk factors and dietary habits that would benefit from further assessment to develop preventive education.
  - Briefly describe how diet relates to oral health.
  - Provide a foundation for the needed additional assessment to tailor education specific to the patient at next scheduled appointment.
- Explain the form
  - Provide written and oral instructions for documenting food and beverage intake and daily oral hygiene care.
  - Provide suggestions for listing various foods and use of household measurements for indicating quantity.
  - Instruction for completing the food record encourages the patient to provide a more accurate portrayal of eating behaviors.
  - If time permits, the first day of the food record can be completed with patient to help illustrate how to itemize and list food and beverages consumed and oral hygiene care.
- General directions
  - Include all foods, beverages, and slow-dissolving foods consumed (i.e., candy, cough drops).
  - Emphasize the importance of completing the food record for each meal as soon after eating as possible to avoid forgetting.
  - Encourage use of typical days, uncomplicated by illness, holidays, or other unusual circumstances that may impact dietary choices.
  - Review details of recording the component parts of a combination dish, such as a sandwich: 2 slices of whole-wheat bread, 4 oz of turkey, 1 teaspoon of mayonnaise, 2 slices tomato with lettuce, and 1 slice of cheddar cheese.

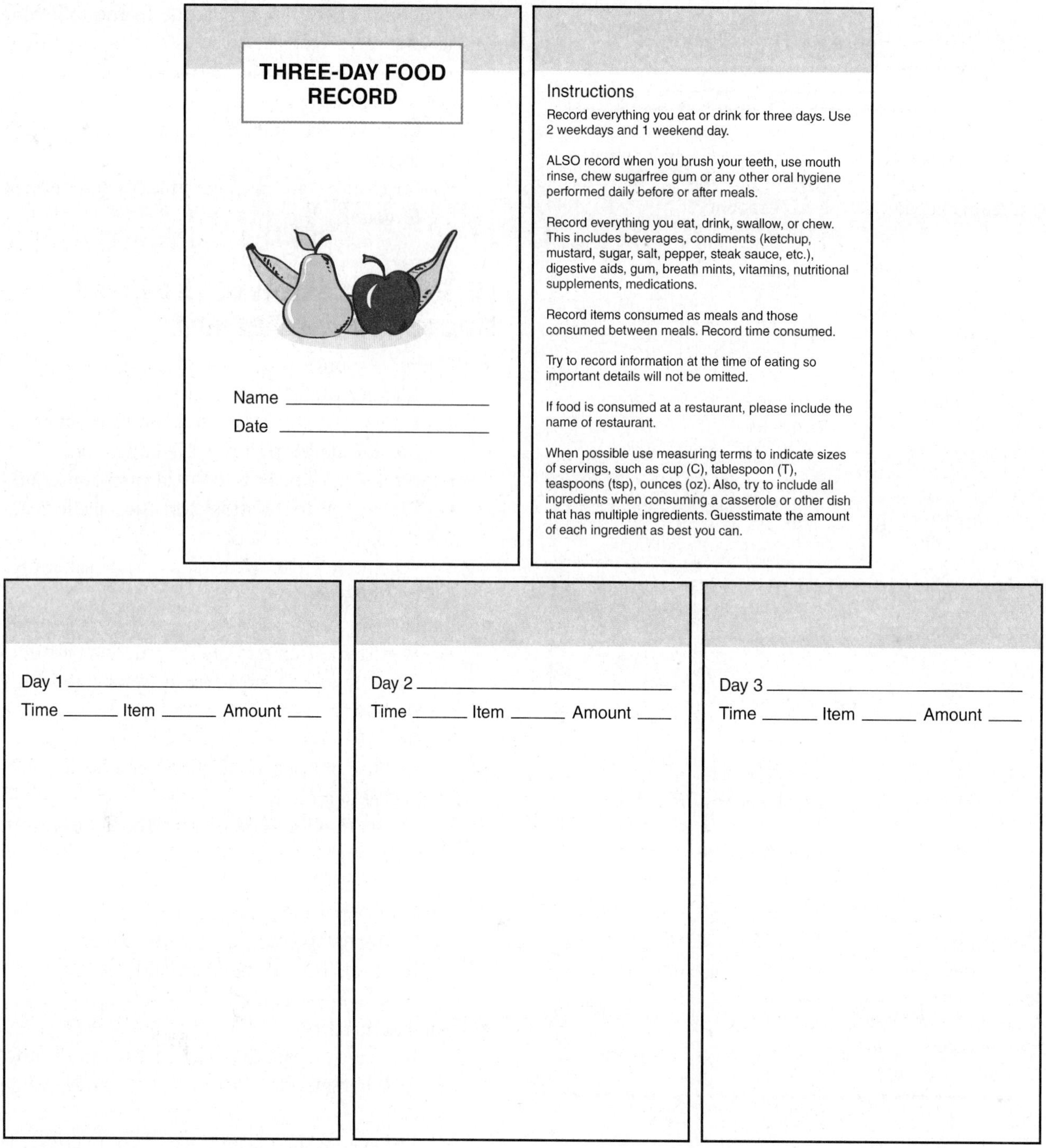

THREE-DAY FOOD RECORD

Name ____________________

Date ____________________

Instructions

Record everything you eat or drink for three days. Use 2 weekdays and 1 weekend day.

ALSO record when you brush your teeth, use mouth rinse, chew sugarfree gum or any other oral hygiene performed daily before or after meals.

Record everything you eat, drink, swallow, or chew. This includes beverages, condiments (ketchup, mustard, sugar, salt, pepper, steak sauce, etc.), digestive aids, gum, breath mints, vitamins, nutritional supplements, medications.

Record items consumed as meals and those consumed between meals. Record time consumed.

Try to record information at the time of eating so important details will not be omitted.

If food is consumed at a restaurant, please include the name of restaurant.

When possible use measuring terms to indicate sizes of servings, such as cup (C), tablespoon (T), teaspoons (tsp), ounces (oz). Also, try to include all ingredients when consuming a casserole or other dish that has multiple ingredients. Guesstimate the amount of each ingredient as best you can.

Day 1 ____________________

Time ______ Item ______ Amount ____

Day 2 ____________________

Time ______ Item ______ Amount ____

Day 3 ____________________

Time ______ Item ______ Amount ____

Figure 33-3 Example of a 3-Day Food Record.

Lisa F. Mallonee, RDH, RD, LD, MPH. Texas A&M School of Dentistry, Caruth School of Dental Hygiene.

- Be accurate in determining the amounts eaten, using household measurements (e.g., 1/2 cup cereal, 1 tsp margarine, 3 oz fish). A 3-oz serving size can be compared to the size of a deck of cards.
  - Record all fluids consumed, including water and alcoholic beverages as well as amounts.
  - Record added sauces, gravies, condiments, and all extras such as sugar and cream in coffee.
- Encourage patient to record intake of daily nutritional supplements.
- Record if food was consumed outside of the home and the location.
- Instruct patient to select consecutive days and at least one weekend day for a realistic representation of diet pattern.
- Encourage patient to include oral hygiene care performed before or after meals.

V. Receiving the Completed Food Record

- Review patient's food record and obtain supplemental information
  - Receive the food record soon after its completion.
  - Question the patient to clarify presented information.
  - Does the record represent typical days or weeks?
  - Identify influences on appetite such as illness or stress.
  - Identify food likes and dislikes, food preferences, intolerances, and food allergies.
  - Note frequency of dining out.
  - Identify special diets being followed at home.
  - Determine average alcohol intake.
  - Which family member is doing the cooking and food shopping?
  - Ask about common food habits, such as snacking at night.
- Common omissions include:
  - Garnishes: frosting, whipped cream, butter or margarine on vegetables, salad dressings, and oil.
  - Beverages: quantity and if pre-sweetened or amount of sweetener added.
  - Snacks: type, brand, and quantity.
  - Chewing gum or mints: sugarless, **noncariogenic** sweetener such as xylitol or other sugar alcohols,[17] aspartame, or sucralose, and quantity.
  - Canned fruit: packed in water, heavy or light syrup, own juices, or sweetened with sugar substitute, and quantity.
  - Fruit and vegetables: canned, fresh, or frozen.
  - Cereal: sugar-coated or low-sugar brand, type of milk and/or sugar added, and quantity.
  - Potato: baked, mashed, or fried.
  - Seasonings or sauces: quantity and type.

VI. Analysis of Dietary Intake

Principal parts of the 24-hour recall or food record to analyze are the number of servings in each food group, frequency of cariogenic foods/acidic beverages, timing of when these foods/beverages are consumed, and consistency of the diet.

A. Nutritional Analysis of 24-Hour Recall Intake

- When time and/or patient compliance are factors, a 24-hour recall analysis is appropriate.
- Compare intake of food groups recorded in the patient's 24-hour food recall with individual needs identified using MyPlate.
- Determine nutritional adequacy.
- Calculate the patient's "sweet score," as outlined in Table 33-5.
- Cariogenic foods are listed and categorized as solid, liquid, or slowly dissolving.
- Totals for the 1 day are multiplied by respective time factors and a score determines patient's caries risk.

B. Nutritional Analysis for Adequacy of Food Intake from the Food Record

- Use the Dietary Analysis Recording Form to summarize adequacy of daily portions of each food group (**Table 33-4**).
- Each food serving recorded by the patient is entered into a food group with number of servings.
- Comparison of intake reported on patient's food record with individual caloric needs for age, sex, height, weight, and activity level identified using MyPlate food guidance system
- Create individualized plans using MyPlate Plan at www.myplate.gov/myplate-plan. Use this information to determine adequacy of intake.
- From the dietary intake form(s) completed by the patient (Table 33-4), each serving is entered as a check in the space beside the appropriate food group
- Totals for the week are added, and the average per day calculated.
- The average is compared to the recommended servings for each food group.
- Assist patient when inadequacies or deficiencies are identified.
- Analysis of cariogenic foods.
  - Identify physical form of carbohydrate.
    - Liquids: sweetened or unsweetened soft drinks; fruit juice with added sugars.
    - Soft solid/sticky and retentive: cakes, cookies, chips, pretzels, jellybeans, and chewy, sticky candies.
    - Hard solid/slowly dissolving: hard candies, mints, and cough drops.
  - Identify frequency of meals and snacks.
    - When snacks are consumed.
    - Number of between-meal snacks consumed daily.

Table 33-4 Dietary Analysis Recording Form

Age: __________ Sex: ____________ Height: __________ Weight: ______________

Activity Level:

- Physically active less than 30 minutes daily
- Physically active 30–60 minutes daily
- Physically active more than 60 minutes daily

									USDA Food Patterns for Five Most Used Caloric Levels (12 Total Levels)					Adequate	
Food Groups	**Day 1**	**2**	**3**	**4**	**5**	**6**	**7**	**Daily Average**	**1,000 kcals**	**1,600 kcals**	**1,800 kcals**	**2,200 kcals**	**2,800 kcals**	**Yes**	**No**
Grains									3 oz-eq	5 oz-eq	6 oz-eq	7 oz-eq	10 oz-eq[a]		
Vegetables									1 cup	2 cups	2.5 cup	3 cups	3.5 cups		
Fruits									1 cup	1.5 cups	1.5 cups	2 cups	2.5 cups		
Dairy									2 cups	3 cups	3 cups	3 cups	3 cups		
Protein foods									2 oz-eq	5 oz-eq	5 oz-eq	6 oz-eq	7 oz-eq		
Oils[b]									15 g/4 tsp	22 g/ tsp	24 g/6 tsp	29 g/7 tsp	36 g/9 tsp		
Forms of Foods Consumed									**Total**						
Liquid						With meal End of meal Between meals			Total all liquid exposures and multiply by 20 minutes and divide by total number of days to equal daily acid attack from liquid. **Total Liquid Minutes**__________						
Soft/solid sticky/retentive						With meal End of meal Between meals			Total all soft and hard solid exposures and multiply by 40 minutes and divide by total number of days to equal daily acid attack from solids. **Total Solid Minutes**__________						
Hard/ solid slowly dissolving						With meal End of meal Between meals			Add both liquid and solid totals to determine the number of minutes per day teeth are under acid attack. **Total Daily Minutes of Acid Attack** __________						

Individualized food group and caloric needs based on age, sex, height, weight and activity levels.
Data from MyPlate Plan at www.myplate.gov/myplate-plan

[a]eq is the abbreviation for the word equivalents.

[b]4.2 grams = 1 teaspoon

    - Circle in red and tally the number of cariogenic foods, both solid and liquids.
    - Frequency more relevant than quantity in caries incidence.
    - High frequency of eating events decreases the ability of calcium and phosphate to remineralize teeth between episodes.
- During counseling appointment, show the patient how to:
    - Select and circle in red the cariogenic forms of foods consumed.
    - Select liquid, soft solid, slow-dissolving foods, and time of eating.
    - Total the number of forms of foods/beverages consumed including both liquid and solids and multiply total by 20 minutes (liquids) and 40 minutes (solids).
    - Divide by number of days (3-, 5-, or 7-day food record).
    - Add both liquid and solid scores to determine total minutes teeth are exposed to sweets and acid attack (**Table 33-5**).

Table 33-5 **Scoring the Sweets (Caries-Promoting Potential)**

Food Items (from patient's 24-hour recall)	Reference Foods Considered Carogenic	Frequency (place a check for each exposure to cariogenic food)	Weighted Score	Total Points Each Category
1. 2. 3. 4.	**Liquid** Soft drinks, fruit drinks, cocoa, sugar and honey in beverages, nondairy creamers, ice cream, sherbet, flavored or frozen yogurt, pudding, custard, Jello	______ ______ ______ ______	X 1	
1. 2. 3. 4. 5. 6.	**Solid and sticky** Cakes, cupcakes, doughnuts, sweet rolls, potato chips, pretzels, pastry, canned fruit in syrup, bananas, cookies, chocolate candy, caramel, toffee, jelly beans, other chewy candy, chewing gum, dried fruit, marshmallows, jelly, jam	______ ______ ______ ______ ______ ______	X 2	
1. 2. 3.	**Slowly dissolving** Hard candies, breath mints, antacid tablets, cough drops	______ ______ ______	X 3	
				Total Score__________

Using the 24-hour recall dietary intake form:

- Classify each sweet into liquid, solid and sticky, or slowly dissolving (use reference food list).
- For each time a sweet was eaten, either at a meal or between meals (at least 20 minutes apart), place a check in the frequency column.
- In each category, tally the number of sweets eaten and multiply by the weighted score. Record the category points in the respective column.
- Tally all the category points to determine the total score.

Sweet Score: (risk for dental caries)	How to Lower Your Risk for CARIES:
0–1 low risk 2–4 5–7 moderate risk 8–9 > 10 high risk	1. Cut down on the frequency of between-meal sweets. 2. Don't sip constantly on sweetened beverages. 3. Avoid using slowly dissolving items like hard candy, cough drops, and so on. 4. Eat more **cariostatic** foods: foods that exert an inhibitory action on the progress of dental caries, such as low-fat cheese, protein-rich foods, raw vegetables, nuts, and popcorn.

Reprinted with permission from Carole A. Palmer, EdD, RD. Division of Nutrition and Oral Health Promotion, Department of General Dentistry, Tufts University School of Dental Medicine.

C. Analysis of Diet Consistency

- Help patient to identify the types of firm and fibrous foods from the food record such as:
  - Uncooked fruits and vegetables.
  - Cooked; crisp–tender vegetables.
- Help patient to identify the frequency of cariogenic food or acidogenic beverage patterns:
  - Daily or occasionally.
  - During meal, end of meal, or between meals.

D. Benefits of Food Record Analysis

- Patient can identify appropriate and inappropriate practices for dental caries control.
- Corroborate findings with clinical findings and patient's oral health problems in preparation for counseling session to provide preventive education.
- Aids in goal setting to modify habits for reduced risk of dental caries.

Preparation for Additional Counseling

I. Define Objectives

- Help the patient understand the individual oral disease risk factors and appreciate the need for changing habits.
- Explain specific alterations in the diet necessary for improved general and oral health.
- Improve dental caries control.
  - Promote minimal consumption of cariogenic foods and acidogenic beverages; suggest methods to cut back on frequency of consumption.
  - Encourage consumption of cariogenic foods and acidogenic beverages with a meal rather than in between meals.
  - Substitute noncariogenic foods or include **anticariogenic** foods, when possible, into the diet

II. Planning Factors

A. Patient Attitude

- Consider patient's willingness and ability to cooperate as evidenced by keeping appointments and following personal oral care procedures.
- Consider patient's cultural and healthcare beliefs, nutrition knowledge, and oral health literacy.

B. Possible Barriers

- Difficulty and resistance to change of normal habits.
- Patient dissatisfaction with suggested modifications to consumption of usual or customary foods.
- Patient may not attempt to make modifications if recommendations are numerous or overwhelming.
- Lack of appreciation of need for change due to limited knowledge of the relationship between diet, nutrition, and oral health.
- Common misconception about concentrated sugar as an indispensable energy source or that natural sugars such as honey, molasses, agave nectar, etc. are a healthy alternative.
- Cultural and religious patterns significant to food selection and preparation.
- Financial considerations in food purchasing.
- Emotional eating patterns and cravings for sweets.
- Parental attitude toward sweets in the diet.
  - Belief that elimination of all sugars would deprive a child of normal childhood pleasures.
  - Alternatively, sugars may be viewed by parents as "bad" foods for children. Foods are not "good" or "bad"; rather it is the form, frequency, amount, and timing of consumption that may be a concern for oral and overall health.

III. Appropriate Teaching Materials

- Information from patient's medical history; dental history; extra/intraoral exam; dental charting; periodontal assessment; caries risk assessment; radiographs; 24-hour recall; and 3-, 5- or 7-day food record.
- Diagram of dental caries factors (Figure 33-2), chart demonstrating the etiology of caries food models, food labels, or charts of dietary standards and requirements.
- Educational leaflets or pamphlets to illustrate patient's special dietary needs or factors in relation to oral health.
- Realistic goals with specific suggestions for modifications of food and beverage habits based on patient preferences in collaboration with the patient.

- A list of snack suggestions to minimize oral disease risk and promote healthy diet habits.

Counseling Procedures

I. Setting

- Ideally, the counseling environment should be free from interruptions and distracting background sounds to promote an environment more conducive to learning.
- If discussion does not occur in a separate clinical treatment room, the patient should be comfortably seated upright in the dental chair.
- Provide limited but pertinent educational information.
  - Avoid overloading with too much new information or extensive goal setting so as not to overwhelm the patient.
  - Posters and pamphlets.
  - Food labels and food models of portion sizes.
- Persons involved in promoting change:
  - For a younger patient, the primary caregiver is present since this individual supervises the child's eating and oral care.
  - Although this may not be ideal, the person preparing meals and grocery shopping needs to be present to learn about appropriate food choices.

II. Setting the Stage for a Successful Counseling Session

- Be prepared.
- Plan for only a few simple visual aids.
- Concentrate on the dietary factors related to the patient's oral disease risk.
- Encourage parents not to bring small children (other than the patient); they may create distractions.
- Develop a friendly atmosphere; establish eye contact with a warm, nonthreatening environment.
- Adequately discuss all questions from patient or caregiver using a conversational tone without lecturing.
- Keep session brief, informative, and engaging for the patient.
- At the close, provide a checklist of identified goals determined by the clinical and patient.

III. Presentation of Findings

A. Review Purpose of the Meeting

- Provide explanation of the relevance between diet and patient's oral disease risk.
- Emphasize health promotion and disease prevention.

B. Clarification of "Cariogenic" Foods

- Calculate the score from the Scoring the Sweets (Table 33-5) or Dietary Analysis Record Form (Table 33-4) to emphasize caries risk.
- Clarify confusion of hidden sugars, added sugars, and natural sugars.
- Clarify the moderation of sugar intake and help patient identify substitutions.
- Clarify the cariogenic potential of refined carbohydrates, such as pretzels, crackers, white breads and pastas.

C. Review of Dental Caries Initiation

- The sucrose from cariogenic food on the tooth surface combines with pathogenic bacteria and can be changed to acid in minutes.
- The pH drops to below 5.5, which is the critical level for demineralization of enamel.
- Acid left undisturbed will be cleared from the mouth from 20 minutes to up to 2 hours, depending primarily on salivary flow. For a patient with xerostomia, clearance takes much longer.

D. Frequency and Time of Exposure

- Each exposure of the tooth surface to acidogenic beverages, sucrose, or other cariogenic food in a meal or snack increases the amount of acid on the tooth.
- The quantity of a cariogenic food is not as significant as when and how often the tooth is exposed to a cariogenic food.[18]
- Prolonged intake of a cariogenic solid or acidogenic liquid, such as continuous sipping of a sucrose-containing beverage or a sugar-free acidic beverage while working at a desk, does not allow for a remineralization period to occur, in which the pH can rise above the critical level.

E. Retention

- Cariogenic foods consumed after brushing and flossing before bedtime are not cleared readily because salivary flow decreases during sleep.
- Cariogenic/acidogenic liquids are cleared from the mouth faster than solids.

- Oral retentiveness of cariogenic foods is related to length of time food debris with fermentable carbohydrate remains on the teeth and exposure to decreased biofilm pH.[19-21]
    - Highly retentive fermentable carbohydrates have a delayed rate of oral clearance, increasing exposure of teeth to a decreased pH and higher potential for demineralization.[19,20,22]
- Sequence of food consumption within a meal pattern is related to caries incidence.[21-24]
    - Eating fermentable carbohydrates at the beginning of a meal or between other noncariogenic foods (protein and fat) is less cumulative in cariogenic potential.
    - Protein and fat are not metabolized by oral bacteria or broken down by salivary amylase and are recommended to be paired with a fermentable carbohydrate within a meal or at the end of a meal. Examples include nuts, natural peanut butter, avocado, cheese, or plain dairy
    - Cheese eaten after sweets or at the end of a meal alters the decrease in pH and production of acids in the oral cavity.[24,25]
- Noncariogenic sweeteners may be incorporated for caries prevention and management of a healthy weight in patients at risk for obesity.[14,26]

IV. Specific Dietary Recommendations

A. Examination of the Patient's Food Record

- After analyzing the diet, assist the patient in identifying the deficiencies of various food groups and sugar intake.
- Try to retain as many as possible of the patient's present food habits.
- Make recommendations that can be adapted to the patient's lifestyle with the overall goal of decreasing oral disease risk.
- Discuss foods from each food group that the patient likes and can be added to the diet.
- Limit the use of cariogenic foods and acidic beverages to mealtimes rather than between meals.
- Assist patient in finding acceptable substitutions for the cariogenic food choices:
    - Unflavored milk.
    - Cheese.
    - Peanut butter (check the label of the peanut butter to choose one without added sugar) on sliced apples.
    - Sugar-free gelatin or pudding.
    - Crunchy vegetables.
- Explore ways to decrease sugar in food preparation and when purchasing ready-made food.
    - Carefully read nutrition labels of prepared foods and choose foods with no added sugar when possible.
    - Add spices to heighten flavor in place of sugar.
    - Decrease the amount of sugar called for in recipes.
- To enhance compliance, help patients create their own **meal plan** for 1 day.
    - Incorporate the principles to reduce oral disease risk discussed during the preventive dietary education.
    - Collaborate on realistic modifications the patient can achieve and is willing to try.
    - Avoid too many changes that may be overwhelming.
    - Determine patient comprehension of information presented and patient's motivational level.
    - Include morning, afternoon, and evening snacks as well as breakfast, lunch, and dinner in a meal plan for a day.
- Encourage daily use of fluoride in water, foods, dentifrices, and rinses.
- When toothbrushing and interdental care are not possible, encourage rinsing with water.

Evaluation of Progress

I. Immediate Evaluation

- Assess the patient's verbal and nonverbal interest, comprehension, and participation in the dietary analysis and counseling session.
- Providing a checklist with agreed upon goals will promote accountability.

II. Three-Month Follow-Up

- Request patient keep a 3-, 5-, or 7-day food record for assessment and evaluation.
- Review personal oral care procedures and provide suggestions as needed.
- Scaling as needed; fluoride varnish application.
- Collaborate on ideas for further modifications when indicated. Smaller goals may need to be established for greater compliance.
- Document progress, additional material reviewed, and plan for continued behavior modification.

III. Six-Month Follow-Up

- Perform examination and clinical procedures.
  - Charting of carious lesions and demineralized areas.
  - Disclose and evaluate biofilm score and educate as needed with new biofilm removal brush, interdental, and tongue-cleaning devices.
  - Scaling as needed; fluoride varnish application if indicated.
- Compare dental caries incidence with previous chartings and completed restorative dentistry.
- Make collaborative dietary recommendations with patient in accord with new assessment.
- Document progress, education provided, and plan.

IV. Overall Evaluation

- Consistent reduction in dental caries rate in the years following the initial counseling shows sustained change in habits.
- Patient's and caregivers' attitudes toward maintaining adequate oral health habits.
- Attempts to maintain a diet containing minimum cariogenic foods.
- Compliance with keeping regular appointments for professional dental care.

Documentation

The following factors are included when documenting patient care that includes diet analysis and patient counseling:

- Rationale for dietary analysis and further education on diet as it pertains to oral health.
- The type of dietary intake utilized for dietary assessment.
- The results of the dietary analysis.
- The results of the sugar score and the level of caries risk.
- Instructions given on completing the food record.
- **Box 33-3** contains an example progress note for a patient receiving dietary analysis and counseling.

Box 33-3 Example Documentation: Patient Receiving a Dietary Analysis and Counseling

- **S**—A 24-year-old, Hispanic female arrived for her annual examination and preventive care appointment. Her medical and dental history were unremarkable.
- **O**—Caries, periodontal, and oral cancer risk assessments were performed. A comprehensive periodontal examination reveals biofilm-induced gingivitis with localized bleeding on probing. Dental examination reveals three new carious lesions.
- **A**—Risk assessment indicates the patient is at high risk for dental caries because of the frequency of cariogenic snacks and regular consumption of diet beverages. A 24-hour recall was performed chairside. Dietary analysis revealed a sweet score of 9, indicating a moderate caries risk. Evaluation of diet for nutritional adequacy revealed an inadequate representation of fruits and vegetables and minimal dairy intake.
- **P**—Preventive education included review of toothbrushing, flossing, and dietary changes to reduce the risk for caries. Reducing the frequency of snacks between meals was discussed. Recommendations include having desserts or sodas (regular or diet) during meals. The patient was encouraged to rinse with water following desserts or sodas consumed between meals to reduce demineralization and subsequent caries risk. The patient was also provided with a prescription for a home fluoride for daily application prior to bedtime. A follow-up appointment was made in 2 weeks.

Signed: ______________________________, RDH
Date: ____________________________________

Factors to Teach the Patient

Medications with Sucrose

- The need to try to avoid liquid or chewable forms containing sucrose.
- Reasons to avoid frequent daily use of medications with sucrose.
- Reasons for rinsing with water after a medication contained in a sucrose mixture.

Medications with Side Effect of Xerostomia

- Drugs the patient is using that cause xerostomia (dry mouth).
- How xerostomia increases the risk of dental caries development.
- Why it is necessary to use saliva substitutes, and avoid candies containing sucrose that slowly dissolve in the mouth.
- Effect of xerostomia on chewing and swallowing.

Facts about Dental Caries

- How dental caries on the tooth surface starts and progresses.
- How a cariogenic diet, host factors/tooth surface, saliva, and microorganisms/biofilm interact, contribute as factors in the dental caries process (Figure 33-2).
- How repeated, frequent acid production and the pH in the dental biofilm promote demineralization and increased risk of caries.
- Why there is a need to avoid frequent episodes of eating or drinking food or beverages that contain sucrose (Figure 33-4).
- Why it is important to limit in between meal snacking on cariogenic/acidogenic foods and beverages.

References

1. Institute of Medicine Subcommittee on Interpretation and Uses of Dietary Reference Intakes; Institute of Medicine Standing Committee on the Scientific Evaluation of Dietary Reference Intakes. *Dietary Reference Intakes: Applications in Dietary Planning*. Washington, DC: National Academies Press; 2003.
2. National Research Council. *Dietary Reference Intakes: The Essential Guide to Nutrient Requirements*. Washington, DC: The National Academies Press; 2006. https://nal.usda.gov/sites/default/files/fnic_uploads/DRIEssentialGuideNutReq.pdf. Accessed April 27, 2022.
3. Institute of Medicine Standing Committee on the Scientific Evaluation of Dietary Reference Intakes and its Panel on Folate, Other B Vitamins, and Choline. *Dietary Reference Intakes for Thiamin, Riboflavin, Niacin, Vitamin B_6, Folate, Vitamin B_{12}, Pantothenic Acid, Biotin, and Choline*. Washington, DC: National Academies Press; 1998.
4. United States Department of Agriculture, Center for Nutrition Policy and Promotion. Choose My Plate guidelines. 2011. http://www.choosemyplate.gov. Accessed April 23, 2022.
5. Varela-López A, Navarro-Hortal MD, Giampieri F, Bullón P, Battino M, Quiles JL. Nutraceuticals in periodontal health: a systematic review on the role of vitamins in periodontal health maintenance. *Molecules*. 2018;23(5):pii:E1226.
6. Ab Malik N, Mohamad Yatim S, Mokhtar KN, et al. Oral health and vitamin D in adult: a systematic review. *Br J Nutr*. 2022;1-29.
7. Miley DD, Garcia MN, Hildebolt CF, et al. Cross-sectional study of vitamin D and calcium supplementation effects on chronic periodontitis. *J Periodontol*. 2009;80(9):1433-1439.
8. Ahmadi-Motamayel F, Falsafi P, Abolsamadi H, Goodarzi MT, Poorolajal J. Evaluation of salivary antioxidants and oxidative stress markers in male smokers. *Comb Chem High Throughput Screen*. 2019;22(7):496-501.
9. Ahmadi-Motamayel F, Falsafi P, Goodarzi MT, Poorolajal J. Evaluation of salivary catalase, vitamin C, and alpha-amylase in smokers and non-smokers: a retrospective cohort study. *J Oral Pathol Med*. 2017;46(5):377-380.
10. Institute of Medicine, Food and Nutrition Board. *Dietary Reference Intakes for Vitamin C, Vitamin E, Selenium, and Carotenoids*. Washington, DC: National Academy Press; 2000.
11. Martinez-Herrera M, Silvestre-Rangil J, Silvestre FJ. Association between obesity and periodontal disease: a systematic review of epidemiological studies and controlled clinical trials. *Med Oral Patol Oral Cir Bucal*. 2017;22(6):e708-e715.
12. Keller A, Rohde JF, Raymond K, Hetiman BL. Association between periodontal disease and overweight and obesity: a systematic review. *J Periodontol*. 2015;86(6):766-776.
13. Akarsu S, Karademir SA. Association between body mass index and dental caries in a Turkish subpopulation of adults: a cross-sectional study. *Oral Health Prev Dent*. 2020;18(1):85-89.

14. Horst JA, Tanzer JM, Milgrom PM. Fluorides and other preventive strategies for tooth decay. *Dent Clin North Am.* 2018;62(2):207-234.
15. Sheiham A, James WP. Diet and dental caries: the pivotal role of free sugars reemphasized. *J Dent Res.* 2015;94(10):1341-1347.
16. Marshall TA. Chairside diet assessment of caries risk. *J Am Dent Assoc.* 2009;140(6):670-674.
17. American Academy of Pediatric Dentistry. Policy on use of xylitol in pediatric dentistry. In: *The Reference Manual of Pediatric Dentistry*. Chicago, IL: American Academy of Pediatric Dentistry; 2021:72-73.
18. Head D, Devine DA, Marsh PD. In silico modelling to differentiate the contribution of sugar frequency versus total amount in driving biofilm dysbiosis in dental caries. *Sci Rep.* 2017;7(1):17413.
19. Bradshaw DJ, Lynch RJ. Diet and the microbial aetiology of dental caries: new paradigms. *Int Dent J.* 2013;63 (suppl 2):64-72.
20. Chankanka O, Marshall TA, Levy SM, et al. Mixed dentition cavitated caries incidence and dietary intake frequencies. *Pediatr Dent.* 2011;33(3):233-240.
21. Botelho JN, Villegas-Salinas M, Troncoso-Gajardo P, Giacaman RA, Cury JA. Enamel and dentine demineralization by a combination of starch and sucrose in a biofilm—caries model. *Braz Oral Res.* 2016;30(1).
22. Halvorsrud K, Lewney J, Craig D, Moynihan PJ. Effects of starch on oral health: systematic review to inform WHO guideline. *J Dent Res.* 2019;98(1):46-53.
23. Rugg-Gunn AJ, Edgar WM, Geddes DA, Jenkins GN. The effect of different meal patterns upon plaque pH in human subjects. *Br Dent J.* 1975;139(9):351-356.
24. Linke HA, Riba HK. Oral clearance and acid production of dairy products during interaction with sweet foods. *Ann Nutr Metab.* 2001;45(5):202-208.
25. Nadelman P, Magno MB, Masterson D, da Cruz AG, Maia LC. Are dairy products containing probiotics beneficial for oral health? A systematic review and meta-analysis. *Clin Oral Investig.* 2018;22(8):2763-2785.
26. Roberts MW, Wright JT. Nonnutritive, low caloric substitutes for food sugars: clinical implications for addressing the incidence of dental caries and overweight/obesity. *Int J Dent.* 2012;2012:625701.

CHAPTER 34

Fluorides

Erin E. Relich, RDH, BSDH, MSA
Lisa F. Mallonee, RDH, RD, LD, MPH

CHAPTER OUTLINE

LEARNING OBJECTIVES

After studying this chapter, the student will be able to:

1. Describe the mechanisms of action of fluoride in the prevention of dental caries.
2. Explain the role of community water fluoridation on the decline of dental caries incidence in a community.
3. Recommend appropriate over-the-counter (OTC) and professionally applied fluoride therapies based on each patient's caries risk assessment.
4. Compare use of fluoride home products (OTC and prescription).
5. Incorporate fluoride into individualized prevention plans for patients of various ages and risk levels.

The use of fluorides provides the most effective method for dental caries prevention and control. Fluoride is necessary for optimum oral health at all ages and is made available at the tooth surface by two general means:

- Systemically, by way of the circulation to developing teeth (pre-eruptive exposure).
- Topically, directly to the exposed surfaces of teeth erupted into the oral cavity[1] (posteruptive exposure).
- Maximum caries inhibiting effect occurs when there is systemic exposure before tooth eruption and frequent topical fluoride exposure throughout life.[2]

Fluoride Metabolism[1,3]

I. Fluoride Intake

- Sources
  - Drinking water that contains fluoride naturally or has been fluoridated.
  - Prescribed dietary supplements.
  - Foods, in small amounts.
  - Foods and beverages prepared at home or processed commercially using water that contains fluoride.
  - Varying small amounts ingested from dentifrices, mouthrinses, supplements, and other fluoride products used by the individual.

II. Absorption

A. Gastrointestinal Tract

- Fluoride is rapidly absorbed as hydrogen fluoride through passive diffusion in the stomach.
  - Rate and amount of absorption depend on the solubility of the fluoride compound and gastric acidity.
  - Most is absorbed within 60 minutes.
- Fluoride that is not absorbed in the stomach will be absorbed by the small intestine.
- There is less absorption when the fluoride is taken with milk and other food.

B. Bloodstream

- Plasma carries the fluoride for its distribution throughout the body and to the kidneys for elimination.
- Maximum blood levels are reached within 30 minutes of intake.
- Normal plasma levels are low and rise and fall according to intake.

III. Distribution and Retention

- **Fluoride** is distributed by the plasma to *all* tissues and organs. There is a strong affinity for mineralized tissues.
- Approximately 99% of fluoride in the body is located within the mineralized tissues.
- Concentrations of fluoride are highest at the surfaces next to the tissue fluid supplying the fluoride.
- The fluoride ion (F) is stored as an integral part of the crystal lattice of teeth and bones.
  - Amount stored varies with the intake, the time of exposure, and the age and stage of the development of the individual.
  - The teeth store small amounts, with highest levels on the tooth surface.
- Fluoride that accumulates in bone can be mobilized slowly from the skeleton due to the constant resorption and remodeling of bone.
- Once tooth enamel is fully matured, the fluoride deposited during development can be altered by cavitated dental caries, erosion, or mechanical abrasion.[1]

IV. Excretion

- Most fluoride is excreted through the kidneys in the urine, with a small amount excreted by the sweat glands and the feces.
- There is limited transfer from plasma to breast milk for excretion by that route.[1]

Fluoride and Tooth Development

- Fluoride is a nutrient essential to the formation of teeth and bones, as are calcium, phosphorus, and other elements obtained from food and water.
- A comprehensive review of the histology of tooth development and mineralization is recommended to supplement the information included here.[4,5]

I. Pre-eruptive: Mineralization Stage

- Fluoride is deposited during the formation of the enamel, starting at the dentinoenamel junction, after the enamel matrix has been laid down by the ameloblasts.
  - **Figure 34-1A** shows the distribution of fluoride in all parts of the teeth during mineralization.

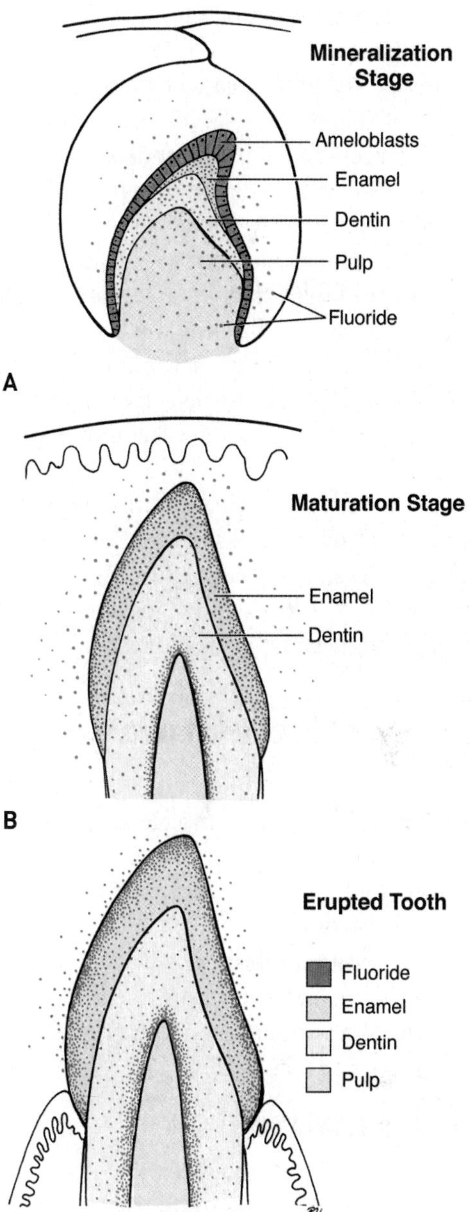

Figure 34-1 Systemic Fluoride. Green dots represent fluoride ions in the tissues and distributed throughout the tooth. **A:** Developing tooth during mineralization shows fluoride from water and other systemic sources deposited in the enamel and dentin. **B:** Maturation stage before eruption when fluoride is taken up from tissue fluids around the crown. **C:** Erupted tooth continues to take up fluoride on the surface from external sources. Note concentrated fluoride deposition on the enamel surface and on the pulpal surface of the dentin.

  - The **hydroxyapatite** crystalline structure becomes **fluorapatite**, which is a less soluble **apatite** crystal.[2]
  - Pre-eruptive fluoride may contribute to shallower occlusal grooves and reduce the risk of fissure caries.[2]

- The hard tissue formation of the primary teeth begins in utero. See Chapter 47.
- The first permanent molars begin to mineralize at birth. See Chapter 16.
- Effect of excess fluoride (**fluorosis**)[6,7]
  - Dental fluorosis is a form of hypomineralization that results from systemic ingestion of an excess amount of fluoride during tooth development.
  - During mineralization, the enamel is highly receptive to free fluoride ions.
  - The normal activity of the ameloblasts may be inhibited, and the defective enamel matrix that can form results in discontinuity of crystal growth.
- Dental fluorosis can appear clinically in varying degrees from white flecks or striations to cosmetically objectionable stained pitting. See Chapter 21.
- Chapter 47 lists the weeks in utero when the hard-tissue formation begins for the primary teeth.

II. Pre-eruptive: Maturation Stage

- After mineralization is complete and before eruption, fluoride deposition continues in the surface of the enamel.
  - **Figure 34-1B** shows fluoride around the crown during **maturation**.
  - Fluoride is taken up from the nutrient tissue fluids surrounding the tooth crown.

III. Posteruptive

- After eruption and throughout the life span of the teeth, the concentration of fluoride on the outermost surface of the enamel is dependent on:
  - Daily topical sources of fluoride to prevent **demineralization** and encourage **remineralization** for prevention of dental caries.
  - Sources for daily topical fluoride include fluoridated drinking water, dentifrices, mouthrinses, and other fluoride preparations used by the patient.
  - The fluoride on the outermost surface is available to inhibit demineralization and enhance remineralization as needed (**Figure 34-1C**).
  - **Figure 34-2A** depicts the areas on the tooth that acquire fluoride after eruption.
  - The continuous daily presence of fluoride provided for the tooth surfaces can inhibit the initiation and progression of dental caries.
  - Uptake is most rapid on the enamel surface during the first years after eruption.

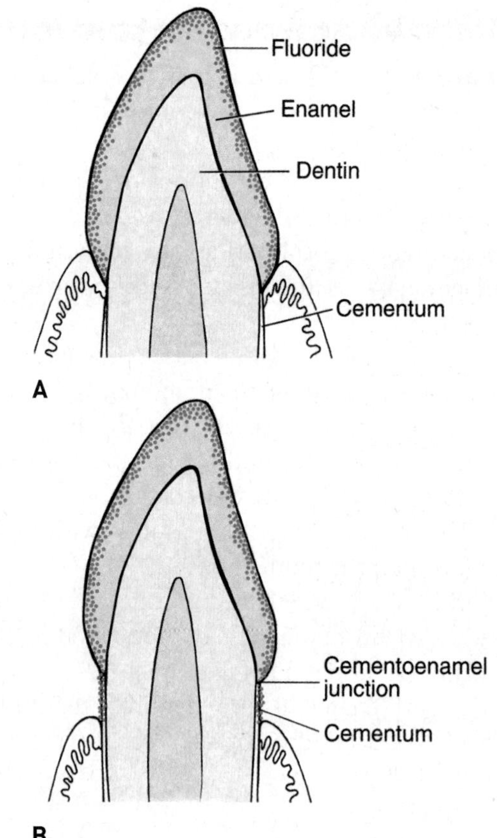

Figure 34-2 Fluoride Acquisition after Eruption. **A:** Fluoride represented by green dots on the enamel surface is taken up from external sources, including dentifrice, rinse, topical application, and fluoridated drinking water passing over the teeth. **B:** Gingival recession exposes the cementum to external sources of fluoride for the prevention of root caries and the alleviation of sensitivity.

  - Repeated daily intake of drinking water with fluoride provides a topical source as it washes over the teeth throughout life.

Tooth Surface Fluoride

Fluoride concentration is greatest on the surface next to the source of fluoride.

- For the enamel of the erupted tooth, highest concentration is at the outer surface exposed to the oral cavity.
- For the dentin, the highest concentration is at the pulpal surface.
- Periodontal attachment loss or gingival recession can often cause the root surface and cementum to become exposed to the oral cavity and external fluoride sources.

I. Fluoride in Enamel

A. Uptake

- Uptake of fluoride depends on the level of fluoride in the oral environment and the length of time of exposure.
- Hypomineralized enamel absorbs fluoride in greater quantities than sound enamel; it incorporates into the hydroxyapatite crystalline structure to become fluorapatite.[6]
- Demineralized enamel that has been remineralized in the presence of fluoride will have a greater concentration of fluoride than sound enamel.

B. Fluoride in the Enamel Surface

- Fluoride is a natural constituent of enamel.
- The intact outer surface has the highest concentration, which falls sharply toward the interior of the tooth.[8]

II. Fluoride in Dentin[9]

- The fluoride level may be greater in dentin than that in enamel.
- A higher concentration is at the pulpal or inner surface, where exchanges take place.
- Newly formed dentin absorbs fluoride rapidly.

III. Fluoride in Cementum[9]

- The level of fluoride in cementum is high and increases with exposure.
  - With recession of the clinical attachment level, the root surface is exposed to the fluids of the oral cavity.
  - **Figure 34-2B** shows fluoride acquisition to exposed cementum.
  - Fluoride is then available to the cementum from the saliva and all the sources used by the patient, including drinking water, dentifrice, and mouthrinse.

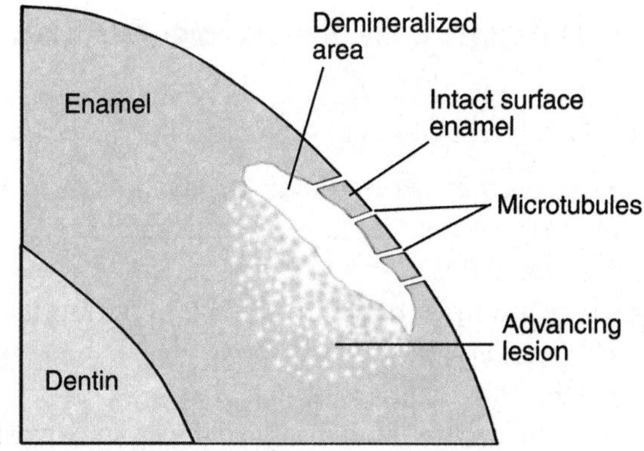

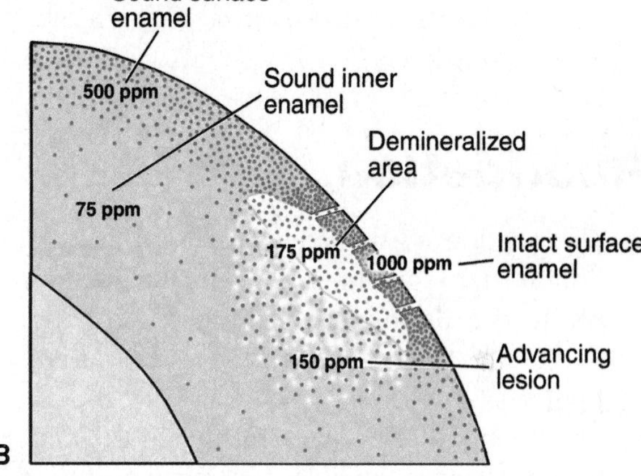

Figure 34-3 Examples of Enamel Fluoride Content.
A: Early stage of dental caries with an intact surface enamel and subsurface demineralized area.
B: A demineralized area readily takes up available fluoride. As shown, the fluoride content (1000 ppm) of the relatively intact surface over a subsurface demineralized white spot is higher than that of the sound surface enamel (500 ppm). The body of the advancing lesion has a higher fluoride content (150 ppm) than does the sound inner enamel (75 ppm).

Demineralization-Remineralization[8]

Figure 34-3 illustrates the comparative levels of fluoride that may be found in the tooth surface and the sublevel lesion in early dental caries.

I. Fluoride in Biofilm and Saliva

- Saliva and biofilm are reservoirs for fluoride; saliva carries minerals available for remineralization when needed.
- Fluoride helps to inhibit demineralization when it is present at the crystal surface during an acid challenge.
- Fluoride enhances remineralization, forming a condensed layer on the crystal surface, which attracts calcium and phosphate ions.
- High concentrations of fluoride can interfere with the growth and metabolism of bacteria.
- Dental biofilm may contain 5–50 **ppm** fluoride. The content varies greatly and is constantly changing.
- Fluoride may be acquired directly from fluoridated water, dentifrice, and other topical sources and brought by the saliva or by an exchange of fluoride in the biofilm to the demineralizing tooth surface under the biofilm.

II. Summary of Fluoride Action

Having fluoride available topically to the tooth posteruptively is key to its effectiveness.

- Frequent exposure to fluoride, such as from fluoridated water, dentifrice, and mouthrinse, is recommended.
- There are three basic topical effects of fluoride to prevent dental caries[8]:
  - Inhibit demineralization.
  - Enhance remineralization of incipient lesions.
  - Inhibit bacterial activity by inhibiting *enolase*, an enzyme needed by bacteria to metabolize carbohydrates.

Fluoridation

- Fluoridation is the adjustment of the natural fluoride ion content in a municipal water supply to the optimum physiologic concentration to maximize caries prevention and limit enamel fluorosis.[10]
- Fluoridation has been established as the most efficient, effective, reliable, and inexpensive means for improving and maintaining oral health for all who use it.
- Fluoridation was named by the U.S. Centers for Disease Control and Prevention (**CDC**) as one of the 10 most significant public health measures of the 20th century.[10]
- The estimated annual cost per person per year is low, with lower cost per person for communities of more than 20,000 people.[11]
- As of 2018, 63.4% of the total U.S. population received fluoridated water, whereas 73.0% of the population served by public (municipal) water systems received fluoridated water. These percentages vary greatly from state to state.[12]

I. Historical Aspects[13]

A. Mottled Enamel and Dental Caries

- Dr. Frederick S. McKay
  - Early in the 20th century, Dr. McKay began his extensive studies to find the cause of "brown stain," which later was called mottled enamel and now is known as *dental fluorosis*.
  - He observed that people in Colorado Springs, Colorado, with mottled enamel had significantly less dental caries.[14] He associated the condition with the drinking water, but tests were inconclusive.
- H.V. Churchill
  - In 1931, H.V. Churchill, a chemist, pinpointed fluorine as the specific element related to the tooth changes that Dr. McKay had been observing clinically.[15]

B. Background for Fluoridation

- Dr. H. Trendley Dean
  - Epidemiologic studies of the 1930s, sponsored by the U.S. Public Health Service (**USPHS**) and directed by Dr. Dean, led to the conclusion the optimum level of fluoride in the water for dental caries prevention averages 1 ppm in moderate climates.
  - Clinically objectionable dental fluorosis is associated with levels well over 2 ppm.[16]
  - From this knowledge and the fact many healthy people had lived long lives in communities where the fluoride content of the water was much greater than 1 ppm, the concept of adding fluoride to the water developed.
  - It was still necessary to show the benefits from controlled fluoridation could parallel those of natural fluoride.

C. Fluoridation—1945

- The first communities were fluoridated in 1945.
- Research in the communities began before fluoridation was started to obtain baseline information.

D. Control Cities

- Aurora, Illinois, where the natural fluoride level was optimum (1.2 ppm), was used to compare the benefits of natural fluoride in the water supply with those of fluoridation, as well as with a fluoride-free city, Rockford, Illinois.
- Original cities with fluoridation and their control cities in the research are shown in **Box 34-1**.
- The research conducted in those cities, as well as throughout the world, has documented the influence of fluoride on oral health.

II. Water Supply Adjustment

A. Fluoride Level

- In 2015, the U.S. Department of Health and Human Services updated the recommendation for the optimal concentration of water fluoridation to 0.7 ppm for all communities, regardless of climate.
  - The decision was substantiated by the fact that Americans have access to many more

Box 34-1 First Fluoridation Research Cities

Research City	Control City
Grand Rapids, Michigan (January 1945)	Muskegon, Michigan
Newburgh, New York (May 1945)	Kingston, New York
Brantford, Ontario (June 1945)	Sarnia, Ontario
Evanston, Illinois (February 1947)	Oak Park, Illinois

sources of fluoride today than they did when water fluoridation was first introduced in the United States.[17]
- The change still provides an effective level of fluoride to reduce the incidence of dental caries while minimizing the rate of fluorosis.

B. Chemicals Used

- All fluoride chemicals must conform to the appropriate American Water Works Association standards to ensure the drinking water is safe.[18]
- Sources
  - Compounds from which the fluoride ion is derived are naturally occurring and are mined in various parts of the world.
  - Examples of common sources are fluorspar, cryolite, and apatite.
- Criteria for acceptance of a fluoride compound for fluoridation include:
  - Solubility to permit regular use in a water plant.
  - Relatively inexpensive.
  - Readily available to prevent interruptions in maintaining the proper fluoride level.
- Compounds used:
  - Dry compounds: sodium fluoride (**NaF**) and sodium silicofluoride.
  - Liquid solution: hydrofluorosilicic acid.

Effects and Benefits of Fluoridation

Fluoridated water is a systemic source of fluoride for developing teeth and a topical source of fluoride on the surfaces of erupted teeth throughout life.[19]

I. Appearance of Teeth

- Teeth exposed to an optimum or slightly higher level of fluoride appear white, shiny, opaque, and without blemishes.
  - When the level is slightly more than optimum, teeth may exhibit mild enamel fluorosis seen as white areas in bands or flecks. Without close examination, such spots blend with the overall appearance.
- Today, the majority of fluorosis is mild and not considered an esthetic problem.[10,20]

II. Dental Caries: Permanent Teeth

A. Overall Benefits

- Maximum benefit is seen with continuous use of fluoridated water from birth.
- Estimates have shown the reduction in caries due to water fluoridation alone (factoring out other sources of topical fluoride) among adults of all ages is 27%.[19]
- The effects are similar to communities with optimum levels of natural fluoride in the water.
- Many more individuals are completely caries free when fluoride is in the water.

B. Distribution

- Anterior teeth, particularly maxillary, receive more protection from fluoride than do posterior teeth.[16]
  - Anterior teeth are contacted by the drinking water as it passes into the mouth.

C. Progression

- Not only are the numbers of carious lesions reduced, but the caries rate is slowed.
- Caries progression is also reduced for the surfaces that receive fluoride for the first time after eruption.[21]

III. Root Caries

- Root caries experience in lifelong residents of a naturally fluoridated community is in direct proportion to the fluoride concentration in the water compared with the experience of residents of a fluoride-free community.[22]
- The incidence of root caries is approximately 50% less for lifelong residents of a fluoridated community.[23]

IV. Dental Caries: Primary Teeth

- With fluoridation from birth, the caries incidence is reduced up to 40% in the primary teeth.[10]
- The introduction of fluoridation into a community significantly increases the proportion of caries-free children and reduces the decayed, missing, and filled teeth (**dmft/DMFT**) scores compared to areas that are nonfluoridated over the same time period.[20]

V. Tooth Loss

- Tooth loss due to dental caries is much greater in both primary and permanent teeth without fluoride because of increased dental caries, which progresses more rapidly.[24]

VI. Adults

- When a person resides in a community with fluoride in the drinking water throughout life, benefits continue.[25,26]

VII. Periodontal Health

- Indirect favorable effects of fluoride on periodontal health can be shown.
  - Fluoride functions to decrease dental caries. The presence of carious lesions favors biofilm retention, which can lead to periodontal infection, particularly adjacent to the gingival margin.

Partial Defluoridation

- Water with an excess of natural fluoride does not meet the requirements of the USPHS.
- Several hundred communities in the United States had water supplies that naturally contained more than twice the optimal level of fluoride.
- **Defluoridation** can be accomplished by one of several chemical systems.[27] The **efficacy** of the methods has been shown.
- Examples: The water supply in Britton, South Dakota, has been reduced from almost 7 to 1.5 ppm since 1948, and in Bartlett, Texas, from 8 to 1.8 ppm since 1952. Examinations have shown a significant reduction in the incidence of objectionable fluorosis in children born since defluoridation.[27,28]

School Fluoridation

- To bring the benefits of fluoridation to children living in rural areas without the possibility for community fluoridation, adding fluoride to a school water supply has been an alternative.
- Because of the intermittent use of the school water (only 5 days each week during the 9-month school year), the amount of fluoride added was increased over the usual 1 ppm.
- Example: In the schools of Elk Lake, Pennsylvania, after 12 years with the fluoride level at 5 ppm in the school drinking water, the children experienced a 39% decrease in DMF surfaces compared with those in the control group.[29]
- Example: In the schools of Seagrove, North Carolina, after 12 years with the fluoride level at 6.3 ppm in the school drinking water, the children experienced a 47.5% decrease in DMF surfaces compared with those in the control group.[29]
- Such systems have significance in the long history of fluoridation efforts for all people in the United States.
- School fluoridation has been phased out in several states, and the current extent of this practice is unknown. Operations and maintenance of small fluoridation systems are problematic.[10]

Discontinued Fluoridation

- When fluoride is removed from a community water supply that had dental caries control by fluoridation, the effects can be clearly shown.
- Example: In Antigo, Wisconsin, the action of antifluoridationists in 1960 brought about the discontinuance of fluoridation, which had been installed in 1949.
  - Examinations in the years following 1960 revealed the marked drop in the number of children who were caries free and the steep increase in caries rates.
  - From 1960 to 1966, the number of caries-free children in the second grade decreased by 67%.[30]
  - Fluoridation was reinstated in 1966 by popular demand.

Fluorides in Foods

I. Foods[31]

- Certain foods contain fluoride, but not enough to constitute a significant part of the day's need for caries prevention.
- Examples: Meat, eggs, vegetables, cereals, and fruit have small but measurable amounts, whereas tea and fish have larger amounts.

- Foods cooked in fluoridated water retain fluoride from the cooking water.

II. Salt[32-34]

- Fluoridated salt has not been promoted in the United States, but is widely available and used in Germany, France, and Switzerland along with other European countries where 30% to 80% of the domestic marketed salt is fluoridated.
- Another 30 countries or more use fluoridated salt worldwide for its effectiveness as a community health program.
- Fluoridated salt results in a reduced incidence of dental caries, but there is insufficient evidence for its overall effectiveness.
- Fluoridated salts currently available supply about one-third to one-half of the amount of fluoride ingested daily from 1 ppm fluoridated water.
- Fluoridated salt is recommended by the World Health Organization as an alternative to fluoridated water to target underprivileged groups.

III. Halo/Diffusion Effect

- Foods and beverages that are commercially processed (cooked or reconstituted) in optimally fluoridated cities can be distributed and consumed in nonfluoridated communities.
- The **halo or diffusion effect** can result in increased fluoride intake by individuals living in nonfluoridated communities, providing them some protection against dental caries.[31]

IV. Bottled Water

- Bottled water usually does not contain optimal fluoride unless it has a label indicating that it is fluoridated.
- Patients need to be advised to fill their drinking water bottles from a fluoridated water supply.

V. Water Filters[35]

- Reverse osmosis and water distillation systems remove fluoride from the water, but water softeners do not.
- Carbon filters (for the end of a faucet or in pitchers) vary in their removal of fluoride.
- Carbon filters with activated alumina remove fluoride.
- Patients need to be warned that water filters may remove fluoride from the drinking water and need to be checked with the manufacturer before purchase.

VI. Infant Formula[36-38]

- There has been an increase in breastfeeding in the United States, but infant formula remains a major source of nutrition for many infants.
- Ready-to-feed formulas do not need to be reconstituted, but water is added to powdered and liquid concentrate formulas.
- Breast milk may contain 0.02 ppm fluoride, and all types of infant formula themselves contain a low amount of fluoride (0.11–0.57 ppm).[37]
- The level of fluoride in the water supply used to reconstitute powdered or liquid concentrate formulas determines the total fluoride intake.
- The American Dental Association (**ADA**) recommends continuing to use optimally fluoridated water to reconstitute infant formula while being aware of the possible risk of mild enamel fluorosis in the primary teeth.[38]

Dietary Fluoride Supplements[10,39,40]

- Prescription fluoride supplements were introduced in the late 1940s and are intended to compensate for fluoride-deficient drinking water.
- The current supplementation dosage schedule developed by the ADA and the American Association of Pediatric Dentistry (**AAPD**) and revised in 2010 includes children aged 6 months through 16 years.
    - **Table 34-1** contains the daily dosage amounts based on the age of the child and the amount of fluoride in the primary water supply.

Table 34-1 **Fluoride Supplements Dose Schedule (Mg NaF/D)[a]**

	Water Fluoride Ion Concentration (ppm)		
Age of Child (Y)	**Less Than 0.3**	**Between 0.3 and 0.6**	**Greater Than 0.6**
Birth–6 mo	0	0	0
6 mo–3 y	0.25 mg	0	0
3–6 y	0.50 mg	0.25 mg	0
6–16 y	1.0 mg	0.50 mg	0

[a]About 2.2 mg of sodium fluoride provides 1 mg of fluoride ion.

Reproduced from American Academy of Pediatric Dentistry. Fluoride therapy. In: *The Reference Manual of Pediatric Dentistry.* Chicago, IL: American Academy of Pediatric Dentistry. 2021; 302-305. https://www.aapd.org/media/Policies_Guidelines/BP_FluorideTherapy.pdf (2018). Accessed March 22, 2022.

- Clinical recommendations from the ADA Council on Scientific Affairs include the use of fluoride supplements for children:
  - At high risk of developing dental caries.
  - Those whose primary source of drinking water is deficient in fluoride.[41]

I. Assess Possible Need

- Review the patient's history to be certain the child is not receiving other fluoride such as vitamin–fluoride supplements.
- Determine if the fluoride level of all sources of drinking water is below 0.6 ppm.
- Refer to the list of fluoridated communities available from state or local health departments.
- Request water analysis when the fluoride level has not been determined, for example, in private well water.
- Determine if the child's risk for dental caries is high or moderately high before considering the use of fluoride supplements.[39]
- Reassess the caries risk at frequent intervals as the status may be affected by the child's development, personal and family situations, and behavioral factors such as changes in oral hygiene practices.[33,41]

II. Available Forms of Supplements

- NaF supplements are available as tablets; lozenges; and drops in 0.25-, 0.50-, and 1.0-mg dosages.
- Prescribed on an individual patient basis for daily use at home.

A. Tablets and Lozenges

- Tablets are chewed thoroughly, swished/rinsed around in the oral cavity, and forced between the teeth before swallowing.
- Lozenges are dissolved for 1–2 minutes in the mouth to provide both pre-eruptive and posteruptive benefits.[41]
- Best taken at bedtime after teeth are brushed.
  - Avoid drinking, eating, or rinsing before going to sleep to gain maximum benefit.

B. Drops

- A liquid concentrate with directions that specify the number of drops for the prescription dose daily.
- Primary use for child aged 6 months to 3 years, and patient of any age unable to use other forms that require chewing and swallowing.

III. Prescription Guidelines

- No more than 264 mg NaF (120 mg fluoride ion) to be dispensed per household at one time.
- Take supplements with food to decrease stomach upset.
- Storage
  - Keep products out of reach of children.
  - Keep tablets in the original container, away from heat and direct light, and away from damp places such as a bathroom or kitchen sink area.
- Missed dose
  - Take as soon as remembered.
  - If near time of next dose, take at the next regular time.

IV. Benefits and Limitations

- Prenatal use by pregnant women
  - Administration of prenatal dietary fluoride supplements is not recommended.
  - Some evidence has shown that fluoride crosses the placenta during the fifth and sixth months of pregnancy and may enter the prenatal deciduous enamel.[42]
  - Overall, there is weak evidence to support the use of fluoride supplements to prevent dental caries in primary teeth.
- Daily fluoride supplements offer caries preventive benefits in permanent teeth. School-aged children who chewed, swished, and swallowed 1-mg fluoride tablets daily on school days had significantly lower caries experience than those who did not use fluoride supplements.
- The use of fluoride supplements in children older than 6 years of age shows a 24% decrease in DMF tooth surfaces in permanent teeth compared to no fluoride supplements.[43]
- Consider the child's age, caries risk, and all sources of fluoride exposure before recommending the use of fluoride supplements.[33,41]

Professional Topical Fluoride Applications

Topical fluorides are an essential part of a total preventive program for patients of all ages.

- Fluoridated water and fluoride toothpaste are the primary sources of topical fluoride for patients of all ages and levels of caries risk.

- Additional topical fluoride sources may be professionally applied and/or self-applied by the patient for those at an elevated caries risk.

I. Historical Perspectives

- Professionally applied fluoride has been instrumental in the reduction of dental caries in the United States and other industrialized countries since the early 1940s.
- Dr. Basil G. Bibby conducted the initial topical NaF study using Brockton, Massachusetts schoolchildren.[44]
- More than one-third fewer new carious lesions resulted from a 0.1% aqueous solution applied at 4-month intervals for 2 years by a dental hygienist.
- The research led to extensive studies by Dr. John W. Knutson and others sponsored by the USPHS.
    - The aim was to determine the most effective concentration of NaF, the minimum time required for application, and procedural details.[45,46]

II. Indications

- The professional application of a high-concentration fluoride preventive agent is based on caries risk assessment for the individual patient.
- Indications for a professional fluoride application are outlined in **Box 34-2**.[47]
- See Chapter 25 for the criteria to determine low, moderate, and high caries risk.

III. Compounds

- **Table 34-2** provides a summary of the available professional fluoride applications.
    - 2.0% NaF as **gel** or foam delivered in trays.
    - 1.23% acidulated phosphate fluoride (**APF**) as a gel or foam delivered in trays.
    - 5% NaF as a varnish brushed on the teeth.
- 2.0% NaF gel
    - NaF, also called "neutral sodium fluoride" due to its neutral pH of 7.0, contains 9050 ppm fluoride ion.
    - Clinical trials demonstrating the efficacy of neutral NaF are based on a series of four or five applications on a weekly basis.[48]

Box 34-2 Indications for Professional Topical Fluoride Application[47]

- Patients at an elevated (moderate or high) risk of developing caries. (Refer to Chapter 25.)
- **5% NaF varnish** at least every 3–6 months (for all ages and adult root caries), or
- **1.23% APF gel** 4-minute trays at least every 3–6 months (for 6 years and older and adult root caries).
- Patients at a low risk of developing caries may not benefit from additional topical fluoride other than **OTC**-fluoridated toothpaste and fluoridated water daily.

Data from American Dental Association Council on Scientific Affairs. Topical fluoride for caries prevention: executive summary of updated clinical recommendations and supporting systematic review. *J Am Dent Assoc*. 2013;144(11):1279-1291.

Table 34-2 Professionally Applied Topical Fluorides

Agent	Form	Concentration	Application Mode/Frequency	Notes
NaF neutral or 7 pH	2% Gel or foam[a]	9050 ppm 0.90% F ion	Tray (4 minutes)/no currently recommended interval	Do not overfill: see Figure 34-5
Acidulated phosphate 3.5 pH	1.23% Gel or foam[a]	12,300 ppm 1.23% F ion	Tray (4 minutes)/at least every 3–6 months	Do not overfill: see Figure 34-5
NaF neutral or 7 pH	5% Varnish	22,600 ppm 2.26% F ion	Apply thin layer with a soft brush (1–2 minutes)/at least every 3–6 months depending on caries risk level	Sets up to a hard film
SDF pH 8–10	5.0–5.9% Fluoride	44,800 ppm 4.48% F ion	Apply a thin layer with a microbrush (1 minute and let dry)/apply at least every 6–12 months[67]	Goes on clear, becomes black/gray upon application to cavitated areas

[a]There is limited published clinical evidence supporting the effectiveness of foam.[47]

F, fluoride; NaF, sodium fluoride; ppm, parts per million; SDF, silver diamine fluoride

Data fom Weyant RJ, Tracy SL, Anselmo T, et al. Topical fluoride for caries prevention: executive summary of the updated clinical recommendations and supporting systemic review. J Am Dent Assoc. 2013;144(11):1279-1291; and Horst J, Ellenikiotis H, Milgrom P. UCSF protocol for cariesarrest using silver diamine fluoride: rationale, indications and consent. J Calif Dent Assoc. 2016;44(1):16-28.

  - Quarterly or semiannual applications are most common in clinical practice.
- 2.0% NaF foam
  - There is limited clinical evidence to demonstrate foam's effectiveness in caries prevention.
- 1.23% APF gel
  - Contains 12,300 ppm fluoride ion.
  - A 4-minute tray application is recommended at least every 3–6 months per year for individuals aged 6 years and older at an elevated risk for dental caries.[47]
  - Widely used because of its storage stability, acceptable taste, and tissue compatibility.
  - Low pH of 3.5 enhances fluoride uptake, which is greatest during the first 4 minutes.[49]
  - APF may etch porcelain and composite restorative materials, so it is not indicated for patients with porcelain, composite restorations, and sealants.[50]
  - The hydrofluoride component of APF can dissolve the filler particles of the composite resin restorations.
  - Macroinorganic filler particles of composite materials demonstrate noticeable etched patterns generated by APF, whereas many of the more recently available microfilled composites/resins are not as sensitive to the APF.[50]
  - The **prevented fraction** of dental caries ranged from 18% to 41% with the use of APF or NaF gels.[51]
  - In 2018, an expert panel from the ADA recommended the prioritized use of 1.23% APF gel (every 3 to 6 months) or 5% sodium fluoride varnish (every 3 to 6 months) to arrest or reverse noncavitated carious lesions on the facial and lingual surfaces of both primary and permanent teeth.[52]
- 1.23% APF foam
  - There is limited clinical evidence to show the effectiveness of foam in caries prevention.
- 5% NaF varnish
  - Fluoride varnishes (FVs) were developed during the late 1960s and early 1970s to prolong contact time of the fluoride with the tooth surface.[53]
  - Varnishes are safe, effective, fast, and easy to apply, and patient acceptance is good.
  - The use of varnish 2–4 times per year is associated with a 43% decrease in DMFT surfaces in permanent teeth and 37% in primary teeth.[54]
  - Varnish has a higher concentration of fluoride than gel or foam (22,600 ppm fluoride ion), but an overall less amount of fluoride is used per application (<7 mg varnish vs. 30 mg of gel for a child).
  - Varnish sets quickly and remains on the teeth for up to several hours, releasing fluoride into the pits and fissures, proximal surfaces, and cervical areas of the tooth where it is needed the most.[55]
  - Application is recommended at least every 3–4 months per year for individuals at an elevated risk for dental caries.[47]
  - Varnish is effective in reversing active pit and fissure enamel lesions in the primary dentition[56] and remineralizing enamel lesions, regardless of whether the varnish is applied over or around the demineralizing lesion.[57]
  - Varnish is also effective in reducing demineralization (white areas) around orthodontic brackets.[58]
  - Varnish received approval from the U.S Food and Drug Administration (**FDA**) for use as a cavity liner and for treatment of dentin hypersensitivity.[59] Varnish may be used for dentin hypersensitivity. (See Chapter 41.)
  - Varnish is the only professional topical fluoride to be used for children younger than 6 years.
  - Its use in the United States as a caries preventive agent is considered off-label but has become a standard of care in practice.[55]
  - Fluoride varnish's highest prevented fractions were 21.3% for caries arrest and 55.7% for caries prevention.[60]
  - In 2018, an expert panel from the ADA recommended the prioritized use of sealants and 5% NaF varnish (every 3 to 6 months), 1.23% APF gel (every 3 to 6 months), or 0.2% sodium fluoride mouthrinse (once per week) to arrest or reverse noncavitated carious lesions on the occlusal surfaces of both primary and permanent teeth.[52]
  - As far as the approximal surfaces of primary and permanent teeth, the expert panel suggested 5% sodium varnish application (every 3 to 6 months).[52]
  - Five percent NaF varnish is now offered with different formulations containing mineral enhancements:
    - Complex of casein phosphopeptide and amorphous calcium phosphate (ACP).
    - ACP.
    - Tri-calcium phosphate modified by fumaric acid.

    - Calcium and phosphate with xylitol.
    - Calcium sodium phosphosilicate.
    - Sodium trimetaphosphate.
  - Some manufacturers are adding mineral additives to the FV formulations with the theory that by making them bioavailable in the saliva, it will increase the overall anticariogenic efficacy.[61]
    - More in vivo research studies with human subjects are needed to determine the efficacy and benefits of mineral enhanced FV formulations.[62]
    - There is no recommendation by the ADA at this time for FV with mineral enhancements.
  - Allergic reactions such as contact dermatitis or stomatitis from exposure to the **rosin/colophony**, a sticky secretion typically made from plants or trees contained in FVs, are uncommon, but have been reported in the literature.[59,63-65]
  - FV formulations that contain synthetic rosin/colophony are now available on market as an alternative for those patients with a known or suspected allergy to traditional plant-based rosins.
- 38% silver diamine fluoride (SDF)[52,60,66-71]
  - No adverse issues have been reported in Japan since SDF was approved over 80 years ago.
  - 24.4% to 28.8% silver (253,870 ppm Ag—antimicrobial effects)
  - 5.0% to 5.9% fluoride (44,800 ppm F—promotes remineralization)
  - 8% ammonia (stabilizing agent/solvent)
  - pH 8–10, both colorless and tinted (blue) formulations available.
  - FDA cleared in 2015 as a Class II medical device for management of dentinal hypersensitivity.
  - Off-label use is caries arrest and prevention for high caries risk patients.
  - SDF's lowest prevented fractions were 96.1% for caries arrest and 70.3% for caries prevention.[60]
  - In 2017, a panel from the AAPD developed conditional recommendations from the evidence for the use of 38% SDF to arrest the carious lesions of children, adolescents, and those with special needs.[68-70]
  - In 2018, an expert panel from the ADA recommended the prioritized use of 38% SDF twice per year to arrest advanced carious lesions on the coronal surfaces of both primary and permanent teeth over 5% sodium fluoride varnish.[52]
  - Application of SDF biannually is more effective than annual application.[52,71]
  - Anterior teeth have a higher rate of caries arrest after SDF placement than posterior teeth.[69,71]
  - Individual state Dental Hygiene Practice Acts determine whether SDF application is permitted by the registered dental hygienist.

Clinical Procedures: Professional Topical Fluoride

I. Objectives

- Prevention of dental caries
  - Identify special problems, including areas adjacent to restorations, orthodontic appliances, xerostomia, and other risk factors.
  - Box 34-2 contains indications for the application of a professional fluoride.
  - Examples: active or secondary caries, exposed root surfaces, current orthodontic treatment, low or no fluoride exposure, or xerostomia.
- Remineralization of demineralized areas
  - Demineralized white areas on the cervical third, especially under dental biofilm.
- Desensitization
  - Fluoride aids in blocking dentinal tubules. (See Chapter 41.)
- Varnish covers and protects a sensitive area, and fluoride is slowly released for uptake.

II. Preparation of the Teeth for Topical Application

- General preparation for tray and varnish applications
  - Most patients will receive a professional topical fluoride application following their routine continuing care appointment.
  - When the fluoride application is to be applied at a time other than following scaling and debridement, rubber cup polishing is not routinely necessary because fluoride will penetrate biofilm and provide the same benefits with or without prior polishing.[47,72]
  - Calculus and stain removal are completed first.
  - After calculus removal, apply principles of selective polishing for stain removal.

- Select an appropriate cleaning or polishing agent that will not harm the tooth surface or the restorative material present.
- A fluoride-containing polishing paste is not effective as a fluoride application.[73]
- Preparation and procedure for gel or foam tray application is included in **Table 34-3**; preparation and procedure for varnish application is described in Table 34-4.

III. Patient and/or Parent Counseling

- Help patients understand the purposes and benefits as well as the limitations of topical applications.
- Fluoride is one part of the total prevention program that includes daily biofilm control and limitation of cariogenic foods.

IV. Tray Technique: Gel or Foam

- Tray application appointment preparation
  - Prepare the patient for any discomfort, for example, the 4-minute timing when tray application is to be used.
  - Explain the need not to swallow and to expectorate immediately after the tray is removed.
- Tray selection and preparation
  - **Figure 34-4** shows tray selection for coverage of all exposed root surfaces.

Table 34-3 Procedure for Topical Gel or Foam Professional Tray

Patient selection	■ Determine need based on caries risk assessment (not to be used for children younger than 6 years of age). ■ Choose the type of fluoride (APF or NaF and gel or foam); data support use of APF gel. ■ Seat upright. ■ Explain procedure including length: 4 minutes. ■ Instruct not to swallow. ■ Tilt head forward slightly.
Tray coverage	■ Choose appropriate size for full coverage. ■ Complete dentition must be covered, including anterior and posterior vertical coverage, distal dam depth, and close fit to teeth. ■ Check for coverage of areas of recession (if unable to cover exposed root surfaces, use varnish application). ■ Proper and improper tray coverage: see Figure 34-4.
Place gel or foam	■ Use minimum amount of gel or foam in the trays, as shown in Figure 34-5. ■ Fill tray one-third full with gel; completely fill, but do not overfill with foam.
Dry the teeth	■ Place a saliva ejector in the mouth during the drying procedure ■ Dry the teeth before insertion of trays starting with the maxillary teeth; facial, occlusal, and palatal surfaces and then the mandibular teeth; lingual, occlusal, and facial surfaces.
Insert trays	■ Place both filled trays in mouth. ■ A two-step procedure (one tray at a time) may be required; if so, patient may not rinse but must expectorate after the removal of each tray to prevent swallowing.
Isolation	■ Use a saliva ejector for suction.
Attention	■ Do not leave patient unattended.
Timing	■ Use a timer; do not estimate (4 minutes). ■ Procedure will take 8 minutes when a two-step procedure is used.
Completion	■ Tilt head forward for removal of tray. ■ Instruct patient to expectorate for several minutes; do not allow swallowing. ■ Wipe excess gel or foam from teeth with gauze sponge. ■ Use high-power suction to draw out saliva and gel. ■ Instruct patient that nothing is to be placed in the mouth for 30 minutes; do not rinse, eat, drink, or brush teeth.

APF, acidulated phosphate fluoride; NaF, sodium fluoride.

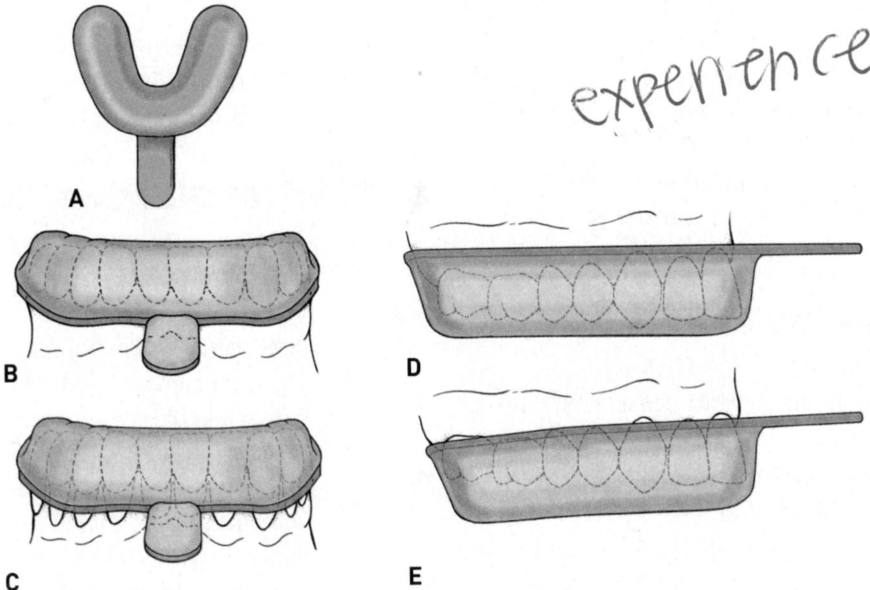

Figure 34-4 Tray Selection. **A:** Mandibular tray held for try-in. **B:** Tray over teeth is deep enough to cover the entire exposed enamel above the gingiva. **C:** In the patient with recession and areas of root surfaces exposed, the tray may not be deep enough to cover the root surfaces where fluoride is needed for prevention of root caries or hypersensitivity. A custom-made tray is needed. **D:** Tray adequately covers the distal surface of the most posterior tooth. **E:** If the tray does not cover the distal surface of the most posterior tooth or the cervical third of canine and central incisor adequately, the tray may need to be repositioned to cover the distal surface, or a larger stock or custom-made tray is needed.

- Design of trays: maxillary and mandibular trays may be hinged together or separated, are of a natural rounded arch shape to hold the gel and prevent ingestion and are available in various sizes and brands.
- **Figure 34-5** shows the amount of gel to be placed in each tray.
- Most gels are **thixotropic** to offer better physical and handling characteristics for use in trays.
- Procedures for a professional gel or foam tray fluoride application are listed in Table 34-3.

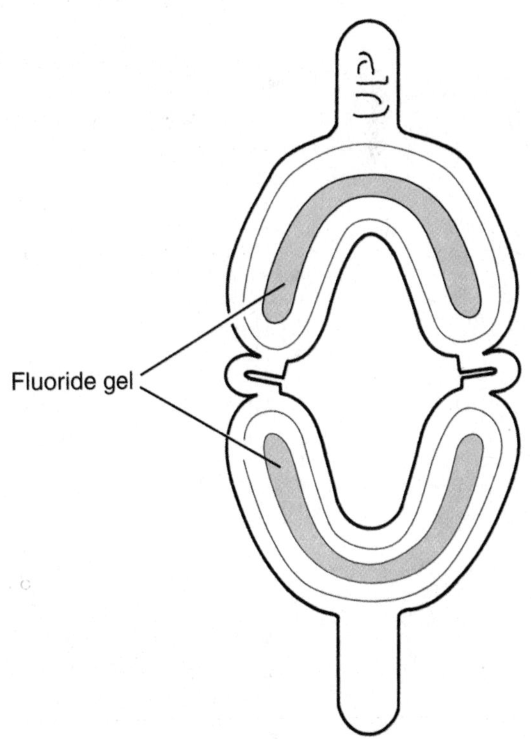

Figure 34-5 Measured Gel in Tray. No more than 2 mL of gel is placed in each tray for children, and no more than 5 mL is placed in each tray for adults. This amount fills each tray size one-third full.

V. Varnish Technique[55]

- Varnish application appointment sequence:
  - Dispense varnish: If dispensed from a tube (rather than a single-dose packet), discard any clear varnish because the ingredients have separated and will contain only a fraction of the intended amount of fluoride.[74]
  - Unit-dosed 5% NaF varnish is available in premeasured wells or individual packets of different dosages with an applicator brush to mix the varnish and then apply.

- Unit dosages are generally 0.25, 0.4, or 0.5 mL for the primary, mixed, and permanent dentitions, respectively, and are available in different flavors and colors (yellow, white, and clear).
- Procedures for a professional varnish fluoride application are listed in **Table 34-4**.

VI. After Application

- Tray application
  - Instruct patients not to rinse, eat, drink, brush, or floss for at least 30 minutes after gel or foam applications.
  - Rinsing immediately after a tray application has been shown to significantly lessen the benefits.[75]
- Varnish application
  - Instruct patients to avoid hot drinks and alcoholic beverages; eating hard, sticky, or crunchy foods; and brushing or flossing the teeth for 4–6 hours after application or until the next morning to allow fluoride uptake to continue undisturbed.
  - Varnish residue is removed by the patient toothbrushing and flossing the next day.

VII. Silver Diamine Fluoride

- Indications[67]
  - Extreme caries risk (xerostomia, severe early childhood caries, or cancer treatments—radiation/chemotherapy).
  - Treatment challenged by behavioral/medical management.
  - Patients with carious lesions that may not all be treated in one visit (stabilize patient).
  - Difficult to treat dental carious lesions.
  - Patients with limited access to dental care (underserved populations).
- Advantages[76]
  - Noninvasive (no needle or drill required).
  - **Cariostatic** agent.
  - Reduces caries risk of adjacent teeth.[66]
  - Reduces dentinal hypersensitivity.

Table 34-4 Procedure for Varnish Application (5% NaF)

Patient selection	▪ Determine need based on caries risk assessment (only professional fluoride recommended for children younger than 6 years of age). ▪ Review the medical history and verify the patient does not have a known rosin/colophony sensitivity or allergy.[59,63-65] ▪ If there is a suspected or known allergy to rosin/colophony, select a varnish formulation that contains synthetic rosin or utilize an alternative topical fluoride application (tray method with 1.23% APF gel for 6 years and older and adult root caries). ▪ Explain procedure. ▪ Seat supine. ▪ For the infant and toddler, the parent and clinician can sit knee to knee with the child held across the knees. ▪ Instruct not to swallow during the procedure.
Prepare product	▪ Dispense from a tube or open a single-dose packet. ▪ Have applicator brush available.
Dry teeth	▪ Varnish sets up in the presence of saliva, but it is recommended to remove excess saliva by wiping the teeth with a gauze square.
Apply varnish	▪ Dip applicator brush in varnish and mix well. Systematically brush a thin layer over all tooth surfaces. For prevention of early childhood caries in the infant, toddler, or very young child, apply to the maxillary anterior teeth first and then proceed to other areas of the dentition if patient is cooperative. For all other patients, use a systematic approach. Begin with mandibular teeth; facial, occlusal, and lingual surfaces and then the maxillary teeth; palatal, occlusal, and facial surfaces. Provide full coverage to all areas of the teeth including areas of recession and the cervical third of facial, lingual, and palatal surfaces and occlusal surfaces. Application time is approximately 1–3 minutes.
Completion	▪ Instruct patient that the teeth will feel like they have a coating or film, but this is not visible if a clear product has been used. Ask the patient to avoid hard foods, drinking hot or alcoholic beverages, brushing, and flossing the teeth until the next day or at least 4–6 hours after application.

- Contraindications[67]
    - Allergy to silver.
    - Pregnancy/breastfeeding.
- Relative contraindications[67,69]
    - Painful sores or raw areas on the gingiva or in the mouth (ulcerative gingivitis or stomatitis).
    - Avoid application on cavitated teeth with suspected pulpal involvement.[69]
- Potential limitations and risks[67]
    - Communicate effectively with the patient/parent/legal guardian/advocate and consider written informed consent form for SDF placement prior to application.
    - Placement of SDF does not eliminate the need for future restorations.
    - SDF needs to be applied one to two times at separate dental hygiene visits for maximum benefit (approximately once every 6–12 months).
    - The affected area of decay will likely stain black/gray permanently upon SDF placement; however, healthy enamel will not stain.
    - If accidentally applied to the skin or gingiva, a brownish stain may appear, which will not wash away immediately (should dissipate within 1–3 weeks).
    - Metallic/bitter taste.
- SDF application appointment sequence[67]
    - Dispense 1 drop in a dappen dish, which will treat up to five surfaces/10 kg per treatment visit, maximum dose 25 μL.
    - Protect the clinical environment by covering the unit with plastic and the counter with a tray cover or plastic lined bib.
    - Provide a plastic bib and protective eyewear for the patient.
    - Isolate the tongue and cheek with gauze/cotton rolls to prevent staining of soft tissues.
    - Dry the lesion.
    - Immerse microsponge brush in SDF, remove excess on the side of the dappen dish.
    - Apply SDF directly to the carious lesion and allow it to absorb for 1–3 minutes; may reapply.
- Allow the area to fully dry for 60 seconds.
- Place gloves, cotton, and microsponge brush in a plastic bag for disposal.
    - Procedures for SDF application are listed in **Table 34-5**.

Self-Applied Fluorides

- Self-applied fluorides (prescription [**Rx**] and OTC products) are available as dentifrices, mouthrinses, and gels.
- Concentrations of 1500 ppm fluoride or less can be sold OTC.[39] However, some products containing less than 1500 ppm of fluoride are available only by Rx.
- May be applied by toothbrushing, rinsing, or trays that are custom made or disposable.

Table 34-5 Procedure for SDF Application[67]

Patient selection	■ Determine indications (e.g., extreme caries risk, xerostomia, severe childhood caries). ■ Review contraindications/relative contraindications. ■ Communicate effectively regarding potential limitations and risks with the patient/parent/guardian and consider written informed consent prior to application. ■ Inform the patient the affected area of decay will likely stain black/gray permanently upon placement of SDF. ■ Provide protective eyewear and a plastic bib to the patient, and isolate both the tongue and cheek with gauze or cotton rolls to prevent staining.
Prepare operatory and product	■ To avoid staining, place a tray cover or a plastic lined bib on the counter and ensure operatory unit is adequately protected with plastic. Dispense 1 drop in a dappen dish/10 kg per treatment visit. ■ Have microsponge brush available.
Dry the carious lesion and apply the SDF	■ Dry the lesion. Immerse the microsponge in the SDF. Remove any excess product on the side of the dappen dish. Apply directly to the carious lesion and allow it to absorb for 1–3 minutes; may reapply as needed.
Completion	■ Allow the area to fully dry for 60 seconds. Place microsponge brush, cotton, and gloves into a plastic bag for disposal. ■ There are no postplacement patient instructions with SDF; however, reevaluation of the area is recommended 2–4 weeks after initial application.[69]

I. Indications

- Patient needs are determined as part of total care planning.
- Indications for use of tray, rinsing, and/or toothbrushing depend on the individual patient prevention needs and caries risk assessment.
- Certain patients need multiple procedures combined with professional applications at their regular continuing care appointments. Special indications are suggested as each method is described in the following sections.

II. Methods

The three methods for self-application are by tray, rinsing, and toothbrushing.

- Tray
  - Custom-made or disposable tray: The tray is selected to fit the individual mouth and completely cover the teeth being treated.
  - Figure 34-4 shows adequate and inadequate tray coverage on the teeth.
  - Instruction is provided not to overfill the tray.
- Rinsing
  - The patient swishes for 1 minute with a measured amount of a fluoride rinse and expectorates.
  - Certain patients will need to learn how to rinse properly to force the solution between the teeth. Chapter 28 lists steps for teaching how to rinse.
- Toothbrushing
  - A fluoride-containing dentifrice is used for regular brushing after breakfast and before going to bed without further eating.
  - Brush-on gel is used after regular brushing to provide additional benefits.
  - Use an interdental brush to apply fluoride to proximal surfaces or open furcations.

Tray Technique: Home Application

- The original gel tray studies using custom-fitted polyvinyl mouthpieces compared the use of 1.1% APF with plain NaF gel.
- The gel was applied daily over a 2-year period by schoolchildren aged 11–14 years during the school years. Dental caries incidence was reduced up to 80%.[77]

I. Indications for Use

- Rampant enamel or root caries in persons of any age to prevent additional new carious lesions and promote remineralization around existing lesions.
- Xerostomia from any cause, particularly loss of salivary gland function.
- Exposure to radiation therapy.
- Root surface hypersensitivity.

II. Gels Used (Available by Prescription)

- Concentrations[39]
  - 1.1% NaF; 5000 ppm fluoride.
  - 1.1% APF; 5000 ppm fluoride.
- Precautions[39]
  - Dispense small quantities.
  - Maximum adult dose is 16 drops per day (4–8 drops on the inner surface of each custom-made tray).
  - Use neutral sodium preparations on porcelain, composites, titanium, or sealants.
  - Patients with mucositis may experience irritation with the APF due to the high acidity.
- Patient instructions
  - Use the gel tray once each day, preferably just before going to bed without further eating and after toothbrushing and flossing.
  - **Box 34-3** outlines the procedures for the patient to follow for a home tray application.
  - A printed copy of the instructions is given to the patient.

Fluoride Mouthrinses

- Mouthrinsing is a practical and effective means for self-application of fluoride for individuals at moderate or high caries risk.
- Do not use for patients aged 6 years or younger, or for those unable to rinse for a physical or other reason.[78]
- Rinsing can be part of an individual care plan or can be included in a group program conducted during school attendance.

I. Indications

- Mouthrinsing with a fluoride preparation may be an additional benefit for the following:
  - Young persons during the high-risk preteen and adolescent years.
  - Patients with areas of demineralization.

- Patients with root exposure following recession and periodontal therapy.
- Participants in a school health group program for children older than 6 years.
- Patients with moderate-to-rampant caries risk who live in a fluoridated or nonfluoridated community.
- Patients whose oral health care is complicated by biofilm-retentive appliances, including orthodontics, partial dentures, or space maintainers.
- Patients with xerostomia from any cause, including head and neck radiation and saliva-depressing drug therapy.
- Patients with hypersensitivity of exposed root surfaces.

Box 34-3 Instructions for Home Tray Application

1. One daily application just before bedtime; do not eat or drink until morning. If applied at another time of day, do not eat or drink for at least 30 minutes.
2. Brush and floss before applying tray to remove biofilm and food debris.
3. Use prepared custom-made polyvinyl trays. Disposable trays can be used if the appropriate fit can be obtained.
4. Distribute no more than 4–8 drops or a thin ribbon of the gel on the inner surface of each tray. Each drop is equivalent to 0.1 mL.
5. Expectorate to minimize saliva in the mouth.
6. Apply one tray at a time. Hold head upright.
7. Apply the mandibular tray first; close gently to hold the tray in place.
8. Time by a clock for 4 minutes. Do not swallow.
9. Expectorate several times when the tray is removed to prevent swallowing gel and then prepare the mouth for the other tray.
10. Apply the maxillary tray and follow steps 7–9 as for the mandibular tray.
11. After tray removal, do not eat, drink, or brush teeth for at least 30 minutes.
12. After both trays are removed, rinse the trays under running water and brush them clean.
13. Keep in open air for drying.

II. Limitations

- Children younger than 6 years of age and those of any age who cannot rinse because of oral and/or facial musculature problems or other disability.
- Alcohol content:
  - Alcohol-based mouthrinses are not recommended; aqueous solutions are available.
  - Alcohol content of commercial preparations is not advisable for children, especially adolescents.
  - Alcohol-containing preparations are never to be recommended for a person recovering from alcohol use disorder (AUD); however, a history of AUD would not necessarily be known to the clinician.
- Compliance is greater with a daily rinse than with a weekly rinse for at home use.

III. Preparations[39]

- Oral rinses are categorized as low-potency/high-frequency rinses or high-potency/low-frequency rinses.
- Most low-potency rinses may be purchased directly OTC, whereas most high-potency rinses are provided by prescription (Rx).
- **Table 34-6** contains the compounds, concentration, and recommended frequency of use for currently available self-applied fluoride rinses.

Table 34-6 Patient-Applied Fluoride Mouthrinses (Age 6 Years and Older)

Type/Percentage (RX or OTC)	Concentration in PPM	Frequency of Use (10 mL or 2 Teaspoons Swished for 1 Min)
0.2% NaF (Rx)	905	Once daily or once weekly
0.044% NaF and APF (Rx and OTC)	200	Once daily
0.05% NaF (OTC)	230	Once daily
0.0221% NaF (OTC)	100	Twice daily

APF, acidulated phosphate fluoride; NaF, sodium fluoride; OTC, over-the-counter; Rx, prescription

- Low potency/high frequency (available OTC)
  - Preparations
    - 0.05% NaF; 230 ppm.
    - 0.044% NaF or APF; 200 ppm (available by Rx or OTC depending on the brand).
    - 0.0221% NaF; 100 ppm.
  - Specifications
    - No more than 264 mg NaF (120 mg of fluoride) can be dispensed at one time.
    - A 500-mL bottle of 0.05% NaF rinse contains 100 mg of fluoride.
    - Bottle is required to have a child-proof cap.
    - Rinses are not to be used by children younger than 6 years of age or by children or adults with a disability involving oral and/or facial musculature.
    - Young children do not have sufficient ability to expectorate, and they tend to swallow quickly.
    - The rinse is to be fully expectorated without swallowing.
  - Procedure for use
    - Low-potency rinses are used once or twice daily with 2 teaspoonfuls (10 mL) after brushing and before bedtime. Follow manufacturer's ADA-approved specifications.
    - The adult and pediatric maximum dose is 10 mL of solution.
    - Swish between teeth with lips tightly closed for 60 seconds; spit out.
    - Have the patient practice rinsing at the dental chair.
    - Instruct patient: Do not eat or drink for 30 minutes after rinsing.
- High potency/low frequency (available by Rx)
  - Preparation
    - 0.20% NaF; 905 ppm.
    - Originally recommended as a weekly rinse, but it can be used up to once per day.[47]
  - Procedure for use: the same as for high-frequency/low-potency rinses.

The prevented fraction of dental caries ranges from 30% to 59%, with the use of 0.2% NaF rinse on various rinsing schedules.[51]

IV. Benefits

- Benefits from fluoride mouthrinsing have been documented many times since the original research using various percentages of different fluoride preparations.[79,80]
- Frequent rinsing with low concentrations of fluoride has the following effects:
  - Primary teeth present in school-aged children benefit by as much as a 42.5% average reduction in dental caries incidence.[81]
  - Greater benefit for smooth surfaces, but some benefit to pits and fissures.
  - Greatest benefit to newly erupted teeth.
  - The program needs to be continued through the teenage years to benefit the second and third permanent molars.
  - Added benefits for a community with water fluoridation.[82]
  - Effective in preventing and reversing root caries.[83]

Brush-On Gel

- Brush-on gel has been used as an adjunct to the daily application of fluoride in a dentifrice and as a supplement to periodic professional applications.
- Regular use has been shown to help control demineralization around orthodontic appliances.[84]
- Provides protection against postirradiation caries in conjunction with other fluoride applications.[85]
- In 2018, an expert panel from the ADA recommended the prioritized use of 5000 ppm fluoride (1.1% NaF) toothpaste or gel at least once per day to arrest or reverse noncavitated and cavitated root surfaces or lesions of permanent teeth over other modalities.[52]

I. Preparations

Table 34-7 contains the type, concentration, and daily usage guidelines for currently available self-applied fluoride gels.

- 1.1% NaF (neutral pH) or 1.1% APF (3.5 pH); 5000 ppm
  - Available as a gel to be used separate from toothbrushing.
- 1.1% neutral NaF is also available as a dentifrice with an **abrasive system** added.
  - The rationale for the dentifrice product is to increase compliance with one step (brushing only) rather than brushing, followed by application of the high-concentration gel with a toothbrush.
  - Requires a prescription.
- Stannous fluoride (**SnF_2**) 0.4% in glycerin base (1000 ppm).
  - Available as a gel to be used separate from toothbrushing.
  - Available OTC.

Table 34-7 Patient-Applied Fluoride Gels: Brush-On or Use in Custom-Made Trays (Age 6 Years or Older)

Type/Percentage (Rx or OTC)	Concentration in PPM	Daily Usage Guidelines
1.1% NaF gel or paste (Rx)	5000	Brush on teeth, twice per day or 4–8 drops on inner surface of custom-made tray or brush on teeth
1.1% APF (Rx)	5000	Brush on teeth, preferably at night or 4–8 drops on inner surface of custom-made tray
0.4% SnF (OTC)	1000	Brush on teeth, preferably at night

APF, acidulated phosphate fluoride; NaF, sodium fluoride; OTC, over-the-counter; Rx, prescription

II. Procedure

- Teeth are cleaned first with thorough brushing and flossing before gel application with a separate toothbrush.
- Use once a day or more as recommended, preferably at night after toothbrushing and flossing.
- Place about 2 mg of the gel over the brush head and spread over all teeth.
- Brush 1 minute, then swish to force the fluid between the teeth several times before expectorating.
- Do not rinse.

Fluoride Dentifrices

I. Development

- Historically tried with various compounds, including stannous fluoride, NaF, sodium monofluorophosphate, and amine fluoride.
- Early research objectives: to find compatible fluoride, abrasive systems, and formulations containing available fluoride for uptake by the tooth surface.
- In 1960, the first fluoride dentifrice gained approval by the ADA, Council on Dental Therapeutics: 0.4% stannous fluoride.[86]

II. Indications

- Dental caries prevention
  - Fluoride dentifrice approved by the ADA is an integral part of a complete preventive program and is a basic caries prevention intervention for all patients.[86]
  - Recommended for all patients regardless of their caries risk.
  - Toothbrushing that covers all the teeth on all surfaces at least twice per day with fluoridated toothpaste is the foundation for all patients' fluoride regimen.
  - Patients with moderate-to-rampant dental caries are advised to brush three or four times each day with a fluoride-containing dentifrice.
  - Expectorate, but do not rinse after toothbrushing, to give the fluoride a longer time to be effective.

III. Preparations

Fluoride dentifrices are available as gels or pastes. Amine fluorides are used in other countries, but not available in the United States.

- Current fluoride constituents[87]
  - NaF 0.24% (1100 ppm).
  - Sodium monofluorophosphate (Na_2PO_3 F) 0.76% (1000 ppm).
  - Stannous fluoride (SnF_2) 0.45% (1000 ppm).
- Guidelines for acceptance
  - Look for ADA Seal of Acceptance. The requirements for acceptance of fluoridated toothpaste by the ADA are described in Chapter 28.

IV. Patient Instruction: Recommended Procedures

Advise the patient in the selection of a fluoride dentifrice, the need for frequent use, the method for application to all the tooth surfaces, and the importance of using a fluoride dentifrice to promote oral health.

- Select an ADA-accepted fluoride-containing dentifrice.
- Place recommended amount of dentifrice on the toothbrush.
- Children (younger than 3 years): twice-daily brushing (morning and night) with no more than a "smear" or the size of a grain of rice of fluoride dentifrice spread along the brushing plane.[88,89] Chapter 47 illustrates a small smear.
  - Daily oral care begins with the eruption of the first primary tooth.

    - The supervision of oral hygiene by parents or family members with attention to daily biofilm removal by toothbrushing can make a significant impact on the small child's oral health.
- The paste is then spread over all the teeth before starting to brush so that all teeth benefit and large amounts of paste are not available for swallowing. Older child (ages 3–6 years): twice-daily brushing (morning and night) with fluoride toothpaste the size of a small pea.
    - Demonstrate spreading this amount over the ends of the toothbrush and explain that the child is not to swallow excess amounts of dentifrice.[88,89]
- Adults: Use 1/2 inch of fluoride dentifrice twice daily.
    - Spread dentifrice over the teeth with a light touch of the brush.
    - Proceed with correct brushing positions for sulcular removal of dental biofilm. (See Chapter 26.)
    - Do not rinse after brushing to keep fluoride in the oral cavity.[88,90]
- Keep dentifrice container out of reach of children.

V. Benefits

- Twice-daily use has greater benefits than once-daily use.[78]
- Patients at moderate and high caries risk and those who live in a nonfluoridated community benefit from using a dentifrice several times per day to maintain salivary fluoride levels.
- The dentifrice is a continuing source of fluoride for the tooth surface in the control of demineralization and the promotion of remineralization.
- The use of a dentifrice with a fluoride concentration of 1000 ppm and above compared to a dentifrice without fluoride can prevent dental caries up to an average of 23%.[91]

Combined Fluoride Program

- All patients, regardless of caries risk, benefit from at least twice-daily use of a fluoridated dentifrice and consumption of fluoridated water multiple times during each day.
- Patients at moderate-to-high caries risk benefit from additional methods of fluoride exposure.
- Additional caries reduction can be expected when another topical fluoride, such as a mouthrinse or gel tray, is combined with a fluoride dentifrice.[92]
- When self-administered methods are chosen, patient cooperation is a significant factor.
- Age and eruption pattern influence the method selected.
- Continuing care appointments are to be scheduled for frequent professional topical applications for those at moderate and high caries risk and for continuing instruction and motivation regarding daily fluoride use for all patients.

Fluoride Safety

- Fluoride preparations and fluoridated water have wide margins of safety.
- Fluoride is beneficial in small amounts, but it can be injurious if used without attention to correct dosage and frequency.
- All dental personnel need to be familiar with the following:
    - Recommended approved procedures for use of products containing fluoride.
    - Potential toxic effects of fluoride.
    - How to administer general emergency measures when accidental overdoses occur. (See the "Internal Poisoning" section of Chapter 9.)

I. Summary of Fluoride Risk Management

- Use professionally and recommend only approved fluoride preparations for patient use.
    - Products may have approval from the FDA and the ADA in the United States.
    - Read about the programs of the ADA Council on Scientific Affairs and the Seal of Approval of Products in Chapter 28.
- Use only researched, recommended amounts and methods for delivery.
- Know potential toxicity of the various products and be prepared to administer emergency measures for treating an accidental toxic response.
- Instruct patients in proper care of fluoride products.
    - Dentist prescribes no more than 120 mg of fluoride at one time (no more than 480 of the 0.25 mg tablets or 240 of the 0.5 mg tablets).[39] Do not store large quantities in the home.
    - Request parental supervision of a child's brushing or other fluoride administration. Rinses, for example, are not to be used by children younger than 6 years of age.
    - Fluoride products have child-proof caps and are to be kept out of reach of small children

and other persons, such as the intellectually challenged, who may not understand limitations.
- In school health programs, dispensing of the fluoride product is to be supervised by responsible adults. Containers are to be stored under lock and key when not in active use.

II. Toxicity

- Acute toxicity refers to rapid intake of an excess dose over a short time.
  - Acute fluoride poisoning is extremely rare.[93]
- Chronic toxicity applies to long-term ingestion of fluoride in amounts that exceed the approved therapeutic levels.
- Accidental ingestion of a concentrated fluoride preparation can lead to a toxic reaction.
- Certainly lethal dose (CLD)[94]
  - A lethal dose is the amount of a drug likely to cause death if not intercepted by antidotal therapy.
  - Adult CLD: about 5–10 g of NaF taken at one time. The fluoride ion equivalent is 32–64 mg of fluoride per kilogram body weight (mg F/kg; **Box 34-4A**).
  - Child CLD: approximately 0.5–1.0 g, variable with size and weight of the child.
- Safely tolerated dose (STD): one-fourth of the CLD
  - Adult STD: about 1.25–2.5 g of NaF (8–16 mg F/kg).
  - Child: **Box 34-4B** shows STDs and CLDs for children.
  - Weights given for each selected age are minimal, and calculations for the doses are conservative.
  - As can be noted in Box 34-5B, less than 1 g (1000 mg) may be fatal for children aged 12 years and younger, and 0.5 g (500 mg) exceeds the STD for all ages shown.
  - For children younger than 6 years of age, however, 500 mg could be lethal.[94]

III. Signs and Symptoms of Acute Toxic Dose

Symptoms begin within 30 minutes of ingestion and may persist for as long as 24 hours.

- Gastrointestinal tract
- Fluoride in the stomach is acted on by the hydrochloric acid to form hydrofluoric acid, an irritant to the stomach lining. Symptoms include:
  - Nausea, vomiting, and diarrhea.
  - Abdominal pain.
  - Increased salivation and thirst.
- Systemic involvements
  - Blood: calcium may be bound by the circulating fluoride, thus causing symptoms of hypocalcemia.
  - Central nervous system: hyperreflexia, convulsions, and paresthesias.
  - Cardiovascular and respiratory depression: if not treated, may lead to death in a few hours from cardiac failure or respiratory paralysis.

Box 34-4 Lethal and Safe Doses of Fluoride

A. Lethal and safe doses of fluoride for a 70-kg adult

CLD
5–10 g NaF
Or
32–64 mg F/kg
STD = 1/4 CLD
1.25–2.5 g NaF
Or
8–16 mg F/kg

B. CLDs and STDs of fluoride (mg F/kg) for selected ages

Age (Years)	Weight (lb/kg)	CLD (mg)	STD (mg)
2	22/10	320	80
4	29/13	422	106
6	37/17	538	135
8	45/20	655	164
10	53/24	771	193
12	64/29	931	233
14	83/38	1206	301
16	92/42	1338	334
18	95/43	1382	346

IV. Emergency Treatment

- Induce vomiting
  - Mechanical: digital stimulation at the back of tongue or in the throat.
- Second person
  - Call emergency service; transport to hospital.

- Administer fluoride-binding liquid when patient is not vomiting
  - Milk.
  - Milk of magnesia.
  - Lime water ($CaOH_2$ solution 0.15%).
- Support respiration and circulation
- Additional therapy indicated at emergency room
  - Calcium gluconate for muscle tremors or tetany.
  - Gastric lavage.
  - Cardiac monitoring.
  - Endotracheal intubation.
  - Blood monitoring (calcium, magnesium, potassium, pH).
  - Intravenous feeding to restore blood volume, calcium.

V. Chronic Toxicity

- Skeletal fluorosis[93]
  - Isolated instances of osteosclerosis, an elevation in bone density, can result from chronic toxicity after long-term (10 years or more) ingestion of water with 8–10 ppm fluoride or from inhalation of industrial fumes or dust.
  - Skeletal fluorosis in its early stages is characterized by stiff and painful joints and becomes crippling in its later stages.
  - It has never been a public health concern in the United States, even in communities that naturally have had high levels of fluoride in the water for generations.
  - Is endemic in certain countries such as China and India with high levels of natural fluoride in the water.
  - Predisposing factors, dietary deficiencies, and population differences with regard to fluoride metabolism may play a role in its development in addition to exposure.
  - Methods for defluoridation have been developed, as described in this chapter.
- Dental fluorosis
  - Ingestion of naturally occurring excess fluoride in the drinking water and/or fluoride dental products can produce visible fluorosis only when used during the years of development of the crowns of the teeth, namely, from birth until age 16 or 18 years, or when the crowns of the third permanent molars are completed.
  - No systemic symptoms result from the fluoride, and the individual has protection against dental caries.
  - Scoring system used to describe dental fluorosis is found in Chapter 21.
- Mild fluorosis
  1. Clinical evaluation
     - Mild and very mild forms, dental fluorosis appears as "**white spots**" or **enamel opacities** in the enamel surface.
     - No esthetic or health problem is involved. Many such white spots are not visible, except when scrutinized under a dental light and the surface is dried.
     - Not all white spots in the enamel are related to fluoride intake; distinction can be made by reviewing the patient's dental and fluoride intake history, by noting the location and distribution of the white spots, and by considering the sequence of tooth development.
  2. Relation to fluoride sources
     - Mild fluorosis may result from inadvertent ingestion of excess fluoride by young children during topical procedures, both self-applied and professional.
     - No problem exists when care is taken to follow basic steps, such as those listed in Table 34-3, Table 34-4, and Table 34-5, for professional applications.
     - Mouthrinses are not indicated for children younger than 6 years of age.
     - Small amounts of dentifrice may be swallowed incidentally at each brushing. A child aged 4 years who lives in a nonfluoridated community uses a daily supplement (0.5 mg) and swallows two or three small amounts of dentifrice ingests far less than the STD of 106 mg.

Documentation

A patient receiving a topical fluoride application and/or counseling regarding fluoride needs the following documented in the permanent record:

- Caries risk level (document as low, moderate, high, or very high).
- Current use of fluoride toothpaste and exposure to fluoridated water.
- Type, concentration, mode of delivery, and postoperative instructions if a professional fluoride application is provided.
- Type, amount, and instructions for the use of any Rx or OTC patient-applied fluoride products recommended.
- A sample documentation using the SOAP format is provided in **Box 34-5**.

Box 34-5 **Example Documentation: Professional Fluoride Application and Prescribing Home Fluoride**

- **S**—A 26-year-old male patient presents for a periodic oral examination, radiographs, and dental prophylaxis. Patient states that he drinks high-sucrose beverages on a frequent, daily basis. He also reports using toothpaste with fluoride twice daily and consumes fluoridated water.
- **O**—Patient presents with medication-induced xerostomia. Two proximal cavitated lesions were discovered on bitewing radiographs.
- Patient was classified as being high risk for caries after conducting a caries risk assessment analysis.
- **P**—Applied 5% NaF varnish to the entire dentition and provided postoperative instructions. Prescribed 1.1% NaF gel (two refills) to apply with a separate toothbrush at night. Discussed the need for an additional varnish application in 3 months to help prevent the future onset of dental caries.

Signed: ______________________________, RDH
Date: ___________________________________

Factors to Teach the Patient

I. Personal Use of Fluorides

- Purposes, action, and expected benefits relative to the specific forms of fluoride treatment the patient will receive based upon individual caries risk.
- Specific instructions concerning self-applied techniques that will be performed at home.

II. Need for Parental Supervision

- Supervise daily care of child's teeth and mouth with the recommended amount of fluoridated toothpaste to prevent excess ingestion of fluoride.
- Keep fluoride products out of reach of small children.

III. Determine Need for Fluoride Supplements

- Must determine child is at high caries risk and consumes fluoride-deficient drinking water.
- Where to send private water source sample for fluoride analysis.

IV. Fluorides Are Part of the Total Preventive Program

- Emphasize fluoride toothpaste and fluoridated water as the cornerstones for prevention of dental caries.
- Regular professional supervision and care.

V. Fluoridation

- How drinking fluoridated water helps people of all ages and need to advocate to keep in community water supplies.
- How to access the CDC Community Water Fluoridation website to obtain reliable information about fluoridation in the United States.

VII. Bottled Drinking Water/Water Filters

- When bottled water does not have a label indicating that it is fluoridated, recommend filling a water bottle from a fluoridated water supply.
- Check with the water filter manufacturer to be certain the fluoride will not be removed through filtration.
- Distillation and reverse osmosis systems remove fluoride from drinking water, but water softeners do not.

VIII. Infant Formula

- Educate parents that powdered or liquid concentrate infant formula and the water used to reconstitute this formula may contain fluoride.

References

1. Ellwood R, Fejerskov O, Cury JA, Clarkson B. Chapter 18: Fluorides in caries control. In: Fejerskov O, Kidd E, eds. *Dental Caries: The Disease and Its Clinical Management*. 2nd ed. Oxford, England: Blackwell Munksgaard; 2008:293-294.
2. Newbrun E. Systemic benefits of fluoride and fluoridation. *J Public Health Dent*. 2004;64(suppl s1):35-39.
3. Ekstrand J. Chapter 4: Fluoride metabolism. In: Fejerskov O, Ekstrand J, Burt BA, eds. *Fluoride in Dentistry*. 2nd ed. Copenhagen, Denmark: Blackwell Munksgaard; 1996:55-67.
4. Bath-Balough M, Fehrenbach M. *Dental Embryology, Histology, and Anatomy*. 2nd ed. St. Louis, MO: Saunders; 2006: 179-189.
5. Melfi RC, Alley KE. *Permar's Oral Embryology and Microscopic Anatomy*. 10th ed. Philadelphia, PA: Lippincott Williams & Wilkins; 2000:43-87.
6. Levy S. An update on fluorides and fluorosis. *J Can Dent Assoc*. 2003;69(5):286-291.
7. Aoba T, Fejerskov O. Dental fluorosis: chemistry and biology. *Crit Rev Oral Biol Med*. 2002;13(2):155-170.
8. Featherstone JD. The science and practice of caries prevention. *J Am Dent Assoc*. 2000;131(7):887-899.
9. Yoon SH, Brudevold F, Gardner DE, Smith FA. Distribution of fluoride in teeth from areas with different levels of fluoride in the water supply. *J Dent Res*. 1960;39:845-856.
10. Centers for Disease Control and Prevention. Recommendations for using fluoride to prevent and control dental caries in the United States. *MMWR Recomm Rep*. 2001;50(RR-14):1-42.
11. Centers for Disease Control and Prevention. Populations receiving optimally fluoridated public drinking water–United States, 1992–1996. *MWWR Morb Mortal Wkly Rep*. 2008;57(27):737-741.
12. Centers for Disease Control and Prevention. Division of Oral Health, National Center for Chronic Disease Prevention and Health Promotion. Community water fluoridation. Atlanta, GA: Water Fluoridation Statistics; 2018. Page last reviewed September 8, 2020. https://www.cdc.gov/fluoridation/statistics/2018stats.htm. Accessed July 23, 2021.
13. Herschfeld JJ. Classics in dental history: Frederick S. McKay and the "Colorado brown stain." *Bull Hist Dent*. 1978;26(2): 118-126.
14. McKay FS. The relation of mottled enamel to caries. *J Am Dent Assoc*. 1928;15:1429-1437.
15. Churchill HV. Occurrence of fluorides in some waters of United States. *J Ind Eng Chem*. 1931;23:996-998.
16. Dean HT, Arnold FA Jr, Elvove E. Domestic water and dental caries. V. Additional studies of the relation of fluoride domestic waters to dental caries experience in 4425 white children, aged 12 to 14 years, of 13 cities in 4 states. *Public Health Rep*. 1942;57:1155-1179.
17. Department of Health and Human Services. U.S. Public Health Service Recommendation for Fluoride Concentration in Drinking Water for the Prevention of Caries. *Public Health Rep*. 2015;130:1-14. http://www.cdc.gov/fluoridation/index.htm. Accessed October 3, 2022.
18. Centers for Disease Control and Prevention. Engineering and administrative recommendations for water fluoridation, 1995. *MMWR Recomm Rep*. 1995;44(RR-13):1-40.
19. Griffin SO, Regnier E, Griffin PM, Huntley V. Effectiveness of fluoride in preventing caries in adults. *J Dent Res*. 2007;86(5): 410-415.
20. Yeung CA. A systematic review of the efficacy and safety of fluoridation. *Evid Based Dent*. 2008;9(2):39-43.
21. Dirks OB, Houwink B, Kwant GW. Some special features of the caries preventive effect of water fluoridation. *Arch Oral Biol*. 1961;4:187-192.
22. Burt BA, Ismail AI, Eklund SA. Root caries in an optimally fluoridated and a high-fluoride community. *J Dent Res*. 1986; 6(9):1154-1158.
23. Stamm JW, Banting DW, Imrey PB. Adult root caries survey of two similar communities with contrasting natural water fluoride levels. *J Am Dent Assoc*. 1990;120(2):143-149.
24. Ast DB, Fitzgerald B. Effectiveness of water fluoridation. *J Am Dent Assoc*. 1962;65:581-587.
25. Russell AL, Elvove E. Domestic water and dental caries. VII. A study of the fluoride-dental caries relationship in an adult population. *Public Health Rep*. 1951;66(43):1389-1401.
26. Englander HR, Wallace DA. Effects of naturally fluoridated water on dental caries in adults: Aurora-Rockford, Illinois, Study III. *Public Health Rep*. 1962;77(10):887-893.
27. Horowitz HS, Maier FJ, Law FE. Partial defluoridation of a community water supply and dental fluorosis. *Public Health Rep*. 1967;82(11):965-972.
28. Horowitz HS, Heifetz SB. The effect of partial defluoridation of a water supply on dental fluorosis—final results in Bartlett, Texas, after 17 years. *Am J Public Health*. 1972;62(6):767-769.
29. Horowitz HS. Effectiveness of school water fluoridation and dietary fluoride supplements in school-aged children. *J Public Health Dent*. 1989;49(5):290-296.
30. Lemke CW, Doherty JM, Arra MC. Controlled fluoridation: the dental effects of discontinuation in Antigo, Wisconsin. *J Am Dent Assoc*. 1979;80(4):782-786.
31. Jackson RD, Brizendine EJ, Kelly SA, Hinesley R, Stookey GK, Dunipace AJ. The fluoride content of foods and beverages from negligibly and optimally fluoridated communities. *Community Dent Oral Epidemiol*. 2002;30(5):382-391.
32. Burt BA, Marthaler TM. Chapter 16: Fluoride tablets, salt fluoridation, and milk fluoridation. In: Fejerskov O, Ekstrand J, Burt BA, eds. *Fluoride in Dentistry*. 2nd ed. Copenhagen, Denmark: Blackwell Munksgaard; 1996:291-310.
33. Espelid I. Caries preventive effect of fluoride in milk, salt and tablets: a literature review. *Eur Arch Paediatr Dent*. 2009; 10(3):149-156.
34. European Academy of Paediatric Dentistry. Guidelines on the use of fluoride in children: an EAPD policy document. *Eur Arch Paediatr Dent*. 2009;10(3):129-135.
35. American Dental Association. *Fluoridation Facts*. Chicago, IL: American Dental Association; 2005.
36. Hujoel PP, Zina LG, Moimaz SA, Cunha-Cruz J. Infant formula and enamel fluorosis: a systematic review. *J Am Dent Assoc*. 2009;140(7):841-854.
37. Siew C, Strock S, Ristic H, et al. Assessing the potential risk factor for enamel fluorosis: a preliminary evaluation of fluoride content in infant formulas. *J Am Dent Assoc*. 2009; 140(10):1228-1236.
38. Berg J, Gerweck C, Hujoel P, et al. Evidence-based clinical recommendations regarding fluoride intake from reconstituted infant formula and enamel fluorosis. *J Am Dent Assoc*. 2011;142(1):79-87.
39. Burrell KH. Chapter 10: Fluorides. In: Mariotti AJ, Burrell KH, eds. *American Dental Association, Council on*

Scientific Affairs: ADA/PDR Guide to Dental Therapeutics. 5th ed. Chicago, IL: American Dental Association and Thomson PDR; 2009:323-337.

40. Ismail AI, Hasson H. Fluoride supplements, dental caries, and fluorosis: a systematic review. *J Am Dent Assoc*. 2008;139(11): 1457-1468.
41. Rozier RG, Adair S, Graham F, et al. Evidence-based clinical recommendations on the prescription of dietary fluoride supplements for caries prevention. *J Am Dent Assoc*. 2010;141(12):1480-1489.
42. Toyama Y, Nakagaki H, Kato S, et al. Fluoride concentrations at and near the neonatal line in human deciduous tooth enamel obtained from a naturally fluoridated and a non-fluoridated area. *Arch Oral Biol*. 2001;46(2):147-153.
43. Tubert-Jeannin S, Auclair C, Amsallem E, et al. Fluoride supplements (tablets, drops, lozenges or chewing gums) for preventing dental caries in children. *Cochrane Database Syst Rev*. 2011;(12):CD007592.
44. Bibby BG. Use of fluorine in the prevention of dental caries. II. The effects of sodium fluoride applications. *J Am Dent Assoc*. 1944;31:317.
45. Knutson JW. Sodium fluoride solutions: technique for application to the teeth. *J Am Dent Assoc*. 1948;36(1):37-39.
46. Galagan DJ, Knutson JW. The effect of topically applied fluorides on dental caries experience; experiments with sodium fluoride and calcium chloride; widely spaced applications; use of different solution concentrations. *Public Health Rep*. 1948;63(38):1215-1221.
47. Weyant RJ, Tracy SL, Anselmo T, et al. Topical fluoride for caries prevention: executive summary of the updated clinical recommendations and supporting systemic review. *J Am Dent Assoc*. 2013;144(11):1279-1291.
48. Warren DP, Chan JT. Topical fluorides: efficacy, administration, and safety. *Gen Dent*. 1997;45(2):134-140, 142.
49. Ripa LW. An evaluation of the use of professionally (operator applied) topical fluorides. *J Dent Res*. 1990;69(Spec No): 786-796.
50. Soeno K, Matsumura H, Atsuta M, Kawasaki K. Influence of acidulated fluoride agents and effectiveness of subsequent polishing on composite material surfaces. *Oper Dent*. 2002; 27(3):305-310.
51. Poulsen S. Fluoride-containing gels, mouthrinses and varnishes: an update of evidence of efficacy. *Eur Arch Paediatr Dent*. 2009;10(3):157-161.
52. Slayton RL, Urquhart O, Araujo MWB, et al. Evidence-based clinical practice guideline on nonrestorative treatments for carious lesions: a report from the American Dental Association. *J Am Dent Assoc* 2018:149(10):837-849.
53. Beltrán-Aguilar ED, Goldstein JW, Lockwood SA. Fluoride varnishes: a review of their clinical use, cariostatic mechanism, efficacy and safety. *J Am Dent Assoc*. 2000;131(5):589-596.
54. Marinho VC, Worthington HV, Walsh T, Clarkson JE. Fluoride varnishes for preventing dental caries in children and adolescents. *Cochrane Database Syst Rev*. 2013;(7):CD002279.
55. Bawden JW. Fluoride varnish: a useful new tool for public health dentistry. *J Public Health Dent*. 1998;58(4):266-269.
56. Autio-Gold JT, Courts F. Assessing the effect of fluoride varnish on early enamel carious lesions in the primary dentition. *J Am Dent Assoc*. 2001;132(9):1247-1253.
57. Castellano JB, Donly KJ. Potential remineralization of de-mineralized enamel after application of fluoride varnish. *Am J Dent*. 2004;17(6):462-464.
58. Demito CF, Vivaldi-Rodrigues G, Ramos AL, Bowman SJ. The efficacy of fluoride varnish in reducing enamel demineralization adjacent to orthodontic brackets: an in vitro study. *Orthod Craniofac Res*. 2004;7(4):205-210.
59. Association of State and Territorial Dental Directors Fluorides Committee. *Fluoride Varnish: An Evidence-Based Approach Research Brief*. https://astdd.org/docs/fl-varnish-brief-september-2014-amended-05-2016.docx. Accessed September 20, 2022.
60. Rosenblatt A, Stamford TC, Niederman R. Silver diamine fluoride: a caries "silver-fluoride bullet." *J Dent Res*. 2009; 88(2):116-125.
61. Shen P, Bagheri R, Walker GD, et al. Effect of calcium phosphate addition to fluoride containing dental varnishes on enamel demineralization. *Aust Dent J*. 2016;61:357-365. doi:10.111/adj.12385
62. Majithia U, Venkataraghavan K, Choudary P, Trivedi K, Shah S, Virda M. Comparative evaluation of application of different fluoride varnishes on artificial early enamel lesion: an in vitro study. *Indian J Dent Res*. 2016;27:521-527.
63. Bruze M. Systemically induced contact dermatitis from rosin. *Scand J Dentv Res*. 1994;102:376-378.
64. Sharma PR. Allergic contact stomatitis from colophony. *Dent Update*. 2006;33:440-442.
65. Isaksson M, Bruze M, Bjorkner B, Niklasson B. Contact allergy to Duraphat. *Scand J Dent Res*. 1993;101:49-51.
66. Chu CH, Lo ECM. Promoting caries arrest in children with silver diamine fluoride: a review. *Oral Health Prev Dent*. 2008;6(4):315-321.
67. Horst J, Ellenikiotis H, Milgrom P. UCSF protocol for caries arrest using silver diamine fluoride: rationale, indications and consent. *J Calif Dent Assoc*. 2016;44(1):16-28.
68. Crystal, YO, Marghalani AA, Ureles SD, et al. Use of silver diamine fluoride for dental caries management in children and adolescents, including those with special health care needs. *Pediatr Dent*. 2017;39(5):E135-E145.
69. American Academy of Pediatric Dentistry. Chairside guide: Silver diamine fluoride in the management of dental caries lesions. Pediatr Dent 2018;40(6):492-3.
70. American Academy of Pediatric Dentistry. Fluoride therapy. In: *The Reference Manual of Pediatric Dentistry*. Chicago, IL: American Academy of Pediatric Dentistry; 2020:288-291.
71. Crystal YO, Niederman R. Evidence-based dentistry update on silver diamine fluoride. *Dent Clin North Am*. 2019;63(1):45-68.
72. Ripa LW. Need for prior tooth cleaning when performing a professional topical fluoride application: review and recommendations for change. *J Am Dent Assoc*. 1984;109(2):281-285.
73. Vrbic V, Brudevold F, McCann HG. Acquisition of fluoride by enamel from fluoride pumice pastes. *Helv Odontol Acta*. 1967; 11(1):21-26.
74. Shen C, Autio-Gold J. Assessing fluoride concentration uniformity and fluoride release from three varnishes. *J Am Dent Assoc*. 2002;133(2):176-182.
75. Stookey GK, Schemehorn BR, Drook CA, Cheetham BL. The effect of rinsing with water immediately after a professional fluoride gel application on fluoride uptake in demineralized enamel: an in vivo study. *Pediatr Dent*. 1986;8(3):153-157.
76. Castillo J, Rivera S, Aparicio T, et al. The short-term effects of diammine silver fluoride on tooth sensitivity: a randomized controlled trial. *J Dent Res*. 2011;90(2):203-208.
77. Englander HR, Keyes PH, Gestwicki M, Sultz HA. Clinical anticaries effect of repeated topical sodium fluoride applications by mouthpieces. *J Am Dent Assoc*. 1967;75(3):638-644.

78. Adair SM. Evidence-based use of fluoride in contemporary pediatric dental practice. *Pediatr Dent.* 2006;28(2):133-142.
79. Torell P, Ericsson Y. The potential benefits derived from fluoride mouthrinses. In: Forrester DJ, Schulz EM, eds. *International Workshop on Fluorides and Dental Caries Reductions.* Baltimore, MD: University of Maryland School of Dentistry; 1974:114-176.
80. Birkeland JM, Torell P. Caries-preventive fluoride mouth-rinses. *Caries Res.* 1978;12(suppl 1):38-51.
81. Ripa LW, Leske GS, Varma A. Effect of mouthrinsing with a 0.2 percent neutral NaF solution on the deciduous dentition of first to third grade school children. *Pediatr Dent.* 1984;6(2):93-97.
82. Driscoll WS, Swango PA, Horowitz AM, Kingman A. Caries-preventive effects of daily and weekly fluoride mouthrinsing in a fluoridated community: final results after 30 months. *J Am Dent Assoc.* 1982;105(6):1010-1013.
83. Heijnsbroek M, Paraskevas S, Vav der Weijden GA. Fluoride interventions for root caries: a review. *Oral Health Prev Dent.* 2007;5(2):145-152.
84. Stratemann MW, Shannon IL. Control of decalcification in orthodontic patients by daily self-administrated application of a water-free 0.4 percent stannous fluoride gel. *Am J Orthod.* 1974;66(3):273-279.
85. Wescott WB, Starcke EN, Shannon IL. Chemical protection against postirradiation dental caries. *Oral Surg Oral Med Oral Pathol.* 1975;40(6):709-719.
86. American Dental Association, Council on Dental Therapeutics. Evaluation of Crest toothpaste. *J Am Dent Assoc.* 1960;61:272.
87. Mariotti MJ, Burrell K. Mouthrinses and dentifrices. In: *American Dental Association, Council on Scientific Affairs: ADA/PDR Guide to Dental Therapeutics.* 5th ed. Chicago, IL: American Dental Association and Thomson PDR; 2009: 305-321.
88. American Academy of Pediatric Dentistry Liaison with Other Groups Committee; and American Academy on Pediatric Dentistry Council on Scientific Affairs. Guideline on fluoride therapy. *Pediatr Dent.* 2013;36:171-174.
89. American Dental Association Council on Scientific Affairs. Fluoride toothpaste use for young children. *J Am Dent Assoc.* 2014;145(2):190-191.
90. Sjogren K, Melin NH. The influence of rinsing routines on fluoride retention after toothbrushing. *Gerodontology.* 2001; 18(1):15-20.
91. Walsh T, Worthington HV, Glenny AM, Appelbe P, Marinho VC, Shi X. Fluoride toothpastes of different concentrations for preventing dental caries in children and adolescents. *Cochrane Database Syst Rev.* 2010;(1):CD007868.
92. Marinho VC. Cochrane reviews of randomized trials of fluoride therapies for preventing dental caries. *Eur Arch Paediatr Dent.* 2009;10(3):183-191.
93. Whitford GM. Acute and chronic fluoride toxicity. *J Dent Res.* 1992;71(5):1249-1254.

CHAPTER 35

Sealants

Jill C. Moore, EdD, MHA, BSDH, RDH

CHAPTER OUTLINE

LEARNING OBJECTIVES

After studying this chapter, the student will be able to:

1. Describe the development and purposes of dental sealant materials.
2. Explain the types of sealant materials and list the criteria of an ideal dental sealant material.
3. List indications and contraindications for placement of dental sealants.
4. Describe the clinical procedures for placement and maintenance of a dental sealant.
5. Explain the factors that affect sealant penetration.
6. Identify factors to document a dental sealant placement in the patient record.

Introduction

A pit and fissure **sealant** is an organic **polymer** (resin) that flows into the pit or fissure of a posterior tooth and bonds by mechanical retention to the tooth.

- Placement of dental sealants is an evidence-based preventive recommendation that can significantly reduce the incidence of dental caries.[1]
- As part of a complete preventive program, pit and fissure sealants are indicated for selected patients.
- Topically applied fluorides protect smooth tooth surfaces more than occlusal surfaces; dental sealants reduce the incidence of occlusal dental caries.
- The incidence of new pit and fissure caries can be lowered by 86% if the sealant is retained at 1 year, 78.6% at 2 years, and 58.6% at 4 years.[2]
- Sealant application is a part of a complete prevention program, not an isolated procedure.
- As an isolated procedure, the patient (and parent) may misunderstand the specific role of sealants in prevention.
- Other surfaces and other teeth still need other methods of preventive protection.

I. Development of Sealants

Sealants were developed by Dr. Michael Buonocore and a group of dental scientists at the Eastman Dental Center in Rochester, New York.[3]

- Early research focused on the need to prepare the enamel surface so a dental material would adhere.
- They demonstrated that, by using an **acid-etchant** process, the enamel could be altered to increase retention.
- The research proved to be a major breakthrough, particularly in esthetic and preventive dentistry.[3,4]

II. Purposes of the Sealant

- Provides a physical barrier to "seal off" the pit or fissure.
- Prevents oral bacteria and their nutrients from collecting within the pit or fissure to create the acid environment necessary for the initiation of dental caries.
- Fills the pit or fissure as deep as possible and provide tight smooth margins at the junction with the enamel surface.[5,6]
- Provides continued protection in the depth of the micropore even when the sealant material is worn or cracked away on the surface around the pit or fissure, and new sealant material can be added for repair and to reseal the enamel/sealant junction.[5]

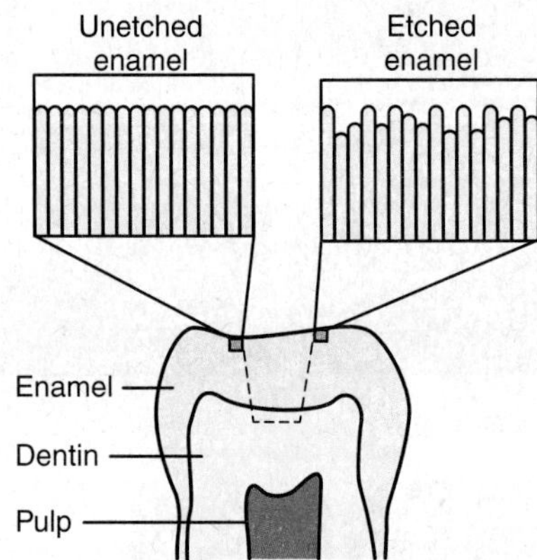

Figure 35-1 Dental Sealant Adhesion.

III. Purposes of the Acid Etch

- To produce irregularities or **micropores** in the enamel.
- To allow the liquid resin to penetrate into the micropores and create a bond or mechanical locking.
- **Figure 35-1** demonstrates the microscopic change of the enamel before and after acid etch is placed.

Sealant Materials

The variety of available sealant materials provides options for both the patient and clinician. The clinician decides which material will be most beneficial depending on:

- An assessment of patient needs and caries risk.
- Sealant placement environment.
- Available supplies.

I. Criteria for the Ideal Sealant[3]

- Achieve prolonged **bonding** to the enamel.
- Be biocompatible with oral tissues.
- Offer a simple application procedure.
- Be a free-flowing, low-**viscosity** material capable of entering narrow fissures.
- Have low solubility in the oral environment.

II. Classification of Sealant Materials

- A majority of sealants in clinical use are made of **Bis-GMA** (bisphenol A–glycidyl methylacrylate).[5] The techniques of application vary slightly among available products; follow manufacturer's directions.
- There is no difference in the preventive effect of resin-based or glass-ionomer cement. Resin-based

application will generate aerosols and glass-ionomer cement can be placed without generating aerosols.[7] Follow updated Centers for Disease Control and Prevention guidance specific to aerosol generating procedures (AGPs). See Chapter 6 for more on AGPs.

A. Classification by the Method of Polymerization

- Self-cured or **autopolymerized**
  - Preparation: material supplied in two parts. When the two are mixed, they quickly polymerize (harden).
  - Advantage: no **curing** light required.
  - Disadvantages: mixing required; working time limited because **polymerization** begins when the material is mixed.
- Visible light-cured or **photopolymerized**
  - Preparation: material hardens when exposed to a special curing light.
  - Advantages: no mixing required; increased working time due to control over start of polymerization.
  - Disadvantages: extra costs and disinfection time required for curing light, protective shields, and/or glasses.

B. Classification by Filler Content

- Filled
  - Purpose of filler: to increase **bond strength** and resistance to abrasion and wear.
  - Fillers: glass and quartz particles give hardness and strength to resist occlusal forces.
  - Effect: viscosity of the sealant is increased. Flow into the depth of a fissure varies.
- Unfilled
  - Clear, does not contain particles.
  - Less resistant to abrasion and wear.
  - May not require occlusal adjustment after placement, so provides an advantage for school and community health programs where sealants are placed.
- Fluoride releasing
- Purpose: to enhance caries resistance.
- Action: remineralization of **incipient caries** at the base of the pit or fissure.

C. Classification by Color

- Available: clear, tinted, and opaque.
- Purpose: quick identification for evaluation during maintenance assessment.
- Effect: clear, tinted, or opaque sealants do not differ in retention.

Indications for Sealant Placement

Individual patient benefit will depend on the following:

- Health, diet, and lifestyle.
- Age of tooth and past caries experience.
- Tooth anatomy.

I. Patients at Risk for Dental Caries (Any Age)

The following risk factors will lead to an increased risk of dental caries:

- Xerostomia: from medications or other reasons.
- Patient undergoing orthodontic treatment.
- Incipient pit and fissure caries (limited to the enamel) with no radiographic evidence of caries on an adjacent proximal surface.
- Low socioeconomic status.
- Diet high in sugars.
- Inadequate daily oral health care.

II. Selection of Teeth

- Newly erupted: place sealant as soon as the tooth is fully erupted.[8]
- Occlusal contour: when pit or fissure is deep and irregular, as illustrated in **Figure 35-2**.

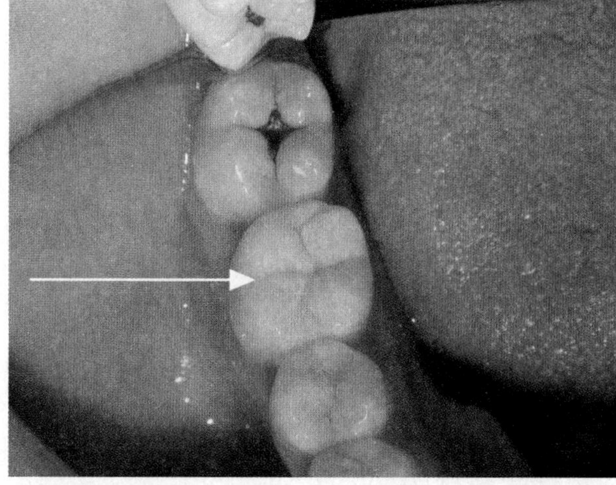

Figure 35-2 Molar Tooth with Pits and Fissures. Tooth #30 with deep fissures is selected for placing a dental sealant. Note the amalgam filling on tooth #31, which is evidence of previous dental caries experience.

Photograph courtesy of Jill Moore, EdD, MHA, BSDH, RDH, School Oral Health Consultant, Michigan Department of Health and Human Services.

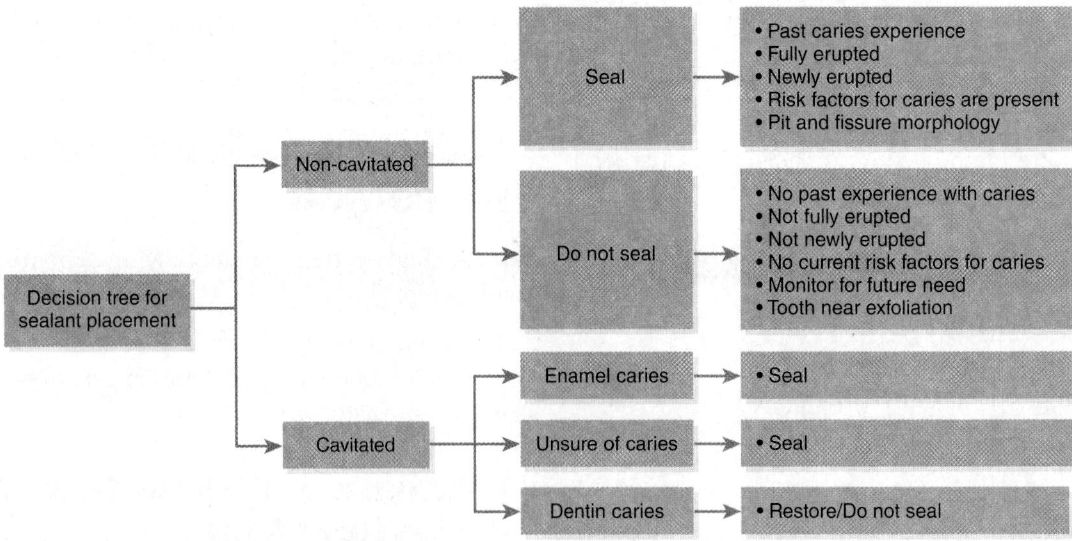

Figure 35-3 Decision Tree for Sealant Placement. Flowchart to assist in decision making for placement of sealants.

Developed by Jill C. Moore, EdD, MHA, BSDH, RDH.

- Caries history: other teeth restored or have carious lesions.
- **Figure 35-3** is a flowchart to assist in decision making.

III. Contraindications for Sealant Placement

- Radiographic evidence of adjacent proximal dental caries.
- Pit and fissures are well coalesced and self-cleansing; low caries risk.
- Tooth not completely erupted.
- Primary tooth near exfoliation.

Penetration of Sealant

Penetration of sealant material to the depth of the fissure depends on the following:

- Configuration of the pit or fissure.
- Presence of deposits and debris within the pit or fissure.
- Properties of the sealant itself.

I. Pit and Fissure Anatomy

The shape and depth of pits and fissures vary considerably even within one tooth. (**Figure 33-4A**) Anatomic differences include:

- Wide V-shaped (**Figure 35-4B**) or narrow V-shaped fissures.
- Long narrow pits and grooves reach, or nearly reach, the dentinoenamel junction (**Figure 35-4C**).
- Long constricted fissures with a bulbous terminal portion (**Figure 35-4D**) that may take a wavy course, which may not lead directly from the outer surface to the dentinoenamel junction.

II. Contents of a Pit or Fissure

A pit or fissure may contain the following:

- Dental biofilm, pellicle, debris.
- Rarely but possibly intact remnants of tooth development.

III. Effect of Cleaning

- Cleaning the tooth prior to acid etching can increase sealant retention.
- Use of an air polisher or laser prior to acid etching is not well supported by the literature, mainly because of added cost.[9]
- Cleaning the tooth with a toothbrush and water is ideal because the narrow, long fissures are difficult to clean completely.[10]
- Removal of pumice used for cleaning and thorough washing are necessary for retention of the sealant.
- Cleaning the tooth with pumice prior to dental sealant placement is avoided; if used, complete removal of pumice is necessary.
- Retained cleaning material can block the sealant from filling the fissure and can also get mixed with the sealant.

IV. Amount of Penetration

- Wide V-shaped and shallow fissures are more apt to be filled by sealants (Figure 35-4B).

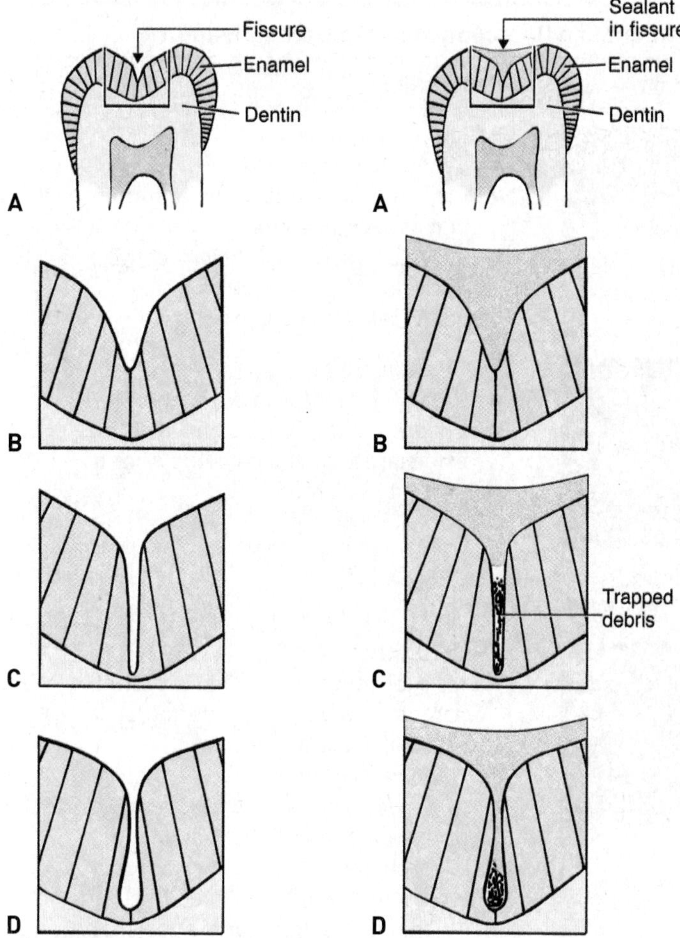

Figure 35-4 Occlusal Fissures. Drawings made from microscopic slides show variations in the shape and depth of fissures both before and after sealant placement. **A:** Tooth with section enlarged for (B–D). **B:** Wide V-shaped fissure shows full sealant penetration. **C:** Long narrow groove that nearly reaches the dentinoenamel junction. **D:** Long constricted form with a bulbous terminal portion.

- Although ideally the sealant penetrates to the bottom of a pit or fissure, such penetration is frequently impossible.
- Microscopic examination of pits and fissures after sealant application has shown the sealant material often does not penetrate to the bottom because residual debris, cleaning agents, and trapped air prevent passage of the material (Figure 35-4C–D).
- The bacteria in incipient dental caries at the base of a well-sealed pit or fissure have no access to nutrients required for survival.

Clinical Procedures

To achieve high dental sealant retention rates:

- Treat each quadrant separately while placing sealants on all eligible teeth.
- Use the four-handed method with an assistant:
  - To ensure moisture control.
  - To work efficiently and save time.
- Follow manufacturer's directions for each product.
- Success of treatment (retention) depends on the precision in each step of the application.
- Retention of sealant depends on maintaining a dry field during etching and sealant placement.
- Step-by-step clinical procedures and equipment/supplies needed for the placement of a dental sealant are illustrated in **Table 35-1**. Additional details for each step are provided in Sections I through IX.

I. Patient Preparation

- Explain the procedure and steps to be performed.
- Provide patient with ultraviolet (UV)-protective safety eyewear for protection from:

Table 35-1 Steps for Placement of a Photopolymerized Dental Sealant

Step	Illustration	Description	Equipment and Supplies
Step 1	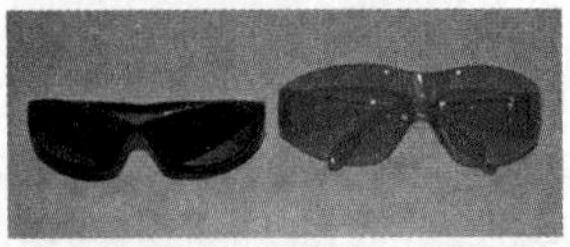 Courtesy of Jill Moore, RDH, BSDH, MHA, EdD, School Oral Health Consultant, Michigan Department of Health and Human Services.	Patient preparation ■ Seat patient comfortably. ■ Provide patient education materials and answer questions. ■ Provide ultraviolet (UV)-protective eyewear for protection from chemicals and curing light.	■ Patient education materials ■ Safety glasses for patient
Step 2	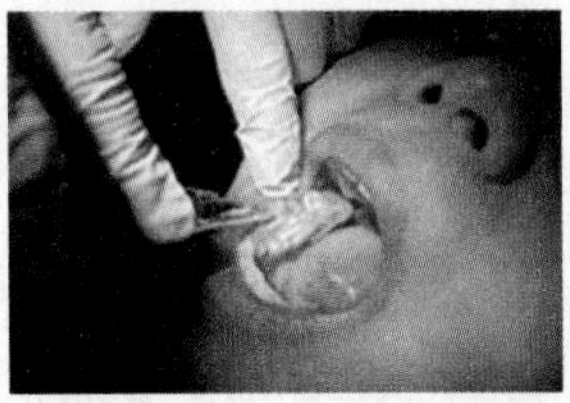 Courtesy of Susan J. Jenkins, RDH, MS, CAGS, Forsyth School of Dental Hygiene, MCPHS University.	Tooth preparation ■ Clean the tooth with a toothbrush. ■ Ensure the tooth is free from debris, external stain, and calculus prior to sealant placement.	■ Toothbrush ■ Examination instruments (mirror and explorer)
Step 3	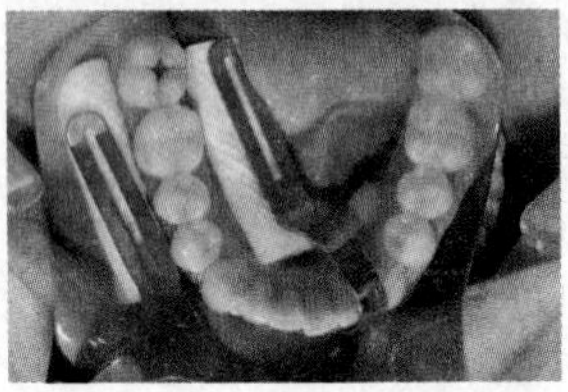 Courtesy of Jill Moore, RDH, BSDH, MHA, EdD, School Oral Health Consultant, Michigan Department of Health and Human Services. 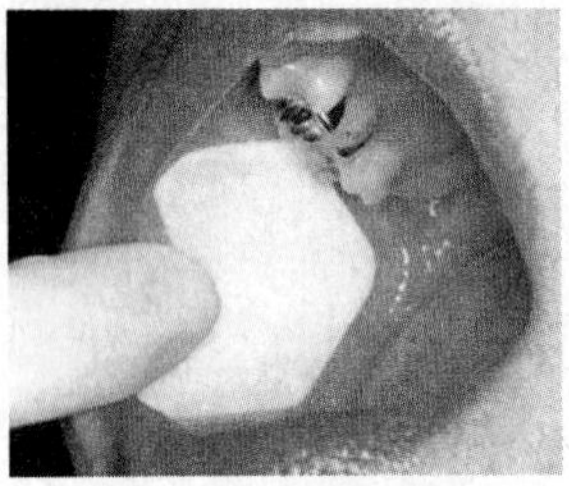 Courtesy of Jill Moore, RDH, BSDH, MHA, EdD, School Oral Health Consultant, Michigan Department of Health and Human Services.	Tooth isolation ■ Maintain a working field that is not contaminated by saliva during all steps of sealant placement. ■ Options include: • Rubber dam (not shown) • Cotton rolls on the mandibular arch (top left) • Triangular bibulous pad to cover the parotid duct for the maxillary arch (lower left) • Commercial isolation system with light and high speed suction (**Figure 35-5A**) • Note: Take care to moisten all cotton prior to removal to avoid sticking to dry mucosa.	■ Rubber dam set up (optional) ■ Cotton rolls and holders (**Figure 35-5B**) ■ Bibulous pads (lower left)
Step 4	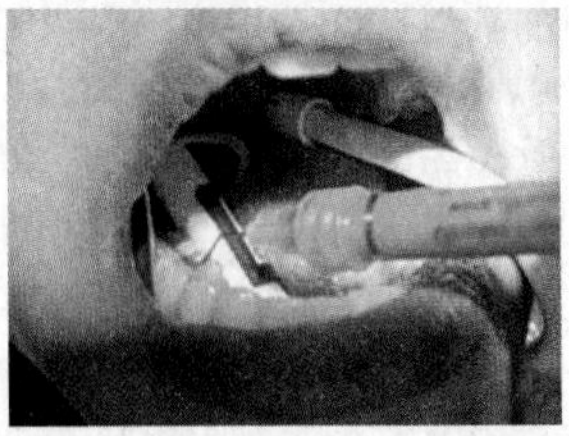 Courtesy of Susan J. Jenkins, RDH, MS, CAGS, Forsyth School of Dental Hygiene, MCPHS University. 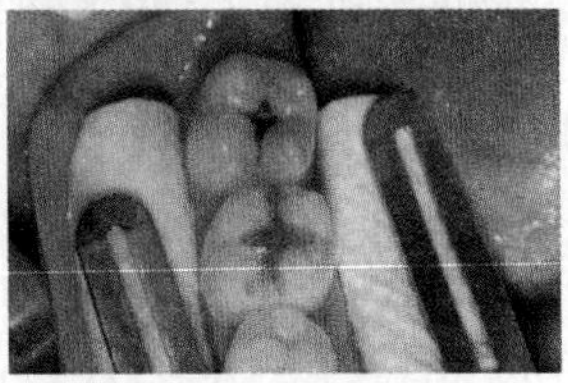 Courtesy of Jill Moore, RDH, BSDH, MHA, EdD, School Oral Health Consultant, Michigan Department of Health and Human Services.	Acid etch ■ Dry entire area for 20–30 sec with air/water syringe. ■ Maintain a dry field. Use a commercial etchant applicator (shown), brush, or cotton pellet to dispense etchant material. ■ Place the acid etch only within the grooves and fissures where the sealant will be placed (shown at lower left). ■ Note: Follow manufacturer's directions for application time; usually between 15 and 60 sec.	■ Air/water syringe ■ Acid-etch material and applicator, brush, or cotton pellet

Step	Illustration	Description	Equipment and Supplies
Step 5	Courtesy of Jill Moore, RDH, BSDH, MHA, EdD, School Oral Health Consultant, Michigan Department of Health and Human Services.	Rinse and air dry tooth ■ Place the high-velocity evacuation system over the tooth. ■ Rinse the tooth with the air/water syringe. ■ Spray water until the surface is free of etch (30–60 sec). ■ Spray air with an air/water syringe until dry. ■ Re-isolate if necessary.	■ High-velocity evacuation system ■ Air/water syringe
Step 6	Courtesy of Jill Moore, RDH, BSDH, MHA, EdD, School Oral Health Consultant, Michigan Department of Health and Human Services.	Evaluate for complete etching ■ A completely etched tooth will have a chalky-white appearance when dry. ■ If the surface does not appear chalky, repeat the acid-etch step.	■ Air/water syringe ■ Mouth mirror for retraction and indirect vision
Step 7	Courtesy of Susan J. Jenkins, RDH, MS, CAGS, Forsyth School of Dental Hygiene, MCPHS University.	Place sealant material ■ Continue to maintain a dry field. ■ Use external fulcrum (fingers resting lightly on patient's chin or cheek). ■ Place the wet sealant material in the prepared pits and fissures. ■ Adjust flow so sealant material is deposited only within the grooves, pits, and fissures.	■ Sealant material and applicator ■ Slow-speed saliva ejector to help maintain dry field
Step 8	Courtesy of Susan J. Jenkins, RDH, MS, CAGS, Forsyth School of Dental Hygiene, MCPHS University.	Cure sealant If using light-polymerized sealant material: ■ Ensure clinician and patient have UV-protective eye protection. ■ Cover entire tooth with light and cure for 20–30 sec in accordance with manufacturer's instructions. If using self-curing sealant material: ■ Maintain dry field and allow drying time as indicated in manufacturer's instructions.	■ UV-protective goggles/glasses for patient and clinicians ■ Curing light ■ Saliva ejector to help maintain dry field
Step 9	Courtesy of Jill Moore, RDH, BSDH, MHA, EdD, School Oral Health Consultant, Michigan Department of Health and Human Services.	Final/cured sealant ■ Gently check for voids in the sealant material with explorer. ■ Additional material can be added if the surface is not contaminated or wet.	■ Mirror and explorer ■ Saliva ejector to help maintain dry field ■ Additional sealant material, if needed, to fill voids

(continues)

Table 35-1 Steps for Placement of a Photopolymerized Dental Sealant *(continued)*

Step	Illustration	Description	Equipment and Supplies
Step 10	Courtesy of Susan J. Jenkins, RDH, MS, CAGS, Forsyth School of Dental Hygiene, MCPHS University	Check occlusion ■ Use articulating paper to locate high spots and adjust as needed. ■ Unfilled sealant material will wear down via normal attrition. ■ Filled sealant material will require occlusal adjustment.	■ Articulating paper ■ Holder
Step 11	Seal Out TOOTH DECAY A BOOKLET FOR PARENTS Courtesy of National Institute of Dental and Craniofacial Research. https://www.nidcr.nih.gov/sites/default/files/2017-11/seal-out-tooth-decay-parents.pdf.	Follow-up ■ Provide patient education materials for the patient to take home. ■ Answer patient's questions. ■ Re-evaluate sealants at each subsequent maintenance appointment.	■ Excellent patient education materials are available for free from the National Institute of Dental and Craniofacial Research website (www.nidcr.nih.gov/orderpublications/).

Photographs in Steps 2, 4A, 7, 8, and 10 courtesy of Susan J. Jenkins, RDH, PhD, Forsyth School of Dental Hygiene, MCPHS University. Photograph in Step 11 courtesy of National Institute of Dental and Craniofacial Research. https://www.nidcr.nih.gov/sites/default/files/2017-11/seal-out-tooth-decay-parents.pdf. Additional photographs courtesy of Jill Moore, EdD, MHA, BSDH, RDH, School Oral Health Consultant, Michigan Department of Health and Human Services.

- Chemicals used during etching and sealant placement.
- The UV light from the curing lamp.

II. Tooth Preparation

A. Purposes

- Remove deposits and debris.
- Permit maximum contact of the etch and the sealant with the enamel surface.
- Encourage sealant penetration into the pit or fissure.

B. Methods

- Examine the tooth surfaces: remove calculus and stain.
- For a patient with no stain or calculus, apply toothbrush filaments straight into occlusal pits and fissures.
- Suction the pits and fissures with a high-velocity evacuator.
- Gently use the explorer tip to remove debris and bacteria from the pit or fissure and suction again to remove loosened material.
- Evaluate the need for additional cleaning; brushing may be sufficient.

III. Tooth Isolation

A. Purposes of Isolation

- Maintaining a dry tooth is the single most important factor in sealant retention.
- Keep the tooth clean and dry for optimal action and bonding of the sealant.
- Eliminate possible contamination by saliva and moisture from the breath.
- Keep the materials from contacting the oral tissues, being swallowed accidentally, or being unpleasant to the patient because of their flavor.

B. Rubber Dam Isolation

- Rubber dam application is the method of choice for complete isolation. This method is especially helpful when more than one tooth in the same quadrant is to be sealed.
- Rubber dam is essential when profuse saliva flow and overactive tongue and oral muscles make retraction and consistent maintenance of a dry, clean field impossible.
- When a quadrant has a rubber dam and anesthesia for restoration of other teeth, teeth indicated for sealant can be treated at the same time.

- Use local anesthesia when application of the clamp cannot be tolerated by the patient.
- Rubber dam may not be possible when a tooth needed to hold the clamp is not fully erupted.

C. Cotton-Roll Isolation

- Patient position: tilt the head to allow saliva to pool on the opposite side of the mouth.
- Position cotton-roll holder. **Figure 35-5A** shows the placement of two types of cotton-roll holders.
- Place a saliva ejector.
- Apply triangular saliva absorber (**bibulous pad**) over the opening of the parotid duct in the cheek.
- Take care to prevent saliva contamination from entering the area to be etched.

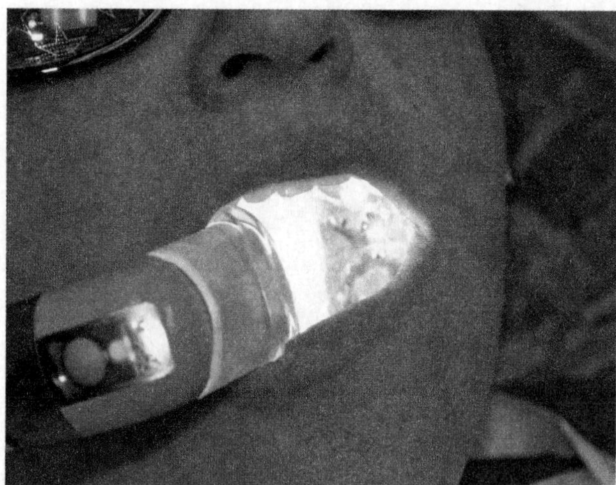

A

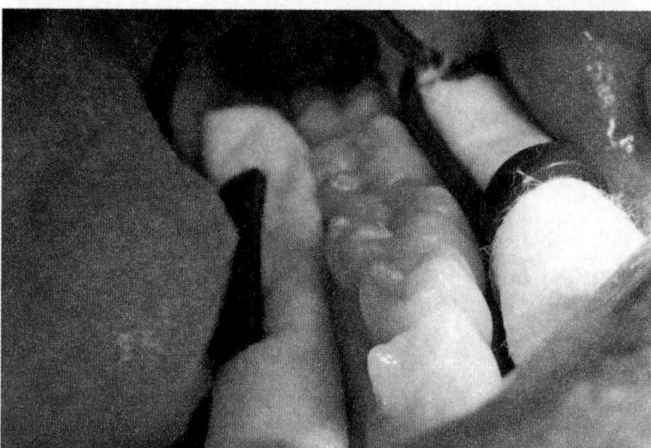

B

Figure 35-5 Tooth Isolation. **A:** Demonstrates a commercial isolation system which has an internal light and high evacuation suction. This system will allow for two-handed sealant placement. **B:** Illustrates a disposable plastic cotton roll holder used to isolate teeth in a mandibular quadrant.

Photographs courtesy of Jill Moore, EdD, MHA, BSDH, RDH, School Oral Health Consultant, Michigan Department of Health and Human Services.

D. Additional Isolation Options

- Commercially available isolation systems (**Figure 35-5B**) that can be attached to the dental unit offer intraoral quadrant isolation, illumination, and suction.

IV. Acid Etch

A. Dry the Tooth

- Purposes
  - Prepare the tooth for acid etch.
  - Eliminate moisture and contamination.
- Use clean, dry air
  - Clear water from the air/water syringe by releasing the spray into a sink.
  - Test for absence of moisture by blowing on a mouth mirror or other dry surface.
- Air dry the tooth for at least 10 seconds.

B. Apply Etchant

- Action
  - Creates micropores to increase the surface area and provide retention for the sealant.
  - Removes contamination from the enamel surface.
  - Provides antibacterial action.
- Etchant solution forms
  - Phosphoric acid: 15% to 50%, depends on the product and manufacturer.
  - Liquid: low viscosity allows good flow into the pit or fissure but may be difficult to control.
  - Gel: tinted gel with thick consistency allows increased visibility and control but may be difficult to rinse off the tooth surface.
  - Semi-gel: tinted, with enough viscosity to allow good visibility, control, and rinsing ease.
- Etchant timing varies from 15 to 60 seconds. Follow manufacturer's instructions for each product.
- Etchant delivery
  - Liquid etch: use a small brush, sponge, or cotton pellet; continuously pat rather than rub, when applying to keep the surface moist.
  - Gel and semi-gel: use a syringe, brush, or manufacturer-supplied single-use cannula.

V. Rinse and Air Dry Tooth

- Rinse thoroughly; apply continuous suction to prevent saliva from reaching the etched surface.
- Dry for 15–20 seconds and maintain a dry field through isolation.

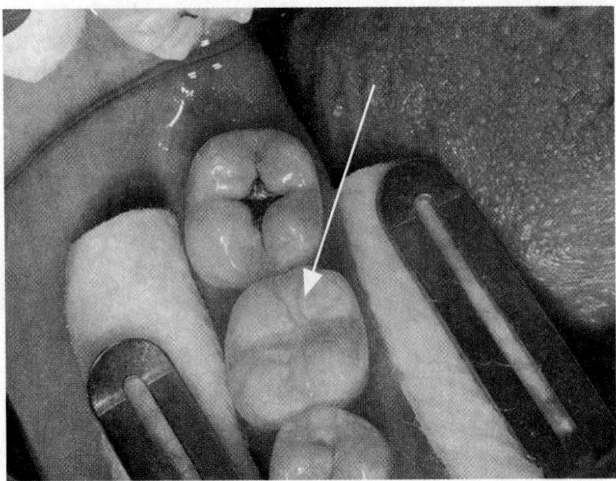

Figure 35-6 Placement of Dental Sealant Material. Appropriate placement of a dental sealant will completely fill pits and fissures, but not compromise occlusion by overfilling to a high, flat surface.

Photograph courtesy of Jill Moore, EdD, MHA, BSDH, RDH, School Oral Health Consultant, Michigan Department of Health and Human Services.

VI. Evaluate for Complete Etching

- Dry and examine the etched surface.
- Repeat etching process if the surface does not appear chalky white.

VII. Place Sealant Material

Follow manufacturer's instructions included in the sealant material package. General instructions include:

- Avoid overmanipulation of sealant materials to prevent producing air bubbles.
- Use the disposable implement supplied in the sealant material package for application.
- Flow minimal amount into all pits and fissures; do not overfill to a high, flat surface.
- **Figure 35-6** illustrates a correctly filled dental sealant surface.

VIII. Cure Sealant

- If using a light-cured sealant material:
  - Leave the liquid sealant material in place for 10 seconds to allow for optimum penetration.
  - Use UV-blocking eye protection for both the clinician and patient.
  - Apply the curing light for 20–30 seconds in accordance with the manufacturer's instructions. Cover the entire tooth surface with the light to ensure complete polymerization.
- If using an autopolymerized sealant material, consult the manufacturer's instructions for curing time.

IX. Evaluate Cured Sealant

- Check for voids gently with explorer: additional sealant material can be added if the surface is not contaminated or wet.

X. Check Occlusion

- Use **articulating paper** to locate high spots; adjust as required.
- Occlusal wear: unfilled sealants wear down via normal attrition to the correct height; **filled sealants** require occlusal adjustment.

XI. Follow-Up

- Educate the patient.
- Administer fluoride treatment.
- Re-evaluate at each subsequent appointment.

Maintenance

Dental sealants need to be in place to prevent caries, and should be checked for the following[11]:

- Retention.
- Need for replacement when sealant is missing or partially retained.

I. Retention

- At each continuing care appointment, or at least every 6 months, each sealant needs to be examined for retention and to identify deficiencies that may have developed.
- Properly placed dental sealants can be retained for many years.[1,2]

II. Factors Affecting Retention

- During placement: precision of technique with exclusion of moisture and contamination.
- Patient self-care: advise patient to avoid biting or chewing on hard surfaces such as a pencil or ice cubes.
- Dental hygiene care: avoid using an air-powder polisher on intact sealants during maintenance appointments.[12]

III. Replacement

- Consult the manufacturer's instructions.
- Tooth preparation: same as for original application.
- Removal of firmly attached sections of retained sealant is not usually necessary.
- Re-etching of the tooth surface prior to replacement of a dental sealant is always essential.

School-Based Dental Sealant Programs

- Healthy People 2030 Objectives call for an increase in children and adolescents who have received dental sealants.
- Many states in the United States are not meeting national goals for delivering dental sealants to low-income children.[13]
- Delivery of dental sealants in school-based settings is a proven strategy[13,14] that can:
  - Effectively increase the percentage of children in communities who receive dental sealants.
  - Reduce the risk for decay for high-risk children.
- Many such school-based programs provide additional preventive services such as screening, prophylaxis, topical fluoride application, and oral health education.[11]
- Programs that provide sealants are an effective adjunct to preventive care provided in traditional dental care settings.[1,2]
- **Figure 35-7** shows a portable dental unit set up in a classroom in a public school The tent is incorporated to assist in controlling aerosols and spatter in a public setting.

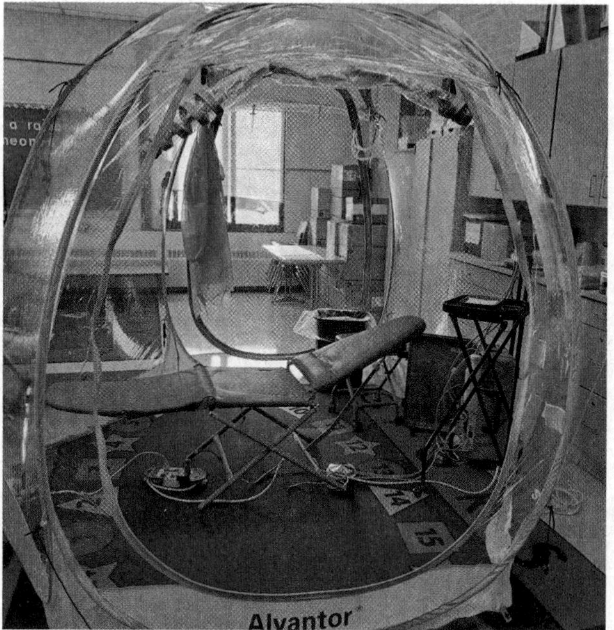

Figure 35-7 Delivery of Dental Sealants in a School-Based Program Using Portable Dental Equipment Set Up in the School Library.

Photograph courtesy of Jill Moore, EdD, MHA, BSDH, RDH , School Oral Health Consultant, Michigan Department of Health and Human Services.

Documentation

Documentation in the record of a patient receiving a sealant contains a minimum of the following:

- Reason for selection of certain teeth for sealants; informed consent of patient, parent, or other caregiver.
- Type of sealant used, preparation of tooth, manner of isolation, patient cooperation during administration; postinsertion instructions given.
- Sample documentation for placement of dental sealants may be reviewed in **Box 35-1**.

Box 35-1 Example Documentation: Placement of Dental Sealants

- **S**—A 12-year-old male patient presents for dental sealant placement.
- **O**—Occlusal contour and previous history of dental caries in primary dentition indicate need for sealant placement for second molars; X-rays indicate no dental caries on proximal surfaces of second molars. Tooth #30 partially erupted with operculum.
- **A**—Need to wait until #30 is completely erupted to place sealant.
- **P**—Reviewed sealant education materials with mother and patient. Mother provided consent for placement of the recommended sealants. Sealants placed on #3-O, 14-O, 14-L, 19-O, 19-B pit using right-side, then left-side isolation. Autopolymerized opaque sealant material used with 15% acid etch, applied as per manufacturer's directions. Patient tolerated treatment well, no gagging, minimal saliva, easy isolation.

Next steps: Schedule in 1 month to re-examine for sealant placement on #30 and retention check on 3, 14, and 19.

Signed: ______________________________, RDH

Date: ______________________________

Factors to Teach the Patient

- Sealants are part of a total preventive program. They are not substitutes for other preventive measures. Limitations of dietary sucrose, refined carbohydrate intake, use of fluorides, and dental biofilm control are major factors along with sealants for prevention of dental caries.
- What a sealant is and why such a meticulous application procedure is required.
- What can be expected from a sealant; how long it may last and how it prevents dental caries.
- Need for examination of the sealant at frequent, scheduled maintenance appointments, and need for replacement when missing or chipped.
- Avoid biting hard items such as a pencil, hard candy, or ice cubes to increase sealant retention.

References

1. Ahovuo-Saloranta A, Forss H, Walsh T, et al. Sealants for preventing dental decay in the permanent teeth. *Cochrane Database Syst Rev*. 2013;(3):CD001830.
2. Beauchamp J, Caufiel PW, Crall JJ, et al. Evidence-based clinical recommendations for the use of pit-and-fissure sealants: a report of the American Dental Association Council on Scientific Affairs. *J Am Dent Assoc*. 2008;139(3):257-268.
3. Handleman SL, Shey Z. Michael Buonocore and the Eastman Dental Center: a historic perspective on sealants. *J Dent Res*. 1996;75(1):529-534.
4. Cueto EI, Buonocore MG. Sealing of pits and fissures with an adhesive resin: its use in caries prevention. *J Am Dent Assoc*. 1967;75(1):121-128.
5. Wright JT, Tampi MP, Graham L, et al. Sealants for preventing and arresting pit-and-fissure occlusal caries in primary and permanent molars. *J Am Dent Assoc*. 2016;147(8):631-645.
6. Wright JT, Crall JJ, Fontana M, et al. Evidence-based clinical practice guideline for the use of pit-and-fissure sealants. A report of the American Dental Association and the American Academy of Pediatric Dentistry. *J Am Dent Assoc*. 2016;147(8):672-682.
7. Eden E, Frencken J, Gao S, Horst JA, Innes N. Managing dental caries against the backdrop of COVID-19: approaches to reduce aerosol generation. *Br Dent J*. 2020;229(7):411-416.
8. Jaafar N, Ragab H, Abedrahman A, Osman E. Performance of fissure sealants on fully erupted permanent molars with incipient carious lesions: a glass-ionomer-based versus a resin-based sealant. *J Dent Res Dent Clin Dent Prospects*. 2020;14(1):61-67.
9. Bagherian A, Sarraf Shirazi A. Preparation before acid etching in fissure sealant therapy: yes or no?: a systemic review and meta-analysis. *J Am Dent Assoc*. 2016;147(12):943-951.
10. Deery C. Brushing as good as handpiece prophylaxis before placing sealants. *Evid Based Dent*. 2010;11:79-80.
11. Sreedevi A, Brizuela M, Mohamed S. Pit and fissure sealants. *StatPearls*; 2021. https://www.ncbi.nlm.nih.gov/books/NBK448116/. Accessed October 3, 2022.
12. Pelka MA, Altmaier K, Petschelt A, Lohbauer U. The effect of air-polishing abrasives on wear of direct restoration materials and sealants. *J Am Dent Assoc*. 2010;141(1):63-70.
13. PEW Center on the States. *States Stalled on Dental Sealant Programs: A 50-State Report*. Washington, DC: The PEW Charitable Trusts; 2015. http://www.pewtrusts.org/~/media/assets/2015/04/dental_sealantreport_final.pdf. Accessed September 9, 2021.
14. Children's Dental Health Project. *Dental Sealants: Proven to Prevent Decay*. Washington, DC: Children's Dental Health Project; 2014:21. https://www.cdhp.org/resources/314-dental-sealants-proven-to-prevent-tooth-decay. Accessed September 9, 2021.

SECTION VII

Implementation: Treatment

Introduction for Section VII

The first objective of dental hygiene treatment is to create an environment in which the oral tissues can return to health.

In the sequence of patient care, introduction to preventive measures occurs first to help ensure the success of dental hygiene treatment. Professional treatment interventions make a limited contribution to arresting the progression of disease without daily biofilm control measures performed by the patient. Dental hygiene treatment interventions include:

- Anxiety and pain control.
- Instrumentation for scaling and subgingival debridement.
- Extrinsic stain removal.
- Care of dental restorations.
- Posttreatment care procedures.
- Placement and removal of dressings.
- Removal of sutures.
- Treatment of hypersensitive teeth.
- Immediate evaluation, short-term follow-up, and maintenance assessment of treatment outcomes.

The Dental Hygiene Process of Care

- Dental hygiene treatment uses nonsurgical periodontal therapy combined with preventive care as a part of the dental hygiene process of care (**Figure VII-1**).
- Dental hygiene care can comprise the total treatment needed for certain patients with uncomplicated disease or the initial nonsurgical phase of treatment for others with more advanced disease.
- General objectives of dental hygiene instrumentation are as follows:
  - Create an environment in which the tissues can return to health and be maintained.
  - Aid in the prevention and control of gingival and periodontal infections by removal of periodontal pathogenic microorganisms and factors that predispose to the retention of dental biofilm.
  - Prepare the teeth and gingiva for dental procedures, including those performed by the restorative dentist, prosthodontist, orthodontist, pedodontist, and oral surgeon.
  - Improve oral esthetics and biofilm control of the oral cavity.

Ethical Applications

- The professional dental hygienist acknowledges the ethical implications of all aspects of providing patient care.
- Many ethical facets of dental hygiene care can:
  - Relate directly to the provider–patient, intraprofessional, or interprofessional relationships.
  - Affect the overall delivery of dental services.
- Practicing a consistent and professional demeanor with all patients and all members of the patient

care team can be achieved and will uphold high standards and quality of care.

- The conduct of the professional dental hygienist prior to, during, and following the dental hygiene appointment is subject to moral assessment.
- Several ethical and professional issues to be considered are listed in **Table VII-1**.

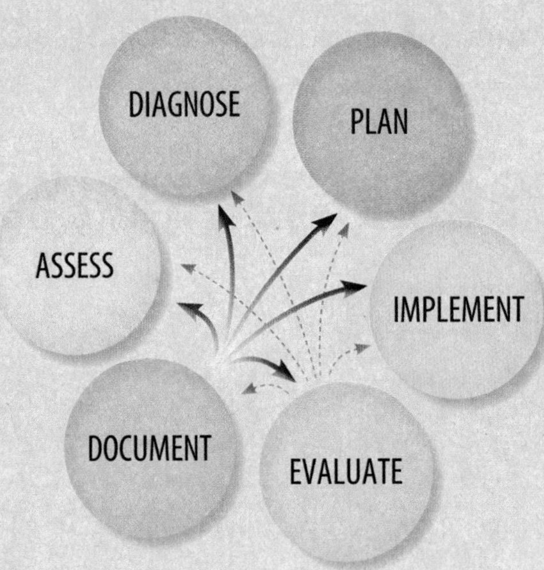

Figure VII-1 The Dental Hygiene Process of Care

Table VII-1 Ethical and Professional Issues

Professional Issues	Explanation	Application Examples
Expressed or implied contracts	A written (third-party payment) or oral agreement (between provider and patient) for specific services or a course of treatment.	Coding of dental hygiene services based on current edition of Current Dental Terminology guidelines.
Whistle-blowing	The disclosure of illegal or immoral wrongs committed by an individual practitioner. May involve negligent acts.	■ Reporting the lack of infection control procedures. ■ Reporting the actions of an impaired colleague to a state dental board.
Privacy rights	Involves the handling of health information through protection of privacy, insurance access, preventing fraud and abuse, and standardization within the healthcare industry.	Health Insurance Portability and Accountability Act (HIPAA): seeks to protect the confidentiality of dental records, especially where computers are used to document patient data.
Supervision	The ethical and legal working relationship among the dentist, dental hygienist, and other healthcare providers.	A dental hygienist in a collaborative practice treating patients who reside in a nursing home.

CHAPTER 36

Anxiety and Pain Control

Debra November-Rider, RDH, MSDH

CHAPTER OUTLINE

LEARNING OBJECTIVES

After studying this chapter, the student will be able to:

1. Describe the components of pain.
2. Summarize the advantages and disadvantages of nitrous oxide–oxygen administration.
3. Define titration and explain application during nitrous oxide–oxygen sedation.
4. List the local anesthetics of short, intermediate, and long duration and indications for use.
5. Give examples of absolute and relative contraindications for local anesthetic administration.
6. Identify items in the local anesthesia armamentarium and describe the purpose of each.
7. Summarize local and systemic complications from the administration of local anesthesia and how to manage them.
8. List the components of a complete patient record entry following the administration of local anesthesia or nitrous oxide–oxygen sedation.

According to the 2020 Oral Health in America: Advances and Challenges, 20% of Americans have moderate to high dental anxiety/fear about visiting the dental office.[1] More recent systematic reviews and meta-analyses reported about 15% of U.S. adults and children have some level of dental anxiety.[2,3] Of these, approximately 3% have severe dental fear/anxiety.[3]

- There are many contributing causes, one of which is the association of pain with dental procedures. Ranking of negative dental stimuli ranges from the sight of the needle (54.1%), use of scaler/curette (56%), having a dental x-ray (61.4%), and getting an injection (68.1%).[4]
- Concern for patient anxiety and pain is an integral part of a dental hygiene appointment.
- Recognizing and managing a patient's anxiety and pain is an essential part of dental hygiene care planning.
- The decision to use a pharmacologic agent for management of anxiety and pain is dependent on a number of factors including the following:
  - Periodontal health status.
  - The treatment being rendered.
  - Patient's **pain threshold**.

Components of Pain

I. Pain Perception

- Relates to the physical process of receiving a painful stimulus and transmitting the information through the nervous system to the brain, where it is interpreted as pain.
- Little variability in pain perception between individuals with intact nervous systems.

II. Pain Reaction

- Pain reaction is a combination of interpretation of and response to the pain message.
- It is highly variable between individuals and even in the same individual at different times.
- Accounts for much of the variability seen between patients in personal pain management needs.
- Many factors influence pain reaction, including age, fatigue, emotional state, and both cultural and ethnic learned behaviors.
- Anxiety has special significance: The anxious patient is predisposed to feel pain. Research has shown an association between individuals with red hair and higher levels of dental fear and anxiety.[5,6]

III. Pain Threshold

- Varies between individuals, with some having a low pain threshold and others having a high pain threshold.
- Highly reproducible.
- May be altered by drugs such as local anesthesia.

Pain Control Mechanisms

- Match the pain control method to the patient's treatment needs and medical status.
- All pain management techniques are more effective if utilized before the patient experiences pain. The following five pain control mechanisms are often combined for optimum effect.

I. Remove the Painful Stimulus

- Affects pain perception.
- Example: clinician repositions fulcrum to avoid pinching the patient's lip during instrumentation.

II. Block the Pathway of the Pain Message

- Affects pain perception.
- Examples: use of local anesthetic, topical anesthetic.

III. Prevent Pain Reaction by Raising Pain Reaction Threshold

- Affects pain reaction.
- Examples: use of nitrous oxide–oxygen conscious sedation; nonopioid analgesics such as nonsteroidal anti-inflammatory drugs (NSAIDs).

IV. Depress Central Nervous System

- Affects pain reaction.
- Example: use of **general anesthesia**.

V. Use Psychosedation Methods (Iatrosedation)

- **Iatrosedation** or psychosedation helps reduce patient anxiety.
- Affects both pain perception and pain reaction.
- Includes any nonpharmacologic technique to reduce patient anxiety.
  - Builds a trust relationship.
  - Allows the patient to feel more in control.
- May be used alone or combined with pharmacologic pain management.
- Examples: explain procedures carefully; allow patient to express concerns; use relaxation or distraction techniques.

Nonopioid Analgesics

Over-the-counter (OTC) analgesics are an effective adjunct for preventing or reducing the mild-to-moderate discomfort that patients experience during dental hygiene therapy or postoperatively.[7-10]

I. Drugs

- NSAIDs.
  - Block **prostaglandin synthesis** at peripheral nerve endings to inhibit generation of pain message.
  - Suppress onset of pain.
  - Decrease pain severity.
  - Drugs of choice for dental pain.
  - If hemostasis is a consideration during treatment or postoperative bleeding is a concern, use caution when recommending NSAIDs.
  - Acetaminophen (e.g., Tylenol).

II. Indications for Use

- Mild-to-moderate pain during treatment and postprocedure healing.

Nitrous Oxide–Oxygen Sedation

- Nitrous oxide–oxygen sedation (N_2O–O_2) has been safely used in dental settings for pain control and anxiety management since the 18th century.[11-13]

- A state of **conscious sedation** is produced with the patient awake, relaxed, responsive to commands, able to cooperate with treatment, and having intact protective reflexes.
- The patient has some degree of **analgesia** and a higher pain reaction threshold.

Characteristics of Nitrous Oxide

- Inhalation sedation with nitrous oxide provides a safe method of pain control, reduces patient anxiety, and produces few adverse reactions.[12,13]
- Gaseous agent (nitrous oxide) is absorbed from the lungs into the cardiovascular system.
- Is not biotransformed in the body; eliminated through the lungs.
  - Recommended to start with 10–15% N_2O (1–1.5 L) and add incrementally as needed to achieve desired result.[12]
  - Onset: rapid, less than 30 seconds; peak effect occurs less than 5 minutes.
  - Duration: terminated as soon as delivery of nitrous is stopped.
  - The clinician has the unique ability to control the amount of sedation based on the patient's psychological needs and level of pain control.
  - U.S. Food and Drug Administration (FDA) pregnancy category: C.

I. Anesthetic, Analgesic, and Anxiolytic Properties

- Produces analgesia.
  - Achieves optimum analgesia and patient cooperation at 20–40% nitrous oxide for most patients.[12]
  - The need for higher or lower concentrations depends on individual biologic variability.
  - Reduces the intensity of pain but does not block it, only mildly potent as an anesthetic gas.
  - Use with local anesthetics when the patient experiences significant discomfort.
- Anxiolytic (sedative) effects.
  - Sedation reduces patient's level of fear and anxiety; has a positive effect on pain threshold.
- Possesses slight amnestic properties.

II. Chemical and Physical Properties

- Gas at room temperature and pressure.
- Heavier than air.
- Colorless; sweet smelling.
- Nonirritating and nonallergenic. No allergic reaction has ever been reported.
- Nonflammable but will support the combustion of flammable substances.

III. Blood Solubility

- Relatively insoluble in blood; primary saturation of blood occurs in 3–5 minutes.
- The gas molecules at the alveoli–blood interface and blood–brain interface pass readily to the tissue with the lowest concentration of nitrous oxide.
- Results in rapid onset and recovery.
- **Diffusion hypoxia** can occur at completion of sedation procedure if 100% oxygen is not administered.

IV. Pharmacology of Nitrous Oxide

- Is not metabolized in the body; remains unchanged in blood and tissues.
- Enters and exits almost entirely through the lungs.

Equipment for Nitrous Oxide–Oxygen

- Available as a portable unit or a central storage system with gas piped to individual treatment rooms.
- Units have several built-in safety features to ensure a minimal level of oxygen is delivered and the two gases cannot be reversed during delivery.
- The equipment can be divided into three basic parts:
  - Gas storage cylinders.
  - A gas delivery system.
  - A scavenger system with the nasal hood (mask) having components of both the gas delivery and scavenger portions.

I. Compressed Gas Cylinders

- Nitrous oxide
  - Color code: blue.
  - Physical state: gas and liquid.
  - Tanks: 95% liquid and 5% vapor; full tanks = 750 psi.
- Oxygen
  - Color code: green (International = white).
  - Physical state: gas.

- Handle carefully
  - Do not use grease, oil, lubricant, or hand cream around the cylinder valves or any fittings that come in contact with the gases.
  - Store vertically on a rack or in another stable and secure manner.
  - Open cylinder valves slowly in a counterclockwise direction.

II. Gas Delivery System

- Regulator or reducing valve
  - Converts high pressure of gas in the cylinders to a usable, lower level.
  - Subject to extreme high temperature if compressed gas cylinders are opened quickly.
- Flow meter
  - Visual indicator of liters per minute (L/min) flow of oxygen and nitrous oxide.
  - Gas flow rates of nitrous oxide and oxygen are adjusted independently and the sum of the two is the total gas flow rate.
  - A total combined gas flow rate is established and respective concentrations of the two gases are adjusted concurrently.
- Reservoir bag
  - Reservoir of gases to accommodate an exceptionally deep breath.
  - Allows for visualization of respirations for monitoring.
  - Degree of inflation can be used to help establish total flow rate of gas needed by the patient for comfortable respirations.
  - May be used to provide oxygen in assisted ventilation if attached to a full-face mask with relief valve.
- Conducting or breathing tubes

III. Nasal Hood, Nose Piece, and Mask

- Deliver gas for patient inhalation.
- Collect exhaled gas and direct it into scavenger system.
- Good fit and seal around patient's nose are essential in size selection.
- Ideally, use a disposable item or sterilize before each use.

IV. Scavenger System

- Removes exhaled gas to keep nitrous oxide levels low in the **ambient air** of the treatment room.
- Connects to the office central evacuation system.
- Vents to outside of building and away from windows and air intakes.

V. Safety Features

- Universal color coding of cylinders, hoses, flow controls for each gas.
- Pin index and diameter index safety systems physically prevent gas cylinders or hoses from being interchanged by mistake between the gases due to incompatible placement of pins (projections) and diameter differences in the couplings.
- Minimum oxygen flow: 30% or 3 L/min.
- Oxygen fail-safe system automatically shuts off nitrous oxide if the oxygen falls below a minimum level.
- Emergency air inlet to provide room air if system shuts down.
- Oxygen flush button to supply 100% oxygen quickly.

VI. Equipment Maintenance

- Function checks
  - Maintain working order and safe practice by periodic checking of equipment.
- Gas leaks
  - All equipment connections and rubber components are subject to leaking. **Figure 36-1** shows the places that need to be examined for tight connections, defects, and wear. Apply soapy water to connections; bubbles will form if leaks are present.

Patient Selection

I. Indications

- Patient with mild-to-moderate **anxiety**.
- Medically compromised patient who would benefit from additional oxygen and/or anxiety reduction.
  - Examples: patient with cardiovascular or cerebrovascular disease, or stress-induced bronchial asthma.
  - Procedures of short duration with low level of pain. The analgesic effect is most pronounced on soft tissues, making it especially useful during dental hygiene procedures.
  - Patient with strong gag reflex.

II. Contraindications

- **Absolute contraindications** include:
  - Chronic respiratory disease should secure a medical consultation first.[12]

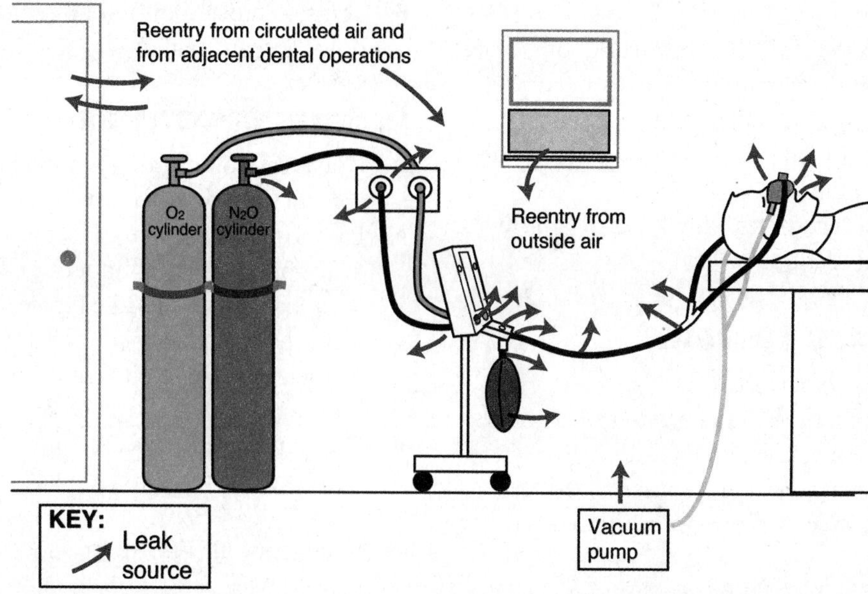

Figure 36-1 Potential Sources of Leaks from Nitrous Oxide–Oxygen Delivery Systems. Arrows show locations where regular inspection and testing is necessary. The most common sites of leakage are high-pressure connections: from the gas delivery cylinders, the wall connectors, the hoses connecting to the anesthetic machine, and the anesthesia machine itself (especially the on-demand valve). Low-pressure connections include from the anesthetic flow meter and the scavenging mask. Look for loose-fitting connections, loosely assembled or deformed slip joints and threaded connections, defective or worn seals, and gaskets. Rubber goods: hoses and reservoir bag. Look for cracks and tears.

National Institute for Occupational Safety and Health (US). Alert: Controlling Exposures to Nitrous Oxide during Anesthetic Administration [Joint Publication of Public Health Service, Centers for Disease Control, National Institute for Occupational Safety and Health]. Cincinnati, OH: U.S. Department of Health, Education, and Welfare; 1994:5. Publication No. 94-100.

    - Chronic respiratory conditions: chronic obstructive pulmonary disease, emphysema, cystic fibrosis, chronic bronchitis, and tuberculosis.
    - Upper respiratory tract infection or other acute respiratory conditions (coronavirus, cold, sinus problems, mouth breather, allergies, bronchitis, and cough)[14]: if nose breathing would be difficult or breathing apparatus cannot be sterilized or replaced.
    - Recent tympanic membrane graft.
    - Recent ophthalmic surgery using intraocular gases: vision damage could result from increased pressure on the eye during healing.[15,16]
    - Pregnancy: first-trimester nitrous oxide crosses the placenta; effects on fetus are inconclusive; not metabolized in the body; however, safest of all anxiety-lowering techniques, so a consult with primary care provider may be required to determine whether it can be safely used.[17]
- **Relative contraindications** include:
    - Current antidepressants or other psychotropic drugs, need to be aware of possible synergistic interaction.
    - Current or recovering drug or alcohol addiction: may trigger an episode or promote addictive behavior.[12]
    - Individuals with certain phobias, such as claustrophobia.
    - Unable to understand directions and procedure (e.g., Alzheimer's disease).
    - Bleomycin therapy.

Clinical Procedures for Nitrous Oxide–Oxygen Administration

Box 36-1 lists the sequence of steps for nitrous oxide–oxygen administration.

I. Patient Preparation

- Inform before appointment
    - No specific food limitations, but generally avoid fasting or heavy meals just before the appointment.
    - Wear comfortable clothing and loosen tight collars.

Box 36-1 Steps in Nitrous Oxide–Oxygen Administration

1. Assess patient's medical status.
2. Take and record pretreatment vital signs.
3. Educate patient and secure informed consent.
4. Prepare delivery equipment (open tanks, select nasal hood).
5. Activate scavenger system.
6. Turn on oxygen to a flow rate of 5–7 L/min.
7. Place nasal hood and adjust to fit.
8. Adjust gas flow rate.
9. Begin nitrous oxide at about 10–20%.
10. Titrate to optimum level.
11. Monitor throughout treatment.
12. Return to 100% oxygen.
13. Take and record posttreatment vital signs.
14. Remove nasal hood when patient feels fully recovered.
15. Record progress notes.

- Inform at time of appointment
  - Explain procedure in positive terms.
  - Stress the pleasant sense of relaxation; the patient will be aware and in control at all times.
  - Obtain informed consent.
- Assess and perform
  - Evaluate patient's medical status; determine the **ASA classification** (American Society of Anesthesiologists). (See Chapter 11.)
  - Take and record vital signs.
  - Place patient in a supine position.

II. Equipment Preparation

- Nasal hood
  - Select the appropriate size for optimum comfort and minimum gas leakage.
  - Attach to tubing.
- Scavenger system
  - Connect, usually to high-speed volume evacuation, and activate system.
  - Adjust setting of scavenger system.
- Turn on gas cylinders
  - Open slowly, first oxygen, then nitrous oxide.
  - Confirm that all equipment is operating correctly.

III. Technique for Gas Delivery

A. Establish Volume of Gas Flow

- Based on patient's size and medical/psychological condition; determine the total liters flow per minute.[12]
- Begin with 6 L 100% oxygen/min for adults.
- Gas flow rate between 6 and 7 L/min for average adults, 4 and 5 L/min for most children.[13]
- Place nasal hood, adjust for comfort; patient may assist in positioning; establish good seal.
- Adjust flow using the inflation of the reservoir bag and feedback from the patient.

B. Titration

Individualized drug dose is determined by increasing the percentage of nitrous oxide in small increments until the optimum sedation level is achieved based on clinical signs and symptoms.

- Initial concentration: Start **titration** at about 10–15% concentration of nitrous oxide.[12]
  - Because of the rapid uptake of nitrous oxide in the lungs and distribution through the body, the effect of each dose can be assessed after 1–2 minutes.
- Patient response: Observe the patient for signs of relaxation or other changes.
  - Ask the patient what is felt. Use the patient's signs and symptoms to determine when the optimum level of sedation has been reached.
  - **Table 36-1** lists signs and symptoms for various levels of nitrous oxide–oxygen sedation.
- Adjust dose: Increase or decrease the nitrous oxide by 5–10% when the optimum individual dose has not been achieved. Wait 1–2 minutes and reassess. Repeat as needed.
  - Distribution of optimum sedation dose for different individuals follows a bell curve. Generally, 20–40% nitrous oxide results in adequate sedation for dental treatment.
  - At high altitudes, greater nitrous oxide concentrations will be needed because of the change in the partial pressure of the gases.
- Time: Allow approximately 5 minutes for titration.
- Monitor: Continue to monitor and adjust the concentration throughout the appointment.
  - As the appointment proceeds or during less anxiety-producing parts of the appointment, a lower dose may be more comfortable.
  - Avoid excessive fluctuations.
- Attend patient: Never leave a sedated patient unattended; sedation can become deeper without some stimulation or interaction.
- Outcome: Titration increases clinical success rate of nitrous oxide–oxygen conscious sedation and decreases adverse responses.
- Advantages: Only the amount of drug required by the patient is given.

Table 36-1 Signs and Symptoms of Nitrous Oxide–Oxygen Sedation

Level of Sedation	Signs and Symptoms
Minimal sedation (ideal)	Comfortable/relaxed; reduced fear and anxiety; tingling of extremities and/or near mouth; body warmth; glazed eyes; responds to directions; intact protective cough and gag reflex; light feeling; vasodilation of neck and face
Oversedation	Disassociation from surroundings; hallucinating; feeling of floating or flying. Inability to follow directions and keep mouth open; dizziness; drowsiness
Oversedation (serious)	Delayed responses; slurred words; agitated and/or combative behavior; vomiting; loss of consciousness

- Allows for individual biovariability.
- Uncovers **idiosyncratic** reactions early.
- Minimizes negative experiences with oversedation.

Box 36-2 Example Documentation: Nitrous Oxide–Oxygen Conscious Sedation

- **S**—Patient presents with gag reflex and anxiety about dental treatment.
- **O**—Medical history nonsignificant. ASA I.
- **A**—No contraindication for use of nitrous oxide–oxygen.
- **P**—Total gas flow rate: 5 L/min; 35% (2 L/min) nitrous oxide and 65% (4 L/min) oxygen for 40 minutes. Patient reports tingling in extremities and relaxed feeling. 100% oxygen administered for 5 minutes following treatment; patient said he felt fully recovered.

Vital Signs	Pretreatment	Posttreatment
Blood pressure	124/84	120/82
Pulse	75	70
Respirations	12	12

Signed: ______________________, RDH
Date: ______________

IV. Completion of Sedation

- Recovery
  - Procedure: At the completion of sedation, return the patient to 100% oxygen for a minimum of 5 minutes, or longer if needed for full recovery.
  - Factors affecting recovery time: Biologic variation, duration of sedation procedure, and concentration of nitrous oxide administration.
  - Signs of recovery: Patient's report of feeling "back to normal" and is alert and able to respond appropriately to questions.
  - Comparable presedation and postsedation vital signs are recorded.
  - Elimination: Within 5–10 minutes, 99% removed completely from the body.
- Diffusion hypoxia occurs when the patient is returned directly to room air rather than 100% oxygen.
  - Nitrous oxide diffuses into an area of lower concentration more rapidly than oxygen, causing inadequate oxygen in the alveoli if the patient is not given supplemental oxygen at the completion of sedation.
  - Hypoxia can result in patient discomfort or syncope.
  - Inadequate postsedation oxygen may result in a feeling of lethargy, headache, or nausea.
  - Prevention: Administer 100% oxygen for no less than 5 minutes.
- Dismissal following full recovery
  - Patients should be fully alert and show no signs of disorientation.
  - Usually, the patient is able to return to all normal activities, including driving.
  - Vital signs should return to baseline readings.
  - Recovery time varies for each patient.
- Record keeping: As with every dental procedure, complete documentation is essential and good practice. The following items need to be included in the patient's record when administering nitrous oxide–oxygen analgesia (see **Box 36-2**):
  - Medical and psychological history review, including determination of the ASA classification.
  - Reason for nitrous oxide use.
  - Presedation and postsedation vital signs.
  - Concentrations of both nitrous oxide and oxygen administered.
  - Total gas flow rate (L/min).
  - Length of time for sedation procedure.
  - Length of time on recovery oxygen.
  - Statement of patient's recovery status and any post care instructions given.

- Any adverse reactions. Summary of patient's response to nitrous oxide can be helpful for subsequent appointments.
- Signature and date.

Potential Hazards of Occupational Exposure

Chronic **occupational exposure** to nitrous oxide may have deleterious effects on healthcare providers. Overexposure must be prevented.

I. Issues of Occupational Exposure

- Potential health problems[12,18-22]
  - Reduced fertility with unscavenged nitrous oxide exposure.
  - Spontaneous abortion.
  - Increased rate of neurologic, renal, and liver disease.
  - Decreased mental performance, audiovisual ability, and manual dexterity.
- Recommended exposure levels
  - Consensus has not been reached on occupational exposure limits; there is currently no exposure standard.
  - National Institute of Occupational Safety and Health recommends no more than 25 parts per million (ppm) during administration.

II. Methods for Minimizing Occupational Exposure

- Use an effective scavenging system that can move 45 L/min of air.
- Maintain equipment and inspect regularly for gas leaks, especially at the locations shown in Figure 36-1. Shut off and secure equipment at the end of each day's use.
- Improve general air quality:
  - Introduce fresh air.
  - Use a nonrecycling air-conditioning system or open a window.
  - Vent the scavenger system gases outside the building and away from windows and air intakes.
- Use an air sweep fan to direct nitrous oxide away from the clinician's breathing zone; periodically monitor air quality in the clinician's breathing zone.
- Minimize patient conversations and mouth breathing; fit the nasal hood carefully to avoid leaks.
- Set conservative limits on the duration and concentration of nitrous oxide use per patient.

Advantages and Disadvantages of Nitrous Oxide–Oxygen Sedation Anesthesia

I. Advantages

- Both a mild analgesic and sedative: reduces patient's reaction to pain by raising pain threshold.
- Increases relaxation and cooperation during treatment.
- Reduces the gag reflex.
- Very safe with few side effects and few medical contraindications. Excellent for management of many medically compromised patients[12,14]:
  - Respiratory disease (asthma): nitrous is nonirritating and will not precipitate an attack.
  - Cerebrovascular disease: elevated level of oxygen given, which is beneficial.
  - Hepatic disease: nitrous not metabolized like other drugs in the body.
  - Epilepsy: does not increase risk of seizure development.
  - Diabetes: no contraindication.
- Allergy: no reported allergy to nitrous oxide.[12]
- Provides oxygen enrichment as well as stress reduction.
- Helps prevent emergencies because of anxiety and pain management.
- Readily absorbed and excreted from the body; rapid onset and recovery from drug effect.
- Able to titrate to optimum level.
- Recovery is complete so patient can be dismissed to return to normal activities.
- Appointments less stressful for clinician because of relaxed, conscious, cooperative patient.

II. Disadvantages

- A low-**potency** analgesic drug.
  - Not effective with all patients because of low potency; does not block all perceptions.
  - Severely distressed or phobic patient may need a more potent drug or combination of drugs.
- Patient must be able and willing to breathe through the nose.
- Equipment and gases are expensive.
- Use of poor techniques such as failure to titrate or use a scavenger system results in undesirable patient experiences and potential staff health risks.[12,18-22]

- Potential for recreational abuse by health professionals.
- May stimulate sexual phenomena in some patients.[23]

Local Anesthesia

- **Local anesthesia** is the main modality for the management of dental pain.
- Blocks sensations, especially of pain, from teeth, soft tissues, and bone in the anesthetized area.
- Root instrumentation without discomfort requires a profound pulpal and periodontal tissue **anesthesia** to increase patient comfort and compliance during the appointment.

Pharmacology of Local Anesthetics

- Local anesthetics are the most frequently used drugs for dental and dental hygiene treatment.
- When administered correctly, local anesthesia is a safe and effective method for pain control.

I. Contents of a Local Anesthetic Cartridge

A dental cartridge is prefilled by the manufacturer. Cartridges contain either 1.7 or 1.8 mL of solution.[24] Anesthetic cartridges include the following:

- Amide anesthetic: blocks the transfer of ions across the nerve membrane, which stops the transmission of pain messages.
- Vasoconstrictor: constricts local blood vessels to offset the vasodilation caused by the amide anesthetic. Provides greater duration, more profound anesthesia, and hemostasis to the immediate area.
- Antioxidant: preservative added to prevent the oxidation of the vasoconstrictor, usually sodium metabisulfite or sodium bisulfite.
- Sterile water: diluting agent.
- Sodium chloride: creates a biocompatible solution with the body.

II. Ester and Amide Anesthetic Drugs

Dental local anesthetic drugs can be divided chemically into two major groups: esters and amides. The first dental anesthetic was procaine (Novocain), an ester, which has not been available in dental cartridges in the United States since 1996.[24]

A. General Characteristics of Ester Anesthetics

- Widely used in topical anesthetic agents.
- Causes vasodilation of local blood vessels.
- High incidence of allergic reactions from by-product, para-aminobenzoic acid (PABA).[24]
- Hydrolyzed in plasma by the enzyme pseudocholinesterase.
- Elimination via the kidneys.
- Atypical plasma cholinesterase may result in slow removal of the drug from the blood resulting in toxicity (see "General Medical Considerations" section).[24]

B. General Characteristics of Amide Anesthetics

- Safe and effective with minimal side effects when administered correctly.[24-29]
- Cause vasodilation of local blood vessels.
- Extremely low incidence of allergic reactions.[24]
- Metabolized by the liver (all amides with the exception of articaine are primarily biotransformed in the liver)[24-28] (see "General Medical Considerations" section).
- Elimination via the kidneys.

C. Duration of Amide Drugs

- There are three categories of duration for dental local anesthetics:
  - Short acting (~30 minutes of pulpal anesthesia).
  - Intermediate acting (~60 minutes of pulpal anesthesia).
  - Long acting (~90 minutes of pulpal anesthesia).
- Factors influencing the duration include:
  - Individual response to the drug.
  - Type of injection administered (supraperiosteal/infiltration versus nerve block).
  - Accuracy of the injection.
  - Anatomic barriers (ligaments, tendons, fascial planes, density of bone).
  - Vascularity at site of injection.
  - Presence of inflammation and/or infection.
  - Injecting a plain local anesthetic versus a local anesthetic with a vasoconstrictor.

III. Specific Characteristics of Amide Drugs

A. Lidocaine Hydrochloride (HCl)

- Properties
  - Proprietary name: Xylocaine.
  - Duration: intermediate acting.

- Considered the "gold standard" of all the local anesthetics.[24]
- Metabolized in the liver and excreted by the kidneys.

- Dosage
  - Concentration: 2%.
  - Vasoconstrictor: epinephrine 1:50,000 (for hemostasis) or 1:100,000.
  - mg/cartridge: 36 mg (1.8 mL), 34 mg (1.7 mL).
- Safety and precautions
  - **MRD (maximum recommended dose)** = 500 mg; 3.2 mg/lb; 7.0 mg/kg.[24]
  - FDA pregnancy category: B (**Box 36-3**).
  - Calculate the MRD, confirm a negative **aspiration** prior to depositing, deposit a full cartridge in no less than 1 minute.
  - *Absolute contraindication:* allergy to the local anesthetic or sodium bisulfite; cocaine or methamphetamine use in the previous 24 hours; current cannabis use and the administration of epinephrine.[25,26]
  - *Relative contraindication:* cardiovascular disease, angina, cerebrovascular accident (CVA), hypertension, hyperthyroidism, significant liver or kidney disease, patients taking beta-blockers or cimetidine on a regular basis, steroid-dependent asthmatics, avoid 1:50,000 for ASA 3 cardiac, CVA, hyperthyroidism, and patients sensitive to **epinephrine**.
  - Recommended for pediatric patients, pregnant women, most procedures and treatment requiring intermediate duration; best choice for bleeding control (1:50,000).

Box 36-3 FDA Pregnancy Categories

Category A
Adequate and well-controlled studies have failed to demonstrate a risk to the fetus in the first trimester of pregnancy (and there is no evidence of risk in later trimesters).

Category B
Animal reproduction studies have failed to demonstrate a risk to the fetus and there are no adequate and well-controlled studies in pregnant women.

Category C
Animal reproduction studies have shown an adverse effect on the fetus and there are no adequate and well-controlled studies in humans, but potential benefits may warrant use of the drug in pregnant women despite potential risks.

Category D
There is positive evidence of human fetal risk based on adverse reaction data from investigational or marketing experience or studies in humans, but potential benefits may warrant use of the drug in pregnant women despite potential risks.

Category X
Studies in animals or humans have demonstrated fetal abnormalities and/or there is positive evidence of human fetal risk based on adverse reaction data from investigational or marketing experience, and the risks involved in use of the drug in pregnant women clearly outweigh potential benefits.

U.S. Department of Health and Human Services; Chemical Hazards Emergency Medical Management. FDA pregnancy categories. April 2017. https://chemm.nlm.nih.gov/pregnancycategories.htm. Accessed 18 July 2019.

B. Mepivacaine HCl

- Properties
  - Proprietary name: Polocaine, Carbocaine.
  - Duration: short acting (3% plain solution); intermediate acting (2% 1:20,000 levonordefrin).
  - Weak vasodilator.
  - Metabolized in the liver and excreted by the kidneys.
- Dosage
  - Concentration: 2% (with vasoconstrictor), 3% (plain).
  - Vasoconstrictor: levonordefrin 1:20,000.
  - mg/cartridge: 2% = 36 mg (1.8 mL); 34 mg (1.7 mL).
  - mg/cartridge: 3% = 54 mg (1.8 mL), 51 mg (1.7 mL).
- Safety and/or precautions
  - MRD = 400 mg; 3.0 mg/lb; 6.6 mg/kg.[24]
  - FDA pregnancy category: C.
  - Calculate the MRD, confirm a negative aspiration prior to depositing, deposit a full cartridge in no less than 1 minute.
  - *Absolute contraindication:* allergy to the local anesthetic or sodium bisulfite; cocaine or methamphetamine use in the previous 24 hours (2% 1:20,000).
  - *Relative contraindication:* patients taking tricyclic antidepressants (TCAs)—interacts with levonordefrin, significant liver or kidney disease.
  - Recommended for short duration (3% plain solution), when a vasoconstrictor is contraindicated (3% plain solution), pediatric patients, patients who are epinephrine sensitive.

C. Prilocaine HCl

- Properties
  - Proprietary name: Citanest.
  - Duration: short acting administered as an infiltration; intermediate acting when administered as a nerve block.[24]
  - Weak vasodilator.
  - Metabolized: liver, small percentage by lungs as alternate site and excreted by the kidneys.
- Dosage
  - Concentration: 4%.
  - Vasoconstrictor: epinephrine 1:200,000.
  - mg/cartridge: 72 mg (1.8 mL); 68 mg (1.7 mL).
- Safety and precautions
  - MRD = 600 mg; 3.6 mg/lb; 8.0 mg/kg.[24]
  - FDA pregnancy category: B.
  - Calculate the MRD, confirm a negative aspiration prior to depositing, deposit a full cartridge in no less than 1 minute; may cause increased risk of paresthesia with an inferior alveolar (IA) nerve block.[29-33]
  - Metabolic by-products may cause acquired methemoglobinemia, a condition that reduces the blood's oxygen-carrying capacity (see "Specific Medical Considerations" section).
  - May cause increased risk of paresthesia with an IA nerve block.[30,31,33]
  - *Absolute contraindication:* allergy to the local anesthetic or sodium bisulfite; cocaine or methamphetamine use in the previous 24 hours (1:200,000), current cannabis use and the administration of epinephrine.[25,26]
  - *Relative contraindication:* significant liver or kidney disease, methemoglobinemia, sickle cell anemia, anemia, respiratory or cardiac failure, patients on acetaminophen long term.
  - Recommended for patients when a vasoconstrictor is contraindicated (4% plain solution). Plain solution provides intermediate duration when administered as a nerve block.

D. Articaine HCl

- Properties
  - Duration: intermediate acting.
  - Shortest **half-life** of all the amide anesthetics; reported to diffuse through soft and hard tissues better than other amides.[24]
- Dosage
  - Concentration: 4%.
  - Vasoconstrictor: epinephrine 1:100,000 and 1:200,000.
  - mg/cartridge: 72 mg (1.8 mL); 68 mg (1.7 mL).
  - MRD = determined by weight; 3.2 mg/lb; 7.0 mg/kg.
  - Metabolized: blood plasma (approx. 90–95%) and the liver (approx. 5–10%).
  - Excreted: kidneys.
  - Half-life: 30–45 minutes; shortest of all amide anesthetics.
  - FDA pregnancy category: C.
  - Calculate the MRD, confirm a negative aspiration prior to depositing, deposit a full cartridge in no less than 1 minute.
  - May cause increased risk of paresthesia with an IA nerve block.[29-32]
  - *Absolute contraindication:* allergy to the local anesthetic or sodium bisulfite; cocaine or methamphetamine use in the previous 24 hours, current cannabis use and the administration of epinephrine.[25,26]
  - *Relative contraindication:* significant liver or kidney disease.
  - Recommended for patients with moderate systemic disease (liver, cardiac). It has the lowest risk of systemic toxicity and shortest half-life allows for safer reinjections.[24]

E. Bupivacaine HCl

- Properties
  - Proprietary name: Marcaine.
  - Duration: long acting; longest onset of all the local anesthetics.
  - Most potent of the local anesthetics.
  - Metabolized by the liver and excreted by the kidneys.
- Dosage
  - Concentration: 0.5%.
  - Vasoconstrictor: epinephrine 1:200,000.
  - mg/cartridge: 9 mg (1.8 mL), 8.5 mg (1.7 mL).
- Safety and precautions
  - MRD = 90 mg; 0.9 mg/lb; 2.0 mg/kg (no mg/lb recommended for the United States, only for Canada).[24]
  - FDA pregnancy category: C.
  - Safety and/or precautions: calculate the MRD, confirm a negative aspiration prior to depositing; deposit a full cartridge in no less than 1 minute; highly toxic, stay below the MRD, use caution with reinjection.

- *Absolute contraindication:* allergy to the local anesthetic or sodium bisulfite; cocaine or methamphetamine use in the previous 24 hours, current cannabis use and the administration of epinephrine.[25,26]
- *Relative contraindication:* children or adults who are prone to self-mutilation post injection.
- Recommended for posttreatment pain control and procedures requiring greater than 60 minutes of pulpal anesthesia.

IV. Vasoconstrictors

A. Reasons for Use

- Safety: Potential for toxic reaction (overdose) to the local anesthetic is reduced by slowing the rate at which it enters circulation.
- Longevity: Duration of anesthetic effect is increased.
- Effectiveness: Depth and profoundness of anesthetic is increased.
- Hemostasis: Only if drug is locally injected directly into the area; epinephrine 1:50,000 is most effective.[24,33]

B. Potential Risks with Use of Vasoconstrictors

- Hypersensitivity to the drugs.
- Medical problems (see "Specific Medical Considerations" section).
- Drug interactions (see "Potential Drug Interactions" section).
- Degree of risk to medically compromised patients, including those with heart disease varies. The use of vasoconstrictors in low doses is considered safe.[24,33]

C. Preservatives

- Sodium bisulfite
  - Preservative added to local anesthetic cartridges that contain a vasoconstrictor.
  - Prevents the oxidation of the vasoconstrictor.
  - Provides a shelf-life of approximately 18 months.
  - Most likely offending agent in a dental cartridge when an allergic reaction occurs.[24,33]
  - Avoid administering any local anesthetic with a vasoconstrictor for patients that have a confirmed bisulfite allergy.
  - Best alternative choice: 4% prilocaine plain as a nerve block or 3% mepivacaine.

D. Drugs

- Epinephrine (Adrenalin)
  - Potent sympathomimetic amine.
  - Allergic reaction is rare because adrenalin is produced endogenously.[24]
  - Concentrations: 1:50,000, 1:100,000, or 1:200,000.
  - MRDs for healthy patients and for medically compromised, especially those with cardiac disease are listed in **Table 36-2**.
  - *Absolute contraindication:* bisulfite allergy; myocardial infarction (MI; within 6 months);

Table 36-2 Vasoconstrictors: Concentrations and Maximum Recommended Dose (MRD)

	MRD in Healthy Patients		MRD in Medically Compromised Patients	
Vasoconstrictors and Concentrations	**MG/APPT**	**Cartridges/APPT**	**MG/APPT**	**CARTRIDGES/APPT**
Epinephrine (based on 1.8 mL)				
1:50,000 (0.036 mg/cart.)	0.2	5.5	0.04	1.1
1:100,000 (0.018 mg/cart.)	0.2	11	0.04	2.2
1:200,000 (0.009 mg/cart.)	0.2	22[a]	0.04	4.4
Levonordefrin (based on 1.8 mL)				
1:20,000 (0.09 mg/cart.)	1.0	11.1	0.2	2.2

[a]Local anesthetic is the limiting drug.
MG/APPT, milligrams per appointment.

Table 36-3 Duration of Local Anesthetics Currently Available in the United States

Local Anesthetic Drugs	Soft Tissue (minutes)	Pulpal (minutes)	Duration Category
4% articaine 1:100,000 epinephrine	180–360	60–75	Intermediate
4% articaine 1:200,000 epinephrine	120–300	45–60	Intermediate
0.5% bupivacaine 1:200,000 epinephrine	240–540	90–180	Long
2% lidocaine 1:50,000 epinephrine	180–300	60	Intermediate
2% lidocaine 1:100,000 epinephrine	180–300	60	Intermediate
3% mepivacaine plain	120–180	20 (infiltration) 40 (nerve block)	Short intermediate
2% mepivacaine 1:20,000 levonordefrin	180–300	60	Intermediate
4% prilocaine plain	90–120 (infiltration) 120–240 (nerve block)	10–15 (infiltration) 40–60 (nerve block)	Short intermediate
4% prilocaine 1:200,000 epinephrine	180–480	60–90	Intermediate

coronary bypass surgery (within 6 months); uncontrolled angina, arrhythmias, hypertension, hyperthyroidism, or diabetes; pheochromocytoma (catecholamine producing tumors); cocaine or methamphetamine use within 24 hours; current cannabis use and the administration of epinephrine.[25,26]
    - *Relative contraindication:* cardiac conditions (ASA 3); taking nonselective beta-blockers or antidepressants; controlled hypertension, hyperthyroidism, or diabetes.
- Levonordefrin (Neo-Cobefrin)
    - About 15% as potent as equal doses of epinephrine and with less cardiac and central nervous system stimulation. Used at higher concentration (1:20,000) to accomplish adequate vasoconstriction.[24]
    - Not a good choice if hemostasis is required.
    - *Absolute contraindications:* bisulfite allergy; uncontrolled angina, arrhythmias, blood pressure, hyperthyroidism, or diabetes; cocaine or methamphetamine within 24 hours.
    - *Relative contraindication:* patients taking TCAs.[24,33]
    - MRDs for healthy patients and for medically compromised, especially those with cardiac disease, are given in Table 36-2.

V. Criteria for Local Anesthetic Selection

- Length of time needed for pain control is a primary criterion for drug selection. **Table 36-3** lists the typical duration of action for common local anesthetics.
- Need for hemostasis.
- Medical status of the patient.
- Potential for prolonged discomfort after treatment.
- Potential for self-inflicted injury before anesthetic wears off.

Indications for Local Anesthesia

- Local anesthesia is indicated for treatment that has the potential to cause discomfort or pain.
- Anesthesia prevents both the patient and clinician from the anticipation of discomfort, reducing stress, and making treatment comfortable.

I. Dental Hygiene Procedures

- Scaling and root debridement in areas with probing depths of 4 mm or greater.
- Extensive instrumentation with either manual or power-driven instruments.

- Treatment in areas of challenging pocket topography, furcation areas, or other difficult root anatomy.
- Instrumentation of sensitive root surfaces.
- Instrumentation in areas of painful, inflamed soft tissue.
- Treatments involving soft-tissue manipulation.
  - Gingival curettage.
  - Suture removal.
  - Removal of subgingival overhanging restoration.
  - Treatment in areas with excessive hemorrhage.

II. Patient Factors

- Extent of patient's oral status and periodontal condition directly influence the extent or rigor of the needed treatment.
- Patient's pain reaction or pain threshold.

Patient Assessment

The goal of patient assessment is to ensure an effective and safe local anesthesia experience. Pretreatment evaluation is the first and most important step for avoiding a medical emergency.

I. Sources of Information for Complete Preanesthetic Assessment

- Chief complaint.
- Vital signs.
- Medical history; ASA status. (See Chapter 11.)
- Current medications.
- Emotional status/anxiety level.
- Dental history related to local anesthesia.
- Presence of infection or inflammation.

II. Treatment Considerations Based on Assessment Findings

Amide local anesthetics and the vasoconstrictor normally incorporated into the dental anesthetic cartridge can be administered safely to almost all patients. Options for treatment include:

- Use local anesthetic without special precautions.
- Avoid use of local anesthetic or of a specific local anesthetic because of high medical risk.
- Select an alternative drug to minimize or avoid risk.
- Limit the dose of drug given at any specific appointment.
- Use local anesthesia combined with stress reduction techniques; use in combination with nitrous oxide–oxygen conscious sedation.
- Seek medical intervention, consult, or additional testing before proceeding.
- Administer **block anesthesia** (sometimes called regional anesthesia) rather than **infiltration** in inflamed tissue which has a low pH that inhibits drug distribution and effectiveness.

III. General Medical Considerations

- Regular utilization of safeguards such as medical history questionnaire, dental history, physical examination, and vital screenings (blood pressure, heart rate, and respiration) can help prevent most medical emergencies in the dental office or clinic.
- The ASA Classification System is a tool to help assess medical risk of a patient receiving anesthesia and undergoing surgical procedures. (See Chapter 11 for more information.)
  - ASA 4 patients and some ASA 3 patients (especially those who are anxious about injections) may not tolerate the injection procedure and the subsequent treatment.
  - Elective treatment for patients who are too medically compromised for local anesthesia (ASA 4 and some ASA 3) is not performed except in the case of emergency procedures until medical status improves; may not be appropriate for any elective dental therapy.
- When performing a risk–benefit analysis for use of local anesthesia, consider the potential for medical distress that can result from inadequate pain control.
- Seek a medical consult when there is doubt about the safety of a local anesthetic choice.
- Calculate the MRD for all patients, especially children or adults weighing less than 150 pounds. Every drug has an MRD in mg/lb and mg/kg that is used for the calculation (**Table 36-4**).
  - Determine and administer the smallest effective dose for each patient.
  - Always use the smallest effective dose.
- Contraindications to local anesthesia administration
  - The clinician may need to either limit (relative contraindication) or completely avoid (absolute contraindication) use of a local anesthetic drug or vasoconstrictor depending on specific medical or psychological considerations of the patient or medications.

Table 36-4 Local Anesthetics Maximum Recommended Dose (MRD)

Local Anesthetic Drug	mg/lb	mg/kg	MRD (mg)
Articaine	3.2	7.0	N/A[a]
Bupivacaine	2.0	0.9	90
Lidocaine	3.2	7.0	500
Mepivacaine	3.0	6.6	400
Prilocaine	3.6	8.0	600

[a]No FDA absolute maximum recommended dose provided.

IV. Specific Medical Considerations

A. Allergy

- Amide anesthetics: True allergy is rare. If confirmed, avoid offending drug, choose a different amide; a slight chance of cross-allergenicity may occur;[24,31] refer to allergist for testing.
- Ester anesthetics: Allergy is fairly common. If confirmed, avoid all ester anesthetics, including topical anesthetics.
- Bisulfites: Sodium bisulfite and sodium metabisulfite are used as the preservatives for the vasoconstrictor. If allergy is known, avoid anesthetics containing vasoconstrictors.[24,29]
- Best choice: 3% mepivacaine or 4% prilocaine plain if sodium bisulfite is the allergen.

B. Hyperthyroidism

- Uncontrolled hyperthryoidism: avoid vasoconstrictor.
- Controlled: can choose local anesthetic with a vasoconstrictor but stay below the MRD and use the weakest vasoconstrictor concentration.[34,35]
- Best choice: 4% prilocaine plain, 3% mepivacaine plain, 2% mepivacaine 1:20,000, or local anesthetic with epinephrine 1:200,000 (articaine, prilocaine, or bupivacaine).

C. Impaired Liver or Kidney Function

- Only severe impairment is clinically relevant (ASA 3 or 4).
- Half-life of amide anesthetic could be prolonged, which could result in overdose.
- Best choice: 4% articaine (1:100,000 or 1:200,000) since very little is biotransformed through the liver.[35]

D. Malignant Hyperthermia (MH)

- Life-threatening complications associated with the administration of general anesthesia.
- Syndrome that is transmitted genetically; defect in the distribution of myoplasmic calcium.
- MH most often occurs after first exposure to general anesthesia.
- Clinical signs: tachycardia, high fever, tachypnea, cardiac dysrhythmias, muscle rigidity, cyanosis, and death.
- Absolute contraindication for patients to receive general anesthesia (succinylcholine).
- Local anesthetics with or without vasoconstrictors can be used. No current evidence to support avoidance of local anesthetics or vasoconstrictors.[29,35]
- Medical consult is recommended prior to treatment.

E. Methemoglobinemia

- A congenital or acquired condition; hemoglobin molecule is converted to methemoglobin, which has less oxygen-carrying capacity. A cyanosis-like state may develop if a high percentage of molecules convert.
- Prilocaine, articaine, and topical benzocaine can cause a dose-related methemoglobinemia.[24,30,31] Avoid their use in patients with a preexisting condition.
- Avoid prilocaine or benzocaine if on long-term acetaminophen use.
- Best choice: lidocaine, mepivacaine, or bupivacaine.

F. Heart Failure

- Reduced circulation resulting from heart failure slows elimination of amide anesthetic, which increases potential for anesthetic overdose.
- Patient is stress intolerant—pain and anxiety must be carefully managed. Consider use of nitrous oxide–oxygen sedation alone or in combination with local anesthesia.[12,35]
- Obtain medical consult and clearance before treating.
- Best choice: 2% lidocaine 1:100,000 (cardiac dosage for epinephrine).

G. Coronary Heart Disease, MI, Recent Heart Surgery, and Stroke

- Do not treat within the first 6 months; higher risk of a subsequent event or complication.[35] Consult with the cardiologist.
- Concern is for the use and amount of vasoconstrictor. Epinephrine cardiac dose = 0.04 mg per appointment; levonordefrin cardiac dose = 0.2 mg per appointment; do not use 1:50,000 epinephrine concentration for these patients.[24]

- Decision based on patient ASA category, procedure to be performed, duration needed for pain control; medical consultation recommended.
- Best choice: plain anesthetic (if adequate depth and duration of pain control can be achieved); 1:200,000 epinephrine concentrations (if hemostasis is not a consideration); 2% mepivacaine 1:20,000.

H. Angina

- *Uncontrolled angina*—avoid all dental procedures; *controlled*—limit amount of vasoconstrictors.[24]
- Best choice: plain local anesthetic*; 2% mepivacaine 1:20,000 or local anesthetics with 1:200,000.

I. Hypertension

- *Uncontrolled hypertension*—avoid all dental procedures; *controlled*—limit amount of vasoconstrictors.[24]
- Best choice: plain anesthetics*; 1:200,000 epinephrine concentrations (if hemostasis is not a consideration); 2% mepivacaine 1:20,000.

J. Hemophilia

- Excessive bleeding may result from needle contact with a blood vessel.
- Decision based on severity of condition can range from treatment in hospital to avoiding injections into highly vascularized areas (e.g., the posterior superior alveolar [PSA]).
- Best choice: local anesthetic with a vasoconstrictor; avoid plain anesthetics.

K. Pregnancy and Lactation

- Local anesthetics and vasoconstrictors are not teratogens and may be safely administered.
- Select a drug in the FDA pregnancy risk category B (lidocaine or prilocaine). The FDA classifies drugs according to their safety for the fetus. Refer to Box 36-3 for FDA pregnancy categories.
- Dental treatment, including use of local anesthetic, can be done during any trimester.[36,37]
- All local anesthetics are expressed in breast milk; use smallest effective dose.
- Best choice (pregnancy): 2% lidocaine 1:100,000; 4% prilocaine plain or 1:200,000 (FDA drug category B).
- Best choice (lactation): articaine 1:200,000 due to its half-life compared to the other anesthetics.

L. Diabetes

- Epinephrine opposes action of insulin and may raise blood glucose levels; should be used with caution.
- Best choice: plain local anesthetic*; 1:200,000 concentrations; 2% mepivacaine 1:20,000.

M. Glaucoma

- Avoid or limit amount of vasoconstrictor, may increase ocular pressure due to vasoconstriction.
- Best choice: plain local anesthetic*; 1:200,000 concentrations; 2% mepivacaine 1:20,000.

N. Atypical Plasma Cholinesterase

- Uncommon, autosomal recessive trait; inability to metabolize ester drugs.
- Relative contraindication: ester drugs; avoid topical benzocaine.
- Best choice: amide topical and local anesthetics.[24]

O. Potential Drug Interactions

- All medications reported in a patient's medical history need to be reviewed for potential drug interactions before selecting the local or topical anesthetic.
- Following are examples of frequently prescribed or OTC drugs that interact with an anesthetic or a vasoconstrictor warranting precautions.
  - Histamine (H_2) receptor blockers (e.g., Tagamet) and lidocaine: reduce ability of liver to metabolize lidocaine; limit amount of lidocaine especially in patients with congestive heart failure (ASA 3) and taking a histamine blocker.[38,39]
  - Nonselective beta-blockers (e.g., Inderal, Corgard) and vasoconstrictors: increased risk of serious hypertension, cardiac dysrhythmias, and a potential cardiac event; use plain anesthetic unless hemostasis is needed.
  - TCAs (tricyclic antidepressants) (e.g., Elavil, Norpramin) and vasoconstrictors: increased risk of hypertension and cardiac dysrhythmias; limit epinephrine and avoid levonordefrin.[39]
  - Phenothiazines (e.g., Thorazine) and vasoconstrictors: possible severe hypotension; be aware of potential postural hypotension; use cardiac dose and avoid 1:50,000 epinephrine.
  - Cocaine, methamphetamine, cannabis, and vasoconstrictors: increased risk of hypertensive crisis, MI, or stroke; avoid all vasoconstrictors for 24 hours of using offending drug.[25,39,40]

*Plain local anesthetics (if can achieve adequate depth and duration of pain control).

Armamentarium for Local Anesthesia

I. Syringe

- Nondisposable types
  - Breech-loading, metallic, aspirating (most frequently used).
  - Breech-loading, metallic, aspirating, petite (smaller thumb ring diameter makes handling easier for clinicians with small hands).
  - Breech-loading, metallic, self-aspirating (easier aspiration for clinicians with small hands).
  - Breech-loading, plastic, aspirating.
  - Pressure syringe for periodontal ligament (PDL) injection.
  - Jet injector (needleless syringe); used for topical anesthesia of the palate.
- Safety syringes (single-use, self-sheathing to prevent needle stick injury) (**Figure 36-2**).
  - Computer-controlled local anesthesia delivery (C-CLAD) system.
- Design features of syringes
  - Durable metal or plastic can be sterilized and reused with the addition of a new needle and cartridge.

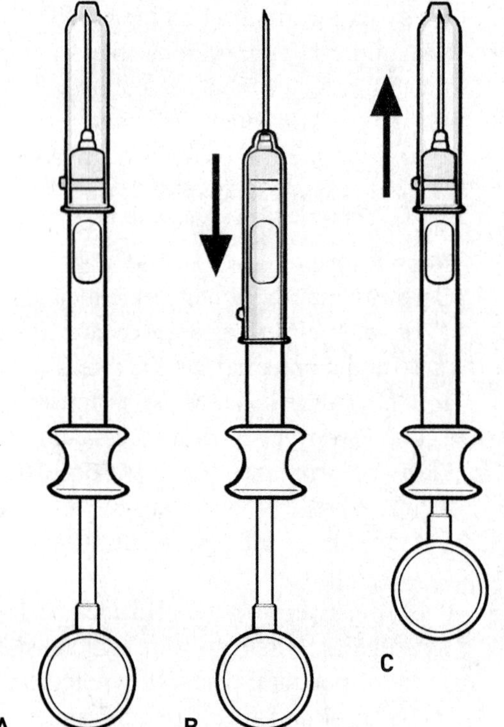

Figure 36-2 Prevention of Percutaneous Injury: Self-Sheathing Safety Needle. **A:** Syringe with protective sheath over the needle. **B:** As the injection is made, the sheath slides back. **C:** After injection, the sheath returns to cover the needle and protect the clinician during disposal.

  - Single-use, disposable safety syringes have features to prevent inadvertent needle stick after use.
  - Provide good visibility of the cartridge to determine whether a positive aspiration has occurred.
- Promote easy aspiration
  - Manual aspiration is the traditional design.
  - Self-aspirating syringe works well for small hands.

II. Needle

- Disposable.
  - Intended only for single-patient use.
- Parts and lengths of the needle (**Figure 36-3**).

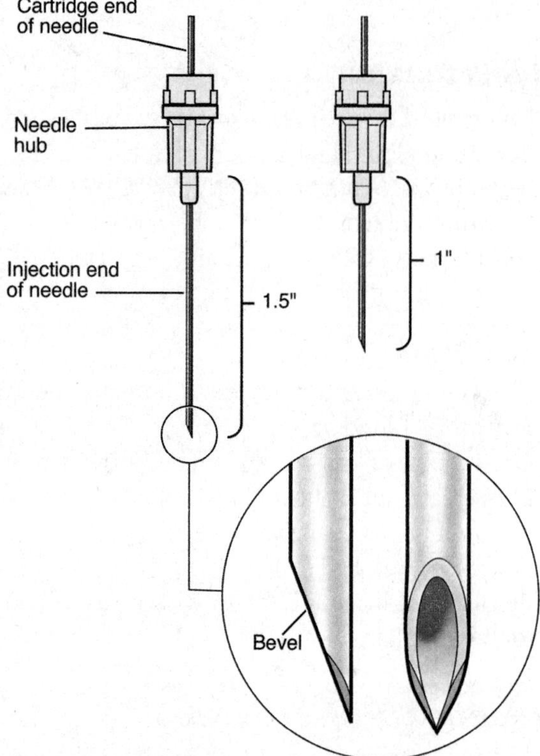

Figure 36-3 The Dental Anesthetic Needle. Dental needles are available in three lengths: long, short, and extra-short. Lengths vary slightly between manufacturers. The components of the needle are cartridge end, which penetrates the rubber diaphragm of the dental cartridge; hub, which attaches the needle to the syringe (made of plastic or metal); and injection end or shank or shaft, which penetrates the oral tissue so that anesthetic solution is deposited at the desired site. Inset: shows an enlargement of the tip of the needle with sharp terminus and bevel. When giving an injection, the needle is oriented so that the bevel is parallel to the bone to help prevent the needle from catching the periosteum, the sensitive covering over the bone. Needles should be changed after three to four uses to prevent unnecessary discomfort to the patient from a dull or barbed needle.

- Needle lengths are not standardized and therefore can vary depending on the manufacturer.
    - Long needle: approximately 30–35 mm (1½ inches).
    - Short needle: approximately 20–25 mm (1 inch).
    - Extra-short needle: approximately 10–12 mm (1/2 inch); used for palatal injections.
- Gauge or needle diameter
    - Size: Ranked from largest to smallest, 25-, 27-, and 30-gauge needles are used in dentistry.
    - Rigidity: 25-gauge needles are stiffer and have less needle deflection as they pass through tissue. Increased accuracy with deep tissue penetration (IA and Gow–Gates [GG] nerve blocks).
    - Aspiration: Larger-gauge needles provide easier and more accurate aspiration.

III. Cartridge or Carpule

- Volume: 1.7 or 1.8 mL of solution.
- Storage:
    - Store at cool room temperature and away from the light.
    - Do not store in an alcohol or disinfectant solution.
- Label on each cartridge: drugs, manufacturer, and expiration date.
- Color coding: Local anesthetic drug is identified by color on cartridge. Color codes are standardized and shown in **Box 36-4**.

IV. Additional Armamentarium

- Topical antiseptic (e.g., povidone–iodine) to prevent postinjection infections.

Box 36-4 Anesthesia Color Code

Color Codes for Local Anesthetics Currently Available in the United States

A uniform system for easy recognition and safety

Anesthetic	Color
Lidocaine 2% with epinephrine 1:100,000	
Lidocaine 2% with epinephrine 1:50,000	
Mepivacaine 2% with levonordefrin 1:20,000	
Mepivacaine 3% plain	
Prilocaine 4% with epinephrine 1:200,000	
Prilocaine 4% plain	
Articaine 4% with epinephrine 1:100,000	
Articaine 4% with epinephrine 1:200,000	
Bupivacaine 0.5% with epinephrine 1:200,000	

- Topical anesthetic to increase patient comfort.
- Cotton gauze to wipe the injection site to clean, dry, and remove the topical anesthetic. May also be used to improve grasp for lip or cheek retraction.
- Needle recapping device if self-sheathing needle is not used.
- Hemostat for broken needle removal from soft tissues if it occurs.
- Sharps disposal system to meet safe practice standards for used needle disposal.

V. Sequence of Syringe Assembly

- **Figure 36-4A** illustrates the assembly of the conventional, metallic, breech-loading anesthetic syringe; sequence makes the attachment between the harpoon and rubber stopper easier without applying excess force to the glass cartridge.

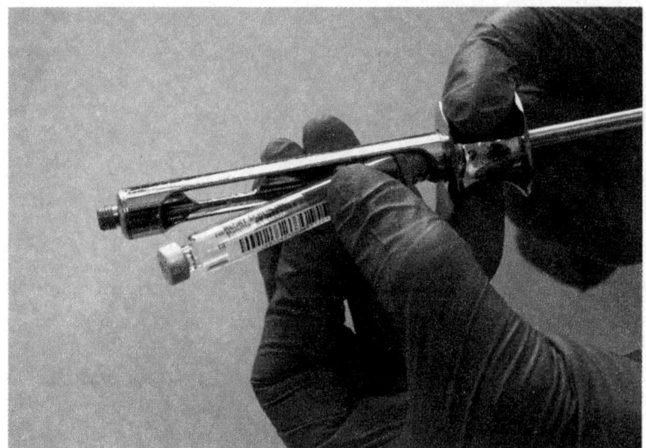

A

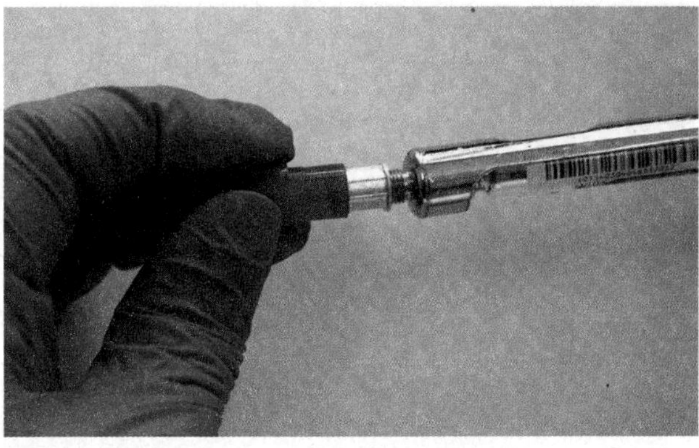

B

Figure 36-4 Sequence for Assembling a Breech-Loading Aspirating Syringe. **A:** 1. Pull back on thumb ring. 2. Insert anesthetic cartridge, rubber stopper end first, toward the thumb ring, then the diaphragm end toward the needle opening. 3. Set harpoon and test for lock into rubber stopper. 4. Remove safety cap from needle. **B:** 5. Screw needle onto the syringe.

- **Figure 36-4B** demonstrates attachment of the dental needle to the needle adapter end of the syringe.

VI. C-CLAD System

- Pressure, volume, and rate of deposit of local anesthetic delivery are precisely regulated by a computer.
- Device includes a light, pen-like handpiece attached to a computer-controlled motor that is activated by a foot or finger control. Any gauge Luer Lock needle and standard anesthetic cartridge may be used.
- Slow, controlled delivery of anesthesia solution promotes more comfortable injections, especially palatal and PDL injections; allows unique injections, the anterior middle superior alveolar and the palatal anterior superior alveolar, as well as all traditional dental injections.
- Good option for needle phobic and pediatric patients.

Clinical Procedures for Local Anesthetic Administration

Administer the most comfortable injections possible by using gentle tissue manipulation, careful needle penetration, slow deposition of solution, and good patient communication. An example progress note for a patient receiving local anesthesia is found in **Box 36-5**.

I. Injection(s) Selection

- Basic injections
  - **Table 36-5** lists injections with hard and soft tissues anesthetized, and the branches of the trigeminal nerve involved.
- Areas anesthetized
  - **Figure 36-5** shows the areas to be anesthetized.

Box 36-5 Example Documentation: Local Anesthesia

- **S**—Patient reported general root sensitivity and gum bleeding when brushing.
- **O**—Reviewed medical history, no contraindications to treatment, ASA I; IOE negative; BP = 115/75, HR = 65.
- **A**—Moderate generalized chronic periodontitis. Plaque score: 50%.
- **P**—NSPT on mandibular left quadrant; 20% benzocaine topical applied; 1:00 PM administered one cartridge of 2% Xylocaine 1:100,000 epinephrine using a 25-gauge long needle; 36 mg lidocaine and 0.018 mg epinephrine given for a left IA and buccal nerve blocks. Patient tolerated procedure well, no adverse reactions. Post-BP = 120/76; HR = 66; written posttreatment instructions given to the patient.

Signed: ______________________, RDH
Date: ________________

Table 36-5 Common Local Anesthetic Injections for Dental Hygiene Procedures

Injection	Tissues Anesthetized	Branch of the Trigeminal Nerve
Maxillary Arch		**Maxillary Division**
Supraperiosteal	*Teeth:* individual teeth *Periodontium and soft tissues:* periodontium of teeth anesthetized including facial or buccal tissue overlying individual teeth	Individual terminal branches
PSA	*Teeth:* second and third molars; first molar including mesiobuccal root (72% completely anesthetized) *Periodontium and soft tissues*: periodontium of teeth anesthetized including overlying buccal tissues	Posterior superior alveolar
MSA	*Teeth:* first and second premolars, mesiobuccal root of first molar (28%) *Periodontium and soft tissues:* periodontium of teeth anesthetized including overlying buccal tissues	Middle superior alveolar
ASA	*Teeth:* canine and incisors *Periodontium and soft tissues:* periodontium of teeth anesthetized and overlying facial tissues and lip	Anterior superior alveolar

Injection	Tissues Anesthetized	Branch of the Trigeminal Nerve
IO	*Teeth:* incisors, canine, premolars, and MB root of first molar if MSA nerve is present (28%) *Periodontium and soft tissues:* periodontium of teeth including overlying facial tissues, including the lower eyelid, side of nose, cheek, and upper lip	Infraorbital (includes both ASA and MSA)
GP	*Teeth:* none *Periodontium and soft tissues:* lingual gingiva and palatal tissue from distal of third molar to mesial of first premolar medial to midline of palate	Greater palatine
NP	*Teeth:* none *Periodontium and soft tissues:* palatal tissues from distal of right canine to distal of left canine	Nasopalatine
Mandibular Arch		**Mandibular Division**
IA	*Teeth:* entire quadrant of teeth *Periodontium and soft tissues:* buccal periosteum and soft tissues from premolars to midline	Inferior alveolar (includes mental and incisive nerves)
L	*Teeth:* none *Periodontium and soft tissues:* lingual gingiva, floor of the mouth, anterior two-thirds of tongue	Lingual
LB	Teeth: none *Periodontium and soft tissues:* buccal periosteum and soft tissues of molars	Long buccal
M	*Teeth:* none *Periodontium and soft tissues:* buccal gingival tissue and mucous membranes from mental foramen to midline, lower lip, skin of chin	Mental
I	*Teeth:* premolars to central incisor in same quadrant *Periodontium and soft tissues:* buccal periosteum, gingival tissue, and mucous membranes from premolars to central incisor in same quadrant, lower lip, skin of chin	Incisive
Gow–Gates technique	*Teeth:* entire mandibular quadrant of teeth *Periodontium and soft tissues:* buccal and lingual tissues; anterior two-thirds of tongue and floor of mouth; lower lip; skin over the zygoma; posterior portion of the cheek and temporal regions	Mandibular nerve—V_3 nerve block (includes IA, mental, incisive, lingual, mylohyoid, auriculotemporal, and buccal nerves)
Either Arch		
Intraseptal	*Teeth:* unreliable; primarily soft-tissue anesthesia; good technique for hemostasis of moderate inflamed tissue (e.g., curettage) *Periodontium and soft tissues:* periosteum and gingiva of anesthetized area	Terminal nerve endings
PDL	*Teeth:* individual tooth *Periodontium and soft tissues:* periosteum, gingiva and mucous membrane associated with anesthetized tooth	Terminal nerve endings

ASA, anterior superior alveolar; GP, greater palatine; I, incisive; IA, inferior alveolar; IO, infraorbital; L, lingual; LB, long buccal; M, mental; MSA, middle superior alveolar; NP, nasopalatine; PDL, periodontal ligament; PSA, posterior superior alveolar

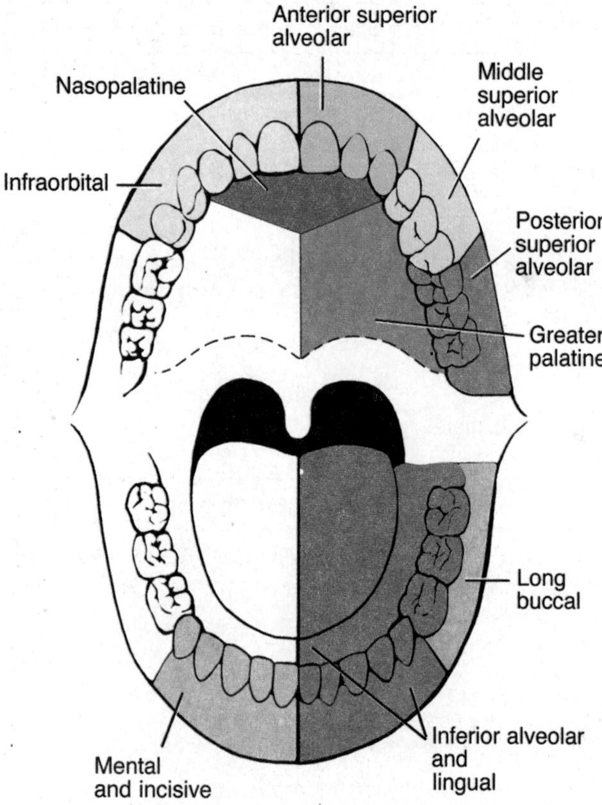

Figure 36-5 Diagrammatic Representation of Teeth and Soft Tissues Anesthetized by Common Dental Injections

- Steps and procedures
  - **Box 36-6** outlines the sequence and procedures for the administration of local anesthesia.

Box 36-6 Steps in the Administration of Local Anesthesia

1. Assess patient medical status, treatment, and pain control needs in order to select safest and most effective injection(s) and anesthetic drug.
2. Assemble and test the syringe setup (Figure 36-3 and Figure 36-4).
   - Orient the needle so the bevel will be toward the bone during the injection (with the exception of palatal injections).
   - Test the assembled syringe.
3. Position patient for good visibility and to prevent syncope with head level with or lower than heart.
4. Use topical anesthetic.
   - Apply topical to dry tissue at the injection site for the appropriate time. For benzocaine, 1–2 minutes is optimal.
   - Remove residual topical anesthetic.
5. Wipe injection site with gauze to dry and clean surface bacteria, saliva, and topical anesthetic from the area before injection.
6. Retract the lip or cheek for good visibility; gently stretch the tissue for easier needle penetration.
7. Keep the syringe out of the patient's sight.
8. Pick up the syringe so that the large window is facing the clinician.
9. Establish a fulcrum or hand rest for stability during the injection.
10. Insert the needle into the tissue and gently advance to desired site for administration of anesthetic.
11. Aspirate before depositing solution; re-aspirate as needed throughout procedure.
12. Deposit the anesthetic solution slowly (1–2 minutes for full cartridge) to prevent patient discomfort and to reduce potential for a toxic reaction.
13. Withdraw the needle carefully at the completion of the injection and recap the needle using a safe technique.
14. Remain with and observe the patient. Adverse drug reactions (ADRs) are most likely to occur during or shortly after the injection.
15. Record injection information in patient chart.
16. Use positive, supportive communication with the patient throughout the procedure.

II. Aspiration

- Purpose
  - To confirm the tip of the needle is not within a blood vessel prior to depositing the local anesthetic.
  - An anesthetic solution must be deposited **extravascular** to be effective and to prevent toxicity.
- When to aspirate
  - Before depositing anesthetic solution.
  - Periodically throughout injection to confirm that the needle has not moved and entered a blood vessel; to slow the rate of deposit.
- Interpretation
  - Any fluid at the tip of the needle will be drawn into the cartridge. If the tip of the needle is in an artery or vein, blood will become visible; it may only be a small amount at the needle end of the cartridge.
  - Negative aspiration: no blood in cartridge; proceed with injection.
  - Positive aspiration: blood in the cartridge.
    - A small amount of blood with most of the cartridge clear: move to a new location and re-aspirate.
    - Diffuse blood in cartridge: withdraw needle, replace cartridge, and repeat injection.

III. Sharps Management

- Needle recapping
  - Needles are recapped immediately following an injection utilizing a needle cap holder

that allows a one-handed recapping technique. Examples of devices are shown in **Figure 36-6**.

- Correct and incorrect methods:
  - One-handed "scoop" technique (**Figure 36-7A–D**).
  - Unsafe recapping of a contaminated needle (**Figure 36-8A–B**).
- Do not manipulate needles; do not bend or break.

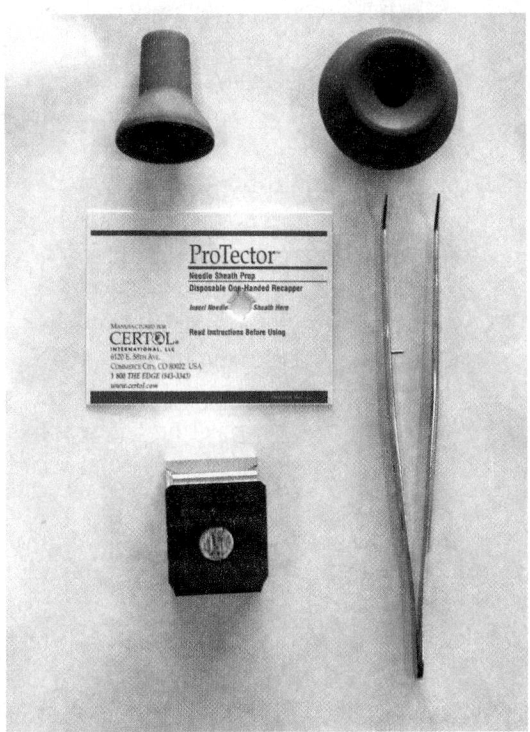

Figure 36-6 Commercially Available Holders for Needle Caps. One-handed capping or recapping with a safety mechanical device to hold the needle sheath is acceptable.

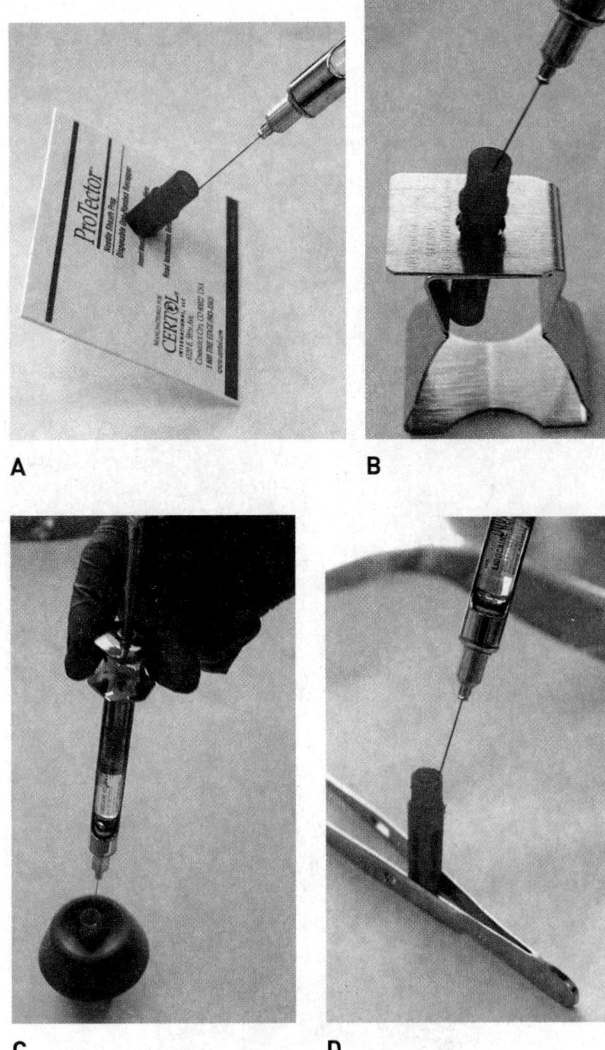

Figure 36-7 Safe Needle Recapping Techniques. **A–D:** Correct utilization of the various needle cap holders will allow for a safe one-handed needle recapping method.

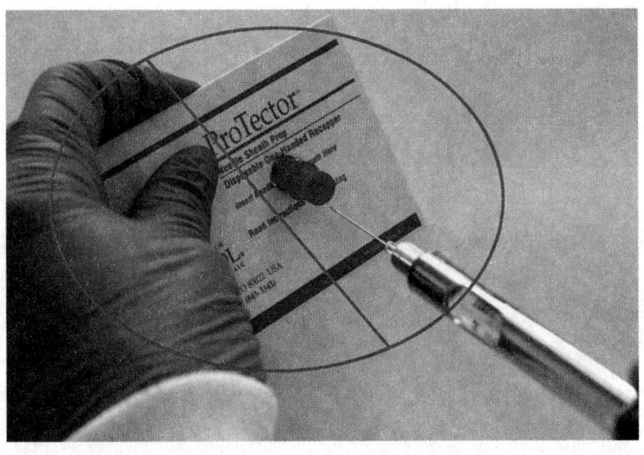

A

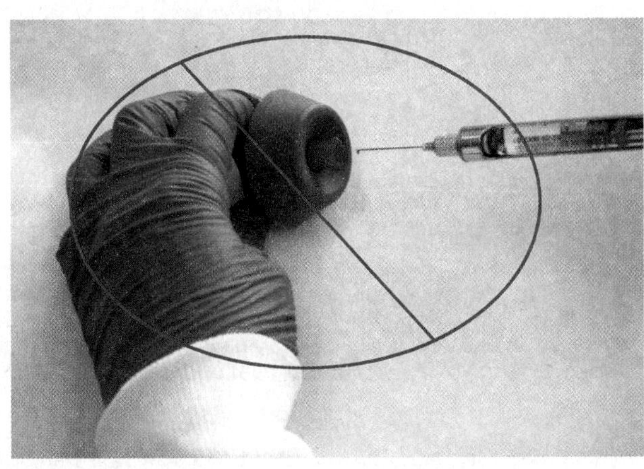

B

Figure 36-8 Unsafe Needle Recapping Techniques. **A** and **B**: Increases risk of needle exposure to the clinician.

- Needle removal
- Disposal containers for contaminated sharps are placed so they are readily accessible and located as close as possible to the area of use (**Figure 36-9A–C**).
    - Discard full sharps containers according to local, state, and federal regulations.

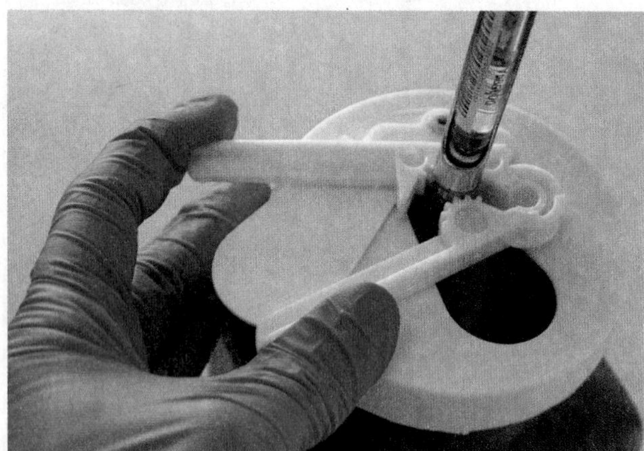

A

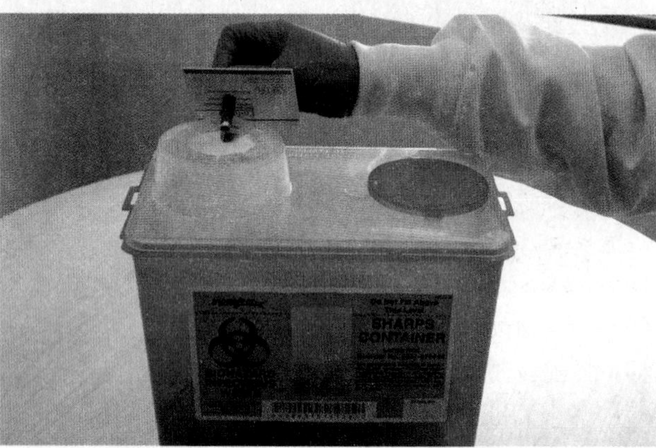

B

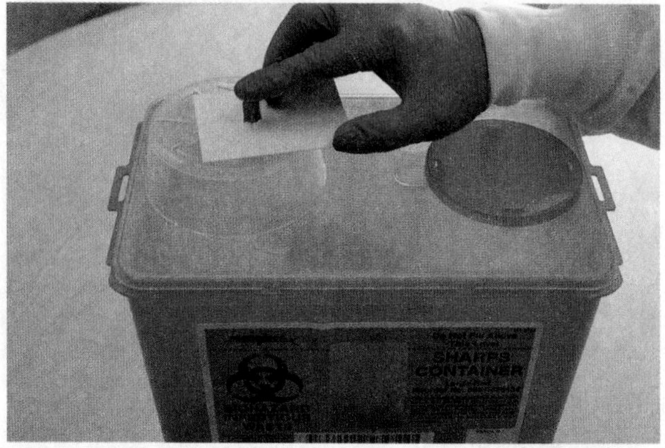

C

Figure 36-9 Needle Disposal Technique. **A–C:** Dental needles must be disposed of in the appropriate sharps containers using a one-handed technique.

Potential Adverse Reactions to Local Anesthesia

I. Adverse Drug Reactions

- Overdose (toxicity)
    - Overdose is the most common adverse drug reaction (ADR).[24]
    - Occurs when the circulating blood level of the drug becomes too high and reaches a toxic level for the individual.
    - Reaction continues as long as the local anesthetic plasma level remains above threshold for overdose.
- Typical causes of overdose
    - Intravascular injection: prevented by aspiration before deposition of the anesthetic drug.
    - Excessive total drug dose: affected by drug volumes; drug choice; patient's weight, age, and physical/medical status.
    - Rapid absorption into the circulatory system: affected by rate of injection, presence or absence of a vasoconstrictor, or vascularity of injection site.
    - Reduced elimination and/or metabolism of drug: reduced kidney or liver function or reduced circulation as a result of congestive heart failure may reduce the rate at which the drug is removed from circulation.
- Reducing risk of overdose in the pediatric population
    - Treat only one quadrant at a time with local anesthesia.
    - Do not administer full cartridges per injection.
    - Avoid using local anesthetic solutions with no vasoconstrictor unless a vasoconstrictor is contraindicated.
    - Choose the lowest effective local anesthetic concentration.
    - Stay below the MRD specific for that patient.
- Primary prevention
    - Thorough review of medical history including any anxiety, fear, or phobias.
    - Limit amount of topical anesthetic.
    - Use vasoconstrictor when not contraindicated.
    - Position patient in a supine or semi-supine position to prevent syncope.
    - Administer lowest concentration and amount necessary to achieve adequate pain control.
    - Aspirate and inject slowly (no less than 1 minute for a full cartridge).

  - Continue to observe patient before, during, and after administration.
- Allergy
  - Incidence: Although often reported, incidence is rare with amide drugs.[24,41,42] (Review allergy in "Specific Medical Considerations" section .)
  - Symptoms: Response may range from mild, such as localized erythema or itching, to life-threatening, such as generalized anaphylaxis or laryngeal edema.
  - Onset: May range from a few seconds to hours.
  - Management: Chapter 9 presents procedures for managing an allergic reaction.

II. Psychogenic Reactions

- Cause
  - A **psychogenic reaction** is an emotional or anxiety response to the injection procedure.
- Symptoms
  - Vasodepressor syncope (fainting) and hyperventilation are most common.[24,35]
  - Symptoms can be highly varied and may mimic drug reactions or other medical conditions.
  - Reactions reported by patients as allergies are often psychogenic in nature.

III. Local Complications

Local and topical anesthetics can cause a variety of local complications ranging from mild to severe; transient to permanent. The clinician is responsible to recognize, prevent, and manage any complications that may arise.

- Trismus: caused from trauma to muscles resulting in spasm of the jaw muscles that restricts opening or is painful; most often results from IA nerve block.
  - Prevention: use aseptic technique; avoid contaminating the needle; avoid repeated insertions into muscle.
  - Management: apply warm, moist cloth to outside of face; warm saline rinses; analgesics for pain; light physiotherapy to exercise jaw.
- Hematoma (bruise): Blood from a nicked artery or vein leaks into the surrounding tissue.
  - Prevention: minimize number of needle penetrations; know the anatomy of the area; do not use needle as a probe.
  - Management: apply ice and pressure to the area immediately, continue over next 6 hours (20 minutes on/20 minutes off) for first day; avoid aspirin for pain.
- Paresthesia: caused from physical trauma to nerve or chemical insult; generally lasts for short period (hours–days), but can be long-term, lasting months to years (permanent).[31-33,43]
  - Prevention: proper infection control (needle sterility) and handling of dental cartridge (do not immerse in solutions, e.g., alcohol); thorough assessment to determine whether to administer 4% solution for an IA nerve block.
  - Evidence has shown an increased risk of paresthesia from injecting with a 4% anesthetic (articaine or prilocaine).[32,44] The risk and benefit of use of a 4% solution must be considered when choosing a local anesthetic.
  - Management: reassure patient; determine extent of paresthesia and document; re-evaluate 1–2 months for any changes; refer to oral surgeon for consult if no improvement.
- Facial paralysis: from injecting anesthetic into parotid gland capsule.
  - Prevention: good IA injection technique; must touch periosteum prior to depositing; use alternative techniques: PDL, GG nerve block.
  - Management: discontinue treatment; manually close patient's eye (have patient remove contact lenses if wearing them) on affected side, place a gauze patch over eye and tape closed; paralysis lasts as long as the duration of soft-tissue anesthesia.
- Broken needle: caused from bending the needle, sudden movement by patient, using smaller gauge needles for deep insertions (e.g., 30 gauge); inserting needle to the hub.
  - Prevention: use larger-gauge needles (25 or 27); do not insert the needle to the hub; do not bend the needle; do not force against resistance.
  - Management: instruct patient to keep mouth open, do not allow the patient to close; if visible, use a hemostat or locking cotton pliers to remove needle from soft tissue; if unable to retrieve, refer to oral surgeon for consult.
- Epithelial desquamation (tissue sloughing): may follow prolonged application of topical anesthetic.
  - Prevention: apply topical anesthetic correctly (follow manufacturer's instructions); avoid high concentrations of vasoconstrictor (1:50,000 on palatal injections).
  - Management: topical analgesics for pain.
- Infection: caused by nonsterile technique; injecting into an area of infection.
  - Prevention: use sterile armamentarium; change needle if injecting into area of infection.

- Management: evaluate as soon as possible; antibiotics may need to be prescribed.
- Pain on injection: caused by careless injection technique; fast rate of deposit; using a dull or barbed needle.
  - Prevention: follow proper injection technique; use topical anesthetic prior to injection; use a sharp needle; slow rate of deposit; anesthetic solutions need to be kept at room temperature.
- Burning on injection: low pH of anesthetic solution containing a vasoconstrictor; contaminated solutions.
  - Prevention: use a higher pH solution; inject small amount of a plain local anesthetic solution prior to injecting local anesthetic with a vasoconstrictor (patient will then not feel burning from the low pH of anesthetic with a vasoconstrictor).
  - Management: reassure patient; will subside by the time the injection is completed. May also consider using a buffered local anesthetic.
- Self-inflicted soft-tissue injury*: occurs mainly in children.*
  - Prevention: use shorter duration local anesthetics; inform parent/caregiver of duration of soft-tissue anesthesia; insert cotton roll to prevent biting of lip.
  - Management: analgesics for pain; lukewarm saline rinses; topical analgesics.

Advantages and Disadvantages of Local Anesthesia

I. Advantages

- Patient experiences no pain or discomfort during treatment procedure.
- Clinician has increased confidence to provide complete treatment when the patient is pain-free.
- Local effect results in loss of sensation in area of treatment without a change in level of consciousness or patient cooperation.
- Completely reversible without residual side effects.
- Rapid onset of action.
- Adequate duration of clinical action that is reasonably predictable and that can be varied by choice of commercially available drugs.
- Relatively free of allergic reactions.
- Achieves hemostasis if injected directly into area where bleeding is a factor.

II. Disadvantages

- Anticipating and receiving dental injections may cause high anxiety for patient. Effects may include:
  - Need for special anxiety reduction technique.
  - Undesirable psychogenic reactions.
  - Avoidance of needed care.
- Significant potential exists for toxicity (overdose).
- There are systemic side effects from both the local anesthetic drug and vasoconstrictor.
- Potential for soft-tissue injury post injection, especially for the pediatric population and mentally challenged adolescents and adults.

Noninjectable Anesthesia

The anesthetic drugs are applied to the surface of the oral tissues including pocket lining tissue making this a topical application of anesthesia. Various formulations for dentistry include gels, creams, liquids and sprays.

- Trade name: Oraqix.
- Drugs: 2.5% lidocaine and 2.5% prilocaine; subgingival liquid-to-gel delivery thermosetting system.
- Indications: adults who require localized anesthesia during scaling and/or root debridement; initial or maintenance treatment of periodontal pockets where profound pulpal anesthesia is not needed; needle phobic adults.
- Onset: ~1 minute; duration: ~20 minutes with a range of 14–31 minutes.
- MRD: five cartridges/appointment.
- Pregnancy category: B (see Box 36-3).
- Contraindicated: allergy to lidocaine or prilocaine; history of methemoglobinemia; children (not approved for use).[34]
- Precautions: do not inject.

I. Armamentarium and Pharmacology

A unique dispenser with a blunt-tipped applicator delivers a gel containing both lidocaine and prilocaine into the periodontal pocket. Both the dispenser and the anesthetic gel are contraindicated for injections.[45]

- Dispenser cartridge and blunt-tipped applicator
  - Packaged together; for single-patient use.
  - For use only with special dispenser and not for injection.

- Blunt-tipped applicator is individually bent by clinician with either a single or double bend.
- Cartridge contains 42.5 mg lidocaine and 42.5 mg prilocaine; 1.7 mL cartridge.
- Store at room temperature.

- Anesthetic gel composition
  - Anesthetics: 2.5% lidocaine and 2.5% prilocaine amide anesthetics.
  - Poloxamers: thermosetting agents.
  - pH adjuster: hydrochloric acid.
  - Purified water.
- Anesthetic gel characteristics
  - Low-viscosity fluid at room temperature.
  - Gel at oral temperature.

Topical Anesthesia

- A topical anesthetic is a drug applied directly to the surface of the mucous membrane to produce a loss of sensation.
- A topical anesthetic is used with varying degrees of success for short-duration desensitization of the gingiva and oral mucosa, but it does not affect pulpal anesthesia.
- Terminal nerve endings 2–5 mm beneath surface are anesthetized.[24,46]
- Topical anesthetic is not a substitute for local anesthetic administered by injection.

I. Indications for Use

A topical anesthetic can be used conservatively for selected dental hygiene and dental services, including the following:

- Reduce discomfort of an injection.
- Prevention of gagging in radiographic techniques and impression taking.
- Temporary relief of pain from localized diseased areas, such as oral ulcers, wounds, or inflammation.
- Suture removal.

II. Action of a Topical Anesthetic

- Purpose
  - The purpose of a topical anesthetic is to desensitize the mucous membrane by anesthetizing the terminal nerve endings.
  - The superficial anesthesia produced is related to the amount of absorption of the drug by the tissue.
- Factors that affect efficacy
  - Type of drug.
  - Duration of application.
  - Site of application: thickness of stratified squamous epithelial covering; degree of keratinization.
    - Highly resistant: skin, lips, palatal mucosa.
    - Slow absorption: attached gingiva, palatal gingiva.
    - Fast absorption: tissue without keratinization, such as vestibular mucosa.

III. Agents Used in Surface Anesthetic Preparations

Table 36-6 provides onset and duration of topical anesthetics.

- Benzocaine (ester)
  - Types and formulations: Used in 6–20% (20% most common in dentistry) formulations;

Table 36-6 Topical and Noninjectable Anesthetic Characteristics

Types	Drug	Maximum Recommended Dose	Onset	Duration
Noninjectable local anesthetic	Amide *2.5% Lidocaine and 2.5% prilocaine*	Five cartridges per appointment	~1 min	14–31 min 20 min average
Topical anesthetics	Ester *Benzocaine* (6–20%)	No established MRD; follow manufacturer's recommendations	30 sec–2 min	5–15 min
	Ester *Tetracaine* (0.25–0.5%); combined with other drugs	20 mg (1 mL of 2% solution)	Slow, up to 20 min	20–60 min
	Amide *Lidocaine ointment* (2% and 5%)	2% and 5%—200 mg	1–2 min	15 min

available as liquid, gel, ointment, spray, and gel patch; most widely used topical agent.
  - Onset: 30 seconds–2 minutes; duration: 5–15 minutes.
  - Not readily absorbed into circulation; potential for toxicity is minimal.
  - May cause allergic reaction at site of application after prolonged or repeated use.
  - Precautions: fast absorption on nonkeratinized tissue—concern for toxicity; can cause methemoglobinemia (dose related); children.
  - Pregnancy category: C (see Box 36-3).
- Tetracaine HCl (ester)
  - Types and formulations: used in 0.25–0.5% formulations; typically available as part of a combination of drugs in liquid, gel, and controlled-dose spray.
  - Most potent; readily absorbed causing deeper penetration, longer effect, and more potential for toxicity. Not to be used over a large area.
  - Onset: slow, within 20 minutes; duration: 20–60 minutes.
  - Precautions: rapid absorption on mucous membranes, abraded tissues; children.
  - Pregnancy category: C (see Box 36-3).
- Lidocaine HCl (amide)
  - Types and formulations: used in 2% or 5% formulations; available in ointment, metered spray, and in combination with prilocaine.
  - The only amide used alone as a topical.
  - Toxicity unlikely from topical alone but would be additive with other amide anesthetics. Greatest risk from sprays.
  - Onset: 1–2 minutes, peak between 5 and 10 minutes; duration: 15 minutes.
  - Precautions: abraded tissues; large areas; children.
  - Pregnancy category: B (see Box 36-3).
- Dyclonine HCl (ketone)
  - Types and formulations: 0.5% or 1% formulation from a compounding pharmacy; available as a liquid, lozenges, and spray.
  - As a gargle is good for gag reflex suppression.
  - Onset: slow, up to 10 minutes; duration: 30 minutes (average), but up to 1 hour.
  - Precautions: abraded tissues; reduce dosage in children and medically compromised adults.
  - Pregnancy category: C (see Box 36-3).

IV. Topical Drug Mixtures

- Eutectic mixture of local anesthetics (EMLA; amide)
  - EMLA is a combination of two or more drugs and provides more rapid onset on intact skin.
  - Types and formulations: 2.5% lidocaine and 2.5% prilocaine; cream; lidocaine and prilocaine periodontal gel (Oraqix).
  - Pregnancy category: B (see Box 36-3).
- Benzocaine, butamben, and tetracaine (ester)
  - Types and formulations: 14% benzocaine, 2% butamben, 2% tetracaine; as a liquid, spray, and gel.
  - Onset: rapid, less than 1 minute; duration: 30–60 minutes.
  - Pregnancy category: C (see Box 36-3).
  - Precautions: fast absorption into tissues—higher risk for toxicity; not to be injected.

V. Adverse Reactions of Topical Anesthetics

- Ester topical anesthetics have a higher incidence of allergic reactions from primary metabolite, PABA.
- Redness.
- Tissue sloughing.
- Edema.
- Pain and burning at site.
- Greater risk of toxicity compared to local anesthetics (higher drug concentrations and no vasoconstrictor).

Application of Topical Anesthetic

I. Patient Preparation

- Consult medical and dental history for pertinent information concerning patient's previous experiences with anesthetics. A patient with an allergy to a local anesthetic may also be allergic to a topical anesthetic.
- Determine the most appropriate anesthetic agent and method of application.
- Explain purpose and anticipated effect to the patient.

II. Application Techniques

Several application techniques are available. Not all methods are applicable to all products. Select the most appropriate method from the following:

- Surface application
  - May be used with liquid, gel, or ointment formulations of any of the available topical agents.

- Topical is applied with a cotton-tipped swab or cotton roll.
- Time before becoming effective varies with the drug used.
- After application, excess topical is removed by rinsing or gentle wiping.

- Aerosol spray
  - Prevent inhalation by avoiding spray preparations when another method would be as effective. A spray must never be directed toward the throat.
  - Use metered- or controlled-dose spray dispensers to prevent overdose.

III. Completion of Topical Anesthetic Application

- Wait appropriate length of time for anesthetic to take effect before proceeding.
- Limit drug exposure.
  - Apply only to the area of need.
  - Use the smallest effective amount.
  - Remove residual drug after application time.
- Apply to a limited area when using a drug with a short duration of action for a long procedure such as scaling.
- Record topical anesthetic drug information in the patient's record.

New Developments in Pain Control

I. Anesthesia Reversal Agent

A. Properties

- Drug: phentolamine mesylate (trade name: OraVerse); nonselective alpha adrenergic blocking agent.
- Formulation: 0.4 mg/1.7 mL.
- Indications: reversal of soft-tissue anesthesia (~50% reduction time).[47-50] Recent research has shown that it may be less effective for reversal of pulpal anesthesia.[47]
- Metabolized by the liver and excreted by the kidneys.
- Onset: rapid; duration: 30–45 minutes.
- Dosage and MRD: 1:1 ratio (local anesthetic cartridge containing a vasoconstrictor).
- Contraindicated: children younger than 3 years of age and/or 33 lb (15 kg); postsurgical patients; post-PDL or intraosseous injections.
- Pregnancy category: C (see Box 36-3).

B. Advantages

- Patients can return to normal function faster.[47-50]
- Decrease risk of soft-tissue injury from prolonged anesthesia.

C. Technique

- Administered by injection in same location and with same technique as the local anesthesia being reversed approximately 20–30 minutes prior to the end of the procedure.
- Dosage:
  - Adult: 1:1 ratio; one cartridge of phentolamine mesylate per cartridge of anesthetic containing a vasoconstrictor, not to exceed two cartridges.
  - Children: (1/2 cartridge MRD).
- Candidates for use: adult patients with no contraindications to use; pediatric patients; geriatric patients; diabetic patients; special needs patient.
- Not candidates: sensitivity to phentolamine mesylate; children younger than 3 years of age or weighing less than 33 lb; postsurgical patients; (increased bleeding); history of MI, angina; coronary artery disease.

II. Buffered Local Anesthetic

A. Properties

- Buffered local anesthetic; sodium bicarbonate (8.4% neutralizing additive solution); Brands: Onset, Anutra.
- Increases the pH of the local anesthetic solution with a vasopressor to a more physiologic range.
- Reduces stinging on injection and provides faster onset.[51-55]
- Higher nerve block injection success and the need for a smaller concentration claims, needs further research.[52,54,55]
- Increased effectiveness in areas of inflammation.

B. Advantages

- Greater patient comfort.
- More rapid onset.
- Decreased postinjection tissue injury.

III. Intranasal Dental Anesthetic

A. Properties

- Drug: trade name: Kovonaze.
- FDA approval 2016.
- Intranasal anesthesia.

- 3% Tetracaine and 0.05% oxymetazoline (vasoconstrictor).
- Provides maxillary pulpal and soft-tissue anesthesia from first premolar to second premolar in the adjacent quadrant.
- Biotransformed: plasma.
- Excreted: kidneys.
- Half-life: 5.2 hours.

B. Advantages

- Anesthesia of maxillary teeth (#4–#13) with no needle.[56-59]
- Good for pediatric (88 lb [40 kg] or more) and needle phobic patients.

C. Contraindications and ADRs

- *Absolute contraindication:* known hypersensitivity to tetracaine, benzyl alcohol, other ester drugs, PABA, oxymetazoline; uncontrolled hypertension or thyroid disease.
- *Relative contraindications:* monoamine oxidase inhibitors, nonselective beta-blockers, TCAs, drugs causing methemoglobinemia, history of frequent nose bleeds.
- Adverse reactions: rhinorrhea, nasal congestion, increased lacrimation, nasal discomfort, oropharyngeal pain; asymptomatic increase in blood pressure.

IV. Periodontal Anesthetic Kit

- Properties
  - HurriPak (Beutlich LP Pharmaceuticals)
  - 20% benzocaine solution; plastic syringe (3 mL) and disposable plastic tips for insertion and deposition in gingival sulcus.
  - Onset of action is 30 seconds and duration of action is ~15 minutes.
  - If duration not adequate, additional injection techniques may be required.[60]

Documentation

Documentation in the permanent record for each appointment when a pain control drug or technique is used includes a minimum of the following factors:

- Date.
- Medical status and vital signs (both pre- and posttreatment). Document any contraindications to the administration of either the local anesthetic or vasoconstrictor.
- Review of dental and psychological history as it pertains to the administration of local anesthesia.
- Informed consent was obtained (oral and/or written).
- Rationale for pain control use.
- Location and type of injection.
- Time of administration.
- Number of cartridges; type and concentration of the local anesthetic including milligram of drugs administered.
- Type and concentration of vasoconstrictor including milligrams administered if applicable.
- Any adverse reactions that occurred.
- Posttreatment instructions given (specify written or oral).
- Full signature.
- Example documentation for a patient receiving nitrous oxide–oxygen conscious sedation is found in Box 36-2 and for a patient receiving local anesthesia in Box 36-5.

Factors to Teach the Patient

I. Nitrous Oxide–Oxygen Conscious Sedation

- Educate the patient about the importance of breathing through their nose while using nitrous oxide for the best result.
- Inform the clinician if the sedation becomes too strong or is too weak so that adjustments can be made. The level of sedation should be adjusted individually for optimum relaxation and comfort.
- Eat normally before treatment; avoid fasting or heavy meals.

II. Local and Topical Anesthesia

- Be careful not to bite lip, cheek, or tongue while tissues are without normal sensations. Warn and watch children to prevent injury. Do not test anesthesia by biting the lip.
- Avoid chewing hard foods and avoid hot food and drinks until normal sensation has returned.

References

1. National Institutes of Health. Oral Health in America: Advances and Challenges. U.S. Department of Health and Human Services, National Institute of Dental and Craniofacial Research, National Institutes of Health; 2021:790. Accessed October 9, 2022. https://www.nidcr.nih.gov/research/oralhealthinamerica
2. Silveira ER, Cademartori MG, Schuch HS, Armfield JA, Demarco FF. Estimated prevalence of dental fear in adults: a systematic review and meta-analysis. *J Dent*. 2021;108:103632.
3. Cianetti S, Lombardo G, Lupatelli E, et al. Dental fear/anxiety among children and adolescents: a systematic review. *Eur J Paediatr Dent*. 2017;18(2):121-130.
4. Doebling S, Rowe MM. Negative perceptions of dental stimuli and their effects on dental fear. *J Dent Hyg*. 2000;74(2):110-116.
5. Binkley CJ, Beacham A, Neace W, Gregg RG, Liem EB, Sessler DI. Genetic variations associated with red hair color and fear of dental pain, anxiety regarding dental care and avoidance of dental care. *J Am Dent Assoc*. 2009;140(7):896-905.
6. Randall CL, McNeil DW, Shaffer JR, Crout RJ, Weyant RJ, Marazita ML. Fear of pain mediates the association between MC1R genotype and dental fear. *J Dent Res*. 2016;95(10):1132-1137.
7. Smith EA, Marshall JG, Selph SS, Barker DR, Sedgley CM. Nonsteroidal anti-inflammatory drugs for managing postoperative endodontic pain in patients who present with preoperative pain: a systematic review and meta-analysis. *J Endod*. 2017;43(1):7-15.
8. Jeske A, Zahrowski J. Good evidence supports ibuprofen as an effective and safe analgesic for postoperative pain. *J Am Dent Assoc*. 2010;141(5):567-568.
9. Moore RA, Derry S, Aldington D, Wiffen PJ. Single dose oral analgesics for acute postoperative pain in adults: an overview of Cochrane reviews. *Cochrane Database Syst Rev*. 2015;(9):CD008659.
10. Moore PA, Ziegler KM, Lipman RD, Aminoshariae A, Carrasco-Labra A, Mariotti A. Benefits and harms associated with analgesic medications used in the management of acute dental pain: an overview of systematic reviews. *J Am Dent Assoc*. 2018;149(4):256-265.e3.
11. Hu L. Beyond nitrous oxide: sedation and anesthesia alternative in the dental office. *J Mass Dent Soc*. 69(4):10-14.
12. Clark MS, Brunick AL. *Handbook of Nitrous Oxide and Oxygen Sedation*. Mosby; 2008.
13. American Dental Association. *Guidelines for Use of Sedation and General Anesthesia by Dentists*. ADA; 2016:15. https://www.ada.org/en/search-results#q=sedation%20guidelines&t=all&sort=relevancy. Accessed October 27, 2021.
14. Sun R, Jia WQ, Zhang P, et al. Nitrous oxide-based techniques versus nitrous oxide-free techniques for general anaesthesia. *Cochrane Database Syst Rev*. 2015;(11):CD008984.
15. Tanchyk A, Tanchyk A. The absolute contraindication for using nitrous oxide with intraocular gases and other dental considerations associated with vitreoretinal surgery. *Gen Dent*. 2013;61(6):e6-7.
16. Lockwood AJ, Yang YF. Nitrous oxide inhalation anaesthesia in the presence of intraocular gas can cause irreversible blindness. *Br Dent J*. 2008;204(5):247-248.
17. Malamed S. *Sedation: A Guide to Patient Management*. 6th ed. Mosby; 2017.
18. National Institute for Occupational Safety and Health. *Control of Nitrous Oxide in Dental Operatories*. US Department of Health and Human Services,Public Health Services, CDC; 1996:4. https://www.cdc.gov/niosh/docs/hazardcontrol/hc3.html. Accessed October 27, 2021.
19. Donaldson M, Donaldson D, Quarnstrom FC. Nitrous oxide-oxygen administration: when safety features no longer are safe. *J Am Dent Assoc*. 2012;143(2):134-143.
20. Rowland AS, Baird DD, Weinberg CR, Shore DL, Shy CM, Wilcox AJ. Reduced fertility among women employed as dental assistants exposed to high levels of nitrous oxide. *N Engl J Med*. 1992;327(14):993-997.
21. Cohen EN, Gift HC, Brown BW, et al. Occupational disease in dentistry and chronic exposure to trace anesthetic gases. *J Am Dent Assoc*. 1980;101(1):21-31.
22. National Institute for Occupational Safety and Health. *Request for Assistance in Controlling Exposures to Nitrous Oxide during Anesthetic Administration*. US Department of Health and Human Services,Public Health Services, CDC; 1994. https://www.cdc.gov/niosh/docs/94-100/default.html. Accessed October 27, 2021.
23. Jastak JT, Malamed SF. Nitrous oxide sedation and sexual phenomena. *Dent Anaesth Sedat*. 1984;13(2):70-73.
24. Malamed SF. *Handbook of Local Anesthesia*. 7th ed. Elsevier Health Sciences; 2014.
25. Feuerstein J, Reimers N, Lerman M, Rosenberg M. What every dentist should know about cannabis. *J Mass Dent Soc*. 2017;66(3):20-26.
26. Patel RS, Manocha P, Patel J, Patel R, Tankersley WE. Cannabis use is an independent predictor for acute myocardial infarction related hospitalization in younger population. *J Adolesc Health*. 2020;66(1):79-85.
27. Moore PA, Hersh EV. Local anesthetics: pharmacology and toxicity. *Dent Clin North Am*. 2010;54(4):587-599.
28. Haas DA. An update on local anesthetics in dentistry. *J Can Dent Assoc*. 2002;68(9):546-551.
29. Rosenberg H, Pollock N, Schiemann A, Bulger T, Stowell K. Malignant hyperthermia: a review. *Orphanet J Rare Dis*. 2015;10(1):93.
30. Taleb M, Ashraf Z, Valavoor S, Tinkel J. Evaluation and management of acquired methemoglobinemia associated with topical benzocaine use. *Am J Cardiovasc Drugs*. 2013;13(5):325-330.
31. Ogle OE, Mahjoubi G. Local anesthesia: agents, techniques, and complications. *Dent Clin North Am*. 2012;56(1):133-148.
32. Haas DA, Lennon D. A 21 year retrospective study of reports of paresthesia following local anesthetic administration. *J Can Dent Assoc*. 1995;61(4):319-330.
33. Garisto GA, Gaffen AS, Lawrence HP, Tenenbaum HC, Haas DA. Occurrence of paresthesia after dental local anesthetic administration in the United States. *J Am Dent Assoc*. 2010;141(7):836-844.
34. Becker DE. Preoperative medical evaluation: part 2: pulmonary, endocrine, renal, and miscellaneous considerations. *Anesth Prog*. 2009;56(4):135-145.
35. Malamed SF. *Medical Emergencies in the Dental Office*. 7th ed. Elsevier Health Sciences; 2014.
36. American College of Obstetricians and Gynecologists. Oral Health care during pregnancy and through the lifespan. Published 2017. https://www.acog.org/en/clinical/clinical-guidance/committee-opinion/articles/2013/08/oral-health-care-during-pregnancy-and-through-the-lifespan. Accessed October 30, 2021.

37. American Dental Association. Pregnancy. Oral health topics. Published May 4, 2021. https://www.ada.org/en/member-center/oral-health-topics/pregnancy. Accessed October 30, 2021.
38. Moore PA. Adverse drug interactions in dental practice: interactions associated with local anesthetics, sedatives and anxiolytics. Part IV of a series. *J Am Dent Assoc*. 1999;130(4):541-554.
39. Becker DE. Adverse drug interactions. *Anesth Prog*. 2011;58(1):31-41.
40. Blanksma CJ, Brand HS. Cocaine abuse: orofacial manifestations and implications for dental treatment. *Int Dent J*. 2005;55(6):365-369.
41. Speca SJ, Boynes SG, Cuddy MA. Allergic reactions to local anesthetic formulations. *Dent Clin North Am*. 2010;54(4):655-664.
42. Bina B, Hersh EV, Hilario M, Alvarez K, McLaughlin B. True allergy to amide local anesthetics: a review and case presentation. *Anesth Prog*. 2018;65(2):119-123.
43. Moore PA, Haas DA. Paresthesias in dentistry. *Dent Clin North Am*. 2010;54(4):715-730.
44. Piccinni C, Gissi DB, Gabusi A, Montebugnoli L, Poluzzi E. Paraesthesia after local anaesthetics: an analysis of reports to the FDA Adverse Event Reporting System. *Basic Clin Pharmacol Toxicol*. 2015;117(1):52-56.
45. Food and Drug Administration. Drug Approval Package: Oraqix (Lidocaine and Prilocaine) NDA #021451. Published 2003. https://www.accessdata.fda.gov/drugsatfda_docs/nda/2003/021451s000_OraqixTOC.cfm. Accessed October 27, 2021.
46. Kumar M, Chawla R, Goyal M. Topical anesthesia. *J Anaesthesiol Clin Pharmacol*. 2015;31(4):450-456.
47. Hersh EV, Lindemeyer RG. Phentolamine mesylate for accelerating recovery from lip and tongue anesthesia. *Dent Clin North Am*. 2010;54(4):631-642.
48. Helmi M, AlDosari M, Tavares M. Phentolamine mesylate may be a safe and effective option to reduce discomfort and time to recovery after dental care with local anesthesia. *J Evid-Based Dent Pract*. 2018;18(2):181-184.
49. Prados-Frutos JC, Rojo R, González-Serrano J, et al. Phentolamine mesylate to reverse oral soft-tissue local anesthesia: a systematic review and meta-analysis. *J Am Dent Assoc*. 2015;146(10):751-759.
50. Elmore S, Nusstein J, Drum M, Reader A, Beck M, Fowler S. Reversal of pulpal and soft tissue anesthesia by using phentolamine: a prospective randomized, single-blind study. *J Endod*. 2013;39(4):429-434.
51. Kattan S, Lee SM, Hersh EV, Karabucak B. Do buffered local anesthetics provide more successful anesthesia than nonbuffered solutions in patients with pulpally involved teeth requiring dental therapy?: a systematic review. *J Am Dent Assoc 1939*. 2019;150(3):165-177.
52. Phero JA, Reside GJ, Turner BH, Phillips C, White R. A comparison of buffered and non-buffered 2% lidocaine with epinephrine, a pilot study. *J Oral Maxillofac Surg*. 2016;74(9):e41.
53. Malamed SF, Tavana S, Falkel M. Faster onset and more comfortable injection with alkalinized 2% lidocaine with epinephrine 1:100,000. *Compend Contin Educ Dent*. 2013;34 Spec No 1:10-20.
54. Saatchi M, Khademi A, Baghaei B, Noormohammadi H. Effect of sodium bicarbonate-buffered lidocaine on the success of inferior alveolar nerve block for teeth with symptomatic irreversible pulpitis: a prospective, randomized double-blind study. *J Endod*. 2015;41(1):33-35.
55. Hobeich P, Simon S, Schneiderman E, He J. A prospective, randomized, double-blind comparison of the injection pain and anesthetic onset of 2% lidocaine with 1:100,000 epinephrine buffered with 5% and 10% sodium bicarbonate in maxillary infiltrations. *J Endod*. 2013;39(5):597-599.
56. Ciancio SG, Hutcheson MC, Ayoub F, et al. Safety and efficacy of a novel nasal spray for maxillary dental anesthesia. *J Dent Res*. 2013;92(suppl 7):S43-S48.
57. Hersh EV, Pinto A, Saraghi M, et al. Double-masked, randomized, placebo-controlled study to evaluate the efficacy and tolerability of intranasal K305 (3% tetracaine plus 0.05% oxymetazoline) in anesthetizing maxillary teeth. *J Am Dent Assoc*. 2016;147(4):278-287.
58. Ciancio SG, Marberger AD, Ayoub F, et al. Comparison of 3 intranasal mists for anesthetizing maxillary teeth in adults: a randomized, double-masked, multicenter phase 3 clinical trial. *J Am Dent Assoc*. 2016;147(5):339-347.
59. Hersh EV, Saraghi M, Moore PA. Intranasal tetracaine and oxymetazoline: a newly approved drug formulation that provides maxillary dental anesthesia without needles. *Curr Med Res Opin*. 2016;32(11):1919-1925.
60. Lee HS. Recent advances in topical anesthesia. *J Dent Anesth Pain Med*. 2016;16(4):237-244.

CHAPTER 37

Instruments and Principles for Instrumentation

Uhlee (Yuri) Oh, RDH, MS
Linda D. Boyd, RDH, RD, EdD
Esther M. Wilkins, BS, RDH, DMD

CHAPTER OUTLINE

LEARNING OBJECTIVES

After studying this chapter, the student will be able to:

1. Identify the three main parts of a periodontal instrument.
2. Differentiate among various types of removal instruments based on their design.
3. State the indications and contraindications for the use of various removal instruments.
4. Describe and demonstrate fundamental techniques for manual and powered instrumentation.
5. Practice exercises designed to develop hand dexterity and prevent trauma.

Instrumentation begins with the knowledge of instrument parts and identification of each instrument during dental hygiene assessment and treatment.

- The fundamentals of instrumentation technique include:
  - Stabilization by means of a correct grasp and **fulcrum**.
  - Instrument **adaptation**, **angulation**, and **activation**.
- A study of oral and dental anatomy and histology needs to accompany learning instrumentation technique.
- Development of a thorough, efficient, and safe procedure for treatment depends on an understanding of the normal, healthy, and disease characteristics of the dental and periodontal tissues being treated.
- A high degree of skill in the care and use of the instruments is required.
- Skill depends on knowledge and understanding of the goals of therapy and how the goals can be reached through application of the fundamental principles of instrumentation.

Overview of Periodontal Instruments

Periodontal instruments refer to instruments used around ("perio") the teeth ("odont"). With the increasing number of periodontal instruments available, it is essential to understand the fundamentals of instrument design and basic principles of periodontal instrumentation.

I. Instrument Classification

Periodontal instruments can be classified into two main categories: assessment and deposit removal instruments. Each category serves a different purpose, which dictates the design of the instrument.

A. Assessment Instruments

- Instruments used for assessment include the mouth mirror, explorers, and periodontal probes. These instruments are described in Chapter 20.
- This chapter focuses on instruments used for scaling and nonsurgical periodontal treatment procedures.

B. Removal Instruments

- Consist of instruments used for **scaling**, or removal of hard and soft dental deposits.
- Includes manual **scalers**, manual **curets**, periodontal files, and powered scalers.

II. Instrument Identification

A. Instrument Design

- Each instrument can be identified at a glance by instrument design.
- The ability to quickly identify instruments contributes to organization of instrument cassettes and efficiency of services rendered.

- In instances when an instrument cannot be quickly identified visually, the clinician can refer to the instrument design name and number labeled on the instrument handle.

B. Design Name

- Instruments are often named after the institution or individual responsible for their design or development.
- Popular instruments named after *institutions* include the UNC-15 probe (University of North Carolina at Chapel Hill), TU-17 explorer (Tufts University), and ODU-11/12 explorer (Old Dominion University).
- Popular instruments named after *individuals* include the Gracey curets (named after Dr. Clayton H. Gracey) and the Nevi scalers (named after craftsman Neville Hammond).

C. Design Number

- Instruments are also designated with a number following the design name.
- This number indicates the specific design of the working end and the area of the dentition indicated for use.
- The same instrument may be made by various manufacturers using the same design number.

Instrument Design

The three major parts of a periodontal instrument include the handle, shank, and working end. The relationship of these parts is illustrated by the curet in **Figure 37-1**.

I. Handle

Instrument handles come in various forms and designs. **Figure 37-2** shows a few types of handles available. Selecting efficient and comfortable, or ergonomic, handles can reduce the risk of developing musculoskeletal disorders of the hand and wrist.

A. Weight

- Handles may be heavy and composed of solid metal, or they may be lightweight and hollow.
- Handles with lighter weight enhance tactile sensitivity and lessen fatigue related to a tighter grasp.
- Ergonomic handles ideally weigh less than 15.0 g.[1]

B. Diameter

- Diameters of instrument handles vary widely from standard handles that are 6.5 mm in diameter to larger handles that are 10 mm in diameter.
- Instruments with thin, small-diameter handles increase muscle activity and pinch force, which over time can lead to musculoskeletal injuries.
- Ergonomic instruments have a 10-mm diameter handle.[1]

C. Texture

- Instrument handles may have either smooth or varying degrees of raised textures.
- A smooth handle may require a tighter grasp to prevent slipping in wet oral environments, which can lessen tactile sensitivity and increase clinician's fatigue.
- The textured handle created by ribbed or knurled patterns and serrations can provide better control with a firm, yet lighter grasp without lessening tactile sensitivity.[1]

II. Shank

- The **shank** is the portion of the instrument which connects the **working end** to the handle, as shown in Figure 37-1.
- The section of the shank between the working end and the first bend in the instrument closest to the working end is called the **terminal shank** or *lower shank*, as labeled in Figure 37-1. With many instruments, the terminal shank can provide a cue for correct working end identification and positioning for treatment.

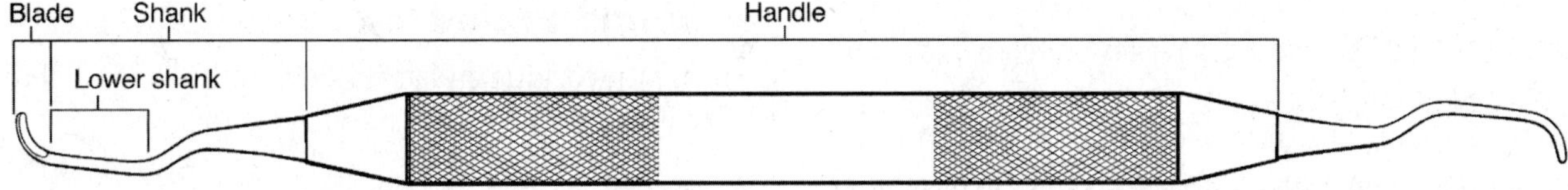

Figure 37-1 Parts of an Instrument. This curet shows the relationship of the working end (blade), shank, and handle. The section of the shank that extends from the blade to the first bend in the shank is referred to as the *terminal* or *lower shank*.

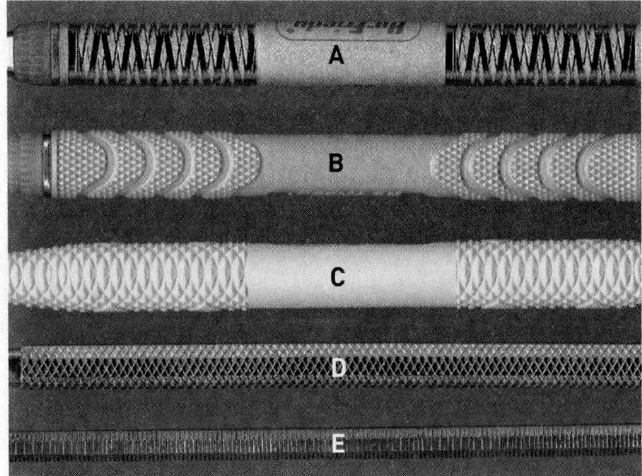

Figure 37-2 Handle Diameter and Texturing. The diameter and texturing of a handle varies greatly from manufacturer to manufacturer. Shown here are examples of the variations in design characteristics of instrument handles. Instruments (**A**, **B**, and **C**) with large diameter handles and raised textures would be easy to hold and reduce muscle fatigue. These instruments have additional texturing on the tapered portion of the handle to reduce muscle strain for short-fingered clinicians who must grip the tapered portion of the handle. Instrument (**D**) has a smaller diameter handle and less pronounced texturing. Instrument (**E**) has a small diameter handle and very limited texturing.

- The shape, length, and rigidity of the shank govern the access of the working end to various teeth and tooth surfaces in the mouth.

A. Shape

- Straight/simple: Fewer bends and flat nature of an instrument shank make it ideal for adaptation to tooth surfaces with easy access, such as anterior teeth.
- Angled/complex: Contains many bends in the shank, which makes it ideal for adaptation to tooth surfaces that are difficult to access, such as proximal surfaces of posterior teeth.
  - In general, the more difficult it is to access the tooth surface, the more and deeper bends there are in the instrument shank.
  - Examples: Gracey curets 11/12, 13/14, and 15/16 are used on posterior teeth and have three bends.
  - Because the distal surfaces of molars and premolars are much less accessible than the mesial surfaces, the angles in the shank of the 13/14 are designed with deeper bends than the 11/12 to make access possible.

B. Length

- The distance from the working end to the junction between the shank and handle in most instruments is 35–40 mm (1.5 inches).
- Too short a distance limits action subgingivally.
- Extended lower shank length:
  - Adding on 3 mm permits the blade to access deep pockets along narrow roots and into furcation areas.[2]
  - Examples: after five, mini-five, and micro-mini five curets.

C. Rigidity

- Instruments are made with shanks of varying degrees of thickness and rigidity appropriate for their purpose.
- Rigid: A thicker shank is stronger and is able to withstand greater pressure applied during instrumentation. More rigid instruments are needed for removal of heavy calculus deposits that are firmly attached to the tooth surface.
- Flexible: A thinner shank may provide more tactile sensitivity and may be used for removal of finer deposits of calculus and for root debridement.

III. Working End

- The working end refers to the part of the instrument used to carry out its purpose and function. Each instrument has a distinctive working end.
- The working end of a scaler or curet is called a **blade**.
- The parts of a blade of a curet are illustrated in **Figure 37-3**. The blades of both a scaler and curet include the following:
  - Face—the inner surface of the blade opposite to the back.
  - Back—the outer surface of the blade opposite to the face.
  - Lateral surfaces—the sides of the blade that converge to form the *back* of the instrument.
  - Cutting edge—where the *face* and the lateral surface meet to form the sharp line or edge of a scaler or curet.

A. Single-Ended

There is a working end attached to only one end of the instrument handle (e.g., mouth mirror).

B. Double-Ended; Unpaired

There are working ends attached to both ends of the instrument handle, but working ends differ in design

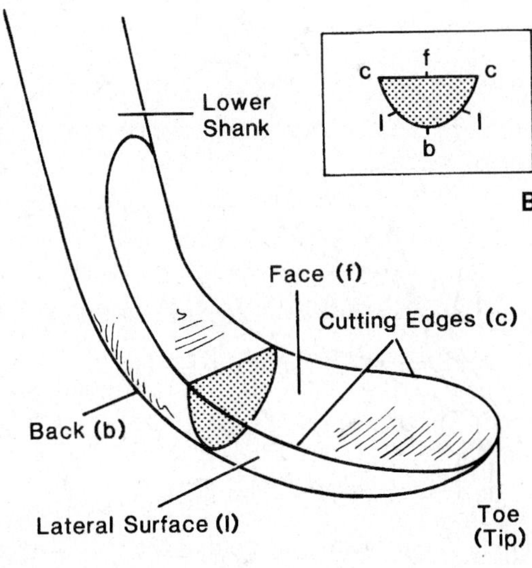

Figure 37-3 Parts of a Curet Blade. **A:** Curet with parts labeled. The curet has a rounded toe, whereas the scaler has a pointed tip. **B:** Semi-circular cross-section of a curet.

and function (e.g., probe on one end and explorer on the other end).

C. Double-Ended; Paired

The working ends attached to both ends of the instrument handle are mirror images of each other. One end is used for access from the facial/buccal and the other end from the lingual/palatal on the same tooth (e.g., universal curet).

Grasps and Fulcrum

I. Dominant Hand

- During periodontal instrumentation, the **dominant hand** is used to grasp and activate the treatment instrument.
- The manner in which the instrument is held influences the entire procedure.
- The appropriate grasp is controlled, displays the confidence of the clinician in the work being done, and provides the following effects:
  - Prevention of fatigue to clinician's fingers, hands, and arms.
  - Positive control of the instrument with balance and flexibility during motion.
  - Decreased hazard of trauma to the dental and periodontal tissues, which in turn results in less post-care discomfort for the patient.
  - Increased fingertip tactile sensitivity.
- A tight grasp lessens the tactile sensitivity and, hence, the effectiveness of instrumentation.

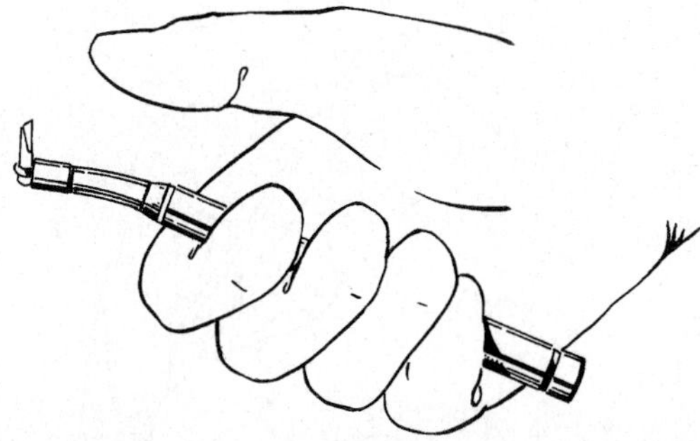

Figure 37-4 Palm Grasp of Instrument. The instrument handle is held in the palm by cupping the index, middle, ring, and little fingers. Thumb is free and serves as the finger rest.

II. Nondominant Hand

- The **nondominant hand** is often used for essential supplementary functions to assist the dominant hand.
- The following are functions of the nondominant hand:
  - To use the mouth mirror for indirect vision, indirect lighting, and retraction.
  - To assist in providing the dominant hand with an auxiliary finger rest.

III. Palm Grasp

- Description: The handle of the instrument is held in the palm of the clinician's dominant or nondominant hand by cupping the index, middle, ring, and little fingers (**Figure 37-4**).
- Used to grasp:
  - Air/water syringe.
  - Periodontal instruments with nondominant hand when adjusting the light with dominant hand.
  - Periodontal instruments with nondominant hand when stabilizing the instrument for sharpening.

IV. Modified Pen Grasp

- The modified pen grasp is a three-finger grasp with specific target points of the thumb, index finger, and middle finger all in contact with the instrument (**Figure 37-5**).
- The instrument is held by the pads of the thumb and index fingers, placed opposite of each other on the handle.
- The inner corner of the middle finger is placed on the upper portion of the shank to guide the movement of the instrument, to prevent the

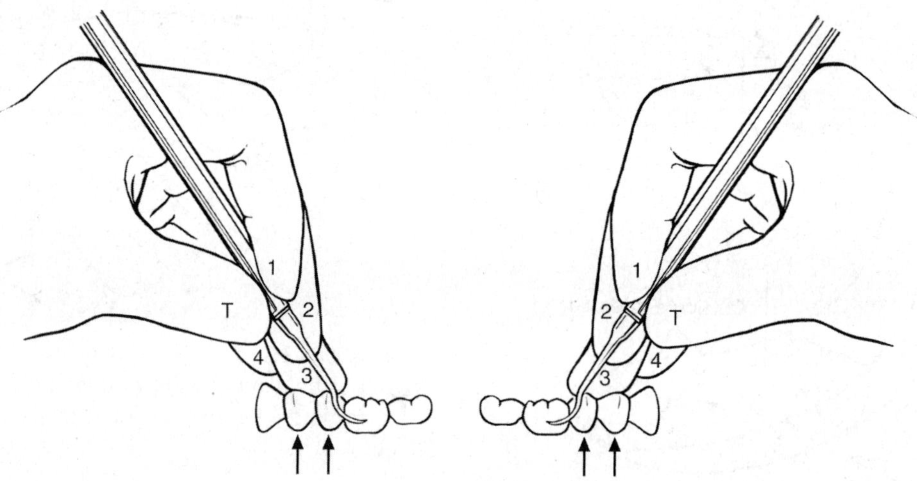

Figure 37-5 Modified Pen Grasp for Left and Right Hands. An instrument is held by the thumb (T), index finger, and (1) the second, or "middle," finger (2), which also provides support. The third, or "ring," finger (3) serves as the finger rest, and the fourth, or "little," finger (4) is positioned beside the ring finger to supplement the finger rest.

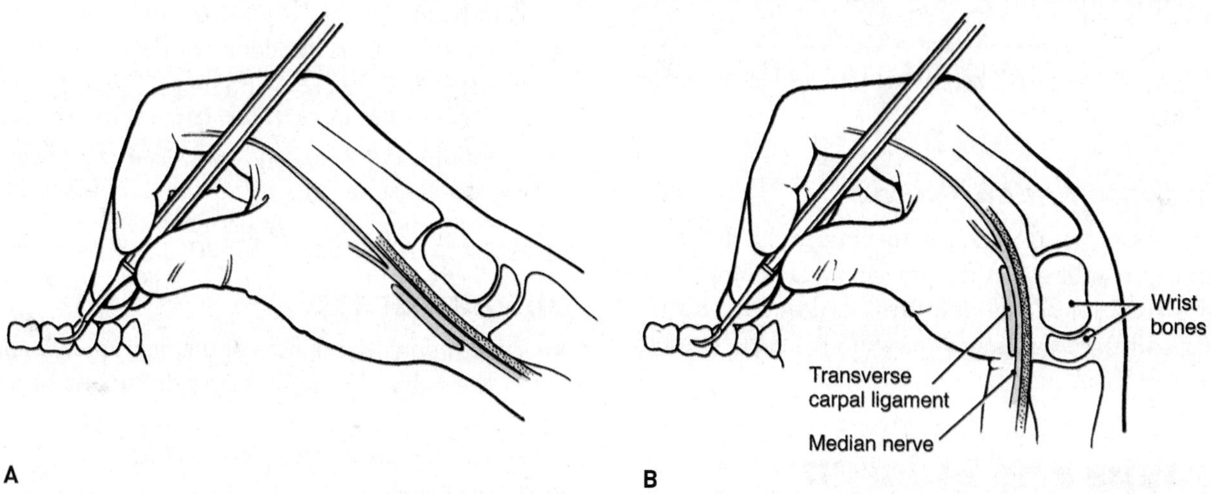

Figure 37-6 Effect of Wrist Position. **A:** Wrist in neutral position in straight line with forearm. **B:** Bent wrist shows cramping of median nerve in the carpal tunnel of the wrist. Repeated pressure on the median nerve can cause carpal tunnel syndrome.

instrument from slipping during adaptation and activation, and to optimize application of lateral pressure.

- The ring finger is used to establish a finger rest/fulcrum.
- The side-to-side contact of the index, middle, and ring fingers allows for greater stability, strength, and control during instrumentation.

V. Neutral Wrist

- A neutral wrist is important to prevent carpal tunnel syndrome, a musculoskeletal disorder brought on by pressure on the median nerve in the carpal tunnel due to inappropriate work habits, such as working with a bent wrist.[3]
- During instrumentation, the wrist should be straight, and the forearm and hand are in the same horizontal plane when in the neutral position.
- **Figure 37-6** illustrates the straight wrist versus a bent wrist.

VI. Fulcrum

A fulcrum is the support, or point of rest, on which a lever turns or pivots.

A. Purpose

- An effective, well-established fulcrum is essential for the following reasons:
  - Stability—provides a focal point from which the whole hand can move as a unit.

- Control of unit and **stroke**—allows controlled action of the instrument and limits instrumentation to where it is needed.
- Prevention of injury—prevents irregular pressure and uncontrolled movement that can cause injury to the patient's oral tissues.
- Patient comfort—patients may sense a securely applied instrument, which may increase their confidence in the clinician's ability.
- Allows for stability and control of instrument during activation (strokes) compared to the patient's chin, lips, and cheeks, which are less reliable because they are mobile and flexible.
- Prevents accidental finger injury during instrumentation if the patient were to move suddenly or the instrument were to slip.
- Promotes an effective grasp.

B. Intraoral Fulcrum

- The intraoral fulcrum is a finger rest inside the patient's mouth that serves to provide stabilization of the hand during instrumentation.
- **Figure 37-7** shows the fingers grouped together with the fulcrum established where the ring finger maintains its position on a tooth adjacent to the tooth being treated.
- The ideal finger rest or fulcrum:
  - Is a firm and stable tooth adjacent to the tooth being treated.
  - Is in the same arch and quadrant as the tooth being instrumented when possible.
  - Allows convenient access to the working area.
  - Allows for easy instrument adaptation.

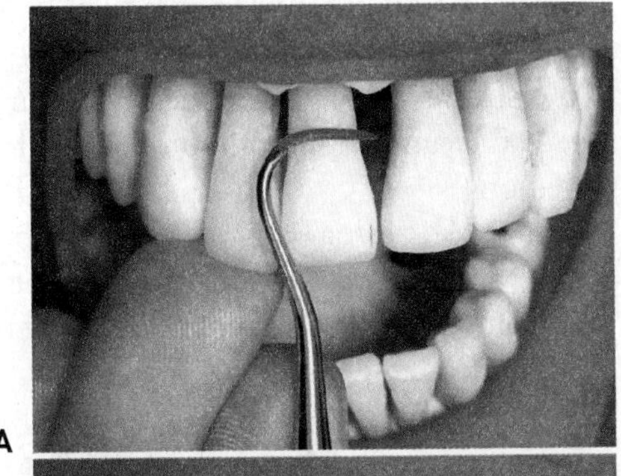

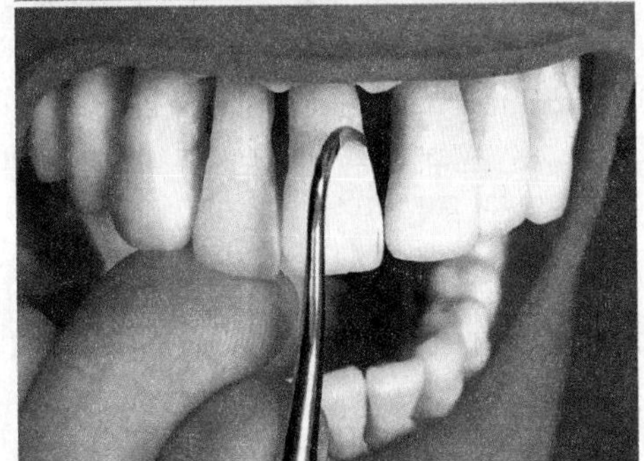

Figure 37-7 Instrument Adaptation. Sickle scaler adaptation at the line angle of an anterior tooth.
A: Incorrect adaptation can result in soft-tissue trauma and discomfort for the patient. **B:** Correct adaptation as a result of rolling the instrument handle.

C. Extraoral Fulcrum

- An intraoral fulcrum cannot always be established. In areas that are difficult to access such as maxillary posterior regions, an extraoral fulcrum may be more effective.[4]
- Entails maximizing the contact of the clinician's instrumentation hand with the patient's face.
- Cheek and chin are most commonly used.
- A secure fulcrum is dependent on pressure against the face and underlying bone.
- The grasp on the instrument will need to be modified so that it is farther from the working end than what is used with a traditional intraoral fulcrum.

D. Alternative Fulcrums

- In some instances, establishing an intraoral or extraoral fulcrum may not be possible or sufficient due to the following reasons:
  - Limited access to posterior teeth.
  - Limited access to tenacious calculus in difficult to reach areas (e.g., deep periodontal pockets) where greater support and pressure are required for instrumentation.[5]
  - Patient's facial musculature.
  - Small mouth (microstomia).
  - Difficulty opening the mouth (trismus).
  - Large tongue (macroglossia).
  - Crowding and malalignment of individual teeth.
  - Physical disabilities interfering with the oral cavity.
- In such cases, an alternative fulcrum may be used; however, basic rules for stability and control are still applied, and fulcrums on movable tissues are avoided.
- Three types of variations are suggested here: substitute, supplementary, and reinforced finger rests.
  - Substitute finger rest: used for missing or mobile teeth.
    - For an edentulous area, a cotton roll or gauze sponge may be packed into the

area to provide a dry finger rest. Otherwise, a rest across the dental arch or in the opposite arch may be required to provide stability.
        - For mobile teeth with inadequate bony support, use only with minimal pressure for brief periods, or avoid altogether for finger rests since they are unstable and undue stress on the tooth could traumatize and tear the periodontal ligament fibers.
        - For areas with inadequate space or visibility, an index finger of the nondominant hand may be placed in the vestibule over a cotton roll or a dry gauze square, and the usual finger rest can be placed on the index finger to aid retraction and visibility, particularly in the mouth of a small child.
    - Supplementary finger rest: also known as a "finger-on-finger" rest.
        - Place the index finger of the nondominant hand on the occlusal surfaces of teeth adjacent to the working area to serve as a fulcrum for the dominant ring finger.
        - Such supplements are helpful for achieving a parallel orientation of the terminal shank to proximal surfaces.
    - Reinforced finger rest: used to provide additional strength and force, particularly for tenacious calculus in pockets.[5]
        - Index finger of nondominant hand can be rested on the tooth adjacent to the one being scaled, while the thumb is placed on the instrument shank (or handle) for reinforcement.
        - When applied correctly, greater control of the instrument can result, and the danger of instrument breakage is reduced.
        - A stable fulcrum for both hands is needed to distribute the pressure.

Instrumentation Basics

I. Adaptation

- With an appropriate grasp and fulcrum, the instrument is ready for application. The working end of the instrument is adapted to the surface of the tooth where instrumentation will take place.
- Select the correct end of a double-ended paired instrument.
- The blade of an instrument is divided into thirds, referred to as the heel-third, the middle-third, and the tip- or toe-third.
- The side of the tip- or toe-third is adapted to the contour of the tooth surface being examined or treated for maximum usefulness.
- About 2–3 mm of the toe-third of a curet may be adaptable to a "flat" tooth surface, whereas less than 2 mm of tooth surface may be adaptable at a line angle or convex surface of a narrow root.
    - As the instrument is activated, it is adapted to changes required by variations in the tooth surface topography.
- All line angles require the instrument be rolled between the fingers as the instrument is activated to turn the working end to keep the toe- or tip-third adapted to the tooth surface.
- At each change of direction around a line angle, the instrument must be rolled.
- Figure 37-7 shows the adaptation of a sickle scaler tip to a line angle.
- Additional areas requiring more attention, time, and careful application of skill include convex/rounded surfaces and concave grooves.
    - A properly adapted instrument should not harm the tooth surface being treated or the surrounding or adjacent tissues.

II. Angulation

- Angulation refers to the angle formed between the working end of an instrument and the tooth surface.
- Each instrument is applied to a tooth surface in a specific manner for optimum adaptation and angulation.
    - Probe: The usual angulation of a probe is to maintain the side of the tip on the tooth, keeping the long axis of the working end parallel to the root surface.
    - Explorer: The side of the explorer tip is kept adapted to the tooth at all times (at an angle of approximately 5° or less) to feel for changes in the tooth surface, such as roughness. Chapter 20 illustrates the use of the subgingival explorer.
    - Scalers and curets: Angulation refers to the angle formed by the face of the blade with the tooth surface to which the instrument is applied.
        - At 0° ("closed") angulation, the face of a curet is flat against the tooth surface (**Figure 37-8A**). This is crucial to prevent soft tissue trauma when inserting the blade beneath the gingival margin.
        - For both curets and scalers, a 70° ("open") angulation between the face of the

instrument and the tooth surface permits effective calculus removal (**Figure 37-8B**).
  - Attempting to remove calculus at a 0° closed angulation uses only the lateral surface of a sharp blade, which can result in the burnishing of calculus.
  - Burnishing produces a smooth veneer, making the calculus difficult or impossible to detect with an explorer.

III. Activation (Stroke)

- A stroke is an unbroken movement made by an instrument; it is the action of an instrument in the performance of the task for which it was designed.
- Stability—during a stroke, the whole hand pivots or rotates on the fulcrum.
- Motion—generated by a unified action of the shoulder, arm, wrist, and hand.
- Length—limited by the extent of calculus deposit and by the anatomic features of the area where the deposit is located.
- There are various types of strokes. Examples are the "probing or walking stroke," "exploratory or assessment stroke," "scaling or calculus removal stroke," or "root debridement stroke."

A. Lateral Pressure

- **Lateral pressure** refers to the pressure of the instrument applied against the tooth surface during activation.
- Types of pressure applied can be light, moderate, or heavy.

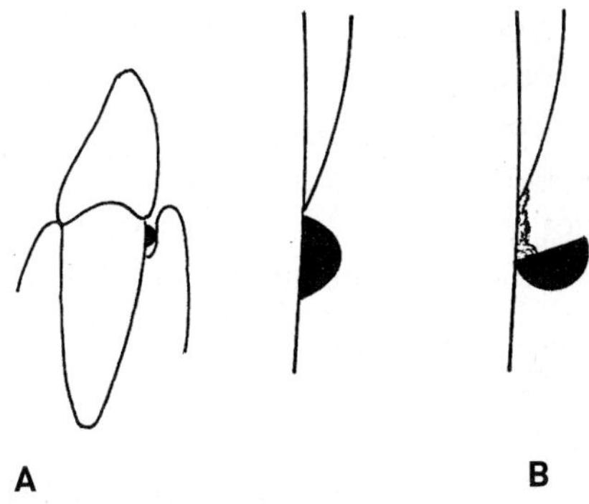

Figure 37-8 Instrument Angulation. Enlargement of pocket area from the tooth on the left shows cross-section of a curet blade in black. **A:** The face of the curet blade is closed, or angulated at 0° with the tooth surface during insertion into the pocket. At 0° the face of the blade is flat against the tooth surface. **B:** The face of the blade is opened or angulated at approximately 70° with the tooth surface for calculus removal.

- Balance of pressure: For control, a balance or an equalization of pressure is established between the pressure applied on the instrument blade against the tooth surface and the pressure on the fulcrum.
  - Keeping the two forces equal will facilitate stable, intentional control of the instrument as it is activated.
- Effects of excessive pressure:
  - Excess removal of tooth structure; gouging of root surfaces.
  - Loss of instrument control.
  - Potential damage to soft tissue, resulting in bleeding and possible laceration.
  - Patient discomfort; discomfort during healing later.
  - Clinician fatigue.

B. Direction

- Vertical: Strokes are parallel to the long axis of the tooth being treated (**Figure 37-9B**).
- Horizontal: Strokes are parallel to the occlusal surface of the tooth being treated (**Figure 37-9C**).
- Oblique: Strokes are diagonal to the long axis of the tooth being treated (**Figure 37-9A**).
- Figure 37-9 shows direction of strokes for various instruments.

C. Walking Stroke

- Used with a probe to move up and down in small increments, gently touching the base of the sulcus or pocket with each down stroke. (See Chapter 20.)
- Consists of a light grasp, light pressure, and vertical movement.

D. Exploratory/Assessment Stroke

- Used with explorers and removal instruments to maximize tactile sensitivity when assessing tooth

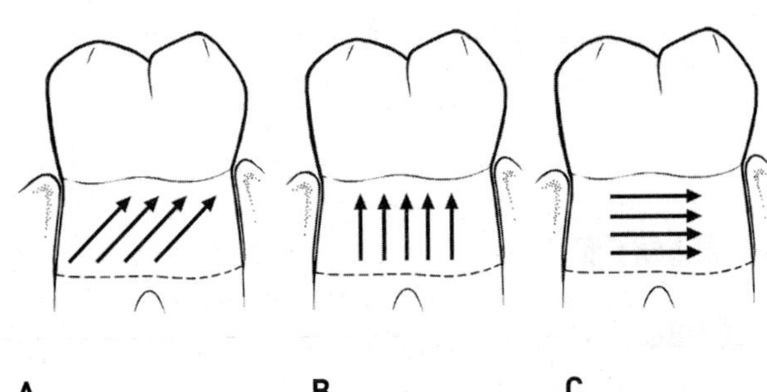

Figure 37-9 Directions of Instrument Strokes. Arrows on root surface represent diagonal or oblique strokes (**A**), vertical strokes (**B**), and horizontal strokes (**C**).

surfaces and detecting irregularities, such as the presence of:
    - Calculus.
    - Carious lesions.
    - Rough overhanging margins of crowns or restorations.
- Also used with manual/powered removal instruments to rehearse the movement of the instrument before activation to confirm correct adaptation.
- Consists of a light grasp, light pressure, and movement in vertical, horizontal, and oblique directions.

E. Scaling/Calculus Removal Stroke

- Used with manual removal instruments to remove calculus deposits.
- Short, well-controlled, and firm pull-stroke (emphasis on movement away from the base of the sulcus or pocket).
- Consists of a firm grasp, moderate-to-heavy pressure, and movement of the blade in vertical, horizontal, and oblique directions while keeping the instrument carefully adapted to the tooth.
- When transitioning from an assessment to removal stroke, the pressure on the tooth and fulcrum increases significantly to achieve stability and control of the instrument as it is activated.

F. Root Debridement Stroke

- Used when removing soft deposits from a tooth surface with minimal deposit.
- The grasp is consistent with the amount of lateral pressure placed on the blade to the tooth.
- Light-to-moderate lateral pressure (depending on the texture and consistency of the deposits encountered) is used in vertical, horizontal, and oblique directions.
    - When the texture of the deposits changes from grainy to heavy, the pressure on both the fulcrum and blade against the root surface will increase in order to remove the deposits.
    - Pressure is, therefore, responsive to the tactile information transmitted as the instrument progresses along the root surface.

Scalers

I. Uses

- **Scalers** are used principally for removal of supragingival calculus.
- May be useful for removal of gross calculus that is slightly below the gingival margin when it is continuous with the supragingival calculus, and when the gingival tissue is spongy and flexible to permit easy insertion of the instrument.[6] Extreme caution must be used since the pointed tip of the blade and back of the sickle scaler can traumatize the tissue.

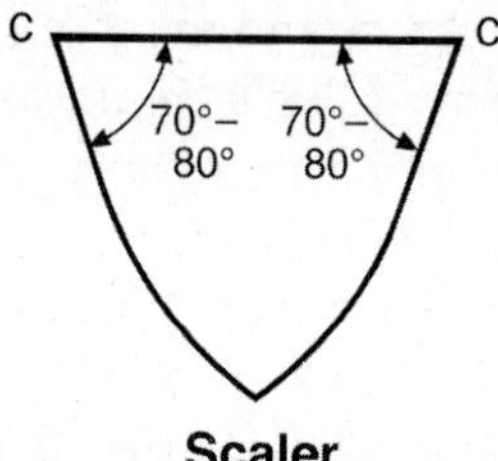

Figure 37-10 Internal Angles of a Scaler. Cross-section of a scaler shows the 70° to 80° internal angles. These angles are restored by sharpening techniques.

II. Instrument Design

A. Blade

- Two cutting edges.
- The face converges with the two lateral surfaces to form the tip of the scaler, which is a sharp point.
- Has a triangular cross-section with a V-shaped back (**Figure 37-10**).
- Internal angles of 70° to 80° are formed where the lateral surfaces meet the face at the cutting edges.

B. Shank

- Straight—unpaired instrument in which the relationships of the shank, blade, and handle are in a flat plane; adaptable primarily for anterior teeth, although may be used for scaling premolars when the lips and cheeks permit retraction for correct angulation.
- Modified or contra-angle—paired instruments are mirror images of each other to provide access to posterior teeth; one end adapts from the buccal and the other from the lingual and palatal aspects.

III. Types

A. Sickles

- A scaler with a curved blade is referred to as a "sickle" (**Figure 37-11**).
- Face of the blade is curved from a lateral view.

B. Jacquettes

- A straight-bladed scaler is referred to as a "Jacquette" (**Figure 37-12**).
- Face of the blade is straight from a lateral view.

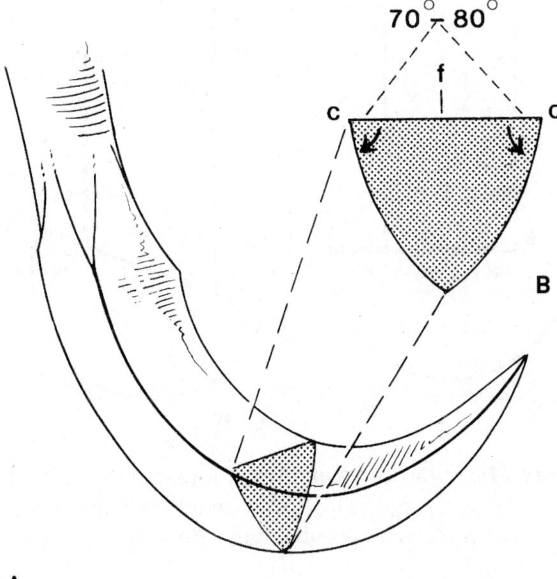

Figure 37-11 Curved Scaler (Sickle Scaler). **A:** The curved blade terminates in a point. **B:** Cross-section shows the face (f) and the two cutting edges (c) formed where the lateral surfaces meet the face at 70° to 80° angles. This type of scaler is also called a sickle scaler.

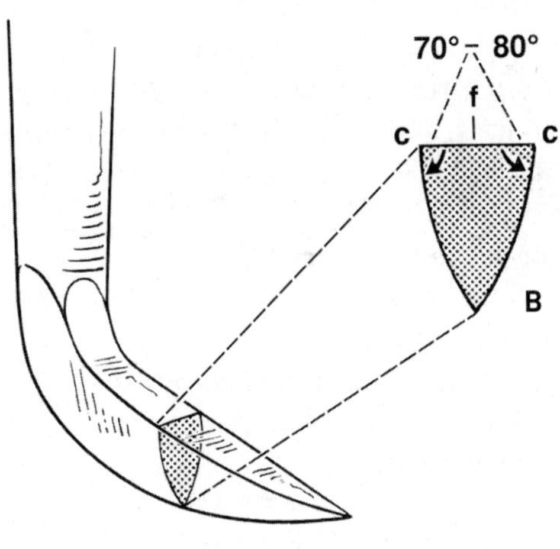

Figure 37-12 Straight Scaler (Jacquette). **A:** The straight blade converges to a point where the two cutting edges meet at the tip. **B:** Cross-section of the scaler shows the face (f), the two cutting edges (c), and the 70° to 80° internal angles. This type of scaler is also known as the Jacquette scaler.

IV. Scaler-Specific Instrumentation

- Adaptation: Tip-third or terminal third of the cutting edge is maintained on the tooth surface at all times. For the line angles, only the terminal 1–2 mm of the tip is used.
- Angulation: The face of the blade is adapted to the tooth surface at an angle of approximately 70°.
- Activation: Both light assessment strokes and heavy calculus removal strokes may be performed.
- Small scalers can be useful for removal of fine supragingival deposits directly under contact areas and between overlapping teeth.
- Tactile sensitivity is decreased with larger, heavier blades.
- The size, thickness, and length of large blades may cause undue trauma to the gingival tissue.
- Pointed tip and straight cutting edges cannot be adapted to the curved root surfaces.
- There is increased risk of gouging or scratching the cemental surface.

Curets

I. Uses

- **Curets** are used for removal of supra- and subgingival calculus and biofilm.
- Rounded back does not traumatize the gingival margin or base of sulcus or pocket when inserted subgingivally.
- Necessary after powered scaling to remove residual deposits or "fine scale" for completion of periodontal debridement.

II. Instrument Design

A. Blade

- Two cutting edges on a curved blade.
- The face converges with the two lateral surfaces to form a rounded toe.
- Has a semicircular cross-section with a rounded back (**Figure 37-13**).
- Internal angles of 70° to 80° are formed where the lateral surfaces meet the face at the cutting edges.
- Figure 37-3 shows a curet blade with each part labeled.

B. Shank

- Angles or curves in the shank are specific to each of the many different curets available.
- Slender shanks allow entrance into the sulcus or pocket with minimal trauma to the gingival margin.

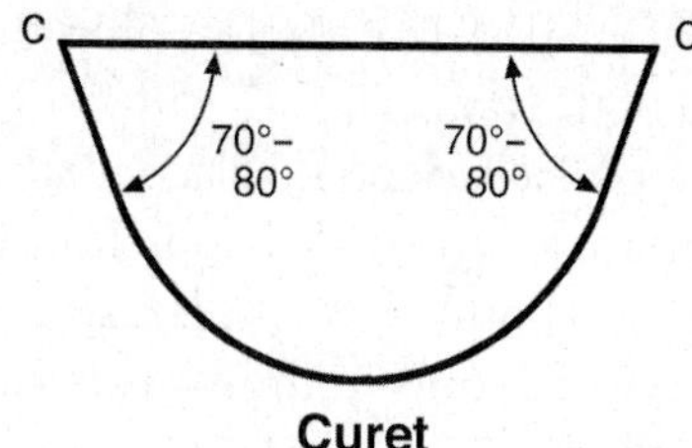

Figure 37-13 Internal Angles of a Curet. Cross-section of a curet shows the 70° to 80° internal angles at the cutting edges. These angles are restored by sharpening techniques.

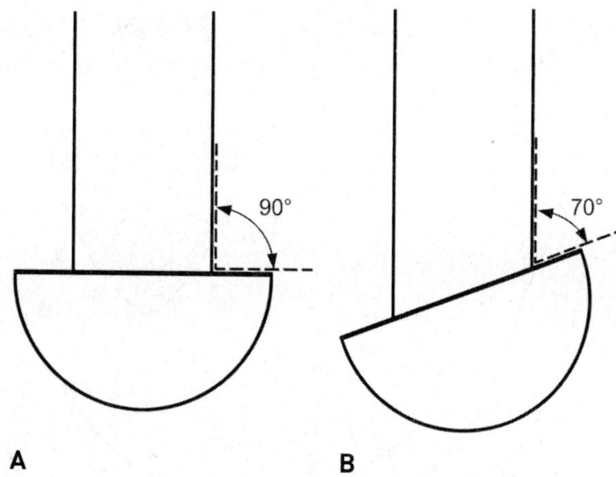

Figure 37-14 Curet Design. **A:** A universal curet with the blade at a 90° angle to the lower shank. **B:** Face of blade of an area-specific curet offset at a 70° angle to the lower shank.

III. Types

A. Universal Curets

- **Universal curets** can be adapted for supra- and subgingival instrumentation on any tooth surface.
- Ideal for removing large deposits quickly and efficiently across multiple teeth.
- Working ends—paired mirror images on a double-ended instrument.
- Face—perpendicular (at a 90° angle) to the lower shank (**Figure 37-14A**).
- Cutting edges—two per working end.
  - Cutting edges are parallel and level with each other.
  - Both cutting edges are used; therefore, blade is sharpened on both sides and around the toe.

B. Area-Specific Curets

- **Area-specific curets** are designed for adaptation to specific surfaces.
- Ideal for fine scaling and root debridement.
- Working ends—paired mirror image on a double-ended instrument. The typical pairs are numbers 1/2, 3/4, 5/6, 7/8, 9/10, 11/12, 13/14, 15/16, and 17/18 (e.g., Gracey curet series).
- Face—at an approximate 70° angle in relation to the lower shank to create an **offset blade** (**Figure 37-14B**).
- Cutting edge—one working lower cutting edge per working-end.
  - The working cutting edge is the lower edge of the blade when the handle is held vertically.
  - Only the lower cutting edge is used; therefore, the blade is sharpened on one side (lower edge) and around the toe.

C. Advanced Area-Specific Curets

- Variations of area-specific curets provide clinicians with greater opportunities to complete advanced instrumentation,[2] such as:
  - In deep pockets.
  - On curvatures of root surfaces with moderate-to-severe attachment loss.
  - On furcations on multirooted teeth.
- Terminal (lower) shank can vary in length and thickness, while the blade can vary in length and width. Some common variations are listed here.
- After-five curet (**Figure 37-15B**)
  - Terminal shank is 3 mm longer than a standard curet.
  - Blade width is decreased by 10%.
  - Allows improved access to pocket depths beyond 5 mm.
- Mini-five curet (**Figure 37-15C**)
  - Terminal shank is 3 mm longer than a standard curet.
  - Blade width is decreased by 10%.
  - Blade length is 50% shorter.
  - Shorter blade length facilitates adaptation to the curved features of root morphology including concavities, longitudinal depressions on proximal surfaces, root surfaces within furcations, and interradicular convexities.
- Micro-mini five curet (**Figure 37-15D**)
  - Terminal shank is 3 mm longer and thicker than a standard curet.

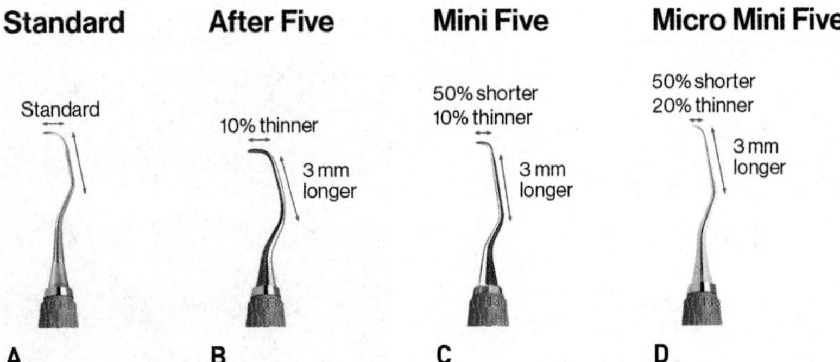

Figure 37-15 Gracey Tip Comparison. **A:** A standard Gracey curet. **B:** The after-five curet has a 3-mm longer shank than (A). **C:** The mini-five curet has a 50% shorter blade and 3-mm longer shank than (A). **D:** The micro-mini five curet has a 50% shorter blade that is narrower and 20% thinner than (A).

B to D: Courtesy of Hu-Friedy.

- Blade width is decreased by 20% compared to a mini-five curet.
- Blade length is 50% shorter than a standard curet.
- The longer and more rigid shank, combined with its narrower and shorter blade, allows application of greater lateral pressure when scaling very deep and tenacious calculus deposits.

IV. Curet-Specific Instrumentation

- Adaptation: Toe-third of the cutting edge is maintained on the tooth surface at all times. For line angles, the terminal 1–2 mm of the toe only may be used.
    - Either cutting edge of a universal curet may be adapted on a tooth surface.
    - Only the lower cutting edge of an area-specific curet may be adapted on a tooth surface.
- Angulation: The face of the blade is adapted to the tooth surface at various angles, depending on the action being performed (Figure 37-8).
    - When deposits are *removed supragingivally*, the blade face-to-tooth angulation is approximately 70°.
    - When the curet is *inserted subgingivally into the sulcus or pocket*, the blade is "closed" with the blade face-to-tooth angulation of approximately 0°.
    - When deposits are *removed subgingivally*, the blade is "opened" with the face-to-tooth angulation of approximately 70°.
- Activation: Light assessment strokes, moderate root debridement strokes, and heavy calculus removal strokes may be performed.

Periodontal Files

I. Working Files

Includes stainless steel Hirshfeld and Orban files.[7]

A. Uses

- Crushes and fractures heavy calculus into fragments prior to use of curets.
- Removes burnished calculus that is impervious to removal with other bladed instruments.
- Removes gross deposits of calculus on patients for whom ultrasonic use is contraindicated.

B. Instrument Design

- Multiple cutting edges lined up as a series of miniature hoes on a round, oval, or rectangular base (**Figure 37-16A**).
- The metal multiple blades are at a 90° angle with the shank (**Figure 37-16B**).
- Reduced tactile sensitivity because of the series of blades.
- Shanks are variously angulated; most are paired instruments.

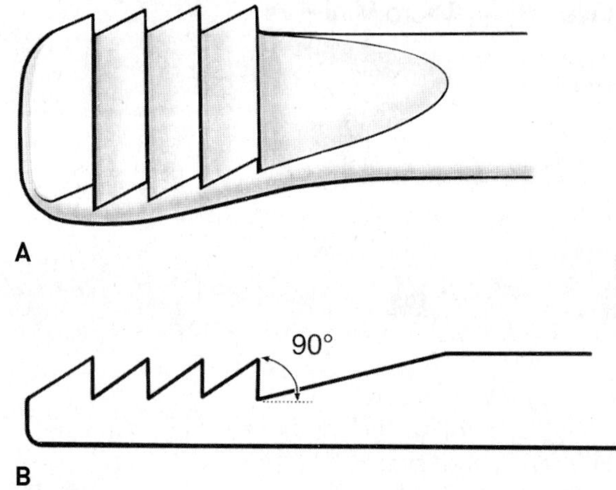

Figure 37-16 Working File Scaler. **A:** A file has multiple cutting edges. **B:** Each blade is at a 90° angle with the shank.

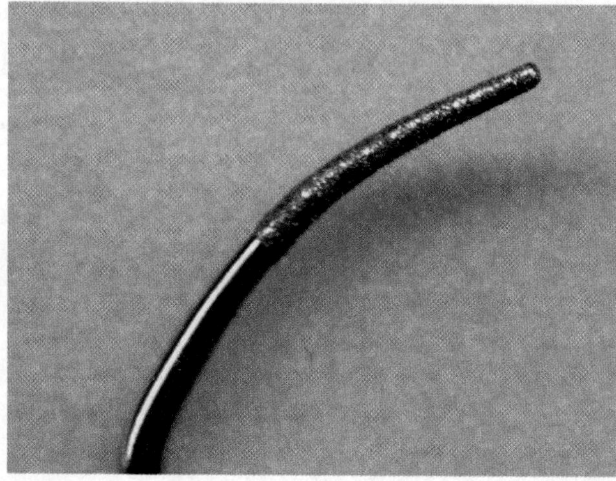

Figure 37-17 Diamond-Coated Finishing File. A close-up view of a working end on a diamond-coated file. Note the textured coating on the working end.

C. Instrumentation

- Can be used supra- and subgingivally.
- Adaptation: Entire working surface is placed flat against the area to be treated.
- Pressure applied permits the cutting edges to grasp the surface.
- Activation—pull-stroke only, using a linear motion.
- File use is always followed by curet instrumentation to smooth surface.

II. Finishing Files

These are not true files, scalers, or curets because there are no blades. These include Bedbug and diamond-coated files.[8]

A. Uses

- Used for finishing of root surfaces and accessing furcation areas.
- Early research suggests that the use of diamond-coated curets after conventional curets may provide a tooth surface more compatible with attachment of periodontal ligament fibroblasts.[8]

B. Instrument Design

- The diamond coating, which is used to remove the calculus, is placed 180° to 360° around the tip depending on the manufacturer (**Figure 37-17**).
- They have paired ends (buccal/lingual and mesial/distal) like other file scalers.

C. Instrumentation

- Adaptation: Working surface is placed flat against the root surface.
- Very light pressure is used to prevent damage to the root surface.
- Activation: Strokes are multidirectional (horizontal, vertical, and oblique) in a push–pull motion.

Powered Instruments

- Manual instrumentation was the only method of calculus removal until powered scalers were introduced in the 1950s.[9]
- The **ultrasonic** power-driven scaling device converted high-frequency electrical energy into mechanical energy in the form of rapid vibrations.
- Later, **sonic scalers** were developed that worked on the same principle but utilized an air turbine as an energy source.
- Technologic advances in powered scalers improved and allowed for rapid calculus removal that resulted in much less hand fatigue for the clinician.
- A number of clinical trials have compared the effectiveness of manual versus powered instruments. Some studies have demonstrated powered and manual instrumentation can produce similar clinical outcomes, such as calculus and biofilm removal, periodontal pocket depth reduction, and clinical attachment gain when instruments are applied correctly and sensitive posttreatment evaluation is made.[10,11] Others have shown manual instrumentation to be more effective than

powered instrumentation in treating moderate (4–6 mm) and deep (>6 mm) pockets.[12]

- The newest EFP (European Federation of Periodontics) clinical practice guidelines for treatment of stage I to III periodontitis suggest evidence supports either powered or hand instrumentation.[13]

I. Mechanism of Action

A. Mechanical Vibration

- Power-driven scaling devices convert electrical energy (ultrasonic) or air pressure (sonic) into high-frequency sound waves.
- Sound waves produce rapid mechanical vibrations in the tip of the powered scaler handpiece (**Figure 37-18**).
- The vibrating tip of the powered scaler is applied to calculus to shatter the hard deposits from the tooth surface.

B. Irrigation

- Water is required in the handpiece to dissipate heat produced by the vibrating tip.
- The water spray also creates a **lavage** that penetrates to the base of the pocket to provide a continuous flushing of blood, debris, microorganisms, and endotoxins.
- Oscillation of the ultrasonic tip causes **acoustic turbulence**, which has a disruptive effect on surface bacteria.[10]
- Ultrasonic debridement following manual instrumentation provides cleansing and rinsing of scaled tooth surfaces, which can promote healing of soft tissues.

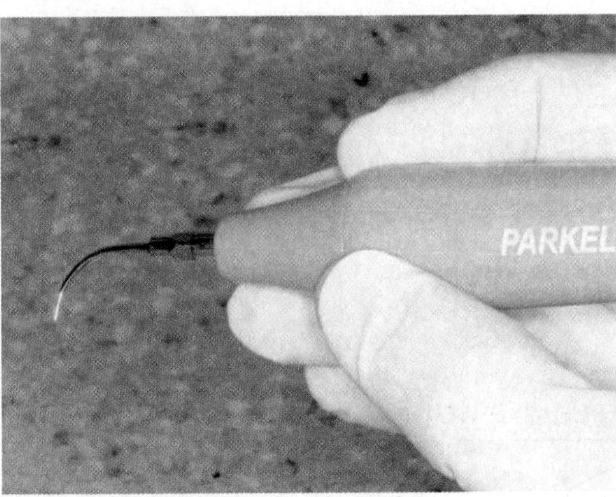

Figure 37-18 Piezoelectric Handpiece and Universal Tip. An example of a piezoelectric ultrasonic handpiece and powered tip.

C. Cavitation

- When the water in the handpiece meets the vibrating tip, **cavitation**, or the formation of microscopic bubbles, occurs.
- When the bubbles collapse, they release energy that creates adverse conditions of pressure and temperature that destroy bacterial cell walls.[10]

D. Variable Elements

- Power-driven scaling devices feature variable elements, such as their amplitude and frequency output.
- **Amplitude**—distance of tip movement measured in micrometers.
  - Determines power output of the instrument.
  - Setting adjustable on all ultrasonic devices.
- **Frequency**—speed of tip movement.
  - Number of cycles per second (cps) the tip moves.
  - Setting adjustable only on manually tuned ultrasonic devices.
  - Majority of available devices have preset or "automatic" tuning.

II. Indications for Use

- Removal of dental biofilm, extrinsic stain, and supra- and subgingival calculus.
- Subgingival periodontal debridement, including:
  - Removal of calculus, attached biofilm, and endotoxins from the root surface.
  - Reduction of bacterial load in the periodontal pocket.
- Debridement of furcation areas.
- Debridement of deposits before oral surgery.

III. Contraindications

A. Systemic Health Conditions

- Communicable disease[14,15]
  - Patient with a communicable disease that can be transmitted by aerosols, such as tuberculosis and coronavirus.
- Susceptibility to infection[16]
  - Compromised patient with marked susceptibility to infection.
  - Examples: Immunosuppression from disease or chemotherapy, uncontrolled diabetes, or kidney or other organ transplant.
- Respiratory risk[17]
  - Patient who may aspirate material and microorganisms from biofilm and periodontal pockets into the lungs.

- Examples: History of chronic obstructive pulmonary disease, asthma, emphysema, or cystic fibrosis.
- Difficulty swallowing or dysphagia[18]
    - Patient with a swallowing problem (dysphagia) or susceptibility to gagging.
    - Dysphagia results in liquids being aspirated into the lungs along with oral bacteria and increases the risk of aspiration pneumonia. Consultation with the primary care provider is needed prior to dental treatment.
    - Examples: Amyotrophic lateral sclerosis, muscular dystrophy, Parkinson's disease, paralysis, multiple sclerosis, and after stroke.
- Cardiac pacemaker[19]
    - Some studies have shown that ultrasonic devices may cause electromagnetic interference with implanted cardiac devices.[18,19]
    - Newer shielded cardiac devices may be less susceptible to interference.
    - Piezoelectric dental scalers may be safer than magnetostrictive scalers.[20,21]
    - Due to conflicting evidence, the clinician should consult with the patient's cardiologist to obtain medical clearance prior to use.

B. Oral Conditions

- Demineralized areas
    - Ultrasonic vibrations can remove the delicate remineralizing layer of a demineralized area.[20,21]
- Exposed dentinal surfaces
    - Applying too much lateral pressure or setting the power too high can damage and remove tooth structure.[20]
    - The smear layer can be removed and dentinal tubules uncovered, which can create and/or increase existing sensitivity.
- Thermal injury
    - Thermal damage to the pulp can occur if the ultrasonic tip overheats because of excess lateral pressure or inadequate water to cool the tip.[14]
    - Gingival tissues can experience thermal injury if water cooling is inadequate.
- Children
    - Young, growing, developing tissues are sensitive to ultrasonic vibrations.
    - Primary and newly erupted permanent teeth have large pulp chambers. Vibrations and heat from the **ultrasonic scaler** may damage pulp tissue.[14]
- Restorations[23]
    - Improper tip application may create roughness due to scratches, chips, pores, or notches in porcelain, composite, and metal restorative materials.
    - May remove the glaze of the porcelain and create pores on the surface where the tip was in contact with the porcelain.
- Titanium implant abutments
    - Ultrasonic instrumentation will damage titanium surfaces unless the insert is designed for use with implants.[22,23]

IV. Risks and Considerations

- Hearing impact
    - Extended exposure to noises above a certain level, such as the noise of a high-speed handpiece or an ultrasonic scaler, may be damaging to the ears.
    - Temporary hearing changes have been demonstrated for both clinicians and patients.[14]
- Cumulative trauma
    - Many dental hygienists suffer from musculoskeletal injuries related to cumulative trauma.
    - Scaling reduces the pinch force and finger–hand muscle activity needed to remove deposits, which can reduce operator fatigue.[9]
    - However, work with instruments that vibrate, such as the ultrasonic scaler, is associated with sensorineural dysfunction that includes temporary loss of tactile sensitivity in the fingertips.[14]
- Magnetic fields
    - Ultrasonic scalers produce weak, time-varying magnetic fields similar to those produced by common household appliances.
    - There is no scientific evidence that cumulative exposure to weak, time-varying magnetic fields has caused any biologic harm to dental personnel.
- Aerosols and spatter[15,16]
    - Aerosols—invisible airborne particles smaller than 50 μm that are dispersed into the surrounding environment by dental equipment.
    - Spatter—droplets of airborne particulate matter larger than 50 μm that fall to the ground.
    - The use of powered scalers creates aerosols and spatter that contain patient's saliva, blood, microorganisms, debris, and other potentially infectious materials.

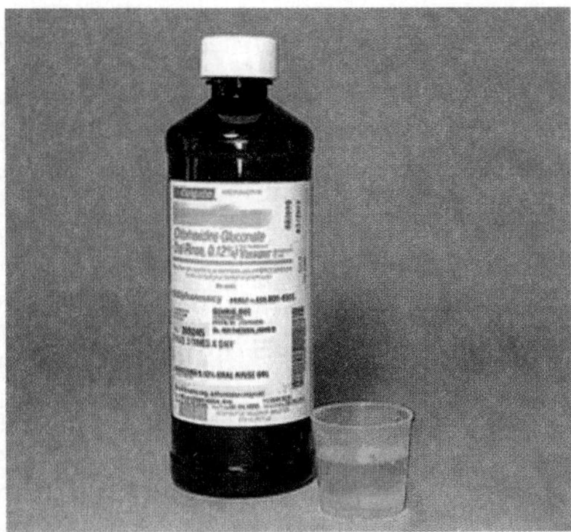

Figure 37-19 Preprocedure Rinse. Administering a preprocedural rinse is recommended to reduce the numbers of bacteria and other oral pathogens in aerosols.

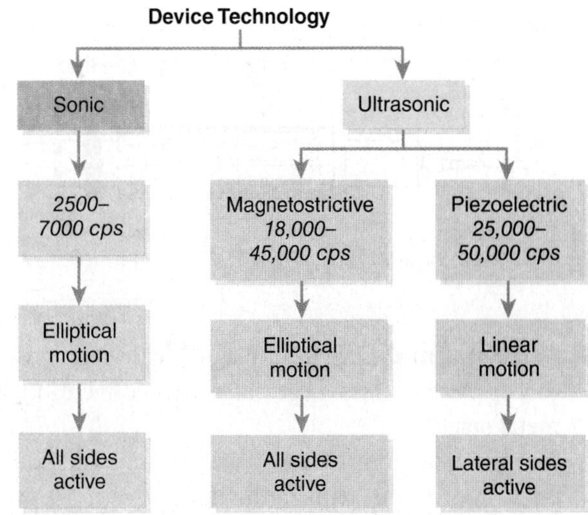

Figure 37-20 Power-Driven Scaling Devices Technology. For sonic and both magnetostrictive and piezoelectric ultrasonic scalers, the speed (cps), motion (linear or elliptical), and active part of the tip (lateral sides only or all sides) are identified.

- Aerosols can remain suspended in the air for up to hours following powered instrumentation.
- It is important to follow the most current infection control guidelines to reduce the risk of contamination and infection from aerosols and spatter, including the use of more stringent personal protective equipment; a preprocedural mouth rinse, such as a chlorhexidine gluconate rinse (see **Figure 37-19**); and use of a high-volume evacuator.[14–16]

V. Types

- Sonic scalers.
- Ultrasonic scalers:
  - **Magnetostrictive**
  - **Piezoelectric**
- These various powered scalers are mainly distinguished by their frequency output and the direction of tip movement, as shown in **Figure 37-20**.

Sonic Scalers

I. Mechanism of Action

- Sonic scalers are driven by compressed air from the dental unit rather than electrical energy.
- Amplitude—less powerful than ultrasonic scalers.
- Frequency—vibrates between 3000 and 8000 cps; fewer vibrations make calculus removal more difficult.
- Tip movement—elliptical pattern, but varies depending on tip and type of sonic scaler.
- Active surface of the tip—all surfaces of the tip are active.
  - Heat is not generated by the active tip.

II. Equipment

A. Unit Parts

- Handpiece.
- Interchangeable scaling tips.
- Handpiece attaches directly to the dental unit and is activated with the conventional handpiece foot control.

B. Unit Preparation

- Flush water lines in slow-speed suction line for 2 minutes.
- Attach sonic handpiece to slow-speed handpiece line.
- Attach the tip onto the handpiece.

Magnetostrictive Ultrasonic Scalers

I. Mechanism of Action

- Magnetostrictive ultrasonic devices are driven by electrical currents.
- Conventional magnetostrictive units utilize inserts, or longitudinal **stacks** of metal strips, in the handpiece (**Figure 37-21**).

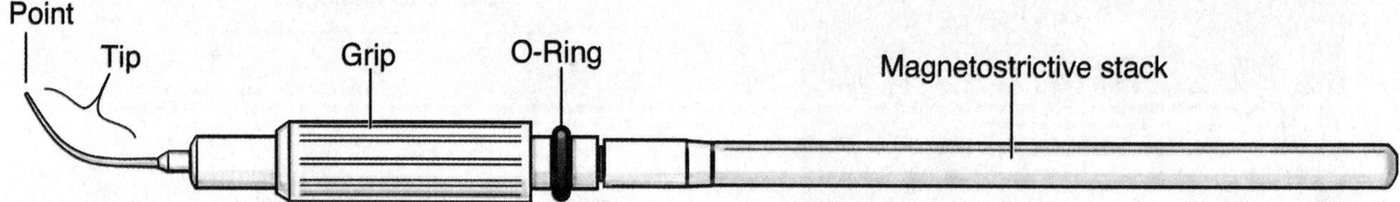

Figure 37-21 Magnetostrictive Ultrasonic Handpiece Insert. With parts labeled.

- **Ferromagnetic units** utilize a fragile ferric rod that generates less heat than the conventional metal stack.
- A magnetic field is created by expansion and contraction of metal strips in the handpiece.
- Amplitude—more powerful than sonic scalers.
- Frequency—conventional units range from 18,000 to 45,000 cps, while ferromagnetic units operate at 42,000 cps.
  - Older conventional units are designed to operate at 25,000 cps and are called 25-**kilohertz (kHz)** machines.
  - Newer conventional units are designed to operate at 30,000 cps and are called 30-kHz machines.
- Tip movement—elliptical pattern.
- Active surfaces of tip—all surfaces of the tip are active.
- Water cools the heat generated in the handpiece and tip.

II. Equipment

A. Unit Parts

- Electric generator.
- Handpiece assembly.
- Set of interchangeable scaling tip inserts.
- Foot control to activate the handpiece.

B. Unit Preparation

- Establish power and water connections.
- Flush water lines for 2 minutes.
- Select the appropriate insert.
  - Insert needs to be compatible with ultrasonic unit.
  - For instance, the metal stacks in the 30-kHz inserts are much shorter than the 25-kHz inserts.
- Hold handpiece upright as it is filled with water.
- Fill completely with water before seating the insert to eliminate trapped air bubbles and reduce heat.
- Select the appropriate power setting according to the task at hand.
- Adjust the water setting.

Piezoelectric Ultrasonic Scalers

I. Mechanism of Action

- **Piezoelectric** ultrasonic devices are driven by electrical currents.
- Use a ceramic rod and crystal **transducers** housed in the handpiece to activate the tip.
- Amplitude—more powerful than sonic scalers.
- Frequency—ranges from 25,000 to 50,000 cps, varies according to manufacturer.
- Tip movement—linear pattern, forward and backward.
- Active surface of tip—only the lateral surfaces of the tip are active.
- Water cools the heat generated at the tip.

II. Equipment

A. Unit Parts

- Electric generator.
- Handpiece assembly.
- Set of interchangeable scaling tips.
- Foot control to activate the handpiece.
- Some piezoelectric ultrasonic units have reservoirs (see **Figure 37-22**) that can hold antimicrobial solutions that can be used as irrigants for lavage.

B. Unit Preparation

- Establish power and water connections.
- Flush water lines for 2 minutes.
- Select the appropriate tip.
- Securely screw the tip onto the handpiece using the tip wrench.
- Select the power setting according to the task at hand.
- Adjust the water setting.

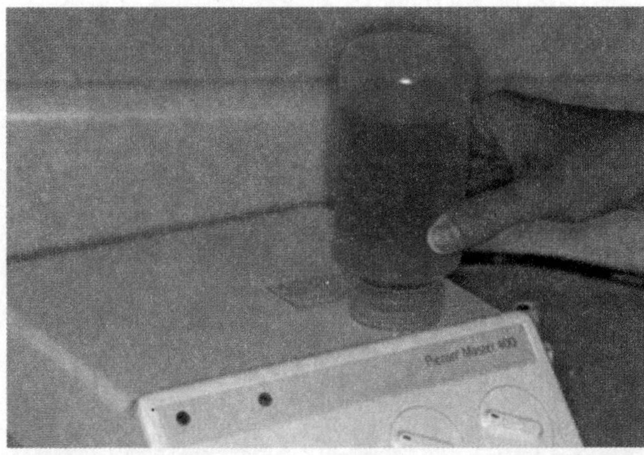

Figure 37-22 Reservoir for Ultrasonic Unit. This ultrasonic device has an optional reservoir system for dispensing irrigant solutions—such as chlorhexidine gluconate—to an ultrasonic tip.

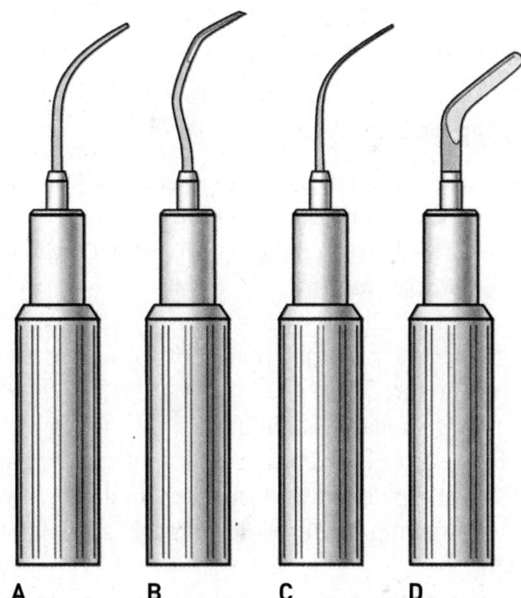

Figure 37-23 Ultrasonic Tip Designs. **A:** Straight, standard-diameter tip. **B:** Triple-bend tip for access to line angles and proximal surfaces. **C:** Thin-diameter tip for access to deep pockets. **D:** Beavertail tip for supragingival surfaces needing removal of heavy calculus or cement.

Powered Instrumentation Technique

I. Insert/Tip Selection

- Selecting the appropriate ultrasonic insert/tip is crucial for effectively and efficiently accomplishing the task at hand.
- Similar to hand instruments, the inserts and tips of powered instruments can vary in design.

A. Size

- Standard-diameter tips: used for moderate-to-heavy calculus removal (**Figure 37-23A**).
- Thin-diameter tips: used for biofilm debridement and light calculus removal. Also ideal for accessing deep periodontal pockets (**Figure 37-23C**).

B. Shape

- Straight design: has a simple shank and is used universally on all tooth surfaces (Figure 37-23A).
- Complex design: has multiple bends in the shank to allow easy access to line angles and proximal surfaces (**Figure 37-23B**).
- Left/right contra-angled inserts: complementary inserts have shanks that are curved to the left/right to better adapt to root concavities (e.g., furcations) and proximal surfaces of posterior teeth.
- Beavertail design: has a flat and wide working end; ideal for use on supragingival surfaces for the removal of heavy calculus, stain, and orthodontic cement (**Figure 37-23D**).

II. Power Setting

- When selecting the appropriate power setting, it is important to consider the task at hand and the insert/tip selected.
- Consistent use of the unit on the lowest power setting for hard deposit removal will burnish the calculus present versus shattering the deposit, making it more difficult to detect and remove.
- Consistent use of the unit on the highest power setting for soft deposit removal will cause unnecessary discomfort to the patient.

A. Low-to-Medium Power

- Used with thin-diameter tips/inserts.
- Ideal for removal of biofilm, other soft deposits, and light-to-moderate calculus.

B. Medium-to-High Power

- Used with standard-diameter tips/inserts.
- Ideal for removal of moderate-to-heavy calculus.

III. Water Setting

- Proper water setting will create a halo of fine mist at the tip of the instrument with or without drips of water.

- If the tip becomes warm or hot, increase the water setting to prevent damage to hard and soft tissues.

IV. Grasp

- Balance the assembled handpiece in the web between the thumb and index fingers.
  - This ensures a lighter grasp farther away from the working end.
  - A light grasp will increase tactile sensitivity and prevent application of excess lateral pressure.
- Establish a feather-light grasp.
- The weight of the cord tends to pull on the handpiece and place additional strain on the wrist. Use the following strategies to manage the weight of cord:
  - Loop the cord and hold it between the ring finger and little finger.
  - Drape the cord over the clinician's shoulder.

V. Fulcrum/Rest

- An intraoral hard-tissue fulcrum is not required because force and pressure against the tooth surface are not indicated.
- A gentle finger rest is used to stabilize and guide the instrument tip in anterior segments.
- Extraoral and soft tissue rests allow for proper access and adaptation to deeper posterior segments.

VI. Adaptation

- Keep the side of the instrument tip closely adapted to the tooth surface.
- Do not hold the tip perpendicular to the tooth surface at any time because damage to the tooth surface can result.
- Narrow periodontal pockets:
  - Narrow subgingival pockets can impede visibility and interfere with proper adaptation.
  - When instrumenting narrow pockets use an insert with appropriate length and limited width.
  - Direct the tip apically and confirm access to the attachment prior to activating the tip.
- Piezoelectric-specific technique:
  - Use the terminal 2–3 mm of the tip's lateral surfaces only (**Figure 37-24**).
  - Position the lateral surface of the tip in contact with the tooth.
  - Keep terminal lateral surface of the tip adapted at all times around curvatures and line angles using wrist pivot.

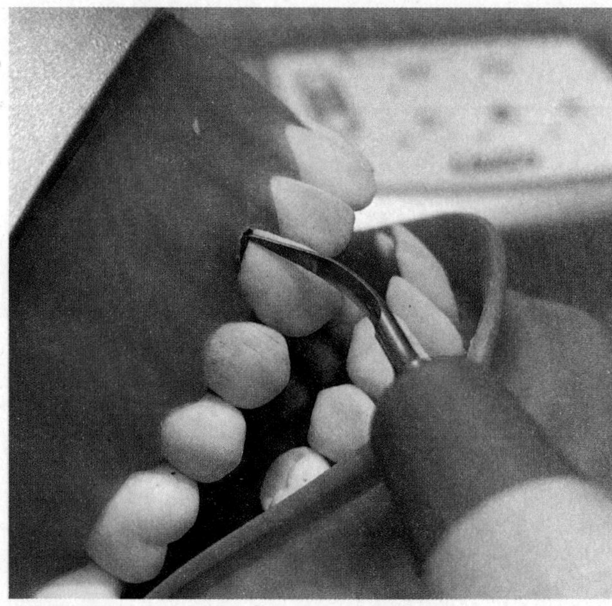

Figure 37-24 Adaptation of Ultrasonic Tip. Placing the point of the tip directly on the tooth surface must be avoided to prevent damage to the tooth structure. Damage occurs when the point is held perpendicular to the surface.

VII. Activation (Stroke)

- Use overlapping vertical, horizontal, and oblique strokes for coverage of all tooth surfaces.
- Keep the instrument tip moving at a slow to moderate pace with feather-light pressure at all times to prevent the following:
  - Damage to the tooth surface.
  - Scratches or gouging on the tooth surface.
  - Dampening and deactivation of the tip vibrations.
  - Burnishing of calculus.
  - Excessive heat buildup.
  - A galvanic shock-like effect to the patient.
- If the tip gets stuck in an embrasure:
  - Deactivate the power; remove the instrument tip from the embrasure.
  - Reposition the instrument by lightly exploring with the tip to get in position and then reactivate the power.

Dexterity Development

- The clinician returning to practice after a temporary leave of absence can perform hand exercises to develop manual dexterity and strength for effective instrumentation.
- In addition, all clinicians need an understanding of preventive measures to preserve the health of

their hands, arms, shoulders, and all muscles and joints involved when undertaking patient care.

- The use of new or unusual instruments requires different hand coordination. Control is essential, and guided strength contributes to control.
- Proficiency during procedures comes from repeated correct use of the instruments.
  - Exercises for the fingers, hands, and arms supplement experience.
  - Directed exercises are needed for both hands, separately and together.
  - During the training period, a regular period of time each day can be set aside for exercises.

I. Squeezing

A. Purpose

- To develop strength and control.

B. Therapy Putty or a Soft Ball

- Hold putty in palm of hand; grip with thumb and all fingers (**Figure 37-25A**).
- Tighten and release grip at regular intervals.
- One hand rests while the other is exercising.
- Use a ball in each hand to exercise at the same time.

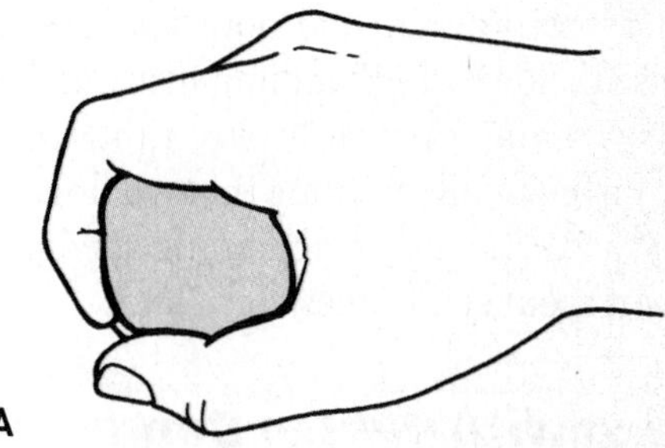

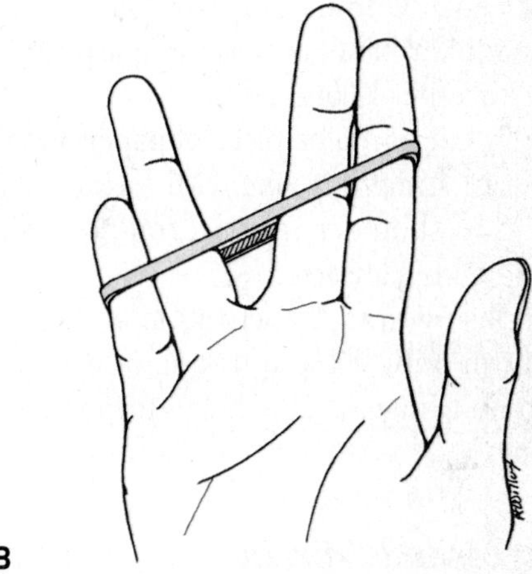

Figure 37-25 Exercises for Dexterity Development. **A:** Squeezing therapy putty can aid in developing strength and control. **B:** A rubber band can be applied at each group of finger and thumb joints and stretched.

II. Stretching

A. Purpose

- To strengthen finger and hand muscles.
- To develop control of finger movements.

B. Rubber Band on Finger Joints

- Place band at joint between first phalanx and second phalanx.
- Stretch band by separating middle and ring fingers (**Figure 37-25B**).
- Place band at joint between second phalanx and third phalanx and proceed as before.
- Place bands on both hands and do exercises together.

C. Rubber Band on Finger Joints with Use of Fulcrum

- Place band on joint between first phalanx and second phalanx.
- Establish fulcrum on tabletop with ring and little fingers closely adjacent to each other; elbow and forearm are free, as they are during instrumentation. Keep wrist straight, in same horizontal line as the forearm, and hold elbow at 90°. Stretch the band by separating middle and ring fingers.
- Touch thumb and index and middle fingers to simulate a modified pen grasp for holding an instrument. Stretch the band by separating middle and ring fingers.

III. Pen/Pencil Exercises

A. Purpose

- To develop correct modified pen grasp.
- To propel instrument by activation from wrist and arm, without moving fingers.
- To practice instrument rolling.
- To develop control and precision.
- To practice use of instruments when indirect vision is required.

B. Everyday Penmanship

- Use modified pen grasp whenever possible for writing.

- Practice writing with the nondominant hand to increase dexterity for handling instruments.
- Practice rolling a pencil between the thumb and index fingers while keeping the two fingers opposite of each other and maintaining adequate space between them at all times.

C. Writing with Rubber Band around Grasp

- Hold a pencil with modified pen grasp.
- Place a rubber band around the grasp to keep the fingers together as one unit.
- Establish fulcrum on a piece of paper on tabletop.
- Keep wrist straight in line with forearm; elbow is at 90°, and shoulder is in neutral position. Forearm and elbow are free.
- Accomplish writing by activation of the wrist and upper arm only, without flexing or extending the thumb and fingers. This helps to prevent digital motions.

C. Using Mouth Mirror

- Hold mouth mirror with modified pen grasp in nondominant hand.
- Hold a pencil with modified pen grasp in the dominant hand.
- While looking only through the mouth mirror, practice writing exercises. Reverse hands.
- You may also practice tracing and outlining drawings or the small squares on a sheet of graph paper via indirect vision to develop precision and accuracy.

IV. Refining Use of Mouth Mirror and Cotton Pliers

A. Purpose

- To develop ability to turn mouth mirror at various angles.
- To develop dexterity in holding objects with cotton pliers.

B. Mouth Mirror

- Hold mouth mirror with modified pen grasp, ring finger on tabletop as fulcrum finger with little finger closely adjacent to it; elbow and forearm are free. The mirror is used most frequently in the nondominant hand.
- Practice turning mirror with fingers, adjusting as to the several surfaces of the tooth.
- Hold a small object in the dominant hand for viewing in mirror held in nondominant hand.
- Practice crossing the mirror over fulcrum finger as in position for retracting lower lip while viewing lingual surfaces of mandibular anterior teeth in mouth mirror.

C. Cotton Pliers

- Make small, tight cotton pellets with thumb and index and middle fingers of each hand, then make one in each hand simultaneously.
- Hold cotton pliers with modified pen grasp and establish fulcrum finger on tabletop; elbow and forearm are free.
- Practice picking up cotton pellets using indirect vision (right hand, then left).
  - Use in wiping motion on tabletop or other object.
  - Move to different area to release pellet.

V. Increasing Tactile Sensitivity

A. Purpose

- To establish desired grasp of the explorer and probe to ensure maximum tactile or touch sensitivity.

B. Explorer

- Mount small pieces of various grades of sandpaper on a card.
- Hold explorer with modified pen grasp, and establish fulcrum finger on tabletop, with upper arm and forearm free. With eyes closed, compare roughness of the various grades of sandpaper. Use a light, exploratory/assessment stroke.
- Various tools and educational aids (e.g., Calculus Detection PRO and Calculus Detection Calibrator) are available commercially to help develop tactile sensitivity required to detect cementum and varying degrees of calculus (see **Figure 37-26**).

C. Probe

- Hold a periodontal probe in the dominant hand using a modified pen grasp.
- Next to a precision scale (e.g., laboratory, kitchen, or food weighing scale), establish a level fulcrum,

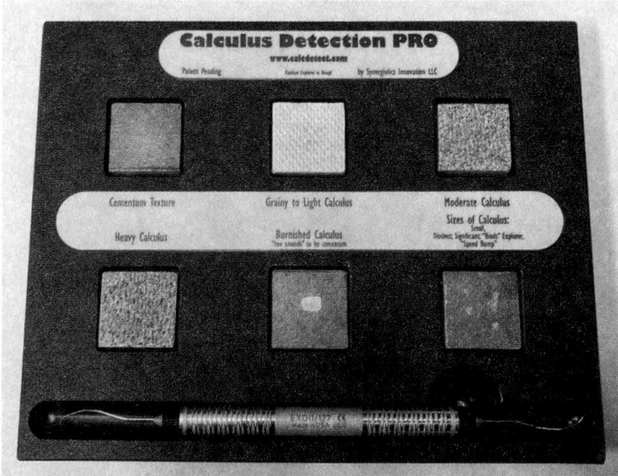

Figure 37-26 Calculus Detection Tool. This tool consists of an explorer and mounted textured tiles that simulate different tooth structures and varying degrees of calculus.
Courtesy of Calculus Detection PRO.

making sure not to fulcrum directly on the scale itself.

- With the probe tip, apply just enough force on the scale to reach the recommended probing force of 0.25 g.[24]
- Repeat multiple times to develop muscle memory of optimal probing force.

Cumulative Trauma

Following proper instrumentation techniques and ergonomic practices will preserve the musculoskeletal well-being of the dental hygienist.

- Primary occupational hazards are related to personal everyday habits during chairside practice.
- The symptoms of carpal tunnel syndrome are caused by compression of the median nerve within the carpal tunnel, as shown in Figure 37-6. Chapter 8 shows the anatomy of the carpel tunnel wrist area.

I. Risk Factors for Trauma

- Poor posture.
- Extended periods of time spent in the same work position.
- Repetitive movements during instrumentation.

II. Preventing Trauma

- Practice prevention, before serious disability can occur.

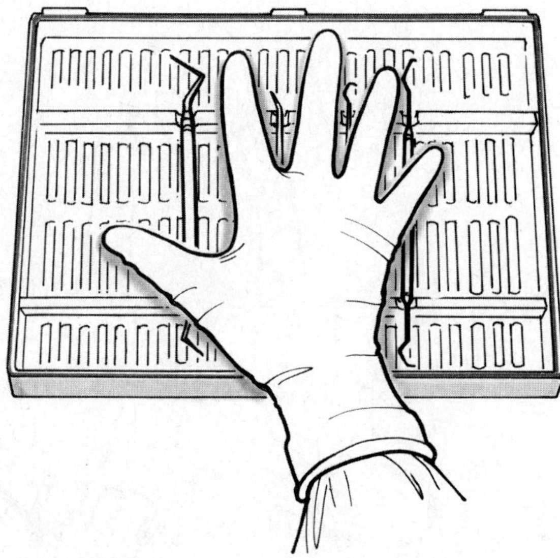

Figure 37-27 Stretching Fingers Prior to Instrument Retrieval. One of the exercises that can be used during everyday clinical practice.

- Exercises performed chairside and between appointments can contribute greatly to long-term prevention.
- One easy and practical exercise that can be performed during patient treatment is stretching the fingers and wrists after returning an instrument to the cassette and before picking up a new one (see **Figure 37-27**).
- Stretching exercises for stress release, improvement of posture, and counteracting repetitive movements used during instrumentation are suggested in **Figure 37-28**.
- Additional exercises are shown in Chapter 8.

Documentation

Documentation of instrument selection and instrumentation techniques in a patient record can provide guidance during subsequent dental hygiene care. For example, notes made in the patient record may include the following:

- Areas of the patient's dentition that require more careful attention or careful application of skill.
- Specific instruments shown to be more effective in specific areas, such as minicurets in a particularly deep pocket.
- Instruments avoided due to patient contraindications or discomfort, such as an ultrasonic scaler due to dentinal hypersensitivity.
- An example progress note is found in **Box 37-1**.

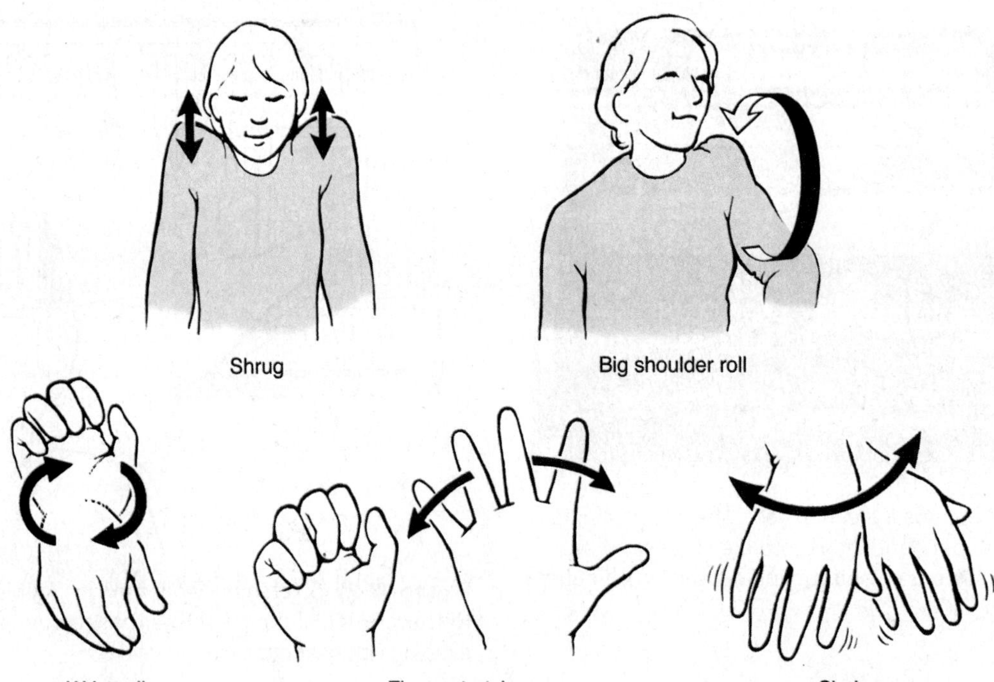

Figure 37-28 Chairside Stretching Exercises. Stretching exercises to relax the back, shoulders, and neck are shown with the shrugging of shoulders and rolling of the head and shoulders. Hand and finger rolls, stretches, and shaking can be performed anytime.

Box 37-1 Example Documentation: Instrumentation

- **S**—Female patient, 32 years old with cerebral palsy and dysphagia, presents to clinic with caregiver for first "long overdue" dental appointment in 5 years.
- **O**—Generalized erythematous and inflamed gingiva with festooned margins and bulbous interdental papillae noted. Heavy, generalized calculus present on all teeth; bridge of calculus noted from #20 to #29 and occlusal calculus noted on all molars and premolars.
- **A**—Unable to perform an accurate comprehensive periodontal examination today due to heavy supragingival calculus overlying soft tissues. Exposed six vertical bitewings using a NOMAD (mobile radiology unit) to assess for caries and bone loss.
- **P**—Completed a full mouth debridement today for gross calculus removal. Did not use ultrasonic scaler due to patient's difficulty swallowing and risk for aspirating water into the lungs. Used the universal and rigid Gracey curets to remove heavy supragingival calculus.

Next steps: Patient to return with caregiver in 1 week for a full comprehensive periodontal examination.

Signed: ______________________________, RDH
Date: ______________

Factors to Teach the Patient

- The benefits and risks of using various types of instruments.
- Why it is necessary to use a variety of instruments for treatment.
- What sensations and experiences to expect during the use of certain instruments.
- How the patient can cooperate to help you instrument more effectively and efficiently.

References

1. Simmer-Beck M, Branson BG. An evidence-based review of ergonomic features of dental hygiene instruments. *Work*. 2010;35(4):477-485.
2. Belano Sanchez J, Nguyen M. Improve nonsurgical periodontal therapy with appropriate instrument choice. *Dimens Dent Hyg*. 2021;19(2):16-18.
3. You D, Smith AH, Rempel D. Meta-analysis: association between wrist posture and carpal tunnel syndrome among workers. *Saf Health Work*. 2014;5(1):27-31.
4. Matsuda S, Pattison GL. Extraoral fulcrums. *Dimens Dent Hyg*. 2004;2(10):21-23.
5. Nguyen M, Pattison AM. Activate alternative fulcrums. *Dimens Dent Hyg*. 2014;12(5):24-28.
6. Pattison AM. The secret use of sickle scalers. *Dimens Dent Hyg*. 2008;6(9):46-47.
7. Pattison AM. Key to effective calculus removal. *Dimens Dent Hyg*. 2011;9(10):50-53.
8. Eick S, Bender P, Flury S, Lussi A, Sculean A. In vitro evaluation of surface roughness, adhesion of periodontal ligament fibroblasts, and *Streptococcus gordonii* following root instrumentation with Gracey curettes and subsequent polishing with diamond-coated curettes. *Clin Oral Investig*. 2013;17(2):397-404.
9. Lea SC, Walmsley AD. Mechano-physical and biophysical properties of power-driven scalers: driving the future of powered instrument design and evaluation. *Periodontol 2000*. 2009;51:63-78.
10. Krishna R, De Stefano JA. Ultrasonic vs. hand instrumentation in periodontal therapy: clinical outcomes. *Periodontol 2000*. 2016;71(1):113-127.
11. Muniz FWMG, Langa GPJ, Pimentel RP, Martins JR, Pereira DH, Rösing CK. Comparison between hand and sonic/ ultrasonic instruments for periodontal treatment: systematic review with meta-analysis. *J Int Acad Periodontol*. 2020;22(4):187-204.
12. Zhang S, Leidner D. From improper to acceptable: how perpetrators neutralize workplace bullying behaviors in the cyber world. *Inf Manage*. 2018;55(7):850-865.
13. Sanz M, Herrera D, Kebschull M, et al. Treatment of stage I-III periodontitis: the EFP S3 level clinical practice guideline. *J Clin Periodontol*. 2020;47(Suppl 22):4-60.
14. Trenter SC, Walmsley AD. Ultrasonic dental scaler: associated hazards. *J Clin Periodontol*. 2003;30(2):95-101.
15. Centers for Disease Control and Prevention (CDC). Interim infection prevention and control recommendations for healthcare personnel during the coronavirus disease 2019 (COVID-19) pandemic. Published September 10, 2021. https://www.cdc.gov/coronavirus/2019-ncov/hcp/infection-control-recommendations.html. Accessed September 17, 2021.
16. Kohn WG, Collins AS, Cleveland JL, et al. Guidelines for infection control in dental health-care settings--2003. *MMWR Recomm Rep*.2003;52(RR-17):1-61.
17. Vilela MCN, Ferreira GZ, Santos PS, Rezende NP. Oral care and nosocomial pneumonia: a systematic review. *Einstein*. 2015;13(2):290-296.
18. Logemann JA, Curro FA, Pauloski B, Gensler G. Aging effects on oropharyngeal swallow and the role of dental care in oropharyngeal dysphagia. *Oral Dis*. 2013;19(8):733-737.
19. Niu Y, Chen Y, Li W, Xie R, Deng X. Electromagnetic interference effect of dental equipment on cardiac implantable electrical devices: a systematic review. *Pacing Clin Electrophysiol*. 2020;43(12):1588-1598.
20. Paramashivaiah R, Prabhuji MLV. Mechanized scaling with ultrasonics: perils and proactive measures. *J Indian Soc Periodontol*. 2013;17(4):423-428.
21. Kaufmann M, Solderer A, Gubler A, Wegehaupt FJ, Attin T, Schmidlin PR. Quantitative measurements of aerosols from air-polishing and ultrasonic devices: (how) can we protect ourselves? *PloS One*. 2020;15(12):e0244020.
22. Mann M, Parmar D, Walmsley AD, Lea SC. Effect of plastic-covered ultrasonic scalers on titanium implant surfaces. *Clin Oral Implants Res*. 2012;23(1):76-82.
23. Renvert S, Hirooka H, Polyzois I, Kelekis-Cholakis A, Wang HL, Working Group 3. Diagnosis and non-surgical treatment of peri-implant diseases and maintenance care of patients with dental implants - Consensus report of working group 3. *Int Dent J*. 2019;69(Suppl 2):12-17.
24. Al Shayeb KNA, Turner W, Gillam DG. Periodontal probing: a review. *Prim Dent J*. 2014;3(3):25-29.

CHAPTER 38

Instrument Care and Sharpening

Esther M. Wilkins, BS, RDH, DMD
Linda D. Boyd, RDH, RD, EdD

CHAPTER OUTLINE

LEARNING OBJECTIVES

After studying this chapter, the student will be able to:

1. Describe the benefits of using sharp instruments.
2. Describe the consequences of using dull instruments.
3. Demonstrate proper technique for sharpening procedures for a variety of periodontal instruments.
4. Explain how to preserve optimal instrument design when sharpening.

Instrument Sharpening

Objectives for techniques of sharpening emphasize the *preservation of the original shape of the blade while restoring a sharp cutting edge.*

- Instruments are designed for a particular purpose.
  - Inaccurate sharpening techniques can distort the blade and render the instrument useless for its intended purpose.
- Sharpening is an essential and integral part of instrumentation.
  - Sharpening procedures are technique-sensitive and require skill and patience to become proficient.
  - The clinician must test instrument **sharpness** at the beginning and during each appointment.
- Successful clinical outcomes with cutting instruments are dependent on correctly contoured and sharpened instruments.
- Maintaining instrument sharpness prevents loss of blade structure to minimize the need to recontour to restore the original shape.

I. Benefits from Use of Sharp Manual Instruments

Instruments must be sharp to efficiently complete scaling and subgingival instrumentation with minimal trauma to the tissues. When the instrument blade is maintained with its original contour and sharp **cutting edges**, the following may be expected[1,2]:

- Increased tactile sensitivity.
- Greater grab force.
- Fewer strokes required with reduced working time.
- Less possibility of **burnishing** rather than removing the calculus.
- Less blade slippage helps prevent trauma to gingival tissues.
- Less pressure on tooth surfaces resulting in less discomfort for the patient.
- Decreased possibility of nicking, grooving, or scratching the tooth surfaces.
- Less fatigue for the clinician.

II. Consequences of Using Dull Manual Instruments

- Stress and frustration of using ineffective instruments resulting in burnished or inadequate removal of calculus.
- Wasted time, effort, and energy.
- Loss of control and increased likelihood of slipping with instrument and lacerating the gingival tissue.
- Less pressure on tooth surfaces may improve patient comfort.
- A dull instrument requires increased pinch force, causing muscle strain that increases the risk of developing work-related musculoskeletal disorders.[3]

III. Dynamics of Sharpening

Instrument sharpening is accomplished by filing the surface or surfaces that form the cutting edge.

A. Cutting Edge

- The cutting edge is a very fine line formed where the face and lateral surface meet at an angle (see **Figure 38-1**).[4]
- The edge becomes dull when pressed against a hard surface (the tooth), or it may be nicked when drawn over a rough surface.
- A dull edge (also called a **beveled** edge) is when the two planes of the blade no longer come to a fine edge and are flattened (**Figure 38-2**). The object in sharpening is to reshape the cutting edge to a fine line while removing a minimal amount of material.[1,4]
  - Approximately 45 scaling strokes create a very rounded cutting edge; even 15 strokes result in a slightly rounded cutting edge.[5]

B. Sharpening Stone Surface

- A sharpening stone acts as an abrasive to reshape a dulled blade by grinding the surface until the cutting edge is restored.
- The surface of the stone is made up of masses of minute crystals, which are the abrasive particles that accomplish the grinding of the instrument.

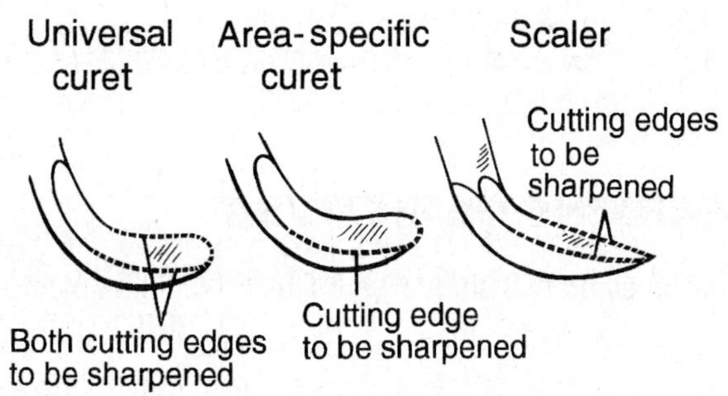

Figure 38-1 Selection of Cutting Edge to Sharpen. Both cutting edges and the rounded toe are sharpened for a universal curet. An area-specific curet is sharpened on the longer cutting edge and the rounded toe. A scaler is sharpened on the two sides, and the tip is brought to a point.

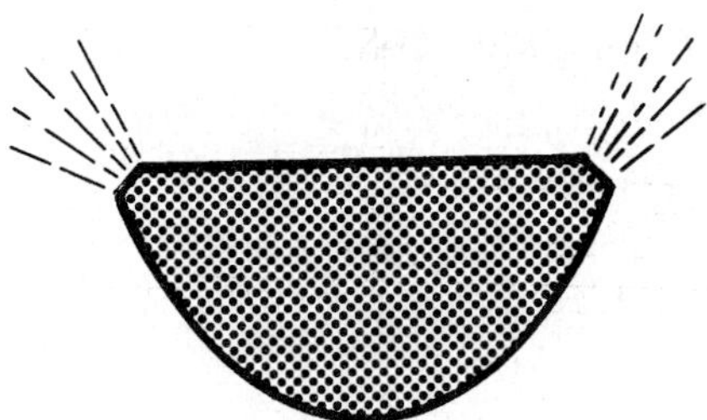

Figure 38-2 Cross Section of a Dull Curet. A sharp curet has a fine line at the cutting edge that will not reflect light. A dull cutting edge is like a beveled or flattened surface and reflects light as shown.

- Average roughness (Ra) indicates a smaller particle size or a finer grit that abrades or reduces more slowly and produces a finer cutting edge.[1]

IV. Types of Sharpening Devices

A. Stones

- Ceramic stone (Ra 1.32 mcg) has small, round, regular abrasive particles (**Figure 38-3C**).
    - Recommended to maintain a cutting edge, but not for sharpening dull or partially dull instruments.[1]
- **Arkansas stones** can vary in particle size (Ra 2.47–4.54 mcg), but are more coarse than ceramic stones (**Figure 38-3A**).[1]
    - Recommended for sharpening partially dull instruments.
- Carborundum (Ra 4.5 mcg) and India stones (Ra 5.6-6 mcg) (**Figure 38-3B**) have the roughest grit with large and irregular particles.[1]
    - Recommended for reshaping and sharpening totally dull instruments.

B. Artificial Materials

- Steel alloys are metals that are harder than most dental instrument steel and, therefore, are capable of sharpening the instrument.
- A diamond-coated stainless steel sharpening card is about the size of a credit card and used in the same way as other sharpening stones (**Figure 38-3D**). However, research suggests they remove significantly more metal than ceramic stones, resulting in the need for more frequent replacement of scalers.[6]

C. Power-Driven or Mechanical Sharpening Devices

- A number of manufacturers offer power-driven sharpening devices.
- Research suggests a better cutting edge is created with manual sharpening.[7]

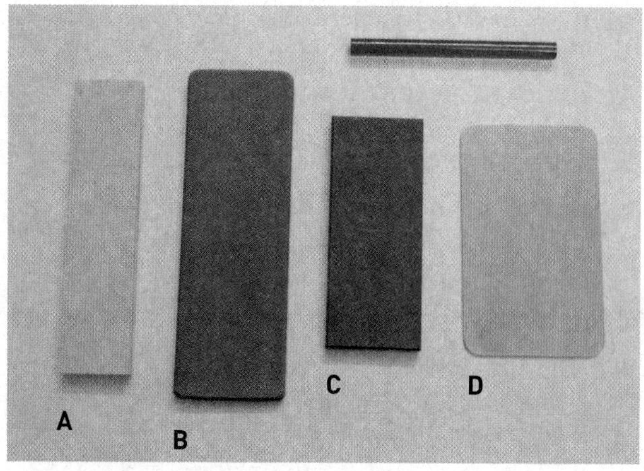

Figure 38-3 Types of Sharpening Stones. **A:** Arkansas stone. **B:** India stone. **C:** Ceramic stone. **D:** Diamond-sharpening card.

Basic Sharpening Principles

I. Sterilization of the Sharpening Stone

- A sterile sharpening stone and acrylic **testing stick** are parts of a basic clinical setup for a scaling appointment.
- Sterilization of stones may be accomplished using any of the acceptable sterilization methods in accordance with specific manufacturer's recommendations. Sterilization methods are discussed in Chapter 7.
- Over time, the steam autoclave may dry out an Arkansas stone and lead to chipping or breakage.[8]

II. Instrument Handling

All instruments must be handled with care to preserve sharpness and prevent accidental damage to the cutting edges.

III. Preparation of Stone for Sharpening

A. Dry Stone

- Advantage: The problems related to maintaining a sterile stone and preventing contamination when oil, tap water, or a lubricant is applied are eliminated.
- A dry stone contributes to the following effects:
    - Sharpens the cutting edge without nicks in the blade; nicks can be created from particles of metal suspended in a lubricant.

- Allows the stone to be completely sterilized without the problem of interference by the oil left in and on the stone.

B. Water on Stone

- Water can be used for lubrication of ceramic stones, but they may also be used dry.

C. Lubricated Stone

- Oil lubrication is recommended with certain quarried stones, such as the Arkansas stone, to prevent drying out.
- Instruments are autoclaved before sharpening, and the stone and instruments are sterilized again after nonsterile lubricant is used.
- The lubricant can facilitate the movement of the instrument blade over the stone to prevent scratching of the stone.
  - Suspend the metallic particles removed during sharpening.
  - Help to prevent clogging of the pores of the stone (glazing).

IV. Sharpening Overview

A. Objectives

The objectives during sharpening are twofold:

- To produce a sharp cutting edge.
- To preserve the original shape of the instrument.
  - The contour of a curet toe is a smooth, continuous curvature with no points or flat edges.

B. When to Sharpen

- Sharpen at the first sign of dullness during an appointment.[8]
  - However, some states, provinces, or workplaces may have policies in place that recommend against chairside sharpening to prevent clinician injury.
- Recontouring an overly dull instrument may result in more frequent instrument replacement.
  - Restoring original contour to a grossly dull instrument often leaves a blade that is not functional.

C. Angulation

- Before starting to sharpen, analyze the cutting edge and establish the proper angle between the stone and the blade surface.
- Maintain the angle through the firm grasp, secure hand rest, moderate pressure, short stroke, and other features of the technique appropriate to the individual instrument.

D. Maintain Control

- Maintain control so that the entire surface is reduced evenly.
- Care must be taken not to create a new bevel at the cutting edge.

E. Care of Sharpening Stone

- Prevent grooving of the sharpening stone by varying the areas for instrument placement.
- Cleaning and stain removal procedures are described in section "Care of Sharpening Equipment" in this chapter.

V. Tests for Instrument Sharpness

Even brand-new instruments need to be tested for sharpness and often need to be sharpened prior to use.[2]

A. Visual or Glare Test

- Examine the cutting edge under adequate light using magnification.
- Because the sharp cutting edge is a fine line, it does not reflect light.
- The dull cutting edge presents a flat, shiny surface, which can reflect light.
  - Figure 38-2 shows the cross section of a dull universal curet.
  - The dull cutting edges are tiny surfaces that reflect light.

B. Plastic Testing Stick

- Use a sterile plastic or acrylic ¼-inch rod, 3 inches long (see **Figure 38-4**).
- Place the fulcrum finger on the end of the stick.
- Apply the heel (shank end) of the cutting edge to the plastic stick, first at 90°, then closed to the correct angle for scaling (70°).
- Press lightly but firmly.
- Roll the cutting edge forward from the shank end to the toe by turning or rolling the instrument handle in the fingers to test the entire length of the blade.

C. Confirming Sharpness Using the Plastic Testing Stick

- The *sharp* cutting edge engages or grips the plastic as the length of the blade is tested. Each portion

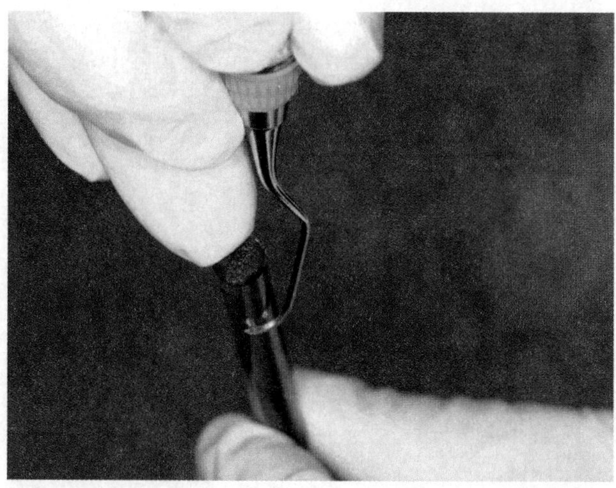

Figure 38-4 Plastic Testing Stick. Sharpness can be evaluated using a test stick. A test stick is a cylindrical rod made of plastic or acrylic.

Reproduced from Nield-Gehrig J. *Fundamentals of Periodontal Instrumentation and Advanced Root Instrumentation.* Philadelphia, PA: Lippincott Williams & Wilkins; 2011.

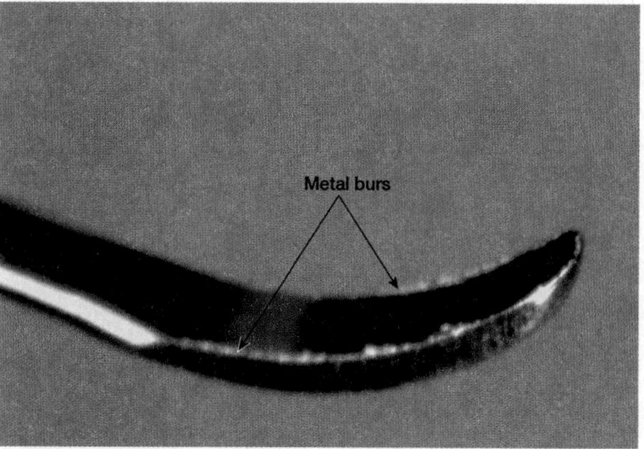

Figure 38-5 Wire Edge after Sharpening. Sharpening can produce minute metal burs that project from the cutting edge.

Reproduced from Nield-Gehrig J. *Fundamentals of Periodontal Instrumentation and Advanced Root Instrumentation.* Philadelphia, PA: Lippincott Williams & Wilkins; 2011.

of the cutting edge will engage the plastic uniformly as the blade advances.
- The *dull* cutting edge does not catch without undue pressure and slides or slips on the surface of the stick.
- Because the edge is not uniformly dulled during use, there will be portions of a blade that exhibit varying degrees of sharpness or dullness.
- As the instrument blade is rolled along the testing stick, the degree of slipping versus engagement will indicate the degree of sharpness or dullness. If only limited portions of the blade exhibit dullness, attempt to note the segments that slip as the blade is rolled along the testing stick.
  - The entire length of the cutting edge is always sharpened to maintain the original form.
  - Awareness of the portion(s) exhibiting dullness can guide pressure and the number of sharpening strokes to minimize oversharpening.

VI. Evaluation of Technique

- Observe closely the stabilization of both the instrument and stone, keep each aligned in a single plane, to evaluate sharpening technique.
  - Self-check: As the stone is activated for sharpening, observe the top of the instrument to ensure it is secure and not moving.
  - Self-check: Observe stone to ensure it remains in a single plane of movement up and down as during sharpening stroke.
- Visually inspect the cutting edge with well-lit magnification.
- A sharp cutting edge results from:
  - Instrument and stone positioned at the correct angle.
  - Movement occurring in a single plane.
- Visually an irregular bevel is revealed by:
  - Breaks in the fine line of the blade edge.
  - Varying facets indicating improper stone placement/movement.

VII. After Sharpening

A. Finishing the Instrument

Newly sharpened instruments are finished by carefully inspecting the edges for a clean consistent bevel with no particles or "wire edge" remaining.

B. How the Wire Edge Is Produced

- During sharpening, some of the metal particles removed during grinding remain attached to the edge of the instrument and create the wire edge (**Figure 38-5**).[4,9]
- If allowed to remain, the tiny particles may damage the root surface when applying the instrument during treatment subgingival instrumentation.[1]

C. Removal of Wire Edge

- Wipe the instrument carefully with a dry gauze square or an alcohol wipe to remove particles.

VIII. Instrument Wear

- As curets are used, the cutting edge wears down, leaving a narrower face and shorter length over a period of time.

- Sharpening also contributes to the size reduction.
- Instruments that become narrow can be reserved for patients with minimal deposit and require primarily biofilm debridement.
- Evaluation during sharpening procedures provides the opportunity for careful evaluation of instrument quality.
- After sufficient reduction, instruments must be discarded and replaced.
  - Blades will no longer access or adapt to the tooth surface.
  - Thinner blades are more susceptible to breakage with lateral pressure and may result in tissue injury.[10]
  - In addition, retrieval of the broken tip can be challenging and even constitute an emergency.[11]

Sharpening Curets and Scalers

Research on the most effective sharpening technique is inconsistent, so the technique that creates a sharp cutting edge with the least clinician effort and minimizes removal of metal from the instrument should be used.[1,4,12,13]

I. Technique Objectives

- Preserve the original contour of the blade.
- Sharpen frequently to maintain sharpness and prevent need for excessive recontouring of the blade.

II. Selection of Cutting Edges to Sharpen

A. Scalers/Sickles

- Most scalers are universal instruments.
- Cutting edges on both sides of the face are sharpened (Figure 38-1).
- A two-step sharpening procedure is used.

B. Curets: Universal

- Cutting edges on both sides of the face and the toe are sharpened (Figure 38-1).
- A three-step sharpening procedure is used.

C. Curets: Area Specific

- Cutting edges on one side of the face and the toe are sharpened.
- Sharpen the longer cutting edge; generally, it will be the one farthest from the handle. In Figure 38-1, it is indicated by the dotted line.
- A two-step sharpening procedure is used: one side of the face and the toe.

Moving Flat Stone: Stationary Instrument

- In this technique, the instrument is held stationary while the sharpening stone if moved up and down.
- The technique described applies to both curets and scalers.
- Because the scaler has a pointed tip and the curet has a round toe end, a variation is necessary in the adaptation of the sharpening stone to that portion of the blade (**Figure 38-6**).

I. Examine the Cutting Edge to Be Sharpened

Test for sharpness to determine specific areas that are dull, but plan to sharpen the whole cutting edge(s) to maintain original contour.

II. Review the Angulation to Be Restored at the Dull Cutting Edge

- Internal angle of the blade at the cutting edge(s) is 70° to 80°. (See Chapter 37.)
- Visible angle at which the stone will be placed will be 110°, as shown in Figure 38-6.

III. Stabilize and Position the Instrument

- Grasp the instrument in the nondominant hand in a palm grasp.
- Lean the hand against the edge of an immovable workbench or table under bright light.
- The instrument is positioned low enough to allow the clinician to see the cutting edges clearly.
- Turn the face of the instrument up and parallel with the floor. Point the curet toe (or scaler tip) toward the clinician to provide better access for moving the stone (**Figure 38-7B**).
- The cutting edges begin at the lower shank.
- The cutting edges are parallel, until they converge.
- For the curet, the cutting edges curve to form the toe.
- For the scaler, the cutting edges taper to make the pointed tip.

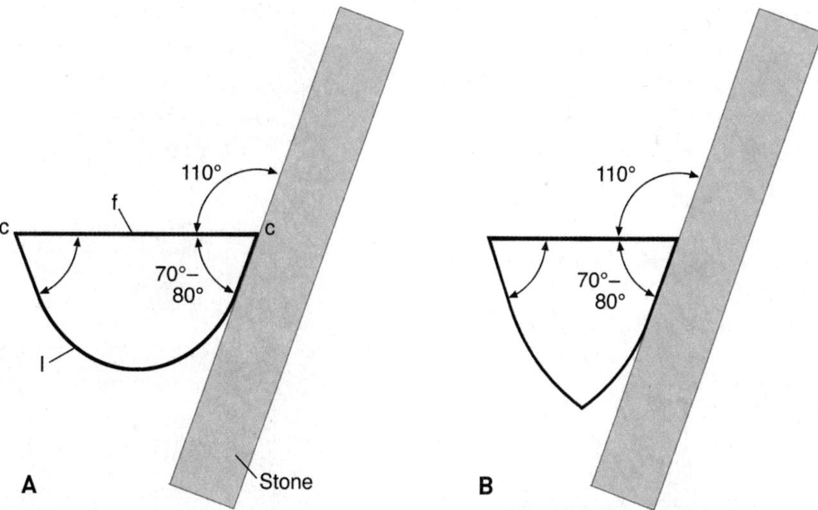

Figure 38-6 Angulation for Sharpening. Cross sections of a curet **(A)** and a scaler **(B)** show correct angulation of the face (f) of the blade with the flat sharpening stone to reproduce the internal angle of the instrument at 70°. Note the cutting edges (c) and the lateral surfaces (l).

IV. Apply the Sharpening Stone

- Hold the stone perpendicular to the floor, at the shank third of the cutting edge.
- From the 90° angle with the face of the instrument, open the stone to make an angle of 110° (**Figures 38-7C, 38-8A-B**).

V. Activate the Sharpening Stone

A. Steps One and Two

- Maintain the stone in contact with the blade and at the proper angle throughout the procedure.
- Tighten the grasp on the instrument (nondominant hand) while applying a smooth, even pressure to the cutting edge to keep the instrument stable and motionless.
- Move the stone up and down with short rhythmical strokes about ½-inch high. Place more pressure on the down stroke. Maintain the 110° angle precisely. Finish each area with a down stroke.[14]
- For the universal curet:
  - Follow the cutting edge to where the curvature for the toe begins, applying three or four down strokes overlapping at each millimeter of the cutting edge.
  - Proceed to the opposite side to sharpen, repeating the steps just described (Figure 38-8).
  - Next, proceed to the third step to sharpen the toe.
- For the area-specific curet: Apply sharpening strokes **only** to the one blade: proceed to the third step to sharpen around the toe.
- For the sickle scaler: Follow the same procedure to where the cutting edge tapers to form the sharp tip and continue in that direction to finish that side of the blade. Proceed to the other side to sharpen the opposite cutting edge.

B. Step Three: The Toe of a Curet

- Tip curet down to make the toe parallel with floor.
- Apply stone to make a 90° angle with the toe.
- Open the stone to make a 110° angle.
- Apply strokes for sharpening as described for the sides of the face of the blade.

VI. Test for Sharpness

- Apply testing stick along the entire cutting edges.
- Repeat sharpening procedures as necessary to retain clean, sharp cutting edges.

Stationary Flat Stone: Moving Instrument

- In this method, the instrument moves and the sharpening stone remains stationary.

I. Curet

- Place the stone flat on a steady surface.
- Examine the cutting edges to be sharpened. Test for sharpness.

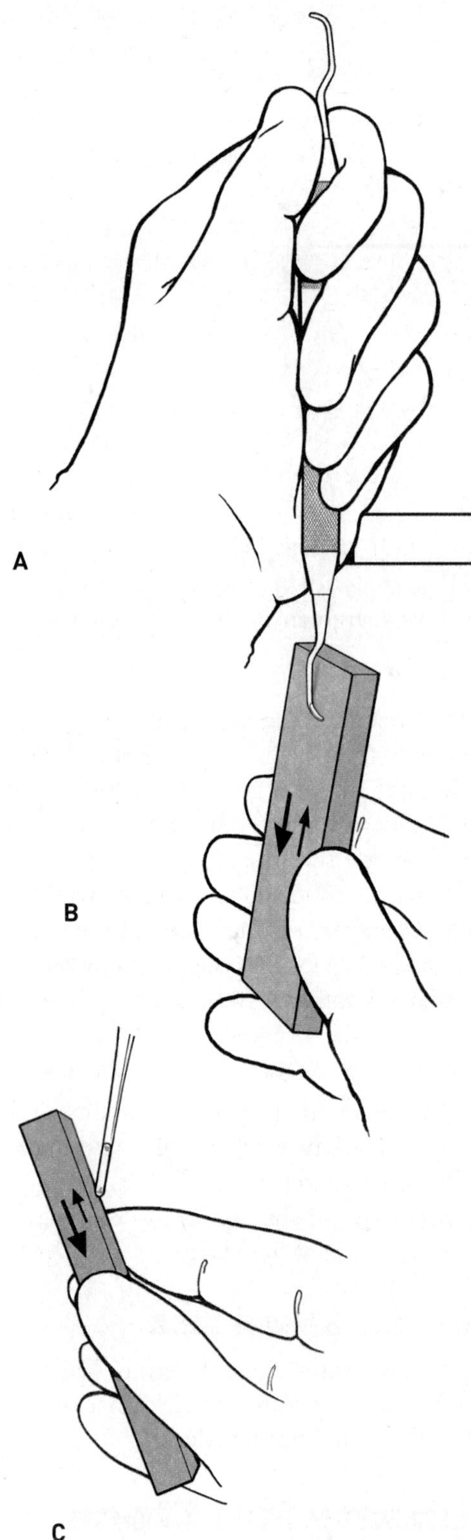

Figure 38-7 Stationary Instrument—Moving Stone Technique. **A:** Grasp the instrument with the nondominant hand. Stabilize the hand on the edge of a stationary table or bench and provide good light on the instrument. **B:** The stone is angled with the face of the instrument at 110° to maintain the internal angle of the blade at 70° to 80°. **C:** Stone reversed to sharpen the opposite cutting edge of a universal curet.

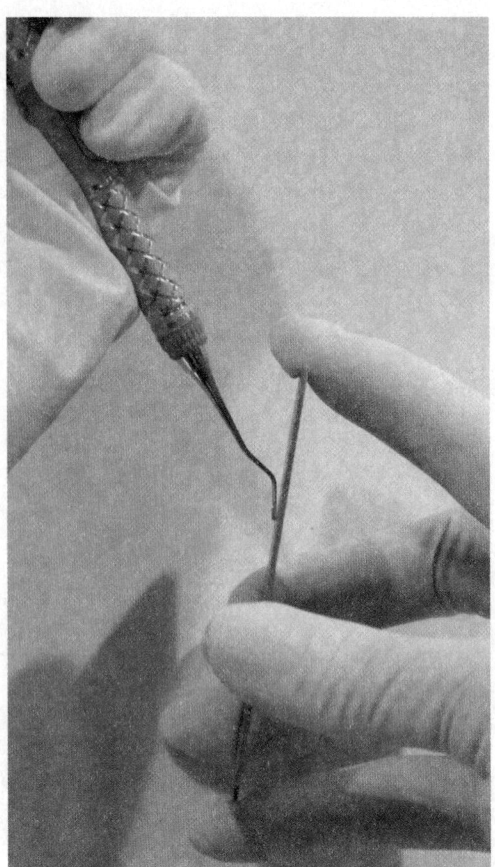

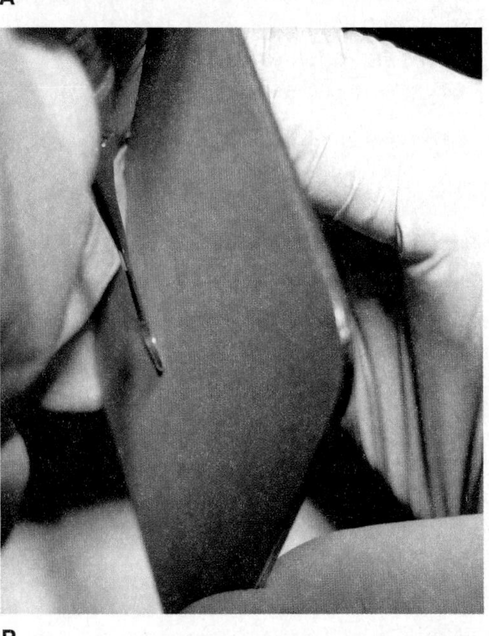

Figure 38-8 Stationary Instrument—Moving Diamond-Sharpening Card. **A** and **B:** Grasp the instrument with the nondominant hand. Stabilize the hand. The card is angled with the face of the instrument at 110° to maintain the internal angle of the blade at 70° to 80°. Image (B) shows how the orientation of the diamond-sharpening card to the instrument face and blade look to the clinician during the sharpening process.

- Hold the instrument in a modified pen grasp, and establish a secure finger rest (**Figure 38-9A**).
- Apply the cutting edge to the stone. An angle of 110° is formed by the stone and face.
  - Because the curet is curved, only a small section of the cutting edge can be applied at one time.
  - Sharpening is performed in a series of applications of the cutting edge to the stone, each overlapping the previous, as the instrument is turned and drawn steadily along the stone.
  - The portion of the cutting edge nearest the shank is applied first (**Figure 38-10A–B**).
- Apply moderate to light but firm pressure while the instrument is activated.
- Use a slow, steady stroke to maintain control and to ensure that each portion of the cutting edge receives equal treatment.
- Move the blade forward into the cutting edge. Turn the instrument continuously until the center of the round end of the blade is reached.

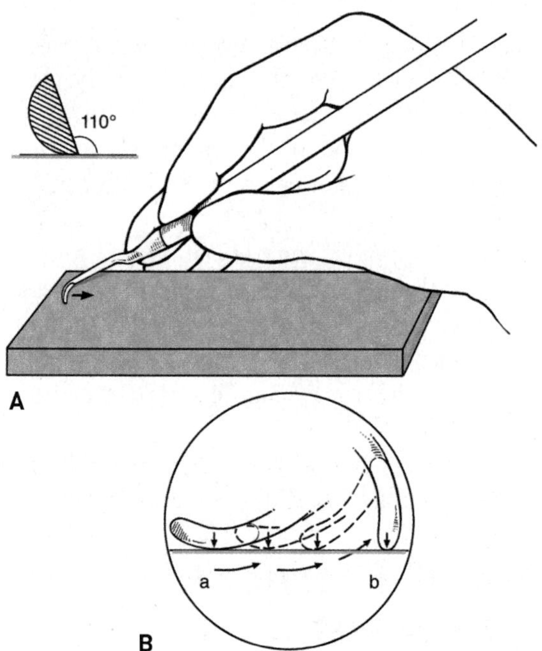

Figure 38-9 Stationary Stone—Moving Instrument Technique for a Curet. **A:** Stone placed flat with blade in position at the beginning of the sharpening stroke. With the finger rest stabilized on the edge of the stone, the cutting edge is maintained at the proper angulation (110°) as the instrument is drawn along the stone with an even, moderate pressure. **B:** The movement of the blade is shown by the arrows, which indicate each portion of the cutting edge as the blade is turned on the stone from the beginning (a) to the completion (b) of the stroke at the center of the round toe of the curet. For a universal curet, the instrument is turned over and the opposite cutting edge is sharpened.

- Test for sharpness along the entire cutting edge; reapply to stone as necessary for ideal sharpness.
- Turn the instrument to sharpen the second cutting edge. Overlap at the center of the round toe. Universal curets are sharpened on both sides and around the toe. The single blade of the Gracey curet and around the toe are sharpened (see Figure 38-9).
- Carefully wipe the instrument with a gauze square or an alcohol wipe to remove the wire edge.

II. Scaler: Sickle or Jacquette

- Place the stone flat on a firm table or bench top under adequate light. Do not tilt the stone while sharpening.
- Examine cutting edges to be sharpened. Test for sharpness.
- Hold the instrument with a firm pen grasp, using the thumb and index and middle (second) fingers to prevent the instrument from rotating or changing angles during sharpening (Figure 38-10A–B).
- Establish finger rest on side of stone using ring and little fingers.
- Stabilize stone with fingers of opposite hand.
- Apply cutting edge to be sharpened to the stone. Maintain 70° to 80° internal angle of the instrument (Figure 38-10B). The portion of the cutting edge nearest the shank is applied first.

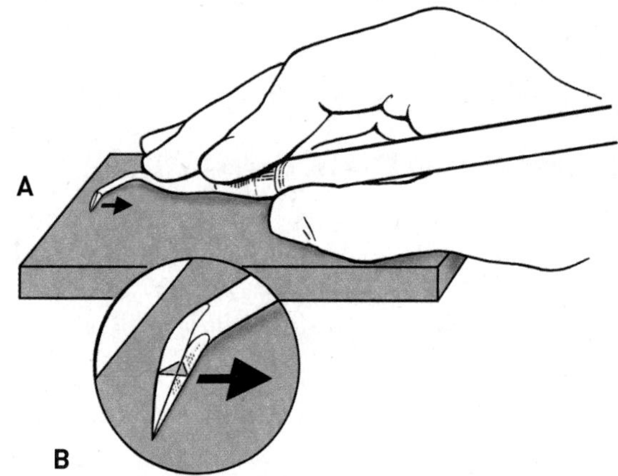

Figure 38-10 Stationary Stone Technique for a Sickle Scaler or Jacquette. **A:** With a modified pen grasp and a finger rest established on the side of the stone, the scaler is positioned for sharpening. **B:** The portion of the cutting edge nearest the lower shank is applied first with an angle of 110° between the face and the stone. The instrument is turned continuously to follow the arclike shape of the blade. The cutting edges are sharpened to the pointed tip.

- Apply moderate to light but firm pressure while instrument is in motion. Heavy pressure can reduce control of instrument, cause scratching of the stone, and produce an unfavorable bevel at the cutting edge.
- Use a short, slow stroke to maintain the exact relation of the cutting edge to the stone.
    - Pull blade forward, toward the cutting edge.
    - All fingers move with the arm as a unit.
    - Use a slow, steady stroke to maintain control and to ensure that each portion of the cutting edge receives equal treatment.
    - Turn the instrument continually to follow the shape of the blade to the pointed tip.
- Test for sharpness after one or two strokes. Repeat as needed for ideal sharpness.
- Turn instrument and proceed to sharpen other lateral surface. When instrument placement is awkward for a modified contra-angle scaler, use a narrow side of the stone.

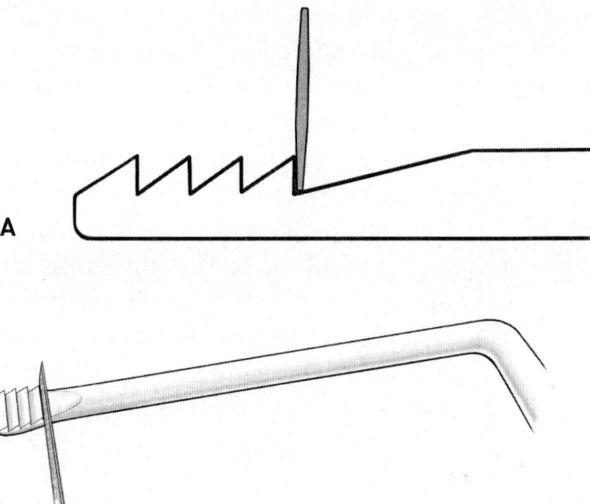

Figure 38-11 Sharpening a File Scaler. **A:** Tanged file in position against one of the several surfaces to be ground. **B:** With the file scaler stabilized to prevent movement, the tanged file is pulled through the channel using a moderate, steady pressure against the surface to be ground.

Sharpening the File Scaler

- Files are sharpened with a flat sharpening instrument called a tanged file.
    - Diamond-coated files are *not* sharpened.
- Use of magnification and good illumination is necessary when sharpening files to ensure correct placement of the tanged file.
- Use a testing stick to check for the degree of sharpness of the file.
- If the file blades do not grasp the plastic testing stick when adapted lightly, they will need to be sharpened.

I. Surface to Be Sharpened

- Examine the file closely with the head of the working end positioned outward (**Figure 38-11A**).
- Note the two angular surfaces that meet to form a "V" shape (**Figure 38-11B**).
- The surface to be contacted with the tanged file and ground during sharpening is the surface of the "V" that is farthest away.

II. Sharpening Procedure

- Prepare a workplace with good illumination and magnification, such as loupes or a magnified light ring.
- Place the sterile file on a clean surface. Secure it with the series of teeth facing up.
- Position the right end of the tanged file in the channel as shown in the illustration (Figure 38-11A). (Left-handed clinicians reverse the process, positioning the left end of the tanged file in the channel.)
- With light-to-moderate steady pressure, pull the tanged file through the channel, moving in a straight line from one end to the other in one direction only.
- Release pressure and reposition the tanged file back at the starting point. Repeat the process. Two or three passes with the tanged file are usually sufficient to bring each edge back to sharpness.
- Sharpen the remaining blades using the same technique.
- Test for sharpness and repeat the sharpening stroke as needed for ideal edge sharpness.

Care of Sharpening Equipment

I. Flat Sharpening Stone

A. Prepare for Sterilization

Submerge in ultrasonic cleaner or scrub with soap and water to remove metal particles left from sharpening.

B. Stain Removal

- Check manufacturer's recommendation.
- Alternate cleaning suggestions: Use powdered cleanser when stone becomes discolored. If the stone becomes "glazed" by metal particles ground into the surface, rub sandpaper over the stone surface.

Box 38-1 Example Documentation: Monitoring of Sharpness of Instruments

- **S**—Female patient, 48 years old and in good health, presents for the third in a series of subgingival instrumentation appointments (maxillary left quadrant).
- **O**—Previously documented assessment findings for maxillary left quadrant include: heavy generalized calculus, generalized 4- to 5-mm probing depths, and 8-mm probing depth on the mesial of #12 and distal of #15 (furcation involvement).
- **A**—Burnished calculus was noted on the quadrants completed.
- **P**—Instrument sharpness carefully monitored. File scaler and power scaler were used to break up burnished calculus and rigid Gracey curettes used for removal. Completed quadrant debridement with power and manual instruments. Extended shank mini curets were used for root debridement in the mesial concavity of #12 and distal furcation of #15.

Next steps: Scheduled for subgingival instrumentation on mandibular left quadrant and re-evaluate completed quadrants, particularly pocket areas >4 mm.
Signed: ____________________, RDH
Date: ________________

C. *Storage*

- Keep in sealed, sterilized packages for sharpening at instrument preparation area.
- A stone and testing stick should be stored with each instrument setup in the cassette for use during the treatment appointment.

II. Care of the Tanged File

Because the tanged file corrodes easily when exposed to moisture, it may require special handling.

- Wipe the tanged file with a sterile gauze soaked with isopropyl alcohol after use.
- Sterilize in a dry heat oven or chemical vapor sterilizer. (See Chapter 7.)

III. Manufacturer's Directions

Follow manufacturer's directions for all artificial stones.

Documentation

- See **Box 38-1** for a sample documentation.

Factors to Teach the Patient

- Benefits of using a finely sharpened instrument for calculus removal.
- Harmful effects of using dull instruments.

References

1. Acevedo RAA, Cardozo AKV, Sampaio JEC. Scanning electron microscopic and profilometric study of different sharpening stones. *Braz Dent J*. 2006;17(3):237-242.
2. Matsui K, Onaka K. Assessing significance of sharpening brand-new scaler. *Bull Tokyo Dent Coll*. 2013;54(1):1-8.
3. Johnson CR, Kanji Z. The impact of occupation-related musculoskeletal disorders on dental hygienists. *Can J Dent Hyg*. 2016;50(2):72-79.
4. Balevi B. Engineering specifics of the periodontal curet's cutting edge. *J Periodontol*. 1996;67(4):374-378.
5. Tal H, Panno JM, Vaidyanathan TK. Scanning electron microscope evaluation of wear of dental curettes during standardized root planing. *J Periodontol*. 1985;56(9):532-536.
6. Hessheimer HM, Payne JB, Shaw LE, Spanyers EM, Beatty MW. A comparison of efficiency and material wear of diamond-plated versus ceramic sharpening stones. *J Dent Hyg*. 2017;91(5):64-67.
7. Nahass HE, Madkour GG. Evaluation of different resharpening techniques on the working edges of periodontal scalers: a scanning electron microscopic study. *Life Sci J*. 2013;10(1):989-993.
8. Wiebe CB, Hoath BJ, Owen G, Bi J, Giannelis G, Larjava HS. Sterilization of ceramic sharpening stones. *J Can Dent Assoc*. 2017;83(h11):1488-2159.
9. Huang CC, Tseng CC. Effect of different sharpening stones on periodontal curettes evaluated by scanning electron microscopy. *J Formosan Med Assoc*. 1991;90(8):782-787.
10. Liu G, Liu X, Li N, et al. Wear and fracture of curettes due to sharpening and scaling processes. *Int J Dent Hyg*. 2021;20(3):564-570.

11. Ingole PD, Ramakrishna RD, Iqbal MA, Bang KO. Retrieval of fractured Gracey's curette from maxillary sinus: a rare case report. *Int J Med Dent Case Rep*. 2018;5(1):1-3.
12. Di Fiore A, Mazzoleni S, Fantin F, Favero L, De Francesco M, Stellini E. Evaluation of three different manual techniques of sharpening curettes through a scanning electron microscope: a randomized controlled experimental study. *Int J Dent Hyg*. 2015;13(2):145-150.
13. Hu-Friedy Mfg. Co., LLC. A timely approach to instrument sharpening. https://www.hufriedygroup.com/sites/default/files/409_SHM_Its_About_Time_Manual__0317.pdf. Accessed January 25, 2022.
14. Andrade Acevedo RA, Cézar Sampaio JE, Shibli JA. Scanning electron microscope assessment of several resharpening techniques on the cutting edges of Gracey curettes. *J Contemp Dent Pract*. 2007;8(7):70-77.

CHAPTER 39

Nonsurgical Periodontal Therapy and Adjunctive Therapy

Linda D. Boyd, RDH, RD, EdD
Uhlee (Yuri) Oh, RDH, BS
Esther M. Wilkins, BS, RDH, DMD

CHAPTER OUTLINE

LEARNING OBJECTIVES

After studying this chapter, the student will be able to:

1. Explain the goals and desirable clinical endpoints or outcomes for nonsurgical periodontal therapy.
2. Devise a care plan for a patient with each of the periodontal classifications.
3. Describe the changes in the subgingival bacteria after periodontal debridement.
4. Describe current evidence related to laser therapy for initial therapy.
5. Develop postoperative instructions for a patient following a nonsurgical periodontal therapy appointment.
6. List the steps in re-evaluation of nonsurgical periodontal therapy and the decisions that must be made based on the clinical outcomes.
7. Compare and contrast the risks and benefits of systemic antibiotics and local delivery antimicrobials.
8. Critically evaluate the benefit of local delivery antimicrobials on changes in pocket depth and clinical attachment level (CAL).

Nonsurgical Periodontal Therapy

I. Introduction to Components of Initial Periodontal Therapy

- **Periodontal debridement** remains the "gold standard" for initial therapy in inflammatory gingival and periodontal infections and includes the following therapeutic interventions[1,2]:
  - Patient education for preventive strategies to control dental biofilm with ongoing evaluation and reinforcement.
  - Management or elimination of modifiable risk factors for periodontal disease such as tobacco, glycemic control in diabetes, and dietary counseling.
  - **Nonsurgical periodontal therapy (NSPT)** or professional mechanical plaque removal (PMPR) to remove dental biofilm, **endotoxins**, other bacterial products, and calculus.
  - Elimination of local factors contributing to periodontal disease such as overhanging margins of restorations, caries, and ill-fitting prostheses.
  - Use of adjunctive agents such as antimicrobial or **antibiotic** agents as appropriate to enhance periodontal treatment outcomes.
  - Re-evaluation of initial therapy to identify the need for surgical periodontal therapy or ongoing periodontal maintenance.

Nonsurgical Periodontal Therapy Goals and Outcomes

- The therapeutic goals of NSPT are to manage or eliminate plaque biofilm and risk factors for periodontitis in order to stop progression of disease and maintain oral health.

I. Interrupt or Arrest the Progress of Disease

- Reduce formation of dental biofilm.
- Delay repopulation of subgingival pathogenic microorganisms.
- Change behavioral and lifestyle habits of the patient to reduce risk factors for periodontal infections.

II. Create an Environment to Support Healing and Resolution of Inflammation

- Facilitate resolution of disease to restore gingival health.
- Reduce pocket depths.[1]
- Eliminate bleeding on probing (BOP).
- Increase attachment level.[1]
- Remove calculus and restorative dentistry irregularities to reduce biofilm retention.[1,2]

III. Induce Positive Changes in Quality and Quantity of Subgingival Biofilm

- Before instrumentation, the predominant microorganisms are anaerobic, gram-negative, motile forms with many spirochetes and rods, high counts of all types of microorganisms, and many leukocytes.[3,4]
- After instrumentation, the composition of the bacterial flora tends to shift to those seen in health with a predominance of aerobic, gram-positive, nonmotile, coccoid forms with lower bacterial load (**Table 39-1**).[3]
    - However, in some individuals, periodontal pathogens may persist after NSPT, and further treatment may be necessary to manage periodontal disease progression.[5]

IV. Educate the Patient about Effective Biofilm Management

- To assume a co-therapist role in maintaining periodontal health following nonsurgical and/or surgical periodontal treatment.
- To make a commitment to perform daily personal biofilm control measures.
- To continue with periodontal maintenance appointments at intervals consistent with patient's individual risk factors to monitor and manage periodontal disease.[2,6]

Table 39-1 Effect of Subgingival Instrumentation on Pocket Microflora

Periodontal Infection before Treatment	Periodontal Health after Treatment
Predominant flora is: Anaerobic Gram negative Motile Spirochetes, motile rods; pathogenic	Predominant flora is: Aerobic Gram positive Nonmotile Coccoid forms; nonpathogenic
Total microbial count: Very high total count of all types of microorganisms	Total microbial count: Much lower total counts of all types of microorganisms
Leukocyte count: Many leukocytes	Leukocyte count: Lower leukocyte counts

V. Provide Initial Preparation (Tissue Conditioning) for Surgical Periodontal Therapy in Advanced Disease

- Reduce or eliminate etiologic and predisposing factors.[2]
- Re-evaluation following initial NSPT allows for identification of those areas requiring surgical intervention.[2]

Nonsurgical Periodontal Therapy Treatment Goals and Components

I. Patient with Gingivitis

A. Therapeutic Goals

- Therapeutic goal: reversal of inflammation to establish gingival health through elimination of etiologic factors.[2]

B. Treatment for Gingivitis

- Step 1 of therapy applies to gingivitis and all stages of periodontitis[2]:
    - Individualized patient education to motivate and provide ongoing support for behavior change in effective daily biofilm removal.

        - See Chapters 24, 26, and 27 for guidance on behavior change and selection of toothbrush and interdental aids.
    - Recommendations for management of individual modifiable risk factors for oral disease based on risk[2] such as:
        - Office and home fluorides. (See Chapter 34.)
        - Smoking cessation support and referral to services as appropriate. (See Chapter 32.)
        - Dietary assessment and counseling. (See Chapter 33.)
        - Desensitization of teeth. (See Chapter 41.)
        - Care for dental implants and prostheses. (See Chapters 30 and 31.)
- Step 2 of therapy:
    - Professional supragingival and subgingival instrumentation for biofilm and calculus removal.[2]
    - Management of restorative biofilm-retentive factors by removal of overhanging margins and rough surfaces of restorations.[2]
    - In nondental plaque–induced gingivitis, patients may need to be referred for additional diagnostics and treatment due to the many possible etiologies of the condition.[7]

II. Patient with Stage I to III Periodontitis

A. Treatment Goals

- Therapeutic goals[1,2]:
    - Reduction in gingival inflammation and BOP.
    - Reduction in pocket depths and number of diseased sites.
    - CALs are stabilized or improved.
    - Decrease in supragingival dental biofilm by the patient to a level consistent with health.

B. Treatment for Stage I to III Periodontitis

- Step 1 of therapy (as described in the treatment for gingivitis section) applies to all stages of periodontitis.
- Step 2 of periodontal therapy[1,2]:
    - Subgingival instrumentation with hand or powered (ultrasonic or piezo) alone or combination of both.
        - Lipopolysaccharides or endotoxins, derived from the cell walls of gram-negative pathogenic microorganisms, trigger an inflammatory host response, leading to destruction of the periodontal attachment.
        - Subgingival instrumentation aids in removing the endotoxins in biofilm and biofilm colonizing calculus.[8,9]
        - However, the cementum should be preserved during subgingival instrumentation as much as possible as it serves as a source of growth factors for **new attachment**.[10]
    - Chlorhexidine mouthrinse may be used for a short period of time following subgingival instrumentation.
    - Sustained-release chlorhexidine may be considered as an adjunct to subgingival instrumentation.
    - Sustained-release locally delivered antibiotics that may be considered as adjuncts to subgingival instrumentation include:
        - Doxycyline hyclate (Atridox)
        - Minocyline HCl (Arestin)
    - In specific patients, systemic antibiotics may be considered.
- Re-evaluation to assess the outcomes of treatment to determine if additional treatment is indicated.

III. Patients with Moderate-to-Severe Periodontitis (Stage III or IV) or Patients with Poor Response to Initial or Maintenance Therapy

A. Treatment Goals

- Therapeutic goal[2]:
    - To gain access to deep pocket sites to regenerate or resect areas negatively impacting management of periodontitis such as bony defects.
- Steps 1 and 2 of periodontal therapy used for Stage I to III periodontitis treatment should be performed prior to considering Step 3 of therapy.[2]
- Step 3 of therapy[2]:
    - Localized subgingival instrumentation with or without adjunctive therapies.
    - Surgical periodontal procedures include[2]:
        - Flap surgery to provide access.
        - Regenerative procedures: bone grafting, guided tissue regeneration.

    - Resective therapy: gingival flaps with or without osseous surgery, root resective therapy, gingivectomy.
- For these patients, thorough NSPT prepares the tissues for the surgical phase of treatment by reducing the bacterial load and inflammation.

Dental Hygiene Treatment Care Plan for Periodontal Debridement

- The needs of the individual patient are identified through patient assessment. (Refer to Chapter 20.)
- The course of treatment is defined by the dental hygiene diagnosis and care plan. (Refer to Chapters 22 and 23.)
- Included in the care plan are the following:
    - Management of individual modifiable risk factors such as tobacco cessation.
    - Periodontal diagnosis, including the distribution and severity of the periodontal infection.
    - Treatment sequence needed for the individual.
    - Length and number of appointments required to complete treatment.
    - Plan for re-evaluation and continuing care. (See Chapters 44 and 45.)

Appointment Planning

- Whether a single or multiple appointment plan is required, the initial step is patient education.
- The overall care plan should be reviewed and discussed to obtain informed consent of the patient, parent, or guardian.
- Treatment begins with the patient taking responsibility for daily removal of biofilm.[2]

I. Single Appointment

- The diagnosis may be gingivitis with minimal inflammation and small deposits near the gingival margin, so local anesthesia may not be needed. (See Chapter 19.)
- If only a few teeth are periodontally involved and require localized NSPT, limited areas of local anesthesia may be required.
- Patient with an acceptable biofilm score and evidence of adequate oral self-care without the need for follow-up instruction.
- The patient is compliant in regular periodontal maintenance.

II. Multiple Appointments

Factors that determine the number of appointments needed include the extent of periodontal involvement as shown by probing measurements, distribution and extent of calculus deposits, and adequacy of biofilm removal.

A. Management of Modifiable Risk Factors

- At the initial appointment, education should begin to manage modifiable risk factors, such as tobacco cessation and biofilm removal. Chapter 24 provides guidance on motivational interviewing to assist with this component of treatment.
- Patient education to assess and refine daily oral self-care techniques for dental biofilm removal is initiated at the first NSPT appointment.
    - Interdental devices to complement the use of a toothbrush can be added as the patient demonstrates readiness. It is important not to overwhelm the patient at the first appointment.
- At each successive appointment, disclose the biofilm and review with the patient.
- Change or add new oral hygiene aids as needed based on patient's preferences and dexterity.
- Typically, inflammation and bleeding will gradually improve at each appointment as a result of improvement in biofilm removal and periodontal debridement.

B. Quadrant Scaling Appointments

- One system for appointment planning is by quadrants or sextants with local anesthesia for moderate-to-severe disease, such as stages III and IV periodontitis, at 1-week intervals.
    - This allows for review of oral self-care and healing of the area(s) treated at the previous appointment(s).
- With less severe periodontitis, such as stage I or II, and a compliant patient, two quadrants on the same side (maxillary and mandibular arches) may be completed at an appointment.
- After subgingival instrumentation is completed, the need for re-evaluation should be reinforced to assess the need for additional care.

- The periodontal maintenance (or supportive periodontal care) interval should be determined based on the patient risk for disease progression.[2]

C. Evaluation

- At each appointment, the healing of the quadrants previously treated should be assessed.
- Any residual calculus can be removed.
- Best done 4–8 weeks following completion of NSPT to allow for connective tissue healing.[11]
- Re-evaluation is important to determine the periodontal maintenance interval and the need for referral and/or surgical therapy.

III. Full-Mouth Disinfection

A. Definition

- System of performing NSPT in two long appointments completed within a 24-hour period with adjunctive chlorhexidine mouthrinse.[2,12]
  - The procedures are best accomplished under local anesthesia with a chairside dental assistant.
- Systematic review of the research on full-mouth disinfection versus traditional NSPT found no clear evidence of a benefit for one approach over another.[2,12]

B. Rationale

- The rationale is completing the procedure in one session or multiple sessions within 24 hours reduces likelihood of re-infection of previously treated sites.[12]

C. Limitations

- Case selection: Many patients would not be able to withstand such intense treatment.
  - The health status of the patient also needs to be considered due to the systemic implications of an acute systemic inflammatory response.[2]
- Eliminates opportunities for review and repeated instruction at the patient's learning pace without a series of appointments with time in between for patient practice of oral self-care.
- The ability to re-evaluate healing of each quadrant is also not possible.

IV. Definitive Nonsurgical Periodontal Therapy

A. Quadrant or Sextant Approach

- Quadrant or sextant treatment to completion is recommended.
- The decision between a quadrant and sextant approach is made according to what can reasonably be completed by the clinician and tolerated by the patient during an appointment.
- Treatment appointments are scheduled accordingly.

B. Factors to Consider in Care Planning

- Access: the relative ease of instrument insertion to the base of the soft-tissue pocket.
  - Tissue tone, such as fibrosity of the free gingiva.
  - Probing depths: attachment pattern around the full circumference of each tooth.
- Deposit on tooth surfaces
  - Extent and distribution of calculus.
  - Age of calculus/degree of mineralization.
  - Strength of attachment of calculus to the tooth.
- Root anatomy
  - Multirooted teeth with furcation involvement.
  - Deep concavities.
- Patient factors
  - Behavioral factors, such as apprehension.
  - Need for local anesthetic or nitrous oxide/oxygen sedation.
  - Limited capacity for opening mouth.

Preparation for Periodontal Therapy

I. Review the Patient's Assessment Record

- Document individual needs: from medical, dental, and psychosocial history along with previous appointment experiences.
- Identify systemic or physical problems with potential for emergency.

II. Review Radiographic Findings

A. Findings Applicable During Instrumentation

- Anatomic features of roots, furcations, and bone level, which may impact selection and adaptation of instruments.
- Overhanging restorations to be removed or scheduled for replacement.

B. Use Radiographs as Guide

- Keep radiographs on lighted viewbox or the computer screen throughout the treatment for reference to observe bone level, root anatomy, and contour of restorations for each area.

III. Review Care Plan and Treatment Records

- Document flow and sequence of planned appointments.
- Document findings related to the instrumentation process.
  - Assess periodontal chart to review attachment topography and access limitations.
  - Assemble procedure tray setup or cassette to include appropriate instruments.
- Review previous appointment progress notes.
  - Read details of prior treatment, noting quadrants or sextants completed, which will be reassessed for healing.
  - Determine how previous treatment appointments have been tolerated by the patient.
  - Plan appropriate local anesthesia for pain management.[13]
- Keep periodontal probing chart within view of the clinician throughout the treatment for reference. Ideally the radiographs and periodontal chart can be viewed side-by-side during patient care.

IV. Patient Preparation

A. Premedication Requirements for High-Risk Patient

- Transient **bacteremia** can occur during and immediately after scaling procedures.
- Flossing and a single quadrant of scaling and root debridement result in the same incidence and magnitude of bacteremia, so only high-risk patients are in need of antibiotic premedication.[14]
- Consult with the primary care provider to determine whether premedication is required. (See Chapter 11 to identify patients who may be at risk for bacterial endocarditis and be in need of prophylactic premedication.)

B. Provide Preprocedural Antimicrobial Rinse

- Preprocedural rinsing with chlorhexidine gluconate lowers bacterial aerosols and contamination produced by ultrasonic instrumentation.[14,15]
- Preprocedural rinsing with chlorhexidine rinse has not been shown to reduce bacteremia, or bacteria in the bloodstream, following NSPT.[14]

C. Prepare for Local Anesthesia

- Adequate pain control tends to facilitate better patient outcomes and higher levels of patient satisfaction with treatment.
- Patients who refuse local anesthesia experience more discomfort, dental anxiety, longer treatment times, greater residual gingival inflammation, and more pocket depths greater than or equal to 5 mm.[13]
  - Rather than asking patients if they "want" local anesthesia, the clinician should state the best treatment option and discuss the impact of pain control on improved outcomes to aid the patient in decision making.

V. Supragingival Examination

A. Visual

- Gross deposits and tooth surface irregularities can be seen by direct vision. Fine, unstained, white, or yellowish calculus is frequently invisible when wet with saliva.
- Observe tooth surfaces closely while applying a gentle stream of compressed air using appropriate measures to manage aerosols.[15] Dry calculus is more visible than wet calculus.

B. Tactile

- An enamel surface without deposits or anatomic irregularities is smooth.
- An explorer tip passed over the surface slides freely, smoothly, and quietly.
- When rough calculus deposits are present, the explorer tip does not slide freely, but meets with resistance over varying textures.
- Deposits can produce a surface that feels like sand paper or a click as the explorer passes over them.

VI. Subgingival Examination

A. Visual

- Gingiva: The clinical appearance suggestive of underlying calculus may include the following:
  - Soft, spongy, bluish-red gingiva, with enlargement of the interdental papillae over proximal surface calculus.
  - Dark-colored area beneath relatively translucent marginal gingiva.

- Calculus
    - A loose, edematous pocket wall can be deflected from the tooth surface with a gentle stream of compressed air.
    - Dark, subgingival calculus can be seen within the pocket on the root surface.

B. Tactile

- Periodontal charting
    - Use probing depth recordings as a basic guide for the depth of insertion of the curet.
    - Study the soft-tissue attachment pattern for instrument selection to provide access to the base of the pocket.
- Identify shallow pockets (sulci)
    - Scaling in shallow pockets may lead to loss of periodontal attachment due to detachment of periodontal ligament fibers, so it must be done with care.[16]
    - Root surfaces free of calculus require minimal lateral pressure for comprehensive biofilm removal.
- Determine distribution and extent of deposits
    - Use an explorer, such as an ODU 11/12, for detection of calculus deposits.
    - The periodontal probe may also detect the presence of moderate to heavy calculus deposits, as shown in **Figure 39-1**.
    - The novice dental hygiene student will benefit from recording the location of calculus.
- Evaluate tooth topography
    - Detect grooves and furcations using a horizontal stroke (Figure 39-1C).
    - Use a Nabers furcation probe to assess furcations. (See Chapter 20.)
    - Note anatomic root and furcation variations (**Figure 39-2**).
- Evaluate restorative margins
    - Detect overhanging restorations that need to be evaluated by the dentist for possible replacement or margination.
    - Detect marginal irregularities that retain biofilm.

VII. Formulate Strategy for Instrumentation

- Combine clinical findings with information documented in the patient's record.
- Review overall treatment objectives for the patient.
- Determine a strategy for instrumentation.

Advanced Instrumentation

I. Definitions

- Scaling and root planing (SRP): removal of calculus and "diseased" cementum was previously considered the desired endpoint necessary in order to achieve periodontal health.
    - Evidence now demonstrates removal of cementum is not necessary to reduce endotoxin levels and cementum needs to be preserved to facilitate new attachment.[9,17,18]

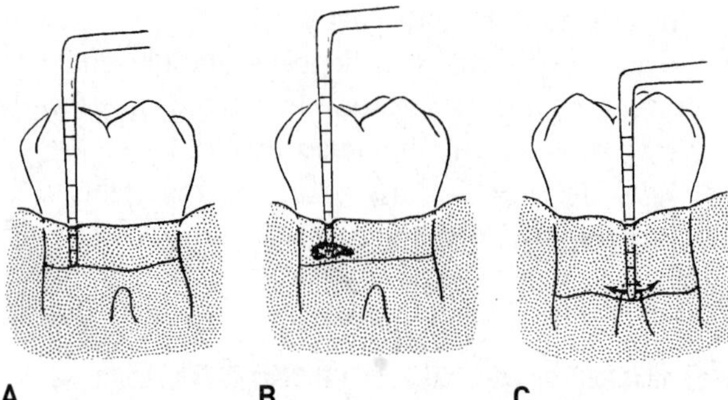

Figure 39-1 Subgingival Examination Using a Probe. **A:** Probe inserted into the bottom of a pocket for complete examination prior to subgingival scaling. **B:** As the probe passes over the root surface, it may be intercepted by a hard mass of calculus. **C:** Using a horizontal probe stroke to examine the topography of a furcation area. Keep the side of the tip of the probe on the tooth surface and slide over one root, into the furcation, and across to the other root.

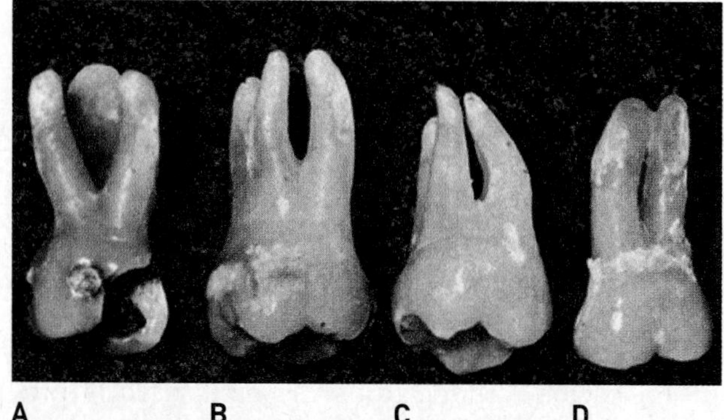

Figure 39-2 Anatomic Variations of Furcations. **A:** Divergent roots with the furcation in the coronal one-third of the root with a short root trunk. **B:** Convergent roots with the furcation in the middle one half of the root with a longer root trunk. **C:** Very convergent roots. **D:** Fused roots with the furcation in the coronal one-third of the root.

- However, SRP continues to be common terminology used in private practice and by insurance companies.
- Subgingival instrumentation *or* periodontal debridement *or* root surface debridement: involves disruption and removal of dental biofilm and associated endotoxins along with calculus from the root. Use of ultrasonic instrumentation, along with avoidance of excessive instrumentation time and pressure, helps to preserve cementum and dentin.[2,18]

II. Subgingival Anatomic Considerations

- Tooth morphology
  - Level of clinical attachment (normal or clinical attachment loss) varies; more attachment loss, resulting in deeper pocket depths exposing additional root concavities and possible furcations, complicates instrumentation.
  - The cementum is thin (0.03–0.06 mm), and care must be taken to minimize removal during instrumentation.[9]
- Soft-tissue pocket wall
  - The pocket is an extremely small area for manipulation of instruments.
  - The pocket narrows in the deeper area next to the clinical attachment.
  - Bleeding during instrumentation can impact visibility.
- Variations in probing depths
  - The periodontal charting is a guide to subgingival instrumentation and will serve as a *road map* to guide instrument depth of insertion.
- Nature of subgingival calculus
  - Location: Calculus may be located on the enamel, the root, or both (**Figure 39-3**).
  - Morphology of calculus: Subgingival calculus is irregularly deposited. It can present as a spicule, ledge, smooth veneer, and other forms. (See Chapter 17.)
  - Burnished calculus: Subgingival calculus that has been partially instrumented and may be smooth, making it difficult to detect when an explorer is used to check the area.

III. Instrumentation Technique

This chapter focuses on the components of advanced instrumentation for deposit removal. **Box 39-1** summarizes the steps. Types of instruments and the basic principles for their use are included in Chapter 37.

A. Instrument Selection and Sequence

- The order in which instruments are selected and used can impact the efficiency and quality of biofilm and calculus removal.
- Instrument selection sequence is recommended as follows (the order may vary depending on the

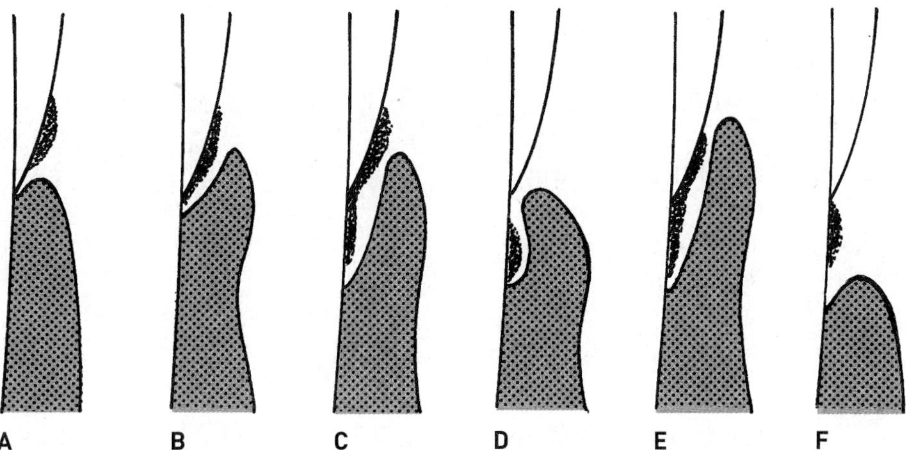

Figure 39-3 Location of Instrumentation. The location of calculus deposits, level of periodontal attachment, depth of pocket, and position of the gingival margin determine the site of instrumentation. **A:** Supragingival calculus on the enamel. **B:** Gingival pocket with both supragingival and subgingival calculus on enamel. **C:** Periodontal pocket with both supragingival and subgingival calculus. **D:** Periodontal pocket with subgingival calculus only on the root surface. **E:** Periodontal pocket with subgingival calculus on both the enamel and the root surface. **F:** Calculus on the root surface exposed by gingival recession.

Box 39-1 Steps for Calculus Removal Using Manual Instruments

Assessment

- Probe to determine pocket/sulcus characteristics and confirm soft-tissue attachment topography.
- Explore to determine location and extent of deposits and tooth surface irregularities.
- Select correct instruments to adapt and conform to concavities and other root morphology characteristics for areas being treated.

Preparation: Instrument Control

- Hold instrument with a modified pen grasp.
- Identify correct cutting edge of blade for surface being scaled.
  - For area-specific curets: terminal shank parallel with surface being scaled.
  - For universal curets: terminal shank less than parallel with surface being scaled (~20°).
- Establish a light finger rest for instrument placement to allow for adjustment and repositioning.
- Insert: use placement or exploratory stroke to locate apical edge of deposit.
- Adjust working angulation (average at 70°).

Action: Strokes

- Secure a stable, functional extraoral finger rest or intraoral fulcrum that can support instrument placement and activation at the correct working stroke angulation.
  - Pressure into the fulcrum equals the pressure against the tooth.
  - Balance fulcrum pressure with lateral pressure of the strokes.
- Activate for working stroke.
  - Apply firm lateral pressure for calculus removal.
  - Apply moderate lateral pressure to smooth the surface.
  - Apply light lateral pressure for biofilm debridement.
  - Control length and direction of stroke with respect to the **instrumentation zone**.
  - Maintain continuous adaptation throughout the stroke.

Channels: Overlap to Completion

- Continue channel scaling with overlapping multidirectional strokes.
  - Use an exploratory stroke to reposition blade for next stroke.
  - Activate instrument circumferentially around tooth.
  - Keep toe adapted around line angles by rolling handle.
  - Cover all surfaces comprehensively to remove all traces of calculus and biofilm.

Evaluation

- Use explorer to determine endpoint of treatment.

depth of the periodontal pocket and tenacity of the calculus):

  - For Stage I and II periodontitis, the following instruments are used in this order:
    1. Straight/universal and triple bend-type ultrasonic tips/inserts used on moderate-to-high power.
    2. Sickle scalers.
    3. Universal curets.
    4. Gracey curets.
    5. Precision-thin ultrasonic tips/inserts for final finishing.
- For Stage III and IV periodontitis, where greater clinical attachment loss is involved, the following instruments may also be needed to access the base of pockets and furcation areas for debridement:
  - Thin left/right ultrasonic tips/inserts used on low-to-moderate power.
  - Mini-bladed area-specific Gracey curets.
  - Micro-mini–bladed Gracey curets.
  - Diamond files—used with light pressure only.
  - Periodontal files.

B. Finger Rest

- Various factors such as tooth position and calculus tenacity may impact the fulcrum chosen.
- Review Chapter 37 for basics on fulcrums, which may include intraoral, extraoral, and alternative fulcrums such as supplementary, substitute, and reinforced.

C. Adaptation

- Keep the working-end closely aligned with the surface of the tooth throughout the stroke.
- Convex surfaces, concavities, and furcations all require precise adaptation (**Figure 39-4**).

D. Lateral Pressure

- Light pressure is needed for exploration to position blade below the calculus deposit and to debride biofilm while preserving cementum.
- Moderate-to-heavy pressure is needed for manual working strokes depending on the degree of mineralization or tenacity of the calculus attachment.
- Factors affecting lateral pressure are as follows:
    - Sharp instrument
        - A minimum degree of pressure allows the cutting edge to "grab" the calculus.
        - Less time, with fewer strokes, is required.
        - Fatigue is kept to a minimum.
    - Dull instrument
        - When dull, the blade cannot engage the deposit and will slide over it, burnishing it on the surface, making it difficult to detect and remove.
        - Stroke control is reduced with the heavier pressure needed to activate a dull blade; this can lead to the instrument slipping and potentially causing trauma to the patient's gingival tissues.
        - Grasp and lateral pressure tend to increase, which may increase operator fatigue.
        - More strokes are needed and result in inefficiency that increases treatment time.

E. Activation/Stroke

- Confine the strokes to the pocket to minimize the need for repeated reinsertion of the curet to prevent trauma to the gingival margin.
- Make strokes in channels (**Figure 39-5**).
    - At the completion of each stroke, move the instrument laterally a very short distance to assure overlap.
    - Maintain the same finger rest.
    - Overlap strokes in channels to ensure complete coverage of subgingival surface for thorough removal of deposits.
    - Repeat strokes until the surface has been completely debrided.

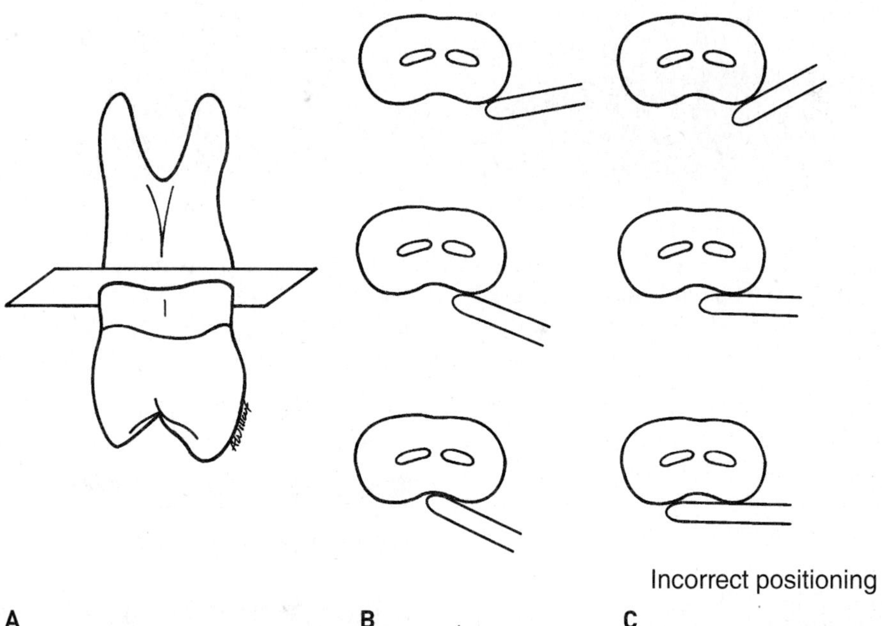

Figure 39-4 Instrument Adaptation. **A:** Maxillary first premolar shows cross section of root drawn for (B) and (C). **B:** Diagram of three positions of a curet shows correct adaptation at a line angle and on the concave mesial surface with toe third of the instrument maintained on the tooth as the instrument is adapted. **C:** Diagram shows incorrect adaptation with toe of curet turned away from the tooth surface.

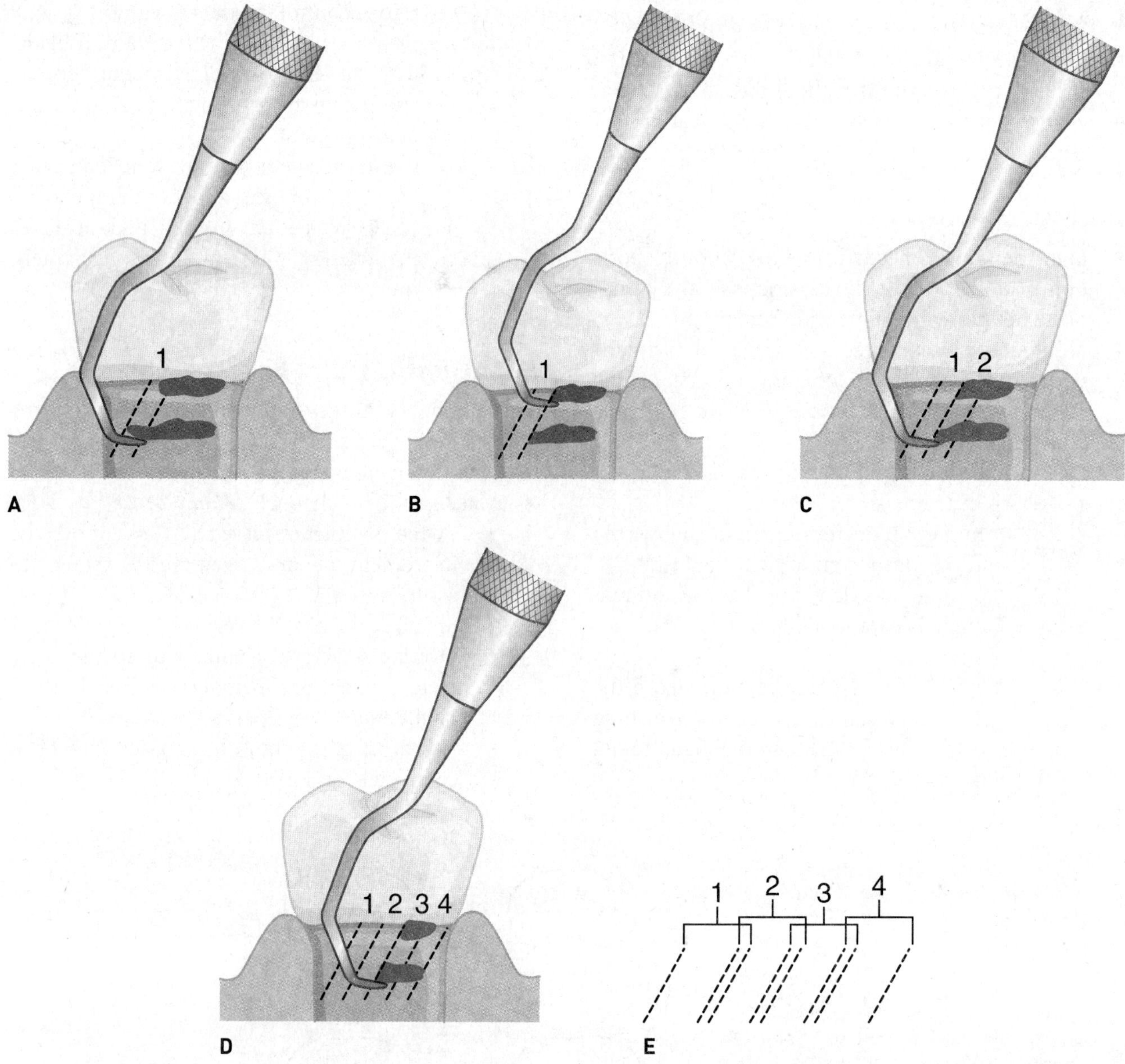

Figure 39-5 Channel Scaling. **A:** Curet adapted in position for channel 1 stroke from the base of the pocket under the calculus deposit. **B:** Completion of stroke for channel 1. **C:** Using an exploratory stroke, the curet is lowered into the pocket and is positioned for calculus removal in channel 2. **D:** Curet positioned for channel 3. Several strokes in each channel may be needed to ensure complete calculus removal. **E:** Strokes of each channel overlap strokes of the previous channel.

F. Channeling

- Overlap strokes in channels to ensure complete coverage of subgingival surface for thorough removal of deposits (Figure 39-5).
- Maintain the same finger rest.
- At the completion of each stroke, move the instrument laterally a very short distance to assure overlap.
- Repeat strokes until surface has been completely debrided.
- As a surface area becomes smooth, a gradual change in the sound of the instrument stroke may occur as the calculus is removed.

Specialized Debridement Instruments

I. Furcation Debridement

- Specialized instruments for furcation debridement include:
  - Precision-thin left/right ultrasonic tips/inserts used at low power may be used alone or in combination with hand instrumentation.
  - Mini-bladed Gracey numbers 5–6, 11–12, 13–14.

- Micro-mini–bladed Gracey numbers 1–2, 11–12, 13–14.
- Diamond files: use only with light pressure.

- Close adaptation of precision ultrasonic insert or blade to the contour of the furcation area.
- Use explorer such as regular or extended ODU 11/12 with light lateral pressure to assess root debridement.

II. Advanced Ultrasonic/ Piezoelectric Tips

- Straight/universal and triple bend-type tips are used for moderate-to-heavy deposit removal on most surfaces; however, periodontal involvement may call for use of more specialized and area-specific tips, such as those listed in the subsequent section.

A. Thin/Periodontal Tip

- Thinner and longer tips provide better access to subgingival surfaces.
- Allow superior coverage of deep pockets and furcations.
- The limitation for magnetostrictive thin tips is they can only be used on low-to-medium power to prevent breakage and may burnish and/or not remove moderate-to-heavy calculus deposits. This limits their use to light calculus and biofilm debridement.
- Piezoelectric thin tips may be used on high power.

B. Plastic, Silicone, or Carbon Composite Tip

- An insert with a plastic, silicone, or carbon composite tip may be used on titanium implants or esthetic materials surfaces.[19]
  - However, all ultrasonic tips resulted in some microscopic alterations in the implant surface.
- A low power, light pressure is all that is needed to remove biofilm and mineralizing deposits.

III. Subgingival Air Polishing

- Subgingival air polishing is an alternative to hand and ultrasonic instrumentation for subgingival biofilm management.[20]
- Subgingival air polishers deliver a stream of compressed air, water, and a nonabrasive powder (e.g., glycine or erythritol powder) through a nozzle to debride biofilm from shallow sulci, periodontal pockets, and around implants (**Figure 39-6A**).
- Subgingival air polishing has been shown to be equally effective as ultrasonic instrumentation in reducing BOP and periodontal probing depths; however, increase in CAL may be greater with erythritol powder air polishing.[21]

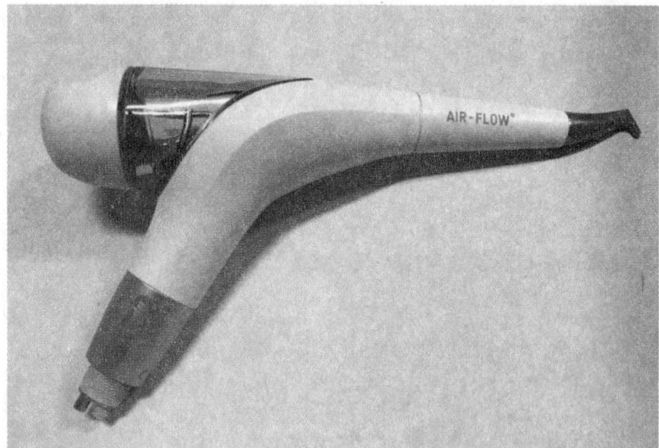

A

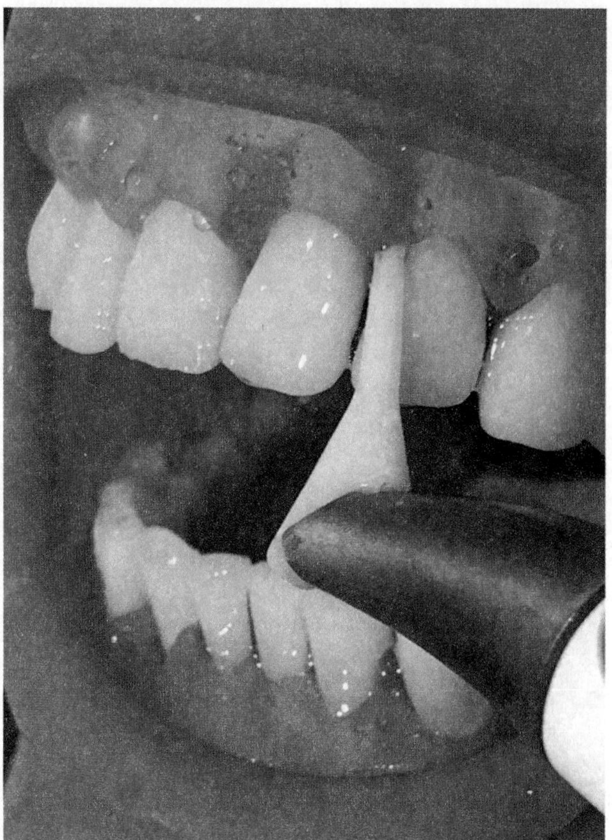

B

Figure 39-6 Air Polisher. **A:** A handheld air polisher that connects to the dental until. Can be filled with appropriate powder and used supragingivally and subgingivally. **B:** Air polisher with a disposable periodontal nozzle that is inserted subgingivally into a deeper pocket to flush out biofilm.

- Research seems to support air polishing as an alternative or adjunct to hand instrumentation during supportive periodontal therapy or maintenance.[20,21]
- Advantages
  - More effective than hand instrumentation at lowering bacterial counts in deep periodontal pockets.[22]
  - Nonabrasive and safe to use on soft tissues, round restorations, and titanium implants.[23]
  - Greater comfort for patients and less perceived pain than hand and ultrasonic instrumentation.[23]

A. Contraindications

Due to the production of water and aerosols, contraindications remain similar to those for the use of an ultrasonic scaler:

- Communicable diseases.
- Immunosuppression.
- Respiratory risk.
- Difficulty swallowing.
- Allergies to powder used.

B. Use

- Infection control protocol is also similar to that used for ultrasonic instrumentation due the high level of contamination from aerosols,[24,25] including the use of:
  - Antimicrobial preprocedural mouthrinse.[15]
  - High-volume evacuator (HVE) or extraoral local extractor IELE).[26]
  - Face shield.
  - Appropriate personal protective equipment (PPE), including a National Institute for Occupational Safety and Health (NIOSH)-approved N95 or equivalent respirator in areas of substantial or high levels of aerosol-borne infectious disease transmission such as COVID-19.[27]
- Technique for debriding shallow sulci:
  - Keeping a distance of 3–5 mm away from the tooth surface, direct the nozzle toward the gingival margin anywhere from 30 to 60°.
  - Press the device pedal for no longer than 5 seconds per site.
  - Make small horizontal or circular strokes.
- Technique for debriding periodontal pockets up to 5 mm using a disposable periodontal nozzle (**Figure 39-6B**):
  - Gently insert nozzle into the periodontal pocket.
  - Once inserted, press the device pedal for 5 seconds per site.
  - Use short vertical strokes.

IV. Laser Therapy

- Use of lasers in periodontal treatment is controversial, but continues to increase despite conflicting research findings.[2,28,29]
  - The American Academy of Periodontology's best evidence consensus summary suggests the evidence to support use of lasers for treatment of chronic periodontitis is weak.[28]
  - Evidence suggests that as an adjunct to conventional NSPT, laser therapy has no significant effect or modest improvement of less than 1 mm in pocket depth and CAL.[28,29]
  - The European Federation of Periodontology (EFP) clinical practice guidelines are not to use lasers as an adjunct to subgingival instrumentation.[2]
- Significantly more well-designed research is needed to further explore the benefit of laser-assisted periodontal therapy.[2,28]

A. Types of Lasers

- Lasers emit light through a process called stimulated emission.
  - When the light reaches the tissue, it is reflected, scattered, absorbed, or transmitted to surrounding tissues.
  - The wavelength of the light influences how the light interacts with the tissue.
- The wavelength of lasers most often used in periodontal treatment is 635–10,600 nm and includes[30]:
  - Semiconductor diode lasers.
  - Solid-state lasers: neodymium-doped yttrium, aluminum, and garnet (Nd:YAG); neodymium-doped yttrium, aluminum, and perovskite (Nd:YAP); erbium-doped yttrium, aluminum, and garnet (Er:YAG); and erbium, chromium-doped yttrium scandium, gallium, and garnet (Er,Cr:YSGG).
  - Gas lasers (CO_2).
- The equipment for laser therapy is expensive, and cost–benefit over traditional periodontal debridement has not been evaluated.
  - Typically each manufacturer requires the purchaser to contract with them for training to use the equipment, which further impacts the cost and standardization of therapy.

B. Purported Benefits of Lasers in Nonsurgical Periodontal Therapy

- Enhances pocket disinfection by reduction of subgingival bacterial load.
- Promotes wound healing.
- Hemostasis.
- Root debridement; however, there is potential for damage to the root surface with hard-tissue lasers.

C. Technique

- For calculus removal:
  - Insert laser fiber into the pocket parallel to the long axis of the tooth.
  - Angulation is 45°.
  - A horizontal and vertical stroke is used as the fiber is advanced around the root surface.
  - Water spray along with high-volume evacuation is used to keep the area clear of debris.
- For reduction of bacterial load (i.e., pocket sterilization) and curettage of granulation tissue (i.e., laser curettage)[31]:
  - Insert laser fiber into the pocket parallel to the long axis of the tooth.
  - The fiber is directed toward the soft-tissue wall of the pocket.
  - Move fiber in a horizontal and apical direction in a sweeping motion at a slow-to-moderate speed.
  - Use moistened gauze to remove debris from the fiber periodically.
  - Use high-volume evacuation for debris and to aspirate fumes.

Postoperative Instruction for Subgingival Instrumentation Appointments

- Instructions following NSPT should include information on:
  - Management of discomfort.
  - Oral self-care.
  - Diet.
  - Where to call in case of a problem or question.

I. Management of Discomfort

- There may be some soft-tissue discomfort when the local anesthesia wears off.
  - Any discomfort can usually be managed with over-the-counter analgesics, including acetaminophen (Tylenol), aspirin, or ibuprofen (Advil).
  - A nonsteroidal anti-inflammatory drug such as ibuprofen can also help reduce inflammation and swelling.
- On occasion, a cold compress or ice pack may help with discomfort.
- If the patient experiences dentin hypersensitivity, a toothpaste for sensitivity, such as a 5% potassium nitrate dentifrice, may be recommended.
  - The patient should understand that it may take several weeks of repeated used for improvement of the dentin hypersensitivity.

II. Oral Self-Care

A. Rinsing

- A warm solution may be soothing to the tissues helping healing.
- Possible solutions for rinsing may include:
  - Hypertonic salt solution: 1/2 teaspoonful of salt in 1/2 cup (4 oz) of warm water.
  - Sodium bicarbonate solution: 1/2 teaspoonful of baking soda in 1 cup (8 oz) of warm water.
  - Rinsing directions: Every 2 hours; after eating; after toothbrushing; before bedtime.
- Chlorhexidine gluconate 0.12% has been shown to provide a small reduction in pocket depths when used in conjunction with periodontal debridement.[2,32] It may be especially helpful in the presence of significant gingival inflammation.
  - Directions: twice daily, after breakfast and before going to bed, without eating after rinsing to take advantage of the substantivity property of chlorhexidine.
  - Rinsing is not a substitute for personal biofilm removal with toothbrush and interdental aids.
  - Limit use to 2 weeks following the final periodontal debridement appointment to minimize tooth staining or other adverse effects of chlorhexidine.

B. Biofilm Management

- The patient needs to understand the significance of daily biofilm disruption/removal, particularly in the quadrant or sextant receiving treatment to support optimal healing.[2]
- A soft toothbrush should be used. The patient may find that moistening the toothbrush with

warm water and brushing without toothpaste initially may be more comfortable for the tissues. The fluoride toothpaste can then be added at the end of brushing.
- There may be slight bleeding during oral self-care, but this should stop as the tissues heal.
- The patient should continue to use the interdental cleaning aid recommended. If an interdental brush will fit interproximally, this can be very helpful to facilitate tissue healing.

III. Diet

- The patient should be instructed to avoid chewing solid food or drinking hot liquids until the local anesthetic has worn off to avoid trauma to the tongue, cheek, and lips.
- If the tissues are tender during healing, consume bland foods without strong, spicy seasonings, as well as nutrient-dense, high-protein foods to promote healing.

IV. Emergency Management

- The patient should be given information about who to call in the following situations:
  - Bleeding that does not stop within a few hours.
  - Pain not managed by use of ibuprofen or Tylenol, particularly pain that wakes the patient during the night.
  - Swelling that increases after the first 1–2 days.

V. Instruction Format

- Instruction format could be:
  - A paper handout with notes specific to the patient.
  - Instructions via email or general instructions on the office/clinic website.
- A phone call or text message the evening or day after the appointment to check on how the patient is doing may also be appreciated, especially for patients who are apprehensive, to build a trusting relationship.

Re-evaluation of Nonsurgical Periodontal Therapy

I. Clinical Endpoints

- BOP: eliminated.
- Probing depths: reduced.
- Clinical attachment levels: unchanged or improved.
- Inflammation: resolved.
- Gingival appearance: size reduced, color normal.
- Subgingival microflora: lowered in numbers, delay in repopulation.
- Dental biofilm control record: improvement in scores approaching 100% biofilm free.
- Tooth surfaces: smooth; no biofilm-retentive irregularities.
- Quality-of-life factors: oral comfort with freedom from pain.

II. Re-evaluation Time Frame

- Recommendations are for the initial therapy re-evaluation to occur 4–8 weeks after NSPT.[11]
  - At least 2 weeks after instrumentation is complete for the re-establishment of the junctional epithelium.[11]
  - Four to 8 weeks are needed for the connective tissue to heal following NSPT.[11]
  - Waiting longer than 2 months may allow the pathogenic bacteria to repopulate the periodontal pockets. In addition, it is necessary to identify and remediate any residual subgingival calculus at the re-evaluation appointment to facilitate continued healing.[11]

III. Re-evaluation Procedure

A. Periodontal Examination

- A comprehensive periodontal examination is performed and documented to compare pre- and posttreatment findings.[2]
  - Changes in BOP, CAL, biofilm, and inflammation in particular are evaluated and discussed with the patient.
  - Assessment for subgingival calculus is also needed. According to the literature, 17% to 69% of surfaces may have residual calculus.[11] Re-instrument as needed.
- Reviewing oral self-care techniques with the patient and offering assistance in continued refinement are essential to aid in continued healing and disease management.[2]

B. Establish Continuing Care Interval

- The patient may have reached the point of being able to be managed under the care of the dental hygienist, and a periodontal maintenance interval should be determined based on the following[2]:
  - Soft-tissue response to instrumentation and degree of healing.

- Changes and/or stabilization in probing depth.
- Patient risk factors: use of tobacco; systemic influences such as control of diabetes.
- Effectiveness of biofilm control efforts; level of skill.
- Motivation and responsibility assumed for daily oral self-care.
- Psychosocial factors; stress, mental health issues impacting oral self-care.

- There may be localized activity, and adjunctive therapy may be considered.
- In case of advanced disease that has not responded adequately to NSPT, a referral to a periodontist is necessary. (See Chapter 45.)

Adjunctive Therapy

- Pharmacologic agents are used as adjuncts to mechanical therapy.

Antimicrobial Treatment

- Objectives of **antimicrobial therapy** include:
  - Arresting of infection using antimicrobials to slow or arrest loss of periodontal attachment and other periodontal tissue destruction caused by microorganisms.
  - Suppression and elimination of pathogenic microorganisms to allow the recolonization of the microbiota compatible with health.

I. Systemic Delivery of Antibiotics

- Systemic administration of antibiotics is highly successful in the world of medical care. Antibiotics have saved the lives of many people with generalized infectious diseases.
- A significant disadvantage to use of systemic antibiotics over the past 50 years is an increase in antibiotic resistance, so they need to be used with caution after a careful risk–benefit analysis.[2,33]

A. Action of Systemically Administered Antibiotic

- In contrast to locally applied agents placed directly into a pocket, antibiotics administered systemically reach the pathogenic organisms in the pocket through blood circulation via the cardiovascular system.
- The antibiotic is absorbed into the circulation from the intestine. From the bloodstream, the drug is passed into the body tissues.
- The antibiotic enters the periodontal tissues and passes into the pocket by way of the gingival crevicular fluid.

B. Selection of Antibiotic

- Systemic antibiotics may be prescribed as an adjunct to NSPT for a patient who does not respond to traditional periodontal therapy and experiences continued loss of attachment; however, evidence is inconsistent on the benefit of their use.[2,34]
- Antibiotics regimens used with periodontal debridement include the following[35]:
  - Metronidazole (MET) and amoxicillin as an adjunct to subgingival instrumentation have shown the greatest benefit with statistically significant reductions in bleeding and pocket depths with gain in clinical attachment.
  - The evidence for the benefit of the use of tetracycline, specifically doxycycline or minocycline, along with subgingival instrumentation is of low.
  - Azithromycin with NSPT has not shown a significant benefit.

C. Limitations

- In addition to the possibility of antibiotic resistance by the organisms, other factors that preclude the widespread use of systemic antibiotics for periodontal treatment include[2,35]:
  - Side effects of certain antibiotics.
  - Potential for the development of resistant strains.
  - Local concentration diluted by the time the drug reaches the pathogens; drug is "wasted" in that it covers a large area not needing the treatment.
  - Superimposed opportunistic infection can develop, such as candidiasis.
  - Low compliance of the patient in following the prescription for the required number of days.

D. Use of Systemic Therapy

- Most periodontal infection responds well to NSPT, meticulous biofilm control, and antimicrobial mouthrinses/dentifrices. However, there are groups of people who do not respond to initial

therapy who would benefit from systemic antibiotics, including those with:
- Continued loss of attachment despite initial therapy and thorough biofilm control.
- Acute periodontal infection, such as necrotizing ulcerative gingivitis or periodontitis, periodontal abscess.
- Generalized Stage III periodontitis in young adults.[2]
- Medical conditions predisposing to periodontal disease, such a poorly controlled diabetes.

II. Systemic Subantimicrobial Dose Antibiotics

- A subantimicrobial dose (SSD) does not have antimicrobial or antibiotic effects, and to date, antibiotic resistance has not been identified.
- Doxycycline in a low dose modulates the host inflammatory response and inhibits the continued breakdown of collagen.[1]
  - The only approved systemic SDD is Periostat.
- SDD (20 mg/twice a day) has been used for moderate-to-severe periodontitis as an adjunct to NSPT for 3–9 months.
- Evidence shows small gains in clinical attachment (an average of 0.35 mm).[1]

III. Local Delivery Antimicrobial Agents

- The concept of a controlled local delivery system for treatment of periodontal pathogens in a pocket infection was developed over many years by Goodson et al. with the introduction of a tetracycline fiber placed subgingivally.[36]
  - Improvements in probing depth, CAL, BOP, and reduction of sites with periodontal pathogenic microorganisms laid the groundwork for continuing research and development in local delivery agents.[36]
- Local delivery means the medication is concentrated at the site of the infection to reduce the bacterial load and inflammation to enhance healing.
- Local drug antimicrobial agents (LDAs) can be divided into two classes[37]:
  - Sustained-release formulations release a drug for a period less than 24 hours and are used in a variety of ways. The nicotine patch, used to assist a person with tobacco cessation, is an example.
  - Controlled delivery refers to providing the medication over an extended period of time that exceeds 1 day.

A. Requirements

A local delivery method can place high concentrations of the antimicrobial in an infected pocket. To be successful, the medication must[38]:

- Provide adequate bactericidal drug concentration.
- Reach site of disease activity, such as the bottom of the pocket and furcation.
- Stay in contact long enough in the effective concentration for the antimicrobial action to take place.
- Be easy to apply.
- Be biocompatible and **biodegradable**.
- Cost and the benefit for the patient must be carefully evaluated, given the average gains in clinical attachment of approximately 0.24 to 0.64 mm.[1,38,39]

B. Advantages of Local Delivery Agents

- Local delivery agents have the potential to enhance therapy at localized sites unresponsive to NSPT.
- Advantages include[38]:
  - Direct placement at site of infection.
  - Reliable drug delivery without reliance on patient compliance.
  - Safer with fewer side effects.
  - Noninvasive and typically painless.

C. Limitations to Local Delivery Agents

- Therapies other than LDAs should be considered in the following situations[40]:
  - Multiple sites with pocket depths greater than or equal to 5 mm in a quadrant.
  - LDAs have been attempted and did not control the localized infection.
  - Intrabony defects are present, which require surgical intervention.

Indications for Use of Local Delivery Agents

I. Nonsurgical Periodontal Therapy

- NSPT is considered the "gold" standard and results in reduction in inflammation and gain in clinical attachment of 0.49 mm.[39]

- The adjunctive use of local antimicrobials may enhance the effect of the mechanical instrumentation.
  - Use of an LDA in addition to NSPT may result in an additional 0.24 to 0.64-mm gain in clinical attachment.[1]

II. Adjunctive Treatment: At Re-evaluation

- At the completion of initial periodontal therapy, a re-evaluation is completed 4–6 weeks later.
  - Residual calculus is removed.
  - Control of dental biofilm is assessed, and reinforcement is provided for the patient.
  - For areas of residual pocket depth and/or BOP, adjunctive therapy may be considered, such as systemic antibiotics or a local delivery antimicrobial agent.

III. Recurrent Disease

- Periodontal disease tends to be cyclical with periods of stability and progression.
- Recurrence or progression of periodontal disease may be due to:
  - Noncompliance with periodontal maintenance schedule.
  - Inadequate daily control of dental biofilm.
  - Inadequate periodontal debridement.
  - Continued tobacco use.
  - Inadequate control of systemic disease such as diabetes.
  - Unknown reasons.
- Recurrence of periodontal infection may be localized, particularly in pockets associated with root concavities, furcations, and areas of complex root morphology, where definitive debridement is most challenging.
  - Burnished calculus is difficult to detect with an explorer and becomes recolonized with pathogenic microbes soon after debridement, which interferes with healing.
  - Bleeding may indicate residual burnished calculus from insufficient instrumentation.
- Localized areas of active disease are candidates for application of an antimicrobial agent.

IV. Peri-implantitis

- Peri-implantitis may respond to a local delivery antimicrobial, but the evidence is weak.[41]

Types of Local Delivery Agents

- Average improvement in clinical attachment with use of adjunctive agents versus periodontal debridement alone ranges from 0.18 to 0.64 mm (**Table 39-2**).[1]

I. Minocycline Hydrochloride

- Bioresorbable minocycline hydrochloride (HCl) is a sustained-release agent delivered in microsphere form and placed in periodontal pockets after periodontal debridement.
- Research indicates the following benefits to use of the minocycline HCl microspheres with NSPT include an average gain in clinical attachment of 0.40 mm.[1]

A. Description

- Unit-dose cartridge contains 1 mg minocycline.
- Once the minocycline microspheres come in contact with gingival crevicular fluid, they hydrolyze, allowing them to adhere to the surrounding surfaces.
- Sustained release for 14 days.
- Does not block the flow of subgingival fluid.
- Contraindications[42]:
  - Patients sensitive to tetracycline.
  - Women who are pregnant or breastfeeding.
  - Do not use in children younger than 8 years of age due to possible enamel hypoplasia or permanent tooth discoloration.
  - Gastrointestinal issues.
  - Photosensitivity may occur, so protect the skin from prolonged sun exposure.
  - Prolonged use can result in fungal or bacterial **superinfection**.

B. Administration

- Site selection:
  - Use as an adjunct to periodontal debridement.
  - Probing depth of at least 5 mm.
- Cartridge loading:
  - Insert unit-dose cartridge into dispenser handle.
  - Exert slight pressure.
  - Twist cartridge until it locks securely into place.
- Tip preparation
  - Cartridge tip can be manipulated to reposition the angle for difficult-to-reach areas.

Table 39-2 Local Delivery Antimicrobials

	Arestin	Atridox	PerioChip
Active ingredient	Minocycline HCl (1 mg)	Doxycycline hyclate (10%)	Chlorhexidine gluconate
Method of delivery	Unit-dose cartridge inserts into cartridge handle.	Doxycycline hyclate (10%); single use syringe suspended in 450 mg of ATRIGEL [poly(dl-lactide): NMP].	Chlorhexidine in a gelatin matrix is used for placement in the periodontal pocket.
Mechanism of action	Exerts antimicrobial activity by inhibiting protein synthesis in the bacterial cell wall that causes leakage and destroys the cell.	Subgingival controlled release; upon contact with crevicular fluid, the liquid product solidifies and then permits controlled release for a period of 7 days.	Controlled release over a 7- to 10-day period; bacteriostatic and bactericidal against gram-negative organisms.
Indications	As an adjunctive therapy to scaling and root debridement for reduction of pocket depth and BOP in patients with adult periodontitis.	For use in the treatment of chronic adult periodontitis for reduction in probing depth, reduction in BOP, and a gain in clinical attachment.	In conjunction with periodontal debridement.
Contraindications	Sensitivity to minocycline and/or tetracycline; children; pregnant or nursing women.	Sensitivity to doxycycline or any of the tetracycline class.	Hypersensitivity to chlorhexidine.

BOP, bleeding on probing.

  - Leave cap covering the cartridge in place prior to manipulating the angle to prevent agent from being inadvertently expelled.
  - Remove cap.
- Delivery of agent:
  - Place cartridge tip into the site selected for treatment.[42]
  - Keep tip parallel to the long axis of the tooth as it enters the periodontal pocket (**Figure 39-7**).
  - Do not force the tip to the base of the pocket.
  - Gently press thumb ring of handle to express the agent while withdrawing cartridge tip coronally from the base of the pocket.
  - With delivery complete, retract thumb ring and remove cartridge with free hand.
  - Discard contaminated cartridge.
  - Sterilize handle prior to reuse.

C. Posttreatment Instructions

Instruct patient on proper care of treated areas. Give written guidelines to prevent misunderstanding.

- Avoid touching treated area(s).[42]
- Do not use interdental cleaners or floss between teeth that have been treated for at least 10 days.[42]
- Avoid eating hard, crunchy, or sticky foods that could disturb retention of the product for 1 week.[42]
- Avoid brushing for 12 hours.
- Some mild-to-moderate sensitivity may be present the first week after scaling and root debridement and placement of minocycline HCl, but the patient needs to contact the dentist if pain or swelling occurs.
- Schedule a follow-up appointment for continuing maintenance care.

II. Doxycycline Hyclate

A. Description

- Biodegradable doxycycline polymer in liquid form is controlled-release agent delivered by **cannula** into a pocket and solidifies on contact with the sulcular fluid.
- Research indicates the following benefits to use of the doxycycline hyclate with NSPT may results in an average gain in clinical attachment of 0.64 mm.[1]

B. Equipment

- Two syringe mixing system consisting of the following[43]:
  - Syringe A contains 450 mg of the **bioabsorbable** polymeric formulation.

  - Syringe B contains 50 mg of doxycycline hyclate.
  - Once combined, the solution contains 10% of doxycycline hyclate.
- Cannula: blunt ended, 23-gauge, narrow diameter.
- **Controlled release** of drug for 7 days.[43]
- Contraindications[43]:
  - Patients sensitive to tetracycline.
  - Women who are pregnant or breastfeeding.
  - Do not use in children younger than 8 years of age due to possible enamel hypoplasia or permanent tooth discoloration.
  - Photosensitivity may occur, so protect the skin from prolonged sun exposure.
  - Prolonged use can result in fungal or bacterial superinfection.

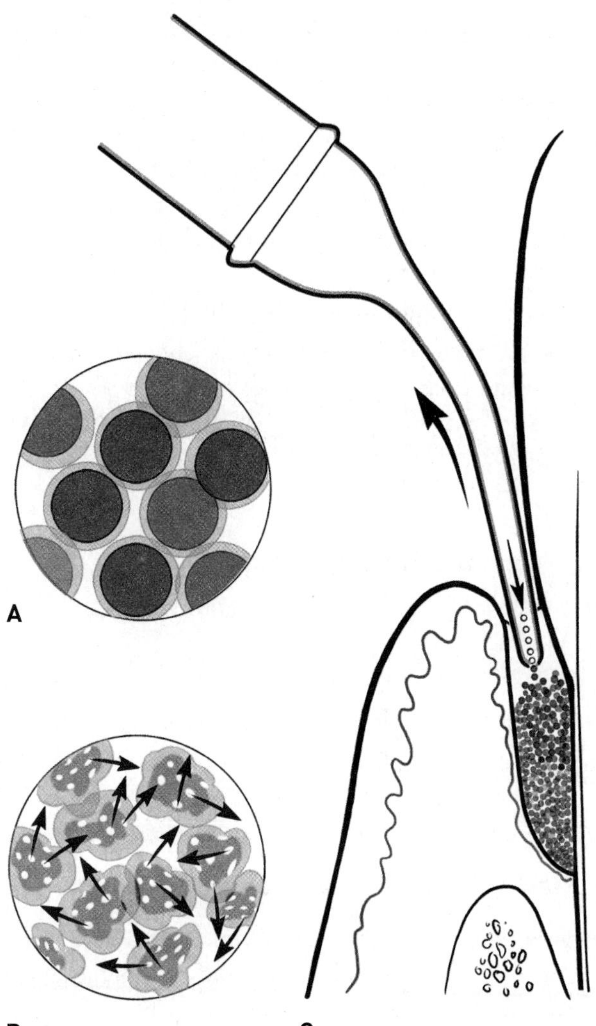

Figure 39-7 Minocycline HCl. **A:** Minocycline microspheres intact within cannula, prior to application. **B:** Deposition: cannula is withdrawn from periodontal pocket as plunger is depressed. **C:** Once deposited, microspheres dissipate, releasing activated minocycline HCl into the subgingival space.

C. Administration

- Site selection
  - Probing depth of at least 5 mm.
- Preparation of agent
  - If refrigerated, take pouches with product out of refrigerator at least 15 minutes before mixing.
  - Mixing: Two syringes are coupled, and the substances are passed back and forth, which is one mixing cycle. Mixing continues for 100 mixing cycles (**Figure 39-8A**). Follow the manufacturer's instructions.[43]
  - Adapt cannula: Attach 23-gauge blunt cannula to syringe. As the cap is removed, the cannula is held part way and bent against the wall of the cover to provide an angle appropriately similar to a periodontal probe for insertion into the periodontal pocket (**Figure 39-8B**).
- Delivery of agent[43]
  - Place cartridge tip into the site selected for treatment.
  - Keep tip parallel to the long axis of the tooth as it enters the periodontal pocket.
  - Do not force the tip to the base of the pocket.

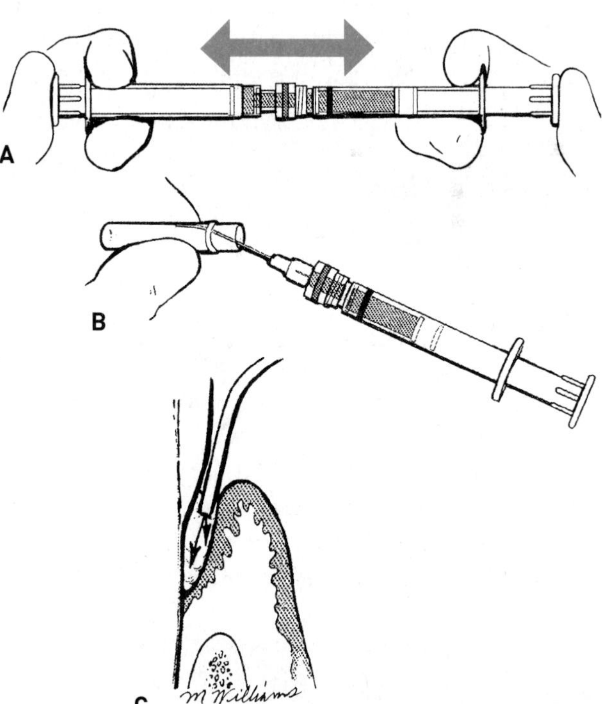

Figure 39-8 Doxycycline Polymer Gel. **A:** Syringes are coupled, and the contents passed back and forth until mixed. **B:** The cannula is attached to the syringe with the agent; as the cap is removed, the cannula is pressed against the side to bend it to an angle appropriate for accessing the pocket to be treated. **C:** The cannula is inserted into the base of the pocket, and the agent is released to fill the pocket.

- Express the agent as the cannula is withdrawn to the gingival margin (**Figure 39-8C**).
- Use a blunt instrument to pack the agent down.
- Placing a periodontal dressing or adhesive over the area to aid retention.

D. Posttreatment Instructions

- Instruct patient on proper care of treated areas, including the following:
  - Prevent accidental removal.
  - Routine brushing and other oral self-care on all other areas, but avoid toothbrushing or use of interdental aids in the treated areas for 7 days.[43]
  - Schedule a follow-up appointment to remove periodontal dressing and evaluate tissue response.
- Schedule periodontal maintenance.

III. Chlorhexidine Gluconate

- The chlorhexidine gluconate chip is biodegradable and intended for use as an adjunctive therapy with periodontal debridement.[1,44]
- Research indicates the benefit to use of the chlorhexidine chip with periodontal debridement is an average gain in clinical attachment of 0.40 mm.[1]

A. Description

- *Size:* 4 mm x 5 mm and 0.35-mm thick (**Figure 39-9**).

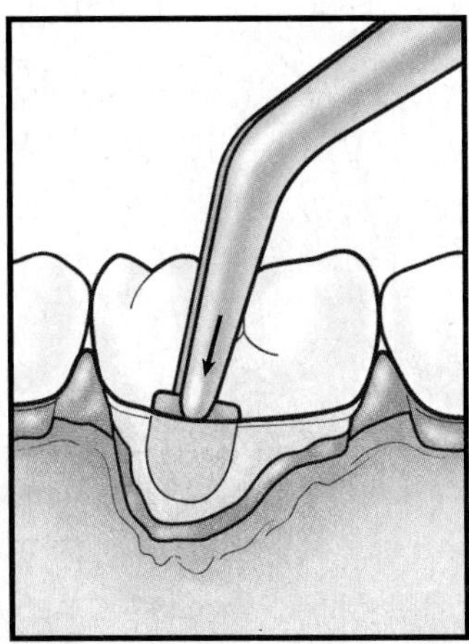

Figure 39-9 Chlorhexidine Gluconate Chip. The gelatin chip is inserted into periodontal pockets greater than or equal to 5 mm. The gelatin chip adheres to the tooth surface and dissolves slowly—releasing the chlorhexidine antimicrobial agent trapped in the gelatin.

- Shape: orange-brown, rectangular, rounded at one end.
- Contents: matrix of hydrolyzed gelatin with 2.5 mg chlorhexidine gluconate.
- Controlled delivery with 40% of dose in first 24 hours and remaining dose is delivered over a period up to 10 days.[44]
- Store product at controlled room temperature 15°C–25°C (59°F–77°F).
- Contraindications:
  - Do not use in acute periodontal abscess.
  - Exercise caution in pregnant or breastfeeding women.

B. Administration

- Site selection
  - Pocket depth: pockets greater than or equal to 5 mm.[44]
  - Chips placed: up to eight chips can be inserted at one appointment.
- Steps in placement[44]
  - Isolate with cotton rolls and dry area prior to chip placement. Chip may start to soften and become more difficult to place if it gets wet before placement in the pocket.
  - Insert by grasping the chip with cotton pliers, positioning chip with round side away from the cotton pliers.
  - Insert the chip, curved end first, to the bottom of the pocket.[44] The chip can be maneuvered with the tips of the cotton pliers or a flat instrument.

C. Posttreatment Instructions

- Instruct patient on proper care of treated areas, including the following:
  - Prevent accidental removal.
  - Avoid interdental care in the treated areas for 10 days.[44]
- Schedule periodontal maintenance.

Documentation

Documentation for the second in a series of appointments for a quadrant of scaling and root debridement with local anesthesia:

- Complete health history and assessment examination findings.
- Record new blood pressure.
- Oral preliminary examination to evaluate progress of healing for the previously treated quadrant(s).

Box 39-2 Example Documentation: Special Attention to Instrument Adaptation on a Compromised Tooth Surface

- **S**—Female patient, 26 years old, presents for routine continuing care after being away for 2 years in the Peace Corps in Africa. Patient states she had tried hard to care for her teeth daily, but safe water was never assured, and she ran out of floss without a place to shop for more. She pointed to the upper left quadrant and said it was sore and bleeding up there. No changes in health history
- **O**—Vital signs normal (BP 121/70). Generalized moderate calculus, with generalized 4-mm probing depths. Tooth #12 mesial has 6-mm pocket, BOP, and calculus (visible on the BW radiograph).
- **A**—Tooth #12 had a mesial concavity requiring careful adaptation with hand and ultrasonic instrument tips.
- **P**—In addition to full mouth debridement, local anesthesia was used to infiltrate #12 with localized subgingival instrumentation on the mesial surface of #12 with moderate subgingival calculus and heavy bleeding. Patient instructed on biofilm management and use of interdental brush, especially on the mesial #12.

Next Steps: Appointment made in 2 weeks for re-evaluation of #12 mesial.
Signed: ______________________, RDH
Date: ________________

- Biofilm index and any additional instruction or aids provided to the patient.
- Treatment completed during the appointment, including description of the amount of bleeding, necrotic tissue, along with amount and tenacity of subgingival calculus. Also note any areas that will need re-evaluation at the next appointment.
- A sample progress note may be reviewed in **Box 39-2**.

Factors to Teach the Patient

- The significance of dental biofilm in periodontal infection.
- The nature, occurrence, and etiology of calculus; its role as a biofilm reservoir.
- The responsibility of the patient in thorough daily removal of biofilm to control and prevent progression of periodontal infection.
- Reasons for multiple appointments to complete the scaling and subgingival instrumentation.
- The rationale for re-evaluation following the completion of scaling and root debridement.
- The importance of the patient's role in maintenance of therapeutic gains.
- The limitation of nonsurgical treatment and the rationale for the possible need for referral to a periodontist depending on the outcomes of nonsurgical treatment.
- The rationale for adjunctive therapy to aid in healing following periodontal debridement.

References

1. Smiley CJ, Tracy SL, Abt E, et al. Systematic review and meta-analysis on the nonsurgical treatment of chronic periodontitis by means of scaling and root planing with or without adjuncts. *J Am Dent Assoc*. 2015;146(7):508-524.e5.
2. Sanz M, Herrera D, Kebschull M, et al. Treatment of stage I-III periodontitis: the EFP S3 level clinical practice guideline. *J Clin Periodontol*. 2020;47(Suppl 22):4-60.
3. Abusleme L, Hoare A, Hong BY, Diaz PI. Microbial signatures of health, gingivitis, and periodontitis. *Periodontol 2000*. 2021;86(1):57-78.
4. Curtis MA, Diaz PI, Van Dyke TE. The role of the microbiota in periodontal disease. *Periodontol 2000*. 2020;83(1):14-25.
5. Eick S, Mathey A, Vollroth K, et al. Persistence of *Porphyromonas gingivalis* is a negative predictor in patients with moderate to severe periodontitis after nonsurgical periodontal therapy. *Clin Oral Investig*. 2017;21(2):665-674.
6. Farooqi OA, Wehler CJ, Gibson G, Jurasic MM, Jones JA. Appropriate recall interval for periodontal maintenance: a systematic review. *J Evid Based Dent Pract*. 2015;15(4):171-181.

7. Chapple ILC, Mealey BL, Van Dyke TE, et al. Periodontal health and gingival diseases and conditions on an intact and a reduced periodontium: consensus report of workgroup 1 of the 2017 World Workshop on the Classification of Periodontal and Peri-Implant Diseases and Conditions. *J Clin Periodontol*. 2018;45(Suppl 20):S68-S77.
8. Strachan A, Harrington Z, McIlwaine C, et al. Subgingival lipid A profile and endotoxin activity in periodontal health and disease. *Clin Oral Investig*. 2019;23(9):3527-3534.
9. Cadosch J, Zimmermann U, Ruppert M, Guindy J, Case D, Zappa U. Root surface debridement and endotoxin removal. *J Periodontal Res*. 2003;38(3):229-236.
10. Bozbay E, Dominici F, Gokbuget AY, et al. Preservation of root cementum: a comparative evaluation of power-driven versus hand instruments. *Int J Dent Hyg*. 2018;16(2):202-209.
11. Segelnick SL, Weinberg MA. Reevaluation of initial therapy: when is the appropriate time? *J Periodontol*. 2006;77(9): 1598-1601.
12. Eberhard J, Jepsen S, Jervøe-Storm PM, Needleman I, Worthington HV. Full-mouth treatment modalities (within 24 hours) for chronic periodontitis in adults. *Cochrane Database Syst Rev*. 2015;(4):CD004622.
13. Leung WK, Duan YR, Dong XX, et al. Perception of non-surgical periodontal treatment in individuals receiving or not receiving local anaesthesia. *Oral Health Prev Dent*. 2016;14(2):165-175.
14. Balejo RDP, Cortelli JR, Costa FO, et al. Effects of chlorhexidine preprocedural rinse on bacteremia in periodontal patients: a randomized clinical trial. *J Appl Oral Sci*. 2017;25(6):586-595.
15. Mohd-Said S, Mohd-Dom TN, Suhaimi N, Rani H, McGrath C. Effectiveness of pre-procedural mouthrinses in reducing aerosol contamination during periodontal prophylaxis: a systematic review. *Front Med*. 2021;8:600769.
16. Drisko CL. Periodontal debridement: still the treatment of choice. *J Evid Based Dent Pract*. 2014;14:33-41.e1.
17. Alexandridi F, Tsantila S, Pepelassi E. Smoking cessation and response to periodontal treatment. *Aust Dent J*. 2018;63(2):140-149.
18. Ciantar M. Time to shift: from scaling and root planing to root surface debridement. *Prim Dent J*. 2014;3(3):38-42.
19. Sahrmann P, Winkler S, Gubler A, Attin T. Assessment of implant surface and instrument insert changes due to instrumentation with different tips for ultrasonic-driven debridement. *BMC Oral Health*. 2021;21(1):25.
20. Nascimento GG, Leite FRM, Pennisi PRC, López R, Paranhos LR. Use of air polishing for supra- and subgingival biofilm removal for treatment of residual periodontal pockets and supportive periodontal care: a systematic review. *Clin Oral Investig*. 2021;25(3):779-795.
21. Abdulbaqi HR, Shaikh MS, Abdulkareem AA, Zafar MS, Gul SS, Sha AM. Efficacy of erythritol powder air-polishing in active and supportive periodontal therapy: a systematic review and meta-analysis. *Int J Dent Hyg*. 2022;20(1):62-74.
22. Flemmig TF, Arushanov D, Daubert D, Rothen M, Mueller G, Leroux BG. Randomized controlled trial assessing efficacy and safety of glycine powder air polishing in moderate-to-deep periodontal pockets. *J Periodontol*. 2012;83(4):444-452.
23. Tan SL, Grewal GK, Mohamed Nazari NS, Mohd-Dom TN, Baharuddin NA. Efficacy of air polishing in comparison with hand instruments and/or power-driven instruments in supportive periodontal therapy and implant maintenance: a systematic review and meta-analysis. *BMC Oral Health*. 2022;22(1):85.
24. Innes N, Johnson IG, Al-Yaseen W, et al. A systematic review of droplet and aerosol generation in dentistry. *J Dent*. 2021;105:103556.
25. Zemouri C, de Soet H, Crielaard W, Laheij A. A scoping review on bio-aerosols in healthcare and the dental environment. *PLoS One*. 2017;12(5):e0178007.
26. Ou Q, Placucci RG, Danielson J, et al. Characterization and mitigation of aerosols and spatters from ultrasonic scalers. *J Am Dent Assoc*. 2021;152(12):981-990.
27. Centers for Disease Control and Pevention (CDC). Interim infection prevention and control recommendations for healthcare personnel during the coronavirus disease 2019 (COVID-19) pandemic. Published September 10, 2021. https://www.cdc.gov/hicpac/recommendations/core-practices.html. Accessed September 17, 2021.
28. Chambrone L, Ramos UD, Reynolds MA. Infrared lasers for the treatment of moderate to severe periodontitis: an American Academy of Periodontology best evidence review. *J Periodontol*. 2018;89(7):743-765.
29. Lin Z, Strauss FJ, Lang NP, Sculean A, Salvi GE, Stähli A. Efficacy of laser monotherapy or non-surgical mechanical instrumentation in the management of untreated periodontitis patients. A systematic review and meta-analysis. *Clin Oral Investig*. 2021;25(2):375-391.
30. Salvi GE, Stähli A, Schmidt JC, Ramseier CA, Sculean A, Walter C. Adjunctive laser or antimicrobial photodynamic therapy to non-surgical mechanical instrumentation in patients with untreated periodontitis: a systematic review and meta-analysis. *J Clin Periodontol*. 2020;47(S22):176-198.
31. Gao YZ, Li Y, Chen SS, Feng B, Wang H, Wang Q. Treatment effects and periodontal status of chronic periodontitis after routine Er:YAG laser-assisted therapy. *World J Clin Cases*. 2021;9(32):9762-9769.
32. da Costa LFNP, Amaral C da SF, Barbirato D da S, Leão ATT, Fogacci MF. Chlorhexidine mouthwash as an adjunct to mechanical therapy in chronic periodontitis: a meta-analysis. *J Am Dent Assoc*. 2017;148(5):308-318.
33. Diallo OO, Baron SA, Abat C, Colson P, Chaudet H, Rolain JM. Antibiotic resistance surveillance systems: a review. *J Glob Antimicrob Resist*. 2020;23:430-438.
34. Khattri S, Kumbargere Nagraj S, Arora A, et al. Adjunctive systemic antimicrobials for the non-surgical treatment of periodontitis. *Cochrane Database Syst Rev*. 2020;11:CD012568.
35. Teughels W, Feres M, Oud V, Martín C, Matesanz P, Herrera D. Adjunctive effect of systemic antimicrobials in periodontitis therapy: A systematic review and meta-analysis. *J Clin Periodontol*. 2020;47 Suppl 22:257-281.
36. Goodson JM, Haffajee A, Socransky SS. Periodontal therapy by local delivery of tetracycline. *J Clin Periodontol*. 1979;6(2):83-92.
37. American Academy of Periodontology. American Academy of Periodontology statement on local delivery of sustained or controlled release antimicrobials as adjunctive therapy in the treatment of periodontitis. *J Periodontol*. 2006;77(8):1458.
38. Steinberg D, Friedman M. Sustained-release delivery of antimicrobial drugs for the treatment of periodontal diseases: fantasy or already reality? *Periodontol 2000*. 2020;84(1):176-187.

39. Smiley CJ, Tracy SL, Abt E, et al. Evidence-based clinical practice guideline on the nonsurgical treatment of chronic periodontitis by means of scaling and root planing with or without adjuncts. *J Am Dent Assoc*. 2015;146(7):525-535.

40. Jepsen K, Jepsen S. Antibiotics/antimicrobials: systemic and local administration in the therapy of mild to moderately advanced periodontitis. *Periodontol 2000*. 2016;71(1):82-112.

41. Ramanauskaite A, Fretwurst T, Schwarz F. Efficacy of alternative or adjunctive measures to conventional non-surgical and surgical treatment of peri-implant mucositis and peri-implantitis: a systematic review and meta-analysis. *Int J Implant Dent*. 2021;7:112.

42. Wynn R. Minocycline hydrochloride. *Lexicomp Online for Dentistry*. Updated February 16, 2022. https://online-lexi-com.ezproxymcp.flo.org/. Accessed March 27, 2022.

43. Wynn R. Doxycycline hyclate. *Lexicomp Online for Dentistry*. Updated March 25, 2022. https://online-lexi-com.ezproxymcp.flo.org/. Accessed March 27, 2022.

44. Food and Drug Administration. PerioChip. Published November 2012. https://www.accessdata.fda.gov/drugsatfda_docs/label/2012/020774s012lbl.pdf. Accessed March 27, 2022.

CHAPTER 40

Sutures and Dressings

Susan J. Jenkins, RDH, PhD

CHAPTER OUTLINE

LEARNING OBJECTIVES

After studying this chapter, the student will be able to:

1. State the functions and purposes of sutures and periodontal dressings.
2. Describe the differences between absorbable and nonabsorbable sutures.
3. Describe the procedure for suture removal.
4. Describe the procedure for periodontal dressing placement and periodontal dressing removal.
5. Explain approaches for managing biofilm with the periodontal dressing in place and upon removal.

Many periodontal surgical procedures require sutures and dressings. The dental hygienist will often participate in the patient's oral self-care instruction at initial placement and during postoperative care.

Sutures

I. The Ideal Suture Material

- A **suture** is a strand of material used to control bleeding, stabilize the wound edges in the proper position, protect the wound, and aid in patient comfort.[1]
  - Sutures are necessary in many oral surgical procedures when a surgical wound must be closed, a flap positioned, or tissue grafted.
- Historically, a wide range of suture materials has been used, including silk, cotton, linen, and animal tendons and intestines.
- The ideal suture material is nonallergenic, easy to handle, and sterile; has adequate **tensile strength**; does not interfere with healing; causes minimal inflammatory reaction; and has some capacity to stretch to allow for wound edema.[1,2]
  - Ultimately, the ideal suture does not exist and each surgeon must select the best suture material based on the surgical procedure to be performed and patient and wound characteristics.[2]

II. Functions of Sutures

- Close periodontal wounds and secure grafts in position.
- Assist in maintaining **hemostasis**.
- Reduce posttreatment discomfort.
- Promote primary intention healing.
- Prevent underlying bone exposure.
- Protect a healing surgical wound from foreign debris and trauma.

III. Characteristics of Suture Materials

A. Biologic Characteristics

The biologic characteristics of suture materials include the following[1]:

- Sterility.
- Reabsorption ability.
- Tolerability: creates minimal inflammatory reaction in the tissue.

B. Physical Characteristics

Physical characteristics of suture materials include the following[1]:

- Tensile strength.
- Flexibility: ability to twist and tie knot without breaking.
- Plasticity: ability to maintain new shape.
- Elasticity: ability of material to stretch and return to original shape.
- Maneuverability: easy to handle and able to create a small knot.
- Fluency: passes through tissue with minimal trauma.
- Length and diameter: various lengths and diameters are available.

IV. Classification of Suture Materials

A. Type of Material Used

- Two types of suture materials are used[1]:
  - Natural: classified into animal origin (i.e., catgut and silk) and vegetal origin (i.e., cotton and linen).
  - Synthetic: developed to reduce tissue reactions and unpredictable rates of absorption commonly found in natural sutures.

B. Absorption Properties

- Absorbable sutures
  - Natural absorbable sutures: digested by body enzymes.
    - Plain gut: monofilamentous, derived from purified collagen of sheep or cattle and lasts about 8 days before beginning to degrade.[1]
    - Chromic gut: contain chromatic salts to delay enzyme resorption for 18 days.[1]
- Synthetic resorbable sutures: broken down by **hydrolysis**, a process in which water slowly penetrates the suture filaments to cause a breakdown of the suture's polymer chain.
  - Example: polyglactin (Vicryl), poliglecaprone (Monocryl), and polydioxanone (PDS II).
- Nonabsorbable sutures: not digested by body enzymes or hydrolyzation; patient returns for removal usually after 1 week.
  - Natural nonabsorbable
    - Silk.
  - Synthetic nonabsorbable
    - Nylon (Ethilon).
    - Polyester (Ethibond).
    - Polypropylene (Prolene).

- Polytetrafluoroethylene (PTFE) (Gore-Tex).
- Coated sutures: Suture material coated with the antibacterial agents chlorhexidine may provide antibacterial efficacy and oral biofilm inhibition, reducing surgical site infections.[1,3,4]
- Although nonabsorbable silk sutures have been widely used, research is showing silk sutures increase inflammation at the suture site due to bacterial accumulation, increasing patient discomfort and increased healing time. All suture material attract bacteria.[5,6]
  - Of the nonabsorbable suture material, nylon sutures have demonstrated the lowest bacterial accumulation.
- Current trends are favoring adsorptive suture materials. Ultimately, suture choice is determined by the provider.

C. Number of Strands

- Monofilament suture: single strand of material; typical of gut, nylon, PTFE, and other synthetic sutures.[1]
- Multifilament suture: several strands twisted or braided together: typical of silk, nylon, polyglycolic acid, polyester, and other synthetic sutures.[1]

D. Diameter of Suture Material

- Numbers range from 1 to 10 and are associated with diameter.
- Thin sutures have the greatest number of zeros from 1-0 to 12-0.

V. Selection of Suture Materials

Choosing the appropriate suture material for a specific procedure is critical both for patient comfort and tissue health. Suture selection is based on the following[2]:

- Preference and experience of the surgeon.
- Characteristics of the tissue and the presence of saliva.
- Characteristics of the wound such as length and tissue type (mucosa vs. attached gingiva).
- Cosmetic implications.
  - Examples of suture types surgeons may use for specific procedures are listed in **Table 40-1**.

Table 40-1 Selection of Suture Material

Suture Types	Specific Dental Procedures
Silk, nonabsorbable, braided	Periodontal flaps and closure
Nylon, monofilament	Periodontal flaps and closure
Polyester, braided	Periodontal flaps and closure
Gut, absorbable	Extraction socket, bone grafting, free-gingival grafting
Absorbable preferred: nonabsorbable used when pain and swelling may be anticipated	Implant flap closure

Needles

Many types of suturing needles are available. Their use and selection are primarily based on specific procedures, location for use, and clinician's preference.

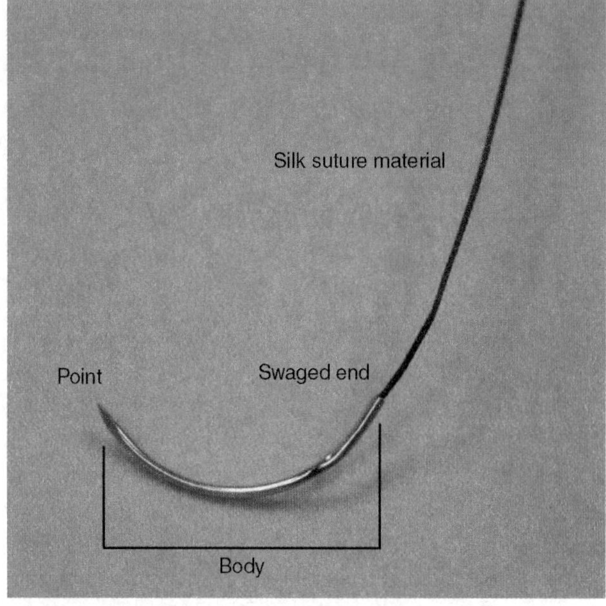

Figure 40-1 Suture Needle Components

Courtesy of Susan Jenkins, MCPHS University Forsyth School of Dental Hygiene.

I. Needle Components

- Swaged end (eyeless)
  - The **swaged** end allows the suture material and needle to act as one unit (**Figure 40-1**).
- Body
  - Shape/curvature
    - Straight.
    - Half-curved.
    - Curved 1/4, 3/8, 1/2, 5/8 (**Figure 40-2**).
  - Diameter
    - Gauge or size; finer for delicate surgeries.

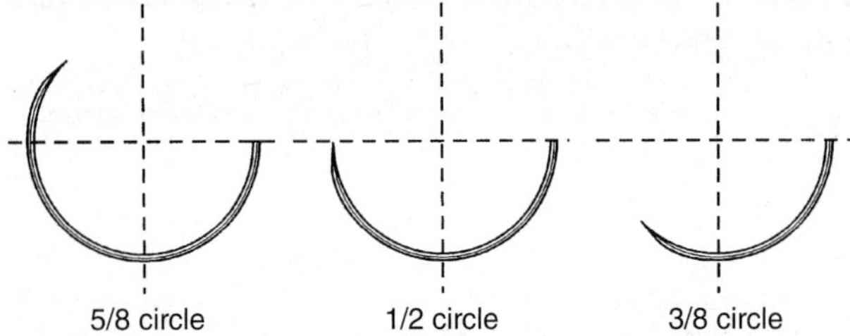

Figure 40-2 Suture Needles. A curved needle is manipulated with a needle holder. The 3/8 curve is most effective for closure of skin and mucous membranes and is a needle of choice in many dental and periodontal surgeries.

- The body is the strongest part of the needle that is grasped with the needleholder during the surgical procedure.
- The swaged end is the weakest part of the body.

- Point
  - Point of the needle extends from the extreme tip of the needle to the widest part of the body.
  - Each needle point is designed and manufactured to penetrate tissue with the highest degree of sharpness.

II. Needle Characteristics

- Material
  - Most needles are made of stainless steel formulated and sterilized for surgical use.
- Attachment
  - Majority of needles are permanently attached to suture material.
  - Eliminates need for threading and unnecessary handling.
- Cutting edge (**Figure 40-3**)
  - Reverse cut: the sharpest needle[3]; has two opposing cutting edges, with a third located on the outer convex curve of needle.
  - Conventional cut: consists of two opposing cutting edges and a third within the concave curvature of the needle.
- Requirements
  - Needle point: designed to meet the needs of specific surgical procedures.
    - Sharp enough to penetrate tissues with minimal resistance.
    - Rigid enough to resist bending, yet are flexible.
    - Sterile and corrosion resistant.
  - Surgical needles: intended to carry suture material through tissues with minimal trauma.

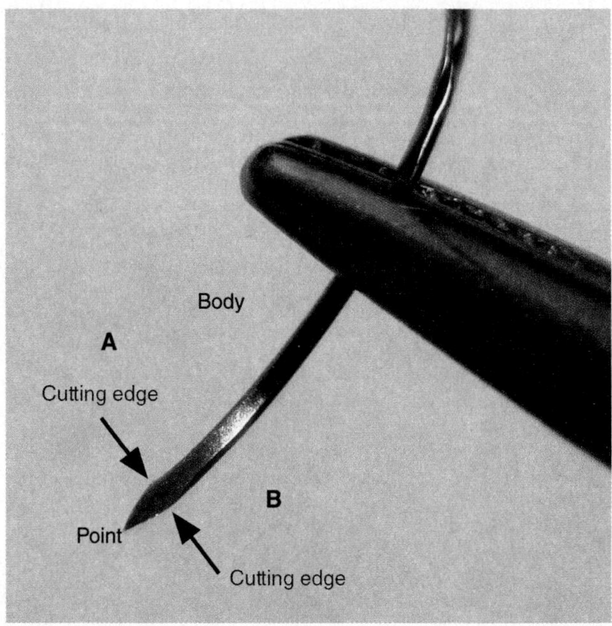

Figure 40-3 Suture Needles. Shapes of Points. Triangle shows cross section of needle point. **A:** Conventional cutting with third cutting edge on the inside of the needle curvature. **B:** Reverse cutting with a third of cutting edge on the outer curvature of the needle, used for difficult-to-penetrate tissue, such as skin.

Courtesy of Susan Jenkins, MCPHS University Forsyth School of Dental Hygiene.

Knots

The book *Surgical Knots and Suturing Techniques*[7] describes a variety of surgical knots. Only a few are used in dentistry.

- Type of knot used will depend on the:
  - Specific procedure.
  - Location of the incision.
  - Amount of stress the wound will endure.
- Square knots are most frequently used in dentistry because they are the easiest and most reliable.

I. Knot Characteristics

- The knot is tied as small as possible.
- Completed knot needs to be firm to reduce slipping.
- Excessive tension should be avoided to prevent breakage or trauma to the tissue.

II. Knot Management

- The knot is tied on the facial aspect for easier access for removal.
- A 2- to 3-mm suture "tail" is left to assist in locating the suture for removal.

Suturing Procedures

- Many different patterns of suturing are used. Assisting and observing during the surgical procedure can be an educational experience for the dental hygienist.
- General types of sutures used in the oral cavity are described next.

I. Blanket (Continuous Lock)

- Each stitch is brought over a loop of the preceding one, thus forming a series of loops on one side of the incision and a series of stitches over the incision (**Figure 40-4A**).
- Uses: to approximate the gingival margins after **alveolectomy**.

II. Interrupted

- **Figure 40-4B** shows a series of interrupted sutures.

III. Continuous Uninterrupted

- A series of stitches tied at one or both ends.
- Examples of sutures that may be applied in a series are the sling or suspension and the blanket.

IV. Circumferential

- Suture that encircles a tooth for suspension and retention of a flap.

V. Interdental

- Flaps are on both the lingual and facial sides; interdental **ligation** joins the two by passing the suture through each interdental area (**Figure 40-4C**). Coverage for the interdental area can be accomplished by **coapting** the edges of the papillae.

VI. Sling or Suspension

- When a flap is only on one side, facial or lingual, the sutures are passed through the interdental papilla, around the tooth, and into the adjacent papilla (**Figure 40-4D**).
- The suture is adjusted so that the flap can be positioned for correct healing.

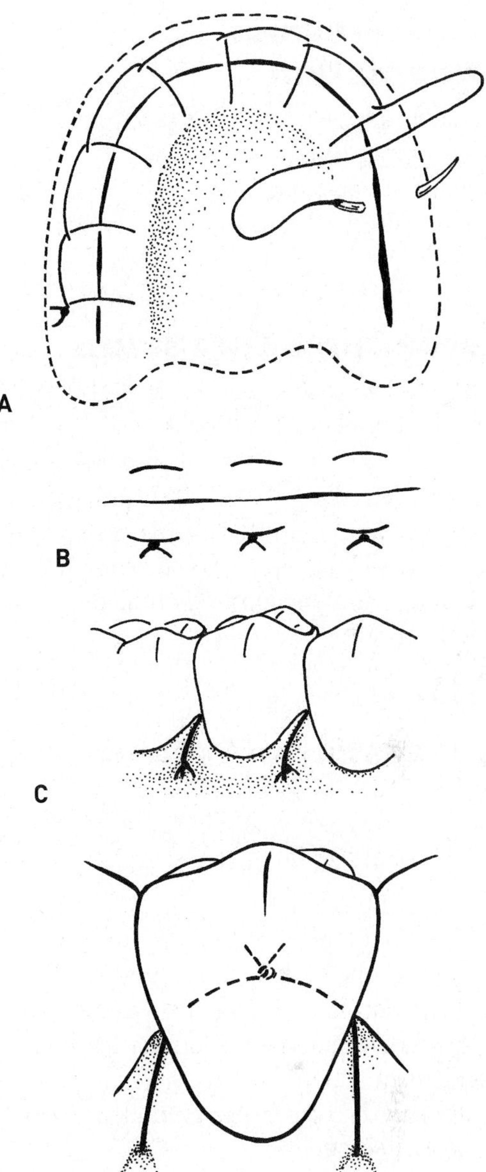

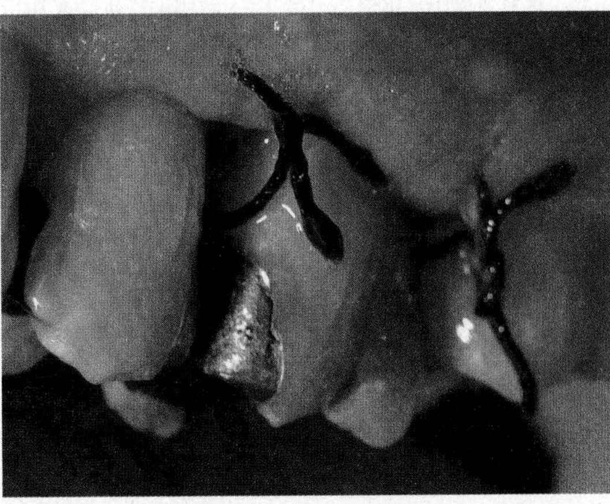

Figure 40-4 Types of Sutures. **A:** Blanket stitch. **B:** Interrupted, individual sutures. **C:** Interdental individual sutures. **D:** Sling or suspension suture tied on the lingual (dotted line) **E:** Interrupted silk sutures in place 1-week postsurgery.

Courtesy of Dr. Robert Lewando, Boston, MA.

Procedure for Suture Removal

- Removal schedule: 7 days after the surgery and no longer than 14 days to prevent tissue infection and promote healing.

I. Review Previous Documentation

- Medical history.
- Surgical procedures.
- Patient reactions to healing.
- Current surgery: number and type of sutures placed.

II. Sterile Clinic Tray Setup

- Sterile mouth mirror.
- Sterile cotton pliers.
- Sterile curved sharp scissors with pointed tip (suture scissors).
- Gauze.
- Topical anesthetic: type that can be applied safely on an abraded or incompletely healed area.
- Cotton pellets.
- Saliva ejector tip.

III. Preparation of Patient

- Patient history check
  - Patients with valvular heart disease require consultation with the cardiologist.[8]
    - Sutures are colonized by bacteria and should be removed as soon as possible once adequate wound healing has occurred.[1,2,9]
    - Suture removal can cause bacteremia.[5,6,10-12]
- Patient examination
  - Observe healing tissue around the suture(s) (**Figure 40-4E**).
  - Record any deviations in color, size, shape of the tissue, adaptation of a flap, or coaptation of an incision healing by first intention.
- Preparation of the sutured area
  - Sutures placed without a dressing may have debris lodged in them at the time of removal.
  - Irrigate and/or swab with a cotton tip applicator or cotton pellet.
  - 0.12% chlorhexidine mouthrinse or 3% peroxide can be used to dip the cotton tip applicator to aid in debris removal.
  - Follow with another rinse or wipe gently with a gauze sponge.
  - Place and adjust saliva ejector.

IV. Steps for Removal

- The suture removal procedure described here and illustrated in **Figure 40-5** is for a single interrupted suture.
- The same principles apply for the ends and each segment of a continuous suture, wherever suture material can pass through the soft tissue.
- Steps
  1. Review the surgeon's chart notes to determine the number of sutures placed and visually locate them prior to beginning suture removal.
  2. Use caution when removing a periodontal dressing to prevent tearing a suture that may have become embedded in the dressing, causing the patient significant discomfort.
  3. Once the sutures are exposed, carefully remove debris by irrigating with water and/or use antiseptic/antimicrobial like 0.12% chlorhexidine mouthrinse on a cotton tip applicator or cotton pellet.
  4. Gently grasp the ends of the suture above the knot with the cotton plier held in the nondominant hand. Gently draw the suture up several millimeters if possible and hold with slight tension (Figure 40-5A). A finger rest is needed for control.
  5. With the scissors in the dominant hand, insert one blade of the scissors just under the suture knot on one thread of the suture material (Figure 40-5B).
  6. Hold knot end up with the cotton plier and pull gently to allow suture to exit through the side opposite where it was cut (Figure 40-5C).
  7. Place each suture on a piece of gauze and proceed to remove the next suture.
  8. Count the total number of sutures removed to ensure they were all removed.
     - During healing, sutures can become loosened, misplaced, or occasionally covered by tissue.
     - A remaining suture can lead to infection and possible abscess.
  9. Irrigate with water or antiseptic. Apply gauze with slight pressure on any bleeding spots.
  10. Provide proper postsuture removal instructions both verbally and in writing.
  11. Observe all tissue and record observations, noting any adverse reactions or bleeding.

Periodontal Dressings

Historically, periodontal dressings were thought to prevent wound infection and enhance healing; however, current evidence does not support this.[13,14] The use of a periodontal dressing is based on the personal preference and judgment of the clinician.

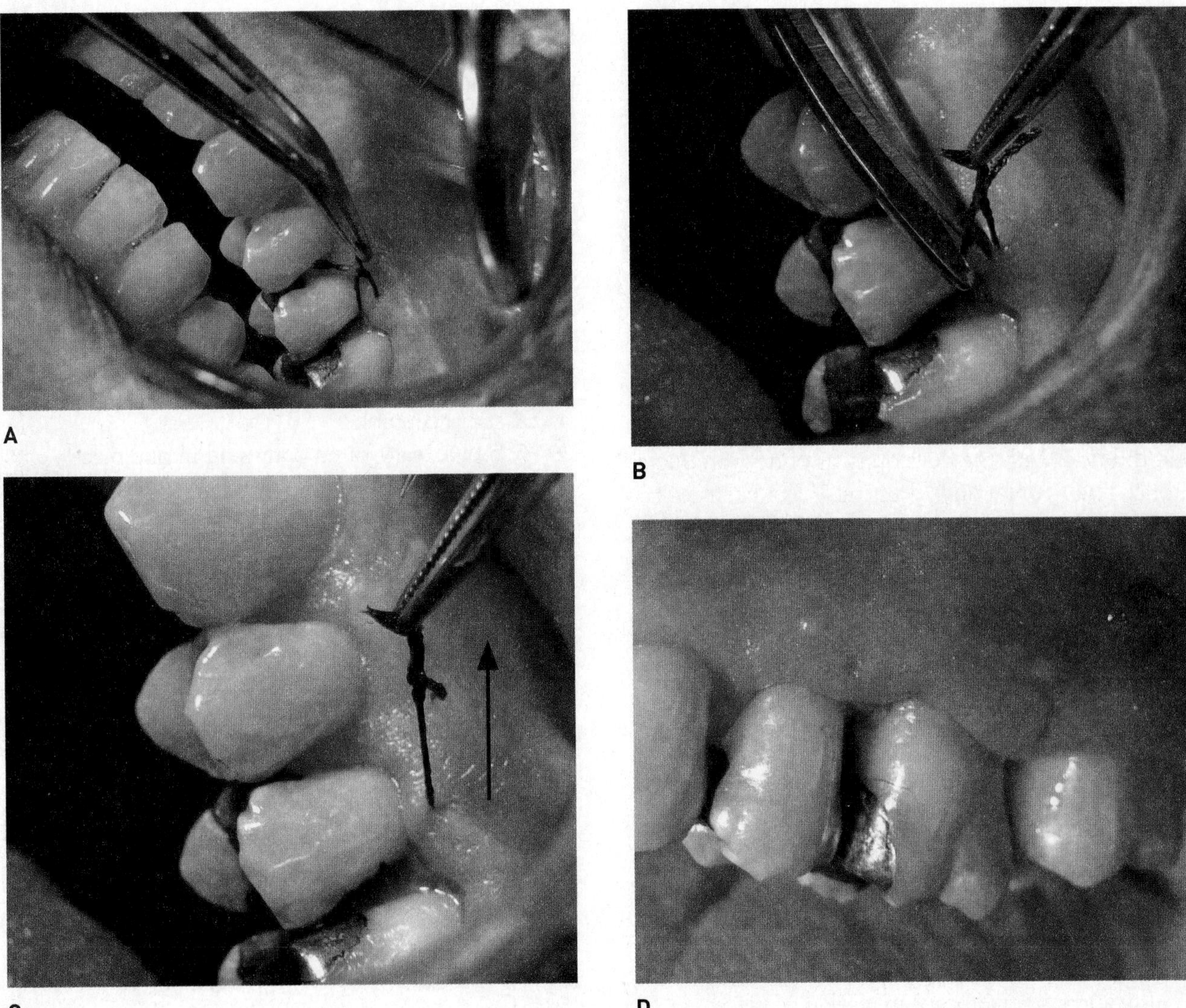

Figure 40-5 Suture Removal. **A:** Suture grasped by pliers near the entrance into tissue. **B:** Suture pulled gently up while scissor is inserted close to the tissue and cut. **C:** Suture is held up for vertical removal. **D:** Suture is pulled gently to bring it out on the side opposite from where it was cut. The object is to prevent the external part of the suture from passing through the tissue and introducing infectious material.

Courtesy of Dr. Robert Lewando, Boston, MA.

I. Purposes and Uses

- The purposes and uses of periodontal dressing include the following[10-15]:
  - Reduce pain following surgery.
  - Provide a physical barrier to external irritation and trauma, and may reduce bacterial colonization of the suture material.
  - Help prevent posttreatment bleeding by securing initial clot formation.
  - Support mobile teeth during healing.
  - Minimize tooth hypersensitivity.
  - Assist in shaping or molding newly formed tissue, in securing a flap, or in immobilizing a graft.
  - Possible use after nonsurgical periodontal therapy has also been proposed to enhance periodontal outcomes, but more research is needed.[16]

II. Characteristics of Acceptable Dressing Material

An acceptable dressing material has the following characteristics:

- Preparation, placement, and removal will take place with minimal discomfort to the patient.
- Material adheres to itself, teeth, and adjacent tissues and maintains retention within interdental areas.

- Provides stability and flexibility to withstand distortion and displacement without fracturing.
- Is nontoxic and nonirritating to oral tissues.
- Possesses a smooth surface that will resist accumulation of dental biofilm.
- Will not traumatize tissue or stain teeth and restorative materials.
- Possesses an aesthetically acceptable appearance.

Types of Dressings

Traditionally, dressings were classified into two groups: those that contained **eugenol** and those that did not. With the development of new products, "noneugenol-containing" dressings have been reclassified into **chemical-cure** and **visible light-cure** (*VLC*) materials. They are available as ready-mix, paste–paste, or paste–gel preparations.

I. Zinc Oxide with Eugenol Dressing

- Example: Kirkland periodontal pack.

A. Advantages

- Consistency: firm and heavy—provides support for tissues and flaps.
- Slow setting: extended working time.
- Preparation and storage: can be prepared in quantity and stored (frozen) in work-size pieces.

B. Disadvantages

- Taste: sharp, unpleasant taste.
- Tissue reaction: irritating; hypersensitivity reactions can occur.
- Consistency: the dressing is rough, hard and brittle, breaks easily, and encourages dental biofilm retention.

II. Chemical-Cured Dressing

- Two examples of chemical-cured dressings are PerioCare and Coe-Pak.

A. Basic Ingredients

- Coe-Pak: most commonly used two-paste system.[15]
  - Base paste: zinc oxide with added oils and gums.
  - Catalyst paste: resins, fatty acids, and chlorothymol as an antibacterial agent.
  - Coe-Pak is available in regular and fast set; hand mix or cartridge delivery.
- PerioCare: two-paste system.[15]
  - One paste contains metal oxides and oil.
  - The other paste contains a gel rosin and fatty acids.

B. Advantages

- Consistency: pliable, easy to place with light pressure.
- Smooth surface: comfortable to patient; resists biofilm and debris deposits.
- Taste: acceptable.
- Removal: easy, often comes off in one piece.

III. Visible Light-Cured (VLC) Dressing

- VLC dressing (Barricaid VLC) is available in a syringe for direct application.
- The same light-curing unit used for composite restorations and sealants is used.

A. Advantages

- Color: more like gingiva than other dressings and often preferred in anterior areas.
- Setting: cured in increments with a light-curing unit.
- Removal: easy, often comes off in one piece.

IV. Collagen Dressing

- Absorbable collagen dressings (e.g., CollaCote) used to promote wound healing.[15]
- Contributes to decreased inflammation and subsequent reduced discomfort.[17]
- Special use in periodontal surgery for a collagen patch dressing: for protection of graft sites of the palate during healing.
- Formed into a bullet shape to use for deep biopsy sites.[15]
- Available in individual unit sterile packages.
- Collagen dressing may be placed on clean moist or bleeding wounds.

V. Alternative Material for Periodontal Dressing

- *Curcumin (Tumeric) Gel*[18]
  - Anti-inflammatory and antioxidant properties reduce inflammation and discomfort and increase healing.
  - Reduces edema.
  - Topical application.

Clinical Application

I. Dressing Placement

- General procedure
  - For all types of dressing, follow the manufacturer's instructions. Each product has unique properties that require special handling.
- Retention
  - Mold the dressing by pressing at each interproximal site to cover interdental tissue (**Figure 40-6A**). Do not extend over the height of contour of each tooth.
  - **Border mold** to prevent displacement by the tongue, cheeks, lips, or frena (**Figure 40-6B–C**).
  - Check the occlusion and remove areas of contact.

II. Characteristics of a Well-Placed Dressing

- Dressings placed in keeping with biologic principles contribute to healing and are more comfortable for the patient.
- A satisfactory dressing (**Figure 40-6D-E**) has the following characteristics:
  - Is secure and rigid. A movable dressing is an irritant and can promote bleeding.
  - Has as little bulk as possible, yet is bulky enough to give strength.
  - Locks mechanically interdentally and cannot be displaced by action of tongue, cheek, or lips.
  - Covers the entire surgical wound without unnecessary overextension.
  - Fills interdental area and adequately covers the treated area to discourage retention of debris and dental biofilm.

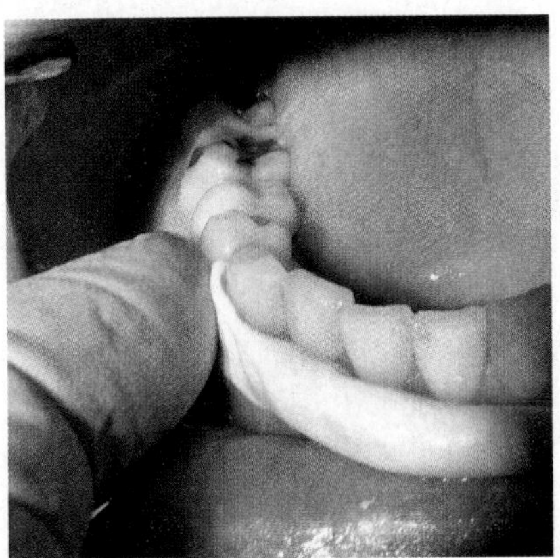
A

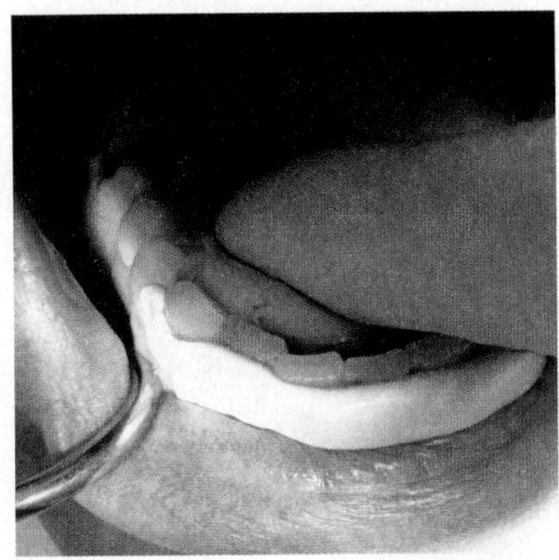
B

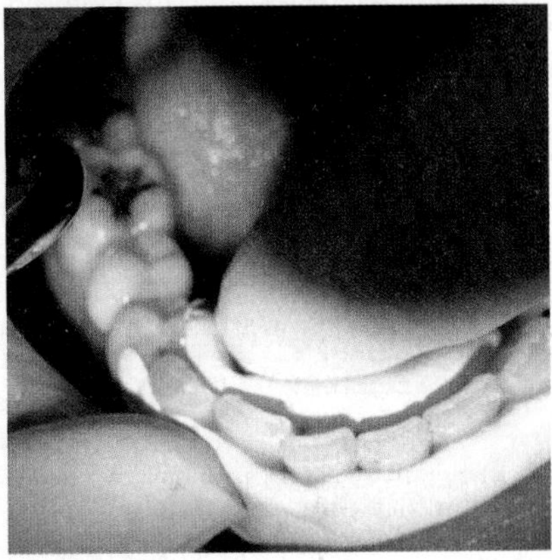
C

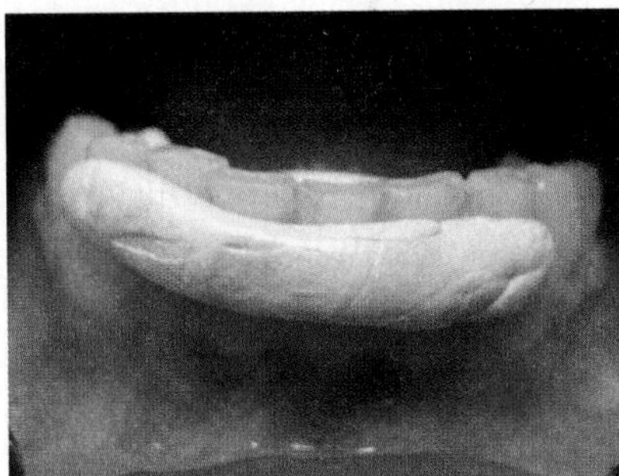
D

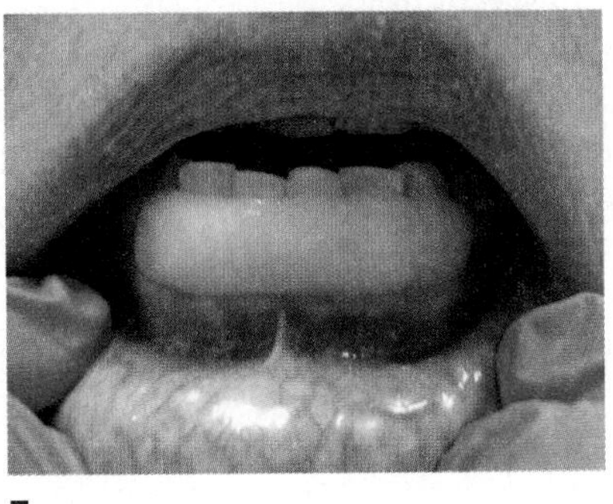
E

Figure 40-6 Periodontal Dressing. **A:** Gently pressing the facial periodontal dressing into the interproximal space. **B:** Gently pushing the lingual periodontal dressing into the interproximal space. **C:** Gently pressing the dressing from the buccal and lingual to help "lock" the dressing in place. **D:** Correct placement of the periodontal dressing. A dressing must cover the surgical wound without unnecessary overextension and fill interdental areas to lock the dressing between the teeth. It is molded in the vestibule and around frena to allow movement of the lips, cheeks, and tongue with no displacement of the dressing. **E:** Reso-Pac (Hager Worldwide), a hydrophilic, more esthetically pleasing periodontal dressing.

Courtesy of Susan Jenkins, MCPHS University Forsyth School of Dental Hygiene.

- Possesses a smooth surface to prevent irritation to cheeks and lips while resisting debris and biofilm retention.

III. Patient Dismissal and Instructions

- Patient is not dismissed until bleeding or oozing from under a dressing has stopped.
- Written instructions are necessary to reinforce those that are provided verbally. **Table 40-2** lists items to discuss with the patient before discharge.

Dressing Removal and Replacement

During healing, epithelium begins to cover a wound in 5–6 days and complete epithelial healing in 7–14 days.[19] The dressing may be left in place for 7 to 10 days, as determined by the surgeon.

Keep the following factors relative to dressings in mind:

- If the dressing becomes dislodged before the removal appointment, the healing tissue needs to be evaluated.

Table 40-2 Instructions for Posttreatment Care

Factor	Instructions to Patient	Purpose of Instruction
Information for the patient about the dressing	■ Dressing will protect the surgical wound. ■ Do not disturb the dressing. ■ Allow it to remain until the next appointment.	■ An informed patient is more likely to be more compliant.
Care during the first few hours	■ Do not eat anything that requires chewing. ■ Use only cool liquids. ■ Stay quiet and rest. ■ If a periodontal dressing was placed, it will not set for a few hours.	■ Do not touch or disturb the surgical area. ■ Dressing will become set or become hard.
Local anesthesia	■ Be careful not to bite lip, cheek, or tongue. ■ Avoid foods that require chewing, hot liquids, and spicy foods until anesthesia has worn off.	■ Prevent trauma to lips, cheeks, and tongue. ■ Rest and be quiet.
Discomfort after local anesthesia wears off	■ Fill any prescriptions provided by the dentist or periodontist and follow directions. ■ Do not take more than directed. ■ Avoid aspirin. ■ Call the dental office if pain persists.	■ Pain control. ■ Aspirin can interfere with blood-clotting mechanisms. ■ The patient will be more prepared to manage any postoperative discomfort when appropriately informed.
Ice pack or cold compress	■ Apply every 30 minutes for 15 minutes; or 15 minutes on, then 15 minutes off. ■ Use as directed only.	■ Prevent swelling from edema.
Bleeding	■ Slight bleeding within the first few hours is not unusual. ■ Blood clot must not be disturbed. ■ Do not suck on the area or use straws.	■ When bleeding seems persistent or excessive, please call the dental office immediately.
Dressing care and retention	■ Avoid disturbing the dressing with the tongue or trying to clean under it. ■ Small particles may chip off, which is not a problem unless sharp edges irritate the tongue or the dressing becomes loose. ■ Call the dentist if the entire dressing or a large portion falls off before the fifth day. ■ Rinse with a saline solution; rinse with chlorhexidine 0.12% morning and evening after brushing teeth.	■ Dressing is needed for wound protection. ■ Epithelium covers wound by fifth or sixth day in normal healing.

Factor	Instructions to Patient	Purpose of Instruction
Use of tobacco and tobacco products	■ Do not smoke; avoid all tobacco products. ■ A heavy smoker must make every effort to decrease quantity of tobacco used. The dental hygienist may suggest a nicotine patch to aid in preventing withdrawal symptoms and aid the patient in abstaining from tobacco use.	■ Heat and smoke irritate the gingiva and delay healing.
Rinsing	■ Do not rinse on the day of treatment. ■ Second day: Use saline solution made with 1/2 teaspoon (measured) in 1/2 cup of warm water every 2–3 hours. ■ Begin chlorhexidine 0.12% b.i.d. (twice a day).	■ Might disturb blood clot. ■ Saline cleanses and aids healing.
Toothbrushing and flossing	■ Continue to maintain optimal personal oral self-care in untreated areas. ■ Lightly brush occlusal surface over dressing material. ■ Use extra soft or soft brush dampened with warm water, and carefully clean film from dressing. ■ Clean the tongue.	■ Dental biofilm control essential to reduce the number of oral microorganisms. ■ Odor and taste control. ■ Oral sanitation.
Diet	■ Use highly nutritious foods for healing. ■ Follow the MyPlate guide. (See Chapter 33.) ■ Use soft-textured diet. ■ Avoid highly seasoned, spicy, hot, sticky, crunchy, and coarse foods.	■ Healing tissue requires a healthy diet and specific comfort foods. ■ Use soft foods to protect the dressing from breakage or displacement.
Mastication	■ Avoid foods that require excessive chewing such as hard, crunchy, or sticky foods. ■ Chew only on the untreated side. ■ Use ground meat or cut meat into small, bite-sized pieces.	■ To protect the dressing while it protects the surgical site.

- When the dressing remains intact for 4 or 5 days, replacement may not be necessary.
- When replacement is indicated, the dressing is replaced in its entirety rather than patched.
- Instruct the patient to proceed with daily biofilm removal and rinsing using an antimicrobial agent.
- Schedule follow-up appointment for the patient.

I. Patient Examination

- Question patient about and record posttreatment effects or discomfort. Record length of time the dressing remained in place.
- Examine the mucosa around the dressing and record its appearance.

II. Procedure for Removal

- Insert a smooth instrument such as a plastic instrument under the border of the dressing and gently apply lateral pressure.
- Watch for sutures lodged in the dressing. If present, cut before removing the dressing.
- Remove fragments of dressing gently with cotton pliers to avoid scratching the thin epithelial covering of the healing tissue.
- Observe tissue and record its appearance. Note any deviations from normal healing that is expected within the number of days.
- Use a scaler for removal of fragments adhering to tooth surfaces and near the gingival margin.
- Use an air–water syringe with a gentle stream of *warm* water. Warm diluted mouthrinse may soothe the healing area.

III. Dressing Replacement Procedure

- Topical anesthetic may be necessary to prevent patient discomfort.
- Use a soft dressing with minimal pressure during application.

IV. Patient Oral Self-Care Instruction

Biofilm control follow-up is essential after final dressing removal.

- Use an extra soft or soft toothbrush on the treated area, paying careful attention to biofilm removal at the gingival margin.
- Increase intensity of care on the treated area each day, with a return to normal oral self-care procedures by day 3 or 4.
- Rinse with 0.12% chlorhexidine gluconate twice daily during the healing period. Gently force liquid between the teeth when swishing.
- Recommend a dentifrice with sodium fluoride for caries prevention and a prescription fluoride may be indicated depending on the patient's caries risk.
- If the patient experiences postsurgical sensitivity, recommend a dentifrice containing a desensitizing agent. Suggestions for coping with sensitivity are found in Chapter 41.

V. Follow-Up

The return for observation of the surgical areas can be scheduled in 1–2 weeks, depending on the patient's progress and treatment planning.

Documentation

Detailed documentation is required at each patient visit. The appointment is dated and signed by the attending clinician.

- At the time of surgical treatment include in the patient's permanent record at least the following:
  - Vital signs.
  - Anesthesia: type, location, number and size of carpules, and patient response to anesthesia.
  - Sutures: type, location, and number placed.
  - Dressing: specific type and area placed.
  - Provide instructions to patient prior to dismissal.
  - Date and signature by attending dentist or periodontist and surgical assistant.
- Dressing and suture removal
  - Tissue examination: tissue response.
  - Patient comments of posttreatment effects, discomfort.
  - Number of sutures removed: compare with number placed.
  - Patient instruction for continued care.
  - Date and signature by attending dental hygienist.
- Sample documentation may be reviewed in **Box 40-1**.

Box 40-1 Example Documentation: Sutures and Dressings

S—Patient presents for postsurgical dressing removal between teeth 11 and 15. Patient states no postsurgical problems.
O—Tissue bled slightly during dressing removal. Removed four sutures; confirmed four sutures were placed during surgery. Patient responded well.
A—Dr. examined area; no additional dressing needed; patient discharged with posttreatment instructions.
P—Patient instructed to call if any problems; patient to return for 2-week follow up appointment.

Signed: ______________________________, RDH
Date: ______________________________

Factors to Teach the Patient

- Provide the posttreatment instructions as outlined in Table 40-2.
- Care of the mouth during the period after treatment while wearing a periodontal dressing.
- Reasons for not using aspirin for pain relief.
- Inform and explain why tobacco use is detrimental and delays healing. Encourage cessation of use of all forms of tobacco.
- Discuss the importance of regular periodontal maintenance after treatment is complete.

References

1. Minozzi F, Bollero P, Unfer V, Dolci A, Galli M. The sutures in dentistry. *Eur Rev Med Pharmacol Sci*. 2009;13(3):217-226.
2. Selvi F, Cakarer S, Can T, et al. Effects of different suture materials on tissue healing. *J Istanb Univ Fac Dent*. 2016;50(1):35-42.
3. Burkhardt R, Lang NP. Influence of suturing on wound healing. *Periodontol 2000*. 2015;68(1):270-281.
4. Ahmed I, Boulton AJ, Rizvi S, et al. The use of triclosan-coated sutures to prevent surgical site infections: a systematic review and meta-analysis of the literature. *BMJ Open*. 2019;9(9):e029727.
5. Asher R, Chacartchi T, Tandlich M, Shapira L, Pollak D. Microbial accumulation on different suture materials

following oral surgery: a randomized controlled study. *Clin Oral Investig.* 2019;23:559-565.

6. Dimova C, Popovaka M, Evrosimovskka B, et al. Various suturing material and wound healing process after oral surgery procedure—a review. *J Hyg Eng Des.* 2020;95-100.
7. Giddings FD. *Book of Surgical Knots and Suturing Techniques.* 3rd ed. Fort Collins, CO: Giddings Studio Publishing; 2009.
8. Nishimura RA, Otto CM, Bonow RO, et al. 2017 AHA/ACC focused update of the 2014 AHA/ACC guideline for the management of patients with valvular heart disease: A report of the American College of Cardiology/American Heart Association Task Force on clinical practice guidelines. *J Am Coll Cardiol.* 2017;70(2):252-289.
9. Giglio JA, Rowland RW, Dalton HP, et al. Suture removal-induced bacteremia: a possible endocarditis risk. *J Am Dent Assoc.* 1992;123(1):65-70.
10. Banche G, Roana J, Mandras N, et al. Microbial adherence on various intraoral suture materials in patients undergoing dental surgery. *J Oral Maxillofac Surg.* 2007;65(8): 1503-1507.
11. Otten JE, Wiedmann-Al-Ahmad M, Jahnke H, Pelz K. Bacterial colonization on different suture materials: a potential risk for intraoral dentoalveolar surgery. *J Biomed Mater Res B Appl Biomater.* 2005;74(1):627-635.
12. King RC, Crawford JJ, Small EW. Bacteremia following intraoral suture removal. *Oral Surg Oral Med Oral Pathol.* 1988;65(1):23-27.
13. Soheilifar S, Bidgoli M, Faradmal J, Soheilifar S. Effect of periodontal dressing on wound healing and patient satisfaction following periodontal flap surgery. *J Dent.* 2015;12(2):151-156.
14. Dumville JC, Gray TA, Walter CJ, et al. Dressings for the prevention of surgical site infection. *Cochrane Database Syst Rev.* 2016;12:CD003091.
15. Kathariya R, Jain H, JadhavT. To pack or not to pack: the current status of periodontal dressings. *J Appl Biomater Funct Mater.* 2015;13(2):e73-e86.
16. Monje A, Kramp AR, Criado E, et al. Effect of periodontal dressing on non-surgical periodontal treatment outcomes: a systematic review. *Int J Dent Hyg.* 2016;14(3):161-167.
17. Vinay Kumar MB, Naraganan V, Jalaluddin M, et al. Assessment of clinical efficacy of different periodontal dressing materials on wound healing: a comparative study. *J Contemp Dent Pract.* 2019;20(8):896-900.
18. Meghana MVS, Deshmukh J, Devarathanamma MV, Asif K, Jyothi L, Sindhura H. Comparison of effect of curcumin gel and noneugenol periodontal dressing in tissue response, early wound healing, and pain assessment following periodontal flap surgery in chronic periodontitis patients. *J Indian Soc Periodontol.* 2020;24(1):54-59.
19. Hämmerle CH, Giannobile WV, Working Group 1 of the European Workshop on Periodontology. Biology of soft tissue wound healing and regeneration: consensus report of Group 1 of the 10th European Workshop on Periodontology. *J Clin Periodontol.* 2014;41(suppl 15):S1-S5.

CHAPTER 41

Dentinal Hypersensitivity

Amy N. Smith, RDH, MPH, PhD

CHAPTER OUTLINE

LEARNING OBJECTIVES

After studying this chapter, the student will be able to:

1. Describe stimuli and pain characteristics specific to hypersensitivity and explain how this relates to differential diagnosis.
2. Describe the factors that contribute to dentin exposure and behavioral changes that could decrease hypersensitivity.
3. Explain the steps in the hydrodynamic theory.
4. Describe two mechanisms of desensitization and their associated treatment interventions for managing dentin hypersensitivity.

The dental hygienist is often the first oral health professional to become aware of the presence of hypersensitive teeth when a patient presents for care. Individuals who have hypersensitivity may be uncomfortable during dental hygiene treatment, since exposure to stimuli such as a cold water spray or contact with metal instruments can elicit the pain of hypersensitive teeth.

- Patients often report activities of daily living such as eating or drinking cold foods or beverages cause pain and request information about causes and treatment for their discomfort.
- Hypersensitivity is often difficult to diagnose because the presenting symptoms can be confused with other types of dental pain with a different etiology.
- Management of hypersensitivity can be a challenge because there are numerous treatment approaches with varying degrees of efficacy.
- Knowledge of the predisposing factors that lead to gingival recession and loss of enamel or cementum and dentin can assist patients in preventing conditions that cause or exacerbate hypersensitivity.

Hypersensitivity Defined

A definitive characteristic associated with **dentinal hypersensitivity** is pain elicited by a stimulus and alleviated upon its removal. Numerous types of stimuli can lead to pain response in individuals with exposed dentin surfaces.

I. Stimuli That Elicit Pain Reaction

- Tactile: contact with toothbrush and other oral hygiene devices, eating utensils, dental instruments, and friction from prosthetic devices such as denture clasps.
- Thermal: temperature change caused by hot and/or cold foods and beverages, and cold air as it contacts the teeth. Cold is the most common stimulus for pain.
- Evaporative: dehydration of oral fluids as from high-volume evacuation or application of air to dry teeth during intraoral procedures.
- **Osmotic**: alteration of pressure in dentinal tubules due to solubility changes in the dentinal fluid.
- Chemical: acids in foods and beverages such as citrus fruits, condiments, spices, wine, and carbonated beverages; acids produced by acidogenic bacteria following carbohydrate exposure; acids from gastroesophageal reflux or vomiting; acidic formulation of whitening agents.

II. Characteristics of Pain from Hypersensitivity

- Sharp, short, or transient pain with rapid onset.
- Cessation of pain upon removal of stimulus.
- Presents as a chronic condition with acute episodes.
- Pain in response to a stimulus that would not normally cause pain or discomfort.
- Discomfort that cannot be ascribed to any other dental defect or pathology.[1]

Etiology of Dentinal Hypersensitivity

A review of tooth anatomy facilitates an understanding of the mechanism of hypersensitivity.

I. Anatomy of Tooth Structures

A. Dentin

- The portion of the tooth covered by enamel on the crown and cementum on the root.
- Composed of fluid-filled dentinal tubules that narrow and branch as they extend from the pulp to the dentinoenamel junction or from the pulp to the dentinocemental junction (**Figure 41-1**).
- Only the portions of the dentinal tubules closest to the pulp are potentially innervated with nerve fiber endings from the pulp chamber.[2]

B. Pulp

- Highly innervated with nerve cell fiber endings that extend just beyond the dentinopulpal interface of the dentinal tubules.[3]
- Body portions of odontoblasts (dentin-producing cells) located within the pulp wall extend their processes from the dentinopulpal junction a short way into each dentinal tubule (Figure 41-1).

C. Nerves

- Nerve fiber endings extend just beyond the dentinopulpal junction and wind around the odontoblastic processes as shown in Figure 41-1.[4] However, not all dentinal tubules contain nerve fiber endings.
- Nerves react via the same **neural depolarization mechanism (sodium-potassium pump)**, which characterizes the response of any nerve to a stimulus.

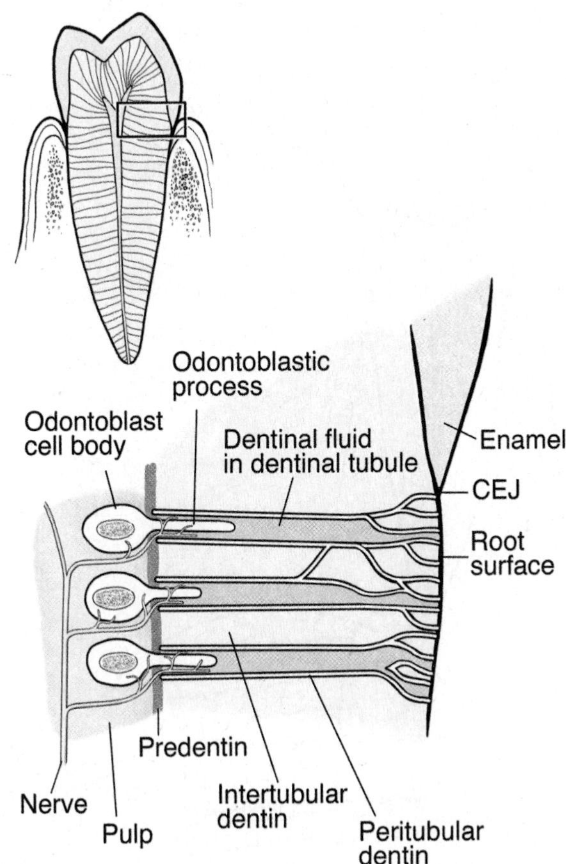

Figure 41-1 Relationship of Dentinal Tubules and Pulpal Nerve Endings. Nerve endings from the pulp wrap themselves around the odontoblasts that extend only a short distance into the tubule. Fluid-filled dentinal tubules transmit fluid disturbances through the mechanism known as hydraulic conductance. CEJ, cementoenamel junction.

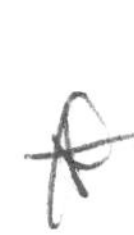

II. Mechanisms of Dentin Exposure

- The sequential events of gingival recession, loss of cementum or enamel, and subsequent dentin exposure, as seen in **Figure 41-2**, can result in hypersensitivity.
- Loss of enamel or cementum can expose dentin gradually or suddenly as in tooth fracture.
- As a result of the lower mineral content of cementum and dentin compared with enamel, demineralization occurs more rapidly and at a lower critical pH.
- Acute hypersensitivity may occur with sudden dentin exposure since gradual exposure allows for the development of natural desensitization mechanisms such as **smear layer** or sclerosis. After many years, secondary or **tertiary/reparative dentin** may form, which also protects the pulp.

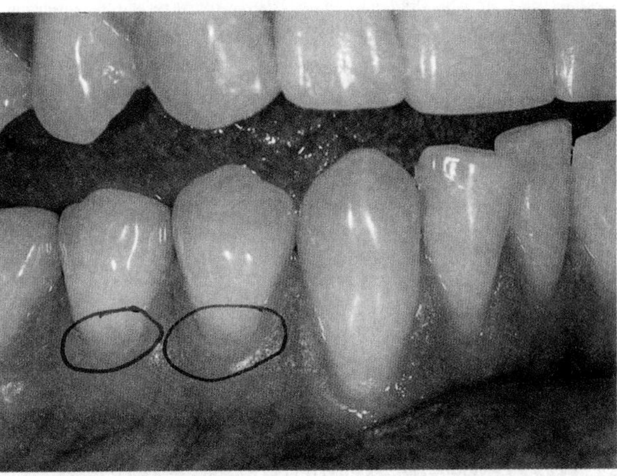

Figure 41-2 Gingival Recession. Note recession from the mandibular right central incisor to the second premolar. If the thin cemental layer of the exposed root surface is lost, dentin hypersensitivity can develop.

A. Factors Contributing to Gingival Recession and Subsequent Root Exposure

The occurrence of gingival recession has a multifactorial etiology. Potential causes include:

- Effects of improper oral self-care:
  - Use of a medium or hard-bristle toothbrush.
  - Frequent, long-term aggressive use of the toothbrush and/or other oral hygiene devices.
- An anatomically narrow zone of attached gingiva is more susceptible to abrasion.
- Facial orientation of one or more teeth.
- A tight and short labial or buccal frenum attachment that pulls on gingival tissues.
- Subgingival instrumentation involving excessive scaling and debridement in shallow sulci.[5]
- Tissue alteration due to apical migration of junctional epithelium from periodontal diseases.
- Periodontal surgical procedures can alter the architecture of gingival tissues resulting in recession.
- Surgical procedures such as crown lengthening, repositioning of gingival tissues, or tooth extractions can affect gingival coverage of adjacent teeth.
- Orthodontic tooth movement may result in loss of periodontal attachment.
- Restorative procedures, such as crown preparation, that abrade marginal gingival tissues.
- Metal jewelry used in an oral piercing of the lip or tongue that repeatedly traumatizes the adjacent facial or lingual gingival tissue.

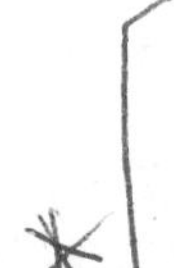

B. Factors Contributing to Loss of Enamel and Cementum

- Loss of tooth structure rarely develops from a single cause but rather from a combination of contributing factors.
- Cementum at the cervical area is thin and easily abrades when exposed.
- Enamel and cementum do not meet at the cementoenamel junction in about 5–10% of teeth, leaving an area of exposed dentin.

C. Attrition, Abrasion, and Erosion

- Attrition can occur due to parafunctional habits such as bruxing.
- Abrasion to sound enamel due to increased toothbrushing forces has not been supported in recent research.[6,7]
- Effects of attrition and abrasion are exacerbated when acid erodes the tooth surface or when the tooth is brushed immediately after consumption of acidic foods and beverages.
- Hypersensitivity may be a clinical outcome of erosion.[8]
- Erosion can occur from dietary acids, such as citrus fruits/juices, wine, and carbonated drinks.[9]
- Dietary acid intake results in an immediate drop in oral pH; after normal salivary neutralization, a physiologic pH of 7 reestablishes within minutes.
- Frequent acid consumption is a critical factor, holding or "swilling" of acidic agents, holding low-pH foods such as citrus fruits against teeth, or continual snacking increases erosion risk.
- Gastric acids from conditions such as gastric reflux, morning sickness, or self-induced vomiting (bulimia) repeatedly expose teeth to a highly acidic environment.

D. Abfraction

- Abfraction, a wedge-shaped cervical lesion, has a questionable etiology.[10-13]
- A cervical lesion caused by lateral/occlusal stresses or tooth flexure from bruxing.
- Microscopic portions of the enamel rods chip away from the cervical area of the tooth, resulting in loss of tooth structure (**Figure 41-3**).
- Lesion appears as a wedge or V-shaped cervical notch.
- A cofactor with abrasion for loss of tooth structure and potential sensitivity.

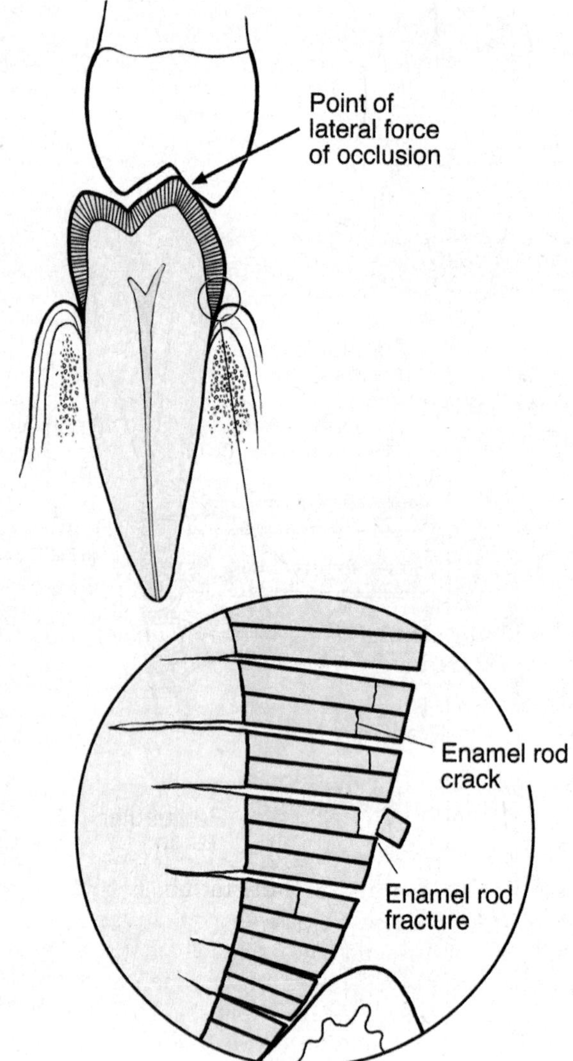

Figure 41-3 Process of Abfraction. Lateral occlusal forces stress the enamel rods at the cervical area, resulting in enamel rod fracture over time. In an advanced stage, a wedge- or V-shaped cervical lesion is visible. Although minute cracks in the enamel rods may not be clinically evident, the tooth can exhibit hypersensitivity.

E. Other Factors

- Crown preparation procedures that remove enamel or cementum can expose dentin at the cervical area.
- Instrumentation during scaling or root debridement procedures on thinning cementum.
- Frequent or improper stain-removal techniques, in which abrasive particles wear away the cementum and dentin.
- Root surface carious lesions.
- Removal of proximal enamel using a sandpaper disk or strip to create additional space for orthodontic movement of crowded teeth, also known as "enamel stripping."

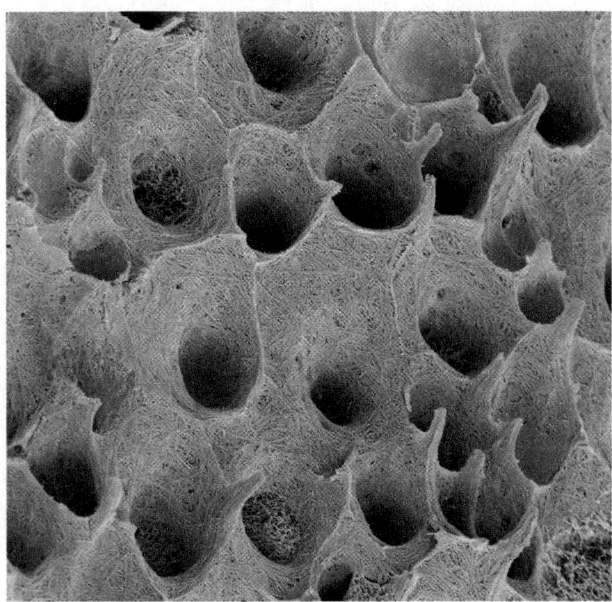

Figure 41-4 Open Dentin Tubules. A acanning electron micrograph (SEM) of dentinal tubules.

III. Hydrodynamic Theory

Hydrodynamic theory is a currently accepted explanation for transmission of stimuli from the outer surface of the dentin to the pulp.

- Described in the 1960s by Brännström, who theorized that a stimulus at the outer aspect of dentin will cause fluid movement within the dentinal tubules.[14]
- Fluid movement creates pressure on the nerve endings within the dentinal tubule, which transmits the pain impulse by stimulating the nerves in the pulp.
- Credibility for this theory is supported by the greater number of widened dentin tubules seen in hypersensitive teeth compared with nonsensitive teeth.[2] **Figure 41-4** depicts open dentinal tubules at the microscopic level. **Figure 41-5** depicts partially occluded dentinal tubules.

Natural Desensitization

- Hypersensitivity can decrease naturally over time, even without treatment interventions.
- These mechanisms include those listed here.

I. Sclerosis of Dentin

- Occurs by mineral deposition within tubules as a result of traumatic stimuli, such as attrition or dental caries.

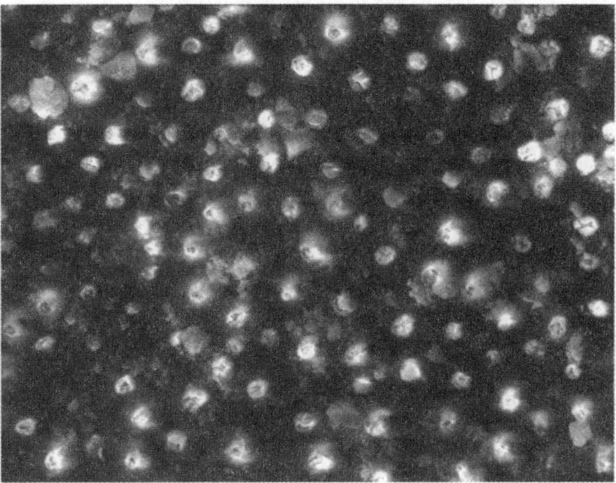

Figure 41-5 Partially Occluded Dentin Tubules. These dentin tubules are nearly filled.

- Creates a thicker, highly mineralized layer of **intratubular or peritubular dentin** (deposited within the periphery of the tubules).
- Results in a smaller-diameter tubule that is less able to transmit stimuli through the dentinal fluid to the nerve fibers at the dentinopulpal interface.

II. Secondary Dentin

- Deposited gradually on the floor and roof of the pulp chamber after the apical foramen is completed.
- Formed more slowly than primary dentin; both types of dentin are created by odontoblasts.
- Creates a "walling off" effect between the dentinal tubules and the pulp to insulate the pulp from dentin fluid disturbances caused by a stimulus such as dental caries.
- With aging, **secondary dentin** accumulates, resulting in a smaller pulp chamber with fewer nerve endings and less sensitivity.

III. Smear Layer

- Consists of organic and inorganic debris that covers the dentinal surface and the tubules.[15]
- Accumulates following scaling and root instrumentation, use of toothpaste (abrasive particles), cutting with a bur, attrition, or abrasion.
- Occludes the dentinal tubule orifices, forming a "smear plug" or a natural "bandage" that blocks stimuli.

- The nature of the smear layer changes constantly since it is subject to effects such as mechanical disruption from ultrasonic debridement, or dissolution from acid exposure.

IV. Calculus

- Provides a protective coating to shield exposed dentin from stimuli.
- Postdebridement sensitivity can occur after removal of heavy calculus deposits; dentinal tubules may become exposed as calculus is removed.

The Pain of Dentin Hypersensitivity

Individuals react differently to pain based on factors such as age, gender, situation and context, previous experiences, pain expectations, and other psychological and physiologic parameters.

I. Patient Profile

The prevalence of reported hypersensitivity varies due to differences in the stimulus, and whether data are gathered by patient report or standardized clinical examination. Patient accounts may not represent true hypersensitivity since the pain can be confused with other conditions.

A. Prevalence of Hypersensitivity

- Current systematic review articles reveal a global prevalence of dental hypersensitivity to be between 3% and 65% with most populations ranging from 10% to 30%.[16-18]
- Most commonly found among 30- to 40-year-olds.[16,17]
- Higher prevalence has been reported in periodontally involved populations.[16,18]
- Incidence and severity decline with advancing age due to the effects of sclerosis and secondary dentin.[16]
- Gingival recession is more prevalent with aging.[19] However, dentinal hypersensitivity is not more prevalent with aging.
- Hypersensitivity, when measured objectively, occurs more often in women.[16,20]

B. Teeth Affected

- Hypersensitivity has been reported to occur primarily at the cervical one-third of the facial surfaces of premolars and mandibular anterior teeth,[21] or on premolars and molars.[16]
- Can occur on any tooth exhibiting predisposing factors.

II. Pain Experience

A. Neural Activity

- Stimuli that affect the fluid flow within the dentinal tubules can activate the terminal nerve endings near to or surrounding the dentinal tubules; activation of these nerve fibers elicits the pain response.
- Occurs via the depolarization/neural discharge mechanism that characterizes all nerve activity.
- The sodium–potassium pump depolarizes the nerve as potassium leaves the nerve cell and sodium enters it.

B. Pain Perception

- The degree of pain is not always proportional to the amount of recession, the percentage of tooth structure loss, or to the quality or quantity of stimulus.
- Individuals experience the subjective phenomenon of pain differently. Many diverse variables such as stress, fatigue, and health beliefs can impact pain perception.

C. Impact of Pain

- Hypersensitivity can manifest as acute or chronic pain; acute pain may result in anxiety, whereas chronic pain may contribute to depression.
- Stress may exacerbate the pain response.
- Persistent discomfort from dentin hypersensitivity may affect quality of life.

Differential Diagnosis

- Etiology of pain can be systemic, pulpal, periapical, restorative, degenerative, or neoplastic.
- A differential diagnosis can rule out other causes of pain before treating for hypersensitivity.
- Skilled interviewing and diagnostics contribute to the differential diagnosis.
- Components to consider in the differential diagnosis of tooth pain are detailed in **Table 41-1**.

I. Differentiation of Pain

- Hypersensitivity pain elicited by a nonnoxious stimulus, such as cold water, can mimic pain elicited by a noxious agent, such as cavitated dental caries.

Table 41-1 Differential Diagnosis of Tooth Pain

Condition	Signs and Symptoms	Clinical Assessment
Dentinal hypersensitivity	Thermal, mechanical, evaporative, osmotic, chemical sensitivity Sharp, sudden, transient pain	Clinical examination: gingival recession and loss of tooth structure
Caries extending into dentin	Thermal sensitivity Pain on pressure Pain with sweets	Clinical examination Radiographic examination
Pulpal caries	Thermal sensitivity Severe, intermittent, or throbbing pain Pain on chewing	Clinical examination Radiographic examination
Fractured restoration	Thermal sensitivity Pain on pressure	Clinical examination
Fractured tooth	Thermal sensitivity Pain on pressure	Occlusal examination Transillumination
Recently placed restoration	Thermal sensitivity Pain on pressure	Dental history Clinical examination Occlusal examination
Occlusal trauma	Chemical sensitivity Thermal sensitivity Pain on pressure Mobility	Occlusal examination
Pulpitis	Severe, intermittent, throbbing pain	Thermal and electric pulp tests Percussion
Sinus infection	"Nondescript" tooth pain Nasal congestion (drainage) Sinus pressure Headache	Clinical examination, including extraoral sinus palpation Radiographic examination
Galvanic pain	Sudden, sharp stabbing pain on tooth-to-tooth contact	Examination for contact between restoration of dissimilar nonprecious metals
Periodontal ligament inflammation	Pain on chewing Clinical examination, including palpation for apical tenderness	Percussion
Abfraction	"Cratered" areas of enamel or dentin at cementoenamel junction in the shape of a wedge or V-shaped notch	Clinical examination Occlusal examination

- The pain of hypersensitivity subsides when the stimulus is removed.
- It is difficult to distinguish between the pain of hypersensitivity and other causes of dental pain when both are in the mild-to-moderate range. Many types of dental pain can be intensified by thermal, sweet, and sour stimuli.
- Chewing pain (occlusal pressure) can be indicative of pulpal pathology.
- Pulpal pain is severe, intermittent, and throbbing. The pain results from deep dental caries, pulpal inflammation, vertical tooth fracture, or infection, and may occur without provocation and persist after stimulus is removed.

II. Data Collection by Interview

- Utilize direct, open-ended, and nonleading questions.
  - Establish the location, degree of pain, onset/duration, source of stimulus, intensity, and alleviating factors related to the painful

Box 41-1 Trigger Questions for Data Collection

- Which tooth or teeth surfaces is/are sensitive?
- On a scale from 1 to 10, with 10 being the most painful, what is your pain intensity?
- How long does the pain last?
- Which words best describe the pain: sharp, dull, shooting, throbbing, persistent, constant, pressure, burning, intermittent?
- Does it hurt when you bite down (pressure)?
- On a scale from 1 to 10, with 10 being a major impact, how much does the pain impact your daily life?
- Is the pain stimulated by certain foods? Sweet? Sour? Acidic?
- Does sensitivity occur with hot or cold food or beverages?
- Does discomfort stop immediately upon removal of the painful stimulus, such as cold food or beverage, or does it linger?
- Have you used whitening products lately?

response; patients may have difficulty characterizing the pain.
  - Ask trigger questions as suggested in **Box 41-1** to elicit detailed information to characterize the pain and assist in the dental hygiene diagnosis.
- Establish rapport, combined with effective listening and counseling skills, to develop collaborative treatment/management strategies.
- Record a thorough dental history, including pain chronology, nature, location, aggravating and alleviating factors, and history of dental treatment/restorations.

III. Diagnostic Techniques and Tests

When patients have difficulty describing and localizing their pain, the following diagnostic techniques and tests can aid in differentiating among the numerous causes of tooth pain.

- Visual assessment of tooth integrity and surrounding tissues.
- Palpation of extra and intraoral soft tissues.
- Evaluation of nasal congestion, drainage, or sinus expressed as tooth pain.
- Occlusal examination with use of marking paper to detect a premature contact or hyperfunction following placement of a new restoration.
- Radiographic assessment to determine signs of pulpal pathology, vertical tooth fracture, or other irregularities of the teeth or surrounding structures.
- Percussion with use of an instrument handle to lightly tap on each tooth. A pain response may indicate pulpitis.
- Mobility testing may detect trauma or periodontal pathology.
- Pain from biting pressure with use of a bite stick to assess pain indicative of tooth fracture.
- Transillumination with a high-intensity, focused light to enhance visualization of a cracked tooth; dye may also indicate a fracture line.
- Pulpal pathology assessment with thermal or electric pulp tests.

Hypersensitivity Management

When the differential diagnosis indicates dentinal hypersensitivity, the dental hygiene care plan includes further assessment and patient counseling combined with treatment interventions.

I. Assessment Components

- Determine extent and severity of pain.
  - Solicit a self-report of symptoms, including the eliciting stimuli.
  - Quantify and record the baseline pain intensity using objective measures such as the visual analog scale (VAS) and/or the verbal rating scale (VRS), as described in **Box 41-2**.
- Determine if oral self-care procedures contribute to loss of gingival attachment or tooth structure.
- Use a diet analysis to assess the frequency of acidic food and beverage intake; correlate intake with timing of toothbrushing.
- Explore parafunctional habits, such as bruxing, that may contribute to abfraction and attrition.

II. Educational Considerations

- Provide education regarding etiology and contributing factors. Explain the natural mechanisms for resolution of hypersensitivity over time.
- Discuss realistic oral self-care measures that the patient is likely to maintain and include technique demonstrations.
- Utilize effective communication and motivational interviewing skills to promote compliance and to decrease patient anxiety. (See Chapter 24.)

Box 41-2 Subjective Pain Assessment Form

Name: ______________
Date: ______________
Teeth: ______________

VAS—Visual Analog Scale
Please place an "X" on the line at a position between the two extremes to represent the level of pain that you experience.

No Discomfort |————————————| Severe Discomfort

Discomfort Scale

VRS—Verbal Rating Scale
0 = No discomfort/pain, but aware of stimulus
1 = Slight discomfort/pain
2 = Significant discomfort/pain
3 = Significant discomfort/pain that lasted more than 10 seconds

III. Treatment Hierarchy

- There are two basic treatment goals:
  - Pain relief.
  - Modification or elimination of contributing factors.
- Address mild-to-moderate pain with conservative approaches or agents; more severe pain may require an aggressive approach.
- Sequence treatment approaches from the most conservative and least invasive measures to more aggressive modalities.
- Prognosis of pain resolution is difficult to predict due to variable success with different treatment options among individuals.
  - Historically, a vast array of treatment approaches have been utilized with varying degrees of success; no one best method has been identified due to lack of quality **randomized controlled trial** (RCT) data, difficulties inherent in dentin hypersensitivity research design, and a significant placebo effect.
  - A trial-and-error approach may be necessary to determine the most effective treatment option.
  - Characteristics of an ideal desensitizing agent are listed in **Box 41-3** and can be useful evaluation criteria when selecting a desensitizing agent.
- Treatment options that include both oral self-care measures and professional interventions with the same objective of reducing hypersensitivity have a synergistic effect.

Box 41-3 The Ideal Desensitizing Agent

- Minimal application time.
- Easy application procedure.
- Does not endanger the soft tissues.
- Acceptable cost.
- Requires few dental appointments.
- Does not cause pulpal irritation or pain.
- Rapid and lasting effect.
- Causes no staining.
- Consistently effective.
- Acceptable taste.

IV. Reassessment

- Evaluate treatment interventions.
  - Allow sufficient time to elapse (2–4 weeks) to evaluate effectiveness of treatment recommendations; assess and reinforce behavioral changes.
  - Repeat the VAS and/or the VRS to compare changes in pain perceptions from baseline.
- If pain persists, a different option may provide relief.

Oral Hygiene Care and Treatment Interventions

I. Mechanisms of Desensitization

- Desensitization agents and oral self-care measures disrupt the pain transmission as described by the hydrodynamic theory in one of two ways[17]:
- Prevent nerve depolarization that interrupts the neural transmission to the pulp. This physiologic process is the mechanism of action for potassium-based products.[22]
- Prevent a stimulus from moving the tubule fluid by occlusion of dentin tubule orifices or reduction in tubule lumen diameter.

II. Behavioral Changes

- Encourage habits that allow tubules to remain occluded or that occlude **patent** tubules.
- Use a motivational interviewing approach to help the patient commit to appropriate oral self-care and dietary habits before or in conjunction with self-applied or professionally applied desensitizing agents. (Motivational interviewing is discussed in Chapter 24.)
- Educate the patient that some products may take 2–4 weeks to decrease sensitivity.

A. Dietary Modifications

- Have patient analyze acidic food and beverage habits that incite pain from dissolution of the smear layer, which covered open dentinal tubules.[23] Examples include citrus fruits and juices, acidic carbonated beverages, sharp flavors and spices, pickled foods, wines, and ciders.
- Counsel patient regarding change in dietary habits.
- Help patient determine if brushing is sequenced immediately after consuming acidic foods and beverages. Advise altering sequence to eliminate combined effects of erosion and abrasion, which can accelerate tooth structure loss.[24]
- Guide patient toward mouthrinses with a nonacidic formulation.
- Provide professional treatment referrals for patients with eating disorders such as bulimia or systemic conditions such as acid reflux that repeatedly create an acidic oral environment.
- The acidic environment created by bulimia and acid reflux can be neutralized by rinsing with water (particularly fluoridated water) or an alkaline rinse such as bicarbonate of soda in water.
- Counsel patient to eliminate or reduce extremes of hot and cold foods and beverages to avoid discomfort.

B. Dental Biofilm Control

- In the presence of dental biofilm, the dentinal tubule orifices increase to three times the original size; with reestablishment of biofilm control measures, there is a 20% decrease in size.[25]
- The presence/amount of dental biofilm on exposed root surfaces does not directly correlate with the degree of dentin sensitivity,[20] suggesting biofilm composition may be a factor.

C. Eliminate Parafunctional Habits

- Help patient evaluate bruxing and clenching behaviors and whether additional treatment is indicated.
- Determine need for occlusal adjustments to reduce destructive forces.
- Coach patient to monitor occurrence of subconscious parafunctional behaviors and levels of stress. Identify whether stress reduction protocols are needed.
- Introduce behavior modification techniques and refer when needed.

D. Toothbrush Type and Technique

- Brush one or two teeth at a time with a soft or ultrasoft toothbrush, rather than using long, horizontal strokes over several teeth to prevent further recession and loss of tooth structure.
- Identify brushing sequence and adjust by beginning in least sensitive areas and ending with more sensitive areas. In the initial phases of brushing, toothbrush filaments are stiffer and brushing is more aggressive.
- Help patient investigate current toothbrush grip. Adjust to a modified pen grasp rather than a traditional palm grasp to reduce the amount of pressure applied.
- Explore receptivity to use of a power toothbrush because it removes dental biofilm effectively with less than half the pressure of a manual toothbrush; an individual using a manual toothbrush typically exerts 200–400 g of pressure; 70–150 g of pressure is usually exerted with a power toothbrush.[26] Some power toothbrushes have a self-limiting mechanism to reduce filament action if too much pressure is applied.
- Recommend and demonstrate dental biofilm control measures that are meticulous, yet gentle, and do not contribute to further abrasion of hard or soft tissues.

III. Desensitizing Agents

- There are study design challenges when researching desensitization due to subjectivity of the pain response, the strong placebo effect, and the process of natural desensitization.
- Despite widespread professional recommendation and use, there is little in vivo scientific evidence validating the efficacy and mechanisms of action of desensitizing agents.
- RCTs are needed to support professional recommendation and treatment. The exception is fluoride, with a substantial body of knowledge validating its usefulness as a desensitizing agent.
- Desensitizing agents can be categorized according to their mechanisms of action, either depolarization of the nerve or occlusion of the dentinal tubule. Potassium salts are the only agents that are theorized to work by depolarization.

A. Potassium Salts

- Formulations containing potassium chloride, potassium nitrate, potassium citrate, or potassium oxalate reduce depolarization of the nerve cell membrane and transmission of the nerve impulse.[24]

- Potassium nitrate dentifrices containing fluoride are widely used[22] and readily available over the counter.

B. Fluorides

- Precipitate calcium fluoride (CaF_2) crystals within the dentinal tubule to decrease the lumen diameter.[24]
- Create a barrier by precipitating CaF_2 at the exposed dentin surface to block open dental tubules.[27]
  - Fluoride varnishes are Food and Drug Administration (FDA)-approved for tooth desensitization and a cavity liner, although they are frequently used "off-label" for dental caries prevention.
  - Fluoride gels and varnishes are most commonly used and are a successful treatment modalilty.[28,29]

C. Oxalates

- Block open dental tubules.[30]
- Oxalate salts such as potassium oxalate and ferric oxalate precipitate calcium oxalate crystals to decrease the lumen diameter.[30]

D. Glutaraldehyde

- Coagulates proteins and amino acids within the dentinal tubule to decrease the dentinal tubule lumen diameter.[30]
- Can be combined with hydroxyethylmethacrylate, a hydrophilic resin, which seals tubules.[30]
- Creates calcium crystals within the dentinal tubule to decrease the lumen diameter.[31]

E. Calcium Phosphate Technology

- Advocated for use as a caries control agent to reduce demineralization and increase remineralization by releasing calcium and phosphate ions into saliva for deposition of new tooth mineral (hydroxyapatite).[32]
  - Calcium phosphates can compromise the bioavailability of fluorides since calcium and fluoride react to form calcium fluoride.[33]
  - May be effective for patients with poor salivary flow and consequent deficient calcium phosphate levels.[34]
- Agents that support remineralization may lessen dentinal hypersensitivity by occluding dentinal tubule openings.
- Most studies in support of calcium phosphate technology are animal, in vitro, or in situ models designed to analyze remineralization rather than hypersensitivity.
  - One in vivo study found a reduction in bleaching-induced sensitivity at days 5 and 14 when amorphous calcium phosphate (ACP) was added to a bleaching gel.[35]
  - Additional research related to calcium phosphate technologies is needed.[36]
- ACP
  - Theorized to plug dentinal tubules with calcium and phosphate *precipitate*; promotes an ACP reservoir within the saliva.
  - Enhances fluoride delivery in calcium and phosphate-deficient saliva.[34]
  - May remineralize areas of acid erosion and abrasion and reduce hypersensitivity.[35]
- Calcium sodium phosphosilicate (CSP)
  - Contains sodium and silica in addition to calcium and phosphorus.
  - Delivered in solid bioactive glass particles that react in the presence of saliva and water to release calcium and phosphate ions and create a calcium phosphate layer that crystallizes to hydroxyapatite.
  - Reacts with saliva; sodium buffers the acid, and calcium and phosphate saturate saliva to fill demineralized areas with new hydroxyapatite.
  - Claims include remineralizing enamel and dentin, positive impact on acid erosion and abrasion, a bactericidal effect, and reduction in hypersensitivity.
  - RCT comparing a CSP and a potassium nitrate toothpaste found, using a VAS, that CSP paste was significantly better at reducing dentin hypersensitivity.[37]
- Casein phosphopeptide (CPP)–ACP
  - CPP is a milk-derived protein that stabilizes ACP and allows it to be released during acidic challenges.
  - Researchers are exploring benefits such as remineralization of acid erosion, caries inhibition, and reduction of dentinal hypersensitivity.
- Tricalcium phosphate (TCP)
  - Developed in an effort to create a calcium material that can coexist with fluoride to provide greater efficacy than fluoride alone.[34] Additional components are added to β-TCP to "functionalize" it. Increased remineralization has been demonstrated in vitro[38]; in vivo evidence is needed.

IV. Self-Applied Measures

A. Dentifrices

- In many OTC sensitivity-reducing dentifrices, 5% potassium nitrate, sodium fluoride, or stannous fluoride separately or in combination are the active desensitizing agents. Studies have suggested that some of the desensitizing effects of dentifrices may be due to the blocking action of the abrasive particles.[24]
- Tartar control dentifrices may contribute to increased tooth sensitivity for some individuals, although the mechanism is unclear.
- Dentifrices containing highly concentrated fluoride (5000 ppm fluoride) combined with an abrasive to facilitate extrinsic stain control are available by prescription. This formulation is also available with the addition of potassium nitrate.

B. Gels

- Gels containing 5000 ppm fluoride are a prescription product brushed on for generalized hypersensitivity or burnished into localized areas of sensitivity.
- Contain no abrasive agents for biofilm and stain control.
- Can be self-applied with custom or commercially available fluoride or whitening trays.

C. Mouthrinses

- Mouthrinse containing 0.63% stannous fluoride can be prescribed for daily use to treat hypersensitivity.
- Short-term use (2–4 weeks) will limit staining concerns.

V. Professionally Applied Measures

A. Tray-Delivered Fluoride Agents

- A tray delivery system can be used to apply a 2% neutral sodium fluoride solution.
- Select trays of adequate height and fill with sufficient fluoride agent to cover the cervical areas of each tooth.

B. Fluoride Varnish

- A 5% sodium fluoride varnish maintains prolonged contact with the tooth surface by serving as a reservoir to release fluoride ions in response to pH changes in saliva and biofilm.[39]
- Does not require a dry tooth surface, which is advantageous since drying the tooth can be a painful procedure for a patient with dentin hypersensitivity.
- Use a microbrush to apply the varnish to the exposed dentin surface.
- Instruct the patient to avoid oral hygiene self-care for several hours to allow the fluoride to stay in contact with the tooth surface for as long as possible, preferably overnight.

C. 5% Glutaraldehyde

- Use a microbrush to apply to the affected tooth surface.
- Prevent excess flow into soft tissues with cotton roll isolation since contact with soft tissues may cause gingival irritation.

D. Oxalates

- Oxalate preparations are applied (burnished) to a dried tooth surface.
- May provide immediate and short-term relief, rather than long-term relief.

E. Unfilled or Partially Filled Resins

- Used to cover patent dentinal tubules.
- Resins are applied following an acid etch step that may remove the smear layer and cause discomfort.
- The tooth surface must be dehydrated before resin application, which can create discomfort.
- Use of local anesthetic may facilitate patient comfort during this procedure.

F. Dentin-Bonding Agents

- Obturates the tubule opening and does not require use of acid etch or dehydration; a single application may protect against further erosion for 3–6 months.
- Methylmethacrylate polymer is a common dentin sealer.

G. Glass Ionomer Sealants/Restorative Materials

- Glass ionomer may be placed in the presence of moisture, which eliminates the need for drying the tooth.

- In addition to the glass ionomer restoration physically blocking the dentinal tubule, there is an added benefit of slow fluoride release.

H. Soft-Tissue Grafts

- Surgical placement of soft-tissue grafts to cover a sensitive dentinal surface.

I. Lasers

- Nd:YAG laser treatment can obliterate dentinal tubules through a process called "melting and resolidification." When used with an appropriate protocol, there is no resulting damage to the pulp or dentin surface cracking.[40,41]
- Low-level diode laser treatments have shown a reduction in dentinal hypersensitivity, but the exact mechanism of action is unclear.[42]
- Diode laser treatments combined with sodium fluoride varnish application have shown an immediate decrease in sensitivity.[43]
- A recent meta-analysis of laser use for dentinal hypersensitivity concluded that diode and YAG lasers both produced immediate and long-term desensitizing effects when compared to the control treatments.[44]
- Long term, in vivo studies are needed to establish safety and efficacy of laser treatment for dentin hypersensitivity. The FDA has not approved these devices for this therapeutic modality.

VI. Additional Considerations

A. Periodontal Debridement Considerations

- Preprocedure
  - Explain potential for sensitivity resulting from calculus removal and/or instrumentation of teeth with areas of exposed cementum or dentin.
  - Patients are likely to respond more favorably to treatment when prepared for what might occur.
  - When multiple teeth in the same treatment area are hypersensitive during scaling and root instrumentation procedures, local anesthetics and/or nitrous oxide analgesia can be utilized.
  - Desensitizing agents that are marketed for immediate relief from severe hypersensitivity can be used.
- Postprocedure
  - Professionally applied desensitization agents can be used.
  - Patient is instructed in daily oral self-care behavior changes and use of self-applied desensitizing agents.

B. Tooth Whitening–Induced Sensitivity

Tooth whitening agents, such as hydrogen peroxide and carbamide peroxide, may contribute to increased dentinal hypersensitivity.

- Thought to result from by-products of 10% carbamide peroxide (3% hydrogen peroxide and 7% urea) readily passing through the enamel and dentin into the pulp; the reversible pulpitis is caused from the dentin fluid flow and pulpal contact of the hydrogen peroxide without apparent harm to the pulp.[45]
- Hypersensitivity may dissipate over time, lasting from a few days to several months.
- Exposed dentin and preexisting dentin hypersensitivity increase hypersensitivity risk secondary to whitening.
- Some whitening products contain fluoride or potassium nitrate to eliminate or minimize the effects of sensitivity.
- Recommendations to prevent or reduce tooth whitening–induced sensitivity include[45]:
  - Use of a potassium nitrate, fluoride, or other desensitization product starting 2 weeks before or concurrently with whitening.
  - Some at-home whitening gels incorporate 5% potassium nitrate, fluoride, and ACP.
  - Home-use whitening products are usually less concentrated than professionally applied in-office treatment options, with less hypersensitivity risk.
  - Allow for a "recovery period" between whitening sessions during which desensitizing agents are used. Decrease frequency of use by whitening every second or third day. (See Chapter 43 for more information.)

C. Research Developments

- The search for the ideal desensitizing agent is ongoing.
- Evidence-based scientific research indicated as new products are developed; in vivo research protocols are needed to support clinical application.

Box 41-4 Example Documentation: Patient with Dentinal Hypersensitivity

- **S**—Patient complains of pain when eating/drinking cold foods/beverages that disappears immediately after.
- **O**—Generalized facial gingival recession of 1–2 mm on all teeth in the mandibular arch.
- **A**—Based on patient symptoms, exposed roots, and no other evidence of dental disease, the working diagnosis is dentinal hypersensitivity.
- **P**—Applied fluoride varnish and gave postoperative instructions; advised patient to avoid acidic beverages, or not to brush immediately after ingestion of citrus fruits or beverages; also advised to rinse with fluoridated water to buffer acidic conditions (to raise pH). Recommended purchase and use of an OTC potassium nitrate–containing dentifrice. Explained that relief from the dentifrice can take between 2 and 4 weeks. Advised to contact the office if pain persists or worsens.

Next Steps: Follow-up at next visit.
Signed: ______________________________, RDH
Date: ________________________________

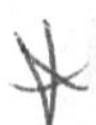

Documentation

The permanent record for a patient with a history of tooth sensitivity needs to include at least the following information:

- Medical and dental history, vital signs, extra and intraoral examinations, consultations, and individual progress notes for each appointment and maintenance appointments.
- For dentin hypersensitivity: identify teeth involved (including measurements of recession, attached gingiva, abfractions, and attrition), differential diagnosis, and all treatments, along with patient instruction for ideal oral self-care, diet, and other for preventive recommendations.
- Outcomes and posttreatment directions.
- A progress note example for the patient with hypersensitive dentin may be reviewed in **Box 41-4**.

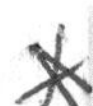

Factors to Teach the Patient

- Etiology and prevention of gingival recession.
- Factors contributing to dentin hypersensitivity.
- Mechanisms of dentin tubule exposure, which can allow various stimuli to trigger pain response.
- Natural desensitization mechanisms that may lessen sensitivity over time.
- Appropriate oral hygiene self-care techniques, such as using a soft toothbrush and avoiding a vigorous brushing technique that may exacerbate current gingival recession and subsequent abrasion of root surfaces.
- Connection between an acidic diet and dentin sensitivity; need to eliminate specific foods and beverages that can trigger sensitivity.
- Toothbrushing is not recommended immediately after consumption of acidic foods or beverages.
- Behavior modifications or treatments for eliminating parafunctional habits.
- The challenges of managing hypersensitivity, hierarchy of treatment measures, and variable effect of treatment options.

References

1. Addy M. Etiology and clinical implications of dentine hypersensitivity. *Dent Clin North Am.* 1990;34(3):503-514.
2. Absi EG, Addy M, Adams D. Dentine hypersensitivity: the development and evaluation of a replica technique to study sensitive and non-sensitive cervical dentine. *J Clin Periodontol.* 1989;16(3):190-195.
3. Frank RM. Attachment sites between the odontoblast process and the intradental nerve fibre. *Arch Oral Biol.* 1968;13(7):833-834.
4. Thomas HF, Carella P. Correlation of scanning and transmission electron microscopy of human dentinal tubules. *Arch Oral Biol.* 1984;29(8):641-646.
5. Dufour LA, Bissell HS. Periodontal attachment loss induced by mechanical subgingival instrumentation in shallow sulci. *J Dent Hyg.* 2002;76(3):207-212.
6. Wiegand A, Burkhard JP, Eggmann F, Attin T. Brushing force of manual and sonic toothbrushes affects dental hard tissue abrasion. *Clin Oral Investig.* 2013;17(3):815-822.

7. Heasman PA, Holliday R, Bryant A, Preshaw PM. Evidence for the occurrence of gingival recession and non-carious cervical lesions as a consequence of traumatic toothbrushing. *J Clin Periodontol*. 2015;42(Suppl 16):S237-S255.
8. Absi EG, Addy M, Adams D. Dentine hypersensitivity: the effect of toothbrushing and dietary compounds on dentine in vitro. *J Oral Rehabil*. 1992;19(2):101-110.
9. Prati C, Montebugnoli L, Suppa P, Valdrè G, Mongiorgi R. Permeability and morphology of dentin after erosion induced by acidic drinks. *J Periodontol*. 2003;74(4):428-436.
10. Staninec M, Nalla RK, Hilton JF, et al. Dentin erosion simulation by cantilever beam fatigue and pH change. *J Dent Res*. 2005;84(4):371-375.
11. Litonjua LA, Andreana S, Bush OJ, et al. Wedged cervical lesions produced by toothbrushing. *Am J Dent*. 2004;17(4):237-240.
12. Estafan A, Furnari PC, Goldstein G, et al. In vivo correlation of noncarious cervical lesions and occlusal wear. *J Prosthet Dent*. 2005;93(3):221-226.
13. Sarode GS, Sarode CS. Abfraction: a review. *J Oral Maxillofac Pathol*. 2013;17(2):222-227.
14. Brännström M, Linden LA, Astrom A. The hydrodynamics of the dental tubule and of pulp fluid: a discussion of its significance in relation to dentinal sensitivity. *Caries Res*. 1967;1(4):310-317.
15. Eldarrat AH, High AS, Kale GM. In vitro analysis of "smear layer" on human dentine using ac-impedance spectroscopy. *J Dent*. 2004;32(7):547-554.
16. Splieth CH, Tachou A. Epidemiology of dentin hypersensitivity. *Clin Oral Invest*. 2013;17(suppl 1):S3-S8.
17. Shiau HJ. Dentin hypersensitivity. *J Evid Base Pract*. 2012; 12(suppl 1):220-228.
18. Kim JW, Park JC. Dentin hypersensitivity and emerging concepts for treatments. *J Oral Bio*. 2017;59(4):211-217.
19. Mantzourani M, Sharma D. Dentine sensitivity: past, present, and future. *J Dent*. 2013;41(suppl 4):S3-S17.
20. Kassaba MM, Cohen RE. The etiology and prevalence of gingival recession. *J Am Dent Assoc*. 2003;134(2):220-225.
21. Gillam DG, Aris A, Bulman JS, et al. Dentine hypersensitivity in subjects recruited for clinical trials: clinical evaluation, prevalence and intraoral distribution. *J Oral Rehabil*. 2002;29(3):226-231.
22. Orchardson R, Gillam DG. The efficacy of potassium salts as agents for treating dentin hypersensitivity. *J Orofac Pain*. 2000;14(1):9-19.
23. Correa FO, Sampaio JE, Rossa C, et al. Influence of natural fruit juices in removing the smear layer from root surfaces—an in vitro study. *J Can Dent Assoc*. 2004;70(10):697-702.
24. Orchardson R, Gilla DC. Managing dentin hypersensitivity. *J Am Dent Assoc*. 2006;137(7):990-998.
25. Kawasaki A, Ishikawa K, Suge T, et al. Effects of plaque control on the patency and occlusion of dentine tubules in situ. *J Oral Rehabil*. 2001;28(5):439-449.
26. Van Der Weijden GA, Timmerman MF, Reijerse E, et al. Toothbrushing force in relation to plaque removal. *J Clin Periodontol*. 1996;23(8):724-729.
27. Suge T, Ishikowa K, Kawasaki A, et al. Effects of fluoride on the calcium phosphate precipitation method for dentinal tubule occlusion. *J Dent Res*. 1995;74(4):1079-1085.
28. Ritter AV, de L Dias W, Miguez P, et al. Treating cervical dentin hypersensitivity with fluoride varnish: a randomized clinical study. *J Am Dent Assoc*. 2006;137(7):1013-1020.
29. Cunha-Cruz J, Wataha JC, Zhou L, et al. Treating dentin hypersensitivity, therapeutic choices made by dentists of the Northwest PRECEDENT network. *J Am Dent Assoc*. 2010;141(9):1097-1105.
30. Haywood VB. Dentine hypersensitivity: bleaching and restorative considerations for successful management. *Int Dent J*. 2002;52(suppl 1):376.
31. Pashley DH, Kalathoor S, Burnham D. The effects of calcium hydroxide on dentin permeability. *J Dent Res*. 1986; 65(3):417-420.
32. Featherstone JD. The continuum of dental caries-evidence for a dynamic disease process. *J Dent Res*. 2004;83(Spec No C):C39-C42.
33. Karlinsey RL, Mackey AC, Walker ER, et al. Surfactant-modified B-TCP: structure, properties, and in vitro remineralization of subsurface enamel lesions. *J Mater Sci Mater Med*. 2010;21(4):2009-2020.
34. Chow L, Wefel JS. The dynamics of de- and remineralization. *Dimensions Dent Hyg*. 2009;7(2):42-46.
35. Giniger M, MacDonald J, Ziemba S, et al. The clinical performance of professionally dispensed bleaching gel with added amorphous calcium phosphate. *J Am Dent Assoc*. 2005;136(3):383-392.
36. Yengopal V, Mickenautsch S. Caries-preventive effect of casein phosphopeptide-amorphous calcium phosphate (CPP-ACP): a meta-analysis. *Acta Odontol Scand*. 2009;21:1-12.
37. Pradeep AR, Sharma A. Comparison of clinical efficacy of a dentifrice containing calcium sodium phosphosilicate to a dentifrice containing potassium nitrate and to a placebo on dentinal hypersensitivity: a randomized clinical trial. *J Periodontol*. 2010;81(8):1167-1173.
38. Karlinsey RL, Mackey AC, Walker ER, et al. Preparation, characterization and in vitro efficacy of an acid-modified β-TCP material for dental hard-tissue remineralization. *Acta Biomater*. 2010;6(3):969-978.
39. Shen C, Autio-Gold J. Assessing fluoride concentration uniformity and fluoride release from 3 varnishes. *J Am Dent Assoc*. 2002;133(2):176-182.
40. Kara C, Orbak R. Comparative evaluation of Nd:YAG laser and fluoride varnish for the treatment of dentinal hypersensitivity. *J Endod*. 2009;35(7):971-974.
41. Lopes AO, Aranha ACC. Comparative evaluation of the effects of Nd:YAG laser and a desensitizer agent on the treatment of dentin hypersensitivity: a clinical study. *Photomed Laser Surg*. 2013;31(3):132-138.
42. Yilmaz H, Kurtulmus-Yilmaz S, Cengiz E. Long-term effect of diode laser irradiation compared to sodium fluoride varnish in the treatment of dentine hypersensitivity in periodontal maintenance patients: a randomized controlled clinical study. *Photomed Laser Surg*. 2011;29(11):721-725.
43. Corona S, Nascimento T, Catirse A, Lizarelli R, Dinelli W, Palma-Dibb R. Clinical evaluation of low-level laser therapy and fluoride varnish for treating cervical dentinal hypersensitivity. *J Oral Rehabil*. 2003;30(12):1183-1189.
44. Hu ML, Zheng G, Han JM, Yang M, Zhang YD, Lin H. Effect of lasers on dentine hypersensitivity: evidence from a meta-analysis. *J Evid Based Dent Pract*. 2019;19(2):115-130.
45. Haywood VB, Sword RJ. Tray bleaching status and insights. *J Esthet Restor Dent*. 2021;33(1):27-38.

CHAPTER 42

Extrinsic Stain Removal

Heather Doucette, DipDH, BSc, MEd
Linda D. Boyd, RDH, RD, EdD

CHAPTER OUTLINE

LEARNING OBJECTIVES

After studying this chapter, the student will be able to:

1. Describe the difference between a cleaning agent and a polishing agent.
2. Explain the basis for selection of the grit of polishing paste for each individual patient.

3. Discuss the rationale for avoiding polishing procedures on areas of demineralization.
4. Explain the effect abrasive particle shape, size, and hardness have on the abrasive qualities of a polishing paste.
5. Explain the types of powdered polishing agents available and their use in the removal of tooth stains.
6. Explain patient conditions that contraindicate the use of air-powder polishing.

Introduction

After treatment by scaling, root debridement, and other dental hygiene care, the teeth are assessed for the presence of remaining dental stains.

- The cleaning or **polishing agents** used must be selected based on the patient's individual needs such as the type, location, and amount of stain present.
- Preliminary examination of each tooth will reveal the surfaces to be treated, which may be tooth structure (enamel, or in the case of recession, cementum, or dentin) or when restored, a variety of dental materials (metal or esthetic, tooth-color restorations).
- Preservation of the surfaces of both the teeth and the restorations is of primary importance during all cleaning and **polishing** procedures.
- Stain removal requires the use of polishing agents with various **abrasive** grits. The smallest, least abrasive **grit** is used.
- Some patients will not consider their teeth "cleaned" unless they have been polished. For this situation when no extrinsic stain is present, use a **cleaning agent** to avoid abrasion of the dental hard tissues and remove dental biofilm.
- Incorrect selection of a prophylaxis paste can worsen hypersensitivity.
- The longevity, esthetic appearance, and smooth surfaces of dental restorations depend on appropriate care by the dental hygienist and the daily oral self-care by the patient.

Purposes for Stain Removal

Stains on the teeth are not etiologic factors for oral disease.

- The removal of stains is for esthetic, not for therapeutic or health, reasons.
- The American Dental Hygienists' Association and the Academy of Periodontology include tooth polishing in their definitions of the term "oral prophylaxis."[1,2]

Science of Polishing

- Polishing is intended to produce intentional, selective and controlled wear. Within the science of **tribology**, polishing is considered to be **two-body abrasion** or **three-body abrasion**.[3]
  - Two-body abrasive polishing involves the abrasive particles attached to a medium, such as a rubber cup impregnated with abrasive particles and does not require a polishing paste.
  - Three-body abrasive polishing is the type most commonly used by dental hygienists, in which loose abrasive particles (like those in prophy polishing paste) form a slurry between the tooth surface and the polishing application device (rubber cup or brush).[3]

Effects of Cleaning and Polishing

Attention must be given to the positive and negative effects of polishing so evidence-based decisions can be made for the treatment of each patient.

I. Precautions

- As with all gingival manipulation, including oral self-care with a toothbrush,[4] bacteremia can be created during the use of power-driven stain removal instruments.
- A thorough medical history is essential before all treatment and must be reviewed and updated at each succeeding appointment.
- Patients at risk due to existing medical conditions may require antibiotic prophylaxis as specified by the patient's medical provider. (See Chapter 11.)

II. Environmental Factors

A. Aerosol Production

- Aerosols, droplets, and spatter are created during the use of some dental instruments, including a slow-speed handpiece with a rubber cup to hold polishing paste, the air-water syringe, and air polishing.[5]

- Polishing with a slow-speed handpiece is considered moderate risk for contamination while air polishing and use of an air-water syringe is high risk.[5]
- The biologic contaminants of aerosols can stay suspended for long periods and contaminate surfaces, particularly the clinician's torso and arm, and the patient's body.[5]
  - These aerosols may provide a means for possible disease transmission to dental personnel, as well as to other patients, but further research is needed.[5]
- Use of aerosol-generating procedures (AGPs) must be avoided if possible when a patient is known to have an infectious disease.[6]
  - AGPs may need to be avoided or limited for those with a chronic respiratory disease or who are immunocompromised.
- Centers for Disease Control and Prevention (CDC), Occupational Safety and Health Administration (OSHA), and local guidelines should be followed during all dental care, including AGPs. (See Chapter 6 and 7.)

B. Spatter

- Serious eye damage and infection have occurred because of spatter from polishing paste or from other dental instruments.[7]

III. Effect on Teeth

A. Removal of Tooth Structure

- The fluoride-rich outer surface of the enamel is necessary for protection against dental caries and care must be taken to preserve it.
- Excessive abrasion from coarse polishing paste results in a surface with more scratches prone to extrinsic stain reformation and retention of plaque biofilm.[8]
- The least abrasive prophylaxis paste or cleaning agents should be used to minimize removal of tooth surface.[8]

B. Areas of Demineralization

- Demineralization: Polishing demineralized white spots of enamel is contraindicated. More surface enamel is lost from abrasive polishing over demineralized white spots than over intact enamel.[8]
- Remineralization: Demineralized areas of enamel can remineralize with exposure to fluoride from saliva, water, dentifrices, and professional fluoride applications along with remineralization agents (e.g., CPP-ACP [casein phosphopeptide-amorphous calcium phosphate]).[9] Polishing procedures can interrupt enamel surface remineralization.

C. Areas of Thin Enamel, Cementum, or Dentin

- Areas of thin enamel are contraindicated for polishing and include:
  - Enamel hypoplasia.
  - Hypomineralization.
  - Amelogenesis imperfecta. (See Chapter 16.)
- Exposed dentin and cementum
  - Exposure of dentinal tubules: Cementum and dentin are softer and more porous than enamel, so greater amounts of their surfaces can be removed during polishing than from enamel.[10] Polishing of exposed cementum and dentin is contraindicated.
  - Abrasion of the dentin may result in dentin hypersensitivity.[11]

D. Care of Restorations and Implants

- Use of coarse abrasives may create deep, irregular scratches in restorative materials. **Figure 42-1** shows a scanning electron photomicrograph of the damaged surface of a composite restoration polished with a rubber cup and coarse prophylaxis paste.
- Select a cleaning agent or a polishing agent recommended by the manufacturer of the restorative materials.[12-14]

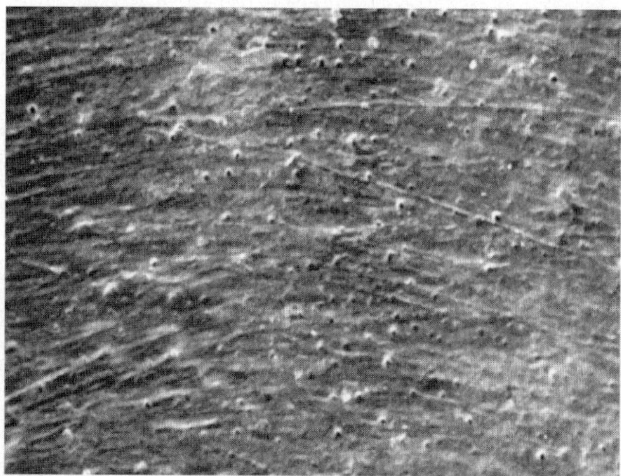

Figure 42-1 Scanning Electron Photomicrograph of a Composite Restoration Polished with Coarse Prophylaxis Paste

E. Heat Production

- Steady pressure with a rapidly revolving rubber cup or bristle brush and a minimum of wet abrasive agent can create sufficient heat to cause pain and discomfort for the patient.
- The pulp chamber in the teeth of children is large and may be more susceptible to heat.
- The rules for the use of cleaning or polishing agents include[8]:
  - Use light pressure (20 psi) at a slow, steady speed (2500–3000 rpm) of the rubber cup.
  - Use a moist cleaning or polishing agent; never use a dry powder due to the heat created.
  - Use a light patting motion and polish the tooth surface for 2–5 seconds.

IV. Effect on Gingiva

- Trauma to the gingival tissue can result, especially when the prophylaxis angle is operated at a high speed with heavy pressure and the rubber cup is applied for an extended period of time adjacent to gingival tissues.
- It may be best to delay stain removal after nonsurgical periodontal treatment (NSPT) to allow for healing of the sulcular tissue. If selective polishing is required, it can be done at the re-evaluation appointment following initial NSPT therapy.

Indications for Stain Removal

I. Removal of Extrinsic Stains

A. Patient Instruction

- Extrinsic stains often attach to the salivary pellicle and plaque biofilm layer of the tooth, so educating the patient on thorough dental biofilm removal is essential.[15]
- Patients who use tobacco should be counseled about cessation to reduce this cause of external stain. Tobacco cessation is described in Chapter 32.
- Components of the diet may also be a source for external stains, such as drinking tea, coffee, or red wine, so educate the patient about possible adjustments in intake to reduce stain.

B. Scaling and Root Debridement

- In addition to the use of cleaning or polishing agents during polishing procedures, stains can also be removed during scaling and root instrumentation.
  - Example: Black line stain has been compared to calculus because it may be elevated from the tooth surface and may need to be removed by instrumentation.[16] (See Chapter 17.)

II. To Prepare the Teeth for Caries-Preventive Procedures

A. Placement of Pit and Fissure Sealant

- Follow manufacturer's directions. Sealants vary in their requirements.
- Avoid commercial oral prophylaxis pastes containing **glycerin**, oils, flavoring substances, or other agents. Glycerin and oils can prevent an optimum acid-etch and interfere with the adherence of the sealant to the tooth surface, causing the sealant to fail.
  - **Air-powder polishing** is one method of choice for preparing tooth surfaces for sealants; however, care must be taken to manage aerosols.[17,18] (See Chapter 35.)
  - An alternative is the use of a plain, fine pumice mixed with water when precleaning is necessary.
- If pumice is used, the tooth surface(s) needs to be rinsed thoroughly to remove the particles.

III. To Contribute to Patient Motivation

- Smooth, polished tooth surfaces may be easier to achieve once the patient has a biofilm and debris-free mouth and may contribute to patient motivation.

Clinical Application of Stain Removal

The decision to polish teeth is based on the individual patient's needs.

I. Summary of Contraindications for Polishing

The following list suggests some of the specific instances in which polishing either can be performed with a cleaning agent or is contraindicated.

A. No Visible Stain Extrinsic Stain

- If no stain is present, polishing with an abrasive polishing agent is not indicated.

B. Patients with Respiratory Problems

- Care must be taken to minimize the aerosols from the air–water syringe when rinsing in general,[5] but specifically for conditions at higher risk for infectious disease such as asthma, emphysema, cystic fibrosis, lung cancer, or patients requiring oxygen.
- This caution also applies to the use of air-powder polishers and spatter from prophylaxis polishing pastes.[5]

C. Tooth Sensitivity

- Abrasive agents can expose dentinal tubules in areas of thin cementum or dentin.
- The polishing of dentin and cementum is contraindicated.

D. Restorations

- Restorations and titanium implants may be scratched by abrasive prophylaxis polishing pastes.
- Tooth-colored restorations need to be polished with a cleaning agent, polishing paste specifically formulated for use on esthetic restorations, or the paste recommended by the manufacturer of the restorative material.[12-14]

II. Suggestions for Clinic Procedure

A. Provide Initial Education

- Daily dental biofilm removal to assist in dental stain control.
- Educate the patient that drinking coffee, tea, or red wine; tobacco; and/or marijuana is responsible for most dental stains.
- Provide patients with information about the types of dentifrices that are safe for stain control and those contraindicated due to excessive abrasiveness or chemical harshness.
- Initiate tobacco cessation when stain is primarily from tobacco use. (See Chapter 32.)

B. Remove Stain by Scaling

- Whenever possible, stains can be removed during scaling and root debridement.

C. Stain Removal Techniques

- Moist cleaning agent or low-abrasive prophylaxis paste.
- Slow-speed handpiece.
- Use the lightest pressure necessary for stain removal.
- Minimal heat production.
- Soft rubber cup at 90° to tooth surface with intermittent light applications.

Cleaning and Polishing Agents

There are two distinct types of agents used for "polishing" teeth: one is a cleaning agent, and the other is a polishing agent.

I. Cleaning Agents

- Unlike polishing agents, cleaning agents are round, flat, nonabrasive particles and do not scratch surface material but produce a higher luster than polishing agents.
    - Feldspar, sodium–aluminum silicate cleaning agent is a powder and can be mixed with water to make a paste for cleaning.

II. Polishing Agents

- Traditionally, abrasive agents have been applied with polishing instruments to remove extrinsic dental stains and leave the enamel surface smooth and shiny.
- Polishing agents act by producing scratches in the surface of the tooth or restoration created by the friction between the abrasive particle and the softer tooth or restorative surface.
- The cleaning and polishing process progresses from coarse abrasion to fine abrasion until the scratches are smaller than the wavelength of visible light, which is 0.05 μm.[8]
- When scratches of this size are created, the surface appears smooth and shiny—the smaller the scratches, the shinier the surface.
- For esthetic restorative surfaces, follow manufacturer instructions to choose the correct polishing agent.[12–14]

III. Factors Affecting Abrasive Action with Polishing Agents

During polishing, sharp edges of abrasive particles are moved along the surface of a material, abrading it by producing microscopic scratches or grooves. The rate of abrasion, or speed with which structural material is removed from the surface being polished, is governed by hardness and shape of the abrasive particles, as well as by the manner in which they are applied.

A. Characteristics of Abrasive Particles

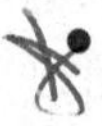

- Shape: Irregularly shaped particles with sharp edges produce deeper grooves and thus abrade faster than do rounded particles with dull edges.

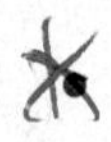

- Hardness: Particles must be harder than the surface to be abraded; harder particles abrade faster.
    - Many of the abrasives used in prophylaxis polishing pastes are 10 times harder than the tooth structure to which they are applied.[8]
    - **Table 42-1** provides a comparison of the Mohs hardness value of dental tissues compared to agents commonly used in prophylaxis polishing pastes and substances used in cleaning agents.

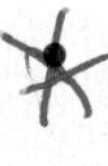

- Body strength: Particles that fracture into smaller sharp-edged particles during use are more abrasive than those that wear down during use and become dull.

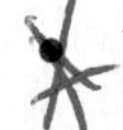

- Particle size (grit)
    - The larger the particles, the more abrasive they are and the less polishing ability they have.
    - Smaller (finer) abrasive particles achieve a glossier finish.
    - Abrasive and polishing agents are graded from coarse to fine based on the size of the holes in a standard sieve through which the particles will pass.[15]

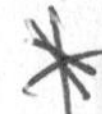

Table 42-1 Mohs Hardness Value of Dental Tissues Compared to Commonly Used Polishing Abrasive Particles

	MOHS Hardness Value
Dental Tissues	
Enamel	5
Dentin	3.0–4.0
Cementum	2.5–3.0
Abrasive Agents in Polishing Pastes	
Zirconium silicate	7.5–8.0
Pumice	6.0–7.0
Silicone carbine	9.5
Boron	9.3
Aluminum oxide	9
Garnet	8.0–9.0
Emery	7.0–9.0
Zirconium oxide	7
Perlite	5.5
Calcium carbonate	3
Aluminum silicates	2
Sodium	0.5
Potassium	0.4

The Mohs hardness value of enamel, cementum, and dentin compared to the Mohs hardness value of abrasive materials commonly used in prophylaxis polishing pastes. The Mohs hardness value is indicative of a material's resistance to scratching. Diamonds have a maximum Mohs value of 10; talc has a minimum of Mohs hardness of 1.

B. Principles for Application of Abrasives

- Quantity applied: The more particles applied per unit of time, the faster the rate of abrasion.
    - Particles are suspended in water or other liquid to reduce heat produced by friction.
    - Frictional heat produced is proportional to the rate of abrasion; therefore, the use of *dry agents* is *contraindicated* for polishing natural teeth because of the potential danger of thermal injury to the dental pulp.
- Speed of application: The greater the speed of application, the faster the rate of abrasion.
    - With increased speed of application, pressure must be reduced.
    - Rapid abrasion also increases frictional heat.
- Pressure of application: The heavier the pressure applied, the faster the rate of abrasion.
    - Heavy pressure *is* contraindicated because it increases frictional heat.

IV. Abrasive Agents

The abrasives listed here are examples of commonly used agents. Some are available in several grades, and the specific use varies with the grade.

- For example, while a superfine grade might be used for polishing enamel surfaces and metallic restorations, a coarser grade would be used only for laboratory purposes.
- Abrasives for use daily in a dentifrice are a finer grade than those used for professional polishing.

A. Silex (Silicon Dioxide)

- XXX Silex: fairly abrasive.
- Superfine Silex: can be used for heavy stain removal from enamel.

B. Pumice

- Powdered pumice is of volcanic origin and consists chiefly of complex silicates of aluminum, potassium, and sodium.
- Pumice is the primary ingredient in commercially prepared prophylaxis pastes. The specifications for particle size are as follows:
  - Pumice flour or superfine pumice: least abrasive and can be used on enamel, dental amalgams, and acrylic resins.[8]
  - Fine pumice: mildly abrasive.
  - Coarse pumice: not for use on natural teeth.

C. Calcium Carbonate (Whiting, Calcite, Chalk)

- Less abrasive than pumice.[8]
- Various grades are used for different polishing techniques.

D. Tin Oxide (Putty Powder, Stannic Oxide)

- Polishing agent for teeth and metallic restorations.

E. Emery (Corundum)

Not used directly on the enamel.

- Aluminum oxide (alumina): the pure form of emery. Used for composite restorations and margins of porcelain restorations.
- Levigated alumina: consists of extremely fine particles of aluminum oxide, which may be used for polishing metals but are destructive to tooth surfaces.

F. Rouge (Jeweler's Rouge)

- Iron oxide is a fine red powder sometimes impregnated on paper discs.
- It is useful for polishing gold and precious metal alloys in the laboratory.

G. Diamond Particles

- Constituent of diamond polishing paste for porcelain surfaces.

V. Cleaning Ingredients

- Particles for cleaning agents differ from abrasive agents in shape and hardness.
- Particles used for cleaning agents include feldspar, alkali, and aluminum silicate.

A. Clinical Applications

Numerous commercial preparations for dental prophylactic cleaning and polishing preparations are available. Clinicians need more than one type available to meet the requirements of individual restorative materials.

B. Packaging

- Commercial preparations are in the form of pastes or powders.
- Some are available in measured amounts contained in individual plastic containers for one-time use to prevent cross contamination.
- Selection of a preparation is based on qualities of abrasiveness, consistency, and/or flavor for patient preference.

C. Enhanced Prophylaxis Polishing Pastes

Additives are included in prophylaxis polishing pastes to provide a specific function, such as enhancing the mineral surface of enamel, diminishing dentin hypersensitivity, or tooth whitening.

- Fluoride prophylaxis pastes
  - Application of fluoride by use of fluoride-containing prophylaxis polishing pastes cannot be considered a substitute for a professionally applied topical fluoride treatment.
  - Enamel surface: The greatest benefit of fluoride as a prophylaxis polishing paste additive occurs when the fluoride ions in the prophylaxis paste are released into the saliva.
    - The fluoride ions that become mixed in the saliva may become incorporated into the hydroxyapatite structure of the tooth, thus aiding in the remineralization of the tooth and improving enamel hardness.[19]
  - Clinical application: Use only an amount sufficient to accomplish stain removal to prevent excessive fluoride intake in a child. The paste may contain 4000–20,000 ppm fluoride ion.[20]
- Amorphous calcium phosphate and other forms of calcium and phosphate
  - Amorphous calcium phosphate and other formulations of calcium and phosphate, as additives to prophylaxis polishing pastes, have been shown to hydrolyze the tooth mineral to form apatite.[21]
  - When prophylaxis polishing pastes containing calcium and phosphate become mixed with saliva, the mineral ions may become incorporated into the hydroxyapatite structure

of the tooth, thus aiding in remineralization the enamel.[21-23]

- Fluoride, calcium, and phosphate
  - Fluoride, calcium, and phosphate prophylaxis pastes have the potential to have all three minerals incorporated into the hydroxyapatite structure of the tooth, thus aiding in remineralization to improve enamel hardness.
- Dentin hypersensitivity
  - The purpose of prophylaxis polishing pastes containing arginine, calcium, and bicarbonate/carbonate is to minimize dentin hypersensitivity.[22,23] Mixing these ingredients produces arginine bicarbonate and calcium carbonate. When applied with a rubber cup, these adjunctive ingredients can aid in temporarily occluding the dentinal tubules.

Procedures for Stain Removal (Coronal Polishing)

I. Patient Preparation for Stain Removal

A. Instruction and Clinical Procedures

- Review medical history to determine premedication requirements.
- Review intraoral charting and radiographs to locate all restorations.
- Provide education and hands-on practice with biofilm control techniques.
- Complete scaling, root debridement, and overhang removal.
- After scaling and other periodontal treatment, an evaluation is made to determine the need for **coronal polishing** for stain removal, polishing restorations, and dental prostheses.
- Inform the patient that polishing is a cosmetic procedure, not a therapeutic one.
- Explain the difference between cleaning and polishing agents.
- Check all restorations to ensure that the correct polishing agent has been selected.

B. Explain the Procedure

- Describe the noise, vibration, and grit of the polishing paste.
- Explain the frequent use of rinsing and evacuation with the saliva ejector.

C. Provide Protection for Patient

- Safety glasses worn for scaling should be kept in place to prevent eye injury or infection from the prophylaxis paste.
- Fluid-resistant bib over patient to keep moisture from skin and clothing.

D. Patient Position

- The patient is positioned for maximum visibility.

E. Patient Breathing

- Encourage the patient to breathe only through the nose.
- Less fogging of mouth mirror.
- Enhanced patient comfort.

II. Environmental Preparation

Environmental factors are described in Chapter 7.

A. Procedures to Lessen Aerosols Created

- Flush water through the tubing for 2 minutes at the beginning of each work period and for 30 seconds after each appointment.
- Request the patient rinse with an antimicrobial mouthrinse to reduce the numbers of oral microorganisms before starting instrumentation.[24]
- Use high-velocity evacuation to minimize droplet spatter and aerosols.[24]

B. Protective Barriers

- Protective eyewear and bib are necessary for the patient.
- The clinician should wear the appropriate personal protective equipment (PPE) per current OSHA and CDC guidelines.[24] (See Chapter 6.)

The Power-Driven Instruments

I. Handpiece

- A handpiece is used to hold rotary instruments.
- The three basic designs are straight, contra-angle, and right-angle.
- Instruments have been classified according to their rotational speeds, designated by revolutions per minute (rpm) as high speed and low (or slow) speed.
- Handpiece must be maintained and sterilized according to manufacturer's directions.

Table 42-2 Comparison of Disposable Prophylaxis Angles and Stainless-Steel Prophylaxis Angles

	Disposable Prophylaxis Angle	Disposable Angle with Abrasive-Impregnated Rubber Cup	Stainless Steel Prophylaxis Angle
Maintenance and care	One-time use, discard	One-time use, discard	Requires maintenance, sterilization
Attachments	Supplied with rubber cup from the manufacturer	Supplied with rubber cup from the manufacturer that is impregnated with one type of abrasive	Accepts variety of attachments: cups, brushes, and cone-shaped rubber points
Screw-in or snap-on rubber cups	Usually screw-in type cup		Will accept screw-in or snap-on cups and brushes
Advantages	Requires no maintenance or sterilization	Requires no additional prophylaxis paste	Can be used hundreds of times if maintained properly
Disadvantages	Not packaged with other attachments Creates refuse that is not biodegradable	Must have water and/or saliva as lubricant Creates refuse that is not biodegradable	Requires time to clean and maintain

A. Slow or Low Speed

- Low-speed handpieces are used for cleaning or polishing the teeth with a prophylaxis angle and rubber cup.
- *Speed*: Typical range is up to 5000 rpm for low-speed handpieces manufactured for dental hygienists. Other low-speed handpieces may have a higher range of rpms; air-driven.

II. Types of Prophylaxis Angles

- Types of prophylaxis angles are described in **Table 42-2**.
- Contra- or right-angle attachments to the handpiece for which polishing devices (rubber cup, bristle brush) are available. Contra-angle prophylaxis angles may have a longer shank and a wider angle between the rubber cup and shank to allow for greater reach when polishing posterior teeth and surfaces.
- Stainless steel with hard chrome, carbon, steel, or brass bearings.
- **Figure 42-2** shows examples of one-time use disposable contra-angle and right-angle prophylaxis angles and a stainless-steel prophylaxis angle.
- Stainless steel prophylaxis angles are sealed to prevent contamination, but there tends to be some leakage, so they need to be sterilized after each use following the manufacturer's instructions for maintenance.[25]
- Unless disposable, only instruments that can be sterilized should be used.

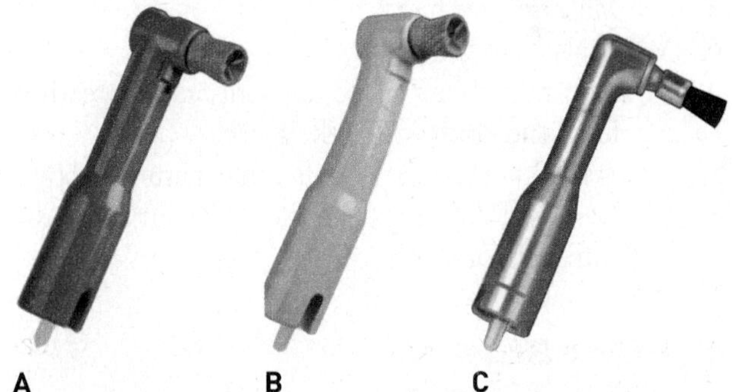

Figure 42-2 Prophylaxis Angles. **A:** Disposable right-angled prophylaxis angle with rubber cup attached. **B:** Disposable contra-angled prophylaxis angle with an attached rubber cup impregnated with a polishing agent (abrasive particles). **C:** Sterilizable stainless steel prophylaxis angle holding a cleaning or polishing brush on a mandrel.

III. Prophylaxis Angle Attachments

A. Rubber Polishing Cups

- Types: **Figure 42-3** shows several types of rubber polishing cups from which to choose. The internal designs and sizes have the same purpose, which is to aid in holding the prophylaxis polishing paste in the rubber cup while polishing. The ideal rubber cup design retains the prophylaxis polishing paste in the cup and releases the paste at a steady rate.
  - Slip-on (snap-on): with ribbed cup to aid in holding polishing agent.

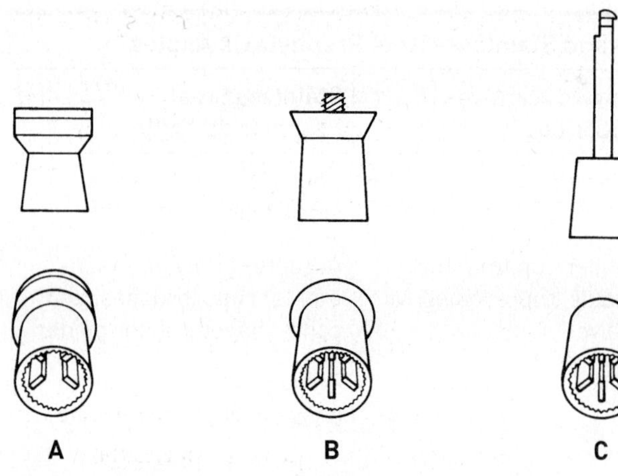

Figure 42-3 Rubber Cup Attachments. **A:** Slip-on or snap-on for button-ended prophylaxis angle. **B:** Threaded for direct insertion in right-angle. **C:** Mandrel stem for latch-type prophylaxis angle.

- Threaded (screw type): with plain ribbed cup or flange (webbed) type.
- Mandrel mounted.
- Materials
  - Natural rubber: more resilient; adapts readily to fit the contours of the teeth.
  - Synthetic (non-latex): stiffer than natural rubber.
- Use: removal of stains from the tooth surfaces and polishing restorations.

B. Bristle Brushes

- Types
  - For prophylaxis angle: slip-on or screw type.
  - For handpiece: mandrel mounted.
- Materials: synthetic.
- Use:
  - Stain removal from deep pits and fissures and enamel surfaces away from the gingival margin.
  - A brush is contraindicated for use on exposed cementum or dentin.

C. Rubber Polishing Points

- **Figure 42-4** shows an example of a rubber point that screws into a prophylaxis angle.
- Material
  - Natural rubber: flexible so that tip adapts to a variety of surfaces.
- Use
  - Stain removal and biofilm from proximal surfaces, embrasures, and around orthodontic bands and brackets.

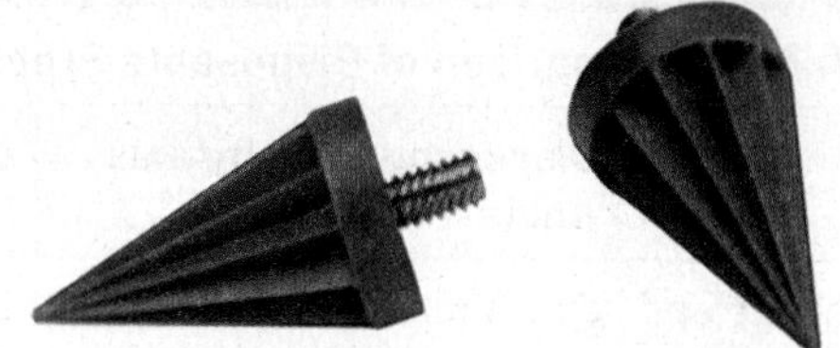

Figure 42-4 Flexible Rubber Point Has Screw Connection for a Prophylaxis Angle. Made with ribs or grooves to carry cleaning or polishing agent to difficult-to-reach areas.

IV. Uses for Attachments

A. Handpiece with Straight Mandrel

- Dixon bristle brush (type C, soft) for polishing removable dentures.
- Rubber cup on mandrel for polishing facial surfaces of anterior teeth.

Use of the Prophylaxis Angle

I. Effects on Tissues: Clinical Considerations

- Can cause discomfort for the patient if care and consideration for the oral tissues are not exercised to prevent unnecessary trauma.
- Tactile sensitivity of the clinician while using a thick, bulky handpiece is diminished and unnecessary pressure may be applied inadvertently.
- The greater the speed of application of a polishing agent, the faster the rate of abrasion. Therefore, the handpiece is applied at a low rpm.
- Trauma to the gingival tissue can result from too high a speed, extended application of the rubber cup, or use of an abrasive polishing agent.

II. Prophylaxis Angle Procedure

- Apply the polishing agent only where it is needed. See section *Contraindications*.

A. Instrument Grasp

- Modified pen grasp. (See Chapter 37.)

B. Finger Rest

- Establish a fulcrum firmly on tooth structure or use an exterior rest.
- Use a wide rest area when practical to aid in the balance of the large instrument. For example,

place pad of rest finger across the occlusal surfaces of premolars while polishing the molars.
- Avoid use of mobile teeth as finger rests.

C. Speed of Handpiece

- Use low speed to minimize frictional heat.
- Adjust rpm as necessary.

D. Use of Rheostat

- Apply steady pressure with foot to produce an even, low speed.

E. Rubber Cup: Stroke and Procedure

- Observe where stain removal is needed to prevent unnecessary rubber cup application.
- Fill rubber cup with polishing agent and distribute agent over tooth surfaces to be polished before activating the power.
- Establish finger rest and bring rubber cup almost in contact with tooth surface before activating power source.
- Using slowest rpm, apply revolving cup at a 90° angle lightly to tooth surfaces for 2 to 5 seconds. Use a light pressure so that the edges of the rubber cup flare slightly. The rubber cup needs to flare slightly underneath the gingival margin and onto the proximal surfaces.
- Move cup to adjacent area on tooth surface; use a patting or brushing motion.
- Replenish supply of polishing agent frequently.
- Turn handpiece to adapt rubber cup to fit each surface of the tooth, including proximal surfaces and gingival surfaces of fixed partial dentures.
- Start with the distal surface of the most posterior tooth of a quadrant and move forward toward the anterior; polish only the teeth that require stain removal. For each tooth, work from the gingival third toward the incisal third of the tooth.
- When two polishing agents of different abrasiveness are to be applied, use a separate rubber cup for each.
- Rubber cups, polishing points, and polishing brushes cannot be sterilized and are used only for one patient and then discarded.

F. Rubber Polishing Points

- Rubber polishing points can be used around orthodontic bands and brackets, on fixed bridges, and in wide interproximal spaces or embrasures.
- Rubber points are loaded with the cleaning or polishing agent in the grooves around the sides. The rubber points will need to be replenished frequently with paste after use on every one to two teeth.

G. Bristle Brush

- Bristle brushes are used selectively and limited to occlusal surfaces.
- Lacerations of the gingiva and grooves and scratches in the tooth surface, particularly the roots and restorations, can result when the brush is not used with caution.
- Soak stiff brush in hot water to soften bristles.
- Distribute mild abrasive polishing agent over occlusal surfaces of teeth to be polished.
- Place fingers of nondominant hand in a position to retract and protect cheek and tongue from the revolving brush.
- Establish a firm finger rest and bring brush almost in contact with the tooth before activating power source.
- Use slowest rpm as the revolving brush is applied lightly to the occlusal surfaces only. Avoid contact of the bristles with the soft tissues.
- Use a short stroke in a brushing motion; follow the inclined planes of the cusps.
- Move from tooth to tooth to prevent generation of excessive frictional heat. Avoid overuse of the brush. Replenish supply of polishing agent frequently.

H. Irrigation

- Irrigate teeth and interdental areas thoroughly several times with water from the syringe to remove abrasive particles. Care must be taken to minimize creation of aerosols.
- The rotary movement of the rubber cup or bristle brush can force the abrasive into the gingival sulci and irritate soft tissues.

Air-Powder Polishing

- Principles of selective stain removal are applied to the use of the air-powder polishing system (**Figure 42-5**). After biofilm control instruction, instrumentation, and periodontal debridement are completed, follow with an evaluation of need for stain removal.

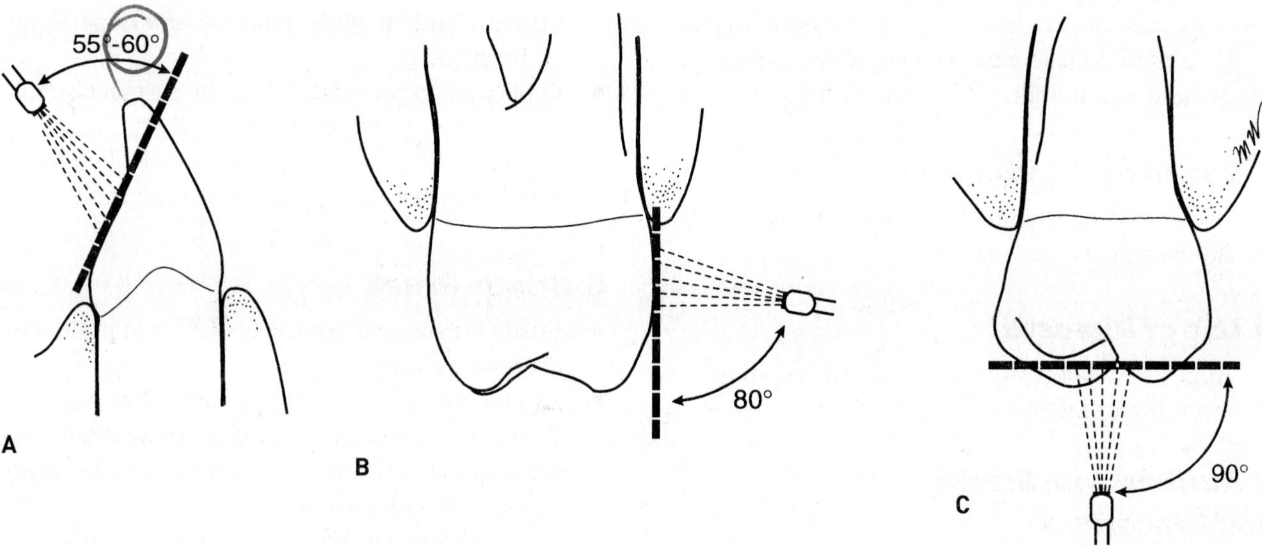

Figure 42-5 Air-Powder Polishing. Direct the aerosolized spray for **(A)** the anterior teeth at a 60° angle. **B:** The posterior teeth facial and lingual or palatal at an 80° angle. **C:** The occlusal surfaces at a 90° angle to the occlusal plane.

I. Principles of Application

- Air-powder systems manufactured by several companies are efficient and effective methods for mechanical removal of stain and biofilm.[26]
- Air-powder polishing systems use air, water, and specially formulated powders to deliver a controlled spray that propels the particles to the tooth surface.
  - Only powders approved by each air-powder polishing manufacturer are used in each brand of air-powder polishing unit.[26] The use of an unapproved powder in an air-powder polishing unit could void the warranty on the unit.
- The handpiece nozzle is moved in a constant circular motion, with the nozzle tip 4–5 mm away from the enamel surface.
- The spray is angled away from the gingival margin.
- The periphery of the spray may be near the gingival margin, but the center is directed at an angle less than 90° away from the margin.
- Complete directions for care of equipment and preparation for use of the device are provided by the individual manufacturer.

II. Specially Formulated Powders for Use in Air-Powder Polishing

Several manufacturers make and sell air-powder polishing powders.

- The abrasiveness of one brand of powder may differ from another brand, even though it is the same type of powder.[27]

A. Sodium Bicarbonate

- Sodium bicarbonate was the original powder used in air-powder polishing.[26]
- It is specially formulated with small amounts of calcium phosphate and silica to keep it free flowing.
- The Mohs hardness number for sodium bicarbonate is 3 and the particles average 74 μm in size.[27]
- The *only* type of sodium bicarbonate that can be used in air-powder polishing units is the type specially formulated for air-powder polishing.
- Sodium bicarbonate air-powder is available with flavorings.

B. Aluminum Trihydroxide

- Aluminum trihydroxide was the first air-powder developed as an alternative to sodium bicarbonate.
- Aluminum trihydroxide has a Mohs hardness value of 4 and the particles range in size from 80 to 325 μm.[27]

C. Glycine

- Glycine is an amino acid. For use in powders, glycine crystals are grown using a solvent of water and sodium salt.

- Glycine particles for use in air polishing have a Mohs hardness number of >4 and are 20–25 µm in size.[28]
- Glycine has been shown to be safe and effective for subgingival biofilm removal.[26,29]

D. Erythritol

- Erythritol is a nontoxic, chemically neutral, highly water-soluble polyol that is used as an artificial sweetener and food additive.
- Erythritol particles for use in air polishing have a Mohs hardness number of <2 and are 14 µm in size.[28]
- Erythritol has been shown to be safe and effective for subgingival biofilm removal.[28]

E. Calcium Carbonate

- Calcium carbonate is a naturally occurring substance that can be found in rocks.
- It is a main ingredient in antacids and is also used as filler for pharmaceutical drugs.
- Calcium carbonate has a Mohs number of 3 and particles are 45 µm in size.[26]

F. Calcium Sodium Phosphosilicate (Novamin)

- Calcium sodium phosphosilicate (Novamin) is a bioactive glass and has a Mohs hardness number of 6, making it the hardest air-polishing particle used in air-powder polishing powders.[27] The particles vary from 25 to 120 µm in size. This powder should not be used on any tooth structure or restorative material.[27]

III. Uses and Advantages of Air-Powder Polishing

- Requires less time, is ergonomically favorable to the clinician, and generates no heat.[26,29]
- Some air-polishing powders are less abrasive than traditional prophylaxis pastes, which makes the air-powder polisher ideal for stain and biofilm removal. However, some are much more abrasive and should only be used on surfaces that they will not damage.[27]
- Removal of heavy, tenacious tobacco stain and chlorhexidine-induced staining.
- Stain and biofilm removal from orthodontically banded and bracketed teeth and dental implants.[26,30]
- Before sealant placement or other bonding procedures.[26]
- Root detoxification for periodontally diseased roots by the periodontist during open periodontal surgery.[31]

IV. Technique

- A preprocedural antimicrobial rinse like 0.12% chlorhexidine is recommended to reduce the bacterial load and dispersion in this AGP.[24,26]
- Use of a high-volume evacuation (HVE) can reduce bacterial contamination up to 94.8%.[32]
- Increasing the water:powder ratio and adjusting the patient's position may also reduce the aerosols created.[32]

A. For Anterior Teeth

- Place the handpiece nozzle at a 60° angle to the facial and lingual surfaces of anterior teeth (**Figure 42-5A**).[26]

B. For Posterior Teeth

- Place the handpiece nozzle at an 80° angle to the facial and lingual surfaces (**Figure 42-5B**).[26]

C. For Occlusal Surfaces

- Place the handpiece nozzle at a 90° angle to the occlusal plane (**Figure 42-5C**).[26]

D. Incorrect Angulation

- Incorrect angulation of the handpiece can result in excessive aerosol production.
- The handpiece nozzle is never directed into the gingival sulcus or into a periodontal pocket with little bony support remaining, as this could result in facial emphysema (also known as a subcutaneous emphysema).[33]
- Facial emphysemas exhibit symptoms such as sudden soft tissue swelling with crepitus. If detected early, patients with facial emphysemas require observation and improve in 2–3 days.[33] There can be rare life-threatening complications so referral to a medical provider may be necessary.
- The closer the nozzle is held to the enamel, the more spray will deflect back into the direction of the clinician.
- When a clinician directs the handpiece at a 90° angle toward a facial, buccal, and some lingual

surfaces, the result is an immediate reflux of the aerosolized spray back onto the clinician.

- Changing the angle to the proper angulations of 60° and 80° will result in a change in the angle of the reflection, thus reducing the amount of reflux of aerosolized spray.

V. Recommendations and Precautions

A. Aerosol Production

- Air polishing is an AGP and therefore requires additional precautions to manage the aerosols and for PPE used by the clinician.[24,34] Suggestions for minimizing contamination and the effects of the aerosols include the following:
  - Patient uses a preprocedural antibacterial mouthrinse, particularly chlorhexidine.[35]
  - High-volume evacuation must be used to minimize aerosol dissemination.[24,36]
- See Chapter 6 for more information.

B. Protective Patient and Clinician Procedures

- Use protective eyewear, appropriate face mask, face shield, protective gown, and hair cover.
- Lubricate patient's lips to prevent the drying effect of the sodium bicarbonate using a nonpetroleum lip lubricant.
- Do not direct the spray toward the gingiva or other soft tissues, which can create patient discomfort and undue tissue trauma.
- Avoid directing the spray into periodontal pockets with bone loss or into extraction sites as a facial emphysema can be induced.

VI. Risk Patients: Air-Powder Polishing Contraindicated

The information from the patient's medical history is used and appropriate applications made. Antibiotic premedication is indicated for all the same patients who are at risk for any dental hygiene procedure. (See Chapter 11.)

A. Contraindications

- Physician-directed sodium-restricted diet (only for sodium bicarbonate powder).
- Respiratory disease or other condition that limits swallowing or breathing, such as chronic obstructive pulmonary disease.
- Patients with end-stage renal disease, Addison's disease, or Cushing's disease.
- Communicable infection that can contaminate the aerosols produced.
- Immunocompromised patients.
- Patients taking potassium, antidiuretics, or steroid therapy.
- Patients who have open oral wounds, such as tooth sockets, from oral surgery procedures.

B. Other Contraindications

- Root surfaces: Avoid routine polishing of cementum and dentin.
  - There is some evidence they can be removed readily during air-powder polishing if a sodium bicarbonate powder is used.[37]
  - However, research indicates that glycine[37] and erythritol[28,29] powders are safe for use subgingivally.
- Soft, spongy gingiva: The air-powder can irritate the free gingival tissue, especially if not used with the recommended technique.
  - Instruct the patient in daily biofilm removal.
  - Following scaling and periodontal debridement, postpone the stain removal until soft tissue has healed.
- Restorative materials: The use of air-powder polishing on composite resins, cements, and other nonmetallic materials can cause removal or pitting if an incorrect air polishing powder is used.[17,27] Manufacturer's recommendations for the use of a particular air polishing powder should be followed.[27]
  - **Table 42-3** provides a guide as to which restorative materials can be safely treated with the air-powder polishing powders containing sodium bicarbonate, aluminum trihydroxide, glycine, and erthyritol.[27,38]
  - Significant damage to margins of dental castings has been shown with incorrect usage of powder.

Polishing Proximal Surfaces

- Take care in the use of floss, tape, and finishing strips.
- Understanding the anatomy of the interdental papillae and relationship to the contact areas and proximal surfaces of the teeth is prerequisite to the prevention of tissue damage.

Table 42-3 Recommendations for Use of Air Polishing on Restorative Materials

	Polishing Powder Containing			
Restorative Material	**Sodium Bicarbonate**	**Aluminum Trihydroxide**	**Glycine**	**Erythritol**
Amalgam	Yes	No	Yes	Yes
Gold	Yes[a]	No	Yes	Yes
Porcelain	Yes[a]	No	Yes	Yes
Hybrid composite	No	No	Yes	Yes
Microfilled composite	No	No	Yes	Yes
Glass ionomer	No	No	Yes	Yes
Compomer	No	No	Yes	Yes
Luting agents	No	No	Yes	Yes

[a]Only if margin is avoided.

- Polish accessible proximal surfaces as much as possible during the use of the rubber cup in the prophylaxis angle.
- This can be followed by the use of dental tape with a polishing agent when indicated.

I. Dental Tape and Floss

A. Uses During Cleaning and Polishing

- Techniques for tape and floss application are described in Chapter 27.
- The same principles apply whether the patient or the clinician is using the floss.
- Finger rests are used to prevent snapping through contact areas.
- Stain removal with dental tape: Polishing agent is applied to the tooth, and the tape is moved gently back and forth and up and down curved over the area where stain was observed.
- Cleaning gingival surface of a fixed partial denture: A floss threader is used to position the floss or tape over the gingival surface. The agent is applied under the pontic, and the floss or tape is moved back and forth with contact on the bridge surface. Floss threaders are described and illustrated in Chapter 30.
- Flossing: Particles of abrasive agent can be removed by rinsing and by using a clean piece of floss applied in the usual manner.
- Rinsing and irrigation: Irrigate with air-water syringe to remove abrasive agent being careful to minimize aerosols.

The Porte Polisher

- Design
    - The porte polisher is a manual instrument designed especially for extrinsic stain removal or application of treatment agents such as for hypersensitive areas.
    - It is constructed to hold a wood point at a contra-angle. The wood points may be cone or wedge-shaped and made of various kinds of wood, preferably orangewood.[39] **Figure 42-6** illustrates a typical porte polisher.

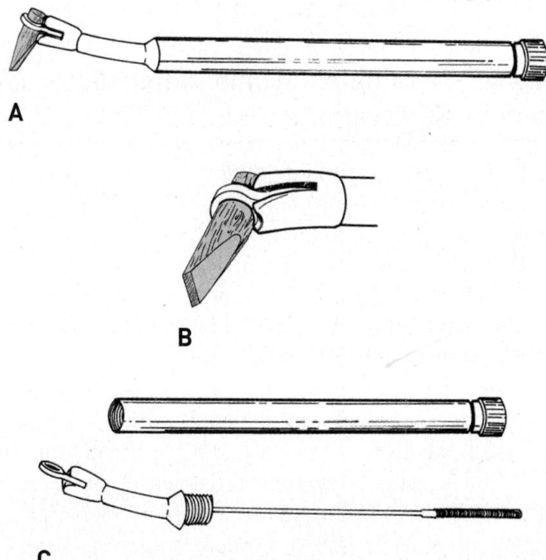

Figure 42-6 Porte Polisher. **A:** Assembled instrument shows position of wood point ready for instrumentation. **B:** Working end shows wedge-shaped wood point inserted. **C:** Disassembled, ready for autoclave.

- Grasp: The instrument is held in a modified pen grasp or palm grasp.
- Application: The wood point is applied to the tooth surface using firm; carefully directed; massaging, circular, or linear strokes to accommodate the anatomy of each tooth.
    - A firm finger rest and a moderate amount of pressure of the wood point provide protection for the gingival margin and efficiency in technique.
- Advantages
    - The porte polisher is useful for instrumentation of difficult-to-access surfaces of the teeth, especially malpositioned teeth.
    - No heat generation, no noise compared with powered handpieces, and minimal production of aerosols.
    - The porte polisher is portable and therefore is useful in any location, for example, for a bedbound patient.
- Disadvantages
    - It is time consuming and requires force.

Documentation

Documentation for a patient receiving tooth stain removal as part of the dental hygiene care plan for a maintenance appointment would include a minimum of the following:

- Review patient medical history with questions to determine health problems, recent medical examinations and treatments, and changes in medications.
- Current clinical examination findings: intraoral, extraoral, periodontal, and dental.
- With dental charting: identification of dental materials used in restorations that can influence choice of polishing agents. Identification would require use of radiographs and the intraoral dental charting.
- Dental hygiene examination for state of patient's personal daily self-care, calculus and biofilm deposits, sources for dental stains, products used for oral care, and dietary factors influencing the dentition and all oral tissues: questions answered about best choices for various products.
- A sample progress note may be reviewed in **Box 42-1**.

Factors to Teach the Patient

- How stains form.
- The importance of biofilm and calculus removal at maintenance appointments.
- The meaning of selective polishing and contraindications for polishing.
- Stains and biofilm removed by polishing can return promptly if biofilm is not removed faithfully on a schedule of two or three times each day.
- The options for stain removal that are appropriate for the patient.

Box 42-1 Example Documentation: Selection of Polishing Agent for a Patient with Esthetic Restorations

- **S**—A 36-year-old male patient presents for regular maintenance appointment. He comments on how pleased he is that his new implant crown and other esthetic restorations are not distinguishable from the color of his natural teeth. Updated medical history, medications, no changes.
- **O**—Blood pressure (115/75); extra-intraoral examinations: no findings; comprehensive periodontal examination: localized 3–4 mm, with bleeding on probing in 4 mm pockets in molar areas; supragingival calculus mand ant.; minimal biofilm with isolated areas of yellowish staining.
- **A**—Confirmed the material used for the various restorations and found that the patient has porcelain crowns on teeth numbers #2, 14, and anterior microhybrid composite restorations in teeth numbers #6, 7, 8, 10, and 11. Patient has an implant and porcelain crown on #9. Note: Microhybrid composite restorations and implant crown match the patient's natural teeth to the extent that it is difficult to identify the restorations.
- **P**—Gave patient new toothbrush with tongue cleaner on back and demonstrated the tongue cleaner. Reviewed oral-self care for areas areas of residual biofilm. Completed debridement. Avoided use of air polishing with sodium bicarbonate and prophy paste. Selected a cleaning agent to remove biofilm and isolated areas of yellowish staining.

Next regular appointment 4 months.
Signed: ______________________, RDH
Date: ________________

References

1. American Dental Hygienists' Association. American Dental Hygienists' Association Position Paper on the Oral Prophylaxis. Published 1998. https://www.adha.org/resources-docs/7115_Prophylaxis_Postion_Paper.pdf. Accessed August 29, 2021.
2. Academy of Periodontology. Glossary of periodontal terms. https://members.perio.org/libraries/glossary. Accessed August 29, 2021.
3. Lanza A, Ruggiero A, Sbordone L. Tribology and dentistry: a commentary. *Lubricants*. 2019;7(6):52.
4. Tomás I, Diz P, Tobías A, Scully C, Donos N. Periodontal health status and bacteraemia from daily oral activities: systematic review/meta-analysis. *J Clin Periodontol*. 2012;39(3):213-228.
5. Innes N, Johnson IG, Al-Yaseen W, et al. A systematic review of droplet and aerosol generation in dentistry. *J Dent*. 2021;105:103556.
6. Centers for Disease Control and Prevention. Healthcare workers. Published February 11, 2020. https://www.cdc.gov/coronavirus/2019-ncov/hcp/infection-control-recommendations.html. Accessed September 11, 2021.
7. Ekmekcioglu H, Unur M. Eye-related trauma and infection in dentistry. *J Istanb Univ Fac Dent*. 2017;51(3):55-63.
8. Sawai MA, Bhardwaj A, Jafri Z, Sultan N, Daing A. Tooth polishing: the current status. *J Indian Soc Periodontol*. 2015;19(4):375-380.
9. Farooq I, Bugshan A. The role of salivary contents and modern technologies in the remineralization of dental enamel: a narrative review. *F1000Res*. 2020;9:171.
10. Pence SD, Chambers DA, van IG, Wolf RC, Pfeiffer DC. Repetitive coronal polishing yields minimal enamel loss. *J Dent Hyg*. 2011;85(4):10.
11. Liu X-X, Tenenbaum HC, Wilder RS, Quock R, Hewlett ER, Ren Y-F. Pathogenesis, diagnosis and management of dentin hypersensitivity: an evidence-based overview for dental practitioners. *BMC Oral Health*. 2020;20:220.
12. Can Say E, Yurdagüven H, Malkondu Ö, Ünlü N, Soyman M, Kazazoğlu E. The effect of prophylactic polishing pastes on surface roughness of indirect restorative materials. *Sci World J*. 2014;2014:e962764.
13. Yap AUJ, Wu SS, Chelvan S, Tan ESF. Effect of hygiene maintenance procedures on surface roughness of composite restoratives. *Oper Dent*. 2005;30(1):99-104.
14. Neme A, Frazier K, Roeder L, Debner T. Effect of prophylactic polishing protocols on the surface roughness of esthetic restorative materials. *Oper Dent*. 27(1):50-58.
15. Prathap S, Rajesh H, Boloor VA, Rao AS. Extrinsic stains and management: a new insight. *J Acad Indus Res*. 2013;1(8):435-442.
16. Żyła T, Kawala B, Antoszewska-Smith J, Kawala M. Black stain and dental caries: a review of the literature. *BioMed Res Int*. 2015;2015:e469392.
17. Cvikl B, Moritz A, Bekes K. Pit and fissure sealants—a comprehensive review. *Dent J*. 2018;6(2):18.
18. Botti R, Bossù M, Zallocco N, Vestri A, Polimeni A. Effectiveness of plaque indicators and air polishing for the sealing of pits and fissures. *Eur J Paediatr Dent*. 2010;11(1):15-18.
19. Mellberg JR, Nicholson CR, Ripa LW, Barenie J. Fluoride deposition in human enamel in vivo from professionally applied fluoride prophylaxis paste. *J Dent Res*. 1976;55(6):976-979.
20. Centers for Disease Control and Prevention (CDC). Recommendations for using fluoride to prevent and control dental caries in the United States. *MMWR Recomm Rep*. 2001;50(RR-14):1-42.
21. Zhao J, Liu Y, Sun W-B, Zhang H. Amorphous calcium phosphate and its application in dentistry. *Chem Cent J*. 2011;5:40.
22. Milleman JL, Milleman KR, Clark CE, Mongiello KA, Simonton TC, Proskin HM. NUPRO sensodyne prophylaxis paste with NovaMin for the treatment of dentin hypersensitivity: a 4-week clinical study. *Am J Dent*. 2012;25(5):262-268.
23. Khijmatgar S, Reddy U, John S, Badavannavar AN, Souza TD. Is there evidence for Novamin application in remineralization?: a systematic review. *J Oral Biol Craniofac Res*. 2020;10(2):87-92.
24. Centers for Disease Control and Prevention (CDC). Interim infection prevention and control guidance for dental settings during the coronavirus disease 2019 (COVID-19) pandemic. Published February 11, 2020. https://www.cdc.gov/coronavirus/2019-ncov/hcp/dental-settings.html. Accessed August 28, 2021.
25. Herd S, Chin J, Palenik CJ, Ofner S. The in vivo contamination of air-driven low-speed handpieces with prophylaxis angles. *J Am Dent Assoc*. 2007;138(10):1360-1365.
26. Dhande SR, Muglikar S, Hegde R, Ghodke P. Air-powder polishing: an update. *Recent Dev Med Med Res*. 2021;14(22):152-167.
27. Barnes CM, Covey D, Watanabe H, Simetich B, Schulte JR, Chen H. An in vitro comparison of the effects of various air polishing powders on enamel and selected esthetic restorative materials. *J Clin Dent*. 2014;25(4):76-87.
28. Kröger JC, Haribyan M, Nergiz I, Schmage P. Air polishing with erythritol powder – In vitro effects on dentin loss. *J Indian Soc Periodontol*. 2020;24(5):433-440.
29. Sultan DA, Hill RG, Gillam DG. Air-polishing in subgingival root debridement: a critical literature review. *J Dent Oral Bio*. 2017;2(10):1065.
30. Tuchscheerer V, Eickholz P, Dannewitz B, Ratka C, Zuhr O, Petsos H. In vitro surgical and non-surgical air-polishing efficacy for implant surface decontamination in three different defect configurations. *Clin Oral Invest*. 2021;25(4):1743-1754.
31. Schmidlin PR, Fujioka-Kobayashi M, Mueller H-D, Sculean A, Lussi A, Miron RJ. Effects of air polishing and an amino acid buffered hypochlorite solution to dentin surfaces and periodontal ligament cell survival, attachment, and spreading. *Clin Oral Invest*. 2017;21(5):1589-1598.
32. Khursheed DA. Managing periodontics patients during the SARS-CoV-2 pandemic. *J Int Oral Health*. 2020;12(8):85-89.
33. Alonso V, García-Caballero L, Couto I, Diniz M, Diz P, Limeres J. Subcutaneous emphysema related to air-powder tooth polishing: a report of three cases. *Aust Dent J*. 2017;62(4):510-515.
34. Centers for Disease Control and Prevention (CDC) HICPAC. Core infection prevention and control practices for safe healthcare delivery in all settings—recommendations of the HICPAC. Published September 10, 2021. https://www.cdc.gov/hicpac/recommendations/core-practices.html. Accessed September 17, 2021.
35. Koletsi D, Belibasakis GN, Eliades T. Interventions to reduce aerosolized microbes in dental practice: a systematic review with network meta-analysis of randomized controlled trials. *J Dent Res*. 2020;99(11):1228-1238.
36. Kumbargere Nagraj S, Eachempati P, Paisi M, Nasser M, Sivaramakrishnan G, Verbeek JH. Interventions to reduce contaminated aerosols produced during dental procedures for preventing infectious diseases. *Cochrane Database Syst Rev*. 2020;10:CD013686.

37. Bühler J, Schmidli F, Weiger R, Walter C. Analysis of the effects of air polishing powders containing sodium bicarbonate and glycine on human teeth. *Clin Oral Invest*. 2015;19(4):877-885.
38. Janiszewska-Olszowska J, Drozdzik A, Tandecka K, Grocholewicz K. Effect of air-polishing on surface roughness of composite dental restorative material—comparison of three different air-polishing powders. *BMC Oral Health*. 2020;20(1):30.
39. Tungare S, Paranjpe AG. Teeth polishing. In: *StatPearls*. StatPearls Publishing; 2021. http://www.ncbi.nlm.nih.gov/books/NBK513328/. Accessed September 22, 2021.

CHAPTER 43

Tooth Bleaching

Heather Hessheimer, RDH, MS

CHAPTER OUTLINE

LEARNING OBJECTIVES

After studying this chapter, the student will be able to:

1. Discuss the mechanism, safety, and efficacy of tooth bleaching agents.
2. Identify specific tooth conditions and staining responses to tooth bleaching.
3. Differentiate reversible and irreversible side effects associated with the tooth bleaching process.
4. Assess appropriate interventions for tooth bleaching side effects.

Overview of Tooth Bleaching

Patients of all ages have concerns about the appearance of their teeth and expect their dental hygienists to guide them in their **esthetic** choices with evidence-based information. Because there are many causes of tooth discoloration, a review of Chapter 17 is recommended.

- Tooth **bleaching** may result in significantly whiter teeth and contribute to an increase in patient's self-confidence.
- A whiter smile may motivate the patient to maintain improved oral health, which is a significant benefit.

I. Bleaching versus Whitening

The terms "bleaching" and "**whitening**" have been used interchangeably, but are not the same:

- Tooth whitening refers to any process to lighten the tooth color.[1]
- Bleaching involves free radicals and the breakdown of chromagens.[1]

II. Vital Tooth Bleaching versus Nonvital Tooth Bleaching

- Teeth can be stained **intrinsically** and **extrinsically**.
- External tooth bleaching is used for both vital and nonvital teeth.
  - Agents for bleaching are applied to the external surfaces of the teeth.
  - Bleaching agents break down chemical bonds into larger pigmented organic molecules, called chromogens, making them refract light and appear lighter.[1]
- **Color** change can extend into the dentin to produce a whitened tooth.
- Nonvital teeth become intrinsically stained by blood breakdown products or agents from root canal therapy.[1]
- Nonvital tooth bleaching is a procedure performed by a dentist after root canal therapy using a rubber dam or other type of isolation.[2]
  - The bleaching agents are introduced into the pulp chamber.
  - The color of a single tooth is lightened to help it blend with the adjacent teeth.

III. History

A. Nonvital Tooth Bleaching History

- Bleaching of discolored, nonvital teeth was first described as early as 1864.[3]
- In 1961, the *walking bleach method* was introduced. The *walking bleach method* sealed a mixture of sodium perborate and water into the pulp chamber and retained it there between the patient's visits.[3]
- By 1963, the *walking bleach method* was modified to use water and 30% to 35% hydrogen peroxide instead of the sodium perborate and water. Result: improved lighter color of nonvital teeth.[3]

B. Vital Tooth Bleaching History

- In the 1960s, tooth lightening was observed after orthodontics used an antiseptic containing carbamide peroxide to promote tissue healing due to gingivitis.[3]
- In the 1980s, lighter tooth color was noted after advising patients to use carbamide peroxide in customized trays for antiseptic purposes following periodontal surgery.
- In 1989, the use of carbamide peroxide for the primary purpose of tooth bleaching was introduced.[3,4]
  - A custom tray was used to maintain the bleaching gel on the tooth surface for an extended time.
  - The procedure was known as nightguard vital bleaching (NGVB) and is a dentist-monitored process.
- No significant, long-term oral or systemic health risks have been associated with professional at-home tooth bleaching materials containing 10% carbamide peroxide or 3.5% hydrogen peroxide when professionally supervised.[5,6]

Vital Tooth Bleaching

The bleaching process is a subject of ongoing research and current theories about the mechanism of action involve a chemical change within the tooth structure.

I. Mechanism of Bleaching Vital Teeth

- Bleaching products penetrate enamel and dentin reaching the pulp within 5–15 minutes.[7-10]
- Bleaching products break down chromogens into smaller, less pigmented constituents that are locked in the enamel matrix and dentinal tubules.[1,9]
- The chemical reactions from bleaching products change the optical qualities of the tooth color.[11]

II. Tooth Color Change with Vital Tooth Bleaching

- The color of the teeth is influenced by thickness of enamel and underlying color of dentin.
- Color of both dentin and enamel are changed; primarily the dentin color is changed.
- Dentin color is either yellow or gray and can be seen through the enamel due to its **translucency**.
- Darker teeth take more time to lighten.
- Each tooth reaches a maximum color change. Additional bleaching product or contact time will not necessarily result in a lighter color.[1,5]
- Bleaching products cause teeth to become dehydrated during and after product administration. A lighter shade can result temporarily.[12]

- Color will stabilize approximately 2 weeks after bleaching.[10]

III. Materials Used for Vital Tooth Bleaching

- Both hydrogen peroxide and carbamide peroxide are used to lighten vital teeth.
- Hydrogen peroxide has a short working time because it begins to break down in 30–60 minutes[10]; carbamide peroxide has an extended working time.
- The chemicals are used alone or in combination.
- Bleaching materials need an appropriate viscosity to flow over the tooth surface, but not so excessive as to spread onto gingival and other oral tissues.

A. Hydrogen Peroxide

- Used directly or produced through a chemical reaction when carbamide peroxide breaks down (see **Figure 43-1**).[11]
- Has a lower pH than carbamide peroxide, which may result in susceptibility to demineralization or erosion when used for longer treatment times than recommended.[1]
  - Takes less time per day, but more days, to change tooth color effectively.[6]
  - Higher concentrations of hydrogen peroxide may result in greater sensitivity and more color relapse after termination of bleaching.[13]

B. Carbamide Peroxide

- Active agent in many bleaching systems in a 10% concentration.
- Breaks down into hydrogen peroxide and urea. As shown in the flowchart (Figure 43-1), urea may further break down into ammonia with high pH to facilitate bleaching.
- Has slow release: 50% of peroxide released in 2 hours and remainder of peroxide in 6 hours, resulting in less sensitivity.[10]
  - At neutral pH, 10% solution safe and has similar efficacy as more concentrated solutions with less sensitivity.[5] A 10% solution has not been shown to affect the hardness of dental enamel.[14]

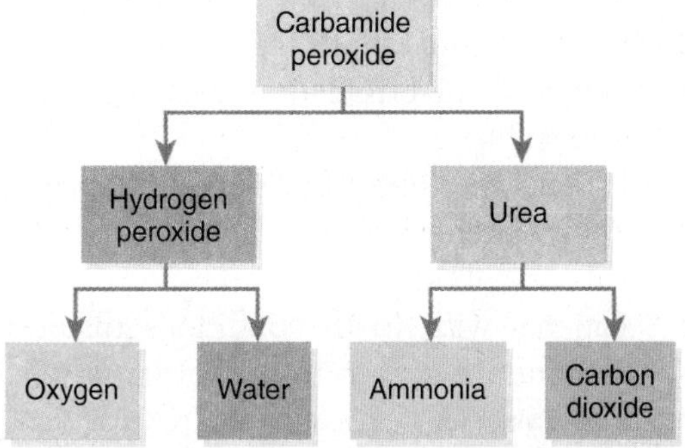

Figure 43-1 Hydrogen Peroxide and Carbamide Peroxide Product Breakdown. Flowchart to show breakdown of bleaching products. Hydrogen peroxide breaks down into oxygen and water; carbamide peroxide breaks down into hydrogen peroxide and urea, which further break down as shown.

C. Desensitizers

- Materials to reduce the sensitivity side effect of bleaching may be added to bleaching systems.
- Materials can be:
  - Incorporated into the bleaching gel.
  - Applied to teeth before bleaching.
  - Given for use in trays before, during, and after treatment.
- Material used:
  - **Potassium nitrate**: creates a calming effect on pulp by affecting the transmission of nerve impulses.[15,16]
  - Sodium fluoride: aids in remineralization and reducing sensitivity.[16]
  - Calcium phosphate and **amorphous calcium phosphate**: aid in reducing sensitivity and remineralization.[17]

D. Other Ingredients

- Carbopol: a water-soluble resin used as a thickening agent
  - Prolongs the release of hydrogen peroxide from carbamide peroxide.
  - Promotes quicker results.
- Glycerin: a gel to thicken and control the flow of bleaching agent to prevent overextending onto gingival tissues.
- Sodium hydroxide: a cleaning agent.
- **Surfactants**: help to lift and remove extrinsic stains.
- Flavoring: aids in patient satisfaction and compliance.

IV. Vital Tooth Bleaching Safety

A. Tooth Structure

- Both hydrogen peroxide 3.5% and carbamide peroxide 10% are considered safe to lighten the color of teeth when professionally monitored.[10]
- Carbamide peroxide 10% will cause fewer changes in the enamel matrix.[14]

- Research is inconsistent in regard to pulpal necrosis from the heat produced during laser-activated treatment.[18,19]

B. Soft Tissue

- Hydrogen peroxide is caustic and may cause burning and bleaching of the gingiva and any exposed oral tissue.[3]
- Hydrogen peroxide 10% concentration or higher has greater incidence of gingival irritation.[6]
- Ill-fitting or overfilled trays may cause product spillage onto soft tissues, resulting in tissue burning.[6]

C. Restorative Materials

- Restorative material color will not be lightened by bleaching.
- Complications with current restorations may include[1]:
  - Increased surface roughness.
  - Change in surface color.
  - Increased microleakage.
- After bleaching, new restorative procedures need to be delayed for 2 weeks to allow for color stabilization.[10,20]
- Bonding needs to be delayed for 2 weeks due to significantly reduced bonding strength associated with recently bleached tooth surface.[10,20]
- Bleaching chemicals containing hydrogen peroxide may:
  - Cause porosity in restorative materials due to the lower pH, resulting in surface changes in surface texture and hardness.[21]
  - Increase mercury release from amalgam restorations, giving off a green hue.[21]
  - Increase solubility of some dental cements.[20]

D. Systemic Factors

- The use of tooth-bleaching products containing hydrogen peroxide or carbamide peroxide has not been shown to increase the risk of oral cancer in the general population, including those persons who abuse alcohol and/or are heavy cigarette smokers.[22]
- The effects of accidental ingestion of hydrogen peroxide or carbamide peroxide depend on the amount and concentration ingested.[3]
  - Effects of small amounts may include sore throat, nausea, vomiting, abdominal distention, and ulcerations of the oral mucosa, esophagus, and stomach.
  - Large amounts can be fatal, so it is essential to keep it out of the reach of children.
- Medications that may be associated with photosensitivity and hyperpigmentation when light-activated bleaching agents are used are listed in **Box 43-1**.

Box 43-1 Medications Associated with Potential Photosensitivity and Hyperpigmentation

- Acne medications
- Antiarrhythmic drugs
- Antibiotics
- Anticancer drugs
- Antidepressants
- Antihistamines
- Antiparasitics
- Antipsychotics
- Antiseizure medications
- Arthritis medications
- Birth control medications
- Coal tar
- Diuretics
- Hypoglycemics
- Nonsteroidal anti-inflammatory drugs
- Phenothiazines[23]
- Retinoids[23]
- Steroids
- Sulfur-containing drugs
- Targeted anticancer therapies (BRAF, EGFR, VEGFR, MEK, and Bcr-Abl tyrosine kinase inhibitors)
- Tranquilizers[23]

E. Cautions and Contraindications Associated with Vital Tooth Bleaching

- Treatment considerations may include:
  - Subjective determination when tooth shade is acceptable.
  - Patients with unrealistic personal expectations.
  - Poor patient compliance with treatment results in suboptimal outcomes.
  - Patients with tooth conditions that do not respond favorably to vital tooth bleaching (see **Table 43-1**).
- Children and adolescents
  - The American Academy of Pediatric Dentistry (AAPD) discourages full-arch cosmetic bleaching for patients with a mixed dentition, but encourages judicious use of vital and nonvital bleaching due to the negative

Table 43-1 Decision Making for Tooth Bleaching

Tooth Condition	Response to Tooth Bleaching	Special Considerations
Yellow color	Normally excellent	Resistant yellow may be tetracycline stain
Enamel white spots	Do not bleach well or may get lighter during bleaching	■ Eventually background color lightens resulting in less noticeable white spots ■ Goes through splotchy stage before background color whitens ■ Microabrasion may lessen white spots if less than one-third through enamel
Brown fluorosis stains	Respond 80% of the time	Microabrasion techniques done after bleaching and color stabilization may improve final result
Nicotine stains	Require longer treatment	May take 2–3 mo of nightly application
Tetracycline stains	Multicolored band may not respond well. ■ Gray most difficult ■ Dark grays only get lighter ■ Dark cervical has poorest prognosis	Requires 3-6 mo of daily bleaching
Minocycline stains	Will respond; will take longer than yellow stain	■ Type of tetracycline stain ■ Gives gray hue
Root exposure	Does not respond to bleaching	Better treated with periodontal coverage
Dentinogenesis imperfecta and amelogenesis imperfecta	No significant improvement with bleaching	Inherited conditions resulting in defective dentin and enamel, respectively
Microcracks	Become whiter than rest of tooth	Bright light or magnification required during assessment to view; may appear streaky during bleaching process
Anterior lingual amalgams	Become more visible after bleaching	Replacement with very light composite restoration before bleaching
Dental caries	Not to be bleached	■ Decay removal ■ Temporary restoration followed by bleaching and final restoration after color stabilization. Carbamide peroxide may increase sensitivity
Dark canines	Require longer bleaching	Isolated canine treatment until color match
Attrition	Incisal edges do not respond	Composite restorations added to incisal edges after bleaching
Aging	Excellent	More youthful appearance; root surfaces exposure likely
Translucent teeth	Bleaching will increase translucency at incisal	Translucent areas will appear darker after bleaching due to contrast

self-image that may arise from a discolored tooth or teeth.[24]

- Current AAPD recommendations for children and adolescent use include[24]:
  - Delaying treatment until after permanent teeth have erupted.
  - Use of a custom-fabricated tray to limit amount of bleaching gel.
  - Close supervision.
- Tooth bleaching is contraindicated in the following patients:
  - Pregnant and lactating women.

Box 43-2 Issues Associated with Light-Activated Bleaching

Light-activated bleaching is contraindicated for patients who are:

- Light sensitive.
- Taking a photosensitive medication.
- Receiving photochemotherapeutic drugs or treatments such as psoralen and ultraviolet radiation.

Exposure to ultraviolet radiation produced by some lights must be avoided for those at increased risk for or with a history of skin cancer, including melanoma.

- Use of photosensitive medications (see Box 43-1).
- Laser light/power bleaching contraindicated for some patients as described in **Box 43-2**.

V. Factors Associated with Efficacy

- Some tooth conditions will not respond to tooth bleaching; other tooth conditions will respond slowly (Table 43-1).[10]
- The initial color of the teeth and type of stain present will affect the final color change.[10]
- Specific indications for bleaching and methods of treatments are listed in **Table 43-2**.
- Attrition: occlusal wear through enamel exposes the darker underlying dentin.
- Concentration of bleaching agent.
- Ability of agent to reach the stain molecules.
- Duration of contact of the active bleaching agent: the longer the duration, the greater the degree of bleaching.
- Number of times the agent is applied to obtain desired results: darker teeth tend to require more treatment applications.
- Temperature of agent: heat will result in faster oxygen release, but speed of color change may not be altered.

A. *Intrinsic*

- Tetracycline and minocycline staining
  - Tetracycline particles incorporate into dentin calcium during mineralization of unerupted teeth. Result: discolored dentin resistant to bleaching.[10]
  - Minocycline, a derivative of tetracycline, can discolor erupted teeth.[10]
  - Tetracycline and minocycline staining severity varies. A comparison of before and after bleaching of brown tetracycline staining is shown in **Figure 43-2**.
    - *First-category staining*: light-yellow to light-gray responds to bleaching.
    - *Second-category staining*: darker and more extensive yellow-gray responds to extended bleaching time.
    - *Third-category staining*: intense dark gray-blue banding stains. Severe third-category staining may require porcelain veneers for satisfactory esthetic result.
    - Some tetracycline stains will require 1–12 months to achieve a satisfactory result.
- Fluorosis
  - Fluorosis results from ingesting excessive fluoride during tooth development resulting in white or brown spots on teeth.
  - Bleaching does not change white spots, but lightens the background color, making the contrast less noticeable.[10]
  - White spots go through a splotchy stage during bleaching but will return to baseline.
  - Amorphous calcium phosphate may be effective in lessening the white spots if lesion is less than one-third through enamel.[25]
  - Brown discoloration responsive to bleach 80% of the time.[10]
  - Resin infiltration or **microabrasion** may be recommended to decrease additional brown discoloration.[10,26]

Table 43-2 Indications for Tooth Bleaching and Methods of Treatment

Indication	Method to Treat
Discolored, endodontically treated tooth	Internal bleaching; in-office or walking
Single or multiple discolored teeth	External bleaching: in-office one to three visits or custom trays worn 2–6 weeks
Surface staining	Dental prophylaxis and brushing with whitening dentifrice
Isolated brown or white discoloration, shallow depth in enamel	Microabrasion followed by neutral sodium fluoride applications
White discoloration on yellowish teeth	Microabrasion followed by custom tray bleaching

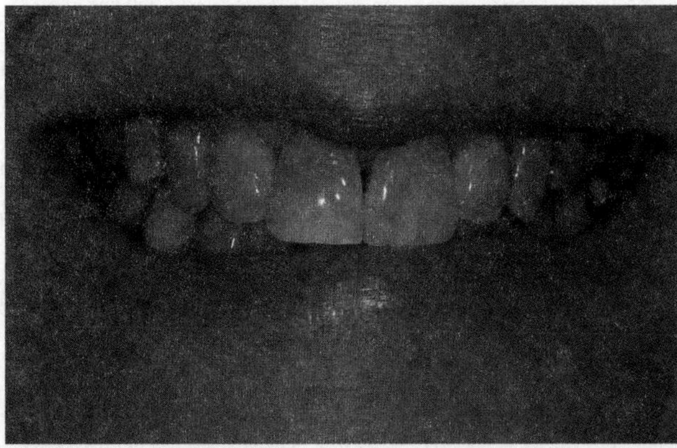

A

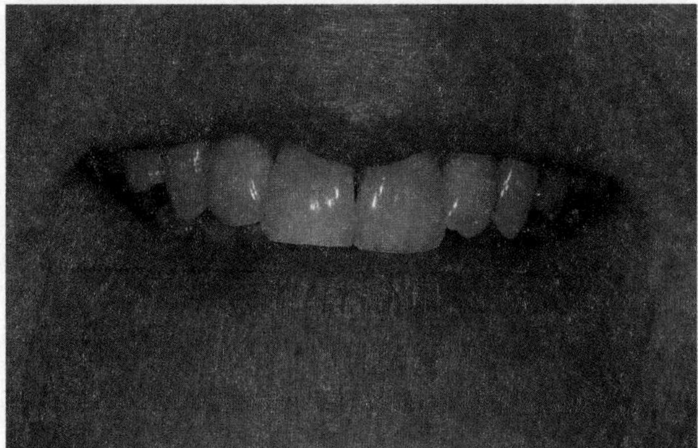

B

Figure 43-2 Before and After Bleaching of Moderate Tetracycline-Stained Teeth. **A:** Patient before treating. **B:** Patient after being treated with 10% carbamide peroxide for 4 months. Some tetracycline-stained teeth will require up to 12 months to achieve improved results. Those with severe gray stain or banded staining may require porcelain veneers to achieve an acceptable cosmetic result.

Images courtesy of Dr. Van B. Haywood, DMD, Professor, Dental College of Georgia, Augusta University.

- Tobacco
  - Tobacco stains: require 1–3 months of nightly treatment due to the tenacity of the stain.

B. Extrinsic

- Interactions with bleaching agents.
  - Staining agents may compromise treatment.[1]
  - Advise patient to avoid:
    - Coffee and tea.
    - Dark sodas or soft drinks.
    - Red wine.
    - Soy sauce.
    - Tobacco.
- Chromogenic bacteria.
- Biofilm accumulation.
- Topical medications.

C. Longevity of Results

- Relapse of shade occurs almost immediately as newly bleached, dehydrated teeth rehydrate.
- As months and years pass, teeth may discolor and darken again, especially if stain-inducing activities continue.
- To maintain shade, periodic bleaching procedures are performed or repeated.

VI. Reversible Side Effects of Vital Bleaching: Sensitivity

The most common side effects of bleaching are tooth tingling and sensitivity. An aching sensation can occur because of the insult of peroxide on nerves: a reversible pulpitis.[10]

- Mild-to-moderate tooth sensitivity is reported in as many as 75% of patients.[3,20]
- Primarily occurs in the first 2 weeks of treatment and may last days to months after cessation of bleaching.
- Side effects resolve completely as teeth become accustomed to bleaching.
- Not correlated with increased wear time.
  - Lower concentrations have been used for up to 12 months (i.e., in bleaching tetracycline stain) and do not exhibit greater sensitivity.[10]
  - Higher concentrations of hydrogen peroxide may result in greater sensitivity.
- Patients with prior history of tooth sensitivity may be more at risk to develop sensitivity during bleaching.[3,10]
- Vulnerable tooth surfaces include:
  - Exposed root surfaces and dentin appear to increase risk of developing sensitivity and need to be protected from bleaching material.
  - Teeth with unrestored abfraction lesions tend to have more sensitivity.
- Addition of desensitizing materials decreases sensitivity.
- Treatments to reduce tooth sensitivity are listed in **Table 43-3**.

VII. Irreversible Tooth Damage

A. Root Resorption

- Can occur after bleaching, particularly after intracoronal, nonvital tooth bleaching when heat is applied during the technique.[3,27]
- Internal and external resorption may become apparent several years after bleaching.[3]

Table 43-3 Desensitization Procedures for Bleaching

Pretreatment	■ Brush on or use the bleaching tray with a desensitizing toothpaste containing potassium nitrate, without sodium lauryl sulfate, which removes the smear layer from dentin, beginning 2 weeks before bleaching. ■ Use toothpaste with prescription strength sodium fluoride. ■ Use toothpaste that includes calcium carbonate.
During treatment	■ Continue to use desensitizing toothpaste, which includes sodium fluoride or potassium nitrate, daily between treatments. Amorphous calcium phosphate may be used as well. ■ Increase time intervals between treatments. ■ Reduce exposure time of bleaching materials. ■ Limit the amount in the tray to prevent tissue contact.
Postbleaching	■ Sensitivity diminishes with time. ■ Continue daily use of desensitizing dentifrice and amorphous calcium phosphate. ■ Have professional fluoride varnish application. ■ Avoid foods and beverages with temperature extremes or that contain acidic elements.

- Occurs usually in cervical third of the tooth.[3]
- Cause may be related to a history of trauma.[3]
- May lead to tooth loss.[3]
- Bleaching agents should not be placed on exposed cementum to avoid complications.

B. Tooth Fracture

- May be related to removal of tooth structure or reduction of the microhardness of dentin and enamel.[28]
- More common with nonvital tooth bleaching.[29]
- May lead to tooth loss.

C. Demineralization

- Demineralization with slight surface pitting can result from a hydrogen peroxide concentration above 15%.[30]
- Patient with over-the-counter (OTC) product may not seek or follow professional advice and attempt to get the teeth whiter by using the product more often than recommended.
- Remineralization should be initiated early and fluoridated carbamide peroxide gels may be a good choice to aid remineralization.[31]
- Remineralization protocols are described in Chapter 25.

D. Erosion

- Products containing acidic pH may result in tooth erosion over time.
- The higher the percentage of hydrogen peroxide, the lower the pH.
- More common with OTC bleaching products.

VIII. Modes of Vital Tooth Bleaching

- A comparison of the advantages and disadvantages of professionally applied and professionally dispensed/professionally monitored systems and the OTC systems is listed in **Table 43-4**.
- The different methods of tooth bleaching can achieve similar, effective results, although the mode of delivery, length of treatment, and ease of treatment vary.

A. Professionally Applied

- Professionally applied bleaching may be performed with high concentrations of 30% to 40% hydrogen peroxide or 35% to 44% carbamide peroxide.
- Bleaching gels are administered by a dental professional and are not for at-home use.
- Some systems use activation or enhancement with a light or heat source (**Figure 43-3**).
    - Local anesthesia should not be used in order to monitor heat-provoked sensitivity.
    - Heat applied or produced by the use of light may cause an adverse effect such as necrosis of the pulp of the tooth.[32]
    - Additional issues associated with the use of a light-activated bleaching are listed in Box 43-2.
- Laser-safe/ultraviolet light protection of eyes for anyone in the treatment room is required.
- Gingival sensitivity or irritation may occur.[10]
    - Rubber dam or an equivalent technique, such as a liquid light-cured resin dam, should be used to isolate the caustic agents from contact with soft tissues.

Table 43-4 Comparisons of Modes of Tooth Bleaching Systems

Methods	Advantages	Disadvantages
Professionally applied utilizing laser/ultraviolet light system procedure	■ Performed as part of comprehensive care ■ Treatment may be combined with trays and professional grade home bleaching materials ■ Professional product selection ■ Patient education. ■ Follow-up, evaluation of effectiveness ■ Sensitivity treatment ■ Compliance guaranteed ■ Quickest result	■ Higher cost ■ Higher risk for sensitivity
Professionally dispensed, includes professional grade product and trays	■ Performed as part of comprehensive care ■ Appropriate patient selection ■ Professional product selection ■ Patient education ■ Follow-up, evaluation of effectiveness ■ Sensitivity treatment; patient can also use less often if sensitive ■ Choice of comfortable time and place for application ■ Potential for best result	■ Cost ■ Longer time to whiten than professionally applied ■ Patient compliance
Over-the-counter	■ Lowest cost ■ Easier access to purchase ■ Immediate start ■ Choice of comfortable time and place for application ■ Short exposure time	■ No comprehensive exam ■ Slowest and least effective results ■ Noncustomized delivery ■ Compliance issues ■ Bulky fit for patient ■ Results and tissue response not monitored ■ Limited effects due to short exposure time ■ Unsupervised

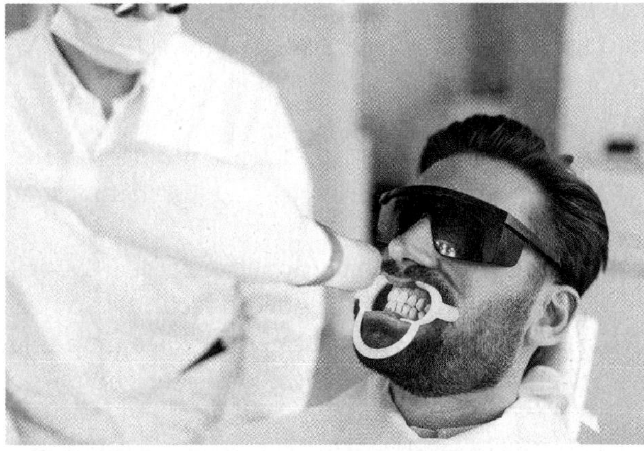

Figure 43-3 Laser Tooth Whitening Treatment

- Take care to assure the liquid light-cured resin dam is in the interproximal spaces to protect gingival tissue.
- Improvements in paint-on rubber dams, cheek, lip retractors, and lower concentrations of peroxide have made in-office bleaching safer for the patient.

- Treatment may take one to six applications for optimal results.
- Time for each application varies between different products; ranges from 30- to 60-minute treatment.
- Laser/power bleaching treatment plan may also involve use of **bleaching trays** for home use.

B. Professionally Dispensed/ Professionally Monitored

- Also called bleaching trays, external bleaching, at-home bleaching.
- Study model preparation
    - An impression of the teeth is taken to prepare the cast for fabrication of the tray.
    - Inspect impression to ensure all anatomy is present without bubbles or voids.
    - Dental stone is poured into the impression with little delay to avoid distortion.

- Place impression on vibration plate while slowly pouring stone mixture in impression to avoid bubbles on the cast surface.
- After entire arch is filled with stone mixture, let solidify for 1 hour. Remove cast from impression and inspect for voids.
- An ideal cast is trimmed into a horseshoe shape with the central incisors perpendicular to the base to allow proper suction during tray formation.
- With a moderate grasp, place the back of cast on model trimmer pushing lightly.
- Hold the cast with the occlusal plane parallel to wheel until vestibule is removed.
- Light-cured block-out resin can be placed on the surfaces of teeth to be bleached. A 1-mm border with no block-out should be maintained to allow proper fit of bleaching tray to the tooth.

- Tray preparation
  - Thin, vacuum-formed custom trays are made for each dental arch to be bleached.
  - Place prepared cast on base of vacuum former and place sheet of thin tray material in holder. Raise to heating element and heat tray material until it sags 1 inch.
  - Lower material to the vacuum base and allow machine to suction material around cast for 1 minute.
  - Carefully remove from base since material may be hot. Cool completely before removing cast from material.
  - Trays should be trimmed with small, sharp scissors in a smooth motion to produce uniform edges.
  - As shown in **Figure 43-4**, trays are either scalloped at gingival margin or unscalloped and trimmed 1–2 mm from deepest portion of gingival margin, taking care to cut around the incisive papilla and frena.
  - Unscalloped trays seal better and result in less gingival irritation.[10]
  - Trays are fitted to the patient and adjusted to ensure bleaching material will not come into contact with soft tissues.
- Digital impressions
  - An intraoral scanner is inserted into the oral cavity and moved over the surface of the teeth to create a digital image.
  - The image is displayed on a computer screen and used for fabrication of bleaching trays.
- Patient instruction
  - Instructions and bleaching materials for use in the trays at home should be provided.

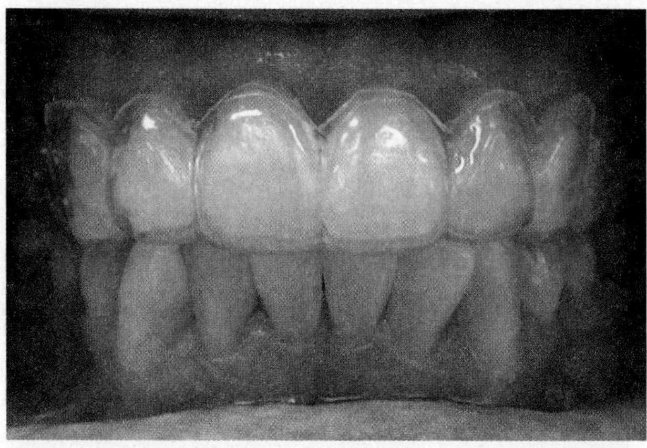

A

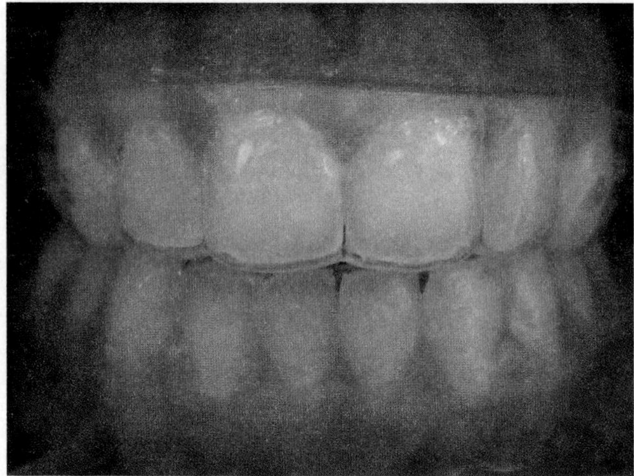

B

Figure 43-4 Scalloped and Unscalloped Bleaching Tray Designs. Either scalloped or unscalloped trays may be used. **A:** Scalloped trays aim to protect the gingiva and exposed root surfaces. **B:** Unscalloped trays are more comfortable and take less preparation time. Patients need to be warned to avoid overfilling trays.

  - Patient should practice placing correct amount of bleaching gel to demonstrate understanding.
  - Once or twice daily application for 1–2 weeks is usually recommended if lack of sensitivity and other side effects permit. Maximum color change obtained with consistent compliance (see **Figure 43-5**).
  - The enamel may become more porous during treatment[13]; therefore, patient should be advised to avoid staining agents.
- Patient retains the trays after completion of bleaching to reuse for touch-ups as needed.
- Professionally dispensed bleaching products are commonly recommended after professionally applied bleaching procedures to maintain and promote results.

C. OTC Products

- OTC products may use generic bleaching trays (**Figure 43-6**).
- When asked about use of the self-directed product, a dental hygienist should stress the need for professional examination and supervision; the products can cause harm if misused, may irritate tissues, or cause systemic illness if ingested.
- May be recommended to help maintain results of professionally applied and professionally dispensed methods of bleaching.
- The dental professional must be informed of patient's proposed use of OTC products to discuss risks and possible interaction with any proposed dental treatment.
- An oral evaluation is recommended before use of the at-home or OTC products, as well as appropriate dental and periodontal treatment including calculus, stain, and biofilm removal.
- Delivered with various packaging, viscosities, and flavors (**Box 43-3**).

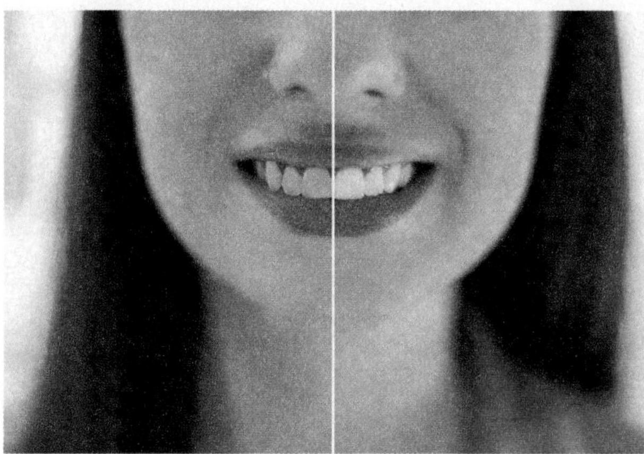

A B

Figure 43-5 Professionally Monitored At-Home Bleaching Tray Treatment. **A:** Before treatment. **B:** After treatment.

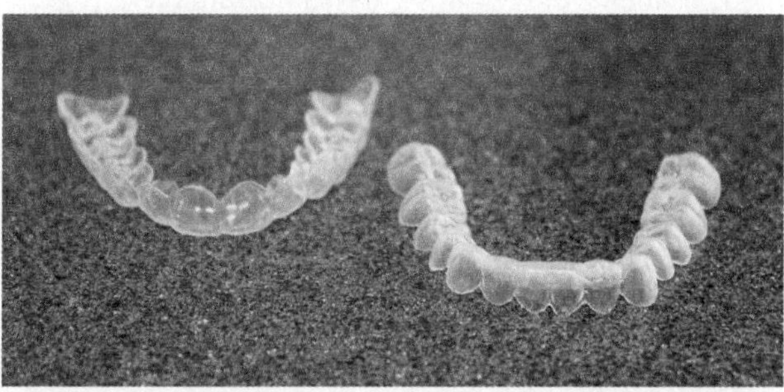

A

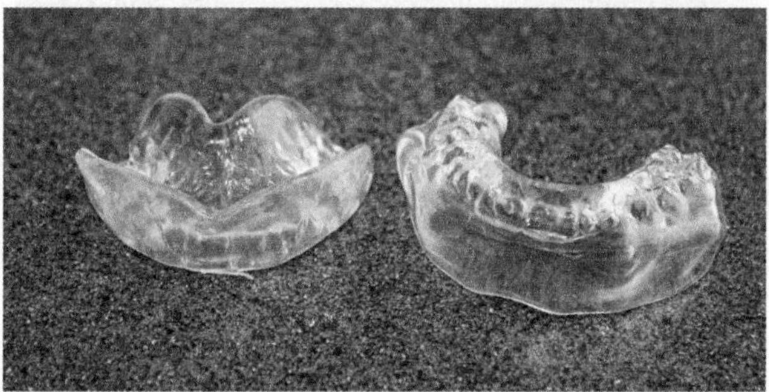

B

Figure 43-6 Comparison of Professional and OTC Bleaching Trays. **A:** Scalloped professionally dispensed bleaching trays. Professionally dispensed trays are fitted to the patient using impressions, casts, and flexible plastic for custom fit. **B:** Over-the-counter (OTC) bleaching trays made by patient at home and are bulkier.

Photo courtesy Heather Hessheimer, RDH, MS.

Box 43-3 Over-the-Counter Bleaching Preparations

Strips

- Hydrogen peroxide is delivered on polyethylene film strips.
- Strips are placed on the teeth up to two times per day for 30 minutes for about 2 weeks.

Prefabricated Trays

- Thin-membrane tray loaded with bleaching agent is adapted to maxillary or mandibular arch.
- Usually worn 30–60 minutes daily for 5–10 days.

Paint-on

- Carbamide peroxide is incorporated into a thick gel that is painted on the teeth selected to be bleached.
- An advantage to this method is that individual teeth may be bleached.

Dentifrice

- Some have more abrasive materials to remove extrinsic stains.
- Owing to short exposure time, the bleaching agent in the dentifrice has little effect on staining.
- Some contain hydrogen peroxide; others contain agents that may deter further attachment of stains to the teeth.

Mouthrinse

- Contain a variety of active ingredients to bleach teeth, remove stains, or prevent stain retention.
- Content of alcohol is avoided in selection of mouthrinse.

Nonvital Tooth Bleaching

Also called *walking bleach method* and *internal bleaching*, nonvital tooth bleaching involves the bleaching of a single, endodontically treated tooth that is discolored.

- Alternative to more invasive correction, such as a post and core with crown.
- Performed by a dentist.
- Requirements for procedure:
  - Healthy periodontium.
  - Successfully obturated root canal filling.
  - Root canal filling is sealed off with a restorative material before treatment to prevent bleaching agent from reaching periapical tissue.

I. Procedure for Bleaching Nonvital Teeth

- Hydrogen peroxide and/or sodium perborate is placed in the pulp chamber, sealed, and left for 3–7 days, as outlined in **Box 43-4**.
- Hydrogen peroxide and sodium perborate may be synergistic and very effective in bleaching the tooth.
- The process is repeated until a satisfactory result is obtained.
- Once a satisfactory result is obtained, the pulp chamber is sealed with glass ionomer cement.
- Appoint patient 2 weeks later to place permanent, bonded, composite-resin restoration in access cavity to allow dissipation of residual oxygen that would interfere with efficacy of bonding agent.
- If unsuccessful after repeated attempts, techniques for vital tooth bleaching or an alternative restorative procedure, such as a post and core with crown, can be attempted.

II. Factors Associated with Efficacy

- Results usually last longer than external tooth bleaching.
- There is no universal standard for what is considered acceptable esthetics.
  - Personal background, culture, and patient's image of esthetics are factors.
  - The dentist initially may not identify a patient's esthetic issues in the same way that the patient identifies them.
- Careful communication and agreement about the course of treatment and the expected result of treatment before the start of bleaching by the patient is essential.

Box 43-4 Procedure for Nonvital Tooth Bleaching

Periodontally healthy, endodontically treated tooth:

1. Photograph of the tooth to be bleached with shade guide.
2. Provide dental hygiene services to remove extrinsic stain and calculus.
3. Probe circumferentially to determine the outline of the cementoenamel junction.
4. Rubber dam isolation is applied to prevent contamination of root canal therapy.
5. Prepare access cavity. Remove all endodontic obturation material, sealer, cement, and necessary restorative material without removing more dentin than necessary.
6. Remove 2–3 mm of obturation material from the root canal to level below the crest of the gingival margin.
7. Irrigate access cavity with copious amount of water and dry well without desiccating.
8. Root canal therapy is sealed off, commonly with glass ionomer cement or other filling material.
9. Medicament is placed in pulp chamber.
10. Pulp chamber is sealed with a temporary restoration.
11. Patient returns in 3–7 days for evaluation.

Aforementioned procedure is repeated several times until desired result is obtained. To finalize procedure:

1. Rubber dam isolation.
2. Temporary restoration on medicament is removed.
3. Pulp chamber is irrigated thoroughly with water.
4. Coronal restoration is placed; generally a composite material.
5. Photograph tooth with corresponding shade guide for records.

Dental Hygiene Process of Care

I. Patient Assessment

- Review of medical history; identify any contraindications for bleaching.
- Complete dental assessment, including the following:
  - Complete extraoral and intraoral examination with oral cancer screening.
  - Updated radiographs.

- Comprehensive dental exam.
    - The presence of cavitated dental caries is a contraindication for bleaching. A lesion is prepared and restored with a temporary restoration to be replaced with permanent matching restoration upon completion of bleaching.
    - To identify abscesses or nonvital teeth, which would require endodontic therapy before bleaching.
- Comprehensive periodontal examination including areas of recession. Cementum needs to be protected from bleaching material to avoid potential internal and/or external resorption.
- Determine initial tooth shade either manually with a shade guide (**Figure 43-7**) or electronically with a spectrophotometer (**Figure 43-8**). **Box 43-5** provides tips for manually selecting a tooth shade.
- Obtain photographic record of tooth shade without lipstick or strong clothing colors that may interfere with accurate assessment. Use the canine

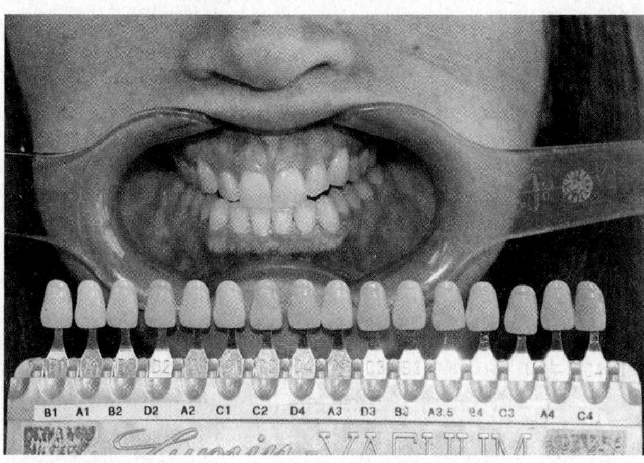

A

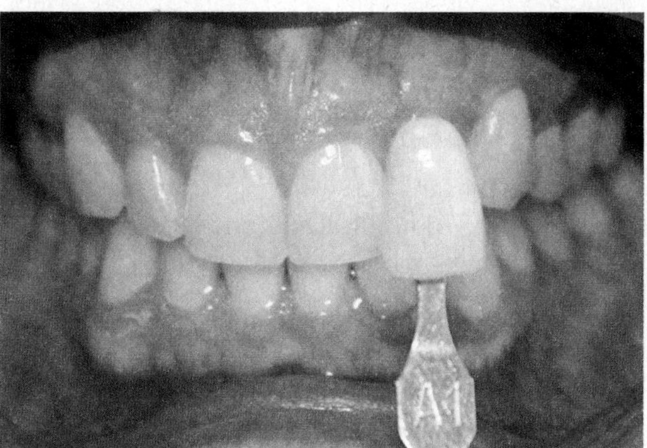

B

Figure 43-7 Manual Selection of Tooth Shade. Patient's shade taken, recorded, and photographed in natural light or color-corrected lighting after extrinsic stain removal before bleaching. **A:** Several manufacturers provide color ranges with as many as 29 shades. **B:** Patient's shade and photograph are recorded at each visit while in bleaching treatment.

Photo courtesy Heather Hessheimer, RDH, MS.

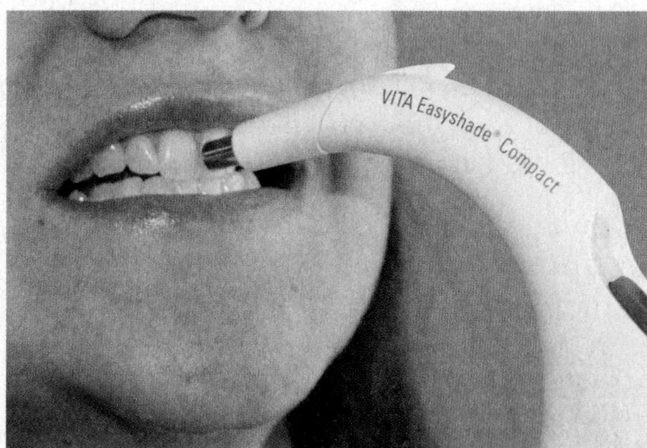

Figure 43-8 Digital Photographic Record of Tooth Shade. Electronic digital shade guides provide objective records.

Photo courtesy Heather Hessheimer, RDH, MS.

Box 43-5 Tips for Manually Selecting Tooth Shade

Three concepts should be considered when determining tooth shade: hue, chroma, and value. *Hue* refers to the color of a tooth. Some teeth are more yellow while others are more red or gray. *Chroma* refers to the saturation, or intensity of the color. *Value* is the lightness or brightness of the color. When selecting tooth shade, it is best to start with selecting the proper *value*.

1. Arrange shade guide on the *value* scale with incisal edges oriented for maxilla.
2. Limit extra light sources in the room. Have patient face natural lighting if possible.
3. Remove any distracting colors from view, such as wiping off lipstick or covering brightly colored clothing.
4. Rest eyes by looking at light-gray color prior to shade matching.
5. Hold shade guide close to patient's teeth so shadow of the upper lip will be similar and select the *value* that best represents their tooth brightness. When debating between two shades, select the lighter of the two.
6. Next select the chroma that best correlates in that *value* range.
7. Finally, confirm the *hue* of the selected shade is appropriate for the tooth being matched.

for base color. Color will be gray or yellow. Confirm with patient.

- Identify those factors that would lead to a guarded prognosis for bleaching, such as:
  - Unrealistic expectations of the patient.
  - History of sensitive teeth.
  - Extremely dark gingival third of tooth visible during a smile.
  - Extensive white spots that are very visible.
  - Temporomandibular joint dysfunction or bruxism that would make wearing bleaching trays uncomfortable and potentially aggravate condition.
  - Inability to tolerate the taste of the product.
- Identify contraindications for at-home bleaching, including the following:
  - Unwillingness or inability to comply with at-home treatment routines.
  - Excessive existing restorations not requiring replacement.
  - Pregnancy or lactation.

II. Dental Hygiene Diagnosis

Distortions in body image can include obsessive teeth whitening so it is important to identify when the request for whitening becomes excessive and make appropriate referral.

III. Dental Hygiene Care Plan

- Plan dental hygiene therapy and preventive procedures.
- Choose appropriate bleaching method.
  - Discussion of procedure, risks, and realistic results.
  - Plan with patient for anticipated needs after bleaching, such as replacement of existing tooth-colored restorations that will not match after bleaching.
- List procedure and risks.
- Encourage questions.
- Obtain informed consent and patient's signature.

IV. Implementation

- Education to aid the patient in optimal biofilm removal as it may also help reduce sensitivity.
- Dental hygiene therapy: debridement of all soft and hard deposits along with extrinsic stains.
- Pretreatment desensitization when indicated. Recommended procedures for pretreatment, during treatment, and post-bleaching are listed in Table 43-3.
- Premedication with anti-inflammatory pain medication when indicated for sensitivity.
- Preparation of trays: impression and construction.
- Provide patient education and instructions for use with an emphasis on the following:
  - Tooth sensitivity treatment and sensitivity prevention.
  - Effective daily biofilm removal before bleaching material use to prevent additional extrinsic stain accumulation.
  - Avoid or minimize foods and beverages that stain teeth such as coffee, red wine, and use of tobacco to maximize results.
  - Use of nonabrasive whitening dentifrice.
  - Avoidance of overfilling tray to protect soft tissue and exposed cementum.
  - Removal of excess bleaching material after use.
  - Avoidance of swallowing bleaching material due to irritation of materials to mucosa.

V. Evaluation and Planning for Maintenance

- Monitor appointments as needed to assess patient compliance, results, and sensitivity.
- At continuing care appointments, compare tooth color with tooth color guide. Take follow-up photos as appropriate for records.
- Tooth color from bleaching relapses with time.
- Plan for repeat of bleaching process at appropriate intervals.

Documentation

Documentation in the patient's permanent record when planning tooth bleaching includes a minimum of the following:

- Current oral conditions.
- Consent to treat related to tooth bleaching.
- Services provided including necessary records for tooth shade.
- Impressions and preparation of the trays.
- Demonstration of tray filling, positioning, timing, and cleaning.
- Instructions given to patient.
- Planned follow-up care and appointments.
- Patient problems or complaints expressed.
- An example documentation is shown in **Box 43-6**.

Box 43-6 Example Documentation: Patient Receiving Vital Tooth Bleaching

- **S**–Patient states she is unhappy with the color of teeth. Patient states she has sensitive teeth.
- **O**–Tooth shade: C-1; appears to have only yellow stain. Patient's medical and dental histories present no contraindications for tooth bleaching. Radiographs and dental examination reveal absence of cavitated caries.
- **A**–Patient presents with a deficit in wholesome body image as evidenced by her statement she is self-conscious of tooth color.
- **P**–Consent for treatment signed and copy given to patient. Completed prophylaxis with all extrinsic stain removed. Intraoral photographs obtained to document tooth color. Impressions and preparation of bleaching trays. Dispensed three syringes of carbamide peroxide 10%. Patient instructed to brush with potassium nitrate product for 2 weeks before beginning bleaching process; after beginning bleaching use of carbamide peroxide 10% every other day.

Patient demonstrated dispensing correct amount of bleaching gel into tray. Patient states tray provides comfortable fit; understanding of sensitivity treatment; and willingness to return for follow-up appointment.
Next steps: Patient scheduled for follow-up appointment 2 weeks after bleaching process initiated.
Signed: ______________________, RDH
Date: ________________

Factors to Teach the Patient

- Why a complete oral cancer screening and dental examination, including radiographs and periodontal evaluation, is performed before any form of bleaching is initiated.
- During bleaching, teeth and gingival tissues may become sensitive for a period of time.
- If sensitivity is experienced, use a desensitizing product, discontinue bleaching, or delay next treatment.
- Regardless of method, color relapse occurs in a relatively short period of time.
- Excessive use of bleaching products may be harmful. Follow manufacturer's directions.
- Existing tooth-colored restorations will not change color, and therefore may not match and may need to be replaced after bleaching.

References

1. Carey CM. Tooth whitening: what we now know. *J Evid-Based Dent Pract*. 2014;14 Suppl:70-76.
2. Coelho AS, Garrido L, Mota M, et al. Non-vital tooth bleaching techniques: a systematic review. *Coatings*. 2020;10(1):61.
3. Dahl JE, Pallesen U. Tooth bleaching—a critical review of the biological aspects. *Crit Rev Oral Biol Med*. 2003;14(4):292-304.
4. Haywood VB. History, safety, and effectiveness of current bleaching techniques and applications of the nightguard vital bleaching technique. *Quintessence Int*. 1992;23(7):471-488.
5. de Geus JL, Wambier LM, Boing TF, Loguercio AD, Reis A. At-home bleaching with 10% vs more concentrated carbamide peroxide gels: a systematic review and meta-analysis. *Oper Dent*. 2018;43(4):E210-E222.
6. American Dental Association. Whitening. Oral Health Topics. Published October 30, 2020. https://www.ada.org/en/member-center/oral-health-topics/whitening. Accessed November 4, 2021.
7. Bharti R, Wadhwani K. Spectrophotometric evaluation of peroxide penetration into the pulp chamber from whitening strips and gel: an in vitro study. *J Conserv Dent JCD*. 2013;16(2):131-134.
8. Llena C, Martínez-Galdón O, Forner L, Gimeno-Mallench L, Rodríguez-Lozano FJ, Gambini J. Hydrogen peroxide diffusion through enamel and dentin. *Materials*. 2018;11(9):1694.
9. Ubaldini ALM, Baesso ML, Medina Neto A, Sato F, Bento AC, Pascotto RC. Hydrogen peroxide diffusion dynamics in dental tissues. *J Dent Res*. 2013;92(7):661-665.
10. Haywood VB, Sword RJ. Tray bleaching status and insights. *J Esthet Restor Dent*. 2021;33(1):27-38.
11. Pereira Sanchez N, Aleksic A, Dramicanin M, Paravina RD. Whitening-dependent changes of fluorescence of extracted human teeth. *J Esthet Restor Dent*. 2017;29(5):352-355.
12. Hatırlı H, Karaarslan EŞ, Yaşa B, Kılıç E, Yaylacı A. Clinical effects of dehydration on tooth color: how much and how long? *J Esthet Restor Dent*. 2021;33(2):364-370.
13. Mokhlis GR, Matis BA, Cochran MA, Eckert GJ. A clinical evaluation of carbamide peroxide and hydrogen peroxide whitening agents during daytime use. *J Am Dent Assoc*. 2000;131(9):1269-1277.
14. Zanolla J, Marques A, da Costa DC, de Souza AS, Coutinho M. Influence of tooth bleaching on dental enamel microhardness: a systematic review and meta-analysis. *Aust Dent J*. 2017;62(3):276-282.

15. Martini EC, Favoreto MW, Rezende M, de Geus JL, Loguercio AD, Reis A. Topical application of a desensitizing agent containing potassium nitrate before dental bleaching: a systematic review and meta-analysis. *Clin Oral Investig*. 2021;25(7):4311-4327.
16. Wang Y, Gao J, Jiang T, Liang S, Zhou Y, Matis BA. Evaluation of the efficacy of potassium nitrate and sodium fluoride as desensitizing agents during tooth bleaching treatment—a systematic review and meta-analysis. *J Dent*. 2015;43(8):913-923.
17. Oldoini G, Bruno A, Genovesi AM, Parisi L. Effects of amorphous calcium phosphate administration on dental sensitivity during in-office and at-home interventions. *Dent J*. 2018;6(4):E52.
18. Sari T, Celik G, Usumez A. Temperature rise in pulp and gel during laser-activated bleaching: in vitro. *Lasers Med Sci*. 2015;30(2):577-582.
19. De Moor RJG, Verheyen J, Verheyen P, et al. Laser teeth bleaching: evaluation of eventual side effects on enamel and the pulp and the efficiency in vitro and in vivo. *Sci World J*. 2015;2015:835405.
20. Tredwin CJ, Naik S, Lewis NJ, Scully C. Hydrogen peroxide tooth-whitening (bleaching) products: review of adverse effects and safety issues. *Br Dent J*. 2006;200(7):371-376.
21. Attin T, Hannig C, Wiegand A, Attin R. Effect of bleaching on restorative materials and restorations—a systematic review. *Dent Mater Off Publ Acad Dent Mater*. 2004;20(9):852-861.
22. Munro IC, Williams GM, Heymann HO, Kroes R. Tooth whitening products and the risk of oral cancer. *Food Chem Toxicol Int J Publ Br Ind Biol Res Assoc*. 2006;44(3):301-315.
23. Lugović-Mihić L, Duvančić T, Ferček I, Vuković P, Japundžić I, Ćesić D. Drug-induced photosensitivity - a continuing diagnostic challenge. *Acta Clin Croat*. 2017;56(2):277-283.
24. American Academy of Pediatric Dentistry. Policy on the use of dental bleaching for child and adolescent patients. *Pediatr Dent*. 2018;40(6):92-94.
25. Abdullah Z, John J. Minimally invasive treatment of white spot lesions—a systematic review. *Oral Health Prev Dent*. 2016;14(3):197-205.
26. Gugnani N, Pandit IK, Gupta M, Gugnani S, Soni S, Goyal V. Comparative evaluation of esthetic changes in nonpitted fluorosis stains when treated with resin infiltration, in-office bleaching, and combination therapies. *J Esthet Restor Dent*. 2017;29(5):317-324.
27. Sulieman M. An overview of bleaching techniques: 2. Night guard vital bleaching and non-vital bleaching. *Dent Update*. 2005;32(1):39-40, 42-44, 46.
28. Elfallah HM, Bertassoni LE, Charadram N, Rathsam C, Swain MV. Effect of tooth bleaching agents on protein content and mechanical properties of dental enamel. *Acta Biomater*. 2015;20:120-128.
29. Kazemipoor M, Azad S, Farahat F. Concurrent effects of bleaching materials and the size of root canal preparation on cervical dentin microhardness. *Iran Endod J*. 2017;12(3):298-302.
30. Grazioli G, Valente LL, Isolan CP, Pinheiro HA, Duarte CG, Münchow EA. Bleaching and enamel surface interactions resulting from the use of highly-concentrated bleaching gels. *Arch Oral Biol*. 2018;87:157-162.
31. Bollineni S, Janga RK, Venugopal L, Reddy IR, Babu PR, Kumar SS. Role of fluoridated carbamide peroxide whitening gel in the remineralization of demineralized enamel: an in vitro study. *J Int Soc Prev Community Dent*. 2014;4(2):117-121.
32. Benetti F, Lemos CAA, de Oliveira Gallinari M, et al. Influence of different types of light on the response of the pulp tissue in dental bleaching: a systematic review. *Clin Oral Investig*. 2018;22(4):1825-1837.

SECTION VIII

Evaluation

Introduction for Section VIII

Evaluation of dental hygiene care is a determination of whether the oral health goals identified in the patient's care plan have been met. The systematic evaluation of dental hygiene prevention and treatment interventions:

- Relies on the careful collection of data and comparison of posttreatment information with baseline data.
- Determines further treatment needs and appropriate periodontal maintenance interval.
- Allows comparison with both previous and future observations to determine changes in the patient's oral health status over time.

The Dental Hygiene Process of Care

- Evaluation is an essential component of every step in the dental hygiene process of care, as illustrated by the arrows in **Figure VIII-1**.
- The dental hygienist who evaluates each step in the process during each patient appointment will assure that attention is paid to any changing circumstance that affects patient care or treatment outcomes.
- As the process of patient care continues:
  - A new care plan, based on evaluation data, will address further treatment or preventive needs and/or determine the proper maintenance interval to support the patient's oral health status.
  - During the maintenance appointment, the process will be used to determine if the patient's needs have changed and to plan and implement interventions that meet those needs.

Ethical Applications

- It is beneficial to evaluate an ethical situation involving treatment outcomes or self-evaluation of professional skills and abilities based on the Standards of Professional Responsibility outlined in the ADHA Code of Ethics and listed in **Box VIII-1**.
- The ethical dental hygienist will:
  - Assess how a particular decision could potentially affect each of the professional roles of a dental hygienist.
  - Evaluate a choice of action that acknowledges each area of professional responsibility.

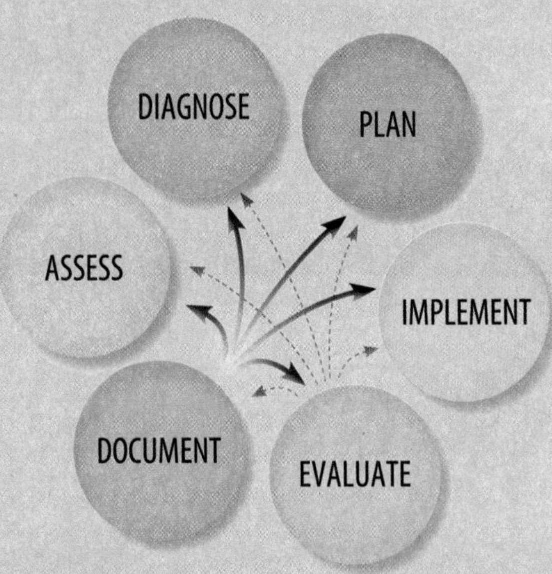

Figure VIII-1 The Dental Hygiene Process of Care

Box VIII-1 Standards of Professional Responsibility

Professional dental hygienists acknowledge the following responsibilities:

- To ourselves as individuals and professionals.
- To family and friends.
- To patients.
- To employers and employees.
- To the dental hygiene profession.
- To the community and society.
- To scientific investigation.

CHAPTER 44

Principles of Evaluation

Linda D. Boyd, RDH, RD, EdD
Charlotte J. Wyche, RDH, MS

CHAPTER OUTLINE

LEARNING OBJECTIVES

After studying this chapter, the student will be able to:

1. Identify and define key terms and concepts related to the evaluation of dental hygiene interventions.
2. Discuss standards for dental hygiene practice.
3. Identify skills related to self-assessment and reflective dental hygiene practice.

Principles of Evaluation

- Evaluation is a systematic determination of worth, value, or significance.[1]
- Ongoing evaluation is an important component of providing evidence-based dental hygiene care.
- Evaluation measures determine whether treatment and oral health education goals outlined in the dental hygiene care plan are achieved.[2-7]
- As illustrated in the dental hygiene process of care (Section VIII Introduction), ongoing evaluation at each step provides **feedback** to determine success or indicate the need to modify procedures throughout the process.

I. Purposes of Evaluation

- Ongoing evaluation measures patient satisfaction with care provided.

- Assessing the outcome of both clinical and preventive interventions at the completion of a treatment cycle identifies need for further treatment and adapted self-care protocols.
- The evaluation process also helps to determine the appropriate continuing care interval to achieve and maintain optimal oral health.

II. Evaluation Design

- The four most common types of **evaluation design** (listed with dental hygiene practice examples in **Table 44-1**) include[8]:
  - **Formative evaluation**
  - **Process evaluation**
  - **Outcome evaluation**
  - **Impact evaluation**
- The dental hygiene evaluation process compares actual to expected treatment outcomes to assess the extent to which preventive and therapeutic interventions have been effective in meeting goals.[3,5-7]

III. Evaluation Process

- When writing the dental hygiene care plan, **indicators** (evaluation measures) that will evaluate each oral health goal and outcome can be determined.
- Following treatment, assessment information is collected again to compare with baseline data.
- An evidence-based decision-making approach is used to determine any necessary modifications to the ongoing treatment sequence or to plan maintenance care.

Table 44-1 Four Most Common Types of Evaluation

Types of Evaluation	Dental Hygiene Practice Examples
Formative evaluation	Information collected during dental hygiene assessment that will allow the dental hygienist to monitor patient needs (e.g., need for pain control) and adapt care to the patient's general health or oral health status
Process evaluation	Immediate: use of explorer to check for residual calculus Ongoing: monitoring of tissue trauma during instrumentation or evaluation of patient self-care during a multi-appointment treatment sequence
Outcome evaluation	Determination at end of treatment sequence to confirm whether oral health goals stated in the patient's treatment plan have been met
Impact evaluation	Assessment of the impact of oral health treatment on the patient's overall health status

Evaluation Based on Goals and Outcomes

- The dental hygiene care plan establishes individualized short- and long-range patient goals for each dental hygiene intervention.
- The treatment, education, and self-care instruction goals listed in the patient's care plan provide the basis for evaluating whether the expected outcomes have been achieved at each level.
- Outcomes that can be evaluated following the completion of dental hygiene treatment and patient education in each area of a three-part plan for care are listed in **Box 44-1**.
- Selected outcomes are used to develop goals for patient care when writing a new dental hygiene care plan.

Box 44-1 Expected Outcomes Following Dental Hygiene Interventions

Gingival/Periodontal Health Outcomes

- Reduced probing depths
- No bleeding on probing, exudate, or suppuration
- Reduced gingival swelling and edema
- No further loss in attachment level
- Decrease or no change in mobility

Dental Caries Risk Outcomes

- No new cavitated lesions
- Demineralized/noncavitated areas arrested
- Reduced intake of cariogenic foods/beverages
- Dental sealants placed
- Increased fluoride use

Prevention Outcomes

- Elimination of iatrogenic factors (calculus, restoration overhangs)
- Reduced dental biofilm
- Patient report of compliance with daily oral self-care recommendations
- Compliance with recommended continuing care interval
- Tobacco-free status achieved
- Modification/management of systemic risk factors

Evaluation of Clinical (Treatment) Outcomes

- Final evaluation of dental hygiene treatment outcomes is performed after initial dental hygiene therapy has been completed.
- When a treatment sequence consists of multiple appointments, evaluation of the previously treated areas at each subsequent appointment allows immediate intervention in an area that shows poor response to the previous treatment.
- The examinations used for initial assessment as well as evaluation assessment are described more completely in Chapters 13, 16, 17, and 20.

I. Visual Examination

- Obtain biofilm score after the soft-tissue visual inspection has been completed so the use of disclosing solution does not interfere with the soft-tissue examination.
- Gingival examination looks for changes in tissue color, size, shape (contour), and consistency and compares them to examination findings documented prior to treatment.
- Visual examination can also determine whether a goal related to caries risk, such as restorative treatment or sealants, has been achieved.

II. Periodontal Examination

- A comprehensive periodontal examination is performed and documented using a form that allows comparison with pretreatment assessment data.
- Current pocket depths, bleeding points, exudate/suppuration, mobility, furcation involvement, and changes in clinical attachment level noted during the comprehensive examination are documented in the periodontal record.
- See Chapter 31 for information about assessment of dental implants.

III. Tactile Evaluation

- All tooth surfaces, particularly in areas demonstrating bleeding points or exudate/suppuration, should be assessed for residual calculus deposits and other iatrogenic factors.
- Difficult-to-access areas require special attention during evaluation and include:
    - Concavities and depressions of the root anatomy.
    - Subgingival margins of crowns, fixed partial denture, or overhanging restoration.
    - Furcation involvement.

Evaluation of Health Behavior Outcomes

- Evaluation of health behavior outcomes provides evidence of:
    - The patient's understanding and compliance with the clinician's counseling and education interventions.
    - Development of oral self-care skills.
- The dental hygiene care plan establishes self-care and health behavior goals developed in collaboration with the patient.
- If the evaluation process indicates goals have not been met or only partially met, the data collected during evaluation can provide a baseline from which the dental hygienist can again collaborate with the patient to develop new goals.
- Methods for evaluating oral self-care and health behavior outcomes are as follows.

I. Visual Examination

- Patient biofilm control is evaluated using the same dental indices used to determine original biofilm levels.
- For areas where the patient is not able to remove the biofilm, oral self-care skills are evaluated by observing a demonstration by the patient and assisting in refining the technique.

II. Interview Evaluation

- Patient interviewing techniques can be used to determine whether each goal established by the patient for health behavior change and daily oral self-care has been met.
- Patient interview and discussion can be used to evaluate:
    - Success of factors associated with patient comfort during treatment.
    - The patient's understanding of recommendations and oral self-care instructions.
    - Effectiveness of the clinician's communication approaches.

Comparison of Assessment Findings

- Evaluation results can be used to determine[2,3,5,6]:
    - The dental hygiene care plan for continuing care.
    - The need for consultation or referral for specialized periodontal care.

Box 44-2 Factors Considered When Determining the Need for Retreatment, Referral, or Maintenance Interval

- Soft-tissue response to instrumentation and degree of healing
- Changes and/or stabilization in probing depth and attachment loss
- Patient health behaviors, such as use of tobacco
- Systemic influences on oral health status, such as diabetes
- Level of skill and effectiveness in biofilm control
- Motivation and responsibility assumed for daily personal oral self-care
- Psychosocial factors that can affect oral status, such as stress

- Additional factors taken into account when determining the next steps for patient care are listed in **Box 44-2**.

Standard of Care

- In addition to evaluating individual patient outcomes at all points in the dental hygiene process of care, the dental hygienist is responsible for evaluating personal adherence to a professional **standard of care** for practice.
- Standards of care in dentistry evolved from early court cases that established a ruling of negligence when healthcare providers failed to possess a minimum standard of special knowledge and ability, or adhere to reasonable and recognized standards while providing patient care.[9]
- The *American Dental Hygienists' Association Standards for Clinical Dental Hygiene Practice*, based on the dental hygiene process of care, provides the standard of care for dental hygienists in the United States.[2]
- Canada and provincial Colleges of Dental Hygienists also provides documents that outline standards for dental hygiene care.[3–7]
- Guidelines published by both dental and dental hygiene professional associations, such as the *American Academy of Pediatric Dentistry Guideline on Caries Risk-Assessment*,[10] are additional sources used for establishing a professional standard of care.
- Three sources for determining standard of care in a legal dispute are listed in **Box 44-3**.
- Failure to provide a minimally acceptable level of patient care is considered to be professional negligence.

Box 44-3 Three Sources for Determining Standard of Care in a Legal Dispute[11-13]

- Opinion of **expert witnesses**
- Evidence-based clinical practice guidelines may be considered the standard of care.
  - Even if a practice is not the standard of care, a jury may ask if it was reasonable.
  - Courts may also compare care to what other professionals in the community would provide.
- Federal, state, or local statutes and/or regulations

Data from Moffett P, Moore G. The standard of care: legal history and definitions: the bad and good news. *West J Emerg Med*. 2011;12(1):109-112; Cooke BK, Worsham E, Reisfield GM. The elusive standard of care. *J Am Acad Psychiatry Law*. 2017;45(3):7; Curley AW. The legal standard of care. *J Am Coll Dent*. 2005;72(4):20-22.

- The professional dental hygienist recognizes that standards of care change based on new evidence and require continuous lifelong learning to maintain competence.[2,3,5-7]

Self-Assessment and Reflective Practice

- Dental hygiene education programs recognize ongoing self-assessment of skills as an essential component of evaluating clinical practice.[8,9]
- Although self-assessment and reflection in healthcare practice have been studied mainly in educational settings, there is evidence to suggest that these skills can:
  - Be successfully taught and developed, mainly through reflective writing.[14-16]
  - Be enhanced with practice.[15–17]
  - Help assure quality and positive outcomes in the delivery of patient care.[18]

I. Purpose

- Self-assessment of personal clinical and communication skills and knowledge can guide the dental hygiene practitioner toward an evidence-based approach to finding new information to support best-practice interventions for patient care.
- Reflecting on clinical experiences contributes to development of critical-thinking skills to help the practitioner determine and implement new and more successful approaches for patient care.[19]
- Self-assessment can assist the dental hygienist to determine a need to enhance specific clinical skills and abilities, or develop a plan for continuing education that supports professional learning goals.

II. Skills and Methods

- Key skills for reflective practice include:
  - Perceptive self-awareness.
  - Judgment and self-assessment.
  - Critical analysis and synthesis.
  - Access to and application of new knowledge.
  - Feedback and evaluation (continued reflection).
- Methods for informal assessment of professional practice include individual reflection (thinking about one's own practice habits) or discussing clinical issues with colleagues.
- Reflective practice can also take on a more formal aspect, as in developing a professional portfolio or maintaining a written "critical incident" journal.[15,20,21]

III. A Critical Incident Technique

Critical incident technique (CTI) is used to evaluate practice in the form of answering questions about a specific situation, often called a critical incident, which prompts the practitioner to reflect on the incident.[22]

- Three steps, sometimes referred to as the "What? So What? Now What?" approach, can be used to structure written reflective journal entries or can also be used to guide a less formal means of thoughtful personal self-assessment.
- The approach to reflective self-assessment includes a basic progression of reflective actions with questions for each step to help guide thinking about the situation from a variety of perspectives.
- The steps and a brief clinical practice example are provided in **Table 44-2**. The same steps

Table 44-2 Components of a Critical Incident Technique to Reflection and Self-Assessment

Step	Summary/Definition	Some Example Questions for Guiding Reflection	Clinical Practice Example
Description "What?"	Brief description of what happened and what effect the situation had on those involved in the incident	What about the situation triggered a need to evaluate what happened? Who was involved? How did those involved feel about or react to the incident? What about this situation is interesting to explore further?	Patient presents for evaluation following scaling and subgingival instrumentation. Residual calculus, resulting in areas of bleeding and need for patient to return for retreatment of those areas. Patient is not happy about the need for retreatment. Dental hygienist is concerned about her personal skill in calculus removal
Analysis "So What?"	Reflective phase that involves analysis and critical thinking to identify potential causes and factors that influenced the outcome, the gaps related to standards of good practice, changes that need to be made in current practice, and new knowledge required	Why did this happen? What gaps in knowledge or skill influenced the outcome? Does the knowledge base need to be updated? Were patient and/or clinician's goals met during this situation? How were values or ethical standards related to or applied during this situation?	The dental hygienist reflects on the situation and realizes that this is not the first time the personal patient care goal for complete calculus removal at each appointment has not been met. Recently, while participating in an advanced instrumentation continuing education course, it became clear that the problem is not deficient scaling and subgingival instrumentation skills. She has not been assessing sharpness of her instrument before the appointment or sharpening during the session
Application "Now What?"	Summary of insights or learning from the situation and a plan for addressing need for new knowledge or alternative action	What was learned? What next steps can be taken to produce a different outcome in a future situation?	The dental hygienist learned that instrumentation skill alone might not be all that is necessary to meet the goal of complete calculus removal. Next steps: find an instrument-sharpening "how-to" booklet to begin practicing sharpening and attend a continuing education workshop related to instrument sharpening at the first opportunity

and similar questions can be used to guide self-assessment reflection about situations involving communication skills, patient education approach, or adherence to ethical and legal standards of practice.

Documentation

I. Patient Care Outcomes

- Evaluation of factors such as patient comfort, communication efforts, and treatment safety and efficacy is ongoing and occurs at each patient appointment. Documentation in the patient record provides guidance for future patient interactions.
- Documentation of outcomes evaluation following clinical dental hygiene treatment is similar to the documentation of clinical data during initial assessment.
- Evaluation data following treatment are recorded in an identical format to the pretreatment assessment data, which facilitates comparison and analysis of outcomes.
- **Box 44-4** has an example progress note that documents evaluation of a patient care situation.

II. Self-Assessment and Reflection

Self-assessment and reflection are key components of continuing to develop competence as a practitioner and are a part of the accreditation standards for dental hygiene programs.[7,15,16,23] Evidence of self-assessment and reflection can be documented in several ways. Two suggestions are as follows:

- Regular written entries in a professional practice reflection journal that describe and critically analyze a variety of clinical, ethical, and professional situations the dental hygienist has found meaningful. Over time, this ongoing record will reflect how the practitioner's professional skills, actions, and knowledge have been enhanced through the process of reflective practice.
- A clinical practice portfolio can be developed to document a variety of factors related to professional development and self-evaluation of dental hygiene practice. A portfolio may contain artifacts such as:
  - Case presentations describing care provided for patients with special needs.
  - A personal practice philosophy describing ethical parameters that impact how the dental hygienist provides care.
  - Goals for future continuing education and courses taken or planned for reaching those goals.

Box 44-4 Example Documentation: Evaluation of Patient Comfort During a Sequence of Treatment Appointments

- **S**–A 79-year-old male patient presents for the third in a series of appointments scheduled for scaling and subgingival instrumentation. Patient states: "Following both of the previous appointments, my back has significantly bothered me because of laying back so far in the dental chair for such a long time. Do we need to have such long appointments?"
- **O**–Patient medical history form indicates history of osteoarthritis, but no previous problem with back pain.
- **A**–Analyzed the problem through discussion with patient about how to balance his needs with the time necessary to complete planned care at each appointment. Decided together that placing a small cushion (or his jacket) beneath his knees as well as briefly bringing the chair to an upright position every 15 minutes could help to alleviate his discomfort.
- **P**–Completed third quadrant nonsurgical periodontal therapy and reviewed flossing technique while using the new "comfort protocol." He indicated that he felt much better during this treatment session.

Next steps: Reevaluate at the next appointment, scheduled in 2 weeks.

Signed: ______________________________, RDH

Date: ______________________________

Factors to Teach the Patient

- The need for evaluation of outcomes from previous treatment to establish the basis for decisions about the "next step" in treatment, maintenance, and possible referral to a specialist.
- Types of evaluation measures and indicators that measure outcomes for each goal.

References

1. Centers for Disease Control and Prevention. *Framework for Program Evaluation*. CDC; 1999:58. https://www.cdc.gov/evaluation/framework/index.htm. Accessed November 10, 2022.
2. American Dental Hygienists' Association. *2016 Revised Standards for Clinical Dental Hygiene Practice*. Published June 2016. https://www.adha.org/resources-docs/2016-Revised-Standards-for-Clinical-Dental-Hygiene-Practice.pdf. Accessed December 11, 2021.
3. College of Dental Hygienists of Ontario. *CDHO-Standards of Practice*. Published January 1, 2012. https://odha.on.ca/wp-content/uploads/2019/08/Handout-CDHO-Standards-of-Practice.pdf. Accessed January 25, 2022.
4. College of Dental Hygienists of British Columbia. *College of Dental Hygienists of British Columbia Scope of Practice Statement*. https://www.cdhbc.com/Practice-Resources/Scope-of-Practice-Statement.aspx. Accessed January 25, 2022.
5. College of Registered Dental Hygienists of Alberta (CRDHA). *College of Registered Dental Hygienists of Alberta (CRDHA) Practice Standards*. Published March 2019. https://www.crdha.ca/public/download/files/133143. Accessed January 25, 2022.
6. Canadian Dental Hygienists Association, Federation of Dental Hygiene Regulatory Authorities, Commission on Dental Accreditation of Canada, National Dental Hygiene Certification Board. *Entry to Practice Competencies and Standards for Canadian Dental Hygienists*. Published January 2010. https://www.cdha.ca/pdfs/Competencies_and_Standards.pdf. Accessed January 25, 2022.
7. Federation of Dental Hygiene Regulators of Canada (FDHRC). *Entry-to-Practice Canadian Competencies for Dental Hygienists*. Published November 2021. https://www.fdhrc.ca/wp/wp-content/uploads/2021/12/EPCCoDH_FDHRC_November_2021.pdf. Accessed January 15, 2022.
8. Centers for Disease Control and Prevention. *Types of evaluation*. https://www.cdc.gov/std/program/pupestd/types%20of%20evaluation.pdf. Accessed January 25, 2022.
9. Graskemper JP. The standard of care in dentistry: Where did it come from? How has it evolved? *J Am Dent Assoc*. 2004;135(10):1449-1455.
10. American Academy of Pediatric Dentistry. Guideline on caries-risk assessment and management for infants, children, and adolescents. *Pediatr Dent*. 2016;38(6):142-149.
11. Moffett P, Moore G. The standard of care: legal history and definitions: the bad and good news. *West J Emerg Med*. 2011;12(1):109-112.
12. Cooke BK, Worsham E, Reisfield GM. The elusive standard of care. *J Am Acad Psychiatry Law*. 2017;45(3):7.
13. Curley AW. The legal standard of care. *J Am Coll Dent*. 2005;72(4):20-22.
14. Mays KA, Branch-Mays GL. A systematic review of the use of self-assessment in preclinical and clinical dental education. *J Dent Educ*. 2016;80(8):902-913.
15. Mann K, Gordon J, MacLeod A. Reflection and reflective practice in health professions education: a systematic review. *Adv Health Sci Educ Theory Pract*. 2009;14(4):595-621.
16. Asadoorian J, Schönwetter DJ, Lavigne SE. Developing reflective health care practitioners: learning from experience in dental hygiene education. *J Dent Educ*. 2011;75(4):472-484.
17. Tabassian LJ, Nagasawa M, Ba AK, et al. Comparing dental student preclinical self-assessment in the United States and Japan. *J Dent Educ*. 2022;86(1):21-28.
18. Jackson SC, Murff EJT. Effectively teaching self-assessment: preparing the dental hygiene student to provide quality care. *J Dent Educ*. 2011;75(2):169-179.
19. Mould MR, Bray KK, Gadbury-Amyot CC. Student self-assessment in dental hygiene education: a cornerstone of critical thinking and problem-solving. *J Dent Educ*. 2011;75(8):1061-1072.
20. Gadbury-Amyot CC, Bray KK, Austin KJ. Fifteen years of portfolio assessment of dental hygiene student competency: lessons learned. *J Dent Hyg*. 2014;88(5):267-274.
21. Gwozdek AE, Springfield EC, Kerschbaum WE. ePortfolio: developing a catalyst for critical self-assessment and evaluation of learning outcomes. *J Allied Health*. 2013;42(1):e11-17.
22. Steven A, Wilson G, Turunen H, et al. Critical incident techniques and reflection in nursing and health professions education: systematic narrative review. *Nurse Educ*. 2020;45(6):E57-E61.
23. Commission on Dental Accreditation, American Dental Association. Current Accreditation Standards. Current accreditation standards. https://www.ada.org/en/coda/current-accreditation-standards. Accessed January 29, 2022.

CHAPTER 45

Continuing Care

Linda D. Boyd, RDH, RD, EdD
Denise Zwicker, BDH, MEd

CHAPTER OUTLINE

LEARNING OBJECTIVES

After studying this chapter, the student will be able to:

1. Describe the goals of a continuing care program in dental hygiene practice.
2. Determine appointment intervals based on an individual patient's risk factors, compliance, and oral health history.
3. Name and discuss the contributing factors in recurrence of periodontal disease.
4. List steps in a continuing care appointment, including assessment, care plan, and therapy.
5. Outline methods for continuing care systems in the dental office or clinic.

Goals of the Continuing Care Program

Following active treatment, the patient enters a new phase of treatment for **continuing care**. Goals of continuing care include[1,2]:

- Development of an individualized plan based on treatment outcomes.
- Maintain the healthy state attained during active therapy.
- Monitor oral self-care behaviors.
    - Offer encouragement for oral self-care. The success of the program depends on **compliance** by the patient with the daily oral self-care and regular professional maintenance.
- Monitor risk and clinical signs of health and disease, including:
    - Periodontal infection.
    - Oral mucosal lesions.
    - Dental caries (noncavitated and continuum to cavitated lesions).
    - Eruption patterns and occlusion.

Box 45-1 Purposes and Outcomes of Periodontal Maintenance[3-5]

- Resolve inflammation
- Reduce bleeding on probing to <10% of sites
- Preserve clinical attachment levels
- Arrest disease progression
- Support behavior change and modify oral self-care techniques as needed to adequately manage plaque biofilm
- Early identification of active periodontal disease for re-treatment
- Monitor changes and address modifiable risk factors
- Monitor patient control of systemic diseases associated with progression of periodontal disease (i.e., diabetes)

- Monitor the need for referral and interprofessional collaboration with medical and other professionals.

I. Periodontal Maintenance

- Patients who comply with regular periodontal maintenance **(PM)** or supportive periodontal therapy (SPT) intervals have less attachment and tooth loss.[3-5]
- Evidence suggests it is optimal for patients with a history of periodontal disease to be seen every 3 to 6 months based on risk factors for disease progression.[3]
- Therapeutic goals of PM (or SPT) include the following (**Box 45-1**)[6]:
  - Prevent the recurrence of disease and maintain the state of periodontal health attained during initial surgical or nonsurgical periodontal therapy.
  - Prevent or reduce the incidence of tooth or implant loss with careful monitoring.
  - Increase timely identification of the need for treatment of other conditions or systemic disease manifested in the oral cavity such as poorly controlled diabetes mellitus.

Continuing Care Appointment Procedures

As with preparation of the diagnosis and initial dental hygiene care plan, the steps in the process of care apply for the dental hygiene continuing care plan. See Chapters 1, 22, and 23 for more information on the dental hygiene process of care.

I. Assessment

- Preparation of assessment data follows the same procedure as for a new patient.
- At every maintenance appointment, regardless of the interval, a patient of any age requires a complete reassessment, diagnosis, and care plan.

A. Review of Patient History

- Supplemental questions are asked to determine the present state of health with emphasis on changes since the previous appointment.
- Recent illnesses; hospitalizations; current medications, including prescription, over-the-counter, and herbals/supplements; and other pertinent new data.
- Date of last physical examination with primary care provider.

B. Vital Signs

- Blood pressure and other vital signs are documented. (See Chapter 12.)

C. Extraoral and Intraoral Examination

- A thorough extraoral and intraoral examination is documented. (This is described in Chapter 13.)

D. Radiographs

- The frequency of radiographic surveys is in accord with the determination of an individual patient's need and recommendations for dental radiographs from the American Dental Association and Food and Drug Administration. (See Chapter 15.)[7]

E. Periodontal Examination

- Observe and record gingival color, size, shape, and texture, and mucogingival changes.
- Complete periodontal examination: pocket depths, bleeding on probing (BOP), exudate or suppuration, attachment levels, furcation involvement, and gingival recession.[8]
  - Compare current findings with previous periodontal assessments to assess changes since treatment was completed.
- Occlusion, fremitus, and mobility.
- Calculus: distribution and amount.
- Biofilm and soft deposits: distribution and amount.

F. Examination of the Teeth

- Integrity of restorations and sealants.
- Dental caries: demineralization, white spot lesions, and cavitated lesions.
- Dentin hypersensitivity: location and severity.

G. Risk Assessment

- Evaluate the presence of systemic disease or other modifiable risk factors such as smoking.

H. Evaluation of Biofilm and Effectiveness of Self-Care Measures

- Apply a disclosing agent to evaluate the quantity of biofilm.

I. Examination of Specific Areas

- Areas of special interest include endodontically treated teeth, postsurgical areas, implants, occlusal factors, and prosthetic appliances.

II. Continuing Care Plan

A care plan is outlined on the basis of the new evaluation of the patient's oral condition and dental hygiene diagnosis.

A. Oral Hygiene Instruction/Motivation

- During continuing care, the patient is considered a co-therapist.
- To keep etiologic factors under control, patient compliance with daily oral self-care is a major component of the total program. (See Chapters 26 and 27.)

B. Periodontal Instrumentation and Debridement

- The periodontal examination findings may indicate presence of active disease requiring nonsurgical periodontal therapy.
- Plan appropriate pain control, such as local anesthesia.
- Plan appropriate number of appointments.
- Local delivery of antimicrobials in isolated periodontal pockets with active disease that fail to respond to nonsurgical therapy. (See Chapter 39.)
- For areas of continued BOP, referral to a periodontist for evaluation for possible surgical therapy.

C. Dental Caries Control

- Prevention needs to address modifiable caries **risk factors** with attention to root caries, appropriate use of professional and home fluorides, and diet modifications.
- Implement or monitor previously introduced remineralization protocol. (See Chapter 25.)

D. Supplemental Care Procedures

- Smoking cessation assistance. (See Chapter 32.)
- Desensitization of dentin hypersensitivity (See Chapter 41.)
- Special care for implants and fixed prostheses (See Chapters 30 and 31.)
- Referral for retreatment evaluation.

III. Criteria for Referral to a Periodontist

A. Referral from General Practice

General practice dentists may include periodontal surgical therapy in their practice, but referral to a periodontist is recommended for care outside the scope of practice of a general dentist. The patient should be co-managed with the periodontal office.

- During patient care in a general practice, the dental hygienist should confer with the dentist to determine the need for referral to a periodontist in the following situations:
  - Initially when a patient new to the practice is examined with the following findings[9]:
    - Stage III or IV periodontitis with furcation involvement.
    - Periodontal abscess and acute periodontal conditions such as necrotizing ulcerative gingivitis or periodontitis.
    - Drug-induced gingival enlargement (such as in Dilantin hyperplasia).
    - Areas of inadequate attached gingiva, especially when gingival margins are rolled, inflamed, and bleed easily.
  - During the reevaluation, following nonsurgical periodontal therapy, consider referral for the following[9]:
    - Clinical attachment loss with unresolved pocket depths >5 mm and bleeding on probing.
    - Radiographic evidence of progressive bone loss.
    - Vertical bone loss.
    - Anatomic gingival defects.

  - Pocket depth or narrow deep pockets that cannot be accessed nonsurgically for complete debridement.
  - Furcations and other complex anatomic areas that cannot be successfully instrumented by nonsurgical methods.
- During periodontal maintenance, consider referral to a periodontist if the following are present[9]:
  - Recurrence of bleeding or suppuration on probing, not managed by re-treatment with subgingival instrumentation.
  - Increasing pocket depths/attachment loss.
  - Increasing mobility or migration of teeth.
  - Recurrent periodontal abscesses.

B. Recurrence of Periodontal Disease

- Recurrence of signs and symptoms of periodontal infection indicates recolonization of periodontal pathogens.
- Recolonization of a pocket can occur in an average of 42 days.[10]
  - Without adequate daily dental biofilm control combined with regular professional maintenance procedures, infection can recur.
  - Colonization depends on the number, frequency of exposure, and virulence of the organisms.
  - Transmission of periodontal microorganisms has been reported between spouses and from mother to child.[11,12]
  - Upon completion of treatment, the rate at which colonization may recur will vary with each patient depending on a number of contributing factors.
- Contributing factors for recurrence:
  - Inadequate biofilm control.
  - Lack of patient compliance with PM appointments.[3,6]
  - Inadequate professional treatment.
    - Inadequate or incomplete debridement, particularly in areas of difficult access such as furcations and deep proximal pockets.
    - Clinician experience and skill level impact the outcomes in addition to patient compliance.[13]
    - Biofilm retention: failure to remove or replace overhanging restorations and other biofilm niches that foster bacterial growth.
  - Failure of tobacco cessation including smoking tobacco, vaping nicotine (electronic nicotine delivery system-ENDS) smokeless tobacco, or waterpipe tobacco smoking.[14-17]
  - Systemic diseases such as diabetes mellitus influence healing and lack of control may be related to bone loss and severity of infections.[18]
  - Genetic factors: Future testing for genetic factors may be used as a component of risk assessment.[19,20]

Appointment Intervals

- Appointment interval planning
  - The frequency of continuing care or maintenance depends on the needs of each individual patient.
  - Appointment intervals may vary from 3 to 6 months.[3]
  - Reevaluate the continuing care interval periodically and modify in accordance with changing needs of the patient.
- Factors to consider in determining continuing care or maintenance interval include:
  - Risk for periodontal disease progression.[21]
  - Risk for dental carious lesions.[22]
  - Risk for oral cancer: frequent tobacco and alcohol users.
  - Predisposing diseases, conditions, and behaviors for periodontal diseases, including diabetes, host genetic factors, smoking, and stress.[18]
  - Compliance: keeping appointments and adequate daily biofilm control.[4,5]
  - Previous treatment: Patient who has a history of disease, either dental caries or periodontal infection, is at a greater risk for recurrence.
  - Restorative complications: implants and prosthetic replacements.
- Special appointment intervals of 2 months may be required for patients with special needs. A few examples include:
  - Cognitive or physical disability
    - Managing the toothbrush and other oral care devices may be difficult; when the disability involves the face, opening the mouth may be challenging.
  - Medically compromised and those with recent hospitalization
    - Those who have been recently hospitalized may find oral self-care tiring and require some modifications to oral self-care routines. Appointments may need to be shorter due to patient fatigue.
    - Patients undergoing chemotherapy or radiotherapy may need more frequent appointments.

- Rampant dental caries
    - More frequent appointments may be needed for caries management including fluoride applications, dietary counseling, and support of oral self-care for biofilm control.
- Orthodontic therapy.
    - Appliances make cleaning and biofilm control difficult; frequent topical fluoride applications may be indicated; response of gingival tissue to biofilm accumulation to be monitored.

Methods for Continuing Care Systems

- The continuing care system is essential for managing the oral health of patients.
- Methods for administration of continuing care include prebooking or prescheduling an appointment; sending a reminder card; or sending a reminder email or cell phone text to schedule an appointment.

I. Prebook or Preschedule Method

- Make each subsequent patient appointment prior to the patient leaving the office or clinic.
- An appointment card may be given to the patient with a reminder to enter it on their calendar.
    - If the patient uses a calendar application on their cell phone or tablet, encourage entering the new appointment before leaving the office or clinic.
- Appointment reminders can be done by:
    - Preparing a postcard for mailing a month or two before the scheduled appointment. The card can be prepared by the patient before leaving the office or postcards and labels can be printed from the patient management system.
    - Sending a reminder via email, text, or other electronic media.

II. Monthly Reminder Method

- If an appointment is not prescheduled, a monthly list of all patients due for maintenance can be generated.
    - For a manual system, postcards can be filed alphabetically by the last name of the patient under the month when the patient is due.
    - Practice management systems can easily create patient-specific postcards or letters to be mailed to the patient. Many systems can be set up to automate the process.

Documentation

For the patient's permanent record, the following information needs to be recorded for a patient who is scheduled for routine continuing care:

- Medical and dental histories updated with each continuing care appointment.
- Significant chief complaints and questions the patient may have concerning the treatment provided and of the personal self-care expected.
- Findings during routine examinations including vital signs, extraoral and intraoral, periodontal, dental, temporomandibular joint, occlusion, and all special examinations following individual treatments for other reasons.
- A sample progress note may be reviewed in **Box 45-2**.

Box 45-2 Example Documentation: Continuing Care Appointment

- **S**—A patient presents for 3-month PM appointment and apologized for not being able to clean her teeth after lunch. She described her daily oral self-care regimen.
- **O**—Medical, dental, and medication reviews, no changes. BP 135/60, extra- and intraoral nothing remarkable. Vertical bitewings for molar areas were exposed based on patient risk factors. Periodontal examination with probing revealed numerous proximal areas of 3- to 4-mm areas with BOP on molars, subgingival calculus, and moderate-to-heavy biofilm suggesting lack of adequate interdental cleaning.
- **A**—Generalized Stage II, Grade B periodontitis. Interdental biofilm accumulation with need for more specific instruction to include interdental brushes.
- **P**—Asked patient to demonstrate current brushing method and provided additional instruction to modify her technique with emphasis on Bass brushing for interdental cleaning. Advised brushing more than once a day with a focus on each tooth. Demonstrated use of interdental brush. Gave her sample interdental brushes and provided suggestions on where to purchase them. Completed subgingival instrumentation for maxillary and mandibular right quadrants.

Next visit: 2 weeks to monitor healing and progress with improvement in oral self-care. Complete NSPT for left quadrants with local anesthesia due to extreme sensitivity in maxillary molars.

Signed: ______________________, RDH
Date: ______________________

Factors to Teach the Patient

- Purpose of follow-up and continuing care or maintenance appointments.
- The importance of the role of the patient and responsibility in their oral self-care along with attendance at regular maintenance appointments.
- Importance of managing chronic disease like diabetes to prevent progression of oral disease.

References

1. American Dental Hygienists' Association. *2016 Revised Standards for Clinical Dental Hygiene Practice*. Published June 2016. https://www.adha.org/resources-docs/2016-Revised-Standards-for-Clinical-Dental-Hygiene-Practice.pdf. Accessed December 11, 2021.
2. Federation of Dental Hygiene Regulators of Canada (FDHRC). *Entry-to-Practice Canadian Competencies for Dental Hygienists*. Published November 2021. https://www.fdhrc.ca/wp/competency-project/. Accessed January 15, 2022.
3. Campos IS, de Freitas MR, Costa FO, Cortelli SC, Rovai ES, Cortelli JR. The effects of patient compliance in supportive periodontal therapy on tooth loss: a systematic review and meta-analysis. *J Int Acad Periodontol*. 2021;23(1):17-30.
4. Fardal Ø, Grytten J. Applying quality assurance in real time to compliant long-term periodontal maintenance patients utilizing cost-effectiveness and cost utility. *J Clin Periodontol*. 2014;41(6):604-611.
5. Sanz M, Herrera D, Kebschull M, et al. Treatment of stage I-III periodontitis: the EFP S3 level clinical practice guideline. *J Clin Periodontol*. 2020;47 (Suppl 22):4-60.
6. Trombelli L, Franceschetti G, Farina R. Effect of professional mechanical plaque removal performed on a long-term, routine basis in the secondary prevention of periodontitis: a systematic review. *J Clin Periodontol*. 2015;42 (Suppl 16):S221-236.
7. American Dental Association, US Department of Health and Human Services, Food and Drug Administration. *The Selection of Patients for Dental Radiographic Examinations*. Published 2012. https://www.fda.gov/radiation-emitting-products/medical-x-ray-imaging/selection-patients-dental-radiographic-examinations. Accessed January 29, 2022.
8. Preshaw PM. Detection and diagnosis of periodontal conditions amenable to prevention. *BMC Oral Health*. 2015;15 (Suppl 1):S5.
9. Krebs KA, Clem DS, American Academy of Periodontology. Guidelines for the management of patients with periodontal diseases. *J Periodontol*. 2006;77(9):1607-1611.
10. Mousquès T, Listgarten MA, Phillips RW. Effect of scaling and root planing on the composition of the human subgingival microbial flora. *J Periodontal Res*. 1980;15(2):144-151.
11. Greenstein G, Lamster I. Bacterial transmission in periodontal diseases: a critical review. *J Periodontol*. 1997;68(5):421-431.
12. Feng X, Zhu L, Xu L, et al. Distribution of 8 periodontal microorganisms in family members of Chinese patients with aggressive periodontitis. *Arch Oral Biol*. 2015;60(3):400-407.
13. Kozlovsky A, Rapaport A, Artzi Z. Influence of operator skill level on the clinical outcome of non-surgical periodontal treatment: a retrospective study. *Clin Oral Investig*. 2018;22(8):2927-2932.
14. Tonetti MS, Eickholz P, Loos BG, et al. Principles in prevention of periodontal diseases: consensus report of group 1 of the 11th European Workshop on Periodontology on effective prevention of periodontal and peri-implant diseases. *J Clin Periodontol*. 2015;42 (Suppl 16):S5-11.
15. Chaffee BW, Couch ET, Vora MV, Holliday RS. Oral and periodontal implications of tobacco and nicotine products. *Periodontol 2000*. 2021;87(1):241-253.
16. Chaffee BW, Couch ET, Ryder MI. The tobacco-using periodontal patient: The role of the dental practitioner in tobacco cessation and periodontal diseases management. *Periodontol 2000*. 2016;71(1):52-64.
17. Ramôa CP, Eissenberg T, Sahingur SE. Increasing popularity of waterpipe tobacco smoking and electronic cigarette use: implications for oral health care. *J Periodontal Res*. 2017;52(5):813-823.
18. Jepsen S, Caton JG, Albandar JM, et al. Periodontal manifestations of systemic diseases and developmental and acquired conditions: consensus report of workgroup 3 of the 2017 World Workshop on the Classification of Periodontal and Peri-Implant Diseases and Conditions. *J Periodontol*. 2018;89 (Suppl 1):S237-S248.
19. Schaefer AS, Bochenek G, Manke T, et al. Validation of reported genetic risk factors for periodontitis in a large-scale replication study. *J Clin Periodontol*. 2013;40(6):563-572.
20. Rudick CP, Lang MS, Miyamoto T. Understanding the pathophysiology behind chairside diagnostics and genetic testing for IL-1 and IL-6. *Oral Dis*. 2019;25(8):1879-1885.
21. Tonetti MS, Greenwell H, Kornman KS. Staging and grading of periodontitis: framework and proposal of a new classification and case definition. *J Periodontol*. 2018;89 (Suppl 1):S159-S172.
22. Featherstone JDB, Crystal YO, Alston P, et al. Evidence-based caries management for all ages-practical guidelines. *Front Oral Health*. 2021;2:14.

SECTION IX

Patients with Special Needs

Introduction for Section IX

The dental hygienist's obligation is to see that no patient needs special rehabilitative dental or periodontal services because of any condition that could have been prevented by dental hygiene care.

- For every patient, dental hygiene interventions are selected and patient management strategies are considered according to individualized needs.
- Patients with special needs that may complicate the plan for dental hygiene care are those with significant concerns related to:
    - Their age group.
    - Specific oral and general systemic conditions.
    - Degree of physical or cognitive disability.
- Dental hygiene care for patients with special needs may require:
    - A modification of treatment based on knowledge of the various special needs conditions and the individual's specific needs to provide optimal care.
    - Pursuit of current evidence-based information about medically complex conditions the individuals may experience is essential for successful patient management.
    - Collaboration with an interprofessional team of both healthcare and home care providers to assure the patient's needs are met.
- Optimum oral health is frequently a contributing factor in maintaining or restoring optimum systemic health and enhancing quality of life.
- Patients with chronic disabling conditions or advanced stages of disease may not be able to perform self-care regimens independently or access dental care in traditional practice settings, which may require care in alternative settings or use of teledentistry to coach and support caregivers.

The Dental Hygiene Process of Care

- The care of patients with special needs integrates learning from other areas of medical and social sciences into the dental hygiene process of care.
- The importance of each step in the process (**Figure IX-1**) is enhanced when providing care for a patient with health concerns that affect patient management or increase risk for poor treatment outcomes.

Ethical Applications

- The complex medical and dental conditions of certain patients may translate into a need to identify innovative treatment approaches that consider:
    - The quality of care provided.
    - The patient's quality of life.
- Increasingly, medically compromised patients are ambulatory and appear in a dental practice or clinic for maintenance and preventive procedures.

- A dental hygienist may also provide care in alternative settings such as a long-term care facility or the patient's home.
- The ethical dental hygienist:
  - Selects dental hygiene interventions consistent with the patient's physical, mental, and personal capabilities.
  - Instructs patients and/or caregivers about oral hygiene problems and needs related to their systemic disorders and medications.
  - Ensures that appropriate persons are included in chairside discussions, if someone other than the patient is responsible for making treatment decisions.
  - Confidently communicates with all healthcare professionals who comprise the patient's interprofessional care team.
- **Table IX-1** provides an overview of some ethical concerns to be considered when presenting treatment options to patients with special needs.

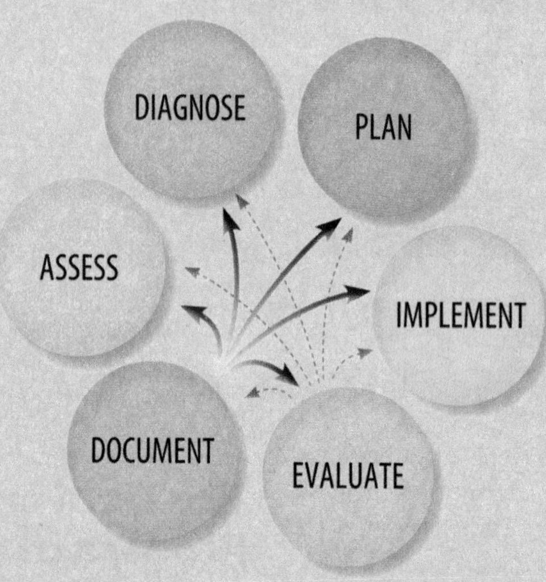

Figure IX-1 The Dental Hygiene Process of Care

Table IX-1 Ethical Concerns for Treatment Options

Quality of Life	Definition	Application Examples
Competency	The patient's ability to make choices about dental and dental hygiene care.	Educates the patient based on intellectual capacity so autonomous consent can be given.
Surrogate	Described as a "substitute" or proxy with regard to healthcare decisions.	Acknowledges a "durable power of attorney" for a patient, where applicable.
Advanced directives	Individuals may write their choices for limiting health care in the event that they are unable to make choices in the future.	Examples include a "living will," "do not resuscitate" order, and "patient values" history.

CHAPTER 46

The Pregnant Patient and Infant

Lori Rainchuso, RDH, MS, DHSc

CHAPTER OUTLINE

LEARNING OBJECTIVES

After studying this chapter, the student will be able to:

1. Describe the oral implications of fetal development in all stages of pregnancy.
2. Identify common oral findings during pregnancy.
3. Recognize the association between periodontal infection and pregnancy.
4. Assess and develop an appropriate dental hygiene care plan for the pregnant patient.
5. Identify considerations that may occur during pregnancy and need referral.
6. Recognize the importance of infant oral health.
7. Describe anticipatory guidance considerations for the infant and caregiver education.
8. Define early childhood caries and recognize methods of bacterial transmission.
9. Describe the components and techniques for conducting an infant oral examination.

Pregnancy is a unique time during a woman's life. Attention is focused on healthy lifestyle practices for both the mother and developing **fetus**.[1]

- *Prenatal care* refers to supervised preparation for childbirth to help a woman enjoy optimum health during and after pregnancy and to maximize chances for the infant to be born healthy.[2]
  - Prenatal care involves the combined efforts of the obstetrician and/or midwife, nurse practitioner, dentist, dental hygienist, dietitian, and expectant parents.
- There is no indication dental and dental hygiene treatment during any trimester of pregnancy can cause harm to the mother or the baby. However, most research indicates weeks 14–20 of the second trimester as most ideal for dental treatment.[3]

Introduction

- Professional guidelines recommend medical providers (prenatal care specialists) refer patients for oral health examinations early in pregnancy.[4]
  - Referrals from medical providers may bring many women to the private dental practice or dental clinic who would not routinely access dental care. Many of these women may not have had education about the value of daily oral self-care and diet related to the health of the oral tissues.[5]
  - Numerous misconceptions can be addressed when providing information about the relationship between pregnancy and oral health.[5]
- Women who do not receive routine oral health care may appear for emergency dental services[6] and once the emergency situation is resolved, they may be receptive to a preventive program of care and instruction.
- The dental hygienist in public health, especially maternal and child health clinics, participates in community educational programs with public health nurses. In these programs, individuals not well informed about oral health may learn of the need for professional dental and dental hygiene care and education during pregnancy.

Fetal Development

- Pregnancy is arbitrarily divided into three periods of 3 months each called the first, second, and third trimesters.[7]
- Physiologic changes in the mother occur in nearly every body system.[8]
- Early development of the embryo is greatly influenced by heredity and the general health of the mother.[8]
- Full-term pregnancy, or period of **gestation**, is approximately 40 weeks. Premature birth refers to a birth before the 37th completed week of gestation.[8]

I. First Trimester

- During the early stages of pregnancy, the embryo is highly susceptible to injuries, malformations, and mortality.[9]
- Teratogenic effects can be produced by many sources, including maternal poor nutrition, infections, and drug intake.
- All organ systems are formed (organogenesis) during the first trimester. By the 8th week the fetus moves, and swallows at approximately the 10–12th week.[8]

A. Oral Cavity Development Includes the Teeth, Lips, and Palate

- Tooth buds develop between the 5th and 6th weeks. Initial mineralization occurs from the 4th to 5th month.[10] (See Table 47-4.)
- Lips form during the 4th–7th week and the palate forms between the 8th and 12th weeks.[10]
- Cleft lip is apparent by the 8th week; cleft palate, by the 12th week. (See Chapter 49.)

II. Second and Third Trimesters

- The organs are completed, and growth and maturation continue.[8]
- Rapid fetal growth and weight changes occur during the second and third trimesters.
- The second trimester is the ideal time for dental treatment.[11]

III. Factors That Can Harm the Fetus

A. Infections

- Studies indicate a strong relationship between periodontal diseases and adverse pregnancy outcomes; however this does not confer causality.[12,13]
- The American Academy of Periodontology recommends women who are planning to become pregnant or currently are pregnant to have a periodontal examination and receive preventive or therapeutic treatment as needed.[14]

- Protection from periodontal infection and infectious diseases is necessary to prevent potential harm to the developing fetus.[14,15]
- Women of childbearing age need to take advantage of all recommended immunizations prior to conception.[15]
- Defects, deformities, and life-threatening infections in the fetus can result from infection acquired during pregnancy or during delivery and after birth.[15]
- Rubella (German measles), measles (rubeola), varicella, herpes viruses, hepatitis B, human immunodeficiency virus (HIV) infection, syphilis (congenital syphilis), and gonorrhea all can have serious effects on the fetus. (See Chapter 5.)

B. Pharmacokinetics

- During pregnancy, normal physiologic changes occur; as a result, drug movement within biologic systems is unique.[16]
- Nearly all drugs pass across the placenta to enter the circulation of the developing fetus and may have teratogenic effects based on factors such as gestational age, route of administration, absorption, dose, and maternal serum levels.[16]
  - However, the majority of medications/drugs prescribed or used by an oral health professional and dispensed during pregnancy are not associated with teratogenic effects or adverse effects of fetal development.[1,17,18]
  - **Table 46-1** lists selected drugs with indications, contraindications, and special considerations for pregnant women.
- Effect of tetracycline
  - Tetracycline is well known for intrinsic staining of tooth structure.[18]
  - The effect occurs during mineralization of the primary teeth beginning at about 4 months of gestation and of the permanent teeth near and after birth. (See Table 47-4.)
  - When an antibiotic is required during pregnancy, the prescribing of tetracycline must be avoided.[1,19]
- Therapy for HIV infection[20]
  - Prevention of perinatal HIV transmission and health for the fetus and newborn are considered with the plan for optimal health care for the expectant mother with HIV/acquired immunodeficiency syndrome (AIDS) infection.
  - Among HIV-infected pregnant women who are eligible, combined antiretroviral therapy (cART) is considered a safe and effective treatment in maternal viral suppression and in decreasing mother-to-child transmission and infant mortality.
  - There are high morbidity and mortality rates among pregnant and postpartum women with HIV infection who have suspended cART.

C. Substance Use Disorders

- Use of tobacco (smoking[21] and electronic cigarettes[22]), alcohol,[23] cannabis,[24] and substances of abuse during pregnancy can have severe influences on the developing fetus, as well as on the child after birth.
- Pregnancy is an ideal time to motivate a patient to quit smoking and avoid the use of other harmful substances.
- Explain increased risks for reduced birth weight, spontaneous abortion, perinatal death, and sudden infant death syndrome (SIDS).[21]
- Explain the effects of second-hand and third-hand smoke on the fetus and child after birth.[25]
- The effects of tobacco use on pregnancy and assistance for smoking cessation are discussed in Chapter 32.
- Information on the effects of alcohol use during pregnancy and fetal alcohol syndrome is included in Chapter 59.

D. Herbal Supplements

- Plant-derived products taken for medicinal purposes. Common perinatal uses are for nausea and vomiting prevention, stretch mark avoidance, upper respiratory infections, labor induction, caffeine substitute, and increased milk production.[26]
- Herbal supplements are not regulated by the Food and Drug Administration as a "conventional food" or drug product, but as a dietary supplement. Dietary supplements are not reviewed for safety or effectiveness prior to being marketed to the public.[27]
- Questions about the use of herbal dietary supplements, their amount, and duration of use are documented when taking a routine medical history. Present to the patient information about possible complications and herb-drug interactions that could potentially harm mother and developing fetus.[26]
- Several of these supplements have oral health implications:
  - Echinacea, used for upper respiratory infections, has been associated with numerous infant complications including cleft lip, heart conditions, hydronephrosis, and trisomy 18.[26]
  - Ginger, used for nausea, can cause dry mouth and dehydration.[26]

Table 46-1 Pharmacologic Considerations for Pregnant Women[a]

Pharmaceutical Agent	Indications, Contraindications, and Special Considerations
Analgesics	
Acetaminophen	May be used during pregnancy. Oral pain can often be managed with nonopioid medication. If opioids are used, prescribe the lowest dose for the shortest duration (usually <3 days), and avoid issuing refills to reduce risk for dependency
Acetaminophen with codeine, hydrocodone, or oxycodone	
Codeine	
Meperidine	
Morphine	
Aspirin	May be used in short duration during pregnancy, 48–72 hours. Avoid in first and third trimesters
Ibuprofen	
Naproxen	
Antibiotics	
Amoxicillin	May be used during pregnancy
Cephalosporins	
Clindamycin	
Metronidazole	
Penicillin	
Ciprofloxacin	Avoid during pregnancy
Clarithromycin	
Levofloxacin	
Moxifloxacin	
Tetracycline	Never use during pregnancy
Anesthetics	Consult with a prenatal care health professional before using intravenous sedation or general anesthesia. Limit duration of exposure to <3 hours in pregnant women in the third trimester
Local anesthetics with epinephrine (e.g., bupivacaine, lidocaine, mepivacaine)	May be used during pregnancy
Nitrous oxide (30%)	May be used during pregnancy when topical or local anesthetics are inadequate. Pregnant women require lower levels of nitrous oxide to achieve sedation; consult with prenatal care health professional
Antimicrobials	Use alcohol-free products during pregnancy
Cetylpyridinium chloride mouthrinse	May be used during pregnancy
Chlorhexidine mouthrinse	
Xylitol	

[a]The pharmacologic agents listed are to be used only for indicated medical conditions and with appropriate supervision.

Oral Findings during Pregnancy

I. Gingival Conditions

- Increased gingival inflammation is a well-documented phenomenon that occurs during pregnancy. However, the findings regarding duration, timeframe of inflammation peak, and the severity of inflammatory response are inconsistent.[28]
- Gingival changes in pregnancy usually appear in the first trimester and can continue throughout gestation.[29]
- When the patient uses adequate oral self-care measures for biofilm control, major adverse gingival changes are not expected.
- Symptoms typically abate after the birth of the child, but may continue after birth if the mother is breast-feeding.[29]

II. Gingivitis

- Considered the most common oral condition associated with pregnancy.[4,30]
- Commonly referred to as pregnancy gingivitis or pregnancy-induced gingivitis.[4]

A. Clinical Appearance

- Shows characteristics of inflamed tissues, including enlargement, redness, smooth and shiny surface.
- Bleeding on probing (BOP).[29]

B. Associated Factors

- The following have been noted as potential factors; however evidence is not conclusive:
  - Increased circulating levels of estrogen (estradiol) and progesterone hormones in pregnancy.[31]
  - Immunologic alterations that cause a weakening of the mother's cell-mediated immune response.[32]
  - Increased proportions of oral microbiota such as *Aggregatibacter actinomycetemcomitans, Porphyromonas gingivalis, Prevotella*, and *Campylobacter rectus* have been found during pregnancy.[33]
  - Increased dental plaque biofilm formation.[29,34]

III. Gingival Enlargement [35-37]

A. Oral "Pyogenic" Granuloma

- Also referred to as pregnancy epulis, granuloma gravidarum, pregnancy granuloma, or a pregnancy tumor.
- The use of the word *tumor* is misleading; the lesion is not a tumor, but a hyperplasia, and may also occur in nonpregnant women.
- Benign, inflammatory lesion; rapid growing gingival mass that reacts to a variety of stimuli.
- When the lesion is removed during pregnancy, there is some tendency for recurrence.

B. Clinical Appearance

- The lesion appears as an isolated, discrete, soft, round enlargement near the gingival margin usually associated with an interdental area, as shown in **Figure 46-1**.
- It forms in a mushroom-like shape with a smooth, glistening surface.
- The pressure of the lip or cheek tends to flatten it.
- The color depends on the age of the lesion, with newer lesions having increased vascularity and may be purplish-red, magenta, or deep blue, sometimes dotted with red; older lesions may have a pinker color.

C. Symptoms[31]

- Bleeds readily with slight trauma.
- Painless unless it becomes large enough to interfere with occlusion and mastication.

D. Significance

- Interference during mastication: can contribute to inadequate nutritive intake for expectant mother and developing fetus because of discomfort when chewing.
- Provides a site for bacterial growth: potential development of periodontal attachment loss and eventual bone destruction.

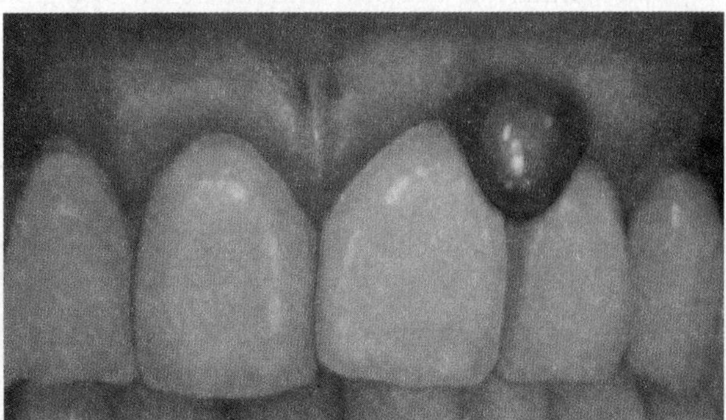

Figure 46-1 "Pyogenic" Granuloma or "Pregnancy Tumor." Isolated, discrete, round, soft enlargement near the gingival margin; smooth, glistening surface, purplish-red in color.

- Results in bleeding and pain: may interfere with routine dental biofilm removal using toothbrush and interdental aids.
- Creates undesirable esthetic effects.
- Lesion must be ruled out for similar appearing malignancies and underlying systemic conditions. Referral for excision and biopsy may be indicated.

IV. Periodontal Infections

- Pregnancy-associated immunologic changes cause a suppression of the mother's cell-mediated immune response, particularly the neutrophil function.[38]
- Although evidence regarding causality is lacking, many epidemiologic studies suggest an association between periodontal infections and several adverse pregnancy outcomes, such as preeclampsia, preterm delivery, and **low birth weight**.[12,39]
- Evidence regarding nonsurgical periodontal treatment and improvement of adverse pregnancy outcomes is not conclusive.[40,41]
- Evidence shows periodontal treatment is safe during pregnancy.[40] The American Academy of Periodontology recommends that a pregnant woman undergo a routine periodontal examination.[14]
- Preventive services such as periodontal maintenance care can be rendered during pregnancy.
- Periodontal therapeutic services can be rendered during pregnancy.[14]

V. Enamel Erosion

A. Development

- Nausea with vomiting over an extended period can lead to demineralization and acid erosion primarily on the maxillary anterior lingual, maxillary and mandibular occlusal, and the posterior region of the mandibular buccal surfaces.[42]

B. Recommendations for the Patient[1,43]

- Eat small amounts of nutritious yet noncariogenic foods throughout the day.
- Use a sodium bicarbonate rinse after vomiting to neutralize acid on teeth: 1 cup of water to 1 teaspoon of sodium bicarbonate.
- Chew gum containing **xylitol** after eating.
- Use a soft toothbrush and low-abrasive fluoride toothpaste to prevent damage to demineralized tooth surfaces.

Aspects of Patient Care

I. Assessment

- Preventive oral health care needs to begin early and continue throughout the pregnancy, to keep the gingival tissues in optimum health and prevent oral infections.[4]

A. Medical History: Health Problems Need Identification during Examination

- **Gestational diabetes**: first recognition during pregnancy; may require insulin and careful supervision.[44] More information is included in Chapter 54.
- Women with hypertension are considered to be at high risk for complications during pregnancy. A consultation with the patient's physician and/or obstetrician is necessary.[1]
- Adolescent health: when the expectant mother is an adolescent, her own special needs differ from those of a mature woman.[45,46]
  - Complications such as delivery of a low-birth-weight baby and increased mortality for both mother and child occur more frequently in adolescent pregnant females.[45,46]
- Aspects of adolescent development are described in Chapters 47 and 53.

B. Consultations

- Treatment approval is not required when providing routine dental care.
- Consultation with the patient's physician and/or obstetrician may be indicated when an abnormal blood pressure or underlying health condition are present.

II. Radiography

A. Universal Safety Factors

- Guidelines for dental radiographs during pregnancy have been established.[47]
- ALARA (as low as reasonably achievable) principles to minimize the patient's exposure to radiation need to be followed. (See Chapter 15.)
- Recommendations advise that dental radiographs are safe throughout pregnancy and X-ray exposure for a diagnostic procedure does not cause harmful effects to the developing embryo or fetus.[47]

- With safety factors of modern radiography, the patient can be assured essential radiographs can be taken safely during pregnancy.[4]
- When radiographs are required during pregnancy, the patient is covered with a lead apron and a thyroid collar.[4]

III. Overall Treatment Considerations

A. Dental Hygiene Care Goal

- The dental hygienist who is well informed about dental care can motivate the patient during her pregnancy and can alleviate fears related to certain services.
- When treating a pregnant patient, the dental hygienist's goal is to optimize the oral health of both the mother and child.

B. Dental Care

- Restorative: Complete restorative needs with permanent restorative materials, such as amalgam or composite materials. Recommended at any time during pregnancy.[4]
- Although silver diamine fluoride has not been specifically tested with pregnant women, protocol does not contraindicate its use. However, the use of potassium iodide to reduce staining from silver diamine fluoride is contraindicated during pregnancy and the first 6 months of breastfeeding.[48]
- Elective esthetic treatment: Postpone until after delivery.[49]

C. Appointment Planning

- Appointment adaptations for the prenatal patient are listed in **Table 46-2**.
- Frequency depends on patient care plan.[1]
    - Monthly appointments or appointments three times during the 9-month period may be required.
    - Appointment frequency depends on the patient's needs as well as ability and motivation to maintain good oral self-care.
- Individual appointments
    - Avoid morning appointments for patients experiencing **hyperemesis gravidarum**.[50]
    - A series of appointments is indicated when calculus deposits are heavy and/or periodontal infection is present.
- Postpartum continuing care appointments
    - Emphasis is placed on motivating the patient to continue routine appointments for dental hygiene and dental care after delivery.

D. Patient Positioning

- Effect of supine position[51]
    - The weight of the developing fetus in the uterus bears down directly on the major vessels, including the aorta and the inferior vena cava.
    - The vessels are pressed between the spinal column and the uterus.
    - Commonly occurs during the third trimester, symptoms of circulatory insufficiency can appear when venous return is decreased.
- Supine hypotensive syndrome: emergency[51]
    - Patient is lying in supine position.
    - Abrupt fall in blood pressure.
    - Bradycardia, sweating, nausea, weakness, air hunger.
    - Symptoms caused by impaired venous return resulting from pressure of the uterus with the developing baby on the inferior vena cava.
    - Leads to decrease in blood pressure, reduced cardiac output, and loss of consciousness.
- Emergency treatment[51]
    - Roll the patient over to left side to relieve pressure of the uterus on vena cava.
    - Blood pressure should return to normal promptly.
- Alternate positions[29] (**Figure 46-2**).
    - Elevate 15° the right hip to displace the uterus to the left.[51] Use a pillow or rolled-up blanket (Figure 46-2A).
    - Patient lies on left side in a semi-supine position[11] (Figure 46-2B).

IV. Dental Hygiene Care

A. Preventive Care and Measures

- Preventive oral health care needs priority attention, beginning with information and motivation.
- Areas of food impaction need to be corrected, and all overhanging restorations reshaped or replaced.
- All nonsurgical periodontal therapy procedures are thoroughly completed.
- When a patient has gingival enlargement and inflammation, instruction in biofilm control and other preventive measures including diet and eating patterns are needed.

Table 46-2 Appointment Adaptations for the Prenatal Patient

Characteristic	Dental Hygiene Implication
Fatigues easily, may even fall asleep	Short appointments; several in series, as needed Work with an assistant to accomplish more at each appointment
General awkwardness because of new shape and weight gain	Attend to details, such as gently lowering and straightening chair for patient Make sure rinsing facilities are convenient; preferably, an assistant assists with high speed suction
Frequent urination	Allow sufficient appointment time for interruptions Suggest at beginning of appointment that patient indicate if a restroom break is needed
Discomfort of remaining in one position too long	Position the patient on her left side and not in supine or Trendelenburg position (Figure 46-2)
Backache	Encourage position changes throughout the appointment Assistance with high speed suction during intraoral instrumentation can shorten appointment time
Faintness and dizziness	Be prepared for emergency (see Chapter 9)
Adverse reaction to strong smells and flavors	Recommend less strong-flavored dentifrice
Exaggerated reactions to odors and flavors of medicaments and other office materials	Determine particularly obnoxious odors for an individual patient and remove them; check office ventilation
Unpleasant taste in mouth	Advise: nonalcoholic mouthrinse; use a neutral sodium fluoride rinse Demonstrate tongue cleaning (see Chapter 26)
Nausea and vomiting	To avoid tooth abrasion, do not brush immediately after vomiting. Rinse generously with fluoridated water or one cup water and a teaspoon of sodium bicarbonate (baking soda) mixture after vomiting to neutralize the acid from the teeth
Gagging	Recommend a small toothbrush Turn head down over sink while brushing; helps to relax throat and allow saliva to flow out Take care in instrument and radiographic film placement
Physician's recommendation for alleviation of nausea symptoms: frequent eating of small amounts of foods	Encourage use of noncariogenic foods
Unusual food cravings	If cravings are for sweets, clearly define relationship of frequent snacking of cariogenic foods to dental caries Conduct a dietary analysis. Provide list of nutritious noncariogenic snacks

- At the follow-up appointments, evaluation of biofilm removal with disclosing agent is done and oral hygiene modifications are made as needed.

B. Instrumentation

- Thorough instrumentation for complete calculus removal is indicated.[52]
- The use of ultrasonic scalers is not contraindicated for reasons related to pregnancy.[3]
- Nonsurgical periodontal therapy may be performed during pregnancy.[40]

C. Anesthesia

- Local anesthetics containing epinephrine are allowed during pregnancy.[1,17]

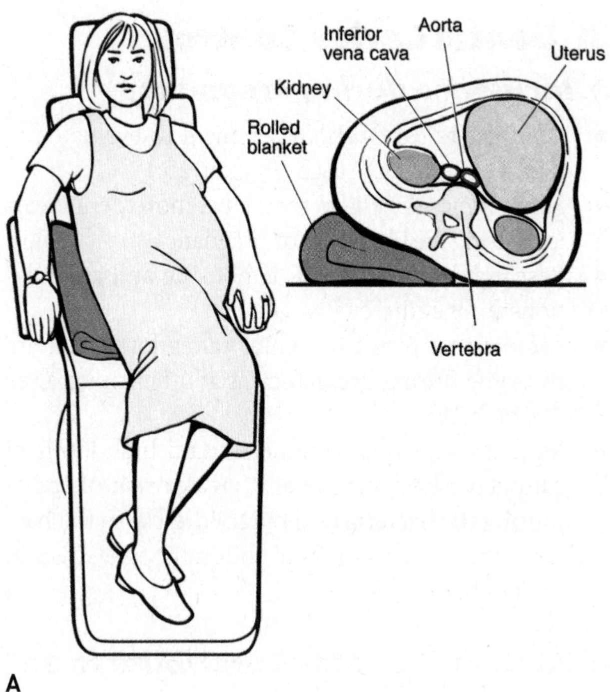

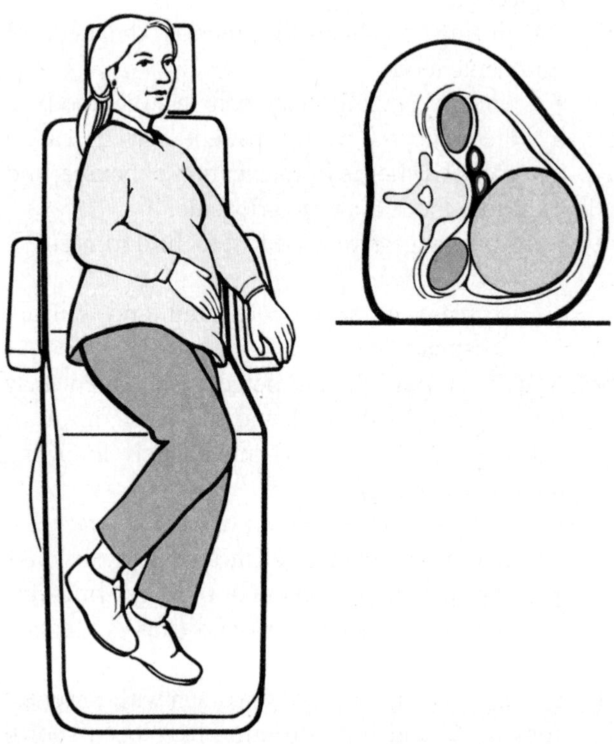

Figure 46-2 Positions during Pregnancy. The supine position allows the weight of the developing fetus to bear down directly on the major vessels. **A:** Patient lies on left side with a pillow or blanket roll to elevate right hip. **B:** Patient turned farther to left. Note position of uterus in cross sections of the abdomen.

- After consultation with the patient's physician, nitrous oxide/oxygen may be used in moderation.[1,53]
- If used in the second or third trimester, precaution is required, including minimizing the length to 30 minutes with oxygen percentage at 50%.[1]

Patient Instruction

- The emphasis on general health during pregnancy provides the ideal setting for instructions relative to many aspects of oral health for the mother, her expected child, and other family members.
- New developments in disease prevention and control need to be explained.
- Helping the mother learn what to expect before infant arrival is essential.[54]

I. Dental Biofilm Control[49]

- A schedule for oral self-care is established and specific methods are outlined and demonstrated. A series of instructional sessions is better for patient learning.
- Gingival changes during pregnancy require daily oral self-care by the patient and periodic professional oral healthcare appointments.

II. Diet and Healthy Lifestyle

- Diet, physical activity, and healthy behaviors aid in promoting optimal weight gain during pregnancy.[55,56]
- Excessive weight gain beyond the recommended range is associated with poor maternal and infant health outcomes.
- The nutritional needs of a woman increase during pregnancy and while breastfeeding to support the physiologic changes and to ensure normal fetal development.[57]
- Consuming a varied diet containing the essential protective food groups, with a minimum intake of cariogenic foods, is necessary.[58] The website www.choosemyplate.gov is a valuable resource with specifics for maternal nutrition. The ChooseMyPlate Food Guide is shown in Chapter 33.
- Instruction is provided for dental caries prevention and to maintain the health of the supporting structures of the teeth.[1]

A. Purposes of Adequate Diet during Pregnancy

- Maintain good health and overall well-being.[59]
- Protect and promote the health of the oral tissues of the mother.[60]

- Provide the essential building materials for the developing fetus.
- Minimize postpartum health problems.

B. Dietary Needs during Pregnancy

- It is essential the mother's dietary needs are met to maintain her own nutritional status as well as the needs of the developing fetus. These particular needs are[56]:
  - Proteins for general tissue construction.
  - Minerals, especially calcium and phosphorus, for bone and tooth mineralization; iron for red blood cells.
  - Vitamins, especially vitamin D, for calcium metabolism; folate to prevent neural tube defects and low birth weight.
  - A multivitamin supplement during pregnancy may be recommended for women with a poor diet and low intake of nutrient-dense foods.[61]

C. Dietary Assessment and Recommendations for Oral and General Health

- Intake from food groups.
  - Consume a healthy diet from the fruit, vegetable, whole grain, protein, and low-fat/fat-free dairy food groups.[58]
  - In addition to eating folate-rich foods (dark green leafy vegetables), take a supplement containing folic acid for a recommended total intake level of 400 mg per day.[61]
  - Low-fat/fat-free calcium-rich foods.[62]
  - Recommended dietary allowance (RDA) of 1300 mg of calcium per day is required for a pregnant adolescent (14–18 years) and 1000 mg for those 19–50 years. The RDAs are the same for breastfeeding mothers.[62]
- Frequency and types of snacks per day.[56]
  - Limit cariogenic food frequency.
  - Increase healthy snacks, such as carrots, fresh fruits, or almonds.
- Intake of sweetened and caffeinated beverages, such as soda or coffee.
  - Limit or avoid drinking beverages sweetened with sugar.[56]
  - Limiting caffeine intake to <200 mg a day or eliminate caffeine intake.[63]
  - Substitute with fluoridated water.[1]
- Avoid sugar-containing chewing gum.[43]
  - Substitute with a sugarless chewing gum containing xylitol.[1]

III. Dental Caries Control

A. Incidence during Pregnancy

- Complete a caries risk assessment to evaluate patient's caries risk.[64] (See Chapter 25.)
- Some patients believe they have more dental caries during and because of pregnancy.
- Research has shown this is not true and any relationship is indirect.[5]
- Factors that result in dental caries formation are the same during pregnancy as at other times. (See Chapter 25.)
- Mothers with poor oral health and high levels of cariogenic bacteria are at a greater risk of transmitting the bacteria to their children with the bacteria and increasing their children's caries risk in infancy.[65]

B. Factors That May Contribute to an Increase in Dental Caries Rate

- Previous neglect: a patient may not have maintained a routine dental care. The existing dental caries during pregnancy may represent years of neglect.
- Diet during pregnancy: may increase the intake of cariogenic foods.
  - Unusual cravings may include sweet foods.
  - Frequency of eating: patient may be eating every few hours for prevention of nausea, and those foods may be cariogenic.[66]
- Salivary changes: from the first to third trimester.[67]
  - Lower salivary pH.
  - Decrease in salivary calcium and salivary phosphate.
- Neglect of oral self-care procedures: patient may lack interest in daily dental biofilm removal or fail to rinse (with water) immediately following intake of a cariogenic food.
  - Vomiting associated with morning sickness may lead to tooth decalcification and erosion.[66]
  - The smell of toothpaste or the act of brushing may precipitate nausea and cause reduction in oral care.
- Low socioeconomic status: women with lower income level and less education have been shown to have a higher rate of dental disease as well as untreated dental caries.[68]

C. Relationship of Fluoride

- There is no evidence prenatal fluoride supplementation intake by the woman influences the rate of early childhood dental caries in their offspring.[69]

IV. Fluoride Program

A. Professional Topical Application

- Professional fluoride varnish application for caries prevention.[70]
- Applications can be indicated, especially for patients with a tendency toward demineralization and those with numerous restorations. Management of caries risk is described in Chapter 25.

B. Self-Applications

- A fluoride dentifrice.
- Drinking fluoridated water is recommended for all patients.[71]
- Other fluoride recommendations are individualized according to patient need.[1]
- A daily fluoride mouthrinse, gel tray, or other mode of application may be indicated for patients who have a high caries risk; review technique for at-home use.

Special Problems Requiring Referral

I. Depression during Pregnancy

- Childbearing years place women at greatest risk for depression.[72]
- Oral healthcare professionals can learn to identify signs and symptoms of depression in pregnant patients. Treatment for depression and dental hygiene care for individuals with depression are described in Chapter 58.

A. Signs of Perinatal Depression[73]

- Sadness; depressed or indifferent mood.
- Insomnia or excessive sleep.
- Loss of appetite or excessive eating.
- Anxiety; panic attacks.
- Feelings of worthlessness and suicidal thoughts.[74]

B. Impact on Health of the Fetus[75]

- Higher tendencies for preeclampsia.
- Fetal growth restriction.
- Low birth weight.
- Preterm delivery.

C. What to Do[73]

- Explain that depression is a medical illness caused by a chemical imbalance in the brain.
- Indicate that depression is treatable, and when treated, can improve the quality of life.
- Refer patient to the primary care provider or a community mental health resource center.

II. Domestic Violence

A. Identification

- Identification, assessment, and intervention with victims of domestic violence[76] can be a significant part of a dental visit. (See Chapter 14.)

B. Common Sites of Injury[77]

- Head.
- Soft tissue.
- Neck.

C. Obstetric and Other Manifestations

- Obstetric: miscarriage, preterm birth, low birth weight, and delayed prenatal care.[78]
- Substance abuse.[79]
- Depression.[79]
- Suicide attempts.[79]

D. What to Do

- Address the issue with the patient.[43]
- Refer to a Domestic Violence Intervention Program in the community when domestic violence is suspected.

Transitioning from Pregnancy to Infancy

- Once the baby is born, the focus shifts to the oral health needs of both mother and child. The next section will address infant oral health and parental guidance through the first year of life.

Infant Oral Health

- To optimize infant oral health, oral health counseling begins during prenatal dental visits.[54]

I. Anticipatory Guidance

- Dental care during pregnancy includes educating the expectant mother about the importance of infant oral health to improve preparedness (**Table 46-3**).

Table 46-3 Anticipatory Guidance: Birth to 12 Months

Area of Concern	Birth to 6 Months	6 to 12 Months
Developmental milestone	■ Eruption of first tooth ■ Pattern of eruption	■ Pattern of eruption ■ Expected new teeth
Nutrition and feeding	■ Relation of improper bottle/ breastfeeding to initiation of dental caries ■ No propping of bottles in bed ■ Avoid use of bottle as pacifier ■ Passage of alcohol and drugs to infant through breast milk	■ Discuss weaning by age 1 year ■ Establish use of sippy cup ■ Avoid at-will access to bottle or sippy cup ■ Discuss use of juice, sweet treats, dried fruit, and retentive carbohydrates (e.g., biscuits; baked snacks or dry cereal; puffs or crunchies; and yogurt/fruit 'melts') for snacks along with their role in and caries initiation ■ Discuss consumption of sugar-sweetened beverages ■ Snacking safety (aspiration) ■ Avoid use of food for behavior modification
Oral hygiene and caries prevention	■ Discuss vertical and horizontal transmission of *Streptococcus mutans* ■ Clean ridges after each feeding (soft, wet cloth or gauze) ■ Positioning of infant for viewing and cleaning oral cavity	■ Use of brush (post-tooth eruption) and appropriate amount of fluoridated toothpaste ■ Review position of infant for brushing ■ Caregiver looks for signs of oral disease ■ Importance of maintaining primary dentition
Fluoride information	■ Explain the relation of fluoride to teeth ■ Anticipate need to supplement ■ Check water supply for fluoride content at home and daycare	■ When water supply is deficient, prescribe supplement (see Table 34-1) ■ Discuss compliance ■ Review manner of storage: cool, dry, out of reach ■ Possible fluoride varnish application
Injury prevention	■ Explain avoidance of over-the-counter benzocaine and homeopathic products for teething. ■ Discuss car seat safety	■ Discuss highest accident rate is 1–2 years ■ Car seat safety ■ Trauma proofing ■ Confirm emergency access to dental provider
Habits/function behaviors	■ Discuss teething ■ Discuss nonnutritive sucking	■ Discuss oral/head and neck signs of child abuse
Environmental (passive) smoke	■ Detrimental at all ages; smoking parents encouraged to start tobacco cessation program	■ Provide smoke-free environment
Dental/dental hygienist visit	■ Provide rationale for timing of baby's first dental visit ■ Explain what happens at first dental visit ■ Encourage parents to make appointments for their own dental care to eliminate *S. mutans* and maintain oral health	■ Schedule first dental visit within 6 months of eruption of first tooth ■ Provide information about how to make the first dental/dental hygiene visit a happy experience ■ Review need for parents to complete their own dental care

- Discussion of a healthy diet and eating practices for early childhood caries prevention.[80]
- **Anticipatory guidance** helps a parent learn what to expect during the infant's early and future developmental stages.[81]
- Eruption patterns vary and are familial in nature; the primary maxillary and mandibular central and lateral incisors generally erupt prior to age 1.[10] This process is known as teething. See Chapter 47 for tooth eruption patterns.

- Teething often causes the infant to experience mild irritability, increased salivation, and a low-grade fever.[54]
- To ease teething discomfort, a cool teething ring[43] or washcloth is recommended.
- Over-the-counter teething products containing anesthetics such as benzocaine are not recommended for children younger than 2 years.[82]
- Over-the-counter teething products containing benzocaine can cause a rare but potentially fatal condition, methemoglobinemia.[82]
- Homeopathic teething tablets and gels pose a risk for infants/children and should be avoided.[83,84]
- It is recommended an infant receive a dental examination at the eruption of the first primary tooth and no later than 12 months.[81]
- Establishment of a **dental home** for infants by no later than 12 months of age is recommended. Early establishment of a dental home is crucial in prevention of **early childhood caries** (ECC) and overall well-being.[85]
- When discussing anticipatory guidance, include the following: normal eruption patterns, infant daily oral hygiene, the role of fluoride, nutrition and diet, nonnutritive oral habits such as pacifier use and thumb sucking, speech development, and dental trauma and injury avoidance[81] (see Table 46-3).
- Developmental milestones to consider when providing patient education are outlined in **Table 46-4**.

II. Infant Daily Oral Hygiene Care

- Advise caregiver to brush the infant's teeth twice daily, with a child-size toothbrush.[81]
- A smear layer (approximately the size of a grain of rice) of fluoridated toothpaste is advised for an infant, up to the age of 3 years.[86]
- Brushing technique involves lifting of the lip to expose the cervical one-third portion of the erupted anterior teeth.[44]
- Advise caregiver to look frequently at the infant's teeth for demineralization (white chalky appearance) and early carious lesions.[81] (See Chapter 47.)

A. Inquire about Fluoride Exposure[87]

- History of exposure to fluoride.
- Fluoride level of current water supply, including childcare environments (check public health department records).
- Well water (have water tested for fluoride level).
- Use of fluoridated or unspecified bottled water.
- Use of fluoride supplementation can begin at 6 months of age.[88] (See Chapter 34.)

III. Feeding Patterns (Birth to 1 Year)

A. Frequency and Method of Feeding

- Explain the cariogenicity of certain foods and beverages, the consequence of frequent consumption of sugary beverages and foods or retentive carbohydrates, and the demineralization process.[89] (See Chapter 33.)
- Problems with feeding and sleeping
  - When the infant falls asleep after sucking, milk collects around teeth and causes demineralization, which can increase the child's risk of ECC.[89]

B. Breastfeeding

- The U.S. Surgeon General endorses exclusive breastfeeding for the first 6 months of life, and up to 12 months of age with additional nutritional supplementation after the first 6 months of life.[90]

Table 46-4 Milestones in Child Development: Birth to Age 12 Months

Areas	Birth to 6 Months	6 to 12 Months
Language	■ 0–2 months: quiets to sound ■ Reflects displeasure at noises ■ Coos and babbles	■ Says dada or mama ■ Understands name ■ Pays attention to verbalization
Motor	■ 2 months: head control ■ 6 months: transfer hand to hand ■ Grasps with forearm (ulnar grasp)	■ 7–9 months: sits ■ 9–10 months: plays pat-a-cake ■ Waves bye-bye
Social/emotional	■ 2 months: gazes at human face ■ Alert to voices	■ Inhibited by word "no" ■ Separation anxiety ■ Stranger awareness

- Evidence suggests breastfeeding can aid in dental caries prevention for at least the first 6 months of life.[91]
- Discourage prolonged, at-will breastfeeding after tooth eruption.[89]
- If the infant sleeps with the mother, discourage nocturnal breastfeeding after the eruption of the first tooth.[89]

C. *Bottle Feeding*

- The American Dental Association supports the use of fluoridated water with liquid or powdered concentrated infant formula.[92]
- Hold the child during feeding.[89]
- Discourage putting the infant to bed with a bottle containing anything other than fluoridated water after the first tooth eruption.[93]
- Avoid use of sweetened milk, juice, or other sweet liquids in a bottle or sippy cup.[89]
- Inquire about the age when other children in the family were weaned.
- Encourage parents to have infant drink from a cup by age 1 year. The American Academy of Pediatric Dentistry recommends children be weaned from the bottle at approximately 12–18 months of age.[93]

IV. Nonnutritive Sucking

- Suggestions for pacifier selection and use:
  - The use of pacifiers has been shown to decrease the incidence of SIDS.[93]
  - The American Academy of Pediatrics Task Force on SIDS recommends the use of a pacifier throughout the first year of life.[94]
  - Choose a pacifier with solid construction that cannot be pulled apart. **Figure 46-3** shows two types of pacifiers: one has an orthodontic nipple and the other a nonorthodontic nipple. The orthodontic nipple is designed to be more like a mother's breast nipple during nursing.
  - The orthodontic nipple is reported to cause less severity of malocclusion when compared to the conventional nipple.[95]
  - Ventilated shield larger than the child's mouth, at least 1–1/2 inches (3.8 cm) wide, to prevent swallowing.[96]
  - Avoid tying to the crib, child's clothing, or around the neck or hand, which could lead to strangulation.[96]

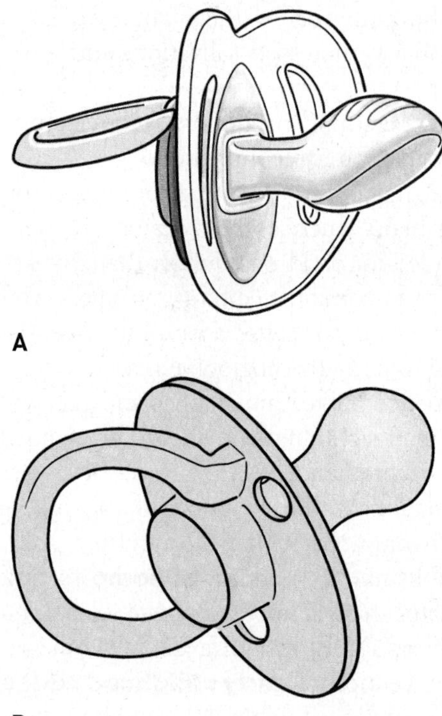

Figure 46-3 Criteria for Selecting Pacifiers. Two styles of pacifier nipples: (**A**) orthodontic and (**B**) conventional. True orthodontic pacifiers expand to support the palate and maintain natural tongue posture. It is important to select the appropriate bulb size for each stage of development (0–2, 3–6, 6–18 months). Criteria for selection of a safe pacifier; size of shield is wider than child's mouth (at least 1.25 inches) in diameter; shield has air vents; plastic portion is of sturdy construction to prevent separation and possible choking; and nipple is checked frequently for cracking and stickiness, at which time pacifier is replaced.

  - Avoid cleaning in the parent's/caregiver's mouth since caries-producing bacteria could be transferred to the infant.[97]
  - Clean in warm, soapy water. Replace with a new pacifier regularly.[96]

V. Components of the First Dental Visit

A first dental visit is recommended at the eruption of the first tooth, and no later than age 1 year.[81]

- One of the major reasons for this first visit is to establish a dental home.[85] (See Chapter 47.)

A. *Components of Dental Visit*

- To ensure patient cooperation, schedule the first visit at a time that is best for baby.

- A thorough medical history is necessary prior to beginning the infant oral examination.
- Explain to caregiver that crying is common during the oral examination.
- Complete a caries risk assessment and discuss potential risk factors for ECC and **severe ECC**.[73] Some of the risk factors include:
  - Diet and feeding patterns.[98]
  - Poor daily oral hygiene care.[89]
  - Limited/no water fluoridation exposure.[71]
  - Poor maternal dental health. Research shows a strong association between maternal caries-producing bacterial loads and ECC development.
  - The process known as vertical transmission occurs when saliva containing *S. mutans* is exchanged from a primary caregiver to an infant. This can occur during kissing, sharing of food, drink, eating utensils, and the cleaning of pacifiers via the caregiver's mouth.[65]
  - The process known as horizontal transmission occurs when saliva containing *S. mutans* is exchanged between siblings and children at daycare.[99]

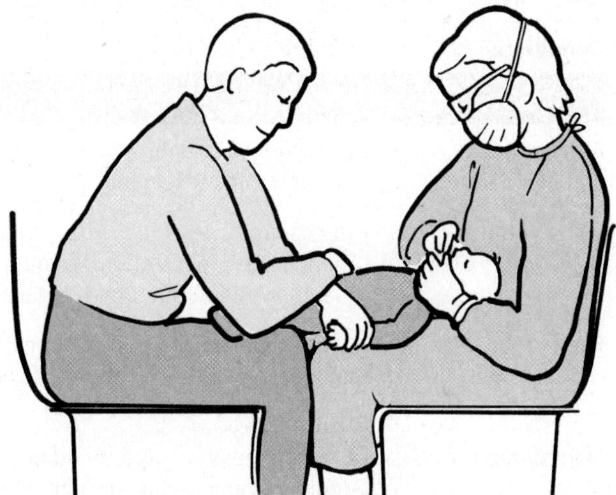

Figure 46-4 Knee-to-Knee Infant Examination. The clinician makes the oral examination, discusses oral findings, and demonstrates proper oral care for the parent. The position of the infant then is reversed so the parent has the opportunity to position the child and demonstrate proper oral care.

B. Oral Examination: Positioning to Access[3]

- Seat parent and clinician knee to knee.
- Place child's head on the lap of the examiner, as seen in **Figure 46-4**.
- Have caregiver crisscross arms gently across the infant's body, stabilizing the infant's hands and feet.

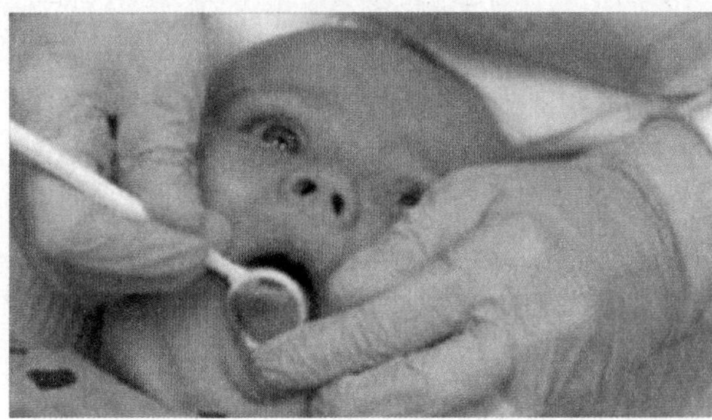

Figure 46-5 Infant Oral Examination. Using a plastic mirror. Looking for presence of carious lesions on primary (deciduous) teeth.

C. Examination Sequence

- Examine the child's head and neck, legs, and arms for evidence of abuse. Signs of abuse are described in Chapter 14.
- When teeth are present, lift the lips away from the gingival margin to observe the condition of the anterior teeth (**Figure 46-5**).
- Examine all teeth for evidence of biofilm, discoloration.[81]
- Look for malformations, dental caries, and white spot lesions. (See Chapter 47.)
- Assess for atypical frenum attachment that may potentially limit tongue mobility and cause feeding issues.[54]
- Show parents oral findings and inform them of the significance.
- Make referral to the dentist if evidence of pathology is noted (Table 46-1 and **Table 46-5**).

D. Treatment

- Biofilm removal: use dampened cloth to clean gums[54] and a soft infant-size toothbrush when teeth are present.[100]
- Fluoride varnish (2.26% fluoride ion/5% sodium fluoride) application is recommended for children younger than 6 years who are moderate-to-high risk for ECC on a quarterly basis or at least biannually.[100]

Table 46-5 Oral Soft and Hard Tissue Conditions/Pathology in Infants (0–6 Months)

Conditions	Findings	Significance/Treatment
Soft Tissue		
Ankyloglossia	Short lingual frenum; may limit tongue mobility; hinder feeding	May resolve with development; surgical correction if interferes with feeding
Bohn nodules	Buccal and lingual aspects of maxillary and mandibular ridges and hard palate; mucous gland remnant; smooth, translucent nodules	No treatment; independently resolves
Cleft	Various classifications of severity (class 1–7); unilateral or bilateral; lip and/or palate	Evaluate for possible submucous palatal cleft; treatment is individualized; surgical closure and rehabilitation
Dental lamina cysts	Crest of maxillary and mandibular ridges; dental lamina origin; smooth, translucent	No treatment; independently resolves
Epstein's pearls	Palate near raphe; keratin-filled cysts; smooth, translucent nodules	No treatment; independently resolves
Oropharyngeal candidiasis (thrush)	Mucosa or tongue; white, curd-like plaques; wiping off leaves red and inflamed area	Discomfort; nystatin to infant and to nipples of breastfeeding mother; symptoms dissipate in approximately 2 weeks
Primary herpetic gingivostomatitis	Erythematous gingiva; mucosal hemorrhages; small cluster vesicles throughout oral cavity	Discomfort; encourage fluids; oral acyclovir may shorten duration of symptoms
Teeth		
Natal/neonatal teeth	85% mandibular primary incisors; natal teeth are present at birth; neonatal erupt first month; attachment is limited to gingival margin	Discomfort; ulceration and bleeding; treatment is individualized; extraction if suspect detachment and aspiration; oral analgesics for discomfort

Data from American Academy of Pediatric Dentistry. Perinatal and infant oral health care. *The Reference Manual of Pediatric Dentistry*. 2021.

Documentation

- Documentation for the pregnant patient includes a minimum of the following:
  - Thorough medical history; medications/supplements taken; use of tobacco, alcohol, or illicit drugs; history of gestational diabetes, miscarriage, hypertension, and morning sickness.
  - Consultations with primary care provider and obstetrician along with their response.
  - Oral examination findings with areas of concern that need treatment and follow-up.
  - Changes from previous examinations with respect to oral self-care by the patient and record types of instruction provided.
- A sample progress note may be found in **Box 46-1**.

Factors to Teach the Patient

- The relationship of oral health of the mother to the general health of the fetus and newborn.
- The serious effects of tobacco and other drugs on the health of the fetus, the infant, and the child.
- Reasons for dental hygiene appointments early during pregnancy, at regular intervals throughout pregnancy, and after birth of the baby.
- Rationale for receiving professional oral health care during pregnancy.
- The rationale for maintaining good oral self-care to control dental biofilm throughout the pregnancy and after the baby's birth.
- Self-examination of the oral cavity to evaluate the effectiveness of daily dental biofilm removal and the health of the soft tissues.
- Reasons for limiting fermentable carbohydrate intake, drinking fluoridated water, and maintaining a healthy diet from the fruit, vegetable, grain, meat and meat alternatives, and dairy food groups.

Box 46-1 Example Documentation: Pregnant Patient

- **S**—A 32-year-old female presents for a 3-month continuing care appointment. Patient is in her second trimester, 15th week of pregnancy. Patient is currently taking folic acid (vitamin B9) supplement, 600 mcg, and prenatal vitamin daily. Patient reports mild nausea "morning sickness" during the morning hours. Patient's chief complaint: mild bleeding when brushing. States she has not been compliant with daily oral self-care, as her 1-year-old requires a lot of attention.
- **O**—Intraoral assessment reveals generalized gingival inflammation, edematous and erythematous, with generalized light biofilm/plaque, new localized subgingival calculus deposits on mandibular posterior molars. Hard tissue examination: cavitated carious lesion on #3. Periodontal examination findings: localized BOP #2, 3, 14, 18, 30, 31; localized 4-mm periodontal pocket depths on #2, 3, 14, 18, 31 were noted in periodontal chart.
- **A**—Patient presents at a high caries risk. Periodontal condition: gingivitis combination of plaque-induced and pregnancy.
- **P**—Patient congratulated on keeping the 3-month maintenance appointment, as last appointment was previously canceled. Frequent bathroom breaks were offered. Dietary analysis completed and resources for improved nutritional intake were given. Relationship of nutritional intake for patient and baby was discussed, as well as dental caries relationship to carbohydrate foods. Patient demonstrated toothbrushing method, and better angulation was suggested. A powered electric toothbrush was advised for improved oral health. Discussed anticipatory guidance for new baby and 1-year-old son.

Next visit: Restorative #3. Additionally, patient scheduled son for 1-year oral health assessment.

Signed: ______________________________, RDH

Date ________________

References

1. Oral Health Care During Pregnancy Expert Workgroup. *Oral health care during pregnancy: A National consensus statement*. 2012. https://www.mchoralhealth.org/PDFs/OralHealthPregnancyConsensus.pdf. Accessed August 19, 2021.
2. U.S. Department of Health and Human Services, Office on Women's Health. Prenatal care. Published April 1, 2019. https://www.womenshealth.gov/a-z-topics/prenatal-care. Accessed August 19, 2021.
3. Barzel R, Holt K, eds. *Oral Health During Pregnancy: A Resource Guide*. 3rd ed. Washington, DC: National Maternal and Child Oral Health Resource Center; 2020.
4. American College of Obstetricians and Gynecologists; Women's Health Care Physicians, Committee on Health Care for Underserved Women. *Committee Opinion Number 569. Oral Health Care during Pregnancy and Through the Lifespan*. August 2013. Reaffirmed 2019. https://www.acog.org/en/clinical/clinical-guidance/committee-opinion/articles/2013/08/oral-health-care-during-pregnancy-and-through-the-lifespan. Accessed August 19, 2021.
5. Rocha JS, Arima L, Chibinski AC, et al. Barriers and facilitators to dental care during pregnancy: a systematic review and meta-synthesis of qualitative studies. *Cad Saude Publica*. 2018;34(8):e00130817.
6. Owens P, Manski R, Weiss A. Emergency department visits involving dental conditions, 2018. In: *Healthcare Cost and Utilization Project (HCUP) Statistical Briefs*. Rockville, MD: Agency for Healthcare Research and Quality; 2006.
7. U.S. Department of Health and Human Services Office on Women's Health. Stages of pregnancy. Published April 18, 2019. https://www.womenshealth.gov/pregnancy/youre-pregnant-now-what/stages-pregnancy. Accessed August 23, 2021.
8. Cunningham FG, Leveno KJ, Bloom SL, et al. *Williams Obstetrics*. 25th ed. McGraw Hill; 2018.
9. Hardy K, Hardy PJ. 1(st) trimester miscarriage: four decades of study. *Transl Pediatr*. 2015;4(2):189-200.
10. Lunt RC, Law DB. A review of the chronology of calcification of deciduous teeth. *J Am Dent Assoc*. 1974;89(3):599-606.
11. Favero V, Bacci C, Volpato A, et al. Pregnancy and dentistry: a literature review on risk management during dental surgical procedures. *Dent J*. 2021;9(4):46.
12. Daalderop LA, Wieland BV, Tomsin K, et al. Periodontal disease and pregnancy outcomes: overview of systematic reviews. *JDR Clin Transl Res*. 2018;3(1):10-27.
13. Komine-Aizawa S, Aizawa S, Hayakawa S. Periodontal diseases and adverse pregnancy outcomes. *J Obstet Gynaecol Res*. 2019;45(1):5-12.
14. American Academy of Periodontology. Statement regarding periodontal management of the pregnant patient. *J Periodontol*. 2004;75(3):495.
15. Advisory Committee on Immunization Practices, Workgroup on the Use of Vaccines during Pregnancy and Breastfeeding. *Guiding principles for development of ACIP recommendations for vaccination during pregnancy and breastfeeding*. https://www.cdc.gov/vaccines/hcp/acip-recs/rec-vac-preg.html?CDC_AA_refVal=https%3A%2F%2Fwww.cdc.gov%2Fvaccines%2Facip%2Fcommittee%2Fguidance%2Frec-vac-preg.html. Accessed August 23, 2021.

16. Pinheiro EA, Stika CS. Drugs in pregnancy: pharmacologic and physiologic changes that affect clinical care. *Semin Perinatol*. 2020;44(3):151221.
17. Lee JM, Shin TJ. Use of local anesthetics for dental treatment during pregnancy: safety for parturient. *J Dent Anesth Pain Med*. 2017;17(2):81-90.
18. Ansari J, Carvalho B, Shafer SL, Flood P. Pharmacokinetics and pharmacodynamics of drugs commonly used in pregnancy and parturition. *Anesth Analg*. 2016;122(3):786-804.
19. Omranipoor A, Kashanian M, Dehghani M, Sadeghi M, Baradaran HR. Association of antibiotics therapy during pregnancy with spontaneous miscarriage: a systematic review and meta-analysis. *Arch Gynecol Obstet*. 2020;302(1):5-22.
20. Chilaka VN, Konje JC. HIV in pregnancy – an update. *Eur J Obstet Gynecol Reprod Biol*. 2021;256:484-491.
21. Avşar TS, McLeod H, Jackson L. Health outcomes of smoking during pregnancy and the postpartum period: an umbrella review. *BMC Pregnancy Childbirth*. 2021;21(1):254.
22. Regan AK, Bombard JM, O'Hegarty MM, Smith RA, Tong VT. Adverse birth outcomes associated with prepregnancy and prenatal electronic cigarette use. *Obstet Gynecol*. 2021;138(1):85-94.
23. Lange S, Probst C, Gmel G, Global prevalence of fetal alcohol spectrum disorder among children and youth: a systematic review and meta-analysis. *JAMA Pediatr*. 2017;171(10): 948-956.
24. Bandoli G, Jelliffe-Pawlowski L, Schumacher B, et al. Cannabis-related diagnosis in pregnancy and adverse maternal and infant outcomes. *Drug Alcohol Depend*. 2021;225: 108757.
25. National Institute on Drug Abuse. *What are the effects of secondhand and thirdhand tobacco smoke?* Published 2021. https://www.drugabuse.gov/publications/research-reports/tobacco-nicotine-e-cigarettes/what-are-effects-secondhand-thirdhand-tobacco-smoke. Accessed August 24, 2021.
26. Muñoz Balbontín Y, Stewart D, Shetty A, Fitton CA, McLay JS. Herbal medicinal product use during pregnancy and the postnatal period: a systematic review. *Obstet Gynecol*. 2019;133(5): 920-932.
27. U.S. Food and Drug Administration, Office of Dietary Supplement Programs. Dietary supplements. Published August 16, 2019. https://www.fda.gov/food/dietary-supplements. Accessed August 24, 2021.
28. Figuero E, Carrillo-de-Albornoz A, Martín C, Tobías A, Herrera D. Effect of pregnancy on gingival inflammation in systemically healthy women: a systematic review. *J Clin Periodontol*. 2013;40(5):457-473.
29. González-Jaranay M, Téllez L, Roa-López A, Gómez-Moreno G, Moreu G. Periodontal status during pregnancy and postpartum. *PloS One*. 2017;12(5):e0178234.
30. Hartnett E, Haber J, Krainovich-Miller B, et al. Oral health in pregnancy. *J Obstet Gynecol Neonatal Nurs*. 2016;45(4): 565-573.
31. Wu M, Chen S-W, Su W-L, et al. Sex hormones enhance gingival inflammation without affecting IL-1β and TNF-α in periodontally healthy women during pregnancy. *Mediators Inflamm*. 2016;2016:4897890.
32. Lasisi TJ, Abdus-Salam RA. Pregnancy-induced periodontal inflammation: influence of salivary cytokines and antimicrobial proteins. *Saudi Dent J*. 2018;30(4):306-311.
33. Jang H, Patoine A, Wu TT, Castillo DA, Xiao J. Oral microflora and pregnancy: a systematic review and meta-analysis. *Sci Rep*. 2021;11(1):16870.
34. Figuero E, Carrillo-de-Albornoz A, Herrera D, Bascones-Martínez A. Gingival changes during pregnancy: I. Influence of hormonal variations on clinical and immunological parameters. *J Clin Periodontol*. 2010;37(3):220-229.
35. Jafarzadeh H, Sanatkhani M, Mohtasham N. Oral pyogenic granuloma: a review. *J Oral Sci*. 2006;48(4):167-175.
36. Silva de Araujo Figueiredo C, Gonçalves Carvalho Rosalem C, Costa Cantanhede AL, Abreu Fonseca Thomaz ÉB, Fontoura Nogueira da Cruz MC. Systemic alterations and their oral manifestations in pregnant women. *J Obstet Gynaecol Res*. 2017;43(1):16-22.
37. Maymone MBC, Greer RO, Burdine LK, et al. Benign oral mucosal lesions: clinical and pathological findings. *J Am Acad Dermatol*. 2019;81(1):43-56.
38. Wu M, Chen S-W, Jiang S-Y. Relationship between gingival inflammation and pregnancy. *Mediators Inflamm*. 2015;2015:623427.
39. Gare J, Kanoute A, Meda N, et al. Periodontal conditions and pathogens associated with pre-eclampsia: a scoping review. *Int J Environ Res Public Health*. 2021;18(13):7194.
40. Govindasamy R, Periyasamy S, Narayanan M, et al. The influence of nonsurgical periodontal therapy on the occurrence of adverse pregnancy outcomes: a systematic review of the current evidence. *J Indian Soc Periodontol*. 2020;24(1):7-14.
41. Lavigne SE, Forrest JL. An umbrella review of systematic reviews of the evidence of a causal relationship between periodontal disease and adverse pregnancy outcomes: a position paper from the Canadian Dental Hygienists Association. *Can J Dent Hyg*. 2020;54(2):92-100.
42. Donovan T, Nguyen-Ngoc C, Abd Alraheam I, Irusa K. Contemporary diagnosis and management of dental erosion. *J Esthet Restor Dent*. 2021;33(1):78-87.
43. Massachusetts Department of Public Health. Massachusetts oral health practice guidelines for pregnancy and early childhood. March 2016. https://www.mass.gov/files/documents/2016/10/ne/oral-health-guidelines.pdf. Accessed August 24, 2021.
44. Sanz M, Ceriello A, Buysschaert M, et al. Scientific evidence on the links between periodontal diseases and diabetes: consensus report and guidelines of the joint workshop on periodontal diseases and diabetes by the International Diabetes Federation and the European Federation of Periodontology. *J Clin Periodontol*. 2018;45(2):138-149.
45. American Academy on Pediatric Dentistry, Council on Clinical Affairs Committee on the Adolescent. Guideline on oral health care for the pregnant adolescent. *Pediatr Dent*. 2016;38(5): 59-66.
46. American Academy of Pediatric Dentistry. Oral health care for the pregnant pediatric dental patient. Published online 2021. https://www.aapd.org/globalassets/media/policies_guidelines/bp_pregnancy.pdf. Accessed August 24, 2021.
47. Committee Opinion No. 723: guidelines for diagnostic imaging during pregnancy and lactation. *Obstet Gynecol*. 2017; 130(4):e210-e216.
48. Horst JA. Silver fluoride as a treatment for dental caries. *Adv Dent Res*. 2018;29(1):135-140.
49. Kurien S, Kattimani VS, Sriram RR, et al. Management of pregnant patient in dentistry. *J Int Oral Health*. 2013;5(1):88-97.
50. Massoth C, Chappell D, Kranke P, Wenk M. Supine hypotensive syndrome of pregnancy: a review of current knowledge. *Eur J Anaesthesiol*. 2022;39(3):236-243.
51. California Dental Association Foundation, American College of Obstetricians and Gynecologists, District IX. Oral health

during pregnancy and early childhood: evidence-based guidelines for health professionals. *J Calif Dent Assoc*. 2010;38(6): 391-403, 405-440.

52. Zafirova Z, Sheehan C, Hosseinian L. Update on nitrous oxide and its use in anesthesia practice. *Best Pract Res Clin Anaesthesiol*. 2018;32(2):113-123.
53. American Academy Pediatric Dentistry. Perinatal and infant oral health care. Published online 2021. https://www.aapd.org/globalassets/media/policies_guidelines/bp_perinataloralhealthcare.pdf. Accessed August 23, 2021.
54. Stang J, Huffman LG. Position of the Academy of Nutrition and Dietetics: obesity, reproduction, and pregnancy outcomes. *J Acad Nutr Diet*. 2016;116(4):677-691.
55. Procter SB, Campbell CG. Position of the Academy of Nutrition and Dietetics: nutrition and lifestyle for a healthy pregnancy outcome. *J Acad Nutr Diet*. 2014;114(7):1099-1103.
56. Jouanne M, Oddoux S, Noël A, Voisin-Chiret AS. Nutrient requirements during pregnancy and lactation. *Nutrients*. 2021;13(2):692.
57. US Department of Agriculture. Pregnancy and breastfeeding. My Plate. https://www.myplate.gov/life-stages/pregnancy-and-breastfeeding. Accessed August 29, 2021.
58. Isola G. The impact of diet, nutrition and nutraceuticals on oral and periodontal health. *Nutrients*. 2020;12(9):E2724.
59. Najeeb S, Zafar MS, Khurshid Z, Zohaib S, Almas K. The role of nutrition in periodontal health: an update. *Nutrients*. 2016;8(9):E530.
60. Brown B, Wright C. Safety and efficacy of supplements in pregnancy. *Nutr Rev*. 2020;78(10):813-826.
61. Office of Dietary Supplements (ODS). Calcium. Published August 17, 2021. https://ods.od.nih.gov/factsheets/Calcium-HealthProfessional/. Accessed August 19, 2021.
62. Frayer NC, Kim Y. Caffeine intake during pregnancy and risk of childhood obesity: a systematic review. *Int J MCH AIDS*. 2020;9(3):364-380.
63. Featherstone JDB, Chaffee BW. The evidence for caries management by risk assessment (CAMBRA®). *Adv Dent Res*. 2018;29(1):9-14.
64. da Silva Bastos Vde V de A, Freitas-Fernandes LB, Fidalgo TK da S, et al. Mother-to-child transmission of *Streptococcus mutans*: a systematic review and meta-analysis. *J Dent*. 2015;43(2):181-191.
65. Jevtić M, Pantelinaci J, Jovanović Ilić T, et al, The role of nutrition in caries prevention and maintenance of oral health during pregnancy. *Med Pregl*. 2015;68(11-12):387-393.
66. Yousefi M, Parvaie P, Riahi SM. Salivary factors related to caries in pregnancy: a systematic review and meta-analysis. *J Am Dent Assoc*. 2020;151(8):576-588.e4.
67. Azofeifa A, Yeung LF, Alverson CJ, Beltrán-Aguilar E. Dental caries and periodontal disease among U.S. pregnant women and nonpregnant women of reproductive age, National Health and Nutrition Examination Survey, 1999-2004. *J Public Health Dent*. 2016;76(4):320-329.
68. Takahashi R, Ota E, Hoshi K, et al. Fluoride supplementation (with tablets, drops, lozenges or chewing gum) in pregnant women for preventing dental caries in the primary teeth of their children. *Cochrane Database Syst Rev*. 2017;10:CD011850.
69. Carey CM. Focus on fluorides: update on the use of fluoride for the prevention of dental caries. *J Evid-Based Dent Pract*. 2014;14 Suppl:95-102.
70. Iheozor-Ejiofor Z, Worthington HV, Walsh T, et al. Water fluoridation for the prevention of dental caries. *Cochrane Database Syst Rev*. 2015;(6):CD010856.
71. Dennis C-L, Falah-Hassani K, Shiri R. Prevalence of antenatal and postnatal anxiety: systematic review and meta-analysis. *Br J Psychiatry J Ment Sci*. 2017;210(5):315-323.
72. Van Niel MS, Payne JL. Perinatal depression: a review. *Cleve Clin J Med*. 2020;87(5):273-277.
73. Okagbue HI, Adamu PI, Bishop SA, Oguntunde PE, Opanuga AA, Akhmetshin EM. Systematic review of prevalence of antepartum depression during the trimesters of pregnancy. *Open Access Maced J Med Sci*. 2019;7(9):1555-1560.
74. Dadi AF, Miller ER, Bisetegn TA, Mwanri L. Global burden of antenatal depression and its association with adverse birth outcomes: an umbrella review. *BMC Public Health*. 2020;20:173.
75. Daley D, McCauley M, van den Broek N. Interventions for women who report domestic violence during and after pregnancy in low- and middle-income countries: a systematic literature review. *BMC Pregnancy Childbirth*. 2020;20(1):141.
76. Petrone P, Jiménez-Morillas P, Axelrad A, Marini CP. Traumatic injuries to the pregnant patient: a critical literature review. *Eur J Trauma Emerg Surg*. 2019;45(3):383-392.
77. Pastor-Moreno G, Ruiz-Pérez I, Henares-Montiel J, et al. Intimate partner violence and perinatal health: a systematic review. *BJOG*. 2020;127(5):537-547.
78. Stubbs A, Szoeke C. The effect of intimate partner violence on the physical health and health-related behaviors of women: A systematic review of the literature. *Trauma Violence Abuse*. 2022;23(4):1157-1172.
79. Riggs E, Kilpatrick N, Slack-Smith L, et al. Interventions with pregnant women, new mothers and other primary caregivers for preventing early childhood caries. *Cochrane Database Syst Rev*. 2019;2019(11).
80. American Academy of Pediatric Dentistry. Periodicity of examination, preventive dental services, anticipatory guidance/counseling, and oral treatment for infants, children, and adolescents. *Pediatr Dent*. 2018;40(6):194-204.
81. U.S. Food and Drug Administration. *Risk of serious and potentially fatal blood disorder prompts FDA action on oral over-the-counter Benzocaine products used for teething and mouth pain and prescription local anesthetics*. Published May 23, 2018. https://www.fda.gov/drugs/drug-safety-and-availability/risk-serious-and-potentially-fatal-blood-disorder-prompts-fda-action-oral-over-counter-benzocaine. Accessed November 3, 2022.
82. U.S. Food & Drug Administration. *FDA warns against the use of homeopathic teething tablets and gels*. Published 2016. https://www.fda.gov/news-events/press-announcements/fda-warns-against-use-homeopathic-teething-tablets-and-gels. Accessed August 31, 2021.
83. U.S. Food & Drug Administration. *FDA warns consumers about homeopathic teething products. FDA*. Published November 4, 2019. https://www.fda.gov/drugs/information-drug-class/fda-warns-consumers-about-homeopathic-teething-products. Accessed August 31, 2021.
84. American Academy of Pediatric Dentistry. *Policy on the dental home*. Published 2020. https://www.aapd.org/globalassets/media/policies_guidelines/p_dentalhome.pdf. Accessed August 31, 2021.
85. American Dental Association Council on Scientific Affairs. Fluoride toothpaste use for young children. *J Am Dent Assoc*. 2014;145(2):190-191.
86. American Dental Association. Fluoridation facts. Published 2018. https://www.ada.org/~/media/ADA/Files/Fluoridation_Facts.pdf?la=en. Accessed September 2, 2021.

87. Rozier RG, Adair S, Graham F, et al. Evidence-based clinical recommendations on the prescription of dietary fluoride supplements for caries prevention: a report of the American Dental Association Council on Scientific Affairs. *J Am Dent Assoc*. 2010;141(12):1480-1489.
88. Kirthiga M, Murugan M, Saikia A, Kirubakaran R. Risk factors for early childhood caries: a systematic review and meta-analysis of case control and cohort studies. *Pediatr Dent*. 2019;41(2):95-112.
89. U.S. Department of Health and Human. Executive summary: the Surgeon General's call to action to support breastfeeding. *Breastfeed Med*. 2011;6(1):3-5.
90. Avila WM, Pordeus IA, Paiva SM, Martins CC. Breast and bottle feeding as risk factors for dental caries: a systematic review and meta-analysis. *PloS One*. 2015;10(11):e0142922.
91. Berg J, Gerweck C, Hujoel PP, et al. Evidence-based clinical recommendations regarding fluoride intake from reconstituted infant formula and enamel fluorosis: a report of the American Dental Association Council on Scientific Affairs. *J Am Dent Assoc*. 2011;142(1):79-87.
92. Policy on Early Childhood Caries (ECC): classifications, consequences, and preventive strategies. *Pediatr Dent*. 2018;40(6): 60-62.
93. Moon RY, Task Force on Sudden Infant Death Syndrome. SIDS and other sleep-related iinfant deaths: evidence base for 2016 updated recommendations for a safe infant sleeping environment. *Pediatrics*. 2016;138(5):e20162940.
94. Lima AADSJ, Alves CMC, Ribeiro CCC, et al. Effects of conventional and orthodontic pacifiers on the dental occlusion of children aged 24-36 months old. *Int J Paediatr Dent*. 2017;27(2):108-119.
95. American Academy of Pediatrics. Pacifier safety. Published November 19, 2018. https://www.healthychildren.org/English/safety-prevention/at-home/Pages/Pacifier-Safety.aspx. Accessed August 31, 2021.
96. Anil S, Anand PS. Early childhood caries: prevalence, risk factors, and prevention. *Front Pediatr*. 2017;5:157.
97. Wong A, Subar PE, Young DA. Dental caries: an update on dental trends and therapy. *Adv Pediatr*. 2017;64(1): 307-330.
98. Manchanda S, Sardana D, Liu P, et al. Horizontal transmission of *Streptococcus mutans* in children and its association with dental caries: a systematic review and meta-analysis. *Pediatr Dent*. 2021;43(1):1E-12E.
99. American Academy of Pediatric Dentistry. Perinatal and infant oral health care. In: *The Reference Manual of Pediatric Dentistry*. Chicago, IL: American Academy of Pediatric Dentistry; 2021:262-266.
100. Weyant RJ, Tracy SL, Anselmo TT, et al. Topical fluoride for caries prevention: executive summary of the updated clinical recommendations and supporting systematic review. *J Am Dent Assoc*. 2013;144(11):1279-1291.

CHAPTER 47

The Pediatric Patient

Dana E. Kleckler, RDH, BS
Lisa F. Mallonee, RDH, RD, LD, MPH

CHAPTER OUTLINE

LEARNING OBJECTIVES

After studying this chapter, the reader will be able to:

1. Describe the specialty of pediatric dentistry.
2. Discuss the use of a caries risk assessment tool to identify an individual patient's risk and preventive factors.

3. Identify age-appropriate anticipatory guidance/counseling factors to educate parents/caregivers of toddlers, school-aged children, and adolescents.
4. Identify preventive and therapeutic oral healthcare interventions based on age and caries risk assessment.
5. Discuss oral health home care needs, adjunct aids, and continuing care recommendations for children.

Oral health for **toddlers**, **preschoolers**, **school-aged children**, and **adolescents** depends primarily on parental intervention for the young child, and gradually transitioning the child through parent involvement to independent management of daily oral self-care. Parents are:

- Provided with education through **anticipatory guidance** before a child's birth and at regular intervals thereafter. (See Chapter 46.)
- Given the information needed to assess their child's oral health status.
- Taught how to intervene and to anticipate the child's oral health needs at various ages and stages of growth and development.

Pediatric Dentistry

I. The Specialty of Pediatric Dentistry

- An age-defined specialty that provides both primary and comprehensive preventive and therapeutic oral health care for **infants** and children through adolescence, including those with special healthcare needs.[1]
- Requires 2 years of additional residency training (after the required 4 years of dental school) in dentistry for infants, children, teens, and children with special needs.[2]

II. The American Academy of Pediatric Dentistry

- The American Academy of Pediatric Dentistry (AAPD), founded in 1947, is the not-for-profit professional membership association representing the specialty of pediatric dentistry.[3]
- Pediatric dentists provide care to millions of our nation's infants, children, adolescents, and persons with special healthcare needs, and are the primary contributors to professional education programs and publications on pediatric oral health.[3]
- The AAPD's mission is to advance optimal oral health for all children by delivering outstanding service that meets and exceeds the needs and expectations of our members, partners, and stakeholders.[4]
- Professional and parental information is available at the AAPD website (www.aapd.org).[5]

The Child as a Patient

The age categories of pediatric patients are[6]:

- Infants: 0–1 year of age. (See Chapter 46.)
- Toddlers: 1–3 years of age.
- Preschoolers: 3–5 years of age.
- School-aged children (middle childhood): 6–11 years of age.
- Adolescents (young teens and teenagers): 12–17 years of age.

I. The Dental Home

- **Dental home**[7] is defined by the AAPD as "an ongoing relationship between the dentist and the patient, inclusive of all aspects of oral health care delivered in a comprehensive, continuously accessible, coordinated, and family-centered way."
- The AAPD, the American Dental Association (ADA), and the American Academy of Pediatrics recommend a dental home should be established no later than 12 months of age and include referral to dental specialties when appropriate.
- Emphasis is placed on oral health counseling and prevention. One out of 10 toddlers already has one or more dental caries.[8]

II. Barriers to Dental Care

- Availability of dental providers that accept patient's insurance, are in the geographic area, with convenient office hours, and/or are willing to see children.
- Financial (income/dental insurance).
- Lack of parental oral health literacy and the importance of oral health.
- Language.
- Transportation.

III. Child Dental Visits

A. Purposes

- The purposes of the dental hygiene visit are to:
  - Establish rapport, teach appropriate behaviors, and prevent management problems.
  - Develop and continue a relationship with the child and the family.
  - Initiate and/or strengthen positive age-appropriate preventive measures, such as fluoride usage, appropriate nutritional practices, and daily dental biofilm removal.
  - Discover, intercept, and recommend changes in any parental practices that may be detrimental to the child's oral health.
- Appointments are planned for clinical oral examination, caries risk assessment, biofilm and calculus removal, professional fluoride application, radiographic assessment, treatment planning of dental disease, evaluation of developing dentition/malocclusion, anticipatory guidance/counseling, and introduction to dental hygiene.

B. Frequency of Continuing Care

- Visits to the dental hygienist and the dentist are scheduled according to the child's specific needs. A common appointment plan for children with little or no oral disease is every 4 or 6 months.
- Some patients may require more frequent intervals based upon the child's risk factors and historical, clinical, and radiographic findings.[9]
- Reevaluation and reinforcement of preventive activities contribute to improved instruction for the parent, child, and adolescent.[9]

C. Scheduling

The best time to schedule dental visits for toddlers and young school-aged children is:

- Early in the morning when the child is well rested and more cooperative.
- After naps when the child is not tired and is more apt to listen and cooperate.

Patient Management Considerations

Cooperation is usually gained with nonverbal communication such as smiling and talking with the child and the parent.

I. Toddlers (1–3 Years of Age)

- Primary teeth are vulnerable to tooth decay upon the eruption of the first tooth, usually between the ages of 6 and 12 months.
- Children who wait to have their first dental visit until 2 or 3 years of age are more likely to require restorative and emergency visits.
- Use child-friendly terms instead of dental terms. See **Box 47-1** for examples of child-friendly terms.

A. Oral Examination: Positioning for Access

- Utilize the knee-to-knee positioning for the oral examination and teach the parent to utilize this position at home to provide thorough biofilm removal with toothbrush and floss. Refer to Chapter 46.
- Prior to performing the examination, explain to the parent proper positioning—child's legs around parent's waist, parent's elbows restrain child's legs, and parent holds child's hands on their stomach.
- It is the clinician's responsibility to control the head during the examination.
- Crying during the examination is normal behavior and can provide better visibility of the child's mouth and throat.

Box 47-1 Child-Friendly Substitution Words for Dental Terminology

Dental Term	Child-Friendly Term
Air/water syringe	Water squirter, wind
Amalgam restoration	Silver star
Dental light	Sunshine light
Explorer, scaler	Tooth counter
Fluoride varnish	Fluoride tooth vitamins
High-speed handpiece	Mr. Whistle
Low-speed handpiece	Tooth tickler, Mr. Bumpy
Mouth mirror	Tooth mirror
Mouth prop	Tooth pillow
Prophy paste	Special toothpaste
Dental hygiene treatment	Teeth cleaning
Saliva ejector	Mrs. Thirsty/special straw
Suction (high-speed)	Vacuum

B. Examination Sequence

- Examine the child's head and neck, legs, and arms for evidence of abuse. Abuse is described in Chapter 14.
- Oral soft tissues are assessed (see **Table 47-1**).[10]
- Lift the upper lip to observe the condition of the anterior teeth.

Table 47-1 Oral Soft and Hard Tissue Conditions/Pathology in Children Approximately 6 Months to 5 Years

Conditions	Findings	Significance
Soft Tissue		
Eruption cysts	Translucent, smooth; may appear blue to blue-black if bleeding in cystic space	No treatment
Mucocele	Lower lip, floor of mouth, buccal mucosa most common in order of occurrence; fluid-filled vesicle or blister; trauma, tearing of minor salivary duct	May resolve or require surgical excision
Traumatic ulcer	Ulceration of the tongue, cheek, or lip after 24 hours of a dental appointment with local anesthesia	Due to patient chewing or biting soft tissue when area is numb; complications are rare, should be seen within 24 hours; clean wound; warm saline mouthrinse; possible suture
Alveolar abscess	Smooth, red or yellowish nodule; tender; primary teeth—more diffuse infections; may be acute or chronic	Radiographic evaluation, drainage, and antibiotic may be required
Acute herpetic gingivostomatitis	Initially, yellow or white fluid-filled vesicles, which in a few days rupture and form painful ulcers; 1–3 mm diameter; whitish gray membrane cover; circumscribed area of inflammation; may have a fever; regional lymphadenopathy; diffuse, swollen erythematous gingiva; poor appetite; dehydration	Urgent care; resolves in 10–14 days; antiviral medication; mild topical anesthetic; systemic analgesics; fluids; monitor for dehydration
Geographic tongue	Red, smooth areas devoid of filiform papillae on dorsum of tongue; margins well developed, slightly raised; pattern changes	No treatment Brush tongue to reduce bacteria
Verruca vulgaris	Multiple white sessile lesions; fingerlike projections, rough surface; human papilloma virus in origin	May resolve spontaneously or require excision
Teeth		
Enamel hypoplasia	Disturbance of enamel matrix during tooth development; irregular to round pits of varying size on enamel, usually in a row; multiple causes	Esthetics
Fluorosis	Infrequent in primary dentition; may be seen in cervical region of second primary molars; appearance ranging from fine white flecks to brown opaque lesions and/or pitting	Esthetics; daily biofilm removal
White-spot lesions	Opaque enamel, usually cervical and proximal areas of teeth at contacts; earliest clinical sign of the carious process; indicates the surface and underlying enamel are demineralized	Twice daily biofilm removal with a fluoride toothpaste; professional topical fluoride treatment every 3 months; diet counseling.
Fused teeth	Usually limited to anterior teeth; union of two independently forming primary tooth buds; familial tendency	Possible caries at point of fusion; may be absence of one of corresponding permanent teeth
Gemination	More common in primary teeth; invagination of single tooth germ; bifid crown on single root; crown appears wide	None

Data from Dean JA. *McDonald and Avery's Dentistry for the Child and Adolescent*. 11th ed. Maryland Heights, MO: Elsevier; 2021.

II. Preschoolers (3–5 Years of Age)

A. Prepare the Child for the Dental Visit

- Make the dental visit as pleasant as possible for the child.
- Children are told that the dental hygienist and dentist help them take good care of their teeth.
- Parents are instructed to avoid using negative words, such as "hurt," "pain," and "don't be scared."
- When the child is not present, parents are asked if the child has any fears or has had any prior negative experiences.

B. Positioning

- For young preschoolers (3 years old) utilization of the knee-to-knee positioning may still be needed.
- May sit in the dental chair without any problems and can be encouraged with "being a big girl or boy."
- The dental chair may be modified by removing the headrest or a portion of the backrest, if possible, to better fit the child.

C. Parental Involvement

- Determine the expected developmental milestones of the child according to the chronologic age, as outlined in **Table 47-2**.[11]
- Ask parents to identify actual developmental milestones so appropriate management can be initiated during the appointment.
- Ask parents to provide a general statement regarding the child's temperament and ability to cooperate.
- Evaluate whether the parent needs to accompany the child into the treatment room.

III. School-Aged Children (6–11 Years of Age)

- Can be an active participant in the dental care visit.
- May still display signs of anxiety or uncooperativeness.
- Typically, once a child is in school full time, having a parent present during their appointments is no longer necessary.
- Child's dentition may be all primary or mixed dentition, or by 11 or 12 years of age all permanent dentition, depending on individual development.
- Examine the need for pit and fissure sealants.
- A periodontal assessment needs to be completed even if there is no bone loss. Child may have pockets, bleeding, and subgingival calculus.
- Child is starting to develop independent skills and ability to perform their own oral care.
- Continue to avoid the use of negative words.
- Avoid lecturing or reprimanding with a negative tone. Suggest, advise, and highlight the positive.
- Use of pictures for explaining proper oral hygiene, calculus, and biofilm may help the child understand.
- When teaching brushing and flossing techniques, demonstrate the techniques to the child and have the child demonstrate their ability to perform; modify as needed.

IV. Adolescents (12–18 Years of Age)

- Dental hygiene services provided during adolescence can impact oral health throughout the patient's lifetime.
- Need to assess for periodontal issues and diseases at each hygiene visit.
- May respond and wish to be treated as adults or as children at different times.
- Are learning to adapt to body changes, sexual impulses, secondary sex characteristics, and independence.
- May exhibit the different characteristics to one degree or another. **Table 47-3** lists factors related to the psychological development of adolescents.
- May have anxiety due to family issues (i.e., divorce), school performance, sexual issues, peer pressures, violence, or substance abuse.
- Concern over physical characteristics and personal appearance. Want to dress/be like their peers.
- Teachers, coaches, and health professionals can have a powerful impact with this age group.
- Additional communication strategies for motivating adolescent patients are discussed in Chapter 3.

Components of the Dental Hygiene Visit

Components of the dental visit are essentially the same for all pediatric patients. A clinical examination and diagnostic tools are utilized during a

Table 47-2 Milestones in Child Development: 12 Months to 5 Years

Areas	12 Months	18 Months	2 Years	3 Years	4 Years	5 Years
Language/ communication	■ Responds to simple spoken requests ■ Uses simple gestures, like shaking head "no" or waving "bye-bye" ■ Makes sounds with changes in tone (sounds more like speech) ■ Says "mama" and "dada" and exclamations like "uh-oh!" ■ Tries to say words you say	■ Says several single words ■ Says and shakes head "no" ■ Points to show someone what they want	■ Points to things or pictures when they are named ■ Know names of familiar people and body parts ■ Says sentences with two to four words ■ Follows simple instructions ■ Repeats words overheard in conversation ■ Points to things in a book	■ Follows instructions with two or three steps ■ Can name most familiar things ■ Understands words like "in," "on," and "under" ■ Says first name, age, and gender ■ Names a friend ■ Says words like "I," "me," "we," and "you," and some plurals (cats, dogs, cars) ■ Talks well enough for strangers to understand most of the time ■ Carries on a conversation using two to three sentences	■ Knows some basic rules of grammar, such as correctly using "he" and "she" ■ Sings a song or says a poem from memory such as the "Itsy Bitsy Spider" or the "Wheels on the Bus" ■ Tells stories ■ Can say first and last name	■ Speaks very clearly ■ Tells a simple story using full sentences ■ Uses future tense; for example, "Grandma will be here" ■ Says name and address
Movement/ physical development	■ Gets to a sitting position without help ■ Pulls up to stand, walks holding on to furniture. May take a few steps without holding on ■ May stand alone	■ Walks alone ■ May walk up steps and run ■ Pulls toys while walking ■ Can help undress self ■ Drinks from a cup ■ Eats with a spoon	■ Stands on tiptoe ■ Kicks a ball ■ Begins to run	■ Climbs well ■ Runs easily ■ Pedals a tricycle (three-wheel bike) ■ Walks up and down stairs, one foot on each step	■ Hops and stands on one foot up to 2 seconds ■ Catches a bounced ball most of the time ■ Pours, cuts with supervision, and mashes own food	■ Stands on one foot for 10 seconds or longer ■ Hops; may be able to skip ■ Can do a somersault ■ Uses a fork and spoon and sometimes a table knife ■ Can use the toilet on their own ■ Swings and climbs

Social/ emotional	■ Shy/nervous with strangers ■ Cries when mom or dad leaves ■ Has favorite things and people ■ Shows fear in some situations ■ Hands you a book when they want to hear a story ■ Repeats sounds or actions to get attention ■ Puts out arm or leg to help with dressing ■ Plays "peak-a-boo" or "pat-a-cake"	■ Likes to hand things to others as play ■ May have temper tantrum ■ May be afraid of strangers ■ Shows affection to familiar people ■ Plays simple pretend, such as feeding a doll ■ May cling to caregivers in new situations ■ Points to show others something interesting ■ Explores alone but with parent close by	■ Copies others, especially adults and older children ■ Gets excited when with other children ■ Shows more and more independence ■ Shows defiant behavior (doing what they have been told not to) ■ Plays mainly beside other children, but is beginning to include other children, such as chase games	■ Copies adults and friends ■ Shows affection for friends without prompting ■ Takes turns in games ■ Shows concern for a crying friend ■ Understands the idea of "mine" and "his" or "hers" ■ Shows a wide range of emotions ■ Separates easily from mom and dad ■ May get upset with major changes in routine ■ Dresses and undresses self	■ Enjoys doing new things ■ Play "Mom" or "Dad" ■ Is more creative with make-believe play ■ Would rather play with other children than alone ■ Cooperates with other children ■ Often cannot tell what is real and what is make-believe ■ Talks about what they like and are interested in	■ Wants to please friends ■ Wants to be like friends ■ More likely to agree with rules ■ Likes to sing, dance, and act ■ Is aware of gender ■ Can tell what is real and what is make-believe ■ Shows more independence (e.g., may visit a next-door neighbor on their own [adult supervision is still needed]) ■ Is sometimes demanding and sometimes very cooperative
Cognitive (learning, thinking, problem-solving)	■ Explores things in different ways, like shaking, banging, throwing ■ Finds hidden things easily ■ Looks at the right picture or thing when it is named ■ Copies gestures ■ Starts to use things correctly: drinks from a cup, brushes hair ■ Bangs two things together ■ Puts things in a container; takes things out of a container ■ Lets things go without help ■ Pokes with index finger ■ Follows simple directions like "pick up the toy"	■ Knows what ordinary things are for (telephone, brush, spoon) ■ Points to get the attention of others ■ Shows interest in a doll or stuffed animal by pretending to feed ■ Points to one body part ■ Scribble on their own ■ Can follow one-step verbal commands without any gestures (sits when you say "sit down")	■ Finds things even when hidden under two or three covers ■ Begins to sort shapes and colors ■ Completes sentences and rhymes in familiar books ■ Plays simple make-believe games ■ Builds towers of four or more blocks ■ Might use one hand more than the other ■ Follow two-step instructions such as "Pick up your shoes and put them in the closet" ■ Names items in a picture book such as a cat, bird, or dog	■ Can work toys with buttons, levers, and moving parts ■ Plays make-believe with dolls, animals, and people ■ Does puzzles with three or four pieces ■ Understands what "two" means ■ Copies a circle with pencil or crayon ■ Turns book pages one at a time ■ Builds towers of more than six blocks ■ Screws and unscrews jar lids or turns door handle	■ Names some colors and some numbers ■ Understands the idea of counting ■ Starts to understand time ■ Remembers parts of a story ■ Understands the idea of "same" and "different" ■ Draws a person with two to four body parts ■ Uses scissors ■ Starts to copy some capital letters ■ Plays board or card games ■ Tells you what he thinks is going to happen next in a book	■ Counts 10 or more things ■ Can draw a person with at least six body parts ■ Can print some letters or numbers ■ Copies a triangle and other geometric shapes ■ Knows about things used every day, like money and food

Data from Centers for Disease Control and Prevention. Learn the signs. Act early. https://www.cdc.gov/ncbddd/actearly/index.html. Published November 3, 2017. Updated February 18, 2021. Accessed.March 30,2022.

Table 47-3 Psychosocial Development of Adolescents

	Early Adolescence Approximately 11–13 Years of Age	Middle Adolescent Approximately 14–17 Years of Age	Late Adolescent Approximately 18–21 Years of Age
Environment	■ Home ■ Middle school ■ Extracurricular activities	■ Home ■ High school ■ Extracurricular activities/ employment	■ Home/dorm ■ Secondary education ■ Employment
Identity/ independence	■ Struggles with identity ■ Increased need for privacy ■ Desire for independence	■ Self-involvement increases, continual change between high expectations and poor self-concept ■ Tendency to distance themselves from parents/parent conflicts peak ■ Continual drive for independence	■ Firmer sense of identity ■ Increased independence or completely independent ■ Self-reliant
Physical	■ Puberty is beginning ■ Physical growth: height and weight ■ Uncertain about changing appearance	■ Puberty is complete ■ Physical growth continues for males, decreases for females as puberty progresses ■ Continued uncertainty regarding physical changes/appearance	■ Females typically fully developed ■ Males continue to physically change (hair, muscle mass, height, weight) ■ Acceptance of pubertal changes
Cognitive	■ Growing abstract thinking ■ Deeper moral thinking ■ Intellectual interests become more important and expand	■ Continued growth of abstract thinking ■ Ability to set goals ■ Interest in moral reasoning	■ Ability to think ideas through ■ Think or be interested about the future ■ Continued interest in moral reasoning
Peers	■ Intense relationships with same-sex friends ■ Increased influences of peer groups ■ Worried about being "normal"	■ Need for friends, reliance of friends, and need to fit in/ popularity ■ Increased sexual activity and experimentation ■ Risk-taking behaviors	■ Peer relationships important ■ Development of intimate/serious relationships

Data from AACAP. Facts for Families. Washington, DC: American Academy of Child & Adolescent Psychiatry; 1952–2013. AACAP Facts for Families: Normal Adolescent Development Part 1, No. 57; December 2015. https://www.aacap.org/AACAP/Families_and_Youth/Facts_for_Families/FFF-Guide/Normal-Adolescent-Development-Part-I-057.aspx; AACAP. Facts for Families. Washington, DC: American Academy of Child & Adolescent Psychiatry; 1952–2013. AACAP Facts for Families: Normal Adolescent Development Part II, No. 58; December 2015;https://www.aacap.org/AACAP/Families_and_Youth/Facts_for_Families/FFF-Guide/Normal-Adolescent-Development-Part-II-058.aspx. Accessed March 28, 2022.

dental hygiene appointment to assess the child's overall oral health based on age and developmental milestones.

I. Initial Interview/New Patient Visit

- Parents are seated in a quiet, private place so they can concentrate and feel comfortable while supplying the information requested.
- As rapport is established with the parent(s), an explanation is given as to why the information is needed.
- The initial medical and family history information is collected and reviewed.

II. Child and Family Medical/Dental History

A. Family Configuration

- Number of people in the household and their relationship to the child.
- Other caregivers, the time periods, and location.
- Socioeconomic status and educational level of parents/guardians.

B. Medical History of the Child

- An accurate, comprehensive, and up-to-date medical history is necessary for correct diagnosis and effective treatment planning.[8]
- Dental caries and periodontal disease infections of parents and other children.
- Other health problems: The child patient with diabetes; cardiovascular disease; a mental, physical, or sensory disability; or other systemic involvement requires special adaptations of procedures. (See the various chapters of Section IX of this text.)
- Refer to Chapter 11 regarding the medical health history process.

III. Intraoral and Extraoral Examination

- Table 47-1 lists pediatric age-specific soft-tissue and hard-tissue conditions/pathology and identifies significance to dental hygiene care.[10]
- Evaluate head and extremities for any abnormalities or signs of child abuse.
- Refer to Chapter 13 for performing the intra- and extraoral examination.

IV. Developing Dentition, Occlusion, and Temporomandibular Joint Disorder

A. Evaluation

- Retract the lips to expose the facial aspect of the teeth to evaluate cervical areas for demineralization.
- Assess and document amount of biofilm present and any discolorations.
- Document tooth eruption delays compared with normal averages (**Table 47-4**).
- Adequate spacing for developing dentition.
- Classification of occlusion.
- Look for malformations (Table 47-1 and **Figure 47-1**) and dental caries (**Figure 47-2**).
- Loss of teeth and condition of present restorations.
- Evaluation of pits and fissures for indication for sealants or repair of previously placed sealants.
- Temporomandibular joint (TMJ) disorder for clicking, popping, grinding, or discomfort upon opening, closing, or mastication.
- Chapter 16 identifies general features to observe when examining the child's teeth.

Table 47-4 Tooth Development and Eruption: Primary Teeth

Tooth	Hard Tissue Formation Begins (Weeks in Utero)	Enamel Completed (Months after Birth)	Eruption (Months)	Root Completed (Year)
Maxillary				
Central incisor	14	1 1/2	10 (8–12)	1 1/2
Lateral incisor	16	2 1/2	11 (9–13)	2
Canine	17	9	19 (16–22)	3 1/4
First molar	15 1/2	6	16 (13–19 in boys; 14–18 in girls)	2 1/2
Second molar	19	11	29 (25–33)	3
Mandibular				
Central incisor	14	2 1/2	8 (6–10)	1 1/2
Lateral incisor	16	3	13 (10–16)	1 1/2
Canine	17	9	20 (17–23)	3 1/4
First molar	15 1/2	5 1/2	16 (14–18)	2 1/4
Second molar	18	10	27 (23–31 in boys; 24–30 in girls)	3

Reprinted with permission from Lunt RC, Law DB. A review of the chronology of deciduous teeth. *J Am Dent Assoc*. 1974; 89:372.

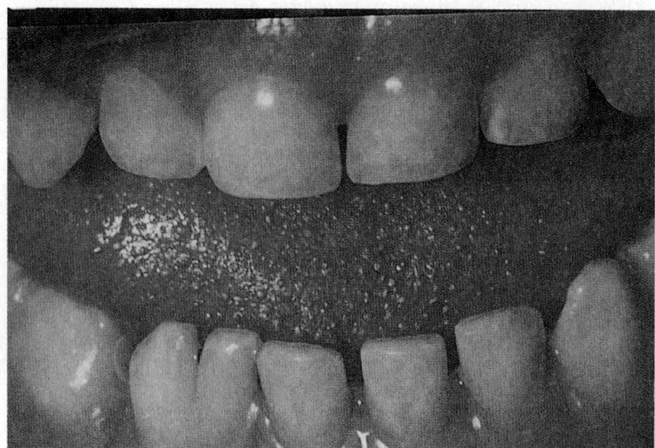

Figure 47-1 Developmental Disturbance of Primary Teeth. Germination of mandibular right lateral incisor caused by invagination of a single tooth germ and resulting in a notched and grooved crown.

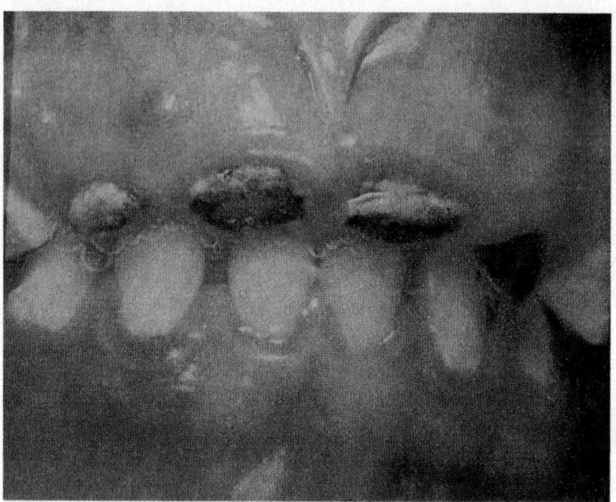

Figure 47-2 Severe Early Childhood Caries. Nearly complete loss of tooth structure of maxillary incisors. Note the abscess on the gingival tissues between the maxillary right central and lateral incisor, and the cervical biofilm on the mandibular incisors.

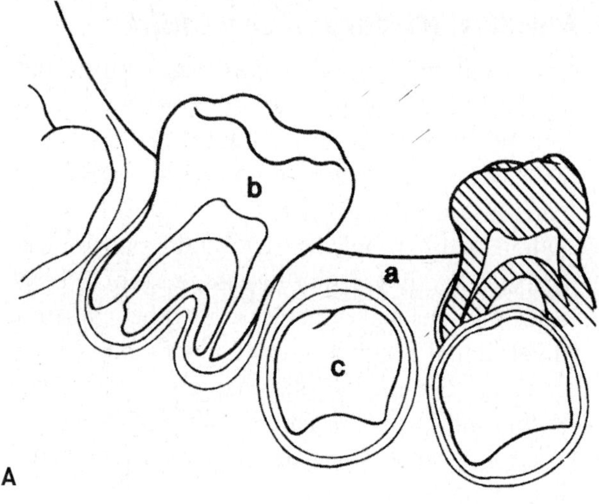

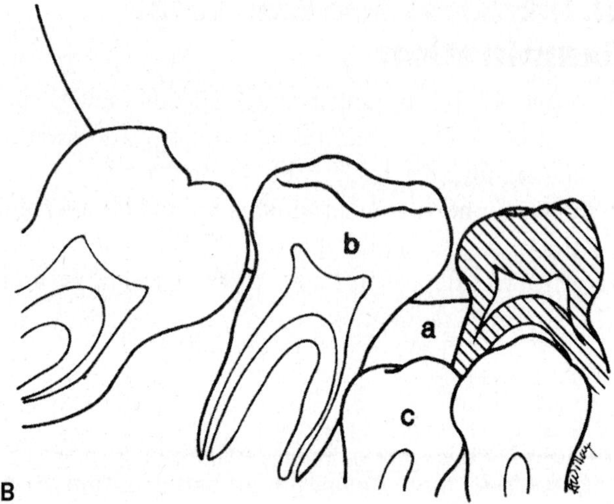

Figure 47-3 Premature Loss of Second Primary Molar. **A:** Developing first permanent molar (b) inclines and drifts mesially into the space (a) from which the second primary molar was removed. Developing second permanent premolar (c) is crowded. **B:** Space from which molar was removed (a) is nearly closed by the mesial drift and eruption of the first permanent molar (b). Developing second premolar (c) is closed in and prevented from eruption. Note that the second permanent molar has impacted against the first molar.

B. Indications for Referral

- Severely crowded, malposed, or congenitally missing teeth.
- Overbite, overjet, crossbites, or other malocclusions requiring intervention.
- Early loss of primary molars: this condition, if untreated, usually disrupts the eruption and alignment of permanent molars and premolars, as depicted in **Figure 47-3**.

V. Radiographic Assessment

Radiographs are a valuable diagnostic tool to aid in the overall oral health and developing an individualized treatment plan of infant, child, or adolescent dental needs.

A. Radiographic Needs

- The dentist's professional judgment and ADA/Food and Drug Administration guidelines are to prescribe needed dental radiographs for the child. (See Chapter 15.)
- A patient's age is not an indicator for initial radiographic needs.
- Each child is unique and the need can only be determined by the dentist after reviewing the patient's medical and dental histories, completing a clinical examination, and assessing the patient's vulnerability to environmental factors that affect oral health.

B. Cooperation

- Each child is different. Cooperation may depend on age and previous dental experiences.
- Use of tell–show–do, assistance of a parent, dental assistant or dentist, and/or using holding devices will aid in taking radiographs. (See Chapter 15.)

VI. Dietary Assessment

- A study of the child's diet and counseling relative to general nutrition and dental caries control can provide important learning experiences for the parent, child, or adolescent.
- When discussing diet with adolescent patients, responsibility is placed on them and their ability to make choices.

A. Diet Instruction Suggestions

- The use of the terms "healthy versus unhealthy" snacks instead of "good versus bad" snacks. The young child may not be able to distinguish the difference between "good" snacks that are "bad" for teeth, such as cookies are "good" tasting, but are "bad" for teeth.
- Advice on food choices from the most recent MyPlate Food Guide is illustrated in Chapter 33.

VII. Dental Hygiene Treatment

A. Purpose

- Removal of biofilm, stain, and calculus for gingival health.
- Educate parents and children regarding proper, daily biofilm control procedures and other preventive measures.

B. Type of Dental Hygiene Treatment

- The type of dental hygiene treatment provided for the child depends on the age and oral findings.
- The use of a disclosing agent is essential for assessment and education for school-aged children and adolescents.
- Perform at beginning of appointment to provide a visual tool for children to understand the presence of biofilm and removal with toothbrushing technique.
- Frequency of dental hygiene treatment is based on assessment of caries risk and periodontal health.

C. Instrumentation

- Presence of calculus is evaluated at each hygiene appointment for all ages.
- Removal of all local irregularities, including inadequate margins of restorations.
- When ultrasonic scaling is utilized for a pediatric patient with mixed dentition, it is only used on permanent teeth, never primary teeth.
- Ultrasonic scaling is effective for localized moderate-to-heavy calculus and orthodontic patients.

VIII. Prevention

A. Fluoride

Fluoride contributes to the prevention, inhibition, and reversal of caries.[12] Refer to Chapter 34 for additional fluoride information.

- *Professional application:*
  - Well water and nonfluoridated city water—have tested for fluoride level.
  - Use of nonfluoridated bottled water or water systems using reverse osmosis.
  - Application of professional fluoride treatment is based on the child's caries risk.
  - Children with moderate caries risk need to receive a professional fluoride application every 6 months; high caries risk receive at a greater frequency of 3–6 months.[9]
- *Supplementation:*
  - Fluoride supplementation may be considered if fluoride exposure is not optimal. The ADA and the AAPD guidelines are used for supplementation recommendations. (See Chapter 34.)
  - For children older than 6 years with moderate caries risk, over-the-counter fluoride rinses can be recommended as a supplement to daily brushing.
- Prescription fluoridated toothpaste is recommended for children with high caries risk or who have numerous carious lesions on proximal surfaces.
- A daily application of a fluoride gel in a custom-made tray may be necessary in select cases.
- *Fluorosis:*
  - Dental fluorosis occurs as a result of excess fluoride ingestion during tooth formation.[13]
  - Enamel fluorosis and primary teeth fluorosis can only occur when teeth are forming.[14]

B. Dental Sealants[15,16]

- As many as 90% of dental caries in school-aged children occurs in pits and fissures.
- Dentition is evaluated periodically for development defects and deep pits and fissures that may contribute to caries risk.

- Dental sealants are evaluated for repair or replacement as part of a periodic dental examination.
- Complete information about dental sealants can be found in Chapter 35.

C. Antibacterial Therapeutic Mouthrinses[17]

- Children younger than 6 years of age should not use mouthrinse, unless directed by a dentist, because they may swallow large amounts of the liquid inadvertently.
- Are available over-the-counter and by prescription, depending on the formulation.
- There are mouthrinses available that help reduce or control dental biofilm, gingivitis, bad breath, and tooth decay.
- With over-the-counter products, look for mouthrinses that have the ADA Seal of Acceptance. The Seal shows a product is safe and effective for the purpose claimed.
- Mouthrinses do not take the place of optimal brushing and flossing.
- Parent/**main caregiver** of the child may rinse at bedtime with a 0.12% chlorhexidine gluconate for 1 week per month to decrease risk of transferring cariogenic bacteria.[18]

Periodontal Risk Assessment

I. Gingival and Periodontal Evaluation

Nondestructive gingival inflammation in childhood without appropriate intervention may progress to more significant periodontal diseases.[19] The risk of periodontal disease is lowered by establishing excellent oral hygiene habits in children, which will carry over to adulthood.

- Periodontal evaluation
    - Significant changes occur in the periodontium as the dentition changes from primary to permanent teeth.[19]
    - Periodontal probing, periodontal charting, and radiographic periodontal diagnosis should be a consideration when caring for the adolescent.[20]
    - The extent and nature of the periodontal evaluation is determined professionally on an individual basis.[20]
    - Routine periodontal screening and probing is indicated following the eruption of permanent incisors and first molars.[21]
    - The use of the **periodontal screening and recording (PSR)** method can facilitate the early detection of periodontal diseases in children and the need for a comprehensive periodontal examination.[22] See Chapter 20 for more information about the PSR.

II. Periodontal Infections

- Significant changes occur in the periodontium as the dentition changes from primary to permanent teeth.[19]
- Adolescents are at risk for periodontal infections and gingival problems.
- Careful periodontal probing and review of radiographs are indicated for each patient.
- Emphasis is placed on preventive measures, early assessment, early treatment, and regular maintenance appointments.
- Development stages of gingivitis and periodontitis are discussed in Chapter 19.

A. Biofilm-Induced Gingivitis

- Most common periodontal disease among children.
- Incidence and severity may increase during puberty.
- Clinical changes and hormonal changes related to increased dental biofilm.
- Exaggerated response to dental biofilm.

B. Risk Factors for Periodontitis[23]

- Genetic factors.
- Host immune factors.
- Infrequent, inadequate dental and dental hygiene care.
- Local factors: supragingival and subgingival calculus; dental biofilm accumulations.
- Oral hygiene personal habits of care.
- Orthodontics—fixed or removable.
- Pathogenic microorganisms, viruses.
- Socioeconomic influences.
- Systemic diseases such as diabetes and hematologic diseases.
- Untreated dental caries and defective restorations.
- Use of tobacco.

Caries Risk Assessment

A caries management by risk assessment (**CAMBRA**) process uses a questionnaire such as the AAPD Caries Assessment Tool (CAT) to interview the parent and/or child in combination with other assessment data to determine caries risk level. See Chapter 25 for more information about caries risk assessment.

I. Purpose

- To identify and decrease contributing factors (biologic and clinical findings).
- Identify current protective factors.

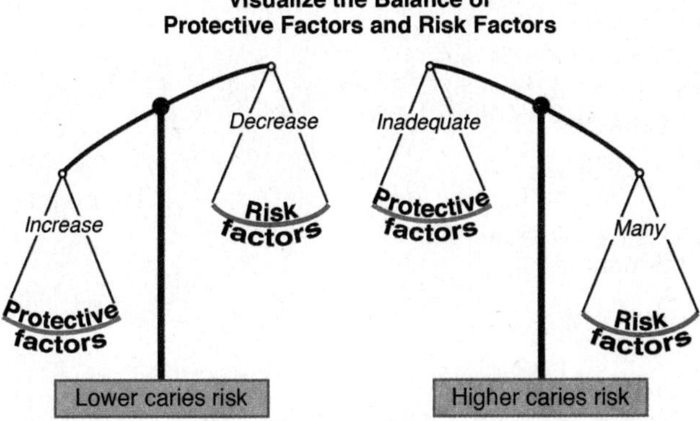

Figure 47-4 Visualize the Caries Balance. Individualized assessment of risk factors can help determine the caries risk level of each patient. Providing interventions that increase protective factors such as adequate biofilm removal and fluoride exposure can change the balance and reduce caries risk.

- Classifies the child's risk level for developing caries.
- A communication tool with the parent and/or age-appropriate child in discussing and eliminating risks.
- A balance of risk factors and protective factors is needed to prevent the progression of caries as visualized in **Figure 47-4**.

II. Principles

- Provide parent and/or patient education.
- Promote remineralization of noncavitated lesions by use of topical fluorides.
- Modify oral flora to favor oral health by use of topical antibacterial therapeutic agents.
- Minimal restoration of cavitated lesions and defective restorations.

III. Steps

- Complete a caries risk assessment based on the child's specific age-related risk and preventive factors. See Chapter 25 for additional information on caries risk assessment.
- Determine level of caries risk.

Diagnostics should be used to develop a treatment plan for caries management based on age specific interventions and restorative care. **Table 47-5** provides

Table 47-5 Caries Management Based on Risk Level for Patients Up to Age 6 Years Old

	Caries Risk Level			
Caries Management System/ Guideline	**Low**	**Moderate**	**High**	**Very High or Extreme**
AAPD	■ Brushing: 2X/day with fluoride toothpaste • smear 0–2 yrs old • pea sized amount 3–5 yrs old ■ Oral health education and anticipatory guidance	■ Brushing: 2X/day with smear of fluoride toothpaste • smear 0–2 yrs old • pea sized amount 3–5 yrs old ■ Fluoride supplements (depending on access to community water fluoridation) ■ Topical fluoride every 6 months	■ Brushing: 2X/day with smear of fluoride toothpaste • smear 0–2 yrs old • pea sized amount 3–5 yrs old ■ Fluoride supplements ■ Topical fluoride every 3 months ■ Oral health education and anticipatory guidance	

(continues)

Table 47-5 Caries Management Based on Risk Level for Patients Up to Age 6 Years Old *(continued)*

Caries Management System/ Guideline	Caries Risk Level			
	Low	**Moderate**	**High**	**Very High or Extreme**
	▪ Diet counseling: age-appropriate feeding practices ▪ Radiographs every 12–24 months ▪ Baseline Salivary mutans streptococci (MS) bacterial levels ▪ Sealants (3–5 yrs old) ▪ Regular dental visits every 6–12 months	▪ Oral health education and anticipatory guidance ▪ Diet counseling: age-appropriate feeding practices ▪ Radiographs every 6–12 months ▪ Baseline Salivary MS bacterial levels ▪ Sealants (3–5 yrs old) ▪ Dental visits every 6 months	▪ Diet counseling: age-appropriate feeding practices/ reduce sugar total intake and frequency ▪ Baseline Salivary MS bacterial levels ▪ Radiographs every 6 months ▪ Sealants (3–5 yrs old) ▪ Dental visits every 3 months	
CAMBRA	▪ Brushing 2X/ day with fluoride toothpaste • smear 0–2 yrs old • pea sized amount 3–5 yrs old ▪ Radiographs: 12–24 months ▪ Dental visits: every 6–12 months	▪ Brushing 2X/ day with fluoride toothpaste • smear 0–2 yrs old • pea sized amount 3–5 yrs old ▪ Fluoride supplements or fluoridated water ▪ Fluoride varnish every 6 months ▪ Diet counseling ▪ Oral health education and anticipatory guidance ▪ Sealants on at-risk pits and fissures ▪ Radiographs 6–12 months ▪ Dental visits every 6 months	▪ Brushing 2X/ day with fluoride toothpaste • smear 0–2 yrs old • pea sized amount 3–5 yrs old ▪ Fluoride supplements or fluoridated water ▪ Fluoride varnish every 3 months ▪ Diet counseling: reduce cariogenic food/beverage intake and frequency ▪ Oral health education and anticipatory guidance ▪ Sealants on enamel defects and at-risk pits and fissures ▪ Radiographs 6 months ▪ Dental visits every 3 months ▪ For early lesions, silver diamine fluoride or ITR (interim therapeutic restoration) may be considered	▪ Supervised brushing 3X/ day with fluoride toothpaste (spitting, but no rinsing of toothpaste) • smear 0–2 yrs old • pea sized amount 3–5 yrs old ▪ Fluoride supplements or fluoridated water ▪ Fluoride varnish every 1–3 months ▪ Diet counseling: reduce cariogenic food/beverage intake and frequency ▪ Oral health education and anticipatory guidance ▪ Sealants on enamel defects and at-risk pits and fissures ▪ Brush or wipe with baking soda or xylitol ▪ Use casein phosphopeptide–amorphous calcium phosphate (ACP/CPP) paste ▪ Home fluoride trays may be needed to manage caries risk ▪ For early lesions, silver diamine fluoride or ITR (interim therapeutic restoration) may be considered ▪ Radiographs 6 months ▪ Dental visits monthly

Data from American Academy of Pediatric Dentistry. Caries-risk assessment and management for infants, children, and adolescents. In: *The Reference Manual of Pediatric Dentistry*. Chicago, IL: American Academy of Pediatric Dentistry; 2021:252–257; and Featherstone JDB, Crystal YO, Alston P, et al. Evidence-based caries management for all ages: practical guidelines. *Front Oral Health*. 2021;2:657518.

management guidelines for children younger than 6 years old. See Chapter 25 for caries management guidelines for children 6 years and older. See Chapter 25 for more information about caries risk assessment.

V. Early Childhood Caries[24]

- The disease of early childhood caries (ECC) is the presence of one or more decayed (noncavitated or cavitated lesions), missing (due to caries), or filled tooth surfaces in any primary tooth in a child younger than 6 years.
- A child younger than 3 years with any smooth-surface caries (white-spot lesion or cavitated lesion) is indicative of severe early childhood caries (S-ECC).
- This form of caries is usually seen in children who routinely have been given a bottle when going to sleep containing a cariogenic liquid (formula, milk, or juice) or have experienced prolonged at-will breastfeeding.
- Nursing bottle caries, baby bottle tooth decay, and rampant caries are older terms. The AAPD adopted the term ECC to reflect the multifactorial etiology (frequency, tooth-adherent-specific bacteria, primarily mutans streptococci [MS] that metabolize sugars to produce acid that, over time, demineralizes tooth structure).
- The consequences of ECC often include a higher risk of new caries lesions in both the primary and permanent dentition, hospitalizations and emergency room visits, high treatment costs, loss of school days, diminished ability to learn, and reduced oral health–related quality of life.[25]
- ECC case definition criteria are found in Chapter 16.

A. Prevalence

- Tooth decay (dental caries) affects children in the United States more than any other chronic infectious disease.[26]
- Tooth decay affects one in four children aged 3–5 and 6–9 years who live in poverty.[27]

B. Microbiology

- Dental caries is a common chronic infectious transmissible disease resulting from tooth-adherent–specific bacteria, primarily MS.[26] Lactobacilli in large numbers are also in the dental biofilm.
- Transfer of MS from parent, caregiver, sibling, or other child by saliva-sharing behaviors to the infant or young child.[28]
- Colonization of MS has been shown to occur before tooth eruption and as early as birth.[29]
- High levels of MS in saliva and dental biofilm are a strong risk indicator for ECC.[30]
- Avoid saliva-sharing behaviors such as kissing on the mouth, tasting food before feeding, cleaning a dropped pacifier by mouth, and sharing of cups, toys, or utensils.[31]

C. Risk Factors

The areas of concern related to disease indicators/risk factors are listed in Table 47-5. Teaching parents about the cause and effects of ECC is a significant part of anticipatory guidance (**Table 47-6**).

Table 47-6 Anticipatory Guidance: 12 Months to 6 Years of Age

Area of Concern	12–24 Months	2–3 Years	4–6 Years
Developmental milestone	■ Check tooth contacts ■ Close contacts: teach parents to floss ■ Normal/abnormal eruption pattern	■ Primary dentition complete ■ Evaluate occlusion for crowding, overbite, overjet ■ Bruxing and occlusal wear ■ Evaluate for sealants on primary teeth based on caries risk	■ Discuss exfoliation of primary teeth ■ Eruption patterns and expected new permanent teeth ■ Evaluate for sealants on first permanent molars
Nutrition and feeding	■ Nutrition, snacking based on child's diet ■ Reduce snacking frequency ■ Review snacking safety ■ Avoid food as reward for behavior modification ■ Avoid dependence on sippy cup	■ Suggest snacks from fruit, vegetable, dairy, and meat groups ■ Limit juice intake to 4 oz	■ Snacking: suggest healthy snacks ■ Limit juice and soda

(continues)

Table 47-6 Anticipatory Guidance: 12 Months to 6 Years of Age *(continued)*

Area of Concern	12–24 Months	2–3 Years	4–6 Years
Oral hygiene and caries prevention	■ Complete caries risk assessment ■ Oral hygiene index (OHI) with parent and daily oral hygiene completed by parent ■ Disclose for dental biofilm ■ Review brushing; continue with a "smear" of fluoridated toothpaste ■ Lift upper lip when brushing ■ Parents are the role models ■ Parents look for signs of disease ■ Review position of child for OH—knee-to-knee	■ Complete caries risk assessment ■ OHI with parents and child. Parent continues with daily oral hygiene and child may "have a turn" ■ Ask about problems ■ Lift upper lip when brushing ■ Brush morning and night ■ Use a "pea"-sized amount of fluoridated toothpaste ■ Review signs of disease ■ Review position of child for OH—standing behind child	■ Complete caries risk assessment ■ OHI including flossing with parents and child; parent continues with daily oral hygiene; child also performs brushing after parent ■ Review signs of disease
Fluoride information	■ Update fluoride status ■ Store fluoride products out of reach of children ■ Use of small, thin smear of fluoride dentifrice on brush ■ Fluoride varnish application	■ Parents control toothpaste ■ Evaluate changes in diet and water ■ Make appropriate fluoride recommendations ■ Fluoride varnish application	■ Parents continue toothpaste control ■ Check fluoride status ■ Varnish applications
Trauma/injury prevention	■ Car seat safety ■ Discuss oral electrical burns and child-proofing home ■ Care of avulsed tooth	■ Provide trauma management plan at day care or preschool ■ Discuss head and neck, oral signs of child abuse ■ Review other safety measures (i.e., bike helmet, car seats)	■ Trauma management plan at school ■ Review need for mouth guard ■ Discuss bike safety ■ Monitor for signs of child abuse ■ Review other safety measures
Habits/function behaviors	■ Effects of continued thumb, finger, or pacifier sucking	■ **Nonnutritive sucking** may still be present ■ Discuss elimination of thumb/finger sucking; possible early orthodontic referral	■ Eliminate thumb/finger sucking; possible orthodontic referral needed
Environmental (passive) smoke	■ Smoke-free environment required	■ Smoke-free environment required	■ Smoke-free environment required
Dental/dental hygiene visit	■ Home preparation for dental visit ■ Frequency depends on caries risk and parent compliance with home preventive measures ■ Parents emphasize helping-caring nature of dentist/dental hygienist ■ Toothbrush dental biofilm removal ■ Radiographic evaluation if indicated ■ Discuss findings and recommendations with parents	■ Frequency of preventive care based on caries risk ■ Use disclosing solution to identify dental biofilm ■ Toothbrush or rubber cup dental biofilm removal ■ Radiographic evaluation if indicated ■ Discuss findings and recommendations with parents	■ Frequency of preventive visits and radiographic evaluation based on risk factors ■ Emphasize helping-caring nature of providers ■ Use disclosing solution to identify dental biofilm ■ Assess for calculus requiring scaling ■ Rubber cup polishing ■ Discuss findings and recommendations with parents

Data from American Academy of Pediatric Dentistry. Periodicity of examination, preventive dental services, anticipatory guidance/ counseling, and oral treatment for infants, children, and adolescents. *The Reference Manual of Pediatric Dentistry*. Chicago, IL.: American Academy of Pediatric Dentistry; 2021:241-251. http://www.aapd.org/media/Policies_Guidelines/G_Periodicity.pdf. Accessed March 10, 2022.

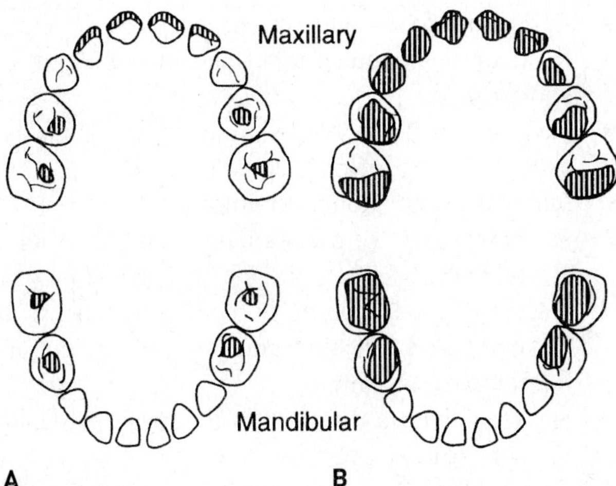

Figure 47-5 Progression of Early Childhood Caries. **A:** Earliest caries affect the maxillary anterior teeth, followed by the molars as they erupt. **B:** Severe extensive lesions develop in all except the mandibular anterior teeth. Protection for the mandibular incisors and canines is provided by the tongue during the sucking process.

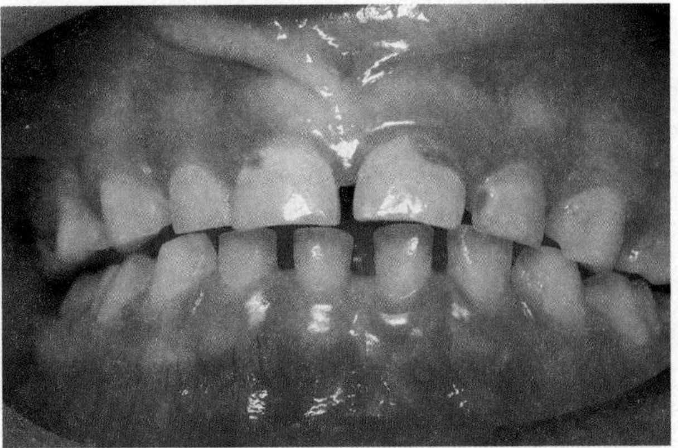

Figure 47-6 White-Spot Lesions and Cavitation of White Lesion Areas. Opaque, chalky enamel areas, usually on cervical or proximal areas of teeth at contacts, indicate that the surface and underlying enamel are demineralized. Subtle white lesions (indicated by the arrows) at the cervical margin of the maxillary lateral incisors provide the earliest clinical sign of the carious process. Cavitation of the white lesion areas results in small brownish-looking cavitated areas (indicated by the arrows). These can be seen adjacent to white-spot lesions on the distal–facial surfaces of the central incisor. A large cavitated carious lesion can be seen on the and the mesial–facial surface of the left lateral incisor. Note additional white-spot lesions at the cervical margins of the maxillary canines, the right maxillary molar and the left mandibular molar.

Photograph courtesy of Dr. Alton McWhorter, DDS, Texas A&M University, School of Dentistry, Department of Pediatrics.

D. Predisposing Factors

- Placing bottle/**sippy cup** in bed.
- Bottle/sippy cup contains milk, formula, or sweetened fluid with sucrose.
- Prolonged at-will breast or bottle feeding as a sleep aid or behavioral control.
- Ineffective or no daily biofilm removal from the teeth.

E. Effects

- Maxillary anterior teeth and primary molars are the first to be affected, as noted in Figure 47-2 and **Figure 47-5**.
- As the child falls asleep, pools of the sweet liquid can collect around the teeth.
- While the sucking is active, the liquid passes beyond the teeth.
- The nipple covers the mandibular anterior teeth; hence, they are rarely affected.

F. Recognition

- Demineralization or white-spot lesions may be noted along the cervical third of the maxillary anterior teeth and proximal surfaces when the upper lip is lifted (**Figure 47-6**).
- At a later stage, cavitation occurs and the lesions appear brown or dark brown (Figure 47-6). Eventually, the crowns may be destroyed to the gum line, abscesses may develop, and the child may suffer severe pain and discomfort. An advanced stage of dental caries is shown in Figure 47-2.

G. Management

- Emphasis is placed on the prevention and arrestment of the disease process.[25]
- Parent engagement to facilitate and promote preventive measures while encouraging the identification and reduction of individual risk factors.[25]
- Active surveillance, which includes monitoring caries progression and implementing prevention programs such as frequent fluoride varnish applications.[25]
- Arrestment of caries with silver diamine fluoride.[25]

Anticipatory Guidance

- Anticipatory guidance is the process of providing practical, developmentally appropriate information about children's health to prepare parents for the significant physical, emotional, and psychological milestones.[9]

- Involves both the parent and the child patient (when age-appropriate).
- Customized patient-centered recommendations presented orally, demonstration provided, and written documentation to be taken home for reference.
- Anticipatory guidance specific to developmental milestones, nutrition and feeding, oral hygiene measures, dental caries prevention, health and safety precautions, and treatment measures are outlined in Table 47-6 and **Table 47-7**.

I. Dietary and Feeding Pattern Recommendations

A. Toddlers and Preschoolers

- Children need a series of small, healthy meals during the day.
- Healthy snacks include noncariogenic foods from the grain, vegetable, fruit, meat/meat alternatives, and dairy groups.
- Sweetened foods and drinks are limited to three or less per day and provided at mealtimes rather than between meals.
- Do not allow the child to sip or graze at will on a bottle or sippy cup containing milk or sweet liquids, which promotes demineralization and ECC.
- Milk and water should be the primary beverages, with no more than 4–6 oz of juice per day with meals.

B. School-Aged

- Educate about healthy snacks and drinks; encourage tooth-healthy choices.
- School-aged children continue to have problems with likes and dislikes.
- Choices are strongly influenced by both their physical and social environments; ease of access, parents' education, time constraints, ethnicity, eating together, TV viewing during meals, and the source of food (e.g., restaurants, schools); family, friends, and the media (especially TV) influence their food choices[32]
- Parents have a direct role in children's eating patterns through their behaviors, attitudes, and feeding styles.[32]

C. Adolescent

- Adolescents' frequency of eating increases due to growth periods, emotional issues, or peer pressures.
- Cariogenic foods and drinks are often selected. Incidence of dental caries may increase during adolescence.
- Highest caries risk of any time in life for males; exceeded only during pregnancy for females.
- Inadequate nutrition is common.
  - Boys: due to over activity and poor food selection.
  - Girls: due to voluntary diet restrictions, with poor food selection and fad diets in the attempt to be trim.
  - Teens with a distorted body image may take concern to extremes.
- Eating disorders
  - Anorexia nervosa and/or bulimia can lead to severe health complications and even death.
  - Successful treatment usually requires an interdisciplinary team approach involving medical care, psychotherapy, and nutrition and family counseling. (See Chapter 58.)
- Iron-deficiency anemia
  - Common among teenage girls, particularly after the onset of menstruation.
  - Treated with iron supplements, changes in diet, or both.

II. Oral Health Considerations for Toddlers/Preschoolers

A. Gaining Cooperation

- At these ages, the child is becoming more independent.
- Parents can provide a fun activity by making up and singing a brushing song.
- For a 2- to 3-year-old, teach the child to take turns with the parent when brushing by using the phrase, "It's your turn to brush," followed by, "It's my turn to brush."
- To gain better cooperation, connect brushing with a fun activity such as first, we brush teeth and then, we read a story.
- Provide or recommend a 2-minute timer to be used for motivation during brushing.

B. Brushing and Flossing

- Establish a routine: make suggestions as to how to establish and maintain a brushing routine.
- Recommend brushing in the morning after breakfast and before bedtime.
- Specify that the most critical time for dental biofilm removal is before bedtime.

Table 47-7 Anticipatory Guidance: 6 Years of Age to Adolescent

Area of Concern	6–12 Years	12 Years and Older
Developmental milestone	■ Eruption patterns; mixed dentition; missing teeth ■ Evaluate orthodontic needs ■ Evaluate for sealants on permanent molars	■ Eruption patterns; permanent dentition; missing teeth ■ Evaluate orthodontic needs ■ Evaluate for sealants on second permanent molars
Nutrition and feeding	■ Snacking: continue with healthy snack choices ■ Limit juice, soda, and sports drinks ■ Discussion with parent and child on hidden sugars, carbohydrate snacks, and frequency	■ Snacking: continue with healthy snack choices ■ Limit juice, soda, and sports drinks ■ Discussion with parent and child on hidden sugars, carbohydrate snacks, and frequency
Oral hygiene and caries prevention	■ Complete caries-risk assessment form ■ OHI with child; parent supervises daily oral hygiene; child performs daily oral hygiene ■ Reinforce brushing for 2 minutes, twice daily ■ Teach flossing and use of floss holders if needed; flossing daily ■ Review need for adjunct hygiene care products (disclosing tablets, fluoride rinses, floss threaders) ■ Review signs of disease	■ Complete caries-risk assessment form ■ OHI with child; consult with parent as necessary ■ Reinforce brushing for 2 minutes, twice daily ■ Teach flossing and use of floss holders if needed; flossing daily ■ Review need for adjunct hygiene care products (disclosing tablets, fluoride rinses, floss threaders) ■ Review signs of disease
Fluoride information	■ Check fluoride status ■ Varnish applications	■ Check fluoride status ■ Varnish applications
Trauma/injury prevention	■ Trauma management plan at school ■ Review need for mouth guard ■ Discuss bike safety ■ Monitor for signs of child abuse ■ Review other safety measures	■ Trauma management plan at school ■ Review need for mouth guard ■ Discuss bike safety ■ Monitor for signs of child abuse ■ Review other safety measures
Habits/function behaviors	■ Evaluation for orthodontic referral	■ Evaluation for orthodontic referral
Environmental (passive) smoke	■ Smoke-free environment required ■ Educate regarding tobacco use	■ Smoke-free environment required ■ Educate regarding tobacco use
Dental/dental hygiene visit	■ Frequency of preventive visits and radiographic evaluation based on risk factors ■ Emphasize helping–caring nature of providers ■ Use disclosing solution to identify dental biofilm ■ Evaluate periodontal status as permanent teeth erupt ■ Assess for calculus requiring scaling ■ Rubber cup polishing ■ Discuss findings and recommendations with parents ■ Age-appropriate counseling for substance abuse and/or smoking	■ Frequency of preventive visits and radiographic evaluation based on risk factors ■ Emphasize helping–caring nature of providers ■ Use disclosing solution to identify dental biofilm ■ Evaluate periodontal status as permanent teeth erupt ■ Assess for calculus requiring scaling ■ Rubber cup polishing ■ Discuss findings and recommendations with parents ■ Assessment for removal of third molars ■ Age-appropriate counseling for: substance abuse, intraoral/perioral piercing, and/or smoking

Data from American Academy of Pediatric Dentistry. (Revised 2018);40(6):104-203. http://www.aapd.org/media/Policies_Guidelines/G_Periodicity.pdf. Accessed March 10, 2022.

C. Parental Involvement and Supervision

- Parents keep fluoride toothpaste out of reach of the child and oversee/place the correct amount of toothpaste on the toothbrush.
- Until the child develops fine motor coordination and can effectively remove biofilm, the parents/caregivers assist the child in cleaning the teeth by doing the brushing and flossing. The time to cease assistance depends on parental/caregiver assessment and varies markedly from child to child.
- Parents teach the child to brush and then evaluate to ensure effective and complete biofilm removal.
- Parents floss closely approximated primary teeth to remove biofilm from proximal surfaces.

D. Toothpaste

- Children's toothpastes manufactured in the United States contain the same amount of fluoride as adult toothpastes, whereas manufacturers in several countries around the world reduce the amount of fluoride in children's toothpastes.
- Parents/caregivers are informed that they need to prevent problems by controlling the amount of toothpaste used and placing it out of the child's reach.
- For children younger than 6 years, regularly ingesting pea-sized amounts or more can lead to mild fluorosis.[33]
- Appropriate amount of fluoridated toothpaste is to be used for children of all ages.[33]
- Children like the taste of toothpaste and may eat a large amount at one time, resulting in acute fluoride toxicity.

E. Instructions for Parents

- An adult can brush the child's teeth with a tiny amount of fluoridated toothpaste as soon as the first tooth comes in.
- Children younger than 3 years use a small "smear" of fluoride toothpaste (an amount about the size of a grain of rice), as illustrated in **Figure 47-7**.[33]
- Children who are 3 years and older use a "pea-size" amount of fluoride toothpaste.[34] See an illustration in Figure 47-7.
- Teach children to spit out toothpaste as soon as they are old enough to do so.[33]
- Continue to control the toothpaste and keep it out of reach.
- Teach parents how to examine the mouth for signs of gingival inflammation, dental caries, and injury.

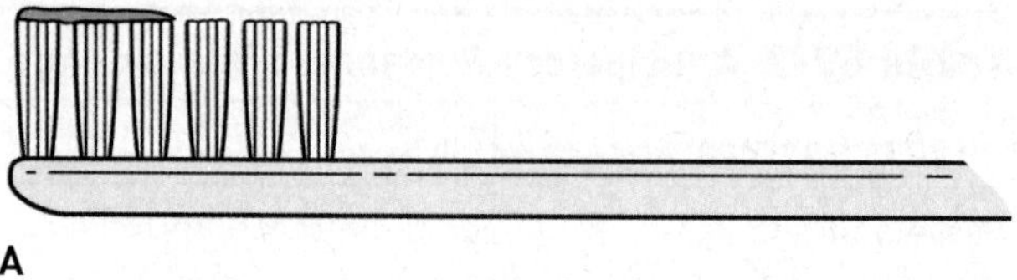

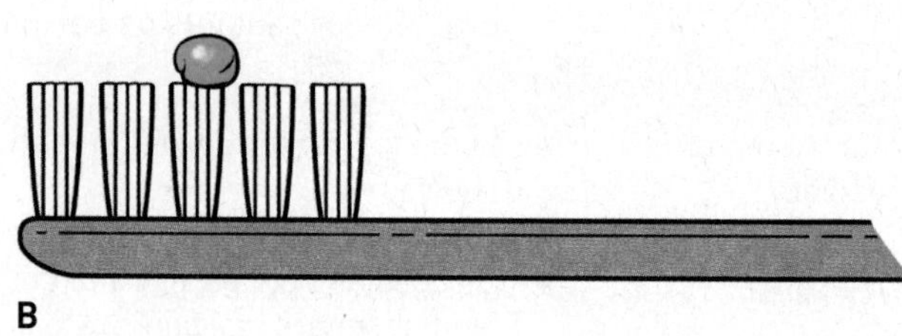

Figure 47-7 Dentifrice for a Child. For children younger than 3 years, the parent is instructed to place a small smear of fluoridated toothpaste on a child-sized brush **(A)**. For all children aged 3–6 years, the appropriate size is that of a small pea **(B)**. The paste is spread in a thin layer over the brush surface and then spread over all of the teeth before brushing.

- Evaluation of pits and fissures for caries-susceptible primary and permanent teeth (molars, premolars, and anterior teeth).

III. Speech and Language Development

- Premature loss of primary teeth, digit habits, and malocclusions can have direct implications on a child's development of speech and language.
- Early detection and referral can help correct speech or language development.

IV. Digit Habits

- Prolonged thumb- and finger-sucking habits have been associated with narrow maxillary arch width, anterior open bite, posterior crossbite, increased overjet, and decreased overbite[34] (see **Figure 47-8**).

V. Accident and Injury Prevention

- Age-appropriate accident and injury prevention counseling for orofacial trauma is provided and/or evaluated at every hygiene visit.
- Written information regarding what to do in the event of a traumatic oral injury makes parents feel more prepared.
- Chapter 9 provides information on a dislocated jaw, facial fracture, and tooth forcibly displaced or avulsed.

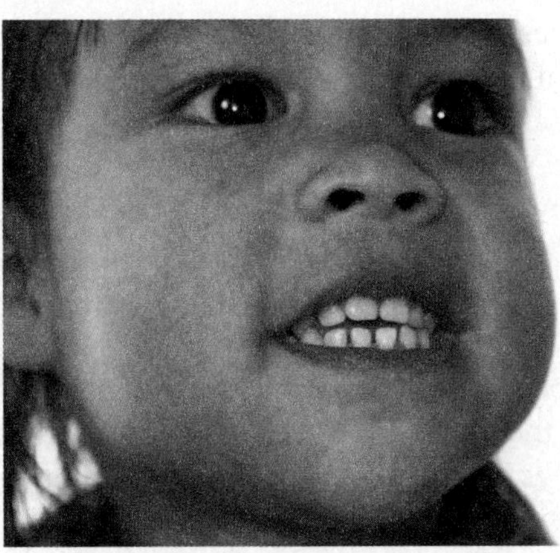

Figure 47-8 Effects of Prolonged Thumb Sucking on Teeth. Anterior open bite.

A. Toddlers

- The greatest incidence of injury to the primary dentition occurs at 2–3 years of age. Toddlers have increased mobility and developing coordination and as a result are subject to injuries.
- Provide counseling regarding play objects, pacifiers, car seats, and electrical cords.

B. School-Aged Children

- House structures/furniture such as floors, steps, tables, and beds are most commonly associated with dental injuries in children younger than 7 years.
- Parents can be taught to protect the child by close supervision, anticipating problems, and making the environment safe by removing dangers.

C. Adolescents

- Common injuries to permanent teeth are related to car accidents, violence, and sports-related trauma.
- Counseling and providing athletic mouth guards for all contact sports and activities can enhance trauma prevention.

VI. Oral Malodor (Halitosis)

A. Causes[35]

- Biofilm accumulation on the tongue and teeth.
- Diet.
- Dry mouth, low levels of saliva inhibit the ability to wash away food debris.
- Health conditions (e.g., infections in the nose, throat, or lungs; chronic sinusitis; postnasal drip; chronic bronchitis; or disturbances in the digestive system).[36]
- Medications.
- Mouth breathing.
- Oral infections (e.g., dental caries, periodontal conditions, draining fistulas, oral surgery, oral sores).
- Smoking.

B. What to Teach Parents

- Explain bacterial causes.
- Emphasize thorough dental biofilm removal through daily brushing of the teeth.
- Teach how to floss their child's teeth.
- Show how to brush gently the dorsum of the tongue (refer to Chapter 26).

VII. Oral Health Considerations for Adolescents[20]

Increased risk for dental caries and periodontal infections during adolescence has already been described in this chapter. Some additional examples of oral problems related to adolescent development and behavior characteristics, including risky health behaviors, are listed here.

- Assess the presence, position, and development of third molars. Provide a referral if the need of removal is indicated.
- Oral manifestations of sexually transmitted infections.
- Potential effects of hormonal fluctuations and use of oral contraceptives on periodontal tissues. (See Chapter 53.)
- Oral findings of anorexia nervosa or bulimia. (See Chapter 58.)
- Traumatic injury to teeth and oral structures.
    - Contact sports and skateboarding are risky behaviors.
    - Automobile and motorcycle accidents can also cause dental injuries.
- If pregnancy and parenting are issues for the adolescent patient, the dental hygienist can use anticipatory guidance to educate about important oral health issues for the mother and infant. (See Chapter 46.)
- Counsel patients, parents, and guardians regarding the human papillomavirus vaccination, in accordance with Centers for Disease Control and Prevention recommendations, as part of anticipatory guidance for adolescent patients.[37]

VIII. Tobacco/Obstructive Sleep Apnea/Piercings/ Substance Abuse

- As the child approaches adolescence, the prevention discussion can be expanded to include the serious health consequences of tobacco use, intraoral/perioral piercings, **obstructive sleep apnea** (OSA), and substance abuse.

- Discussion of tobacco use includes:
  - Smoking, smokeless tobacco, and exposure to second-hand smoke.
  - Current tobacco use trends (i.e., electric cigarettes, hookah).
  - Oral effects of tobacco, including leukoplakia, periodontal disease, and oral cancer. (See Chapter 32.)
- Discussion of identifiable signs, symptoms, and evaluation of OSA is a part of a child's regular clinical examination.
  - **Pediatric OSA** is a disorder of breathing characterized by prolonged episodes of complete or partial upper airway obstruction during sleep, often resulting in gas exchange abnormalities and arousals that cause disrupted sleep.[38]
  - Signs and symptoms of OSA include[38]:
    - Excessive daytime sleepiness.
    - Loud snoring three or more nights per week.
    - Episodes of breathing cessation witnessed by another person.
    - Abrupt awakenings accompanied by shortness of breath.
    - Awakening with dry mouth or sore throat.
    - Morning headache.
    - Difficulty staying asleep.
    - Unusual sleep positions (seat or neck hyperextended).
    - Attention problems.
    - Mouth breathing.
    - Sweating.
    - Restlessness.
    - Waking up a lot.
    - Bed wetting (after at least 6 months of continence).
    - Poor school performance due to misdiagnosed attention deficit-hyperactivity disorder, aggressive behavior, or developmental delay.
  - Referral to child's pediatrician if suspected of being at risk for OSA.
  - Comorbidities with OSA can be cardiovascular problems, impaired growth, learning problems, and behavioral problems.
  - Untreated OSA in combination with insulin resistance and obesity in a child sets the stage for heart disease and endocrinopathies.[39]
  - The inclusion of sleep questions on the health history form may further help identify patients at risk.[38] Questions may include:
    - Does your child snore loudly when sleeping?
    - Does your child have trouble breathing while sleeping?
    - Does your child stop breathing while sleeping?
    - Does your child occasionally wet the bed at night?
    - Is your child hard to wake up in the morning?
    - Does your child complain of headaches in the morning?
    - Does your child tend to breathe through their mouth during the day?
    - Have you or the teacher commented your child appears sleepy during the day?
    - Does your child fall asleep quickly?
  - Treatment of OSA may be accomplished with either surgical or non-surgical options, depending on the severity and etiology.[38]
  - Nonsurgical treatment includes[38]:
    - Treatment of nasal allergies.
    - Continuous positive airway pressure (CPAP)
    - Weight reduction.
    - Changes in sleeping position.
  - Discussion of complications and nonreversible conditions that can result from intraoral/perioral piercings includes[40-47]:
    - Oral piercings, including the tongue, lips, cheeks, and uvula, have been associated with pathologic conditions, including pain, infection, scar formation, tooth fractures, metal hypersensitivity reactions, localized periodontal disease, speech impediment, Ludwig angina, hepatitis, and nerve damage.
    - Increased dental biofilm levels, gingival inflammation and/or recession, caries, diminished articulation, and metal allergy.
    - Life-threatening complications have been reported, including bleeding, edema, endocarditis, and airway obstructions.
    - Use of dental jewelry (e.g., grills) has been documented to cause dental caries and periodontal problems.[47]
  - The patient who has or is considering an oral piercing must be:
    - Educated regarding daily hygiene of the piercing site to avoid infection.
    - Counseled at every dental hygiene visit regarding possible complications.
    - Encouraged to remove the piercings.
- A complete discussion about oral complications related to the use of cocaine and other street drugs is found in Chapter 59.

IX. Referral

- Appropriate referrals are made when problems that require intervention by other health providers are identified.
- Conditions requiring referral include:
  - Evidence of systemic illness and pathology.
  - Child abuse or neglect and evidence of poor parenting skills.[48]
  - Failure to provide safety measures.
  - Substance abuse in the family.[48]
- Understand the reporting and licensing requirements for child abuse and neglect specific to your state.

Role of Teledentistry

- Teledentistry is defined as the "provision of real time and offline dental care such as diagnosis, treatment planning, consulting, and follow-up."[49]
- Studies find teledentistry to be as reliable as visual clinical examinations for screenings, orthognathic evaluations, indications for oral surgery, and managing odontogenic infections.[49]
- As a result of the COVID-19 pandemic, teledentistry has been utilized more frequently due to social distancing regulations.[49]
- The AAPD encourages the use of teledentistry as an adjunct to in-person clinical care to improve access to care for infants, children, adolescents, and individuals with special healthcare needs.[49]

Treatment Planning and Consent

- The dental hygiene diagnosis is used to develop the dental hygiene care plan. (See Chapters 22 and 23.)
- Before treatment, the care plan is discussed with the dentist to integrate the dental hygiene plan into the comprehensive dental treatment plan.
- Inform parent/guardian of findings from the assessment and present the care plan both orally and in writing.
- Have parent/guardian sign an informed consent before treatment. (See Chapter 23.)
- *Medical clearance*: the parent/guardian will need to consent to medical clearance for conditions requiring antibiotic coverage, local anesthesia, or other medication for a patient under legal age.
- *Parental approval*: the dental hygienist care plan requires approval by the parent/guardian.

Documentation

The following items are documented in the progress notes of pediatric patients:

- Overall appraisal of physical status and key health history findings.
- Existing pathology: soft tissue, gingiva, caries, occlusal status.
- Oral hygiene status and caries risk assessment.
- Anticipatory guidance provided, parent/patient recommendation, and any adjunct hygiene aids provided (disclosing tablets, home fluoride prescriptions, interdental brush, and floss threader).
- Procedures completed: initial examination, recall examination, scaling and polishing, radiographs taken, type of fluoride provided.
- Child's behavior throughout the appointment and level of cooperation (e.g., patient's behavior quiet during appointment but cooperative with all aspects of the appointment).
- Treatment planned for next visit.
- **Box 47-2** provides an example of documentation for a child's dental visit.

Box 47-2 Example Documentation: Preventive Dental Hygiene Visit by Child Patient

- **S**—An 8-year-old male presents for continuing care visit. Medical history reviewed with mother. No health concerns, no medications, no chief complaint. Home care: brushing one time per day in the morning and does not floss.
- **O**—Intraoral/extraoral examination: within normal limits; buccal mucosa: bilateral linea alba; tongue: coated. Class II occlusion, 50% overbite, 3 mm overjet, lower anterior crowding. Clinical findings: sealants on #3, 14, 19, and 30 sound. Radiographic findings: no caries. Oral hygiene: generalized moderate biofilm, localized light calculus: supragingival mandibular anteriors—all surfaces, subgingival mandibular posterior linguals, and supra/subgingival facial of maxillary first molars. Periodontal evaluation of permanent teeth: 1–2 mm with bleeding on probing.

(continues)

Box 47-2 Example Documentation: Preventive Dental Hygiene Visit by Child Patient *(continued)*

- **A**—Generalized gingivitis due to moderate biofilm, localized calculus, and generalized slight/moderate bleeding. OH is poor, "plaque-free score" = 20%, no improvement same as last visit, caries risk = low.
- **P**—Scaled, polished, and flossed. Applied 5% sodium fluoride varnish. OHI and recommendations: using modified bass technique, two times per day brushing for 2 minutes w/fluoridated toothpaste, daily flossing using a floss holder, use of disclosing tablets every other day.

Goal for next appointment: "plaque-free score" improvement, and reduced areas of calculus present. Patient was well behaved and had genuine interest in improving his oral health care. Parent advised to supervise care at home.

Signed: ______________________________, RDH
Date: ______________

Factors to Teach the Parents

- How the parents' own oral health affects their child's oral health.
- How the bacteria that cause dental caries can be transferred to the baby's mouth from parents or from other family members.
- How fluoride makes enamel stronger and more resistant to the bacteria that cause dental caries.
- Methods to prevent dental caries from developing in a young child's mouth.
- How feeding methods and snacking patterns can contribute to dental caries.
- How the parent can examine the infant's/child's mouth and what to look for during the examination.
- Reasons why the baby's mouth needs to be examined by an oral health professional at 6 months of age or as soon as the first tooth erupts.
- Reasons why maintenance of primary teeth is necessary for oral health, growth, and development.
- Ways parents can prepare their young children for visits to the dentist and dental hygienist.
- How parents can prevent accidents and injury in their infants and children.

References

1. American Academy of Pediatric Dentistry. Overview. In: *The Reference Manual of Pediatric Dentistry*. Chicago, IL: American Academy of Pediatric Dentistry; 2021:7-9. https://www.aapd.org/globalassets/media/policies_guidelines/i_overview.pdf. Accessed March 31, 2022.
2. HealthyChildren.org. What is a pediatric dentist? Published February 10, 2016. Updated March 17, 2022. https://www.healthychildren.org/English/family-life/health-management/pediatric-specialists/Pages/What-is-a-Pediatric-Dentist.aspx. Accessed March 30, 2022.
3. American Academy of Pediatric Dentistry. About AAPD. https://www.aapd.org/about/about-aapd/who-is-aapd. Accessed March 31, 2022.
4. American Academy of Pediatric Dentistry. Mission statement. https://www.aapd.org/about/about-aapd/who-is-aapd. Accessed March 31, 2022.
5. American Academy of Pediatric Dentistry. https://www.aapd.org. Accessed March 31, 2022.
6. Centers for Disease Control and Prevention. Child development. Published January 3, 2017. Updated February 22, 2021. https://www.cdc.gov/ncbddd/childdevelopment/positiveparenting/index.html. Accessed March 30, 2022.
7. American Academy of Pediatric Dentistry. Definition of a dental home. *Pediatr Dent*. 2015;39(6):12.
8. Shelov SP, Altmann TR, Hannermann RE. Part 1. In: *Caring for Your Baby and Young Child, Birth to Age 5*. 6th ed. Elk Grove Village, IL: American Academy of Pediatrics; 2014:395.
9. American Academy of Pediatric Dentistry. Guideline on periodicity of examination, preventive dental services, anticipatory guidance/counseling, and oral treatments for infant, children, and adolescents. *Pediatr Dent*. 2013;39(6):188-195.
10. McDonald RE, Avery DR, Dean JA. *Dentistry for the Child and Adolescent*. 10th ed. Maryland Heights, MO: Mosby Elsevier; 2016.
11. Centers for Disease Control and Prevention. Learn the signs. Act early. Published November 3, 2017. Updated February 18, 2021. https://www.cdc.gov/ncbddd/actearly/index.html. Accessed March 30,2022.
12. American Academy of Pediatric Dentistry. Guideline on fluoride therapy. *Pediatr Dent*. 2014;39(6):242-245.
13. Wong MC, Glenny AM, Tsang BW, Lo EC, Worthington HV, Marinho VC. Cochrane review: topical fluoride as a cause of dental fluorosis in children. *Evid Based Child Health*. 2011;6(2):388-439.
14. DenBesten P, Li W. Chronic fluoride toxicity: dental fluorosis. *Monogr Oral Sci*. 2011;22:81-96.
15. American Academy of Pediatric Dentistry. Policy on third-party reimbursement of fees related to dental sealants. *Pediatr Dent*. 2017;39(6):120-121.
16. Wright JT, Crall JJ, Fontana M, et al. Evidence-based clinical practice guideline for the use of pit-and-fissure sealants: a report of the American Dental Association and the American Academy of Pediatric Dentistry. *J Am Dent Assoc*. 2016;147(8):672-682.e12.

17. American Dental Association. Mouthwash (mouthrinse). Published September 13, 2017. http://www.ada.org/en/member-center/oral-health-topics/mouthrinse. Accessed March 30, 2022.
18. American Academy of Pediatric Dentistry. Caries-risk assessment and management for infants, children, and adolescents. In: *The Reference Manual of Pediatric Dentistry*. Chicago, IL: American Academy of Pediatric Dentistry; 2021:252-257.
19. Carranza FA, Newman MG. *Carranza's Clinical Periodontology*. 11th ed. St. Louis, MO: Elsevier Saunders; 2012:104-110.
20. American Academy of Pediatric Dentistry. Guideline on adolescent oral health care. *Pediatr Dent*. 2013;35(6):142-149.
21. Clerehugh V, Tugnait A. Diagnosis and management of periodontal diseases in children and adolescents. *Periodontol 2000*. 2001;26(1):146-168.
22. Clerehugh V, Tugnait A. Periodontal diseases in children and adolescents: I. aetiology and diagnosis. *Dent Update*. 2001;28(5):222-230, 232.
23. Albandar JM, Rams TE. Risk factors for periodontitis in children and young persons. *Periodontol 2000*. 2002;29(1):207-222.
24. American Academy of Pediatric Dentistry. Policy on early childhood caries (ECC): classifications, consequences, and preventive strategies. *Pediatr Dent*. 2016;39(6):59-61.
25. American Academy of Pediatric Dentistry. Policy on Early Childhood Caries (ECC): Unique Challenges and Treatment Options. https://www.aapd.org/globalassets/media/policies_guidelines/p_eccuniquechallenges.pdf. Accessed August 1, 2021.
26. Centers for Disease Control and Prevention. Oral health. https://www.cdc.gov/healthywater/hygiene/disease/dental_caries.html. Accessed March 31, 2022.
27. Dye BA, Li X, Thorton-Evans G. NCHS data briefs. National Center for Health Statistics, Centers for Disease Control and Prevention. Published August 2012. https://www.cdc.gov/nchs/data/databriefs/db197.pdf. Accessed March 13, 2022.
28. Berkowitz RJ. Mutans streptococci: acquisition and transmission. *Pediatr Dent*. 2006;28(2):106-109.
29. Wan AK, Seow WK, Purdie DM, Bird PS, Walsh LJ, Tudehope DI. Oral colonization of *Streptococcus mutans* in six-month-old predentate infants. *J Dent Res*. 2001;90(12):2060-2065.
30. Parisotto TM, Steiner-Oliveira C, Silva CM, Rodrigues LK, Nobre-dos-Santos M. Early childhood caries and mutans streptococci: a systematic review. *Oral Health Prev Dent*. 2010;8(1):59-70.
31. California Dental Association Foundation; American College of Obstetricians and Gynecologists, IX District. Oral health during pregnancy and early childhood: evidence-based guideline for health professional. *J Calif Dent Assoc*. 2010;38(6):391-426.
32. Patrick H, Nicklas TA. A review of family and social determinants of children's eating patterns and diet quality. *J Am Coll Nutr*. 2005;24(2):83-92.
33. Wright JT, Hanson N, Ristic H, et al. Fluoride toothpaste efficacy and safety in children younger than 6 years. *J Am Dent Assoc*. 2014;145(2):182-189.
34. American Academy of Pediatric Dentistry. Management of the developing dentition and occlusion in pediatric dentistry. *Pediatr Dent*. 2014;39(6):334-347.
35. Bad breath: causes and tips for controlling it. *J Am Dent Assoc*. 2012;143(9):1053.
36. Kinberg S, Stein M, Zion N, Shaoul R. The gastrointestinal aspects of halitosis. *Can J Gastroenterol*. 2010;24(9):552-556.
37. American Academy of Pediatric Dentistry. Policy on human papilloma virus vaccinations. https://www.aapd.org/research/oral-health-policies--recommendations/human-papilloma-virus-vaccinations/. Accessed August 25,2021
38. American Academy of Pediatric Dentistry. Policy on obstructive sleep apnea. https://www.aapd.org/research/oral-health-policies--recommendations/obstructive-sleep-apnea/. Accessed August 25, 2021.
39. Trosman I. Childhood obstructive sleep apnea syndrome: a review of the 2012 American Academy of Pediatrics guidelines. *Pediatr Ann*. 2013;42(10):195-199.
40. Titus P, Titus S, Frances G, Alani MM, George AJ. Ornamental dentistry—an overview. *J Evol Med Dent Sci*. 2013;2(7):666-676.
41. Durosaro O, El-Axhary R. A 10-year retrospective study on palladium sensitivity. *Dermatitis*. 2009;20(4):208-213.
42. Ziebolz D, Hildebrand A, Proff P, Rinke S, Hornecker E, Mausberg R. Long-term effects of tongue piercing—a case-control study. *Clin Oral Investig*. 2012;16(1):231-237.
43. Plessa A, Pepelassi E. Dental and periodontal complications of lip and tongue piercing: prevalence and influencing factors. *Aust Dent J*. 2012;57(1):71-78.
44. Hennequin-Hoenderdos NL, Slot DE, Van der Weijden GA. The incidence of complications associated with lip and/or tongue piercings: a systematic review. *Int J Dent Hyg*. 2016;14(1):62-73.
45. Reyes P. Hole-y mouth jewelry! Piercings could lead to anterior tooth loss. *J Calif Dent Assoc*. 2008;36(9):651, 655.
46. Centers for Disease Control and Prevention, Division of Viral Hepatitis. Hepatitis C FAQs for health professionals. https://www.cdc.gov/Hepatitis/HCV/HCVfaq.htm. Accessed March 31, 2022.
47. Hollowell W, Childers N. A new threat to adolescent oral health: the grill. *Pediatr Dent*. 2007;29(4):320-322.
48. American Academy of Pediatric Dentistry. Guideline on oral and dental aspects of child abuse and neglect. *Pediatr Dent*. 2017;39(6):235-241.
49. American Academy of Pediatric Dentistry. Teledentistry policy. https://www.aapd.org/globalassets/media/policies_guidelines/p_teledentistry.pdf. Accessed August 25, 2022.

CHAPTER 48

The Older Adult Patient

Lisa M. LaSpina, RDH, DHSc

CHAPTER OUTLINE

AGING
- **I.** Biologic and Chronologic Age
- **II.** Classification by Function
- **III.** Primary, Secondary, and Optimal Aging

NORMAL PHYSIOLOGIC AGING
- **I.** Musculoskeletal System
- **II.** Cardiovascular System
- **III.** Respiratory System
- **IV.** Gastrointestinal System
- **V.** Central Nervous System
- **VI.** Peripheral Nervous System
- **VII.** Sensory Systems
- **VIII.** Endocrine System
- **IX.** Immune System
- **X.** Cognitive Change

PATHOLOGY AND DISEASE
- **I.** Factors that Influence Disease
- **II.** Response to Disease

CHRONIC CONDITIONS ASSOCIATED WITH AGING
- **I.** Alzheimer's Disease
- **II.** Osteoarthritis
- **III.** Alcoholism
- **IV.** Osteoporosis
- **V.** Sexually Transmitted Diseases
- **VI.** Respiratory Disease
- **VII.** Cardiovascular Disease

ORAL CHANGES ASSOCIATED WITH AGING
- **I.** Soft Tissues
- **II.** Teeth
- **III.** The Periodontium

DENTAL HYGIENE CARE FOR THE OLDER ADULT PATIENT
- **I.** Barriers to Care
- **II.** Assessment
- **III.** Preventive Care Plan
- **IV.** Dental Biofilm Control
- **V.** Relief for Xerostomia
- **VI.** Periodontal Care
- **VII.** Dental Caries Control
- **VIII.** Diet and Nutrition

DOCUMENTATION

FACTORS TO TEACH THE PATIENT

REFERENCES

LEARNING OBJECTIVES

After studying the chapter, the student will be able to:

1. Describe physiologic and cognitive changes associated with aging.
2. Explain common chronic conditions associated with aging.
3. Identify common oral changes associated with aging.
4. Demonstrate best practices for communicating with the older adult patient.
5. Explain and document the dental hygiene process of care for the older adult patient.

The trend for the number of adults older than 65 years continues to increase in the United States and is projected to grow to 95 million in 2060.[1] The aging population is becoming racially and ethnically diverse.[1] The first of the "baby boom" generation, adults born between the years 1946 and 1964, turned 65 in 2011. They are the first generation to benefit from systemic fluoride in community water supplies and topically in toothpastes.

- The older adult population is:
    - Retaining more natural teeth, many with full dentitions.[2]
    - Motivated to maintain and improve oral health.[2]
    - Seeking more preventive procedures for oral health than in previous years.[2]
- Dental hygienists will be challenged by the complex needs of the **aging** population.
- As the lifespan of individuals increases, so does the incidence of chronic diseases.
- Dental hygienists need to be competent in providing safe, preventive, and therapeutic services for the older adult patient in all types of dental settings.
- An increasing number of dental hygienists will specialize in the care of older adults and be employed in long-term care, home health care, and assisted living facilities.
- Tooth loss increases with age, but not because of the aging process.
- Dental caries and periodontal diseases are the major causes of tooth loss.
- Periodontal diseases in the older adult population represent the cumulative effects of long-standing, undiagnosed, untreated, or neglected chronic infection.
- Dental caries in the older adult population is associated with:
    - Gingival recession.
    - Salivary hypofunction.
    - Use of xerostomia-inducing medications.
    - Diet high in fermentable carbohydrates.
    - Poor oral hygiene.
- The use of fluoride can provide valuable protection to teeth and exposed root surfaces for all ages. It is unfortunate some older adults believe fluoride is only for children.

Aging

I. Biologic and Chronologic Age

- From a biopsychosocial viewpoint, 65 years of age is the entry point for "old age." **Gerontology** has divided the period of 65 and older into subgroups[2,3]:
    - Young-old, adults between the ages of 65 and 74 years.
    - Old-old, adults between the ages of 75 and 84 years.
    - Oldest-old, adults between the ages of 85 and 99 years.
    - Centenarians, adults between the ages of 100 and 109 years.
    - Supercentenarians, adults older than 110 years.
- **Biologic age** is not synonymous with **chronologic age**:
    - Signs of aging appear at different chronologic ages in different individuals.
    - Aging is a process with many physiologic changes.
    - A person can be biologically old at age 65; others can be physically fit at age 75.

II. Classification by Function

- The degree of general health and physical activity provides a classification system, **functional age**, not based on chronologic age but on how the older adults actually perform various activities.
- Relative to the degree of impairment, older adults' functional ability may be categorized as robust, frail, or dependent.
- Classification by function is defined by activities of daily living (ADLs). ADLs are skills, such as eating, bathing, and mobility, required for individuals to independently care for themselves. ADLs are described in Chapter 22.

III. Primary, Secondary, and Optimal Aging

- Primary aging (also referred to as normal aging): age-related changes that occur in the body's systems advancing at an individual rate. These age-related changes are universal, intrinsic, and progressive. Example: skin wrinkling.[3]
- Secondary aging (also referred to as impaired aging): age-related changes due to disease that leads to impairment. These age-related changes are associated with trauma and chronic diseases. Example: heart disease.[3]
- Optimal aging (also referred to as successful aging): aging is slowed or altered due to preventive measures to avoid negative changes. Example: eating a healthy diet and daily physical activity.[2,3]

Normal Physiologic Aging

- Primary normal changes with aging are physiologic.
- Secondary pathologic aging influences and accelerates the aging process.
  - Each age level brings changes in body metabolism, activity of the cells, endocrine balance, and mental processes.
  - In a healthy person, free of chronic diseases and medications with their potential side effects, the tissue changes of aging may be more subtle, appear at a later age, and be influenced by the person's **lifestyle**.
- Skin: thin, wrinkled, and dry, with pigmented spots, and loss of tone.
- Reduced tolerance to temperature extremes and solar exposure.
- Normal physiologic changes that occur as the individual ages are universal, progressive, intrinsic, and unavoidable. These changes vary among individuals and the body's systems.
- During aging, an overall gradual reduction in functional capacities occurs in most organs, with a decrease in cell metabolism and numbers of active cells.
- The following provides a summary of physiologic changes that occur due to the normal aging process.

I. Musculoskeletal System

- Bone volume (mass) decreases gradually after the age of 40 years.
- Loss of muscle function: diminished muscular strength and speed of response.
- Curvature of cervical vertebrae due to a decrease in bone density and atrophic changes to cartilage and muscle.
- Joints may stiffen because of loss of elasticity in the ligaments.

II. Cardiovascular System

- Decrease in cardiovascular reserve; increase stiffness of the left ventricle.[4]
- Blood vessels become less elastic and flexible.[4]
  - Lumen of vessels decreases in size with resultant reduction of blood supply to organs, especially the liver and kidneys.
  - Increased peripheral resistance.
- Atherosclerosis (fatty deposits on inner walls of arteries) is associated with aging; diet, smoking, and lack of exercise can be an influence.
- Changes in cardiovasculature do not affect function under normal, nonstressful conditions.

III. Respiratory System

- Vital capacity is progressively diminished, leading to decreased efficiency of oxygen–carbon dioxide exchange.[5]
- Skeletal changes weaken respiratory muscles, which limits chest expansion and reduces effective ventilation.[5]
- Less effective cough reflex; increased risk for respiratory infections.[5]

IV. Gastrointestinal System

- Production of hydrochloric acid and other secretions gradually decreases.
- Peristalsis is slowed.
- Decreased absorptive functions can affect nutrition and medications.

V. Central Nervous System

- Intellectual or cognitive function is slowed, not lost.
- Complex tasks may be more difficult.
- Short-term memory declines; long-term memory remains constant.

VI. Peripheral Nervous System

- Decrease in tactile sensitivity.
- Decreased proprioception (sense of one's position in space); risk for falls.

VII. Sensory Systems

- Age-related vision changes include[6]:
  - Presbyopia.
  - Decreases in visual acuity (more light needed), peripheral vision, color clarity (problems with blues and greens).
  - Decreased dilation and constriction of pupils results in difficulty adjusting to changes in light and problems with glare.
- Age-related hearing changes include[7]:
  - **Presbycusis**.
  - Thicker and dryer cerumen (wax) contributes to hearing loss.
  - Decrease in the ability to hear high-frequency tones.
  - **Tinnitus**.
- Management of a dental hygiene patient with vision and hearing impairment is discussed in Chapter 51.

VIII. Endocrine System

- Decrease in thyroid efficiency; decreased basal metabolic rate.
- Altered thermoregulatory system; sensitive to cold; may not respond to infection with increased temperature.

IX. Immune System

- The immune system declines with age. Among individuals, the degree of decline varies greatly. Age-related changes are labeled as immunosenescence.[8]
- Age-related changes in the skin and mucous membranes decrease effectiveness of the first line of defense against invading substances.
- Persistent low-grade inflammation.
- Increased incidence of autoimmune disorders and impaired wound repair.
- Changes in the immune system result in increased incidence of infections. Older adults need to seek immunizations for coronavirus disease (COVID-19), influenza, varicella–zoster virus, and pneumococcal pneumonia. Vaccinations for hepatitis A, hepatitis B, hepatitis C, varicella, and meningococcal infection are recommended.

X. Cognitive Change

- Cognitive change can distract the individual's attention away from their activities of daily living.[9]
- The older adult patient struggles with numerous demands, which can affect the ability to function, especially the ability to concentrate.
- Factors such as excess light and noise can distract the older adult from perceiving relevant information.
- Supportive interventions to aid an older adult with cognitive changes to maintain normal life activities are listed in **Table 48-1**.
- Tooth loss and gingival inflammation are associated with lower cognitive performance.[10]

Table 48-1 Supportive Interventions to Aid an Older Adult with Cognitive Changes

Situation	Supportive Intervention
Physical surroundings–environmental	▪ Reduce clutter.
Informational	▪ Use 14-point font for paper and online reading materials. ▪ Avoid unnecessary medical and legal jargon in patient reading materials. ▪ Facilitate use of reminder devices and lists.
Behavioral	▪ When possible, alter situations that restrict behaviors, including transportation and mobility problems. ▪ Provide assistive devices to promote independence and control.
Affective	▪ Assess for personal concerns and worries. ▪ Manage to decrease anxiety.

Pathology and Disease

I. Factors that Influence Disease

- An older person's health status is influenced by many factors. Biologic, environmental, psychosocial, psychological, and lifestyle factors influence longevity.
- Genetically, a person may belong to a family that has exhibited resistance to disease factors.
- Healthy dietary habits and regular exercise can prevent or minimize disease.
- The following risk factors influence disease states:
  - Tobacco use: all forms.
  - Use of alcohol.
  - Substance use.
  - Obesity and overweight.
- Decreased immunologic functioning in aging is a factor for increased susceptibility of both men and women to human immunodeficiency virus (HIV) infection, acquired immunodeficiency syndrome (AIDS), and other sexually transmitted diseases (STDs).
- Associations between periodontitis and specific systemic diseases include[11-14]:
  - Atherosclerotic diseases.[11,13,14]
  - Diabetes mellitus.[11,12,14]
  - Respiratory infections.[11,14]
  - Rheumatoid arthritis.[11,14]
- The incidence of oral disease is cumulative: periodontitis and caries occurs over one's lifetime[15]

II. Response to Disease

- The diseases that affect the older adult age group also occur in younger people; however:
  - There are differences, such as a lessened reserve capacity.

Box 48-1 Characteristics of Altered Response to Disease in the Older Adult

- *Course and severity:* disease may occur with greater severity and have a longer course, with slower recovery.
- *Pain sensitivity:* may be lessened.
- *Body temperature response:* may be altered so that a patient may be very ill without the expected increase in body temperature.
- *Healing response:*
  - Decreased healing capacity.
  - More prone to secondary infection.

  - An older adult may not present with the classic symptoms of disease as would a younger person.
- Characteristics of the altered response of the older adult to disease are listed in **Box 48-1**.

Chronic Conditions Associated with Aging

- Although many older adults function well and live independently in the community, the incidence of chronic diseases increases with advancing age.
- Individuals may have more than one chronic illness.
- The most common chronic conditions are osteoarthritis, visual and hearing impairments, cardiovascular diseases, and diabetes.
- Because of the number of chronic conditions, patients may be taking a large number of medications (**polypharmacy**), which can exacerbate xerostomia and increase the possibility of drug interactions.

I. Alzheimer's Disease

- **Dementia** is severe impairment of cognitive abilities, notably thinking, memory, and judgment. **Alzheimer's disease** is a nonreversible type of dementia and the most common of all dementias.

A. Etiology

- Two types:
  - Early onset: rare, reported in individuals in their 30s and 40s.
  - Late onset: most common, in people older than 65 years.
- Etiology unknown: theories include genetics, environment, nutrition, free radicals, and infectious agents.
- Average duration is 8–10 years from the onset of symptoms to death.

B. Symptoms and Stages

- The common impairments of Alzheimer's disease may be divided into overlapping stages and may extend up to 20 years.
- **Box 48-2** illustrates the progression of Alzheimer's disease symptoms through stages that describes how a person's abilities change from normal function through advanced disability.
- Keep in mind the stages are general guides; symptoms vary greatly. Not every individual with Alzheimer's disease will experience the same symptoms or progress at the same rate.

C. Treatment

- There is no proven treatment to prevent or cure the disease.
- Treatment is designed to support the family as well as the patient.
- Requires a prolonged multidisciplinary effort.
- Medications are prescribed for patients with mild-to-moderate symptoms.
- Medications prescribed to address behavioral problems include:
  - Antidepressants.
  - Antianxiety medications.
  - Antipsychotics.
  - Anticonvulsants may be prescribed for the small percentage of individuals who have seizures.

D. Dental Hygiene Management Considerations

- **Box 48-3** illustrates guidelines for caregivers of persons with Alzheimer's disease.
- Specific dental hygiene care considerations for the patient with early and later stages of Alzheimer's disease are listed in **Box 48-4**.
- Link between periodontal disease and Alzheimer's disease; brain inflammation can result from periodontal bacteria and the entry of pathogen products into the brain.[16]
- Goals of dental hygiene care:
  - Preserve oral health and function.
  - Prevent future oral and systemic disease.
  - Provide comfort.

Box 48-2 Stages of Alzheimer's Disease

Stage 1: Normal Function

- No memory problems.

Stage 2: Very Mild

- Memory lapses; personal awareness of forgetting familiar words or the location of everyday objects.
- No medical diagnosis of dementia.

Stage 3: Mild

- Memory lapses; family members/friends begin to notice problems in memory or concentration.
- Observable difficulties include:
  - Trouble remembering names or the right words.
  - Performing tasks.
  - Losing objects.
  - Trouble organizing.

Stage 4: Moderate

- Able to clearly detect that there are problems.
- Observable difficulties include:
  - Forgetting events and personal history.
  - Increasing difficulty with complex tasks.
  - Withdrawn.

Stage 5: Moderately Severe

- Noticeable lapses in memory and thinking.
- Does not remember own address/phone number.
- Confused; does not know what day it is.
- Still self-sufficient with eating or using the toilet.

Stage 6: Severe

- Memory worsens/personality changes.
- Observable difficulties include:
  - Cannot recall recent experience.
  - Trouble remembering the names of family members.
  - Changes in sleep patterns.
  - Needs assistance with toileting/unable to control bladder or bowels.
  - Personality and behavior changes such as being more suspicious.
  - Compulsive/repetitive behavior (e.g., shredding facial tissue).
  - Wanders easily/can become lost.

Stage 7: Very Severe

- Loss of ability to respond to environment.
- Cannot carry on a conversation or easily control movement.
- Observable difficulties include:
  - Eating.
  - Using the toilet.
  - Smiling.
  - Holding head upright.
  - Swallowing.

Data from Stages of Alzheimer's Disease. Alzheimer's Association Website: https://www.alz.org/alzheimers-dementia/stages#overview. Accessed August 29, 2021.

Box 48-3 Alzheimer's Disease: Guidelines for Caregivers

- Keep the same daily routine. Keep the environment calm.
- Promote the use of clocks, calendars, and newspapers to maintain the patient's orientation.
- Watch the patient's medical and oral health. Encourage exercise and regular dental visits.
- Keep communication open. Use laughter as a tool.
- Use positive reinforcement.

Data from Saxon SV, Etten M, Perkins, EA. *Physical Change and Aging: A Guide for Helping Professions*. 7th ed. New York: Springer Publishing Company; 2021:66.

Box 48-4 Dental Hygiene Care Considerations for a Patient with Alzheimer's Disease

Early Stages

- Review of the patient's medical and dental history at each maintenance appointment may reveal lapses in memory and other signs of early disease.
- An early sign may be a slow decline of interest in oral hygiene and personal care.
- Provide routine care with initiation of aggressive preventive regimens.
- Three-month intervals for maintenance appointments are recommended.
- Topical fluoride applications; fluoride varnish.
- Oral hygiene instruction; involve caregivers early in the disease process.

Later Stages

- Routine intraoral examination to assess lesions due to cancer, medications, or injury.
- Sedation may be required.
- Possible need for mouth prop and physical restraint.
- Caregivers assume daily oral care. Power toothbrushes may improve dental biofilm removal for caregivers to use.
- Patient may reside in a long-term care facility. Dental hygienists who specialize in the treatment of this population may oversee care.

- The dental hygiene care plan:
  - Considers the current stage of the patient's disease.
  - Provides a plan for comprehensive care in anticipation of future decline in oral health.
- Undiagnosed patients: when patient's behavior is suspect, a referral to the patient's primary care provider is made.

II. Osteoarthritis

- Osteoarthritis is the most common form of arthritis and involves a progressive loss of articular cartilage. Management of the patient with arthritis is discussed in more detail in Chapter 52.

A. Symptoms

- Intermittent joint pain.
- Stiffness upon arising.
- Crepitation (creaking joints).

B. Treatment

- Physical therapy.
- Exercise.
- Rest.
- Reduced stress on joints.
- Dietary modifications.
- Drug therapy.

C. Dental Hygiene Management Considerations

- Keep appointments short.
- Schedule afternoon appointments.
- Allow breaks to rest the jaw.

III. Alcoholism

A. Effects of Alcohol Use

- Owing to age-related primary physiologic changes, older drinkers may experience more detrimental health-related effects compared with younger drinkers.
- Older adults require less alcohol for adverse effects to occur.
- Excessive use of alcohol by older adults may[17]:
  - Result in more severe health-related consequences.
  - Exacerbate medical and emotional problems associated with aging.
  - Predispose to adverse drug reactions with prescription and over-the-counter medications.
  - Be associated with major depressive disorder.

B. Dental Hygiene Management Considerations

- Management of a dental hygiene patient with a substance-related disorder is discussed more completely in Chapter 59.

IV. Osteoporosis

- **Osteoporosis** is a bone disease involving loss of mineral content and bone mass.
- It is common in individuals older than age 60, and the incidence increases with age.
- Although most prominent in postmenopausal women, the condition may also occur at other ages and in men.

A. Causes

- Endocrine: hormonal disturbances; depletion of estrogen after menopause.
- Inadequate intake of calcium and/or vitamin D or defective absorption of calcium or vitamin D metabolism.

B. Prevention

- Prevention is the first line of defense against osteoporosis.
- Adequate calcium and vitamin D intake during adolescence and early adulthood is critical to forming peak bone mass.
- The minimum requirements for both calcium and vitamin D increase with age.
- Load-bearing exercise is necessary to maintain bone mass.

C. Risk Factors

A number of risk factors have been identified; some of which work together. From the risk factors, a list of methods for long-term prevention can be derived:

- Female gender; positive family history.
- White or Asian ethnicity (worldwide, Blacks are least affected).
- Low calcium and vitamin D intake (lifelong).
- Early menopause or early surgical removal of ovaries; use of corticosteroids; eating disorders.
- Sedentary lifestyle; lack of exercise.
- Alcohol abuse; tobacco use; high caffeine intake.
- High sodium intake.
- Low body mass index.

D. Relationship to Periodontal Disease

- A relationship exists between the reduced bone mineral density of osteoporosis and oral bone loss in skeletal and mandibular bone; oral bone loss in the edentulous person pertains to[18]:
  - Periodontal bone destruction.
  - Residual ridge loss.

- Mutual risk factors of osteoporosis and periodontal disease
  - Smoking.
  - Nutritional deficiencies.
  - Alcohol use.
  - Hormonal status.
- Osteoporotic bone is:
  - Less dense.
  - More readily absorbed.

E. Symptoms

Osteoporosis develops over many years; a long asymptomatic period of bone change can occur with no clinical symptoms.[19]

- Clinical symptoms may include:
  - Backache: stooping posture. **Figure 48-1** illustrates the posture of an older adult with osteoporosis.
  - Vertebral fractures or compression fractures that cause the spine to curve.
  - Fractures: hip, compression fractures of spine, ends of long bones.
  - Evidence of bone changes in the mandible: residual ridge resorption.

F. Treatment/Medications

- A number of medications, with various mechanisms of action, decrease bone resorption, increase bone formation, or both.
- Whichever regimen of medications is prescribed, successful treatment and prevention requires simultaneous intake of calcium and vitamin D.

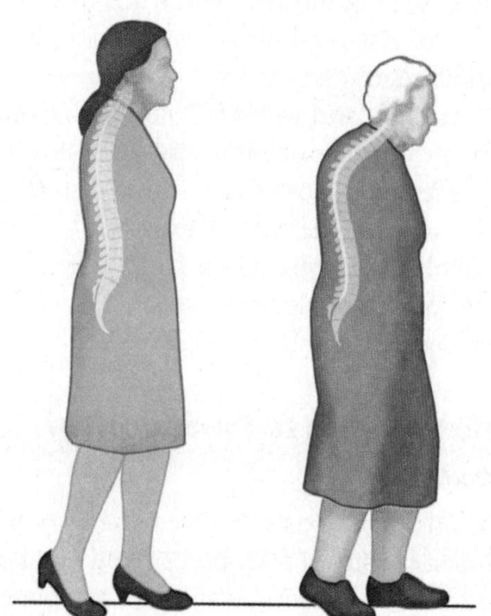

Figure 48-1 Example of an Older Adult's Posture with Osteoporosis. Vertebral fractures or compression fractures cause the spine to curve.

- Bisphosphonates: slows bone metabolism/increasing bone density.
- Selective estrogen receptor modulators: inhibits bone resorption.
- Calcitonin: inhibits bone resorption.
- Parathyroid hormone: stimulates bone formation.

G. Treatment and Prevention

- Weight-bearing physical activity, such as walking, has a beneficial effect on bone mass.
- Activities of daily living and physical activity require caution and preventive measures to avoid accidental falls.
- Avoid smoking and excessive alcohol intake.
- Severe involvement of the spine may require orthopedic support and medication for pain.
- Dental hygiene management considerations:
  - Do not rush; try to prevent falls.
  - Provide extra time for positioning; provide cushioning.
  - Taking bisphosphonates may be a contraindication for dental surgery due to increased risk for osteonecrosis (bone destruction) of the jaw and consultation with the primary care provider is needed.
  - Health promotion opportunities exist for long-term prevention. Encourage:
    - Smoking cessation.
    - Limiting alcohol consumption.
    - Healthy lifestyles involving adequate calcium and vitamin D intake and regular physical activity.

V. Sexually Transmitted Diseases

- The most common STDs include:
  - Chlamydia.
  - Syphilis.
  - HIV/AIDS.
  - Genital herpes.
  - Gonorrhea.
  - Human papillomavirus.
- STDs are on the rise in the older adult populations.

A. Incidence in Older Populations

The most common STD in this demographic is HIV/AIDS, with an increase of new HIV/AIDS cases in the 50 years and older age group.[20]

- Factors that influence the increase in numbers include:
  - Increased use of medications to treat erectile dysfunction.

- Increased divorce rate.
- People living longer and generally in better health.
- Sexually active senior women are more prone to acquiring STDs due to:
  - Thinning of the epithelium of the vaginal area.
  - Diminished immune system.
- Increased number of older adults living in assisted living centers or senior housing communities.
- Cultural and generational differences may explain why older adults are not as knowledgeable about the need for safe-sex practices.
- Older adults might not practice safe sex since there is no risk of pregnancy.

B. Dental Hygiene Management Considerations

- Medical referral or consultation.
- An appointment with the patient's physician is necessary to determine what medication is needed to treat the STD.
- Goals of dental hygiene care include:
  - Open, nonjudgmental communication.[21]
  - Increased patient awareness of the transmission of STDs.
  - Importance of communication with the patient's physician.

VI. Respiratory Disease

- Older adults are at higher risk for respiratory disease.[22]
- Good oral hygiene practices can reduce the progression or occurrence of respiratory diseases among older adult patients.
- Chapter 60 provides more information regarding dental hygiene care for patients with respiratory disease.

A. Age-Related Disorders of the Respiratory System

- Pneumonia.
- Chronic obstructive pulmonary disease.
- Asthma.

B. Dental Hygiene Management Considerations

- Monitor vital signs.
- Adjust seating position as needed for comfortable breathing. Refer to Chapter 4 for information related to patient positioning.

VII. Cardiovascular Disease

- Heart disease is a common cause of death for the older adult patient over age 65 years.
- Health promotion and healthy behaviors initiated early can prevent heart disease.
- Age-related disorders of the cardiovascular system include:
  - Arteriosclerosis and atherosclerosis.
  - Hypertension and postural hypotension.
  - Angina pectoris.
  - Myocardial infarction.
  - Congestive heart failure.
  - Heart valve disease.
  - Transient ischemic attack (ministroke).
  - Cerebrovascular accident (stroke).
- Dental hygiene management considerations:
  - Monitor blood pressure.
  - Use of relaxation techniques.
  - Lifestyle changes.
- Chapter 61 provides more information regarding dental hygiene care for patients with cardiovascular disease.

Oral Changes Associated with Aging

- Healthy tissue features of primary aging need to be separated from the long-term effects of secondary aging due to chronic disease and medications.

I. Soft Tissues

A. Lips

- Tissue changes: dry, purse-string opening results from dehydration and loss of elasticity within the tissues.
- Angular cheilitis is not specifically an age-related lesion, but it is seen frequently among older adults.[23]
  - Etiologic factors may be candidiasis and vitamin B deficiency.
  - Appears as skin folds with fissuring at the angles of the mouth and can be related to reduced vertical dimension or inadequate support of the lips.
  - Cheilitis in conjunction with dentures is described in Chapter 30.

B. Oral Mucosa

- Atrophic changes: the tissue may become thinner and less vascular, with a loss of elasticity;

a smooth, shiny appearance is related to thinning of the epithelium.
- Hyperkeratosis: white, patchy appearance of tissue may develop because of irritation from sharp edges of broken teeth, restorations, or dentures, and from use of tobacco.
- Capillary fragility: facial bruises and petechiae of the mucosa are common.

C. Tongue

- Atrophic glossitis (burning tongue)
  - The tongue appears smooth and shiny with atrophied papillae.
  - The condition is usually related to anemia that results from a deficiency of iron or combinations of deficiencies.
  - Deficiency anemia results from nutritional factors.
- Taste sensations
  - Taste buds decrease in number and size.[24]
  - The acuity of the perception for salt declines with age.
  - The perception of sweet and sour does not decline with age.
  - Olfactory acuity, which significantly affects taste, declines more than taste.
  - Flavoring agents and spices can be added to foods instead of salt and sugar to enhance taste.
  - Tongue cleaning increases taste perception.
- Sublingual varicosities
  - Clinical appearance: deep, red or bluish nodular dilated vessels on either side of the midline on the ventral surface of the tongue.
  - Significance: varicosities do not have a direct relation to systemic conditions.

D. Xerostomia

- Xerostomia, dryness of the mouth
  - Characterized by the absence or diminished quantity of saliva.[25]
  - Prevalent in the older adult.[26]
  - A symptom, not a disease entity.
- Lack of saliva and the effect of a dry mouth are significant contributing factors to oral discomfort and disease, particularly dental caries.
- Causes of xerostomia include:
  - Systemic medications, which provide the most common influence. Many drugs that are common prescription items produce dry mouth as a side effect.
  - Autoimmune diseases such as **Sjögren's syndrome**, rheumatoid arthritis, or systemic lupus erythematosus.
  - Diabetes.
  - Radiation to head and neck for cancer therapy: permanent damage to the salivary glands can result.
- Clinical symptoms include:
  - Feeling of oral dryness; tongue sticks to the palate.
  - Difficulty with mastication, swallowing, and speech.
  - Impaired taste.
  - Burning, and soreness of mucosa and tongue.
- Oral effects of xerostomia
  - Heavy dental biofilm, material alba, and debris accumulation can lead to increased:
    - Severity of periodontal infection and demineralization of tooth surface.
    - Predisposition to dental caries, particularly root caries.
    - Problems of denture wearing.
    - Dietary changes during eating; may use increased quantities of liquid to soften food for swallowing.
- See **Box 48-5** for a partial list of drug groups that may decrease salivary function.

E. Oral Candidiasis

- Oral candidiasis is an infection of the oral mucosal tissues.
- Candidiasis is associated with the use of antibiotics, head and neck radiation therapy, chemotherapy, steroids, and other immunosuppressive drugs.
- Medical conditions that alter the immune system, including diabetes and HIV infection, permit overgrowth of the *Candida* organisms.
- Patients with xerostomia have an increased incidence of candidiasis.

Box 48-5 Partial List of Classes of Drugs That Decrease Salivary Function

- Anticholinergics
- Antihistamines
- Antihypertensives
- Antianxiety
- Anticonvulsants
- Diuretics
- Antidepressants (tricyclic)
- Nonsteroidal anti-inflammatory drugs

- Denture stomatitis and angular cheilitis represent the two common forms, as described in Chapter 30.

II. Teeth

A. Color

- Darkening or yellowing is the result of changes in the underlying dentin.
- Color changes result from long use of tobacco and beverages such as tea and coffee.
- Dark intrinsic stains from dental restorations.

B. Dental Pulp

- Pulpal changes develop as reactions to wear, dental caries, restorations, bruxism, and other assaults during the elderly person's long life.[27]
- Narrowing of pulp chambers and root canals; increased deposition of secondary and tertiary dentin. **Figure 48-2** provides examples of radiographs showing the narrowing of pulp canals with age.
- Progressive deposition of calcified masses (pulp stones or denticles).

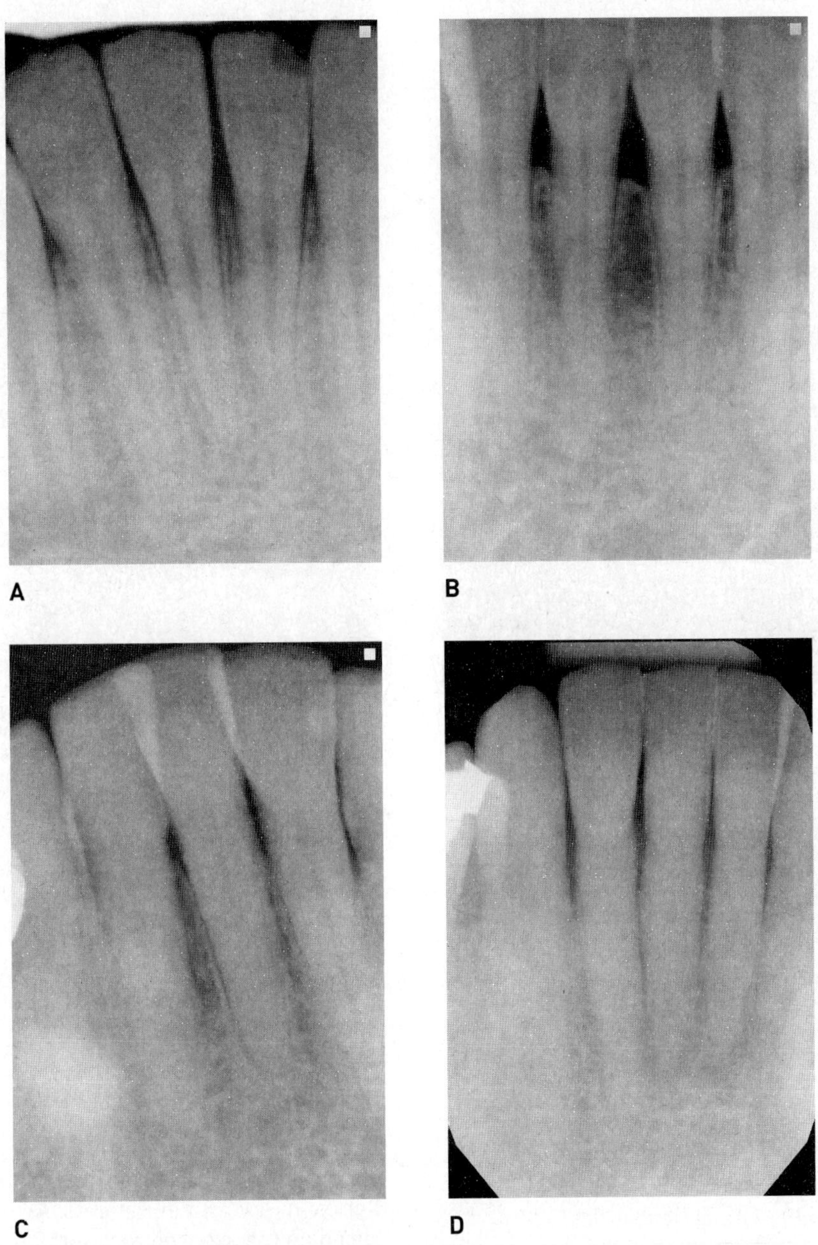

Figure 48-2 Radiographs Provide an Example of Narrowing Pulp Canals with Age. The radiograph of an 11-year-old boy **(A)** illustrates pulp canals common in youth; radiographs **(B)** and **(C)** illustrate narrowing with advancing age; and the radiograph of a 97-year-old woman **(D)** shows pulp canals, which are significantly diminished.

C. Attrition

- Signs of wear, which may be long-term effects of diet, occupational factors, or bruxism.
- Attrition may be accompanied by chipping and teeth may seem more brittle.

D. Abrasion

- Abrasion at the cervical third of a tooth may result from extended use of a hard toothbrush in a horizontal direction with an abrasive dentifrice.
- With current preventive measures, use of soft-textured brushes, and attention to abrasiveness of dentifrices, future generations will be less likely to exhibit such tooth alterations.
- **Figure 48-3** provides photographic and radiographic images of abrasion.

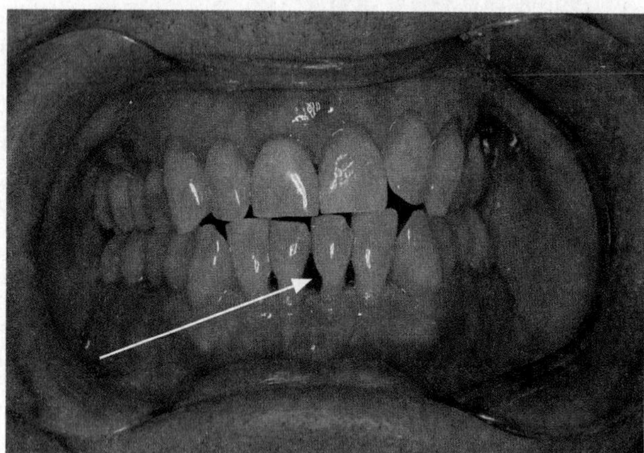

A

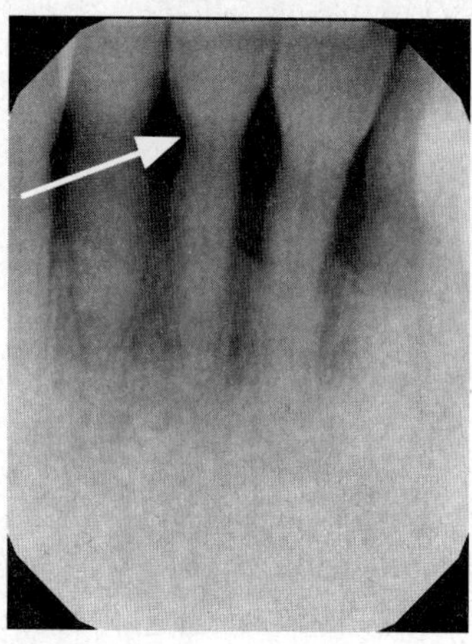

B

Figure 48-3 In both the photograph **(A)** and the radiograph **(B)**, the arrow points to areas of abrasion present in the lower anterior teeth of a 66-year-old man.

Photograph courtesy of Dr. Paul Epstein, DMD.

E. Root Caries

- Prevalence: older adults have more root caries than any other age group, except in communities with natural fluoride or community water fluoridation.[28]
    - A photograph in **Figure 48-4** provides examples of root caries.

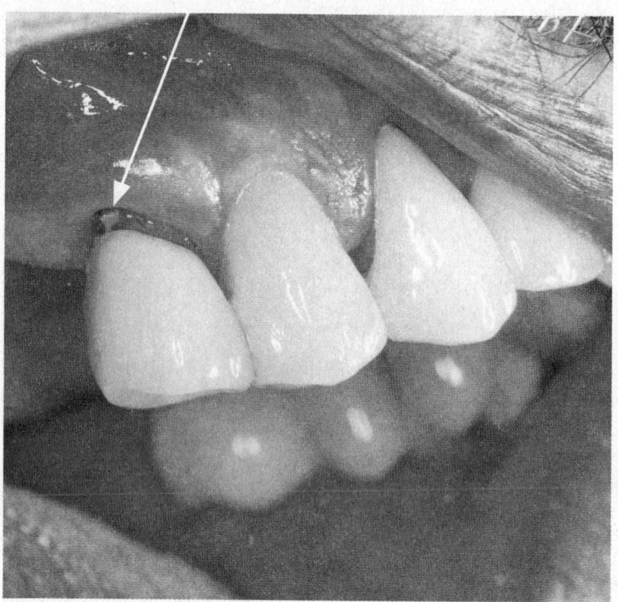

A

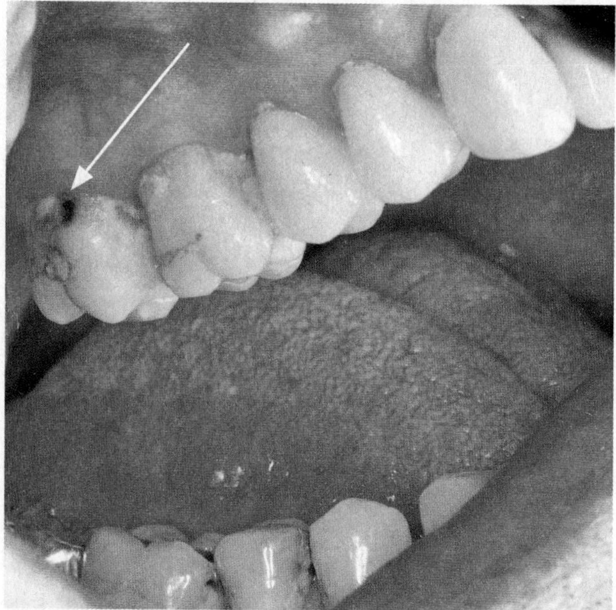

B

Figure 48-4 Two Photographs Provide Examples of Root Caries in Older Adult Patients. **A:** Illustrates a cavitated lesion on the exposed root surface apical to the margin of a crown on tooth number 4. The arrow in photograph **(B)** points to dental caries apical to the cementoenamel junction on tooth number 3. Notice the previously restored areas on adjacent teeth.

Photograph courtesy of Dr. Paul Epstein, DMD.

- Chlorhexidine rinses periodically for individuals with high bacterial counts; effective against *Streptococcus mutans.* (See Chapter 25.)
- Xylitol chewing gum after meals and snacks for patients without chewing and swallowing difficulties.

VIII. Diet and Nutrition

- Dietary and resulting nutritional deficiencies are common in older people.
- Characteristic changes, such as burning tongue, angular cheilitis, and atrophic glossitis, may be related to vitamin B deficiencies.
- Factors contributing to dietary and nutritional deficiencies include:
  - Limited budget.
  - Not eating regular meals; frequently eating non-nutritious snacks.
  - Lack of interest in shopping for or preparing food.
  - Acuteness of senses (taste, smell) lowered; may seek highly seasoned or sweetened foods.
  - Inadequate masticatory efficiency because of tooth loss or dentures that no longer fit properly.
  - Adverse food selection may result from social embarrassment over inability to chew.
  - Following dietary fads that provide only a limited and unbalanced diet.
  - Difficulty in swallowing.
  - Alcohol use disorder.
- Dietary/nutritional considerations for older adults include:
  - Reduced need for calorie intake as a result of decreased energy needs; to avoid overweight or obesity.
  - Protein, vitamins, minerals, and water are particularly important for body function, repair, and resistance to disease.
  - Increased need for protein, calcium, vitamin D, and folate.
- A necessary objective in geriatric nutrition is to slow or prevent the progression of diet-induced chronic diseases. Examples are:
  - Atherosclerosis related to high dietary fat diets.
  - Anemias related to iron and vitamin B_{12} deficiencies.
  - Osteoporosis resulting from inadequate intake of calcium and vitamin D.
- Fluoride intake over the years is beneficial in the prevention of osteoporosis and bone fractures, and water fluoridation is beneficial for direct application to the teeth.
- Instructions in diet and oral health:
  - Dietary analysis by means of a 3- or 5-day record of the patient's diet can provide information to guide recommended changes. (See Chapter 33.)
  - Patients with cognitive and/or memory deficits may be unable to provide an accurate food diary. When possible, enlist the help of family members or caretakers.
  - Minimally, an accurate 24-hour food recall needs to be obtained. (See Chapter 33.)
  - Recommendations for older adult patients are based on establishing a well-balanced diet with limited amounts of cariogenic foods for dental caries prevention.
  - Provide patient with dietary educational materials.
  - Refer older adults with complex medical conditions to a registered dietitian nutritionist.
- Patient motivation may be enhanced by discussing the relationship of dietary deficiencies to:
  - Lowered resistance to disease.
  - Appearance (weight control).
  - Premature aging.

Documentation

The permanent record for an older adult needs a complete personal health history followed from an initial appointment to include a minimum of the following:

- Detailed medical history.
- Current vital signs.
- History of medications.
- Current radiographs with exposure records.
- Extraoral and intraoral examination with particular emphasis on oral cancer and all pathologies.
- Dental history.
- Detailed dental charting and periodontal clinical examination including record of probing depths, clinical attachment level, furcations, mobility, occlusion, calculus classification, and biofilm control record.
- For each professional visit, a summary of current findings and planned treatment as well as outcomes from previous appointment treatments.
- A sample of documentation for an older adult dental visit may be reviewed in **Box 48-6.**

Box 48-6 Example Documentation: Older Adult Patient with Xerostomia

- **S**—A 78-year-old female presents for a 6-month continuing care appointment. Patient stated "I wake up in the middle of the night with my tongue sticking to the roof of my mouth. My tongue becomes sore."
- **O**—Updating the medical health history, a new antihypertensive medication called hydrochlorothiazide is noted. During the intraoral examination, decreased flow of saliva is observed.
- **A**—Significant decrease in salivary flow is most likely due to the new antihypertensive medication. No previous clinical notes have documentation of complaints of xerostomia from the patient or noted findings of xerostomia from the intraoral examination. Patient is at high risk for caries based on the ADA caries risk assessment tool.
- **P**—Patient was given instructions for the management of xerostomia such as the use of a saliva substitute and drinking plenty of water. Additional instructions were provided specifically for biofilm control and 5% sodium fluoride gel was prescribed with instructions for use to manage increased risk of dental caries. Fluoride varnish was applied due to high caries risk.

Next step: Reevaluate at the 3-month continuing care appointment.

Signed: ______________________________, RDH

Date: ________________

Factors to Teach the Patient

- Remind patient of the importance of telling the dentist and dental hygienist about all changes in personal health, medical care received since the last appointment, and all changes in prescriptions.
- The interrelationship of systemic and oral health.
- The dentition can last a lifetime. Daily preventive measures and a healthy lifestyle are essential.
- The value of a well-balanced diet with reduced calories and regular exercise for successful aging.
- Importance of drinking fluoridated water when it is available.
- Dental caries is a transmissible disease; therefore, it is urgent to have all cavitated lesions restored and dental biofilm removed from the teeth daily.

References

1. Population Reference Bureau. Fact sheet: aging in the United States. https://www.prb.org/resources/fact-sheet-aging-in-the-united-states/. Accessed August 1, 2021.
2. Calabrese JM, Rawal K. Demographics and oral health care utilization for older adults. *Dent Clin N Am*. 2021;65:241-255.
3. Whitbourne SK, Whitbourne SB. *Adult Development and Aging Biopsychosocial Perspectives*. 7th ed. Hoboken, NJ: John Wiley & Sons Inc; 2020:8-10.
4. Govindaraju DR, Pencina KM, Raj DS, Massaro JM, Carnes BA, D'Agostino RB. A systems analysis of age-related changes in some cardiac aging traits. *Biogerontology*. 2014;15(2):139-152.
5. Lowery EM, Brubaker AL, Kuhlmann E, Kovacs EJ. The aging lung. *Clin Interv Aging*. 2013;8:1489-1496.
6. Chader GJ, Tayloe A. Preface: the aging eye: normal changes, age-related diseases, and sight-saving approaches. *Invest Opthalmol Vis Sci*. 2013;54(14):ORSF1-ORSF4.
7. Bainbridge KE, Wallhagen MI. Hearing loss in an aging American population: extent, impact, and management. *Annu Rev Public Health*. 2014;35:139-152.
8. Sadighi Akha, AA. Aging and the immune system: An overview. *J Immunol Methods*. 2018;463:21-26.
9. Yam A, Marsiske M. Cognitive longitudinal predictors of older adults' self-reported IADL function. *J Aging Health*. 2013;25(suppl 8):163S-185S.
10. Rozas NS, Sadowsky JM, Jeter CB. Strategies to improve dental health in elderly patients with cognitive impairment: a systematic review. *J Am Dent Assoc*. 2017;148(4):236-245.
11. Bui FQ, Coutinho Almeida-da-Silva CL, Huynh B, et al. Association between periodontal pathogens and systemic disease. *Biomed J*. 2019;42:27-35.
12. Hetal O, Gostemeyer G, Joachim K. Predictors for tooth loss in periodontitis patients: systematic review and meta-analysis. *J Clin Periodontal*. 2019;46:699-712.
13. Sanz M, Del Castillo AM, Jepsen S. Periodontitis and cardiovascular disease: consensus report. *J Clin Periodontol*. 2020;47(3):268-288.
14. Berkey D, Scannapieco F. Medical considerations relating to the oral health of older adults. *Spec Care Dentist*. 2013;33(4):164-178.
15. Tonetti MS, Bottenberg P, Conrads G, et al. Dental caries and periodontal diseases in the ageing population: call to action to protect and enhance oral health and well-being as an essential component of healthy ageing: consensus report of

group 4 of the joint EFP/ORCA workshop on the boundaries between caries and periodontal diseases. *J Clin Periodonotol*. 2017;44(Suppl 18):S135-S144.

16. Liccardo D, Marzano F, Carraturo F, et al. Potential bidirectional relationship between periodontitis and Alzheimer's disease. *Front Physiol*. 2020;11:1-13.
17. Loscalzo E, Sterling RC, Weinstein SP. Alcohol and other drug use in older adults: results from a community needs assessment. *Aging Clin Exp Res*. 2017;29:1149-1155.
18. Wang C, McCauley LK. Osteoporosis and periodontitis. *Curr Osteoporos Rep*. 2016;14:284-291.
19. Anil S, Preethanath RS, Almoharib HS, Kamath KP, Anand PS. Impact of osteoporosis and its treatment on oral health. *Am J Med Sci*. 2013;346(5):396-401.
20. Centers for Disease Control and Prevention. HIV among older Americans. https://www.cdc.gov/hiv/group/age/olderamericans/. Accessed August 29, 2021
21. Guneri P, Epstein J, Botto RW. Breaking bad medical news in a dental care setting. *J Am Dent Assoc*. 2013;144(4):381-386.
22. Vadiraj S, Nayak R, Choudhary GK, Kudyar N, Spoorthi BR. Periodontal pathogens and respiratory diseases—evaluating their potential association: a clinical and microbiological study. *J Contemp Dent Pract*. 2013;14(4):610-615.
23. Stoopler ET, Nadeau S, Sollecito TP. How do I manage a patient with angular cheilitis? *J Can Dent Assoc*. 2013;79:d68.
24. Toffanello ED, Inelmen EM, Imoscopi A, et al. Taste loss in hospitalized multimorbid elderly subjects. *Clin Interv Aging*. 2013;8:167-174.
25. Wiener C, Wu B, Crout R, et al. Hyposalivation and xerostomia in dentate older adults. *J Am Dent Assoc*. 2010;141(3): 279-284.
26. Villa A, Nordio F, Gohel A. A risk prediction model for xerostomia: a retrospective cohort study. *J Gerontol*. 2016;33: 562-568.
27. Iezzi I, Pagella P, Mattioli-Belmonte M. The effects of ageing on dental pulp stem cells, the tooth longevity elixir. *Eur Cell Mater*. 2019;37:175-185.
28. Heasman PA, Ritchie M, Asuni A, et al. Gingival recession and root caries in the ageing population: a critical evaluation of treatments. *J Clin Periodontal*. 2017;44(Suppl 18):S178-S193. 29. Ghezzi EM. Developing pathways for oral care in elders: evidence-based interventions for dental caries prevention in dentate elders. *Gerodontology*. 2014;31(suppl 1):31-36.
29. Zander HA, Hurzeler B. Continuous cementum apposition. *J Dent Res*. 1958;37(6):1035-1044.

CHAPTER 49

The Patient with a Cleft Lip and/or Palate

Linda D. Boyd, RDH, RD, EdD
Sara L. Beres, RDH, MSDH

CHAPTER OUTLINE

LEARNING OBJECTIVES

After studying this chapter, the student will be able to:

1. Describe the types of cleft lip and palate that result from developmental disturbances.
2. Identify and describe the roles of the professionals on the interdisciplinary team for the treatment of a patient with cleft lip and/or palate.
3. Recognize the oral characteristics a patient with cleft lip and/or palate may experience.
4. Explain how to adapt the dental hygiene appointment sequence for a patient with cleft lip and/or palate.

Overview of Cleft Lip and Palate

Cleft lip and **cleft palate** are the most common of the many types of congenital **craniofacial** anomalies.[1]

- Cleft lip and palate may occur as isolated conditions, but frequently occur as part of a **syndrome** with other birth defects.
- Cleft lip and palate can significantly impact speech, hearing, adequate nutrition, oral health, mental and social development, and quality of life.[1]
- Global prevalence[1]:
  - Cleft lip or palate ranges from 0.03 to 0.033 per 1000 births.
  - Cleft lip and palate (CL/P) prevalence is 0.45 per 1000 births.
- Prevalence varies by country and by ethnicity with CL/P, from 1/500 in Asian populations to 1/1000 in European and 1/2500 in African populations.[2]

Classification of Clefts

- Classification is based on disturbances in the embryologic formation of the lip and palate as they develop from the **premaxillary** region toward the uvula in a definite pattern.
- Clefts are described based on the following[3]:
  - Structures involved.
  - Unilateral or bilateral.
  - Severity.
- There is not a universally agreed upon classification system for clefts, but **Figure 49-1** illustrates one method of classifying cleft lip and palate.[4,5]

Etiology

I. Embryology

- Cleft lip and palate represent a failure of normal fusion of embryonic processes during development in the first trimester of pregnancy.[2]
- **Figure 49-2** shows the locations of the globular process and the right and left maxillary processes.
- With normal fusion, no cleft of the lip results.
- Fusion begins in the premaxillary region and continues backward toward the uvula.
- Formation of the lip[2]:
  - Occurs between the fourth and eighth weeks *in utero*.
  - A cleft lip becomes apparent by the end of the second month *in utero*.
- Development of the palate[2]:
  - Takes place during the 5th to 12th weeks.
  - A cleft palate is evident by the end of the third month.

II. Risk Factors

Multifactorial genetic and environmental factors can be significant etiology of CL/P.

- Genetics—Present or past members of a family increase the risk, as well as increased maternal age.[2]

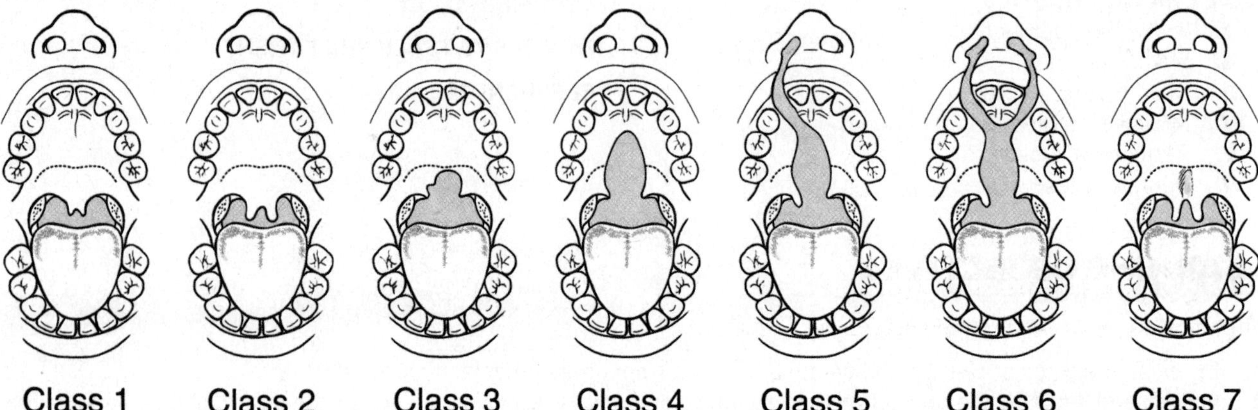

Figure 49-1 Classification of Cleft Lip and Cleft Palate. Class 1: cleft of the tip of the uvula; Class 2: cleft of the uvula (bifid uvula); Class 3: cleft of the soft palate; Class 4: cleft of the soft and hard palates; Class 5: cleft of the soft and hard palates that continues through the alveolar ridge on one side of the premaxilla, usually associated with cleft lip of the same side; Class 6: cleft of the soft and hard palates that continues through the alveolar ridge on both sides, leaving a free premaxilla, usually associated with bilateral cleft lip; and Class 7: submucous cleft in which the muscle union is imperfect across the soft palate. The palate is short, the uvula is often bifid, a groove is situated at the midline of the soft palate, and the closure to the pharynx is incompetent.

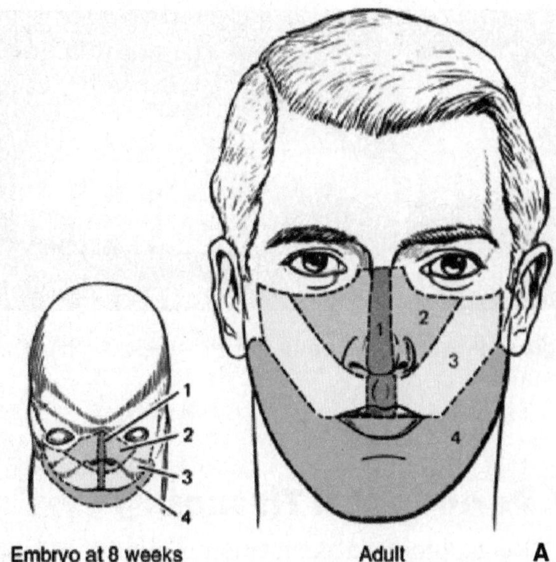

Figure 49-2 Developmental Processes of the Face. **A:** The nose, eyes, and mouth form between the fourth and sixth weeks of development. **B:** Development of the face illustrating derivatives of embryologic development. (1) Median nasal process; (2) lateral nasal process; (3) maxillary process; and (4) mandibular process. Clefts can occur at the midline of the maxillary and/or the mandibular process if fusion fails during development.

- Nutritional factors[2]
  - Folic acid (folate) in adequate amounts may reduce the risk for CL/P by 40%.
  - Zinc deficiency increases risk of clefts.
  - Vitamin A (retinoid compounds) have inconsistent findings in regard to whether it increases the risk for CL/P, so a balanced diet is recommended without exceeding the upper tolerable levels of Dietary Reference Intake.
- Drugs, including both recreational and prescription medications[2]
  - Cocaine.
  - Tobacco smoking (10 cigarettes or more/day).
  - Alcohol use.
  - Anticonvulsants such as phenytoin, valproic acid, and phenobarbital.
  - Corticosteroids.
- Metabolic diseases[2]
  - Diabetes, including gestational diabetes.
  - Maternal weight and obesity.
- Ionizing radiation[2]

General Physical Characteristics

I. Other Congenital Anomalies

- Incidence of multiple **congenital** anomalies is high with cleft lip and/or palate.

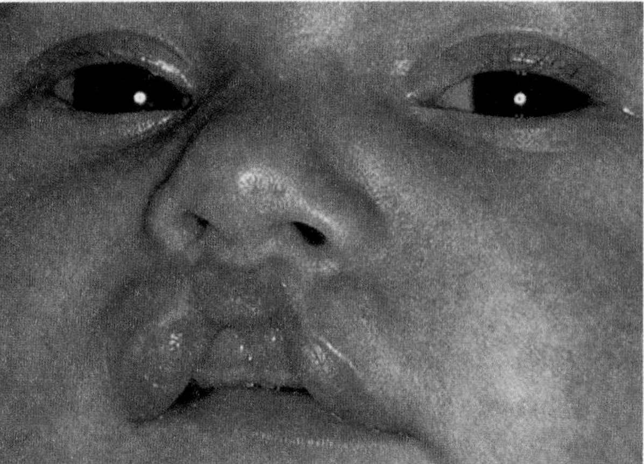

A

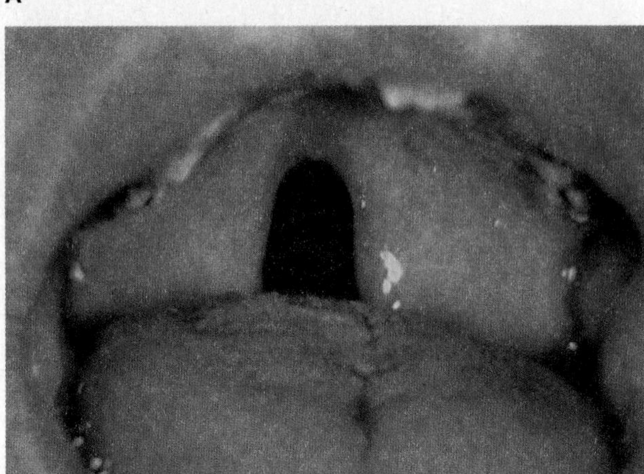

B

Figure 49-3 A: Cleft lip. **B:** Cleft palate.

- At least 400 syndromes have been identified in which clefting is the primary feature.[6]

II. Facial Deformities

Facial deformities may include (see **Figure 49-3**):

- Depression of the nostril on the side with the cleft lip.
- Deficiency of upper lip, which may be short or displaced backward.
- Overprominent lower lip.

III. Infections

- Predisposition to middle-ear infections is common.[7]

IV. Feeding Issues

- Infants with cleft lip and palate are unable to create the negative intraoral pressure to suck milk from a bottle or breastfeed and need a special feeding device.[7]
- Careful attention must be paid to adequate weight gain to support growth.

V. Speech

- Patients with cleft lip and/or cleft palate have difficulty making certain sounds and may produce weak, hypernasal tones, and may sound muffled.[7]
- Children may also experience language delays.[8]

VI. Hearing Loss

- The incidence of mild to moderate hearing loss is significantly higher in individuals with cleft palate than in the noncleft population.[7]
- Hearing loss may be associated with delayed speech development.

Oral Characteristics

I. Tooth Development

- Disturbances in the normal development of the tooth buds occur more frequently in patients with clefts than in the general population.
- There is a higher incidence of missing teeth (agenesis), supernumerary teeth, developmental enamel defects, and microdontia or peg-shaped anterior teeth.[9]
- Common missing teeth include[10]:
  - Maxillary lateral incisors.
  - Mandibular second premolars.
  - Usually correspond to the side of the mouth that has the cleft.

II. Malocclusion

- The majority of children with cleft lip and palate require orthodontic care.[7]
- Orthodontic treatment may be required after each stage of surgical treatment for cleft palate.

III. Open Palate

- Before surgical correction, an open palate provides direct communication with the nasal cavity.
- A cleft palate may cause formula or breast milk to pass into the nasal cavity. A prosthetic palatal **obturator** may be constructed to aid during drinking and eating (**Figure 49-4**).

IV. Muscle Coordination

- A lack of coordinated movements of lips, tongue, cheeks, floor of mouth, and throat may exist.
- Compensatory habits may be formed by the patient in the attempt to produce normal sounds while speaking.

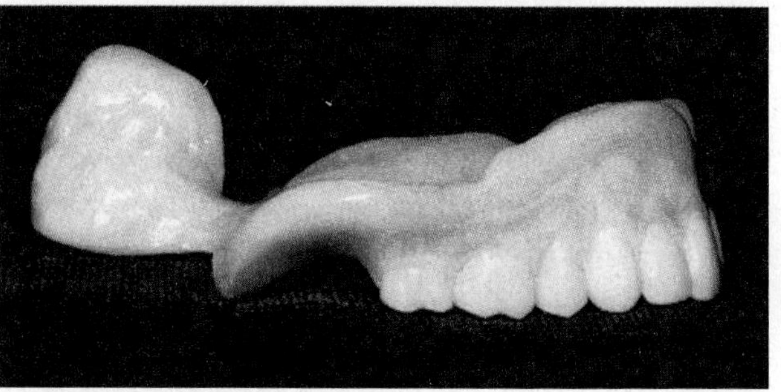

Figure 49-4 Maxillary Obturator Prosthesis with Denture.

V. Periodontal Tissues

- Dental biofilm accumulation is influenced by the irregularly positioned teeth, inability to keep lips closed, mouth breathing, and the difficulties in accomplishing adequate biofilm removal, especially around the cleft areas.
- Patients with cleft palate and lip have increased plaque indices, pocket depths, and slightly greater attachment loss.[9]

VI. Dental Caries

- Children with a cleft lip and/or palate are at higher risk for dental caries.[11]
- Risk factors include:
  - Malpositioned teeth.
  - Problems of mastication.
  - Longer oral clearance time when eating.
  - Diet selection.
  - Difficulty with adequate removal of dental biofilm.
- Feeding difficulties of infants and toddlers also contribute to early childhood caries (ECC). (See Chapters 25 and 47.)

Treatment

- The American Cleft Palate-Craniofacial Association provides standards for approval of teams.[12]
- Members of the interdisciplinary patient care team are listed in **Box 49-1**.
- The team is responsible for providing integrated case management to ensure the quality and continuity of care.[13]
- Intraoral and/or extraoral appliances can be used in preparation for primary lip and palate surgery, including active and passive appliances, lip tapping/lip strapping, and the semi-active **nasoalveolar molding appliance**.[14]

Box 49-1 Interdisciplinary Team for Treatment of Patient with Cleft Lip and/or Palate[12,13]

Dental Profession

- Oral and maxillofacial surgery
- Orthodontics
- Pediatric dentistry
- Dental hygiene
- Prosthodontics
- Implantology
- Periodontics

Medical Profession

- Anesthesiology
- Genetics/dysmorphology
- Imaging/radiology
- Neurology
- Neurosurgery
- Ophthalmology
- Otolaryngology
- Pediatrics
- Physical anthropology
- Plastic surgery
- Psychiatry

Allied Medical

- Audiology
- Registered Dietitian/Registered Dietitian Nutritionist
- Nursing
- Genetic counseling
- Psychology
- Social work
- Speech–language pathology
- Vocational counseling

I. Cleft Lip

- Surgical repair of the cleft lip is usually done at 2.5–6 months of age and before 12 months of age.[7,13] A general rule for scheduling surgery is the rule of 10s: when the child is approximately 10 weeks of age, weighs 10 pounds, and has achieved a serum hemoglobin of 10 mg/mL.[15]
- The infant's general health is a determining factor regarding when it is safe to perform the surgery.

A. Rationale for Early Treatment

- Aid in feeding.
- Encourage development of the premaxilla.
- Help partial closure of the palatal cleft.
- Assist families in adjusting to the birth of a child with cleft lip and/or palate.

B. Orthodontics and Dentofacial Orthopedics

- In preparation for cleft closure, orthodontic, and **orthopedic** treatment may be needed to reduce the protrusion and stabilize the premaxilla.[14]

II. Cleft Palate

- Primary surgery to close the palate is usually undertaken by 18 months of age, or earlier when possible.[13]
- The combined efforts of many specialists are required, as listed in Box 49-1.

A. Goals for Treatment

- Produce anatomic closure.
- Maximize maxillary growth and development.
- Achieve normal function, particularly normal speech.
- Relieve problems of airway and breathing.
- Establish good dental esthetics and functional occlusion.

B. Types of Secondary Surgical Procedures

- Secondary surgical care (**Box 49-2**) refers to additional surgical procedures after primary closure of the clefts.
- Secondary surgery may involve the lips, nose, palate, and jaws.
  - Objectives are to improve function for coherent communication, improve appearance, or both.
- Treatment plans are individualized to fit the needs of the patient.
- Team evaluations on a periodic basis determine the effects of treatment and outline the next phase.

C. Use of Bone Grafting

Bone **grafting** is used to repair residual alveolar and hard palate clefts.

- Alveolar graft[16,17]
  - Placed before eruption of maxillary teeth at the cleft site.
  - Creates a normal architecture through which the teeth can erupt.
  - Provides bony support for orthodontic treatment.

Box 49-2 Types of Secondary Surgical Procedures[13]

- **Rhinoplasty** and nasal septal surgery for an airway problem.
- Velopharyngeal flap or other pharyngoplasty.
- Closure of palatal fistulae.
- Tonsillectomy and/or adenoidectomy.
- Bone grafting for alveolar cleft.

    - Provides bone for placement of dental implants if needed.
    - Support is provided for teeth adjacent to the cleft areas to minimize movement.
- Hard palate graft[18]
    - Provides closure of oronasal fistulae.
    - The alveolar and hard palate clefts may be grafted simultaneously during surgery.
    - Helps to relieve a compromised airway.
- Sources for autogenous bone for graft[19]
    - Rib, iliac crest, skull, mandible, or bone morphogenetic proteins.

D. Use of Osseointegrated Implant

After bone grafting, implants can be used to replace individual teeth.

- Implants also provide support for a complete **prosthesis**.

III. Prosthodontics

A. Types of Appliances

- Obturator: a removable prosthesis may be designed to provide closure of the palatal opening (Figure 49-4).[20]
- Speech-aid prosthesis: a removable appliance to complete the palatopharyngeal valving required for speech.[20]

B. Purposes and Functions of a Prosthesis

The prosthesis may be designed to accomplish one or all of the following[20]:

- Closure of the palate.
- Replacement of missing teeth.
- Scaffolding to fill out the upper lip.
- Masticatory function.
- Restoration of vertical dimension.
- Post-orthodontic retainer.

IV. Orthodontics

- Treatment may be initiated as early as 3 years of age, depending on dentofacial development. However, the orthodontist may be involved much earlier as part of the cleft palate interdisciplinary team.[13]
- Each stage of surgery and treatment may require orthodontic intervention and follow-up.
- Final formal orthodontic treatment for realigning the teeth and gaining a functional occlusion may start during the mixed dentition years or later.
- During the orthodontic treatment period, an intensive program for dental caries prevention and gingival health is maintained.

V. Speech–Language Therapy

- Ongoing evaluation is started in very young children for early identification and treatment of communication disorders.[13]

VI. Restorative Dentistry

- A major problem can be dental caries, leading to tooth loss.
    - Loss of teeth may result in major difficulties in all phases of treatment.
- Preservation of primary teeth has special significance.
- The dental hygienist is a member of the team with responsibilities to coordinate preventive dental and periodontal care.

Dental Hygiene Care

- Preventive measures for the preservation of the teeth and their supporting structures are essential to the success of the special care needed for the habilitation of the patient with a cleft lip and/or palate.
- Teeth will often be poorly formed, lack enamel, and be at risk for loss due to decay.[9]
- Each phase of dental hygiene care and instruction takes on greater significance in light of the magnified problems of the patient with a cleft lip and/or palate.
- Every attempt is made to avoid the need to remove teeth, especially around the cleft area. In an area already weakened by lack of bone, removal of teeth creates further complications.
- The presence of teeth encourages optimum arch growth.

I. Parental Counseling: Anticipatory Guidance

- Understanding the value of preventive procedures by the patient and the parents (or caregiver) is necessary to support the patient.
- When the patient has not had specialized care, the dental team has a responsibility to arrange referral to an available agency, clinic, or private practice specialist.
- Primary concerns are daily dental biofilm removal and prevention of ECC.

II. Objectives for Appointment Planning

- Frequent appointments, scheduled every 3 or 4 months, are usually needed during the maintenance phase of the patient's care.
- Objectives include the following:
  - To review dental biofilm control measures.
  - To provide encouragement for the patient to maintain the health of the supporting structures and cleanliness of the removable prostheses. (See Chapter 30.)
  - To remove all calculus and biofilm as a supplement to the patient's daily oral self-care procedures.
  - To supervise a dental caries prevention program for both primary and permanent dentitions with fluorides and sealants. (See Chapters 34 and 35.)

III. Appointment Considerations

A. Patient Apprehension and Self-Esteem

- A patient who has had multiple surgeries and medical visits may become anxious about dental and dental hygiene care.
- Lower self-esteem, difficulties in social interaction, and bullying have also been noted in patients with cleft lip and/or palate.[21]
  - In addition to the child, parents may also experience psychological effects unless they have adequate social support.

B. Communication

- Speech: speech may be difficult to understand. With repeated contact, understanding can be developed. Referral for speech assessment, if not already done, is recommended.
- Hearing: depending on the severity of hearing loss, the approach is similar to that for speech difficulties. Suggestions for care of patients with hearing problems are described in Chapter 51.

C. Provide Motivation

- Use of a motivational interviewing approach can help patients and parents feel like active participants in decision making and goal setting. (See Chapter 24.)

IV. Patient Instruction

A. Personal Oral Care Procedures

- For a small child, the caretakers may be afraid of damaging the deformed areas or hurting the child if cleaning methods are employed.
- An empathetic approach and plan for continued instruction over a long period is needed.
  - Personal daily care: select toothbrush, brushing method, and auxiliary aids according to the individual needs.
  - Fluoride: initiate daily self-application of fluoride by way of a fluoride dentifrice, and diet supplements for a young child in a nonfluoridated community. Additional fluoride recommendations depend on modifiable risk factors identified for caries. (See Chapter 34.)
  - Prosthesis or speech aid: halitosis may be a problem because mucus secreted in the nasal cavity, as well as biofilm, accumulates on the prosthesis and must be thoroughly cleaned on a regular basis. (See Chapter 30.)

B. Diet

- Need for a varied diet: include adequate proportions of all essential food groups. (See Chapter 33.)
- Need for prevention of dental caries: limit cariogenic foods and beverages, particularly for between-meal snacks.

C. Smoking Cessation

- The patient or family member who smokes or uses any form of smokeless tobacco should be informed about the effects of tobacco on the oral tissues.[22]
- Emphasis on the potential damage to the periodontal tissues can have special significance for the patient with a cleft palate.
- Offer assistance with a smoking cessation program.

V. Dental Hygiene Care Related to Oral Surgery

A. Presurgery

- Treatment objectives have particular significance because the patient with a cleft palate is more susceptible to infections of the upper respiratory area and middle ear. (See Chapter 56.)

B. Postsurgery Personal Oral Care

- After each feeding (liquid diet for several days, soft diet for the next week), the mouth is rinsed carefully.
- Oral care is needed and accomplished carefully, usually by the parent or caregiver, to avoid damage to the healing suture lines.
- In selected cases, a toothbrush with suction attachment may be useful.

Documentation

The documentation of care the patient with cleft lip or palate receives over the individual's lifetime is imperative. Documentation includes the following:

- Description of location, classification, and extent of cleft.
- History and status of surgical interventions.
- Missing teeth and related recommendations for self-care regimens.
- Description of prosthetic appliances and recommendations for daily care regimens.
- A documentation example for a patient appointment is found in **Box 49-3**.

Box 49-3 Example Documentation: Patient with Cleft Lip and/or Palate

- **S**—A 12-year-old patient presented for routine maintenance appointment. Reviewed medical history: patient has recently started full mouth orthodontic treatment. All vital signs are normal.
- **O**—Extraoral examination: bilateral scarring on maxillary lip from cleft lip surgery at age 3 months. Intraoral examination: missing #D and G (permanent teeth are not present on recent pano). Dental biofilm free score: 50% primarily interproximally.
- **A**—Bilateral cleft lip.
- **P**—Disclosing solution used to show biofilm, demonstrated modified Bass toothbrushing. Showed patient and mother how to use floss threader to floss between wires and brackets. Showed patient and his mother how to use an interdental brush. Hand scaled all four quads and applied 5% sodium fluoride varnish. Gave postoperative instructions. Patient tolerated appointment well. Three-month continuing care appointment scheduled.

Signed: ______________________, RDH
Date: ____________

Factors to Teach the Patient

- Provide the parents with anticipatory guidance for management of risk factors for oral disease. (See Chapters 47 and 48.)
- Individualized biofilm removal, especially for cleft areas.
- Proper cleaning of tongue and removable appliances.
- Necessity for regular dental hygiene appointments to prevent oral infection and caries.
- Resources with addresses for team treatment clinics specializing in craniofacial developmental defects.

References

1. Salari N, Darvishi N, Heydari M, Bokaee S, Darvishi F, Mohammadi M. Global prevalence of cleft palate, cleft lip and cleft palate and lip: a comprehensive systematic review and meta-analysis. *J Stomatol Oral Maxillofac Surg*. 2002;123(2):110-120.
2. Nasreddine G, El Hajj J, Ghassibe-Sabbagh M. Orofacial clefts embryology, classification, epidemiology, and genetics. *Mutat Res Rev Mutat Res*. 2021;787:108373.
3. American Speech-Language-Hearing Association. Cleft Lip and Palate. American Speech-Language-Hearing Association.

https://www.asha.org/practice-portal/clinical-topics/cleft-lip-and-palate/. Accessed January 29, 2022.

4. Khan M. A revised classification of the cleft lip and palate. *Plastic Surg*. 2013;21(1):3.
5. Allori AC, Mulliken JB, Meara JG, Shusterman S, Marcus JR. Classification of cleft lip/palate: then and now. *Cleft Palate Craniofac J*. 2017;54(2):175-188.
6. Johnson MM. Prenatal imaging for cleft lip and palate. *Radiol Technol*. 2019;90(6):581-596.
7. Lewis CW, Jacob LS, Lehmann CU, et al. The primary care pediatrician and the care of children with cleft lip and/or cleft palate. *Pediatrics*. 2017;139(5):e20170628.
8. van Eeden S, Stringer H. Linguistic and auditory processing skills in non-syndromic children with cleft palate: a scoping review. *J Commun Disord*. 2020;87:106029.
9. Marzouk T, Alves IL, Wong CL, et al. Association between dental anomalies and orofacial clefts: a meta-analysis. *JDR Clin Trans Res*. 2021;6(4):368-381.
10. Bazrafkan L, Hayat AA, Tabei SZ, Amirsalari L. Clinical teachers as positive and negative role models: an explanatory sequential mixed method design. *J Med Ethics Hist Med*. 2019;12.
11. Worth V, Perry R, Ireland T, Wills AK, Sandy J, Ness A. Are people with an orofacial cleft at a higher risk of dental caries? A systematic review and meta-analysis. *Br Dent J*. 2017;223(1):37-47.
12. American Cleft Palate-Craniofacial Association. Standards of Approval for Team Care. ACPA. Published February 2019. https://acpa-cpf.org/team-care/standardscat/standards-of-approval-for-team-care/. Accessed January 30, 2022.
13. American Cleft Palate-Craniofacial Association. Parameters of Care. Published online February 2018. https://acpa-cpf.org/team-care/standardscat/parameters-of-care/. Accessed January 30, 2022.
14. Maillard S, Retrouvey JM, Ahmed MK, Taub PJ. Correlation between nasoalveolar molding and surgical, aesthetic, functional and socioeconomic outcomes following primary repair surgery: a systematic review. *J Oral Maxillofac Res*. 2017;8(3):e2.
15. Walker NJ, Anand S, Podda S. Cleft lip. In: *StatPearls*. StatPearls Publishing; 2022. http://www.ncbi.nlm.nih.gov/books/NBK482262/. Accessed January 30, 2022.
16. Wu C, Pan W, Feng C, et al. Grafting materials for alveolar cleft reconstruction: a systematic review and best-evidence synthesis. *Int J Oral Maxillofac Surg*. 2018;47(3):345-356.
17. Mundra LS, Lowe KM, Khechoyan DY. Alveolar bone graft timing in patients with cleft lip and palate. *J Craniofac Surg*. 2022;33(1):206-210.
18. Kim EN, Tuncer FB, Mehta ST, Yamashiro D, Siddiqi F, Gociman B. Simultaneous closure of alveolus and hard palate with concomitant bone grafting. *Plast Reconstr Surg Glob Open*. 2019;7(7S):3-4.
19. Francisco I, Paula AB, Oliveiros B, et al. Regenerative strategies in cleft palate: an umbrella review. *Bioengineering*. 2021;8(6):76.
20. Reisberg DJ. Dental and prosthodontic care for patients with cleft or craniofacial conditions. *Cleft Palate Craniofac J*. 2000;37(6):534-537.
21. Al-Namankany A, Alhubaishi A. Effects of cleft lip and palate on children's psychological health: a systematic review. *J Taibah Univ Med Sci*. 2018;13(4):311-318.
22. Chaffee BW, Couch ET, Ryder MI. The tobacco-using periodontal patient: The role of the dental practitioner in tobacco cessation and periodontal diseases management. *Periodontol 2000*. 2016;71(1):52-64.

CHAPTER 50

The Patient with a Neurodevelopmental Disorder

Linda D. Boyd, RDH, RD, EdD
Charlotte J. Wyche, RDH, MS

CHAPTER OUTLINE

NEURODEVELOPMENTAL DISORDERS OVERVIEW

INTELLECTUAL DISABILITY

- **I.** Definition
- **II.** Model of Human Functioning and Disability
- **III.** Supportive Services
- **IV.** Classification of Intellectual Disabilities
- **V.** Etiology
- **VI.** Components of Support
- **VII.** General Characteristics
- **VIII.** Factors Significant for Dental Hygiene Care

DOWN SYNDROME

- **I.** Physical Characteristics
- **II.** Cognitive and Behavioral Characteristics
- **III.** Comorbidity and Health Considerations
- **IV.** Oral Findings
- **V.** Factors Significant for Dental Hygiene Care

FRAGILE X SYNDROME

- **I.** Physical Characteristics
- **II.** Cognitive and Behavioral Characteristics
- **III.** Comorbidity and Health Considerations
- **IV.** Oral Findings
- **V.** Factors Significant for Dental Hygiene Care

AUTISM SPECTRUM DISORDER

- **I.** Prevalence
- **II.** Etiology
- **III.** Characteristics
- **IV.** Treatment Approaches
- **V.** Factors Significant for Dental Hygiene Care
- **VI.** Approaches to Dental Care for Patients with Autism

DENTAL HYGIENE CARE

- **I.** Oral Health Problems
- **II.** Dental Staff Preparation
- **III.** Dental Hygiene Care Plan
- **IV.** Appointment Considerations

DOCUMENTATION

FACTORS TO TEACH THE PATIENT

FACTORS TO TEACH THE CAREGIVER

REFERENCES

LEARNING OBJECTIVES

After studying this chapter, the student will be able to:

1. Define and describe neurodevelopmental disorders.
2. Give examples of the characteristics, oral findings, and health problems significant for providing dental hygiene care for patients with neurodevelopmental disorders, including intellectual disabilities, Down syndrome, and autism spectrum disorder.
3. Recognize adaptations necessary for providing dental hygiene care for a patient with a neurodevelopmental disorder.

Neurodevelopmental Disorders Overview

- Neurodevelopmental disorders are a diverse group of chronic and potentially severe conditions that:
  - Typically manifest in the early developmental period.
  - Usually last throughout a person's lifetime.
  - Lead to intellectual, social, and/or physical impairments.
  - Create problems with major life activities such as language, mobility, learning, self-help, and independent living.
- Down syndrome (DS) and **autism spectrum disorder** (ASD) are two major categories of patients with **neurodevelopmental disorders** that dental professionals encounter in standard dental settings. **Box 50-1** lists the major diagnostic categories of neurodevelopmental disorders.

Box 50-1 An Overview of Neurodevelopmental Disorders[1]

Intellectual Developmental Disorders with Deficits in Intellectual and Adaptive Functioning

- **Global developmental delay**: diagnosis used for individuals younger than 5 years when assessment of reasons for not meeting developmental milestones is difficult.
- **Unspecified intellectual disability**: used in exceptional circumstances for individuals older than 5 years when diagnosis is impossible because of the associated sensory deficits, physical impairments, severe behavioral problems, or mental disorders.

Communication Disorders

- **Language disorder**: difficulty in acquisition and use of language, functional limitations in effective communication.
- **Speech sound disorder**: persistent difficulty with sound production and speech intelligibility.
- **Childhood-onset fluency disorder (stuttering)**: disturbances in fluency, timing, and repetition patterns of speech.
- **Social (pragmatic) communication disorder**: difficulty using verbal and nonverbal communication in a manner that is appropriate for the social context.
- **Autism spectrum disorder**: severity of the condition is based on the level of social communication impairment and restrictive, repetitive behavior patterns.
- **Attention deficit-hyperactivity disorder**: persistent inattention, hyperactivity, and impulsivity.
- **Specific learning disorder**: impairments in one or more academic domains (reading, writing, or mathematics).
- **Developmental coordination disorder**: characterized by clumsiness, slowness, and inaccuracy of expected performance level of motor skills.
- **Stereotypic movement disorder**: characterized by repetitive purposeless movements, with or without self-injurious behaviors.
- **Tic disorders**: characterized by sudden rapid motor movement or vocalizations.
  - Tourette disorder: both motor and vocal tics.
  - Persistent (chronic) motor or vocal tic disorder: either motor or vocal tics, but not both, that have persisted for more than 1 year.
  - Provisional tic disorder: motor and/or vocal tics present for less than 1 year since first onset.

Intellectual Disability

I. Definition

Intellectual disabilities (IDs) are characterized by[1-3]:

- Limitations in individual's ability to learn at a level needed to engage in activities of daily living.
- Limitations in adaptive behavior related to conceptual (e.g., reading and writing), social (e.g., interpersonal), and practical (e.g., dressing, managing money) skills.
- Symptoms may begin at birth, but include any intellectual disability before the age of 18 years.
- Disabilities related to IDs are a symptom in well over 200 different conditions.

II. Models of Human Functioning and Disability

Several models of human functioning or disability have been proposed to better understand the interactions of disability with individual and environmental characteristics.[2] Based on these, a model has been proposed to assess and support those with ID, which includes the following components[2]:

- Diagnosis is based on three criteria[4]:
    - Intelligence testing (problem solving, abstract thinking, judgment, academic learning abilities, ability to plan ahead, etc.)
    - Assessment of adaptive behaviors.
    - Age of onset.
- Assessment of functioning: establish baseline information for behavioral, social, and functional problems.
- Assessment of support needs.
- Planning and developing individual supports.
- Assessment of personal outcomes including quality of life.

III. Supportive Services

- Supportive services include[5]:
    - Avoid preventable causes of ID, such as fetal alcohol syndrome from maternal alcohol consumption, and limit negative effects of conditions resulting in ID.
    - Early intervention to support the development and growth of the individual as well as the family.
    - Individualized education plans to support development of autonomy, self-determination, and self-advocacy.
    - Positive behavioral supports to improve quality of life and reduce negative behaviors.
    - Identify and provide individual supports such as assistive technology to enhance the ability to perform activities of daily living and community participation.
    - Provide long-term family and individual support to help individuals with ID to transition to community living.
- Dental care is one of the supportive services needed for the individual with ID to ensure[5]:
    - Freedom from oral discomfort and pain.
    - Attain and maintain oral health.
    - Improved quality of life.

IV. Classification of Intellectual Disabilities

- The traditional levels of **intellectual functioning** have included *mild, moderate, severe*, and *profound.*[1] However, the International Classification of Diseases 11 (ICD-11) added the following classifications: *provisional* and *unspecified.*[6]
- Standardized intelligence tests are used to assess the overall **intelligence quotient (IQ)** consisting of fluid (ability to think logically and solve problems) and crystalized (the ability to use experience and knowledge) intelligence.[7]
- Onset of the ID is before age 18 years.[1,3]
- A diagnostic category of *unspecified* is used when standardized tests cannot be performed because of lack of cooperation, severe impairment, or infancy.

A. Mild Intellectual Disability

- IQ approximate range 50–69 (in adults, mental age from 9 to less than 12 years).
- Impairment of **adaptive behavior**[6,8]:
    - Slower in acquisition and comprehension of complex language, academic, social, and daily living skills.
    - Practical life skills such as basic personal self-care and domestic activities can be learned and these individuals can function with minimal support. They often can live independently and maintain employment as adults with minimal support.

B. Moderate Intellectual Disability

- IQ approximate range 35–49 (adult mental age from 6 to less than 9 years).
- Impairment of adaptive behavior[6,8]:
    - A marked developmental delay occurs in the early years; child can be trained in personal care and hygiene with moderate support.

- Capacity for language and academic skills is limited to basic skills and they may not learn to read and write.
- Can live independently in a group home setting with moderate support and maintain employment as an adult.

C. Severe Intellectual Disability

- IQ approximate range 20–34 (adult mental age from 3 to younger than 6 years).
- Impairment of adaptive behavior[6,8]:
  - Very limited language and communication skills. Limited capacity for academic skills.
  - Motor impairments require daily support in a supervised setting; however, with extensive training they may be able to acquire basic self-care skills.

D. Profound Intellectual Disability

- IQ under 20 (adult mental age younger than 3 years).
- Impairment of adaptive behavior[6,8]:
  - Severe limitation in self-care, continence, communication, and mobility.
  - Close supervision and assistance with self-care and activities of daily living are necessary.
  - These individuals are not able to live independently.

E. Provisional Intellectual Disability

- This diagnosis is assigned when there is evidence of an ID, but the individual is an infant or child younger than 4 years, so it is not possible to conduct an assessment of intellectual functioning or adaptive behavior because of sensory or physical impairments or severe behavioral or mental disorders.[6]

V. Etiology

Anything that interferes with normal brain development can result in ID. There are prenatal, perinatal, and postnatal causes of ID that may include the following[3,8,9]:

- Prenatal:
  - DS is the most common genetic cause of ID.
  - Fragile X syndrome (FXS) is the most common inherited cause of ID in males.
  - Maternal infections (e.g., rubella, cytomegalovirus).
  - Environmental exposure to substances such as alcohol or drugs.
  - Nutritional deficiencies (e.g., iodine deficiency).
- Perinatal:
  - Delivery complications.
- Postnatal:
  - Exposure to toxic substances (e.g., lead exposure).
  - Brain radiation.
  - Childhood brain infections.
  - Traumatic brain injury.
  - Complications of prematurity (e.g., hypoxemia or periventricular hemorrhage).
- Etiologies of many IDs are unknown.

VI. Components of Support

Early diagnosis is essential to identify any comorbid medical, behavioral, or mental health disorders and determine services necessary to maximize potential and quality of life. Components of support fall into three categories[8,10]:

- Professional interventions:
  - Address or manage any underlying causes of ID such as the need to restrict phenylalanine in someone with phenylketonuria.
  - Management of comorbid physical or mental health disorders to improve functioning and life skills.
  - Early behavioral and cognitive interventions, special education, and psychosocial support to optimize functioning.
- Inclusive environments:
  - Support individuals' growth and development.
  - Supported living, work, and inclusive education.
- Support strategies include:
  - Assistive devices and technology.
  - Reasonable accommodations.
  - Build on personal strengths.
  - Treatment with dignity and respect.

VII. General Characteristics

A. Physical Features

- Many individuals with ID may not have unusual physical characteristics.
- Delays in physical and motor functioning, such as walking, running, and jumping, are often associated with a lower IQ in this population.[11]
- Physical characteristics are most prominent in DS and FXS and may include[12]:
  - Facial or other characteristics may be **pathognomonic** for a particular condition or syndrome (e.g., DS, described later in this chapter).

- Skull anomalies include **microcephalus** (smaller), hydrocephalus (larger, contains fluid), spherical, conical, or otherwise asymmetric shapes.
- **Dysmorphic** features, such as asymmetries of the face, malformations of the outer ear, anomalies of the eyes, or unusual shape of the nose, may become apparent as the child develops.

B. Oral Findings

- Higher levels of dental biofilm are present.[13,14]
- Gingivitis of those with ID is higher than those without ID, and more than half of adults with ID have more severe periodontal disease.[14,15]
- Dental caries
  - Research on the caries rates of those with ID do not agree, and at this time evidence suggests the risk for caries is similar to the general population.[13,16]
  - However, the rate of untreated caries is higher with more missing permanent teeth due to caries.[13-15]
  - Level of functioning, medication-induced xerostomia, and ability to perform oral self-care along with feeding issues (e.g., chewing and swallowing disorders, use of sugary foods as rewards, gastroesophageal reflux [GER]) are risk factors for dental caries.[17,18]
- Oral developmental malformations such as malocclusion; protruding tongue with **macroglossia**; narrow, short palate; microstomia; and delayed tooth development.[18]
- Oral habits: clenching, bruxing, mouth breathing, or tongue thrusting.
- Oral hypersensitivities, hyperactive bite or gag reflex.[18]

VIII. Factors Significant for Dental Hygiene Care

- Patients with ID often experience significant barriers to accessing dental care.[19]
- Personal and lifestyle factors impacting oral care include[19]:
  - Cognitive impairment may impact understanding of oral self-care procedures.
  - Oral motor conditions may make oral self-care difficult (e.g., the individual may bite down on the toothbrush), or make it difficult for a caregiver to assist with oral care.
  - Oral tactile sensitivity such as gagging may make oral care difficult for those who support the individual.
  - Challenging or obstructive behaviors making it difficult to perform oral care at home and in a dental setting.
  - Affective factors such as mood, fear, or distress may impact ability to perform oral care.
  - Lifestyle factors, such as intake of high sugar foods and medication use, increase caries risk.
- Social and environmental factors affecting oral care include[19]:
  - Caregiver education and support for regular home and professional oral care.
  - Oral care equipment and/or assistive devices influence oral care.
  - Individualized oral care routines support home care.
  - Transportation for professional care.

Down Syndrome

- Unique group of individuals with ID caused by a chromosomal abnormality; also referred to as trisomy 21 syndrome (**Figure 50-1**).

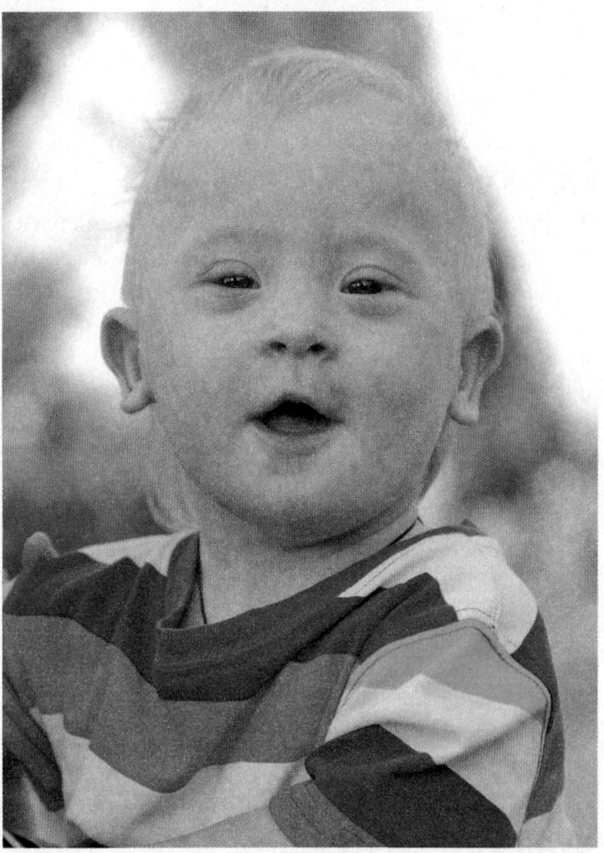

Figure 50-1 Child with Down Syndrome. Common features in children with Down syndrome. Note the child's small rounded skull, small open mouth, slanting almond-shaped eyes, flattened nose bridge, small lower set ears, and short neck.

Types of Epicanthal Folds

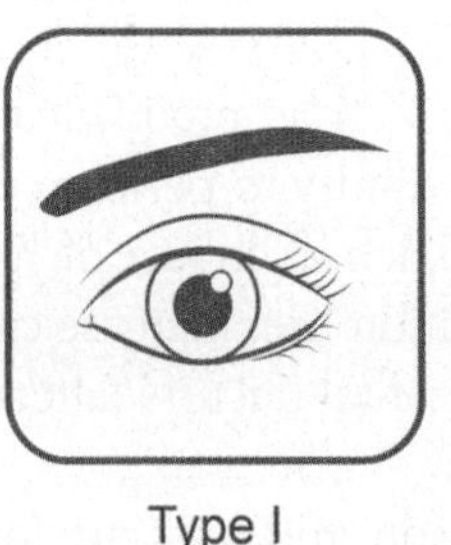
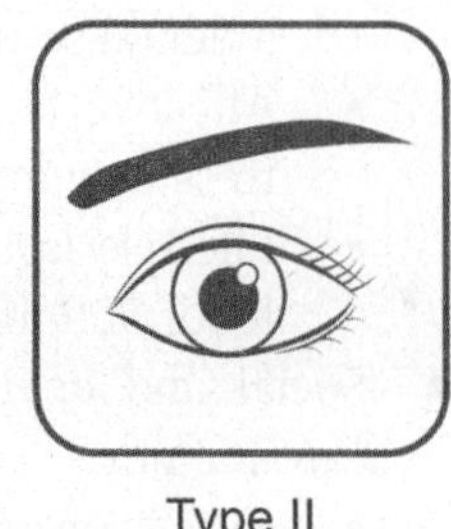
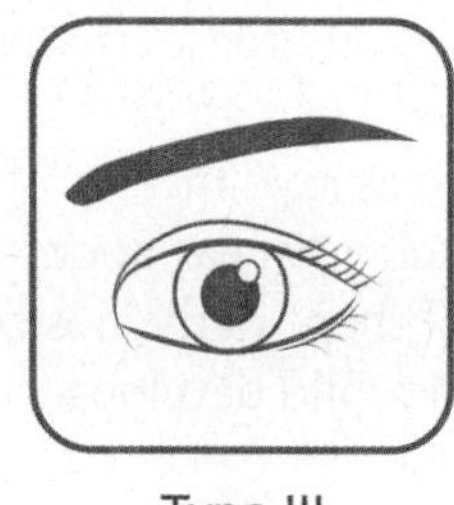
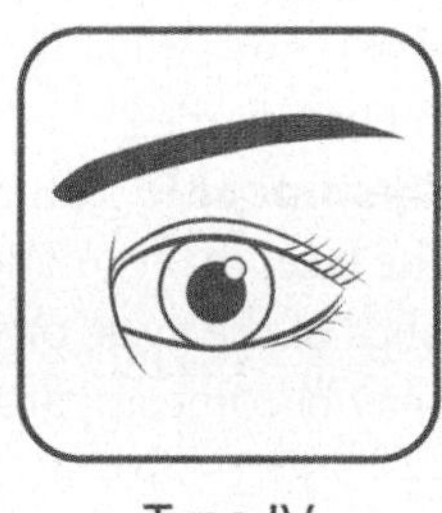

Type I Type II Type III Type IV

Figure 50-2 Down Syndrome: Eye Characteristics. Type I: absence of an epicanthic fold. Type IV: epicanthic fold of a person with Down syndrome.

- Live birth prevalence is about 14.4 in 10,000 in the United State and the rate is increasing, while it shows a decline in Europe with a prevalence of 10.1 per 10,000 live births.[20,21]
- Life expectancy has increased dramatically from the 10 years in 1960 to 47 years in 2007 due to advancements in medical treatment and social support.[22]
- Most live with family in private homes or settings such as group residential homes and access health care as well as dental care services within their communities.

I. Physical Characteristics

- Poor muscle tone and altered gait (e.g., decreased walking speed, reduced step length, wider base of support to compensate for differences in muscle tone).[11,23]
- Short neck.[24]
- Flattened facial profile with a flat nasal bridge.[24]
- Slanted eyes with the **epicanthic fold** of skin continuing from the upper eyelid over the inner angle of the eye (**Figure 50-2**).
- Small mouth and large tongue (macroglossia).[25]
- Small hands with short fingers and the palm has a single, transverse palmar crease.[24]
- Shorter in height.[24]
- Common characteristics of Down syndrome can be seen in **Figure 50-3**.

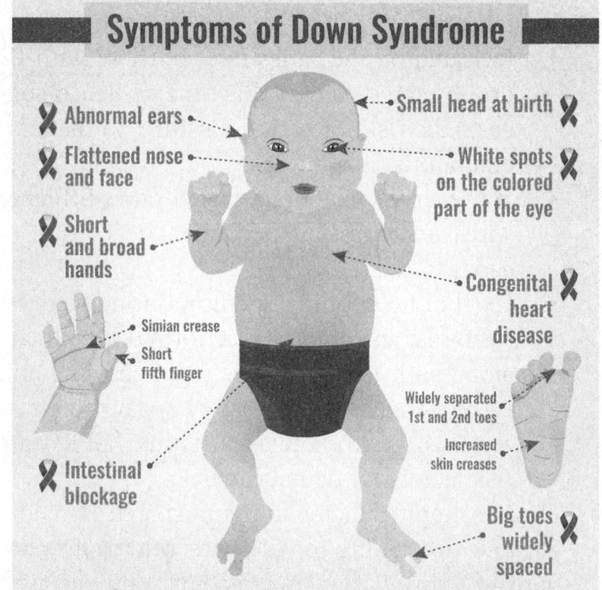

Figure 50-3 Common Characteristics (Symptoms) of Down Syndrome

II. Cognitive and Behavioral Characteristics

Typical characteristics listed here may influence management approaches for dental and dental hygiene appointments.

- The majority of individuals with DS have mild to moderate ID.[26,27]
- Common cognitive functioning characteristics include[26,28]:
  - Short attention span.
  - Delayed language and speech development, especially expressive language.
  - Impaired executive functioning includes:
    - Reduced working memory (temporary memory) and long-term memory for explicit (factual) memory.
    - Poor self-control resulting in impulsive behavior.
    - Difficulty handling emotion.
    - Poorer ability to follow directions.
  - Slower to gain new skills with more difficulty with maintenance of these new skills over time.
  - May have higher nonverbal reasoning (ability to understand, interpret, and analyze visual

information) and ability to solve problems using visual reasoning.

- Individuals with DS are at high risk of Alzheimer's disease, with a prevalence of 13%, and the average age of onset is 55 years. In those older than 60 years, the prevalence is 80%.[27]

III. Comorbidity and Health Considerations

Although improvements in health care and immunizations have resulted in a longer life expectancy, many patients with DS also present with additional special needs and **comorbid** health concerns. Common medical problems include:

- Immune dysregulation results in increased risk for infection and worse clinical outcomes.[29]
- Cardiac problems.[30]
  - In adults with DS, about 33% had evidence of congenital heart disease.
- Neurologic conditions include[27,30]:
  - Epilepsy.
  - Autism spectrum disorder.
  - Cerebrovascular disease.
  - Hypotonia (low muscle tone), which leads to gross motor skill delays.
  - Visual impairment.
    - Nearsightedness, eyes crossing inward, and congenital cataracts are common.
    - White spots (Brushfield spots) on the colored part of the eye.
  - Hearing impairment prevalence in individuals with DS is as high as 73%.
    - This may be a result of chronic ear infections due to congenital ear abnormalities.
  - Early-onset Alzheimer's disease.
  - Cervical spine instability resulting in degenerative changes or spondylosis.
  - Neuropsychiatric disease such as attention deficit-hyperactivity disorder (ADHD), depression.
- Overweight and obesity.[30]
- Thyroid disease: prevalence of hypothyroidism is 27%.[30]
- Osteopenia-osteoporosis.[30]
- Respiratory problems may include[30,31]:
  - Obstructive sleep apnea and airway obstruction are common in DS due to airway anomalies.
  - Dysphagia prevalence is 70% to 90% and poses a risk for aspiration and resulting aspiration pneumonia.
  - Respiratory tract infection with a higher prevalence of respiratory syncytial virus (RSV) and bronchitis.
- Gastrointestinal reflux disease (GERD) due to reduced muscle tone is found in at least one-half of those with DS.[32]

IV. Oral Findings

- Anatomic anomalies[25]:
  - Macroglossia with protruding tongue.
  - Macrosomia.
  - Narrow, vaulted palate.
- Dental anomalies[25]:
  - Delayed or irregular sequence of eruption.
  - Congenitally missing teeth.
  - Irregularities in tooth formation (hypoplastic enamel): microdontia fused teeth.
  - Class III malocclusion, mandibular prognathism, deep overbite, and posterior crossbite are common and relate to the flat face and underdevelopment of the midfacial region (prognathic appearance).
  - Teeth may be spaced because certain anomalous teeth take up less space.
  - Anterior open bite and lip incompetence.
- Temporomandibular joint dysfunction in about 77% of DS patients.[25]
- Mouth breathing is common.
- Periodontal infections are more prevalent and often more severe in people with DS.[33]
- Poor oral hygiene.[33]
- Bruxism.[25]
- Children and young adults with DS have a lower prevalence of dental caries.[16] Factors that may contribute include:
  - Delayed eruption.
  - Congenitally missing teeth and microdontia (small teeth) may result in wider interdental spaces, reducing food accumulation.

V. Factors Significant for Dental Hygiene Care

- Individual factors may include:
  - Review the medical and medication history with the caregiver and carefully investigate any medical conditions in order to plan safe dental/dental hygiene treatment. Consultation with a medical provider may be necessary.
  - Careful attention by the dental hygienist to effective communication by using simple, clear language along with visual aids to help educate the patient and caregiver. In addition, repetition will be necessary due to memory issues.

- Behavior is typically not an issue for children with DS, but talk to the caregiver to determine the most effective way to manage any negative behaviors.
- Minimize stimuli (i.e., noise).
- Positioning of the chair may need to be adjusted if the patient has dysphagia or respiratory problems.
- Visual cues or supports may be helpful for remembering to perform daily oral care. For example, a "story strip" with a picture of each task the individual needs to complete for brushing their teeth.[34] For an individual with visual impairment, auditory cues may be helpful.
- More frequent periodontal maintenance may be necessary.

- Social factors:
  - Children with DS may have access to occupational therapy (OT). OT assists people with self-care tasks and may be a resource to assist with oral hygiene skills.
  - Caregiver education and support for routine oral care will be important to prevent and manage oral disease.
- Environmental factors:
  - Determine living arrangement as those living in a residential center may have more difficulty finding transportation for routine dental care.

Fragile X Syndrome

FXS is the most common genetic cause of inherited ID.[8]

- The most common single-gene cause of ASD.
- Boys are more severely affected because this condition is associated with the X chromosome (**Figure 50-4**).
  - Girls are often carriers (carry the gene on one X chromosome), but will not exhibit the characteristics unless both X chromosomes are affected.

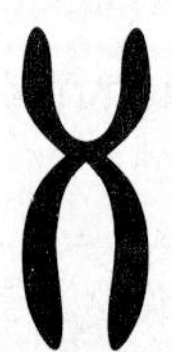

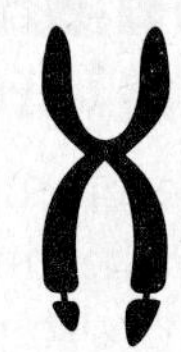

Figure 50-4 Fragile X Chromosome. Fragile X syndrome is a genetic condition with a mutation in the X chromosome.

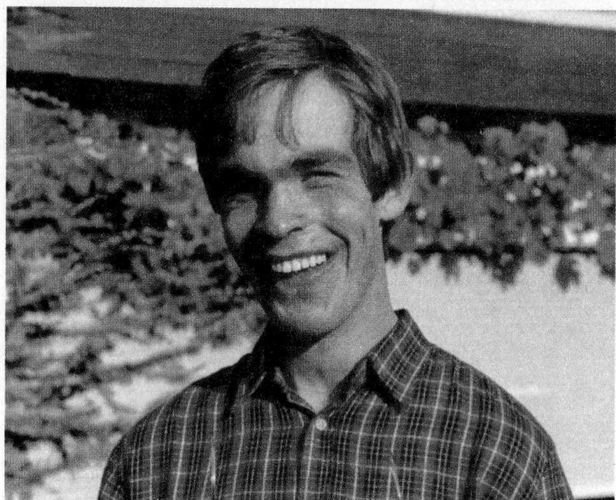

Figure 50-5 Fragile X Syndrome. Fragile X syndrome in a 28-year-old man: broad nose, prognathism, and large ears.

I. Physical Characteristics

In addition to ID, the following are often present (**Figure 50-5**)[35]:

- Prominent forehead.
- Narrow, long face.
- Protruding ears.
- Connective tissue dysplasia results in hyperflexibility of joints.

II. Cognitive and Behavioral Characteristics

Common cognitive and behavioral considerations[35,36]:

- Intellectual disabilities.
- **Hyperactivity** disorder.
- Autism spectrum disorder.
- Weaknesses in short-term and working memory limit the ability to retain and process new information.
- Language processing disorders.
- Attention disorders related to impairment of executive functioning.
- Difficulty with visual-motor coordination, which means they may have trouble with motor skills like toothbrushing.

- Relative strengths include verbal reasoning (ability to understand and logically work through problems) and simultaneous processing (ability to see the "big picture" and understand relationships).

III. Comorbidity and Health Considerations

- Over one-half of individuals with fragile X experience recurrent otitis media because of collapsible Eustachian tubes.[37]
- Neurologic conditions[37]:
  - Seizures.
  - Movement disorders such as hand flapping is common in FXS.
- Gastrointestinal issues[37]:
  - GERD.
  - Diarrhea.
- Ocular disorders are common and many individuals with FXS require glasses for correction.[37]
- Sleep problems occur in one-third of children and teens with FXS.[37]
  - Individuals with FXS are also at risk for obstructive sleep apnea.

IV. Oral Findings

Common oral findings[38]:

- High arched palate.
- Mandibular prognathism.
- Macroglossia.
- Enamel hypoplasia.
- Malocclusion.
- Gingivitis.
- Poor oral hygiene.
- Medication-induced xerostomia.

V. Factors Significant for Dental Hygiene Care

- Individual factors:
  - The dental hygienist needs to carefully investigate the medical history and medications along with questioning the caregiver on behavioral considerations.
  - Explore cognitive and behavioral limitations as well as any vision or hearing issues prior to the first visit.
  - Behavior may result in lack of cooperation with caregivers for oral care.
  - Understand issues with short-term and working memory and adjust oral hygiene education accordingly.
  - Visual-motor coordination may make it more difficult for the patient to learn oral self-care techniques.
  - If GERD is present along with medication-induced xerostomia, additional strategies will be needed to manage caries risk, such as prescription fluoride.
- Social factors:
  - Caregiver education and support for routine oral care will be an important part of preventing and managing oral disease in the FXS patient.

Autism Spectrum Disorder

Autism, first described by Dr. Leo Kanner in 1943, is a complex spectrum of developmental disorders marked by limitations in the ability to understand and communicate. Dr. Hans Asperger published a paper on children with autism who were higher functioning.[39]

- Usually appears during early childhood and persists throughout life, although many individuals with ASD can learn coping behaviors to enhance daily functioning.
- Manifests as a range of disorders, as listed in **Box 50-2**, rather than by the presence or absence of a single behavior or symptom.
- Comorbidity with other disabling and medical conditions is common.

I. Prevalence

- Prevalence has increased in the past two decades; the prevalence of ASD, according to the Autism and Developmental Disabilities Monitoring Network, in 2018 was estimated to be 1 in 44 children.[40]
- The prevalence in 2000 was 1 in 150 children and some of the increase in prevalence may be attributable to better diagnostic criteria and more frequent screening.[41]
- Occurs in all racial, ethnic, and social groups worldwide.[40]
- Frequency of occurrence is almost four times greater in males than in females.[41]

II. Etiology

- The etiology is multifactorial with genetic and environmental factors playing a role.[39,42]
  - Genetic factors are estimated to be 30% of risk for autism.[39]

Box 50-2 Autism Spectrum Disorders

Autistic Disorder

- Impairments in verbal and nonverbal communication and social (i.e., classic autism) interaction, and restrictive or repetitive patterns of behavior, interests, and activities.
- Symptoms are usually measurable by 18 months of age; formal diagnosis is usually made between ages 2 and 3 years, when delays in language development are apparent.

Asperger Disorder

- Three to four times more likely in males.
- Characterized by impairments in social interactions and restricted interests and activities, without clinically significant delays in language, cognitive ability, or developmental age-appropriate skills.

Pervasive Developmental Disorder, not Otherwise Specified (PDD-NOS)

- Severe and **pervasive** impairment in specified behaviors, without meeting all of the criteria for a specific diagnosis (i.e., atypical autism).

Rett Disorder

- An autism-like genetic disorder, which occurs only in girls, causing the development of autism-like symptoms after a period of seemingly normal development.
- Purposeful use of hands is lost and replaced by repetitive hand movements beginning between ages 1 and 4 years.

Childhood Disintegrative Disorder

- Rare autism-like disorder characterized by normal development for at least the first 2 years, followed by a significant loss of previously acquired skills.

- There are about 40 prenatal, perinatal, and postnatal risk factors that may increase the risk for autism, but more research needs to be done to understand how the risk factors work in combination in the development of autism.[39,43]
- Prenatal risk factors[43]:
    - Advanced maternal or paternal age greater than or equal to 35 years.
    - Mother or father's race: white or Asian.
    - Maternal and paternal education level college graduate+.
    - Gestational diabetes.
    - Gestational hypertension.
    - Antepartum hemorrhage (vaginal bleeding between the 20th and 24th week of pregnancy and birth of the baby).
    - Threatened miscarriage (bleeding and abdominal cramping).
- Perinatal risk factors[43]:
    - Cesarean delivery.
    - Gestational age less than or equal to 36 weeks.
    - Breech birth.
    - Preeclampsia.
    - Fetal distress.
    - Induced labor.
- Postnatal risk factors[43]:
    - Low birth weight.
    - Postpartum hemorrhage.
    - Male gender.
    - Brain anomaly.

III. Characteristics

- The onset of autism is typically by age 2 years and some parents may notice signs in the first year of life. Signs may include delays or abnormal responses in the following[44]:
    - Social interaction such as limited interest in other children or caregivers and avoidance of eye contact.
    - Limited use of language.
    - Gets easily upset by minor changes in routine.
    - Symbolic or imaginative play.
- Persistent challenges with social communication and interactions such as the following[1]:
    - Impairment in nonverbal communication for social interaction (e.g., eye-to-eye gaze, facial expression, gestures).
    - Difficulty in developing, maintaining, and understanding peer relationships appropriate for the child's level of development (e.g., unable to make friends or does not show interest in peers).
    - Lack of social or emotional reciprocity or inability to initiate and respond to social interaction.
- Extremely limited interests and repetitive behaviors such as[1,44]:
    - Intense or obsessive focus on a limited number of items or activities (e.g., stacking blocks in the same order every time).
    - Inability to cope with changes in routines (e.g., gets extremely upset when the order of blocks is changed when blocks are stacked).
    - Tends to perform body movements or speech repeatedly (e.g., repeats words or phrases again and again or flaps hands).
    - Overreacts or fails to react to sensory input (e.g., atypical response to sounds or textures).

Box 50-3 Autism Spectrum Disorders: Levels of Severity[1]

Level 3: Requires Very Substantial Support

- Severe verbal and nonverbal communication issues.
- Social interactions are only to meet immediate needs.
- Limited understandable speech.
- Coping with change is extremely difficult.
- Repetitive behaviors significantly limit the ability to function normally.

Level 2: Requires Substantial Support

- Social interactions are limited and the individual may not respond to efforts of others to engage with them.
- Difficulty with the ways they exhibit or interpret nonverbal communication/behavior.
- Difficulty coping with change in routines or activities.

Level 1: Requiring Support

- Some difficulty in the ability to engage with others and may respond in unexpected ways to attempts of others to engage with them.
- Behavior patterns tend to be rigid; difficulty changing focus to new activities.
- Problems with organization and planning.

- The severity designation is based on the level of need for support for communication impairments and behavior patterns (see **Box 50-3**).
- Comorbidities may include other intellectual impairments (e.g., fragile X), language disorders, ADHD, learning disabilities, and epilepsy.[1]

IV. Treatment Approaches

- There is no "cure," in the medical sense, for autism.
- Types of treatment include the following approaches[45]:
  - Behavioral.
  - Developmental.
  - Educational.
  - Social.
  - Pharmacologic.
  - Psychological.
  - Complementary and alternative.
- Treatment is individualized and typically includes multiple approaches.

A. Cognitive-Behavioral Approaches

- Behavioral approaches target behavior change with a focus on what happens before and after a behavior and rewarding desired behaviors while discouraging undesirable behaviors.[45]
- No one behavior-based or educational approach is effective in alleviating symptoms in all cases of autism because of the spectrum nature of the condition and the many behavior combinations that can occur.
- An evidence-based behavioral approach in ASD is the **applied behavior analysis (ABA)**.[46]
  - ABA has been shown to be effective to improve basic communication, social engagement, activities of daily living, and ability to adapt to change.
  - This approach also works with caregivers to improve their ability to recognize cues from the child and be more responsive.
- Naturalistic development behaviors interventions (NDBI) is an approach in which the person conducting the intervention encourages an interactive flow of social engagement that responds to the child's interest, communication, etc.[47]

B. Developmental Approaches

- Early intervention targets children from birth to 3 years old to provide services to improve development in the following areas[47]:
  - Physical, such as walking, crawling, etc.
  - Cognitive, such as learning, problem solving, etc.
  - Communication, such as speech.
  - Social/emotional, such as play.
  - Self-help, such as eating and dressing.
- OT, physical therapy (PT), and speech-language therapy are key to providing developmental therapy.
- Coaching of parents/caregivers is an integral part of this approach in concert with rehabilitative providers (e.g., OT)

C. Educational Approaches

- Educational approaches are delivered in a classroom setting.
- TEACCH (Treatment and Education of Autistic and Related Communication-Handicapped Children) is an example of this approach. It was developed in the 1970s and uses a structured approach with parents and teachers working collaboratively.[48]

D. Social-Relational Approaches

- These approaches focus on improving social skills and making emotional connections with others.[45]
- An example of this approach is "social stories" about what to expect when going to the dentist.

E. Pharmacologic Approaches

- There is no pharmacologic treatment for ASD, but medications are used to manage co-occurring medical (e.g., epilepsy) and psychological (e.g., hyperactivity or anxiety) conditions.
- Risperidone and aripiprazole are antipsychotics approved by the Food and Drug Administration for treatment of irritability, including tantrums, aggression, and self-injury.[49]
- Selective serotonin reuptake inhibitors (SSRIs) such as fluoxetine are used for repetitive or compulsive behaviors; however, the dose has to be carefully monitored as some individuals can become more agitated, with worsening of behavior.[49]
- Stimulants and anti-ADHD agents like Ritalin (methylphenidate) may be used for the management of hyperactivity, impulsivity, and inattention, but like SSRIs, individuals need to be closely monitored to titrate the dose to minimize worsening of behavior.[49]

F. Complementary and Alternative Approaches

- Complementary refers to use of approaches that are not mainstream along with conventional medicine, whereas an alternative approach is used to replace conventional medicine.[50]
- Use of complementary and alternative medicine (CAM) approaches has increased as parents look for non-traditional ways to manage ASD symptoms and minimize the side effects of medications. However, some CAM approaches have little or no evidence to support their use.
    - A common approach used by many parents is a modified/special diet such as restriction of gluten, casein, lactose, and sugar.[51]
        - Evidence does not support the value of a gluten-free, casein-free diet for management of behavior issues associated with ASD.
        - Caregivers should be discouraged from restricting diet choices without oversight by a medical provider because important nutrients may be eliminated, such as calcium and vitamin D.
- Mind-body therapies such as acupuncture, massage, meditation, tai chi, and yoga have been investigated for management of ASD symptoms, but the evidence is limited and more research is needed.[52]

V. Factors Significant for Dental Hygiene Care

- Patience, a consistent approach, and patient preparation prior to the appointment can enhance the probability of a successful dental visit.
- The dental hygienist needs to carefully investigate the medical history and medication along with questioning the caregiver on behavioral considerations.
- Poor oral hygiene and gingivitis are common.
- Impairment in social interaction and difficulty in shifting focus of attention make traditional oral health education approaches difficult.
- Repetitive body movements and mannerisms may compromise patient safety and impact infection control protocols.

VI. Approaches to Dental Care for Patients with Autism

A. D-Termined Program (DTP) of Familiarization and Repetitive Tasking

- DTP is a behavior guidance approach based on ABA for dental professionals, which was developed for use specifically for patients with ASD.[53]
    - Pretreatment assessment form to gather information about behavior challenges and what motivates the child.
    - Familiarization visits.
    - Practicing and learning cooperation skills.
- Benefits of DTP include[53]:
    - Improvement in behavior.
    - Fewer referrals for dental treatment under general anesthesia, resulting in lower costs for dental care.
- Cooperation skills to be learned include:
    - Positioning oneself in the dental chair.
    - Sitting with legs straight and hands at sides or on the tummy.
    - Making eye contact as instructions are given.
    - Opening the mouth and remaining consistently open.
    - Allowing instrumentation and responding appropriately to instructions.

- The five "D" steps for learning cooperation skills[53]:
  - Divide the skill into smaller parts: the key for people with autism is to take each small step of a dental appointment one at a time, and master it before moving ahead.
  - Demonstrate the skill: use the tell–show–do technique.
  - Drill the skill: repeat/practice the skill many times until it becomes second nature.
  - Delight the learner: reward successful attainment of any small portion of the task with reinforcers.
  - Delegate the repetition: involve other members of the dental staff in reinforcing the skills, and have parents and caregivers rehearse/practice at home.

B. Autism Speaks Dental Tool Kit

- The tool kit is designed to[54]:
  - Provide tips to dental professionals for patient care.
  - Teach families how to prepare for the visit to the dentist.
  - Decrease anxiety about the dental visit.
  - Provide information for good oral health for a lifetime.
- Resources include a pre-visit assessment form, a dental professionals tool kit, video, information for caregivers to prepare the child for the dental visit, and instructions for brushing their child's teeth.
  - The pre-visit assessment and interview is particularly important to learn what behaviors might be encountered and what reinforcement for positive behavior might be effective.
  - Home-based preparation may include familiarization with procedures the child will encounter such as "open your mouth" and "counting teeth."

C. Additional Strategies for Dental Care

- In addition to the previously mentioned programs, there are a variety of strategies for preparing to have a positive experience at the dental visit.[55]
  - Desensitization with short familiarization visits may be planned.
  - The initial appointment is to build trust and will aid in learning what the patient is capable of doing.
  - Visual pedagogy is a way to educate the child with ASD through pictures.
  - Create a personalized picture book of the steps in the dental visit to be reviewed at home in preparation for the visit.
  - Teledentistry may be used to introduce the dental office and give the child and parent a chance to ask questions prior to coming to the dental appointment.
  - Social stories are a widely used strategy for ASD and focus on a short story to provide an understanding of the social information for a dental visit and the behavioral expectations.
  - Video modeling to teach behaviors related to the dental visit as well as to educate on oral care at home.

Dental Hygiene Care

- Appointments for medical or dental health care may be overwhelming because of the unfamiliar stimuli for many patients with neurodevelopmental disorders, especially for patients with ASD.
- Dental care may have been neglected due to problems with social interactions, language and communication problems, or difficult behaviors.
- Severity of symptoms dictates the appropriate setting for the delivery of dental care services for these patients.
- With some modifications to the treatment plan and implementation of appropriate behavior guidance techniques, patients with mild-to-moderate manifestations of the condition may be treated successfully in the general dental setting.
- Patients with more severe symptoms may require sedation, general anesthesia, or immobilization in a hospital or specialized setting.

I. Oral Health Problems

Several factors can contribute to poor oral health for individuals with a neurodevelopmental disorder.

A. Previous Dental Care

- Dental care may have been a low priority due to challenges the caregiver encounters in completing the activities of daily living.
- Reasons for unmet dental needs:
  - The child's behavior and parent's embarrassment about the behavior are major barriers to dental care.[56]
  - Cost of treatment, particularly if general anesthesia is recommended.[33]

- Parents may be resistant to the use of protective stabilization or restraints in children unable to follow direction or with behaviors that may cause them harm in the dental chair.[55]
- Unpleasant experiences from previous dental visits.

B. Dental Caries

- Children with ASD tend to have a high level of oral sensory sensitivity, which leads to food selectivity limiting food based on preferred taste, smell, and texture, often resulting in a limited range of diet selections.[57]
  - The foods avoided may include whole grains, meat, fresh fruits, and vegetables.
  - In addition, the preference for "sameness" may result in significant limitations on what the child will eat.
- Feeding problems can lead to parents offering foods that will be eaten by the child, without regard for nutrient content or caries risk.
- Reinforcement for rewards in therapy and in class may be sweet foods such as candy, but increasingly other sorts of tokens are used to earn rewards due the recognition of health risks associated with excess sugar intake, including caries, obesity, and diabetes.
  - The dental hygienist should consult with parents and other healthcare providers (e.g., occupational therapists) to educate them on the importance of avoiding sweet treats as frequent rewards to reduce the caries risk for the child.

C. Oral Hygiene

- Daily oral care procedures may be inadequate for the uncooperative individual, even when delivered by an informed caregiver.
  - Strategies suggested in the resources for the child with autism such as those provided by Autism Speaks can be useful for most children with neurodevelopmental disorders.[54]
- Occupational therapists may be able to assist with the sensory issues some individuals may experience to familiarize them with the sensations associated with routine oral home care.

II. Dental Staff Preparation

- Be familiar with the various neurodevelopmental disorders and prepare for the visit by doing the following:
  - Review medical, dental, and personal histories with the caregiver by telephone interview or teledentistry in advance of the first office appointment. The Autism Speaks resources previously discussed have a form that could be used to gather specific information about behavior, sensitivities, etc.
  - Discuss information with the parent/caregiver, primary care provider, or other healthcare provider associated with the patient.
  - Gather specific information about appropriate motivators and rewards that are safe and effective reinforcers for the individual.
- Consider some of the strategies previously mentioned for those with ASD for preappointment familiarization the parents/caregiver can do at home such as:
  - Place a plastic mirror and flashlight in and out of the mouth.
  - Follow commands such as "Hands on your tummy."… "Feet out straight."
- Plan several short orientation and familiarization appointments initially with not more than a week between visits.
- Involve the same members of the dental team at each appointment to avoid distressing the patient and losing time for reorientation.

III. Dental Hygiene Care Plan

- Plan four-handed dental hygiene for the resistant patient.
- Frequent appointments to prevent oral disease are recommended. As the patient becomes more cooperative, increase the preventive services they will tolerate, which may include:
  - Dental biofilm control for the patient and the caregiver.
  - Debridement as needed.
  - Fluoride varnish therapy: simple, easy-to-do procedure that can be especially helpful for patients unable to cooperate with biofilm control. (See Chapter 34.)
    - Be cautious about oral sensitivities as taste may be a trigger so engage the parent and child in choosing the flavor.
  - Dental sealants. (See Chapter 35.)

IV. Appointment Considerations

- Provide a predictable and consistent experience.
- Create a quiet environment with minimal sensory stimuli; patients with autism may have sensitivity to light, sounds, touch, and smell.

- Avoid loud, inconsistent background music, noisy dental equipment, and conversation not connected to interests of the child or to care.
- Avoid unnecessary touching during treatment.
- Provide sunglasses for patients with light sensitivity.
- Placing the lead apron on the patient to induce deep pressure touch stimulation to help the patient feel more secure and stay calm.

- Desensitization/practice
  - Begin with orientation to the setting and each part of the equipment.
  - If the patient is not ready, instrumentation may not be included at the first appointment.
  - Instruction takes the form of tell–show–do repeated many times. Patience and firmness are necessary elements.
  - Have the caregiver help condition the patient by giving a plastic mouth mirror and a few dental films to take home for practice in the mouth each day.
- Use behavior guidance procedures when the patient condition is appropriate.
  - Involve caregiver(s) while presenting preventive measures in a simple step-by-step manner.
  - Ask the caregiver or parent if the ABA therapist could attend the first dental visit to provide guidance.
  - Provide reinforcing rewards immediately following each success.
  - Use non-food rewards (stickers, picture cards, child-safe tokens, or toys) and explain the rationale against cariogenic food rewards.
- Protective stabilization[58]
  - Protective stabilization is considered an advanced behavior guidance technique in dental settings and the clinician must have adequate training in appropriate, safe, and effective use for a patient who is unable to cooperate.
  - Other, less-restrictive approaches to behavior management should be attempted prior to using protective stabilization.
  - The risks and benefits must be explained prior to asking the parent/guardian for informed consent.
  - Written informed parental/guardian consent is required from the parent or guardian prior to beginning treatment.
  - Parental presence in the operatory may be helpful for both the parent and child.

Documentation

Factors to document include:

- Chronologic age versus developmental age.
- Communication strengths and weaknesses with patient and caregiver.
- Helpful behavioral supports and guidance techniques.
- Treatment completed and modifications that were helpful.
- Recommended home oral hygiene techniques.

Box 50-4 provides an example documentation for a patient with an ID.

Box 50-4 Example Documentation: Patient with an ID

- **S**—Patient presented as a 10-year-old boy with a developmental age of approximately 4 years. Used three to-four-word simple sentences and caregivers presented a picture board that showed the steps of the appointment. This helped the patient recognize how many more steps were needed until the end of the appointment. Patient needs to have his hands held to remind him not to touch and finds comfort in holding his favorite toy that he brought from home. He also loves to hear quiet singing and counting throughout the appointment.
- **O**—Mirror-only examination performed. Biofilm score was approximately 50%. No visual dental caries noted.
- **A**—Dental hygiene diagnosis: biofilm-induced gingivitis.
- **P**—Oral hygiene instruction with patient and caregiver. Rubber cup prophy completed. Flossing of entire mouth. Fluoride varnish applied to entire dentition. Caregivers congratulated on preparing the patient for the visit; patient congratulated on a successful visit.

Next steps: 3 months recall-examination with explorer and biofilm removal with toothbrush.

Signed: ______________________, RDH

Date: ________________

Factors to Teach the Patient

When the patient is able to perform oral self-care skills independently and can expectorate, then proceed with instruction using language and methods appropriate to the intellectual level and abilities of each patient.

- Use a disclosing agent to show the biofilm to the patient and have the patient use the toothbrush or other appropriate oral hygiene aid to remove the biofilm. For someone who is visual, seeing the biofilm may be a helpful educational tool.
- Help the patient to refine their oral hygiene technique and identify which oral hygiene aids may be most appropriate based on the patient's dexterity.
- If the patient is unable to adequately remove dental biofilm, encourage the patient to accept assistance from the parents or caregiver.
- When needed, include the parent or caregiver in the oral self-care instruction.
- Identify ways to support the patient at home with the parent or caregiver, such as providing a reminder or pictures of the technique that can be attached to the bathroom mirror.
- Identify what reinforcers work best for the patient, such as putting a sticker on the calendar each time they perform their oral self-care.

Factors to Teach the Caregiver

- Benefit of frequent intervals for oral health services to prevent disease and make the visits shorter and easier.
- Educate the parent or caregiver about the specific oral hygiene aids and techniques appropriate for the individual patient.
- Provide guidance on assistance of patients with limited abilities, such as:
  - Approach to stabilize the patient's head.
  - Effective retraction of the patient's lips to insert and adapt the toothbrush.
- How to incorporate behavior modification into oral care procedures.
- Emphasize the necessity of repeating tell–show–do instructions often.
- Discuss the need for coordination of the patient's medical and dental team to provide appropriate care.

References

1. American Psychiatric Association. Section II: diagnostic criteria and codes: neurodevelopmental disorders. In: *Diagnostic and Statistical Manual of Mental Disorders*. 5th ed. APA; 2013: 31-86. https://www.psychiatry.org/psychiatrists/practice/dsm. Accessed February 2, 2022.
2. American Association on Intellectual and Development Disabilities. Frequently asked questions on intellectual disability and the AAIDD definition. Published online 2008. https://www.aaidd.org/docs/default-source/sis-docs/aaiddfaqonid_template.pdf?sfvrsn=9a63a874_2. Accessed February 2, 2022.
3. Centers for Disease Control and Prevention. Facts about intellectual disability. Published August 24, 2021. https://www.cdc.gov/ncbddd/childdevelopment/facts-about-intellectual-disability.html. Accessed February 2, 2022.
4. Buntinx WHE, Schalock RL. Models of disability, quality of life, and individualized supports: implications for professional practice in intellectual disability. *J Policy Pract Intellect Disabil*. 2010;7(4):283-294.
5. American Association on Intellectual and Developmental Disabilities. Position statements. https://www.aaidd.org/news-policy/policy/position-statements
6. World Health Organization. ICD-11 for mortality and morbidity statistics. Published May 2021. https://icd.who.int/browse11/l-m/en. Accessed February 2, 2022.
7. Checa P, Fernández-Berrocal P. The role of intelligence quotient and emotional intelligence in cognitive control processes. *Front Psychol*. 2015;6.
8. Boat TF, Wu JT, Committee to Evaluate the Supplemental Security Income Disability Program for Children with Mental Disorders, et al. Clinical characteristics of intellectual disabilities. In: *Mental Disorders and Disabilities Among Low-Income Children*. National Academies Press; 2015. https://www.ncbi.nlm.nih.gov/books/NBK332877/. Accessed February 4, 2022.
9. American Speech-Language-Hearing Association. Intellectual disability: causes. https://www2.asha.org/PRPSpecificTopic.aspx?folderid=8589942540§ion=Causes. Accessed February 4, 2022.
10. Schalock RL, Thompson JR, Tassé MJ. Changes in the field regarding personal support plans. Published online 2018. https://www.aaidd.org/docs/default-source/sis-docs/changes-in-the-field.pdf?sfvrsn=cd8b3021_0. Accessed February 5, 2022.

11. Almuhtaseb S, Oppewal A, Hilgenkamp TIM. Gait characteristics in individuals with intellectual disabilities: a literature review. *Res Dev Disabil*. 2014;35(11):2858-2883.
12. Lee K, Cascella M, Marwaha R. Intellectual disability. In: *StatPearls*. StatPearls Publishing; 2022. http://www.ncbi.nlm.nih.gov/books/NBK547654/. Accessed February 5, 2022.
13. Zhou N, Wong HM, Wen YF, McGrath C. Oral health status of children and adolescents with intellectual disabilities: a systematic review and meta-analysis. *Dev Med Child Neurol*. 2017;59(10):1019-1026.
14. Ward LM, Cooper SA, Hughes-McCormack L, Macpherson L, Kinnear D. Oral health of adults with intellectual disabilities: a systematic review. *J Intellect Disabil Res*. 2019;63(11):1359-1378.
15. Morgan JP, Minihan PM, Stark PC, et al. The oral health status of 4,732 adults with intellectual and developmental disabilities. *J Am Dent Assoc*. 2012;143(8):838-846.
16. Bhoopathi V, Tellez M. Limited quality evidence suggests children and adolescents with Down syndrome have lower prevalence of dental caries compared to non-syndromic children. *J Evid Based Dent Pract*. 2021;21(2):101571.
17. Bakry NS, Alaki SM. Risk factors associated with caries experience in children and adolescents with intellectual disabilities. *J Clin Pediatr Dent*. 2012;36(3):319-323.
18. Ziegler J, Spivack E. Nutritional and dental issues in patients with intellectual and developmental disabilities. *J Am Dent Assoc*. 2018;149(4):317-321.
19. Chadwick D, Chapman M, Davies G. Factors affecting access to daily oral and dental care among adults with intellectual disabilities. *J Appl Res Intellect Disabil*. 2018;31(3):379-394.
20. de Graaf G, Buckley F, Skotko BG. Estimation of the number of people with Down syndrome in Europe. *Eur J Hum Genet*. 2021;29(3):402-410.
21. Mai CT, Isenburg JL, Canfield MA, et al. National population-based estimates for major birth defects, 2010–2014. *Birth Defects Res*. 2019;111(18):1420-1435.
22. Centers for Disease Control and Prevention. Data and statistics on Down Syndrome. Published December 4, 2019. https://www.cdc.gov/ncbddd/birthdefects/downsyndrome/data.html. Accessed February 5, 2022.
23. Zago M, Duarte NAC, Grecco LAC, Condoluci C, Oliveira CS, Galli M. Gait and postural control patterns and rehabilitation in Down syndrome: a systematic review. *J Phys Ther Sci*. 2020;32(4):303-314.
24. Centers for Disease Control and Prevention. Facts about Down Syndrome. Published April 6, 2021. https://www.cdc.gov/ncbddd/birthdefects/downsyndrome.html. Accessed February 5, 2022.
25. Kaczorowska N, Kaczorowski K, Laskowska J, Mikulewicz M. Down syndrome as a cause of abnormalities in the craniofacial region: a systematic literature review. *Adv Clin Exp Med*. 2019;28(11):1587-1592.
26. Hamburg S, Lowe B, Startin CM, et al. Assessing general cognitive and adaptive abilities in adults with Down syndrome: a systematic review. *J Neurodev Disord*. 2019;11(1):20.
27. Santoro JD, Pagarkar D, Chu DT, et al. Neurologic complications of Down syndrome: a systematic review. *J Neurol*. 2021;268(12):4495-4509.
28. Eunice Kennedy Shriver National Institute of Child Health and Human Development. What are common symptoms of Down syndrome? https://www.nichd.nih.gov/health/topics/down/conditioninfo/symptoms. Published January 31, 2017. https://www.nichd.nih.gov/health/topics/down/conditioninfo/symptoms. Accessed February 5, 2022.
29. Huggard D, Doherty DG, Molloy EJ. Immune dysregulation in children with Down syndrome. *Front Pediatr*. 2020;8:73.
30. Capone GT, Chicoine B, Bulova P, et al. Co-occurring medical conditions in adults with Down syndrome: a systematic review toward the development of health care guidelines. *Am J Med Genet Part A*. 2018;176(1):116-133.
31. De Lausnay M, Ides K, Wojciechowski M, Boudewyns A, Verhulst S, Van Hoorenbeeck K. Pulmonary complications in children with Down syndrome: a scoping review. *Paediatr Respir Rev*. 2021;40:65-72.
32. Ravel A, Mircher C, Rebillat AS, Cieuta-Walti C, Megarbane A. Feeding problems and gastrointestinal diseases in Down syndrome. *Arch Pediatr*. 2020;27(1):53-60.
33. Scalioni FAR, Carrada CF, Martins CC, Ribeiro RA, Paiva SM. Periodontal disease in patients with Down syndrome: a systematic review. *J Am Dent Assoc*. 2018;149(7):628-639.e11.
34. Frank K. The use of visual supports for individuals with Down syndrome. Published online February 17, 2017. https://www.advocatehealth.com/assets/documents/subsites/luth/downsyndrome/use-of-visual-supports.pdf. Accessed February 5, 2022.
35. Eunice Kennedy Shriver National Institute of Child Health and Human Development. What are the symptoms of Fragile X syndrome? Published August 5, 2021. https://www.nichd.nih.gov/health/topics/fragilex/conditioninfo/commonsymptoms. Accessed February 5, 2022.
36. Huddleston LB, Visootsak J, Sherman SL. Cognitive aspects of Fragile X syndrome. *Wiley Interdiscip Rev Cogn Sci*. 2014;5(4):501-508.
37. Kidd SA, Lachiewicz A, Barbouth D, et al. Fragile X syndrome: a review of associated medical problems. *Pediatrics*. 2014;134(5):995-1005.
38. Montez ARH, Bizarra M de F, Graça SR. Evaluation of oral characteristics and oral health of individuals with fragile X syndrome and related guardians perceptions. *Spec Care Dentist*. 2021;41(1):13-19.
39. Masi A, DeMayo MM, Glozier N, Guastella AJ. An overview of autism spectrum disorder, heterogeneity and treatment options. *Neurosci Bull*. 2017;33(2):183-193.
40. Maenner MJ. Prevalence and characteristics of autism spectrum disorder among children aged 8 years — autism and developmental disabilities monitoring network, 11 sites, United States, 2018. *MMWR Surveill Summ*. 2021;70.
41. Centers for Disease Control and Prevention. Data and statistics on autism spectrum disorder. Published December 2, 2021. https://www.cdc.gov/ncbddd/autism/data.html. Accessed February 5, 2022.
42. Bhandari R, Paliwal JK, Kuhad A. Neuropsychopathology of autism spectrum disorder: complex interplay of genetic, epigenetic, and environmental factors. In: Essa MM, Qoronfleh MW, eds. *Personalized Food Intervention and Therapy for Autism Spectrum Disorder Management*. Vol 24. *Advances in Neurobiology*. Springer International Publishing; 2020:97-141.
43. Wang C, Geng H, Liu W, Zhang G. Prenatal, perinatal, and postnatal factors associated with autism: a meta-analysis. *Medicine*. 2017;96(18):e6696.
44. Centers for Disease Control and Prevention. Autism spectrum disorder: Screening and diagnosis. Published March 13, 2020. https://www.cdc.gov/ncbddd/autism/screening.html. Accessed February 5, 2022.

45. Centers for Disease Control and Prevention. Treatment and intervention services for autism spectrum disorder. Published January 28, 2022. https://www.cdc.gov/ncbddd/autism/treatment.html. Accessed February 6, 2022.
46. Yu Q, Li E, Li L, Liang W. Efficacy of interventions based on applied behavior analysis for autism spectrum disorder: a meta-analysis. *Psychiatry Investig*. 2020;17(5):432-443.
47. Landa RJ. Efficacy of early interventions for infants and young children with, and at risk for, autism spectrum disorders. *Int Rev Psychiatry*. 2018;30(1):25-39.
48. Panerai S, Zingale M, Trubia G, et al. Special education versus inclusive education: the role of the TEACCH program. *J Autism Dev Disord*. 2009;39(6):874-882.
49. Persico AM, Ricciardello A, Lamberti M, et al. The pediatric psychopharmacology of autism spectrum disorder: a systematic review - Part I: the past and the present. *Prog Neuropsychopharmacol Biol Psychiatry*. 2021;110:110326.
50. National Center for Complementary and Integrative Health. Complementary, alternative, or integrative health: what's in a name? https://www.nccih.nih.gov/health/complementary-alternative-or-integrative-health-whats-in-a-name. Accessed February 6, 2022.
51. DeFilippis M. The use of complementary alternative medicine in children and adolescents with autism spectrum disorder. *Psychopharmacol Bull*. 2018;48(1):40-63.
52. Hourston S, Atchley R. Autism and mind-body therapies: a systematic review. *J Altern Complement Med*. 2017;23(5):331-339.
53. AlHumaid J, Tesini D, Finkelman M, Loo CY. Effectiveness of the D-TERMINED program of repetitive tasking for children with autism spectrum disorder. *J Dent Child*. 2016;83(1):16-21.
54. Autism Speaks. Dental Tool Kit. https://www.autismspeaks.org/tool-kit/dentist-for-kids-with-autism. Accessed February 6, 2022.
55. Chandrashekhar S, Bommangoudar JS. Management of autistic patients in dental office: a clinical update. *Int J Clin Pediatr Dent*. 2018;11(3):219-227.
56. Alshatrat SM, Al-Bakri IA, Al-Omari WM. Dental service utilization and barriers to dental care for individuals with autism spectrum disorder in Jordan: a case-control study. *Int J Dent*. 2020;2020:3035463.
57. Chistol LT, Bandini LG, Must A, Phillips S, Cermak SA, Curtin C. Sensory sensitivity and food selectivity in children with autism spectrum disorder. *J Autism Dev Disord*. 2018;48(2):583-591.
58. American Academy of Pediatric Dentistry. Use of protective stabilization for pediatric dental patients. Published online 2020. https://www.aapd.org/research/oral-health-policies--recommendations/protective-stabilization-for-the-pediatric-dental-patients/. Accessed February 6, 2022.

CHAPTER 51

The Patient with a Disability

S. Kimberly Haslam, RDH, BA, MEd
Charlotte J. Wyche, RDH, MS

CHAPTER OUTLINE

LEARNING OBJECTIVES

After studying this chapter, the student will be able to:

1. Describe the purpose of the Americans with Disabilities Act.
2. Identify and define key terms and concepts relating to individuals with disabilities.
3. Identify risk factors for oral disease associated with disabling conditions.
4. Describe factors that enhance the prevention of oral disease for individuals with disabilities and their caregivers.
5. Explain procedures and factors that contribute to safe and successful management of individuals with disabilities during dental hygiene care.
6. Outline a plan for continuing care for a patient with a disability.

Disabilities Overview

This chapter provides general guidelines for modifying dental hygiene care for a patient with a **disability**. People with disabilities may require a modified approach to oral health care in order to achieve and maintain oral health and prevent rampant dental disease.[1]

- The World Health Organization estimates over 1 billion people worldwide live with some type of disability.[2] In the United States, an estimated 5.6% of children aged 5–17 years, 10.3% of individuals aged 17–64 years, and 33.5% of people older than 65 years are affected by a disability.[3]
- Progress in medical care has increased initial survival of those born with a disability and increased the **survival rate** of those experiencing a disabling condition.[4]
- Advances in medicine have increased the life span of people with **comorbidities**.[4]
- As life expectancy increases, so does the likelihood of acquiring a disability.[4]
- Individuals with disabilities often have less access to oral health services due to challenges for the patient, caregiver, and dental personnel.[5,6]
- The patient may need to overcome numerous obstacles in daily living before the additional issues of oral self-care and access to dental care are addressed.[5,6]
- Imagination, ingenuity, flexibility, persistence, and patience are necessary in order to individualize and modify dental hygiene interventions when caring for people with disabilities.[5,6]
- "People with disabilities" is not a homogenous population; instead, this is a diverse group of people with a variety of abilities and needs.[7]
- Successful management and treatment of patients depend largely on the interpersonal communication between the patient and the clinician.[6]
- Services are provided in a patient-centered manner to focus on the needs of individuals and not their differences.[8]

I. Americans with Disabilities Act

- Purpose
  - The Americans with Disabilities Act (ADA) is civil rights legislation enacted into law on July 26, 1990 "that prohibits discrimination against individuals with disabilities in all areas of public life, including jobs, schools, transportation, and all public and private places that are open to the general public."[9]
- Definition
  - ADA defines an individual with a disability as a person who[10]:
    - Has a physical or mental **impairment** that substantially limits one or more major life activities.
    - Has a history or record of such impairment.
    - Is perceived by others as having such an impairment.

II. Definitions and Classifications

- Disability is an umbrella term for impairment, activity limitations, and participation restrictions.[11]
  - Impairment refers to a problem with body structure or function or mental function (i.e., loss of limb, loss of vision, or memory loss).[12]
  - Disabilities can involve physical impairment, **sensory impairment**, **communication disorders**, cognitive impairment, intellectual impairment, mental illness, and various types of chronic disease.[7]
  - Chronic conditions may result in musculoskeletal disorders and **neurologic disabilities**.

- Activity limitations are when an individual has difficulty in executing a task associated with daily living, such as eating, sleeping, breathing, walking, standing, thinking, concentrating, seeing, hearing, working, reading, communicating, and the operation of major body functions.[12,13]
- Participation is a person's involvement in a life situation, such as employment, education, domestic life, or relationships.[12]

- The term "handicap" is no longer used, as it implies there is a barrier that makes an individual with impairment disadvantaged.[7]
- *Person-first language* is important to emphasize the person and not the disability. The disability is not a defining characteristic of an individual, but rather part of the whole person.[7]
  - Avoid the term "disabled child"; use "child with a disability " instead.
  - When possible, avoid the term "handicapped parking"; use accessible parking instead.
- **Table 51-1** outlines a classification system for disability and health that provides a standard language and framework for the description of health and health-related states.[14]

III. Types of Conditions

- Types of disabilities include:
  - Developmental: hereditary conditions that begin during the development and symptoms manifest before age 21 years and last throughout the individuals' lifespan.[15] Examples: cerebral palsy, autism spectrum disorder, learning disabilities.[15]
  - Acquired: caused by disease, acute medical conditions, or trauma after birth; not caused by hereditary or development. It is a reaction to environmental factors. Examples: accident-related (spinal cord injury, head trauma) arthritis, multiple sclerosis.[16]
  - Age-associated: usually occur after 65 years of age and often related to a chronic health condition. Examples: diabetes mellitus, osteoarthritis, dementia.[17]
- Some types of impairment can manifest as a stable condition, a relapsing and remitting disorder (multiple sclerosis), or a progressive disorder where there is no relief (osteoarthritis, Parkinson's disease).[12,18]
- A temporary disability can result from a physical impairment that only occurs for a short period of time, such as a broken leg, or because of a physiologic condition, such as limitations that may occur during pregnancy.
- A variety of impairments are found among persons with disabilities, and an individual may have more than one type of disability.
- Many diseases and syndromes with associated symptoms of disability or impairment are described in various chapters throughout Section IX of this text.

IV. Physical and Intellectual Disabilities

- Specific physical disabilities. (See Chapter 52.)
- Neurodevelopmental disorders. (See Chapter 50.)

V. Sensory Disabilities

- Sensory disabilities are impairments of one of the senses: **vision**, **hearing**, touch, smell, and spatial awareness.[19]
- When a patient has either a vision or **hearing impairment**, modifications to the dental hygiene process of care, especially communication, are essential.

A. Visual Impairment

- Globally, 2.2 billion people have a near or distance vision impairment.[20]
- In the United States, 12 million people older than 40 years have vision impairment and 1 million are blind.[21]
- Limitations of sight cover a broad spectrum from the slightly affected to totally blind, which is having no perception of light.[22]
- Blindness may be secondary to another primary condition or chronic disease.
- **Legal blindness** is defined as having vision acuity of not more than 20/200 in the better eye with correction (glasses) or having peripheral fields (side vision) of no more than 20° diameter.[22,23]
- Individuals who are blind or visually impaired may use a white cane to aid them while walking and for identification purposes.[24]
- Technology and assistive devices available for the visual impaired include:
  - **Computer screen readers** that allow the individual to read displayed data with a speech synthesizer.
  - Screen magnifiers are available to help the user with low vision by enlarging the text and graphics on the screen.
  - **Braille** wristwatches and printers.[25,26]

Table 51-1 International Classification of Functioning, Disability, and Health[14]

Part 1: Functioning and Disability	
Body Functions	
Mental functions	The brain: both global mental functions, such as consciousness, energy, and drive, and specific mental functions, such as memory, language, and calculation
Sensory functions	Seeing, hearing, tasting, and touch, as well as the sensation of pain
Voice and speech functions	Producing sounds and speech
Functions of the cardiovascular, hematologic, immunologic, and respiratory systems	The heart and blood vessels, blood production, immunity, respiration, and exercise tolerance.
Functions of the digestive, metabolic, and endocrine systems	Ingestion, digestion, and elimination, as well as metabolism and the endocrine glands
Genitourinary and reproductive functions	Urination and reproduction, including sexual and procreative functions
Neuromusculoskeletal and movement-related functions	Movement and mobility, including functions of joints, bones, reflexes, and muscles
Functions of the skin and related structures	Skin, skin glands, nails, hair, and related structures
Body Structures	
Structures of the nervous system	Brain, spinal cord, meninges, and nervous system, including sympathetic and parasympathetic nervous systems
The eye, ear, and related structures	Eye socket, eyeball, external ear, middle ear, inner ear, and related structures
Structures involved in voice and speech	Nose, mouth, pharynx, larynx, and related structures
Structures of the cardiovascular, immunologic, and respiratory systems	Heart, arteries, veins, and capillaries; central lymphoid tissue (bone marrow, thymus) and peripheral lymphoid tissue (lymph nodes, spleen, mucosa-associated lymphoid tissue); and pharynx, trachea, bronchi, and lungs
Structures related to the digestive, metabolic, and endocrine systems	Salivary glands, esophagus, stomach, intestines, pancreas, liver, gallbladder and ducts, endocrine glands, and related structures
Structures related to the genitourinary and reproductive systems	Kidneys, ureter, bladder, pelvic floor, and male and female reproductive structures
Structures related to movement	Head, neck, shoulder, upper and lower extremities, pelvic regions, trunk, musculoskeletal system, and other structures related to movement
Skin and related structures	Skin, skin glands, nails, hair, and related structures
Part 2: Contextual Factors	
Activities and Participation	
Learning and applying knowledge	Learning, applying the knowledge that is learned, thinking, solving problems, and making decisions
General tasks and demands	Carrying out specific single or multiple tasks, organizing routines, and handling stress; identifying the underlying features of the execution of tasks under different circumstances

Communication	General and specific features of communicating by language, signs, and symbols, including receiving and producing messages, carrying on conversations, and using communication devices and techniques
Mobility	Moving by changing body position or location or by transferring from one place to another by carrying, moving, or manipulating objects; by walking, running, or climbing; and by using various forms of transportation
Self-care	Caring for oneself and washing and drying oneself; caring for one's body and body parts; dressing, eating, and drinking; and looking after one's health
Domestic life	Carrying out domestic and everyday actions and tasks; acquiring a place to live, food, clothing, and other necessities; household cleaning and repairing; caring for personal and other household objects; and assisting others
Interpersonal interactions and relationships	Carrying out the actions and tasks required for basic and complex interactions with people (strangers, friends, relatives, family members, and lovers) in a contextually and socially appropriate manner
Major life areas	Carrying out the tasks and actions required to engage in education, work, and employment and to conduct economic transactions
Community, social, and civic life	Actions and tasks required to engage in organized social life outside the family in community, social, and civic areas of life
Environmental Factors That Influence Functioning	
Products and technology	Natural or human-made products or systems of products, equipment, and technology in an individual's immediate environment that are gathered, created, produced, or manufactured
Natural and human-made changes to environment	Animate and inanimate elements of the natural or physical environment, and components of that environment that have been modified by people, as well as characteristics of human populations within that environment
Support and relationships	People or animals that provide practical physical or emotional support, nurturing, protection, assistance, and relationships to other persons in their home, place of work, school, at play, or in other aspects of their daily activities
Attitudes	The observable consequences of customs, practices, ideologies, values, norms, factual beliefs, and religious beliefs that influence individual behavior and social life; individual or societal attitudes about a person's value as a human being that may motivate positive, honorific practices, or negative and discriminatory practices
Services, systems, and policies	Governmental and private programs, infrastructure, regulations, and standards designed to meet the needs of individuals

B. Causes of Visual Impairment

- In the United States, the leading causes of low vision and blindness are primarily age-related eye disease such as macular degeneration, **cataracts**, diabetic retinopathy, and **glaucoma**.[20,21]
- Macular degeneration affects the viewing of fine details and can interfere with reading, driving, and performing daily tasks.[21]
- Blindness in children is prenatal in origin, resulting from maternal infections such as rubella, syphilis, and toxoplasmosis.[27]
- Other causes in childhood are neoplasms and **retinopathy of prematurity**.[27]
- The incidence of retinopathy of prematurity has increased as premature babies' survival rates have increased.[28]
- A major cause of unilateral blindness in North America is ocular trauma related to sport, work, assaults, traffic, and contact lens–induced keratitis.[29-31]
- Sport-related eye injuries are the leading cause of blindness in school-age children in the United States.[30]

- Current preventable strategies need to be implemented,[30,32] including wearing safety glasses during dental hygiene care.

C. Hearing Impairment

- 430 million people worldwide have disabling hearing loss, of which 34 million are children.[33]
- Five out of 1000 children in the United States are born with a detectable level of hearing loss in one or both ears.[34]
- An estimated 6500 newborns have hearing loss.[34]
- Approximately 37.5 million American adults, aged 18 or older, have hearing loss.[35]
- Hearing loss is an umbrella term that means a person cannot hear as well as someone with normal hearing; it can be mild to severe or profound and can affect one or both ears.[33]
- *Hard of hearing* refers to people with mild to severe hearing loss; who communicate through spoken language; and who can benefit from hearing aids, cochlear implants, and other assistive devices such as assistive listening headsets, text telephone devices readers, videotext displays, hearing aids, and closed captioning.[33]
- *Deaf* individuals have profound hearing loss, meaning little or no hearing, and often use sign language and qualified interpreters for communication; they may benefit from the assistive devices listed previously.[33]

D. Causes of Hearing Impairment

- The cause of hearing loss may be associated with the outer-, middle-, or inner-ear mechanisms, singly or in combination. Many factors may contribute to deafness, including[33]:
  - Prenatal: intrauterine infections such as rubella and cytomegalovirus.[33]
  - Perinatal: low birth weight, birth asphyxia (lack of oxygen at birth), inappropriate use of medications during pregnancy, and hyperbilirubinemia (severe jaundice in the neonatal period).
  - Childhood and adolescence: chronic ear infections, fluid in the ear, meningitis and other infections.
  - Adulthood: chronic diseases, smoking, otosclerosis, age-related sensorineural degeneration, sudden sensorineural hearing loss.
  - Other factors: cerumen impaction (impacted ear wax), injury to the head or ear, noise-induced hearing loss (workplace and recreation), medication, chemicals, nutritional deficiencies, viral infections.
- Newborn screening: spread of these universal programs prevents future psychosocial, education, and linguistic implications related to hearing loss.[33,36]
- Partial deafness may not be diagnosed, or certain patients, particularly elderly individuals, may not admit hearing limitation.[37] Clues to the identification of a hearing problem include[37]:
  - Lack of attention—fails to respond to conversation.
  - Focused, strained facial expression or stares when others are talking.
  - Turns head to one side—hearing may be good on one side only.
  - Answers are unrelated to the question.
  - Does one thing when told to do another.
  - Frequently asks others to repeat what was said.
  - Unusual speech quality.

VI. Access to Oral Health Services

- There is disparity between oral health care in people with disabilities and those without. People with disabilities are at greater risk for oral health problems.[38,39]
- Progress is being made to ensure adequate access to dental care, but barriers exist related to the patient, family, caregivers, guardians, and dental professionals (**Table 51-2**).
- Having adequate access to dental and dental hygiene services can make a significant contribution to the oral and overall health, well-being, independence, and sense of personal esteem of a patient with disabilities.[1,38,39]
- Although providing care for patients with disabilities is challenging, training, experience, empathy, patience, and a desire to be successful can help.[38,39]

VII. Trends in Community-Based Delivery of Services

A. Overview

- Individuals with disabilities may be self-sufficient or may have community-based living, educational, and work arrangements.[40]
- Barrier-free or assisted-living housing for individuals and staffed community-based residential facilities for group living are available for those who need daily assistance.
- Many homecare and community-based services are available for individuals with disabilities; however, access to dental and dental hygiene services is often limited by traditional office-based delivery systems.[13,41]

Table 51-2 Examples of Barriers to Access for Dental Care

	Patient	Family, Caregiver, and Guardian	Dental Professional
Attitude barriers	▪ May not comprehend importance of oral health ▪ May not be aware of needing oral care ▪ May not want to or be able to cooperate	▪ May not care for own oral health ▪ May lack dental literacy ▪ May be overstressed with other patient health issues that seem more important than oral needs	▪ May not feel adequately trained to or want to or be able to safely treat a physically, cognitively, or medically compromised patient
Health literacy barriers	▪ May not understand the relationship of oral health to systemic health ▪ May have difficulty understanding insurance coverage, locating a provider, making appointments, or completing paperwork	▪ May not understand the relationship of oral health to systemic health ▪ May have difficulty understanding insurance coverage, locating a provider, making appointments, or completing paperwork	▪ May not understand that the patient has many barriers to accessing oral care ▪ May not have adequately assessed the patient's health literacy when providing previous care
Physical barriers	▪ Fear of not being able to cope with architectural barriers ▪ Fear of falling ▪ Fear of attracting attention and being embarrassed	▪ May not be able to transport patient with wheelchair ▪ May not be able to lift or support patient in car or dental chair	▪ Office facility or treatment rooms may not provide a barrier-free environment
Financial barriers	▪ May have limited income ▪ May not have adequate dental insurance coverage or cannot find a provider who accepts specific insurance	▪ May not be able to take time from employment to accompany patient to appointments	▪ Cost of building accessible features or buying specialized equipment ▪ Lack of reimbursement for the additional cost of longer appointment times needed for care

- New healthcare delivery system models are being proposed to provide access to dental services where people live, work, play, go to school, or receive other social services.[41-43]
- Expansion of "direct access" regulations increase the ability of dental hygienists to provide preventive services in alternative settings and function as members of interprofessional patient care teams.[42]
- See Chapter 4 for information about providing dental hygiene care as a direct access dental hygienist in alternative settings.

Barrier-Free Environment

- Healthcare facilities are required to follow guidelines and specifications for a barrier-free physical environment based on the ADA: Standards for Accessible Design.[43]
- A **barrier-free** facility for a patient in a wheelchair, who requires more space for turning and positioning, is deemed accessible to all individuals.
- Additional features for other specific disabilities are:
  - Braille floor indicators on elevators
  - Doorways, steps, and stairways can be outlined with bright colors to contrast with the background for people with limited vision.

I. External Features

A. Parking

- A reserved area, clearly marked, near the building entrance and 13 feet wide (8-foot car space with 5-foot access aisle permits opening car doors for exiting and reboarding).
- Curb ramps (cuts) from the street and from the parking area.

B. Walkways

- A 3-foot-wide walkway is needed for wheelchair accommodation.
- The surface is solid and nonslip, without irregularities.

C. Entrance

- At least one entrance to the building on ground level accessible by a gently sloping ramp (rise of 1 inch for every 12 inches).
- An easily grasped handrail (height 30–34 inches) is needed on both sides to accommodate left- and right-handed cane and one-crutch users.

D. Door

- The lightweight door with a lever type of handle opens at least 32 inches to accommodate a wheelchair.

II. Internal Features

Official regulations specify dimensions for accessibility of all aspects, including passageways, floors, drinking fountains, and restrooms. A few are described here.[43]

A. Passageways

- Passageways must be at least 3 feet wide.
- Passageways must be free from obstructions, such as hanging signs, chairs, and large plants.

B. Floors

- Level floors with nonslip surfaces.
- Movable rugs or mats are obstacles or hazards for patients who use wheelchairs, walkers, or canes; are elderly; or are blind.

C. Reception Area

- Chairs should permit easy access during seating and rising.
- Eighteen-inch-high, flat, firm seats and arms to provide support when pushing oneself up by the arms.
- Should not slide or tip as the person rises.

III. The Treatment Room

- Doorways are at least 32 inches wide.
- Enough room beside the dental chair to allow for turning the wheelchair.
- Dental chair should lower to 19 inches from the floor and be accessible from both sides for wheelchair transfer.
- An X-ray machine in the same treatment room or a portable or handheld X-ray unit[44] can simplify the problems of moving the patient into a separate radiography room.
- For the patient with visual impairment, move equipment, such as the bracket tray and clinician's stool, from the pathway to the operatory chair and lower the chair before seating the patient.

Risk Assessment

Patients with disabilities may be at higher risk for oral disease due to characteristics related to the specific disability or disease.

- Assessment of oral disease risk factors for a patient with a disability includes assessment of oral conditions, functional ability, and medical status.[45]
- Risk factors associated with specific disabilities and medical conditions are described in the chapters in Section 9 of this text devoted to the specific conditions.

I. Oral Manifestations

- People with disabilities have an increased risk for oral problems.
  - Dental caries is common, often associated with diet and poor oral hygiene.
  - Periodontal disease can occur more often and develop at an earlier age.
  - Malocclusion is associated with muscular abnormalities, developmental delays, delayed tooth eruption, and oral habits such as bruxism or tongue thrusting.[46-48]
  - Oral and craniofacial anomalies may be present, particularly in individuals with developmental disabilities. Examples include:
    - Enamel defects.
    - High lip lines and dry gingiva due to air exposure.
    - Variations in number, size, or shape of teeth.
    - Facial asymmetry and hypoplasia of the midfacial region.[1,48]
    - Cleft lip or palate. (See Chapter 49.)
  - Damaging oral habits can affect both soft and hard oral tissues. Examples include:
    - Bruxism.
    - **Food pouching**.
    - Mouth breathing.
    - Tongue thrusting.
    - Self-injurious behavior.
    - Rumination (regurgitation of chewed food).
    - Pica (eating unusual objects and substances such as cigarette butts or gravel).[48]
  - Evidence of trauma or injury may be present, especially in individuals with a seizure disorder or physical disability.[49]
  - Weakness or paralysis of facial muscles can compromise mastication and self-cleaning

motion of the tongue and may result in food pocketing.[50,51]

- Drooling or impaired swallowing of saliva is a common feature of some disabling conditions involving head and neck musculature, such as cerebral palsy, Parkinson's disease, and stroke.[52,53]
- Potential oral side effects of medications include:
  - Increased dental caries risk due to medication-induced xerostomia.
  - Medications that diminish appetite as a side effect influence eating an adequate diet.
  - Sucrose-based liquid medications contribute to dental caries incidence.[54]
  - Drug-induced gingival enlargement, a potential side-effect of treatment with phenytoin or other antiepileptic medication. (See Chapter 57.)
  - Oral ulcerations, mucositis, and susceptibility to infection and frequent manifestations following chemotherapy, cancer treatment, or radiation to head and neck area. (See Chapter 55.)

II. Functional Ability

- Functional ability refers to the ability of an individual to accomplish daily living skills (bathing, toothbrushing, dressing, answering the phone, etc.).[55,56]
  - In children, functional ability may also include fine motor skills such as coloring a picture or playing with blocks.[57]
- Assessment of functional ability determines what oral self-care tasks an individual can do independently, what range or degree of assistance is needed, or whether the person depends on others for complete care.[57]
- An individual patient's functional level may be affected by:
  - Decrease in cognitive capability.
  - Behavioral problems.
  - Mobility problems.
  - Uncontrolled body movements.[56,58]
  - Children with blindness are limited in terms of learning by imitation.[59,60]
  - A child with blindness may learn to speak later than a child with average vision and may start school later.[59]
  - The earlier the hearing loss in a child, the more serious impact on the child's development.[61,62]
  - Communication delays may impact on social interactions and vocational choices.[61,62]
- Functioning levels and implications for oral self-care are described in **Box 51-1**. (See also Chapter 22.)

Box 51-1 Level of Function and Implications for Oral Self-Care

Activities of Daily Living (ADL)/Instrumental Activities of Daily Living (IADL) Level 0

- Individuals who are capable of flossing and brushing their own teeth.
- Children and those of all ages need varying degrees of encouragement, motivation, and supervision.

ADL/IADL Levels 1 and 2

- Individuals capable of carrying out at least part of their oral hygiene needs but who require considerable training, assistance, and direct supervision.
- The assistance may be verbal, gestural, or hand-over-hand.

ADL/IADL Level 3

- Individuals who are unable to perform their own care and are therefore dependent.
- Patients in this group may be confined to bed and nonambulatory, although others may be confined to wheelchairs. With training, some may be able to attempt some aspects of their own care.

III. Medical Status

- Assistance in completing the health history questionnaire may be needed, especially for the individual with cognitive or visual impairment.[63]
- Specific details of the patient's limitations are recorded so adaptations can be made during the current and future appointments.
- Having extensive knowledge of every health condition and side effects of medications patients are taking is impossible; however, having the knowledge about when to gather and apply additional information is essential.[45,64]
- Assessment and monitoring of the patient's medical status during treatment can reduce the risk of a medical emergency.[64]
- Individuals with a disability may experience additional medical comorbidities and health challenges such as:
  - Cardiac disorders.
  - Gastroesophageal reflux.
  - Seizures.
  - Visual and hearing impairments.

Latex allergies (individuals with spina bifida or who have undergone frequent surgeries).[65]

Oral Disease Prevention and Control

I. Objectives

Whether care is being delivered in a traditional or an alternative practice, the dental hygienist's objectives are to:

- Provide regular professional examinations and treatment at appropriate intervals to maintain patient's oral health.
- Determine patients' ability for oral self-care and need for caregiver intervention.[66]
- Motivate the patient and caregiver to establish and maintain healthy oral tissue.
- Contribute to the patient's general health through preventing tooth loss, thus maintaining ability to masticate food, preventing malnutrition, and maintaining resistance to infection.
- Prevent extensive dental and periodontal treatment the patient may not tolerate because of lowered physical stamina or the inability to cooperate.
- Prevent the need for dentures or other removable prostheses, which can be hazardous, difficult, or impossible for certain patients to tolerate.

II. Preventive Care Introduction

- Preventive interventions are selected based on individualized risk factors and level of assistance needed for daily oral care.[45,49,66]
- Depending on the disability and level of function, the patient may need[1,45,66]
  - Complete assistance.
  - Partial assistance.
  - No assistance with daily biofilm removal.
- Daily personal oral hygiene care can be compromised due to patient or caregiver[1,45,66]
  - Lack of knowledge and understanding about oral disease prevention and how it is accomplished.
  - Lack of motivation to carry out the necessary daily routines.
  - Lack of the necessary cognitive and/or physical coordination to carry out oral hygiene measures.

III. Dental Biofilm Removal

A. Provide Basic Information

- Individualized instruction according to the patient's unique needs and functional ability.
- Determine the current daily care routine to identify if modifications are required.
- Biofilm formation and disease development are described on a level at which the patient and caregiver can learn and be motivated.[1,38,45,66]
- Approaches for motivating the patient or caregiver's health behavior change are described in Chapter 24.

B. Toothbrushing

- Provide clear and concise instructions.
- Biofilm removal is more important than the specific technique used, unless it causes damage to the oral cavity.
- Use of a soft toothbrush and a scrub-brush or circular Fones method may be appropriate and within the capability of certain patients.
- Encourage independence in daily oral care.
- Although a caregiver may be willing to brush the patient's teeth, as much as possible should be carried out by the patient.
- Demonstrate toothbrushing in the patient's mouth and describe the feeling of the filament tips on and under the gingival margin and the feeling of clean teeth.
- Guide patient with hand-over-hand toothbrush technique to help with placement of the toothbrush in the mouth.[1,45,66]
- Adaptations for toothbrush handles
- Basic information about toothbrushes and methods is found in Chapter 26.

C. Adaptive Aids

- For patients whose main barrier to oral self-care is related to grasp, manipulation, or control of a toothbrush, adaptations can help accommodate specific needs.
- Benefits to the patient may include feelings of self-esteem and accomplishment when able to manage the important task of brushing, particularly for patients who have a physical but no cognitive disability.
- General prerequisites for an adaptive aid include:
  - Disinfectable.
  - Durable: can withstand exposure to water and saliva.
  - Resistant to absorption of oral fluids.
  - Replaceable.
  - Inexpensive.

D. Adapted Manual Toothbrush

- **Figure 51-1** illustrates attachments to insert and hold the brush handle against the patient's hand. This attachment is useful for a patient:
  - With fingers permanently fixed in a fist.
  - Who are unable to grasp and hold.
- Aids to enlarge the diameter of the handle of an oral care implement, useful for a patient with limited hand closure, are illustrated in **Figure 51-2** and **Figure 51-3**.
- For a patient with limited shoulder or elbow movement, lengthen handle of the brush using a material strong or rigid enough to provide sufficient lateral pressure to remove biofilm from the tooth surfaces. Examples include:
  - Attach a handle of a kitchen utensil, such as a wooden spoon, to the brush handle with glue or tape (see **Figure 51-4**).
  - Tongue depressors taped to the brush handle, then one or two other tongue depressors taped to overlap and provide an extension.
  - Use other means by wrapping the object securely to the brush handle for elongation.[66]
- A specially designed toothbrush with curved outer filaments and a short stiff center row of filaments

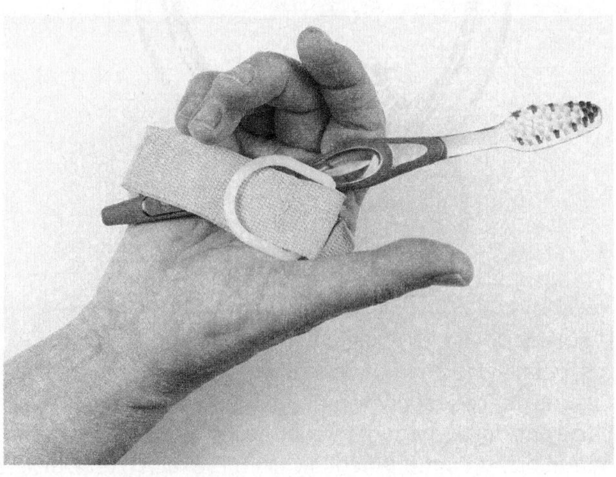

A

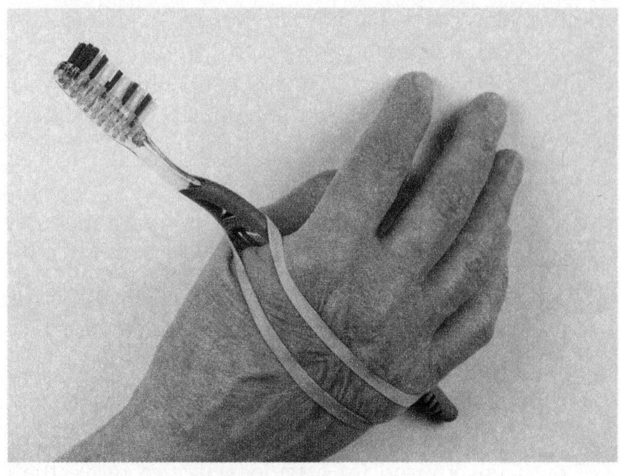

B

Figure 51-1 Aids for Patient Who Cannot Grasp and Hold. Adjustable Velcro strap **(A)** or simple rubber band **(B)** around toothbrush handle enables patient to secure brush firmly across the palm of the hand. A floss holder also may be held by these methods.

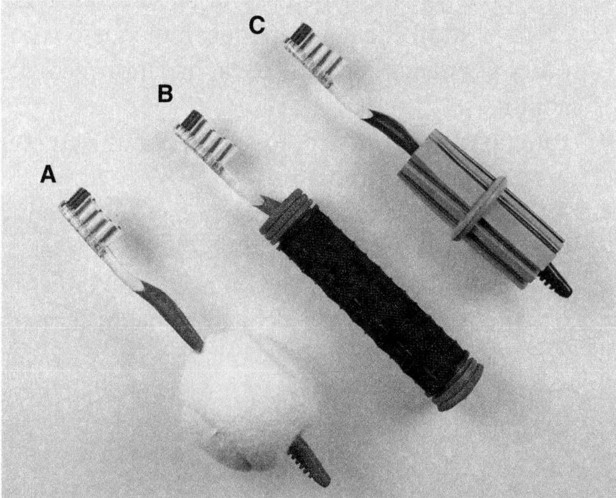

Figure 51-2 Aids for Patient with Limited Grasp.
A: Toothbrush inserted into tennis ball or other soft rubber ball. **B:** Toothbrush inserted into a bicycle handle grip. **C:** Toothbrush inserted into a clean, unused rubber pet toy.

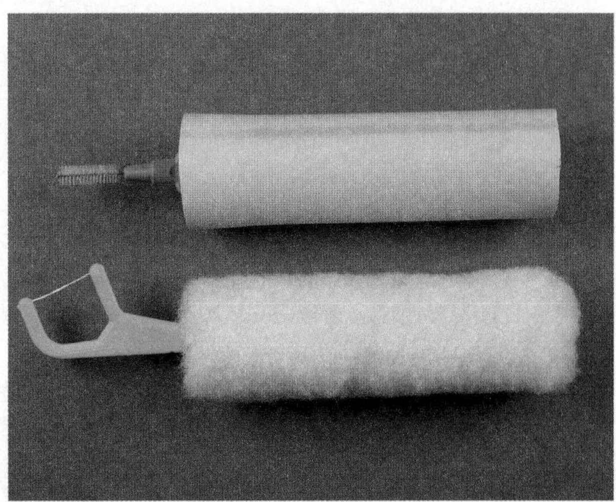

Figure 51-3 Interdental Cleaning Aids for Patient with Limited Grasp. Floss aids and interdental cleaners can be inserted into commercially available foam tubing or the open end of a clean mini-sized paint roller cover.

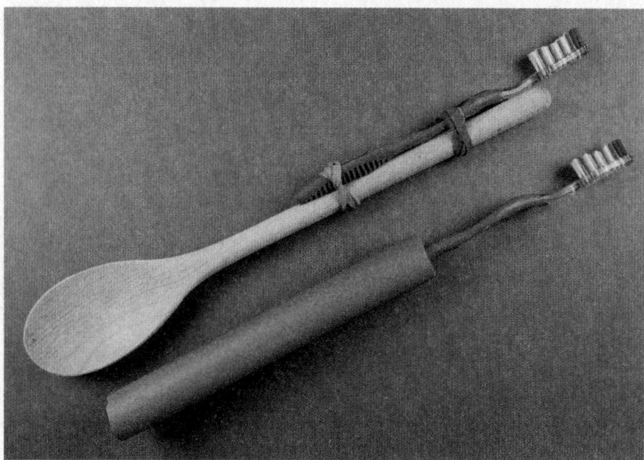

Figure 51-4 Aid for Patient with Limited Shoulder or Elbow Movement. Toothbrush with added handle extension can be created using commercially available foam tubing or by securing a toothbrush to a long-handled wooden spoon with tape or an elastic band.

that brush exposed tooth surfaces simultaneously is shown in **Figure 51-5**.

- For a patient who can hold and position the toothbrush but cannot make strokes for biofilm removal.
- For a patient with hand tremors, such as with Parkinson's disease.
- Can be used for a patient able to move their head side-to-side and up-and-down instead of moving their hand.
- Can be used by a caregiver who provides toothbrushing assistance.
- Provides similar reduction in biofilm compared with use of a conventional brush.[67]

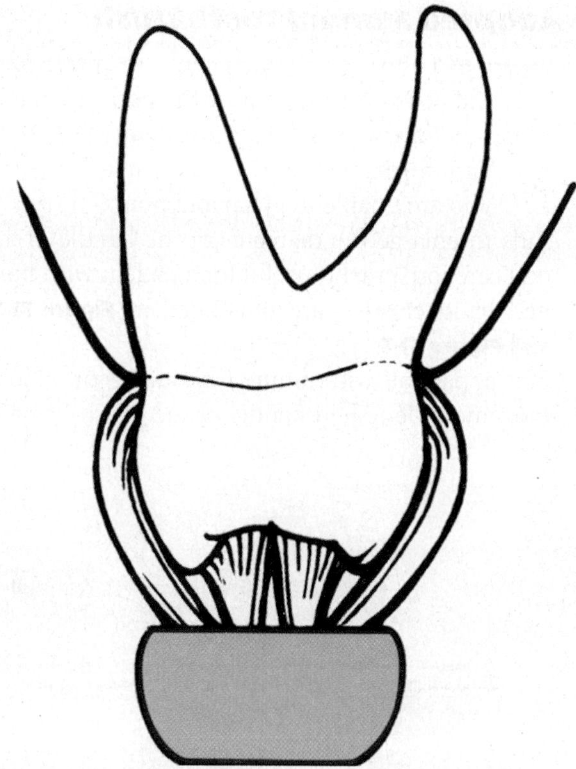

Figure 51-5 Aid for Patient with a Brushing Problem. A specially designed toothbrush is shown on the mesial of a maxillary second primary molar. Used with a back-and-forth motion, the filaments remove debris and dental biofilm simultaneously from the facial, lingual (palatal), and occlusal tooth surfaces.

E. Power-Aided Devices

- Use of a power toothbrush can provide independence and effective biofilm removal for many patients and can motivate patients who have difficulty with a manual toothbrush.[68,69]
  - Can cause trauma if used incorrectly, especially for those who cannot comprehend how it is used.
  - The extra size and weight of the handle may be advantageous for some patients or difficult for others with limited strength.
  - The on/off mechanism may be difficult to use for those lacking finger strength and coordination.
  - The larger handle can aid those who have difficulty grasping objects.
  - The vibrations created during use may not be tolerated by certain patients.
  - Additional cost of the brush may be a consideration for some patients.
- Additional power-aided devices, such as flossers, are available and are recommended based on assessment of an individual patient's need and abilities.
- Patients are instructed to follow manufacturers' instructions for proper use.
- A patient with limited grasp can adapt a cuff around the handle to aid in holding the power-aided brush, similar to those shown in Figure 51-1.
- Cross-contamination can be a problem, particularly in group-living situations. Ensure each patient has a separate marked toothbrush and is kept apart from others.

F. Dentifrice

- A dentifrice containing fluoride is recommended for patients who can use a dentifrice.
- When a patient cannot control saliva, rinse, or expectorate, use of a dentifrice may be contraindicated.
- A dentifrice may increase a gag reflex for certain patients.

- When a parent or other caregiver is assisting, the paste may limit visibility for thorough biofilm removal.
- When a paste is used, only a small, pea-sized amount is placed on the brush.
    - Dentifrice is not essential for biofilm removal, and another method of daily fluoride application may be more appropriate.
- The person who is severely disabled may be treated with a suction brush to help prevent aspiration. (See Chapter 4.)

G. Interdental Cleaning

- If standard use of dental floss is not possible, due to limited dexterity or use of only one hand, the use of a floss holder or other interdental aid can make interdental cleaning possible for the patient or caregiver.
- Methods for increasing the size of a toothbrush handle may be adapted for the handle of a floss holder.
- Careful instruction for use and supervision are needed to prevent tissue damage.
- Other interdental aids are described in Chapter 27.

H. Cleaning Removable Dental Prostheses

- For the patient with difficulty grasping or holding the brush, a denture brush handle may be adapted by any of the methods described for the regular toothbrush.
- A fingernail brush may be used instead of a standard denture brush provided all denture surfaces can be reached for biofilm removal.
- For the patient with use of only one hand or who needs to grasp the denture with two hands to prevent accidents, the following are recommended:
    - Fingernail brush with suction cups.
    - Denture brush, as shown in **Figure 51-6A**.
    - Denture brush with suction cups, as shown in **Figure 51-6B**, can attach low inside the sink bowl.
- The details for cleaning removable prostheses are described in Chapter 30.

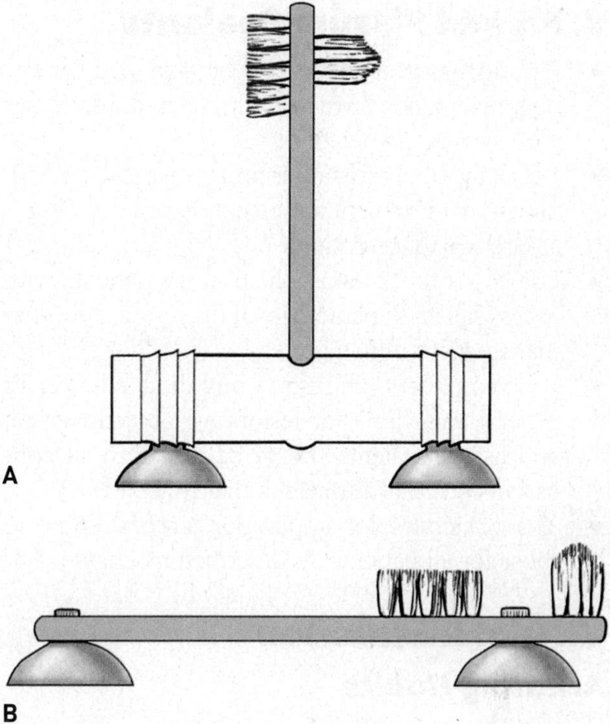

Figure 51-6 Denture Brushes with Suction Cups. **A:** Denture brush in a commercially available mounting. **B:** Suction cups attached directly to a denture brush. Either brush may be positioned in a sink to aid the person who has one hand or who needs to grasp the denture with two hands to prevent accidental dropping and breakage.

IV. Fluorides

- Selection of a fluoride program for any patient depends on the assessment of the individual's caries risk status. (See Chapter 25.)
- The patient with a disability may be at increased risk for caries due to barriers that limit access to preventive services, decreased ability to provide or cooperate with assistance for self-care, and side effects of medications.
- Risk-based fluoride recommendations include:
    - Encouragement to drink fluoridated tap water where available.
    - Use of dentifrice with fluoride.
    - Dietary supplements for young children, when fluoride is below optimum level in the community water supply. (See Chapter 34 for guidelines.)
    - Fluoride varnishes because they are quick and do not need isolation, are tolerated better than fluoride trays for many people with disabilities.[70,71]
    - Self-applied home fluoride gel or toothpaste.
    - See Chapter 34 for additional information.
- For a dependent, low-functioning person, brushing with a fluoride gel or the toothbrush soaked in a fluoridated mouthrinse rather than a toothpaste can be recommended.[70]
- Silver diamine fluoride is beneficial for people with disabilities, as it is noninvasive and could reduce or delay the need for surgical-restorative work.[72,73]

V. Pit and Fissure Sealants

- Pit and fissure sealants can be provided for cooperative patients with developmental disabilities with satisfactory results.
- Use of a dental assistant is imperative to help with patient management and to maintain a dry field to assure sealant retention.
- Use of a rubber dam is helpful for patients with excess saliva, hyperactivity of the tongue, or other management difficulties.
- When a patient who is severely disabled receives general anesthesia for restorative procedures, pit and fissure sealants should be placed in all noncarious occlusal surfaces at that time.
- The principles for application are the same as those for all patients, as described in Chapter 35.

VI. Diet Instruction

A. Eating Habits

- Current dietary requirements, eating and snack habits, extent of oral health knowledge, family customs, and economic status are considered before specific dietary recommendations are made.
- Difficulty of food preparation and dependence on others for grocery shopping can be a major limitation to diet selection for some adults with disabilities.
- Sweets are sometimes used as rewards or bribes by unsuspecting family members or teachers using applied behavioral analysis (ABA) as a teaching tool, and the introduction of sugarless snacks and nonfoods as rewards and teaching tools is especially important.[74]
- A high-functioning patient or the parent/caregiver may be able to keep a food diary.
- With the aid of the daily food record and information from the medical and dental histories, items for counseling can be selected, such as caries prevention.

B. Oral Factors

- Problems with mastication and swallowing can lead to use of a soft diet, often composed mainly of carbohydrates.
- Conditions affecting the integrity of facial musculature can compromise self-cleansing of oral structures and contribute to food pocketing in the buccal vestibule.

C. Recommendations

- Adaptations involve long-range planning for gradual modification of the patient's diet.
- The person who selects and prepares the food for the patient is involved in the planning.
- In an institutional setting, the dental hygienist can work as a member of the interprofessional patient care team with the administrative and medical personnel, teachers, dietitians, and aides to introduce dietary modifications.
- General procedures for dietary assessment, analysis, and counseling are described in Chapter 33.

Patient Management

- With a few modifications and attention to managing specific factors related to each individual's situation, most patients with disabilities can be treated in a clinical setting.
- Only a relatively small number of patients need hospitalization due to difficulties in management or a systemic condition that requires special medical supervision.

I. Objectives

- Increase the efficacy, efficiency, and safety of dental and dental hygiene treatment.
- Make patient appointments pleasant and comfortable.

II. Modes of Communication

- Unless the patient has an extreme cognitive impairment, the patient is always addressed first and the caregiver second.
- Address the patient in *person-first language*, describing them by their abilities rather than labeling them by their disability.
- Parents and/or caregivers can explain how best to communicate with the patient, help interpret the changing moods of the patient, identify problems, and note changes in behavior that may indicate a dental problem.
- Basic behavioral guidance strategies, such as tell–show–do, positive previsit imagery, ask–tell–ask, modeling, distraction, positive reinforcement, and desensitization, can be adapted to address the unique needs of the patient with a disability.[75,76]
- Using nonverbal communication, facial expressions, pointing, body language, and demonstration helps certain patients to respond.
- Kindness, patience, and empathy will help the clinician build trust.
- A person who is totally blind is more likely to accept a new experience if discussed in detail beforehand.

- A person with hearing loss may prefer a particular way of communication.
  - Choices include speaking, **speechreading**, writing, manual, or a combination.
  - Manual communication includes using sign language or "signing" and fingerspelling.
  - *Always ask the patient which means of communication is preferred and how communication can be improved.*

A. American Sign Language

- **American Sign Language** (ASL) is a visual/gestural language with a unique grammar and syntax.
- Many people who are deaf prefer this mode of communication as they grew up using ASL and consider themselves part of a cultural group.
- Individuals who have become deaf in later years may learn sign language and use the signs in English word order, meaning the subject comes before the verb and the verb comes before the object in a sentence structure.
- Some people with deafness prefer to communicate using ASL in medical or dental situations and can request the services of an ASL interpreter.
- A universal sign language has not been recognized, and many countries have their own.

B. American Manual Alphabet

- Fingerspelling "in the air" is often combined with sign language.
- When making an introduction, for example, the name may be fingerspelled.
- New words often do not have signs and are fingerspelled.
- The American Society for Deaf Children (ASDC) has resources for learning ASL, including online classes at https://deafchildren.org.
  - The ASL alphabet can be found at https://deafchildren.org/2019/06/free-asl-alphabet-chart/
  - An ASL fingerspelling app for the cell phone.
  - YouTube also has a number of videos to help learn sign language.

C. Oral Communication

- Oral communication by a person with deafness or severe hearing impairment may require a combination of speech, residual hearing, and speechreading.

D. Speechreading

- Speechreading consists of recognizing spoken words by watching the lips, face, and gestures.
- Many of the mouth movements for spoken words have the same appearance as one or more other words, so speechreading may need to be combined with another method of communication.
- Speechreading is not a reliable means of communication for extended, complex discussions for most people with hearing loss.
- Speechreading is not a choice when the clinician must wear a mask.[77]

E. Writing

- Writing may be an alternative when the patient is hard of hearing or when other methods are not satisfactory.
- Have a single-use writing pad available with pen or pencil for communication purposes.[77]

III. Pretreatment Planning

A. Preliminary Contact

- Information may be obtained from the patient, or with legal authority from the guardian, parent, relative, advocate, or other person responsible for the patient.[78]
- The essential information can be obtained in advance by telephone or telehealth/teledentistry interview.
  - Medical forms also can be mailed to the home for completion.
- Advanced information permits the dental team to be prepared to make the appointment a successful and positive experience for the patient and clinician.

B. Legal Guardianship

- When a person is declared incapacitated by a legal process, a guardian is appointed.[78]
- Documented proof of legal guardianship is kept in the patient record.
- When the patient is unable to sign informed consent for treatment, the legal guardian provides this service.[78]

C. Information to Obtain

- In addition to the usual topics covered by the medical, personal, and dental histories, additional information is requested, using questions listed in **Box 51-2**.
- To avoid unpleasant situations and misunderstanding, ask direct questions about a patient's disability, rather than making assumptions.

Box 51-2 Patient with a Disability: Additional Information to Obtain before the Appointment

Basic Information

- Has a guardian been legally appointed? Obtain written documentation.
- Is there a caregiver, case worker, or counselor who works with the patient?
- Will someone accompany the patient to appointments?
- Does the patient give consent to discuss care with other individuals?
- Degree of independence, self-care, and communication preferences of the patient.

Medical History

- Specific list of disabilities or disabling conditions.
- When diagnosed.
- History of treatments and hospitalizations.
- Current medications and other therapy.
- Names and addresses of specialists.
- Any restrictions, such as dietary or for safety (leg braces, helmet).

Dental History

- Previous dental experiences and patient's attitude.
- Barriers to previous dental care.
- Most recent care: procedures, setting, success.
- History of oral infections and oral habits.
- Fluoride history, including fluoridation levels in drinking water and self- or professionally applied topical methods.
- Current homecare methods: aids and special devices, frequency, degree of self-care.
- Concepts of perceived needs, attitudes, and apparent emphasis on oral care.
- Modifications and successful techniques used before and during appointments.

Supplemental Information

Are any of the following affected by disability?

- Muscular coordination, mobility, walking.
- Sitting tolerance.
- Sitting position.
- Ability to cooperate/involuntary movements.
- Communication: speech, hearing, vision.
- Breathing, including when reclined.
- Swallowing, control of saliva.
- Bowel or bladder control.
- Cognitive abilities, such as memory (short and long term) and executive functioning.
- Dexterity, ability to brush and floss teeth.
- Ability to chew or eat.

Open-Ended Other Information

- Does patient require any additional assistance or have any other issues of concern?

D. Consultation with Interprofessional Care Team

- Management of a patient with disabilities can be very complex due to medical complications.
- Need to prevent negative effects on a medical condition while rendering care.[79]
- Consultation with physicians, social worker, and other medical providers who form the patient's interprofessional care team may be required to help determine an oral health plan.[79]
- Extra time may be required to access information about the conditions and medications before an appointment.

E. Interaction with Caregiver

- A patient with a disability may depend on a caregiver for daily life activities.
- Caregivers may or may not be the legal guardian of the patient or the contact person to plan appointments.[78]
- If the caregiver is not the legal guardian, the adult patient or guardian must be consulted to determine the limits of the caregiver's role.[78]
- Caregivers can be an excellent source of information, help prepare the patient for the appointment, and offer suggestions for gaining cooperation from the patient.
- Invite the caregiver to the office before the appointment to see the facility and become familiar with the surroundings and staff.[78,80]

IV. Appointment Scheduling

A. Special Requirements

- Allow time in the schedule for preparation needed before appointment, for example, to move furniture or retrieve and set up special equipment such as paper to write on for a patient with a hearing impairment.
- Arrangements should be made if the patient requires antibiotic prophylaxis.
- Identify special aids the patient is asked to bring to the appointment, such as a transfer board for transfer into the dental chair, hearing aid, dental prostheses, and biofilm control devices currently in use.
- Individuals who are deaf may require an ASL interpreter.
- Some individuals with disabilities are accompanied by service dogs, such as guide dogs for the visual, hearing, and other disabilities, which are allowed by law into all public buildings and on public transportation.

- When a patient brings a guide dog to the appointment[81]:
  - Do not distract a dog on duty by touching, speaking, or making eye contact.
  - Do not walk on the dog's left side, which can distract the dog.
  - Do not offer the dog food.
  - Do not lead or grab the patient while the dog is guiding.
  - Ask the patient the best place for the dog to stay during the appointment.
- Service dogs are well-trained animals and will lie quietly as directed by the patient.
  - If you want to pet the dog, ask the guide dog-user first. Often the user will remove the harness before allowing someone to pet the dog.[81]

B. Transportation

- A patient may rely on the caregiver or another source for transport to appointment.
- A patient using a wheelchair may need to reserve wheelchair accessible transportation and be limited by the availability of transportation.
- The transportation service may need to be contacted when the patient has completed the appointment; forms may need to be completed.

C. Time Considerations

- Determine how the patient's daily schedule influences time selection for scheduling appointments.
- Inquire about the schedule of the caregiver who accompanies the patient.
- The cooperation of the patient may be decreased if basic routines are disturbed, for example:
  - The appointment for the patient with diabetes cannot interfere with medication, meal, or between-meal eating schedules.
  - The elderly person who rises early may want a morning appointment.
  - Patients with arthritis may have greater mobility later in the day.
  - Child's nap schedule should not be disrupted.
  - Early morning appointment may be difficult for a patient who requires a long time for morning preparation, such as a patient with a spinal cord injury or colostomy.
- Arrange a time when the patient will not have a long wait.
- Allow sufficient time so the patient is not rushed; many persons with disabilities require more time.
- Consider incontinence issues, including time needed for restroom visits.

D. Patient Reception: The Initial Appointment

- The orientation of a patient with a disability paves the way for long-term success of dental and dental hygiene supervision and care.
- The first appointment includes and, when necessary, may be devoted entirely to, a basic orientation to the facilities, the dental chair, and the personnel.
- Several orientation visits may be necessary to acclimate the patient to surroundings and to desensitize.
- **Desensitization techniques** and other basic behavior guidance approaches can help reduce anxiety, particularly for a patient with cognitive impairment or one who is fearful.[75]
- Assessment procedures and preventive personal care instructions are initiated, and participation of the caregiver is solicited as indicated.

V. Introduction of Clinical Settings

- Create a casual and relaxed environment.
- Create unique ways to communicate during treatment, explain the procedure step-by-step, and always face the person when explaining the clinical procedures.[48,63]
- Describe each step in detail before proceeding.[48,63]
- Introduce the patient to the dental office by utilizing their senses.[48,63,79]
- Start the oral examination slowly; use fingers first before introducing instruments.[48,63,79]
- Explain instruments, materials, and how each will be applied using a behavior guidance technique such as the tell–show–do approach.[76]
- Prepare patient for power-driven instruments; avoid surprise applications of compressed air or water from syringe.
- Allow the patient to hear the equipment, such as the saliva ejector, that will be used during the appointment and give a warning prior to using it.[63,76,79]
- Introduce unusual smells or taste utilized during the different treatment.[63,79]
- Apply rubber cup to person's fingernail so they can experience how polishing feels.

A. Patient with a Visual Impairment

- For the patient with a visual impairment, ask their preference for how to guide them to the dental chair. Many prefer to hold the clinician's arm and follow them (**Figure 51-7**).

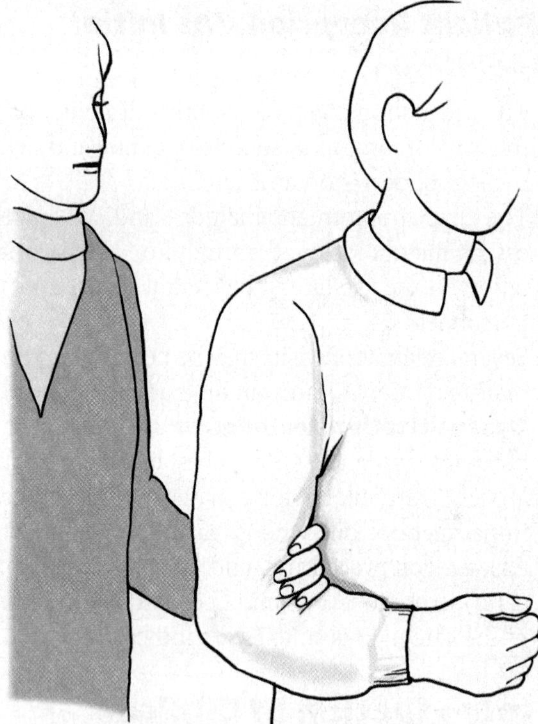

Figure 51-7 Escorting a Visually Impaired Individual. A visually impaired person holds the arm of the guide just above the elbow and walks beside and slightly behind. The guide verbally gives advance notice of approaching changes. The blind person can sense the body movement of the guide and anticipate changes.

- Provide forewarning of potential hazards in the way.
- Because of a visual impairment, the patient may tend to rely more on other senses such as touch and hearing.
- A person with total blindness tries to be neat and orderly. Avoid moving items belonging to the person without alerting them.
- A person with total blindness learns to interpret and rely on tone of voice more than persons with sight, who can watch facial expressions.
- Protective eyewear: the patient may prefer to wear their own glasses.
- Light: avoid directing the dental light in the patient's eyes as sensitivity to light is characteristic of many eye conditions.[63,79]
- Position the patient for best vision. For example, a patient with glaucoma has no peripheral vision; thus, instruction must be given directly in front of the patient.[63]
- Do not expect a patient to see fine detail, such as a radiograph without enlargement.
- Inform the patient when leaving the treatment room to prevent embarrassment of the patient speaking to someone who is not present.

B. Patient with a Hearing Impairment

- Full visibility is essential for communicating with a patient who is hearing impaired or deaf.[77]
  - Wear a Food and Drug Administration (FDA)–approved clear mask.
  - Remove mask when talking if also wearing a clear face shield.
  - Wear a clear face shield.
  - Do not demonstrate oral hygiene techniques out of the patient's field of view.
- Be careful not to touch a hearing aid when it is turned on.
- Adjust patient's head so ears are not compressed against the headrest or pillow, which can cause discomfort.
- Eliminate or minimize background noise.[77]
- Use visual tools, posters, brochures, and so on, to help explain procedures.[77]

VI. Continuing Care Appointments

The frequency of continuing care appointments for all patients is individualized, but more frequent appointments are encouraged for some persons with a disability for the following reasons:

- To decrease the length of a single appointment.
- To assist the patient who has limited ability to perform personal oral self-care adequately.
- To provide motivation through monitoring biofilm and review of procedures for the patient and the caregiver involved.
- To provide preventive procedures such as fluoride.

VII. Assistance for the Patient Who Is Ambulatory

- Ask patient how much and what kind of assistance is needed.
- A patient may walk with one or more assistive aids such as braces, a cane, crutches, or a walker.
- Certain patients do not require assistance because they have developed their own method of balancing; however, many patients gain balance by holding both hands on the partially flexed forearm of a person walking beside them.

A. Seating the Patient

- Raise chair slightly above the patient's knee level and move chair arm out of the way.

- Stand aside or assist while patient moves until the back of legs touch chair and they bend their knees to lower into dental chair.
- If assistance is needed after patient is in the chair, grasp ankles, lift legs, and turn patient into dental chair.
- Remove assistive aids and store out of the way.
- For patients who are blind, lead to chair and have the patient feel the chair, especially the seat and the back prior to seating themselves.

B. The Seated Patient

- Give advance warning to the patient and then tilt chair back slowly.
- If necessary, position supportive padding to maintain patient comfort.

C. Rising from the Chair

- After telling the patient, slowly raise the chair to upright position, with the seat slightly higher than the patient's knee level to minimize need to bend their knees when rising.
- Allow time for adjustment to upright position to avoid the effects of postural (orthostatic) hypertension.
- Ask or assist patient with moving their feet to the floor.
- Retrieve assistive aids and hold them for patient to grasp with the dominant hand.
- Ask patient if assistance is needed to rise from the chair and offer support if needed by placing the clinician's arm under the patient's arm on the non-dominant side until balance is obtained for walking.

VIII. Patient Positioning

- The objectives for patient positioning during treatment are to let the patient feel comfortable while giving the clinician adequate illumination, visibility, and accessibility.
- Extreme care should be given to positioning of any patient with a swallowing defect (dysphagia) or respiratory compromise.
  - The patient may be unable to prevent aspiration of fluids or object placed in the mouth during treatment and a semi-supine position may be required.

A. Adapt Chair Position

- A patient with a respiratory or cardiac complication is positioned with the chair back raised to a level that is comfortable for the patient.
- The patient can be asked, "How many pillows do you use at night?" and the chair can be adjusted accordingly.

B. Body Adjustments

- Patients with a spinal cord injury should do a "push up" and patients with quadriplegia shift their weight every 20 minutes for 10–15 seconds to maintain good circulation in the tissues that do not have sensation, such as the buttocks.[82]
- Allowing movement prevents decubitus ulcers—this is a particular consideration during long procedures.
- Ensure the patient is in center of chair.
- Do not move limbs into unnatural positions.
- Allow patient to settle into a comfortable position.
- Place patient's chin in a neutral or downward position to prevent the gag reflex.[83]

IX. Supportive and Protective Stabilization

- Always obtain a signed informed consent from patient, guardian, or parent before any form of stabilization is performed.[78,84]
- Protective stabilization or medical immobilization techniques described next can help prevent injury to the patient, the caregiver, and the dental practitioner; however, the use of restraint is controversial and has the risk of causing injury or resulting in legal action.[84]
- The method of stabilization is decided after communication-based or desensitizing techniques are tried and is individualized for each patient.
- When the patient is a child, the parent should be present to recognize immobilization protects their child from harm.[84]
- With basic knowledge of methods for maintaining patient stability, adequate visibility of working area, secure instrument grasps and finger rests, and well-controlled strokes, instrumentation can be effectively accomplished.
- Supportive stabilization, such as padding under flexed knees or bite block positioned to rest jaw muscles, can be used to facilitate patient comfort.[84]
- Protective stabilization is never used as a form of punishment.

A. Extremity Movement

- A team member, parent, or caregiver employs a hand guarding or holding the patient's hands.

- If hand guarding is unsuccessful, wrist restraints may be used (Posey straps, Velcro straps, seat belts).[84]

B. Body Enclosure

- Although a small patient may be held by a parent, such positioning can be tiring for the parent, be insecure, and may not provide good body mechanics for the clinician.
- Pediwrap or Papoose Board: adjustable arm or leg immobilizer wraps with Velcro closures or a padded board with wide fabric wraps around upper body, middle body, and legs are available in adult and pediatric sizes, but not recommended unless the clinician has specialized training and informed consent has been obtained.[78,84]

C. Head Stabilization

- Arm of clinician: from a working position at 12 o'clock (top of the patient's head), the nondominant arm is placed around the patient's head to stabilize it in position.
- Head positioner or another person may also stabilize the head.[84]

D. Oral Stabilization

A mouth prop can be used to assist the patient who has difficulty maintaining an open mouth.[84] Training on the technique for safe use of mouth props is required. Patience and a gentle but firm touch are essential. Verbal encouragement should continue throughout the appointment.

- The most stable mouth prop is a sterilized ratchet type (Molt adjustable mouth prop) that can be nearly closed for insertion between the teeth.[85]
  - It can be opened gradually to hold the jaws to the necessary position.
  - The tips are covered with rubber tubing and are positioned over the maxillary and mandibular teeth on one side while the clinician treats the opposite side.
  - However, this form of mouth prop may intimidate children and should be introduced appropriately.
- Different types of rubber bite blocks are available; for example, **Figure 51-8** shows one that allows for placement of a suction tip.
- A long piece of dental floss can be tied through the holes in a commercially available rubber mouth prop, in case of a sudden respiratory change, the prop can be quickly pulled out and breathing normalized.

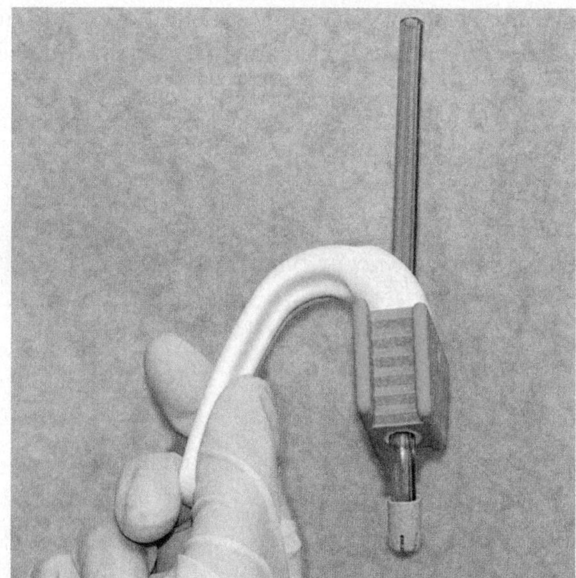

Figure 51-8 Rubber Bite Block Mouth Prop with Saliva Ejector

E. Precautions for Stabilization

- Patient and caregivers are informed of the risks and reassured all stabilization devices are for comfort and to make the work easier and they are in no way meant to hurt or punish.
- Ongoing monitoring of patient's physical and psychological well-being is necessary during stabilization.[86]
- Mobile teeth can be dislodged and swallowed or aspirated.[86]
- Fatigue of the patient's facial and masticatory muscles and temporomandibular joint.

X. Four-Handed Dental Hygiene

- The use of a dental hygiene assistant during the appointment can enhance:
  - Efficiency.
  - Patient management.
  - Patient safety and comfort.
  - Safety and comfort for clinician.
  - Visibility during intraoral procedures.
- Observation and providing continuous suction to maintain a clear visual field for instrumentation and to decrease the risk of aspiration for patients with disabilities that cause excess drooling/salivation, have impaired respiratory function, swallowing, or gag reflex.
- Ensures the patient's safety glasses are in place and provides continuous suction when the patient's disorder involves orofacial muscles and nerves, which increases the risk of splashing of aerosols into the eye.

XI. Instrumentation

- Introduce each procedure and sound to prevent startling a patient; follow the basic instruction rule to tell-show-do[76]
- Biofilm control instruction should precede scaling to reduce the bacterial load during instrumentation.
- Unbreakable plastic mirrors are recommended for use with a patient subject to spasm or sudden closure.
- Use single-end sharp instruments to prevent accidents as the nonworking end of an instrument can be a hazard when an unrestrained patient moves involuntarily.
- Use of power instruments is contraindicated for a patient at risk for aspiration and for patients who overreact to sensory stimuli, such as a patient with autism.
- Finger rests: firm, dependable finger rests are needed. Supplemental or reinforced rests can contribute to instrument stability. An external finger rest and hand rest may be safer for the clinician.
- The occurrence of generalized heavy calculus deposits in patients with disabilities is not unusual due to factors related to the disabling condition.

XII. Pain and Anxiety Control

- Some patients with behavioral or cognitive dysfunction may need intervention beyond standard communication techniques and local anesthesia in order to receive dental care.
- Alternative methods of pain and anxiety control for patients who are unable to cooperate during dental treatment include[1]:
  - Pharmacologically induced sedation: minimal, moderate, or deep sedation; provided by trained dentist or anesthesiologist.
  - General anesthesia: delivered in hospital, surgery centers, or dental offices; provided by trained anesthesiologists.

Wheelchair Transfer

There are several steps to ensure safety for both the patient and the people assisting in the transfer.[76,87]

I. Preparation for Wheelchair Transfer

A. Determine the Patient's Needs[87]

- Always inform the patient of intended actions before starting.
- Ask patient or caregiver the preferred transfer method.
- Determine patient's ability to help.
- Selection of a transfer technique is influenced by the size, weight, and mobility of the patient, along with any special physical conditions and patient's preferences.
- The patient may prefer to transfer from the left or the right side of the dental chair, depending on which side of the body is stronger.
- Transfer from the wheelchair can be a frightening experience to the patient owing to fear of falling and injury.

B. Prepare the Area

- Before starting a transfer, clear the area: move the clinician's stool, bracket tray, foot controls, and operatory light.
- Remove or move the operatory chair armrest out of the transfer area.[87]

C. Special Needs of Patient

- Chair padding: Special padding is used in a wheelchair as protection from pressure sores. Depending on the length of the appointment, the patient will decide whether the padding is moved to the dental chair. Pressure sores (decubitus ulcers) are described in Chapter 52.
- Bags and catheters: For patients wearing a urinary or **colostomy bag**, care must be taken during transfer and after transfer to ensure tubing is not bent or twisted.
- Spasms: Ask the patient about susceptibility to spasms and about procedures to follow for prevention.
- Advice concerning transfer: Ask the patient, family member, or caregiver how best the clinician can help during the transfer. The patient is encouraged to do as much as possible.

II. Transfer of Patient Who Can Assist

When a patient can support their own weight, the "stand and pivot" technique can be used, as shown in **Figure 51-9**.

A. Position the Wheelchair

- Face the wheelchair in the same direction as the dental chair at approximately an angle of 30°, set brakes, and remove footrests and wheelchair armrests.

B. Prepare Dental Chair

- Adjust the chair to the same height as or lower than the wheelchair; clear a path for transfer by lifting or removing the chair arm.
- Always have a second person in the treatment room to help if required.

C. Approach to Patient

- Detach the safety belt, if patient is wearing one.
- Face the patient and place feet outside the patient's feet for pivoting.
- Clinician's knees should be placed close to or against the patient's knees to prevent buckling.
- Place hands under the patient's arms and grasp the waist belt in back. Patient places arms around clinician's neck or places hands on wheelchair to push up.
- Clinician lifts patient to standing position, as in **Figure 51-9B**.

D. Pivot to Dental Chair

- Pivot together slowly until the patient is backed up to the side of the chair, with the backs of the legs touching.
- The patient is gently lowered to a sitting position.
- Reposition the arm of the chair.
- Grasp the patient's legs together between the ankles and knees, and lift them onto the chair, as shown in **Figure 51-9C**.

E. After the Wheelchair Transfer

- Release the wheelchair brake to move it aside.
- In a small treatment room, the wheelchair may be folded and set aside.
- After the appointment, return the patient to the wheelchair in the reverse order of procedure.

III. Transfer of Patient Who Is Immobile

When the patient is unable to support their own weight, two aides are required. The parent or other caregiver may serve as the second person. Never attempt to do this alone.[87]

A. Position the Wheelchair

- Position the wheelchair in the same direction and parallel with the dental chair, set wheelchair brakes, and remove footrests.
- Adjust the dental chair to the same height as or lower than the seat of the wheelchair.
- Move the arm of the dental chair out of the transfer area and remove the arm of the wheelchair.

B. Clinician 1

- Is positioned behind the wheelchair.
- Helps patient cross arms across chest.
- Will place arms under the patient's upper arms and grasp the patient's wrists.

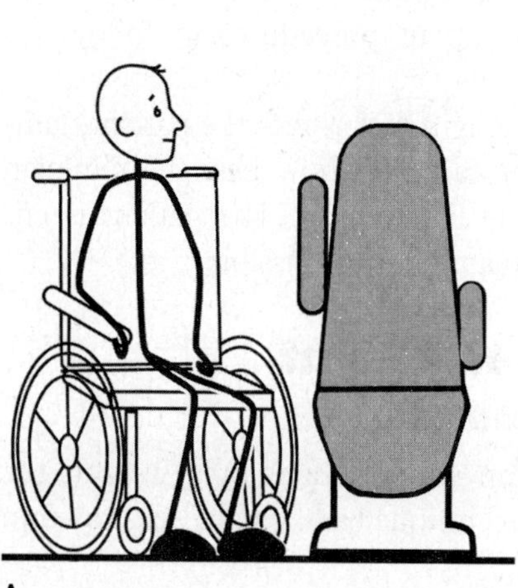

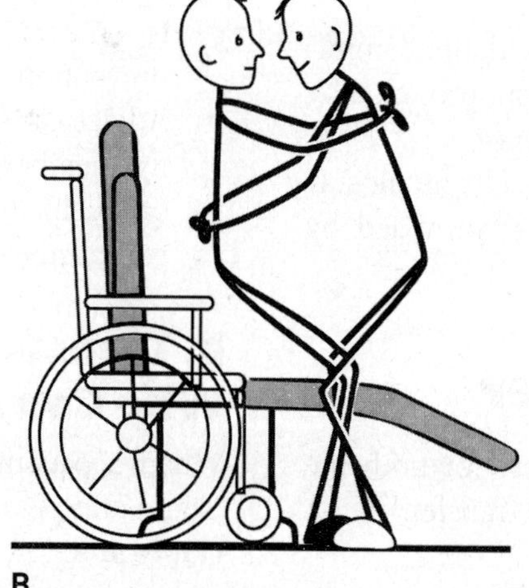

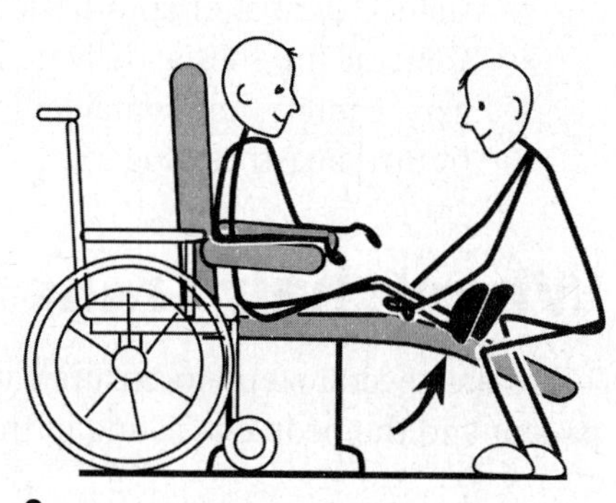

Figure 51-9 Wheelchair Transfer for a Mobile Patient. **A:** Position the wheelchair at level of or lower than the dental chair; set wheelchair brakes, remove footrests and armrests, and raise the dental chair arm. **B:** Clinician places feet outside of the patient's feet, grasps the patient around the waist under the arms, locks hands, or grasps belt in back; patient holds clinician around shoulders or neck; and patient is lifted and pivoted to dental chair side. **C:** Patient is gently lowered to sitting position; dental chair arm is lowered; and clinician grasps legs together to lift onto dental chair.

C. Clinician 2

- Face patient and place both hands under patient's lower thighs.

D. Transfer

- On a prearranged signal and a steady motion, clinician 2 will initiate and lead the lift.
- Both clinicians should use their leg and arm muscles to lift the patient's torso and legs at the same time.
- Gently transfer the patient to the dental chair.
- Secure patient in chair and replace armrest.

E. Repeat in Reverse

- After the appointment, the patient is returned to the wheelchair in the reverse order of procedure.

IV. Sliding Board Transfer

- A patient may bring a sliding board, or one may be kept in the office or clinic. A transfer board is shown in **Figure 51-10**. Two persons are recommended during transfer and are required when the patient is heavy or less mobile.

A. Position the Wheelchair

- Position the wheelchair in the same direction as and parallel with the dental chair, set the brakes, and remove the footrests.
- Adjust the seat of the dental chair to slightly lower than the wheelchair seat.
- Move the arm of the dental chair out of the transfer area and remove the arm of the wheelchair.

B. Adjust the Sliding Board

- Patient or clinician places the sliding board under the hip of the patient.
- The board is extended across the dental chair.

C. Transfer

- Patient shifts weight, balances on hands, and walks the buttocks across the board. The clinician can assist or do the transfer by holding the patient under the axilla (armpit).
- Board is removed and replaced after the appointment.

D. Repeat in Reverse

- Dental chair is positioned slightly higher than the wheelchair seat for the return transfer.

V. Wheelchair Used during Treatment

When the patient is in a total-support wheelchair, transfer to the dental chair may not be advisable. The wheelchair can be positioned for direct utilization.

- Some wheelchairs are self-reclining and have headrests. (See Chapter 4.)
- A portable headrest may be attached to the wheelchair handles, as shown in **Figure 51-11**.
- The dental chair can be swiveled to permit the wheelchair to be placed so the dental light can be directed into the patient's oral cavity.
- An automatic wheelchair lift that tilts the chair back can be obtained for a clinical facility where patients in wheelchairs are treated frequently (**Figure 51-12**).

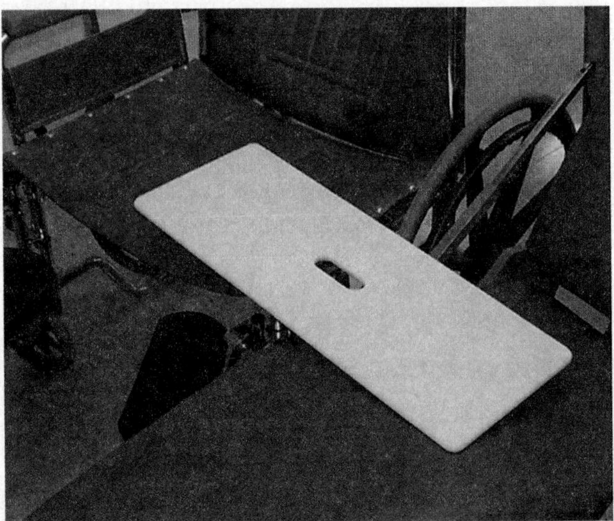

Figure 51-10 Transfer Board. Transfer board placement between wheelchair and dental chair.

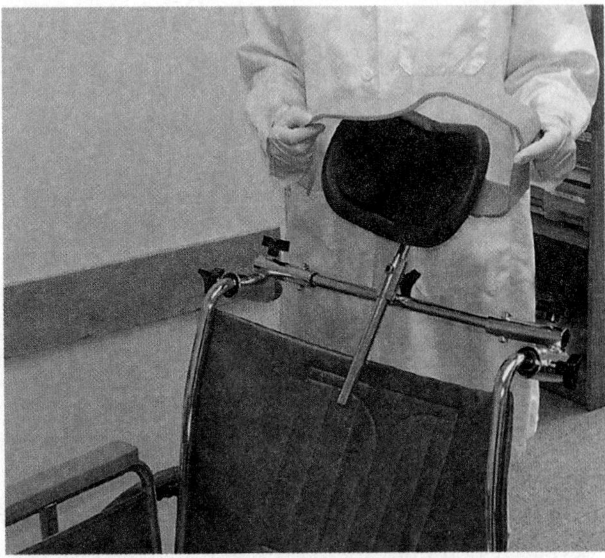

Figure 51-11 Portable Headrest Attached to Wheelchair

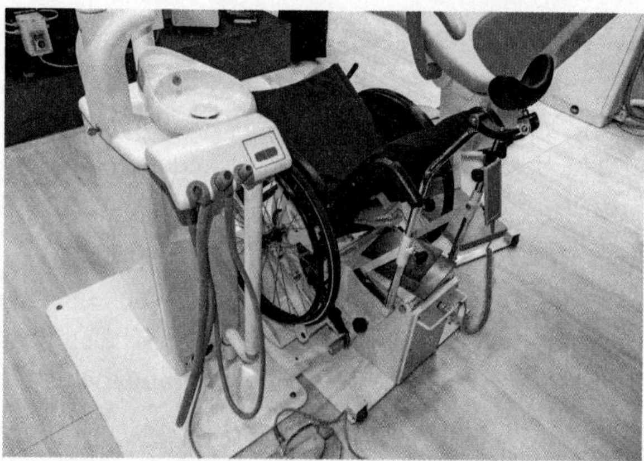

Figure 51-12 Wheelchair Lift Tilts the Wheelchair and Patient to Provide Access to the Clinician.

VI. Position of Patient after Transfer

- Center the patient in the patient chair.
- For patient comfort, reposition special padding and safety belt.
- Ensure any devices and tubing is placed properly.[87]

Instruction for Caregivers

- Individuals who need partial or total care present with varying degrees of ability to cooperate, depending on the type of disability.
- The size of the patient and whether the patient is ambulatory or in a wheelchair (limited to no mobility) are among the factors that influence the technique for management.
- The instructions for the caregiver are given where the specific techniques can actually be demonstrated as they will be done at home.
- Time and repeated practice sessions may be needed for successful biofilm removal.

I. Self-Care and Attitude

- Whenever possible, instruction for the parents, family members, or other caregivers begins with their own oral self-care.
- Success comes when those who care for the patient have knowledge and understanding of the purposes and techniques.

II. General Suggestions

A. Place

- The biofilm removal procedures are accomplished best when both the patient and the caregiver are comfortable and relaxed.
- A small bathroom may be the least desirable place because positioning the patient may be awkward, except when a standing position can be used.[80]
- Good light for visibility of the teeth and control of the head of the person with the disability are prerequisites.

B. Teaching Techniques for Biofilm Removal

- Use of finger rest and hand rest: the person performing the biofilm removal balances the toothbrush, interdental cleaning aid, or any other implement with a finger or hand rest on the side of the patient's face or chin. Such contact contributes to patient control and effective use of the biofilm-removal device.
- Use of a mouth prop: for certain patients, biofilm removal is impossible without a mouth prop, and demonstration for insertion on both sides is needed. For home use, a rolled and moist washcloth may be appropriate.

III. Positions

A. Caregiver Standing

- With the caregiver standing from behind, the arm is brought around the patient's head and the chin is cupped while using the thumb and index finger to retract the lips and cheeks.
- The other hand applies the toothbrush, interdental care aid, or other device.
- This technique requires the patient be able to lean the head back so the parent or caregiver can see the maxillary teeth.
- The procedure may be applicable for the following:
  - Shorter patient standing in front of and backed up to the caregiver.
  - Taller patient seated in a chair with the head tipped back to lean against the caregiver or seated in a large chair or sofa with the head stabilized against the top of chair back.
  - Patient in a wheelchair leaning back against the caregiver or headrest. Wheelchair brakes are set.[66]

B. Caregiver Seated

- Patient seated on pillow on floor in front of caregiver, with back close to the chair and head turned back into caregiver's lap, as shown in **Figure 51-13A**. The caregiver may place their legs over the shoulders of the patient to restrain arms and body movements, as shown in **Figure 51-13B**.

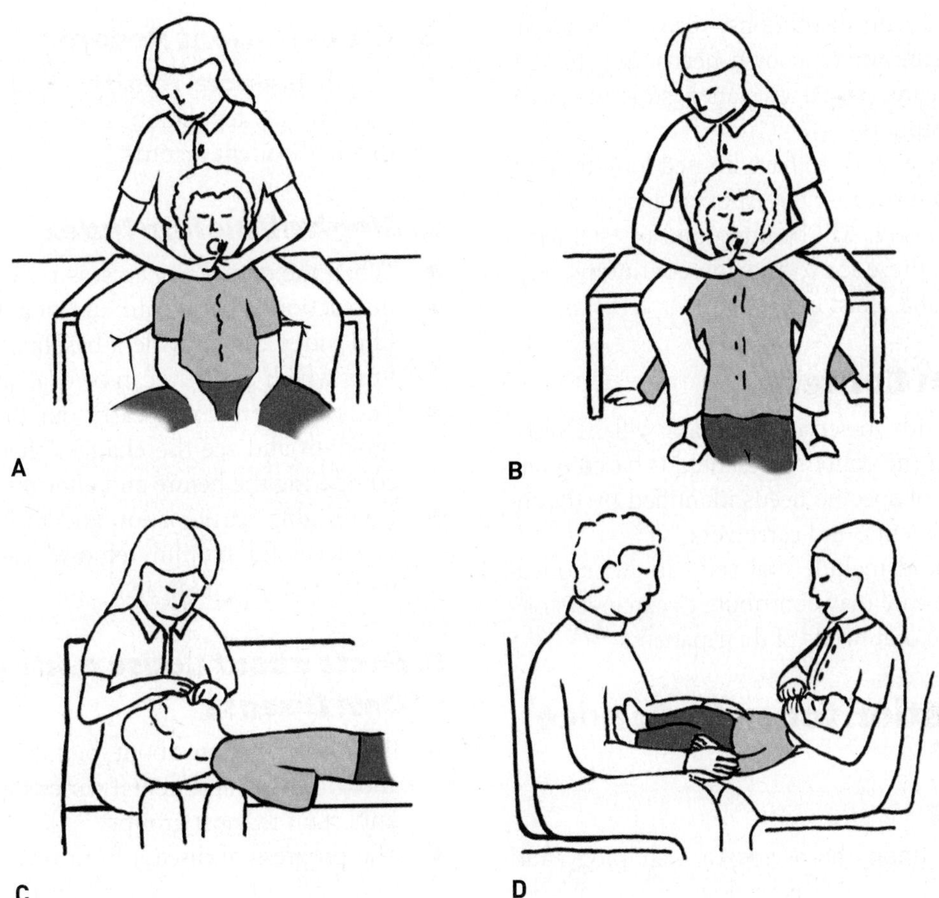

Figure 51-13 Positions for Child or Disabled Patient During Biofilm Removal. **A:** Patient seated on floor with head turned back into the lap of the caregiver. **B:** Patient's arms restrained by legs of caregiver. **C:** Patient reclining on couch with head in lap of caregiver. **D:** Two people participating with small child between. One holds patient for stabilization while the other holds the head for toothbrushing and interdental cleaning.

- Caregiver is seated at the end of a sofa or couch, and patient is lying down with the head in caregiver's lap, as shown in **Figure 51-13C**.
- For a patient who is confined to bed, the caregiver may sit at the patient's head and place the head in the lap. When body and arm movements need to be controlled, the caregiver can sit beside the patient, lean across the patient's chest, and hold the patient's arm against the body with the elbow. The hand of the clinician's restraining arm can hold the mouth prop, retract, or do whatever is necessary.

C. Two People

- In any of the positions previously mentioned, the parent may need the assistance of a second person to hold the hands and arms or otherwise restrain the patient.
- A small child may be placed across the laps of two persons seated facing each other. One stabilizes the head and brushes and performs the toothbrushing and interdental cleaning, while the other person holds hands, arms, and legs as needed, as shown in **Figure 51-13D**.

Group In-Service Education

- Dental hygienists can provide in-service education sessions on oral health measures for those who provide daily personal care for others.[88]
  - Telehealth/teledentistry is an emerging resource for reaching parents and caregivers of those with special needs to provide education and even individual sessions to improve access.[89]
- In-service programs can be provided for teachers, registered nurses, other health professionals, parents, and volunteers in school and community preventive programs.[90]

- In extended care institutions, many patients are unable to care for their own needs and may require total care, partial assistance, supervision, or regular reminders.
  - In-service tends to have limited long-term effect often because of turnover of caregivers in facilities so it will be important to establish a regular presence to provide continuing education and assist caregivers.[91]

I. Program Content

- An oral health in-service program will be more successful if the content presented is based on an assessment of specific needs identified by the institution, patients, and caregivers.
- Content could include oral self-care, as motivation for self-care may contribute to caregivers prioritizing the oral needs of their patients.

II. Preparation for an In-Service Program

A. Planning

- Dependent upon the access to technology and comfort with use of technology, a virtual program may be most effective at providing access to attendees.
  - It could also be recorded for review for those not able to attend.
  - Telehealth/teledentistry has significant potential for health promotion to populations that have difficulty accessing care.[89]
- The dental hygienist can arrange a preworkshop visit to observe and get to know the caregivers and the patient's needs.
- An in-service program needs careful planning based on patient and caregiver needs.
- Objectives are defined in writing and serve as a guide to preparation and evaluation.
- Caregiver or staff concerns are recognized and addressed during the program.
- Effective learning materials are clear and to the point, interestingly presented with appropriate visual aids, and stimulating for learning.
- Initially, basic preparation includes learning about the functioning levels of the patient and assessing the procedures used for oral care.
- A survey of the biofilm control materials and devices available and in current use, methods for labeling or storing individual brushes, and the frequency of use is important.

B. Use of Patient Records

- Health Insurance Portability and Accountability Act (HIPAA) regulations may restrict access to individual patient records.

C. Gingival/Biofilm Index

- When the dental hygienist is providing hands-on instruction for oral care, use of a gingival or biofilm index can provide a baseline of information from which progress can be evaluated.
- The caregivers could carry out the daily biofilm program and see the changes that take place by comparing the before and after results.
- Continuing participation and receiving feedback of successful biofilm removal can provide real motivation to caregivers.

D. Facts about Cause and Prevention of Oral Disease

- Basic information about biofilm, its formation, and gingivitis and dental caries development are important to most groups.
- The progress of disease from reversible gingivitis to periodontitis can be explained, as can the process of dental caries.
- The concept of prevention through biofilm control, fluoride, dietary controls, sealants, and early treatment for restorations is carefully presented.
- Handout materials and colorful visual aids supplement learning.

E. Oral Inspection

- Caregivers can be trained to notice changes to the oral mucosa during daily cleaning and to report to the appropriate person.

F. Techniques of Mouth Care and Oral Disease Control

- Caregivers working in pairs can be more efficient, particularly in the care of challenging patients.
- Individualized plans can be developed, and training provided for caregivers to address specific problems relative to each patient's needs.[88,91]
- Xerostomia relief: Instruction for caregivers includes how to use a swab with saliva substitute to provide relief for certain patients.
- Information to teach caregivers about biofilm control is discussed in Chapters 26 and 27.

- The use of a portable or bedside suction unit for removing debris from a patient's mouth is described in Chapter 4.
- Fluoride application techniques are outlined in Chapter 34.
- Procedures for care of dentures and of the mucosa under the denture are shown in Chapter 30.

G. Denture Marking Procedure

- All dentures must be marked for patient identification.
- The techniques for denture marking are outlined in Chapter 30.

III. Records

- Oral care documentation for each patient is essential to evaluate the success of the in-service presentation.
- During instruction, the staff can learn appropriate information to include in each patient's record.
- Documentation for oral care provided by a caregiver may include implements and materials used, self-care instruction provided, successful techniques, and suggestions for future instruction.

IV. Follow-Up

- After caregivers have tried their newly learned procedures, an opportunity to have questions answered should be provided.
- Direct observation of techniques performed with and for the patients is ideal so specific advice concerning oral problems of patients and modifications can be made to benefit the patient and caregiver.
- The hygienist disclosing and recording the biofilm for comparison of scores before and after the program can show the progress being made both for patient and caregiver motivation as well as for documentation.

V. Continuing Education

- In residential care facilities, individual instruction should be provided for each new employee during the orientation period.
- Periodic in-service presentations for updating all employees can be provided.
- Questions and problems can be discussed, and plans can be introduced for changing a certain procedure based on new research evidence.

The Dental Hygienist with a Disability

- Most disabilities are not an obstacle to dental hygiene licensure and provision of clinical patient care.[92,93]
- Adaptive technology, tax incentives for accessibility construction, and creative thinking can facilitate necessary workplace modifications.
- Additional dental hygiene roles, such as manager, advocate, educator or researcher, may provide employment opportunities for the dental hygienist with a disability.

Documentation

In addition to the standard information recorded for a patient visit, documentation of care provided for a patient who has a disability includes:

- Individualized information about the patient's condition or level of functioning that will affect modifications needed during dental hygiene care. Some suggestions for information needed are listed in **Box 51-3**.
- Specific details related to patient management or communication strategies used during the

Box 51-3 Basic Planning Questions for a Patient with Disability

- What is the patient's functioning level?
- Is the patient capable of all or part of the daily biofilm removal independently or will the patient require partial or total assistance?
- Is the patient involved in any community oral health programs (home, school, or day activity), and can the oral care provider in such a program be contacted to coordinate the instruction given?
- Which disabilities have the greatest influence on oral self-care abilities? What is the anticipated success of the overall preventive program?
- Which techniques and procedures will best fit the situation of the patient and the caregiver?
- How can the patient be helped to be as independent as possible?

dental hygiene appointment, and an indication of whether those strategies were successful.

- Identification of self-care aids, modifications to standard oral hygiene instructions and aids, and details of any recommendations or instructions provided for caregivers.
- **Box 51-4** provides an example of documentation for an appointment with a patient with a disability.

Box 51-4 Example Documentation: Self-Care Management for Patient with a Disability

- **S**—A 25-year-old male patient with Down syndrome, who lives in an assisted-living group home, presents for routine 3-month continuing care appointment. Both the patient and his caregiver state the curved bristle toothbrush, introduced at the last appointment, is working quite well for him and his caregiver has attached a rubber band to the handle in order to help stabilize the toothbrush in his hand.
- **O**—No changes in medical history. His biofilm index is now below 20%.
- **A**—Next step in patient's care plan is to help develop a system that will help patient take more personal responsibility for his own oral self-care with less need for caregiver assistance.
- **P**—Congratulated patient and caregiver on their successful reduction in biofilm. Worked with caregiver to develop a personal "Daily Oral Care" list to identify all the steps and materials necessary for his daily oral care regimen. Caregiver will make up a large poster of the steps using pictures and will laminate and hang the poster by the bathroom sink in order to help the patient be more independent with his daily oral care regimen. Maintenance debridement was completed. Used a "tell–show–do" approach to provide basic instructions for using a floss holder. First time efforts were clumsy, but patient is motivated to practice.

Next steps: Evaluate success at next visit scheduled in 3 months.
Signed: ______________________, RDH
Date: ______________________

Factors to Teach the Patient and Caregiver

- Seek regular dental and medical examinations.
- Have knowledge of current medical health status, names and doses of medications including over-the-counter medications.
- Recognize the early warnings of complications from a disease, condition, or syndrome.
- Recognize the side effects of medical treatments and medications.
- Seek immediate medical attention for any complications.
- Practice a healthy lifestyle, including healthy diet, daily exercise, no tobacco products, alcohol and substance avoidance, attainment and maintenance of ideal weight, and stress reduction. Accept assistance for smoking cessation.
- Practice meticulous oral hygiene to prevent dental and periodontal diseases and adapt techniques as needed.
- Ways to overcome barriers to dental care.

References

1. National Institute of Dental and Craniofacial Research. Developmental disabilities & oral health. Published October 2020. https://www.nidcr.nih.gov/health-info/developmental-disabilities/more-info. Accessed August 11, 2021.
2. World Health Organization. Disability and health. https://www.who.int/news-room/fact-sheets/detail/disability-and-health. Accessed August 11, 2021.
3. Paul S, Rafal M, Houtenville A. *Annual Report on People with Disabilities in America 2020*. Institute of Disability/UCED, University of New Hampshire; 2020. https://disabilitycompendium.org/sites/default/files/user-uploads/Annual%20Report%20for%20Print.pdf. Accessed August 11, 2021.
4. Lee J, Lau S, Meijer E, Hu P. Living longer, with or without disability? A global and longitudinal perspective. *J Gerontol Series A*. 2020;75(1):162-167.
5. Naseem M, Shah AH, Khiyani MF, et al. Access to oral health care services among adults with learning disabilities: a scoping review. *Ann Stomatol (Roma)*. 2016;7(3):52-59.
6. Wilson NJ, Lin Z, Villarosa A, et al. Countering the poor oral health of people with intellectual and developmental disability: a scoping literature review. *BMC Public Health*. 2019;19(1):1530.
7. USDA Forest Service, Technology and Development. Accessibility Tools: Disabled or handicapped or ??? Which terms

should be used? Published March 24, 2013. https://www.fs.fed.us/eng/toolbox/acc/acc02.htm. Accessed August 12, 2021.

8. Northridge ME, Kumar A, Kaur R. Disparities in access to oral health care. *Annu Rev Public Health*. 2020;41:513-535.
9. U.S. Department of Justice. *American with Disabilities Act Amendments Act of 2008*. 2009:51. https://www.ada.gov/pubs/adastatute08.pdf. Accessed August 11, 2021.
10. ADA National Network. What is the Americans with Disabilities Act (ADA)? https://adata.org/learn-about-ada. Accessed August 12, 2021.
11. World Health Organization. Disabilities: Health topics. http://www.emro.who.int/health-topics/disabilities/index.html. Accessed August 12, 2021.
12. Centers for Disease Control and Prevention. Disability and health overview. Published September 15, 2020. https://www.cdc.gov/ncbddd/disabilityandhealth/disability.html. Accessed August 12, 2021.
13. U.S. Department of Justice. The Americans with Disabilities Act. https://beta.ada.gov/. Accessed August 12, 2021.
14. World Health Organization. International Classification of Functioning, Disability and Health (ICF). https://www.who.int/standards/classifications/international-classification-of-functioning-disability-and-health. Accessed August 11, 2021.
15. Centers for Disease Control and Prevention. Facts about developmental disabilities. Published September 26, 2019. https://www.cdc.gov/ncbddd/developmentaldisabilities/facts.html. Accessed August 12, 2021.
16. Peer Connect, National Disability Insurance Scheme. Role changes after acquired disability. https://www.peerconnect.org.au/stuff-peer-networks-talk-about/life-issues/role-changes-after-acquired-disability/. Accessed August 14, 2021.
17. Jaul E, Barron J. Age-related diseases and clinical and public health implications for the 85 years old and over population. *Front Public Health*. 2017;5:335.
18. Jacques E. How coping with progressive disorders can be difficult. *Verywell Health*. Published May 3, 2020. https://www.verywellhealth.com/what-is-a-progressive-disorder-2564690. Accessed August 14, 2021.
19. National Disability Insurance Agency. Sensory disabilities. *Disability Support Guide*. https://www.disabilitysupportguide.com.au/information/article/sensory-disabilities. Accessed August 14, 2021.
20. World Health Organization. Vision impairment and blindness. https://www.who.int/news-room/fact-sheets/detail/blindness-and-visual-impairment. Accessed August 14, 2021.
21. Centers for Disease Control and Prevention. Common eye disorders and diseases. Published June 4, 2020. https://www.cdc.gov/visionhealth/basics/ced/index.html. Accessed August 15, 2021.
22. The American Foundation for the Blind. Key definitions. https://www.afb.org/research-and-initiatives/statistics/key-definitions-statistical-terms. Accessed August 11, 2021.
23. CNIB Canada. What is blindness? https://cnib.ca/en/sight-loss-info/blindness/what-blindness. Accessed August 15, 2021.
24. Wisconsin Department of Health Services. OBVI: Why would someone need a white cane? Published August 25, 2014. https://www.dhs.wisconsin.gov/obvi/whitecane/information.htm. Accessed January 1, 2022.
25. The American Foundation for the Blind. Braille. https://www.afb.org/blindness-and-low-vision/braille. Accessed August 15, 2021.
26. The American Foundation for the Blind. Using technology. https://www.afb.org/blindness-and-low-vision/using-technology. Accessed August 15, 2021.
27. Gilbert C, Foster A. Childhood blindness in the context of VISION 2020 — The Right to Sight. *Bull World Health Org*. 2001:6.
28. National Eye Institute, National Institute of Health. Retinopathy of prematurity. Published July 10, 2019. https://www.nei.nih.gov/learn-about-eye-health/eye-conditions-and-diseases/retinopathy-prematurity. Accessed August 15, 2021.
29. Gilbert C, Foster A. Childhood blindness in the context of VISION 2020 — The Right to Sight. *Bull World Health Org*. 2001;79:227-232.
30. National Eye Institute. Sports and your eyes. https://www.nei.nih.gov/learn-about-eye-health/nei-for-kids/sports-and-your-eyes. Accessed August 15, 2021.
31. Aghadoost D. Ocular trauma: an overview. *Arch Trauma Res*. 2014;3(2):e21639.
32. American Academy of Ophthalmology. Sports eye safety. Published March 8, 2021. https://www.aao.org/eye-health/tips-prevention/injuries-sports. Accessed August 11, 2021.
33. World Health Organization. Deafness and hearing loss. https://www.who.int/news-room/fact-sheets/detail/deafness-and-hearing-loss. Accessed August 15, 2021.
34. Centers for Disease Control and Prevention. About hearing loss in children. Published May 27, 2020. https://www.cdc.gov/ncbddd/hearingloss/data.html. Accessed August 15, 2021.
35. National Institute on Deafness and Other Communication Disorders. Quick statistics about hearing. Published March 25, 2021. https://www.nidcd.nih.gov/health/statistics/quick-statistics-hearing. Accessed August 15, 2021.
36. Centers for Disease Control and Prevention. Hearing loss in children: baby hearing screening. Published June 21, 2021. https://www.cdc.gov/ncbddd/hearingloss/features/baby-hearing-screening.html. Accessed December 31, 2021.
37. Identify the Signs. Signs of hearing loss. https://identifythesigns.org/signs-of-hearing-loss/. Accessed August 15, 2021.
38. Wilson NJ, Lin Z, Villarosa A, et al. Countering the poor oral health of people with intellectual and developmental disability: a scoping literature review. *BMC Public Health*. 2019;19(1):1530.
39. da Rosa SV, Moysés SJ, Theis LC, et al. Barriers in access to dental services hindering the treatment of people with disabilities: a systematic review. *Int J Dent*. 2020;2020:9074618.
40. Centers for Disease Control and Prevention. Disability and health promotion: disability and health overview. Published September 16, 2020. https://www.cdc.gov/ncbddd/disabilityandhealth/disability.html. Accessed December 31, 2021.
41. Canadian Dental Association. *Position Paper on Access to Oral Health Care for all Canadians*. https://www.cda-adc.ca/en/about/position_statements/accesstocarePaper/. Accessed August 16, 2021.
42. National Governors Association. *The Role of Dental Hygienists in Providing Access to Oral Health Care*. https://www.nga.org/wp-content/uploads/2019/08/1401DentalHealthCare.pdf. Accessed August 16, 2021.
43. *2010 ADA Standards for Accessible Design*. https://www.ada.gov/regs2010/2010ADAStandards/2010ADAstandards.htm. Accessed August 16, 2021.
44. Jogezai U. Introduction of NOMAD Pro in a special care dental setting. *J Disabil Oral Health*. 2016;17:78-91.

45. American Dental Hygienists' Association. *2016 Revised Standards for Clinical Dental Hygiene Practice*. https://www.adha.org/resources-docs/2016-Revised-Standards-for-Clinical-Dental-Hygiene-Practice.pdf. Accessed August 16, 2021.
46. Silva KD, Farmer JW, Quiñonez C. *Access to Oral Health Care for Individuals with Developmental Disabilities: An Umbrella Review*. Federal-Provincial-Territorial Dental Directors Working Group; 2017:48.
47. Cabrita JP, Bizarra M de F, Graça SR. Prevalence of malocclusion in individuals with and without intellectual disability: A comparative study. *Spec Care Dentist*. 2017;37(4):181-186.
48. National institute of Dental and Craniofacial Research. Practical oral care for people with intellectual disability. Published online July 2009. https://www.nidcr.nih.gov/sites/default/files/2017-09/practical-oral-care-intellectual-care.pdf. Accessed August 16, 2021.
49. Moreira Falci SG, Duarte-Rodrigues L, Primo-Miranda EF, Furtado Gonçalves P, Lanza Galvão E. Association between epilepsy and oral maxillofacial trauma: a systematic review and meta-analysis. *Spec Care Dentist*. 2019;39(4):362-374.
50. Levin DS, Volkert VM, Piazza CC. A multi-component treatment to reduce packing in children with feeding and autism spectrum disorders. *Behav Modif*. 2014;38(6):940-963.
51. Ney DM, Weiss JM, Kind AJH, Robbins J. Senescent swallowing: impact, strategies, and interventions. *Nutr Clin Pract*. 2009;24(3):395-413.
52. Silva RA, da Silva VM, Lopes MVO, Guedes NG, Oliveira-Kumakura AR. Clinical indicators of impaired swallowing in children with neurological disorders. *Int J Nurs Knowled*. 2020;31(3):194-204.
53. Arboleda-Montealegre GY, Cano-de-la-Cuerda R, Fernández-de-Las-Peñas C, Sanchez-Camarero C, Ortega-Santiago R. Drooling, swallowing difficulties and health related quality of life in Parkinson's disease patients. *Int J Environ Res Public Health*. 2021;18(15):8138.
54. Al Humaid J. Sweetener content and cariogenic potential of pediatric oral medications: a literature. *Int J Health Sci*. 2018;12(3):75-82.
55. Portela D, Almada M, Midão L, Costa E. Instrumental Activities of Daily Living (IADL) limitations in Europe: an assessment of SHARE data. *Int J Environ Res Public Health*. 2020;17(20):E7387.
56. World Health Organization. International Classification of Functioning, Disability and Health (ICF). https://www.who.int/standards/classifications/international-classification-of-functioning-disability-and-health. Accessed August 11, 2021.
57. Tuuliainen E, Autonen-Honko Nen K, Nihtilä A, et al. Oral health and hygiene and association of functional ability: a cross-sectional study among old home care clients. *Oral Health Prev Dent*. 2020;18(1):253-262.
58. Khochen M, British Council. The needs of visually impaired (VI) learners in education: key issues and principles. https://www.teachingenglish.org.uk/article/needs-visually-impaired-vi-learners-education-key-issues-principles. Accessed August 16, 2021.
59. Mosca R, Kritzinger A, van der Linde J. Language and communication development in preschool children with visual impairment: a systematic review. *S Afr J Commun Disord*. 2015;62(1):e1-e10.
60. American Speech Language Hearing Association. Effects of hearing loss on development. https://www.asha.org/public/hearing/effects-of-hearing-loss-on-development/. Accessed August 16, 2021.
61. American Speech Language Hearing Association. Students who are deaf or hard of hearing in the school setting. https://www.asha.org/slp/schools/prof-consult/deaf-or-hard-of-hearing/. Accessed August 16, 2021.
62. U.S. Department of Health and Human Services, Centers for Medicare & Medicaid Services. Improving communication access for individuals who are blind or have low vision. https://www.cms.gov/files/document/audio-sensory-disabilities-brochure-508c.pdf. Accessed August 16, 2021.
63. Jevon P. Medical emergencies in the dental practice poster: revised and updated. *Br Dent J*. 2020;229(2):97-104.
64. Meneses V, Parenti S, Burns H, Adams R. Latex allergy guidelines for people with spina bifida. *J Pediatr Rehabil Med*. 2020;13(4):601-609.
65. National institute of Dental and Craniofacial Research. Dental care everyday-a caregiver's guide. Published online February 2012. https://www.nidcr.nih.gov/sites/default/files/2017-09/dental-care-every-day-caregiver.pdf. Accessed August 16, 2021.
66. Wiener RC, Dinsmore RR, Meckstroth R, Marshall W. Providing daily oral infection control to persons dependent on others for activities of daily living: a semi-qualitative descriptive study. *J Dent Craniofac Res*. 2016;1(1):1.
67. Zhou N, Wong HM, Wen YF, McGrath C. Efficacy of caries and gingivitis prevention strategies among children and adolescents with intellectual disabilities: a systematic review and meta-analysis. *J Intellect Disabil Res*. 2019;63(6):507-518.
68. Lai YYL, Zafar S, Leonard HM, Walsh LJ, Downs JA. Oral health education and promotion in special needs children: Systematic review and meta-analysis. *Oral Dis*. 2022;28(1):66-75.
69. Baygin O, Tuzuner T, Kusgoz A, Senel AC, Tanriver M, Arslan I. Antibacterial effects of fluoride varnish compared with chlorhexidine plus fluoride in disabled children. *Oral Health Prev Dent*. 2014;12(4):373-382.
70. Northridge ME, Kumar A, Kaur R. Disparities in access to oral health care. *Annu Rev Public Health*. 2020;41:513-535.
71. Oliveira BH, Rajendra A, Veitz-Keenan A, Niederman R. The effect of silver diamine fluoride in preventing caries in the primary dentition: a systematic review and meta-analysis. *Caries Res*. 2019;53(1):24-32.
72. Subbiah GK, Gopinathan NM. Is silver diamine fluoride effective in preventing and arresting caries in elderly adults? A systematic review. *J Int Soc Prev Community Dent*. 2018;8(3):191-199.
73. Wilder DA, Ertel HM, Cymbal DJ. A review of recent research on the manipulation of response effort in Applied Behavior Analysis. *Behav Modif*. 2021;45(5):740-768.
74. Radhakrishna S, Srinivasan I, Setty JV, Murali Krishna DR, Melwani A, Hegde KM. Comparison of three behavior modification techniques for management of anxious children aged 4–8 years. *J Dent Anesth Pain Med*. 2019;19(1):29-36.
75. American Academy of Pediatric Dentistry. *Behavior Guidance for the Pediatric Dental Patient*. American Academy of Pediatric Dentistry; 2020:19. https://www.aapd.org/globalassets/media/policies_guidelines/bp_behavguide.pdf. Accessed August 18, 2021.
76. University of Washington, School of Dentistry, Washington State Oral Health Program. Oral health fact sheet for dental professionals: adults with hearing impairment. http://dental

.washington.edu/wp-content/media/sp_need_pdfs/Hearing-Adult.pdf. Accessed August 17, 2021.

77. Shah P, Thornton I, Turrin D, Hipskind JE. Informed consent. In: *StatPearls*. StatPearls Publishing; 2021. http://www.ncbi.nlm.nih.gov/books/NBK430827/. Accessed August 17, 2021.
78. American Academy of Pediatric Dentistry. *Management of Dental Patients with Special Health Care Needs*. AAPD; 2021:8. https://www.aapd.org/media/Policies_Guidelines/BP_SHCN.pdf. Accessed August 17, 2021.
79. Mark AM. Oral health care tips for caregivers. *J Am Dent Assoc*. 2019;150(5):480.
80. Guide Dogs of America. Best practices when around a service dog. Published March 19, 2019. https://www.guidedogsofamerica.org/best-practices-when-around-a-service-dog/. Accessed August 17, 2021.
81. Vos-Draper TL, Morrow MMB. Seating-related pressure injury prevention in spinal cord injury: a review of compensatory technologies to improve in-seat movement behavior. *Curr Phys Med Rehabil Rep*. 2016;4(4):320-328.
82. Quek HC, Lee YS. Dentistry considerations for the dysphagic patient: recognition of condition and management. *Proc Singapore Healthcare*. 2019;28(4):288-292.
83. American Academy of Pediatric Dentistry. *Use of Protective Stabilization for Pediatric Dental Patients.* American Academy of Pediatric Dentistry; 2020:7. https://www.aapd.org/globalassets/media/policies_guidelines/bp_protective.pdf. Accessed August 18, 2021.
84. Lofters A, Clarkson E. Mouth gags: advantages and disadvantages. *Oral Maxillofac Surg Clin North Am*. 2021;33(2):287-294.
85. Townsend JA, Wells MH. Behavior guidance of the pediatric dental patient. In: Nowak AJ, Christensen JR, Mabry TR, Townsend JA, Wells MH, eds. *Pediatric Dentistry*. 6th ed. Elsevier; 2019:352-370. https://www.sciencedirect.com/science/article/pii/B9780323608268000249. Accessed August 18, 2021.
86. National Institute of Dental and Craniofacial Research. Wheelchair transfer: a health care provider's guide. Published online July 2009. https://www.nidcr.nih.gov/sites/default/files/2017-09/wheelchair-transfer-provider-guide.pdf. Accessed January 1, 2022.
87. McNally M. *Oral Care in Continuing Care Settings: Brushing Up on Mouth Care*. Dalhousie University; 2011:69.
88. Fernández CE, Maturana CA, Coloma SI, Carrasco-Labra A, Giacaman RA. Teledentistry and mhealth for promotion and prevention of oral health: a systematic review and meta-analysis. *J Dent Res*. 2021;100(9):914-927.
89. Hummel J, Phillips KE, Holt B, Hayes C. Oral health: an essential component of primary care. Published online June 2015. https://www.safetynetmedicalhome.org/sites/default/files/White-Paper-Oral-Health-Primary-Care.pdf. Accessed January 2, 2022.
90. Wang TF, Huang CM, Chou C, Yu S. Effect of oral health education programs for caregivers on oral hygiene of the elderly: a systemic review and meta-analysis. *Int J Nurs Stud*. 2015;52(6):1090-1096.
91. Bulk LY, Tikhonova J, Gagnon JM, et al. Disabled healthcare professionals' diverse, embodied, and socially embedded experiences. *Adv Health Sci Educ*. 2020;25(1):111-129.
92. Shrewsbury D, Mogensen L, Hu W. Problematizing medical students with disabilities: a critical policy analysis. *MedEdPublish*. 2018;7:1-15.

CHAPTER 52

Neurologic Disorders and Stroke

Lisa F. Mallonee, RDH, RD, LD, MPH

CHAPTER OUTLINE

LEARNING OBJECTIVES

After studying this chapter, the student will be able to:

1. Identify and define key terms and concepts related to physical impairment.
2. Describe the characteristics, complications, occurrence, and medical treatment of a variety of physical impairments.
3. Identify oral factors and findings related to physical impairments.
4. Describe modifications for dental hygiene care based on assessment of needs specific to a patient's physical impairment.

Introduction

- Many conditions related to the neuromuscular system, joints, or connective tissue have as a symptom, or leave as a chronic after effect, loss of function in the form of a physical impairment.
- Dental hygiene treatment modalities and oral care recommendations are adapted to the unique situations created by each disorder.
- This chapter contains descriptions of selected diseases or conditions and describes modifications and adaptations needed by the patient during oral self-care, as well as by the dental hygienist during treatment.
- General suggestions that may be adapted to a variety of patients with disabilities are described in Chapter 51.

Neurologic Disorders Associated with Physical Disability

Most of the disabling conditions described in this chapter are considered neurologic disorders.

- A characteristic of many neurologic disorders is **apoptosis**, the death of cells, specifically the nerve cells in the central nervous system.[1]
- Disruption of sensory or motor neuron signals is the cause of partial or complete **paralysis** associated with neurologic disorders.
- Acute **ischemia** or traumatic injury to the brain or spinal cord causes necrotic (immediate) death of nerve cells in the most severely affected areas and immediate/complete destruction of transmission of neurologic signals.
- Apoptotic cell death, a slower biochemical or metabolic destruction of the nerve cell, occurs in chronic or degenerative neurologic conditions.

I. Acute Disorders

- Acute neurologic disorders can be caused when one or more neurons are injured by trauma or biologic assault or when there is disruption of blood flow to an area of the brain.
- Complete or partial loss of motor ability, sensory perception, or cognitive function can result.
- Acute neurologic disorders discussed in more detail in this chapter include spinal cord injury (SCI), stroke, and **Bell's palsy**.

II. Degenerative Disorders

- Degenerative neural disorders are a result of progressive destruction of nerve cells.
- Patients with these disorders typically become increasingly disabled and dependent on caregivers to help them with everyday activities and personal care as their disease progresses over time.
- Degenerative neural disorders discussed in this chapter include amyotrophic lateral sclerosis (ALS), Parkinson's disease, and postpolio syndrome.

III. Developmental Disorders

- Developmental impairments have their onset early in life, around the time of birth or before a child is 18 years old.
- Depending on the disorder, either a stable or a progressive impairment can result.
- Developmental disorders highlighted in this chapter include cerebral palsy, muscular dystrophies, and myelomeningocele.

Other Conditions That Limit Physical Ability

- Joint and connective tissue diseases, such as arthritis, can affect a patient's ability to provide oral self-care and require adaptations during delivery of dental hygiene care.
- Autoimmune diseases, such as myasthenia gravis, scleroderma, and rheumatoid arthritis, which can limit physical ability, are discussed in Chapter 63.

Spinal Cord Injury

- The spinal cord extends down the middle of the back and carries both motor and sensory nerves that branch to send messages between the brain and specific areas of the body.
- External traumatic force can cause partial or complete loss of sensory and/or motor function related to the spinal cord level and the extent of the injury.

I. Occurrence

- There are more than 294,000 people in the United States living with spinal cord injury (SCI) approximately 17,810 new cases each year.[2]
- More than one-third of trauma cases result from motor vehicle accidents; other causes are falls, diving accidents, violence, and combat injuries.
- Over three-quarters (78%) of all injuries involve males aged between 16 and 30 years, but as the population ages, there has been an increase in average age of injury.

II. Characteristics/Effects of SCI

- The signs and symptoms of paralysis depend on the nature and level of injury to the spinal cord.

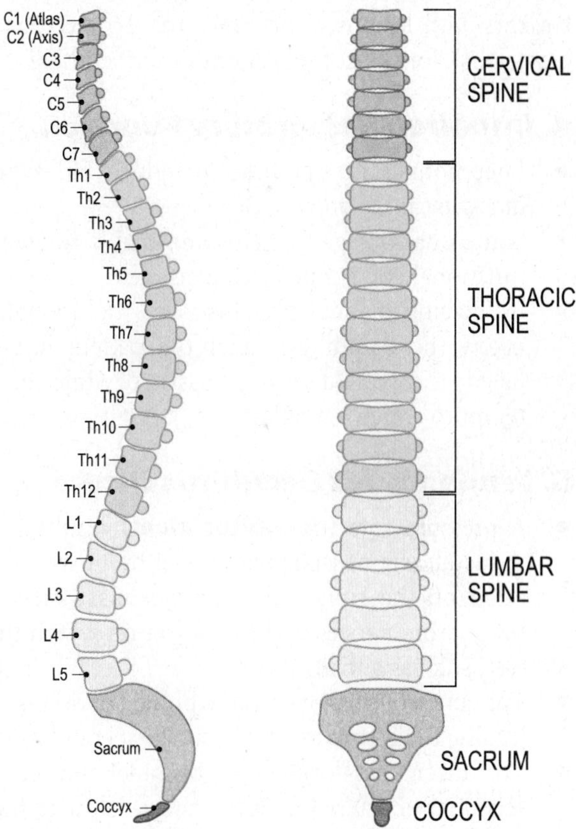

Figure 52-1 Levels of Spinal Cord Injury (SCI). On the left, the vertebrae are designated as C (cervical), Th (thoracic), and L (lumbar). The effects of SCI depend on the level of injury.

- There are 7 cervical (C), 12 thoracic (T), 5 lumbar (L), and 5 sacral (S) vertebrae, with paired spinal nerves extending from each; the areas of the body affected by injury at the different levels are illustrated in **Figure 52-1**.
  - Complete lesion: a complete transection or compression of the spinal cord leaves no sensation or motor function below the level of the lesion.
  - Incomplete lesion: partial transection or injury of the spinal cord leaves some evidence of sensation or motor function below the level of the lesion. Some sensation and motor function may return within a few hours after injury, and maximum return may occur in 6–18 months.
  - Other possible effects: impairment of bladder and bowel control and sexual function; impairment of vasomotor and body temperature regulatory mechanisms.

III. Potential Secondary Complications

Patients with lesions at or above the T6 level are at greater risk for the complications described here.

A. Impaired Respiratory Function

- Pneumonia can significantly reduce life expectancy for a person with SCI.[2]
- Some quadriplegic patients are unable to elicit a functional cough and need assistance.
- By placing manual pressure over the abdomen, below the diaphragm, after the patient has inhaled, the patient may be assisted while an attempt to cough is made.[3]

B. Tendency for Decubitus Ulcers

- A pressure sore (**decubitus ulcer**) results from tissue anoxia or ischemia caused by pressure exerted on the skin and subcutaneous tissues by bony prominences and the object on which they rest, such as a mattress.[4]
- The cutaneous tissue becomes broken or destroyed, leading to destruction in the subcutaneous tissue.
- The ulcer that forms may become infected by secondary bacterial invasion and be slow to heal; anemia and poor nutrition may also contribute.[4]

C. Spasticity

- As **spinal shock** subsides following a traumatic injury, muscle-reflex spasticity develops from a slight to a severe degree.
- Stimuli, such as decubitus ulcers, infections, and sensory irritation, may bring on a spasm.

D. Body Temperature

- High-level quadriplegic patients are unable to regulate body temperature, requiring careful monitoring and intervention to warm or cool the patient as necessary.

E. Vulnerability to Infection

- Complications related to elimination, urinary tract infections, renal stones, secondary infection of decubitus ulcers, and respiratory infections occur more commonly in this population.

F. Cardiovascular Instability

- Bradycardia and hypotension are common because of the loss of the sympathetic autonomic nervous system.
- Deep vein thrombosis is another potentially serious complication.

G. Neurogenic Bladder and Bowel

- Complications related to dysfunction in bladder and bowel emptying require planning to avoid the complications of autonomic dysreflexia.

H. Autonomic Dysreflexia

- Definition
  - Autonomic dysreflexia, or hyperreflexia, is a life-threatening *emergency* condition in which the blood pressure increases sharply.[5]
  - It may occur in patients with lesions at T6 or above.
  - A variety of stimuli may precipitate dysreflexia, including irritation to the bowel or bladder distention.
  - Patients who require manual bowel or bladder management techniques are more susceptible.[6]
- Symptoms
  - Increased blood pressure with slowed pulse rate. Blood pressure may rise to 300/160 mm Hg.
  - Pounding headache.
  - Flushing, chills, perspiration, and stuffy nose.
  - Restlessness; increased spasticity.
- Prevention
  - Consult with the primary care provider when the patient has a history of recurrent difficulties.
  - Avoid abrupt changes in body position and maintain a semi-upright chair position.
  - Monitor bladder outflow catheter tubing, outflow of urine into catheter bag, and bladder distention.
  - Schedule appointments that allow the patient to maintain the regular schedule for the bowel elimination program at home.
- Emergency care
  - Position chair upright gradually.
  - Do *not* recline the chair because increased blood pressure in the brain could result.
  - Check bladder distention and straighten catheter if clamped.
  - Monitor the blood pressure and vital signs using a medical emergency report form. (See Chapter 9.)
  - Call for medical aid if blood pressure does not begin to drop within 2–3 minutes.

IV. Mouth-Held Assistive Devices

The patient with a high-level SCI who does not have strong function of hands and arms may use mouth-held appliances to perform many tasks and the teeth for holding objects. Optimum oral health and effective biofilm control has special significance because many functions cannot be accomplished by an edentulous mouth.

A. Uses

Fabrication of mouth-held appliances contributes to increased independence and makes possible such activities as operating an electric wheelchair, typing on a computer, or turning the pages of a book.

B. Criteria

- Does not harm the oral tissues.[7,8]
  - Stabilization of occlusion with contact for all fully erupted teeth and the biting forces distributed to as many teeth as possible.
  - Is not traumatic to the periodontal supporting structures.
  - Does not prevent eruption of teeth.
- Is comfortable and does not cause fatigue.[7,8]
  - Patient can talk, swallow, and moisten the lips.
  - **Orthosis** can be inserted and removed by the patient.
  - Orthosis is adaptable for the various needs of the quadriplegic patient.
- Can be cleaned and cared for easily.
- Is relatively easy to construct; inexpensive.

V. Dental Hygiene Care

Factors to consider when planning dental hygiene care for the patient with an SCI include:

- Impaired motor and sensory ability.
- Risk for secondary complications during treatment; autonomic dysreflexia and aspiration due to decreased respiratory function.
- Risk for pressure sores, potential for spasticity, poor control of body temperature.
- Use of mouth-held assistive devices.

Cerebrovascular Accident (Stroke)

- **Cerebrovascular accident (CVA)** is sudden loss of brain function resulting from interference of the blood supply to a part of the brain.
- The clinical manifestation of cerebrovascular disease.
- Frequent disability caused by changes in motor function, communication, and perception or **hemiparesis** is common.
- The third leading cause of death, following heart disease and cancer, in the United States.
- The stroke may be severe and death can occur within minutes; a less severe attack leaves the patient with residual and chronic effects.

I. Etiologic Factors

- The blood flow decreases to an area of the brain and shuts off the oxygen supply to the portion of the brain supplied by that vessel, resulting in cerebral infarction.
- The two main causes or types of stroke are ischemic and hemorrhagic.[9]

A. Ischemic Stroke

- Occurs when a blood vessel to the brain is blocked.
- Can be caused by atherosclerotic plaque build-up in a blood vessel.
- A thrombotic stroke is caused when a clot within a blood vessel of the brain or neck closes or occludes an already narrowed vessel.
- An embolic stroke happens when a blood vessel is blocked by a clot or other material carried through the circulation from another part of the body.

B. Hemorrhagic Stroke

- Occurs when a cerebral blood vessel ruptures and bleeds into the brain tissues.
- Common causes include:
  - Defects in blood vessels, such as aneurysm or malformation.
  - Very high blood pressure.
  - Use of blood thinner medication.
  - An ischemic stroke that develops a burst blood vessel and causes bleeding.

C. Predisposing Factors

Early diagnosis and treatment for control of the following predisposing factors are necessary in the prevention of stroke and its devastating effects.

- Atherosclerosis. (See Chapter 61.)
- Hypertension, the greatest risk factor for stroke. (See Chapter 61.)

- **Hypercholesterolemia**, **hypertriglyceridemia**.
- Tobacco use, smoking.
- Cardiovascular disease (rheumatic heart disease, congestive heart failure, history of **transient ischemic attacks**).
- Diabetes mellitus.
- Use of oral contraceptives (enhanced by hypertension, tobacco use, age older than 35).
- Drug abuse (especially in adolescents and young adults).

II. Signs and Symptoms

The effects of a stroke depend on the location of the damage to the brain, as well as on the degree or extent of involvement. Acute symptoms and emergency procedures are included in Chapter 9.

A. Transient Ischemic Attack

- A brief event where the blood supply to a localized area of the brain is interrupted and the patient may have transient signs or symptoms of a stroke.
- These "little strokes" may last a few minutes to an hour and may leave no permanent damage.
- A history of transient attacks is a possible risk factor or warning for a stroke.

B. Residual or Chronic Effects

- Approximately two-thirds of those who survive have some degree of permanent disability.
- Temporary or permanent loss of thought, memory, speech, sensation, or motion results.
- The side of the face and body affected is opposite that of the brain injury (**Figure 52-2**).
- Persons with right **hemiplegia** have more difficulty with verbal communication and are more apt to be cautious, anxious, and disorganized.
- Patients with left hemiplegia have difficulty with action requiring physical coordination and may respond impulsively with overconfidence.
- Common signs and symptoms observed following a stroke are described in **Box 52-1**.

C. Disease Risk Detection

- Calcifications in the carotid artery are observable on a panoramic radiograph.[10,11] If present, the patient should be referred for medical evaluation.
- Radiation therapy is associated with an accelerated form of atherosclerosis formation and risk of stroke.[12]

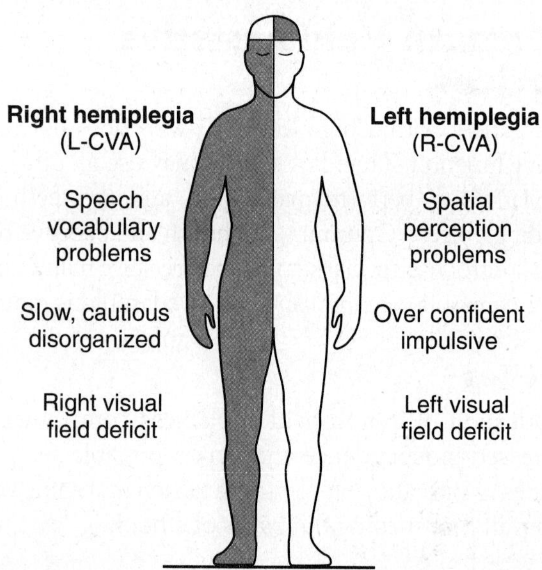

Figure 52-2 Cerebrovascular Accident (CVA) (Stroke). Right hemiplegia is the result of left-sided brain damage, and left hemiplegia results from right-sided brain damage.

Box 52-1 Description of Signs and Symptoms Following Stroke

- **Paralysis:** hemiplegia (one side of the body) or portions, such as an arm, leg, or the face.
- **Articulation:** difficulty of speech, which may be caused by involvement of the tongue, mouth, or throat, as well as **aphasia** by brain damage related to the speech centers, and the patient may have difficulty finding the right word.
- **Salivation:** difficulty in control of saliva complicated by difficulty in swallowing; aspiration.
- **Sensory:** loss in affected parts may result in superficial anesthesia, or the opposite may occur with resultant increased sensitivity to pain and touch.
- **Visual impairment:** blurred vision or diminished visual acuity.
- **Mental function:** may be unaffected, but slowness, poor memory, and loss of initiative are common. Brain deterioration may occur over a period of time.
- **Personal factors:** personality changes relate to emotional trauma, fear, discouragement, and dependency. Anxiety neuroses and periods of depression, which are common, may require assistance from a psychiatrist, psychologist, or social worker.

III. Medical Treatment

- Surgical correction of aneurysms, clots, or malformations may include removal of microscopic clots in the intracranial arteries or minute grafting

Box 52-2 Categories and Purposes of Medications Used to Treat Strokes

- **Anticoagulant:** to thin the blood.
- **Antihypertensive:** to lower the blood pressure.
- **Thrombolytic:** to dissolve clots.
- **Vasodilator:** to relax the blood vessels of the brain.
- **Steroid:** to control brain swelling.
- **Antiepileptic:** to help to control seizures.

to bypass blocked vessels and provide collateral circulation.

- Physical and occupational therapy and rehabilitation techniques are vital to the patient's recovery and functioning.
- Careful recording of the medical history includes the listing of medications. The patient who has experienced a stroke may be taking a variety of drugs for some or all of the purposes found in **Box 52-2**.

IV. Dental Hygiene Care

Particular factors to consider when planning dental hygiene care for the patient with a stroke-related disability:

- Impaired motor and/or cognitive ability.
- Hemiplegia; particularly if the dominant hand is affected. Adjunct aids for oral home care should be considered.
- Facial paralysis; decreased self-cleansing action of the tongue and lips; decreased control of saliva; risk for aerosol in eye during treatment.
- Medication for treatment of the condition: anticoagulant use is common following a stroke.

Bell's Palsy (Idiopathic Temporary Facial Paralysis)

- Bell's palsy is paralysis of the facial muscles innervated by the facial or seventh cranial nerve.
- Although the cause is not known, various possible agents have been implicated, including:
  - Bacterial and viral infections; particularly herpes simplex.
  - Injury, trauma from tooth removal or oral surgery such as the removal of a tumor in the parotid gland area.

I. Occurrence

- Although relatively rare, the incidence increases with each decade of life.
- In younger age groups, women are more frequently affected than are men.
- After 50 years of age, the disorder is more common in men.

II. Characteristics[13]

A. Signs and Symptoms

Abrupt weakness or paralysis of facial muscles, usually without preceding pain, occurs on one side of the face.

- Mouth: the corner of the mouth droops, and salivation with drooling is uncontrollable.
- Eye: eyelid on the affected side may not close; watering and drooping of the lower lid invites infection.
- When only the seventh nerve is affected, sensory responses are still intact.

B. Functional Problems

- Speech and mastication may be impaired.

C. Prognosis

- A majority of patients experience a return to normal within a month with a spontaneous recovery.
- Others may have lasting residual effects or permanent paralysis.

III. Medical Treatment

A. Palliative

- Eye protection such as an eye patch during sleep and eye drops for lubrication during waking hours.
- Hot compresses and massaging the involved muscles provides some relief.
- Analgesics may relieve pain.

B. Drugs

- Corticosteroids, administered within the first 72 hours, have been used to improve the prognosis.
- Antiviral drugs are sometimes prescribed, but the efficacy of these drugs when taken alone is unclear.[14]
- Combining corticosteroid and antiviral treatment is not clearly indicated for standard treatment but may be considered for patients with severe cases.[15]

C. Surgical

- Surgical procedures to relieve pressure on the nerve or reduce deformities have been used but are controversial and seldom recommended.[16]

IV. Dental Hygiene Care

Particular factors to consider when planning dental hygiene care for the patient with Bell's palsy:

- Facial paralysis; decreased self-cleansing action of the tongue and lips; decreased control of saliva; risk for aerosol in eye during treatment.
- Medications used for treatment of the condition.

Amyotrophic Lateral Sclerosis

ALS (often referred to as Lou Gehrig's disease) is a progressive neurodegenerative disorder characterized by a progressive loss of motor neuron function.

I. Occurrence

- Prevalence is approximately 5 per 100,000 population; more than 16,000 people in the United States.[17]
- Men are more often affected than women; Caucasians more frequently than other ethnic groups.
- Onset usually occurs at middle age or later; prevalence highest in those aged 60–69 years and lowest in those aged 18–39 years.[17]

II. Diagnosis

- There are no diagnostic tests for ALS.
- Diagnosis is usually made after ruling out other disorders with similar symptoms.
- Clinically diagnosed with both upper and lower neuron dysfunction, although variants include a pure upper motor and pure lower motor syndrome.[18]

III. Etiology and Pathogenesis

- Unknown cause.
- About 90% of cases are sporadic.
- About 5–10% are familial (predominantly autosomal dominant).
- Average life expectancy is 3–5 years, but the range is broad and some live much longer.
- Typically progressive degeneration of both upper and lower motor neurons with no periods of remission.
- More areas of the body are affected over time; nearly all systems eventually become involved.
- Respiratory failure is the usual cause of death.

IV. Two Forms of ALS

- Spinal form[19]
  - About two-thirds of patients.
  - Early symptoms include muscle weakness in upper and lower limbs and muscle wasting.
- Bulbar onset form[19]
  - About one-third of patients
  - Initially presents with dysarthria.
  - Sometimes dysphagia with solids or liquids is initial symptom.
  - Facial weakness and wasting/spasticity of the tongue are common.
  - Limb symptoms may develop simultaneously or can happen later as the disease progresses.
  - **Sialorrhea** (excessive secretion of saliva; drooling) develops in almost all who have the bulbar-onset form of the disease.

V. Symptoms

- Symptoms include[20]:
  - Cramps and spasticity.
  - Muscle weakness, particularly in extremities.
  - Increasing respiratory difficulty.
  - Difficulty swallowing and chewing.
  - Excessive saliva.[21,22]
  - Depression and anxiety.
  - Cognitive and behavioral changes that can affect compliance with recommendations.[23]

VI. Treatment

- There is only one Food and Drug Administration–approved treatment (riluzole); treatment only extends survival about 2 months.[20]
- Palliative treatment is provided by interprofessional teams.[24]
- Treatment focused on progressive management of symptoms.
- Sialorrhea managed with medications, but in later stages treatment can include radiation or Botox injection into salivary glands.[22]

VII. Dental Hygiene Care

Factors to consider when planning dental hygiene care for the patient with ALS:

- Increased motor impairment over time.
- Need for body stabilization and support.

- Risk for respiratory difficulties.
- Effects of facial paralysis.
- Effects of treatment for sialorrhea.

Parkinson's Disease

- Progressive disorder of the central nervous system characterized by four primary symptoms[25]:
    - Tremor in hands, arms, legs, jaw, and face.
    - Rigidity of limbs and trunk.
    - **Bradykinesia** or slowness of movement.
    - Postural instability.
- It is also known as paralysis agitans and Parkinson's syndrome.
- Although the cause is not known, the basis for the specific group of symptoms is degeneration of certain neurons in the substantia nigra of the basal ganglia, where posture, support, and voluntary motion are controlled.
- In addition, a severe deficiency of dopamine, one of the substances that participates in nerve transmission, occurs.

I. Occurrence[26]

- Parkinson's disease affects almost 1 million middle-aged and older persons in the United States; more than 10 million people worldwide.
- Incidence increases with age; only about 4% are diagnosed before age 50.
- Approximately 60,000 new cases are diagnosed each year.
- One and half times higher incidence in men than in women.

II. Characteristics

- The signs and symptoms center around tremor, rigidity, and loss or impairment of motor function (**akinesia**).
- These factors also occur in other conditions, which are differentiated when a diagnosis is made.
- The disease progresses through stages; from mild/early to severe/advanced with increasing impairment of motor function.

A. General Manifestations

- Body posture bent, with bent head and general stiffness.
- Motion and responses slowed; difficulty in keeping balance and turning.
- Gait slow and shuffling.
- Speech is monotone and slow.
- Resting tremor of one or both hands is common; the tremor can be reduced or stopped when the person engages in a purposeful action such as toothbrushing.
- The fingers may be involved in a "pill-rolling" motion in which the thumb and index finger are rubbed together in a circular movement.
- Nonmotor symptoms include variations in blood pressure, cardiac dysrhythmias, excessive sweating, bowel and bladder dysfunction, and sleep disorders.
- Cognitive ability is seldom affected, except in the advanced stages.
- Eventually, after 10–20 years, the person may become incapacitated and may require complete care.

B. Face and Oral Cavity

- Expression is fixed and mask-like, with diminished eye blinking.
- Tremor or exaggerated movement in lips, tongue, and neck, and difficulty in swallowing.
- Excess salivation and drooling.

III. Treatment

- No known cure for Parkinson's disease.
- Symptomatic control is treated by administration of levodopa combined with carbidopa; this helps delay the alteration of levodopa until it reaches the brain.
    - Side effects can include dizziness and confusion.
- Maintenance of good general health is encouraged, including plenty of rest and nutritious meals.
- Professional physical therapy and occupational therapy have particular significance for a patient's well-being.
- Surgical relief for symptoms is sometimes accomplished by deep brain stimulation (DBS) or **pallidotomy**.

IV. Dental Hygiene Care

Particular factors to consider when planning dental hygiene care for the patient with Parkinson's disease include[27]:

- Increased motor impairment, tremor, and rigidity over time, which interferes with daily activities.
- Rigid, uncontrolled facial muscles; poor control of eyes, lips, tongue, and swallowing muscles.
- Increased drooling of saliva.

- Need for short appointments.
- Potential for cognitive deficits over time.
- Adverse drug interactions and reactions.
- Need for caregiver education.

Postpolio Syndrome (PPS)

I. Description[28]

- Condition that affects adults, years after recovery from an initial attack of the poliomyelitis virus when they were children.
- Cause is unknown; occurs in individuals that were more acutely affected with polio, or poliomyelitis.
- Prevalence is currently unknown, but appears to be growing.
- Treatment focus is mainly palliative, with exercise often prescribed to strengthen specific muscle groups.
- Characterized by slow progressive muscle weakness, fatigue, muscle and joint pain, and potential muscle **atrophy** in muscles originally affected by the poliomyelitis as well as other muscles, including orofacial muscles.

II. Dental Hygiene Care

Particular factors to consider when planning dental hygiene care for the patient with postpolio syndrome:[29]

- Morning appointments.
- Avoid long appointments.
- Impaired motor ability.
- Weakness in respiratory and swallowing muscles.

Cerebral Palsy

I. Description

- A group of disorders that involve the cerebral cortex, the part of the brain that directs motor function.[30]
- Damage to the developing brain can occur, such as:
  - During fetal development, usually (congenital).
  - Natally or postnatally (acquired).
- In many cases the cause is unknown, but can be related to:
  - Abnormal development of the brain.
  - Bleeding in the brain.
  - Severe lack of oxygen.
- Risk factors include[30]:
  - Maternal infections, thyroid abnormalities, or seizures during pregnancy.
  - Maternal exposure to toxic substances during pregnancy.
  - Blood type incompatibility between mother and child.
  - Complicated labor and delivery, breech position of baby during birth, or multiple births.
  - Infant jaundice, infection, or seizures after birth.
  - Severe head injury after birth.
- Symptoms usually can be observed during the first year after birth, but if symptoms are mild, it may not be noticed for several years.
- Cerebral palsy is not progressive.

II. Classifications

Cerebral palsy is classified into four types according to associated motor impairment.[30,31]

A. Spastic Palsy

- Most common type.
- Muscles have increased tone, tension; can be in one limb or all four; sometimes includes oral structures.
- Condition characterized by spasms (sudden, involuntary contractions of single muscles or groups of muscles) and stiff, rigid muscles resistant to movement.
- Complete or partial loss of ability to control muscular movement; movements are awkward and stiff with resistance to movement. Lack of control may cause patient to fall easily.

B. Dyskinetic or Athetoid Palsy

- Characterized by constant, slow, involuntary writhing movements with frequent changes of muscle tone.
- Lack of ability to direct muscles in the motions desired.
- Grimacing, drooling, and speech defects are common.
- Factors influencing movements:
  - Difficult to sit straight or walk.
  - May be initiated and aggravated by stimuli outside the body, such as sudden noises, bright lights, or quick movements by people or things in the area.
  - Intensity influenced by emotional factors; patient is least in control in an emotionally charged environment, such as the dental office or clinic.

C. Ataxic Palsy

- Loss of equilibrium, balance, and depth perception; walk uncertain.
- Lack of coordination; needs time to execute changes.
- Difficulty with precise movements such as writing or buttoning a shirt.
- Involuntary muscle quivering may affect part or all of the body; placing gentle firm pressure on the affected muscles will help calm the tremor.

D. Combined Palsy

- A combination of the three named types.

III. Accompanying Conditions

A. Primitive Reflexes and Abnormal Response to Stimuli[30]

- Asymmetric tonic neck reflex: when head is turned, same side extremities extend and stiffen, while opposite side extremities flex.
- Tonic labyrinthine reflex: if the neck is extended back, extremities also extend back and the back is arched.
- Startle reflex: any surprising stimuli can trigger uncontrolled body movement.

B. Contractures

- Muscles fixed in abnormal positions.
- Increase in muscle spasticity and joint deformities.

C. Seizures

- As many as one-half have seizures and those with seizure disorder are more likely to have an intellectual disability.[30]

D. Sensory Disorders

- Visual impairments and hearing loss are common.

E. Speech and Language Disorders

- Speech may be slow and difficult to understand due to lack of control of mouth and throat muscles (**dysarthria**).
- Difficulty processing auditory information.

F. Cognitive Impairment

- Some individuals with cerebral palsy also have significant cognitive impairment.
- More than 50% *do not* have intellectual or cognitive disabilities; therefore, an inability to communicate does not necessarily mean lack of comprehension.
- Individuals with cerebral palsy may learn more slowly because of sensory impairments, perceptive-cognitive deficiencies, and speech difficulties.

G. Gastroesophageal Reflux

- Some individuals with cerebral palsy may experience reflux; affects individuals that are tube fed as well.
- Should seat patient in upright position.
- Encourage daily use of fluoridated toothpaste, fluoride gel, or rinse.
- Rinsing mouth with plain water or water with ¼ tsp baking soda at least four times a day may help reduce effect of gastric acid.[31,32]

IV. Medical Treatment

- Interprofessional teams of healthcare providers caring for the individual with cerebral palsy can include medical, surgical, orthopedic, and dental providers, as well as speech, physical, recreational, and occupational therapists.
- Orthotic devices to support the lower limbs and the use of cane, crutches, walker, or wheelchair may help to increase function.
- Surgery may be needed for addressing orthopedic deformities, correcting eye or ear difficulties, or severing nerves to relax muscles and reduce chronic pain.
- Oral medications may be used to reduce tension in affected muscles, aid in pain management, or control seizures.

V. Oral Characteristics

A. Disturbances of Musculature

- Facial grimacing, facial asymmetry, and abnormal function of muscles of mastication, swallowing, and speech are common.
- Spasticity of orofacial muscles can interfere with daily oral care.
- Inability to close lips contributes to increased drooling.
- Hyperactive bite and gag reflexes can present difficulties during dental and dental hygiene therapy, as well as during biofilm control at home.

B. Malocclusion

- The incidence of malocclusion is high; often a musculoskeletal abnormality rather than only misaligned teeth.[31]
- Oral habits of mouth breathing, tongue thrusting, and faulty swallowing contribute to open bite with protruding anterior teeth.[32]

C. Attrition and Erosion

- Severe, constant, involuntary bruxism is common and can severely wear down tooth structure and restorations.
- Gastroesophageal reflux can cause erosion of oral tissues.

D. Oral Injury

- Patients may fall frequently, which can damage and fracture teeth and jaws.

E. Dental Caries

- Increased risk of gum disease and caries due to poor oral hygiene.[30]
- Difficulties in maintaining biofilm control and problems of mastication can lead to consumption of a soft diet, which increases risk for dental caries.
- Medications such as seizure drugs can heighten risk of oral disease.

F. Periodontal Infections

- Periodontal or gingival infections are found in a high percentage of patients with cerebral palsy.[32]
- Phenytoin-induced gingival overgrowth: when phenytoin is used for the prevention of seizures, the patient is susceptible to gingival enlargement.
- Risk factors for periodontal involvement: mechanical difficulties related to biofilm control, mouth breathing, and increased food retention because of ineffective self-cleansing all lead to increased periodontal involvement and biofilm collection.
- Many patients with cerebral palsy have heavy calculus deposits.

VI. Dental Hygiene Care

Particular factors to consider when planning dental hygiene care for the patient with cerebral palsy:

- Numerous associated oral characteristics and predisposing factors for oral disease.
- Impaired motor ability; uncontrolled movements, reflexive reactions.
- Compromised ventilatory capacity.[33]
- Involvement of muscles in head and neck.
- Need for body stabilization and support due to joint contractures.
- Potential cognitive impairment and compromised communication.[33]
- Increased risk for seizure.

Muscular Dystrophies

- The muscular dystrophies are a group of more than 30 genetic myopathies characterized by progressive severe weakness and loss of use of groups of muscles.[34]
- The term *dystrophy* means degeneration and is associated with atrophy and dysfunction.
- The syndromes of muscular dystrophy have been separated by clinical and genetic means and range from mild (Becker type) with a later onset to more severe types (Duchenne, facioscapulohumeral).
- All types of muscular dystrophy are genetically inherited and the underlying pathologic processes do not differ.
- Generally, the diseases are limited to skeletal muscles, with rare involvement of the cardiac muscle.
- In the United States, more than 50,000 children and adults are affected with some form of muscular dystrophy.[34]

I. Duchenne Muscular Dystrophy (Pseudohypertrophic)

A. Occurrence

- The Duchenne muscular dystrophy (DMD) type is most common.
- Primarily affects males and transmitted by female carriers of the defective gene.
- Prevalence of approximately 1:7250 males 5–24 years of age.[35]

B. Age of Onset

- The condition is present at birth and becomes apparent during early childhood, usually diagnosed at an average age of 5 years.[35]

C. Characteristics

- Musculature: enlargement (pseudohypertrophy) of certain muscles, particularly the calves, is present in early years.
- Weakness of hips: child falls frequently, has increasing difficulty in standing erect.

- Lordosis: with an abdominal protuberance.
- Waddling: either walks on toes or flat foot because of muscle contracture.
- Precarious balance: patient arches back in attempt to find center of gravity; gait is slow because balance needs to be sustained during each step.
- Progressive muscular wasting:
    - Eventual involvement of thighs, shoulders, trunk; weakness of respiratory muscles.
    - Inactivity is detrimental and increases the individual's helplessness and dependency.
- Intellectual impairment: a mild degree of mental impairment is noted in some persons with DMD.
- Cardiac abnormalities: arrhythmia and cardiomyopathy are common.

D. Prognosis

- Disability may be more severe by puberty; child is confined to a wheelchair.
- Patients rarely live to reach their third decade.

II. Facioscapulohumeral Muscular Dystrophy

A. Occurrence

- Males and females are equally affected.
- Incidence is approximately 1 in 20,000.[36]

B. Age of Onset

- Between 6 and 20 years, with an average at 13 years, after puberty.
- Mild symptoms may appear at later ages, with rare cases occurring during infancy.[36]

C. Characteristics

- Facial muscles involved, particularly the orbicularis oris. The effect of gaping lips on oral tissues is similar to mouth breathing.
- Malocclusion and temporomandibular disorder problems have been noted.
- Scapulae prominent; shoulder muscles weak; difficulty in raising the arms.
- Difficulty in closing eyes completely.
- Cardiac involvement is rare.

D. Prognosis

- Progression is slower than that of the Duchenne type and progress may become arrested.
- Most patients live a normal life span and become incapacitated late in life.

III. Myotonic Muscular Dystrophy (Steinert Disease)

- Most common form in adults; can appear any time from early childhood to adulthood.[37]
- Affects both men and women.
- Prolonged spasm of muscles after use; usually worse in cold temperatures.
- Also affects central nervous system, heart, gastrointestinal tract, eyes, and hormone-producing glands.

IV. Other Types of Muscular Dystrophy

Other, less common types of muscular dystrophy include[38,39]:

- Becker: onset adolescence to early adulthood; similar to Duchenne type, but more benign with a later onset; primarily affects males.
- Emery–Dreifuss: onset childhood to early teens; generally benign, but severe cardiomyopathy and risk for sudden death is a feature.
- Limb-girdle: most severely affects muscles of the hips and shoulders; manifests in late childhood to middle age; progression is slow; death may result due to cardiopulmonary complications.
- Oculopharyngeal and myotonic dystrophies: each is relatively rare, has onset between 40 and 70 years of age, is slowly progressive, and features extensive involvement of orofacial muscles.

V. Medical Treatment

- Supportive treatments consist of[39]:
    - Physical, occupational, and speech therapy.
    - Respiratory therapy.
- Drug therapy includes[39]:
    - Glucocorticoids.
    - Anticonvulsants.
    - Immunosuppressants.
    - Beta blockers, angiotensin-converting enzyme (ACE) inhibitors (for treating heart problems).
- Preventive treatment consists of prenatal diagnosis, carrier detection, and genetic counseling.

VI. Dental Hygiene Care

Particular factors to consider when planning dental hygiene care for the patient with muscular dystrophy[40]:

- Impaired motor ability.
- Potential need for body stabilization and support.
- Some types involve orofacial muscles.

Myelomeningocele

- Spina bifida is a congenital defect or opening in the spinal column. A portion of the spinal membranes may protrude through the opening with or without spinal cord tissue.
- When the spinal cord protrudes through the spina bifida, the condition is called myelomeningocele.
- Anticipatory guidance prior to conception includes the use of multivitamins containing recommended levels of folic acid. A reduced risk of offspring with spina bifida and other neural tube defects has been shown when mothers received folic acid.[41]
- Patients with spina bifida appear to be specifically at risk for latex hypersensitivity.[42] Precautions and management of latex hypersensitivity are discussed in Chapter 6.

I. Description

- Embryologically, a neural tube forms during the first month of pregnancy.
- From the neural tube, the brain, brain stem, and spinal cord arise, and, eventually, the vertebrae form and enclose the spinal cord.
- When a place in the spinal column fails to close, the result is an open defect in the spinal canal, which is called a spina bifida.

II. Types of Deformities[43]

A. Myelomeningocele

- A myelomeningocele is a protrusion or outpouching of the spinal cord and its covering (meninges) through an opening in the bony spinal column.
- Because part of the spinal cord and nerve roots protrude, flaccid paralysis of the legs and part of the trunk results, depending on the level of the protrusion (herniation).

B. Meningocele

- A meningocele is a protrusion of the meninges through a defect in the skull or spinal column.
- No neural elements are contained in the protrusion, but it can cause minor disabilities.

C. Closed Neural Tube Defect

- Malformations in fat, bone, or meninges of spinal cord.
- Few or no symptom in most instances; sometimes causes incomplete paralysis with urinary and bowel dysfunction.

D. Spina Bifida Occulta

- Spina bifida occulta is a congenital cleft in the bony encasement of the spinal cord in which no outpouching of the meninges or spinal cord exists.
- Usually, spina bifida occulta has no symptoms.

III. Physical Characteristics

Depending on the level of the myelomeningocele, some or all of the following signs and physical characteristics may be found.[44]

A. Bony Deformities

- Muscle imbalance from paralysis can cause dislocation of the hip, club foot, and spinal curvatures, such as humpback (**kyphosis**), curvature (scoliosis), or swayback (lordosis).

B. Loss of Sensation

- Lack of skin sensitivity to pain, temperature, and other sensations can lead to problems of inadvertent burn or trauma unrecognized by the patient or caregiver or to pressure sores.
- Frequent position changes are necessary during dental hygiene care.

C. Bladder and Bowel Paralysis

- The nerve supplies to the bladder and bowel are usually affected.
- Lack of bowel and bladder control requires continual attention.
- Kidney infection with loss of kidney function is one cause of shorter life expectancy.

D. Hydrocephalus

- A high percentage of children with myelomeningocele have hydrocephalus, a condition characterized by an excessive accumulation of fluid in the brain. The fluid dilates the cerebral ventricles, causes compression of brain tissues, and separates the cranial bones as the head enlarges (**Figure 52-3**).
- Development is slowed, and intellectual disability may be present.
- Many of these patients have seizures.

IV. Medical Treatment

Surgical, orthopedic, and urologic treatment as well as physical and occupational therapy may constitute a minimum of specialties involved in the care of a patient with myelomeningocele.

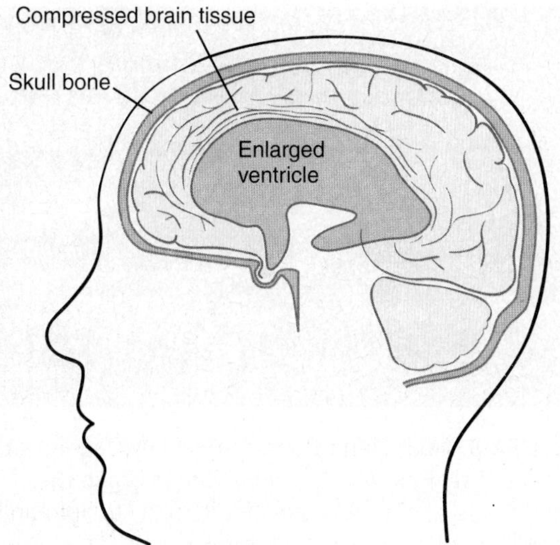

Figure 52-3 Hydrocephalus. The ventricle is enlarged because of the accumulation of fluid. Brain tissues are compressed.

A. Neurosurgery

- Closure of the myelomeningocele: surgical closure helps to prevent infections that may otherwise enter into the spinal cord. Paralysis is not lessened by surgery.
  - Treatment of the hydrocephalus: permanent drainage systems may be accomplished in the form of a **ventriculoatrial shunt** between the cerebral ventricle and the atrium of the heart. Sometimes, drainage by way of the abdomen in the form of a **ventriculoperitoneal shunt** is used (**Figure 52-4**).
- Individuals who have a cerebrospinal fluid **shunt** are at increased risk for transient infections. Need for premedication during dental treatment is established by medical consultation.[45]

B. Orthopedic Surgery

- Orthopedic surgical procedures can assist by reducing or correcting deformities.
- Bracing to support the trunk and lower limbs is used in accord with the extent of the individual's paralysis.
- Ambulation varies from dependency on a wheelchair, walker, crutches, or cane to near normal with only foot problems.

V. Dental Hygiene Care

Particular factors to consider when planning dental hygiene care for the patient with myelomeningocele:

- Impaired motor ability.
- Potential need for body stabilization and support.

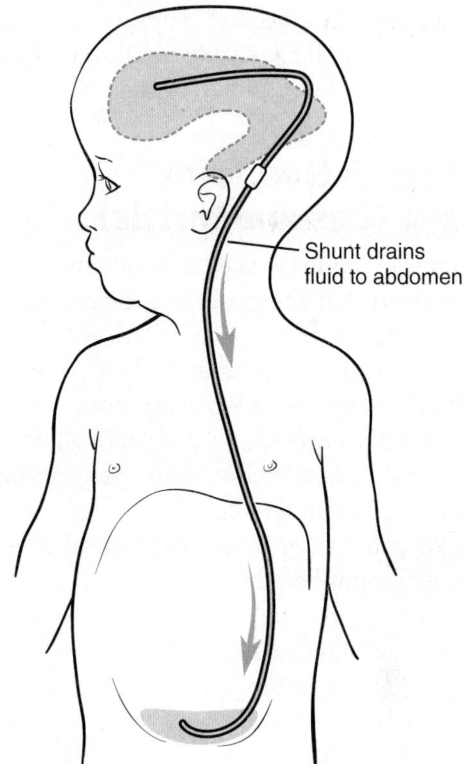

Figure 52-4 Shunt for Hydrocephalus Treatment. Fluid is drained by way of a ventriculoatrial or ventriculoperitoneal shunt.

- Increased risk for latex allergy and transient infections related to a cerebrospinal fluid shunt.

Arthritis

Diseases of the joints, including arthritis, are among the most common causes of chronic illness in the United States. In addition to arthritis as a disease entity, arthritic manifestations may occur as a symptom of various other chronic diseases. A person may suffer from more than one type at a time.

- Arthritis means inflammation in a joint. When many joints are involved, the term polyarthritis may be applied.
  - It may occur in an acute or chronic form and may be localized or generalized.
  - The resulting disability may be temporary or permanent, partial or complete.
- Factors implicated in the cause of rheumatic and arthritic diseases include infectious agents, traumatic disorders, endocrine abnormalities, tumors, allergy and drug reactions, and inherited or congenital conditions. When the cause is

known, specific medical, physical, and surgical therapies may be available to alleviate pain and disability.

I. Degenerative Joint Disease (Osteoarthritis)

- Chronic condition related to breakdown and progressive loss of the hyaline cartilage cushion in the joints.[46]
- Eventually changes in underlying bone are noted.
- Inflammation is not a key symptom.
- Particularly affects the weight-bearing joints.
- No specific cause known, but predisposing risk factors may include:
  - Repeated trauma and mechanical stresses to the weight-bearing joints.
  - Obesity.
  - Age-related changes in the joint tissues.
  - Genetic predisposition.
  - Estrogen deficiency and high bone density may be factors.

A. Occurrence[46]

- Affects 32.5 million US adults
- Incidence increases with age.
- Women, particularly those older than 50 years, have higher rates than men.

B. Symptoms

- At first insidious, the condition leads to pain, deformity, and limitation of movement.
- Hips, knees, fingers, and vertebrae affected most frequently.
- Swelling and inflammation rare; **ankylosis** does not occur.
- Stiffness in the morning on rising and after periods of inactivity; diminishes with exercise.
- Pain aggravated by temperature changes, bearing body weight, and strenuous activity.
- Temporomandibular joint usually without pain or other clinical symptoms, although crepitation, clicking, or snapping may occur when the joints are exercised.

C. Medical Treatment

- Treatments to reduce symptoms include:
  - Physical therapy and regular, moderate exercise.
  - Pain-relieving drug therapy.
  - Weight reduction for obese patients.

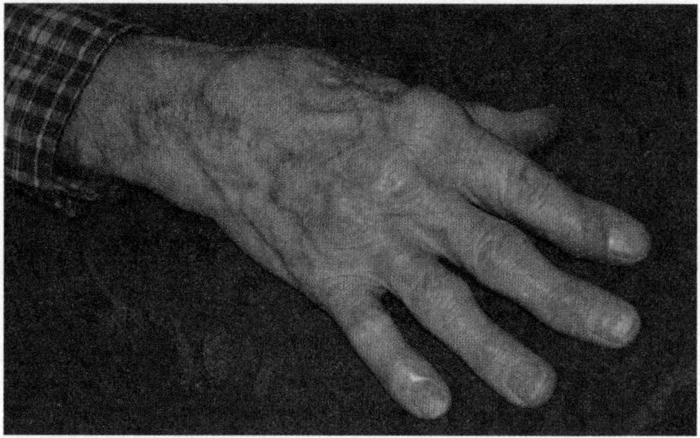

Figure 52-5 Adult Hand Compromised by Degenerative Joint Disease. Pain and lack of ability to grasp the small handle of a toothbrush affect ability to hold and maneuver oral self-care implements.

- Total joint replacement has proved satisfactory for many patients.

II. Dental Hygiene Care

Particular factors to consider when planning dental hygiene care for the patient with arthritis include:

- Joint pain contributes to impaired motor function and difficulty performing everyday activities of living. (See Chapter 51.)
- Affected areas, degree of impairment, and adaptations to provide for patient comfort are considered when planning care and providing instructions for oral self-care.
- The effect of osteoarthritis on the hands of an older patient is considered when planning for self-care procedures (see **Figure 52-5**).

Summary of Considerations for Dental Hygiene Care

- High cost, dental anxiety, and physical barriers are three main reasons individuals with physical disabilities experience difficulty accessing dental care in traditional settings.[47]
- Not being aware of oral health needs is another important barrier to oral care.[47]
- Dental professionals are essential members of the interprofessional patient care team for a patient with a physical impairment.[48,49]
- Early dental hygiene intervention and regular preventive care will aid in optimizing oral health status and minimizing oral problems.

- Knowledge and understanding of the specifics of a patient's particular condition will help the clinician become confident in managing adaptations needed during the dental hygiene appointment.
- Communication to determine and support the patient's wishes in adapting patient care procedures is essential, particularly when the patient is unable to perform daily life activities independently and is dependent on others.
- Most patients with a physical impairment do not have an intellectual impairment.
- Information provided in Chapter 51 is useful for planning dental hygiene care for a patient with a physical impairment, either in a dental clinic or in an alternative practice setting.
- General suggestions for the older adult patient in Chapter 48 may also be useful.

I. Preparation for Appointments

- Communication with the patient or caregiver prior to appointment to assess specific needs will help the clinician to identify and prepare for modifications necessary to provide care based on the individual patient's needs.
- Essential information, such as a completed health history and description of the patient's physical abilities and limitations, can be obtained by telephone.
- Ask specific questions about abilities and limitations in performing activities of everyday living.
  - Information about assistance needed from caregivers.
  - Adaptive aids the patient is currently using for oral self-care or other personal hygiene tasks.
- Determine factors related to the best time of day for dental appointments, for example:
  - Schedule of urinary/bowel management program for a patient with SCI.
  - The time of day when symptoms associated with the particular condition are most likely to be relieved or diminished.
- Assess methods preferred by the patient to communicate with healthcare providers or caregiver.
- Determine adaptations needed for the patient's comfort or safety during the appointment.
  - Blankets or increased air circulation if body temperature control is compromised.
  - Positioning and padding needed for stabilization.
  - Procedures for stress reduction.
- Identify medications that may put the patient at risk for:
  - Xerostomia.
  - Increased bleeding.
  - Potential interactions with local anesthesia.
- Information for appointment scheduling and providing a barrier-free environment is found in Chapter 51.

II. Additional Considerations during Clinical Care

- Frequent, short appointments in a warm, quiet, comfortable atmosphere lessen patient fatigue and emotional stress.
- Emergency care may be needed during the period of recovery, such as immediately following a stroke or traumatic spinal injury; nonemergency care is delayed until the patient is stabilized.
- When the patient's condition involves partial or complete paralysis of facial muscles:
  - Decreased self-cleaning action of the tongue increases potential for collecting dental biofilm on oral surfaces.
  - Rinsing may be difficult or impossible.
  - When anesthesia is used, the affected cheek and lip may be at higher risk for biting injury until the anesthesia has worn off.
  - If the eyelid lacks natural ability to close for protection, care is taken to ensure that calculus, polishing agent, or other foreign material does not splash into the eye by assuring that protective eyewear and suction are used during treatment.
- Potential effects from interactions with medications taken for many disorders and conditions require particular care when administering anesthetics.
  - For example, epinephrine interaction with levodopa, often prescribed for Parkinson's disease, may cause the patient to experience an exaggerated effect on blood pressure and heart rate.
- Dental hygiene care is complicated if the patient has a disorder that involves involuntary movement; for example, athetoid movements in a patient with cerebral palsy.
  - Involuntary movement is not interpreted as lack of cooperation.
  - Ask the patient or caregiver for suggestions about assistance or management.
  - Sedation through premedication may be possible.

III. Assistance for the Ambulatory Patient

- Ask patients how best to provide assistance.
- Suggestions for how to aid patients who walk with one or more assistive aids such as braces, a cane, crutches, or a walker are found in Chapter 51.

IV. Wheelchair Transfer

- Most patients who use wheelchairs can be treated in a traditional clinical setting.
- Detailed information about wheelchair to dental chair transfer is available in Chapter 51.

V. Patient Positioning and Body Stabilization

- Danger for the patient and dental personnel can result from the uncontrolled movement of the patient.
- Communication with patient or caregiver prior to appointment to assess specific needs related to body positioning and use of specific measures such as padding, warm coverings, or other supportive devices will help enhance safety, patient comfort, and clinician efficiency.
- The patient is asked to provide direction for correct, individualized procedures.
- Slow and incremental adjustments of the patient chair during treatment will help maintain comfort and patient stability.
- Prevention of decubitus ulcers can be accomplished by:
  - Appropriate positioning of the dental chair.
  - Use of padding.
  - Periodic repositioning to prevent or reduce pressure.
- Before dental hygiene treatment, the patient is asked about susceptibility to spasms and to describe the procedure to follow should one occur.
- Suggestions for body stabilization and use of mouth props are found in Chapter 51.
- Chapter 4 provides ideas for treatment adaptations when the patient is bed-bound or if care is provided in a nonclinical setting.

VI. Four-Handed Dental Hygiene

- Continuous assistance when providing dental hygiene care for patients with a physical impairment is essential.
- Use of a dental hygiene assistant will:
  - Enhance the clinician's efficiency.
  - Ensure the patient's comfort and safety.

VII. Personal Factors That Affect Self-Care

- Depression from limitations or discouragement from the pain and pressure of treatment and rehabilitation can affect attitude toward oral self-care practices for the patient who has a physical impairment.
- Daily oral care can become a part of the personal hygiene routine accomplished as independently as the patient's ability allows. Physical and occupational therapists provide self-care training to enable as much independence as possible for personal care.
- Paralysis or muscle contractions may make grasping and manipulating a toothbrush difficult or impossible.
- Adaptations that may assist in maintaining daily oral care include:
  - Toothbrush handle modifications. (See Chapter 51.)
  - A specially designed toothbrush. (See Chapter 51.)[50]
  - A lightweight power-driven toothbrush.
  - Instruction for the caregiver assistance, provided on the basis of patient ability and limitations.
- Hemiplegia, common after a stroke, can require helping the patient develop dexterity in the nondominant hand in order to manipulate biofilm removal implements.

VIII. Residence-Based Delivery of Care

- People with physical disabilities may benefit from oral health service delivery models that provide care in their place of residence.
- Delivery of dental hygiene care in alternative settings is discussed in Chapter 4.

Documentation

Documentation in the permanent record for each appointment with a physically impaired patient includes a minimum of the following factors:

- Description of the patient's impairment level and ability to provide oral self-care, with changes/updates noted for each dental hygiene visit, particularly if the patient has a degenerative condition.
- Recommendations for adaptive aids and modifications to daily oral care regimens.

- Description of oral hygiene care instructions provided to the caregiver.
- Description of patient position modifications and other adaptations during patient care.
- An example of documentation for an appointment with a patient with a physical disability is in **Box 52-3**.

Box 52-3 Example Documentation: Maintenance Appointment for Patient with a Physical Impairment

- **S**—A 32-year-old female patient presents for routine 3 month maintenance appointment. Patient is ambulatory with a walker and prefers no assistance at this time, but padding under knees helps her relax and enhances her comfort during treatment.
- **O**—Medical history includes diagnosis of MS 2 years ago. Update today indicates no changes in health history or medications. Decreased ability to grasp a regular toothbrush was noted during oral hygiene instruction. No changes in oral status. Biofilm scores less than 20%.
- **A**—Routine 3 months maintenance care today with the use of padding for patient comfort and reassessment of daily oral self-care procedures are indicated.
- **P**—Full-mouth scaling/root debridement, polish, fluoride varnish application. Several options for modifying/enlarging a toothbrush handle to facilitate better grasp during oral care were discussed with patient. At patient request, instruction for using a power toothbrush was provided. The use of a floss holder was demonstrated and ideas for enlarging the handle were given to the patient.

Signed: ______________________, RDH
Date: ________________

Factors to Teach the Patient

- The need to communicate is key to successful dental treatment and oral health and is achieved by speaking openly about medical history, patient limitations, and adaptations needed for safe dental treatment and effective oral care.
- Daily thorough biofilm removal is necessary to reduce the occurrence of oral disease.
- Regular maintenance appointments are needed to promote oral health.
- Why maintaining periodontal health can help maintain teeth that are necessary as abutments in order to tolerate a mouth-held adaptive aid.
- How to clean and maintain a mouth-held aid.

References

1. Wu HJ, Pu JL, Krafft PR, Zhang JM, Chen S. The molecular mechanisms between autophagy and apoptosis: potential role in central nervous system disorders. *Cell Mol Neurobiol.* 2015;35(1):85-99.
2. National Spinal Cord Injury Statistical Center. *Spinal Cord Injury: Facts and Figures at a Glance*. Birmingham, AL: University of Alabama at Birmingham. 2020. https://www.nscisc.uab.edu/Public/Facts%20and%20Figures%202019%20-%20Final.pdf. Accessed April 21, 2022
3. Berlowitz DJ, Wadsworth B, Ross J. Respiratory problems and management in people with spinal cord injury. *Breathe.* 2016;12(4):328-340.
4. Remaley DT, Jaeblon T. Pressure ulcers in orthopaedics. *J Am Acad Orthop Surg.* 2010;18(9):568-575.
5. Stephenson RO, Berliner J, Klein MG. Autonomic dysreflexia in spinal cord injury. *Medscape.* http://emedicine.medscape.com/article/322809-overview. Updated January 6, 2022. Accessed April 21, 2022.
6. Furusawa K, Tokuhiro A, Sugiyama H, et al. Incidence of symptomatic autonomic dysreflexia varies according to the bowel and bladder management techniques in patients with spinal cord injury. *Spinal Cord.* 2011;49(1):49-54.
7. Berger VM, Pölzer S, Nussbaum G, Ernst W, Major Z. Process development for the design and manufacturing of personalizable mouth sticks. *Stud Health Technol Inform.* 2017;242:437-444.
8. Ruff JC. Selection criteria for static and dynamic mouthsticks. *Gen Dent.* 1990;38(6):414-416.
9. U.S. National Library of Medicine, National Institutes of Health. Stroke. *Medline Plus.* Updated April 1, 2022. http://www.nlm.nih.gov/medlineplus/ency/article/000726.htm. Accessed April 21, 2022.

10. Moshfeghi M, Taheri JB, Bahemmat N, Evazzadeh ME, Hadian H. Relationship between carotid artery calcification detected in dental panoramic images and hypertension and myocardial infarction. *Iran J Radiol*. 2014;11(3):e8714.
11. Lim LZ, Koh PSF, Cao S, Wong RCW. Can carotid artery calcifications on dental radiographs predict adverse vascular events? A systematic review. *Clin Oral Investig*. 2021;25(1): 37-53. doi:10.1007/s00784-020-03696-5
12. Simonetto C, Mayinger M, Ahmed T, et al. Longitudinal atherosclerotic changes after radio(chemo)therapy of hypopharyngeal carcinoma. *Radiat Oncol*. 2020;15(1):102.
13. Warner MJ, Hutchison J, Varacallo M. Bell palsy. *StatPearls*. Treasure Island, FL. StatPearls Publishing; 2022. https://www.ncbi.nlm.nih.gov/books/NBK482290/#_NBK482290_pubdet. Accessed April 21, 2022
14. Gagyor I, Madhok VB, Daly F, Sullivan F. Antiviral treatment for Bell's palsy (idiopathic facial paralysis). *Cochrane Database Syst Rev*. 2019;9(9):CD001869.
15. Gagyor I, Madhok VB, Daly F, et al. Antiviral treatment for Bell's palsy (idiopathic facial paralysis). *Cochrane Database Syst Rev*. 2015;(11):CD001869.
16. National Institute of Neurological Disorders and Stroke. Bell's palsy fact sheet. Updated November 15, 2021. https://www.ninds.nih.gov/Disorders/Patient-Caregiver-Education/Fact-Sheets/Bells-Palsy-Fact-Sheet. NIH Publication Publication No. 18-NS-5114. Accessed April 22, 2022.
17. Mehta P, Raymond J, Punjani R, et al. Prevalence of amyotrophic lateral sclerosis (ALS), United States, 2016, *Amyotroph Lateral Scler Frontotemporal Degener*. 2021;1-6.
18. Holecek V, Rokyta R. Possible etiology and treatment of amyotrophic lateral sclerosis. *Neuro Endocrinol Lett*. 2018;38(8):528-531.
19. Norris SP, Likanje MN, Andrews JA. Amyotrophic lateral sclerosis: update on clinical management. *Curr Opin Neurol*. 2020;33(5):641-648.
20. National Institute of Neurological Disorders and Stroke. Amyotrophic lateral sclerosis (ALS) fact sheets. Updated March 1, 2022. https://www.ninds.nih.gov/Disorders/Patient-Caregiver-Education/Fact-Sheets/Amyotrophic-Lateral-Sclerosis-ALS-Fact-Sheet. NIH Publication No. 16-916. Accessed April 22, 2022.
21. Nakayama R, Nishiyama A, Matsuda C, Nakayama Y, Hakuta C, Shimada M. Oral health status of hospitalized amyotrophic lateral scle. Oral health status of hospitalized amyotrophic lateral sclerosis patients: a single-centre observational study. *Acta Odontol Scand*. 2017;26:1-5.
22. Wang Y, Yang X, Han Q, Liu M, Zhou C. Prevalence of sialorrhea among amyotrophic lateral sclerosis patients: a systematic review and meta-analysis. *J Pain Symptom Manage*. 2022;63(4):e387-e396.
23. Russo M, Bonanno C, Profazio C, et al. Which are the factors influencing NIV adaptation and tolerance in ALS patients? *Neurol Sci*. 2021;42(3):1023-1029.
24. Hogden A, Foley G, Henderson RD, James N, Aoun SM. Amyotrophic lateral sclerosis: improving care with a multidisciplinary approach. *J Multidiscip Healthc*. 2017;10:205-215.
25. National Institute of Neurological Disorders and Stroke. NINDS Parkinson's disease information page. Updated June 24, 2021. https://www.ninds.nih.gov/Disorders/All-Disorders/Parkinsons-Disease-Information-Page. Accessed April 21, 2022.
26. Parkinson's Disease Foundation. Understanding Parkinson's: Statistics. https://www.parkinson.org/Understanding-Parkinsons/Statistics. Accessed April 21, 2022.
27. Bollero P, Franco R, Cecchetti F, et al. Oral health and implant therapy in Parkinson's patients: review. *Oral Implantol*. 2017;10(2):105-111.
28. National Institute of Neurological Disorders and Strokes. Post-polio syndrome fact sheet. https://www.ninds.nih.gov/Disorders/Patient-Caregiver-Education/Fact-Sheets/Post-Polio-Syndrome-Fact-Sheet. NIH Publication No. 12-4030. Accessed April 21, 2022.
29. Haberle CB, Van Stewart A, Staat RH, Gettleman L, Sleamaker TF. Special considerations for treating dental patients exhibiting the "post-polio syndrome". *Spec Care Dentist*. 2001;21(5):167-171
30. National Institute of Neurological Disorders and Stroke. Cerebral palsy: hope through research. Updated September 29, 2021. https://www.ninds.nih.gov/Disorders/Patient-Caregiver-Education/Hope-Through-Research/Cerebral-Palsy-Hope-Through-Research. NIH Publication No. 13-159. 2013. Accessed April 21, 2022.
31. National Institutes of Health, National Institute of Dental and Craniofacial Research. Practical oral care for people with cerebral palsy. 2009. NIH Publication No. 09–519. https://www.nidcr.nih.gov/sites/default/files/2017-09/practical-oral-care-cerebral-palsy.pdf?_ga=2.207835090.1185165932.1522030188-79043338.1522030188. Accessed April 21, 2022.
32. Bensi C, Costacurta M, Docimo R. Oral health in children with cerebral palsy: a systematic review and meta-analysis. *Spec Care Dentist*. 2020;40(5):401-411.
33. Dougherty NJ. A review of cerebral palsy for the oral health professional. *Dent Clin North Am*. 2009;53(2):329-338.
34. National Institute of Neurological Disorders and Stroke. NINDS muscular dystrophy information page. Updated February 26, 2021. https://www.ninds.nih.gov/Disorders/All-Disorders/Muscular-Dystrophy-Information-Page. Accessed April 21, 2022.
35. Centers for Disease Control and Prevention. Muscular dystrophy: data and statistics. *MD STARnet data and statistics*. Reviewed October 27, 2020. https://www.cdc.gov/ncbddd/musculardystrophy/data.html. Accessed April 21, 2022.
36. U.S. National Library of Medicine, National Institutes of Health, Department of Health and Human Services: Genetics Home Reference Website. Facioscapulohumeral muscular dystrophy. Updated September 8, 2020. https://ghr.nlm.nih.gov/condition/facioscapulohumeral-muscular-dystrophy. Accessed April 21, 2022.
37. Muscular Dystrophy Association. Muscular dystrophy (DM). https://www.mda.org/disease/myotonic-dystrophy. Accessed April 21, 2022.
38. John Hopkins Medicine. Types of muscular dystrophy and neuromuscular diseases. https://www.hopkinsmedicine.org/health/conditions-and-diseases/types-of-muscular-dystrophy-and-neuromuscular-diseases. Accessed April 24, 2022.
39. National Institutes for Health, Eunice Kennedy Shriver National Institute of Child Health and Human Development. What are the treatments for muscular dystrophy? Reviewed November 9, 2020. https://www.nichd.nih.gov/health/topics/musculardys/conditioninfo/treatment. Accessed April 21, 2022.
40. Balasubramaniam R, Sollecito TP, Stoopler ET. Oral health considerations in muscular dystrophies. *Spec Care Dentist*. 2008;28(6):243-253.
41. Deavenport-Saman A, Britt A, Smith K, Jacobs RA. Milestones and controversies in maternal and child health: examining a brief history of micronutrient fortification in the US. *J Perinatol*. 2017;3(11):1180-1184.

42. Garg A, Utreja A, Singh SP, Angurana SK. Neural tube defects and their significance in clinical dentistry: a mini review. *J Investig Clin Dent*. 2013;4(1):3-8.
43. National Institute of Neurological Disorders and Stroke. Spina bifida fact sheet. https://www.ninds.nih.gov/Disorders/Patient-Caregiver-Education/Fact-Sheets/Spina-Bifida-Fact-Sheet. NIH Publication No. 21-NS-309. Accessed April 21, 2022.
44. U.S. National Library of Medicine, National Institutes of Health, MedlinePlus. Myelomeningocele. Updated April 1, 2022. http://www.nlm.nih.gov/medlineplus/ency/article/001558.htm. Accessed April 21, 2022.
45. American Academy of Pediatric Dentistry. Antibiotic prophylaxis for dental patients at risk for infection. In: *The Reference Manual of Pediatric Dentistry*. Chicago, IL: American Academy of Pediatric Dentistry; 2021:465-470. http://www.aapd.org/media/Policies_Guidelines/G_AntibioticProphylaxis.pdf. Accessed April 21, 2022.
46. Centers for Disease Control and Prevention. Osteoarthritis. Updated July 27, 2020. http://www.cdc.gov/arthritis/basics/osteoarthritis.htm. Accessed April 21, 2022.
47. Alfaraj A, Halawany HS, Al-Hinai MT, Al-Badr AH, Alalshaikh M, Al-Khalifa KS. Barriers to dental care in individuals with special healthcare needs in Qatif, Saudi Arabia: a caregiver's perspective. *Patient Prefer Adherence*. 2021;15:69-76.
48. Greig V, Sweeney P. Special care dentistry for general dental practice. *Dent Update*. 2013;40(6):452-454, 456-458, 460.
49. American Academy of Pediatric Dentistry. Management of dental patients with special health care needs. In: *The Reference Manual of Pediatric Dentistry*. Chicago, IL: American Academy of Pediatric Dentistry; 2021:287-294. https://www.aapd.org/globalassets/media/policies_guidelines/bp_shcn.pdf. Accessed April 21, 2022
50. Yitzhak M, Sarnat H, Rakocz M, Yaish Y, Ashkenazi M. The effect of toothbrush design on the ability of nurses to brush the teeth of institutionalized cerebral palsy patients. *Spec Care Dentist*. 2013;33(1):20-27.

CHAPTER 53

The Patient with an Endocrine Condition

Mary V. Tolentino, RDH, MS

CHAPTER OUTLINE

LEARNING OBJECTIVES

After studying this chapter, the student will be able to:

1. Identify the major endocrine glands and describe the functions of each.
2. Explain signs, symptoms, and potential oral manifestations of each endocrine gland disorder.
3. Describe hormonal effects and oral health risk factors commonly associated with puberty, menses, contraceptives, and menopause.

Overview of the Endocrine System

Endocrine **glands** secrete substances directly into the blood or lymph system. They secrete highly specialized substances (**hormones**) that, with the nervous system, maintain body **homeostasis**. Influences of the endocrine system on oral health and patient care are discussed in this chapter.

I. Glands of the Endocrine System

- The major endocrine glands, shown in **Figure 53-1**, are the pineal, pituitary, thyroid, parathyroid, and adrenal glands; hypothalamus; thymus; pancreas; and **gonads** (ovaries and testes).
- The anterior pituitary is called the master gland because it regulates the output of hormones by other glands.
- In turn, the pituitary itself is regulated by the hormones produced by the other endocrine glands.
- The endocrine glands and the hormones produced by each are listed in **Table 53-1**.

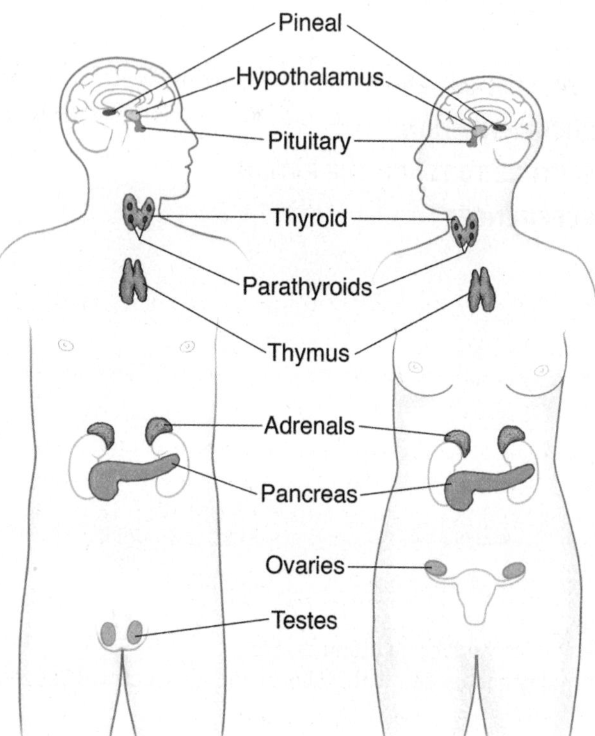

Figure 53-1 The Major Endocrine Glands. Illustrated here for both male and female, these glands produce hormones that regulate body systems.

Table 53-1 Endocrine Glands and the Hormones

Endocrine Gland	Hormone(s) Produced
Pineal	Melatonin
Hypothalamus	Controls hormone production in the pituitary gland
Pituitary	
Anterior	Prolactin Growth hormone Adrenocorticotropin Thyroid-stimulating hormone Luteinizing hormone Follicle-stimulating hormone
Posterior	Oxytocin Antidiuretic hormone (also called vasopressin)
Thyroid	Triiodothyronine (T_3) Thyroxin (T4)
Parathyroid	Parathyroid hormone
Thymus	Humoral factor hormones
Adrenals	
Adrenal cortex (outer portion)	Glucocorticoids (such as cortisol) Mineral corticoids (such as aldosterone)
Adrenal medulla (inner portion)	**Epinephrine** (adrenaline) **Norepinephrine**
Pancreas	Insulin
Gonads	
Testes (males)	Testosterone
Ovaries (females)	Estrogen Progesterone Inhibin

II. Hormones and Their Functions

- Hormones affect a number of major functions and are transported by the blood or lymph.
- Hormones may act directly on body cells or indirectly to control the hormones of other glands.
- Complex and unified actions of hormones produced by endocrine glands augment and regulate many vital functions, including[1]:
    - Growth and development.
    - Energy production.

- Food metabolism.
- Reproductive processes.
- Responses of the body to stress and temperature.

III. Regulation of Hormones

- Regulation of hormonal secretion is complex, and the mechanisms are not fully understood. Normally, hormones are secreted when needed.
- The stimulus for hormone secretion is often a chemical signal in the blood.
  - When the hormone is released, the signal disappears.
  - As more hormone is required, the signal reappears.
- This system of negative feedback works to provide hormones in optimal amounts and only in response to a need.
- Both hyposecretion and hypersecretion of a hormone can cause physical and mental disturbances.

Endocrine Gland Disorders

- When diseases affect the glands, hormones may be underproduced or overproduced, causing physical and biochemical changes that may have profound effects on the body, including the oral cavity.
- Presence or absence of a particular hormone may affect oral structures and may cause the host response to infection, healing, or stress to vary.[2]
- Many systemic diseases and disorders are risk indicators or risk factors for periodontal disease.
- Hormonal fluctuations associated with puberty, pregnancy, and menopause can affect the periodontium and directly modify the tissue's response to local factors.

Pituitary Gland

- The pituitary gland is composed of two functionally distinct portions:
  - Anterior pituitary.
  - Posterior pituitary.
- Each portion of the pituitary secretes different hormones.
- Excess or inadequate secretion of any of these hormones can cause severe problems for body functions.
- The anterior pituitary is called the "master gland" because of its great influence on body organs, other endocrine glands, and overall well-being.

I. Pituitary Tumors

- Adenomas are the most common pituitary tumors.
- These benign tumors:
  - Usually secrete too much of one hormone.
  - Can develop at any age.
- Types of pituitary adenomas include[3]:
  - Functioning tumor: causes the other endocrine glands to secrete excess hormones.
  - Nonfunctioning tumor: secretes excess hormones that are inactive due to cell development process and may not be detectable in blood tests.
- Other types of pituitary disorders include:
  - Craniopharyngiomas: benign tumors that grow near the pituitary gland; most common in children, teenagers, and adults older than 50.
  - Rathke cleft cysts: benign cysts in the pituitary gland.

II. Common Symptoms of Pituitary Disorders

- Headaches.
- Vision problems.
- Mood swings or behavioral changes.
- Weight change.
- Reproductive problems.
- Hypertension.

III. Oral Health Risk Assessment

During oral health assessment, the dental hygienist should recognize the patient with a pituitary gland disorder is at increased risk for:

- **Macrocephaly**.
- **Macrognathia**.
- Disproportionate mandibular growth: mandibular prognathism.
- Open anterior bite.
- Large pulp chambers.
- Delayed eruption of primary and secondary teeth.[2]
- Increased risk for periodontal disease due to growth factors and hormone imbalances.[4]

IV. Patient Management Considerations

- Orthodontic evaluation.
- Increased risk of hypertension.
- Increased risk of developing insulin resistance or type 2 diabetes.
- General anesthesia may be contraindicated due to electrolyte imbalance.

Thyroid Gland

- Thyroid hormone receptors are present in almost every tissue in the body.
- This hormone plays a big role in normal physiologic function in the body including growth and development and energy metabolism.[5]
- Levothyroxine (Synthroid), used to treat thyroid gland disorders, is the third most common drug prescribed in the United States.[6]

I. Hypothyroidism

- Hypothyroidism, the most common thyroid disorder, occurs when the thyroid does not produce enough thyroid hormone.[7]
- It is more common in women than in men. Hypothyroidism develops slowly and is more common in people older than 60 years.
- Untreated or inadequately controlled hypothyroidism may cause an increased susceptibility to infections.
- The most common cause is an autoimmune disorder called Hashimoto disease.
- Characteristics and oral manifestations of hypothyroidism[8] are listed in **Table 53-2**.
- Oral health risk assessment: because of the autoimmune response, patients with hypothyroidism are at an increased risk for:
  - Periodontitis.[8]
  - Oral candidiasis.
  - Easily bleeding gingiva.
  - Poor wound healing.
- Medical management: treatment is levothyroxine with lifelong monitoring.
- Patient management considerations:
  - Monitor vitals: blood pressure and pulse.
  - Avoid aspirin due to increased gingival bleeding and poor wound healing.
  - Increased risk for **myxedema coma** due to long-standing low levels of thyroid hormone in the blood.
  - Myxedema coma is a life-threatening emergency. Triggers for myxedema coma are listed in **Box 53-1**.

II. Hyperthyroidism

- When the thyroid gland produces too much thyroid hormone, also referred to as overactive thyroid, it is called hyperthyroidism.[7,8]
- This can occur over a short or long period of time.

Table 53-2 Characteristics of Thyroid Disorders

Hypothyroidism	
Hashimoto **thyroiditis** **Congenital hypothyroidism**	
General Characteristics	**Oral Manifestations**
▪ Fatigue ▪ Intolerant to cold ▪ Weight gain—decreased metabolic rate ▪ Constipation ▪ Decreased concentration ▪ Bradycardia ▪ Muscle cramps and pain ▪ **Myxedema**	▪ Macroglossia ▪ Salivary gland enlargement ▪ Facial myxedema ▪ Increased dental caries ▪ Compromised periodontal health ▪ Delayed tooth eruption ▪ Delayed wound healing ▪ Hoarse voice ▪ Burning mouth syndrome ▪ Xerostomia ▪ Lichen planus
Hyperthyroidism	
Graves' disease—autoimmune Thyroid storm (**thyrotoxic crisis**)	
General Characteristics	**Oral Manifestations**
▪ Fatigue ▪ Intolerant to heat ▪ Increased appetite ▪ Weight loss ▪ Tremor ▪ Protrusion of the eyes ▪ Excess sweating ▪ Enlargement of thyroid gland	▪ Difficulty swallowing ▪ Increased dental caries ▪ Increased periodontal disease ▪ Macroglossia ▪ Accelerated development of teeth and jaws

- Causes include:
  - Excess of iodine in the diet.
  - Graves' disease (autoimmune disorder that affects the thyroid).
  - Viral infection.
  - Taking too much thyroid hormone medication.
- Characteristics and oral manifestations of hyperthyroidism are listed in Table 53-2.
- Oral health risk assessment:
  - Accelerated tooth development, potential for malocclusion.
  - Analgesics can increase the amount of thyroid hormones, making it more difficult to control hyperthyroidism.

Box 53-1 Triggers for Myxedema Coma in a Patient with Hypothyroidism

- Drugs (especially sedatives, narcotics, anesthesia).
- Infections.
- Stroke.
- Trauma.
- Heart failure.
- Gastrointestinal bleeding.
- Hypothermia.
- Failure to take thyroid medications.

  - Vasoconstrictors are used with caution in patients with uncontrolled hyperthyroidism, as these may increase symptoms of tachycardia.[7]
- Patient management considerations:
  - Check vitals: blood pressure and pulse.
  - **Thyroid crisis (thyroid storm)** is a sudden worsening of hyperthyroidism symptoms, which can be caused by an infection or stress. Immediate hospitalization is necessary.

Parathyroid Glands

As the parathyroid glands develop, they become embedded in the thyroid gland. Secretion of the parathyroid hormone (PTH) is in response to the serum-ionized calcium.[9,10]

- The hormone controls calcium, phosphorus, and vitamin D levels in the blood and bone.
- All parathyroid gland disorders are rare. The most common cause of hypoparathyroidism is when the glands are accidently removed during a thyroidectomy.

I. Hyperparathyroidism

- Occurs when the parathyroid glands produce too much PTH.
- Can cause long-standing hypercalcemia, which may result in osteoporosis.
- Symptoms of hyperparathyroidism:
  - Bone pain.
  - Depression.
  - Fatigue.
  - Frequent broken bones.
  - Kidney stones.
  - Nausea.
  - Loss of appetite.
- Oral health risk assessment:
  - Loss of alveolar bone evident in dental images.
  - Spontaneous mandibular fracture.
  - Widened pulp chambers.
  - Demineralized teeth.
- Patient management considerations:
  - Home fluoride therapy.
  - Increased risk of osteoporosis.

II. Hypoparathyroidism

- Hypoparathyroidism occurs when the glands produce insufficient PTH.
  - Causes the blood calcium levels to decrease and phosphorus levels to increase.
  - Most common cause is injury to the parathyroid glands during thyroid and neck surgery.
- Symptoms[11]:
  - Abdominal pain.
  - Brittle nails.
  - Dry hair.
  - Muscle cramps.
  - Muscle spasms (tetany).
  - Increased muscular and peripheral nerve irritability.
- Oral care risk assessment[8]:
  - Delayed teeth eruption.
  - Congenitally missing teeth.
  - Shortened roots.
  - Delay or cessation of dental development.
  - Enamel hypoplasia.
  - Poorly calcified dentin.
  - Widened pulp chambers.
  - Mandibular tori.
  - Chronic candidiasis.
  - Paresthesia of the tongue or lips.
  - Twitching or spasm of the facial muscles.
- Medical management: calcium supplements needed.
- Patient management considerations:
  - Home fluoride therapy.
  - Antifungal medication to treat chronic candidiasis.

Adrenal Glands

- The adrenal glands consist of a pair of glands that sit at the top of each kidney.
- The glands are composed of an outer cortex and an inner medulla.

- The adrenal glands work with the hypothalamus and the pituitary gland to produce adrenaline, noradrenaline, dopamine, progesterone, and glucocorticoids.
- Treatment for adrenal gland disorders is corticosteroids.

I. Hyperadrenalism/Cushing's Syndrome

Cushing's syndrome, also called hypercortisolism, is caused by too much cortisol production. Increased production of cortisol can be caused by a tumor in the anterior pituitary, a tumor in the adrenal gland, or exogenous administration of steroids.

- Symptoms[11]:
  - Weight gain.
  - Broad, round face.
  - "Buffalo hump."
  - Hypertension.
  - Impaired healing.
  - **Hypokalemia**.
  - Hyperglycemia, glycosuria, polydipsia (mimics diabetes mellitus).
  - Increased bone fractures.
  - Mood swings and depression.
- Oral health risk assessment:
  - Increased melanotic pigmentation may develop black-bluish areas affecting the buccal mucosa, palate, tongue, and lips.
  - Delayed wound healing.
  - Loss of collagen.
  - Skin and oral tissues are fragile.
  - Oral candidiasis.
- Medical management: surgery or radiation.
- Patient management considerations:
  - Antifungal treatment.
  - Antiviral medication.

II. Hypoadrenalism/Addison's Disease/Adrenal Insufficiency

- Hypoadrenalism is divided into three categories:
  - Primary acute (adrenal crisis) failure of the gland to produce cortisol and aldosterone.
  - Primary chronic adrenocortical insufficiency: Addison's disease (an autoimmune disease), also called adrenal insufficiency or hypocortisolism.
  - Secondary adrenocortical insufficiency: rapid withdrawal of steroids or insufficient steroid supplements combined with acute stress (infections, trauma, or surgical procedures) may precipitate an adrenal crisis.
- Symptoms of adrenal crisis, a life-threatening emergency, are listed in **Box 53-2**.
- Symptoms of hypoadrenalism include:
  - Progressive weakness, fatigue.
  - Gastrointestinal disturbances (anorexia, nausea, vomiting, diarrhea).
  - **Hyperkalemia**.
  - **Hypernatremia**.
  - Hypotension.
  - Diaphoresis.
  - Weight loss.
  - Hypoglycemia.
- Oral health risk assessment[11,12]:
  - Hyperpigmentation of the skin and mucosal surfaces.
  - Long-term immune suppression may lead to Kaposi sarcoma, lymphoma, or lip cancer.[6]
  - Oral candidiasis.
- Medical management: treatment is long-term steroid use, which is important to patient management due to increased risk for infection, increased bleeding, and poor healing.
- Patient management considerations:
  - Monitor vital signs: blood pressure and pulse.
  - Provide antifungal medications to treat candidiasis.
  - Provide pain control to avoid stress and invoking an adrenal crisis.
  - Consider antianxiety medications prior to dental treatment.
  - Delay nonemergency dental treatment until condition is stable or well-controlled by medication.

Box 53-2 Symptoms of Adrenal Crisis

- Abdominal pain.
- High fever.
- Loss of appetite.
- Nausea.
- Excessive sweating on face or palms.
- Rapid respiratory rate.
- Darkening of the skin.
- Confusion.
- Dizziness.
- Low blood pressure.
- Rapid heart rate.
- Vomiting.
- Joint pain.
- Dehydration.

Pancreas

- Produces insulin to regulate blood glucose by way of the islets of Langerhans.
- Dysfunction of these cells leads to **insulin resistance** and diabetes.[13,14]
- Diabetes is a disease of metabolism with inadequate production or inferior processing of the hormone insulin.[13,14]
- There is strong evidence that prevalence of thyroid disease is higher in individuals who also have diabetes.[15]
- Diabetes, the most common disorder of the pancreas, is covered in Chapter 54.

Puberty

I. Stages of Adolescence

- The period of life considered **adolescence** is represented by the years between ages 11 and 21.
- The adolescent years, which include puberty, are marked by hormonal fluctuations as well as many physical and psychosocial changes. (See Chapter 47.)
- From a psychosocial aspect, this period can be divided into three overlapping phases:
  - Early adolescence, approximately ages 11–13 years.
  - Middle adolescence, approximately ages 14–17 years.
  - Late adolescence, approximately ages 18–21 years.

II. Pubertal Changes

- **Puberty** is a dynamic period of development marked by rapid changes in body size, shape, and composition.[13]
- Some individuals go through changes earlier and faster than others.
- Physiologic changes occur due to hormone production and secretion by the **endocrine** glands, especially the gonads.
- In males, the testes produce testosterone hormones, and in females, the ovaries produce estrogen, progesterone, and inhibin hormones.
- Onset of **menarche** in females varies, but more commonly occurs during puberty.

A. Hormonal Influences

- Pituitary hormones control the hormones produced by the ovaries and the testes.
- The several hormones produced by the ovaries are known collectively as estrogens, and those produced by the testes are called androgens.
- Responsible for the development of the sex organs, the accessory sex organs, and the secondary sex characteristics.
- As the levels of these hormones fluctuate during adolescence, they have strong physical, mental, and emotional influences throughout the body.

B. Oral Health Risk Assessment[14]

- Gingival inflammation due to the release of increased sex hormones.
- Diet analysis recommended to explore dietary-related dental disease patterns.
- Hyperplastic gingiva related to orthodontic appliances.
- Acute intraoral infections involving the periodontium require immediate treatment.
- Periodontal infection may be localized or generalized. (See Chapter 19.)

III. Patient Management Considerations

Additional information about oral health risk factors and patient management considerations for the adolescent patient are found in Chapter 47.

Women's Health

I. Menstrual Cycle

- The menstrual cycle, illustrated in **Figure 53-2**, is the period from the beginning of one menstrual flow to the beginning of the next menstrual flow.[15]
- The average cycle takes approximately 28 days.
- Menstruation or **menses** occurs in a cyclical manner (lasting 4–6 days) from puberty to menopause.
- The rise and fall of hormone levels during the month control the menstrual cycle.

A. Characteristics

- Estrogen levels rise during the first half of the cycle to prepare the **endometrium** for pregnancy.
- If conception does not occur, estrogen levels decrease and menstruation begins.
- Variations in the cycle are common.
- Factors affecting the cycle: changes in climate, changes in work schedule, emotional trauma,

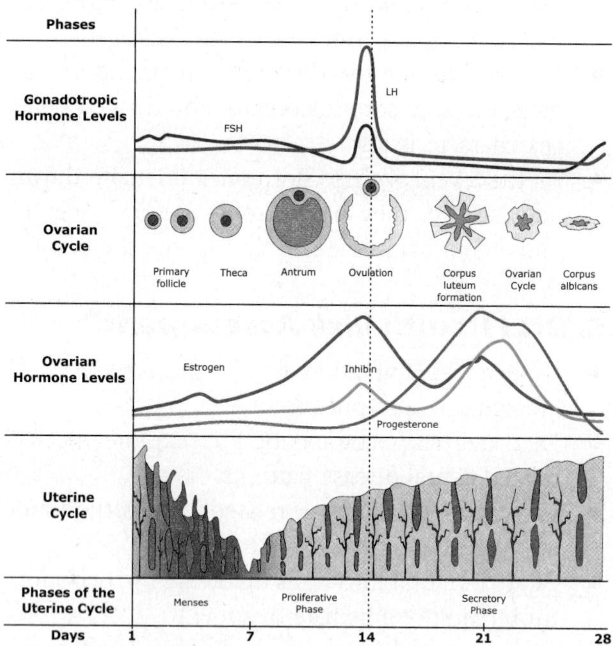

Figure 53-2 Changes during the Menstrual Cycle. The 28 days of a normal cycle are shown, with ovulation between days 12 and 15 and menstrual flow between days 1 and 5 and again at day 28. Hormonal levels **(A)** show the estrogen peak shortly before ovulation during the follicular phase **(B)** of the ovary and the proliferative phase **(C)** of the uterus. The endometrium **(D)** builds up at the end of each menstrual flow. This prepares the area for possible implantation of a fertilized ovum.

acute or chronic illnesses, weight loss, or excessive exercise.

- **Premenstrual syndrome** may occur 7–10 days before menstruation. Symptoms may include fatigue, headache, bloating, **mastalgia**, skin breakouts, cramps, food cravings, depression, anxiety, irritability, hostility, tearfulness, mood changes, reduced ability to concentrate.[16]

B. Oral Health Risk Assessment

- Exaggerated response to local irritants or unusual gingival bleeding may be noted.[17]
- Patient may experience no specific gingival changes.

C. Patient Management Considerations

- Menstruation is normal and shows the body is healthy and functioning normally.
- Question women on the regularity of their menstrual cycle. Irregularity may reflect general health problems.
- Prevention through dental biofilm control, oral self-care measures, and removal of calculus at regular maintenance appointments can reduce oral effects of hormone imbalance during menstruation.

II. Hormonal Contraceptives

A variety of effective forms of hormonal contraceptives containing estrogen and progestin is available by prescription.[18] Delivery methods include:

- Oral contraceptives (birth control pills).
- Implantable rod: contains hormones to prevent pregnancy; commonly implanted under the skin inside the upper arm.
- Intramuscular injection: contains hormones to prevent pregnancy; one shot lasts for 12 weeks.
- Patch: a transdermal patch applied to the skin releases hormones to prevent pregnancy.
- Ring: a small, flexible ring that releases hormones to prevent pregnancy inserted into the vagina once a month.
- Sponge: a round piece of plastic foam inserted into the vagina to block sperm from entering the uterus. Also contains a spermicide.

A. Estrogen and Progestin

- A combination of synthetic hormones estrogen and progestin is nearly 100% effective in preventing pregnancy when taken appropriately.
- Oral contraceptives inhibit the release of gonadotropin-releasing hormones, without which the ovum cannot be released from the ovary.

B. Oral Health Risk Assessment

- An exaggerated response to dental biofilm and other local irritants has been noted in patients who use any type of contraceptive.[19] The gingival response is similar to that described for pregnancy. (See Chapter 46.)
- Record the use of oral contraceptives each time the medical history is updated.

III. Menopause[20]

- **Menopause** is the complete and permanent cessation of menstrual flow.
- Menopause generally occurs between the ages of 47 and 55 years.
- Signals the end of fertility due to decreased production of estrogen and progesterone by the ovaries.

- Menopause is usually confirmed when a woman has no menstrual period for 12 consecutive months and there is no other cause for this change.

A. Characteristics

- Before menopause, menstruation changes in frequency, duration, and amount of flow over a period of about 12–24 months.
- Menopause is accompanied by a number of characteristic physiologic hormonal-based changes.
- Many women experience only minor symptoms; a small percentage have increased symptoms during menopause.

B. General Symptoms

As ovarian function declines with diminishing estrogen, physiologic changes in body function include[20,21]:

- Vasomotor reactions:
  - Hot flashes, defined as periodic surges of heat involving the whole body; may be accompanied by drenching sweats.
  - Hot flash may begin with a headache; proceed to a flushing of the face, with heart palpitations, and dizziness; followed by a chill.
  - Episodes may last a few minutes or more than 30 minutes.
  - Night sweats and sleeping problems may lead to feeling tired, stressed, or tense.
- Mucosal changes:
  - Associated with fluctuating and decreasing estrogen levels.
  - Dryness, irritation, and thinning of tissue may occur.
  - Frequent vaginal infections may occur.
- Emotional disturbances:
  - Alterations in estrogen level may result in mood swings, depression, irritability, and difficulty with concentration or memory.
  - Decreased **libido** and changes in sexual response.
  - Some women experience anxiety, tension, and irritability and feel useless.
  - Weight gain or increase of body fat around the waist.

C. Postmenopausal Effects

- Reproductive organs atrophy.
- Osteopenia and osteoporosis have been associated with menopause.
- Skin and mucous membranes decrease in thickness and keratinization, becoming fragile and easily injured.
- Predisposition to conditions including atherosclerosis, diabetes, and hypothyroidism.

D. Burning Mouth Syndrome

- Burning sensation in the mouth with the absence of an identifiable oral lesion.[22]
- Described as burning, tingling, hot, scalding, numbness.[22]
- Cause is unknown. Very common in menopausal women.
- Treatment includes benzodiazepines, antidepressants, or analgesics.

E. Oral Health Risk Assessment

- Oral changes can be related to menopause, but they are not a common feature.
- Gingival changes[21,23]:
  - Gingival changes associated with menopause usually represent an exaggerated response to dental biofilm.
  - Hormonal changes influence oral tissue response.
  - Menopausal gingivostomatitis may develop. It may also occur after removal of, or radiation therapy to, the ovaries.
- Changes to mucous membranes and tongue[24]
  - Tissue may appear shiny and may vary in color from abnormal paleness to redness. Dryness with burning sensations may be present.
  - Burning mouth syndrome may occur.
  - Altered salivary composition in some menopausal women may be due to psychological stress.
  - Epithelium may become thin and atrophic with decreased keratinization; tolerance for removable prostheses may lessen, especially with **xerostomia**.
  - Taste perception may be altered, described as salty, peppery, or sour.
  - Inadequate diet and eating habits may contribute to adverse changes of the mucosal tissues. The appearance and symptoms frequently resemble those associated with vitamin deficiencies, particularly B vitamins.
- Alveolar bone loss
  - As a result of systemic osteoporosis, ridge resorption and loss of teeth can occur.[25]
  - Osteoporotic jaws may be unsuitable for conventional prosthetic devices or dental implants.

IV. Patient Management Considerations

- During patient education, the relationship of oral conditions to endocrine disorders or hormonal fluctuation is considered.
- Emphasize the need for oral self-care measures due to hormonal fluctuations or imbalances.
- Consider oral effects of medications used to treat endocrine disorders and conditions.
- Control of local factors through preventive dental hygiene appointments will supplement daily personal oral care.
- Create an environment that decreases the stress level for the patient.

A. Patient Approach

- Review and update the patient's health history.
- Rapport begins with the clinician's courtesy; personal attention; and friendly, unhurried manner.
- Give particular attention to details, such as seating the patient promptly, handling materials and instruments efficiently and with calm assurance.

B. Instruction of Patient

- Saliva substitute may be needed to provide relief from xerostomia and aid in the prevention of dental caries.
- Measures for the prevention of periodontal infections can be carefully explained.
- Emphasize reasons for frequent calculus removal as a supplement to meticulous daily self-care.
- Explain the relationship between good general health and oral health.

C. Diet

- Dietary assessment may help the patient identify and make healthy food choices. (Refer to Chapter 33.)
- Recommend whole grain products, vegetables, and fruits. Choose foods low in fat and cholesterol. Recommend calcium to keep bones strong. Limit alcohol intake.
- Caries prevention through selection of nutritious and noncariogenic foods is especially important for the patient who snacks frequently.

D. Fluoride Therapy

- Fluoride recommendations are based on assessment of the patient's dental caries risk status. (Refer to Chapter 25.)

Documentation

When documenting care for a patient with oral manifestations related to hormonal fluctuations, factors to document include:

- Patient's age and gender.
- Description of the patient's health status related to any endocrine disorder or hormone fluctuations.
- Symptoms and oral manifestations related to hormonal fluctuations.
- **Box 53-3** provides an example documentation for a patient with an oral manifestation related to a reproductive hormone fluctuation.

Box 53-3 Example Documentation: Female Patient with Gingivitis due to Hormonal Fluctuation

- **S**—A 13-year-old female patient reports for routine dental hygiene care. Patient stated she has stopped flossing because her gums have been bleeding every time she does.
- **O**—Health history review with patient and parent indicates recent onset of menarche. Examination findings include increased biofilm levels compared to previous findings, extreme maxillary anterior gingivitis, moderate bleeding, and increased sensitivity to instrumentation.
- **A**—Gingival health appears to be exacerbated by hormonal fluctuations related to patient's irregular menstrual cycle as well as her recent reluctance to provide adequate self-care.
- **P**—Motivational interviewing approach to patient education discovers that patient values her beautiful smile. Patient agreed to concentrate on careful, complete daily biofilm removal in order to reduce what she called "disgusting and ugly" gingival redness, swelling, and bleeding. Flossing instruction provided.

Next steps: Patient scheduled for 3-month follow-up maintenance appointment.

Signed: ______________________, RDH

Date: ______________________

Factors to Teach the Patient

- Self-care procedures necessary to maintain good oral health.
- The long-term impact of health behaviors, including lifestyle choices and risk reduction.
- The benefits of fluoride throughout life.
- The importance of nutrition, exercise, and sleep for good health.
- The value of seeking professional help when problems arise.

References

1. Melmed S, Koenig R, Rosen C, Auchus R, Goldfine A. *Williams Textbook of Endocrinology*. 14th ed. Philadelphia, PA: Elsevier Health Sciences; 2019.
2. Scaramucci T, Guglielmi CAB, Fonoff RD, Zardetto CG. Oral manifestations associated with multiple pituitary hormone deficiency and ectopic neurohypophysis. *J Clin Pediatr Dent*. 2011;35(4):409-414.
3. Johns Hopkins Medicine. *Types of pituitary tumors*. Boston, MA: Johns Hopkins. http://www.hopkinsmedicine.org/neurology_neurosurgery/specialty_areas/pituitary_center/pituitary-tumor/types/. Accessed October, 4, 2021.
4. Britto IMPA, Aguiar-Oliveira MH, Oliveira-Neto LA, et al. Periodontal disease in adults with untreated congenital growth hormone deficiency: a case control study. *J Clin Periodontol*. 2011;38:525-531.
5. Little JW. Thyroid disorders. Part II: hypothyroidism and thyroiditis. *Oral Surg Oral Med Oral Pathol Oral Radiol Endod*. 2006;102(2):148-153.
6. Centers for Disease Control and Prevention, National Center for Health Statistics. National ambulatory medical care survey: 2018 state and national summary tables. Updated 2018. https://www.cdc.gov/nchs/data/ahcd/namcs_summary/2018-namcs-web-tables-508.pdf. Accessed October 4, 2021.
7. Rodgers GP. Hypothroidism: symptoms, diagnosis & treatment. *NIH Medline Plus*. 2012;7(1):24-25.
8. Zahid TM, Want BY, Cohen RE. The effects of thyroid hormone abnormalities on periodontal disease status. *J Int Acad Periodontol*. 2011;13(3):80-85.
9. Jain M, Krasne DL, Singer FR, Giuliano AE. Recurrent primary hyperparathyroidism due to type 1 parathyromatosis. *Endocrine*. 2017;55(2):643-650.
10. Rees TD. Endocrine and metabolic disorders. In: Patton LL, Glick M, ed. *The ADA Practical Guide to Patients with Medical Conditions*. 2nd ed. Wiley Blackwell; 2016:71-99.
11. Fabue LC, Soriano YJ, Perex MGS. Dental management of patients with endocrine disorders. *J Clin Exp Dent*. 2010;2(4):e196-e203.
12. Bornstein SR. Predisposing factors for adrenal insufficiency. *N Engl J Med*. 2009;360:2328-2339.
13. National Center for Chronic Disease Prevention and Health Promotion, Division of Diabetes Translation. *National diabetes statistics report, 2020. Estimates of diabetes and its burden in the United States*. Atlanta, GA: Centers for Disease Control and Prevention; 2020. https://www.cdc.gov/diabetes/pdfs/data/statistics/national-diabetes-statistics-report.pdf. Accessed October 4, 2021.
14. National Institute of Diabetes and Digestive and Kidney Diseases. Diabetes overview. What is diabetes? https://www.niddk.nih.gov/health-information/diabetes/overview/what-is-diabetes. Accessed October 4, 2021.
15. Wang C. The relationship between type 2 diabetes mellitus and related thyroid diseases. *J Diabetes Res*. 2013:2013;1-9.
16. U.S. National Library of Medicine. Puberty. *Medline Plus*. Updated March 29, 2022. https://medlineplus.gov/puberty.html. Accessed April 7, 2022
17. American Academy of Pediatric Dentistry. Adolescent oral health care. In: *The Reference Manual of Pediatric Dentistry*. Chicago, IL: American Academy of Pediatric Dentistry; 2021: 267-276.
18. U.S. Food and Drug Administration. Birth Control. For consumers. Birth control. https://www.fda.gov/media/150299/download. Accessed October 15, 2021.
19. Farhad SZ, Esfahanian V, Mafi M, et al. Association between oral contraceptive use and interleukin-6 levels and periodontal health. *J Periodontol Implant Dent*. 2014;6(1):13-17.
20. Yonkers KA, Casper RF. Clinical manifestations and diagnosis of premenstrual syndrome and premenstrual dysphoric disorder. *UpToDate*. Updated March 25, 2022. http://www.uptodate.com/contents/clinical-manifestations-and-diagnosis-of-premenstrual-syndrome-and-premenstrual-dysphoric-disorder. Accessed April 7, 2022.
21. U.S. Department of Health and Human Services. *Menopause*. Updated March 18, 2019. http://womenshealth.gov/menopause/menopause-basics/. Accessed October 15, 2021.
22. Teruel A, Patel S. Burning mouth syndrome: a review of etiology, diagnosis, and management. *Gen Dent*. 2019;67(2): 24-29.
23. American Academy of Periodontology. *Gum disease and women*. Chicago, IL: American Academy of Periodontology. http://www.perio.org/consumer/women.htm. Accessed April 7, 2022.
24. Meurman JH, Tarkkila L, Tiitinen A. The menopause and oral health. *Maturitas*. 2009;63:56-62.
25. Juluri R, Prashanth E, Gopalakrishnan D, et al. Association of postmenopausal osteoporosis and periodontal disease: a double-blind case-control study. *J Int Oral Health*. 2015;7(9): 119-123.

CHAPTER 54

The Patient with Diabetes Mellitus

Linda D. Boyd, RDH, RD, EdD

CHAPTER OUTLINE

LEARNING OBJECTIVES

After studying this chapter, the student will be able to:

1. Describe the types of diabetes mellitus and major characteristics of each.
2. Explain current knowledge about the oral health–diabetes link.
3. Describe the risk factors and criteria used for diagnosis of prediabetes and diabetes.
4. Summarize the lifestyle modifications and medications used to prevent and manage diabetes.
5. Identify the key messages dental hygienists need to convey to patients with diabetes.

Dental professionals have a significant responsibility to:

- Recognize signs and symptoms of diabetes to promote early diagnosis in order to reduce life-threatening complications of the disease and improve quality of life.
- Assess the management and control of diabetes to determine the impact on dental treatment and oral health of the patient.
- Work with the patient and interprofessional collaboration to provide preventive oral care aimed at maintaining health and preventing infections and emergencies.
- Understand the presence of infection, including periodontitis, may make it more difficult to control the blood glucose levels in diabetes.
- Identify and treat acute emergencies.

Diabetes Mellitus

I. Definition

- Diabetes mellitus is a group of metabolic diseases associated with dysregulation of blood glucose.[1]
- Hyperglycemia results from an absolute **insulin** deficiency, inadequate secretion of insulin, and/or resistance to insulin action.[1]
- People with poorly controlled diabetes mellitus are at risk of complications including[1]:
  - **Retinopathy** (loss of vision).
  - Kidney failure.
  - Atherosclerotic cardiovascular disease (i.e., coronary heart disease), cerebrovascular disease (stroke), and peripheral arterial disease.
  - Peripheral neuropathy (nerve damage of extremities) with increased risk for amputation of toes, feet, and legs.

II. Diabetes Impact

A. Prediabetes Prevalence

- In the United States, 96 million adults, more than 1 in 3, have prediabetes.[2]
  - Nearly half (48.8%) of those aged 65 years and older have prediabetes.
  - Prediabetes prevalence is similar among racial and ethnic groups.

B. Diabetes Mellitus Prevalence

- In the United States, 37.3 million adults (11.3% of the population) have diabetes.[2]
  - Approximately 23 million people (8.5% of the population), or 1 in 4, with diabetes are undiagnosed.
  - American Indian/Alaska Natives (14.5%), non-Hispanic blacks (12.1%), and Hispanics (11.8%) have the highest prevalence of diabetes.
  - The southern states and the Appalachian regions have the highest prevalence of diagnosed diabetes.[3]
  - 283,000 children and adolescents younger than 20 years have been diagnosed with diabetes.[2]
- As the population ages and with increases in obesity, diabetes has become more prevalent.
- Diabetes is the most expensive of chronic conditions with an annual total cost of $327 billion in the United States (US). The US spends $1 of every $4 in healthcare costs on diabetes care.[4]
- Globally, 537 million adults or 1 in 10 adults have diabetes.[5]
  - Health expenditures due to diabetes globally are estimated to be 996 billion in US dollars.

Oral Health Implications of Diabetes Mellitus

- Infection that does not respond to treatment and/or tissues that do not heal may be a sign of undiagnosed diabetes.
- Oral findings associated with diabetes can be found in **Table 54-1**.

- Conducting a Prediabetes Risk Test (www.cdc.gov/prediabetes/takethetest/) or Diabetes Risk Test (www.diabetes.org/risk-test or www.healthycanadians.gc.ca/en/canrisk) may help to identify those patients needing referral to a primary care provider for evaluation and diagnosis.[6-8]

Table 54-1 Extraoral/Intraoral Findings Associated with Diabetes[9,10]

Location	Findings
Gingiva	Increased gingival inflammation
Periodontium	Periodontitis: more frequent, severe, longer duration Attachment loss: more frequent, more extensive Probing depths: more teeth with deep pockets Tooth mobility and migration: increased Healing: delayed, increased infection after surgery
Teeth	Poorly controlled diabetes: increased risk of caries (including root caries) related to decreased saliva, diet, and less successful resolution of endodontic therapy related to decreased resistance to infection
Saliva	Glucose in sulcular fluid Xerostomia: contributes to opportunistic infection such as oral candidiasis
Mucosa	Edematous and red color Oral candidiasis Burning mouth and/or tongue, burning mouth syndrome Poor tolerance for removable prostheses Delayed healing May have increased prevalence of lichen planus and aphthous stomatitis
Taste	**Hypogeusia** (diminished taste perception)
Neck	Acanthosis nigricans is a skin condition with a light brown to black appearance in the creases on the neck and in other areas

I. Relationship between Diabetes and Periodontal Disease

- The association of diabetes mellitus with periodontal disease is hypothesized to be related to the inflammatory process involved in the pathogenesis of both diseases.[11,12]

A. Diabetes as a Risk Factor for Periodontitis

- Systematic review suggests patients with diabetes are at a two to four times greater risk for more severe periodontal disease than individuals without diabetes.[12]

B. Effect of Periodontitis on Glycemic Control

- Evidence indicates individuals with diabetes had more severe periodontal disease and a higher **A1c** than healthy individuals.[11,12]

C. Effect of Periodontal Treatment on Diabetes

- Nonsurgical periodontal therapy and management of periodontal disease have resulted in an average decrease in A1c of 0.02% to 1.18% after 6 months.[11]
  - This is roughly equivalent to decreases seen with increased physical activity (–0.15%) and weight loss (–1.1 to –1.6%) in intervention studies.[13,14]
  - Antihyperglycemic medications lower A1c from 0.5% to 1.4%.[15]
  - Management of periodontitis along with lifestyle changes may have an additive effect in lowering A1c.

II. Dental Caries

- Adolescents with diabetes are at two to three times higher risk of dental caries than those without diabetes.[16]
- In adults with diabetes, there is also a higher risk for caries, including root caries.[17]

III. Endodontic Infections

- Patients with diabetes have increased periodontal disease in teeth involved endodontically and have a reduced likelihood of success of root canal treatment.[18]

IV. Dental Implants

- A meta-analysis found the failure rate for dental implants was similar between individuals with and without diabetes.[19]

Basics about Insulin

I. Definition

- Insulin is a hormone produced by **beta cells** in the pancreas.
- Insulin directly or indirectly affects every organ in the body.

II. Description

- The beta cells of the pancreas are responsible for releasing insulin when stimulated by nutrients, primarily glucose.
- Insulin acts like a key to unlock the cell to allow uptake of glucose to use as energy.
- **Figure 54-1A** shows the healthy pancreas and the action of insulin as it is taken up by the body cells.

III. Functions

The functions of insulin are listed in **Box 54-1**. Without insulin, glucose accumulates in the blood, resulting in hyperglycemia, which in the long term results in damage to the cells and tissues throughout the body.

- The normal fasting blood glucose levels in healthy individuals is below 100 mg/dL (<5.4 mmol/L), and the hemoglobin A1c is less than 5.7%.[1]

Box 54-1 Functions of Insulin

1. Facilitates glucose uptake from blood into tissues, which lowers blood glucose level.
2. Speeds the oxidation of glucose within the cells to use for energy.
3. Speeds the conversion of glucose to glycogen to store in the liver and skeletal muscles and to prevent the conversion of glycogen back to glucose.
4. Facilitates the conversion of glucose to fat in adipose tissue.

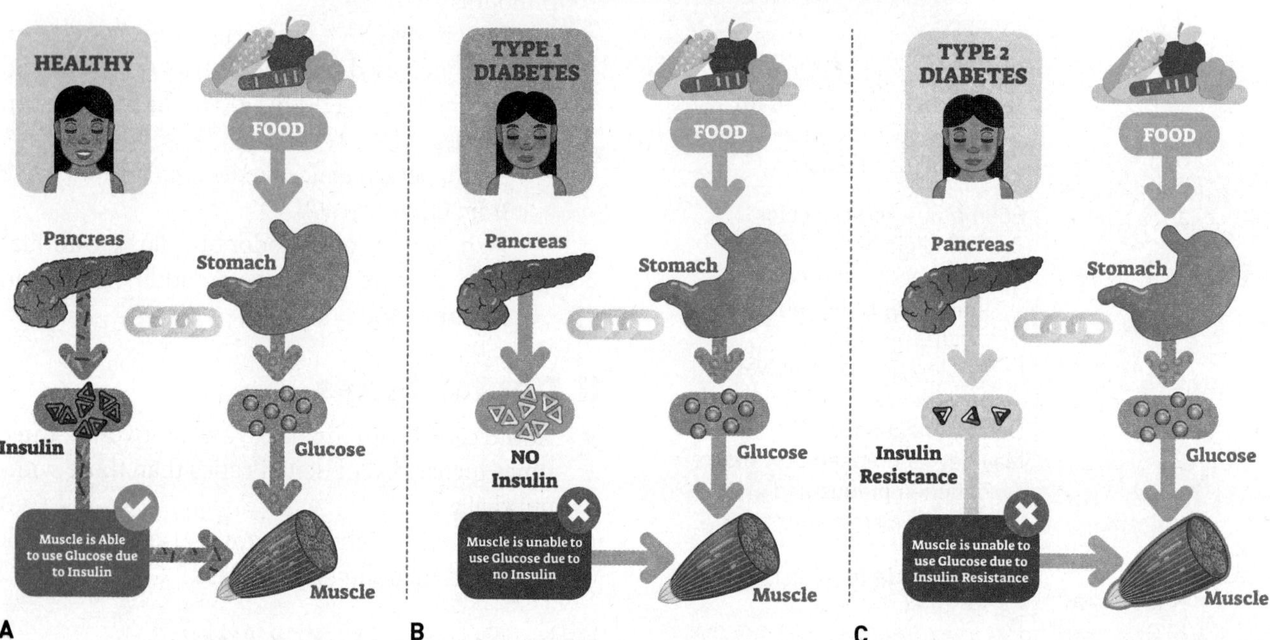

Figure 54-1 Pancreas and Action of Insulin on Muscle in Health, and Type 1 and Type 2 Diabetes. **A:** Healthy pancreas excretes insulin into bloodstream that enables glucose uptake by muscle cell. **B:** Type 1 diabetes shows no insulin produced by pancreas and no glucose uptake by muscle cell. **C:** Type 2 diabetes shows normal, increased, or decreased insulin production by pancreas and the defective receptor on the muscle cell hampers insulin uptake.

IV. Effects of Absolute Insulin Deficiency (Type 1 Diabetes)

Glucose increases in the circulating blood (hyperglycemia) until a threshold is reached and glucose spills over into the urine (glycosuria).

- Increased glycosuria induces osmotic diuresis with excretion of large amounts of urine (polyuria). Water and electrolytes are lost and there is a risk of dehydration.[20]
- Fluid loss signals excessive thirst to the brain (polydipsia).[20]
- Cells starving for glucose may cause the patient to increase food intake (polyphagia), but weight loss is common.[20]
- Without glucose to use for energy, the body metabolizes fat for energy.[21]
  - End products of fat metabolism are harmful **ketones** that accumulate in the blood.
  - Ketones are acidic, and when they accumulate, they are usually neutralized in the blood.
  - When large quantities of ketones are present, the neutralizing effect of the blood is depleted rapidly and an acidic condition (metabolic acidosis) results.
  - Metabolic acidosis (**diabetic ketoacidosis [DKA]**) leads to a diabetic coma if not treated promptly.
  - DKA is most common in Type 1 diabetes, but can also occur in gestational and Type 2 diabetes.
- **Figure 54-1B** shows changes in insulin secretion by the pancreas in Type 1 and Type 2 diabetes.

V. Effects of Impaired Secretion or Action of Insulin (Type 2 Diabetes)

- Deficient insulin action results from inadequate insulin secretion and/or diminished tissue responses to insulin.[22]
  - Cell surface insulin receptors develop defects, and glucose cannot be transmitted into the cells.
  - Blood glucose level increases as the insulin resistance of the cells increases. This stimulates more insulin to be released.
- Over time, insulin secretion may also decline and lead to both decrease of insulin in the blood and increased insulin resistance of the cells.
- **Figure 54-1C** shows the effects of decreased insulin and action of insulin that can occur in type 2 diabetes.

VI. Insulin Complications

- Earlier diagnosis; improved treatment; and better informed patients, family, and friends have reduced the occurrence of emergency insulin complications.
- Constant verbal and visual contact needs to be maintained with a patient during treatment to identify early behavioral and physical changes indicative of a developing medical emergency.

A. Hypoglycemia/Insulin Shock

- Too much insulin (**hyperinsulinemia**) lowers the level of blood glucose, resulting in **hypoglycemia** (low blood glucose).[23]
- Hypoglycemia is an emergency likely to occur in the dental setting for a variety of reasons, including dental anxiety, delays in meals/snacks, and time of day (e.g., afternoon appointments when glucose may be low and insulin levels high).
- See **Box 54-2** for symptoms of hypoglycemia.
- Individuals with a longer duration of diabetes, taking insulin for longer than 5 years, and a history of severe hypoglycemia are more likely to experience hypoglycemic events.[23]
- Hypoglycemic unawareness is the inability of the patient to identify symptoms of low blood glucose and can rapidly become a medical emergency.[23]

B. Hyperglycemic Reaction/Diabetic Coma (Ketoacidosis)

- Too little insulin (**hypoinsulinemia**) with increased levels of blood glucose (**hyperglycemia**).
- **Table 54-2** compares the characteristics of hyperglycemic and hypoglycemic reactions, along with the respective treatment procedures.

Box 54-2 Symptoms of Low and High Blood Glucose

HYPOGLYCEMIA	HYPERGLYCEMIA
▪ Mental confusion	▪ Polyuria
▪ Sweating	▪ Polydipsia
▪ Irritability	▪ Weight loss
▪ Palpitations	▪ Polyphagia
▪ Shakiness	▪ Blurred vision
▪ Pallor	▪ Increased susceptibility to infections
▪ Headache	▪ Impaired growth
▪ Seizure	▪ Ketoacidosis
▪ Coma and death (if untreated)	

Table 54-2 Comparison of Hypoglycemia (Insulin Shock) and Hyperglycemia (Diabetic Coma)[24–26]

	Hypoglycemia/Insulin Shock	Diabetic Coma/Ketoacidosis
History/ predisposing factors	Too much insulin Too little food: omitted or delayed Excessive exercise Stress	Too little insulin: omission of dose or failure to increase dose when requirements increased Too much food Less exercise than planned Infection, illness of any sort Trauma, drugs, alcohol abuse Stress
Occurrence	More common complication than ketoacidosis, especially with less stable type 1 diabetes	Type 1 diabetes, especially if poorly controlled, unstable
Onset	Sudden	Develops slowly over hours/days
Behavioral changes	Confusion, stupor Drowsy, restless Anxious, irritable, agitated Incoordination, weakness	Any hypoglycemic behavioral change
Physical findings	Skin: moist, sweaty, perspiration Hunger Headache Tremor, shakiness, weakness Pallor Dilated pupils, blurry vision Dizziness, staggering gait	Skin: flushed, dry Abdominal pain Nausea, vomiting Lack of appetite Dry mouth, thirst Fruity smelling breath Increased urination
Vital signs	Temperature: normal or below Respiration: normal Pulse: fast, irregular Blood pressure: normal or slightly elevated	Temperature: elevated when infection Respiration: **hyperpnea**, rapid and labored with acetone or fruity smelling breath Pulse: rapid, weak Blood pressure: lowered, person may go into shock
Glucose readings[25]	Level 1 hypoglycemia: 54–69 mg/dL (3.0–3.8 mmol/L)	Level 1 hyperglycemia: 181–250 mg/dL (10.1–13.9 mmol/L)
	Level 2 hypoglycemia: <54 mg/dL (<3.0 mmol/L)	Level 2 hyperglycemia: >250 mg/dL (>13.0 mmol/L)
If left untreated	Possible convulsions, eventual coma, and death	Eventual coma and death
Treatment[25]	Glucose gel (15–20 g) is the preferred treatment for the conscious individual with hypoglycemia After 15 minutes of treatment, if blood glucose shows continued hypoglycemia, the treatment should be repeated. Once blood glucose returns to normal, the individual should consume a meal or snack to prevent recurrence of hypoglycemia If unconscious/unresponsive: injection of glucagon or intravenous glucose	Immediate professional care Activate emergency medical system Monitor vital signs Keep patient warm Fluids for conscious patient Insulin injection after medical assessment
Prevention	Monitoring and regulation of blood sugar and frequent blood glucose monitoring	Monitoring and regulation of blood sugar and frequent blood glucose monitoring

SMBG, self-monitoring of blood glucose

Identification of Individuals at Risk for Development of Diabetes

I. Diabetes Risk Factors

- Genetic risk factors[1,22,27]
  - Family history, such as first-degree relative with diabetes.
  - High-risk race/ethnicity such as African American, Hispanic/Latino, Asian, Native American/Alaska Native/Indigenous People or Pacific Islander.
- Metabolic risk factors[1,22,27,28]
  - Hypertension (>140/90 mm Hg) or taking antihypertensive medications.
  - Women with **polycystic ovarian syndrome (PCOS)**.
  - Age: type 1 is most common in childhood while prediabetes/type 2 diabetes risk is being 45 years or older.
  - History of cardiovascular disease.
  - Overweight with a body mass index (BMI) greater than 25 kg/m.
  - Women who have delivered a baby that weighs over 9 pounds or had gestational diabetes during pregnancy.
  - History of prediabetes.
  - A1c greater than 5.7% (**impaired glucose tolerance** (IGT) or **impaired fasting glucose** (IFG).
- Environmental risk factors[1,22,27]
  - Physical inactivity.
  - Unhealthy diet.

II. Prediabetes

- Individuals who have blood glucose levels above normal but do not meet the criteria for diagnosis of diabetes are considered to have **prediabetes**. (Diagnostic criteria are provided later in this chapter.)
  - Prediabetes means the individual is at high risk for developing diabetes and cardiovascular disease.[1]
  - The Diabetes Prevention Program (DPP) showed a 27% reduction in progression to diabetes in those with prediabetes with lifestyle changes, including modest weight loss of 7% and a minimum of 150 minutes/week of physical activity.[29]
  - The most frequent medication used to manage blood glucose level in prediabetes is metformin.

Classification of Diabetes Mellitus

- Classification is based on the etiology of the disease.
- The type of diabetes is based on the circumstances at the time of diagnosis, such as gestational diabetes during pregnancy.[1]
- A comparison of type 1 and 2 diabetes is found in **Table 54-3**.

Table 54-3 Comparison of Type 1 and Type 2 Diabetes Mellitus[1,27-29]

Characteristic	Prediabetes	Type 1 Diabetes Mellitus (T1DM)	Type 2 Diabetes Mellitus (T2DM)
Age of onset	≥45 years of age	Typically in children, teens, and young adults Peak onset is age 13–14 years	≥45 years of age (in Canada ≥40 years of age)
Body weight	Overweight or obese (BMI ≥25 kg/m^2)	Underweight or normal weight	Overweight or obese (BMI ≥25 kg/m^2)
Ethnicity	Higher risk race/ethnicity (e.g., Black/African American, Hispanic, Latino, Indigenous/Native American, Pacific Islander)	More common in Whites	Higher risk race/ethnicity (e.g. Black/African American, Hispanic, Latino, Indigenous/Native American, Pacific Islander, some Asian Americans)
Hereditary	First-degree family member with diabetes	May inherit a predisposition to develop T1DM Greater risk with parent or sibling with T1DM	First-degree family member with T2DM

(continues)

Table 54-3 Comparison of Type 1 and Type 2 Diabetes Mellitus[1,27-29] *(continued)*

Characteristic	Prediabetes	Type 1 Diabetes Mellitus (T1DM)	Type 2 Diabetes Mellitus (T2DM)
Lifestyle	Physical inactivity	Not considered a risk factor for development	Overweight or obese Physical inactivity High-fat diet
Onset of symptoms	May progress slowly and go undiagnosed	Onset may be in weeks or months	Onset varies, but is typically slow to develop
Symptoms	Seldom have symptoms	Weight loss, weakness Polyuria Frequent/recurrent infections, slow healing Polydipsia Polyuria Polyphagia Blurred vision Fatigue Mood changes, irritability	Polyuria Frequent/recurrent infections, slow healing Polydipsia Polyuria Polyphagia Blurred vision Extreme fatigue Tingling or numbness in hands/feet
Severity	Mild	Life threatening	Severity at onset varies
Complications	Increased risk of cardiovascular disease and stroke	Diabetic ketoacidosis Retinopathy Neuropathy Nephropathy Sleep apnea Cardiovascular disease Stroke Periodontal disease	Same as in T1DM
Ketoacidosis		Common	Less common than in T1DM
Stability		Requires diligence to self-management Can be difficult to control during times of growth	Requires diligence to self-management Lifestyle modifications (i.e., weight loss, healthy diet, and physical activity)
Insulin secretion	Insulin is produced by the pancreas	No insulin production by pancreas, exogenous insulin required	Insulin levels may be normal, elevated, or low along with insulin resistance
Prevention	Prevent progression to diabetes with lifestyle modification (i.e., weight loss, healthy diet, and physical activity)	Onset is not possible to prevent at this time	Remission is possible with lifestyle modifications (i.e., increased physical activity, healthy diet, and weight loss)

I. Type 1 Diabetes Mellitus

A. Description

- Accounts for 5% to 10% of those with diabetes.
- Results from the destruction of insulin-producing beta cells in the pancreas for one of the following reasons[1]:
  - Autoantibodies.
  - No known etiology.
- Results in an absolute insulin deficiency requiring **exogenous insulin** to sustain life.
  - Figure 54-1B illustrates the changes in pancreas function in type 1 diabetes.
- Patients are prone to ketoacidosis.[1]

- Typically arises in childhood or adolescence, but may appear in adulthood depending on the rate of beta-cell destruction.[1]
- Individuals with type 1 diabetes are also prone to other autoimmune disorders such as Graves' disease or Hashimoto thyroiditis.[1]

B. Former Names

- **Insulin-dependent diabetes mellitus**, juvenile diabetes, or juvenile-onset diabetes.

II. Type 2 Diabetes Mellitus

A. Description

- Most prevalent type of diabetes, accounts for 90% to 95% of all patients with diabetes.[1]
- Pancreatic insulin secretion may be low, normal, or even higher than normal, but the patient exhibits an **insulin resistance** that impairs the use of insulin.[1]
  - Figure 54-1C shows changes that occur in type 2 diabetes.
- Onset typically occurs in adulthood, and the risk increases with age, obesity, and lack of physical activity.[1]
- Although traditionally thought of as occurring in adults, the incidence has increased in children and adolescents due to physical inactivity, overabundance of fast food, and obesity.[30]
  - In youth aged 10–19 years, there was an increase of 95% from 2001 to 2017 in cases of type 2 diabetes mellitus.[30]

B. Screening

- Type 2 diabetes is usually identified after acute symptoms of hyperglycemia prompt evaluation.
- Screening in asymptomatic adults is recommended for prediabetes and type 2 diabetes.[1]
  - For all individuals, screening should begin at age 35 (age 40 based on Diabetes Canada guidelines[28]) and be repeated a minimum of every 3 years if test results are normal.
  - Screening begins earlier and more frequently if the patient is overweight or obese (BMI >25 kg/m^2) and has one or more additional risk factors.
- Screening should be done in children and adolescents who are overweight or obese (BMI >85th percentile for age and sex) and have other risk factors for diabetes.[1]

C. Former Names

- **Noninsulin-dependent diabetes mellitus** or adult-onset diabetes.

III. Gestational Diabetes Mellitus

- The prevalence of **gestational diabetes mellitus (GDM)** is 7.1% of pregnancies in the North American and 14% worldwide.[31]
- Defined as any degree of glucose intolerance first recognized during pregnancy.[1]
- Onset is related to genetics, obesity, and hormones causing insulin resistance.
- Insulin adjustment, carefully supervised prenatal care, and improved obstetric practices have lessened much of the potential danger for the mother.
- Infants are larger, premature births are more frequent, and incidence of congenital malformations and perinatal death is high; rates are lower with improved prenatal care.[1]
- Women with a history of GDM have a 10-fold risk for developing type 2 diabetes.[32]

A. Screening

- Pregnant women with risk factors for diabetes should be screened at the initial prenatal visit.[1,28]
- Women with no history of diabetes prior to pregnancy should be screened at 24–28 weeks of gestation.[1,28]
- Women with gestational diabetes should have lifelong screening for diabetes or prediabetes.[1,28]

IV. Other Specific Types of Diabetes Mellitus

A. Monogenic Diabetes Syndromes

- Neonatal diabetes occurs before the age of 6 months and is typically of genetic origin.[1]
- Maturity-onset diabetes of the young (MODY) typically occurs before the age of 25 years and does not exhibit the characteristics of type 1 and 2 diabetes.[1]

B. Cystic Fibrosis-Related Diabetes

- Occurs in 20% of teens and 40% to 50% of adults with cystic fibrosis.[1]
- Insufficient production of insulin from the pancreas is the primary cause and is related to poor nutritional status, more severe inflammatory lung disease, and greater mortality.[1]

C. Posttransplantation Diabetes Mellitus (PTDM)

- Also called new-onset diabetes after transplantation.[1]
- Immunosuppressants and glucocorticoid steroid used posttransplant are the major causes of PTDM.[1]

Diagnosis of Diabetes

I. Diabetes Symptoms

Careful review of the medical history with follow-up questions is used to identify risk factors and symptoms (Table 54-3) of diabetes.

- The classic symptoms of diabetes include the 3 Ps:
  - **Polyphagia** (excessive hunger).
  - **Polydipsia** (excessive thirst).
  - **Polyuria** (excessive urination).

II. Diagnostic Tests

A. Glycated Hemoglobin Assay (HbA1c or A1c)

- A1c measures the quantity of the end product of high glucose bound to a hemoglobin molecule (**glycated or glycosylated hemoglobin**).
  - An easy way to remember this is to think of the red blood cell as your "donut" and the product of high glucose as the "glaze" on your "donut." The higher the level of end-products of high glucose in the blood, the more "glazed" the "donut" (red blood cell).
- A1c value provides an average of **glycemia** (blood glucose levels) over a 3-month period.
- The **HbA1c** test is used to diagnose prediabetes and diabetes.[1,28]
  - Prediabetes is diagnosed with an A1c value of 5.7% to 6.4%.
  - A1c greater than or equal to 6.5% is used to diagnose diabetes.
- The A1c is also used to *monitor* diabetes control[25,28]:
  - Testing is recommended twice a year for individuals with good glycemic control.
  - Patients with unstable glycemic control may require testing every 3 months.
- A1c goal may vary slightly for an individual based on risk for hypoglycemia, but the goal for most nonpregnant adults is less than 7%.[25,28]
  - However, the A1c target is individualized based on many factors and may be less stringent for individuals such as those with a history of severe hypoglycemia, a short life expectancy, or limited resources and support, as well as frail elderly and/or those with dementia may have targets of approximately 8.5%, so consultation with the provider is necessary.

B. Fasting Plasma Glucose

- Measurement for **fasting plasma glucose (FPG)** is taken after fasting at least 8 hours and used for diagnosis in the following ways:
  - FPG of 100–125 mg/dL (5.6–6.9 mmol/L) is used to diagnose prediabetes.
  - FPG ≥126 mg/dL (7.0 mmol/L) is the criterion used for diagnosis of diabetes.
  - Repeat testing is recommended to confirm a diagnosis.

C. 2-Hour Plasma Glucose

Typically measured during an **oral glucose tolerance test**[1,28]:

- A 2-hour plasma glucose (PG) of 140–199 mg/dL (7.8–11 mmol/L) is also used to diagnose prediabetes.
- A 2-hour PG ≥200 mg/dL (11.1 mmol/L) is used as a criterion for the diagnosis of diabetes.
- Repeat testing is recommended to confirm a diagnosis.

III. Diabetes Screening in the Dental Setting

- Dental visits provide an opportunity to screen patients for undiagnosed diabetes (see **Figure 54-2**).[1,33–35]
  - Screening tools for prediabetes, gestational diabetes, and type 2 diabetes are available on the American Diabetes Association and Diabetes Canada websites and could be used chairside in the dental office for screening.[6,8]
  - Screening may also include point-of-care (POC) A1c testing using fingersticks or gingival crevicular bleeding.[36]

Standards of Medical Care for Diabetes Mellitus

- Medical management depends on the severity of the disease and on individual characteristics.
  - Consideration is given to individualized needs related to age, activities, vocation, lifestyle,

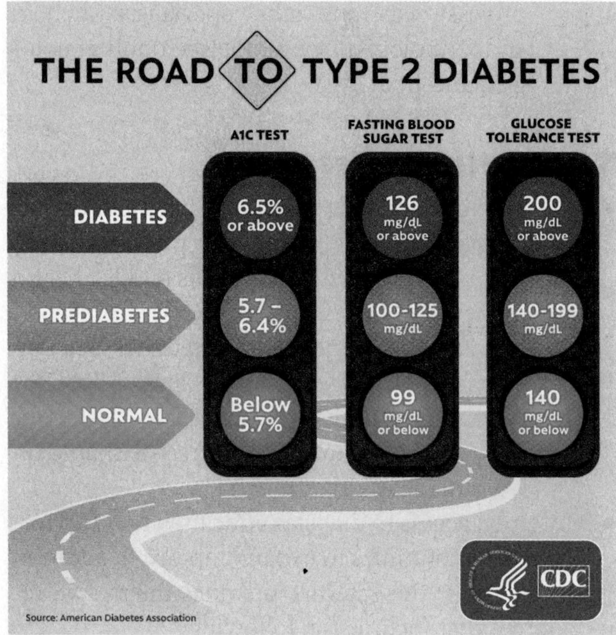

Figure 54-2 The Road to Type 2 Diabetes

Centers for Disease Control and Prevention. https://www.cdc.gov/diabetes/pdfs/library/socialmedia/road-to-diabetes-infographic.pdf. Reference to specific commercial products, manufacturers, companies, or trademarks does not constitute its endorsement or recommendation by the U.S. Government, Department of Health and Human Services, or Centers for Disease Control and Prevention.

knowledge, attitudes, personality, culture, emotional and psychological needs, as well as the health and nutritional status and weight issues of the patient.

I. Early Diagnosis

- Identify individuals with prediabetes and undiagnosed diabetes through regular screening and/or monitoring.[1,28,29]
- Assess risk factors and refer for evaluation.

II. Management of Prediabetes

- The DPP study demonstrated that lifestyle changes including physical activity, attaining and maintaining a healthy weight, and making wise food choices were effective in preventing or delaying the onset of diabetes.[29]

III. Diabetes Self-Management Education

- The National Standards for Diabetes Education and Support guidelines indicate diabetes self-management education is essential for those at risk for developing diabetes as well as for those individuals who are newly diagnosed.[37]
    - Diabetes self-management education and support has been shown to reduce HbA1c by 0.6%, which is equivalent to some medications.[37]

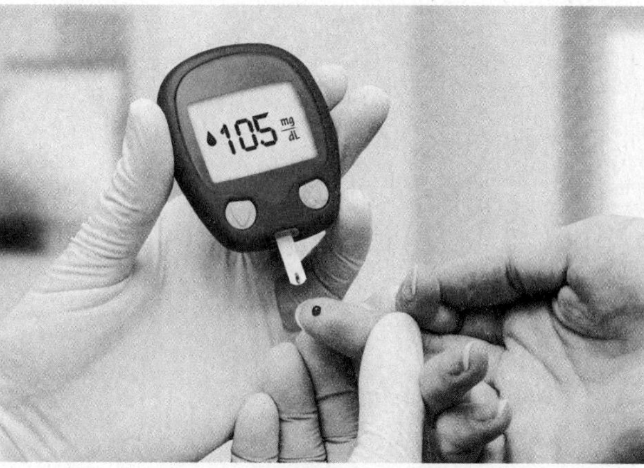

Figure 54-3 Glucometer (Glucose Monitor).
A glucometer is used by individuals with diabetes to use a drop of blood to monitor blood glucose to aid in self-management.

- Maintain tight glycemic control to reduce the complications of diabetes through regular **self-monitoring of blood glucose (SMBG)** at home.[25,28]
    - Frequency and timing are individualized to patient needs, but are often recommended before breakfast, prior to meals, and prior to bedtime.
    - More frequent monitoring is associated with better glycemic control and a lower A1c.
    - Hypoglycemia is a limiting factor in setting a glycemic target.
- Monitoring devices for home may include the following:
    - Glucose meter (or glucometer) is a device that requires a fingerstick to obtain a drop of blood for measurement of blood glucose (**Figure 54-3**).
    - Continuous glucose monitoring (CGM) is done automatically with a device such as FreeStyle Libre or Dexcom throughout the day and night and may have an alarm for hypoglycemia and hyperglycemia.
        - Depending on the device, a sensor is placed on the abdomen or back of the upper arm, and a thin filament is inserted under the skin to measure the interstitial fluid glucose level.
        - A handheld reader is then used to scan the sensor and provide the current blood glucose and an 8-hour history to help the individual understand and manage his or her blood glucose (**Figure 54-4**).

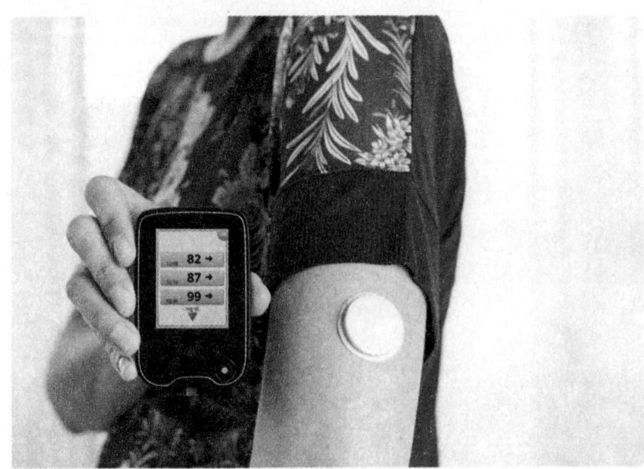

Figure 54-4 Continuous Glucose Monitoring. A blood glucose sensor is worn on the arm or abdomen and a scanner is used to show blood glucose levels.

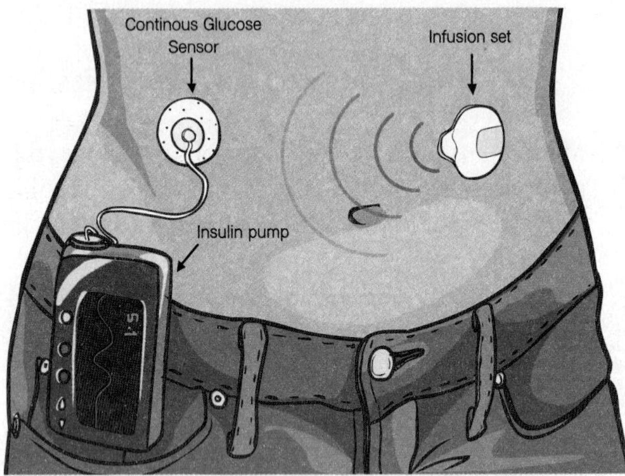

Figure 54-5 Insulin Pump. Insulin pumps may be used for insulin delivery. The blood glucose level is continuously monitored and insulin is delivered as needed.

- Some devices may send the information to a cell phone, and the information can be downloaded to a computer.
- CGM is being used with increasing frequency so during the medical history review, the clinician should ask questions about what tools are being used for checking blood glucose (**Figure 54-5**).

A. Interprofessional Healthcare Team

- Initial and ongoing individualized education is provided by the interprofessional team.
  - Members include physicians; registered nurses; nurse practitioners; physician assistants; registered dietitians; nutritionists; pharmacists; mental health professionals; dental professionals; and other specialists, such as endocrinologist, cardiologist, ophthalmologist, and podiatrist.

B. Educational Resources

- Books and journals: a number of excellent books, professional journals, and other printed materials have been prepared for patients and for health professionals.
  - Annually, the American Diabetes Association publishes evidence-based Clinical Practice Recommendations in the *Diabetes Care* journal. These can be accessed free of charge on www.diabetes.org.
- Internet: access to diabetes education and support resources continues to expand rapidly. In addition to websites, the Internet provides interactive resources that include the following:
  - Interactive behavior change programs.
  - Peer support through social media networks such as Facebook, blogs, and chat rooms.[38]
  - Review strategies to determine the validity of information on websites in Chapter 2.
- Technology and telehealth: Cell phone applications and smartwatch devices for tracking food intake, physical activity, weight, blood glucose, and blood pressure can be used to assist the individual with self-monitoring and can be shared with the healthcare team.[39–41]

IV. Medical Nutrition Therapy

- Medical nutrition therapy (MNT) is individualized to meet the needs of the patients to manage and control diabetes.[28,42]
- The American Diabetes Association and Diabetes Canada recommend nutrition therapy be provided by a registered dietitian/nutritionist.[28,42]
- Goals for MNT include the following[28,42]:
  - A variety of eating patterns are acceptable and should be individualized to meet overall health goals. The Mediterranean diet and Dietary Approaches to Stop Hypertension (DASH) are examples of healthy eating patterns.
  - Energy balance for modest weight loss (5–10 pounds) and weight maintenance.
  - Carbohydrate intake should be evenly distributed throughout the day, with focus on vegetables, fruits, whole grains, beans, and low-fat dairy products and an emphasis on higher fiber and lower glycemic loads over foods with added sugars.

- Similar to the *Dietary Guidelines for Americans* and *Eating Well with Canada's Food Guide*, individuals with diabetes need to limit or avoid added sugar and refined carbohydrates.
- Limit intake of saturated fat, trans fat, and cholesterol. Include foods rich in omega-3 fatty acids such as fatty fish, nuts, and seeds.
- Recommendations for sodium intake of less than 2300 mg/day are the same as for the general population. (See Chapter 33.)
- Alcohol should be in moderation with an understanding about how it may increase the risk for hypoglycemia.

V. Physical Activity

- Adults are encouraged to engage in 150 minutes/week of moderate-intensity physical activity spread over at least 3 days/week.[28,42]
- Children and adolescents are encouraged to engage in 60 minutes/day of moderate- or vigorous-intensity physical activity at least 3 days/week.[42]
- Contributes to lowering insulin requirements by increasing the muscle sensitivity to insulin.

VI. Habits

A. Tobacco

- Patients must avoid all types of tobacco and e-cigarettes.[42] (See Chapter 32.)
  - Tobacco use increases the risk of heart disease, stroke, myocardial infarction, limb amputations, periodontal disease, and numerous other health problems.

B. Alcohol

- Avoid excessive alcohol; alcohol can raise blood pressure and contribute to other health problems as well as difficulty with diabetes management.[42]

VII. Psychosocial Issues

- Screening for diabetes distress (DD) should be done routinely by the primary care provider and requires interprofessional collaboration to manage.[42]
  - DD refers to the psychological challenges of managing a chronic disease like diabetes.

Pharmacologic Therapy

I. Insulin Therapy

- All patients with type 1 diabetes require exogenous insulin for survival. Patients with type 2 diabetes may need to use insulin in combination with other medications for glycemic control.[28,43]

A. Types of Insulin

- Insulin is classified as rapid acting, regular or short acting, intermediate acting, or long acting based on the onset, peak, and duration of action. The types of insulin and range of peak action are found in **Table 54-4**.

B. Dosage

- Objective: attain optimum utilization of glucose throughout each 24 hours.
- Factors affecting the need for insulin: food intake, illness, stress, variations in exercise, or infections.
- "Sick Day Rules": insulin dose is adjusted if there are any factors that affect the need for insulin.

C. Methods for Insulin Administration

- Subcutaneous injection with syringe: a syringe is filled from a vial of insulin. Injection sites are rotated usually on the abdomen, thigh, or upper arm.

Table 54-4 Types and Action of Insulin[44]

Class of Insulin	Type/Name	Onset of Action	Peak Effect	Duration
Rapid acting	Lispro (Humalog), Aspart (NovoLog)	15–30 minutes	2 to 3 hours	4½–7 hours
Regular or short acting	Humulin R, Novolin R	30 minutes	30 minutes to 2½ hours	8 hours
Intermediate acting	NPH (Humulin N, Novolin N)	1–2 hrs	4–12 hours	14–24 hours
Long acting	Detemir (Levemir), Glargine (Lantus)	3–4 hrs	3-9 hours	6–23 hours
Inhaled, rapid acting	Afrezza	12 minutes	35-55 minutes	1½–4½ hours

- Insulin pen: prefilled cartridge of single type of insulin injected with an attached needle. May be disposable or a reusable type.
- Continuous subcutaneous insulin infusion with a battery-operated insulin pump[28,45]:
  - The insulin pump delivers a preprogrammed continuous basal rate of insulin and bolus doses when needed.
  - Offers greater flexibility and control of glycemia to reduce risk of long term complications, but may increase the risk of hypoglycemia.
  - The small cell phone–sized pump can be worn in a pocket or on a belt or a waistband, as shown in Figure 54-5.
- Inhalable insulin[46]:
  - Contraindicated for those who have long-term (chronic) lung problems such as asthma or chronic obstructive pulmonary disease (COPD).
  - Rapid-acting, "mealtime" insulin is taken with an inhaler.
  - Side effects include lower lung function, cough, dry mouth, bronchospasm, or chest discomfort.
  - Brand name: Afrezza.
- Future modes for insulin administration include an insulin patch and implantable insulin pumps.

II. Antihyperglycemic Therapy

- The medications listed in **Table 54-5** may be used individually or in combinations.[15,43]
- The most common medication used in prediabetes is metformin.
- Monotherapy is considered first-line therapy for T2DM: lifestyle management + metformin.[15,43]
- Dual therapy: lifestyle management + metformin + additional agent.[15,43]
  - A1c 1.5% greater than target.
- Triple therapy: lifestyle management + metformin + two additional agents.
- For those with an A1c greater than 10%, insulin may be initiated.[43]

Table 54-5 Antihyperglycemic Agents Used for Treatment of Type 2 Diabetes[15,43]

Agent	Example	Action/Function
Biguanides	Metformin (Glucophage)	■ Prevent liver glycogen breakdown to glucose ■ Increase tissue sensitivity to insulin
Sulfonylureas	Glyburide (Diabeta, Micronase) Glipizide (Glucotrol)	■ Stimulate pancreas to release more insulin after a meal ■ May cause hypoglycemia
Meglitinides	Repaglinide (Prandin) Nateglinide (Starlix)	■ Stimulate pancreas to release more insulin after a meal ■ May cause hypoglycemia
Thiazolidinediones	Pioglitazone (Actos)	■ Increase tissue sensitivity to insulin
Dipeptidyl peptidase-4 inhibitors (DPP-4 inhibitors)	Sitagliptin (Januvia)	■ Improve insulin level after meals and lowers glucose production
Alpha-glucosidase inhibitors	Acarbose (Precose)	■ Slow digestion and absorption of glucose into bloodstream after eating
Bile acid sequestrants	Colesevelam (Welchol)	■ Bind bile acids in intestinal tract, increasing hepatic bile production
Sodium-glucose cotransporter-2 (SGLT2) inhibitors	Canagliflozin (Invokana) Dapagliflozin (Farxiga)	■ Block glucose reabsorption in kidney
Glucagon-like peptide-1 (GLP-1) receptor agonists	Exenatide (Byetta) Liraglutide (Victoza)	■ Increase insulin secretion ■ Decrease glucagon secretion ■ Slow gastric emptying ■ Increase satiety
Dopamine-2 agonists	Bromocriptine (Cycloset)	■ Increase insulin secretion

- The takeaway message for dental professionals is that when a patient is on multiple medications, it means the diabetes is not well controlled.

Complications of Diabetes

Patients with well-controlled blood glucose levels tend to develop fewer complications later in life than those whose diabetes is less well controlled.[25,28]

I. Infection

- Individuals with poorly controlled diabetes are more susceptible to infections and impaired healing, which can worsen prognosis.[47]
- The presence of stress, trauma, and infection affects blood glucose levels.
- Failure to treat an infection intensifies the symptoms and increases the severity of diabetes, which can progress to life-threatening infections or precipitate DKA.[1]
- Diabetes is associated with a nearly three-fold increase in severity of coronavirus disease 2019 (COVID-19), along with two-fold increase in mortality.[48]
- Insulin requirements may need adjustment because of infection, inflammation, trauma, bleeding, pain, or stress, so blood glucose should be monitored regularly.[49]
- Numerous factors are involved including impaired immune response, alterations in metabolism of carbohydrate and protein, vascular changes and impaired circulation, and altered nutritional state.

II. Neuropathy

- Neuropathy can cause pain, numbness, or tingling of mouth, face, and extremities.[28,50]

A. Peripheral Neuropathy

- Symptoms vary based on the sensory nerve fibers affected and may result in loss of sensation in the feet, hands, and fingers.[28,50]
- Numbness in the hands and fingers may make effective oral self-care difficult.
- As many as 50% of people with peripheral neuropathy may be asymptomatic and not recognize the loss of sensation, which can put them at risk for injury and resulting infection.[50]
- Leads to increased incidence of amputations and **Charcot joints**.[50]

B. Autonomic Neuropathy

- Manifestations include tachycardia, orthostatic hypotension, **gastroparesis**, and hypoglycemic unawareness.[28,50]
  - Cardiovascular autonomic neuropathy can be asymptomatic other than changes in the heart rate.
  - Gastroparesis is a slowing of digestion and motility of the gastrointestinal tract.
  - Hypoglycemic unawareness can quickly become an emergency situation because the patient is not able to recognize the usual symptoms of low blood glucose.
- Early management to maintain glycemic levels near normal can be effective in preventing or delaying neuropathy.[28,50]

III. Nephropathy

- Diabetes is a leading cause of renal disease and the most common cause of end-stage renal disease in the United States and Europe. Dialysis or kidney transplant is needed.[28,51]
- Patients diagnosed with diabetes should be screened at least annually for microalbuminuria (protein in the urine).[51]

IV. Retinopathy

- Diabetes is a leading cause of new cases of blindness through the progression of diabetic retinopathy.[28,50]
- Patients are more likely to have glaucoma and cataracts.[28,50]

V. Cardiovascular Disease

- Individuals with diabetes are at high risk for cardiovascular disease, a major cause of morbidity and mortality. Conditions common in people with diabetes include the following[28,52]:
  - Hypertension.
  - Dyslipidemia (high total cholesterol and **low-density lipoprotein [LDL]**).
  - Hypertriglyceridemia (high triglycerides).
- May lead to myocardial infarction and stroke.
- Owing to the excessive risk of coronary heart disease, aggressive treatment for dyslipidemia and hypertriglyceridemia is recommended.[28,52]

VI. Amputation

- Diabetes is a major cause of limb amputation (usually foot) from possible complications of neuropathy and vascular disease.[28,50]

VII. Pregnancy Complications

- Patients with diabetes are at higher risk for spontaneous miscarriages and having babies with birth defects and increased weight.[1,28]

VIII. Mental Health

- Due to complications of diabetes, the daily life of the patient as well as those close to the patient are significantly affected. Diabetes distress (DD) was discussed in the previous section regarding psychosocial issues. However, mental health issues common in those with diabetes include the following[42,53]:
  - Anxiety disorders.
  - Depression affects approximately 1 in 4 adults with type 1 or 2 diabetes.
  - Disordered eating behavior characterized by omission of insulin to lose weight.
- Treatment regimens may be challenging to cope with and lead to emotional and social problems, including depression.
- A suggestion for the patient to discuss psychosocial issues with the primary diabetes care provider may improve patient's compliance with treatment and daily oral personal care.

Dental Hygiene Care Plan

- The control of oral infection is vital. Infections can progress more quickly and can alter the management of diabetes.
- Frequent, thorough oral care requires the patient's cooperation along with regular professional care.
- The patient with diabetes is prone to life-threatening emergencies.
- Emergency practice drills can help the dental team prevent an emergency, identify early indications of a developing emergency, and act swiftly and appropriately.

I. Appointment Planning

Stress, including stress created during a dental or dental hygiene appointment, can affect blood sugar levels. Appointment planning needs to center around many factors, including stress prevention.

A. Time

- Treat patient after a meal, preferably containing protein and fat to slow carbohydrate absorption.
- Avoid peak insulin levels for appointments as noted in Table 54-4.
- Ideal time of appointment varies with individual patient's lifestyle and method of insulin intake or other antihyperglycemic medications.
- Preferred time of appointment may be morning, soon after the patient's normal breakfast and medication.[54]

B. Precautions: Prevent/Prepare for Emergency

- Do not keep the patient waiting.
- Do not interfere with the patient's regular meal and between-meal eating schedule.
- Avoid long, stressful procedures; dental and dental hygiene care can be divided into short appointments appropriate to the individual's needs.
- Take additional precautions indicated for the patient with long-term diabetes with complications related to atherosclerosis and other cardiovascular diseases.
- Prevent and treat all infections promptly.
- Monitor for symptoms of hypoglycemia, including dizziness, sweating (diaphoresis), mental confusion, shakiness, pallor, palpitations, and irritability.[54] The symptoms of hypoglycemia and hyperglycemia are listed in Box 54-2.
- Prepare for hypoglycemic emergency.[55]
  - Keep glucose gel as part of the office emergency kit for the conscious patient.
  - A glucometer should also be part of the emergency supplies to allow testing to identify hypoglycemia and monitor the effect of the glucose gel.

C. Emergency Management

- Recognize any change in patient behavior that signals a diabetes emergency.
  - If in doubt, it is safer to treat for hypoglycemia since it will only cause a brief increase in blood glucose whereas doing nothing may result in the need for 911 and hospitalization.
  - Follow the *Rule of 15s* (see the flowchart in **Figure 54-6** for the management of hypoglycemia).[25]

II. Patient History

A. Medical History

- Questions regarding signs and symptoms of diabetes are included in a standard medical history questionnaire. Appropriate questions to ask are listed in **Box 54-3**.

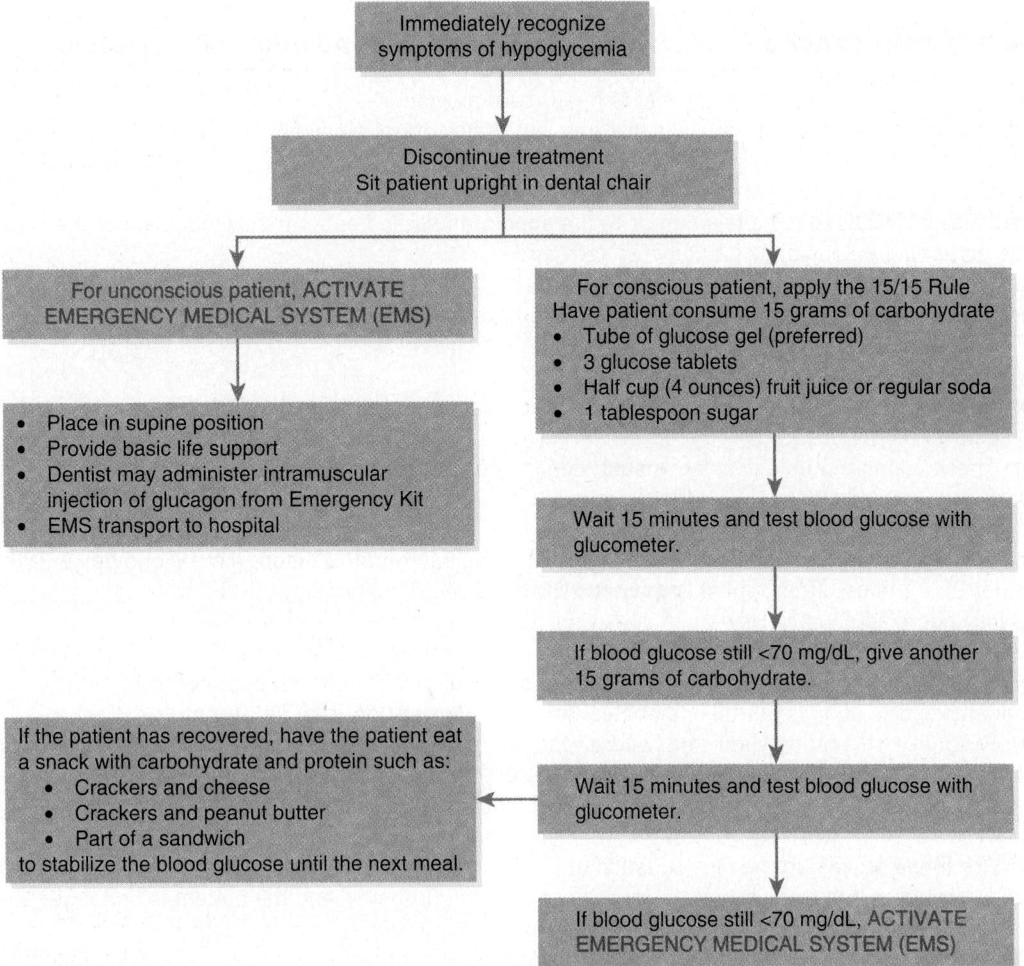

Figure 54-6 Managing Hypoglycemia (Rule of 15s). Flowchart to show steps to take when the patient exhibits symptoms of hypoglycemia (insulin shock).

Box 54-3 Common Medical History Questions to Screen for Diabetes

■ Have you ever been diagnosed with prediabetes, borderline diabetes, or diabetes?	Yes	No
■ Have any members of your family ever been diagnosed with diabetes?	Yes	No
■ Do you urinate frequently? How many times per day?	Yes	No
■ Are you frequently thirsty?	Yes	No
■ Does your mouth feel dry?	Yes	No
■ Have you had any unexplained weight loss?	Yes	No
■ Do you experience excessive hunger?	Yes	No
■ Did you have recent blurred vision?	Yes	No

Gather detailed information on all current prescribed and over-the-counter medications, including recommended dose. Gather information on vitamins and homeopathic or herbal supplements.

Box 54-4 Questions to Ask a Patient with Diabetes to Gather Additional Information

- When was your last visit to your diabetes care healthcare provider?
  Answer: It is recommended individuals with stable glycemic control be seen twice per year and those with poor glycemic control at least quarterly.
- What medications and dose have you taken today?
  Answer: Medications need to be taken prior to the appointment, and patient knowledge about medications suggests personal responsibility for diabetes self-care.
- When did you eat last? What did you eat?
  Answer: Foods containing complex carbohydrates and protein and/or fat 1–2 hours before the appointment to prevent hypoglycemia is ideal.
- Do you monitor your blood sugar at home?
  Answer: Self-monitoring of blood glucose is critical for diabetes self-care management.
- How often do you monitor your blood glucose?
  Answer: Those taking multiple doses of insulin need to check the blood glucose levels three or more times daily. Once or twice daily is typical for those using oral medications.
- What is your usual fasting blood sugar in the morning?
  Answer: Glucose levels between 80 and 130 mg/dL (4.4 and 7.3 mmol/L) before a meal and below 180 mg/dL (10.0 mmol/L) 1–2 hours after a meal (**postprandial**) are recommended.
- What is your hemoglobin A1c? How often does your primary care provider check the A1c?
  Answer: Less than 7% (although there are exceptions) and preferably less than 6.5%; A1c testing recommended twice per year in those with good glycemic control and quarterly in those with poor control.
- (If the patient reports poorly controlled diabetes) Are you experiencing frequent urination?
  Answer: Response of "yes" may indicate hyperglycemia and poor diabetes control and requires referral. The patient will not heal, and it is best to postpone treatment as healing will be suboptimal.
- Do you have frequent episodes of hypoglycemia (low blood sugar)? Can you tell when your blood sugar is getting low?
  Answer: Response of "yes" to the first question and "no" to the second identifies a patient at risk for a medical emergency. Hypoglycemic unawareness occurs because of neuropathy, and the patient is no longer able to identify when the blood sugar has dropped to dangerously low levels.
- (For those with a history of hypoglycemia, ask this question) What time of day does it usually happen and how do you treat it?
  Answer: If the appointment is during a critical time of day for hypoglycemia, precautions must be taken to prevent and treat it or the appointment should be rescheduled. Midafternoon is typically when some types of insulin and oral medications reach their peak action and glucose from the midday meal reaches a low, resulting in a dangerous combination putting the patient at risk for hypoglycemia.
- Have you been hospitalized for hypoglycemia?
  Answer: Response of "yes" indicates extreme risk, and preparation needs to be made to rapidly treat hypoglycemia. Place a glucometer and glucose source near the treatment area for quick access.
- Are you having problems with your eyes, feet, hands, or legs? If so, what kind of problems are you experiencing?
  Answer: A patient experiencing complications may be poorly controlled, and a medical consult is advised.

Data from Boyd LD. Commentary on survey of diabetes knowledge and practices of dental hygienists. *Access*. 2008;22(8):40-43.

  - Supplement the basic medical history with additional questions to obtain information about diabetes (suggested questions along with answers can be found in **Box 54-4**).
  - If an unexplained positive response is present suggesting symptoms of diabetes, the patient should be referred to a primary care provider for evaluation.
- Ask about physical activity and tobacco use; review effects on health.
- Update medical history at each appointment.
- Identify health problems or complications of diabetes that may influence dental treatment.

B. Screening for Diabetes

- The American Diabetes Association offers a prediabetes and diabetes risk test and Diabetes Canada offers a diabetes risk test. These can be used to identify those at risk for diabetes who need referral for further evaluation.[6,8]
- Using POC devices to test HbA1c and blood glucose has been shown to be a cost-effective approach to identifying undiagnosed and at-risk patients needing referral for further evaluation.[33,36]
  - Note: Using these devices is not the same as laboratory tests, and verification is needed by a blood sample evaluated by a certified laboratory.

III. Consultation with Primary Care Provider

- Consultation with the primary care provider to obtain A1c values can be initiated either prior to or at the first visit.
  - **Figure 54-7** provides a conversion for the A1c values to average blood glucose levels.
- Further consultation may be necessary in more advanced periodontal disease to obtain clearance for treatment.

IV. Dental Hygiene Assessment and Treatment

A. Extraoral/Intraoral Examination

- Acanthosis nigricans appears as a light brown to black discoloration of the skin in the creases of the neck and can indicate risk for diabetes (**Figure 54-8**).[56]

B. Dental Biofilm Control Instruction

- Because of the impact of diabetes on periodontal health and the effect of oral infection on diabetes status, daily meticulous oral self-care is crucial.
- Disclosing the biofilm and individualized self-care measures for biofilm control should be conducted at each visit until good control is demonstrated by the patient.

C. Tobacco Cessation

- Refer patient to tobacco cessation programs. (See Chapter 32.)

D. Instrumentation

- Nonsurgical periodontal therapy: definitive nonsurgical periodontal therapy reduces the possibility of periodontal abscess formation. Allow several short appointments if needed for stress management.
- Healing: avoid undue trauma to tissues to minimize the risk for complications associated with healing.

E. Fluoride

- Fluoride treatments, varnishes, and home use of fluoride should be recommended based on caries risk.
- Methods for daily self-fluoride application are described in Chapter 34.

HbA1c %	Scale (HbA1c)	Level	Scale (mg/dl)	Average Blood Glucose mean plasma equivalent (mg/dl)
10.5 and above	12, 11	Seriously Elevated Levels	298, 269	253 and above
8.5 - 10.4	10, 9	Elevated Levels	240, 212	196 - 252
7.1 - 8.4	8	Monitor Closely	185	156 - 195
6.1 - 7.0	7	In Control	154	127 - 155
5.6 - 6.0	6	Non-Diabetic Levels	126	101 - 126
5.1 - 5.5	5		97	
4.0 - 5.0	4		68	68 - 100

Figure 54-7 Average Blood Glucose to HbA1c Conversion.

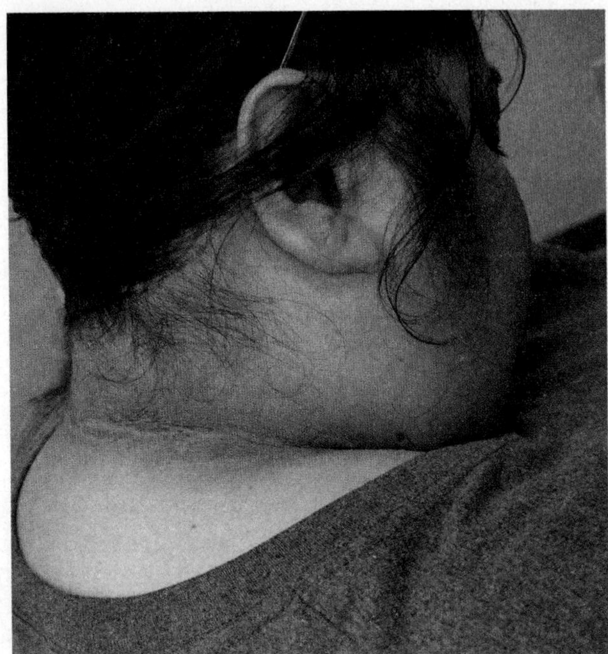

Figure 54-8 Acanthosis Nigricans. This skin condition is seen in patients at risk for diabetes and typically appears on the creases in the neck as a light brown to black discoloration.

Reproduced from DeLong L, Burkhart N. *General and Oral Pathology for the Dental Hygienist.* Philadelphia: Lippincott Williams & Wilkins; 2015.

Box 54-5 Example Documentation: Patient with Diabetes Mellitus

- **S**—A 66-year-old Hispanic female who presents for a periodontal maintenance. She reports bleeding when she flosses for the last couple of weeks. She was recently diagnosed with type 2 diabetes and is taking metformin and glipizide. Her initial HbA1c was 8.5, and she will have a follow-up test next month. She reports checking her blood glucose when she gets up in the morning and before dinner. Her fasting blood glucose this morning was 120. Patient reports taking her medications this morning.
- **O**—Blood pressure: 131/79. Pulse: 88. Respirations: 24. Risk assessment for caries was moderate, periodontal disease was high, and oral cancer was moderate. Periodontal examination reveals localized bleeding on probing, and 1- to 2-mm pocket depth increases primarily in maxillary molar areas. Radiographic bone loss is 1–2 mm in maxillary posterior areas. Biofilm score: 30%. No new dental caries.
- **A**—Localized periodontitis Stage 1, Grade 3 due to poorly controlled diabetes mellitus.
- **P**—Discussed the association of periodontal infection with diabetes and need for meticulous oral self-care and regular professional periodontal maintenance appointments. Reviewed use of interdental brushes for molar areas where biofilm was located. The patient had difficulty removing biofilm on the lingual line angles of the molars, so careful wrapping of the floss was also reviewed. Complete periodontal debridement was performed. Applied 5% sodium fluoride varnish and provided a prescription for 0.12% chlorhexidine gluconate mouthrinse to use twice a day for 2 weeks to assist with healing.

Signed: ______________________________, RDH
Date: ________________

V. Continuing Care

- Appointment for supervision and examination on a regular 3- to 6-month basis as needed.
- Evaluate periodontal health for signs of active disease (e.g., bleeding on probing, clinical attachment loss, etc.).
- Assess soft tissue with attention to areas of irritation related to fixed and removable prostheses.
- Identify any changes requiring consultation or referral to the patient's primary care provider, dietitian, mental health professional, or other specialist.
- Evaluate dental biofilm control and review control with the patient at each appointment. Stress importance of preventing and managing periodontal disease to support diabetes control.

Documentation

- Record status of blood glucose control, including most recent HbA1c and other daily monitoring such as fasting blood glucose levels the patient has performed.
- Update current medications and doses.
- Confirm compliance with medication intake and food consumption.
- Record discussion about relationship between oral health status, oral hygiene status, risk factors, and diabetes.
- **Box 54-5** contains an example progress note for a patient with diabetes.

Factors to Teach the Patient

Factors to Teach Patients with Diabetes

- Importance of regular medical and dental care; eye examinations; blood pressure checks; blood tests for cholesterol, lipids, and kidney readings; and practicing self-examination, particularly of feet, for nerve involvement or delayed healing to prevent complications.
- Connection between oral health and diabetes and need for meticulous oral self-care.
- The patient's role in self-management of diabetes with an emphasis on the need to be compliant with lifestyle modifications including healthy eating, physical activity, weight management, glucose monitoring, tobacco cessation, good oral self-care, limiting or avoiding alcohol, stress management, and use of prescribed medications.
- The value of seeking immediate medical attention for any signs of complications from diabetes.

Factors to Teach Patients at Risk for Diabetes

- Need for regular medical examinations and screening for diabetes.
- How to recognize the early warning signs of diabetes and seek medical consult.
- Factors that affect a healthy lifestyle, including healthy diet, daily exercise, no tobacco products, avoiding alcohol, and maintaining ideal weight.
- How to practice meticulous oral hygiene to prevent dental caries and periodontal disease.
- Stress reduction techniques.

References

1. American Diabetes Association Professional Practice Committee. Classification and diagnosis of diabetes: standards of medical care in diabetes—2022. *Diabetes Care*. 2021;45(suppl 1):S17-S38.
2. Centers for Disease Control and Prevention. National Diabetes Statistics Report. Published January 18, 2022. https://www.cdc.gov/diabetes/data/statistics-report/index.html. Accessed February 23, 2022.
3. Centers for Disease Control and Prevention. National and State Diabetes Trends. Published January 4, 2021. https://www.cdc.gov/diabetes/library/reports/reportcard/national-state-diabetes-trends.html. Accessed February 23, 2022.
4. Centers for Disease Control and Prevention. Cost-effectiveness of diabetes interventions. Published May 17, 2021. https://www.cdc.gov/chronicdisease/programs-impact/pop/diabetes.htm. Accessed February 23, 2022.
5. International Diabetes Federation. *IDF Diabetes Atlas*, 10th edition; 2021. https://diabetesatlas.org/. Accessed February 23, 2022.
6. Health Canada, Government of Canada. The Canadian Diabetes Risk questionnaire (CanRisk). Published October 9, 2012. https://www.healthycanadians.gc.ca/en/canrisk. Accessed February 26, 2022.
7. Centers for Disease Control and Prevention, American Diabetes Association. Could you have prediabetes? Take the test. https://www.cdc.gov/prediabetes/takethetest/. Accessed February 23, 2022.
8. American Diabetes Association. Our 60-second type 2 diabetes risk test: take the risk test today. https://donations.diabetes.org/site/SPageServer?pagename=Diabetes_Risk_Test&source=ada&cate=share&loca=fb. Accessed February 23, 2022.
9. Mauri-Obradors E, Estrugo-Devesa A, Jané-Salas E, Viñas M, López-López J. Oral manifestations of diabetes mellitus: a systematic review. *Med Oral Patol Oral Cir Bucal*. 2017;22(5):e586-e594.
10. Rohani B. Oral manifestations in patients with diabetes mellitus. *World J Diabetes*. 2019;10(9):485-489.
11. Genco RJ, Graziani F, Hasturk H. Effects of periodontal disease on glycemic control, complications, and incidence of diabetes mellitus. *Periodontol 2000*. 2020;83(1):59-65.
12. Sanz M, Ceriello A, Buysschaert M, et al. Scientific evidence on the links between periodontal diseases and diabetes: consensus report and guidelines of the joint workshop on periodontal diseases and diabetes by the International Diabetes Federation and the European Federation of Periodontology. *J Clin Periodontol*. 2018;45(2):138-149.
13. Benham JL, Booth JE, Dunbar MJ, et al. Significant dose-response between exercise adherence and hemoglobin A1c change. *Med Sci Sports Exerc*. 2020;52(9):1960-1965.
14. Blonde L, Pencek R, MacConell L. Association among weight change, glycemic control, and markers of cardiovascular risk with exenatide once weekly: a pooled analysis of patients with type 2 diabetes. *Cardiovasc Diabetol*. 2015;14(1):12.
15. Lipscombe L, Butalia S, Dasgupta K, et al. Pharmacologic glycemic management of type 2 diabetes in adults: 2020 update. *Can J Diabetes*. 2020;44(7):575-591.
16. Beheshti M, Badner V, Shah P, Margulis KS, Yeroshalmi F. Association of diabetes and dental caries among US adolescents in the NHANES dataset. *Pediatr Dent*. 2021;43(2):123-128.
17. Ribeiro BA, Vieira Lima CP, Alves LS, Damé-Teixeira N. Impact of detection criteria on coronal and root caries estimates in adults with and without type 2 diabetes mellitus. *Clin Oral Investig*. 2022;26(4):3687-3695.
18. Gupta A, Aggarwal V, Mehta N, Abraham D, Singh A. Diabetes mellitus and the healing of periapical lesions in root filled teeth: a systematic review and meta-analysis. *Int Endod J*. 2020;53(11):1472-1484.
19. Jiang X, Zhu Y, Liu Z, Tian Z, Zhu S. Association between diabetes and dental implant complications: a systematic review and meta-analysis. *Acta Odontol Scand*. 2021;79(1):9-18.
20. Los E, Wilt AS. Diabetes mellitus type 1 in children. In: *StatPearls*. StatPearls Publishing; 2022. http://www.ncbi.nlm.nih.gov/books/NBK441918/. Accessed February 26, 2022.
21. Dhatariya KK. Defining and characterising diabetic ketoacidosis in adults. *Diabetes Res Clin Prac*. 2019;155:107797.
22. Galicia-Garcia U, Benito-Vicente A, Jebari S, et al. Pathophysiology of Type 2 diabetes mellitus. *Int J Molec Sci*. 2020;21(17):6275.
23. Heller SR, Peyrot M, Oates SK, Taylor AD. Hypoglycemia in patient with type 2 diabetes treated with insulin: it can happen. *BMJ Open Diabetes Res Care*. 2020;8(1):e001194.
24. Centers for Disease Control and Prevention. Diabetes testing. Published May 15, 2019. https://www.cdc.gov/diabetes/basics/getting-tested.html. Accessed February 26, 2022.
25. American Diabetes Association Professional Practice Committee, Draznin B, Aroda VR, et al. Glycemic targets: standards of medical care in diabetes-2022. *Diabetes Care*. 2022;45(suppl 1):S83-S96.
26. Goguen J, Gilbert J. Hyperglycemic emergencies in adults. *Can J Diabetes*. 2018;42:S109-S114.
27. Centers for Disease Control and Prevention. Diabetes basics. Published December 21, 2021. https://www.cdc.gov/diabetes/basics/index.html. Accessed February 26, 2022.

28. Diabetes Canada. Diabetes Canada: Clinical practice guidelines. https://guidelines.diabetes.ca/. Accessed February 26, 2022.
29. Diabetes Prevention Program Research Group. Long-term effects of lifestyle intervention or metformin on diabetes development and microvascular complications over 15-year follow-up: the Diabetes Prevention Program Outcomes Study. *Lancet Diabetes Endocrinol*. 2015;3(11):866-875.
30. Lawrence JM, Divers J, Isom S, et al. Trends in prevalence of Type 1 and Type 2 diabetes in children and adolescents in the US, 2001-2017. *JAMA*. 2021;326(8):717-727.
31. Wang H, Li N, Chivese T, et al. IDF diabetes atlas: estimation of global and regional gestational diabetes mellitus prevalence for 2021 by International Association of Diabetes in Pregnancy study group's criteria. *Diabetes Res Clin Prac*. 2022;183. https://www.diabetesresearchclinicalpractice.com/article/S0168-8227(21)00409-5/fulltext. Accessed February 27, 2022.
32. Vounzoulaki E, Khunti K, Abner SC, Tan BK, Davies MJ, Gillies CL. Progression to type 2 diabetes in women with a known history of gestational diabetes: systematic review and meta-analysis. *BMJ*. 2020;369:m1361.
33. Estrich CG, Araujo MWB, Lipman RD. Prediabetes and diabetes screening in dental care settings: NHANES 2013 to 2016. *JDR Clin Trans Res*. 2019;4(1):76-85.
34. Su N, Teeuw WJ, Loos BG, Kosho MXF, van der Heijden GJMG. Development and validation of a screening model for diabetes mellitus in patients with periodontitis in dental settings. *Clin Oral Investig*. 2020;24(11):4089-4100.
35. Neidell M, Lamster IB, Shearer B. Cost-effectiveness of diabetes screening initiated through a dental visit. *Community Dent Oral Epidemiol*. 2017;45(3):275-280.
36. Suwattipong M, Thuramonwong T, Tantipoj C, et al. Comparison of point-of-care testing and hospital-based methods in screening for potential type 2 diabetes mellitus and abnormal glucose regulation in a dental setting. *Int J Environ Res Public Health*. 2021;18(12):6459.
37. Davis J, Fischl AH, Beck J, et al. 2022 National Standards for Diabetes Self-Management Education and Support. *Sci Diabetes Self Manag Care*. 2022;48(1):44-59.
38. Elaheebocus SMRA, Weal M, Morrison L, Yardley L. Peer-based social media features in behavior change interventions: systematic review. *J Med Internet Res*. 2018;20(2):e20.
39. Wang SY, Yeh HC, Stein AA, Miller ER. Use of health information technology by adults with diabetes in the United States: cross-sectional analysis of National Health Interview Survey data (2016-2018). *JMIR Diabetes*. 2022;7(1):e27220.
40. Sabharwal M, Misra A, Ghosh A, Chopra G. Efficacy of digitally supported and real-time self-monitoring of blood glucose-driven counseling in patients with type 2 diabetes mellitus: a real-world, retrospective study in north India. *Diabetes Metab Syndr Obes*. 2022;15:23-33.
41. American Diabetes Association Professional Practice Committee. Diabetes technology: Standards of Medical Care in Diabetes—2022. *Diabetes Care*. 2021;45:S97-S112.
42. American Diabetes Association Professional Practice Committee. Facilitating behavior change and well-being to improve health outcomes: Standards of Medical Care in Diabetes—2022. *Diabetes Care*. 2021;45(suppl 1):S60-S82.
43. American Diabetes Association. Pharmacologic approaches to glycemic treatment. *Diabetes Care*. 2017;40(suppl 1):S64-S74.
44. Wynn RL, Meiller TF, Crossley HL. Insulin. In: *Lexicomp for Dentistry Online*. 37th ed. 2022:1910.
45. Rodbard D. Continuous glucose monitoring: a review of recent studies demonstrating improved glycemic outcomes. *Diabetes Technol Ther*. 2017;19(S3):S25-S37.
46. Liu H, Shan X, Yu J, Li X, Hu L. Recent advances in inhaled formulations and pulmonary insulin delivery systems. *Curr Pharm Biotechnol*. 2020;21(3):180-193.
47. Dasari N, Jiang A, Skochdopole A, et al. Updates in diabetic wound healing, inflammation, and scarring. *Semin Plast Surg*. 2021;35(3):153-158.
48. Kumar A, Arora A, Sharma P, et al. Is diabetes mellitus associated with mortality and severity of COVID-19? A meta-analysis. *Diabetes Metab Syndr*. 2020;14(4):535-545.
49. Centers for Disease Control and Prevention. Living with diabetes: managing sick days. Published July 23, 2020. https://www.cdc.gov/diabetes/managing/flu-sick-days.html. Accessed February 27, 2022.
50. American Diabetes Association Professional Practice Committee. Retinopathy, neuropathy, and foot care: standards of medical care in diabetes—2022. *Diabetes Care*. 2022; 45(suppl 1):S185-S194.
51. American Diabetes Association Professional Practice Committee. Chronic kidney disease and risk management: Standards of Medical Care in Diabetes—2022. *Diabetes Care*. 2021;45(suppl 1):S175-S184.
52. American Diabetes Association, Professional Practice Committee. Cardiovascular Disease and risk management: Standards of Medical Care in Diabetes—2022. *Diabetes Care*. 2022;45(S1):S1440S174.
53. Heilbrun A, Drossos T. Evidence for mental health contributions to medical care in diabetes management: economic and professional considerations. *Curr Diab Rep*. 2020;20(12):79.
54. Miller A, Ouanounou A. Diagnosis, management, and dental considerations for the diabetic patient. *J Can Dent Assoc*. 2020;86:k8.
55. American Dental Association Council on Scientific Affairs. Diabetes. Published January 24, 2022. https://www.ada.org/resources/research/science-and-research-institute/oral-health-topics/diabetes. Accessed February 27, 2022.
56. Svoboda SA, Shields BE. Cutaneous manifestations of nutritional excess: pathophysiologic effects of hyperglycemia and hyperinsulinemia on the skin. *Cutis*. 2021;107(2): 74-78.

CHAPTER 55

The Patient with Cancer

Jane C. Cotter, BSDH, MS, CTTS, FAADH

CHAPTER OUTLINE

LEARNING OBJECTIVES

After studying this chapter, the student will be able to:

1. Identify healthcare professionals involved in the multidisciplinary oncology team.
2. Explain several systemic medical treatment options utilized in cancer management.
3. Describe common oral complications secondary to cancer treatment.
4. Provide examples of evidence-based dental hygiene care strategies for common oral complications of cancer treatment.

Dental hygiene care of the patient with cancer before, during, and after therapy strives to not only attain, but also maintain a patient's oral health at the highest possible level. This contributes to the patient's general health and overall quality of life.

- Cancer treatment modalities (**radiation therapy**, **chemotherapy**, surgery, and hematopoietic cell transplantation) have the potential to significantly affect the oral cavity.
- The patient will be under the care of a team of multidisciplinary specialists. **Box 55-1** lists the members of the multidisciplinary team.

Box 55-1 Multidisciplinary Team for the Care of the Patient with Cancer

Cancer Specialists

- Medical oncologist: provides cancer management utilizing chemotherapeutic modalities.
- Radiation oncologist: responsible for the planning, delivery, and follow-up of radiation therapy.
- Oncology surgeon (all subspecialties): biopsy and/or excision of cancer.
- **Oncology** nurse: provides clinical support in the medical, surgical, and/or radiation management of the cancer patient.
- Oncology dietitian: specializes in developing a plan for good nutrition during cancer therapy and proper food selection for tube feeding.
- Oncology social worker: provides psychosocial support and is often a liaison between clinical staff and patient/family.
- Oral care specialists: play a role in initial diagnosis and management of oral complications during cancer therapy. Provide dental clearance prior to cancer therapy.
  - Dental hygienist.
  - Dentist.
  - Oral maxillofacial surgeon.
  - Periodontist.
  - Endodontist.
  - Oral maxillofacial prosthodontist.
  - Oral pathologist.

Other Health Specialists

- Speech pathologist.
- Physical therapist.
- Occupational therapist.
- Psychologist/psychiatrist.

Description

- Cancer refers to:
  - A disease in which the normal cell division process (mitosis) malfunctions. Abnormal or damaged DNA result in cells that grow and multiply to form a **neoplasm**.[1]
  - **Benign** neoplasms are slow growing and do not invade surrounding tissue.[1]
  - **Malignant** neoplasms grow rapidly and invade surrounding tissues. Malignant cells that break away may spread to distant locations via the lymph or circulatory system (**metastasis**).[1]
- Cancers are classified based on the tissue origin.[1]
  - Epithelial tissue—**carcinomas**
  - Connective tissue—**sarcomas**
- Categories of cancer[1]
  - Hematologic (blood) cancers
  - Solid tumor cancers
    - Benign
    - Malignant
- The characteristics of benign and malignant neoplasms are compared in **Table 55-1**.[2]
- **Staging**[1]:
  - A succinct, standardized description based on origin, size, and extent of the tumor.
  - Made up of three components: *T* (tumor size), *N* (presence or absence of lymph nodes), and *M* (presence or absence of distant metastases).
- Common signs and symptoms of cancer are listed in **Box 55-2**.

I. Incidence and Survival

Cancer is the second leading cause of death in the United States for adults younger than 85 years.[3] Survival depends on the following:

- Type of cancer.
- Location and size of the tumor.
- Presence of distant metastases.
- Tumor sensitivity to treatment.
- Physical condition: comorbidities and age.

II. Risk Factors

Modifiable and nonmodifiable risk factors for cancer[4]

- Modifiable:
  - Tobacco use
    - Smoked
    - Smokeless

Table 55-1 Characteristics of Benign and Malignant Neoplasms

Characteristic	Benign	Malignant
Cell characteristics	Well-differentiated cells of the tissue from which the tumor originated	Cells are undifferentiated. **Anaplastic** features (lack of differentiation)
Mode of growth	Tumor grows by expansion and does not infiltrate the surrounding tissues; encapsulated	Tumor grows at the periphery and sends out processes that infiltrate and destroy the surrounding tissues.
Rate of growth	Rate of growth is usually slow.	Rate of growth is usually relatively rapid and is dependent on the level of differentiation; the more anaplastic the tumor, the more rapid the rate of growth.
Metastasis	Does not spread by metastasis	Gains access to the blood and lymph systems to metastasize to other organs.
Destruction of tissue	Does not usually cause tissue damage unless location interferes with blood flow	Often causes extensive tissue damage as the tumor outgrows its blood supply or encroaches on blood flow to the area; may also produce substances that cause cell damage.

Reproduced from Norris TL, Tuan RL. *Porth's Pathophysiology: Concepts of Altered Health States*. 10th ed. Philadelphia, PA: Wolters Kluwer; 2019.

Box 55-2 Common Signs and Symptoms of Cancer

- **C:** A change in bowel or bladder habits (colon)
- **A:** A sore that doesn't heal on skin or inside mouth (skin or oral)
- **U:** Unusual bleeding or discharge (uterine, lung, and colon)
- **T:** Thickening or lump in breast tissue or anywhere on the body (breast and testicle)
- **I:** Indigestion/difficulty swallowing
- **O:** Obvious change in wart or mole (skin)
- **N:** Nagging cough or hoarseness (lung or throat)
- **U:** Unexplained anemia
- **S:** Sudden weight loss

Data from American Cancer Society. https://www.cancer.org/treatment/understanding-your-diagnosis/signs-and-symptoms-of-cancer.html. Updated November 6, 2020. Accessed March 12, 2022.

- Alcohol abuse
- Sun exposure
- Immune system deficits
  - Disease states—human immunodeficiency virus (HIV), diabetes
  - Therapeutic intervention—after organ transplant
- Environmental exposure
  - Chemicals—pollution, pesticides, asbestos
- Viruses
  - Human papilloma virus 16 and 18
  - Epstein-Barr virus
  - Hepatitis B or C
  - Herpes virus

- Nonmodifiable:
  - Age
  - Gender
  - Genetics

III. Types of Cancer

Most common cancer types[5]:

- Men
  - Prostate.
  - Lung and bronchus.
  - Colon and rectum.
- Women
  - Breast.
  - Lung and bronchus.
  - Colon and rectum.

IV. How Cancer Is Treated

Cancer treatment may include one or more treatment modalities and is selected based on the size, location, and if there is any metastasis.[6]

- Treatment approaches
  - Curative.
  - Control the spread.

- Palliative care.
- Clinical trials.
- Types of cancer treatment
  - Surgery (excisional or debulking).
  - Chemotherapy.
  - Radiation therapy.
  - Targeted therapy.
  - Immunotherapy.
  - Stem cell or bone marrow transplant.
  - Hormone therapy.
  - Proton therapy.
  - Biologic therapy.
  - Bisphosphonates.
  - Low-dose chemotherapy.

Surgery

- Surgery is the most common form of treatment for solid tumors, both malignant and benign.

I. Indications

- Tumors that are small in size, localized, and easy to remove.[7]
- Debulk or remove portions of large tumors before treatment (chemotherapy or radiation therapy).[7]
- Provide pain relief or prolong life when there is no chance of cure (**palliative/palliation**).[7]

Chemotherapy

I. Objectives

- To destroy cancer cells and prevent metastasis.
- To prevent cancer from recurring.
- To provide an improved quality of life.

II. Indications

- Eliminate a localized tumor too large for surgical removal.
- Treat cancer that has metastasized to other parts of the body.
- Prevent cancer recurrence with maintenance therapy.
- Use before surgery to make a tumor easier to remove completely.
- Palliative.
- Treatment of "liquid tumors" such as **leukemia**.

III. Types

Box 55-3 lists the types of agents used for chemotherapy.

Box 55-3 Types of Agents Used for Chemotherapy

1. Alkylating agents
2. Antitumor antibiotics
3. Monoclonal antibodies
4. Antimetabolites
5. Plant alkaloids
6. Antiangiogenics
7. Hormones
8. Bisphosphonates

IV. Systemic Side Effects

Chemotherapy affects both rapidly dividing cancer cells and rapidly dividing normal cells (hair, oral/gastrointestinal mucosa, and bone marrow). Halting cell division of normal cells may cause side effects that range from mild to life threatening. The most common include the following:

- **Alopecia** (hair loss).
- Myelosuppression (bone marrow suppression causing a reduction in blood counts leading to anemia, leukopenia, and thrombocytopenia).
- Immunosuppression (inhibition of antibody responses resulting from leukopenia).
- Nausea, vomiting, and diarrhea.
- Loss of appetite.
- Gastrointestinal mucositis.

V. Oral Complications

The following are oral complications resulting from chemotherapy[6,8]:

- **Oral mucositis/stomatitis**: an inflammation of the oral mucosa characterized by erythema, ulceration, and pain.
- **Xerostomia**: subjective report of oral dryness.
- **Salivary gland hypofunction**: objective reduction in saliva production.
- Neurosensory: taste alteration, taste loss (dysgeusia)
- Infections:
  - Bacterial.
  - Viral: herpes simplex, varicella zoster, and cytomegalovirus.
  - Fungal: *Candida albicans*.
- Bleeding: anywhere in the mouth; spontaneous or induced.
- Neurotoxicity: mimics toothache; usually bilateral.
- **Osteonecrosis of the jaw (ONJ)**: exposed bone of at least 8 weeks duration in either the maxilla or mandible secondary to use of systemic

bisphosphonates and/or other antiresorptive medication/therapies.[9]

- Also referenced as *medication-related osteonecrosis of the jaw* (MRONJ).

Radiation Therapy

- Radiation therapy uses ionizing radiation to treat cancer.[10]
- Radiation impacts the cancer cell's ability to replicate and survive.
- Not all tumors are radiosensitive (ability of the radiation therapy to kill the tumor).
- Head and neck radiation therapy produces acute short-term and chronic long-term effects in the oral cavity.

I. Indications

- Treat a small localized tumor that is radiosensitive.
- Shrink a large tumor before surgery.
- Increase the effectiveness of chemotherapy when used concurrently.
- Prevent the spread of cancer or control residual tumor.
- Prevent a recurrence of the cancer.
- Provide symptom/pain relief for bone metastases or palliative therapy.

II. Types

A. External Beam

Conventional use of ionizing radiation applied outside the body.

- Intensity-modulated radiation therapy (IMRT)
  - Developed in the late 1990s.
  - Considered a high-precision delivery of radiation.
  - Accomplished via computer-guided images of target anatomy with radiation produced by a linear accelerator.
  - Used in treatment of head and neck cancer.
  - Radiation dose is elevated at the site of the gross tumor while simultaneously sparing the surrounding normal tissue.
  - Results in decreased side effects, better tumor targeting as compared to conventional external beam radiation.
  - **Figure 55-1** illustrates the patient preparation prior to IMRT.
- Intensity modulated proton beam therapy (IMPBT)[11,12]
  - New method of radiation delivery, used in some head and neck cancer patients.
  - Technique is considered more precise than IMRT with less damage to the surrounding oral structures, thus producing less acute and chronic oral complications.
  - Not widely available, more expensive to deliver care.
  - Recent research shows a decrease in mucositis, nausea, and dysgeusia with IMPBT.

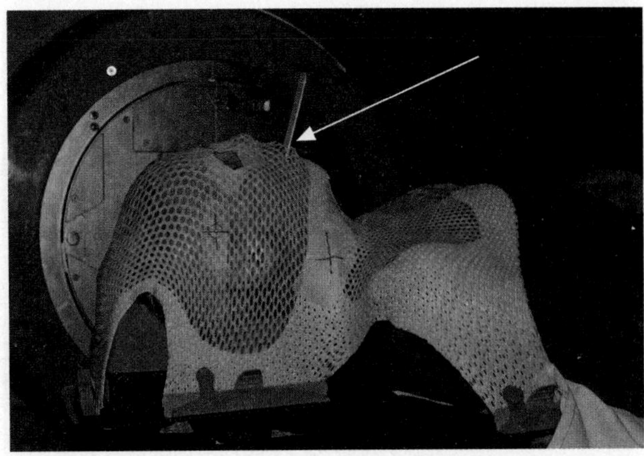

Figure 55-1 Custom Patient Mask. This is worn by the patient at each radiation appointment. The mask, made out of firm mesh, snaps into the treatment table to assist in immobilizing the patient for precise radiation delivery throughout the course of radiation therapy. A bite block is placed intraorally (arrow) to maintain the mouth in a static position. The linear accelerator (source of radiation) is seen in the background.

B. Internal Source

- Radiation source (such as **radium** implants or seeds) is placed within the body.
- Less radiation is delivered to the surrounding tissues than when an external source is utilized.

III. Doses

- Total dose given depends on the type of tumor, treatment goals, and patient's ability to tolerate treatment.
- Total radiation dose can range from 30–70 Gy.
- It is divided into equal doses (conventional) or modulated fractions (IMRT) per day.
- It is given once a day, 5 days a week, for 5–8 weeks.

IV. Systemic Effects

- Skin reactions: looks like a bad sunburn.
- Fatigue.
- Nausea, vomiting, diarrhea, and constipation.
- Immunosuppression.
- Alopecia.

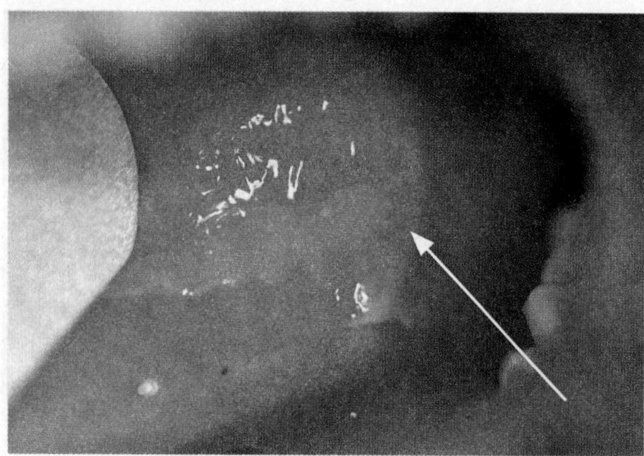

Figure 55-2 Mucositis Left Lateral Border of Tongue, Secondary to Radiation to the Head and Neck Tissue. Note erythema distal to the ulcerated area (arrow). This lesion is characterized by pain, complicating the patient's ability to eat, speak, or swallow.

V. Oral Complications

- Concurrent oral complications
  - Mucositis[13,14] (See **Figure 55-2**)
  - Dysgeusia[15]
  - Xerostomia[16]
  - Infections[13]
    - Bacterial
    - Viral
    - Fungal
- Posttreatment oral complications
  - Xerostomia (lifetime)[16-18]
  - **Dysgeusia**[15,17]
  - **Postradiation caries (PRC)**[17-19]
  - **Trismus**[17,20]
  - **Osteoradionecrosis**[20]

Hematopoietic Stem Cell Transplantation

Bone marrow manufactures stem cells that differentiate into the cells of the blood and immune system. Cancer of the blood and immune system, including leukemia, multiple myeloma, and lymphoma, may be treated with **hematopoietic** stem cell transplantation (HPSCT). Healthy bone marrow stem cells are collected from the patient or a compatible donor.[21]

I. Types

- Autologous: self.
- Allogeneic: human leukocyte antigen–matched donor, either related or unrelated.
- **Syngeneic**: identical twin.

A. Patient Selection

- Indications: patient not responsive to chemotherapy alone; **relapse** occurs after one or more **remissions**.
- Evaluation: medical and dental assessments completed to ensure the patient is free of infection and physically able to undergo the preparative regimen.

B. Conditioning of Patient to Receive Bone Marrow Graft

- Preparative high-dose immunosuppressive regimen: chemotherapy alone or with total body irradiation.
- Purposes:
  - Kill malignant cells.
  - Suppress immune system so new stem cells/marrow will engraft.

C. Transplantation

- Intravenous infusion of donor's marrow/stem cells.

D. Pancytopenia

- **Pancytopenia** is a reduction in all cellular elements of the blood, which includes white blood cells, red blood cells, and platelets.
- Protective isolation for the patient is required; the patient is highly susceptible to infection.
- Function of new marrow (to produce peripheral blood elements) begins after 10–20 days.

E. Recovery

- Immune recovery: 3–12 months; long-term recovery: 1–3 years.
- Autogenic or syngenetic stem cell transplantation has fewer side effects or complications.
- Allogenic stem cell transplantation may have acute and/or chronic complications.

II. Acute Complications

- Acute graft-versus-host disease (GVHD)[22]:
  - Description: The donor's T-lymphocytes see the host cell antigens as foreign and react against the host tissue.
- Symptoms:
  - Present during the first 100 days posttransplant.
  - Painful red skin rash starting on the palms of hands and soles of feet and progressing to the upper trunk.
  - Severe, persistent diarrhea.

    - Jaundice, elevated liver enzymes, liver tenderness.
- Infection:
    - Bacterial.
    - Viral: herpes simplex, varicella zoster, and cytomegalovirus.
    - Fungal: *C. albicans*.
- Gastrointestinal, hepatic, cardiac, pulmonary, hematologic, and neurologic complications.
- Oral complications:
    - Oral mucositis: appears 10–14 days posttransplant.
    - Xerostomia.
    - Viral and fungal infections: herpes simplex virus and *C. albicans*.

III. Chronic Complications

- Chronic GVHD[22,23]:
    - May affect all organs of the body.
    - Can appear up to 2 years posttransplant.
- Oral complications:
    - Oral mucositis.
    - Lichen planus.
    - Oral squamous cell carcinoma.
    - Sjogren syndrome.
    - Rampant caries.

Mucositis Management

I. Prevention/Oral Health Maintenance[24]

- Basic oral care using a soft toothbrush.
- As dental flossing is technique sensitive, use may be precluded during cytotoxic treatment.
- Use of a bland mouthrinse such as normal saline, three to four times/day.
- Modify diet to avoid rough or sharp foods.
- Avoid alcohol and tobacco.
- Cryotherapy (ice chips):
    - Recommended for selected patient populations such as multiple myeloma patients receiving high-dose Melphalan and head and neck cancer patients receiving bolus dosing of 5-fluorouracil.
    - Instruct patient to hold ice chips in mouth immediately prior to and during the administration of chemotherapy agent.
- Palifermin (a human recombinant keratinocyte growth factor)[25]:
    - Intravenous infusion in selected populations prior to peripheral blood stem cell transplant.
    - Given for 3 consecutive days before and after myelotoxic therapy for a total of six doses.

II. Treatment of Established Mucositis[26,27]

- Mouthrinse containing diphenhydramine hydrochloric acid in combination with other agents (usually coating agent and topical anesthetic)
    - Evidence does not support a direct effect of this antihistamine on the prevention or treatment of mucositis lesions.
    - This type of rinse is often used to palliate pain topically.
- Systemic pain medication: patient-controlled analgesia with morphine for the management of pain due to oral mucositis in patients undergoing hematopoietic stem cell transplant.
- Transdermal fentanyl patch may be effective in the management of mucositis pain due to conventional and high-dose chemotherapy with or without total body irradiation.
- Morphine mouthrinse may reduce the severity and duration of mucositis pain in patients undergoing head and neck area radiation therapy.
- Doxepin mouthrinse (0.5%) may be effective for the management of pain due to oral mucositis.

Dental Hygiene Care Plan

I. Objectives

- It is recommended patients be in optimal oral health before starting any type of cancer therapy. Overall objectives include the following[6]:
    - Assess the oral cavity for any signs of hard or soft tissue infection.
    - Eliminate or minimize sources of dental/periodontal or soft tissue infection.
    - Eliminate or minimize any areas of chronic trauma or tissue irritation.
    - Provide preventive oral care education to the patient and/or the caregiver.

II. Personal Factors

The very word *cancer* brings fear and anxiety to the patient, and many times it is viewed by the patient as *cancer equals death*. This will impact anything taught to the patient. Suggestions include the following:

- Encourage the patient to bring a friend or a family member along to take notes during teaching visits.

- Provide written instructions appropriate to the reading level of the patient. Make sure they are written in the patient's native language.
- Provide positive reinforcement and be creative in helping the patient maintain optimal oral health.
- Show acceptance and empathy. Acknowledge the appropriateness of the patient's concerns.
- Practice active listening skills.

III. Oral Care Protocol

The following sections are adapted from the *Oral Complications of Cancer Treatment: What the Oral Health Team Can Do* from the National Institute of Dental and Craniofacial Research (National Institutes of Health publication no. 09-4372).

- Similarities exist among the three forms of treatment (radiation therapy, chemotherapy, and hematopoietic stem cell transplantation).
- There are differences that dental hygienists need to know to provide appropriate oral care.
- Numerous grading scales have been developed to assess the severity of oral mucositis, but none for the other oral complications.
- **Table 55-2** lists an example of one mucositis scale. Scales are useful to:
  - Measure mucositis in the nursing/medical setting.
  - Document treatment toxicity in the clinical and/or research setting.
  - Communicate interprofessionally.

Table 55-2 World Health Organization's Oral Mucositis Scale

Grade	Clinical Features
0	No oral mucositis
1	Mild: soreness, erythema
2	Moderate: oral ulcers, solid foods tolerated
3	Severe: oral ulcers, liquid diet only (due to mucositis)
4	Life threatening: oral ulcers, **alimentation** impossible (due to mucositis)

Data from Lalla R, Sonis S, Peterson D. Management of oral mucositis in patients with cancer. *Dent Clin North Am*. 2008;52(1):61-68; Sonis ST, Eilers JP, Epstein JB, et al. Validation of a new scoring system for the assessment of clinical trial research of oral mucositis induced by radiation or chemotherapy. Mucositis Study Group. *Cancer*. 1999;85(10):2103-2113. doi:10.1002/(sici)1097-0142(19990515)85:10<2103::aid-cncr2>3.0.co;2-0; World Health Organization. Published 1979. *WHO Handbook for Reporting Results of Cancer Treatment*. http://apps.who.int/iris/bitstream/handle/10665/37200/WHO_OFFSET_48.pdf?sequence=1&isAllowed=y. Accessed April 4, 2022.

A. Pretreatment Therapy

- Patients who do intensive personal oral care in preparation for and during their cancer therapy have a reduced risk for the development of oral complications.
- **Box 55-4** provides examples of dental hygiene/dental treatment options that may be beneficial before the start of cancer therapy.

Box 55-4 Dental Hygiene/Dental Pretreatment Guidelines for Patients Planning to Undergo Cancer Therapy

Dental

- Conduct a pretreatment oral health examination.
- Schedule dental treatment in consultation with the oncologist (medical or radiation).
- Extract teeth with a poor or questionable prognosis at least 2 weeks before the start of cancer therapy.
- Restore or repair indicated teeth before the start of cancer therapy.
- Perform other necessary oral surgery procedures at least 2 weeks before the start of cancer therapy.

Dental Hygiene

- Conduct a pretreatment oral health assessment.
- Schedule dental hygiene treatment in consultation with the oncologist (medical or radiation).
- Perform dental hygiene treatment (nonsurgical periodontal debridement, polishing, and fluoride applications) before the start of cancer treatment.
- Evaluate the patient's oral health knowledge and provide an appropriate oral hygiene regimen based on the cancer management.
- Prevent tooth demineralization and dental caries:
  - Instruct the patient in the daily application of fluoride gel at home.
  - If receiving head and neck radiation therapy, fabricate custom gel-applicator trays for the patient.
  - Demonstrate application of a 1.1% neutral pH sodium fluoride gel or a 0.4% stannous unflavored gel for use in the trays or brush-on when tray insertion may not be tolerated.
  - Use only a neutral pH sodium fluoride gel for porcelain crowns or glass or resin ionomer restorations.
  - The trays cover all tooth surfaces and are left in the mouth for 5 minutes. Instruct the patient to have nothing to eat or drink for 30 minutes after using the fluoride.

B. Head and Neck Radiation Therapy[17-19]

- Patients receiving radiation therapy to the head and neck are at high risk for developing severe oral complications that will affect the patient in the short and long term.
- **Box 55-5** lists an example oral care protocol to be followed during treatment.

Box 55-5 Oral Care Protocol during Treatment

Daily Biofilm Removal

- Gently brush teeth with a soft toothbrush and fluoride toothpaste after every meal and at bedtime. The tongue may be brushed with a soft toothbrush and water.
- Use interdental aids to gently, but thoroughly clean between teeth before brushing at least once a day.

Mouthrinsing

- Every 2–3 hours during the day, rinse the mouth with a baking soda, salt, and water solution, followed by a plain water rinse. (Use one-fourth teaspoon baking soda and one-eighth teaspoon salt in a cup of lukewarm water.)
- Use of fluoridated water when available.

Xerostomia

- Sip water frequently.
- Suck on ice chips or use sugar-free gum or candy.
- Use saliva substitute spray or gel or a prescribed saliva stimulant.
- Avoid lemon glycerin swabs.
- Avoid hot, spicy, salty, sharp, or high-sucrose foods.
- Moisten foods with gravy or liquids before eating.

Dental Caries Prevention

- Use fluoride toothpaste every day.
- If prescribed, brush teeth with 1.1% neutral sodium fluoride gel for 60 seconds after usual tooth cleaning, just before going to bed. Do not eat, drink, or rinse for a minimum of 30 minutes afterward.
- If using custom-made polyvinyl trays, place gel in trays, apply to teeth, close mouth, and hold in place for 5 minutes. Set timer. Remove trays, expectorate several times, and do not eat or drink for at least 30 minutes afterward.

Oral Pain Management

- Swish and spit a prescribed mouthrinse containing topical anesthetic solution 30 minutes before eating.

- During radiation therapy:
  - Encourage daily oral care, including biofilm removal at least twice daily.
  - Encourage daily fluoride use in any form (i.e., tray, brush-on, rinse).
  - Monitor the patient for trismus; check for pain or weakness in masticating muscles in the radiation field.
  - Instruct the patient to exercise three times a day, opening and closing the mouth as far as possible without pain; repeat 20 times.
- After radiation therapy:
  - For the first 6 months after cancer treatment, recall the patient every 4–8 weeks as needed for nonsurgical periodontal therapy.
  - Review instructions for daily oral self-care.
  - Reinforce the importance of daily oral self-care.
  - After mucositis subsides, consult with the radiation/medical oncologist regarding timing of denture/appliance fabrication.
  - Observe for trismus, demineralization, and caries.
  - Lifelong, daily applications of prescription fluoride (in any form) are recommended for patients with chronic salivary gland hypofunction.
  - Advise against oral surgery on irradiated bone because of the risk of osteoradionecrosis.
  - Tooth extraction, if unavoidable, is conservative.
  - Prophylaxis against possible osteoradionecrosis is accomplished with pentoxifylline 400 mg pre- and postextraction.[27]

C. Chemotherapy

- The extent of oral complications of chemotherapy depends on the following[6,7,10,18,19]:
  - The degree of preexisting dental and oral disease.
  - The chemotherapy drugs used and their dosages.
  - The use of concurrent or adjuvant radiation therapy to the head/neck.
  - The patient's daily oral self-care.
- Before any dental or dental hygiene clinical procedures during chemotherapy:
  - Consult the medical oncologist.
  - Ask the medical oncologist to order blood work 24 hours before oral surgery or other invasive procedures (such as nonsurgical periodontal debridement). Postpone when the platelet count is less than 50,000/mm^3 or abnormal clotting factors are present and/or neutrophil count is less than 1000/mm^3.
  - In patients with fever of unknown origin as determined by the medical oncologist,

check for oral source of viral, bacterial, or fungal infection.
  - Encourage thorough oral self-care.
  - Review indications for use of antibiotic premedication for patients with central venous catheters or peripherally inserted catheters (also known as central lines). There is no evidence suggesting this is beneficial and as such varies from practitioner to practitioner.
  - Consult the medical oncologist for preference on using the American Heart Association's prophylactic antibiotic regimen or another antibiotic regimen.
- Refer to Box 55-5 for a suggested oral care protocol during treatment.
- After chemotherapy: place the patient on a dental hygiene continuing care schedule once treatment is complete and all side effects, including immunosuppression, have resolved.

D. Hematopoietic Stem Cell Transplantation

Some hematopoietic stem cell transplant patients develop acute oral complications, especially patients who had an allogeneic stem cell transplant and develop GVHD.

- After transplantation[21,22]
  - Monitor for oral infections of the soft tissues. Herpes simplex and *C. albicans* are common oral infections.
  - Delay elective dental procedures (such as implants) for 1 year.
  - Follow patients for long-term oral complications (changes in taste, xerostomia, and dental caries). Such problems are strong indicators of chronic GVHD.
  - Continue to monitor the patient's oral health for biofilm control, tooth demineralization, dental caries, and oral infection.
  - Follow transplant patients carefully for secondary malignancies in the oral region.

E. Special Care for Children

Children receiving chemotherapy and/or radiation therapy are at risk for the same oral complications as adults. Other actions to consider in managing pediatric patients include the following[28,29]:

- Extract loose primary teeth and any teeth expected to exfoliate during cancer treatment.
- Remove orthodontic bands and brackets if myelosuppressive chemotherapy is planned or if the appliances will be in the radiation field.
- Continually monitor craniofacial and dental structures for abnormal growth and development.
- Encourage routine daily personal oral care including biofilm removal and fluoride application.
- Avoid cariogenic foods and drinks. If these are necessary to improve a child's weight, then have the child rinse with fluoridated water after eating or drinking.

Documentation

Each patient appointment is carefully documented to include at least the following:

- Cancer diagnosis, type of treatment, treatment start and completion dates.
- Oncologists' names and contact information; note any consults done with the oncologists.
- Oral assessment, clinical care provided, patient teaching on each visit.
- Any oral complications present, grade of oral mucositis indicating severity and type of symptom management prescribed.
- Planned follow-up visit and plan of care with proposed symptom management treatment outcomes.
- **Box 55-6** shows an example of a documentation for a patient with oral lesions related to cancer therapy.

Box 55-6 Example Documentation: Patient with Oral Lesions Related to Cancer Treatment

- **S**—The patient presents for 3-month periodontal maintenance appointment; medical history changes include diagnosis of stage IV floor of mouth (FOM) cancer; lesion found at previous periodontal maintenance visit and the patient evaluated by otolaryngology 3 months ago, surgery completed 10 weeks ago followed by 6 weeks of radiation therapy (total of 62 Gy) ending last week.
- **O**—Complete oral examination performed; unable to perform periodontal maintenance due to severe oral ulcerations and inflammation involving the tongue bilaterally as well as the mandibular labial mucosa and vestibule; saliva appears thick and ropey; reviewed oral hygiene; the patient is not currently using fluoride.
- **A**—Oral mucositis grade 4 and severe xerostomia following radiation to the oral cavity for squamous cell carcinoma of the FOM. Current health status precludes dental hygiene instrumentation today.

- **P**—Recommend:
  1. Discuss the above findings and today's recommendations with oncology team (primary oncologist and oncology nurse).
  2. Use of extra-soft toothbrush after meals and at bedtime.
  3. Interproximal cleansing with appropriate aid.
  4. Neutral sodium fluoride gel applied with brush 1× day following dental biofilm removal.
  5. Baking soda mouthrinse—mix one-fourth teaspoon baking soda and one-eighth teaspoon salt in 8 oz of warm water; rinse with 20 mL 3× day.
  6. Avoid mouthrinses containing alcohol.

Will follow 1× week until oral mucositis resolves; on next visit, assess xerostomia and make treatment recommendations as needed.

Signed: ______________________________, RDH
Date: ____________________

Factors to Teach the Patient

- How to exercise the jaw muscles three times a day to prevent and treat jaw stiffness from head and neck radiation therapy.
- Why to avoid candy, gum, and soda unless they are sugar free.
- Why to avoid spicy or acidic foods and the use of toothpicks.
- Why to avoid the use of tobacco products and alcohol.
- Why the dental hygienist needs to conduct an oral soft tissue screening and complete oral examination at regular frequent intervals.
- How and when to use dental biofilm control methods, gel-tray application, use of saliva substitute, and all other details of personal oral care to reduce oral side effects caused by the disease and/or cancer treatment.
- Ideas for remembering to follow the instructions to keep the mouth healthier and more comfortable during cancer treatment.
- The reasons why a routine schedule of preventive periodontal scaling, fluoride application, and oral hygiene assessment by a dental hygienist contributes to the success of the cancer treatment.

Factors to Teach the Caregiver

- How maintaining optimal oral health throughout the treatment will contribute to the successful outcome of cancer therapy.
- The need to report any changes in the oral cavity to the oncologist and/or dentist/dental hygienist.
- Why it is necessary for the patient to receive preventive periodontal scaling, polishing if indicated, fluoride application, and oral hygiene assessment by a dental hygienist on a regular frequent basis.
- Why it is important to support the patient in stopping tobacco and alcohol use.

References

1. National Cancer Institute. What Is Cancer? National Cancer Institute. Published May 5, 2021. https://www.cancer.gov/about-cancer/understanding/what-is-cancer. Accessed November 21, 2021.
2. Norris TL, Tuan RL. *Porth's Pathophysiology: Concepts of Altered Health States*. 10th ed. Wolters Kluwer; 2019.
3. Heron M. Deaths: leading causes for 2019. *National Vital Statistics Report*. 70(9):1-114. https://www.cdc.gov/nchs/nvss/leading-causes-of-death.htm#publications. Accessed November 21, 2021.
4. National Cancer Institute. Risk factors. Published 2015. https://www.cancer.gov/about-cancer/causes-prevention/risk. Accessed November 21, 2021
5. National Cancer Institute. Cancer statistics. Published September 25, 2020. https://www.cancer.gov/about-cancer/understanding/statistics. Accessed November 21, 2021.

6. National Cancer Institute. Types of cancer treatment. Published January 1, 2017. https://www.cancer.gov/about-cancer/treatment/types. Accessed November 21, 2021.
7. MD Anderson Cancer Center. Surgery. https://www.mdanderson.org/treatment-options/surgery.html%20Accessed%2010.18.202. Accessed October 18, 2021.
8. Frowen J, Hughes R, Skeat J. The prevalence of patient-reported dysphagia and oral complications in cancer patients. *Support Care Cancer*. 2019;28(3):1141-1150.
9. Yarom N, Shapiro CL, Peterson DE, et al. Medication-related osteonecrosis of the jaw: MASCC/ISOO/ASCO Clinical Practice Guideline. *J Clin Oncol*. 2019;37(25):2270-2290.
10. Hunter M, Kellett J, Toohey K, et al. Toxicities caused by head and neck cancer treatments and their influence on the development of malnutrition: review of the literature. *Eur J Investig Health, Psychol Educ*. 2020;10(4):935-949.
11. Williams VM, Parvathaneni U, Laramore GE, Aljabab S, Wong TP, Liao JJ. Intensity-modulated proton therapy for nasopharynx cancer: 2-year outcomes from a single institution. *Int J of Part Ther*. 2021;8(2):28-40.
12. Lee A, Kitpanit S, Chilov M, Langendijk JA, Lu J, Lee NY. A systematic review of proton therapy for the management of nasopharyngeal cancer. *Int J of Part Ther*. 2021;8(1):119-130.
13. Nishii M, Soutome S, Kawakita A, et al. Factors associated with severe oral mucositis and candidiasis in patients undergoing radiotherapy for oral and oropharyngeal carcinomas: a retrospective multicenter study of 326 patients. *Support Care Cancer*. 2019;28(3):1069-1075.
14. Hansen CR, Bertelsen A, Zukauskaite R, et al. Prediction of radiation-induced mucositis of H&N cancer patients based on a large patient cohort. *Radiother Oncol*. 2020;147:15-21.
15. Asif M, Moore A, Yarom N, et al. The effect of radiotherapy on taste sensation in head and neck cancer patients - a prospective study. *Radiat Oncol*. 2020;15(1):144
16. Martinez AC, Silva IMV, Berti Couto SA, et al. Late oral complications caused by head and neck radiotherapy: clinical and laboratory study. *J Oral Maxillofac Res*. 2020;11(3):e3.
17. Bhandari S, Soni BW, Bahl A, et al. Radiotherapy-induced oral morbidities in head and neck cancer patients. *Support Care Cancer.* 2020;40(3):238-250.
18. Oba MK, Innocentini LM., Viani G, et al. Evaluation of the correlation between side effects to oral mucosa, salivary glands, and general health status with quality of life during intensity-modulated radiotherapy for head and neck cancer. *Support Care Cancer.* 2021;29;127-134.
19. Watson E, Eason B, Kreher M, et al. The DMFTS160: a new index for measuring post-radiation caries. *Oral Onc*. 2020; 108:104823.
20. Khoo SC, Nabil S, Fauzi AA, et al. Predictors of osteoradionecrosis following irradiated tooth extraction. *Radiat Oncol*. 2021;16(1):1-12.
21. Khaddour K, Hana CK, Mewawalla P. Hematopoietic stem cell transplantation. *StatPearls*. Updated June 27, 2022. https://www.ncbi.nlm.nih.gov/books/NBK536951/. Accessed December 5, 2022.
22. Justiz Vaillant AA, Modi P, et al. Graft versus host disease. *StatPearls*. Updated October 20, 2022. https://www.ncbi.nlm.nih.gov/books/NBK538235/. Accessed December 5, 2022.
23. Elas S, Aljitawi O, Zadik Y. Oral graft-versus-host disease: a pictorial review and a guide for dental practitioners. *Inter Dent J*. 2021;71(1):9-20.
24. Brown TJ, Gupta A. Management of cancer therapy-associated oral mucositis. *JCO J Onco Prac*. 2020;16(3):103-109.
25. Pulito C, Cristaudo A, Porta CL, et al. Oral mucositis: the hidden side of cancer therapy. *J Exp Clin Cancer Res*. 2020;39:210.
26. Sio TT, Le-Rademacher JG, Leenstra JL, et al. Effect of doxepin mouthwash or diphenhydramine-lidocaine-antacid mouthwash vs placebo on radiotherapy-related oral mucositis pain: the Alliance A221304 Randomized Clinical Trial. *JAMA*. 2019;321(15):1481-1490.
27. Aggarwal K, Goutam M, Singh M, et al. Prophylactic use of pentoxifylline and tocopherol in patients undergoing dental extractions following radiotherapy for head and neck cancer. *Niger J Surg*. 2017;23(2):130-133.
28. Ritwik P, Chrisentery-Singleton TE. Oral and dental considerations in pediatric cancers. *Cancer Metastasis Rev*. 2020; 39:43-53.
29. Alkhuwaiter S. Parents' awareness and oral health care measurese of pediatric patient receiving chemotherapy. *J Pediatr Dent*. 2021;7(1).

CHAPTER 56

The Oral and Maxillofacial Surgery Patient

Evie F. Jesin, RRDH, BSc
Lisa F. Mallonee, RDH, RD, LD, MPH

CHAPTER OUTLINE

LEARNING OBJECTIVES

After studying this chapter, the student will be able to:

1. Discuss the role of the dental hygienist in the pre- and postsurgery care of the oral and maxillofacial surgery patient.
2. Discuss the pre- and postsurgical care planning for the maxillofacial surgery patient.

3. Identify the types of maxillary and mandibular fractures and discuss treatment options.
4. Describe the modifications for dental hygiene treatment, diet, and personal oral care procedures needed after maxillofacial surgery.
5. Explain the dental hygiene care needed before and after general surgery.

Introduction

Oral and maxillofacial surgery is the specialty of dentistry that includes diagnostic, surgical, and adjunctive treatment of diseases, injuries, and defects involving both functional and aesthetic aspects of the hard and soft tissues in the oral and maxillofacial regions.[1] **Box 56-1** lists the types of treatment included in this specialty.

Box 56-1 Categories of Oral and Maxillofacial Treatments

Dentoalveolar Surgery

Exodontics

- Impacted tooth removal
- Alveolar bone surgery: alveoloplasty, bone grafting, ridge augmentation

Infection

- Abscesses
- Osteomyelitis

Traumatic Injury Treatment

- Fractures of jaws, zygoma
- Fracture of teeth, alveolar bone

Neoplasm and Oral Pathology

- Cysts
- Tumors

Biopsy

- **Incisional biopsy**
- **Excisional biopsy**
- **Exfoliative biopsy**

Dental Implant Placement

Preprosthetic Reconstruction

- **Maxillofacial prosthetics**
- Immediate denture

Orthognathic Surgery

- Prognathism correction
- Facial aesthetics

Cleft Lip/Palate

Temporomandibular Disorders

Salivary Gland Obstruction

- The oral surgeon may be based in a group clinical setting, in a hospital, or in a private practice with outpatient hospital facilities available.
- The oral surgeon is part of a team of specially trained individuals that includes surgical assistants, anesthetists, registered nurses, and dental hygienists.
- The oral surgeon may coordinate the surgical procedures with various dental practitioners, including general dentists, laboratory technicians, prosthodontists, orthodontists, dental implant specialists, and other specialists caring for the patient.
- Surgery for treatment of diseases and correction of defects of the periodontal tissues is categorized specifically as periodontal surgery.
    - Within the scope of periodontal surgery are procedures for pocket elimination, gingivoplasty, treatment of furcation involvements, correction of mucogingival defects, treatment for bony defects about the teeth, and placing implants.
    - Preparation for periodontal surgery is not specifically described in this chapter. Many of the surgical instruments are used by both a periodontist and an oral surgeon (**Figure 56-1**).

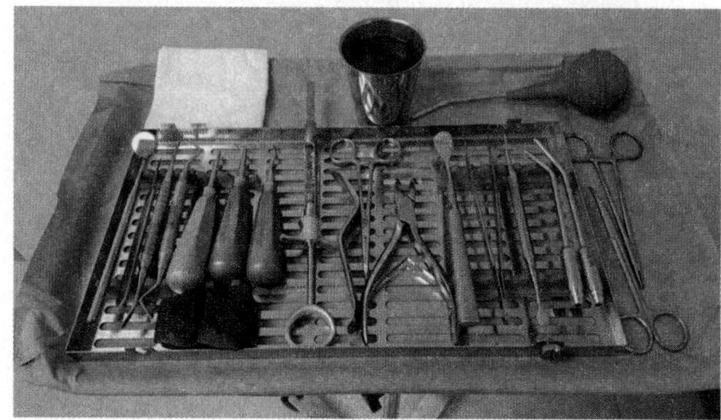

Figure 56-1 Tray Setup for Routine Extraction of Teeth. Instrument identification from left to right: dental mirror, surgical scalpel, periosteal elevator, surgical curette, elevators (three), bite-blocks, syringe with needle, Minnesota retractor, hemostat, rongeurs, retractor, forceps, bone file, surgical aspirating tip, scissors, needle holder, cups with saline solution, and bulb syringe.

Evie F. Jesin, RRDH, BSc, Professor, Toronto, ON, Canada: George Brown College.

Patient Preparation

I. Objectives

Dental hygiene care and instruction before oral and **maxillofacial** surgery may improve a patient's health and well-being by one or more of the following.

A. Reduce Oral Bacterial Count

- Aid in the preparation of an aseptic field for the surgery.
- The human oral cavity harbors a variety of microbes. Recent investigative data indicate more than 400 species of microorganisms exist in the microflora of the human oropharynx.[2]
- Make postsurgical infection less likely or less severe.

B. Reduce Inflammation of the Gingiva and Improve Tissue Tone

- Lessen local bleeding at the time of the surgery.
- Promote postsurgical healing.

C. Remove Calculus Deposits

- Remove a source of dental biofilm retention and thus improve health of gingival tissue.
- Prevent interference with placement of surgical instruments.
- Reduce risks that may result if calculus breaks off during a surgical procedure such as:
  - Danger of inhalation, particularly when a general anesthetic is used.
  - Possibility of calculus lodging in a tooth socket or other surgical area and inhibiting healing.

D. Instruct in Presurgical Personal Oral Care Procedures

- Reduce inflammation and thus improve tissue tone.
- Help to prepare the patient for postsurgical care.

E. Instruct in Appropriate Food Choices

- Foods that provide the nutrients essential to tissue building and repair during pre- and postsurgical periods.
- For the patient who will have teeth removed and immediate complete or partial dentures inserted, the importance of a diet containing all essential food groups is emphasized.

F. Reinforce Pre- and Postsurgery Directions

- Explanation is needed for the immediate presurgical preparation with respect to rest and dietary limitations, particularly when a general anesthetic is to be administered.

G. Motivate the Patient Who Will Have Teeth Remaining

- Motivation to prevent further tooth loss through routine dental and dental hygiene professional care and oral self-care.

II. Personal Factors

- Extent of the surgery to be performed and previous experiences affect patient attitude.
- Many patients in greatest need of presurgical dental hygiene care and instruction may have neglected their mouths for many years. They may have been indifferent to or unaware of the importance of obtaining adequate oral care.
- Visits to a dentist may have been an emergency for a toothache or extraction. Patient oral health literacy may be limited.
- A few possible patient traits are suggested here.

A. Apprehensive and Fearful

- Apprehensive and indifferent toward need for personal care of teeth.
- Fearful of all dental procedures, particularly oral surgery and anesthesia.
- Fearful of personal appearance after surgery.

B. Resigned

- Feeling the situation is unavoidable.
- Lack of appreciation for preserving natural teeth.

C. Discouraged

- Over tooth loss or development of soft-tissue lesions.
- Toward time lost from work.
- By the financial aspects of dental care.
- About inconvenience and discomfort.

Dental Hygiene Care

I. Presurgery Treatment Planning

A. Initial Oral Preparation

- The pending date of surgery and the patient's attitude may limit the time spent.

- Complete medical and dental history, extra- and intraoral examination, vital signs, and photographs.
- Complete radiographs including the use of **cone beam computed tomography (CBCT)**.[3]
- CBCT is more accurate in predicting implant length and width and the need for bone grafting procedures.
- For routine unguided implant placement in sites where anatomic structures and bone grafting are not a concern, the use of a panoramic radiograph could be adequate for determining the length and width of the implant.[4]
- Determine the need for prophylactic premedication. (See Chapter 11.)
- Antibiotics are not required as prophylaxis after third molar surgery. The standard of care after extraction of mandibular third molar surgery for all healthy patients should be an anti-inflammatory regimen.[5] Antibiotic use should be limited to minimize the risk of antibiotic resistance.[6]
- Develop rapport; explain purpose of presurgical appointments.
- Explain and demonstrate dental biofilm control principles. Demonstrate appropriate technique using new soft toothbrush and appropriate adjunctive interdental aids.
- Perform debridement to prepare for tissue healing; local anesthesia is used as needed.
- Provide postsurgical instruction for rinsing with basic saline or with chlorhexidine 0.12% for tissue conditioning.
- For a patient using tobacco products, encourage participation in a tobacco cessation program.

B. Follow-Up Evaluation

- Complete or continue the debridement.
- More appointments may be needed for patients who will have surgery for oral cancer or who have a cardiovascular or other condition for which all periodontal and dental treatment is completed before surgery.
- When radiation or chemotherapy will be used following surgery for oral cancer, or when a prosthetic heart valve or total joint replacement will be involved, complete oral care is needed before surgery.
- Debridement is planned for a few weeks after oral surgery. Emphasis is placed on review and demonstration of daily oral self-care. The patient's oral self-care plan may require modification based on the oral surgery performed.
- Continue to provide support for patients participating in a tobacco cessation program.

II. Patient Instruction: Diet Selection

- Nutritional status can influence the resistance to infection and wound healing, as well as general recovery.
- Nutritional inadequacy or deficiency can occur because of the inability to consume adequate nutrients orally.
- Specific recommendations of what to include and not to include in the diet need to be provided.
- Postsurgical suggestions may differ from presurgical suggestions; for example, when difficulty in chewing is a postsurgical problem, a liquid or soft diet may be required for a short time.
- When major oral surgery requires hospitalization, nasogastric tube feeding may be used during the initial healing period.

A. Nutritional and Dietary Needs

Recommendations for food choices are designed to include the essential nutrients from key food groups from the current food guidance system, MyPlate. (See Chapter 33.)

- Essential for promotion of healing: proteins and vitamins, particularly vitamin A, vitamin C, and riboflavin.
- Essential for healthy gingival tissue: a varied diet that includes adequate portions of all essential food groups.
- Essential for dental caries prevention: noncariogenic foods. When a patient is not able to masticate properly, the diet frequently includes intake of the following:
  - Soft, more processed foods with higher cariogenic potential.
  - Intake of high-sucrose calorie-dense beverages.

B. Suggestions for Instruction

- Provide take-home instruction sheets that recommend specific pre- and postsurgery food options. Foods for liquid and soft diets are listed in the "Dental Hygiene Care" section of this chapter.
- Express nutritional needs in terms of quantity or servings of foods so that the patient clearly understands.
- For the patient who will receive dentures, careful instruction will need to be provided over a period

of time. Information for the patient with new dentures is described in Chapter 30.

- When the patient loses teeth because of dental caries, the diet may have been highly cariogenic. Emphasis needs to be placed on helping the patient include nutritious foods for the general health of the body and, more specifically, the health of the oral soft and hard tissues, which will support the dentures.

III. Presurgical Instructions

- The objective of presurgical instruction is to educate the patient on what to expect during the oral surgery appointment and immediately afterward.[7]
- The patient may have concerns about the anesthesia, the surgical procedure, and/or the outcome.
- For surgery in a hospital setting, the presurgical instructions are often mailed or sent via the electronic health record system to the patient.
- When surgery is done in the dental office, the dental hygienist may be responsible to deliver the instructions.
- Verbal instructions are supplemented with printed information.
- Instructions may include explanation of:
    - Food and liquid restrictions before surgery: specify the number of hours before the time of the surgery when patient should stop further intake of food and fluids.
    - Alcohol and medication restrictions: the patient may be instructed to discontinue use of certain medications (prescribed and over-the-counter), supplements, herbal remedies, and alcohol, which are not compatible with the anesthetic and drugs to be used during and following the surgical procedure.
    - Smoking or vaping: the patient may be instructed to stop smoking or limit smoking well in advance of the surgery date.
    - Recreational drugs: discontinue at least 48-72 hours prior to surgery as instructed by the surgeon.
    - Clothing: the patient may be instructed to wear loose fitting clothing around the neck and upper arms for intravenous delivery and assessment of vital signs throughout the surgical procedure.
    - Makeup: the patient should not wear lipstick or excessive makeup, and nail polish color should be removed.
    - Transport to and from the appointment: when general anesthetic or light sedation is used, the patient is instructed not to drive. Plans for someone to accompany and assist the patient should be made.
    - Ice packs: the patient may be instructed to prepare ice packs or frozen gel packs well in advance of surgery. Ice cubes may be placed in a plastic bag. Ice packs are beneficial for the first 36 hours following the surgical procedure.

IV. Postsurgical Care

A. Immediate Instructions

Printed postsurgical instructions are provided following all oral surgery procedures. The prepared material is reviewed with the patient and/or caregiver or family member after surgery. Specific details vary, but basic information for postsurgical instruction sheets includes the following:

- Management of bleeding:
    - Keep the gauze square in the mouth over the surgical area for half an hour and then discard it.
    - When bleeding persists at home, place a gauze square or cold wet tea bag over the area and bite firmly for 30 minutes.
- Mouthrinsing:
    - Do not rinse for 24 hours after the surgical appointment.
    - Then use warm salt water (one-half teaspoonful salt in one-half cup [4 ounces] of warm water) after toothbrushing and every 2 hours.
- Dental biofilm control: brush the teeth and use interdental aids carefully. Follow instructions for debriding the surgery site provided by the surgeon. Often at a follow-up appointment to assess healing, the patient will be provided with additional information
- Rest: get plenty of rest; at least 8 hours of sleep each night. Avoid strenuous exercise during the first 24 hours, and keep the mouth from excessive movement.
- Diet: use a liquid or soft diet high in protein. Drink water, warm soups (not hot), and fruit juices freely. Avoid spicy, hard, hot, or chewy foods.
- Smoking or vaping: the patient should avoid smoking or vaping for at least 2 weeks postsurgery to allow for initial healing of the surgical site.
- Pain: if needed, use a pain-relieving preparation prescribed by the oral surgeon or general dentist. Prescribed medication will vary from nonsteroidal anti-inflammatory drugs to opioid-containing compounds depending on the procedure. Adhere to directions.

    - Pain relief medication may include ibuprofen and/or acetaminophen for atraumatic removal of teeth; acetaminophen with 30 mg of codeine or a compound using oxycodone may be prescribed for more invasive procedures.[8]
- Limited opening: limited mouth opening will be present—two-finger opening is expected on the third day following surgery.
- Exercise: limit strenuous exercises for the first few days after surgery.
- Ice pack:
    - When swelling is possible, apply ice pack for 15 minutes, followed by 15 minutes off, or as directed by the oral surgeon for the first 36 hours after surgery.
    - Heat is not used for swelling.
- Complications: include the telephone number to call after office hours, should complications arise. Complications may include:
    - Uncontrolled pain, uncontrolled bleeding.
    - Temperature of 101°F or higher.
    - Difficulty in opening the mouth (**trismus**).
    - Unusual or excessive swelling after the surgery.
    - Nerve damage.
    - Infection in the surgical site or area.
    - Possible **alveolitis** or dry socket, especially in lower posterior molars. Alveolitis is extremely painful and usually occurs 2–4 days after tooth extraction if the blood clot is dislodged from the tooth socket exposing bone. The surgical site is irrigated with saline solution or 0.12% chlorhexidine gluconate followed by the placement of iodoform gauze in the socket. The patient returns in 1–2 days to have the iodoform gauze changed and a new one placed, and the site is reevaluated for healing.
- **Box 56-2** identifies important habits for patients to avoid following surgery.

B. Follow-Up Care

- The dental hygienist may participate in suture removal, irrigation of sockets, and other postsurgical procedures when the patient returns.

Box 56-2 Five Ss for Patients to Avoid

- No vigorous swishing.
- No vigorous spitting.
- No smoking or vaping.
- No drinking from a straw.
- No eating of solid food for the first 24 hours.

- Instruction concerning biofilm control, rinsing, oral irrigation, and other oral self-care, as well as diet supervision, can be continued as appropriate.

Patient with Intermaxillary Fixation

- Limited access for oral self-care procedures and the effect of the liquid diet required for most cases define the need for special dental hygiene care for the patient with **intermaxillary fixation (IMF)**.
- Attention to rehabilitation of oral tissues during the period following removal of fixation appliances takes on particular significance to prevent permanent tissue damage and inadequate oral care habits.
- Descriptions in this section are related to a fractured jaw, but IMF may be required for a variety of corrective surgeries and other conditions, including temporomandibular joint treatment and reconstructive and **orthognathic surgeries**.
- Regardless of the reason for IMF, instructions for dental hygiene care are similar, and the patient's problems are much the same.

Fractured Jaw

- The patient with a fractured jaw may be hospitalized.
- A dental hygienist employed in a hospital would be called upon to assume part of the responsibility for patient care or to give oral hygiene instruction to direct care personnel.
- After dismissal from the hospital, the patient may require special attention in the private dental office for a long period.
- Treatment of a fractured jaw can be complex, and the patient may suffer considerably, both physically and mentally.
- Basic knowledge of the nature of fractures and treatment is helpful in understanding the patient's needs.

I. Causes of Fractured Jaws

A. Traumatic

- Domestic violence, gunshots, sporting injuries, falls, road traffic accidents (including motorcycles and bicycles), and industrial accidents.

B. Predisposing

- Pathologic conditions, such as tumors, cysts, osteoporosis, or osteomyelitis, weaken the bone; thus, slight trauma or even tooth removal can cause fracture.

II. Emergency Care

- Immediate attention is paid to care of the patient's general condition.
- Monitor breathing, airway, and circulation, and prepare for possible basic life support measures. (See Chapter 9.)
- Hemorrhage, shock, and skull or internal head injuries are next in the sequence of concern so be prepared for emergency care. (See Chapter 9.)
- Although treatment for the fractured jaw cannot be postponed for any great length of time, its immediate care takes second place to any life threatening condition.

III. Recognition

A. History

- Except for a pathologic fracture, a history of trauma is usually the cause.

B. Clinical Signs

- Pain, especially on movement, and tenderness on slight pressure over the area of the fracture.
- Teeth may be displaced, fractured, or mobile. Because of muscle pull or contraction, segments of the bones may be displaced and the occlusion of the teeth may be irregular.
- Muscle spasm is a common finding, particularly when the fracture is at the angle or ramus of the mandible.
- Crepitation can be heard if the parts of bone are moved.
- Soft tissue in the area of the fracture may show laceration and bleeding, discoloration (**ecchymosis**), and enlargement.

IV. Types of Fractures

- A fracture is classified by using a combination of descriptive words for its *location*, *direction*, *nature*, and *severity*. Fractures may be single or multiple, bilateral or unilateral, and complete or incomplete.

A. Classification by Nature of the Fracture

- Simple: has no communication with outside.
- Compound: has communication with outside.
- Comminuted: shattered.

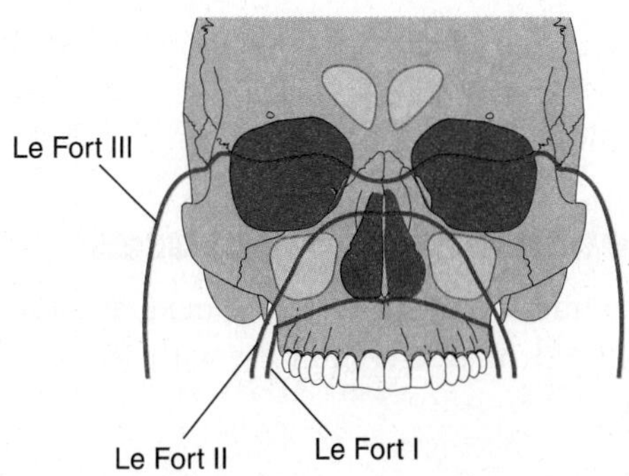

Figure 56-2 Le Fort Classification of Facial Fractures. Le Fort I, horizontal fracture above the roots of the teeth, below the zygomatic process, and across the pterygoid plates. Le Fort II, midface fracture over the middle of the nose and across the intraorbital rims. Le Fort III, transversely across the bridge of the nose and across the orbits and the zygomatic bone.

- Incomplete: "greenstick" fracture has one side of a bone broken and the other side bent.
  - It occurs in incompletely calcified bones (young children, usually).
  - The fibers tend to bend rather than break.

B. Mandibular (Described by Location)

- Alveolar process.
- Condyle.
- Angle.
- Body.
- Symphysis.

C. Midfacial

- Alveolar process: the alveolar process fracture does not extend to the midline of the palate.
- The Le Fort classification is used widely to identify the three general levels of maxillary fractures,[9] as shown in **Figure 56-2**.
  - *Le Fort I*: a horizontal fracture line extends above the roots of the teeth, above the palate, across the maxillary sinus, below the zygomatic process, and across the pterygoid plates.
  - *Le Fort II*: the midface fracture extends over the middle of the nose, down the medial wall of the orbits, across the infraorbital rims, and posteriorly across the pterygoid plates.
  - *Le Fort III*: the high-level craniofacial fracture extends transversely across the bridge of the nose, across the orbits and the zygomatic arches, and across the pterygoid plates.

- *Le Fort combination*: a combination of two levels is also possible such as a right Le Fort I and a left Le Fort II.

V. Treatment of Fractures

- Each fracture differs from the next, and the methods used in treatment vary with the individual case.[10,11]

A. Treatment Planning

- Many factors are involved when the oral surgeon selects the methods to be used, particularly the location of the fracture or fractures, the presence or absence of teeth, existing injuries to the teeth, other head injuries, and the general health and condition of the patient.
- All fractures do not require active intervention. Examples are fractures of the condylar and coronoid processes, nondisplaced fractures of an edentulous mandible, and greenstick fractures of children.

B. Basic Treatment

- Reduction (open or closed) restores normal position of the bones.
- Fixation of the fragments.
- Immobilization for healing.
- Control of treatment complications centers around prevention of infections, misalignment of the parts, and malocclusion of the dentition.

C. Healing

- Union is affected by the location and character of the fracture.
- Depends on the patient's general health and resistance, as well as on cooperation.
- Six weeks is considered the average for the uncomplicated mandibular fracture, and 4–6 weeks for a maxillary fracture.
- Major cause of complication is infection.

Mandibular Fractures

Reduction means the positioning of the parts on either side of the fracture so they are in apposition for healing and restoration of function.

- *Open reduction* refers to the use of a surgical flap procedure to expose the fracture ends and bring them together for healing.
- *Closed reduction* is accomplished by manipulation of the parts without surgery.

I. Closed Reduction

- The closure of the teeth in normal occlusion for the individual is the usual guide for position of the fracture parts in the dentulous patient.
- To identify the customary relation of the teeth can be difficult, especially in the partially edentulous mouth.

II. Intermaxillary Fixation

- After reduction, intermaxillary fixation (IMF) is a method of fixation and immobilization used for many years. It still is indicated under certain circumstances and in certain parts of the world.

A. Description

- IMF is accomplished by applying wires and/or elastic bands between the maxillary and mandibular arches.
- Arch bars: ready-made, contoured arch bars are adapted to fit accurately to each tooth and provide hooks for connecting the arches. A small horizontal elastic may be positioned across the fracture to reduce the lateral displacement.

B. Evaluation: Advantages

- Relative simplicity without surgical requirement: noninvasive.
- Lower cost; shorter hospital stay (depending on other injuries).
- Resources and trained surgeons may be limited in less developed countries.
- Patient can return to activity and work sooner; can use outpatient facility for follow-up.

C. Evaluation: Contraindications and Disadvantages

- Patients with chronic airway diseases who cough and expectorate: asthma and chronic obstructive pulmonary diseases.
- Patients who vomit regularly; notably, during pregnancy.
- Patients with a mental illness.
- Dietary problems: patients lose weight with the liquid, monotonous diet, often with cariogenic content.
- Oral hygiene and dietary limitations lead to increased dental caries and periodontal infection.

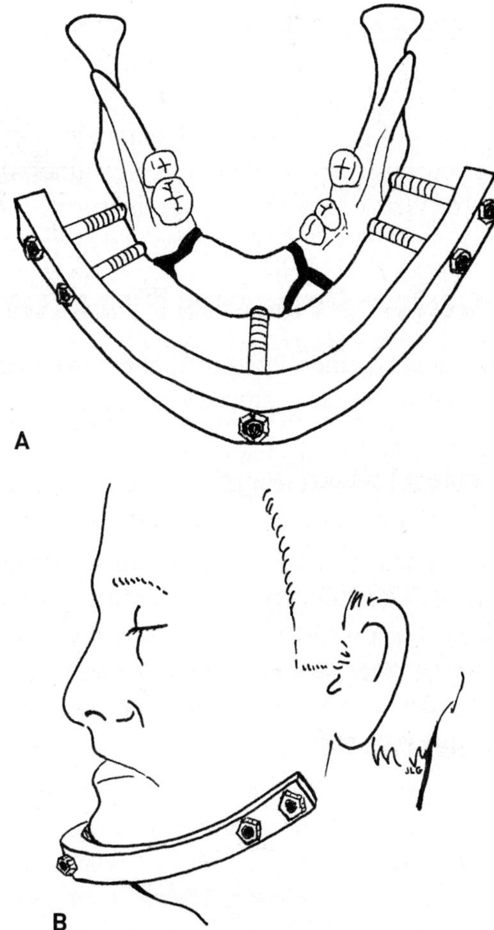

Figure 56-3 External Skeletal Fixation **A:** Precision bone screws placed on either side of the fractures shown by heavy black lines. **B:** Molded acrylic bar positioned over the bone screws and locked into position with nuts.

III. External Skeletal Fixation (External Pin Fixation)

A. Description

- Precision bone screws are placed via skin incisions on either side of the fracture (**Figure 56-3A**).
- An acrylic bar is molded and, while still pliable, is pressed over the threads of the bone screws and locked into position with the screw nuts (**Figure 56-3B**).

B. Indications

Management of a fracture cannot always be accomplished satisfactorily by intermaxillary fixation alone. The following are indications for external fixation:

- Insufficient number of teeth in good condition for IMF.
- As a supplement to IMF when no teeth are present in the fractured portion of the mandible.
- Loss of bone substance.
  - When bone substance is lost because of an accident, a gunshot wound, or a pathologic condition, a bone graft may be indicated.[12]
  - The extraoral fixation is used first to hold the fractured parts in a normal relationship and then to immobilize the area during healing following the bone graft surgery.
- Some patients may be unable to have the jaws closed for a long period. Examples of these are:
  - Patient with a vomiting problem, such as during pregnancy.
  - Patient with a mental or physical disability, such as cerebral palsy, epilepsy, or intellectual disability.
- Edentulous mandible when the fracture fragments are greatly displaced, when the fracture is at the angle of the mandible, or when the mandible is atrophic or thinned.

IV. Open Reduction

A. Principles for Treating Skeletal Fractures

- Anatomic reduction.
- Functionally stable fixation.
- Atraumatic surgical technique.
- Active function.
- Prevention of infection.

B. Description

- Surgical approach to bring the fracture parts together.
- Anesthesia selected in accord with patient history.
- Types of systems used for immobilization include:
  - Transosseous wiring (**osteosynthesis**).
  - Plates of various sizes.
  - Titanium mesh.
  - Bone clamps, staples, and screws.
  - Materials used may include: miniplates, screws, and other parts made of biodegradable or resorbable synthetic materials.

C. Clinical Example

- **Figure 56-4** illustrates various positions for **miniplate osteosynthesis** to provide stability for the reduced fracture parts.
- Care is needed so the screws are not placed over a fracture line or over the roots of teeth and do not infringe on the mandibular canal.

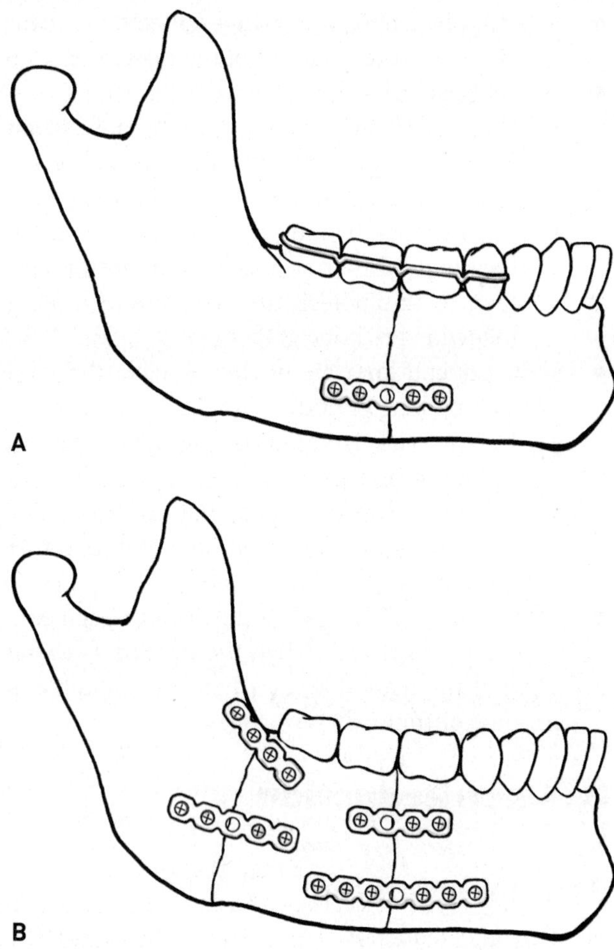

Figure 56-4 Miniplates for Immobilization of Fracture. **A:** Tension band on the teeth to aid in maintaining correct occlusion, while miniplate holds fracture ends in apposition. **B:** Examples of possible positions for miniplates.

Midfacial Fractures

I. Principles

- Maxillary fractures are more difficult to manage because of the number of bones, the associated anatomy, and the complications of basal skull fractures.
- Not all midface fractures need fixation following reduction.
- Both function and cosmetics are involved.

II. Description

A. Older Methods

- Internal wire suspension.
- External cranial suspension to a stable bone, such as uninvolved zygoma.
- Head caps.

B. Current Therapeutic Interventions

- Open reduction with internal fixation.
- Use of bone plates of various sizes.
- Grafts for reconstruction of midface defects.
- Early reconstruction before scarring and soft-tissue contracture deform the surrounding area.

Alveolar Process Fracture

- The most common fracture is of the maxillary or mandibular alveolar process.

I. Clinical Findings

- Face: bruising, areas of swelling.
- Teeth: fractures, mobility, avulsion, displacement.
- Lips and gingiva: bruising, bleeding lacerations from contact with teeth at the time of impact.
- Bone fracture: most frequently in anterior.

II. Treatment

- Replantation of displaced teeth.
- Immobilization with interdental wiring
    - A temporary fixed splint of acrylic may be placed over the wires. The teeth are tested periodically for vitality.
- Endodontic therapy may be required later.

Dental Hygiene Care

I. Problems

- Fixation apparatus, however carefully placed to prevent tissue irritation, interferes with normal function.
- Identification of possible effects of treatment provides the basis for planning dental hygiene care.

A. Development of Gingivitis or Periodontal Complications

- Thick biofilm formation and food debris accumulation provide sources of irritation to the gingiva, resulting in gingivitis.
- Lack of normal stimulation of the periodontium and of cleansing effects usually provided by the action of the tongue, lips, and facial muscles contributes to stagnation of saliva and accumulation of debris and bacteria.
- Tender, sensitive gingiva makes biofilm control more difficult, even on available surfaces.

B. Initiation of Demineralization

- An appetizing and nutritious soft or liquid diet is difficult to plan using limited cariogenic foods for dental caries prevention.

C. Loss of Appetite

- Loss of appetite related to monotonous liquid or soft diet may lead to weight loss and lowered physical resistance.
- Secondary infections, including those of the oral tissues, may result.

D. Difficulty in Opening the Mouth

- When there has been trauma to bony and/or soft tissues of the jaw that require fixation, there is going to be a degree of trismus following release of fixation.
- After removal of appliances, all patients have a degree of muscular trismus that limits personal oral self-care and mastication.

II. Instrumentation

A. Presurgical

- Gross calculus is removed, as much possible, before open reduction procedures. Trauma to surrounding soft tissues of lip, tongue, and cheeks limits accessibility.

B. During Treatment

- Periodic debridement contributes to oral health. Although access is only from the facial aspect for a patient with intermaxillary fixation, some benefit can be obtained. An assistant is needed to provide continual suction during treatment.

C. After Removal of Appliances

- A few weeks after removal of appliances, when the patient can open the mouth normally and resume usual oral self-care, complete debridement can be provided.

III. Diet

- Many patients with fractured jaws tend to lose weight, which is generally related to an inadequate nutrient and caloric intake. Objectives in planning the diet are to:
  - Help the patient maintain an adequate nutritional state.
  - Promote healing.
  - Increase resistance to infection.
  - Prevent new carious lesions. While it is important to manage caries risk, the overall health and nutrition status of the patient must be the first priority. Referral to a registered dietitian may be indicated to ensure adequate nutrition for healing.
- Attention is given to the patient's willingness and ability to follow recommendations.
  - The patient may be in the hospital for a few days to a few weeks, depending on the severity of other injuries.
  - If more in-depth dietary supervision is necessary, the patient may require additional outpatient follow-up appointments.
  - The patient's understanding of dietary instructions, need for adherence to these instructions is essential for adequate healing.

A. Nutritional Needs

After a surgical fixation procedure, a consultation with a registered dietitian may be necessary to ensure adequate nutrition to promote tissue repair and healing.

- Progression from a nutrient dense liquid diet to a soft, protein rich diet is indicated until patient can resume consumption of a healthy eating plan.
- Emphasis on protein; vitamins, particularly A, C, and D; and minerals, particularly calcium and phosphorus.
- MyPlate can be used to help identify dietary requirements for patient's age, taking into consideration lack of physical exercise and loss of appetite when ill.

B. Methods of Feeding

- Plastic straw: liquid is sucked through the teeth or through an edentulous area. Straw can be bent to accommodate a patient who cannot sit up.
- Spoon feeding: when a patient's arms are not functional, direct assistance is needed. The mouth may have injuries that prevent sucking food through a straw.
- Tube feeding: tube feeding may be indicated following various types of extensive oral surgery, facial trauma, burns, immobilized fractured jaw, and other conditions that prevent ingesting sufficient calories and nutritional foods by way of the mouth.
  - A nasogastric tube may be used. Blenderized food can be purchased or prepared, and special tube formulas are available commercially.

- When commercial preparations are used, contents can be selected to meet the specific nutritional and caloric requirements of an individual patient.
- It is ideal to work with a registered dietitian nutritionist (RDN) to determine how best to meet the patient's individual needs.

C. Liquid Diet

A *clear liquid* diet to help prevent dehydration may be prescribed initially, but it can be nutritionally inadequate. A *full liquid* diet to provide high protein and other healing nutrients is of a consistency to be taken by a cup. A *blenderized liquid* diet can be passed through a straw.

- Indications
  - All patients with jaws wired together.
  - Patients with no appliance or single-jaw appliance who have difficulty opening the mouth because of a condition, such as temporomandibular joint involvement or tongue or lip injury, that hinders insertion of food or manipulation of food in the mouth.
- Examples of foods: milk, protein shakes eggnog, smoothies, meat juices and soups, cooked thin cereals, and canned baby foods. Strained vegetables and meats (baby foods) may be added to meat juices and soups.
- Use of a blender: regular table foods can be mixed in a food blender. With liquid, such as clear soup or milk, added, a fluid consistency can be obtained that will pass through a straw (**Figure 56-5**).

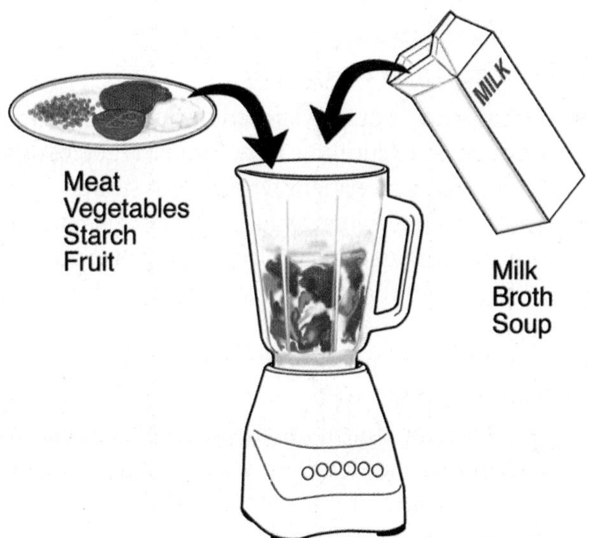

Figure 56-5 Preparation of a Liquid or Soft Diet. Regular table foods can be blended with milk or other nutritious liquid.

D. Soft Diet

- Indications
  - Patient with no appliance or with single-jaw appliance without complications in opening the mouth or in movement of the lips and tongue.
  - Patient who has been maintained on liquid diet throughout treatment period.
    - After appliances are removed, the soft diet is recommended for several days to 1 week to provide the stomach with foods that are readily digestible rather than making a drastic change to a regular diet.
    - A soft diet can also aid by protecting tender oral tissues from the rough textures of a regular diet until the tissues have had a chance to respond to softer foods.
- Examples of foods
  - Soft-poached, scrambled, or boiled eggs; fruit and yogurt smoothies, cooked cereals; mashed soft-cooked vegetables, including potato; mashed fresh or canned fruits; soft, finely divided meats; custards; plain ice cream.

E. Suggestions for Diet Planning with the Nonhospitalized Patient

- Provide instruction sheets with specific food suggestions.
- Express nutritional needs in quantities or servings of foods.
- Show methods of varying the diet. A liquid or soft diet is monotonous due to similarity in texture.
- When possible, encourage limitation of cariogenic foods as an aid to prevention of dental caries.

IV. Personal Oral Self-Care Procedures

- Every attempt is made to keep the patient's mouth as clean as possible for comfort and reduction of bacterial load for disease prevention.
- The extent of possible care depends on the appliances; the condition of the lips, tongue, and other oral tissues; and the dexterity and cooperation of the patient.
- The patient is encouraged to begin toothbrushing as soon as possible after the surgical procedure, but until the patient is able, a plan for care is outlined for a caregiver.

A. Irrigation

- Indications: during the first few days after the surgical procedure, while the mouth may be too tender for brushing, frequent irrigations are required; irrigation also serves as an adjunct to toothbrushing.
- Method: in a hospital, irrigations with suction are possible. At home, the patient irrigates with the head lowered over a sink. (See Chapter 27.)
- Mouthrinse selection: the oral surgeon is consulted for specific instructions. Suggestions include:
  - Physiologic saline (1 tsp [5 g] of salt to 1 cup [250 mL] of warm water).
  - Chlorhexidine gluconate.
  - Fluoride rinse.

B. Early Mouth Cleansing

- While the patient is in the hospital, a soft toothbrush with suction can be used. The toothbrush with suction is described in Chapter 4.

C. Oral Self-Care by the Patient

- As soon as possible, the patient is instructed in oral self-care.
- A toothbrushing method and other aids, such as those used for orthodontic appliances, may be recommended and demonstrated. (See Chapter 29.)
- Interdental and proximal tooth surface care is restricted to access only from the facial approach, making the choice of oral care devices limited.[13]
- Some spaces permit insertion of an interdental brush. With instruction, most patients can use a toothpick in a holder (Perio Aid) to disturb biofilm around and just under the free gingival margin. (See Chapter 27.)
- The ambulatory patient can use a water irrigator. A low-pressure setting is used, and the spray is directed carefully to prevent tissue injury. (See Chapter 27.)

D. After Appliances Are Removed

- Demineralization and dental caries can result from biofilm retention around the appliances.
- Except for the patient who had practiced good oral self-care before the accident, a step-by-step series of lessons is necessary.
- A method for daily self-applied fluoride, such as a mouthrinse or brush-on gel, can be introduced along with the use of a fluoride dentifrice.

Dental Hygiene Care before General Surgery

- When emergency surgery is performed, preparation of the mouth is not possible, and postsurgical examination and care may be complicated by various limitations.
- When surgery is elective, or planned in advance, the patient can be encouraged to have complete dental and periodontal treatment prior to surgery.
- Types of patients are described briefly here. Other examples are found in the various special patient chapters throughout this section of the text.

I. Patient Risk Management

- Patients who receive chemotherapeutic agents following surgery for various types of cancer, and others who use immunosuppressant drugs, require special management to prevent complications during dental and dental hygiene appointments.
- Antibiotic premedication to prevent infective endocarditis and other infections is may be necessary for certain patients. (See Chapter 11.)
- Before surgery for prostheses, transplants, cancer, and other serious conditions, patients are informed of the need for completing oral care treatments and practicing daily oral self-care.

II. Preparation of the Mouth before General Inhalation Anesthesia

- Because the mouth is an entryway to the respiratory system, the possibility always exists that bacteria, debris, and fluids from the mouth may be inhaled or aspirated.
- Aspiration could occur during the administration of an anesthetic or when the patient coughs.

III. Patient with a Long Convalescence

- Patients whose surgery requires a long convalescence may be unable to keep a regular continuing care appointment.
- When the patient has a healthy mouth before hospitalization and convalescence, the problems of postsurgical oral care are lessened, but not eliminated.

- Instruction for the caregiver may be needed. A home visit by the dental hygienist may be possible depending on the state or province practice act. (See Chapter 4.)

IV. Maxillofacial Surgery and COVID-19

- Oral and maxillofacial surgical interventions are high-risk aerosol generating procedures. When community transmission rates are high for a respiratory virus like COVID-19, it is ideal to delay nonemergency surgery where necessary. If oral surgery cannot be delayed, the following recommendations are suggested:
  - Use current recommended personal protective equipment (PPE) for aerosol-generating procedures.
  - Perform several symptom-screening opportunities utilizing teledentistry in advance of the appointment and in person, focusing on presence of symptoms, exposure risk, and travel history.
  - Temperature screening when the patient presents for the appointment.
  - Use preprocedural mouthwashes and PPE for patient and staff in the office.
    - Povidone iodine as a preprocedural rinse has been shown to be effective to reduce the load of coronaviruses in saliva if used by the patient and staff prior to any surgical procedure.[14]
  - Use appropriate ventilation, PPE, high-volume suction, and the appropriate **fallow period**.
  - Utilize extraoral radiographic imaging, such as panoramic or CBCT if possible, to minimize the risk of coughing due to stimulation of the gag reflex with intraoral radiographic films.
  - Utilize absorbable sutures, if possible, to minimize the number of visits to the dental office.
  - Family members who will be accompanying the client home should wait outside the dental office or be contacted just prior to the discharge time of the client.
  - Patients who have symptoms of a transmissible disease such as COVID-19 should have elective surgery postponed for 3 weeks.
- In the event a patient with an active respiratory infection such as COVID-19 requires urgent surgery, a negative-pressure room must be available.[15]
  - Emergency surgery includes conditions involving trauma, airway management, and severe bleeding; conditions requiring drainage, such as Ludwig's angina; and oncosurgery, whereby a delay would seriously impair the patient's outcome.[14]

Documentation

The permanent oral care record for most maxillofacial patients needs to include a summary of the hospital care when available, but may start when the patient returns to the general practice. At that time, the initial documentation needs a minimum of the following:

- Health history, radiograph interpretation, extra- and intraoral findings, and vital signs.
- Comprehensive periodontal examination and summary of current needs.
- Risk factors and dental caries review; complete examination for demineralization.
- Care planning for maintenance.
- A sample progress note is available for review in **Box 56-3**.

Box 56-3 Example Documentation: Postsurgical Dental Hygiene Appointment

- **S**—A 20-year-old college student presents for first dental hygiene appointment following a mandibular fracture due to a motorcycle accident. Stabilizing interdental wiring and fixed splint were removed yesterday. Patient's chief complaint is "My mouth feels dirty and it smells bad." Past medical history: patient admits to smoking a pack of cigarettes a day and an occasional beer on the weekends; otherwise unremarkable.
- **O**—Healthy looking young male in no obvious distress. Oral cavity is remarkable for heavy dental biofilm and calculus buildup; tissues are inflamed, bleeding, and edematous. No pocket depths greater than 4mm. Mandibular fracture appeared completely healed.
- **A**—A 20-year-old male status post-wire removal from motorcycle accident with poor oral hygiene.
- **P**—Complete periodontal debridement × 4 quadrants; detailed oral hygiene instructions; tobacco cessation education; 4-week follow-up to assess healing and patient compliance to oral care instructions and success with tobacco cessation.

Signed: ______________________, RDH
Date: ______________

Factors to Teach the Patient

Accident Prevention

- Always use seat belts in automobiles and other vehicles.
- Use mouthguards and all safety devices during contact sports.
- Wear helmets when using a skateboard, scooter, bicycle, or motorcycle.
- Helmets protect against facial injuries in totality and appear to be more effective at preventing midfacial fractures when compared with mandible fractures.[16]

For the Patient Who Will Have General Surgery

- Significance of a clean mouth during general anesthesia.
- Postsurgery oral problems related to specific diseases.

References

1. National Commission on Recognition of Dental Specialties and Certifying Boards. https://ncrdscb.ada.org/recognized-dental-specialties. Accessed April 11, 2022.
2. Ferneini EM, Goldberg MH. Management of oral and maxillofacial infections. *J Oral Maxillofac Surg*. 2018;76(3):469-473.
3. Carter JB, Stone JD, Clark RS, Mercer JE. Applications of cone-beam computed tomography in oral and maxillofacial surgery: an overview of published indications and clinical usage in United States Academic Centers and Oral and Maxillofacial Surgery Practices. *J Oral Maxillofac Surg*. 2016;74(4):668-679.
4. Deeb G, Antonos L, Tack S, Carolein C, Laskin D, Deeb JG. Is cone-beam computed tomography always necessary for dental implant placement? *J Oral Maxillofac Surg*. 2017;75(2):285-289.
5. Menon RK, Kar Yan L, Gopinath D, Botelho MG. Is there a need for postoperative antibiotics after third molar surgery? A 5-year retrospective study. *J Investig Clin Dent*. 2019;10(4):e12460.
6. Dammling C, Abramowicz S, Kinard B. Current concepts in prophylactic antibiotics in oral and maxillofacial surgery. *Oral Maxillofac Surg Clin North Am*. 2022;34(1):157-167.
7. Hupp JR. Principals of management of impacted teeth. In: Hupp JR, Ellis E, Tucker M, eds. *Contemporary Oral and Maxillofacial Surgery*. 7th ed. Philadelphia, PA: Elsevier; 2019:160-184.
8. Dowell D, Haegerich TM, Chou R. CDC guideline for prescribing opioids for chronic pain—United States, 2016. *JAMA*. 2016;315(15):1624-1645.
9. Haskell R. Applied surgical anatomy. In: Rowe NL, Williams JL, eds. *Maxillofacial Injuries*. London: Churchill Livingstone; 1985:21-24.
10. Bell RB. Contemporary management of mandibular fractures. In: Miloro M, Ghali GE, Larsen PE, Waite PD, eds. *Peterson's Principals of Oral and Maxillofacial Surgery*. 3rd ed. Philadelphia, PA: Lippincott; 2011:407-439
11. Perry M, Brown A, Banks P. Treatment of fractures of the mandible. In: *Fractures of the Facial Skeleton*. 2nd ed. Chichester, West Sussex: Wiley-Blackwell; 2015:69-96.
12. Boyne PJ, Peetz M. Bone grafts. In: *Osseous Reconstruction of the Maxilla and the Mandible: Surgical Techniques using Titanium Mesh and Bone Mineral*. Chicago, IL: Quintessence; 1997:64-74.
13. Phelps-Sandall BA, Oxford SJ. Effectiveness of oral hygiene techniques on plaque and gingivitis in patients placed in intermaxillary fixation. *Oral Surg Oral Med Oral Pathol*. 1983;56(5):487-490.
14. Bali RK, Chaudhry K. Maxillofacial surgery and COVID-19, the pandemic. *J Maxillofac Oral Surg*. 2020;19(2): 159-161.
15. Alterman M, Nassar M, Rushinek H, et al. The efficacy of a protective protocol for oral and maxillofacial surgery procedures in a COVID-19 pandemic area - results from 1471 patients. *Clin Oral Investig*. 2021;35(8):5001-5008.
16. Christian JM, Thomas RF, Scarbecz M. The incidence and pattern of maxillofacial injuries in helmeted versus non helmeted motorcycle accident patients. *J Oral Maxillofac Surg*. 2014;72(12):2503-2506.

CHAPTER 57

The Patient with a Seizure Disorder

Linda D. Boyd, RDH, RD, EdD
Sharon M. Grisanti, RDH, MCOH

CHAPTER OUTLINE

LEARNING OBJECTIVES

After studying this chapter, the student will be able to:

1. Define each term associated with the type of seizure disorder.
2. Describe the etiology of seizure disorders.
3. Discuss clinical manifestations of seizure disorders.
4. Develop a dental hygiene care plan, including patient education prevention strategies, for working with patients with seizure disorders.
5. Prepare an emergency care protocol for a patient having a seizure.

Introduction

- The most common cause of seizures is **epilepsy**, a term used to describe a group of functional disorders of the brain characterized by predisposition to recurrent seizures.[1]
  - Seizures are a symptom of epilepsy, but those who experience a seizure may not have epilepsy. Other causes include high fever, head trauma, stroke, and Alzheimer's disease.[2,3]
- According to the Centers for Disease Control and Prevention, there are approximately 3 million adults and 470,000 children in the United States with active epilepsy.[4] The World Health Organization estimates that, globally, more than 50 million people have epilepsy.[3]
  - Incidence of epilepsy is higher in low-income countries and low socioeconomic groups in high-income countries.[1]

Seizures

I. Seizure Overview

- A **seizure** is a **paroxysmal** event resulting from abnormal brain activity. A seizure may involve loss of consciousness or awareness or impaired awareness with or without convulsive movements or **spasms**.[1]
- Seizures are generally unprovoked and involuntary, but **triggers** may precipitate an epileptic seizure.
- Important characteristics of a seizure to aid in diagnosis of the classification include[5]:
  - Onset: focal or generalized.
  - Level of awareness: with or without awareness.
  - Motor or nonmotor onset symptoms: motor symptoms may include emotional (fear), sensory (aura), and/or cognitive.
- Other terms sometimes used include **convulsion**, fit, spell, and ictus.

A. Seizure Etiology

In addition to epilepsy, seizures can be a symptom of many different conditions. The causes can be genetic, structural/metabolic, or unknown.[1,2,4]

- Genetic
  - Genetic predisposition to seizures or to other neurologic abnormalities for which the seizure may be a symptom.
- Structural/metabolic
  - Seizures can arise during many neurologic and nonneurologic medical conditions:
    - Congenital conditions, such as maternal infection (rubella); toxemia of pregnancy.
    - Maternal drug use.
    - Perinatal injuries.
    - Brain tumor.
    - Cerebrovascular disease (stroke).
    - Trauma (head injury).
    - Infection (meningitis, encephalitis, opportunistic infections of human immunodeficiency virus).
    - Degenerative brain disease such as Alzheimer's disease.
    - Metabolic and toxic disorders, including lead exposure, alcoholism, and other drug addictions; seizures are common during alcohol and/or drug withdrawal.
    - Complication of cancer.
- Immune
  - Autoimmune diseases such as systemic lupus erythematosus, type 1 diabetes mellitus, myasthenia gravis, celiac disease, rheumatoid arthritis, Hashimoto's encephalopathy, psoriasis, and multiple sclerosis.[6]
- Unknown cause
  - The onset and cause of the epileptic seizure are unknown.
  - A neurologic examination may diagnose the reason.

B. Precipitating Factors or Trigger for Seizures

- The patient or caregiver can provide helpful information to prepare dental personnel in the management of an emergency.
- Triggers may occur frequently and are in response to specific stimuli. The dental hygienist should be prepared to eliminate or minimize these stimuli.
- Factors that may precipitate a seizure include[7,8]:
  - Hormonal fluctuation such as in estrogen, progesterone, and cortisol (stress).
  - Emotional stress.
  - Fatigue; sleep deprivation.
  - Alcohol or drug use.
  - Flashing/bright lights or noises.
  - Fever.
  - Noncompliance with antiseizure medications.
  - Physical exercise/physical trauma.

C. Seizure Phases or Stages

- Prodromal stage (preictal period)
  - Some individuals may experience signs a seizure is imminent, including[9]:
    - Behavior changes.
    - Cognitive disturbances.
    - Anxiety and mood changes.
    - Fatigue.
    - Sleep disturbances.
- Aural phase
  - An aura is the early signs of a focal seizure and may include the following[10]:
    - A sense of déjà vu.
    - Abnormal taste or smell.
    - Visual changes such as blurring.
    - Dizziness, light-headedness.
    - Headache.
  - However, not all patients have warning signs, or auras, before a seizure.
- Ictal phase
  - The ictal phase includes the time from the first symptoms to the end of the seizure. The symptoms vary by the seizure classification as outlined in the next section.
  - Seizures last a few second to minutes, but are typically less than 1 minute.[10]
- Postictal phase
  - This is the time following the seizure when the individual is recovering and may include the following symptoms[10]:
    - Confusion.
    - Altered mental status.
    - Sleepiness.
    - Injuries may occur as a result of the seizure.
    - Headache.

II. Classification of Seizures

A. Generalized Onset Seizures

- Motor (tonic-clonic) category[2,4,5]:
  - Affecting both sides of the brain at the same time.
  - Also known as **grand mal** seizures.
  - Muscles of the chest and pharynx may contract at the same time, forcing air out and a sound known as the "epileptic cry."
  - Loss of consciousness or awareness is sudden and complete; the patient becomes stiff and falls or may slide out of the dental chair.
  - Musculature contraction: with tonic phase body becomes rigid, with clonic phase there is intermittent muscular contraction and relaxation.
  - Atonic refers to weakened muscles.
  - Skin color turns pale to bluish; breathing is shallow or stops briefly.
  - Possible loss of bladder and, rarely, bowel control.
  - Tongue may be bitten.
  - Incident usually lasts 1–3 minutes.
  - Respiration returns.
  - Saliva, which previously could not be swallowed, may mix with air and appears foamy.
  - Patient begins to recover, may be confused, tired, complain of muscle soreness or injury; falls into a deep sleep.
  - Stages of a seizure are **aura (prodromal)**, **ictus (tonic-clonic)**, and **postictal** (**Figure 57-1**).
  - Seizure may continue without recovery and progress to ***status epilepticus***, meaning lasting more than 5 minutes or experiencing two or more seizures within a 5-minute period.

Stages of a Seizure

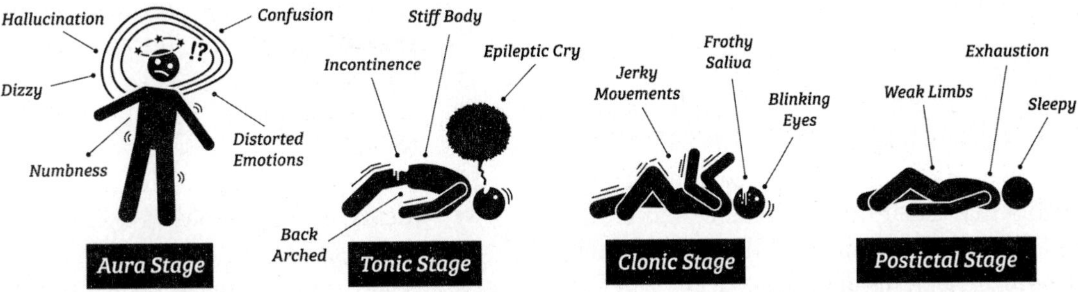

Figure 57-1 Stages of a Motor (Tonic-Clonic) Seizure

- Nonmotor or **absence seizure**[2,4,5]:
  - Previously known as **petit mal**.
  - Loss of consciousness or awareness begins and ends abruptly in about 5–30 seconds.
  - Most common in children, and may lead to learning difficulties if not identified.
  - Patient has a blank stare, usually does not fall, posture becomes fixed, may drop whatever is being held.
  - May become pale.
  - **Myoclonus** may occur: patient may have rhythmic twitching of the eyelids, eyebrows, head, or chewing movements.
  - Attack ends as abruptly as it begins. Patient quickly returns to full awareness, resumes activities, unaware of what occurred.

B. Focal Onset Seizures

- Focal seizures can be simple, complex, or secondary to a generalized seizure.[4,5]
- Focal seizures start with one group of cells in one part of the brain.[4,5]
  - **Focal onset aware** means patient is aware during the seizure.
  - Focal onset impaired awareness means the patient is confused.

C. Unknown Onset Seizures

- Start of seizures is unknown and may be motor or nonmotor.[2]
  - Motor seizures may be tonic-clonic or spasms.
  - Nonmotor seizures may exhibit "behavior arrest," meaning the individual stares without making any movement.
- Seizure has not been witnessed.
- A summary of the classification of seizures is outlined in **Table 57-1**.

III. Diagnosis of a Seizure

Diagnosis includes the following components:

- Medical history
  - The medical history is the first step in the diagnosis of epilepsy seizures.
  - Documentation of initial onset, preliminary factors that led up to the seizure, and a description of what happened during and after the seizure is necessary.
- Physical examination
  - The examination and laboratory tests help to eliminate other possible causes for the seizure.
- Neurologic examination
  - The neurologic exam is likely to include an **electroencephalography (EEG)** to evaluate patterns of normal and abnormal brain activity and the parts of the brain involved.

Treatment

I. Medications

- Antiepileptic drugs (AEDs) are the primary method used to prevent and control seizures.[11-15]

A. Choices

- Patients may be placed on one (monotherapy) or a combination of AEDs.[11]
  - Monotherapy is preferred to minimize adverse side effects and possible drug interactions.
  - Polytherapy is used when seizures cannot be controlled with monotherapy.
- Choice of therapy affected by the classification of seizure, minimization of side effects, and efficacy at reducing seizure frequency.[11]
  - Some AEDs (e.g., valproate) are not recommended for women of childbearing age because of risk for possible birth defects such as spina bifida.[11,12]
- The guidelines for AEDs based on the evidence for managing individuals with new seizures and those with treatment-resistant epilepsy are listed in **Table 57-2**.

B. Side Effects

- Each medication has side effects a patient may experience to varying degrees. It is imperative for patients to follow directions for the use of **antiseizure** medications from their primary care provider.
- Side effects may include the following[11,15,16]:
  - Allergic reaction, rash.
  - Fatigue, dizziness, drowsiness, weakness, **ataxia**, headache, slurred speech, blurred vision.
  - Changes in weight: weight loss or weight gain.
  - Nausea.
  - Memory loss; behavioral and cognitive deficits.
  - Mental health disorders (i.e., psychosis and depression).
  - Behavioral changes: aggressive behavior, irritability.
  - Damage to the kidneys (nephrotoxicity) and liver (hepatotoxicity).

Table 57-1 **Classifications of Seizure Types[3,5]**

Classifications	Definition	Seizure Types
Focal onset ■ Aware ■ Impaired awareness	Involving one side of the brain ■ Aware • Patient aware of surroundings and self • Able to recall events of seizure ■ Impaired awareness • Patient is confused about surroundings	Motor onset ■ Spasms ■ Epileptic ■ **Automatisms** ■ Atonic ■ Clonic ■ Hyperkinetic ■ **Myoclonic** ■ Tonic Nonmotor onset ■ Sensory ■ Emotional ■ **Autonomic** ■ **Behavior arrest** ■ Cognitive Focal to bilateral ■ Tonic-clonic
Generalized onset ■ Impaired awareness	Affecting both sides of the brain ■ Impaired awareness • Patient is confused about surroundings	Motor ■ **Epileptic spasms** ■ Clonic ■ Tonic ■ Tonic-clonic ■ Myoclonic ■ Myoclonic-tonic-clonic ■ Myoclonic-atonic ■ Atonic Nonmotor (absence) ■ Eyelid myoclonic ■ Typical ■ **Atypical** ■ Myoclonic
Unknown onset	Start of seizure is unknown ■ Seizure not witnessed	Motor ■ Tonic-clonic ■ Epileptic spasms ■ Nonmotor ■ Behavior arrest ■ Unclassified

Data from World Health Organization. Epilepsy. Published June 20, 2019. Accessed January 2, 2022. https://www.who.int/news-room/fact-sheets/detail/epilepsy; Fisher RS, Cross JH, French JA, et al. Operational classification of seizure types by the International League Against Epilepsy: position paper of the ILAE Commission for Classification and Terminology. *Epilepsia.* 2017;58(4):522-530.

- Osteopenia: long-term use of valproate and phenytoin.
- Increased risk of birth defects (sodium valproate).
- Induction of systemic lupus erythematosus (SLE).
- Hair loss.
- Gingival hyperplasia (gingival enlargement) is most common with phenytoin.
- Numerous drug interactions, including other AEDs, acetaminophen, nonsteroidal anti-inflammatory drugs, erythromycins, and reduction in the efficacy of oral contraceptives.

Table 57-2 American Academy of Neurology (AAN) and American Epilepsy Society (AES) Guidelines for First-Line Antiepileptic Drugs (AEDs)[13,14]

Generic Name	Brand Name
New-Onset Epilepsy	
Lamotrigine	Lamictal
Levetiracetam	Keppra
Zonisamide	Zonegran
Carbamazepine	Tegretol, Carbatrol
Treatment-Resistant Epilepsy	
Pregabalin	Lyrica
Perampanel	Fycompa
Lacosamide	Vimpat
Eslicarbazepine	Aptiom
Topiramate	Topamax
Other AEDs Prescribed in Specific Seizure Classifications	
Clonazepam (extended release)	Klonopin
Ethosuximide	Zarontin
Gabapentin	Neurontin
Oxcarbazepine	Trileptal
Phenobarbital	Luminal
Phenytoin	Dilantin
Tiagabine	Gabitril
Sodium valproate	Depakote

- Elderly and children
  - Both age groups are more sensitive to side effects such as weakness, unsteadiness, and cognitive alterations.
  - Elderly patients are more likely to be on other medications with possible drug interactions and may forget to take medications.

II. Alternative Therapies for Epilepsy

- Care must be taken to work with a medical provider in using alternative therapies or combining them with typical medications used for treatment.[17,18]
  - Alternative therapies may not have the same level of experimental research related to safety and efficacy so further research is needed.
- Individuals may turn to "natural" medicine due to the cost of AEDs, side effects of drugs, and inability to control seizures with medications.[17]

A. Traditional Chinese Medicine

- Chinese medicine has been used for centuries to treat seizures.[17]
  - Medicine (herbs) are combined with diet to treat disease to provide a holistic approach to health.
- Traditional Chinese medicine herbs used may come from plants (e.g., *Gastrodia elat* and *Uncaria rhychopylla*), fungus (e.g., *Ganoderma lucidum*), and/or animals (e.g., *Olivierus martensii*).[17]

B. Traditional Healers

- Traditional healers in many countries in Latin America, Asia, and Africa use a variety of herbal remedies along with rituals and dietary restrictions for treatment. With the increasing diversity of the population, these individuals may be patients.
- The herbal remedies with the most research include *Acorus calamus* and *Bacopa monnieri* (L.) Wettst. However, more clinical research is needed.[19]

C. Herbal Supplements

- Certain over-the-counter herbal supplements are used as self-medications to help prevent seizures such as ginseng, St. John's wort, melatonin, gingko, and garlic.[18]
  - Ginkgo may increase seizure activity (proconvulsant).
- Herbal supplements have not been shown to effectively treat epileptic seizures and may make seizures worse.[18]

D. Marijuana/Cannabinoids

- Medical marijuana or oral cannabinoids (CBD) have been increasingly used to manage seizure activity in treatment-resistant epilepsy; however, there is inconsistent evidence to show it reduces seizure frequency with the exception of two very specific type of seizure disorders in children.[20-22]
- In some pediatric seizure disorders, well-controlled studies have been conducted, leading to Food and

Drug Administration approval of CBD under the name Epidiolex.[21,22]

E. Ketogenic Diet

- The goal of the ketogenic diet is to induce fat metabolism through ketosis by maintaining a diet high in fat and low in carbohydrates. The exact mechanism by which this reduces seizure activity is under investigation.
- The ketogenic diet has been shown to be an effective treatment for patients with epilepsy, particularly children.[23]

III. Surgery

A variety of surgical interventions are available and indicated when epilepsy is refractory to traditional AED therapy.[24,25] Surgical intervention has become more precise through advances in identifying the epileptogenic area with magnetic resonance imaging, tomography, electroencephalographic studies, neuropsychological testing, and other analyses.

- Surgical options:
    - Resection of parts of the brain, sometimes in conjunction with radiation, is used to manage focal epilepsy.[25]
    - A pacemaker-like device for vagus nerve stimulation delivers signals to the vagus nerve to reduce seizure activity.[24]

Oral Findings

- Epilepsy in itself produces no oral changes.
- Specific oral changes are related to:
    - Side effects of AEDs.
    - Oral accidents during a seizure.
    - Side effects of the epilepsy, such as depression leading to poor oral hygiene and neglect.[26]

I. Effects of Accidents with Seizures

- The head is one of the most common sites for injury during a seizure.[26]

A. Scars of Lips and Tongue

- Oral tissues, particularly tongue, cheek, or lip, may be bitten.
    - Soft-tissue injuries may require sutures.
- Scars may be observed during the extraoral/intraoral examination; cause may be differentiated from other types of healed wounds.

B. Fractured Teeth

- Clenching and bruxing may be forceful enough to fracture teeth.
- In childhood epilepsy, about 14% of children will experience broken teeth from seizures.[26]
- Fractures may extend into the pulp of the tooth, allowing bacterial infection; may require root canal therapy or extraction.

II. Gingival Overgrowth/ Gingival Hyperplasia

- Gingival hyperplasia is a side effect of many medications used to manage epilepsy; approximate prevalences are as follows[27]:
    - 50% with phenytoin.
    - 44% with valproic acid.
    - 71% with oxcarbazepine.
    - 61% with lamotrigine.
- Gingival overgrowth tends to be more significant in polytherapy (meaning more than one medication for seizures) versus monotherapy.[27]

A. Mechanism

- Uptake of folate by fibroblasts may be impaired, resulting in failure to activate collagenase. This, in turn, leads to a decrease in degradation of connective tissue, which presents as gingival overgrowth.[28]
- Tissue color and texture are generally within normal limits, with interdental papilla taking on a lobular shape.
- Based on research, it is believed that inflammation from dental biofilm is a factor in the initiation and severity of gingival hyperplasia.[27–29]

B. Occurrence

- The gingiva may start to enlarge within 3–6 months following initial administration of drug therapy, and it is recommended that preventive dental care and adequate biofilm control begin within 10 days of starting phenytoin therapy.[28,30,31]
- The anterior gingiva are more affected than posterior, and the maxillary more than the mandibular arch.
- Facial and proximal areas are more affected than lingual or palatal areas.

C. Effects of Gingival Hyperplasia

- Quality of life may be impacted by the gingival hyperplasia along with the following[31]:
    - Impairs ability for thorough dental biofilm removal.[29]

- May affect mastication.
- May alter tooth eruption or position.
- When associated with periodontitis and attachment loss, teeth may be mobile.
- May interfere with speech.
- May cause serious esthetic concerns.

D. Clinical Classification of Gingival Hyperplasia

- A grading system can be used to describe the extent of gingival overgrowth from 0 to 3, with 0 being no signs of enlargement.[32]
- Lesions may be localized or generalized.
- Grade 1:
  - Hyperplasia is confined to interdental papilla.
- Grade 2:
  - Tissue increases in size, extends to include the marginal gingiva, and may cover a large portion of the anatomic crown (**Figure 57-2A**).
  - Cleft-like grooves may occur between the lobules.
  - Eventually, the tissue becomes fibrotic, pink, and stippled, with a mulberry or cauliflower-like appearance, as in **Figure 57-2B**.
- Grade 3:
  - Covers three-fourths or more of crown. Large, bulbous interdental papilla may wedge the teeth apart and interfere with mastication and oral self-care.

E. Risk Factors for Gingival Hyperplasia

- Dental biofilm
  - Biofilm appears to be a significant determinant in the severity of phenytoin-induced gingival enlargement.[29]
  - Adequate biofilm control, particularly if started prior to the administration of phenytoin, may help control the extent of gingival overgrowth.
  - Factors impacting adequate biofilm control include:
    - Defective restorations and over- or under-contoured restoration margins.
    - Untreated carious lesions.
    - Calculus provides a site for bacterial accumulation.
    - Crowded or malaligned teeth may complicate biofilm removal.
- Drug dose and other medications the patient may be taking.[29]

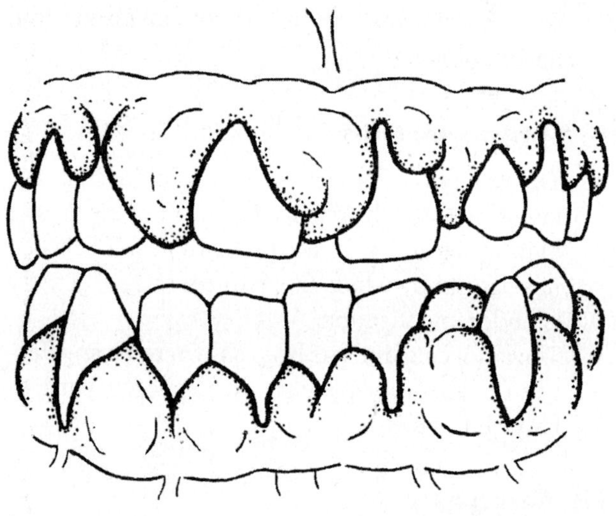

A

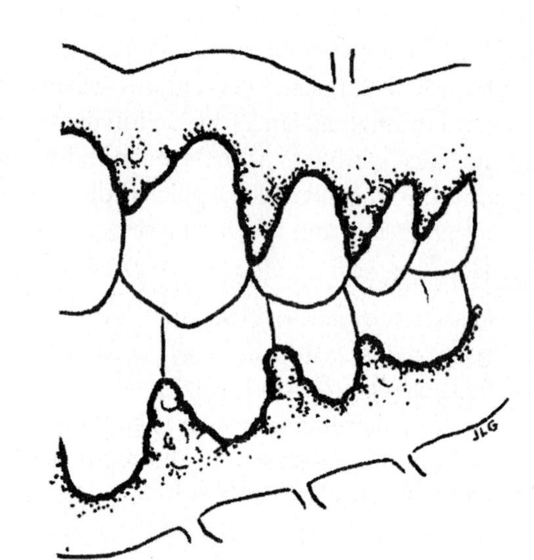

B

Figure 57-2 Phenytoin-Induced Gingival Enlargement. **A:** Papillary enlargement with cleft-like grooves. Note the effect of the pressure of the fibrotic tissue on the position of teeth. Maxillary incisors and the mandibular left canine have been wedged away from normal positions. **B:** Mulberry-like shape of interdental papillae. An illustration shows phenytoin-induced gingival enlargement.

- Gender: men are more likely to develop gingival hyperplasia.[29]
- Genetic susceptibility may influence gingival overgrowth.[29]

F. Treatment

Possible approaches to treatment of gingival hyperplasia include:

- Change in seizure medication:
  - Collaboration with the primary care physician to determine the possibility of choosing

a different AED with lower risk for gingival enlargement.

- Nonsurgical treatment:
  - Periodontal debridement along with strict biofilm control within 10 days of beginning AED.[30]
  - Once the tissue has become fibrotic, resolution of overgrowth is unlikely to occur.
  - Short-term use of 0.12% chlorhexidine gluconate rinse may be used as an adjunct to mechanical biofilm management of gingival overgrowth from AEDs.[33]
- Surgical removal:
  - Nonsurgical therapy along with meticulous oral self-care must be initiated prior to surgical intervention.
  - Gingivectomy is the most common approach for removal of excess tissue and recontouring of the gingiva.
  - Meticulous oral hygiene is required to minimize gingival overgrowth.
  - Despite treatment and continuing maintenance, recurrence of gingiva overgrowth occurs in 34% to 47% of individuals.[33]

Dental Hygiene Care Plan

- Interprofessional collaboration plays an important role in the development of the dental hygiene care plan.

I. Patient History

- Contact the primary care provider when the patient or caregiver is unable to provide needed information, is noncompliant, if seizure activity has increased or changed, or if treatment for epilepsy is impacting the patient's oral health.
- Seizure disorder may co-occur with other conditions such as autism and fragile X syndrome.[34,35]
- A well-controlled patient with epilepsy may still be at risk to have a seizure.
- For seizure-prone patients: advise wearing medical alert jewelry.

II. Information to Obtain

- Information to obtain from a patient with a history of seizures is listed in **Box 57-1**.

III. Patient Approach

- Provide a calm, reassuring atmosphere and treat with patience and empathy.
- Use a motivational interviewing approach to patient education, enabling patients to be partners in the decision-making process. (See Chapter 24.)
- Encourage self-expression, particularly if the patient tends to be quiet and withdrawn or has a narrow range of interests.
- Recognize possible impairment of memory when reviewing oral self-care procedures.
- Encourage patient with positive reinforcement for successes.

Box 57-1 Risk Assessment for Dental Hygiene Treatment: Information to Obtain from Patient with a History of a Seizure Disorder

Basic Information

- Thorough medical history review, including date of last physical examination, other medical conditions or risk factors present.
- Primary care provider: name and phone number.
- Emergency contact person with phone number.

Additional Factors

- Inquire about recent illness, stress, alcohol use, sleep issues, menstrual cycle, fatigue, or pain as factors that may provoke a seizure.
- General well-being; refer for evaluation if patient presents with signs or symptoms of other conditions such as depression.
- Ask if the patient has changed any aspect of their activities of daily living.

Treatment

- Medication list, surgery, or diet.
- Effectiveness of seizure control treatment.
- Investigate each medication for possible interaction with the proposed dental treatment and side effects.
- Nonprescription, herbal supplement use.
- Medication compliance.

About the Seizures

- The frequency and date of last seizure.
- The precipitating/trigger factors or cause of seizure if known.
- Whether the patient experiences **prodrome** or aura signs of an impending seizure.
- The most common characteristics experienced during the seizure (i.e., level of consciousness, respiratory state, and type of motor movements).
- History of injuries, including oral injuries, broken teeth, tongue lacerations.
- Postictal symptoms such as fatigue and confusion.

- Medications used for treatment of seizures may make the patient drowsy. Do not mistake drowsiness (effect of drugs) for inattentiveness.
- Work with the patient to schedule appointments during the best time of day to minimize risk of seizures.

IV. Care Plan: Instrumentation

- Complete removal of all deposits on teeth, and thorough nonsurgical periodontal therapy is essential for patients who plan to take or are taking an antiseizure medication.

A. Prior to and at the Start of Using Antiepileptic Drugs

- A thorough biofilm control program and complete periodontal debridement are needed in preparation for AED therapy.
- The patient (and caregivers) needs to be educated about the importance of an effective daily biofilm control program in preventing or minimizing gingival overgrowth from AEDs.

B. Treatment for the Patient Using Antiepileptic Drugs

1. Slight or mild gingival overgrowth
   - Nonsurgical treatment, including frequent continuing care for maintenance, along with daily oral self-care may minimize gingival overgrowth.
   - Consider short-term use of 0.12% chlorhexidine mouthrinse to manage biofilm.[33]
2. Moderate gingival overgrowth
   - Care must be taken for instrument adaptation during subgingival debridement to prevent tissue trauma (see Figure 57-2A).
   - Evaluate oral self-care effectiveness to individualize and adapt oral health aids to meet the patient's needs and minimize trauma to gingival overgrowth.
   - Reevaluate gingival tissues to determine the need for further treatment.
   - Consultation with the primary care provider about possible alternative medications may be necessary to prevent further gingival overgrowth.
3. Severe fibrotic overgrowth
   - The gingival overgrowth (see Figure 57-2A) can make instrumentation and oral self-care without tissue trauma difficult.
   - Nonsurgical periodontal therapy and biofilm control precedes surgical removal of gingival overgrowth.
   - Consult with the primary care provider about modifying or altering the dose of the AED to limit gingival overgrowth if medically safe.

C. Continuing Care Intervals

- Frequent appointments on 1-, 2-, or 3-month intervals may be indicated, depending on the severity of gingival enlargement as well as the ability and motivation of the patient in maintaining their oral health.

Seizure Emergency First Aid in the Dental Office

I. Preparation for Appointment

- When the patient's medical history indicates susceptibility to seizures, advance preparation may prevent complications should a seizure occur.
- Place emergency materials in a convenient location.
- Provide a calm and reassuring atmosphere.
- Have the patient remove partial denture(s) or denture(s) for the duration of the appointment.
- Have other dental personnel available in case of an emergency.

II. Differential Diagnosis of Seizure

Other diseases or conditions with similar signs or symptoms include:

- Syncope.
- Migraine headache.
- Transient ischemic attack.
- Cerebrovascular accident, stroke.
- Sleep disorder such as narcolepsy.
- Movement disorders such as dyskinesia (common in patients with cerebral palsy or multiple sclerosis).
- Overdose of local anesthetic.
- Hypoglycemia or insulin overdose in a patient with diabetes.
- Hyperventilation.

III. Emergency Procedure

Initiation of management for a seizure emergency follows medical emergency protocols as practiced by the dental team (**Figure 57-3**), including the following[2,4]:

- Terminate the clinical procedure; call the dental team for assistance.

EPILEPSY
First Aid
Stay Safe Side
Do
Remain calm
Keep the person safe from harmful objects
Look at a watch and time the seizure
Make the person as comfortable as possible
When seizure ends, turn the person onto their side
If seizure more than 5 minutes call 911
Stay with them until they awake
Do Not
Do not panic
Do not restrain
Do not put anything in their mouth

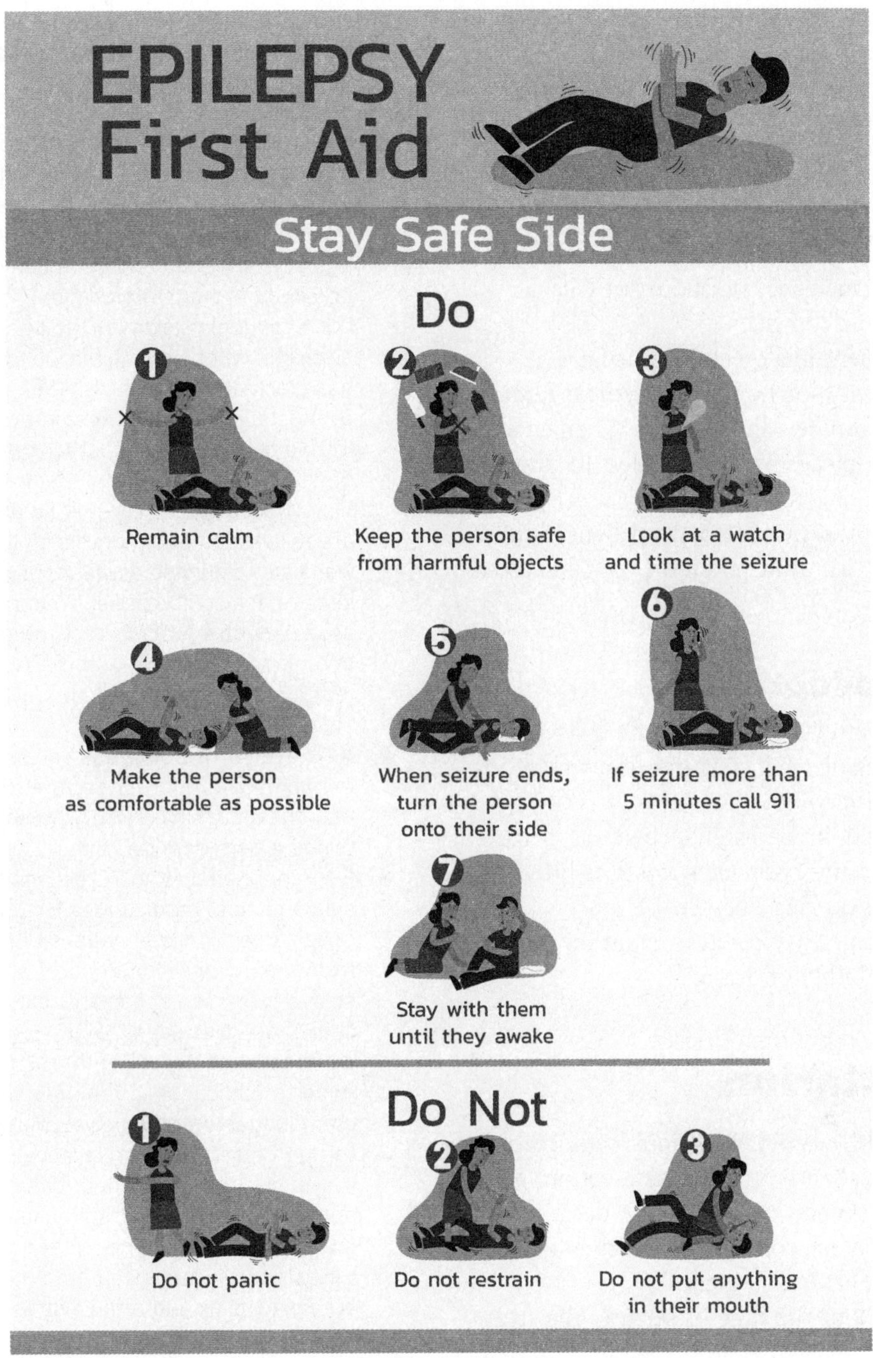

Figure 57-3 Seizure First Aid. **STAY** with the individual. Keep them **SAFE** from harmful objects in the dental environment such as handpieces and instruments. When the seizure has ended, turn the individual on their **SIDE** and stay with them until they have recovered.

- Protect patient from injury.
  - Push aside sharp objects, movable equipment, instrument trays, and remove eyeglasses or protective eyewear.
  - Stay beside the patient to prevent personal injury and reassure.
- Do not hold the person down or try to stop their movements.
- If possible, place the patient on their side and elevate the feet.
- Loosen tight clothing such as a necktie.
- Do *not* place (or force) anything between the teeth.
- Time the seizure and call 911 to activate emergency medical services (EMS) for seizures longer than 5 minutes.[4]
- Monitor and provide basic life support as needed.

- Once the seizure ends, reassure the patient and allow them to recover and monitor vital signs.
  - Check for the level of consciousness and determine if emergency medical assistance is required.

IV. Postictal Phase

- Document the emergency situation. (See Chapter 9.)
- Allow the patient to rest.
- Talk to the patient in a quiet, reassuring tone.
- Check oral cavity for trauma to teeth or tissues. Palliative care can be administered. When a tooth is broken, the piece must be located to prevent aspiration.
- With patient's consent, contact the patient's family/friend or call for transportation to take them home.

V. Status Epilepticus

- Status epilepticus is when a seizure lasts longer than 5 minutes or when seizures occur close together without recovery.[36]
- EMS is notified immediately when the seizure lasts 5 minutes and basic life support is provided until EMS arrives. (See Chapter 9.)
- Prolonged seizure may result in brain injury and long-term morbidity or death.[36]

Documentation

- Complete health history, vital signs, radiographs, findings of extra- and intraoral examination; periodontal history, charting, and tissue description; dental caries history, charting, and current demineralization and carious lesions.
- Information about the type of seizure, the treatment patient is receiving, and what steps to take in the event of an emergency
- Progress notes for each appointment with abbreviated history and current clinical findings.
- A sample progress note may be reviewed in **Box 57-2**.

Box 57-2 Example Documentation: Patient with a Seizure Disorder

- **S**—Steve, a healthy-appearing 55-year-old man, presents for the first of four scheduled periodontal scaling appointments. He stated he recently had a seizure at work when his arms and legs stiffened and he felt confused. When pressed for more information, he stated that he had seen a physician for the seizure. He also states he will be losing his job in 1 month and has started looking for another.
- **O**—Vitals: BP: 120/79, Respiration: 20, Pulse: 80. No chief complaint, other than being upset due to impending job loss. Reassessed medical history and added Tegretol; no other medications are taken. Contacted physician to confirm it was safe to provide dental care with the new seizure activity the patient reported. Periodontal assessment reveals 4- to 5-mm pocket depths in molar areas with 3–4 mm CAL, 70% plaque index, and 30% bleeding on probing. No gingival enlargement found.
- **A**—Need for use of stress-reduction protocols to minimize trigger for seizure. Be prepared to manage a possible seizure. Localized Stage II Grade A periodontitis.
- **P**—Patient education—Discussed potential side effects of medications for the treatment of seizures. Provided patient with information from the Epilepsy Foundation, also on local stress-reduction and exercise classes. Oral self-care—Disclosed biofilm and patient demonstrated use of toothbrush and floss with minor modifications. Patient also educated on management of gingival overgrowth through careful biofilm removal. Treatment provided—Completed debridement with hand and ultrasonic instruments using high-speed evacuation on the upper right quadrant. Patient tolerated treatment well but required frequent breaks to relax and reduce stress.

Next visit: Assess tissue response to debridement of upper right quadrant; reassess plaque score and oral self-care technique, modify as needed. Monitor stress-reduction progress.

Signed: ______________________, RDH
Date: ______________

Factors to Teach the Patient

- Relationship of systemic health to oral health.
- Significance of daily biofilm removal to minimizing gingival overgrowth from antiseizure medication.
- Importance of compliance with taking antiepileptic drug as prescribed.
- Need for providing complete medical history information for dental appointments.
- Seek immediate care if any oral change or injury is suspected.

References

1. Beghi E. The epidemiology of epilepsy. *Neuroepidemiology*. 2020;54(2):185-191.
2. Epilepsy Foundation. Causes of epilepsy and seizures. Published March 19, 2014. https://www.epilepsy.com/learn/about-epilepsy-basics/what-causes-epilepsy-and-seizures. Accessed January 2, 2022.
3. World Health Organization. Epilepsy. Published June 20, 2019. https://www.who.int/news-room/fact-sheets/detail/epilepsy. Accessed January 2, 2022.
4. Centers for Disease Control and Prevention. Epilepsy. Published December 1, 2021. https://www.cdc.gov/epilepsy/index.html. Accessed January 2, 2022.
5. Fisher RS, Cross JH, French JA, et al. Operational classification of seizure types by the International League Against Epilepsy: position paper of the ILAE Commission for Classification and Terminology. *Epilepsia*. 2017;58(4):522-530.
6. Amanat M, Thijs RD, Salehi M, Sander JW. Seizures as a clinical manifestation in somatic autoimmune disorders. *Seizure*. 2019;64:59-64.
7. Nakken KO, Solaas MH, Kjeldsen MJ, et al. Which seizure-precipitating factors do patients with epilepsy most frequently report? *Epilepsy Behav*. 2005;6(1):85-89.
8. Stirling RE, Cook MJ, Grayden DB, Karoly PJ. Seizure forecasting and cyclic control of seizures. *Epilepsia*. 2021;62 (Suppl 1):S2-S14.
9. Scaramelli A, Braga P, Avellanal A, et al. Prodromal symptoms in epileptic patients: clinical characterization of the pre-ictal phase. *Seizure*. 2009;18(4):246-250.
10. Johnson C, Huff JS. Evaluation of seizures and seizure-like activity in the emergency department: part 1. *Emerg Med*. 2018;50(6):127-131.
11. National Institute for Health and Care Excellence. *Epilepsies: Diagnosis and Management*. Published 2021. http://www.ncbi.nlm.nih.gov/books/NBK553536/. Accessed January 6, 2022.
12. Medicines and Healthcare Products Regulatory Agency. Valproate use by women and girls. Published March 23, 2018. https://www.gov.uk/guidance/valproate-use-by-women-and-girls. Accessed January 6, 2022.
13. Kanner AM, Ashman E, Gloss D, et al. Practice guideline update summary: efficacy and tolerability of the new antiepileptic drugs I: treatment of new-onset epilepsy: report of the Guideline Development, Dissemination, and Implementation Subcommittee of the American Academy of Neurology and the American Epilepsy Society. *Neurology*. 2018;91(2):74-81.
14. American Academy of Neurology, American Epilepsy Society. Practice guideline update summary: efficacy and tolerability of the new antiepileptic drugs II: treatment-resistant epilepsy: report of the Guideline Development, Dissemination, and Implementation Subcommittee of the American Academy of Neurology and the American Epilepsy Society. *Neurology*. 2018;91(24):1117.
15. Walia KS, Khan EA, Ko DH, Raza SS, Khan YN. Side effects of antiepileptics--a review. *Pain Pract*. 2004;4(3):194-203.
16. Johnson EL. Seizures and epilepsy. *Med Clin North Am*. 2019; 103(2):309-324.
17. Lin CH, Hsieh CL. Chinese herbal medicine for treating epilepsy. *Front Neurosci*. 2021;15:682821.
18. Schachter SC. Botanicals and herbs: A traditional approach to treating epilepsy. *Neurotherapeutics*. 2009;6(2):415-420.
19. Auditeau E, Chassagne F, Bourdy G, et al. Herbal medicine for epilepsy seizures in Asia, Africa and Latin America: a systematic review. *J Ethnopharmacol*. 2019;234:119-153.
20. Koppel BS, Brust JCM, Fife T, et al. Systematic review: efficacy and safety of medical marijuana in selected neurologic disorders: report of the Guideline Development Subcommittee of the American Academy of Neurology. *Neurology*. 2014;82(17):1556-1563.
21. Nabbout R, Thiele EA. The role of cannabinoids in epilepsy treatment: a critical review of efficacy results from clinical trials. *Epileptic Disord*. 2020;22(S1):S23-S28.
22. O'Connell BK, Gloss D, Devinsky O. Cannabinoids in treatment-resistant epilepsy: a review. *Epilepsy Behav*. 2017; 70(Pt B):341-348.
23. Sourbron J, Klinkenberg S, van Kuijk SMJ, et al. Ketogenic diet for the treatment of pediatric epilepsy: review and meta-analysis. *Childs Nerv Syst*. 2020;36(6):1099-1109.
24. Pérez-Carbonell L, Faulkner H, Higgins S, Koutroumanidis M, Leschziner G. Vagus nerve stimulation for drug-resistant epilepsy. *Pract Neurol*. 2020;20(3):189-198.
25. Rugg-Gunn F, Miserocchi A, McEvoy A. Epilepsy surgery. *Pract Neurol*. 2020;20(1):4-14.
26. Mesraoua B, Deleu D, Hassan AH, et al. Dramatic outcomes in epilepsy: depression, suicide, injuries, and mortality. *Curr Med Res Opin*. 2020;36(9):1473-1480.
27. Gallo C, Bonvento G, Zagotto G, Mucignat-Caretta C. Gingival overgrowth induced by anticonvulsant drugs: a cross-sectional study on epileptic patients. *J Periodontal Res*. 2021;56(2):363-369.
28. Brown RS, Arany PR. Mechanism of drug-induced gingival overgrowth revisited: a unifying hypothesis. *Oral Dis*. 2015;21(1):e51-61.
29. Zoheir N, Hughes FJ. The management of drug-influenced gingival enlargement. *Prim Dent J*. 2019;8(4):34-39.
30. Wynn RL, Meiller TF, Crossley HL. Phenytoin. In: *Lexicomp for Dentistry Online*. 27th ed. Wolter Kluwer; 2021:1910. www.lexi.com. Accessed January 9, 2022.
31. Hatahira H, Abe J, Hane Y, et al. Drug-induced gingival hyperplasia: a retrospective study using spontaneous reporting system databases. *J Pharm Health Care Sci*. 2017; 3(1):19.
32. Beaumont J, Chesterman J, Kellett M, Durey K. Gingival overgrowth: Part 1: aetiology and clinical diagnosis. *Br Dent J*. 2017;222(2):85-91.
33. Mawardi H, Alsubhi A, Salem N, et al. Management of medication-induced gingival hyperplasia: a systematic review. *Oral Surg Oral Med Oral Pathol Oral Radiol*. 2021;131(1): 62-72.
34. Lukmanji S, Manji SA, Kadhim S, et al. The co-occurrence of epilepsy and autism: a systematic review. *Epilepsy Behav*. 2019;98(Pt A):238-248.
35. Stone WL, Basit H, Los E. Fragile X syndrome. *StatPearls*. 2022. Last updated June 29, 2022. http://www.ncbi.nlm.nih.gov/books/NBK459243/. Accessed December 5, 2022.
36. Trinka E, Cock H, Hesdorffer D, et al. A definition and classification of status epilepticus--Report of the ILAE Task Force on Classification of Status Epilepticus. *Epilepsia*. 2015;56(10):1515-1523.

CHAPTER 58

The Patient with a Mental Health Disorder

Linda D. Boyd, RDH, RD, EdD

CHAPTER OUTLINE

LEARNING OBJECTIVES

After studying this chapter, the student will be able to:

1. Describe the various types of mental health disorders and major symptoms.
2. Summarize the side effects of treatment for mental health disorders that may have oral health implications.
3. Explain dental hygiene treatment considerations for each major category of mental health disorder.

Overview of Mental Disorders

A psychiatric or mental health disorder is a complex, clinically significant behavioral or psychological syndrome that may impact the individual's ability to engage in daily activities of living.[1] The causes may be related to behavioral, psychological, or biologic dysfunction in the individual.

- The American Psychiatric Association has classified more than 200 types of mental disorders in the document *Diagnostic and Statistical Manual of Mental Disorders* (*DSM-5*).
- Each disorder has characteristic signs and symptoms.
- This chapter provides descriptions of common mental disorders, including anxiety, mood, and eating disorders, along with schizophrenia.
    - Additional disorders are described in other chapters; for example, alcohol use disorder (see Chapter 59), Alzheimer's disease (see Chapter 48), and autism spectrum disorder and attention-deficit disorder (see Chapter 50).
- With the current policies of deinstitutionalization, more individuals with mental disorders are seeking dental and dental hygiene care in dental offices and clinics.
- *Person-first language* is used to refer to someone with a mental disorder, chronic disease, or disability.[2] The person is emphasized first and not the disorder, disease, or disability.
    - For example, refer to the patient as "an individual with schizophrenia," not as "a schizophrenic."
    - There may be exceptions to this as some individuals may choose to use identity-first language. Therefore, it is important to ask an individual how they would like to be referred to.

I. Prevalence of Mental Disorders

- Globally, 970 million people have a mental health disorder, and the prevalence in North America is 15,446 per 100,000.[3]
    - The most common mental disorders globally are anxiety and depressive disorders.
    - Women had higher prevalence of mood and anxiety disorders, while men had higher rates of attention-deficit hyperactivity and conduct disorders.

Anxiety Disorders

- Anxiety disorders are the most common class of mental disorders.
    - Anxiety disorders are common, with a global prevalence of around 32%.[4]
    - In healthcare workers during the COVID-19 pandemic, the prevalence of anxiety was 40%.[5]
    - The COVID-19 pandemic and associated social distancing, isolation, and quarantine resulted in an increase in anxiety of 25.6% globally.[6]
- Anxiety is a normal reaction to stress.
    - In anxiety disorders, the anxiety is exaggerated resulting in excess worry and avoidance behavior that can impact day-to-day functioning.
    - For formal diagnosis, the symptoms must be present for at least 6 months.[1]
- Some individuals may have secondary problems of alcohol and other substance abuse.
    - The abuse may be the result of an attempt to self-medicate.
- Individuals with anxiety disorders often have comorbid conditions, including other mental health disorders (e.g., major depressive disorder), thyroid disease, cardiovascular conditions, migraine headaches, and/or a respiratory disease.[7]

I. Types and Symptoms of Anxiety Disorders

A. Generalized Anxiety Disorder

- Persistent, pervasive anxiety and excessive worry that are not associated with life-threatening fears or "attacks."[1,8]
- May be complicated by depression, alcohol abuse, or anxiety related to a general medical condition.
- Symptoms include[1,8]:
    - Feeling restless, on-edge, irritable.
    - Sleep disturbances.
    - Difficulty concentrating.
    - Muscle tension.
    - Gastrointestinal symptoms such as abdominal distress.

B. Obsessive-Compulsive Disorder

- Frequent upsetting thoughts (obsessions), and when the individual tries to control them, there is an overwhelming urge (compulsion) to repeat routines or rituals over and over.[8]

- Symptoms include[8]:
  - Spend at least 1 hour a day with obsessive thoughts and rituals that cause distress and interfere with normal daily functioning.
  - Thoughts or obsessions might include fear of germs, dirt, or intruders.
  - Rituals might include washing hands, locking and unlocking doors, or keeping unneeded items (hoarding).

C. Panic Disorder

- Panic disorder is characterized by sudden and repeated episodes of extreme fear (panic attacks).[8]
- Symptoms center on panic attacks[8]:
  - A panic attack may be unexpected (uncued) or "situationally bound" (cued). A situationally bound panic attack invariably results from exposure to a specific trigger, such as the dental office.
  - Fear of being out of control during a panic attack.
  - Physical symptoms during an attack may include pounding or racing heart, sweating, difficulty breathing, numbness, chest palpitations or pain, or dizziness.

D. Posttraumatic Stress Disorder

- All individuals experience stressful or traumatic events, yet not everyone responds in the same way. Some people will develop posttraumatic stress disorder (PTSD), while others are resilient, manage the adversity, and adapt.
- PTSD develops within 3 months of experiencing a terrifying ordeal involving a traumatic event.[8]
- Onset may be triggered by destruction to the home or family or may result from a manmade disaster, such as war; imprisonment; torture; rape; physical or sexual abuse; or other exposure associated with intense fear or serious threat to life.
  - In healthcare workers, nearly one-half reported posttraumatic stress during the COVID-19 pandemic.[5]
  - In survivors of severe COVID-19, it is estimated as many as 30% will experience PTSD.[9,10]
  - It is important for dental providers to be aware of the possible long-term mental health effects on individuals who have survived COVID-19 as well as healthcare providers on the frontline of caring for patients with COVID-19.
- Signs and symptoms include[8]:
  - Flashbacks of the traumatic experience and terror may be triggered by a stimulus that can be readily associated with the original event.
  - Dreams or recollections may cause the individual to feel they are reliving the event.
  - Avoidance of places, events, or objects that are reminders of the triggering event.
  - Loss of interest in activities that were enjoyable in the past.
  - **Hyperarousal** symptoms including feeling tense, difficulty sleeping, angry outbursts, intense fear, and may be easily startled.
  - There may also be cultural differences in symptoms exhibited.
  - In children, symptoms may be slightly different and include bedwetting, acting out the scary event during playtime, or being unusually clingy to a parent or other adult.
- Risk factors for PTSD are related to the intensity of the traumatic event and the susceptibility of the individual[11]:
  - Female gender.
  - Childhood trauma.
  - Exposure to four or more traumatic events.
  - A history of mental illness or substance abuse.
  - Exposure to death, injury, torture, or disfigurement.
- Protective factors for PTSD include[12]:
  - Social support.
  - Secure attachment to family and friends.
  - Resilience
  - Optimism.
  - Self-efficacy.
  - Ability to function despite feelings of fear.

II. Treatment

A. Basic Therapeutic Approach

- Lifestyle modifications include regular physical activity, adequate sleep, stress management, and avoidance of drugs and alcohol.[13,14]
- Diagnose and treat other medical and psychiatric problems.

B. Pharmacologic Treatment

- Antidepressants: antidepressants are preferred as first-line treatment of anxiety disorders.[13,15,16]
  - Examples include fluoxetine (Prozac), paroxetine (Paxil), and sertraline (Zoloft).
  - Side effects: headache, weight gain, tremor, irritability, and xerostomia.

- **Anxiolytics**: These are used only short term because of the risk of dependency and possible cognitive impairment.[13,15,16]
    - Examples include benzodiazepines (diazepam [Valium], lorazepam [Ativan]). These are highly addictive and must be carefully monitored.
    - Side effects: confusion, dizziness, muscle weakness, memory impairment, difficulty in speaking, skin rash, and xerostomia.
- Beta-blockers: taken on a short-term basis for anxiety, these medication help to relieve the physical symptoms of anxiety such as trembling, shaking, and rapid heartbeat.[13]

B. Psychotherapy

- Cognitive behavioral therapy (CBT)[13-15,17]
    - CBT is a combination of strategies to address the **cognitive**, behavioral, and emotional components of the anxiety disorder and PTSD.
    - May be conducted in individual or group sessions.
    - Support groups are also helpful.
- Prolonged exposure (PE) therapy[7,12]
    - PE therapy is used in treatment of PTSD and gradually exposes an individual to the traumatic event in a safe way and helps them to cope with their feelings.
- Cognitive processing therapy (CPT)[14,17]
    - CPT is also used to treat PTSD and helps people to make sense of the traumatic event they experienced.

III. Dental Hygiene Care

A. Personal Factors

- Each anxiety disorder has its own characteristics.
- Relationships with other people can be strained.
- Physical complaints, such as rapid heartbeat, hyperventilation, tightness in the throat, and constant fatigue, are common.

B. Oral Implications

- Xerostomia related to medications put the patient at high risk for dental caries.[18]
- Individuals with a diagnosis of an anxiety disorder are at higher risk of tooth loss.[18]
- Individuals with mental health disorders have a 25% higher caries risk.[18]
- There is a significant association between periodontal disease and emotional disorders (anxiety and depression).[19]
- A patient with obsessive-compulsive disorder may perform excessive, vigorous toothbrushing resulting in gingival and tooth abrasion.

C. Appointment Considerations

- Review medical history and medications carefully.
- Enhance the patient's sense of control.
    - One technique is to establish a "stop signal," which may consist of the patient raising the left hand when they are uncomfortable or need to stop treatment.
    - Explain each step to the patient and keep communication as open as possible.
- Cognitive distraction involves encouraging the patient to think about something besides the dental treatment.
    - Headphones or earbuds for music and relaxation can help to reduce stress.
- Environmental changes can help reduce anxiety.
    - An example would be the smell of lavender in the waiting room to relax the patient in addition to the previously mentioned techniques.
- Nitrous oxide sedation may be helpful to relax the patient. (See Chapter 36.)
- Effective pain control is needed.
    - Use local anesthesia for nonsurgical periodontal therapy (NSPT).
    - Attention to technique to minimize discomfort is essential.
- Schedule appointments in the morning; eliminate unnecessary waiting in the reception area; length of appointment can be minimized to prevent stress.
- Be alert to symptoms of a panic attack, such as sweating or hyperventilation. Allow the patient to sit up and take short breaks.

Depressive Disorders

Mood disorders that include depressive disorders are another common classification of mental disorder.

- The global prevalence of depression was 28% in January to June 2020.[20]
    - Prevalence of depression in the Americas was 34%.
- Risk factors for depressive disorders include[21]:
    - Gender (women are more likely to experience mood disorders).

- History (personal or family) of depression.
- Major life changes and stress.
- Onset is usually in the mid-20s, but it can occur at any age.

I. Types of Depressive Disorders

A. Major Depressive Disorder

- Transient depressed moods occur in the lives of most people due to unforeseen tragic events, illnesses, death, or disappointments in career or other life plans.
- However, major depressive disorder interferes with ability to function in daily life.[8]
- Some individuals experience only one episode of major depression in their lifetime, but it is more common to have recurrent episodes.[8]

B. Perinatal Depression

During pregnancy (prenatal) and in the postpartum period, many physiologic and psychological stresses are related to the changes taking place in the mother's life, which may result in perinatal depression.[22]

- Perinatal depression occurs during pregnancy and can increase risk of adverse pregnancy outcomes such as preeclampsia and low birth weight.[23]
- Postpartum depression (PPD) is mild-to-severe depression within the first month postpartum, but the incidence for PPD tends to peak 3 months after delivery.[24]
  - The prevalence of PPD is estimated to be 12% globally in healthy mothers, with a prevalence in North America of 16%.[24]
  - Recent research suggests that maternal PPD is a strong risk factor for fathers to also experience paternal PPD, with 24% to 50% affected.[24]
- It is critical to identify women with PPD because it can lead to negative mother–infant bonding and interactions that include maternal withdrawal, disengagement, and abuse.[24]
  - The mother may be less likely to engage in preventive care and is less responsive to providing care to the infant; this may include engaging in appropriate feeding practices and oral health care for the infant/children.[24,25]
  - PPD may impact developmental milestones such as cognitive scores and nonverbal communication of the infant/toddler.[25]
  - Infants may also exhibit increased dysregulation of sleep and feeding.[25]
  - Negative infant behaviors are also typical, including excessive infant crying and fusiness.[25]

II. Signs and Symptoms of Depression

- Symptoms vary between individuals, but cause significant distress and daily functioning. Common symptoms include[1,26]:
  - Depressed mood or loss of interest or pleasure in activities present for at least 2 weeks.
  - Feelings of hopelessness, worthlessness, or guilt.
  - Fatigue and lack of energy.
  - Difficulty with memory and concentration.
  - Weight loss or gain.
  - **Insomnia**, early-morning wakefulness.
  - Thoughts of suicide.

III. Treatment

- In the case of depression, one of the first things assessed is suicide risk. Hospitalization may be indicated when potential danger of suicide or harm to others exists.[26]

A. Basic Therapeutic Approach

- Lifestyle modifications include regular physical activity, adequate sleep, and avoidance of drugs and alcohol.
- Diagnose and treat other medical and psychiatric problems.

B. Pharmacotherapy

Second-generation antidepressants are preferred as an initial treatment of depressive disorders.[27] However, they take 2–4 weeks to reach therapeutic levels.

- Selective serotonin reuptake inhibitors[27]
  - Advantages: tolerability better than earlier drugs; better compliance; safety in overdose.
  - Examples: fluoxetine (Prozac), paroxetine (Paxil), and sertraline (Zoloft).
- Serotonin and noradrenergic reuptake inhibitors[27]
  - Examples: duloxetine (Cymbalta) and venlafaxine (Effexor).
- Complementary and alternative therapy[27]
  - St. John's Wort may have similar effects as second-generation antidepressants.

C. Psychotherapy

Psychotherapy combined with pharmacotherapy is more effective than either one alone for treating depressive disorders.[27] Examples of psychotherapy include:

- Behavioral therapy.
- Cognitive behavioral and mindfulness-based cognitive therapy.
- Psychodynamic therapy.
- Interpersonal psychotherapy.

IV. Dental Hygiene Care

A. Personal Factors

- Self-care impairment and lack of motivation negatively impact oral health.[28]
- Symptoms not controlled by medication, such as difficulties with memory, may need to be considered when planning dental hygiene care.
- Individuals with depression may have poor diet quality, such as higher intakes of energy-dense foods that tend to be higher in sugar, which may increase the risk of dental caries and impact healing after periodontal therapy.[29]

B. Oral Health Implications

- Side effects of medications: xerostomia along with poor dietary choices encourages growth of dental biofilm and increases the risk for dental caries.[29]
- Omission of general health habits and neglect of oral care make the person susceptible to oral diseases.
  - Adults with a diagnosis of depression are at a higher risk for dental caries (27%), tooth loss (31%), and being edentulous (17%).[30]
- Taste perception changes may contribute to a preference for sweets and refined sugars, resulting in an intake almost twice that of those without depression.[31]

C. Appointment Interventions

- Assessment
  - Monitor the medical and medication histories closely; note side effects and contraindications related to new drug therapies.
  - Review consultations with medical/psychiatric specialists caring for the patient.
  - Intraoral/extraoral examination: check for signs of xerostomia.
- Approach
  - Provide positive reinforcement and reassurance. Avoid negative guilt-inducing words due to the tendency for individuals to feel guilty and worthless.
  - Show genuine interest in the patient to build rapport.
- Preventive instruction
  - Dental biofilm control: educate the patient and caregivers about the need for daily oral self-care to manage the risk of oral disease.
  - Xerostomia: management of caries risk will depend on the level of risk, but may include dietary counseling, office and home fluorides, rinsing with baking soda solution, and chlorhexidine rinse for those at high or extreme caries risk.[32]
- Implementation of care plan
  - For patients with photosensitivity from medication, provide tinted protective eyewear.
  - Profound local anesthesia when needed for pain control.
  - Provide in-office fluoride varnish after instrumentation.
  - Use care to prevent postural hypotension. Sit the patient up slowly from a reclined position and have the patient remain seated a few moments before standing.

Bipolar Disorder

- Bipolar disorder (BD) was formerly known as manic-depressive disorder and involves mood changes from extreme highs (mania) to extreme lows (depression).[1,8]
  - Globally, 46 million people have BD. The prevalence in the United States is approximately 0.7% and 0.9% in Canada.[33]
  - It is more prevalent in women.[33]
  - Those with BD have the highest risk of suicide for psychiatric conditions (20–30 times higher than the general population).[34]
- BD is the 16th leading cause of years lost to disability (YLD) globally of all diseases because of poor treatment adherence, relapse, and high rates of comorbidities such as anxiety disorder, metabolic syndrome, substance abuse, and attention-deficit disorder.[35]

I. Signs and Symptoms

- Manic episode symptoms include behaviors that are not consistent with the patient's usual behavior, including the following[8,35]:
  - Inflated self-esteem.
  - Decreased need for sleep.
  - Irritable.
  - Attention gets focused on unimportant activities.
  - Excessive involvement in risky activities.
  - Extreme changes in energy, activity, sleep, and behavior based on the large swings in mood.

- Major depressive episode symptoms are the same as those described for depressive disorders.

II. Treatment

- Both pharmacotherapy and psychotherapy are used during all phases of the disorder. Initially, hospitalization may be needed to protect the individual from harm to self or others.

A. Pharmacotherapy

First-line treatments may include single medication, but combination therapies tend to be most effective.[35-37]

- Mood stabilizers
  - Example: lithium.
  - Side effects: xerostomia, restlessness, joint and muscle pain, salivary gland swelling, indigestion, and bloating.
- Atypical antipsychotics are sometimes used in conjunction with antidepressants.
  - Examples: quetiapine (Seroquel), risperidone (Risperdal), and aripiprazole (Abilify).
  - Side effects: dizziness, blurred vision, rapid heartbeat, skin rashes, and drowsiness.

B. Psychotherapy

- Psychoeducation is a first-line treatment and educates the patient and family about BD and coping strategies.[35]
- Second-line therapies include[35]:
  - CBT helps patients learn to change harmful or negative thought patterns and behaviors.
  - Family-focused therapy improves communication and coping strategies to aid in early recognition of manic or depressive episodes.
- Third-line therapies include[35]:
  - Interpersonal and social rhythm therapy (IPSRT) is typically used in conjunction with other psychotherapies and is helpful in the maintenance phase of BD. IPSRT focuses on helping individuals to maintain consistent daily routines such as oral self-care to promote stability in mood.
  - Peer support.

III. Dental Hygiene Care

A. Personal Factors

- In a manic episode:
  - Many patients talk quickly, jump from thought to thought, and have a short attention span.
  - A tendency to argue and become irritable may be apparent.
- In a depressive episode:
  - The patient may not be interested in oral self-care and be unmotivated.

B. Oral Health Implications

- Poor oral hygiene, as often oral self-care is not a priority to the patient.[38]
- Gingival tissues may appear abraded and lacerated because of overzealous toothbrushing with excessive pressure.
- Higher risk for caries and periodontal disease.[38]
- Severe tooth wear.[38]
- Vasoconstrictors should be used with caution with risperidone and consultation with the primary care provider is recommended.[37]

C. Appointment Interventions

- Carefully review medical and medication history; consult with patient's physician/psychiatrist as needed.
- Simplify the surroundings; provide a comfortable, calm environment.
- Patient instruction may be difficult due to a short attention span. Prioritize risk factors and use direct, simple instructions so the patient is not overwhelmed.
  - When applicable, help the patient's caregiver to learn procedures for dental caries prevention and periodontal health.
- Based on caries and periodontal risk assessment, prioritize and implement management strategies such as office and home fluoride application, dietary counseling, and chlorhexidine mouthrinse.[32]
- Shorter continuing care appointments may be needed to prevent and manage oral disease.

Feeding and Eating Disorders

Feeding and eating disorders are serious disturbances in the amounts and types of foods consumed.

- Global prevalence is 0.1% to 1%, with 16 million people having been diagnosed with anorexia or bulimia nervosa.[33]
  - In the United States and Canada, the prevalence is approximately 0.5%, with binge-eating disorder being more common than anorexia.[39]
- Prevalence of other feeding disorders such as pica and rumination disorder is unclear.

- Identification and referral of a patient suspected of having an eating disorder for medical evaluation may be lifesaving because serious medical problems may exist and psychiatric therapy is indicated.
- An interdisciplinary team approach for successful rehabilitation of an individual with an eating disorder involves, at the least, medical, psychiatric, nutritional, dental, and dental hygiene professionals.

I. Types and Symptoms

A. Pica

- Consumption of nonfood items typically occurs in children, but it also common in adults, particularly those with mental disorders and/or intellectual disabilities.[1]
- Diagnostic criteria include[1,8]:
    - Persistent eating of nonfood substances such as dirt, clay, starch, gum, or ice for at least 1 month.
    - Consumption of nonfood items may replace healthy foods and lead to nutrient deficiencies that can impact immune response and healing.

B. Anorexia Nervosa

Anorexia nervosa is characterized by a refusal of the individual to maintain body weight over the minimal normal weight for age and height. The restrictive eating results in life-threatening weight loss.[1,8]

- Anorexia nervosa has the highest mortality rate of any mental disorder.[36]
- Commonly begins in adolescence or young adulthood.
- Signs and symptoms include[1,8,33]:
    - Restriction of energy intake resulting in severe weight loss with emaciation; "waiflike" appearance.
    - Intense fear of weight gain or becoming fat.
    - Body image distortion (**Figure 58-1**).
    - Purging by vomiting, laxatives, and excessive exercise.
    - Malnutrition can have long-term impact on bone mineral density (osteopenia or osteoporosis).
    - Vital signs: low pulse rate, hypotension, decreased respiratory rate, and low body temperature.
    - Metabolic changes: gastrointestinal, cardiovascular, hematologic, and renal system disturbances.
    - Amenorrhea (missed menstrual periods).

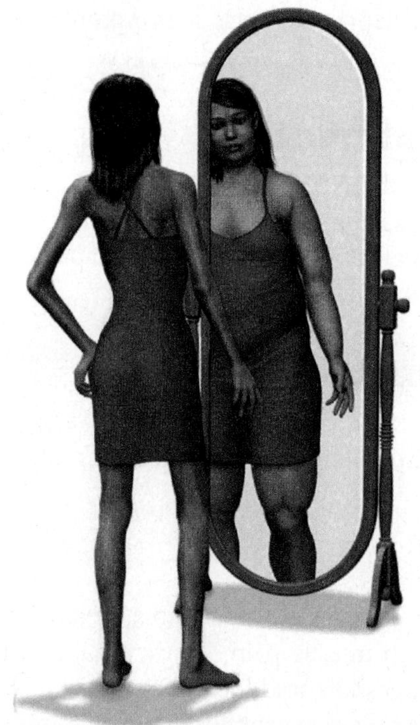

Figure 58-1 Anorexia Nervosa. The person with anorexia typically has a distorted body self-image. Although small and waiflike in real life, the mirror image appears as an overweight individual.

Reproduced from Werner R. *Massage Therapist's Guide to Pathology*. Philadelphia, PA: Lippincott Williams & Wilkins; 2012.

C. Bulimia Nervosa

- Bulimia nervosa is a mental disorder marked by recurrent episodes of uncontrollable binge eating that occur an average of once a week for at least 1 month.[8]
    - Binges involve eating large amounts of food, often in secret, in a short time period of time.
- Two types of **compensatory behaviors** are seen in individuals with bulimia nervosa, known as the purging type and the nonpurging type.
    - Because of the fear of becoming overweight, self-induced vomiting after eating or the use of laxatives or diuretics is characteristic of the purging type (**Figure 58-2**).
    - The nonpurging type uses strict dieting, fasting, and/or vigorous exercise.
- Signs and symptoms include[8,40]:
    - Normal body weight or slightly overweight is typical, in contrast to the person with anorexia, who is underweight.
    - Comorbidity with other mental disorders.
    - At increased risk for substance abuse, suicide, and health complications.
    - Chronically inflamed and sore throat.
    - Parotid gland enlargement.

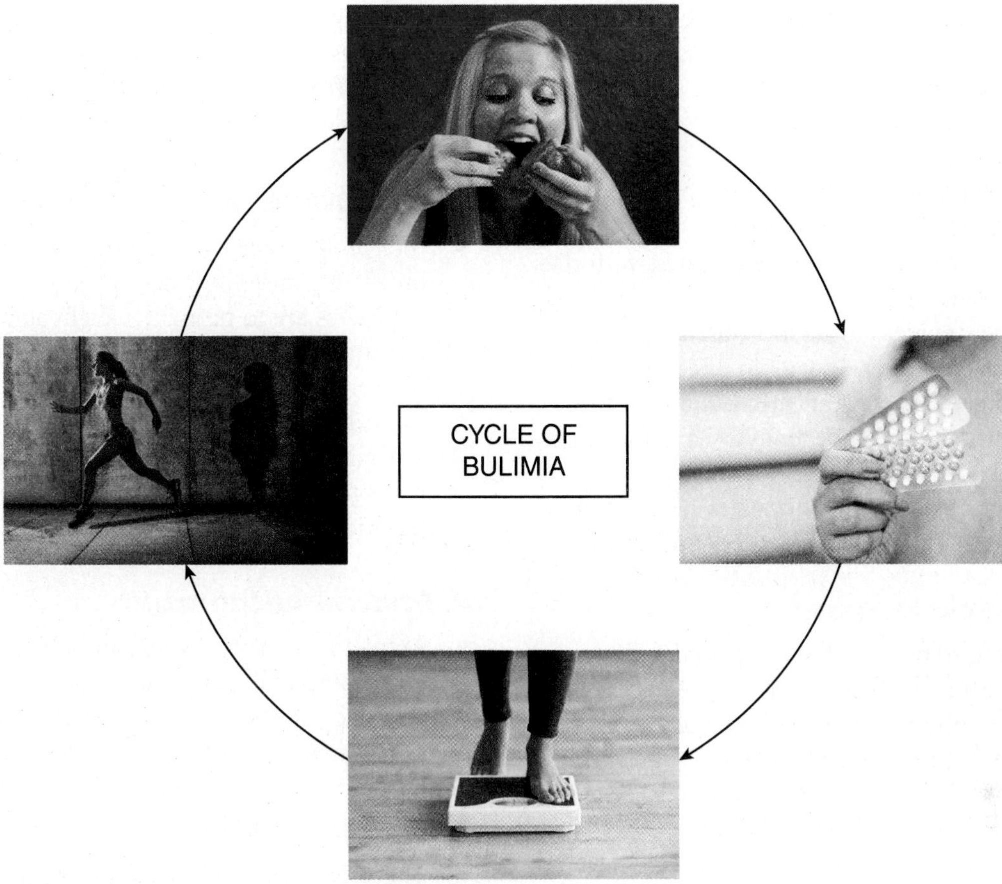

Figure 58-2 Bulimia Nervosa. The person with bulimia becomes trapped in recurring behaviors involving food and weight management. They ingest a vast number of calories at once and then take measures to purge themselves of their binge (e.g., abuse of laxatives, diet pills, and diuretics). They monitor their weight several times a day; some exercise obsessively to burn off the calories.

A: © Carolyn Dietrich/Shutterstock; B: © Poom jung/Shutterstock; C: © Prostock-studio/Shutterstock; D: © Lassedesignen/Shutterstock

- Enamel erosion and dentin hypersensitivity due to frequent exposure to acid gastric fluids.
- Severe dehydration may result from purging.
- Foods consumed during a binge include breads/pasta (65%), sweets (56%), and salty snacks (40%), which may be more cariogenic.[41]

D. Binge-Eating Disorder

- Binge-eating disorder (BED) is defined as recurrent episodes of binge eating without compensatory behaviors, such as self-induced vomiting, seen in bulimia nervosa at least once a week for 3 months.[1,8]
- Signs and symptoms include[1,8]:
  - Occurs in normal weight, overweight, and obese individuals.
  - Binge eating is associated with feeling a loss of control over eating associated with guilt, shame, and embarrassment that impact daily functioning.
  - Comorbid disorders include mental health disorders such as bipolar, depressive, and anxiety disorders.
  - Eating large amounts of food quickly in a 2-hour time period.
  - Eating alone or in secret.
  - Frequent dieting.

E. Type 1 Disordered Eating

- Type 1 disordered eating (T1DE) is also called diabulimia and defined as the restriction or omission of insulin in an individual with type 1 diabetes mellitus in order to lose weight or prevent weight gain.[42]
  - This condition has been documented since the 1970s, but there are no recognized diagnostic criteria in the *DSM-5*.
  - Diabulimia is most often seen in adolescent and young women.

    - These individuals are at increased risk of microvascular complications such as renal failure, neuropathy, heart attack, stroke, and death.
- Signs and symptoms include[43]:
    - Rapid weight loss.
    - Obsession with body size and shape and dissatisfaction with body image.
    - Ketone or "fruity" smell associated with diabetic ketoacidosis.
    - Thirst, frequent urination, and fatigue.
    - Persistent high hemoglobin A1c.
    - Eating behaviors similar to bulimia nervosa.
    - Frequent emergency room visits or admission for diabetic ketoacidosis.
    - Often associated with mental health comorbidities such as anxiety and depression.

F. Orthorexia Nervosa

- Characterized by pathologic or disordered healthy eating with a rigid focus on control and restriction of healthy food choices, such as eliminating all preservatives, coloring, flavoring, and excess fat and sugar.[40] Extreme restriction may result in malnutrition.
- This condition is not recognized by the American Psychiatric Association in the *DSM-5* and did not appear in the peer-reviewed literature until 2004. Some believe it is a subtype of anorexia nervosa.
- Proposed diagnostic criteria include[44]:
    - Compulsive behavior or preoccupation with restrictive dietary practices believed to promote health.
    - Dietary restriction tends to escalate over time with elimination of entire food groups and may engage in "cleanses" (partial fasts) to detoxify.
    - Violation of dietary restriction causes anxiety and shame.
    - Malnutrition or medical complications from the restricted diet.
    - Impairment of social, academic, and/or vocational functioning.

II. Medical Complications

Medical complications are primarily associated with anorexia nervosa and people with bulimia who engage in purging behaviors.[45,46]

- Problems include dehydration, electrolyte imbalance, protein malnutrition, and cardiac arrhythmia.
- Self-medications include abuse of laxatives and diuretics, which contribute to gastrointestinal disturbances.
- Esophageal tears.
- Gastroesophageal reflux disease (GERD).
- Amenorrhea or menstrual irregularities.
- Increased risk for suicide.

III. Treatment

- Interprofessional team treatment for eating disorders is considered best practice. The primary objectives are to promote weight gain and restore nutritional status. Treatment may require months or even years.
- Typically, outpatient treatment is recommended, so if someone has been hospitalized for treatment, it suggests they are at high risk for medical complications and a medical consult is needed.[47]

A. Pharmacotherapy

- Antidepressants (primarily in bulimia nervosa)[47]
    - Example: fluoxetine (Prozac).
    - Side effects: headache, weight gain, tremor, irritability, and xerostomia.

B. Psychotherapy

- The goal of therapy is to help the individual discover the underlying causes of the problems and source of the disordered eating behavior.[47]
    - CBT is the first line of treatment in bulimia nervosa and diabulimia.
    - Interpersonal therapy.
    - Family-based therapy is recommended for younger patients.

C. Nutrition Therapy

- Registered dietitian nutritionists with advanced training in eating disorders work as part of the interprofessional team to conduct a full nutrition assessment, make a diagnosis, and individualize a plan for medical nutrition therapy in collaboration with the team.[48]
- This in-depth type of nutrition counseling is beyond the scope of practice for dental professionals.

IV. Dental Hygiene Care

A. Oral Implications

- Dental erosion (**perimolysis**): the chemical erosion of the tooth surfaces by acid from the regurgitation of stomach contents during vomiting and GERD.[40,49]
    - Individuals who engage in self-induced vomiting have five times greater risk of dental erosion.

- Due to the dental erosion, the earliest evidence of bulimia or binge-eating/purging type of anorexia may be on the smooth palatal surfaces of the teeth.
- The lingual surfaces of the maxillary anterior teeth appear translucent and glasslike (**Figure 58-3B**).
- With time, the erosion extends over the occlusal and incisal surfaces and chipping may occur.
- Restorations in posterior teeth may appear raised because of erosion of the enamel around the margins.

- Dental caries: an increase in caries incidence is found, particularly in cervical caries. Demineralization results from pH changes in the saliva, from xerostomia, and from the large quantities of cariogenic and acidic foods ingested during binges.[40]
- Mucosal lesions: nutrient deficiencies, especially in the B vitamins, may result in angular cheilitis (**Figure 58-4**), glossitis, inflammation of the pharynx (**Figure 58-3A**), and a burning sensation.[49]
- Gingival trauma from compulsive toothbrushing may predispose to recession and bone loss.[49]
- Periodontal manifestations: nutritional deficiencies with inadequate control of dental biofilm due to depression may predispose the patient to gingivitis.[49]
- Saliva: the decrease in quantity, quality, and pH of the saliva limits its buffering and lubricating properties.[44] Dehydration of the oral soft tissues occurs.
  - Body fluid is lost from vomiting and the use of diuretics may result in dehydration and xerostomia.
  - Xerostomia is also a side effect of antidepressant medication prescribed for patients with bulimia and anorexia.
- Hypersensitive teeth: the loss of enamel and the exposure of dentin results in sensitivity, which can be especially noticeable for the maxillary anterior teeth.[40,49]
- Trauma:
  - The soft palate can be traumatized by the finger or toothbrush used to induce vomiting.[40] The same implement may injure the mouth at the commissures.
  - Pharyngeal trauma is caused by a large food bolus that is swallowed or regurgitated (Figure 58-3A).

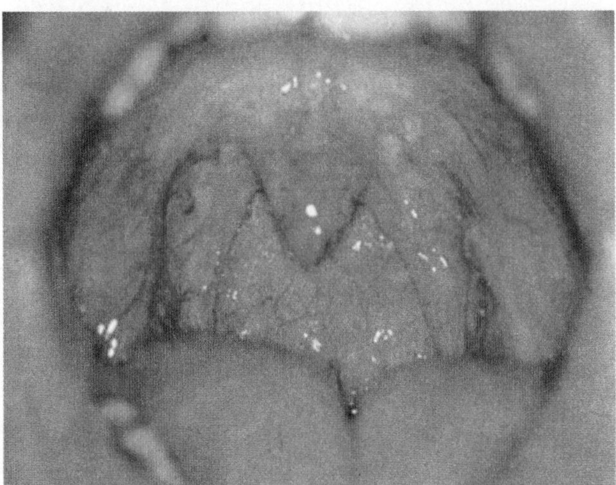

A

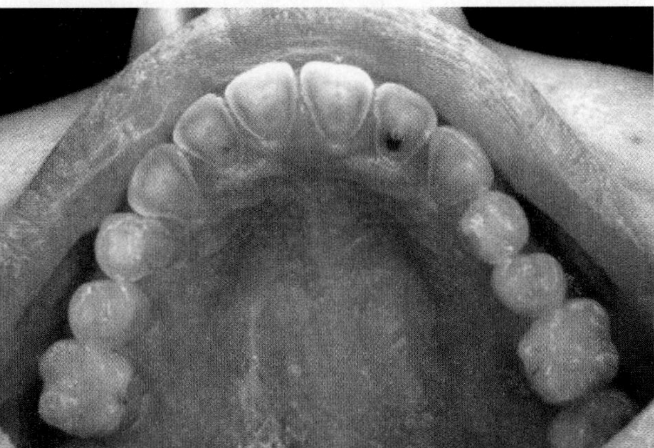

B

Figure 58-3 Oral Manifestations of Purging-Type Eating Disorders. Signs of purging include **(A)** irritation and inflammation of the pharynx as well as the esophagus from chronic vomiting and **(B)** erosion of the lingual surface of the teeth, loss of dental enamel, periodontal disease, and extensive dental caries.

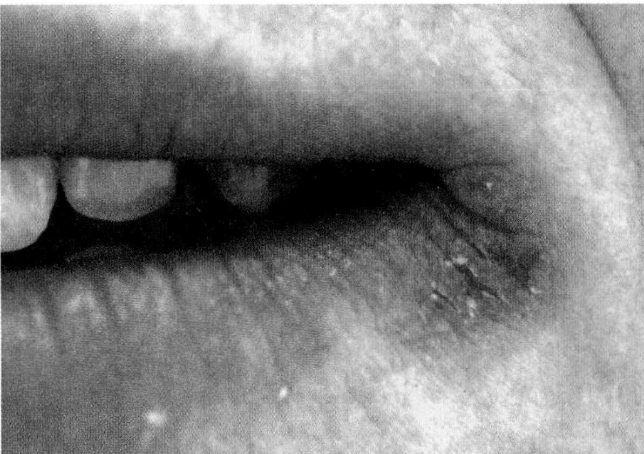

Figure 58-4 Angular Cheilitis. Angular cheilitis may occur in vitamin B deficiencies, which can occur in patients with eating disorders.

- Callus formation or scars on fingers or knuckles used for self-induced vomiting may be observed.
- Parotid gland: enlargement may occur within days after a binge-purge event.[40,49] The cause of enlargement is not known.
  - The degree of enlargement increases with the frequency of vomiting. The gland functions normally and is not sensitive to palpation.
- Bruxism: tooth wear may be associated with GERD.[43]
- Taste: taste perception may be impaired.
- Temporomandibular joint disorders (TMD): self-induced vomiting may cause dislocation or subluxation of the mandibular condyle due to excessive opening and result in symptoms of TMD, including headaches, facial pain, and sensitivity to palpation.[49]

C. Appointment Interventions

- Approach the patient with a nonthreatening, nonjudgmental demeanor. Develop rapport through mutual respect and a trusting relationship.
- Recognize that denial of an eating disorder is common.
- Be aware of answers to medical and personal history questions concerning diet, medications, use of laxatives and diuretics, and weight and weight loss that may provide strong suspicions of a feeding or eating disorder.
- Assess the nutritional status through use of a dietary assessment.
- Record vital signs.
- Perimolysis and dental caries prevention strategies include:
  - Reduction in consumption of cariogenic foods; provide list of suggestions for substitutions.
  - Improvement in oral self-care. Show use of appropriate brushing and flossing with additional interdental aids if required for biofilm removal. Clean the tongue. (See Chapter 26.)
    - A power toothbrush may aid the patient in avoiding application of excess pressure when brushing.
  - Avoidance of brushing after vomiting. Demineralization of the tooth surface by the acid from the stomach starts immediately on contact. Brushing may remove additional enamel/dentin.
  - Remineralization after vomiting with an alkaline rinse of sodium bicarbonate solution to neutralize the acid.
- Management of dental hypersensitivity. (See Chapter 41.)
- Xerostomia management may include:
  - Oral moisturizers.
  - Sipping water.
  - Saliva substitutes.

Schizophrenia

- Schizophrenia is a complex, chronic mental disorder with disturbances in feeling, thinking, cognition, affect, motivation, and behavior that significantly impair function to a level below normal for the individual.[8]
  - Global prevalence of schizophrenia is 0.3%, with 20 million people affected.[33]
- The onset for men is usually in the early to mid-20s and in the late 20s for females.[8]
- Prevalence of substance-use disorder (SUD) is high among patients with schizophrenia.[50]
  - Prevalence of any SUD was approximately 42%, with over 27% using illicit drugs, 26% using cannabis, 24% using alcohol, and 7% using stimulants.
  - Over 60% of patients with schizophrenia use tobacco, and tobacco may be associated with cognitive impairment such as attention, working memory, learning, and problem solving.[51]
- Those with schizophrenia have higher rates of premature mortality and suicide is a common cause of death, with more than one-third (34.5%) exhibiting a lifetime prevalence of suicide ideation and nearly one-half (44.3%) planning suicide.[52]
- Risk factors for schizophrenia are both genetic and environmental.
  - Genetics is a strong contributor to risk for schizophrenia.[53]
  - Environmental factors may contribute to disruption of brain development and include[53]:
    - Obstetric complications.
    - Childhood trauma.
    - Cannabis use (increases the risk five-fold).
    - First-generation immigrant.
    - Living in poverty in an urban setting.

I. Signs and Symptoms

Symptoms fall into two main categories: positive and negative symptoms.

- Positive symptoms are those that reflect unusual, exaggerated behavior and include[8,54]:
  - **Hallucinations** such as voices with the belief an outside entity has power over the individual.
  - Paranoid **delusions**.

    - Disorganized thinking characterized by the person having difficulty organizing thoughts or connecting them logically.
    - Movement disorders such as agitated body movements.
    - People with positive symptoms may "lose touch" with reality and the symptoms may come and go.
- Negative symptoms are associated with an absence of feelings, cognition, or goal directed behavior. Symptoms include[8,54]:
    - The individual may have a "flat **affect**," meaning the person shows no emotion.
    - Lack of pleasure in activities once enjoyed.
    - Inability to start and carry out tasks.
    - Little communication even when forced to interact.
    - These individuals have difficulty with everyday tasks such as oral self-care.
    - Poor executive functioning, meaning difficulty with understanding information and using it to make decisions.
    - Difficulty paying attention.
    - Challenges with working memory or the ability to use information immediately after it is learned.

II. Treatment

- The response to initial treatment can be a predictor of the long-term prognosis.

A. Pharmacotherapy

- The objectives of treatment are to reduce or alleviate the delusions, hallucinations, and other symptoms and to enable the patient to function in daily living while reducing morbidity and mortality.[55]
- Typical antipsychotics are used to block dopamine receptors and are effective against positive symptoms with less effect on negative symptoms.[53]
    - Examples: chlorpromazine (Thorazine), haloperidol (Haldol), and perphenazine (Etrafon, Trilafon).
    - Side effects: xerostomia, persistent muscle spasms, orthostatic hypotension, tremors, confusion, memory loss, and restlessness. Long-term use can lead to **tardive dyskinesia** (uncontrolled muscle movements).[56]
- Atypical antipsychotics were developed in the 1990s and are second-generation antipsychotics recommended for treatment-resistant schizophrenia[55]:
    - Examples: clozapine (Clozaril), quetiapine (Seroquel), risperidone (Risperdal), olanzapine (Zyprexa), and aripiprazole (Abilify).
    - Side effects: xerostomia or sialorrhea (hypersalivation), orthostatic hypotension, dizziness, blurred vision, rapid heartbeat, confusion, skin rashes, drug-induced movement disorders (tardive dyskinesia), and drowsiness.[37,57]
- **Table 58-1** lists a few of the many side effects of antipsychotic medications, with implications that may require adaptations.

B. Psychosocial Intervention

- Psychosocial interventions are utilized once the patient is stabilized on antipsychotic medication.[55]
    - Treatment is to help give general support in dealing with the challenges of the illness such as self-care, work, interpersonal relationships, and communication.
    - Rehabilitation, once stabilized includes, social and vocational training, so a person with schizophrenia can function in the community.
    - Family education is also essential to help them learn coping strategies and problem-solving skills to support their loved one.
- CBT focuses on thinking and behavior and helps the person with schizophrenia manage symptoms that remain despite medication.

III. Dental Hygiene Care

A. Oral Implications

- Overall degeneration of health may have occurred because of neglect of diet, exercise, sleep, general cleanliness, and oral care.
- Concurrent alcohol and/or other drug abuse, as well as smoking, can influence dental and periodontal health.
- Individuals with schizophrenia have higher rates of dental caries, more missing teeth, and fewer filled teeth, suggesting either a lack of access to dental care or a failure to seek dental care.[58]
- Xerostomia coupled with lack of attention to self-care may lead to an increase in dental caries.[59]
- Those with schizophrenia may have greater attachment loss, which may be a result of lack of self-care coupled with lack of dental care and tobacco use.[59]

B. Appointment Planning

- Elective dental and dental hygiene treatment cannot be carried out until the schizophrenia is stabilized.

Table 58-1 Effects of Antipsychotic Medication

Side Effects	Implications For Dental Hygiene Care
Dystonia	
Muscle contractions	Laryngeal spasm; coughing Unable to turn head
Dysarthria	
Difficult speech	Communication difficulty
Parkinson-like syndrome	
Shuffling gait Muscular rigidity Resting tremor (pill rolling) Facial grimacing **Bradykinesia**	Cooperation may be difficult Patient positioning Instrument positioning; retraction
Akathisia	
Restlessness, pacing	Plan short appointments
Akinesia	
Loss of voluntary movement Lethargy, fatigue feelings	Adjust patient position
Tardive dyskinesia	
Involuntary mouth and jaw movements	Difficulty in instrumentation Wearing dentures difficult or impossible Muscle fatigue; may need mouth prop and/or shorter appointments
Anticholinergic effects	
Xerostomia Blurred vision	Dental caries prevention Fluoride dentifrice; saliva substitute Difficulty seeing visual aids
Cardiovascular	
Postural hypotension Tachycardia, palpitations	Have patient sit up slowly and wait before standing Monitor vital signs
Sedation	
Drowsiness	Interfere with patient's daily routine Patient may be late; needs reminders
Blood	
Reduced leukocytes Agranulocytosis	Increased susceptibility to infection Oral candidiasis may be present

- If the patient **decompensates**, such as hallucinates or exhibits bizarre behavior, during a dental or dental hygiene appointment, immediate referral is needed.
- Telephone numbers of the patient's mental healthcare provider should be kept in an easily accessible location for quick referrals.

C. Appointment Interventions

- Because schizophrenia is often a lifelong disorder, planning for future oral health is essential.
- Review medical and medication history; analyze drugs for possible side effects that require appointment modifications (Table 58-1).

- Consult with the mental health provider relative to medications, alcohol or other substance use, and medicolegal competence for informed consent.
- Negative symptoms are associated with poor oral health and a greater need for periodontal treatment.
- Plan a simple routine. For a series of appointments and maintenance, use a familiar, organized routine that is comfortable for the patient.
- Decrease stimulation; create a calm atmosphere; if background music is present, keep it low and soft.
- Management of the risk for caries, periodontal disease, and oral cancer includes the following:
    - Oral self-care instruction to improve biofilm removal on a daily basis.
    - When applicable, evaluate the patient's personal caregiver for attitude and knowledge and provide information and instruction.
    - Diet assessment and counseling to assist patient in making noncariogenic food choices. (See Chapter 33.)
    - Encourage use of xylitol-containing gum or mints when cariogenic snacks or beverages are consumed between meals.
    - Office and home fluorides. (See Chapter 34.)
    - Saliva substitutes may be helpful in patients with severe medication-induced xerostomia.
    - Tobacco cessation may be more difficult for people with schizophrenia because nicotine withdrawal may cause psychotic symptoms to worsen, so the dental professional must collaborate with the medical treatment team to closely monitor the patient.[60] (See Chapter 32.)
- Use a mouth prop to assist the patient with tardive dyskinesia. The patient who does not have control of mouth movements might appreciate the stability.

Mental Health Emergency

I. Psychiatric Emergency

- A psychiatric emergency in a dental clinic or private dental practice would be rare. The most common causes of emergency include a panic attack, atypical drug reaction, and schizophrenic or manic decompensation.

II. Patients at Risk for Emergencies

- Patient with a significant psychiatric history.
- Patient with a known substance abuse history.
- Patient new to the clinic or office; not known by the practitioners.

III. Prevention of Emergencies

- Prepare a complete medical history; collect as much information as possible; consult with the patient's primary care provider and psychiatrist.
- Be alert to risks and characteristic symptoms of each disorder.
- Apply all the principles of stress management.
- Know the patient's medications and when they are taken.
- Request the patient (or caregiver if accompanied) has medication readily available that may be effective during an emergency.
- Develop rapport with each patient; avoid confronting the patient and present a nonthreatening demeanor.

IV. Preparation for an Emergency

- Be mindful of surroundings, such as door access, objects in the room.
- Arrange for colleagues to be aware of the possible needs of a special patient appointment; when possible, plan for an assistant to participate in clinical procedures.
- Review characteristics of possible emergencies; have necessary equipment ready.
- Keep names and contact information of the patient's case manager, psychiatrist, and responsible family member in the record in a prominent position for ready reference.

V. Intervention

- Stay with the patient; request colleague contact patient's case manager, psychiatrist, or other responsible person.
- Maintain a calm, serene manner; talk quietly but firmly.
- Move the patient to a quiet, less stimulating environment. The dental equipment and environment may have contributed to the patient's disturbance.
- If you think the patient might be suicidal because the individual mentions wanting to die or kill themselves, try to remain calm and implement the five action steps of **#BeThe1To**[61]:
    1. **#BeThe1To** *ASK*: Directly ask the patient "Are you thinking about suicide?" Asking in a direct

manner can open the door for the individual to share their feelings.

2. **#BeThe1To** *KEEP THEM SAFE*: Showing support for someone can put time and distance between the person and their chosen suicide method.
3. **#BeThe1To** *BE THERE*: Being present shows support for the person at risk, this can be lifesaving.
4. **#BeThe1To** *HELP THEM CONNECT*: Call the Suicide Prevention Lifeline at 1-800-273-TALK (8255). Your call will be routed to a local call center and they will walk you through resources available to assist and if the patient is willing have them talk to a mental health professional.
5. **#BeThe1To** *FOLLOW-UP:* Following up to see how the individual is doing has been shown to reduce the number of suicide deaths.

- In some areas in the United States, you can dial 988 and be connected to the National Suicide Prevention Lifeline.
- In Canada, call 1-833-456-4566 or text 45645.[62]

Documentation

- The patient with a mental health disorder must complete a health history with details of the medical problem and medication history at the initial appointment.
- Follow-up with progress notes at each succeeding appointment to review all procedures and medications for changes.
- The following list suggests the minimum information to include in the permanent record:
  - Resources for assistance in a convenient place in the event of need to contact: telephone numbers, e-mail addresses and working addresses for physicians, psychiatrist, family, and emergency sources.
  - Progress notes for each appointment and other contacts to update all personal data and treatment.
  - Contacts and correspondence with specialists and others.
  - A sample progress note may be reviewed in **Box 58-1**.

Box 58-1 Example Documentation: Patient with a Mental Disorder

- **S**—Mary is a 23-year-old. Sporadic dental care mainly for emergency root canals and extractions. She presents for an examination and "cleaning" because her physician recommended she seek dental care for obvious decay.
- **O**—Medical history: She reports trouble sleeping and waking at 2 or 3 every morning and not being able to get back to sleep. Mary reports hallucinations of neon people walking down the hallway. She said when she was at work she experienced high levels of anxiety. Her psychiatrist has diagnosed Mary as suffering from panic attacks. She also reported a previous history of being hospitalized for schizophrenia. She has smoked one pack of cigarettes/day since she was 13 years old. Medications: risperidone (Risperdal). Dental examination: Caries noted MOD-#2, 14, 15, 18, 30; M & D #7–10 and #22–27. Leukoplakia noted in vestibule buccal to #28–29. Generalized pocket depths 4–5 mm with bleeding on probing, indicating generalized Stage II, Grade B periodontitis. Biofilm score: 95%. Generalized moderate supra- and subgingival calculus.
- **A**—Patient education to include oral self-care along with strategies to manage risk factors for caries and periodontal disease. Consult with primary care provider to coordinate tobacco cessation based on her history of schizophrenia. Disease control treatment phase to include restoration of carious lesions and NSPT.
- **P**—Disclosed biofilm and patient demonstrated oral self-care techniques. Mary seems to have good toothbrushing and flossing technique, but motivation seems to be her main problem. Suggested putting a sticky note on her bathroom mirror to remind her to perform oral self-care. Another suggestion was to make it a family affair and brush and floss with her children to be a role model to them. Mary was anxious at the beginning of the appointment, but seemed calmer toward the end. Nutrition counseling focused on reducing the frequency of sugar-sweetened snacks and beverages with recommendations to use xylitol gum or mints when she snacks between meals and cannot brush. She was given a prescription for 1.1% sodium fluoride paste to begin using at home. There was not adequate time to begin NSPT at today's appointment.

Next visit: Review oral self-care. Follow-up on diet and tobacco cessation. NSPT maxillary and mandibular right quadrants with two carpules, 2% lidocaine with 1:100,000 epinephrine for an inferior alveolar (IA), posterior superior alveolar (PSA), middle superior alveolar (MSA), and greater palatine (GP) injections.

Signed: ______________________________, RDH
Date: ________________

Factors to Teach the Patient

- The significance of daily oral self-care of the oral cavity.
- How medications cause dry mouth and how it increases the risk for caries.
- The importance of minimizing sweets such as cake, candy, and sugar-sweetened drinks to prevent dental caries.
- The use of saliva substitutes to make a dry mouth feel more comfortable.
- For the patient with bulimia or the binge-eating/purging type of anorexia:
  - The causes and effects of enamel erosion; the high acidity of the vomitus from the stomach.
  - The importance of rinsing after vomiting but not brushing immediately; demineralization begins promptly after the acid from the stomach reaches the teeth. Brushing can cause abrasion of the demineralizing enamel.
  - The need for multiple fluoride applications through office and home fluoride containing dentifrice, rinse, and brush-on gel, as well as professional application of varnish at regular dental hygiene appointments.

References

1. American Psychiatric Association. *Diagnostic and Statistical Manual of Mental Disorders: DSM-5*. Vol 5. American Psychiatric Association; 2013.
2. Special Olympics. Inclusive language for talking about people with intellectual disabilities. Published July 27, 2020. https://www.specialolympics.org/about/intellectual-disabilities/inclusive-language-for-talking-about-people-with-intellectual-disabilities. Accessed March 3, 2022.
3. Global Burden of Disease 2019 Mental Disorders Collaborators. Global, regional, and national burden of 12 mental disorders in 204 countries and territories, 1990–2019: a systematic analysis for the Global Burden of Disease Study 2019. *Lancet Psychiatry*. 2022;9(2):137-150.
4. Wu T, Jia X, Shi H, et al. Prevalence of mental health problems during the COVID-19 pandemic: a systematic review and meta-analysis. *J Affect Disord*. 2021;281:91-98.
5. Saragih ID, Tonapa SI, Saragih IS, et al. Global prevalence of mental health problems among healthcare workers during the Covid-19 pandemic: a systematic review and meta-analysis. *Int J Nurs Stud*. 2021;121:104002.
6. COVID-19 Mental Disorders Collaborators. Global prevalence and burden of depressive and anxiety disorders in 204 countries and territories in 2020 due to the COVID-19 pandemic. *Lancet*. 2021;398(10312):1700-1712.
7. Penninx BW, Pine DS, Holmes EA, Reif A. Anxiety disorders. *Lancet*. 2021;397(10277):914-927.
8. World Health Organization. *ICD-11 for Mortality and Morbidity Statistics*. Published February 2022. https://icd.who.int/browse11/l-m/en#/http%3a%2f%2fid.who.int%2ficd%2fentity%2f1336943699. Accessed March 3, 2022.
9. Greene T, El-Leithy S, Billings J, et al. Anticipating PTSD in severe COVID survivors: the case for screen-and-treat. *Eur J Psychotraumatol*. 2022;13(1):1959707.
10. Crook H, Raza S, Nowell J, Young M, Edison P. Long covid-mechanisms, risk factors, and management. *BMJ*. 2021; 374:n1648.
11. Shalev A, Liberzon I, Marmar C. Post-traumatic stress disorder. Longo DL, ed. *N Engl J Med*. 2017;376(25):2459-2469.
12. Campodonico C, Berry K, Haddock G, Varese F. Protective factors associated with post-traumatic outcomes in individuals with experiences of psychosis. *Fron Psychiatry*. 2021;12.
13. National Institute of Mental Health. Anxiety disorders. https://www.nimh.nih.gov/health/topics/anxiety-disorders. Accessed March 3, 2022.
14. National Institute of Mental Health. Post-traumatic stress disorder. Published May 2019. https://www.nimh.nih.gov/health/topics/post-traumatic-stress-disorder-ptsd. Accessed March 3, 2022.
15. Katzman MA, Bleau P, Blier P, Chokka P, Kjernisted K, Ameringen MV. Canadian clinical practice guidelines for the management of anxiety, posttraumatic stress and obsessive-compulsive disorders. *BMC Psychiatry*. 2014;14(Suppl 1):S1.
16. Andrews G, Bell C, Boyce P, et al. Royal Australian and New Zealand College of Psychiatrists clinical practice guidelines for the treatment of panic disorder, social anxiety disorder and generalised anxiety disorder. *Aust N Z J Psychiatry*. 2018;52(12):1109-1172.
17. American Psychiatric Association. Clinical practice guideline for the treatment of posttraumatic stress disorder (PTSD) in adults. Published 2017. https://www.apa.org/ptsd-guideline. Accessed March 3, 2022.
18. Kisely S, Sawyer E, Siskind D, Lalloo R. The oral health of people with anxiety and depressive disorders - a systematic review and meta-analysis. *J Affect Disord*. 2016;200:119-132.
19. Liu F, Wen YF, Zhou Y, Lei G, Guo QY, Dang YH. A meta-analysis of emotional disorders as possible risk factors for chronic periodontitis. *Medicine*. 2018;97(28):e11434.
20. Nochaiwong S, Ruengorn C, Thavorn K, et al. Global prevalence of mental health issues among the general population during the coronavirus disease-2019 pandemic: a systematic review and meta-analysis. *Sci Rep*. 2021;11(1):10173.
21. National Institute of Mental Health. Depression. https://www.nimh.nih.gov/health/topics/depression. Accessed March 3, 2022.
22. National Institute of Mental Healh. Perinatal depression. https://www.nimh.nih.gov/health/publications/perinatal-depression. Accessed March 5, 2022.
23. Bhat A, Nanda A, Murphy L, Ball AL, Fortney J, Katon J. A systematic review of screening for perinatal depression and anxiety in community-based settings. *Arch Womens Ment Health*. 2022;25(1):33-49.

24. Shorey S, Chee CYI, Ng ED, et al. Prevalence and incidence of postpartum depression among healthy mothers: a systematic review and meta-analysis. *J Psychiatr Res*. 2018;104:235-248.
25. Oyetunji A, Chandra P. Postpartum stress and infant outcome: a review of current literature. *Psychiatry Res*. 2020; 284:112769.
26. McCarron RM, Shapiro B, Rawles J, Luo J. Depression. *Ann Intern Med*. 2021;174(5):ITC65-ITC80.
27. American Psychological Association, Guideline Development Panel for the Treatment of Depressive Disorders. *APA Clinical Practice Guideline for the Treatment of Depression across Three Age Cohorts*. American Psychological Association; 2019.
28. Barbosa AC da S, Pinho RCM, Vasconcelos MMVB, Magalhães BG, Dos Santos MTBR, de França Caldas Júnior A. Association between symptoms of depression and oral health conditions. *Spec Care Dentist*. 2018;38(2):65-72.
29. Camilleri GM, Méjean C, Kesse-Guyot E, et al. The associations between emotional eating and consumption of energy-dense snack foods are modified by sex and depressive symptomatology. *J Nutr*. 2014;144(8):1264-1273.
30. Cademartori MG, Gastal MT, Nascimento GG, Demarco FF, Corrêa MB. Is depression associated with oral health outcomes in adults and elders? A systematic review and meta-analysis. *Clin Oral Investig*. 2018;22(8):2685-2702.
31. Grases G, Colom MA, Sanchis P, Grases F. Possible relation between consumption of different food groups and depression. *BMC Psychol*. 2019;7(1):14.
32. Featherstone JDB, Crystal YO, Alston P, et al. Evidence-based caries management for all ages-practical guidelines. *Fron Oral Health*. 2021;2:14.
33. Dattani S, Ritchie H, Roser M. Mental health. *Our World in Data*. Published August 20, 2021. https://ourworldindata.org/mental-health. Accessed March 5, 2022.
34. Miller JN, Black DW. Bipolar disorder and suicide: a review. *Curr Psychiatry Rep*. 2020;22(2):6.
35. Yatham LN, Kennedy SH, Parikh SV, et al. Canadian Network for Mood and Anxiety Treatments (CANMAT) and International Society for Bipolar Disorders (ISBD) 2018 guidelines for the management of patients with bipolar disorder. *Bipolar Disord*. 2018;20(2):97-170.
36. Wynn RL, Meiller TF, Crossley HL. Lithium. In: *Lexicomp for Dentistry Online*. 39th ed. Wolter Kluwer; 2022:1910.
37. Wynn RL, Meiller TF, Crossley HL. Risperidone. In: *Lexicomp for Dentistry Online*. 39th ed. Wolter Kluwer; 2022:1910.
38. Gurbuz Oflezer O, Altinbas K, Delice M, Oflezer C, Kurt E. Oral health among patients with bipolar disorder. *Oral Health Prev Dent*. 2018;16(6):509-516.
39. Udo T, Grilo CM. Prevalence and correlates of DSM-5 eating disorders in nationally representative sample of United States adults. *Biol Psychiatry*. 2018;84(5):345-354.
40. Lin JA, Woods ER, Bern EM. Common and emergent oral and gastrointestinal manifestations of eating disorders. *Gastroenterol Hepatol (N Y)*. 2021;17(4):157-167.
41. Allison S, Timmerman GM. Anatomy of a binge: food environment and characteristics of nonpurge binge episodes. *Eat Behav*. 2007;8(1):31-38.
42. Cainer A. Recognising and managing type 1 disordered eating in children and young people with diabetes. *Nurs Child Young People*. 2022;34(2):28-32.
43. Hall R, Keeble L, Sünram-Lea SI, To M. A review of risk factors associated with insulin omission for weight loss in type 1 diabetes. *Clin Child Psychol Psychiatry*. 2021;26(3):606-616.
44. Dunn TM, Bratman S. On orthorexia nervosa: a review of the literature and proposed diagnostic criteria. *Eat Behav*. 2016;21:11-17.
45. Puckett L, Grayeb D, Khatri V, Cass K, Mehler P. A comprehensive review of complications and new findings associated with anorexia nervosa. *J Clin Med*. 2021;10(12):2555.
46. Nitsch A, Dlugosz H, Gibson D, Mehler PS. Medical complications of bulimia nervosa. *Cleve Clin J Med*. 2021;88(6): 333-343.
47. Hilbert A, Hoek HW, Schmidt R. Evidence-based clinical guidelines for eating disorders: international comparison. *Curr Opin Psychiatry*. 2017;30(6):423-437.
48. Heafala A, Ball L, Rayner J, Mitchell LJ. What role do dietitians have in providing nutrition care for eating disorder treatment? An integrative review. *J Human Nutr Diet*. 2021;34(4):724-735.
49. Rangé H, Colon P, Godart N, Kapila Y, Bouchard P. Eating disorders through the periodontal lens. *Periodontol 2000*. 2021;87(1):17-31.
50. Hunt GE, Large MM, Cleary M, Lai HMX, Saunders JB. Prevalence of comorbid substance use in schizophrenia spectrum disorders in community and clinical settings, 1990-2017: systematic review and meta-analysis. *Drug Alcohol Depend*. 2018;191:234-258.
51. Coustals N, Martelli C, Brunet-Lecomte M, Petillion A, Romeo B, Benyamina A. Chronic smoking and cognition in patients with schizophrenia: a meta-analysis. *Schizophr Res*. 2020;222:113-121.
52. Bai W, Liu ZH, Jiang YY, et al. Worldwide prevalence of suicidal ideation and suicide plan among people with schizophrenia: a meta-analysis and systematic review of epidemiological surveys. *Transl Psychiatr*. 2021;11(1):552.
53. McCutcheon RA, Reis Marques T, Howes OD. Schizophrenia-an overview. *JAMA Psychiatry*. 2020;77(2):201-210.
54. Batinic B. Cognitive models of positive and negative symptoms of schizophrenia and implications for treatment. *Psychiatr Danub*. 2019;31(Suppl 2):181-184.
55. Keepers GA, Fochtmann LJ, Anzia JM, et al. The American Psychiatric Association practice guideline for the treatment of patients with schizophrenia. *AJP*. 2020;177(9):868-872.
56. Wynn RL, Meiller TF, Crossley HL. Thorazine (and Haldol). In: *Lexicomp for Dentistry Online*. 39th ed. Wolter Kluwer; 2022:1910.
57. Wynn RL, Meiller TF, Crossley HL. Clozapine. In: *Lexicomp for Dentistry Online*. 39th ed. Wolter Kluwer; 2022:1910.
58. Yang M, Chen P, He MX, et al. Poor oral health in patients with schizophrenia: a systematic review and meta-analysis. *Schizophr Res*. 2018;201:3-9.
59. Agarwal D, Kumar A, Manjunath BC, Kumar V, Sethi S. Oral health perception and plight of patients of schizophrenia. *Int J Dent Hyg*. 2021;19(1):121-126.
60. Sagud M, Mihaljevic Peles A, Pivac N. Smoking in schizophrenia: recent findings about an old problem. *Curr Opin Psychiatry*. 2019;32(5):402-408.
61. National Suicide Prevention Lifeline. How the 5 steps can help someone who is suicidal. #BeThe1To. https://www.bethe1to.com/bethe1to-steps-evidence/. Accessed March 6, 2022.
62. Canada Suicide Prevention Service, Crisis Services Canada. https://www.crisisservicescanada.ca/en/. Accessed March 6, 2022.

CHAPTER 59

The Patient with a Substance-Related Disorder

Danielle Collins, CDA, RDH, MS
Linda D. Boyd, RDH, RD, EdD

CHAPTER OUTLINE

LEARNING OBJECTIVES

After studying this chapter, the student will be able to:

1. Explain key terms and concepts related to the metabolism, intoxication effects, and use patterns of alcohol.
2. Identify physical health hazards, medical effects, and oral manifestations associated with alcohol and substances of abuse.
3. Interpret names of the most commonly abused drugs and describe their intoxication effects and methods of use.
4. Discuss modifications for the dental hygiene process of care for patients with substance use disorder. Recognize patients who are cognitively impaired and cannot provide informed consent and be treated in a safe manner.
5. Employ the National Institute on Drug Abuse Quick Screen to assess patients who are at risk for alcohol or substance abuse and provide resources for the patient to seek help.

Introduction

- Substance addiction is the abuse of drugs or alcohol consumed in large amounts over a period of time.
- When an individual consumes a substance such as drugs or alcohol, their brain produces large amounts of dopamine.[1]
  - Dopamine is a neurotransmitter that triggers the brain's reward system.
  - After repeated drug or alcohol use, the brain produces fewer dopamine receptors, reducing the ability to feel pleasure or reward and resulting in the individual increasing use of the substance, leading to an **addiction**.[1]
- The brain also produces endorphins, which is one of the body's natural opioids, to give a feeling of pleasure and **euphoria**.
  - When opioid drugs are taken, they use receptors normally accessed by endorphins to activate powerful reward centers in the brain.
  - Endorphins muffle perceptions of pain and boost feelings of pleasure, creating a temporary sense of well-being.[2]
- Substance use is an illness that can affect anyone. There is no classic cultural, socioeconomic, or educational profile for one who has a **substance abuse disorder (SUD)**.

Alcohol Consumption

I. Clinical Pattern of Alcohol Use

- Drinking in moderation for women is defined as no more than one drink on any single day and for men, it is defined as no more than two drinks on any single day.[3,4] **Figure 59-1** shows what constitutes a standard drink.
- **Binge drinking** occurs when an individual excessively drinks in a short period, typically four drinks for women and five drinks for men in about a 2-hour period, increasing **blood alcohol concentration (BAC)** levels to 0.08 g/dL.[4]
- The National Institute on Alcohol Abuse and Alcoholism (NIAAA) defines heavy drinking as more than 4 drinks in a day or 14 drinks or more per week for men and 3 drinks in a day or more than 7 drinks per week for women.[3]

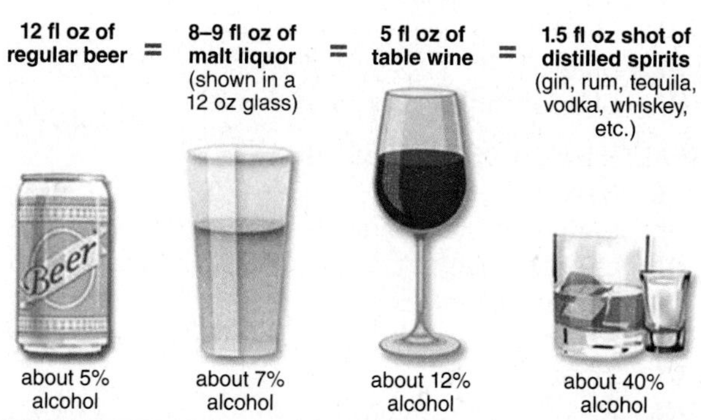

Figure 59-1 What Is a Standard Drink? In the United States, one "standard" drink contains roughly 14 g of pure alcohol, which is found in 12 ounces of regular beer, which is usually about 5% alcohol; 5 ounces of wine, which is typically about 12% alcohol; and 1.5 ounces of distilled spirits, which is about 40% alcohol.

Graphic was designed by Anthony Portillo, adapted from the National Institute on Alcohol Abuse and Alcoholism. (From National Institute on Alcohol Abuse and Alcoholism. https://www.niaaa.nih.gov/alcohol-health/overview-alcohol-consumption/what-standard-drink.)

    - SAMSHA (Substance Abuse and Mental Health Services Administration) defines heavy drinking as binge drinking 5 or more days in the past month.
- Underage drinking is considered excessive alcohol use.[4]
    - Those younger than 21 years who use alcohol are six times more likely to become alcohol dependent.
    - Young people drink less often than adults, but 90% of alcohol is consumed as part of binge drinking.[5]
- Underage drinking results in risk for[5,6]:
    - Impairment of brain growth and development.
    - Alcohol-related injury and death such as motor vehicle accidents, alcohol overdose, fall, etc.
    - Suicide.
    - Impairment of judgement leading to risky behaviors such as unsafe sexual behavior.
    - Physical and sexual assault.
    - Alcohol-induced mental impairment.
- **Alcohol use disorder (AUD)**, also known as alcoholism, is a pattern of alcohol use in which one has difficulty controlling their drinking with changes in the areas of the brain.[4,7,8]
    - AUD is considered a brain disorder and can vary in severity.
    - Only about 10% of those who use excessive alcohol meet the clinical definition for AUD.

A. Effects of Alcohol Overdose

- Alcohol overdose is also referred to as alcohol poisoning.
    - Alcohol poisoning occurs most often in middle-aged adults, and 76% who die are men.[9]
- The following are the effects of **alcohol overdose (intoxication)**[9]:
    - Behavioral changes: aggressiveness, mood instability, impaired judgment; impaired social or occupational functioning; impaired attention and memory; stupor or coma.
    - Physical characteristics: slurred speech, lack of coordination, slow heart rate, mental confusion, unsteady gait, and **nystagmus**.
    - Complications: irresponsible actions in work and family settings.
    - Accidents with resultant bruises, fractures, brain trauma, or death.
    - Vehicular accidents.

B. Symptoms of AUD

- AUD is diagnosed when an individual meets at least 2 of 11 DSM (Diagnostic and Statistical Manual for Mental Disorders) criteria.[8]
- Some overall symptoms of AUD include[7,8]:
    - Craving: a strong need or compulsion to drink.
    - Loss of control: the inability to limit one's drinking to a safe level despite the negative impact it may be having on one's responsibilities to work, school, or family/relationships.
    - **Physical dependence**: withdrawal symptoms, such as nausea, sweating, shakiness, and anxiousness, when alcohol use is stopped after a period of heavy drinking.
    - **Tolerance**: the need to drink greater amounts of alcohol to reach a level of desired intoxication. Other signs include **amnesia** and binge drinking.
    - Continuing to drink despite negative effects on personal relationships and work.

II. Etiology

A. Genetics

- Gene influence on alcohol metabolism impacts response to alcohol and constitutes up to 60% of the risk for developing AUD.[7,10]

B. Individual Characteristics

- The individual characteristics putting individual at risk for AUD include[10]:
    - Behavioral undercontrol such as impulsivity, sensation seeking, and disinhibition.
    - Antisocial behavior and conduct disorder.

C. Environmental

- Environmental factors may include[7,10]:
    - Cultural influences include societal beliefs about alcohol use.
    - Family environment, including parental or sibling use or abuse of alcohol.
    - Childhood trauma such as psychological or sexual abuse.

Metabolism of Alcohol

I. Ingestion and Absorption

- Upon intake, alcohol is absorbed promptly from the stomach and small intestine into the bloodstream.
- Transported to the liver for metabolism.[11]

II. Liver Metabolism

- Alcohol is converted into acetaldehyde by liver enzymes (e.g., dehydrogenase) to acetate, which circulates to the tissues where it is further metabolized to acetyl CoA much like other carbohydrates.[11]
  - Dehydrogenase in the liver is zinc and niacin dependent.[11]

III. Diffusion

- Rate of absorption depends on the alcohol concentration in the drink(s), presence of food in the stomach, gender, body weight, etc.[12]
  - On an empty stomach, blood alcohol levels peak in about 1 hour.
  - Depending on the amount consumed, normal functioning can be impaired the next morning.
- Alcohol is distributed throughout the body and all cells are exposed to the same concentration as what is found in the blood.
- About 2% to 5% is excreted directly through the lungs, skin, and kidney (breath, sweat, and urine).[12]
- A person's alcohol level can be determined by several tests of the blood, urine, saliva, or water vapor in the breath.

IV. Blood Alcohol Level (BAC)

- Alcohol-impaired driving accounted for 28% of the traffic-related fatalities in 2019 in the United States.[13,14]
- A driver is considered alcohol impaired when their BAC (blood alcohol concentration) is 0.08 g/dL or higher.[14]
- The characteristic effects exhibited at various levels of blood alcohol can be seen in **Figure 59-2**.

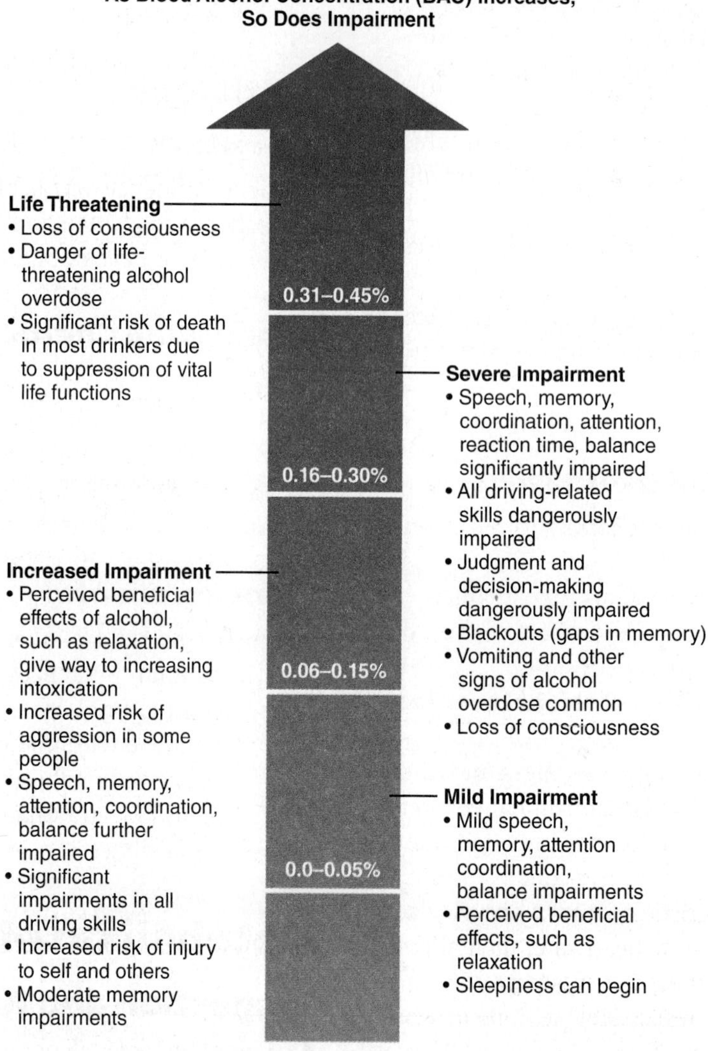

Figure 59-2 Blood Alcohol Concentration (BAC) Levels and Associated Impairment

National Institutes of Health. https://www.niaaa.nih.gov/publications/brochures-and-fact-sheets/understanding-dangers-of-alcohol-overdose

Health Hazards of Alcohol

- Prolonged alcohol use causes many serious medical disorders.
- Alcohol consumption has been identified as a cause for more than 200 diseases, health conditions, or injuries that can affect various organs or body systems. A great way to learn more about the effects on the body are to go to the www.collegedrinkingprevention.gov site where there is an Alcohol and You: An Interactive Body, where you can click on the various organs to learn the effects of alcohol.
- A few are mentioned here.

I. Nervous System

A. Central and Peripheral

- Alcohol interferes with the brain's communication pathways, slowing down the transfer of neurotransmitters.[15]
- While light alcohol use may be protective against cognitive impairment and dementia, in heavy alcohol use, the risk for cognitive impairment and dementia increases.[4,16]
- Prospective memory (remembering to do something in the future) is also negatively impacted by alcohol use.[17]
- Long-term alcohol abuse combined with malnutrition can lead to damage of both central and peripheral nervous systems.

B. Wernicke–Korsakoff's Syndrome

- Wernicke–Korsakoff's syndrome (WKS) is a degenerative brain disorder associated with vitamin B_1 (thiamine) deficiency.[18] It occurs in about 12% of those who abuse alcohol and in 2% of the general population.[19] WKS is two related disorders[18,19]:
  - *Wernicke encephalopathy* (WE) causes brain damage in lower parts of the brain (thalamus and hypothalamus), leading to symptoms of mental confusion, vision problems, and ataxia (lack of muscle coordination). It has been suggested WE is the acute state of WKS.
  - *Korsakoff's psychosis* results in permanent brain damage, including persistent knowledge and memory problems characterized by amnesia, tremor, vision problems, and disorientation. This is considered the chronic stage of WKS.

II. Cardiovascular System

- Drinking excessively for a long period will lead to damage to the heart such as cardiomyopathy, atrial fibrillation, stroke, and hypertension.[4,20]

III. Liver Disease

Chronic alcohol abuse is the most frequent cause of morbidity and mortality from liver diseases. Alcoholic liver disease (ALD) includes the following conditions[4]:

- Fatty liver: early stages are reversible with abstinence.
- Alcoholic hepatitis: inflammation of the liver.
- Early fibrosis: healthy cells replaced by scar tissue.
- Cirrhosis: scarring of the liver with irreversible damage.
- Individuals with hepatitis C virus (HCV) are more susceptible to ALD.

IV. Gastrointestinal System

- Individuals who abuse alcohol are at three times the risk for chronic pancreatitis when compared to light drinkers or those who do not drink.[21]
- Alcohol impairs the intestinal mucosa and causes an increase in permeability, also called leaky gut, which can cause maldigestion and nutrient malabsorption.
- Excessive alcohol intake also changes the gut microbiome to those types that are not protective of the gastrointestinal tract.[22]
- Alcohol also tends to replace the calories in food for an individual with AUD, which results in inadequate intake of nutritious food and subsequent nutrient deficiencies, such as in thiamine.[19,23]

V. Cancer

- Excessive alcohol use can increase the risk of developing certain cancers, including cancers of the[4]:
  - Head and neck (i.e., oral cavity, larynx, and pharyngeal cancer).
  - Esophagus.
  - Colorectal.
  - Liver.
  - Breast.

VI. Immunity

- Those who abuse alcohol have a diminished immune response and suppression of immune system defense.[22]

VII. Reproductive System

- Alcohol affects every branch of the endocrine system, directly and indirectly, through the body's organization of the endocrine hormones.[24]
  - Female: increased risk for menstrual disturbances and decreased fertility.[24]
  - Male: testicular cell damage, decreased testosterone, reduced sperm production, and impotence.[24]

Fetal Alcohol Spectrum Disorders (FASDs)

- FASDs are a group of conditions that can occur in an individual when alcohol is consumed during pregnancy.[25]
  - These conditions include issues with the individual's cognitive, physical, and/or behavioral functioning.[25]
- Prenatal alcohol exposure is the leading preventable cause of birth defects and neurodevelopmental conditions.[26]

I. Alcohol Use during Pregnancy

- Twenty to 30% of women report drinking at some point in their pregnancy, most frequently during the first trimester.[26]
- There is no safe amount of alcohol use during pregnancy. There is no safe form of alcohol during pregnancy; all forms of alcohol are harmful.[26]
- Complete abstinence during pregnancy is safest to prevent FASD.

A. Why Alcohol Is Dangerous during Pregnancy

- Alcohol passes freely across the placenta.
- Increased incidence of spontaneous abortions and stillbirths associated with alcohol consumption.
- Alcohol consumption any time during pregnancy can inhibit the fetus from growing properly (low birth weight) and negatively affect proper development of the brain or central nervous system (CNS).[25,26]
  - Consumption during the first 3 months of pregnancy can cause the infant to have facial dysmorphology,[26] as shown in **Figure 59-3**.
- An infant born with FASD will have many challenges to overcome and manage, including physical, social, psychological, and intellectual disabilities.[25,26]
- Common characteristics associated with FASD are listed in **Box 59-1**.

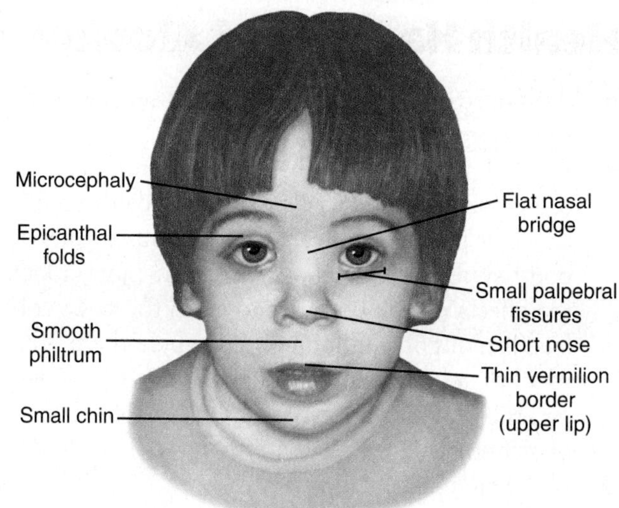

Figure 59-3 Facial Features of Fetal Alcohol Syndrome. Child presenting with the characteristic pattern of abnormal facial features diagnostic for fetal alcohol spectrum disorders, including short palpebral fissure lengths, smooth philtrum, and thin upper lip.

Reproduced from Porth CM. *Essentials of Pathophysiology: Concepts of Altered Health States.* 4th ed. Lippincott Williams & Wilkins; 2014.

Box 59-1 Characteristics and Comorbidities of an Individual with Fetal Alcohol Spectrum Disorder[25,26]

Growth	Low body weight Abnormal facial features, such as a smooth philtrum and thin upper lip Small head size Shorter-than-average height Dysmorphic features
Cognition	Intellectual disability Speech and language delays Poor reasoning and judgment skills Difficulty in school (especially with math) Developmental cognitive delays
Behavioral	Conduct disorders Impulsivity Attention deficit-hyperactivity disorder
Physical	Vision problems, including blindness Chronic otitis media and hearing loss Problems with the heart, kidneys, or bones Congenital malformations of the spine
Mental health	Increased risk for substance use disorders

Data from Popova S, Lange S, Shield K, et al. Comorbidity of fetal alcohol spectrum disorder: a systematic review and meta-analysis. *Lancet.* 2016;387(10022):978-987. doi:10.1016/S0140-6736(15)01345-8; National Institute on Alcohol Abuse and Alcoholism (NIAAA). Fetal Alcohol Exposure. Accessed November 14, 2021. https://www.niaaa.nih.gov/publications/brochures-and-fact-sheets/fetal-alcohol-exposure

Alcohol Withdrawal Syndrome

- **Withdrawal syndrome** consists of disturbances that occur after abrupt cessation of alcohol intake in the alcohol-dependent person.[27]
- Onset and severity of withdrawal symptoms vary.

I. Signs and Symptoms

- Mild symptoms can occur as soon as 6 hours after cessation of alcohol use and include[27]:
  - Insomnia, anxiety, headache, nausea/vomiting, elevated blood pressure, hyperflexia (e.g., twitching), and trembling.
- Moderate symptoms can occur in 12–24 hours and include[27]:
  - Seizures and **hallucinations**.
- Severe form of withdrawal is **delirium tremens**, which is fatal in 15% of cases without treatment. Symptoms include[27]:
  - Vital sign abnormalities, such as tachycardia (rapid heartbeat) and hypertension.
  - Hyperthermia.
  - Agitation.
  - Visual hallucinations.
  - Diaphoresis (sweating)

Treatment for AUD

I. Types of Treatment

There are different types of treatment for AUD.

- Behavioral treatments
  - Individual therapy to help the patient develop skills to stop drinking as well as coping skills to avoid relapse.
  - Marital and family counseling to help the patient build a strong social support system.
- Pharmacologic treatment
  - With moderate to severe AUD, naltrexone (ReVia), acamprosate (Campral), and disulfiram (**Antabuse**) can assist with abstinence.[28,29]
  - Alcohol cannot be used within 12 hours of taking disulfiram or unpleasant side effects result, including flushing, headache, and nausea. This reaction can occur up to 2 weeks after use of the medication.
- Pharmacologic treatments to manage alcohol withdrawal symptoms include benzodiazepines, anticonvulsants, baclofen, GHB (gamma-hydroxybutyric acid), or PAN (psychotropic analgesic nitrous oxide).[29]
- Mutual-support groups
  - Alcoholics Anonymous and other 12-step programs provide peer support for individuals who are trying to quit drinking or have quit and are trying not to relapse.

II. Treatment Settings

- There are both inpatient and outpatient treatment settings.
- Patients with AUD should start with their primary care provider for overall health assessment and assistance in determining the appropriate treatment option and resources.[20]

Abuse of Prescription and Street Drugs

- With the legalization of medical and recreational marijuana in many states and the US **opioid** epidemic,[30] every dental hygienist will encounter a patient with a **chemical dependence** issue and should be able to assess and provide safe patient care.
- Dental professionals need to screen for substance use in the clinical setting.[31]

Risk Management for Prescription Drugs of Abuse

- A major problem facing health care is the **diversion** of prescription medications with a high potential for abuse.
- Substances are classified in the U.S. **Drug Enforcement Administration drug schedule** according to use and abuse potential. In Canada, both Health Canada and the National Association of Pharmacy Regulatory Authorities (NAPRA) have roles related to drug scheduling.[32]

I. Prevention of Opioid Addiction in the Dental Office

- All members of the dental team should take responsibility to prevent opioid addiction.[2]
- Dentists should register with and utilize **prescription drug monitoring programs** (PDMPs) to promote the appropriate use of controlled substances. Prescription pads are not recommended for use to avoid alterations and abuse.

    - The PDMP is an electronic database that tracks controlled substance prescriptions in a state in the United States.[33] Canada has a similar provincial prescription monitoring program.[34]
    - These prescription monitoring programs provide health authorities timely information about prescribing and patient behaviors that contribute to the epidemic and facilitate a quick, targeted response.[33,34]
- Patients should be educated regarding their responsibilities for preventing misuse, abuse, storage, and disposal of prescription opioids.
- All members of the dental team should have continuing education about substance use to raise awareness and understand the clinical management of patients with substance use issues.[31,35]

Most Common Drugs of Abuse

- The most common drugs of abuse are alcohol and those found in the categories in this section. Examples of the substance names in each category and the commercial and street names are listed in **Table 59-1**.

I. Cannabinoids (Marijuana)

- Despite cannabis use being illegal at the federal level, as of November 2021, 36 states legalized marijuana for medical use and 18 states allow nonmedical or recreational use.[37]
- The three basic types of cannabis, used for recreational or medicinal purposes, are called marijuana/weed, hash, or hash oil.[38]

Table 59-1 Most Commonly Used Drugs[36]

Drug Classification	Drug Category	Street Name and Commercial Name	How Utilized	Health Risks
Cannabis	Cannabinoids (marijuana)	Blunt, Bud, Dope, Ganja, Grass, Green, Herb, Joint, Mary Jane, Pot, Reefer, Sinsemilla, Skunk, Smoke, Trees, Weed; Hashish: Boom, Gangster, Hash, Hemp	Smoked/ vaped, Edibles Pill form Topical	Short term: enhanced sensory perception and euphoria followed by drowsiness/relaxation; slowed reaction time; problems with balance and coordination; increased heart rate and appetite; problems with learning and memory; anxiety Long term: mental health problems, chronic cough, frequent respiratory infections
Central Nervous System Depressants	Barbiturates: pentobarbital	Barbs, Phennies, Red Birds, Reds, Tooies, Yellow Jackets, Yellows Nembutal	Pill Capsule Liquid	Drowsiness, slurred speech, poor concentration, confusion, dizziness, problems with movement and memory, lowered blood pressure, slowed breathing
	Benzodiazepines: alprazolam	Candy, Downers, Benzos, Tranks Xanax, Valium, Ativan, Rohypnol		
	Sleep medications	Forget-me-Pill, Tic-Tacs, Sleepeasy, Zombie flip Lunesta, Sonata, Ambien		
Hallucinogens and Dissociative Drugs	Ketamine	Cat Valium, K, Special K, Vitamin K Ketalar	Injected, snorted, smoked (powder added to tobacco or marijuana cigarettes), swallowed	Short term: problems with attention, learning, and memory; dream-like states, hallucinations; sedation; confusion; loss of memory; raised blood pressure; unconsciousness; dangerously slowed breathing Long term: ulcers and pain in the bladder; kidney problems; stomach pain; depression; poor memory.

Drug Classification	Drug Category	Street Name and Commercial Name	How Utilized	Health Risks
	LSD (lysergic acid diethylamide)	Acid, Blotter, Blue Heaven, Cubes, Microdot, Yellow Sunshine *No commercial uses	Swallowed, absorbed through mouth tissues (paper squares)	Short term: rapid emotional swings; distortion of a person's ability to recognize reality, think rationally, or communicate with others; raised blood pressure, heart rate, body temperature; dizziness; loss of appetite; tremors; enlarged pupils Long term: frightening flashbacks (called hallucinogen persisting perception disorder); ongoing visual disturbances, disorganized thinking, paranoia, and mood swings
	MDMA (Ecstasy/ Molly) 3,4-methylenedioxy-methamphetamine	Adam, Clarity, Eve, Lover's Speed, Peace, Uppers *No commercial uses	Swallowed, snorted	Lowered inhibition; enhanced sensory perception; increased heart rate and blood pressure; muscle tension; nausea; faintness; chills or sweating; sharp rise in body temperature leading to kidney failure or death.
Opioids	Fentanyl	Apache, China Girl, China Town, Dance Fever, Friend, Goodfellas, Great Bear, He-Man, Jackpot, King Ivory, Murder 8, and Tango & Cash	Injected, snorted/ sniffed, smoked, taken orally by pill or tablet, and spiked onto blotter paper	Relaxation, euphoria, pain relief, sedation, confusion, drowsiness, dizziness, nausea, vomiting, urinary retention, pupillary constriction, and respiratory depression
	Heroin	Brown Sugar, China White, Dope, H, Horse, Junk, Skag, Skunk, Smack, White Horse *No commercial uses	Injected, smoked, snorted	Short term: euphoria; dry mouth; itching; nausea; vomiting; analgesia; slowed breathing and heart rate Long term: collapsed veins; abscesses (swollen tissue with pus); infection of the lining and valves in the heart; constipation and stomach cramps; liver or kidney disease; pneumonia
	Prescription opioids	Captain Cody, Coties, Schoolboy, Vikes, Dones, Dillies, Demmies, Needle Candy, Fizzies, Monkey, Pers, Roxy, Codeine Duragesic Vicodin Dilaudid Demerol OxyContin, Percodan, Percocet	Injected, swallowed, snorted, suppositories	Short term: drowsiness, nausea, constipation, euphoria, slowed breathing Long term: risk of addiction and overdose

(*continues*)

Table 59-1 Most Commonly Used Drugs[36] *(continued)*

Drug Classification	Drug Category	Street Name and Commercial Name	How Utilized	Health Risks
Stimulants	Cocaine	Blow, Bump, C, Candy, Charlie, Coke, Crack, Flake, Rock, Snow, Toot Cocaine hydrochloride topical solution	Smoked, snorted, injected, inhaled	Short-term: hypersensitive to sensory input (sight, sound); agitated; dilated pupils; increased blood pressure, temperature, and heart rate; restlessness, irritability, anxiety, and paranoia Long-term: cardiovascular effects (heart attacks), neurologic (headaches, seizures, stoke) and gastrointestinal complications
	Methamphetamine	Crank, Chalk, Crystal, Fire, Glass, Go Fast, Ice, Meth, Speed Desoxyn	Swallowed, snorted, smoked, injected	Short term: increased wakefulness and physical activity; decreased appetite; increased breathing, heart rate, blood pressure, temperature; irregular heartbeat Long term: anxiety, confusion, insomnia, mood problems, violent behavior, paranoia, hallucinations, delusions, weight loss, severe dental problems (meth mouth), intense itching leading to skin sores from scratching.
	Synthetic cathinones "bath salts"	Bloom, Cloud Nine, Cosmic Blast, Flakka, Ivory Wave, Lunar Wave, Scarface, Vanilla Sky, White Lightning No commercial uses for ingested "bath salts"	Swallowed, snorted, injected	Short term: increased heart rate and blood pressure; euphoria; increased sociability and sex drive; paranoia, agitation, and hallucinations; violent behavior; sweating; nausea, vomiting; insomnia; irritability; dizziness; depression; panic attacks; reduced motor control; cloudy thinking Long term: death
Inhalants	Various household products (e.g., paint thinner, permanent markers, glue)	Poppers, snappers, whippets, laughing gas	Inhaled through the nose or mouth	Confusion; nausea; slurred speech; lack of coordination; euphoria; dizziness; drowsiness; light-headedness, hallucinations/ delusions; headaches; sudden sniffing death due to heart failure (from butane, propane, and other chemicals in aerosols); death from asphyxiation, suffocation, convulsions or seizures, coma, or choking

Data from National Institute on Drug Abuse. Commonly Used Drugs Charts. Published August 20, 2020. Accessed November 28, 2021. https://www.drugabuse.gov/drug-topics/commonly-used-drugs-charts

- All three types contain more than 100 cannabinoids found within the plant, with tetrahydrocannabinol (THC) and cannabidiol (CBD) being the two best known cannabinoids.[38]
  - THC is the primary psychoactive compound of the plant with effects on anxiety, pain, cognition, and perception of reality.[38]
  - CBD is nonpsychoactive, so patients do not feel "high" using cannabis with this strain.

A. Medical Marijuana Use

- Patients use medical marijuana for a number of purposes, including[39]:

- Management of chronic pain.
- Synthetic oral (THC) medications such as nabilone (Cesamet) and dronabinol (Marinol) are used to reduce nausea and vomiting symptoms related to chemotherapy treatment or acquired immunodeficiency syndrome (AIDS)-related conditions.
- Dronabinol (Marinol) has also been used as an appetite stimulant in human immunodeficiency virus (HIV)/AIDS to promote weight gain.

- Nabiximol oromucosal sprays (Sativex) containing THC can help reduce pain and muscle spasticity in patients suffering from multiple sclerosis, spinal cord injuries, fibromyalgia, or rheumatoid arthritis.
- Children and adolescents with drug-resistant epilepsy have experienced a decrease in seizure occurrences with CBD added into their therapy.[40]

B. Different Forms of Marijuana

- Inhaled[29,30]
  - Cigarette forms called *joints*.
  - Cigars hollowed out and filled with cannabis called *blunts*.
  - Can use a hookah pipe or bong, which filters the smoke through water.
  - Vaping—a fine mist is inhaled instead of smoking the cannabis.
  - Dabbing uses hash oil (most potent type) in a wax form.
- Oral
  - Edibles are when marijuana is added to foods or beverages.[41]
    - The high variability of absorption of edibles and delay in onset of effects can result in overconsumption with adverse effects such as intoxication and gastrointestinal symptoms.
    - A high rate of emergency room visits is associated with edibles.
  - Pill or capsule forms of marijuana (discussed in "Medical Marijuana Use" section).
  - Oral tinctures (liquid cannabis) or oromucosal sprays (also discussed in the "Medical Marijuana Use" section) are applied sublingually for a rapid response.[42]
- Individuals who utilize the inhalation forms of marijuana, similar to tobacco use, are associated with increased risk of cancer, lung damage, and oral health disease, such as oral cancers and periodontitis.[38]

II. Depressants

- A drug that suppresses the central nervous system to calm or sedate the patient.
- Depressants are taken to relieve anxiety, promote sleep, and manage seizure activity.
- Examples are *downers, sleeping pills, ludes, alcohol*.

III. Hallucinogens and Dissociative Drugs

- Chemical substances that produce mind-altering or mental perception-altering properties.
  - Examples include ketamine, LSD (lysergic acid diethylamide), and MDMA (*Molly*).
- These drugs act on the central nervous system, leading to the user seeing and hearing phenomena that do not exist.
- A disorder associated with the use of these substances is hallucinogen persisting perception disorder, commonly known as "flashbacks."

A. Dissociative Drugs

- Ketamine considered a novel psychoactive substance (NPS) and is a dissociative drug used as an anesthetic.[43,44]
- In the past few decades, ketamine has gained popularity as a club drug due to its euphoric qualities. Street names: angel dust, Special K.
- Psychotic adverse effects include vivid, visual, and auditory hallucinations.[43]

B. MDMA

- 3,4-methylenedioxymethamphetamine (*MDMA*) or *Ecstasy* or *Molly* is a popular drug among teens and young adults, widely used at nightclubs and bars (also used as a club drug).
- Molly, which is slang for *molecular*, refers to the pure crystalline powder form of Ecstasy.
- *MDMA* is classified as a stimulant, but is known for its hallucinogenic effects.

IV. Opioids and Morphine Derivatives

- In 2019, 1.6 million people had an opioid use disorder with over 70,000 people dying from a drug overdose.[30]
- Opioids are made from the Asian poppy or produced as synthetic drugs with the effects of opium; they result in analgesic and euphoric effects.

- Opioids are most commonly prescribed as analgesics, anesthetics, antidiarrheal agents, and cough suppressants.

A. Heroin

- Heroin is one of the most commonly abused drugs of this class; it can be injected, smoked, or snorted.
- Once in the bloodstream, it reaches the brain in 15–20 seconds.[45]
- Heroin use results in CNS effects, such as euphoria, analgesia, respiratory depression, and reduced gastrointestinal mobility.[45]

B. Prescription Opioids

- Although these opioids are prescribed legally for medical use to treat pain, use of these medications can lead to addiction and dependence, resulting in harmful consequences similar to illegal heroin use.
    - Between one-quarter and one-third of people who use prescription opioids for chronic pain misuse them, with about 10% developing an opioid use disorder.[30]
- Prescription opioid drugs include oxycodone (OxyContin, Percodan, Percocet), and hydrocodone (Vicodin).
    - Morphine (Avinza) is used to manage severe pain that requires around the clock and long-term pain management.
    - Vicodin (hydrocodone) is an analgesic and pain reliever.
    - OxyContin (oxycodone) is a narcotic pain reliever to treat moderate to severe pain.
    - Percodan (oxycodone/aspirin) is a nonsteroidal anti-inflammatory drug, narcotic, and analgesic used to treat moderate to severe pain.
    - Percocet (oxycodone/acetaminophen) is a pain reliever to treat moderate to severe pain.
    - Fentanyl is a synthetic opioid that is 80–100 times more potent than morphine and prescribed as transdermal or transmucosal patches or lozenges for use with severe pain in individuals resistant to other opioids.[46,47]
        - Duragesic is a fentanyl transdermal patch used to manage chronic pain by slowly releasing fentanyl through the skin into the bloodstream over 48–72 hours.[48]
        - Actiq dissolves quickly and is absorbed through the sublingual mucosa to provide rapid **analgesia**. This is especially beneficial for patients undergoing cancer treatment to treat pain that has a rapid onset with intensity.[49]
- Illegal fentanyl is primarily from China and trafficked through Mexico into the United States. However, India is emerging as a source of fentanyl as well.[46]
    - Even a few grains of fentanyl can be deadly and increasingly is a cause of overdose.[50,51]
    - Fentanyl is found as a contaminant in other illegal drugs like heroin.[51]
    - Fentanyl users do not fit the typical illicit drug user characteristic, since many were prescribed fentanyl following a surgical procedure or to treat chronic pain conditions and became addicted to opioids as a result.
- Naloxone (Narcan) is a nasal spray that counteracts the effects of opioids in overdose situations. It has no abuse potential and is used as a rescue drug for opioid overdose.
    - Narcan is available without a prescription with a request to the pharmacist in the United States and Canada.[52,53]
    - Many dental offices are adding it to their emergency kit and staff should seek training to administer it.[54]
        - Good Samaritan laws in a 40 states limit liability in administering Narcan to someone exhibiting overdose symptoms.[52]
    - Individuals or families with a family member battling an opioid addiction are encouraged to carry Narcan to counter an opioid overdose situation.
    - Withdrawal symptoms from Narcan occur within minutes after administration. Symptoms may include violence, headaches, changes in blood pressure, rapid heart rate, sweating, nausea, vomiting, and tremors. While this may be uncomfortable, it is usually not life threatening.
    - It is essential that emergency medical services (EMS) be activated when Narcan is administered as the individual will need medical assistance.

C. Codeine

- Codeine is an opioid medication used to treat mild to moderately severe pain. It can also be found in prescription cough syrup.
- Codeine is derived from the opium poppy plant (similar to morphine) and is one of the weaker opioids; however, it is still highly addictive with risk for overdose and death.
- Codeine in prescription cough syrup has emerged as a drug of abuse among young people and involves the mixing of codeine- and promethazine-containing cough syrup with soda

and hard candy. The mixture is called "Lean," along with a number of other names.

- *Lean* was initially a popular drink among blues musicians in Houston who mixed Robitussin with beer. Then, in the 1980s, Houston rappers opted to instead use codeine, soda, and a piece of hard candy (commonly a Jolly Rancher) for sweetness.[55]
    - Hip-hop music often incorporates *Lean* into the lyrics of songs with other names such as *sizurp*, *dirty Sprite*, and *purple drank*. Song lyrics also include use of *lean* with other drugs.[55]
    - *Lean* is responsible for the deaths of a number of hip-hop entertainers and is widely popular among young people around the globe.[55]
- *Lean* is so named because of the effect it has on people who drink it as they tend to slouch or lean to one side the more they consume of the substance.

- The effects of codeine are similar to those of other addictive opioids (such as oxycodone and heroin).
    - Effects begin within 30 to 45 minutes, though differing amounts of codeine in *Lean* can shorten onset time.
    - Peak effects begin 1 to 2 hours after ingestion and last about 4 to 6 hours.

V. Stimulants

- A class of drugs that enhances brain activity.
    - Stimulants cause an increase in mental alertness, attention, and energy; they improve motor skills and elicit a general sense of well-being.
    - They increase cardiac and respiratory function and speed up metabolism.
    - Stimulants include drugs such as cocaine, crack cocaine, amphetamine, and methamphetamine.
- Cocaine hydrochloride powder can be "snorted" through the nostrils or, when mixed with water, can be injected intravenously.[56]
    - Crack cocaine is a cocaine alkaloid in the form of a small rock.
    - Crack is cocaine that has been processed from cocaine hydrochloride to a free base for smoking. It is easily vaporized and inhaled and exhibits an extremely rapid onset of effects.
- Overdose deaths from cocaine use tripled from 2012 to 2018.[57]
- Prescription stimulants are used to treat attention deficit-hyperactivity disorder and narcolepsy. They increase alertness, focus, and energy.[58]
    - Common prescription stimulants are dextroamphetamine (Dexedrine), dextroamphetamine/amphetamine (Adderall), methylphenidate (Ritalin, Concerta).[58]
    - Slang terms for prescription stimulants include *Speed*, *Uppers*, and *Vitamin R.*
- Methamphetamine (meth, speed) is taken orally, intranasally (snorting the powder), by intravenous injection, or by smoking.
    - One of the most widely misused drugs; overdose deaths due to meth have increased nearly fivefold from 2012–2018.[57]
    - Ice, a very pure form of methamphetamine (seen as crystals under high magnification), produces an immediate and powerful stimulant effect when smoked.
    - Methamphetamines cause changes to the brain in areas related to emotion and memory and some of these changes may be long term, with a possible increased risk for Parkinson's disease.[59]

A. Synthetic Cathinones (Bath Salts)

- Synthetic cathinones are part of a group of drugs called NPSs.[43]
- Bath salts contain two man-made stimulants, mephedrone and methylone, which affect the brain much like MDMA (Ecstasy).
    - Bath salts are usually in the form of white or brown crystal-like powder which can be swallowed, snorted, smoked, or injected.[60]
- Bath salts' effects can include paranoia (unreasonable distrust of others), hallucinations, increased sex drive, panic attacks, or excited delirium (agitation to violent behavior).[60]
    - Adverse effects from toxicity can include cardiovascular (e.g., cardiac arrest, palpitations), neurologic (e.g., confusion, nausea, and seizures), psychotic, renal, and respiratory effects.[43]
- Synthetic cathinones: can be purchased online and in drug paraphernalia stores under a variety of brand names, which include Bliss, Cloud Nine, Lunar Wave, Vanilla Sky, or White Lightning.

VI. Inhalants

- Inhalants tend to be legal, everyday products such as paint thinners, gasoline, glue, spray paint, computer cleaning dusters, and felt tip markers.[61]
    - Nitrous oxide used in medical and dental settings also presents a risk for abuse.

- A breathable chemical vapor inhaled and absorbed through the lungs to produce psychoactive effects.[61]
- Causes relaxation of the smooth muscle and a decrease in oxygen-carrying capacity of the blood.
- A substance-soaked cloth (called huffing) or substance placed in a paper or plastic bag (called bagging) is applied to the nose and mouth and vapors are inhaled.[62]
- Adolescents are the primary users of inhalants, which can have a major adverse effect is on growth (weight and height).[61,62]
  - The effect on weight during this critical growth period can result in failure to thrive.[62]
- Capable of producing intoxication, abuse, dependence, and even death.
- Intoxication is characterized by mild euphoria and a change in the perception of time.

Medical Effects of Drug Abuse

I. Cardiovascular Effects

- Studies show illicit drug abuse has an adverse effect on the cardiovascular system.
- Intravenous drug use can lead to collapsed veins and bacterial infections of the arterial system and heart valves.[1]
- Cocaine in particular causes vasoconstriction in the coronary arteries, increasing blood pressure and risk of cardiomyopathy, coronary artery disease, arrhythmias, and myocardial infarction.[63]

II. Neurologic Effects

- All addictive drugs target the reward centers in the brain, allowing the user to experience euphoria.[1]
- Repeated drug abuse will alter the structure of the brain, making it more difficult for the user to reach euphoric levels; the user then requires increased levels of the drug, which increases the dependency.[64] These alterations in the brain can lead to[64]:
  - Increased negative mood, stress reactivity, and anxiety.
  - Decision-making or attention problems.
  - Lack of impulse control.
  - Increased sensation-seeking behavior.
  - decreased Cognitive functioning such as memory, reaction time, attention, and information processing.[65]
  - Co-occurring mental health issues, which include depression, suicidal ideation, anxiety, schizophrenia, and personality disorders.[66]
  - Chronic abuse of volatile solvents, such as toluene, damages the protective sheath around certain nerve fibers in the brain and peripheral nervous system. This extensive destruction of nerve fibers is clinically similar to that seen with neurologic diseases such as multiple sclerosis.[67]

III. Gastrointestinal Effects

- Cocaine in particular has been associated with abdominal pain, gastric ulcerations, perforations, and intestinal ischemia due to the extreme vasoconstriction of blood vessels.[68]
- Many drugs of abuse have been known to cause nausea and vomiting leading to appetite loss, malnourishment, and significant weight loss.[36]

IV. Kidney Damage

- Drugs can affect renal function either through the toxic effects of the drug or by a reduction in kidney function.
- Cocaine use has been associated with elevated blood pressure, which can lead to chronic kidney disease.[69]

V. Liver Damage

- The liver detoxifies drugs, chemicals, and alcohol that are ingested, placing it at risk for damage in substance use disorders.
  - Alcohol abuse effects include alcoholic hepatitis, fatty liver disease (steatosis), fibrosis, and cirrhosis.[70]
  - Cannabis is a risk factor for progressive liver fibrosis.[70]
  - Amphetamines like MDMA can induce hepatotoxicity.[70]
  - Cocaine use can range from mild liver abnormalities to severe liver failure.[70]
  - Opioid abuse has increased hepatitis B and C in intravenous drug users, resulting in liver damage.[71]
- Changes in liver function due to drug abuse decrease the metabolism of drugs and may result in toxic levels.

VI. Pulmonary Effects

- Drug abuse can lead to a variety of respiratory problems:
  - Smoking or vaping of cannabis has an increased risk for chronic bronchitis. However,

more research is needed to determine if there is a link between marijuana smoking and lung cancer.[65]
- THC is a cannabinoid found in marijuana and associated with an outbreak of EVALI (electronic-cigarette, or vaping, product use–associated lung injury) cases in 2019. The cause of EVALI was determined to be vitamin E acetate, which is used in the illicit market as an additive to THC oil.[72]
- Smoking crack cocaine can result in acute lung damage as well as subclinical hemorrhage.[73]
- Use of stimulants intravenously can result in a variety of effects including pulmonary granuloma and pulmonary hypertension.[73]

VII. Prenatal Effects

- Prenatal drug abuse has been associated with the following[74]:
  - Miscarriage.
  - Postpartum hemorrhage.
  - Premature birth.
  - Low birth weight.
  - Congenital anomalies.
  - Increase of behavioral and cognitive problems in the child.
  - Respiratory distress syndrome and/or increased respiratory infections, asthma, and ear infections.
- Opioid use during pregnancy can result in a condition in the infant called neonatal abstinence syndrome (NAS) or neonatal withdrawal syndrome.
  - The infant will experience symptoms within 1 to 4 days after birth due to sudden lack of exposure to the opioid of abuse.[75]
  - Symptoms will vary depending on the type of opioid the mother abused and may include irritability, tremors, feeding difficulties, diarrhea, excessive crying, and poor sleep. A small percentage of infants will have seizures.[75]
  - Infants at risk for NAS should be evaluated and monitored by medical providers.

VIII. Infections

- Infections and bloodborne diseases have been recognized as one of the most serious complications among drug users.[76]
- There are many reasons why drug users are at greater risk for infections, such as the following:
  - Engaging in risky behaviors due to impaired self-control, impulsivity, and poor judgment.[76]
  - Unsterile injection techniques, contaminated drug paraphernalia, and sharing of needles.[76]
  - Adulterants (or cutting agents) may be deliberately added to street drugs to enhance their effects, resulting in lower purity of the drug. This will also increase cutaneous abscesses in the drug users.
  - Unsafe sex practices and/or multiple sex partners.
  - Living conditions such as overcrowded housing or homeless shelters or in unsanitary environments such as living on the streets.
  - Malnourishment in conjunction with the effect of the drugs on the body leads to a weakened immune system.
  - Poor personal hygiene.
- The types of infections drug users are at risk for vary widely. The following are a few examples:
  - Infective endocarditis.[77]
  - Skin and soft tissue—abscesses, *Staphylococcus aureus*, and/or cellulitis located at injection sites.[76,77]
  - Central nervous system—abscesses.[77]
  - Bone and joint—septic arthritis and osteomyelitis (an extension of soft-tissue infection).[77]
  - Sexually transmitted infections (STIs)—chlamydia, gonorrhea, chancroid, syphilis, herpes simplex virus-2, human papillomavirus (HPV), HIV/AIDS, hepatitis B, and HCV.[76,78]

Treatment Methods

Chronic drug addiction causes changes in the brain involved in reward and motivation, learning and memory, and control over behavior.

- Drug addiction can be treated but it is complex. Successful treatment should include the following steps[79]:
  - **Detoxification**.
  - Drug rehab or treatment program (inpatient or outpatient).
  - Behavioral therapies.
  - Medication (for opioid, tobacco, or alcohol addiction).
  - Evaluation and treatment for co-occurring mental health issues such as depression and anxiety.
  - Long-term follow-up to prevent relapse.
- The principles that characterize the most effective drug abuse treatment can be found in **Box 59-2**.

Box 59-2 Principles of Drug Addiction Treatment

1. Addiction is a complex but treatable disease that affects brain function and behavior.
2. No single treatment is appropriate for everyone.
3. Treatment needs to be readily available.
4. Effective treatment attends to multiple needs of the individual, not just their drug abuse.
5. Remaining in treatment for an adequate period of time is critical.
6. Behavioral therapies—including individual, family, or group counseling—are the most commonly used forms of drug abuse treatment.
7. Medications are an important element of treatment for many patients, especially when combined with counseling and other behavioral therapies.
8. An individual's treatment and services plan must be assessed continually and modified as necessary to ensure that it meets their changing needs.
9. Many drug-addicted individuals also have other mental disorders.
10. Medically assisted detoxification is only the first stage of addiction treatment and by itself does little to change long-term drug abuse.
11. Treatment does not need to be voluntary to be effective.
12. Drug use during treatment must be monitored continuously, as lapses during treatment do occur.
13. Treatment programs should test patients for the presence of HIV/AIDS, hepatitis B and C, tuberculosis, and other infectious diseases as well as provide targeted risk-reduction counseling, linking patients to treatment if necessary.

National Institute on Drug Abuse. Principles of effective treatment. September 18, 2020. https://www.drugabuse.gov/publications/principles-drug-addiction-treatment-research-based-guide-third-edition/principles-effective-treatment. Accessed December 2, 2021.

I. Behavioral Therapies

- Behavioral therapies help patients modify their attitudes and behaviors toward drug use and encourage healthier life choices.
- Behavioral therapy sessions can be provided in an outpatient or inpatient setting. Inpatient settings are more structured and supervised. Behavioral therapies may also be combined based on individual needs. The following are examples of behavioral therapies[79-81]:
  - Motivational interviewing involves a structured approach to guiding the patient towards abstinence.
  - Cognitive-behavioral therapy (CBT) takes many forms, but involves a cognitive component to identify ways of thinking about substance use along with a behavioral component to develop skills to avoid substance use.
  - Family behavioral therapies may use one of five models that involve the family and support system to encourage healthy behaviors.
  - Contingency management uses positive reinforcement to meet goals.
  - Psychoeducation involves education about the harm of substance use.
  - Peer group therapy provides a supervised setting for interaction with peers to form social support.
  - Intensive case management for SUD co-occurring with another mental health disorder.

II. Pharmacologic Interventions

- Medications help suppress withdrawal symptoms during the detoxification process and prevent relapse. Each type of substance has different pharmacologic therapies and they are used in combination with behavioral therapies.

A. Methamphetamine Dependence Pharmacologic Treatment

- Pharmacologic treatments with the most positive outcomes include[82]:
  - Stimulant agonist treatment, such as dexamphetamine and methylphenidate.
  - Opioid agonists, such as naltrexone.
  - Anticonvulsants (i.e., Topiramate).
- Other treatments such as antidepressants (bupropion) may be used, although they appear less effective in some research.[82]

B. Opioid Use Disorder Pharmacologic Treatment

- Methadone (Dolophine, Methadose)
  - Methadone is a full opioid agonist, meaning it activates opioid receptors in the brain to reduce withdrawal symptoms without producing euphoria.[80,83]
  - Methadone is not a first-line choice in the Canadian guidelines for opioid use disorder because of its addiction potential.[84]
- Buprenorphine (Subutex), buprenorphine/naloxone (Suboxone)

- A partial opioid agonist meaning it is an opioid that can activate and block opioid receptors in the brain to reduce or eliminate withdrawal symptoms without producing euphoria.[80,83]
- Often used for maintenance to prevent relapse.[83]
- Buprenorphine/naloxone is the first-line choice for treatment of opioid use disorder in Canada.[84]

- Naltrexone (Vivitrol/ReVia)
  - This medication is not an opioid; it is an **opioid antagonist**, blocking the brain's opioid receptors preventing the user from reaching the euphoric phase.
  - It is used for those no longer dependent on opioids for preventing relapse.[83]

Dental Hygiene Process of Care

- Every patient appreciates an atmosphere with nonjudgmental, open communication, but this is especially important in caring for patients with SUDs. The patient needs to understand that safe care depends on the clinician knowing the substances in the patient's system.

I. Assessment

A. Patient History

- The medical health history questionnaire should inquire about substances used, how patient administers the substance (i.e., intravenously, smoked), quantity, and time of the last dosage.[54]
- Identify all current medications (both prescription and substances) in order to investigate drug–drug interactions with any medications that may be used in the oral health setting such as local anesthesia. (See Chapter 11.)
- A medical consult with the patient's physician and/or addiction specialist should be conducted prior to any dental care to determine the patient's readiness for treatment.[54]
- Conduct the medical health history examination utilizing a motivational interviewing approach to establish a nonjudgmental environment and encourage open communication. (See Chapter 24.)

B. Screening for Substance Use

- As healthcare professionals, it is our responsibility to screen patients for possible SUDs and work collaboratively with the interprofessional team to refer and support patients in their treatment and recovery.[54]
- The National Institute of Drug Abuse website (www.drugabuse.gov/) provides a list of screening tools for health professionals to assess a patient's drug use, along with interactive platforms to enter patient responses. The results then identify the level of risk and provide guidance for the clinician on next steps.
- Tools for screening for substance use in adolescents include:
  - The Screening to Brief Intervention (S2BI) asks about frequency of use for tobacco, alcohol, and marijuana, which are commonly used by adolescents.[85]
  - Brief Screener for Tobacco, Alcohol, and other Drugs (BSTAD) is also used with adolescents and assesses the same three substances as the S2BI; depending on responses, questions will be generated to gather information about additional substance use.[85]
- Tools for screening adults for substance use include:
  - TAPS (Tobacco, Alcohol, Prescription medication, and other Substance use) Tool, which has two components. The first component screens for tobacco, alcohol, illicit drugs, and prescription drugs. For someone who screens positive on the first part, a second part will determine the risk level for each substance the individual uses.[85]

C. Vital Signs

- All vital signs are likely to show changes from normal with substance use. The following are samples[36]:
  - Blood pressure frequently is increased with alcohol, stimulants, and cannabis; fluctuations can be particularly significant.
  - Irregularity and increases in heart rate occur with drugs like methamphetamine and cannabis. However, heart rate may decrease with use of other substances like opioids.
  - Breathing rate may change, such as slowed breathing with opioid use.
  - Body temperature may also be outside the normal range, such as increases seen with use of methamphetamines.

D. Clinical Examination

- Information in the patient history may not reveal the extent of a patient's drug use.

- Clinical observations along with the medical history may provide a high degree of suspicion.
- Observations to note during the interview could include:
    - Inability to focus or recall simple concepts like phone number or address.
    - May exhibit rapid mood swings or display paranoia or disorientation.
    - May start to complain about dental pain, requesting a prescription for specific pain medications.
- Depression, suicidal/homicidal thoughts, or agitation could indicate a drug overdose and requires immediate emergency care.

E. Extraoral Examination

- Skin changes/lesions may include jaundice, urticaria, **pruritus**, cutaneous fibrosis, granulomas, flushing to name a few.[86]
- Personal appearance
    - Does the patient look much older than their age stated on their health history form?
    - Lack of interest in proper dress and personal hygiene.
    - Wears long sleeves to cover needle marks.
    - Dramatic weight loss and/or emaciated appearance.
- Head and neck
    - Patients smoking or vaping substances are at greater risk for cancers in the head and neck region.
- Eyes. (See **Figure 59-4**)
    - Wears sunglasses to conceal dilated or constricted pupils and eye redness, or to avoid bright light because of eye sensitivity.
    - Pupils dilated (e.g., LSD, cocaine, methamphetamine, benzodiazepines) (Figure 59-4).[36,87]
    - Pupils constricted (heroin, morphine).[87]
- Nose
    - Inhaled or snorted substances can damage nasal structures, causing frequent nosebleeds, or patients may constantly be sniffing or wiping their noses.
    - Nasal septum perforation (cocaine snorting).
- Arms
    - The most common site for drug injection is the antecubital fossa along with the forearm, so be alert for needle marks when assessing vital signs.[86]
    - Injection of illicit drugs can cause subcutaneous abscesses called "popping" that result in scarring.[86]

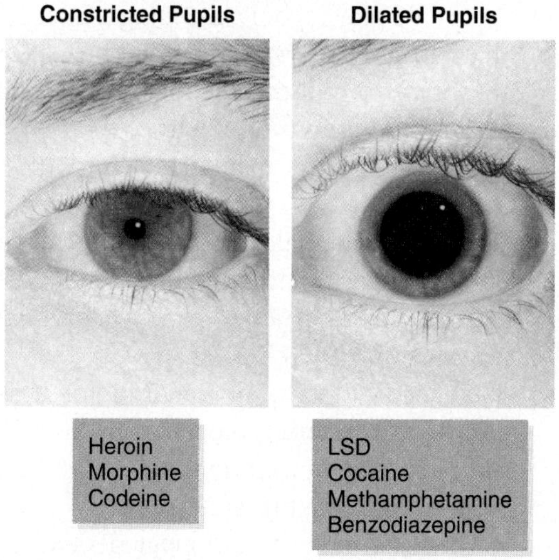

Figure 59-4 Drug Effects on the Pupils. Pupil on left: pinpoint or constricted; occurs in the use of morphine, opioids, and heroin. Pupil on the right: dilated; in the use of hallucinogens, cocaine, methamphetamines, and amphetamines.

- Behavior
    - Sneezing, itching.
    - Tendency to gaze into space; moodiness.
    - Drowsiness, yawning; may sleep long hours.
    - Nodding.
    - Appearance of intoxication or lethargic with or without the odor of alcohol.
    - Slurred speech.
    - Changes in habits, such as irregular attendance at appointments by one who was previously prompt.
    - Hallucinations or convulsions indicate need for immediate emergency care.

II. Intraoral Examination

Specific oral manifestations are associated with particular drugs. Examples can be found in **Box 59-3**.

- Mucosa, lips, tongue[86]
    - Glossitis related to nutritional deficiencies.
    - Angular cheilitis.
    - Burns and sores on lips from smoking crack or meth.
    - Underside of tongue is one of the earliest places jaundice may appear.
- Salivary glands
    - Parotid gland swelling.[86]
    - Xerostomia.[54,86,88]
- Biofilm: poor oral hygiene and heavy biofilm accumulations.[38,89]

Box 59-3 Oral Manifestations of Commonly Abused Substances

a. "Meth mouth"
   - Meth smoker swirls heated, vaporized substances in the mouth.
   - Rampant caries resembling early childhood caries with distinctive pattern of caries on the buccal and lingual cervical smooth tooth surfaces.[90]
   - Severe xerostomia.[88]
   - Bruxism, cracked teeth, excessive wear, tooth sensitivity, and trismus.[90]
   - Periodontal disease.[89,90]
   - Poor oral hygiene.[90]
   - Tooth loss.[88,90]

b. Cocaine abuse
   - Cocaine snorting is associated with perforation of the nasal septum and/or perforation of the palate to form an orofacial defect.[88,91]
   - Facial midline destructive lesions, such as **saddlenose deformity**.[91]
   - Dental attrition from bruxism.[88,91]
   - Xerostomia.[91]
   - Erosive carious lesions from low pH level of cocaine powder.[88]
   - Oral administration may result in gingival lesions and recession due to tissue necrosis.[54,91]
   - Aguesia (loss of taste).[91]

c. Lysergic acid diethylamide and "Ecstasy," hallucinogenic drugs[92]
   - Xerostomia.
   - Temporomandibular joint tenderness.
   - Bruxism leading to tooth wear.
   - Rampant dental caries much like that seen in "meth mouth."
   - Lichenoid and hypertropic lesions.
   - Dentin hypersensitivity.
   - Topical use of Ecstasy may result in tissue necrosis and mucosal fenestration.
   - Poor oral hygiene and bleeding on probing.

d. Cannabis users
   - Xerostomia.[38]
   - Increased risk for periodontal disease.[93]
   - Leukoedema.[38]
   - Stomatitis.[38]

- Gingiva
  - Moderate to severe gingival inflammation.[86]
  - Gingival enlargement.[54]
  - Higher incidence of periodontal disease, particularly severe periodontitis.[88,89]
- Palate
  - Oronasal defect (perforation) in palate due to chronic cocaine snorting.[88]

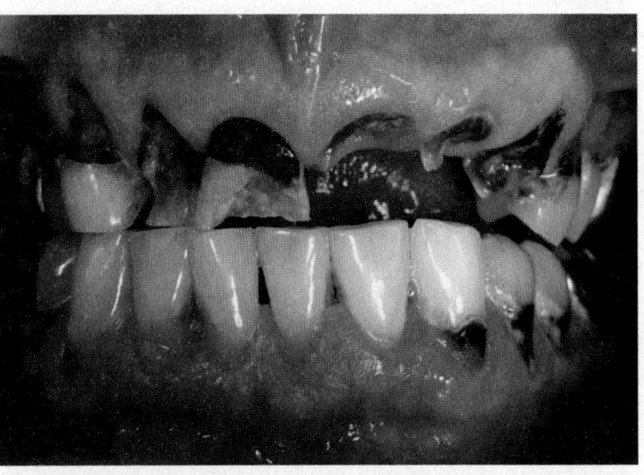

Figure 59-5 Rampant Dental Caries Due to Methamphetamine

- Teeth
  - Attrition secondary to bruxism, especially among cocaine and meth users.[54,86,88,89]
  - Erosion from oral application of substances like cocaine.[88]
  - Dental caries
    - Diet high in cariogenic substances such as sweets and sugar-sweetened beverages.[88]
    - Characteristic "meth mouth" pattern of dental caries on buccal surfaces with fewer restorations suggesting lack of access to regular dental care (**Figure 59-5**).[54,86,88]
    - Tooth loss.[88,89]
- Oral pathologies
  - Leukoplakia and stomatitis (referred as cannabis stomatitis).[38,54,86]
  - Higher incidence of *Candida albicans* infection.[38]
- Temporomandibular joint (TMJ): trismus.[86]

III. Dental Hygiene Diagnosis

- Once the patient is in recovery, careful risk assessment and identification of modifiable risk factors will be essential to manage oral disease.

IV. Care Planning

- For modifiable risk factors, preventive services must be planned to meet the individual needs of the patient.
- Care must be taken to avoid recommending oral health care products with alcohol for those in recovery.
- Preventive services:
  - Oral self-care education. (See Chapter 26, Chapter 27, and Chapter 28.)

- Dietary counseling to aid the patient in making healthy choices and need to stay hydrated to help manage xerostomia. (See Chapter 33.)
- Fluoride will be necessary to mitigate the caries risk. The type and frequency of fluoride will be dependent on caries risk level.[94] (See Chapter 25 and Chapter 34.)
- Chlorhexidine may also be part of management of caries risk.[94,95] (See Chapter 25.)
- Silver diamine fluoride may be helpful in arresting dental caries in those with rampant caries.[95,96]

- Nonsurgical periodontal therapy as required by the periodontal examination.
- Referral for more advanced periodontal disease may be necessary.
- Short appointments may be needed for anxious patients.

V. Implementation

- If the patient is cognitively impaired by a substance, legally the patient cannot provide informed consent to care and cannot be treated.
- The patient should understand the importance of informing the clinician of any substances in their system that could potentially have a negative interaction with local anesthesia (e.g., epinephrine) or other therapeutics the clinician may provide to the patient.[95]
- Anesthesia and pain control may be more difficult to achieve because many substance abusers build up tolerance to various pain reducing effects.
- The dental hygienist should implement good stress reduction protocols for patients who are experiencing anxiety.

A. Preparation for Treatment

- Caution is needed for potential drug–drug interactions.
- When choosing preprocedural rinses, avoid those containing alcohol for patients with a past history or current alcohol use problem.
  - The smallest amount of alcohol ingested by a patient being treated with disulfiram can cause an emergency.
  - Additionally, any patient suffering from xerostomia should avoid any product containing alcohol.

B. Periodontal Debridement

- Use of local anesthesia: use of epinephrine should have been approved during the consultation with the patient's primary care provider prior to treatment.
  - Contraindications for the use of nitrous oxide/oxygen and medical considerations for local anesthesia with or without epinephrine are provided in Chapter 36.
- Careful periodontal debridement to reduce the bacterial load and support healing is essential.

C. Response to Therapy

- The usual oral tissue response expected following periodontal instrumentation may be limited by the following:
  - Prolonged bleeding time; impaired clotting mechanism from chronic liver disease.
  - Inability to obtain profound anesthesia limiting thorough periodontal debridement.
  - Impaired healing.
  - Interference with collagen formation and deposition.
  - Decreased immune system function.
  - Increased susceptibility to postoperative infection.

VI. Evaluation

- The evaluation of dental hygiene care occurs 6–8 weeks after initial debridement.
- Evaluate treatment plans and goals with the patient.
- Make changes according to the patient's progress.
- Evaluate to determine the frequency of continuing care appointments; typically set at 3 months but should depend on many factors such as tissue response and patient's level of motivation.

Documentation

- In patient record document possible substance abuse to alert dental personnel to:
  - Use a mouthrinse without alcohol.
  - Any alerts or contraindications for treatment (e.g., epinephrine in local anesthetic).
  - Inappropriate behavior during appointments, such as aggressive or belligerent behavior.
- Document early oral signs/symptoms of substance abuse such as:
  - Oral examination: ulcerations, infections, and xerostomia.
  - Dental examination: dental caries in unusual sites or more extensive than previously documented.

- Periodontal examination: unexplained rapid changes in periodontal status.
- Patient education: relapse of previously good oral hygiene.
- Psychological reactions and/or aggressive behavior.

- Example documentation for a patient with substance abuse is found in **Box 59-4**.

Box 59-4 Example Documentation: Patient with Substance Abuse

- **S**—A 65-year-old male patient presents for nonsurgical periodontal therapy with local anesthesia appointment. Patient admitted to daily marijuana use to control his arthritic pain, and drinks four to five beers most nights to relax.
- **O**—BP 205/110 mmHg, pulse 89 bpm, and patient stated he has not seen his primary care provider in years.
- **A**—Possible hypertension. The quick results of the TAPS (Tobacco, Alcohol, Prescription medication, and other Substance use) reveals Mr. Keile is an at-risk drinker. The patient is also at risk for illegal drug use with marijuana use that is not prescribed by his medical provider.
- **P**—Referred patient for medical consult to discuss possible hypertension and substance use disorder. Patient became upset upon finding out that no treatment could be initiated today with the patient's blood pressure significantly elevated. Patient stormed out of the operatory and building before the medical consultation referral could be completed or any follow-up appointments could be scheduled.

Signed: ______________________________, RDH
Date: __________________

Factors to Teach the Patient

- Explain how the substance use has affected the patient's oral and general health. Discuss in a positive manner what the patient can do to improve their oral and general health.
- Emphasize the importance of regular dental and dental hygiene care. Also, point out their important role in daily biofilm removal at home.
- Encourage the patient to maintain a healthy diet. Proper nutrition will be crucial to their healing process. Discuss ways to modify diet to reduce caries risk such as replacing some or all sugar-sweetened beverages with water, use of xylitol-containing mints or gum, and rinsing with water after a snack or sugar-sweetened beverage if brushing is not possible.
- Explain the value of using fluoride and chlorhexidine as prescribed for caries prevention.
- Illicit drug use during pregnancy can pose serious risks for unborn babies.

References

1. National Institute on Drug Abuse. *Drugs, Brains, and Behavior: The Science of Addiction*; 2021:32. https://www.drugabuse.gov/publications/drugs-brains-behavior-science-addiction/preface. Accessed November 11, 2021.
2. Wang S. Historical review: opiate addiction and opioid receptors. *Cell Transplant*. 2019;28(3):233-238.
3. National Institute on Alcohol Abuse and Alcoholism (NIAAA). Drinking levels defined. https://www.niaaa.nih.gov/alcohol-health/overview-alcohol-consumption/moderate-binge-drinking. Accessed November 11, 2021.
4. Centers for Disease Control and Prevention. Alcohol and public health: drinking patterns. Published February 16, 2021. https://www.cdc.gov/alcohol/faqs.htm. Accessed November 11, 2021.
5. National Institute on Alcohol Abuse and Alcoholism (NIAAA). Underage drinking. Published May 2021. https://www.niaaa.nih.gov/publications/brochures-and-fact-sheets/underage-drinking. Accessed November 14, 2021.
6. Sullivan EV, Brumback T, Tapert SF, et al. Disturbed cerebellar growth trajectories in adolescents who initiate alcohol drinking. *Biol Psychiatry*. 2020;87(7):632-644.
7. National Institute on Alcohol Abuse and Alcoholism (NIAAA). Understanding alcohol use disorder. Published April 2021. https://www.niaaa.nih.gov/publications/brochures-and-fact-sheets/understanding-alcohol-use-disorder. Accessed November 11, 2021.
8. Witkiewitz K, Litten RZ, Leggio. Advances in the science and treatment of alcohol use disorder. *Sci Adv*. 2019;5(9):eaax4043.
9. National Institute on Alcohol Abuse and Alcoholism (NIAAA). Understanding the dangers of alcohol overdose. https://www.niaaa.nih.gov/publications/brochures-and-fact-sheets/understanding-dangers-of-alcohol-overdose. Accessed November 14, 2021.
10. Wall TL, Luczak SE, Hiller-Sturmhöfel S. Biology, genetics, and environment: underlying factors influencing alcohol metabolism. *Alcohol Res Curr Rev*. 2016;38(1):59-68.

11. Cederbaum AI. Alcohol metabolism. *Clin Liver Dis.* 2012;16(4):667-685.
12. Paton A. Alcohol in the body. *BMJ*. 2005;330(7482):85-87.
13. National Institute on Alcohol Abuse and Alcoholism (NIAAA). Alcohol facts and statistics. Published June 2021. https://www.niaaa.nih.gov/publications/brochures-and-fact-sheets/alcohol-facts-and-statistics. Accessed November 14, 2021.
14. National Highway Traffic Safety Administration. Drunk driving. https://www.nhtsa.gov/risky-driving/drunk-driving. Accessed November 14, 2021.
15. National Institute on Alcohol Abuse and Alcoholism (NIAAA). Alcohol's effects on the body. https://www.niaaa.nih.gov/alcohols-effects-health/alcohols-effects-body. Accessed November 14, 2021.
16. Rehm J, Hasan OSM, Black SE, Shield KD, Schwarzinger M. Alcohol use and dementia: a systematic scoping review. *Alzheimers Res Ther*. 2019;11(1):1.
17. Kyriacou A, Smith-Spark JH, Senar J, Moss AC, Dyer KR. The effects of alcohol use on prospective memory: a systematic literature review. *Subst Use Misuse*. 2021;56(3):359-369.
18. National Institute of Neurological Disorders and Stroke. Wernicke-Korsakoff syndrome. Published March 27, 2019. https://www.ninds.nih.gov/Disorders/All-Disorders/Wernicke-Korsakoff-Syndrome-Information-Page. Accessed November 14, 2021.
19. Isenberg-Grzeda E, Kutner HE, Nicolson SE. Wernicke-Korsakoff-Syndrome: under-recognized and under-treated. *Psychosomatics*. 2012;53(6):507-516.
20. O'Keefe EL, DiNicolantonio JJ, O'Keefe JH, Lavie CJ. Alcohol and CV health: Jekyll and Hyde J-curves. *Prog Cardiovasc Dis*. 2018;61(1):68-75.
21. Singh VK, Yadav D, Garg PK. Diagnosis and management of chronic pancreatitis: a review. *JAMA*. 2019; 322(24):2422-2434.
22. Kany S, Janicova A, Relja B. Innate immunity and alcohol. *J Clin Med*. 2019;8(11):E1981.
23. Wang SC, Chen YC, Chen SJ, Lee CH, Cheng CM. Alcohol addiction, gut microbiota, and alcoholism treatment: a review. *Int J Mol Sci*. 2020;21(17):E6413.
24. Rachdaoui N, Sarkar DK. Pathophysiology of the effects of alcohol abuse on the endocrine system. *Alcohol Res Curr Rev*. 2017;38(2):255-276.
25. Popova S, Lange S, Shield K, et al. Comorbidity of fetal alcohol spectrum disorder: a systematic review and meta-analysis. *Lancet*. 2016;387(10022):978-987.
26. National Institute on Alcohol Abuse and Alcoholism (NIAAA). Fetal alcohol exposure. https://www.niaaa.nih.gov/publications/brochures-and-fact-sheets/fetal-alcohol-exposure. Accessed November 14, 2021.
27. Newman RK, Stobart Gallagher MA, Gomez AE. Alcohol withdrawal. *StatPearls*. Updated August 29, 2022. http://www.ncbi.nlm.nih.gov/books/NBK441882/. Accessed December 5, 2022.
28. American Psychiatric Association. Guideline Summary Statement. In: *The American Psychiatric Association Practice Guideline for the Pharmacological Treatment of Patients With Alcohol Use Disorder*. *Practice Guidelines*. American Psychiatric Association Publishing; 2018:226.
29. Amato L, Minozzi S, Davoli M. Efficacy and safety of pharmacological interventions for the treatment of the Alcohol Withdrawal Syndrome. *Cochrane Database Syst Rev*. 2011;(6):CD008537.
30. US Department of Health and Humans Services. What is the U.S. opioid epidemic? Published October 27, 2021. https://www.hhs.gov/opioids/about-the-epidemic/index.html. Accessed November 18, 2021.
31. National Institute of Drug Abuse. Screening for substance use in the dental setting. Published May 3, 2021. https://www.drugabuse.gov/nidamed-medical-health-professionals/science-to-medicine/screening-substance-use/in-dental-setting. Accessed November 18, 2021.
32. National Association of Pharmacy Regulatory Authorities (NAPRA). Drug scheduling in Canada - general overview. https://napra.ca/drug-scheduling-canada-general-overview. Accessed November 20, 2021.
33. Centers for Disease Control and Pevention. Drug overdose: prescription drug monitoring programs (PDMPs). Published May 19, 2021. https://www.cdc.gov/drugoverdose/pdmp/index.html. Accessed November 18, 2021.
34. Canadian Institute for Health Information. *Opioid Prescribing in Canada: How Are Practices Changing?* 2019:42. https://www.cihi.ca/sites/default/files/document/opioid-prescribing-canada-trends-en-web.pdf. Accessed December 5, 2022.
35. Parish CL, Pereyra MR, Pollack HA, et al. Screening for substance misuse in the dental care setting: findings from a nationally representative survey of dentists. *Addiction*. 2015;110(9):1516-1523.
36. National Institute on Drug Abuse. Commonly used drugs charts. Published August 20, 2020. https://www.drugabuse.gov/drug-topics/commonly-used-drugs-charts. Accessed November 28, 2021.
37. National Conference of State Legislatures. State medical marijuana laws. Published August 23, 2021. https://www.ncsl.org/research/health/state-medical-marijuana-laws.aspx. Accessed November 18, 2021.
38. Bellocchio L, Inchingolo AD, Inchingolo AM, et al. Cannabinoids drugs and oral health—from recreational side-effects to medicinal purposes: a systematic review. *Int J Mol Sci*. 2021;22(15):8329.
39. Whiting PF, Wolff RF, Deshpande S, et al. Cannabinoids for medical use: a systematic review and meta-analysis. *JAMA*. 2015;313(24):2456-2473.
40. Devinsky O, Marsh E, Friedman D, et al. Cannabidiol in patients with treatment-resistant epilepsy: an open-label interventional trial. *Lancet Neurol*. 2016;15(3):270-278.
41. Poyatos L, Pérez-Acevedo AP, Papaseit E, et al. Oral administration of cannabis and δ-9-tetrahydrocannabinol (thc) preparations: a systematic review. *Med Kaunas Lith*. 2020; 56(6):E309.
42. Maccarrone M, Maldonado R, Casas M, Henze T, Centonze D. Cannabinoids therapeutic use: what is our current understanding following the introduction of THC, THC:CBD oromucosal spray and others? *Expert Rev Clin Pharmacol*. 2017;10(4):443-455.
43. Assi S, Gulyamova N, Ibrahim K, Kneller P, Osselton D. Profile, effects, and toxicity of novel psychoactive substances: a systematic review of quantitative studies. *Hum Psychopharmacol*. 2017;32(3).
44. National Institute on Drug Abuse. What are the effects of common dissociative drugs on the brain and body? https://www.drugabuse.gov/publications/research-reports/hallucinogens-dissociative-drugs/what-are-effects-common-dissociative-drugs-brain-body. Accessed November 18, 2021.

45. Huecker MR, Koutsothanasis GA, Abbasy MSU, Marraffa J. Heroin. *StatPearls*. Updated September 9, 2022. http://www.ncbi.nlm.nih.gov/books/NBK441876/. Accessed December 5, 2022.
46. US Drug Enforcement Administration. Fentanyl. https://www.dea.gov/factsheets/fentanyl. Accessed November 20, 2021.
47. National Institute on Drug Abuse. Fentanyl. Published June 6, 2016. https://www.drugabuse.gov/drug-topics/fentanyl. Accessed November 20, 2021.
48. Center for Drug Evaluation and Research. Fentanyl Transdermal System (marketed as Duragesic) Information. *FDA*. Published online November 3, 2018. https://www.fda.gov/drugs/postmarket-drug-safety-information-patients-and-providers/fentanyl-transdermal-system-marketed-duragesic-information. Accessed November 20, 2021.
49. Center for Drug Evaluation and Research. Transmucosal Immediate-Release Fentanyl (TIRF) Medicines. *FDA*. Published online December 29, 2020. https://www.fda.gov/drugs/information-drug-class/transmucosal-immediate-release-fentanyl-tirf-medicines. Accessed November 20, 2021.
50. Mattson CL. Trends and geographic patterns in drug and synthetic opioid overdose deaths — United States, 2013–2019. *MMWR Morb Mortal Wkly Rep*. 2021;70.
51. Health Canada. Fentanyl. Published November 14, 2018. https://www.canada.ca/en/health-canada/services/substance-use/controlled-illegal-drugs/fentanyl.html. Accessed November 20, 2021.
52. National Conference of State Legislatures. Drug overdose immunity and Good Samaritan Laws. Published 2021. https://www.ncsl.org/research/civil-and-criminal-justice/drug-overdose-immunity-good-samaritan-laws.aspx. Accessed November 21, 2021.
53. Health Canada. Frequently Asked Questions: Access to naloxone in Canada (including NARCAN™ Nasal Spray). Published July 6, 2016. https://www.canada.ca/en/health-canada/services/drugs-health-products/drug-products/announcements/narcan-nasal-spray-frequently-asked-questions.html. Accessed November 21, 2021.
54. Viswanath A, Barreveld AM, Fortino M. Assessment and management of the high-risk dental patient with active substance use disorder. *Dent Clin North Am*. 2020;64(3):547-558.
55. Tettey NS, Siddiqui K, Llamoca H, Nagamine S, Ahn S. Purple drank, sizurp, and lean: hip-hop music and codeine use, a call to action for public health educators. *Int J Psychol Stud*. 2020;12(1):42.
56. National Institute on Drug Abuse. What is cocaine? https://www.drugabuse.gov/publications/research-reports/cocaine/what-cocaine. Accessed November 21, 2021.
57. Hedegaard H, Minino AM, Warner M. *Drug Overdose Deaths in the United States, 1999–2018*. National Center for Health Statistics; 2020:8. https://www.cdc.gov/nchs/data/databriefs/db356-h.pdf
58. National Institute on Drug Abuse. Prescription Stimulants DrugFacts. Published June 6, 2018. https://www.drugabuse.gov/publications/drugfacts/prescription-stimulants. Accessed November 21, 2021.
59. National Institute on Drug Abuse. Methamphetamine DrugFacts. Published May 16, 2019. https://www.drugabuse.gov/publications/drugfacts/methamphetamine. Accessed November 21, 2021.
60. National Institute on Drug Abuse. Synthetic Cathinones ("Bath Salts") DrugFacts. Published July 6, 2020. https://www.drugabuse.gov/publications/drugfacts/synthetic-cathinones-bath-salts. Accessed November 18, 2021.
61. Lipari RN. Understanding adolescent inhalant use. In: *The CBHSQ Report*. Substance Abuse and Mental Health Services Administration; 2013. http://www.ncbi.nlm.nih.gov/books/NBK441821/. Accessed November 28, 2021.
62. Crossin R, Lawrence AJ, Andrews ZB, Churilov L, Duncan JR. Growth changes after inhalant abuse and toluene exposure: a systematic review and meta-analysis of human and animal studies. *Hum Exp Toxicol*. 2019;38(2):157-172.
63. Pergolizzi JV, Magnusson P, LeQuang JAK, Breve F, Varrassi G. Cocaine and cardiotoxicity: a literature review. *Cureus*. 2021;13(4):e14594.
64. Volkow ND, Boyle M. Neuroscience of addiction: relevance to prevention and treatment. *Am J Psychiatry*. 2018;175(8):729-740.
65. Cohen K, Weizman A, Weinstein A. Positive and negative effects of cannabis and cannabinoids on health. *Clin Pharmacol Ther*. 2019;105(5):1139-1147.
66. National Institute of Mental Health, U.S. Department of Health and Human Services. Mental health and substance use disorders. Published March 22, 2019. https://www.mentalhealth.gov/what-to-look-for/mental-health-substance-use-disorders. Accessed November 28, 2021.
67. National Institute on Drug Abuse. What are the other medical consequences of inhalant abuse? https://www.drugabuse.gov/publications/research-reports/inhalants/what-are-other-medical-consequences-inhalant-abuse. Accessed November 28, 2021.
68. Farooq I, Bugshan A. The role of salivary contents and modern technologies in the remineralization of dental enamel: a narrative review. *F1000Research*. 2020;9:171.
69. Akkina SK, Ricardo AC, Patel A, et al. Illicit drug use, hypertension, and chronic kidney disease in the US adult population. *Transl Res J Lab Clin Med*. 2012;160(6):391-398.
70. Pateria P, de Boer B, MacQuillan G. Liver abnormalities in drug and substance abusers. *Best Pract Res Clin Gastroenterol*. 2013;27(4):577-596.
71. Verna EC, Schluger A, Brown RS. Opioid epidemic and liver disease. *JHEP Rep Innov Hepatol*. 2019;1(3):240-255.
72. Blount BC, Karwowski MP, Shields PG, et al. Vitamin E acetate in bronchoalveolar-lavage fluid associated with EVALI. *N Engl J Med*. 2020;382(8):697-705.
73. Wurcel AG, Merchant EA, Clark RP, Stone DR. Emerging and underrecognized complications of illicit drug use. *Clin Infect Dis Off Publ Infect Dis Soc Am*. 2015;61(12):1840-1849.
74. Narkowicz S, Płotka J, Polkowska Ż, Biziuk M, Namieśnik J. Prenatal exposure to substance of abuse: a worldwide problem. *Environ Int*. 2013;54:141-163.
75. Khan L. Neonatal abstinence syndrome. *Pediatr Ann*. 2020;49(1):e3-e7.
76. Wang SC, Maher B. Substance use disorder, intravenous injection, and HIV infection: a review. *Cell Transplant*. 2019;28(12):1465-1471.
77. McCarthy NL, Baggs J, See I, et al. Bacterial infections associated with substance use disorders, large cohort of United States hospitals, 2012–2017. *Clin Infect Dis*. 2020;71(7):e37-e44.
78. Haider MR, Kingori C, Brown MJ, Battle-Fisher M, Chertok IA. Illicit drug use and sexually transmitted infections among young adults in the US: evidence from a nationally representative survey. *Int J STD AIDS*. 2020;31(13):1238-1246.
79. National Institute on Drug Abuse. Treatment Approaches for Drug Addiction DrugFacts. Published January 17, 2019. https://www.drugabuse.gov/publications/drugfacts/treatment-approaches-drug-addiction. Accessed December 2, 2021.

80. Hadland SE, Yule AM, Levy SJ, Hallett E, Silverstein M, Bagley SM. Evidence-based treatment of young adults with substance use disorders. *Pediatrics*. 2021;147 (Supplement 2):S204-S214.
81. Steele DW, Becker SJ, Danko KJ, et al. *Interventions for Substance Use Disorders in Adolescents: A Systematic Review*. Agency for Healthcare Research and Quality; 2020. http://www.ncbi.nlm.nih.gov/books/NBK557291/. Accessed December 2, 2021.
82. Siefried KJ, Acheson LS, Lintzeris N, Ezard N. Pharmacological treatment of methamphetamine/amphetamine dependence: a systematic review. *CNS Drugs*. 2020;34(4):337-365.
83. American Society of Addiction Medicine. The ASAM national practice guideline for the treatment of opioid use disorder: 2020 focused update. *J Addict Med*. 2020;14(2S):1-91.
84. Bruneau J, Ahamad K, Goyer MÈ, et al. Management of opioid use disorders: a national clinical practice guideline. *Can Med Assoc J*. 2018;190(9):E247-E257.
85. National Institute on Drug Abuse. Screening tools and prevention. Published January 10, 2019. https://www.drugabuse.gov/nidamed-medical-health-professionals/screening-tools-prevention. Accessed December 2, 2021.
86. Jain NP, Shao K, Stewart C, Grant-Kels JM. The effects of alcohol and illicit drug use on the skin. *Clin Dermatol*. 2021;39(5):772-783.
87. Dhingra D, Kaur S, Ram J. Illicit drugs: effects on eye. *Indian J Med Res*. 2019;150(3):228-238.
88. Baghaie H, Kisely S, Forbes M, Sawyer E, Siskind DJ. A systematic review and meta-analysis of the association between poor oral health and substance abuse. *Addiction*. 2017;112(5):765-779.
89. Yazdanian M, Armoon B, Noroozi A, et al. Dental caries and periodontal disease among people who use drugs: a systematic review and meta-analysis. *BMC Oral Health*. 2020;20(1):44.
90. Hegazi F, Alhazmi H, Abdullah A, et al. Prevalence of oral conditions among methamphetamine users: NHANES 2009-2014. *J Public Health Dent*. 2021;81(1):21-28.
91. Melo CAA, Guimarães HRG, Medeiros RCF, Souza GC de A, Santos PBDD, Tôrres ACSP. Oral changes in cocaine abusers: an integrative review. *Braz J Otorhinolaryngol*. Published online May 14, 2021:S1808-8694(21)00083-5.
92. Taghi KM, Arghavan T, Maryam A, Pourya B, Elham MG, Gelareh T. Drug addiction and oral health; a comparison of hallucinogen and non-hallucinogen drug users. *Int J Dent Oral Health*. 2016;2(6).
93. Chisini LA, Cademartori MG, Francia A, et al. Is the use of Cannabis associated with periodontitis? A systematic review and meta-analysis. *J Periodontal Res*. 2019;54(4):311-317.
94. Featherstone JDB, Crystal YO, Alston P, et al. Evidence-based caries management for all ages-practical guidelines. *Front Oral Health*. 2021;2:14.
95. Cuberos M, Chatah EM, Baquerizo HZ, Weinstein G. Dental management of patients with substance use disorder. *Clin Dent Rev*. 2020;4(1):1-8.
96. Urquhart O, Tampi MP, Pilcher L, et al. Nonrestorative treatments for caries: systematic review and network meta-analysis. *J Dent Res*. 2019;98(1):14-26.

CHAPTER 60

The Patient with a Respiratory Disease

Lisa F. Mallonee, RDH, RD, LD, MPH
Naquilla Thomas, RDH, EdD
Linda D. Boyd, RDH, RD, EdD

CHAPTER OUTLINE

LEARNING OBJECTIVES

After studying the chapter, the student will be able to:

1. Identify and define key terms and concepts related to respiratory diseases.
2. Differentiate between upper and lower respiratory diseases.
3. Describe the etiology, symptoms, and management of respiratory diseases.
4. Plan and document dental hygiene care and oral hygiene instructions for patients with compromised respiratory function.

Respiratory Disease and Oral-Systemic Link

- Scientific evidence shows dental biofilm and microorganisms from periodontal infections are associated with respiratory infections, such as asthma, chronic obstructive pulmonary disease, and pneumonia.[1]
- The dental hygienist's role in the prevention and control of periodontal infections may have a major influence on reducing the bacterial load to aid in the overall health of the patient.

The Respiratory System

I. Anatomy

- Upper respiratory structures: nose, larynx, and pharynx.
- Lower respiratory structures: trachea, bronchi, bronchioles, lungs, and alveolar duct (**Figure 60-1A**).[2]

II. Physiology

The respiratory tract from nasal cavity to lungs serves as a passageway for air exchange (Figure 60-1A).

- Inhaled fresh air: warmed and filtered in the nasal cavity, enters the lungs.
- Exhaled air: with carbon dioxide, leaves the body.
- Gas exchange: at the cellular level, occurs in the alveoli at the ends of the bronchioles, as shown in **Figure 60-1B**.
- Cardiovascular system: functions with the respiratory system to pump oxygenated blood from the lungs to every cell in the body and deoxygenated blood back to the lungs for exhalation.

III. Function of the Respiratory Mucosa

Figure 60-2 shows ciliated epithelial cells and **mucus**-secreting **goblet cells** that line the respiratory tract to make up the respiratory mucosa.

- Mucus secreted from goblet cells moistens inspired air, prevents delicate alveolar walls from becoming dry, and traps dust and other airborne particles.
- Cilia assist in removing foreign material and contaminated mucus with a constant wavelike motion that propels this material back into the larger bronchi and trachea, where it can be coughed up and expectorated or swallowed.
- Lack of function results when the inflammatory process of asthma and **chronic** bronchitis initiates an overabundance of mucus. Congestion is created, and the cilia are prevented from assisting with normal breathing.

IV. Respiratory Assessment

- Respiratory disease assessment includes several objective measures.

A. Vital Signs

- Determination of vital signs (body temperature, pulse, respiratory rate, blood pressure) and also smoking status is considered standard procedure in dental patient care.
- Methods of determining vital signs are described in Chapter 12. Tobacco use is discussed in Chapter 32.

B. Spirometry

- Medical test that measures various aspects of breathing and lung function.
- Used to diagnose and monitor many lower respiratory tract diseases.
- Performed with a **spirometer**, a device that registers the amount of air a person inhales or exhales and the rate at which air is moved in and out of the lungs.
- **Figure 60-3** shows the use of a portable spirometer to evaluate lung function.

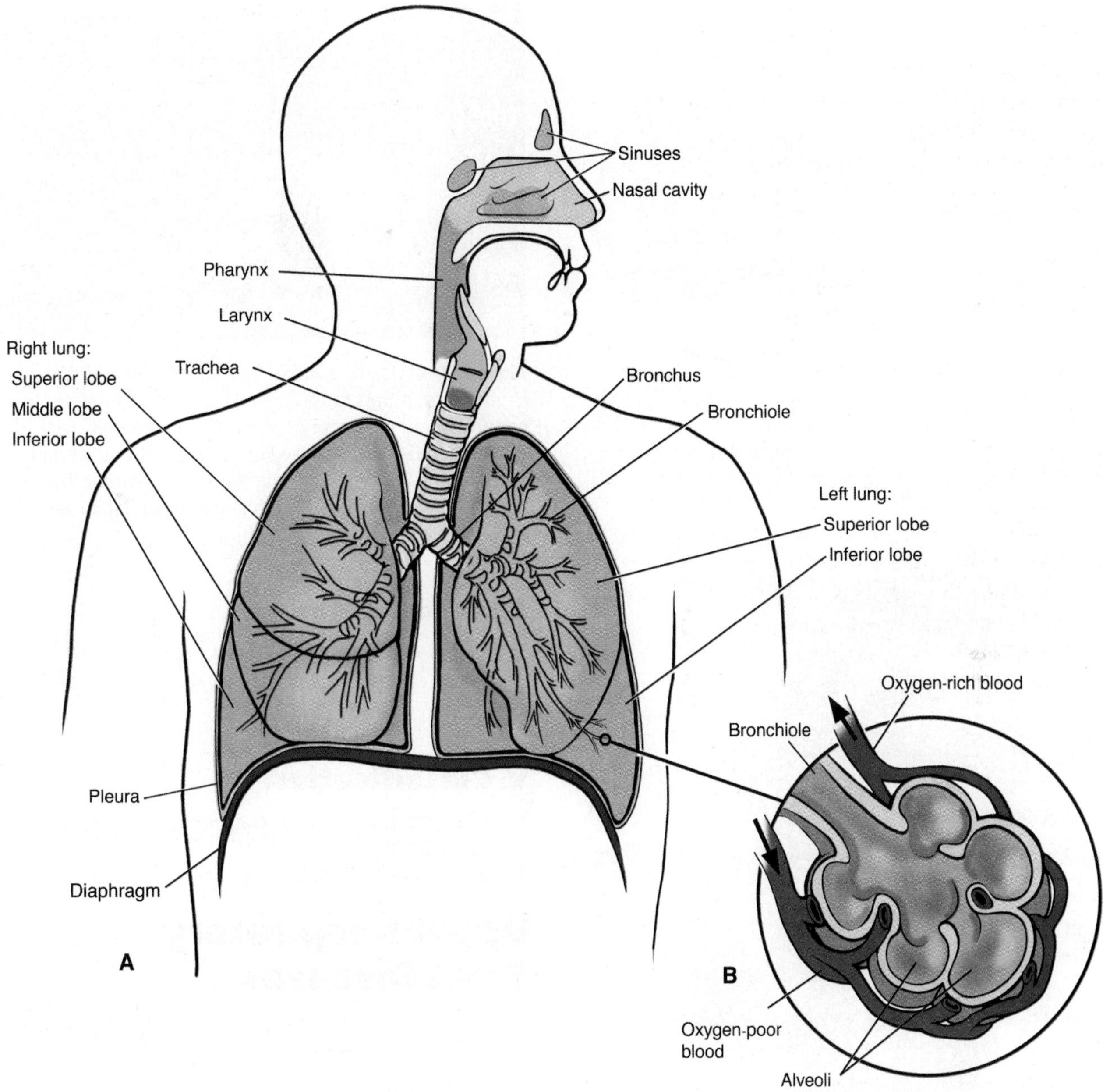

Figure 60-1 Structures of the Respiratory System. **A:** Structures. The major anatomic structures of the respiratory system are shown. Each bronchus branches out to the bronchioles. **B:** Gas exchange. Exchange of oxygen and carbon dioxide occurs in the alveoli of the bronchioles.

C. Pulse Oximetry

- Noninvasive medical test that measures blood oxygen saturation (SpO_2) levels.[1]
- Performed with a pulse oximeter.
  - Color of blood varies depending upon the amount of oxygen it contains.
  - Pulse oximeter emits a light through the finger to calculate the percentage of oxygen.
  - Any finger (excluding the thumb) can be used. A skin callus may interfere with reading.
  - Intended only as an adjunct in patient assessment along with other methods of assessing clinical signs and symptoms.
  - Not accurate in assessing SpO_2 values below 90%.[3]
  - Healthy patients have an oxygen saturation of 95% or higher.[4]
  - Saturation below 90% signifies poor oxygen exchange or hypoxemia.[3]
- **Figure 60-4** shows the use of a pulse oximeter to measure blood oxygen saturation levels.

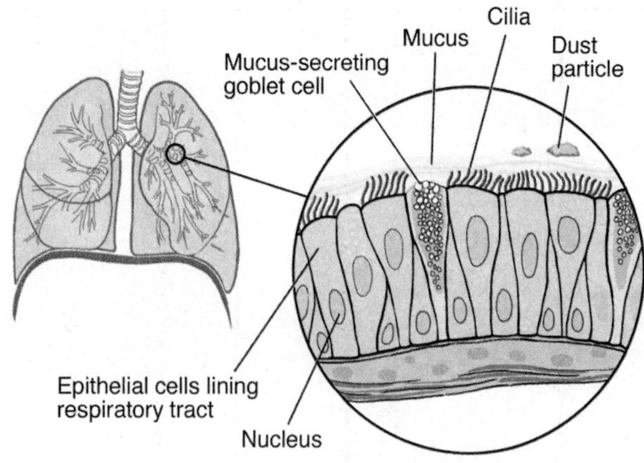

Figure 60-2 Lining of the Respiratory Mucosa. Ciliated epithelial cells and mucus secreted by goblet cells help to remove foreign objects (dust particles). The material is coughed up and either expectorated or swallowed.

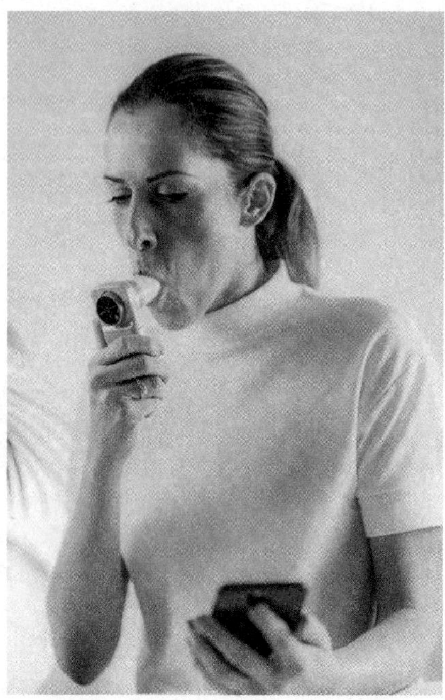

Figure 60-3 Use of a Spirometer to Evaluate Lung Function. Person being tested takes in a full breath, seals their lips over the mouthpiece of the spirometer, and then blows out as hard and as fast as possible for at least 6 seconds. Nose clips may be applied to ensure no air escapes through the nose.

D. Chest Radiography (Imaging)

- Indicates presence of pathologic density (radiopacity) in the lungs.
- Standard chest radiograph: shows a two-dimensional view of lung tissues.
- Computed axial tomography radiograph or computed tomography (CT) scan: shows a three-dimensional cross section of lung tissues.

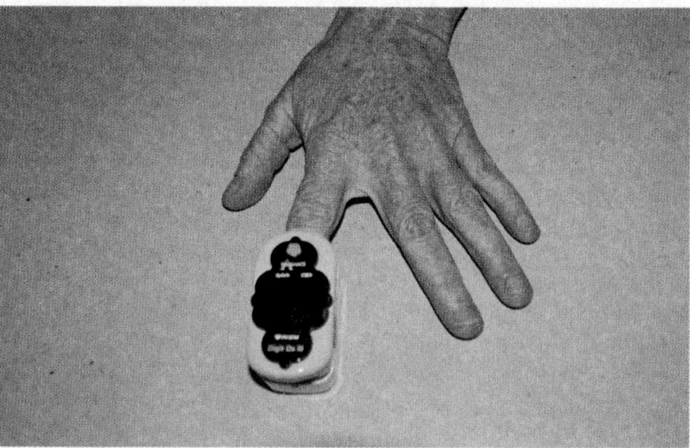

Figure 60-4 Use of a Pulse Oximeter to Measure Blood Oxygen Saturation Level. Color of blood varies depending on the amount of oxygen it contains. The pulse oximeter clips on any finger (except the thumb) and emits a light through the finger to calculate the percentage of oxygen in the blood. Nail polish or a skin callus may interfere with reading.

E. Blood Gas Analysis

- Blood test to determine acid–base balance, alveolar ventilation, arterial oxygen saturation, and carbon dioxide elimination.

V. Classification

- Classification of respiratory diseases is listed in **Table 60-1**.[5-8]

Upper Respiratory Tract Diseases

The more common disorders of the upper respiratory tract are caused by infections or allergic reactions that result in inflammation.

- Signs and symptoms, etiology, medical treatment, and clinical evaluation assessment are summarized in **Table 60-2**.[9-15]

I. Modes of Transmission

- Inhalation of airborne droplets or aerosols.[16]
- Indirect contact with contaminated items.[16]
- Direct contact with an infected person.[16]

II. Dental Hygiene Care

A. Disease Prevention

- All healthcare professionals are encouraged to obtain immunizations for seasonal viral influenza.[17]
- Observe standard precautions including respiratory hygiene and cough etiquette as listed in **Table 60-3**

Table 60-1 Classification of Respiratory Diseases[5–8]

Location/Structures	Acute	Chronic
Upper respiratory tract Diseases of the nose, sinuses, pharynx, larynx	Nonallergic rhinitis (common cold) Sinusitis Pharyngitis/tonsillitis Influenza (flu) ■ Seasonal ■ Viral	Allergic rhinitis (hay fever)
Lower respiratory tract Diseases of the trachea, lungs	Acute bronchitis Pneumonia Pertussis (whooping cough) Respiratory syncytial virus (RSV) Severe acute respiratory syndrome (SARS)	TB Asthma COPD ■ Chronic bronchitis ■ Emphysema Cystic fibrosis (genetic) Occupational lung diseases

COPD, chronic obstructive pulmonary disease; TB, tuberculosis.

Data from Centers for Disease Control and Prevention. National Center for Immunization and Respiratory Diseases (NCIRD). Published March 4, 2022. Accessed March 31, 2022. https://www.cdc.gov/ncird/overview/websites.html; World Health Organization. Chronic respiratory diseases. Accessed March 31, 2022. https://www.who.int/westernpacific/health-topics/chronic-respiratory-diseases; Centers for Disease Control and Prevention. Tuberculosis (TB)- Basic TB Facts. Centers for Disease Control and Prevention. Published June 19, 2019. Accessed March 31, 2022. https://www.cdc.gov/tb/topic/basics/default.htm; Turcios NL. Cystic fibrosis lung disease: an overview. *Respir Care*. 2020;65(2):233-251.

Table 60-2 Summary of Upper Respiratory Diseases: Signs/Symptoms, Etiology, Medical Management, and Dental Hygiene Care—Clinical Evaluation Assessment

Clinical Manifestations	Etiology	Medical Management	Oral Manifestations
Upper Respiratory Infections—Nonallergic Rhinitis (Common Cold)[9,10]			
■ Sneezing and/or coughing ■ Nasal ■ Congestion ■ Nasal discharge (**coryza**) ■ Sore throat ■ Fever in children	■ Viral	■ **Analgesic** ■ *Nasal decongestant ■ *Antihistamine ■ Fluids *(not recommended for children less than 4 years old)	■ Medications and mouth breathing may cause dry mouth
Allergic Rhinitis (Hay Fever)[11,12]			
■ Conjunctivitis ■ Itching (nose, eyes, or mouth) ■ Sneezing ■ Rhinorrhea (runny nose) ■ Nasal and sinus congestion	■ Seasonal triggers (grass, trees, pollen) ■ Perennial triggers (dust mites, mold spores, animal dander) result in immunoglobulin E-mediated hypersensitivity reactions	■ Avoidance of allergen ■ Antihistamines ■ Decongestants ■ Nasal corticosteroids ■ Immunotherapy	■ Drug-induced dry mouth ■ Oral candidiasis from long-term use of corticosteroids ■ Itchy tongue
Sinusitis[13]			
■ Nasal obstruction ■ Purulent rhinorrhea ■ Facial pain and pressure ■ Fever, chills ■ Malaise ■ Cough, especially at night ■ Hyposmia (reduced ability to smell)	■ Bacterial infection ■ Viral in immunocompromised patients ■ Can be secondary to a dental abscess	■ Steam ■ Topical vasoconstrictors via nasal spray ■ Antibiotics only used if other measures are not effective ■ Fluids	■ Dry mouth ■ Maxillary sinusitis may cause toothaches or pain

(continues)

Table 60-2 Summary of Upper Respiratory Diseases: Signs/Symptoms, Etiology, Medical Management, and Dental Hygiene Care—Clinical Evaluation Assessment *(continued)*

Clinical Manifestations	Etiology	Medical Management	Oral Manifestations
Tonsillopharyngitis (Pharyngitis/Tonsillitis)[14]			
■ Sore throat ■ Cervical lymphadenopathy (swollen glands) ■ Exudate from tonsils ■ Fever ■ Odynophagia (painful swallowing)	■ Usually viral ■ Rarely bacterial: Group A beta-hemolytic streptococcus (GABHS) infection	■ Viral: analgesia, hydration, and rest ■ Topical analgesics in lozenges ■ Bacterial: antibiotics	■ Enlarged tonsils ■ Erythematous tissues ■ Palatal petechiae
Influenza (Flu)[15]			
■ Fever ■ Chills ■ Headache ■ Coryza ■ Nonproductive dry cough ■ **Myalgia** ■ **Malaise** ■ Gastrointestinal symptoms such as nausea and vomiting occur in some flu strains	■ Viral ■ Mode of transmission: airborne, direct, or contact with contaminated item	■ Rapid diagnostic test can be used ■ Bed rest, fluids ■ Analgesic ■ Antivirals in first 2 days ■ Monitor for secondary bacterial infection ■ Prevent with annual vaccine	

Data from Fried M. Nonallergic Rhinitis. Merck Manuals Professional Edition. Published December 2021. Accessed March 31, 2022. https://www.merckmanuals.com/professional/ear,-nose,-and-throat-disorders/nose-and-paranasal-sinus-disorders/nonallergic-rhinitis; Pappas DE. The common cold. Principles and Practice of Pediatric Infectious Diseases. Published online 2018:199-202.e1.; Delves PJ. Allergic Rhinitis. Merck Manuals Professional Edition. Accessed March 31, 2022. https://www.merckmanuals.com/professional/immunology-allergic-disorders/allergic,-autoimmune,-and-other-hypersensitivity-disorders/allergic-rhinitis?query=allergic%20rhinitis; Hussein H, Mensah RK, Brown RS. Diagnosis and management of oral allergy syndrome, the itchy tongue allergic reaction. *Compend Contin Educ Dent.* 2019;40(8):502-506.; Fried M. Sinusitis. Merck Manuals Professional Edition. Published December 2021. Accessed March 31, 2022. https://www.merckmanuals.com/professional/ear,-nose,-and-throat-disorders/nose-and-paranasal-sinus-disorders/sinusitis?query=sinusitis; Cheng AG. Tonsillopharyngitis. Merck Manuals Professional Edition. Published March 2022. Accessed March 31, 2022. https://www.merckmanuals.com/professional/ear,-nose,-and-throat-disorders/oral-and-pharyngeal-disorders/tonsillopharyngitis?query=pharyngitis; Tesini BL. Influenza. Merck Manuals Professional Edition. Published September 2021. Accessed March 31, 2022. https://www.merckmanuals.com/professional/infectious-diseases/respiratory-viruses/influenza?query=influenza

Table 60-3 Respiratory Hygiene and Cough Etiquette in Healthcare Settings

To prevent transmission of all respiratory infections in healthcare settings, incorporate the following infection control practices as one component of standard precautions:

Visual alerts	■ Post visual alerts: symptoms of respiratory infection and respiratory hygiene and cough etiquette.
Respiratory hygiene and cough etiquette	■ Use tissue to cover coughs and sneezes and discard in no-touch receptacle. ■ Perform hand hygiene (hand washing with nonantimicrobial soap and water, alcohol-based rub, or antiseptic hand wash) after contact with respiratory secretions or contaminated objects.
Masking and separation of persons with respiratory symptoms	■ Offer masks to persons who are coughing and encourage coughing persons to sit at least 3 feet away from others in common waiting areas.
Droplet precautions	■ Observe droplet precautions (wearing a surgical or procedure mask for close contact) in addition to standard precautions when examining a patient with symptoms of a respiratory infection, particularly when a fever is present.

Data from Centers for Disease Control and Prevention. *Respiratory Hygiene/Cough Etiquette.* Atlanta, GA: Centers for Disease Control. https://www.cdc.gov/oralhealth/infectioncontrol/faqs/respiratory-hygiene.html. Updated March 25, 2016. Accessed March 28, 2022.

to prevent transmission of pathogens from patient to clinician and to prevent healthcare-associated infections to the patient.[18]

B. Appointment Management

- Delay nonemergent treatment until patient is no longer infectious.[19]
- Noninfectious status is determined by temperature returning to normal and regression of symptoms and oral lesions.

C. Bacterial Resistance to Antibiotics

- Due to possible antibiotic resistance, for patients currently prescribed an antibiotic for a non-dental condition (such as acute bacterial bronchitis or sinus infection): a different category of antibiotic will be necessary to treat an odontogenic (dental origin) infection.[20]

Lower Respiratory Tract Diseases

- Considered to be a more serious infection.
- Diseases of the lower respiratory tract are listed in Table 60-1.

Acute Bronchitis

- An **acute** respiratory infection that involves large airways (trachea, bronchi).[21]
- Typically accompanied by or preceded by URI (upper respiratory infection) symptoms.[21]
- Primary symptom: nonproductive or mildly productive cough; may last 2–3 weeks.[21]
- Lower respiratory tract disease symptoms: wheezing, shortness of breath, or chest tightness.
- A comparison of acute viral and bacterial bronchitis is listed in **Table 60-4**.

Severe Acute Respiratory Syndrome-Coronavirus-2 (SARS-CoV-2)

- Severe acute respiratory syndrome (SARS) is a severe form of the coronavirus that progressively leads to severe respiratory insufficiency.[22]
- Exposure to the virus and the onset of symptoms (**incubation period**) vary from person to person, with an average of 11.5 days after exposure This average may differ with emerging variants.[23]

Table 60-4 Comparison of Acute Viral and Bacterial Bronchitis[21]

Item	Viral	Bacterial
Occurrence	▪ Most prevalent	▪ Least prevalent (<5% of cases)
Medical treatment	▪ Symptom relief: acetaminophen, fluids ▪ Inhaled bronchodilators for wheezing ▪ Cough suppressant if interfering with sleep	▪ Limited use of antibiotics

Data from Sethi S. Acute Bronchitis - Pulmonary Disorders. Merck Manuals Professional Edition. Published July 2021. Accessed March 31, 2022. https://www.merckmanuals.com/professional/pulmonary-disorders/acute-bronchitis/acute-bronchitis

I. Etiology

- SARS-CoV-2 is a single-strand RNA virus that causes COVID-19 and triggers an inflammatory response.[23,24]
- Nasal and bronchial epithelial cells are targeted.[23]
- There is ongoing investigation as to the origin of the virus, bats have been identified as reservoirs.[23]

II. Transmission

- Respiratory droplets resulting from sneezing, coughing, or talking.[22,23]
- Infection can be spread via persons who are asymptomatic, presymptomatic, or symptomatic; however, the viral load and shedding begin 2–3 days before symptoms appear.[23]
- Close contact (fewer than 6 feet) with a person infected with the virus for a 15 minutes or more.[22,23]
- Aerosols that remain suspended in the air.[23]

III. Dental Hygiene Care

- Patients who are symptomatic should postpone elective dental treatment.
- Focus on management of dental biofilm.
- Minimize use of aerosol-generating procedures (AGPs) and use appropriate personal protective equipment (PPE) and equipment to mitigate aerosols. (See Chapter 6 and Chapter 7.)
- See **Table 60-5** for additional information.[22-27]

Table 60-5 Summary of SARS-CoV-2: Symptoms, Comorbidities, Medical Management, and Implications for Dental Hygiene Care[22-27]

Initial Symptoms	Long-Term Symptoms (post-COVID-19)	Most Frequent Comorbidities	Medical Management	Implications for Dental Hygiene Care
▪ Fever ▪ Dry cough ▪ Shortness of breath ▪ Loss of smell and/or taste ▪ Fatigue ▪ Diarrhea, nausea, vomiting ▪ Myalgia	▪ Shortness of breath (dyspnea) ▪ Fatigue ▪ Cough ▪ Cardiac abnormalities ▪ Cognitive impairment ▪ Muscle pain ▪ Headache ▪ Multiorgan involvement: respiratory, cardiovascular, neurologic, gastrointestinal, musculoskeletal ▪ Bleeding and coagulation abnormalities	▪ Obesity ▪ Diabetes mellitus ▪ Cardiovascular disease ▪ Chronic pulmonary disease ▪ Hypertension ▪ Chronic kidney disease ▪ Chronic liver disease	▪ Diagnosis: polymerase chain reaction (PCR) testing via nasal swab ▪ Vaccination is recommended to prevent and reduce severity ▪ Treatment depends on severity and ranges from at home quarantine to hospitalization ▪ Antiviral drugs (i.e., remdesivir) ▪ Monoclonal antibodies	▪ Avoid nonemergent care in active disease ▪ Consider teledentistry for initial history gathering, including treatment and long-term symptoms of COVID-19 and impact on organ systems ▪ Adjust care based on long-term symptoms and impact on organ systems ▪ Carefully monitor bleeding ▪ For dyspnea, may want an oximeter to assess oxygen saturation ▪ May require an upright or semi-supine chair position ▪ Assess for opportunistic fungal infection ▪ Possible active periodontal disease ▪ Malnutrition may be a concern for those with extended hospitalization

Data from Tesini BL. COVID-19. Merck Manuals Professional Edition. Published March 2022. Accessed March 31, 2022. https://www.merckmanuals.com/professional/infectious-diseases/covid-19/covid-19?query=COVID-19; Wiersinga WJ, Rhodes A, Cheng AC, Peacock SJ, Prescott HC. Pathophysiology, transmission, diagnosis, and treatment of coronavirus disease 2019 (COVID-19): a review. *JAMA*. 2020;324(8):782-793; Forchette L, Sebastian W, Liu T. A comprehensive review of COVID-19 virology, vaccines, variants, and therapeutics. *Curr Med Sci*. 2021;41(6):1037-1051; La Rosa GRM, Libra M, De Pasquale R, Ferlito S, Pedullà E. Association of viral infections with oral cavity lesions: role of SARS-CoV-2 infection. *Front Med*. 2021;7:571214; Crook H, Raza S, Nowell J, Young M, Edison P. Long covid-mechanisms, risk factors, and management. *BMJ*. 2021;374:n1648; Chakraborty T, Jamal RF, Battineni G, Teja KV, Marto CM, Spagnuolo G. A review of prolonged post-COVID-19 symptoms and their implications on dental management. *Int J Environ Res Public Health*. 2021;18(10):5131.

Pneumonia

- An infection of the alveoli and distal bronchial tree in the lungs caused by viruses, bacteria, fungi, **mycoplasma**, or parasites.[28]
- The respiratory tract of a healthy person is able to defend against organisms aspirated into the lungs.
- Pneumonia develops when immunocompromised, when the bacteria aspirated overwhelms host defenses, or when a virulent pathogen is introduced.[29]

I. Classification of Pneumonia

A. Community-Acquired Pneumonia (CAP)

- Infection occurring in an individual in the community (not in a healthcare facility).[28]
- Transmission via direct or indirect contact, droplets, and aerosols.
- Highest rate is in adults aged 65–79 years.[28]

B. Hospital-Acquired Pneumonia (HAP)

- Infection occurring at least 2 days after admission to a healthcare facility.[28]
- Globally, HAP is a leading cause of death due to hospital-acquired infection.[28]
- Most common in immunocompromised and postsurgical patients, and those 80 years or older.[28]
- Ventilator-associated pneumonia (VAP)
  - Ventilator-associated pneumonia: mechanically ventilated patients in the immediate care unit with no ability to clear oral secretions by swallowing or coughing.
  - VAP affects 10% to 25% of those on mechanical ventilation.[28]
  - In the intensive care unit, VAP is the most common cause of **nosocomial** infection and death, particularly in those with other comorbidities.[28]

C. Aspiration Pneumonia

- Aspiration pneumonia is part of the continuum of CAP and HAP.[28]
- **Dysphagia** and impaired cough reflex increase risk for aspiration pneumonia.
- Oral and periodontal bacteria may be associated with CAP and HAP, but whether they cause aspiration pneumonia needs more research as not all studies agree.[30]

II. Etiology

A. Community-Acquired Pneumonia

- The most frequent pathogen in CAP is *Streptococcus pneumoniae*.
- Methicillin-resistant *Staphylococcus aureus* (MRSA) and other gram-negative bacteria resistant to antibiotics are responsible for a smaller portion of CAP.

B. Hospital-Acquired Pneumonia

- HAP and VAP have a similar etiology from *Pseudomonas aeruginosa* and *S. aureus*.
- Oropharyngeal colonization is a primary etiology of HAP.[28]
- More than one-third (38%) of HAP cases are colonized by antibiotic-resistant organisms.[28]

III. Symptoms

- Clinical symptoms may include[28]:
  - Fever.
  - Cough.
  - Sputum production.
  - Chest pain.
  - Shortness of breath.
  - Fatigue
- Confirmation by chest radiograph is needed for diagnosis.

IV. Medical Management

A. Prevention of Hospital-Acquired and Ventilator-Associated Pneumonia

- Hand hygiene.
- Oral hygiene with antiseptic solution.
  - Evidence is unclear if there may be negative effects from use of chlorhexidine, so this needs more research and care must be taken to avoid aspiration.[28,31]
- Semi-supine position.

B. Pharmacologic Treatment of Pneumonia

- Diagnostic testing must identify the pathogen to identify the appropriate antibiotic therapy.[28]

V. Dental Hygiene Care

- Dependent individuals in nursing homes and hospitals could benefit from including a dental hygienist as part of the interprofessional approach to help prevent aspiration pneumonia.[32]
- For compromised individuals in the dental office:
  - Use 0.12% chlorhexidine gluconate rinse prior to beginning treatment to reduce the bacterial load.
  - Carefully assess patient risk for dysphagia and, if present, avoid use of ultrasonic scalers due to the production of aerosols and use caution when rinsing or using air.

Tuberculosis

- **Tuberculosis (TB)** is a chronic, infectious, and **communicable disease** with worldwide public health significance as a major cause of disability and death, especially in developing countries.[33,34]
- Groups at high risk for exposure to TB include those who have been recently infected with TB bacteria or persons with medical conditions that weaken the immune system. Risk factors include[35]:
  - Close contact with people infected with TB.
  - Living conditions leading to overcrowding, homelessness, and congregate settings (e.g., prisons and long-term care).
  - Residing in countries with a high TB incidence/prevalence.
  - Socioeconomic status, healthcare access, and health disparities.
  - Substance use/abuse, including intravenous drugs, alcohol, and tobacco.
  - Comorbidities such as diabetes, HIV, rheumatoid arthritis, and immunosuppression therapy/immunocompromised.
  - Malnutrition.
  - Medical/dental care providers for any of the aforementioned high-risk groups.

I. Etiology

- *Mycobacterium tuberculosis*, a rod-shaped bacterium (tubercle bacillus), is the most common causative agent.

II. Transmission

- Tubercle bacilli travel in airborne droplet nuclei in infected saliva or mucus from persons with pulmonary or laryngeal TB during forceful expirations (coughing, sneezing, talking, singing).[7]
- Inhalation and other modes of transmission are described in Chapter 5.

III. Disease Development

A. Active Tuberculosis

- Inhaled tubercle bacilli travel to the lung alveoli, where local infection begins.
- While TB can affect any organ or tissue, *M. tuberculosis* is an aerobe and survives best in an environment of high oxygen tension, such as the lungs.
- It may develop quickly after exposure or may not develop for some time after the initial infection.
- Active TB develops when the infectious agent multiplies and compromises the immune system.[36]
- Symptoms include excessive coughing, chest pain, weight loss, fever, and fatigue.

B. Latent Tuberculosis Infection (LTBI)

- Two billion globally and 13 million in the United States are infected with tuberculosis and of these most are asymptomatic and classified as having latent tuberculosis infection (LTBI).
  - Of those with LTBI, only 5% to 10% of progress to active TB in their lifetime.[37]
- Comparison of LTBI and active TB disease including signs/symptoms, diagnosis, and medical treatment with TB drugs is listed in **Table 60-6**.
  - Note treatment guidelines vary and in LBTI it is based on the risk of the patient developing active TB.

IV. Diagnosis

A. Active TB Disease

- Physical examination and evaluation of signs and symptoms.

Table 60-6 Comparison of LTBI and Active TB Disease: Signs/Symptoms, Diagnosis, and Medical Management with TB Drugs[7,34,36-38]

Item	LTBI	Active TB Disease
Signs and symptoms of pulmonary TB	Asymptomatic	■ Bad cough lasting 3 weeks or longer ■ Fatigue ■ Unexplained weight loss ■ Sweating at night ■ Fever or chills ■ **Hemoptysis** ■ Chest pain
Infectivity	Cannot infect others	Can infect others
Diagnostic testing	■ Mantoux skin test (TST) ■ IGRA blood (TB (T-Spot) and QuantiFERON-TB Gold Plus (QFT-Plus)	■ Mantoux skin test (TST) ■ IGRA blood test ■ Sputum smear microscopy ■ Nucleic-acid amplification tests (NAATs)—rapid test ■ Chest radiograph
Treatment	■ 3 months of isoniazid (**INH**) and rifapentine once weekly OR ■ 4 months of rifampin (**RIF**) daily ■ Other regimens may be prescribed based on HIV status and patient tolerance	■ 6-month regimen of four first-line drugs: INH, rifampicin, ethambutol (**EMB**), and pyrazinamide (**PZA**) ■ Therapy for multidrug-resistant TB (i.e., bedaquiline and fluoroquinolones)

IGRA, interferon-gamma release assay; LTBI, latent tuberculosis infection; TST, tuberculin skin test.

Data from Centers for Disease Control and Prevention. Treatment for TB Disease. Atlanta, GA: Centers for Disease Control and Prevention. https://www.cdc.gov/tb/topic/treatment/tbdisease.htm. Updated April 5, 2016. Accessed February 2, 2019; Centers for Disease Control and Prevention, National Center for HIV Viral Hepatitis STD and TB Prevention. Fact Sheet: Treatment Options for Latent Tuberculosis Infection. Atlanta, GA: Center for Disease Control and Prevention; 2016. https://www.cdc.gov/tb/publications/factsheets/treatment/ltbitreatmentoptions_revised.pdf. Accessed February 28, 2019.

- Diagnostic testing has continued to advance and may include[7,34]:
  - Tuberculin skin test (**TST**).
    - Also known as Mantoux test, purified protein derivative (**PPD**) test.
    - PPD is injected under the skin on the forearm. After 72 hours, the circumference of induration (hard swelling) is measured to determine exposure.
  - Interferon-gamma release assay (**IGRA**).
    - Blood test to determine exposure to *M. tuberculosis*.
  - Nucleic-acid amplification tests (NAATs)—rapid test: reduce the time to diagnosis.
  - Sputum smear microscopy
- In the United States, the mainstay of diagnosis is the TST and IGRA blood test according to the Centers for Disease Control and Prevention (CDC),[7] but the World Health Organization highly recommends use of the emerging rapid tests (NAATs) for initial diagnosis.[34]
- The sputum smear microscopy or a rapid molecular test are considered to have a confirmed diagnosis of TB.[34]
- Chest radiograph may aid in ruling out TB in someone with a positive TST or blood test.[7]

B. Latent Tuberculosis Infection

- Tuberculin skin test (TST).
  - A negative TST does not exclude LTBI disease.
- Interferon-gamma release assay (IGRA).
  - IGRA blood test, as with TST, cannot differentiate LTBI from active TB disease. Laboratory sputum smear and culture is required.

V. Medical Management

A. Commonly Prescribed Drugs

- Commonly prescribed TB drugs are included in Table 60-6.

B. Directly Observed Therapy (DOT)

- Directly Observed Therapy (DOT) is key to TB management and consists of a trained observer dispensing and watching as the patient swallows the anti-TB medications.
- Benefits include:
  - High medication compliance.
  - Prevention of multidrug-resistant TB (MDR-TB) disease, which is more severe and difficult to treat.
- Use of telehealth technology via mobile phone, computer, or tablet have allowed for e-DOT (electronic DOT).[39]

C. Drug Resistance

- TB bacteria can become resistant (drugs are no longer effective in killing the bacteria).[34]
- **MDR-TB** is defined as resistance to at least two of the first-line (most preferred) drugs for treatment, isoniazid and rifampin.[34]
  - This requires use of more expensive second-line drugs for treatment.
- Preextensively drug-resistant TB (pre-XDR-TB) is resistant to rifampin and any fluoroquinolone.
- Extensively drug-resistant TB (XDR-TB) is defined as bacterial resistance to rifampin, any fluoroquinolone, and at least of bedaquiline or linezolid and is much harder to treat.

VI. Oral Manifestations

- TB infrequently appears in the oral cavity from pulmonary organisms in infected sputum brought to the mouth by coughing.[40]
- Lesions can be in several forms such as ulcers, nodules, tuberculomas, and periapical granulomas.[40]
  - Classic mucosal lesion: painful, deep, irregular ulcer on dorsum of the tongue as seen in **Figure 60-5**.
  - Lesions can also occur on palate, lips, buccal mucosa, and gingiva.
- A biopsy and laboratory culture of an oral lesion that reveals *M. tuberculosis* confirms a diagnosis of TB.
- Glandular swelling: cervical or submandibular lymph nodes infected with TB. Nodes may become enlarged.

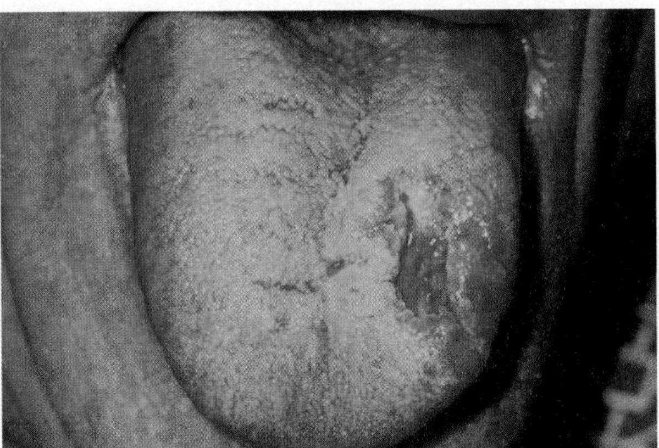

Figure 60-5 Oral Ulcer on Tongue Caused by *Mycobacterium tuberculosis*. The classic oral mucosal lesion is a painful, deep, irregular ulcer on the dorsum of the tongue.

Reproduced from United States Department of Veteran's Affairs. From DeLong L, Burkhart N. *General and Oral Pathology for Dental Hygienists*. Baltimore, MD: Lippincott Williams & Wilkins; 2008.

VII. Dental Hygiene Care

A. Implementation of Infection Control Measures

- Update medical history.
- Recognize signs and symptoms of TB as listed in Table 60-6.
- Consult the web resource for CDC guidelines on infection control and prevention of transmission of TB in healthcare settings.
- Create and routinely update written office/clinic protocols for[41]:
  - Educating and training staff.
  - Instrument reprocessing and operatory cleanup.
  - Appropriate PPE and management of aerosol producing procedures.
  - Identifying, managing, and referring patients with active TB disease.
  - Assessing, managing, and investigating dental staff with positive TST (PPD).

B. Management of Patients with Symptoms or History of TB

- Potential infectivity dictates decisions regarding whether to treat a patient or refer to a physician for medical clearance.
- Active TB disease
  - Do not treat in the dental office or any outpatient facility until after TB therapy is complete for elective treatment.[41]
    - Risk of infection is reduced after completion of 2 weeks of TB therapy.
  - Emergency treatment needs to be performed in a hospital with appropriate isolation, sterilization, and engineering controls such as a positive pressure.
- History of TB
  - Use caution, obtain history of disease and treatment duration, and discuss signs and symptoms of disease.
  - Consult with primary care provider before treatment to verify LTBI is present.
  - Also consult with the primary care provider if adequate treatment time/appropriate medical follow-up is unclear or patient presents with signs or symptoms of relapse.

Asthma

- Asthma is associated with airway hyperresponsiveness and chronic inflammation with recurrent episodes of **dyspnea**, coughing (particularly early in the morning or at night), wheezing, and chest tightness.[42,43]

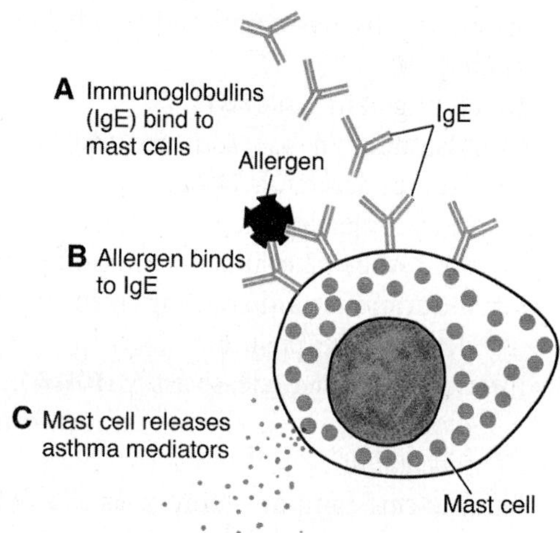

Figure 60-6 Steps of an Immunoglobulin E (IgE)-mediated Hypersensitivity Reaction. **A:** Initial exposure. On initial exposure to an allergen (dust, pollen), immunoglobulins (IgE) are produced and bind to mast cells. **B:** Subsequent exposure. On subsequent exposures, allergen binds to IgE on the mast cell. **C:** Mast cells respond by releasing asthma mediators (histamines, leukotrienes, prostaglandins). The asthma mediators cause bronchoconstriction, vasodilation, and mucus production, resulting in coughing, wheezing, and dyspnea.

I. Etiology

The exact cause of asthma is not completely understood, but the following play a role in the etiology[42,44]:

- Genetics may be responsible for 40% to 85% of susceptibility to asthma.
- Environment
  - Allergic sensitization such as exposure to indoor (e.g., mold, pets) and outdoor (e.g., pollen) allergens may increase risk of developing asthma 4- to 20-fold.
    - Steps of an immunoglobulin E (IgE)-mediated hypersensitivity reaction are shown in **Figure 60-6**.
  - Air pollution.
- Immunization
- *In utero* exposures such as prenatal exposure to tobacco smoke.
- Th2 immunity, which is related to the function of T-cells in humoral immunity and antibody production.

II. Asthma Attack

A. Triggers for Exacerbation of Asthma

- Intrinsic triggers[43,45]:
  - Viral respiratory infection is the most common trigger.
  - **Gastroesophageal reflux disease (GERD)**.

- Chronic rhinosinusitis.
- Emotional stress
- Extrinsic triggers[43,45]:
  - Environmental allergens.
  - Pollen, dust, animal dander.
- Drug- or food-induced[43,45]:
  - Aspirin or nonsteroidal anti-inflammatory drugs (NSAIDs).
  - Beta-blockers or ACE inhibitors
  - Nuts, shellfish, strawberries.
  - Sulfites.
  - Overuse of short-acting beta-2 agonist (SABA).
  - Inadequate inhaled corticosteroid (ICS) use.
- Exercise-induced[45]:
  - Physical activity.
  - Inhalation of cold air.

B. Signs and Symptoms of Severe or Worsening Asthma Attack

- An asthma attack is rapid worsening of asthma and can be life threatening. Classic signs and symptoms may include[45]:
  - Chest tightness, sense of suffocation.
  - Wheezing, coughing.
  - Shortness of breath.
  - Inability to complete a sentence in one breath.
  - **Tachypnea**.
  - **Tachycardia**.
- Life-threatening signs and symptoms[45]:
  - Confusion.
  - Cyanosis.
  - Ineffectiveness of **bronchodilator** to relieve dyspnea.
  - Bradycardia.

C. Prepare for Possible Emergency Care

- Recognize signs and symptoms early.
- Stop dental hygiene treatment.
- Rule out foreign-body obstruction.
- Position in upright position.[45]
- Administer two puffs of short-acting bronchodilator inhaler (preferably the patient's inhaler). Repeat bronchodilator as needed.[45]
- Assess ABCs (airway, breathing, and circulation).
- Administer supplemental oxygen.
- If the attack is not resolved, activate EMS (emergency medical services) and initiate emergency procedures. (See Chapter 9.)
- Assist with the administration of subcutaneous injection or inhalation of epinephrine.[45]
- Monitor vital signs and ABCs until EMS arrives.

III. Medical Management

A. Diagnosis

- Conduct physical examination and lung function assessment (spirometry).

B. Achieve and Maintain Asthma Control

- Assess and monitor asthma severity and asthma control.
- The National Asthma Education and Prevention Program classification is based on four levels of severity and frequency of symptoms as well as pulmonary function assessment (spirometry).[46]
  - Intermittent.
  - Persistent–mild.
  - Persistent–moderate.
  - Persistent–severe.
- Education: patients are advised to have an asthma action plan from the primary care provider explaining the process of disease, treatment options, and how to treat **exacerbations** (worsening of symptoms).
- Control of environmental factors (pollutants and allergens) and **comorbid** conditions that affect asthma (GERD, obesity, obstructive sleep apnea [OSA], rhinitis/sinusitis, stress/depression).
- Medications
  - Treatment is complex and for those with more severe asthma may involve multiple approaches for management.[43,46,47]
    - Inhaled and systemic corticosteroids reduce airway inflammation.
    - Beta agonists (short-acting, long-acting, and ultra-long-acting): relax bronchial smooth muscle.
    - Anticholinergics also relax bronchial smooth muscle.
    - Mast cell stabilizers: inhibit histamine release and reduce airway hyper responsiveness.
    - Leukotriene modifiers: prevent constriction of the bronchial tubes.
    - Methylxanthines: relax bronchial smooth muscle.
    - Immunomodulators: inhibit cytokine production.
- People with asthma are advised to get seasonal influenza vaccinations and may also benefit from immunotherapy (allergy injections).
- Asthma triggers: avoid drugs with known potential to trigger asthma:

    - Aspirin (use acetaminophen).
    - Sulfite-containing local anesthetic solution, such as epinephrine.
    - NSAIDs.
- Avoid drugs that decrease respiratory function, such as narcotics and barbiturates.
- Avoid harmful drug-to-drug interactions.
    - Macrolide antibiotics (such as erythromycin) if patient takes theophylline.
    - Erythromycin inhibits metabolism of theophylline, which can result in an increase in serum level and possible overdose.
    - Discontinue cimetidine 24 hours before intravenous sedation in patients taking theophylline.

IV. Oral Manifestations

- In children, there may be dentofacial deformities such as[48]:
    - Higher palatal vaults.
    - Greater overjet and posterior crossbite.
    - Increased anterior facial height.
- Increased caries risk due to xerostomia due to mouthbreathing and medications such as beta-2 agonist and corticosteroid inhalers.[45]
- Increase in GERD with use of beta-2 agonists and theophylline, which may contribute to enamel erosion.[49]
- Oral candidiasis may occur with high dosage or frequency of inhaled corticosteroids.[49]
- Evidence suggests an association between periodontal disease, particularly gingivitis, and asthma in adults.[50]

V. Dental Hygiene Care

- **Table 60-7** summarizes dental hygiene care before, during, and after treatment.

Chronic Obstructive Pulmonary Disease

- The term chronic obstructive pulmonary disease (COPD) is used to describe persistent respiratory symptoms that result in airflow limitations.[51-53]
- COPD is preventable, but once initiated it tends to be progressive and is not reversible.[53]
- Two of the most common forms of COPD are chronic bronchitis and emphysema.
    - Chronic bronchitis is defined as excessive respiratory tract mucus production sufficient to cause a cough, with expectoration (coughing up mucus) for at least 3 months of the year for 2 years or more.[54]
        - Obstruction caused by narrowing of small airways, increased sputum (phlegm), and mucus plugging.
        - Difficulty breathing present on **inspiration** (breathing in) and **expiration** (breathing out).
    - Emphysema is a small airway disease resulting in pronounced lung hyperinflation from large, dilated alveoli.[52,53]
        - Difficulty breathing only on expiration.

I. Etiology

- The primary etiology is inhaling tobacco smoke with occupational and environmental pollutants as contributing factors.[53]
    - Tobacco use accounts for 80% of COPD cases.[53]
- Genetic abnormalities of lung development may also predispose to COPD.[55]
- Asthma may be a risk for COPD.[55]
- History of severe respiratory disease in childhood.[55]
- Tuberculosis.[55]

II. Signs and Symptoms

- Chronic and progressive dyspnea.[55]
- Chronic cough is often the first symptom.[55]
- Persistent sputum production.[55]
- Wheezing and chest tightness.[55]
- In severe disease, individuals may experience fatigue, weight loss, and anorexia.[55]
- In chronic bronchitis, the patient may experience cyanosis, leading to the term "blue bloater."
- In emphysema, the term "pink puffer" has been used to describe the patient who purses their lips to forcibly expel air.

III. Medical Management

- Medical management depends on the symptoms and exacerbations and may include the following.[52,53]

A. Assess and Monitor Disease

- A thorough medical history and examination is essential to planning care.
- Confirm diagnosis with spirometry and severity of airflow obstruction.[52,55]

Table 60-7 Dental Hygiene Care for the Patient with Asthma[45,48]

Time	Dental Hygiene Care
Prior to Appointment	■ Remind the patient to bring inhaler (rescue drug) and/or other medications. ■ Schedule appointments at times when asthma attacks are less likely which may vary for each patient. ■ Schedule short appointments to minimize stress.
Examination	■ Assess control level: review medical history, frequency/severity of acute episodes, and triggering agents. ■ Questions to ask: in the past 2 weeks, how many times have you: • Had problems with coughing, wheezing, shortness of breath, or chest tightness during the day? • Awakened at night from sleep because of coughing or other asthma symptoms? • Awakened in the morning with asthma symptoms? • Had asthma symptoms that did not improve within 15 minutes of using inhaled medication? • Had symptoms while exercising or playing? ■ Reappoint if symptoms are not well controlled and consult with medical provider. ■ Review current medications used regularly as well as those used for acute asthma attacks and consult a current drug reference to assess potential oral implications and need to modify care plan. ■ Confirm all prescription medication has been taken as prescribed. ■ Assess for gastroesophageal reflux (GERD) and refer for follow up with a medical provider if suspected. ■ Minimize stress and maintain a calm environment. ■ Have bronchodilator and oxygen available. Consider using patient's bronchodilator as a preventive measure before the appointment in those with moderate to severe asthma. ■ Consultation with medical provider may be indicated if the patient is on corticosteroid to determine necessity of steroid replacement.
During patient care	■ Plan preventive care to address risk factors, which may include, but not be limited to: • Advise patient to rinse mouth with water after using inhaler to decrease oral candidiasis. • Use of at home fluorides to reduce caries risk. ■ Prevent triggering a hyperresponsive airway by properly placing cotton rolls, fluoride trays, and suction tip. ■ Avoid triggers. ■ Use local anesthetic without sulfites. ■ Fluoride treatment for all patients with asthma, especially those using inhalers. ■ If asthma attack occurs, stop treatment, and initiate management as described in previous section.
Posttreatment	■ Analgesic drug of choice is acetaminophen (aspirin or nonsteroidal anti-inflammatory drugs may trigger attack).

Data from Baghani E, Ouanounou A. The dental management of the asthmatic patients. *Spec Care Dentist.* 2021;41(3):309-318; Chhabra K, Sood S, Sharma N, Singh A, Nigam S. Dental management of pediatric patients with bronchial asthma. *Int J Clin Pediatr Dent.* 2021;14(5):715-718. doi:10.5005/jp-journals-10005-2024

B. Reduce Risk Factors

- Tobacco cessation.
- Reduction of exposure to environmental indoor/outdoor pollutants.
  - Examples: ozone and industrial air pollution, automobile emissions, household cleaning products.
- Vaccinations for influenza and pneumococcal disease.[55]
- Education on self-management.
- Evidence suggests an association between periodontal disease and COPD, but more research is needed to determine if periodontal therapy will reduce the risk for exacerbation.[56]
  - However, reducing the biofilm load with periodontal therapy has the potential to minimize the risk for aspiration of bacteria.

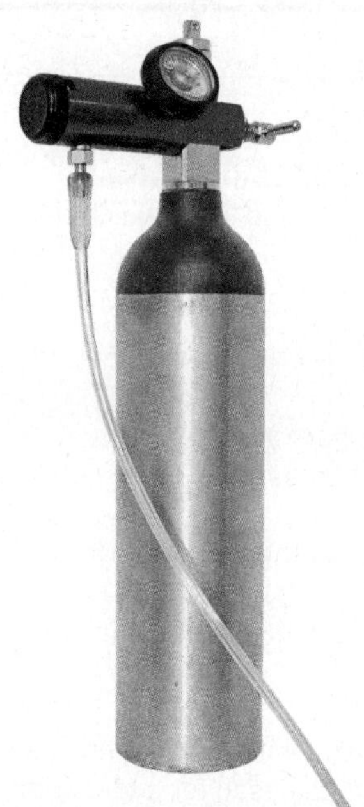

Figure 60-7 Portable Oxygen Tank. A patient who uses oxygen to improve breathing function may hold a portable unit during treatment.

C. COPD Treatment

- Initial pharmacologic treatment depends on the frequency of exacerbations and my include a single medication or dual therapy with the following[52]:
  - Inhaled corticosteroids (ICS) such as Pulmicort and Flovent.
  - Long-acting beta-agonist (LAMA) such as Arcapta or Serevent.
  - Long-acting muscarinic antagonist (LABA) such as Spiriva or Ellipta.
- If initial pharmacologic treatment is not successful in maintaining COPD, triple therapy may be initiated.
- Antibiotics for infectious exacerbations, but with caution to minimize risk of bacterial resistance development.[55]
- If pharmacologic therapy does not manage the COPD or has continued exacerbations, oxygen therapy may be considered and consists of two types (**Figure 60-7**):
  - Continuous flow: oxygen flows at a determined rate of liters per minute.
  - On demand: oxygen flows during inhalation only, extending the period of time between oxygen tank refills.
- Pulmonary rehabilitation, including a structured exercise program, may help relieve symptoms and improve quality of life.

IV. Oral Manifestations

- Oral candidiasis resulting from corticosteroid inhaler use.
- Drug-induced xerostomia.
- Oral manifestations related to tobacco use may also be present. (See Chapter 32.)
- More tooth loss is found in those with COPD.[57]

V. Dental Hygiene Care

- Carefully review the medical history and medications to determine whether a consultation is needed with the primary care provider.
- Identify patients who may experience exacerbation of symptoms under emotional stress.
- Carefully assess vital signs, particularly breathing.
- Chair positioning: an upright or semi-upright position may be necessary to facilitate breathing.
- Appointment length may need to be modified based on patient comfort and tolerance for treatment.
- Educate the patient about the oral–systemic link between periodontitis and COPD.
- Encourage tobacco cessation in patients who smoke. (See Chapter 32.)
- Educate patient about oral self-care to manage oral bacteria.
- Use antimicrobial preprocedural rinse to help reduce the bacterial load in aerosols.
- Minimize aerosols; it may be necessary to avoid the use of power-driven scalers and air polishers to minimize the risk for aspiration pneumonia.[58]
- Nitrous oxide–oxygen inhalation sedation: consult with the medical provider to ensure safety.
- Schedule continuing care based on the periodontal status and patient's ability to maintain adequate oral self-care.

Cystic Fibrosis

Cystic fibrosis (CF) is an autosomal recessive gene disorder. Both parents must carry the genetic mutation for the disease to be transmitted to their children.[59]

- CF is progressive and ultimately fatal.
- With intensive medical treatment and follow up, many people now live into adulthood.

I. Disease Characteristics

- The gene disorder affects the movement of salt and water in and out of epithelial cells in the respiratory tract and exocrine glands (respiratory, pancreas, gastrointestinal) and results in thickened secretions.

A. Respiratory Tract

- Clinical manifestations of the lungs/airway include[60,61]:
  - Cough with sputum production.
  - Chronic sinusitis.
  - Recurrent bacterial and fungal lung infection, such as bronchitis or pneumonia.
  - Pneumothorax.
  - Hemoptysis.
  - May lead to respiratory failure.

B. Pancreas

- Thick mucus clogs pancreatic ducts, resulting in pancreatic insufficiency.[60,61]
  - Clogged ducts prevent the release of pancreatic enzymes into the intestinal tract that break down fats, carbohydrates, and proteins, leading to malnutrition and fat-soluble vitamin deficiency.
- Pancreatitis.[60,61]
- CF-related diabetes.[60,61]

C. Gastrointestinal Tract

- Malabsorption, which may result in failure to thrive in children.[60,61]
- Intestinal obstruction.[60,61]
- Increased gastroesophageal reflux.[61]

D. Other

- Fatty liver, cirrhosis, and liver failure.[60,61]
- Clubbed fingers.[61]
- Arthritis.[61]
- Osteopenia/osteoporosis due to vitamin D deficiency.[60,61]
- Peripheral neuropathy and hemolysis due to vitamin E deficiency.[61]
- Risk for dehydration due to electrolyte imbalances.[60,61]
- Mental health challenges such as depression and anxiety.[61]

II. Medical Management

- CF is a multiorgan system disease, but the core of treatment revolves around nutrition support and management of the respiratory system.

A. Nutrition Support

- Pancreatic enzyme replacement therapy (PERT) such as Creon is taken with each meal and snack.
  - PERT includes lipase, protease, amylase, and a bicarbonate buffer to aid in breakdown and absorption of nutrients.
- Traditionally, CF patients may be advised to consume a high-calorie, high-protein, high-fat diet.[62]
  - However, patients may choose high cariogenic, energy-dense foods like sweets and sweetened beverages.[63]
- Due to increased life span, overweight and obesity is emerging as an issue, so it is important to encourage lifestyle modifications like regular physical activity and consultation with a registered dietitian nutritionist (RDN).[62]
- Those with CF-related diabetes will need referral to an RDN or certified diabetes educator (CDE) to aid in managing their diet; this is beyond the scope of a dental hygienist.

B. Pulmonary Therapy

- Antibiotics, including inhalation solution: tobramycin sulfate nebulizer and low-dose azithromycin.[61]
- Bronchodilators and anti-inflammatory agents.
- Airway clearance therapy (ACT) includes[61]:
  - Chest physiotherapy with chest percussion and having the patient in a variety of positions to allow mucus to drain from the airway.
  - Positive expiratory pressure devices.

III. Oral Manifestations

- Enamel defects in permanent dentition.[63]
- Evidence is inconsistent for the following and needs more research[63]:
  - Possible reduced salivary flow and buffering capacity.
  - Caries incidence.
  - Gingival bleeding and periodontal disease appears lower in CF, possibly due the chronic use of antibiotics and anti-inflammatory medications.

IV. Dental Hygiene Care

- Patient education on oral-self care to manage dental biofilm.
- Adapt chair positioning to aid breathing, possibly in a semi-supine position.
- Preprocedure chlorhexidine rinse to reduce bacterial load.[64]
- Avoid use of rubber dam.
- Minimize or avoid AGPs to reduce risk of aspiration pneumonia.[63,64]

- Management of aerosols during AGPs, such as use of high-volume evacuation (HVE).
- Regular continuing care.

Sleep-Related Breathing Disorders

- There are three categories of sleep-related breathing disorders (SRBDs)[65]:
  - OSA includes pediatric and adult types.
  - Central sleep apnea syndromes.
  - Sleep-related hypoventilation disorders.
- OSA prevalence is about 27% in men and 9% in women aged 30–39, but increases to 43% in men and 28% in women aged 50 to 70 years.[66]

I. Etiology of Obstructive Sleep Apnea

- Repetitive partial or complete collapse of the upper airway during sleep causing reduction or cessation of airflow.[66]
  - Fat deposition as a result in overweight or obesity can result in a narrow upper airway.[66]
- In children, risk factors include tonsillar or adenoid hypertrophy, craniofacial abnormalities, neuromuscular disorders, and obesity.[67]

II. Signs and Symptoms

- Common signs and symptoms may include[66]:
  - Interruption in sleep patterns with excessive sleeplessness and fatigue.
  - Nighttime awakening with or without gasping or choking.
  - Chronic snoring.
  - Witnessed apnea (when a partner witnesses the patient stop breathing), which may be an interruption in snoring followed by a snort.
  - Chronic morning headache.
  - Nocturnal gastroesophageal reflux.

III. Medical Management

- Treatment may include behavioral interventions, medical devices, and surgery as described later.[66]

A. Behavior Interventions

- Weight loss.
- Physical activity.
- Adjustment of sleep position.

B. Medical Devices

- Positive airway pressure (PAP) is the primary therapy for those with OSA.
  - There are several types of PAP devices, including[68]:
    - Continuous positive airway pressure (CPAP) machine (shown in **Figure 60-8**) increases air pressure in the throat so that the airway does not collapse when inhaling.
    - Bilevel positive airway pressure (BPAP) which adjusts the pressure for inspiratory and expiratory pressure based on the patient's respiratory efforts.
    - Adaptive seroventilation (ASV) is more of an on-demand system for pressure support of respiration.
- Oral appliance therapy (OAT) is an effective treatment for mild-to-moderate sleep apnea and for severe sleep apnea when a CPAP is not tolerated by the patient.[29,30]
  - The mandibular repositioning device shown in **Figure 60-9** is the most common form of oral appliance used in clinical practice.
  - The mandibular advancement splint moves the mandible slightly forward and tightens the soft tissue and muscles of the upper airway to prevent obstruction of the airway during sleep.[30-32]
  - Contraindications to OAT include periodontal disease, temporomandibular disorders, and insufficient number of teeth.[33]

C. Surgery

- Uvulopalatopharyngoplasty: resection of the uvula and part of the soft palate.
- Maxillomandibular advancement: resection of bone from the maxilla and mandible.

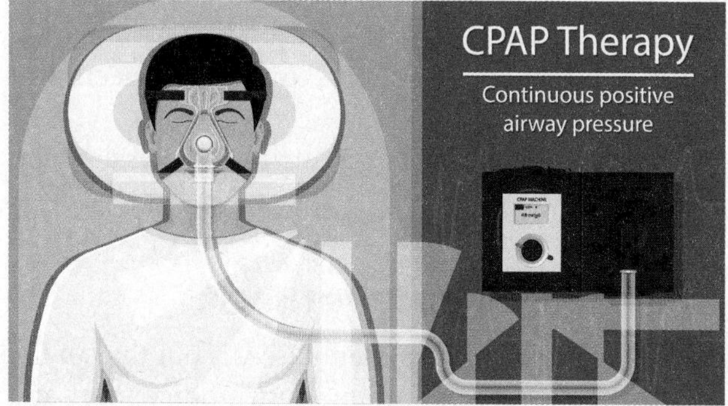

Figure 60-8 Continuous Positive Airway Pressure (CPAP). This machine is attached by a hose to the nose mask that is held in place while sleeping by straps. The CPAP machine increases the air pressure in the throat so the airway does not collapse when inhaling.

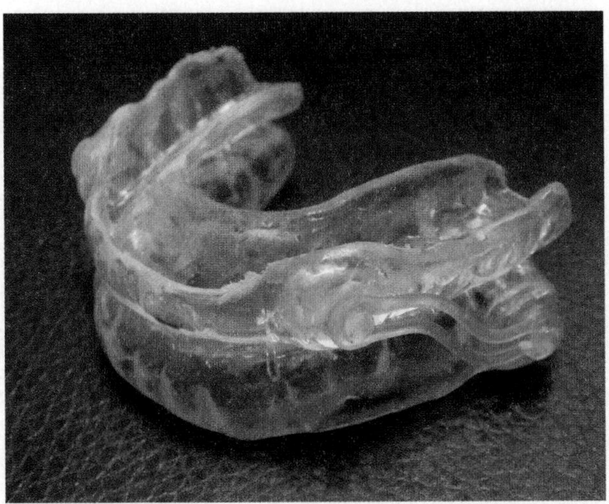

Figure 60-9 Mandibular Advancement Splint (MAS). A splint that moves the mandible slightly forward that tightens the soft tissue and muscles of the upper airway to prevent obstruction of the airway during sleep.

IV. Oral Manifestations

- Craniofacial abnormalities in children.[67]
- Enlarged tonsils.[67]
- Mouth breathing.[69]
- Poor oral hygiene.[69]
- More dental caries in children.[69,70]
- Periodontitis with increases in bleeding on probing, pocket depths, and clinical attachment loss.[70-72]

V. Dental Hygiene Care

- Careful medical history review and consider screening for those at risk or who report symptoms of OSA.[73]
  - There are a number of instruments for OSA screening. The STOP-BANG questionnaire (SBQ; www.stopbang.ca/osa/screening.php) is an easy approach to screen and identify those needing referral for further evaluation.[74]
- Head and neck examination for abnormalities, particularly in children.
- Education for management of dental biofilm and other risk factors for caries and periodontal disease.
- Preventive services should address risk factors for oral disease.
- For patients with a mandibular positioning device, they should be reminded to bring it to each continuing care appointment for evaluation.
- Continuing care needs to be individualized based on the patient's needs and level of oral disease.
- Patients who have had surgical interventions such as maxillomandibular procedures should be encouraged to follow the advice in Chapter 56.

Documentation

Include in the patient's permanent record:

- Alerts for dental personnel to the possibility of disease transmission or a medical emergency due to medical condition or allergy.
  - Paper records: to protect patient confidentiality, place the medical alert box inside front cover.
  - Electronic records: insert in a prominent area.
- Medical consultation: file written reports and document telephone conversations.
- Patient's current health status: especially related to signs and symptoms of respiratory disease, known allergies, current medications.
- Vital signs: including pulse oximetry.
- Oral examination: with attention to oral cancer screening and periodontal evaluation.
- Patient education: especially issues about dry mouth, tobacco cessation, and medication compliance.
- Changes in respiratory signs and symptoms during treatment and interventions performed.
- A sample progress note for a patient with a positive for tuberculosis is shown in **Box 60-1**.

Box 60-1 Example Documentation: Patient with a Positive TST

- **S**—A 36-year-old patient presents for new patient examination. Patient reports she had a positive test for tuberculosis 1 year ago. She states that she was treated and is not contagious.
- **O**—Called patient's physician (Dr. Roberts). Spoke with nurse (Becky) who provided verbal summary and will also send written report to include in the patient's record. Patient successfully completed regime of isoniazid for 9 months. Latest medical examination findings:
  - Chest radiograph—negative
  - Sputum smear and culture—negative
  - Signs and symptoms—none
- **A**—No signs of active TB disease; patient may receive dental treatment without restriction.
- **P**—Proceeded with patient assessment and dental prophylaxis.

Signed: ____________________, RDH
Date: ________________

Factors to Teach the Patient

- Attention to respiratory hygiene and cough etiquette.
- The need for frequent handwashing to help prevent transmission of respiratory disease.
- The need for thorough daily cleaning and drying of toothbrushes to help prevent spread of infections.
- Importance of using a new toothbrush and cleaning dentures/orthodontic appliances after bacterial infections to decrease possibility of reinfection.
- For elderly patients and those with chronic respiratory or cardiovascular disease, diabetes, or immunosuppressed conditions, the need for pneumonia and seasonal influenza immunization.
- To improve compliance in taking all prescribed medications, maintain a medication list and use pill containers that open easily and are labeled with large type.
- Options to combat medication-induced dry mouth.
- Educate the patient to help avoid antibiotic resistance.

References

1. Gomes-Filho IS, Cruz SS da, Trindade SC, et al. Periodontitis and respiratory diseases: a systematic review with meta-analysis. *Oral Dis*. 2020;26(2):439-446.
2. Patwa A, Shah A. Anatomy and physiology of respiratory system relevant to anaesthesia. *Indian J Anaesth*. 2015;59(9):533-541.
3. Rauniyar NK, Pujari S, Shrestha P. Study of oxygen saturation by pulse oximetry and arterial blood gas in ICU patients: a descriptive cross-sectional study. *J Nepal Med Assoc*. 2020;58(230):789-793.
4. Minnesota Department of Health. Oxygen levels, pulse oximeters, and COVID-19. https://www.health.state.mn.us/diseases/coronavirus/pulseoximeter.html. Accessed March 31, 2022.
5. Centers for Disease Control and Prevention. National Center for Immunization and Respiratory Diseases (NCIRD). Published March 4, 2022. https://www.cdc.gov/ncird/overview/websites.html. Accessed March 31, 2022.
6. World Health Organization. Chronic respiratory diseases. https://www.who.int/westernpacific/health-topics/chronic-respiratory-diseases. Accessed March 31, 2022.
7. Centers for Disease Control and Prevention. Tuberculosis (TB): Basic TB facts. Published June 19, 2019. https://www.cdc.gov/tb/topic/basics/default.htm. Accessed March 31, 2022.
8. Turcios NL. Cystic fibrosis lung disease: an overview. *Respir Care*. 2020;65(2):233-251.
9. Fried M. Nonallergic Rhinitis. *Merck Manuals Professional Edition*. Published December 2021. https://www.merckmanuals.com/professional/ear,-nose,-and-throat-disorders/nose-and-paranasal-sinus-disorders/nonallergic-rhinitis. Accessed March 31, 2022.
10. Pappas DE. The common cold. In: *Principles and Practice of Pediatric Infectious Diseases*. 2018:199-202.e1.
11. Delves PJ. Allergic rhinitis. *Merck Manuals Professional Edition*. https://www.merckmanuals.com/professional/immunology-allergic-disorders/allergic,-autoimmune,-and-other-hypersensitivity-disorders/allergic-rhinitis?query=allergic%20rhinitis. Accessed March 31, 2022.
12. Hussein H, Mensah RK, Brown RS. Diagnosis and management of oral allergy syndrome, the itchy tongue allergic reaction. *Compend Contin Educ Dent*. 2019;40(8):502-506.
13. Fried M. Sinusitis. *Merck Manuals Professional Edition*. Published December 2021. https://www.merckmanuals.com/professional/ear,-nose,-and-throat-disorders/nose-and-paranasal-sinus-disorders/sinusitis?query=sinusitis. Accessed March 31, 2022.
14. Cheng AG. Tonsillopharyngitis. *Merck Manuals Professional Edition*. Published March 2022. https://www.merckmanuals.com/professional/ear,-nose,-and-throat-disorders/oral-and-pharyngeal-disorders/tonsillopharyngitis?query=pharyngitis. Accessed March 31, 2022.
15. Tesini BL. Influenza. *Merck Manuals Professional Edition*. Published September 2021. https://www.merckmanuals.com/professional/infectious-diseases/respiratory-viruses/influenza?query=influenza. Accessed March 31, 2022.
16. Thomas M, Bomar PA. Upper respiratory tract infection. *Stat Pearls*. 2022. http://www.ncbi.nlm.nih.gov/books/NBK532961/. Accessed March 31, 2022.
17. Centers for Disease Control and Prevention. Influenza vaccination coverage among health care personnel — United States, 2018–19 influenza season. Published September 24, 2019. https://www.cdc.gov/flu/fluvaxview/hcp-coverage_1819estimates.htm. Accessed March 31, 2022.
18. Centers for Disease Control and Pevention (CDC). Respiratory hygiene/cough etiquette in healthcare settings. Published April 17, 2019. https://www.cdc.gov/flu/professionals/infectioncontrol/resphygiene.htm. Accessed September 17, 2021.
19. American Dental Association. CDC updates COVID-19 guidance for health care personnel. Published January 4, 2022. https://www.ada.org/publications/ada-news/2022/january/cdc-updates-covid-19-guidance-for-health-care-personnel. Accessed March 31, 2022.
20. American Dental Association. Antibiotic prophylaxis prior to dental procedures. Published November 8, 2021. https://www.ada.org/resources/research/science-and-research-institute/oral-health-topics/antibiotic-prophylaxis. Accessed December 24, 2021.
21. Sethi S. Acute bronchitis - pulmonary disorders. *Merck Manuals Professional Edition*. Published July 2021. https://www.merckmanuals.com/professional/pulmonary-disorders

/acute-bronchitis/acute-bronchitis?query=acute%20bronchitis. Accessed March 31, 2022.

22. Tesini BL. COVID-19. *Merck Manuals Professional Edition*. Published March 2022. https://www.merckmanuals.com/professional/infectious-diseases/covid-19/covid-19?query=COVID-19. Accessed March 31, 2022.
23. Wiersinga WJ, Rhodes A, Cheng AC, Peacock SJ, Prescott HC. Pathophysiology, transmission, diagnosis, and treatment of coronavirus disease 2019 (COVID-19): a review. *JAMA*. 2020;324(8):782-793.
24. Forchette L, Sebastian W, Liu T. A comprehensive review of COVID-19 virology, vaccines, variants, and therapeutics. *Curr Med Sci*. 2021;41(6):1037-1051.
25. La Rosa GRM, Libra M, De Pasquale R, Ferlito S, Pedullà E. Association of viral infections with oral cavity lesions: role of SARS-CoV-2 infection. *Front Med*. 2021;7:571214.
26. Crook H, Raza S, Nowell J, Young M, Edison P. Long covid-mechanisms, risk factors, and management. *BMJ*. 2021; 374:n1648.
27. Chakraborty T, Jamal RF, Battineni G, Teja KV, Marto CM, Spagnuolo G. A review of prolonged post-COVID-19 symptoms and their implications on dental management. *Int J Environ Res Public Health*. 2021;18(10):5131.
28. Torres A, Cilloniz C, Niederman MS, et al. Pneumonia. *Nat Rev Dis Primers*. 2021;7(1):25.
29. Sethi S. Overview of pneumonia. *Merck Manuals Professional Edition*. Published December 2020. https://www.merckmanuals.com/professional/pulmonary-disorders/pneumonia/overview-of-pneumonia?query=pneumonia. Accessed March 31, 2022.
30. Kouanda B, Sattar Z, Geraghty P. Periodontal diseases: major exacerbators of pulmonary diseases? *Pulm Med*. 2021;2021:4712406.
31. Zhao T, Wu X, Zhang Q, Li C, Worthington HV, Hua F. Oral hygiene care for critically ill patients to prevent ventilator-associated pneumonia. *Cochrane Database Syst Rev*. 2020;12:CD008367.
32. Barnes CM. Dental hygiene intervention to prevent nosocomial pneumonias. *J Evid Based Dent Pract*. 2014;14 Suppl:103-114.
33. Filardo TD. Tuberculosis — United States, 2021. *Morb Mortal Wkly Rep*. 2022;71.
34. World Health Organization. Global Tuberculosis Report 2021. Published October 14, 2021. https://www.who.int/teams/global-tuberculosis-programme/tb-reports/global-tuberculosis-report-2021. Accessed April 7, 2022.
35. Duarte R, Lönnroth K, Carvalho C, et al. Tuberculosis, social determinants and co-morbidities (including HIV). *Pulmonology*. 2018;24(2):115-119.
36. Brett K, Dulong C, Severn M. *Treatment of Tuberculosis: A Review of Guidelines*. Canadian Agency for Drugs and Technologies in Health; 2020.
37. Sterling TR, Njie G, Zenner D, et al. Guidelines for the treatment of latent tuberculosis infection: recommendations from the National Tuberculosis Controllers Association and CDC, 2020. *MMWR Recomm Rep*. 2020;69(1):1-11.
38. National Tuberculosis Controllers Association. Testing and Treatment of Latent Tuberculosis in the United States: Clinical recommendations. Published online February 2021. https://www.tbcontrollers.org/docs/resources/tb-infection/LTBI_Clinical_Recommendations_Version_002052021.pdf. Accessed April 7, 2022.
39. Centers for Disease Control and Prevention. Electronic directly observed therapy for active TB disease. Published February 15, 2022. https://www.cdc.gov/nchhstp/highimpactprevention/promising-hip-intervention.html. Accessed April 7, 2022.
40. Jain P, Jain I. Oral manifestations of tuberculosis: step towards early diagnosis. *J Clin Diagn Res*. 2014;8(12):ZE18-ZE21.
41. Clough S, Shaw A, Morgan C. Tuberculosis and oral health-care provision. *Br Dent J*. 2018;224(12):931-936.
42. Stern J, Pier J, Litonjua AA. Asthma epidemiology and risk factors. *Semin Immunopathol*. 2020;42(1):5-15.
43. Reddel HK, Bacharier LB, Bateman ED, et al. Global initiative for asthma strategy 2021: executive summary and rationale for key changes. *Am J Respir Crit Care Med*. 2022;205(1):17-35.
44. Yang IV, Lozupone CA, Schwartz DA. The environment, the epigenome, and asthma. *J Allergy Clin Immunol*. 2017;140(1):14-23.
45. Baghani E, Ouanounou A. The dental management of the asthmatic patients. *Spec Care Dentist*. 2021;41(3):309-318.
46. US Department of Health and Human Services, National Heart, Lung, and Blood Institute. *2020 Focused Updates to the Asthma Management Guidelines: A Report from the National Asthma Education and Prevention Program Coordinating Committee Expert Panel Working Group*. National Heart, Lung, and Blood Institute; 2020:322. https://www.nhlbi.nih.gov/health-topics/all-publications-and-resources/2020-focused-updates-asthma-management-guidelines. Accessed April 7, 2022.
47. Ortega VE, Izquierdo M. Drug Treatment of asthma - pulmonary disorders. *Merck Manuals Professional Edition*. Published March 2022. https://www.merckmanuals.com/professional/pulmonary-disorders/asthma-and-related-disorders/drug-treatment-of-asthma. Accessed April 10, 2022.
48. Chhabra K, Sood S, Sharma N, Singh A, Nigam S. Dental management of pediatric patients with bronchial asthma. *Int J Clin Pediatr Dent*. 2021;14(5):715-718.
49. Gani F, Caminati M, Bellavia F, et al. Oral health in asthmatic patients: a review : asthma and its therapy may impact on oral health. *Clin Mol Allergy*. 2020;18(1):22.
50. Ferreira MKM, Ferreira R de O, Castro MML, et al. Is there an association between asthma and periodontal disease among adults? Systematic review and meta-analysis. *Life Sciences*. 2019;223:74-87.
51. Nici L, Mammen MJ, Charbek E, et al. Pharmacologic management of chronic obstructive pulmonary disease. An official American Thoracic Society clinical practice guideline. *Am J Respir Crit Care Med*. 2020;201(9):e56-e69.
52. Singh D, Agusti A, Anzueto A, et al. Global strategy for the diagnosis, management, and prevention of chronic obstructive lung disease: the gold science committee report 2019. *Eur Respir J*. 2019;53(5):1900164.
53. Department of Veterans Affairs, Department of Defense. *VA/DoD Clinical Practice Guideline for the Management of Chronic Obstructive Pulmonary Disease*. Department of Veterans Affairs; 2021:94. https://www.healthquality.va.gov/guidelines/CD/copd/VADoDCOPDCPGFinal508.pdf. Accessed April 10, 2022.
54. Corlateanu A, Mendez Y, Wang Y, et al. Chronic obstructive pulmonary disease and phenotypes: a state-of-the-art. *Pulmonology*. 2020;26(2):95-100.
55. Vogelmeier CF, Criner GJ, Martinez FJ, et al. Global strategy for the diagnosis, management and prevention of chronic obstructive lung disease 2017 report: GOLD executive summary. *Respirology*. 2017;22(3):575-601.
56. Apessos I, Voulgaris A, Agrafiotis M, Andreadis D, Steiropoulos P. Effect of periodontal therapy on COPD outcomes: a systematic review. *BMC Pulm Med*. 2021;21(1):92.

57. Dwibedi N, Wiener RC, Findley PA, Shen C, Sambamoorthi U. Asthma, chronic obstructive pulmonary disease, tooth loss, and edentulism among adults in the United States: 2016 Behavioral Risk Factor Surveillance System survey. *J Am Dent Assoc*. 2020;151(10):735-744.e1.
58. Devlin J. Patients with chronic obstructive pulmonary disease: management considerations for the dental team. *Br Dent J*. 2014;217(5):235-237.
59. De Boeck K. Cystic fibrosis in the year 2020: a disease with a new face. *Acta Paediatr*. 2020;109(5):893-899.
60. Shteinberg M, Haq IJ, Polineni D, Davies JC. Cystic fibrosis. *Lancet*. 2021;397(10290):2195-2211.
61. Goetz D, Ren CL. Review of cystic fibrosis. *Pediatric Annals*. 2019;48(4):154-161.
62. Bailey J, Krick S, Fontaine KR. The changing landscape of nutrition in cystic fibrosis: the emergence of overweight and obesity. *Nutrients*. 2022;14(6):1216.
63. Pawlaczyk-Kamieńska T, Borysewicz-Lewicka M, Śniatała R, Batura-Gabryel H, Cofta S. Dental and periodontal manifestations in patients with cystic fibrosis - a systematic review. *J Cystic Fibrosis*. 2019;18(6):762-771.
64. Koletsi D, Belibasakis GN, Eliades T. Interventions to reduce aerosolized microbes in dental practice: a systematic review with network meta-analysis of randomized controlled trials. *J Dent Res*. 2020;99(11):1228-1238.
65. Sateia MJ. International Classification of Sleep Disorders-Third Edition. *Chest*. 2014;146(5):1387-1394.
66. Gottlieb DJ, Punjabi NM. Diagnosis and management of obstructive sleep apnea: a review. *JAMA*. 2020;323(14):1389-1400.
67. Xu Z, Wu Y, Tai J, et al. Risk factors of obstructive sleep apnea syndrome in children. *J Otolaryngol Head Neck Surg*. 2020;49(1):11.
68. Selim B, Ramar K. Sleep-related breathing disorders: when CPAP is not enough. *Neurotherapeutics*. 2021;18(1):81-90.
69. Davidovich E, Hevroni A, Gadassi LT, Spierer-Weil A, Yitschaky O, Polak D. Dental, oral pH, orthodontic and salivary values in children with obstructive sleep apnea. *Clin Oral Investig*. 2022;26(3):2503-2511.
70. Tamasas B, Nelson T, Chen M. Oral health and oral health-related quality of life in children with obstructive sleep apnea. *J Clin Sleep Med*. 2019;15(3):445-452.
71. Mukherjee S, Galgali SR. Obstructive sleep apnea and periodontitis: a cross-sectional study. *Indian J Dent Res*. 2021;32(1):44-50.
72. Stazić P, Roguljić M, Đogaš Z, et al. Periodontitis severity in obstructive sleep apnea patients. *Clin Oral Investig*. 2022;26(1):407-415.
73. Lavigne GJ, Herrero Babiloni A, Beetz G, et al. Critical issues in dental and medical management of obstructive sleep apnea. *J Dent Res*. 2020;99(1):26-35.
74. Chiu HY, Chen PY, Chuang LP, et al. Diagnostic accuracy of the Berlin questionnaire, STOP-BANG, STOP, and Epworth sleepiness scale in detecting obstructive sleep apnea: a bivariate meta-analysis. *Sleep Med Rev*. 2017;36:57-70.

CHAPTER 61

The Patient with Cardiovascular Disease

Linda D. Boyd, RDH, RD, EdD
Dianne Smallidge, RDH, EdD

CHAPTER OUTLINE

DOCUMENTATION

FACTORS TO TEACH THE PATIENT

REFERENCES

LEARNING OBJECTIVES

After studying this chapter, the student will be able to:

1. Identify the cardiovascular conditions that may be encountered in patients seeking oral health care.
2. Discuss the etiology, symptoms, and risk factors associated with cardiovascular conditions.
3. Discuss the impact of cardiovascular diseases on the oral cavity and their relationship to oral health.
4. Plan dental hygiene treatment modifications for the patient with cardiovascular disease.

Introduction

Cardiovascular disease (CVD) includes conditions and diseases affecting the heart and blood vessels.

- Patients with cardiovascular conditions are encountered frequently in a dental office or clinic and may be from any age group, although the highest incidence is among older people.
- Although a causal relationship between periodontal disease and **coronary heart disease** (CHD) or CVD has not been proven, current data suggest the risk for CVD is modestly higher in those with periodontal disease, suggesting it may be a marker for CHD risk.[1,2]
- Dental hygienists need to take responsibility to inform patients of the significant relationship between oral and systemic health and the related need for maintenance of healthy oral tissues and prevention of periodontal disease.
- The major CVDs are included in this chapter, with their principal symptoms and treatments as well as applications for dental hygiene care.
- Emerging evidence suggests 20% to 30% of those who had COVID-19 (SARS-CoV-2) may have myocardial injury and arrhythmias, so these patients should be questioned about any possible cardiovascular effects of the disease.[3]

Classification

- Anatomic classification
  - Diseases of the heart: pericardium, **myocardium**, endocardium, and heart valves.
  - Diseases of the blood vessels and peripheral circulation.
- Etiologic classification
  - Congenital anomalies.
  - **Atherosclerosis**, hypertension.
  - Infectious agents, immunologic mechanisms.

Infective Endocarditis

- Infective endocarditis (IE) is a microbial infection of the heart valves or endocardium with a high mortality rate.

I. Description

- IE is a serious disease, the prognosis of which depends on the degree of cardiac damage, the valves involved, duration of the infection, and treatment.
  - IE is characterized by the formation of bacterial vegetations on the heart valves or surface of the heart lining (endocardium).
  - When IE develops, it directly affects the function of the heart.
- Incidence of IE is 15 per 100,000.[4]

II. Etiology

- Microorganisms involved may include:[4,5]
  - *Staphylococcus aureus* followed by *Streptococcus viridans* are responsible for IE in most cases.
  - As yeast, fungi, and viruses have been implicated, the choice of the name "infective" endocarditis is more inclusive than "bacterial" endocarditis.
  - Incidence related to dental procedures: the majority of IE cases related to oral microflora are random bacteremias resulting from routine daily activities. An exceedingly small number of cases are believed to result from dental procedures.
    - Recent research suggests no increase in the incidence of IE in North America since the changes in the antibiotic prophylaxis guidelines were made by the American Heart Association in 2007.[6]

- Risk factors[5]
  - Preexisting cardiac abnormalities: bacteria collect on the endocardial (valvular) surface during bacteremia.
  - Prosthetic (artificial) heart valve or implanted cardiac device: there is an increased number of patients who have had valve replacement surgery who are susceptible. Patients who have had prosthetic valve replacements have a risk of developing prosthetic valve endocarditis.
  - History of previous endocarditis.
  - Chronic hemodialysis.
  - Intravenous drug abuse: infected material is injected directly into the bloodstream by contaminated needles. Intravenous drug abusers are at high risk for endocarditis.
  - Comorbidities such as hypertension and poorly controlled diabetes.
- Precipitating factors
  - Self-induced bacteremia: in the oral cavity, self-induced bacteremia may result from eating, bruxism, chewing gum, or any activity that can force bacteria through the wall of a diseased sulcus or pocket.
    - Toothbrushing and flossing for oral hygiene can also cause self-induced transient bacteremia.[7-10]
  - Infection at portals of entry: infections at sites where microorganisms may enter the circulating blood provide a constant source of potentially infectious microorganisms.
    - In the oral cavity, organisms enter the blood by way of periodontal and gingival pockets.
    - An open area of infection, such as an ulcer caused by an ill-fitting denture, may also provide a site of entry.
  - Trauma to tissues by instrumentation: a bacteremia can be created during general or oral surgery, endodontic procedures, periodontal therapy, scaling, and any therapy that results in bleeding.

III. Disease Process

- Transient bacteremia initiated[10]
  - Trauma to a mucosal surface such as the gingival sulcus during instrumentation releases bacteria into the bloodstream.
  - Ease of entry of organisms directly relates to the severity of tissue trauma, quantity of bacterial biofilm, and the severity of inflammation or infection such as periodontitis.
- Bacterial adherence[10]
  - Circulating microorganisms attach to a damaged heart valve, prosthetic valve, or other susceptible area on the endocardium.
- Proliferation of bacteria[10]
  - Microorganisms proliferate to form vegetative lesions containing masses of plasma cells, fibrin, and bacteria.
  - Heart valve becomes inflamed, and function is diminished.
  - Clumps of microorganisms (emboli) may break off and spread by way of the general circulation (**embolism**); complications result.
- Clinical course[11,12]
  - Acute IE develops suddenly and can be life threatening. Subacute IE develops gradually over weeks or months.
  - Severe symptoms of fever, loss of appetite and weight loss, weakness, **arthralgia**, and heart **murmurs** require hospitalization. Diagnosis is based on symptoms, **echocardiography**, blood cell count, and positive blood cultures.
  - Complications may lead to susceptibility to reinfection with IE, congestive heart failure (CHF), and cerebrovascular disease.

IV. Prevention

To prevent IE from dental and dental hygiene treatment, the following need to be addressed:

- Patient history
  - Special content: specific questions need to be directed to elicit any history of congenital heart defects, cardiac transplant, presence of prosthetic valves, acquired valvular defects, or previous episode of IE.
  - Consultation with patient's primary care provider: consultation is necessary for all patients with a history of heart defects and any other conditions suggesting the need for prophylactic antibiotic premedication.
  - Withhold instrumentation: the use of a probe or explorer subgingivally during assessment of the patient should be delayed until the medical clearance is obtained for high-risk individuals.
- Prophylactic antibiotic premedication
  - There exists no conclusive evidence that confirms the effectiveness or ineffectiveness of antibiotic premedication for the prevention of IE.[6,10,12]
  - Recommended regimens: follow the current recommendations of the American Heart Association.[13]

    - When antibiotic prophylaxis is required, verify the antibiotic was taken as prescribed. In the patient record, document the name of the antibiotic, time, and dosage taken by the patient.
    - Specific information can be found in Chapter 11.
- Dental hygiene care
    - Oral health: prevention and management of oral disease is necessary for each patient susceptible to IE.[14]
    - Education: instruction in oral self-care such as brushing and interdental cleaning at initial appointments is essential to reduce the bacterial load.
    - Sequence of treatment: biofilm removal instruction precedes instrumentation for scaling to bring the tissues to a healthy state. The more severe the gingival or periodontal inflammation, the higher the risk of bacteremia during and following instrumentation.
    - Instrumentation: reduce the microbial population about the teeth and on the oral mucosa prior to instrumentation by having the patient brush, floss, and rinse thoroughly with an antimicrobial mouth rinse such as 0.12% chlorhexidine.

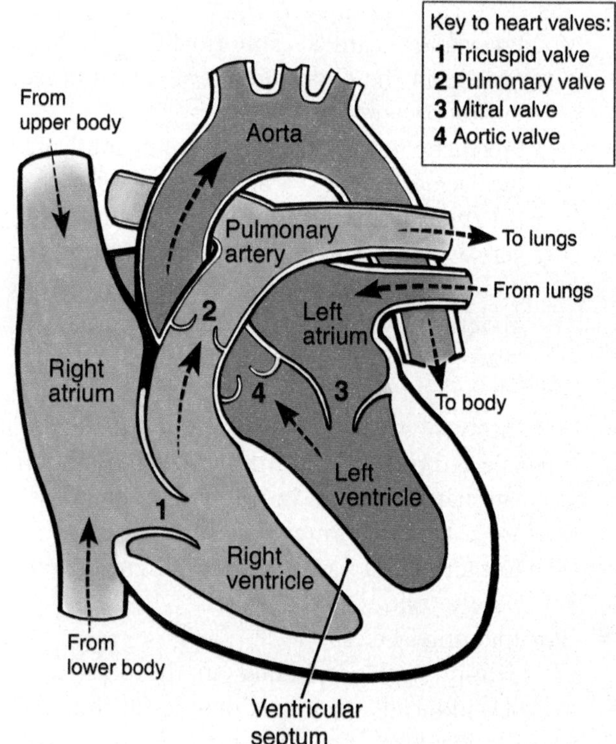

Figure 61-1 The Normal Heart. The major vessels and the location of the tricuspid, pulmonary, aortic, and mitral valves are shown.

Congenital Heart Diseases

I. The Normal Healthy Heart

- A diagram of the normal heart is shown in **Figure 61-1** to provide a comparison with the anatomic changes that may appear in a defective heart.
- In the healthy heart, the blood flows in one direction as each chamber contracts, with the valves acting as trap doors that snap shut after each contraction to prevent backflow of blood.
- The right side of the heart contains deoxygenated blood from the body cells on its way to the lungs for reoxygenation. The left side of the heart contains oxygenated blood from the lungs being pumped out to the aorta on its way to the cells of the body. The septal wall divides the left and right sides of the heart.

II. Anomalies

- Anomalies of the anatomic structure of the heart or major blood vessels result following irregularities of development during the first 9 weeks *in utero*.
- The fetal heart is completely developed by the ninth week.
- Early diagnosis is necessary, but not all defects require treatment.
- Treatment usually involves surgical correction.

III. Etiology

Causes may be genetic or environmental or a combination of both. Many are unknown.

- Genetic[15,16]
    - Heredity is apparent in about 15% of cases.
    - An example of a chromosomal defect is Down syndrome, in which congenital heart anomalies occur frequently.
- Environmental[16]
    - Environmental factors impact fetal heart development during the second and third weeks *in utero* and account for about 30% of cases.
    - Maternal diseases such as rubella, cytomegalovirus, diabetes, and obesity.
    - Maternal medications such as anticonvulsants, antidepressants, and thalidomide.
    - Maternal use of alcohol, tobacco, and illicit drugs.
    - Maternal air pollution exposure.

- Paternal exposure to chemicals, radiation, and heavy metals.
- Maternal exposure to industrial chemical solvents.

IV. Types of Defects

- The types of heart defects that occur most frequently are ventricular septal defect, atrial septal defect, pulmonary **stenosis**, and patent ductus arteriosis.[17]
- Defects (openings) in the septal wall cause a mixing of oxygenated and deoxygenated blood.
- Atrial and/or ventricular septal defects result in mixing of the blood from the left and right sides of the heart.
- Other defects include a passageway between the great arteries and veins, which also causes mixing of oxygenated and deoxygenated blood. Two of the more common congenital heart defects are described here.
- Ventricular septal defect[17]
    - In this type of defect, the left and right ventricles exchange blood through an opening in their dividing wall (septum).
    - The oxygenated blood from the lung, which is normally pumped by the left ventricle to the aorta and then to the entire body, can pass across to the right ventricle through the septal defect, as shown in **Figure 61-2**.
    - The severity of symptoms is directly related to the specific location and size of the defect. Small defects may close without surgical correction.
- Patent ductus arteriosus[17]
    - A patent ductus arteriosus means the passageway (**shunt**) is open between the two great arteries that arise from the heart—namely, the aorta and the pulmonary artery.
    - Normally, the opening closes during the first few weeks after birth.
    - When the opening does not close, blood from the aorta can pass back to the lungs, as shown in **Figure 61-3**.
    - The heart compensates in the attempt to provide the body with oxygenated blood and becomes overburdened.

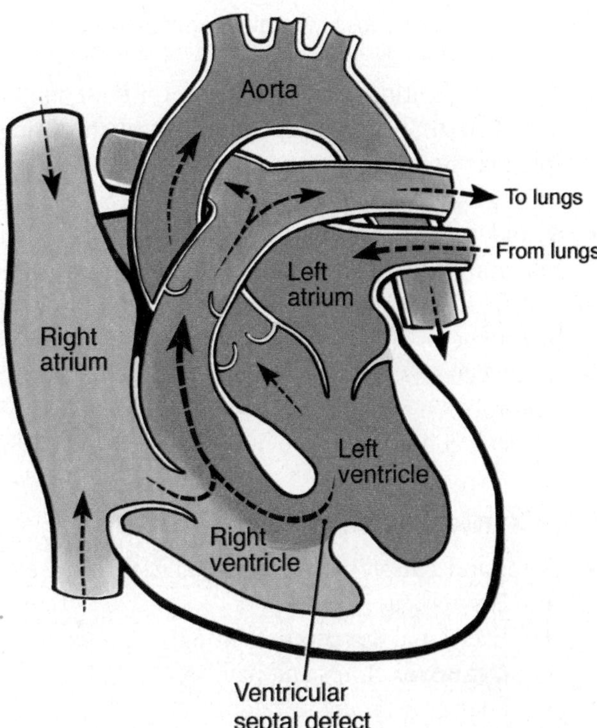

Figure 61-2 Ventricular Septal Defect. The right and left ventricles are connected by an opening that permits oxygenated blood from the left ventricle to shunt across to the right ventricle and then recirculate to the lungs. Compare with Figure 61-1, in which the septum separates the ventricles.

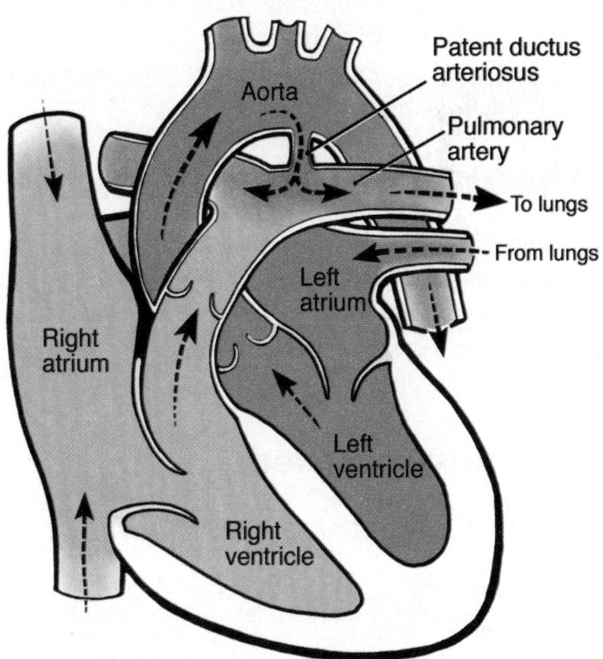

Figure 61-3 Patent Ductus Arteriosus. An open passageway between the aorta and the pulmonary artery permits oxygenated blood from the aorta to pass back into the lungs. Arrows show directions of flow through the patent ductus. Compare with normal anatomy in Figure 61-1.

V. Prevention

Prevention of congenital heart defects includes:

- Rubella vaccination for women of childbearing age is highly advised for those not vaccinated in

childhood or those without confirmation of immunity by a laboratory test.
- No medications, including over-the-counter and herbal medications, should be taken during pregnancy without prior consultation with the physician.
- Avoid tobacco, alcohol, and illicit drugs when planning a pregnancy and throughout pregnancy.
- Attain and maintain a healthy weight prior to pregnancy.
- If diabetes is present, maintain good glycemic control.
- Genetic counseling.

VI. Clinical Considerations

- Signs and symptoms of congenital heart disease[17]:
  - Easy fatigue.
  - Exertional **dyspnea**, fainting.
  - **Cyanosis** of lips and nail beds.
  - Poor growth and development.
  - Heart murmurs.
  - CHF.
- Dental hygiene concerns
  - Prevention of IE: certain defective heart valves are at risk for endocarditis from bacteremia produced during oral treatments. The American Heart Association recommendations for antibiotic prophylaxis must be consulted for procedure with this group of patients.[13]
  - Elimination of oral disease: prevention and management of oral disease.

Rheumatic Heart Disease

- Rheumatic heart disease is a complication following rheumatic fever. A rather high percentage of patients with a history of rheumatic fever have permanent heart valve damage, particularly the mitral valve.[18]

I. Rheumatic Fever

- Incidence[18]
  - Frequency of this condition in developed countries has declined significantly in the past several decades and is not common in the United States.
  - Primarily affects children between the ages of 5 and 17 years.
  - Native Americans have a 7.6 times higher risk of rheumatic fever and Alaska Natives have 4.3 times greater risk.
- Etiology
  - Group A streptococci are the primary etiologic agent.[18]
- Prevention[18]
  - Hand washing is a primary prevention.
  - Early diagnosis and treatment of streptococcal throat and pharyngeal infections are necessary to prevent progression to rheumatic fever.
  - In 60% of cases, the patient may develop recurrent or chronic rheumatic heart disease.
- Symptoms of acute rheumatic fever[18]
  - Arthritis: joint pain in multiple larger joints such as the ankles, knees, elbows, and wrists, as well as joint swelling with redness and warmth.
  - Carditis (heart inflammation).
  - Low-grade fever.
  - Pink skin rash with rounded lesions on trunk and extremities.
  - A later symptom may be muscle weakness with quick involuntary jerky movements while awake.

II. The Course of Rheumatic Heart Disease

Following the acute stage of rheumatic fever, symptoms do not usually persist, except the effects of the valvular deformity.

- Symptoms[18]
  - Stenosis or incompetence of valves; most commonly, the aortic and mitral valves.
  - Heart murmur is influenced by the amount of scarring of the valves and myocardium.
  - Increased risk for cardiac arrhythmias and heart failure.
  - Higher risk of stroke.
  - Increased risk of bacterial endocarditis.
- Practice applications
  - The American Heart Association no longer recommends antibiotic prophylaxis prior to dental treatment for patients with this condition due to minimal risk of developing IE.[13]

Mitral Valve Prolapse

I. Description

- The mitral valve is between the left atrium and the left ventricle (Figure 61-1).
- Oxygenated blood from the lungs passes from the pulmonary vein into the left ventricle, where it is pumped through the aortic valve and into the aorta for distribution to the body cells.

- When the mitral valve leaflets are damaged, the closure is imperfect and the leaflet (or flap) may flop or bulge backward into the left atrium, allowing oxygenated blood to backflow or regurgitate.[19]

II. Symptoms

- Most patients with mitral valve prolapse are asymptomatic.[19]
  - A small number of cases will have symptoms of palpitations, fatigue, atypical chest pain, and a late systolic murmur.
- When there is more severe involvement, an increase in frequency of palpitations and progressive mitral regurgitation is apparent, along with a systolic click and murmur.[19]
- The American Heart Association no longer recommends antibiotic prophylaxis during dental treatment for patients with this condition.[13]

Hypertension

Hypertension means an abnormal elevation of **arterial blood pressure**; it is often called the "silent killer." Hypertension is responsible for more deaths from CVD than any other modifiable risk factor for CVD.[20]

- Detection of blood pressure for dental and dental hygiene patients has become an essential step in patient assessment prior to treatment.
- Early detection, with referral for additional diagnosis and treatment when indicated, can prove to be lifesaving for certain people.
- Knowledge of the health problems of patients is needed to ensure it is safe to provide treatment, such as administration of local anesthesia, and to minimize risk for medical emergencies.

I. Etiology

A. Primary Hypertension

- Prevalence: the lifetime prevalence for high blood pressure is 84% to 93%, with the highest rates in Black/African American (93%) and Hispanic (92%) groups.[20]
- Predisposing or risk factors: combinations of the factors listed are more significant than any one alone[20]:
  - Tobacco use.
  - Genetic predisposition.
  - Overweight and obesity.
  - Excess sodium intake.
  - Physical inactivity.
  - Inadequate potassium intake.
  - Excessive alcohol intake.

B. Secondary Hypertension

- Incidence: about 10% of all hypertension is secondary to other underlying medical conditions.[20]
- Causes of secondary hypertension may include[20]:
  - Renal disease.
  - Obstructive sleep **apnea**.
  - Endocrine conditions, such as Cushing's syndrome, hypothyroidism, hyperthyroidism, and hyperparathyroidism.
  - Drug or alcohol use, such as amphetamines, antidepressants, caffeine, herbal supplements (e.g., ephedra), immunosuppressants, oral contraceptives, and recreational drugs.

II. Blood Pressure Levels

- Classification of blood pressure requires two or more readings at different times.[20]

A. Low Blood Pressure

- Many healthy people, with no evident clinical problems, have a normal systolic pressure under 90 mm Hg.
- A marked sudden drop in blood pressure is usually associated with an emergency, such as severe blood loss, shock, **myocardial infarction**, sepsis, or other medical problem.
- Procedures to follow during specific medical emergencies can be found in Chapter 9.

B. Normal Blood Pressure

- Normal blood pressure for adults older than 18 years is defined as being less than 120/80 mm Hg.[20]
- Elevated blood pressure for adults is defined as having a diastolic blood pressure below 80 with the systolic in the range of 120–129 mm Hg.[20]

C. High Blood Pressure

- Stage 1 hypertension in adults is classified as a diastolic blood pressure of 130 to 139 with systolic pressure of 80 to 89 mm Hg.[20]
- Stage 2 hypertension in adults ranges is a blood pressure of greater than or equal to 140/90 mm Hg.[20]
- These classifications are based on the level of risk for cardiovascular disease.[20]

III. Clinical Symptoms of Hypertension

Hypertension is frequently recognized only by blood pressure readings and may go unrecognized because of the lack of clinical symptoms.

- Major sequelae of long-standing elevation of blood pressure[20]:
  - Cerebrovascular accident or stroke.
  - End-stage renal disease.
  - CHD.
  - Heart failure.
- Hypertension crisis[10]
  - Malignant hypertension is life threatening, sudden, and characterized by extremely high blood pressure over 180/120 mm Hg.[20]
  - Activate emergency procedures as the situation can be fatal if not treated immediately or may result in damage to multiple body systems.

IV. Treatment

Treatment depends on risk factors and stage of hypertension.

- Patients diagnosed or at risk for CVD should target a blood pressure below 130/80 mm Hg.[20]
- In Stage 1 hypertension, those with a low risk for CVD should implement lifestyle modifications for 6 months. If blood pressure does not meet the goal (<130/80), pharmacologic therapy must be initiated.[21]
- Pharmacotherapy is recommended for patients with a systolic reading greater than or equal to 140, or a diastolic reading of greater than or equal to 90.[20]
  - Medications to treat hypertension may include diuretics, calcium channel blockers, beta-blockers, and/or angiotensin-converting enzyme (ACE) inhibitors.

A. Goals

- Primary hypertension
  - Achieve and maintain diastolic pressure level below 80 mm Hg to reduce the risk of serious complications and premature death.

B. Lifestyle Changes

- Weight: achieve and maintain a healthy weight.[20,22]
  - Even modest weight loss of 5% to 10% can lower blood pressure.
- Physical activity: the public health recommendation is 30–60 minutes 4 to 7 days per week (Canada) of moderate intensity aerobic physical activity along with flexibility and resistance exercise.[22-24]
  - Hypertension risk can be decreased by 6%; may help those with hypertension to lower blood pressure and achieve a healthy weight.[23]
- Diet:
  - Sodium restriction, in those who are salt sensitive, may modestly lower blood pressure.
  - A heart-healthy diet like the Mediterranean Diet or DASH (Dietary Approaches to Stop Hypertension) eating plan.[20,22,25]
    - These eating plans tend to be high in whole grains, fruits, vegetables, beans, nuts, fish, and chicken.
    - These plans result in lower sodium and saturated fat intake and are higher in calcium, potassium, magnesium, fiber, and monounsaturated fats.
- Tobacco use: eliminate all forms of tobacco.
- Stress management.[22]
- Moderation in alcohol intake to no more than two "standard" drinks per day; standard drink equals one 12-ounce beer, 1.5 ounces distilled spirits, or 5 ounces of wine.[20,22]

V. Hypertension in Children

- Children aged 3 years and older need to have blood pressure determinations made at least annually.
- Prevalence of hypertension is higher in children who suffer from obesity, sleep disorders, kidney disease, and those who were born prematurely.[26]
- If the blood pressure of a child or adolescent is greater than or equal to the 90th percentile (95th percentile in Canada), the blood pressure measurement should be repeated and the cardiovascular risk assessed.[22,26] (See Chapter 12 for blood pressure values for children and adolescents.)

Ischemic Heart Disease

Ischemic heart disease is an acute and chronic cardiac disability, arising from reduction or arrest of blood supply to the myocardium.[27,28]

- The heart muscle (myocardium) is supplied through the coronary arteries, which are branches of the descending aorta.
- Because of the relationship to the coronary arteries, the disease is often referred to as CHD or coronary artery disease (CAD).

- **Ischemia** is defined as oxygen deprivation in a local area from a reduced passage of blood into the area.
- Ischemic heart disease is the result of an imbalance of the oxygen supply and demand of the myocardium resulting from a narrowing or blocking of the **lumen** of the coronary arteries.

I. Etiology

Other factors may be involved, but the principal cause of reduction of blood flow to the heart muscle is **atherosclerosis** of the vessel walls, which narrows the lumen, thus obstructing the flow of blood.[28]

- Definition of atherosclerosis[27]
  - Atherosclerosis is an inflammatory disease of medium and large arteries driven by lipids, in which **atheromas** deposit and thicken the intimal layer of the involved blood vessel.
  - An atheroma is a fibro-fatty deposit or plaque containing several lipids, especially cholesterol.
  - With time, the plaques continue to thicken and, eventually, close the vessel (**Figure 61-4**).
  - Some plaques calcify, whereas others may develop an overlying **thrombus**.
- Risk factors for atherosclerosis[27,29]:
  - Elevated levels of blood lipids.
  - Hypertension.
  - Diabetes mellitus.
  - Male gender.
  - Inflammation.
  - Tobacco use.
  - Overweight or obesity.
  - Physical inactivity.
  - Older age.
  - Family history of heart disease before age 55.
  - Sleep apnea.
  - Heavy alcohol use.
  - Stress.

II. Manifestations of Ischemic Heart Disease

- Angina pectoris.
- Myocardial infarction.
- CHF.

Angina Pectoris

- Angina pectoris is chest pain, the most common symptom of coronary atherosclerotic heart disease; however, it can also be present in the absence of ischemic heart disease.[30]

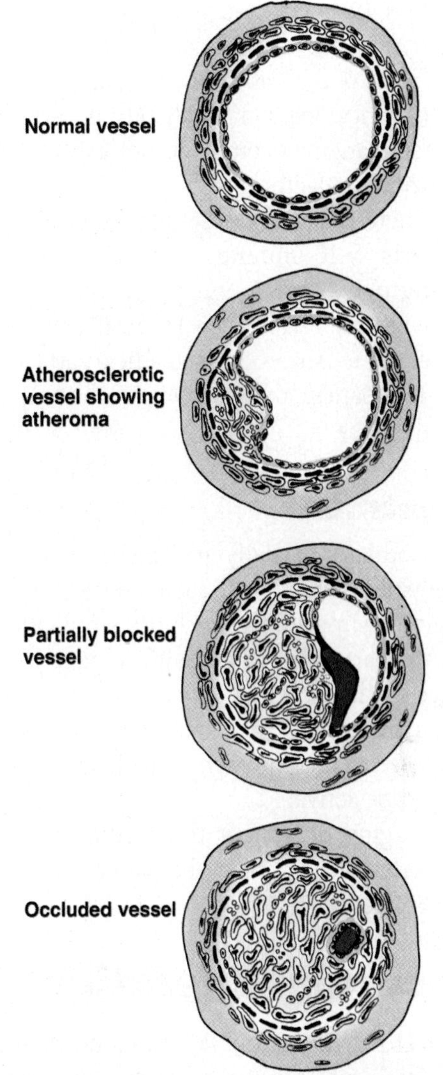

Figure 61-4 Atherosclerosis. An atheroma develops within the lining of the normal blood vessel. The atheroma is made of a fatty deposit containing cholesterol. At first, the atheroma is small, and no symptoms are apparent, but eventually, it enlarges and completely blocks the vessel, thus depriving the area served by the vessel of oxygen.

National Institutes of Health. *Report of the Working Group on Arteriosclerosis of the National Heart, Lung, and Blood Institute, National Institutes of Health, United States Department of Health and Human Services.* Bethesda, MD: National Institutes of Health; 1981. NIH Publication No. 81-2034.

- Symptoms include[30]:
  - The pain is described as a heavy, squeezing pressure or tightness in the mid-chest region and may radiate to the arms, neck, shoulder, or the mandible.
  - Occurs as a result of physical exertion.
  - The symptoms are relieved by rest or by sublingual nitroglycerin within 5 minutes.

I. Precipitating Factors

- Stable angina occurs in a pattern that is consistent for at least 2 months.[31]

- May be precipitated by exertion or exercise, stress, or a heavy meal.
- In the dental office or clinic, an atmosphere of calmness and quiet can help minimize stress.

- Unstable angina occurs without exertion or other precipitating factors.[27,31]
    - There is sudden onset of prolonged pain that lasts >20 minutes and is not relieved by nitroglycerin.
    - Unstable angina is a medical emergency because it can progress to a heart attack.
    - The patient may also experience nausea and dyspnea.

II. Treatment

- A vasodilator, usually nitroglycerin, is administered sublingually.[30] (See Chapter 9.)
- Basic life support that includes supplemental oxygen is part of the treatment provided in a dental office or clinic.
- If the patient does not report relief from the nitroglycerin, the emergency medical system (911) should be activated.
- Thoroughly document the events that occurred and assessment data in the patient's chart for future reference.

Myocardial Infarction

- Myocardial infarction (MI) and unstable angina are considered acute coronary syndrome.[27]
- Other names include: heart attack, coronary **occlusion**, or coronary thrombosis.
- The infarction results from a sudden reduction or arrest of coronary blood flow. However, it can also occur due to a persistent vasospasm in a coronary artery.[27,28]

I. Etiology

- The typical cause is rupture of an atherosclerotic plaque, resulting in creation of a thrombus that partially or completely blocks blood flow through the artery.[27]
    - In some cases, a severe spasm of the coronary artery can precipitate the MI.[27]
- The blockage creates an **infarct**, leading to tissue necrosis.
- Necrosis of the area can occur within a few hours.
- A few patients die immediately or within a few hours.
- COVID-19 has been implicated as an emerging risk factor for acute coronary syndrome.[32]

II. Symptoms

- Pain[16]
    - Location: pain symptoms may start under the sternum, with feelings of indigestion, or in the middle to upper sternum. Pain may last for extended periods, even hours.
        - When the pain is severe, it gives a pressing or crushing heavy sensation and is not relieved by rest or nitroglycerin.
    - One-third of individuals with an MI may not experience chest pain, particularly females.[33]
        - A patient with diabetes may have no symptoms or mild pain.
    - Onset: the pain may have a sudden onset, sometimes during sleep or following exercise. The pain may be radial, similar to angina pectoris, which extends to the left or right arm, neck, and mandible.
- Other symptoms[16]
    - Cold sweat, weakness and faintness, shortness of breath, unexplained weakness, nausea, and vomiting may occur.[33,34]
    - Blood pressure falls below baseline.
    - Women do not always present with symptoms similar to men and may not experience chest pain. Chief symptoms include fainting, pain in the upper back and lower abdomen, and extreme fatigue.[33]

III. Management during an Attack

- Terminate treatment.
    - Sit the patient up for comfortable breathing.
    - Remain calm, give nitroglycerin, and reassure the patient.
- Activate EMS.
    - Apply basic life support measures, if indicated, while waiting for medical assistance.
- Review Chapter 9 for medical management of a heart attack.

IV. Treatment after Acute Symptoms

- Medical supervision[34]
    - Treatment choices are complex, but many patients will be placed on antithrombotic therapy such as anticoagulant or antiplatelet agents.
- Lifestyle changes[34]
    - Cardiac rehabilitation in a medically supervised program is required to learn about the

lifestyle changes needed, which include supervised exercise training and education on heart-healthy choices, including diet, quitting use of tobacco, blood pressure management, and management of stress.

- Subsequent appointments
  - Consultation with the cardiologist is needed to determine when the patient can have routine dental treatment.
  - Traditionally, routine dental treatment has been postponed for at least 6 months following a heart attack; however, more recent guidelines suggest postponing noncardiac surgery (e.g., routine dental care) a minimum of 60 days after an MI.[35]
  - This is in part due to the reduction in mortality rate after an MI.[35]

Heart Failure

- Heart failure, also referred to as CHF, is a syndrome in which an abnormality of cardiac function is responsible for the inability or failure of the heart to pump blood at a rate necessary to meet the oxygen needs of the body tissues.[36]

I. Etiology

- CHF is a chronic, progressive condition resulting from many forms of CVDs and can be related to a number of other systemic conditions, including[36]:
  - Coronary heart disease.
  - MI (heart attack).
  - Hypertension.
  - Diabetes.
  - Arrhythmias.
  - Congenital heart disease.

II. Clinical Manifestations

- The clinical manifestations coincide with the parts of the heart involved.
- Signs and symptoms are different depending, in general, on whether the left or the right side of the heart, or both, are affected.

A. Left Heart Failure

- The left side of the heart receives oxygenated blood from the lungs and pumps the blood into the aorta to the rest of the body. The left ventricle is larger because it supplies most of the heart's pumping power.[37]
  - Left heart failure is a pathologic condition of the left ventricle, resulting in the heart not being capable of pumping oxygen-rich blood to the body or being unable to relax and fill with blood during the rest period between heartbeats.[38]
- Signs and symptoms of left heart failure include the following[38]:
  - Weakness, fatigue.
  - Dyspnea, particularly evident on exertion.
  - Shortness of breath when lying supine, relieved when sitting up.
  - Nocturnal dyspnea may cause the patient to wake up gasping for breath and wheezing.

B. Right Heart Failure

- The right heart receives the **venous blood** from the vena cava and pumps it to the lungs for oxygenation.
- Right heart failure usually occurs as a result of left heart failure.[38]
  - Loss of pumping power by the left ventricle results in blood (fluid) backing up into the lungs and eventually damages the right ventricle.
- Signs and symptoms of right heart failure include the following[38]:
  - Weakness, fatigue.
  - Swelling of the feet and/or ankles. The edema progresses to the thighs and abdomen (ascites) in advanced stages of heart failure.
  - Nausea, bloating, and appetite loss.
  - Weight loss and cachexia (muscle loss).
  - Distended jugular veins.

III. Treatment during Chronic Stages

A patient with an appointment in a dental office or clinic may be receiving a variety of medical treatments. Questioning the patient during review of the medical history to gather more information and consultation with the cardiologist or primary care provider are recommended. Heart failure patients may be using one or more of the following approaches to treatment[20,21]:

- Drug therapy[39]
  - ACE inhibitors, such as lisinopril (Prinivil) or enalapril (Vasotec).
  - Angiotensin receptor blockers, such as losartan (Cozaar) or valsartan (Diovan).
  - Beta-blockers, such as metoprolol (Toprol).
  - Digoxin.

    - Diuretics, such as furosemide (Lasix).
    - Aldosterone antagonists, such as spironolactone (Aldactone).
- Lifestyle modifications[40]
    - Obesity makes the heart work harder so a key goal is to achieve or maintain a healthy weight.
    - Track fluid intake.
    - Limit sodium intake.
    - Make healthy diet choices, preferably with greater consumption of plant-based foods.
    - Tobacco cessation.
    - Stress management.
    - Maintain blood pressure and blood glucose in target range as determined by medical provider.
    - Adequate sleep and management of any sleep-disordered breathing (sleep apnea).
    - Physical activity under medical supervision.
- Surgery may be indicated and include one of the following[39]:
    - Pacemaker.
    - Heart transplant.

IV. Emergency Care for Heart Failure and Acute Pulmonary Edema

- A patient with heart failure or acute pulmonary edema is usually conscious at the time a cardiac medical emergency occurs. See Chapter 9 for emergency procedures to follow.

Cardiac Arrhythmias

- The contractions of the heart are controlled by a complex electronic circuitry system. Impulses within this system send messages to the heart muscle, triggering contraction. The interruption of the conduction of the impulse, causing a delay or block, results in an abnormal heart rhythm or **arrhythmia**.[41]

I. Etiology

- Arrhythmias such as atrial fibrillation (AF) may result from a number of causes, including[41]:
    - Changes to the heart and/or blood flow.
        - Heart failure or a heart attack may damage the heart muscle.
        - Congenital heart conditions.
    - Exertion or strain.
        - Stress, anxiety, anger, pain or a sudden surprise.
    - Excess or deficiency of electrolytes (e.g., deficiency of potassium), hormones (e.g., hypo- or hyperthyroidism), or fluid (e.g., dehydration).
    - Medications such as antihypertensive drugs.
    - Changes in the electrical signaling in the heart.

II. Symptoms

- An arrhythmia may be symptomatic or asymptomatic; patients with an asymptomatic arrhythmia may still be at risk for stroke and sudden cardiac death.[42]
- Symptoms of an arrhythmia may include the following[41]:
    - Heart palpitations.
    - Slow or irregular heartbeat.
    - Dizziness or light-headedness.
    - Feeling faint/syncope.
    - Fatigue.
    - Dyspnea.
    - Sweating.

III. Treatment

- Most arrhythmias do not require treatment.
- Drug therapy for AF may include[41,42]:
    - Beta-blockers, such as atenolol and metoprolol.
    - Calcium channel blockers, such as diltiazem.
    - Digoxin.
    - **Anticoagulants** such as warfarin (Coumadin) and antiplatelets may be used to reduce risk of blood clots and for stroke prevention.
- Lifestyle modifications[43]:
    - Achieve and maintain a healthy weight.
    - Be physically active, with 150 minutes per week of moderate-intensity activity.
        - Physical inactivity is an independent risk factor for AF.
    - Manage sleep-disordered breathing (sleep apnea).
    - Maintain good glycemic control in diabetes mellitus.
    - Monitor and manage blood pressure to reach targets set by medical provider.
    - Consume a heart-healthy diet (e.g., the DASH diet:
        - High in vegetables, fruits, whole grains, low-fat dairy, lean poultry and fish, legumes, and nuts.
        - Limit sodium, added sugars, solid fats, and refined grains.

    - Monitor and manage hyperlipidemia (high cholesterol).
    - Tobacco cessation.
- Medical procedures[42]:
    - Placement of a pacemaker, which is also called an implantable cardioverter defibrillator (ICD).
    - Catheter ablation (a thin tube is inserted in an arm or groin blood vessel and guided to the heart).

Lifestyle Management for the Patient with Cardiovascular Disease

- Nearly 90% of the risk for MI and stroke are modifiable risk factors.[44]
- The recommendations for prevention and management of CVD in all patients include the following[44,45]:
    - Education on lifestyle modifications to reduce the risk of recurrence of cardiovascular events such as a heart attack.
    - Lifestyle modifications include:
        - Weight loss for patients who are obese or overweight to achieve a healthy weight and maintain it.
        - Consume a heart-healthy diet, including fruits, vegetables, whole grains, low-fat dairy products, poultry, fish, legumes, and nuts. DASH diet and Mediterranean diet patterns are recommended.
        - Limit added sugars, saturated fat, trans fat, and red meats.
        - For those with diabetes mellitus, maintain glycemic control with HbA1c <7.0%.
        - For those with hypertension, consume no more than 2400 mg of sodium.
        - Engage in moderate intensity physical activity 150 minutes/week.
        - Limit alcohol to less than two drinks per day for men and one drink per day for women.
        - Tobacco cessation.

Surgical Treatment

I. Revascularization

- Revascularization in CAD is done primarily to relieve symptoms of angina and medical therapy remains the treatment of choice.[46–48]

A. Percutaneous Coronary Intervention

- Also known as coronary angioplasty, it is a nonsurgical procedure to open the coronary arteries.
- A contrast dye is injected, and a catheter is inserted through either a wrist or groin blood vessel and guided to the blocked coronary blood vessel, where an inflatable balloon at the end of the catheter widens the narrowed lumen.
- A stent may be inserted into the artery to provide a semi-rigid scaffolding within the lumen, which helps prevent **restenosis** or re-narrowing of the lumen.
    - The stent may be impregnated with a drug to prevent return of the coronary blockage; this is called a drug-eluting stent.

B. Coronary Artery Bypass Grafting

- Coronary bypass is recommended in patients with more complex multivessel CAD and those with CAD and diabetes.[49]
- A healthy artery or vein is grafted to go around or bypass the blocked portion of an artery.
- The beneficial effects are reduced mortality, relief from angina pain, reduced workload for the heart, and an increase in oxygen and blood supply to the myocardium.[49]
- **Figure 61-5** shows the use of a saphenous vein graft and the internal mammary artery for bypasses.

II. Cardiac Resynchronization Therapy

For those with heart failure or an arrhythmia (irregular heartbeat), cardiac resynchronization therapy (CRT) may be indicated. CRT helps to improve the heart rhythm and involves surgically implanting a pacemaker or defibrillator.[50]

- Natural pacemaker function
    - The natural pacemaker, or center where the normal heartbeat is initiated, is the sinoatrial node, which is located in the right atrium.
    - From that node, impulses are sent along the muscle walls to stimulate and regulate the contractions of the ventricles, which pump the blood throughout the body.
    - When the natural pacemaker cells are not able to maintain a reliable rhythm, or when the impulses are interrupted because of heart block, cardiac arrest, various arrhythmias, or other disease conditions, treatment by a cardiologist may include the placement of an artificial pacemaker.

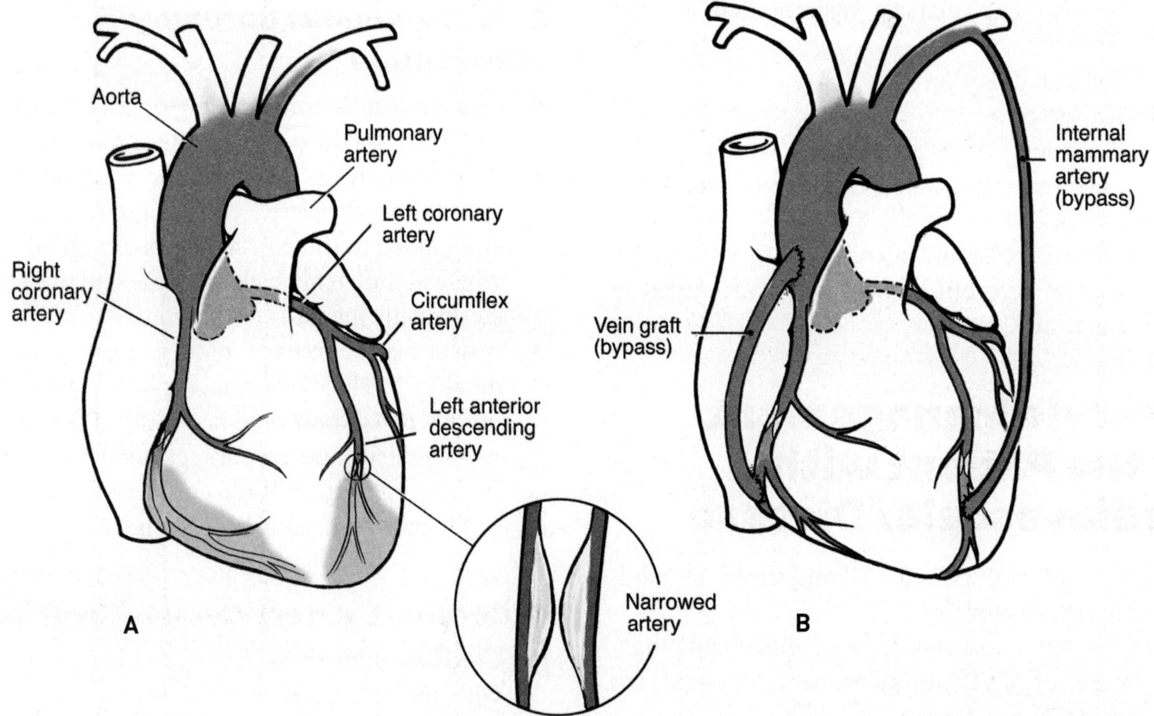

Figure 61-5 Coronary Bypass Surgery. **A:** Heart showing infarcted (shaded) areas created by coronary arteries narrowed by atherosclerosis. **B:** Vein graft from saphenous vein connected with aorta to bypass narrowed area of right coronary artery, and internal mammary artery used to bypass narrowed left anterior descending artery.

A. Cardiac Pacemaker

- Cardiac pacemaker is used in heart failure.[50]
  - A cardiac pacemaker is an electronic stimulator used to send a specified electrical current to the myocardium to monitor heart rate irregularities, and tiny electrical pulses are emitted to correct the heart rate.
  - The pulse generator is a half dollar–size device implanted under the skin just below the collarbone. The area selected depends on the individual condition as determined by the cardiologist (**Figure 61-6**).

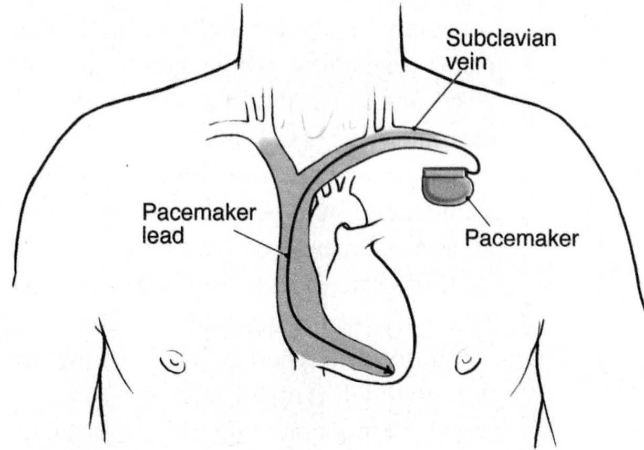

Figure 61-6 Cardiac Pacemaker. The pulse generator is implanted under the skin in the thorax or upper abdomen. The lead electrodes may go to the ventricle, to the atrium, or both to provide the necessary stimulus for regulation of the heartbeat.

B. Implantable Cardioverter Defibrillator

- The ICD detects abnormal heart rhythms and delivers a shock (defibrillation) to return the heart rhythm to normal.[51]
- An ICD is indicated to prevent sudden cardiac death.[52]
- An ICD is a battery-powered pulse generator about the size of a pocket watch surgically placed in the chest or abdomen, often just below the collarbone.[51]
- The ICD may be single (defibrillator only) or dual chamber (pacemaker and defibrillator).[53]
  - A dual-chamber ICD can detect when the heartbeat is too slow and deliver an electric signal to the heart as well as deliver defibrillation shocks for an abnormal rhythm to normalize it.

C. Devices That May Interfere with CRT Devices

- Devices emitting electromagnetic waves may affect the function of pacemaker or ICD devices.
- The American Heart Association lists ultrasonic scalers, cleaners, and drills as posing limited risk.[54]
- However, the dental literature remains inconsistent.
  - Ultrasonic scalers may cause minor electromagnetic interference, but not affect the defibrillator pacing or sensing functions when used at least 15 inches from the ICD.[55-57]
  - Risk for interference also varied by the type and model of CRT device, with newer shielded devices finding less interference.[58]
- The American Dental Association (ADA) recommends consultation with the cardiologist for patients with pacemakers or ICDs to determine whether ultrasonic devices can be used safely.[56]
  - If it is determined that ultrasonic equipment can be used, the ADA recommends they not be waved over the implant area and the equipment should be turned off when not in use.

D. Prophylactic Antibiotic Premedication

- The American Heart Association does not recommend use of antibiotic prophylaxis for those with cardiac implantable electronic devices.[13]
- Although evidence suggests the patient with a pacemaker is at low risk for endocarditis, consult with the cardiologist to verify whether they choose to use prophylactic antibiotics for dental and dental hygiene procedures.

III. Dental Considerations

- Patients in dental offices and clinics who have had or will have cardiac surgery such as coronary artery bypass grafting or heart transplantation need to have their oral health evaluated and managed prior to surgery.

A. Presurgical Dental Care

- Before elective cardiac surgery, the patient should have a comprehensive dental and periodontal examination.
- All active disease should be treated to resolve any sources of acute or chronic infection, and any nonrestorable teeth should be removed.
- Elimination of potential sources of infection is essential to minimize the risk for IE postsurgery.

B. Postsurgical Dental Care

- Adherence to a regular preventive maintenance program to manage dental biofilm and maintain optimal oral health is essential to minimize risk for oral infections.

Antithrombotic Therapy

- Antithrombotic therapy prevents embolus or thrombus formation and may include antiplatelet or anticoagulant drugs.[59]

I. Anticoagulant Therapy

- Anticoagulants are used to prevent occurrence or recurrence of blood clots or thrombus causing a myocardial infarction or stroke.
- Traditional anticoagulant drugs[60]
  - **Heparin** (hospital-administered intravenously).
    - Heparin inhibits several clotting factors.
  - Vitamin K antagonists include coumarin derivatives such as warfarin.
    - Warfarin (Coumadin) blocks the vitamin K–dependent clotting pathway.
    - The most significant adverse event related to warfarin is excessive bleeding or hemorrhage.
- Indications for use[60]
  - Traditionally, warfarin (Coumadin) has been used for long-term anticoagulation following MI to prevent recurrent MI; however, evidence is inconsistent about its effectiveness given newer options for treatment.
- Monitoring of anticoagulant therapy
  - The international normalized ratio (INR) is used to monitor therapy with anticoagulants; a target therapeutic range is between 2.0 and 3.0.[61]
  - The prothrombin time may also be used.

A. Dental Management of Patients Taking Anticoagulants

- Medical history and medication review.
- Consultation with cardiologist and/or primary care provider regarding bleeding risk during dental/dental hygiene procedures.
  - Obtain the most current INR.
  - For a surgical or invasive procedure, the INR may need to be done 24 hours prior to the appointment.

- Discontinuation of anticoagulant therapy is *not* recommended for dental procedures.[60,62]
- Treatment should begin with oral self-care education to ensure adequate biofilm removal to minimize bleeding.
- Local anesthetic with a vasoconstrictor for infiltration is recommended, if there are no contraindications to use of a vasoconstrictor, to minimize bleeding. Use of nerve blocks should be minimized to avoid hemorrhage.
- Following nonsurgical periodontal therapy (NSPT), local hemostasis may include[60]:
  - Minimize tissue trauma.
  - Apply pressure with gauze or sponges against the bleeding area or pack interdentally until bleeding is controlled. If the bleeding is not controlled, the dentist may use a hemostatic dressing like Gelfoam.
  - Do *not* dismiss the patient until bleeding has stopped.
- Postprocedural instructions may include the following:
  - Contact the patient the evening after the procedures to follow up.
  - Avoid rinsing for 24 hours.
  - Advise to avoid vigorous toothbrushing for several hours or until the next day.
  - Provide the patient with extra gauze or sponges to use to apply pressure should bleeding resume.
  - Avoid hot liquid and hard foods for the rest of the day. A soft diet may be suggested, but typically, this is not necessary for NSPT.
  - Provide contact information for the dentist or emergency contact if there is excessive or prolonged bleeding.

II. Direct Oral Anticoagulants

- The newest classification of anticoagulants is direct oral anticoagulants (DOACs); they have more targeted action and less risk of life-threatening bleeding events than the older anticoagulant drugs like warfarin.[63] The mechanism of action varies for each drug.
- Common DOAC drugs[60,62]
  - Dabigatran (Pradaxa).
  - Rivaroxaban (Xarelto).
  - Apixaban (Eliquis).
  - Edoxaban (Savaysa, Lixiana).
- Indications for use[60,62]
  - Prevention of deep venous thromboembolism (DVT).
  - Prevention of stroke in the patient with AF.
- Monitoring of DOAC therapy[60]
  - Routine monitoring is not required.
  - At this time, no established therapeutic ranges have been identified for these drugs.

A. Dental Management of Patients Taking Direct Oral Anticoagulants

- Medical history and medication review.
- Consultation with cardiologist and/or primary care provider regarding bleeding risk during dental/dental hygiene procedures.
- Discontinuation of DOAC therapy is *not* generally recommended for dental procedures.[60,62]
- Treatment should begin with oral self-care education to ensure adequate biofilm removal to minimize bleeding.
- Local measures to manage bleeding and maintain homeostasis may include local anesthesia with a vasoconstrictor for infiltration, minimize tissue trauma, apply pressure to control bleeding, and monitor patient prior to dismissing.

III. Antiplatelet Therapy

- Antiplatelet medications impact aggregation of platelets, which affects the ability of the blood to clot.
- Antiplatelet drugs may be used in combination such as aspirin and clopidogrel.
- Common antiplatelet drugs[60,62,63]
  - Aspirin is used for those at risk to prevent cardiovascular events as well as in dual-antiplatelet therapy.
  - Clopidogrel (Plavix).
  - Ticlopidine (Ticlid).
  - Ticagrelor (Brilinta).
- Indications for use[60]
  - Established CAD.
  - Coronary stenosis.
  - Evidence of cardiac ischemia.
- Monitoring of antiplatelet therapy
  - Platelet function testing is used to evaluate the effectiveness of antiplatelet therapy, but there are no recommendations to assess this prior to most routine dental treatment.[62]

A. Dental Management of Patients Taking Antiplatelet Therapy

- Medical history and medication review.
- Consultation with the cardiologist and/or primary care provider regarding bleeding risk during dental/dental hygiene procedures may be indicated in a

patient taking multiple antiplatelet medications and/or with complex medical conditions.

- Discontinuation of antiplatelet therapy is *not* recommended for most dental procedures.[60,62-64]
- Education to attain optimal oral self-care to ensure adequate biofilm removal to minimize bleeding is an important part of the treatment plan.
- Local measures to manage hemostasis should be implemented as previously noted for anticoagulants and DOACs.

Documentation

Documentation for a routine dental hygiene continuing care or periodontal maintenance appointment for a patient with a cardiovascular illness would need to include a minimum of the following items:

- Record the responses to health history review questions about visitations to the cardiologist, the patient's reported state of health, and physician updates that could influence dental procedures.
- Record all findings and compare to previous assessment outcomes regarding vital signs, extraoral and intraoral examination, and gingival and periodontal clinical examinations.
- An example documentation note may be reviewed in **Box 61-1**.

Box 61-1 Example Documentation: Patient with Uncontrolled Hypertension

- **S**—A 46-year-old African American patient arrives in the dental office for a 3-month periodontal continuing care appointment. He reports he has been diagnosed with high blood pressure (BP) and is taking Procardia.
- **O**—Vital signs: blood pressure: 180/100. Patient reports he cannot afford his medication so he takes it every other day. Contacted his primary care provider to ensure it is safe to proceed with treatment. The provider gave permission, but recommended no vasoconstrictor in the local anesthetic until the BP is under control.
- **A**—A comprehensive periodontal and caries examination; findings include localized Stage II, Grade B periodontitis with bleeding on probing in molar areas along with recurrent caries MO-#14, MO-#15.
- **P**—Oral self-care is reviewed with a focus on use of an interdental brush in posterior interproximal areas. Periodontal maintenance is completed, except for in the area of #14–15 where localized nonsurgical periodontal therapy (NSPT) with local anesthesia is recommended. Patient to follow up with his primary care provider and return for localized NSPT once BP is controlled. Office will follow up in 2 weeks.

Signed: ______________________, RDH

Date: ______________________

Factors to Teach the Patient

- Encourage patients to take their medications as prescribed.
- Assess level of dental anxiety using an assessment tool such as the Modified Dental Anxiety Scale to help the patient identify the things that create anxiety and develop a plan for management. Establishing rapport and building trust is an important part of managing dental anxiety.
- Good communication about treatment options and what the patient can expect can help to minimize anxiety.
- If dental anxiety is moderate to high, the following are suggested as part of a stress-reduction protocol:
  - Select an optimum appointment for the patient with respect to the time of the day that might work best for the patient.
  - Encourage patient to get adequate sleep and rest.
  - Eat meals and snacks on usual schedule, and take medications as directed.
  - If a sedative is prescribed, the patient should follow the directions carefully and will require someone to drive them to and from the appointment.
  - Allow time to get to the dental office or clinic so they do not feel rushed.
  - Suggest bringing their own headphones or ear buds and a cell phone or other portable device to listen to music while waiting for and during the appointment. Some offices have headphones and media such as movies the patient can use as an audiovisual distraction.
  - Nitrous oxide may also be a part of stress reduction.
  - Ensure patient knows how to signal the dental clinician during treatment in the case of a problem.

References

1. Larvin H, Kang J, Aggarwal VR, Pavitt S, Wu J. Risk of incident cardiovascular disease in people with periodontal disease: a systematic review and meta-analysis. *Clin Exp Dent Res*. 2021;7(1):109-122.
2. Humphrey LL, Fu R, Buckley DI, Freeman M, Helfand M. Periodontal disease and coronary heart disease incidence: a systematic review and meta-analysis. *J Gen Intern Med*. 2008;23(12):2079.
3. Mitrani RD, Dabas N, Goldberger JJ. COVID-19 cardiac injury: Implications for long-term surveillance and outcomes in survivors. *Heart Rhythm*. 2020;17(11):1984-1990.
4. Hubers SA, DeSimone DC, Gersh BJ, Anavekar NS. Infective endocarditis: a contemporary review. *Mayo Clinic Proc*. 2020;95(5):982-997.
5. Vincent LL, Otto CM. Infective endocarditis: update on epidemiology, outcomes, and management. *Curr Cardiol Rep*. 2018;20(10):86.
6. Williams ML, Doyle MP, McNamara N, Tardo D, Mathew M, Robinson B. Epidemiology of infective endocarditis before versus after change of international guidelines: a systematic review. *Ther Adv Cardiovasc Dis*. 2021;15:17539447211002688.
7. Carroll GC, Sebor RJ. Dental flossing and its relationship to transient bacteremia. *J Periodontol*. 1980;51(12):691-692.
8. Bhanji S, Williams B, Sheller B, Elwood T, Mancl L. Transient bacteremia induced by toothbrushing a comparison of the Sonicare toothbrush with a conventional toothbrush. *Pediatr Dent*. 2002;24(4):295-299.
9. Dubey R, Jalili VP, Jain S, Dubey A. Transient bacteremia consequent to tooth brushing in orthodontic patients. *Prog Orthod*. 2012;13(3):237-245.
10. Glenny AM, Oliver R, Roberts GJ, Hooper L, Worthington HV. Antibiotics for the prophylaxis of bacterial endocarditis in dentistry. *Cochrane Database Syst Rev*. 2013;(10):CD003813.
11. Armstrong GP. Infective endocarditis - heart and blood vessel disorders. *Merck Manuals*. https://www.merckmanuals.com/home/heart-and-blood-vessel-disorders/endocarditis/infective-endocarditis. Accessed February 17, 2022.
12. Suda KJ, Calip GS, Zhou J, et al. Assessment of the appropriateness of antibiotic prescriptions for infection prophylaxis before dental procedures, 2011 to 2015. *JAMA Netw Open*. 2019;2(5):e193909.
13. Wilson WR, Gewitz M, Lockhart PB, et al. Prevention of viridans group streptococcal infective endocarditis: a scientific statement from the American Heart Association. *Circulation*. 2021;143(20):e963-e978.
14. Carinci F, Martinelli M, Contaldo M, et al. Focus on periodontal disease and development of endocarditis. *J Biol Regul Homeost Agents*. 2018;32(2 Suppl. 1):143-147.
15. Pierpont ME, Brueckner M, Chung WK, et al. Genetic basis for congenital heart disease: revisited. *Circulation*. 2018;138(21):e653-e711.
16. Boyd R, McMullen H, Beqaj H, Kalfa D. Environmental exposures and congenital heart disease. *Pediatrics*. 2022;149(1):e2021052151.
17. Centers for Disease Control and Prevention. What are congenital heart defects? Published January 24, 2022. https://www.cdc.gov/ncbddd/heartdefects/facts.html. Accessed February 17, 2022.
18. de Loizaga SR, Beaton AZ. Rheumatic fever and rheumatic heart disease in the United States. *Pediatr Ann*. 2021;50(3): e98-e104.
19. National Heart, Lung, and Blood Institute. Mitral valve prolapse. https://www.nhlbi.nih.gov/health-topics/mitral-valve-prolapse. Accessed February 17, 2022.
20. Whelton PK, Carey RM, Aronow WS, et al. 2017 ACC/AHA/AAPA/ABC/ACPM/AGS/APhA/ASH/ASPC/NMA/PCNA Guideline for the prevention, detection, evaluation, and management of high blood pressure in adults. *J Am Coll Cardiol*. 2018;71(19):e127-e248.
21. Jones DW, Whelton PK, Allen N, et al. Management of stage 1 hypertension in adults with a low 10-year risk for cardiovascular disease: filling a guidance gap: a scientific statement from the American Heart Association. *Hypertension*. 2021;77(6):e58-e67.
22. Rabi D, McBrien K, Sapir-Pichhadze R, et al. Hypertension Canada's 2020 comprehensive guidelines for the prevention, diagnosis, risk assessment, and treatment of hypertension in adults and children. *Can J Cardiol*. 2020;36:596-624.
23. Liu X, Zhang D, Liu Y, et al. Dose-response association between physical activity and incident hypertension: a systematic review and meta-analysis of cohort studies. *Hypertension*. 2017;69(5):813-820.
24. Pescatello LS, Buchner DM, Jakicic JM, et al. Physical activity to prevent and treat hypertension: a systematic review. *Med Sci Sports Exerc*. 2019;51(6):1314-1323.
25. Filippou C, Tatakis F, Polyzos D, et al. Overview of salt restriction in the dietary approaches to stop hypertension (DASH) and the mediterranean diet for blood pressure reduction. *Rev Cardiovasc Med*. 2022;23(1):36.
26. Flynn JT, Kaelber DC, Baker-Smith CM, et al. Clinical practice guideline for screening and management of high blood pressure in children and adolescents. *Pediatrics*. 2017;140(3).
27. Jensen RV, Hjortbak MV, Bøtker HE. Ischemic heart disease: an update. *Semin Nucl Med*. 2020;50(3):195-207.
28. Kaski JC, Crea F, Gersh BJ, Camici PG. Reappraisal of ischemic heart disease. *Circulation*. 2018;138(14):1463-1480.
29. National Heart, Lung, and Blood Institute. Atherosclerosis. https://www.nhlbi.nih.gov/health-topics/atherosclerosis. Accessed February 17, 2022.
30. Ford TJ, Berry C. Angina: contemporary diagnosis and management. *Heart*. 2020;106(5):387-398.
31. National Heart, Lung, and Blood Institute. Angina. https://www.nhlbi.nih.gov/health-topics/angina. Accessed February 19, 2022.
32. Bikdeli B, Madhavan MV, Jimenez D, et al. COVID-19 and thrombotic or thromboembolic disease: implications for prevention, antithrombotic therapy, and follow-up: JACC state-of-the-art review. *J Am Coll Cardiol*. 2020;75(23): 2950-2973.
33. National Heart, Lung, and Blood Institute. Heart attack. https://www.nhlbi.nih.gov/health-topics/heart-attack. Accessed February 19, 2022.
34. Anderson JL, Morrow DA. Acute myocardial infarction. *N Engl J Med*. 2017;376(21):2053-2064.
35. Fleisher LA, Fleischmann KE, Auerbach AD, et al. 2014 ACC/AHA guideline on perioperative cardiovascular evaluation and management of patients undergoing noncardiac surgery. *Circulation*. 2014;130(24):e278-e333.
36. Malik A, Brito D, Vaqar S, Chhabra L. Congestive heart failure. *StatPearls*. Updated November 7, 2022. http://www.ncbi.nlm.nih.gov/books/NBK430873/. Accessed December 14, 2022.

37. American Heart Association. Types of heart failure. Published May 31, 2017. https://www.heart.org/en/health-topics/heart-failure/what-is-heart-failure/types-of-heart-failure. Accessed February 20, 2022.
38. Fine NM. Heart failure. *Merck Manuals.* Published April 2021. https://www.merckmanuals.com/home/heart-and-blood-vessel-disorders/heart-failure/heart-failure-hf. Accessed February 20, 2022.
39. Yancy CW, Jessup M, Bozkurt B, et al. 2017 ACC/AHA/HFSA focused update of the 2013 ACCF/AHA guideline for the management of heart failure: A report of the American College of Cardiology/American Heart Association Task Force on Clinical Practice Guidelines and the Heart Failure Society of America. *Circulation*. 2017;136(6):e137-e161.
40. Aggarwal M, Bozkurt B, Panjrath G, et al. Lifestyle modifications for preventing and treating heart failure. *J Am Coll Cardiol*. 2018;72(19):2391-2405.
41. National Heart, Lung, and Blood Institute. Arrhythmia. https://www.nhlbi.nih.gov/health-topics/arrhythmia. Accessed February 21, 2022.
42. Al-Khatib SM, Stevenson WG, Ackerman MJ, et al. 2017 AHA/ACC/HRS guideline for management of patients with ventricular arrhythmias and the prevention of sudden cardiac death: a report of the American College of Cardiology/American Heart Association Task Force on Clinical Practice Guidelines and the Heart Rhythm Society. *J Am Coll Cardiol*. 2018;72(14):e91-e220.
43. Chung MK, Eckhardt LL, Chen LY, et al. Lifestyle and risk factor modification for reduction of atrial fibrillation: a scientific statement from the American Heart Association. *Circulation*. 2020;141(16):e750-e772.
44. Franklin BA, Myers J, Kokkinos P. Importance of lifestyle modification on cardiovascular risk reduction: counseling strategies to maximize patient outcomes. *J Cardiopulm Rehab Prev*. 2020;40(3):138-143.
45. Arnett DK, Blumenthal RS, Albert MA, et al. 2019 ACC/AHA guideline on the primary prevention of cardiovascular disease: executive summary: a report of the American College of Cardiology/American Heart Association Task Force on clinical practice guidelines. *Circulation*. 2019; 140(11):e563-e595.
46. Teoh Z, Al-Lamee RK. COURAGE, ORBITA, and ISCHEMIA: Percutaneous coronary intervention for stable coronary artery disease. *Interv Cardiol Clin*. 2020;9(4):469-482.
47. Leong DP, Joseph PG, McKee M, et al. Reducing the global burden of cardiovascular disease, part 2. *Circ Res*. 2017;121(6):695-710.
48. Lawton JS, Tamis-Holland JE, Bangalore S, et al. 2021 ACC/AHA/SCAI guideline for coronary artery revascularization. *J Am Coll Cardiol*. 2022;79(2):e21-e129.
49. Tam DY, Dharma C, Rocha R, et al. Long-term survival after surgical or percutaneous revascularization in patients with diabetes and multivessel coronary disease. *J Am Coll Cardiol*. 2020;76(10):1153-1164.
50. Nakai T, Ikeya Y, Kogawa R, Okumura Y. Cardiac resynchronization therapy: current status and near-future prospects. *J Cardiol*. 2022;79(3):352-357.
51. Medline Plus. Pacemakers and implantable defibrillators. https://medlineplus.gov/pacemakersandimplantabledefibrillators.html. Accessed February 21, 2022.
52. Steffel J. The subcutaneous ICD for prevention of sudden cardiac death: current evidence and future directions. *Pacing Clin Electrophysiol*. 2020;43(12):1421-1427.
53. Borne RT, Masoudi FA, Curtis JP, et al. Use and outcomes of dual chamber or cardiac resynchronization therapy defibrillators among older patients requiring ventricular pacing in the National Cardiovascular Data Registry Implantable Cardioverter Defibrillator registry. *JAMA Network Open*. 2021;4(1):e2035470.
54. American Heart Association. Devices that may interfere with ICDs and pacemakers. https://www.heart.org/en/health-topics/arrhythmia/prevention--treatment-of-arrhythmia/devices-that-may-interfere-with-icds-and-pacemakers. Accessed February 21, 2022.
55. Elayi CS, Lusher S, Meeks Nyquist JL, Darrat Y, Morales GX, Miller CS. Interference between dental electrical devices and pacemakers or defibrillators: results from a prospective clinical study. *J Am Dent Assoc*. 2015;146(2):121-128.
56. American Dental Association. Cardiac implanted devices and electronic dental instruments. Published May 14, 2021. https://www.ada.org/resources/research/science-and-research-institute/oral-health-topics/cardiac-implanted-devices-and-electronic-dental-instruments. Accessed February 21, 2022.
57. Lahor-Soler E, Miranda-Rius J, Brunet-Llobet L, Sabaté de la Cruz X. Capacity of dental equipment to interfere with cardiac implantable electrical devices. *Eur J Oral Sci*. 2015;123(3):194-201.
58. Miranda-Rius J, Lahor-Soler E, Brunet-Llobet L, Sabaté X. Risk of electromagnetic interference induced by dental equipment on cardiac implantable electrical devices. *Eur J Oral Sci*. 2016;124(6):559-565.
59. Weitz JI, Chan NC. Advances in antithrombotic therapy. *Arterioscler Thromb Vasc Biol*. 2019;39(1):7-12.
60. Wynn RL, Meiller TF, Crossley HL. Antiplatelet and anticoagulation considerations in dentistry. Lexicomp for Dentistry Online. Waltham, MA: UpToDate, Inc. 2023.
61. Shikdar S, Vashisht R, Bhattacharya PT. International normalized ratio (INR). *StatPearls*. Updated May 8, 2022. http://www.ncbi.nlm.nih.gov/books/NBK507707/. Accessed December 14, 2022.
62. American Dental Association. Oral anticoagulant and antiplatelet medications and dental procedures. Published September 14, 2020. https://www.ada.org/resources/research/science-and-research-institute/oral-health-topics/oral-anticoagulant-and-antiplatelet-medications-and-dental-procedures. Accessed February 21, 2022.
63. Lee JK. Dental management of patients on anti-thrombotic agents. *J Korean Assoc Oral Maxillofac Surg*. 2018;44(4): 143-150.
64. Ockerman A, Bornstein MM, Leung YY, Li SKY, Politis C, Jacobs R. Incidence of bleeding after minor oral surgery in patients on dual antiplatelet therapy: a systematic review and meta-analysis. *Int J Oral Maxillofac Surg*. 2020;49(1): 90-98.

CHAPTER 62

The Patient with a Blood Disorder

Lisa Welch, RDH, MSDH, EdD

CHAPTER OUTLINE

LEARNING OBJECTIVES

After studying this chapter, the student will be able to:

1. Describe the major types of blood disorders.
2. Explain the general and oral signs and symptoms of the major types of blood disorders.
3. Identify clinical implications of selected blood values, including the INR (international normalized ratio), platelet count, and neutrophil count.
4. Provide examples of dental hygiene treatment modifications necessary for the patient with a blood disorder.

Normal Blood

- Major factors to consider for a patient with a blood disorder are oral soft tissue changes, lowered resistance to infection, and bleeding tendencies.
- Oral manifestations of blood disorders are generally exaggerated in the presence of dental biofilm and local predisposing factors.

I. Composition

- Blood is composed of 45% formed elements and 55% fluid, termed plasma.[1]
- The 45% formed elements consist of[1]:
  - 44% erythrocytes (red blood cells or corpuscles): biconcave discs devoid of a nucleus.
  - 1% leukocytes (white blood cells) and platelets.
- **Figure 62-1** shows the types of red and white blood cells

II. Origin of Blood Cells

- Adult blood cells originate in bone marrow.
- Hemocytoblasts are the stem cells of origin.
- Erythrocytes and granulocytes leave the bone marrow as mature cells and enter the circulating blood.
- Agranulocytes (lymphocytes and monocytes) leave the bone marrow as immature cells and migrate to the lymphoid tissues to mature.
- Certain blood diseases and cancers are characterized by the predominance of immature cells.

Plasma

- Blood is a connective tissue; thus, plasma has similar constituents to that of connective tissue fluid.
- Plasma is composed of 90% water.
- Plasma proteins make up the other 10% and include:
  - Albumin (functions to maintain tissue fluid balance within the vascular system).
  - Gamma globulins (circulating antibodies essential to the immune system).
  - Beta globulins (aid in transport of hormones, metallic ions, and lipids).
  - Fibrinogen and prothrombin (essential for blood clotting).
- Inorganic salts include sodium, potassium, calcium, bicarbonate, and chloride.
- Gases include dissolved oxygen, carbon dioxide, and nitrogen.
- Substances being transported include hormones, nutrients, waste products, and enzymes.
- If either plasma or whole blood is allowed to clot, the remaining fluid devoid of clotting factors is termed *serum*.

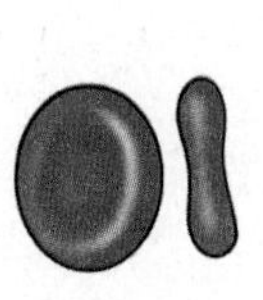

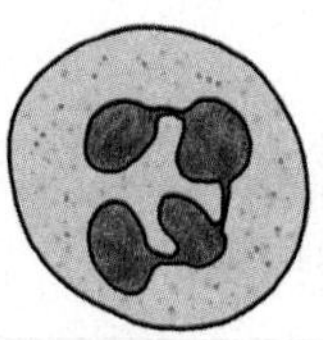

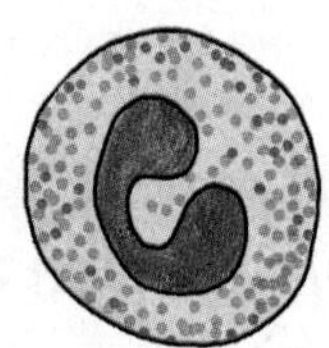

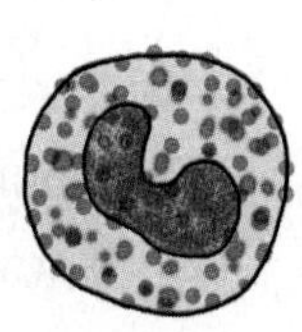

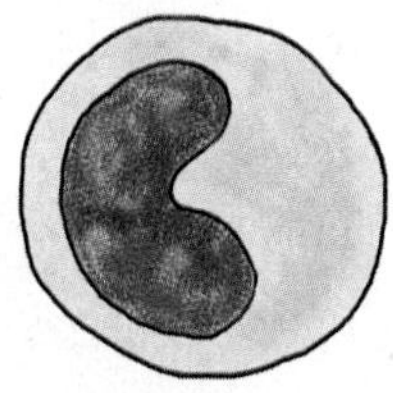

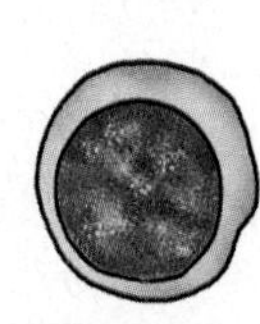

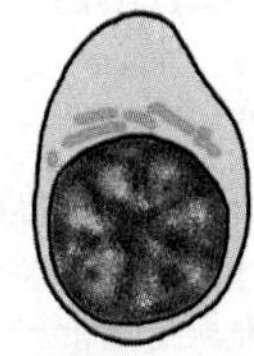

Figure 62-1 Red and White Blood Cells. Diagram shows normal cell forms drawn to scale for comparison of cell size. Note the shape of nuclei in each of the white blood cells. The erythrocyte or red blood cell does not have a nucleus; its biconcave disc shape is shown in the lateral view second from the left.

Red Blood Cells (Erythrocytes)

I. Description

- Red blood cells are more properly termed "corpuscles" because they have no nuclei (Figure 62-1).
- They are flexible biconcave discs containing **hemoglobin**, which can change shape as they pass through small capillaries.
- **Hematocrit**, a test commonly used in health examinations, indicates the amount of blood cells present in a sample of blood expressed as a percentage (**Table 62-1**).
  - Reference values for blood cell counts are listed in **Table 62-2** with examples of conditions in which increases and decreases in the normal values occur.

II. Functions

- Transport hemoglobin, which facilitates the transport of oxygen to the cells in the form of oxyhemoglobin and waste carbon dioxide from the cells in the form of carbaminohemoglobin.

III. Hemoglobin

- Hemoglobin is the iron-containing protein in red blood cells.
- Measured in grams (g) per deciliter (dL) or per 100 milliliters (mL).
- Reference values for adults (18–60 years) range from 12 to 18 g/dL depending on sex (Table 62-1).[2,3]
- Values below reference values may reflect an anemic state; pathologic conditions may result when values increase above reference levels.

Table 62-1 Laboratory Values and Clinical Implications

Test	Reference Range[a]	Clinical Implications	Causes of Deviations
Prothrombin time (PT)	11–15 seconds	Routine care can be performed when PT is <20 seconds	Prolonged in: Prothrombin deficiency Anticoagulant therapy Vitamin K deficiency Liver diseases Aspirin use
International normalized ratio (INR)	<2.5	Routine care can be performed when INR 2–3; medical consult required when INR >3.0	Prolonged in: Polycythemia vera Prothrombin deficiency Anticoagulant therapy Vitamin K deficiency Liver diseases Aspirin use
Activated partial thromboplastin time (aPTT)	25–35 seconds	Routine care when a PTT is <1.5 × normal; medical consult required when >57 sec	Prolonged in: Hemophilia and von Willebrand disease Anticoagulant therapy
Platelet count	140,000–450,000/mm^3	Routine care can be provided when values are >50,000/mm^3 medical consult needed when values <10,000/mm^3—potentially life threatening	Thrombocytopenia: <20,000 mm^3
Hemoglobin (g/dL)	Males: 14-18 g/dL Females: 12–16 g/dL	Delivers oxygen through circulation to body tissues and returns carbon dioxide from tissues to lungs	Increased in: Polycythemia Dehydration Decreased in: Anemias Hemorrhage Leukemias

(continues)

Table 62-1 Laboratory Values and Clinical Implications *(continued)*

Test	Reference Range[a]	Clinical Implications	Causes of Deviations
Hematocrit (volume of packed red cells) (percentage)	Males: 39% to 49% Females: 33% to 43%	Indicates relative proportions of plasma and red blood cells	Increased in: Polycythemia Dehydration Decreased in: Anemias Hemorrhage Leukemias
Absolute neutrophil count (ANC)	Normal ANC: 2500–6000	Measure of the number of infection fighting white blood cells. Routine care 50,000/mm^3; <500/mm^3—potentially life threatening	Decreased in: Anemias Chemotherapy

[a] Ranges vary among health facilities and laboratories. The reference ranges of the facility providing the results are used in interpreting the test result.

Table 62-2 Blood Cell Reference Values

An examination of a blood smear (or film) may be requested by a physician in response to abnormality in blood counts.

Cell Type	Reference Value	Causes of Increase	Causes of Decrease
Red blood cells (erythrocytes)	Males: 4.5–5.9 million/mm^3 Females: 4.5–5.1 million/mm^3	Polycythemia dehydration	Anemias Leukemias Hemorrhage
Platelets (thrombocytes) essential for the process of blood clotting	150,000–450,000/mm^3	Polycythemia vera Chronic myelocytic leukemia Sickle cell anemia Rheumatic fever Hemolytic anemias Bone fractures	Acute severe infections Cirrhosis of the liver Thrombocytopenic purpura Acute leukemias Aplastic anemias Pernicious anemia
White blood cells (leukocytes)	4000–11,000/mm^3	Inflammation Overexertion Polycythemia vera Leukemia	Aplastic anemia Granulocytopenia Drug poisoning Thrombocytopenia Radiation Severe infections (HIV/AIDS) Chemotherapy
Differential White Cell Count			
Neutrophils	40% to 70%	Acute infections Myelogenous leukemia	Aplastic anemia Sepsis Autoimmune disorder
Lymphocytes	22% to 44%	Acute viral infections Bacterial infections (TB) Lymphoma	Bone marrow damage Chemotherapy Immune deficiency HIV infection
Monocytes	0% to 7%	Chronic infections TB Fungal infections Monocytic leukemia	Isolated low count not clinically significant; must repeat low values Bone marrow injury Hairy-cell leukemia

Cell Type	Reference Value	Causes of Increase	Causes of Decrease
Eosinophils	0% to 4%	Asthma Allergies Inflammation Parasitic infections	Eosinopenia Difficult to determine due to low number in the blood; isolated low counts are not clinically significant

Abbreviations: AIDS, acquired immunodeficiency syndrome; HIV, human immunodeficiency virus; TB, tuberculosis

White Blood Cells (Leukocytes)

I. Types of Leukocytes

- White blood cells are divided into two general groups, the granulocytes and the agranulocytes.
- Granulocytes have granules in their cytoplasm, whereas the agranulocytes do not.
- They are further subdivided into the following categories:
  - Granulocytes: neutrophils, eosinophils, and basophils.
  - Agranulocytes: lymphocytes, monocytes.

II. Functions

- Phagocytic, immunologic, and other functions related to the inflammatory process in the connective tissue.
- Blood functions as a transport medium for the white cells as they pass to areas in the connective tissue where they are needed.
- They pass through the walls at the terminal ends of capillaries and into the connective tissue.
- Numbers and proportions in the blood maintain a constant level in health, listed in Table 62-2.
- **Differential cell count** of the white blood cells is used in the detection and monitoring of disease states. Increases and decreases of each cell type can be associated with certain conditions.
- A large number of cells will migrate into the area of an injury.
- Neutrophils arrive first and are active in the **phagocytosis** of foreign material and microorganisms.

III. Agranulocytes

- Lymphocytes
  - Small round cells with a large round nucleus surrounded with a narrow rim of cytoplasm (Figure 62-1).
  - Can move back and forth between the vessels and the extravascular tissues.
  - Capable of reverting to blast-like cells of origin and then multiplying as the immunologic need arises.
- Monocytes
  - Large cells with a bean-shaped or indented nucleus.
  - Actively phagocytic.
  - In connective tissue, monocytes differentiate into macrophages, which are important in immunologic processes.

IV. Granulocytes

- Neutrophils
  - Also called polymorphonuclear leukocytes.
  - Most numerous of all the white blood cells.
  - Nucleus has three to five lobes connected by thin chromatin threads.
  - Cells are round in circulation.
  - Amoeboid (move and change shape) in the tissues and function in phagocytosis.
  - Part of the first line of defense of the body.
- Eosinophils
  - Two-lobed nucleus and larger, coarser granules than those of a neutrophil.
  - Microscopically, the cells stain a distinct bright pink; are readily recognized.
  - Few in number; increase during allergic conditions.
- Basophils
  - Nucleus has a “U” or “S” form.
  - Function is to increase vascular permeability during inflammation so phagocytic cells can pass into the area.

Platelets (Thrombocytes)

- Small round or oval formed element without a nucleus.
- Approximately one-fourth the size of a red blood cell.

- Active in blood clotting mechanisms.
- Essential in the maintenance of the integrity of blood capillaries by repairing them at the time of injury.
- Participate in clot dissolution after healing.

Anemia

- Anemia is the reduction in the number and/or the amount of hemoglobin present in red blood cells such that oxygen-carrying capacity of the blood is diminished.[4]

I. Classification by Cause

A. Caused by Blood Loss

- Acute: blood loss from trauma or disease.
- Chronic: an internal lesion with constant slow bleeding, usually of gastrointestinal or gynecologic origin, can lead to a chronic loss of blood. Iron deficiency anemia can result.

B. Caused by Increased Hemolysis

Hemolysis means the destruction of red blood cells; also called **hemolytic** anemia because it is attributed to cell destruction.

- Hereditary hemolytic disorders
  - Sickle cell disease (SCD), which belongs to the group of hereditary disorders called hemoglobinopathies.
- Acquired hemolytic disorders
  - Drugs, infections, and certain physical and chemical agents may cause red cell destruction.
  - Erythroblastosis fetalis (hemolytic disease of the newborn), a form of antibody-mediated anemia that occurs when an expectant mother is Rh positive and the fetus is Rh negative.

C. Caused by Diminished Production of Red Blood Cells

- Nutritional deficiency
  - Inadequate intake of necessary nutrients for erythrocyte production.
  - Defective absorption from the gastrointestinal tract.
  - Examples: iron deficiency anemia, which may occur during pregnancy or during a growth spurt; celiac disease (sprue), which results from sensitivity to dietary gluten; and pernicious anemia, which results from a B_{12} vitamin absorption deficiency.
  - Increased demand for nutrients such as in growth or pregnancy.
- Bone marrow failure
  - Aplastic anemia (which can be inherited) can occur without apparent cause or when the bone marrow is injured by medications, radiation, chemotherapy, or infection.
  - In aplastic anemia, a combination of anemia, **neutropenia** (reduction in white blood cells), and thrombocytopenia (reduction in number of platelets) occurs, which leads to a quantitative decrease in all cells formed in the bone marrow.
  - Consult with physician to determine if antibiotic premedication is indicated.

D. Anemia of Chronic Diseases

- Second most prevalent anemia after iron deficiency anemia.[5]
- Anemia is associated with many chronic systemic diseases.[5]

E. Caused by Genetic Blood Disorders

- Thalassemia is a diverse group of genetic blood disorders characterized by defects in the synthesis of normal hemoglobin.[6]
- It typically affects people of Mediterranean, African, Middle Eastern, and Southeast Asian descent.
- The condition can range in severity from mild to life threatening.
- The most severe form is beta thalassemia major (Cooley anemia).
- Blood counts are evaluated and monitored for delayed wound healing.
- Treatment[6]:
  - May require periodic and lifelong blood transfusions and chelation therapy.
  - Folic acid supplements.
  - Bone marrow transplant and hematopoietic (blood forming) stem cell transplantation have the potential to cure thalassemia.
  - Novel treatments including gene therapy are under investigation.[6]

II. Clinical Characteristics of Anemia

When a patient's medical history shows the presence of anemia, certain general signs and symptoms may be identified through additional questions or clinical observation including[4]:

- Pale skin, nails, buccal mucosa.
- Weakness, malaise, easy fatigability.
- Dyspnea on slight exertion, faintness.
- Brittle nails with loss of convexity referred to as spooning of the nails.

Iron Deficiency Anemia

I. Characteristics

- Iron deficiency anemia is a hypochromic microcytic anemia, which means that:
  - Hemoglobin content is deficient (hypochromic).
  - Red blood cells are smaller than normal (microcytic).
- Occurs more in younger than older people and more in females than in males.
- Diagnosis is by laboratory test that shows low hemoglobin and a reduced hematocrit value.

II. Causes

The cause of low hemoglobin may include[6-8]:

- Low intake.
  - Malnutrition.
  - Vegans.
- Chronic infection.
- Decreased intestinal absorption.
  - Bariatric surgery (gastric bypass).
  - Celiac disease.
  - Inflammatory bowel diseases (e.g., Crohn disease).
- Increased body demand for iron over and above the daily intake (e.g., during pregnancy).
- Acute or chronic blood loss due to:
  - Excessive menstrual flow.
  - Frequent blood donations.
  - Bleeding disorders.
  - Major surgery.
  - Malignancy.
- Internal bleeding due to:
  - Gastrointestinal diseases, such as ulcer and colon or stomach cancer.
  - Drugs, notably aspirin.
  - Hemorrhoids.
  - Chronic alcoholism.

III. Signs and Symptoms

- General
  - General weakness, pallor.
  - Fatigue on slight exertion.
  - Decreased immune function and increased risk for infection.
- Oral findings
  - Pallor of the mucosa and gingiva.
  - Tongue changes: atrophic **glossitis** with loss of filiform papillae. In moderate and severe anemia, the tongue may be smooth and shiny. The patient may have burning, painful sensations (**glossodynia**).
  - Secondary irritations to the thinned, atrophic mucosa may result from smoking, mechanical trauma, or hot, spicy foods.
  - Angular cheilitis.
  - Increased risk of candidiasis.

IV. Therapy

- Treatment of underlying cause to prevent further blood loss.
- Treated with oral ferrous iron tablets with vitamin C to aid absorption; to be taken on empty stomach for best absorption rates.
- Intravenous (IV) iron therapy may be indicated for certain patients.[7]
- Folic acid supplements may be indicated if there is an underlying folate deficiency.
- Nutritional counseling: recommend foods high in iron.
- Liquid iron preparations, which are sometimes used for children, may stain the teeth. Administering the medicine by way of a straw is advised.

Megaloblastic Anemia

- Characterized by abnormally large (*megalo-*) red blood cells, many of which are oval shaped resulting from a deficiency of vitamin B_{12} (cobalamin) and/or folate, both necessary for the production of healthy red blood cells.

I. Pernicious Anemia

- Etiologic factors[9-13]
  - Considered an autoimmune disease, causing atrophy of the gastric mucosa and destruction of stomach parietal cells.
  - Stomach parietal cells produce **intrinsic factor (IF)** necessary for the absorption of vitamin B_{12}.
  - Deficiency of vitamin B_{12} can also be caused by:
    - Malabsorption due to gastrointestinal disorders such as celiac disease and Crohn's disease.

   - Inadequate intake due to dietary choices may cause deficiency, for example, strict vegans who do not consume animal sources.
   - Chronic atrophic gastritis (e.g., older adults) or surgical removal of part or all of the stomach (e.g., gastric bypass) decreased hydrochloric acid production, decreasing absorption.
   - Long-term use of histamine (H_2) receptor antagonists, proton pump inhibitors, or metformin.[13]
- Age characteristics
  - Pernicious anemia is primarily a disease of adults and occurs with increasing frequency in those older than 60 years, although about one-half of patients are younger than 60 years.[9]
- Signs and symptoms: general
  - Fatigue and weakness.
  - Loss of appetite and weight loss.
  - Poor memory.
- Signs and symptoms: neurologic involvement[9]
  - Sclerosis of the spinal cord.
  - Peripheral neuropathy (numbness and painful tingling of hands and feet).
  - Optical neuropathy.
  - Psychiatric manifestations.
  - Autonomic dysfunction, which may include dizziness or fainting on standing (orthostatic hypotension).
- Signs and symptoms: oral findings
  - Glossitis (Hunter's glossitis), slick or bald tongue, loss of filiform papillae, and burning sensation with certain foods.
  - Sensitivity to hot or spicy foods.
  - Gingiva and mucosa: pale, atrophic similar to vitamin B deficiency.
- Treatment
  - For individuals with IF deficiency and/or malabsorption, vitamin B_{12} is administered by injection daily until the condition is controlled.
  - Once controlled, administration will continue monthly for life or until the underlying condition causing the deficiency is managed.
  - For patients with inadequate IF production, oral supplementation of vitamin B_{12} is the treatment of choice.
  - Vitamin B_{12} is only found in foods from animal sources and fortified foods. Good dietary sources of vitamin B_{12} are meat, clams, liver, fortified breakfast cereals, fish, poultry, milk, cheese, and eggs.

II. Folate-Deficiency Anemia

Folate-deficiency anemia has the same characteristics as pernicious anemia, except no clinical neurologic changes are evident.[14]

- Etiologic factors
  - Decreased intake.
  - Inadequate intake: severely restricted diets or diets influenced by such factors as poverty, food faddism, or alcoholism, when the use of alcohol takes precedence over food.
  - Impaired absorption.
- Individuals at risk of folate inadequacy:
  - Women of childbearing age.
  - Pregnant women.
  - Patients with alcohol dependence.
  - Individuals with malabsorption disorders (e.g., postgastric surgery, celiac disease, and inflammatory bowel disease).
  - Certain treatment regimens impair the utilization of folate (e.g., cancer chemotherapy, rheumatoid arthritis, and medications such as methotrexate and dilantin).
- Dietary factors:
  - In 1998, the Food and Drug Administration required fortification of cereals, breads, flours, pastas, and other grain products with folate.
  - Dietary sources can be found in Chapter 33.
- Fetal development
  - Women with inadequate folic acid intake are at increased risk of having a baby with neural tube defects.
  - Spina bifida (myelomeningocele): a severe condition affecting the formation of the nerves of the spinal cord and resulting in infant paralysis. Spina bifida is described in Chapter 50.

Sickle Cell Disease

- SCD is a hereditary form of hemolytic anemia, resulting from a defective hemoglobin molecule.[15,16]
- The name is derived from the crescent or "sickle" shape assumed by the erythrocytes when the defective hemoglobin loses oxygen (**Figure 62-2**).[15,16]
- It is an autosomal recessive trait. Those with sickle cell trait demonstrate few symptoms unless placed under severe stress.[15,16]

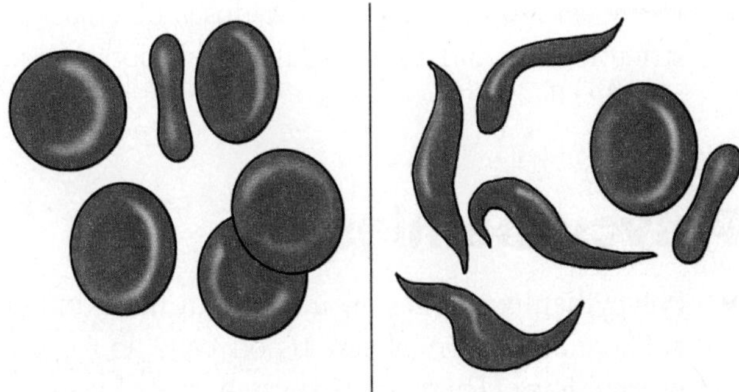

Figure 62-2 Sickle Cell Disease. Left, diagrammatic drawing of normal red blood cells. Right, sickle shapes of red blood cells of a patient with sickle cell disease.

I. Disease Process

Occurs primarily in the African American population and to a lesser degree in Hispanic, Middle Eastern, or Asian Indian populations.[15]

- Diagnosis[15,16]
  - Prenatal diagnosis can be made with 100% accuracy and genetic counseling provided for the parents.
  - A simple blood test will detect SCD or sickle cell trait (parental carrier). Newborn screening is mandatory in most states in the United States.

II. Clinical Course

- Anemia[15]
  - Life span of red blood cells is significantly reduced from a normal life span of approximately 90–120 days to about 10–15 days.
  - Anemia appears within the first 6 months.
  - Growth and development may be impaired during the early years.
  - Increased susceptibility to severe bacterial infection, especially pneumococcal infections in young children.
  - Multiple blood transfusions put patients at risk of blood-borne pathogens (e.g., hepatitis C).
- **Vaso-occlusion**
  - Mortality is primarily from repeated vaso-occlusions (blood vessel blockage), resulting in infarctions, organ damage, and/or stroke.
  - Progressive changes to blood vessels as a result of damage by the sickle-shaped red blood cells that result in the blood vessel blockage.
  - Progressive organ damage resulting in a shortened life expectancy, with an average life expectancy of 54 years and quality of life expectancy being 33 years.[17]
- Pain crises (sickle cell crisis)
  - Repeated episodes of unpredictable acute pain, which results in hospitalization.
  - Often preceded by a viral or bacterial infection.
- Most people with SCD will experience progressive organ damage.
  - Neurologic damage results in impaired cognition and hemorrhagic strokes.
  - Cardiopulmonary damage impairs lung function and results in dilation of the left ventricle of the heart and heart murmurs.
  - Hepatobiliary damage results in abnormal liver function and increases the likelihood of gallstones.
  - Genitourinary damage may result in kidney failure.
  - Skeletal damage may result in necrosis of the hips and shoulders, with a need for joint replacement.
  - Skin effects may result in chronic ulceration.
  - Ocular damage in sickle cell anemia is the leading cause of blindness in patients of African ancestry.

III. Treatment and Disease Management

Treatment and disease management may include the following[15,16]:

- Supportive
  - Management of pain crises remains challenging.
- Oxygen is a mainstay of treatment to minimize **hypoxia**.
- Pain relief without depressing breathing.
- Avoid substance abuse.
- Management of febrile episodes.
- Antibiotics for infectious diseases to avoid sepsis.
- Prevention of sickling.
  - Pharmacologic therapy using a chemotherapy agent (hydroxyurea) to increase hemoglobin F and decrease the permanent formation of sickle cells.
  - Stem cell transplant may be an option.
  - Use of prophylactic penicillin to prevent pneumonia and meningococcal sepsis.

    - Regular blood transfusions.
    - Chemotherapy and gene therapy show promise in the future.

IV. Oral Implications

- Radiographic findings[18]
    - Coarse trabecular pattern appearing as horizontal rows between teeth ("step ladder"), with large marrow spaces.
    - Osteoporotic changes.
- Oral manifestations[18]
    - Necrosis of the dental pulp.
    - Osteomyelitis of the mandible.
    - Enamel hypomineralization.
    - Overgrowth of the facial bones, resulting in protrusion of the maxilla causing malocclusion.
    - Pallor of oral mucosa.
    - Numb chin syndrome (mental nerve neuropathy).
    - Facial and dental pain.
    - Atrophy of papillae on the tongue.

V. Appointment Management

- Thoroughly review the comprehensive medical history. Gather patient information regarding:
    - Related complications specific to organ damage and other problems since birth.
    - Characteristics of pain control (frequency, duration, average number, date of last crisis).
    - Past and current medical treatment (surgeries, transfusions, medications, allergies).
    - Presence of venous access catheters and joint replacement.
    - Growth and development issues.
- Consultation with the patient's primary care provider recommended to determine disease control, including complete blood count.
- Determine if the antibiotic prophylaxis is indicated before any form of tissue manipulation, which could create a bacteremia, is performed because the patient is highly susceptible to infection.[18]
- A stress reduction protocol is necessary to prevent precipitation of a sickle cell crisis.
- Implement a comprehensive preventive program to minimize oral infection and control oral disease risk factors.
- Avoid long, complicated dental appointments by maintaining good oral health with frequent preventive care appointments with the dental hygienist.
- Use local anesthesia with low doses of vasoconstrictors to avoid intravascular occlusion of red blood cells.[18]

Polycythemias

- Polycythemia implies an increase in the number and concentration of red blood cells above the normal level. There are two categories of polycythemia: primary and secondary.

I. Polycythemia Vera (Primary Polycythemia)[19,20]

- Cause
    - Polycythemia vera is a neoplasm caused by a genetic mutation increasing the sensitivity of bone marrow cells to erythropoietin, resulting in an increased production of red blood cells.[19,20]
    - Blood viscosity increases, affecting oxygen transport to tissues.
- Clinical signs and symptoms[19,20]
    - Average age at diagnosis is 60 years.
    - Increased bleeding risk with spontaneous bleeding of the gingiva.
    - Bruise easily, resulting in submucosal **petechiae** and hematoma formation.
    - Risk of fatal and nonfatal blood clot formation, leading to heart attack, stroke, and pulmonary embolism.
    - Migraines.
    - **Vertigo**.
    - Fatigue.
    - Purplish or red areas on the oral mucosa, gingiva, lips, or tongue.
- Treatment[19,20]
    - Chemotherapy.
    - Phlebotomy (blood drawing) to reduce the total volume, particularly the red cell volume, of the blood.
    - Low-dose aspirin (<100 mg/daily) as an antiplatelet.
- Dental hygiene treatment considerations
    - Thorough review of the medical history due to the increased risk of bleeding, bruising, cerebrovascular accident, and myocardial infarction.
    - Consult with the hematologist and/or primary care provider about disease management and patient's blood test results, especially hemoglobin and hematocrit.

- Careful attention to oral self-care and preventive maintenance is required to maintain good oral health.
- Carefully monitor bleeding and monitor clotting during and following instrumentation.
- Provide careful postoperative instructions for early identification of bleeding that does not stop after applying pressure.

II. Secondary Polycythemia[20]

- Secondary polycythemia is also called erythrocytosis (an increase in the number of red blood cells).
- Increased red cell production can result from hypoxia due to chronic obstructive pulmonary disease, cyanotic heart disease, emphysema, tobacco smoking, or residing at high altitudes.
- Bleeding tendencies may be partially controlled with control of gingival irritants.

Disorders of White Blood Cells

- Disorders may occur because of a decrease (**leukopenia**) or an increase (**leukocytosis**) of numbers of white blood cells.
- The types of white blood cells are described in Table 62-2 and illustrated in Figure 62-1.

I. Neutropenia

- A decrease in the total number of neutrophils results when cell production cannot keep pace with the turnover rate or when there is an accelerated rate of removal of cells, as in certain disease states.[21]

A. Etiology[21]

- Defects in myeloid cells possibly due to genetics.
- Secondary neutropenia may develop in the following conditions: alcohol abuse, autoimmune disease (e.g., human immunodeficiency virus [HIV]/acquired immunodeficiency syndrome [AIDS]), chemotherapy or radiation therapy, folate or vitamin B_{12} deficiency, infection, or bone marrow transplant.

B. Signs and Symptoms[21]

- Oral stomatitis and lymph node enlargement may present in patients with neutropenias, resulting from defects in myeloid cells.
- Frequent, severe, or unusual infections such as pneumonia.

C. Diagnosis[21]

- Moderate neutropenia (500–1,000/μL of blood)
- Severe neutropenia (<500/μL)
  - When values drop below 500/μL, even normal microbial flora in the mouth can cause infection.

D. Dental Treatment Considerations

- Thorough review of the medical history is essential.
- Consultation with the primary care provider is necessary to determine if neutrophil count is at a safe level.
- Antibiotic prophylaxis may be needed.

II. Lymphocytopenia

- Abnormally low number of lymphocytes in the blood.

A. Etiology[21]

- Acquired lymphocytopenia may be caused by protein–energy malnutrition, AIDS, chemotherapy, radiation therapy, or infectious disease such as hepatitis, influenza, and tuberculosis.
- Hereditary lymphocytopenia may be associated with inherited immunodeficiency disorders.

B. Signs and Symptoms[21]

- Pallor.
- Bruising (petechiae).
- Mouth ulcers.

C. Dental Treatment Considerations

- The same as for neutropenia.

III. Leukocytosis

Leukocytosis is an increase in the number of circulating white blood cells.

- Caused by inflammatory and infectious states, trauma, exertion, and other conditions listed in Table 62-2.
- The most extreme cause of leukocytosis is leukemia.[22]
  - Leukemias are malignant neoplasms of immature white blood cells that multiply uncontrollably.

- Cancer cells located within the circulating blood and in bone marrow infiltrate into other body tissues and organs such as the spleen and lymph nodes.
- Leukemias can be acute, such as acute lymphocytic leukemia, or chronic, such as chronic lymphocytic leukemia.
- Oral manifestations may include bruising and bleeding of the gingiva.

Platelet Disorders

- Platelets function in the clotting system.
- Disorders include abnormal increases or decreases in numbers of platelets and/or platelet dysfunction.[23]
- When the number of platelets decreases, the risk for bleeding increases.
  - Risk of bleeding increases when platelet count is below 50,000/μL.

I. Thrombocytopenia (Decrease in Platelets)

- Causes of decreases in platelets may include:[23]
  - Decreased production in the bone marrow.
  - Bone marrow depression may be due to drugs, such as hydrochlorothiazide (used to treat high blood pressure) and acetaminophen, infections like HIV and hepatitis, or blood transfusions.
  - If severe, a platelet transfusion may be necessary.

II. Reactive Thrombocytosis (Overproduction of Platelets)

- Overproduction is due to another disorder.
- Causes include acute infection, chronic inflammatory disorders, iron deficiency, and certain cancers.
- Does not usually increase risk of thrombosis.

III. Platelet Dysfunction

- Acquired platelet dysfunction
  - Causes of acquired platelet dysfunction include cirrhosis, systemic lupus erythematosus, and certain drugs.
- Hereditary platelet dysfunction
  - Dysfunction may occur because of a disease such as von Willebrand disease (a coagulation disorder).

Bleeding or Coagulation Disorders

- Blood clotting or hemostasis is the body's mechanism for stopping bleeding from injured blood vessels while preventing intravascular clots, which can cause serious health problems.[24]
- The three main processes of blood clotting include constriction of bleeding vessels, activity of platelets, and activity of blood clotting factors.
- A history or suspicion of a bleeding problem requires careful evaluation before treatment can be started.
- Spontaneous bleeding occurs as small hemorrhages into the skin or mucous membranes and other tissues and appears as petechiae or **purpura**.
- People with bleeding disorders have the tendency to exhibit spontaneous bleeding and moderate to excessive bleeding following trauma, surgical procedure, or dental hygiene therapy, including nonsurgical instrumentation.

I. Oral Findings Suggestive of Bleeding Disorders

- Early signs of systemic conditions frequently appear in the oral soft tissues and clinical examination may identify these changes.
- Referral for medical examination may lead to diagnosis and treatment of a serious disease.
- Laboratory blood tests may provide essential information for safe and effective dental hygiene care.
- Oral soft tissue changes observed in patients with blood diseases are not necessarily exclusive to systemic blood disorders.
- It is necessary to recognize change in a previously healthy patient or an exaggerated response in a patient being examined at an initial appointment.
- Findings suggesting a blood disorder include the following[25-27]:
  - Gingival bleeding, spontaneously or excessive bleeding on gentle probing.
  - History of difficulty in controlling bleeding by usual procedures.
  - History of bruising easily, with large ecchymoses.
  - Numerous petechiae.
  - Marked pallor of the mucous membranes.
  - Atrophy of the papillae of the tongue (atrophic glossitis) or magenta tongue.
  - Angular stomatitis.
  - Persistent sore or painful tongue (glossodynia).

- Acute or chronic infections, such as candidiasis, that do not respond to usual treatment.
- Severe ulcerations associated with a lack of response to treatment.
- Exaggerated gingival response to local irritants, sometimes with characteristics of necrotizing ulcerative gingivitis (ulceration, necrosis, bleeding, pseudomembrane).
- Vascular fragility is increased; petechial and purpuric hemorrhages appear in the skin or mucous membranes, including the gingiva.

II. Disorders of Coagulation

- Abnormal bleeding can be due to acquired, drug-related, or hereditary factors including disorders of the coagulation system, of platelets, and/or of blood vessels.

A. Acquired Bleeding Disorders

- Vitamin K deficiency
  - Vitamin K is essential in the synthesis of prothrombin and clotting factors VII, IX, and X.
  - Vitamin K stores at birth are low and can result in vitamin K deficiency bleeding if prophylactic vitamin K is not administered.[25]
  - Vitamin K is produced in the alimentary tract by intestinal bacteria. Food sources of vitamin K may be found in Chapter 33.
  - Excessive exposure to antibiotic therapy or prolonged gastrointestinal disturbances may affect vitamin K production.
- Liver disease: most clotting factors are produced in the liver. When the liver is not functioning properly, production of clotting factors may be altered.[26,27]
  - May occur in cirrhosis.
- Renal disease: erythropoietin is produced by the kidneys; it is involved in the stimulation of red blood cell production in bone marrow.[26,27]
- Bone marrow disorders: impact red and white blood cell production.[27]

B. Drug-Related Acquired Bleeding Disorders

- Anticoagulation drugs such as warfarin (Coumadin) are vitamin K antagonists and require monitoring of bleeding time with an INR.[28]
- Direct-acting oral anticoagulants (DOACs) such as dabigatran (Pradaxa), rivaroxaban (Zarelto), and apixaban (Eliquis). DOACs do not require regular monitoring with an INR.[28]
- Antiplatelet drugs are meant to prevent thrombus formation and include aspirin.

C. Hereditary Bleeding Disorders

At least 30 hereditary coagulation disorders exist, each resulting from a deficiency or abnormality of a plasma protein.

- Hemophilia
  - Hemophilias are the oldest known hereditary bleeding disorders caused by low levels or complete absence of blood proteins essential for clotting.
- Etiology[29]
  - Results from mutation or deletion affecting the factor VIII or IX gene.
  - Hemophilia is an X-linked recessive genetic disease. The defective gene is located on the X chromosome; thus, the disorder occurs primarily in males.
- Treatment[29]
  - In the 1970s, self-treatment to administer coagulation factors prophylactically to prevent bleeding became the standard of care.
  - Treatment continues to evolve due to creation of coagulation factors with a longer half-life and gene therapy.
- Effects and long-term complications[29]
  - Bleeding and bruising from minor trauma vary depending on the severity of the disease.
  - Bleeding into the soft tissue of joints (**hemarthroses**) of knees, ankles, and elbows begins in the very young with severe hemophilia.
  - Hemorrhage into the muscles (intramuscular hemorrhage) is accompanied by pain and limitation of motion.
  - Bleeding from the gingiva is common and more extensive when periodontal infection is more severe.
- Dental management[30]
  - The hematologist should be consulted prior to performing dental procedures with a risk of bleeding.
  - Injections for local anesthesia such as the inferior alveolar block and alternative routes for delivery may be indicated to reduce the risk of bleeding.
  - Antifibrinolytic agents may be necessary for some dental hygiene therapies including subgingival debridement.
  - In someone with mild bleeding disorders, if clotting does not occur within a few minutes, apply digital pressure to area with sterile gauze.

- If needed, local hemostatic agents can be applied, such as absorbable gelatin sponge. Absorbs for 3–5 days.
- Medical attention required if bleeding is not controlled.

Dental Hygiene Care Plan

I. Preparation for Clinical Appointment

- Certain blood tests may be needed prior to treatment and should be documented.
  - Prothrombin time.
  - **International Normalized Ratio (INR)** ideally should be measured within 24–72 hours of any invasive procedure for those taking anticoagulation drugs.[28]
  - DOACs do not require an INR.[28]
- Basic tests are listed in Table 62-1 with their ranges or values.
- Indications for screening and pre-appointment tests:
  - When the patient reports a history of a bleeding problem.
  - Clinical examination reveals signs of a bleeding disorder.
  - Patient is being treated with anticoagulants, chemotherapy, or corticosteroids.

II. Patient History

A. Medical History Review

The medical history needs to include information regarding the type, severity, medical treatment, medications, and family history of the blood clotting defect.

- Question patient specifically regarding bleeding after previous clinical and surgical procedures, such as tooth extractions.
- Question about blood or plasma transfusions, as individuals who received them prior to 1990 are at risk for hepatitis B and C as well as HIV.[29]
- Patients with bleeding disorders have many emotional stresses related to the condition, including ongoing anxiety, so it is important to understand the patient's psychosocial situation.

B. Medication Review

A careful review of a patient's drug, supplements, and herbal remedy use is critical to determine potential oral and physiologic effects.

- The primary purpose of the drug and potential side effects needs careful review in a current drug reference guide.
- A variety of drugs and herbs may be factors in increased bleeding.
  - Common herbs, supplements, and vitamins associated with increased bleeding are listed in **Box 62-1**.[31,32]
  - It is recommended to carefully review any herbal remedies and supplements the patient may be using that could be associated with an increased risk of bleeding and to discontinue for at least a week prior to receiving invasive surgical procedures.
- Patients taking warfarin (Coumadin; for prevention of recurrent thrombosis), heparin (for short-term use following a total joint replacement procedure), or medication for long-term anticoagulation (such as aspirin) may need special consultation.
  - The most common side effect of both warfarin and heparin is hemorrhage.
  - Hemorrhages may present as gingival bleeding or submucosal bleeding with hematoma formation.
- Cancer chemotherapeutic agents may secondarily induce profound thrombocytopenia (<20,000 mm^3) or neutropenia (<500 mm^3).
- Antithrombotic agents such as aspirin and clopidogrel (Plavix) alter the ability of platelets to stick or clump together and form a clot.

C. Dental History Review

- Discuss previous dental care and perceived treatment needs when developing the current care plan with the patient.

D. Risk Assessment

- The patient with a bleeding disorder may be at high risk for dental caries and periodontal disease, so modifiable risk factors need to be addressed in the treatment care plan.
- Early prevention of oral disease at a young age, including regular professional preventive care, meticulous oral self-care, appropriate use of fluorides, and pit and fissure sealants, is recommended.

III. Consultation with Primary Care Provider/Hematologist

- Consultation with the primary care provider/hematologist is necessary to develop a plan for hemostasis management.[30]
- Anticoagulant therapy is seldom discontinued for most dental treatments because the risk for

Box 62-1 Herbal Supplements and Vitamin Supplements Associated with Increased Bleeding[31,32]

Herbs/Supplements with Antiplatelet Properties	Herbs/Supplements with Anticoagulant Properties	Herbs/Supplements with Both Antiplatelet and Anticoagulant Properties	Herbs/Supplements That Interfere with Clotting via Other Mechanisms	Vitamins That May Increase Bleeding
Aloe	Chamomile	Dong Quai	Flaxseed	Vitamin C
Cranberry	Fenugreek	Evening primrose	Grapefruit	Vitamin E
Feverfew	Red clover	Ginseng	Green tea	
Garlic		Fish oil	Oregano	
Ginger		Omega-3 fatty acids	Saw palmento	
Ginkgo				
Meadowsweet				
Turmeric				
White willow				

Data from Abebe W. Review of herbal medications with the potential to cause bleeding: dental implications, and risk prediction and prevention avenues. *EPMA J.* 2019;10(1):51-64; Violi F, Pignatelli P, Basili S. Nutrition, supplements, and vitamins in platelet function and bleeding. *Circulation.* 2010;121(8):1033-1044

intravascular clot formation is greater than the risk for hemorrhage.[28]

- A joint policy advising health care providers who perform invasive or surgical procedures to contact the cardiologist and discuss patient management before discontinuing antiplatelet drugs was developed by[33]:
  - American Dental Association.
  - American Heart Association.
  - American College of Cardiology.
  - Society for Cardiovascular Angiography and Interventions.
  - American College of Surgeons.
- Consult primary care provider/hematologist to determine whether antibiotic prophylaxis is required during dental procedures to prevent infection in joint prostheses and/or indwelling catheter.[34,35]
- In inherited bleeding disorder, many procedures require factor replacement therapy immediately preceding the dental appointment.[30]
- Request reports of current blood tests.

IV. Examination

- Use a preprocedural chlorhexidine mouthrinse to reduce the bacterial load prior to beginning examination or treatment.
- Radiographic imaging: films/sensor (infection control barriers) can cut and press on the mucous membranes. Exercise care in placement to avoid bleeding and/or a hematoma.
- The dental and periodontal examination can be conducted once a consultation with the primary care provider or specialist has assessed the need for antibiotic prophylaxis or pretreatment to prevent bleeding.

V. Treatment Care Plan

- Select age-appropriate preventive measures based on risk assessment including, but not limited to:
  - Oral self-care instruction.
  - Nutrition counseling.
  - Preventive agents including fluoride treatments, remineralizing agents, and/or sealants.
  - Prophylaxis or nonsurgical periodontal therapy (NSPT).
  - Restorative care.
  - Referral as needed.
  - Continuing care recommendations.

VI. Treatment

- Stress reduction protocol: prevention or reduction of stress begins before the appointment and throughout treatment.

- Provide patient education to enhance oral self-care at the initial appointment and reinforce at each session to prevent oral disease and complications.[30]
  - A soft or medium toothbrush is recommended.[30] If patient prefers using a power brush, proper demonstration of technique is necessary.
  - Choose the appropriate interdental aid(s) and teach the patient correct use to prevent tissue injury.
  - Patients with limited manual dexterity or restrictions to mobility of the elbow or shoulder may benefit from adaptive oral hygiene aids.
- Local anesthesia can be used with caution to avoid block anesthesia (inferior alveolar and posterior superior alveolar) and instead use infiltration injections.
  - Use local anesthesia with a vasoconstrictor to minimize the need to re-inject.
- In those with active periodontal disease with significant gingival inflammation, a consult with the medical provider may be required prior to NSPT to ensure the patient is managed properly to prevent bleeding.
  - Minimize tissue trauma as much as possible.
  - Exercise caution with the use of suction to prevent trauma and hematomas to the buccal, sublingual, or other mucosal tissues.
- Postoperative: monitor to ensure bleeding has stopped postoperatively.
  - Never recommend aspirin or nonsteroidal anti-inflammatory drugs (NSAIDs) for a patient with a bleeding disorder.
  - Ideally call the patient the evening after treatment to ensure they are having no bleeding issues.
- Frequency of continuing care: frequent appointments can aid in keeping the oral tissues in an optimum state of health and help to prevent the need for complex or lengthy dental appointments.

Documentation

Documentation in the permanent record for each appointment with a blood disorder includes a minimum of the following factors:

- Review or update medical history thoroughly. Document laboratory findings.
- Document extra- and intraoral examination findings. Use written description and an intraoral picture when possible.
- Note treatment planning considerations such as shorter appointments, stress reduction protocols that need to be implemented, and oral hygiene considerations.
- Note consultations with other health professionals involved in the patient's care.
- Reference any difficulties with bleeding control during appointment.
- A sample progress note is provided in **Box 62-2**.

Box 62-2 Example Documentation: Patient with a Blood Disorder

- **S**—A 70-year-old white man presents for a new patient examination. He reports having a stroke a year ago and currently taking Coumadin (warfarin). Patient states that his INR last week was 2.8.
- **O**—Oral cancer examination: all tissues appear normal. Full-mouth series of radiographs and caries examination reveal no new caries. Periodontal examination: generalized 4–5 mm pocket depths with localized bleeding on probing. Plaque score: 50%.
- **A**—Increased risk for oral bleeding following dental hygiene treatment.
- **P**—Disclosed plaque biofilm and reviewed technique for oral hygiene aids. Stressed need for meticulous oral self-care to prevent infection and associated bleeding. NSPT completed maxillary and mandibular right quadrants with 2 carpules of 2% xylocaine with 1:100,000 epinephrine. Areas monitored to verify bleeding had stopped within 5 minutes following completion of instrumentation. Postoperative instruction given to contact the office should he be unable to stop bleeding.

Next appointment: Complete NSPT with local anesthesia and apply fluoride varnish.
Signed: ____________________, RDH
Date: ______________

Factors to Teach the Patient

- Need to carefully and thoroughly remove plaque biofilm daily to minimize the risk for oral infection and associated bleeding.
- Brush at least twice per day with daily interdental cleaning and other appropriate oral hygiene aids.[30]
- How to self-evaluate the oral cavity for deviations from normal. Watching for changes in size, shape, and color and contacting oral health professional when lesions last longer than 2 weeks.
- Selection of noncariogenic foods to prevent caries and knowledge about the diet's relationship to health.
- Avoid use of salicylates (aspirin) and NSAIDs.
- Importance of informing the dental provider of any changes to the medical history, including drugs, herbs, supplements, and hospitalizations and providing recent laboratory values before beginning treatment.

References

1. Mescher AL. Blood. In: Mescher AL., ed. *Junqueira's Basic Histology*. 16th ed. New York, NY: McGraw-Hill; 2021.
2. Clinical Laboratory Reference 2021-2022. Table of Reference Intervals. https://www.clr-online.com/CLR_2021-22_Reference_Intervals.pdf. Accessed August 31, 2021
3. Greer JP, Smock MK. Examination of the blood and bone. In: Greer JP, ed. *Wintrobe's Clinical Hematology*. 14th ed. Philadelphia, PA: Wolters Kluwer; 2018. https://labtestsonline.org/tests/white-blood-cell-wbc-differential. Accessed online August 31, 2021
4. Buhn FH. Introduction to anemia and red cell disorders. In: Aster JC, Bunn H, eds. *Pathophysiology of Blood Disorders*. 2nd ed. New York, NY: McGraw-Hill; 2017.
5. Damon LE, Andreadis C. Blood disorders. In: Papadakis MA, McPhee SJ, Rabow MW, eds. *Current Medical Diagnosis & Treatment 2018*. New York, NY: McGraw-Hill; 2018:chap 13.
6. Rund D. Thalassemia 2016: modern medicine battles an ancient disease. *Am J Hematol*. 2016;91(1):15-21.
7. Camaschella C. New insights into iron deficiency and iron deficiency anemia. *Blood Rev*. 2017;31(4):225-233.
8. Office of Dietary Supplements. Iron: Fact sheet for health professionals. Bethesda, MD: National Institutes of Health. http://ods.od.nih.gov/factsheets/Iron-HealthProfessional/. Accessed August 31, 2021.
9. Rojas Hernandez CM, Oo TH. Advances in mechanisms, diagnosis, and treatment of pernicious anemia. *Discov Med*. 2015;19(104):159-168.
10. Office of Dietary Supplements. Vitamin B_{12}: Fact sheet for health professionals. Bethesda, MD: National Institutes of Health. http://ods.od.nih.gov/factsheets/VitaminB12-HealthProfessional/. Accessed August 31, 2021.
11. Green R, Datta Mitra A. Megaloblastic anemias: nutritional and other causes. *Med Clin North Am*. 2017;101(2):297-317. doi:10.1016/j.mcna.2016.09.013
12. Jung SB, Nagaraja V, Kapur A, Eslick GD. Association between vitamin B12 deficiency and long-term use of acid-lowering agents: a systematic review and meta-analysis. *Intern Med J*. 2015;45(4):409-416.
13. Ahmed MA. Metformin and vitamin B12 deficiency: where do we stand? *J Pharm Pharm Sci*. 2016;19(3):382-398.
14. Office of Dietary Supplements. Folate: dietary supplement fact sheet. Bethesda, MD: National Institutes of Health. http://ods.od.nih.gov/factsheets/Folate-HealthProfessional/. Accessed August 31, 2021.
15. Yawn BP, Buchanan GR, Afenyi-Annan AN, et al. Management of sickle cell disease: summary of the 2014 evidence-based report by expert panel members. *JAMA*. 2014;312(10):1033-1048.
16. Sheth S, Licursi M, Bhatia M. Sickle cell disease: time for a closer look at treatment options? *Br J Haematol*. 2013;162(4):455-464.
17. Lubeck D, Agodoa I, Bhakta N, et al. Estimated life expectancy and income of patients with sickle cell disease compared with those without sickle cell disease. *JAMA Netw Open*. 2019;2(11):e1915374.
18. Chekroun M, Chérifi H, Fournier B, et al. Oral manifestations of sickle cell disease. *Br Dent J*. 2019;226(1):27-31.
19. Squizzato A, Romualdi E, Passamonti F, et al. Antiplatelet drugs for polycythaemia vera and essential thrombocythaemia. *Cochrane Database Syst Rev*. 2013;(4):CD006503.
20. Tefferi A, Barbui T. Polycythemia vera and essential thrombocythemia: 2015 update on diagnosis, risk stratification and management. *Am J Hematology*. 2015;90(2):162-173.
21. Territo M. Overview of white blood cell disorders. *The Merck Manual—Professional Edition*. https://www.merckmanuals.com/home/blood-disorders/white-blood-cell-disorders/overview-of-white-blood-cell-disorders. Accessed November 13, 2021.
22. Jabbour E, Kantarjian H. Chronic myeloid leukemia: 2018 update on diagnosis, therapy and monitoring. *Am J Hematol*. 2018;93(3):442-459.
23. Haley KM. Platelet disorders. *Pediatr Rev*. 2020;41(5):224-235.
24. Moak JL. Overview of hemostasis. *The Merck Manual—Professional Edition*. https://www.merckmanuals.com/professional/hematology-and-oncology/hemostasis/overview-of-hemostasis. Accessed November 13, 2021.
25. Sankar MJ, Chandrasekaran A, Kumar P, Thukral A, Agarwal R, Paul VK. Vitamin K prophylaxis for prevention of vitamin K deficiency bleeding: a systematic review. *J Perinatol*. 2016;36(Suppl 1):S29-S35.

26. Hurwitz A, Massone R, Lopez BL. Acquired bleeding disorders. *Hematol Oncol Clin North Am*. 2017;31(6): 1123-1145.
27. Moosajee S, Rafique S. Dental management of patients with acquired and congenital bleeding disorders. *Prim Dent J*. 2020;9(2):47-55.
28. Felix J, Chaban P, Ouanounou A. dental management of patients undergoing antithrombotic therapy. *J Can Dent Assoc*. 2020;86(k17):1488-2159.
29. Mannucci PM. Hemophilia therapy: the future has begun. *Haematologica*. 2020;105(3):545-553.
30. Srivastava A, Santagostino E, Dougall A, et al. WFH guidelines for the management of hemophilia, 3rd edition. *Haemophilia*. 2020;26(Suppl 6):1-158.
31. Abebe W. Review of herbal medications with the potential to cause bleeding: dental implications, and risk prediction and prevention avenues. *EPMA J*. 2019;10(1):51-64.
32. Violi F, Pignatelli P, Basili S. Nutrition, supplements, and vitamins in platelet function and bleeding. *Circulation*. 2010;121(8):1033-1044.
33. American Dental Association. Oral health topics, anticoagulant and antiplatelet medications and dental procedures. Updated September 28, 2022. https://www.ada.org/resources/research/science-and-research-institute/oral-health-topics/oral-anticoagulant-and-antiplatelet-medications-and-dental-procedures Accessed February 2, 2023.
34. Sollecito TP, Abt E, Lockhart PB, et al. The use of prophylactic antibiotics prior to dental procedures in patients with prosthetic joints: evidence-based clinical practice guideline for dental practitioners—a report of the American Dental Association Council on Scientific Affairs. *J Am Dent Assoc*. 2015;146(1):11-16.
35. Abed H, Ainousa A. Dental management of patients with inherited bleeding disorders: a multidisciplinary approach. *Gen Dent*. 2017;65(6):56-60.

CHAPTER 63

The Patient with an Autoimmune Disease

Robin L. Kerkstra, RDH, MSDH
Linda D. Boyd, RDH, RD, EdD

CHAPTER OUTLINE

LEARNING OBJECTIVES

After studying this chapter, the student should be able to:

1. Describe how autoimmune diseases affect the immune system.
2. Identify various types of autoimmune diseases and the identifying symptoms and treatment.
3. Plan dental hygiene care modifications for the patient with an autoimmune disease.

Overview of Autoimmune Diseases

- Autoimmune diseases occur when the immune system has problems fighting viruses, bacteria, and infection because immune cells attack parts of the body instead of protecting it.

I. Immune System Basics

- The immune system consists of two parts, called the acquired and innate immune systems (**Figure 63-1**).
  - As a person grows, so does their acquired immune system and its ability to recognize invaders in the body and remember them for future immune response.
  - Acquired immune cells activate antibodies that attach themselves to invaders to be destroyed.
- Immune cells associated with adaptive immunity, called lymphocytes, develop in the bone marrow and specialize in protecting the body against any foreign invader.
  - There are two major types of lymphocytes: B lymphocytes, which mature in the bone marrow, and T lymphocytes that mature in the thymus.

II. Prevalence of Autoimmune Diseases

- Worldwide prevalence of autoimmune diseases is between 7.6 and 9.4%.[1]
  - Annual increase in prevalence globally ranges from 3.7 to 7.1% for specific autoimmune conditions, including rheumatoid arthritis, celiac disease, and type 1 diabetes.[2]

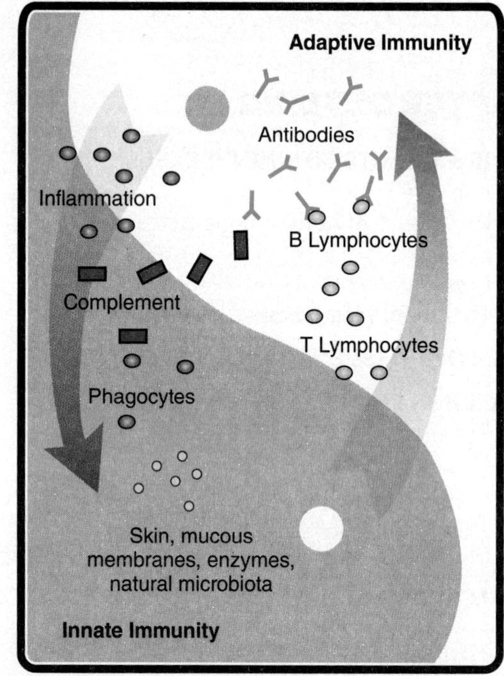

Figure 63-1 Overview of the Immune System. As part of the innate immunity, the human body has natural measures to prevent entry of microbes. When these barriers are overcome, a foreign invader first encounters phagocytes. Inflammation may develop. If the innate immune system cannot destroy the invader, the adaptive immune system is activated with T and B lymphocytes. Although the innate and adaptive immune systems are characterized by contrasting functions and timing, they work closely together and rely on each other to succeed in removing the invading pathogens.

- Immune diseases affect an estimated 4.5% (14.7 million) of the US population.[3]
  - Of individuals with autoimmune diseases, 78% are women.[4]

- Women also are at increased risk of **polyautoimmunity**.[4]
- Female hormonal changes during puberty, pregnancy, and menopause tend to be associated with onset of autoimmune diseases.[4]
- The most common age of onset of autoimmune diseases is 40–50 years.[3]

III. Etiology

- Multifactorial etiology includes a genetic predisposition for activation of self-antigen–specific T lymphocytes resulting in the formation of **autoantibodies**.
- Factors that may modify the autoimmune response include biologic (e.g., sex, pregnancy, and age) and environmental variables (e.g., infectious agents, diet, tobacco, and chemicals).[4,5]
- Autoantibodies cause damage and dysfunction of tissues target tissues and/or organs.
- Some autoimmune diseases tend to co-occur and may have a genetic predisposition, such as type 1 diabetes, rheumatoid arthritis (RA), and thyroiditis.[6]

IV. Classification

- There are 80–100 autoimmune diseases; the most common ones can be found in **Table 63-1**, along with the organ system affected.[5]
- Various classification systems have been proposed and will likely be refined in future years.

A. Organ-Specific Autoimmune Diseases

- In organ-specific diseases, the antibodies and T cells react with self-antigens in specific tissue.[5]
- Examples include:
  - Gastrointestinal (GI) autoimmune diseases: Crohn's disease, celiac disease (CD), and ulcerative colitis (UC).
  - Connective tissue autoimmune diseases: RA and scleroderma. These two autoimmune diseases may also be systemic if they extend beyond their target tissue/organ.
  - Neurologic system autoimmune diseases: multiple sclerosis (MS) and myasthenia gravis.

Table 63-1 **Types of Autoimmune Diseases**

	Organ Affected	Examples of Autoimmune Diseases
Organ-specific autoimmune diseases	Skin	Psoriasis Pemphigus
	Pancreas	Type 1 diabetes mellitus Autoimmune pancreatitis
	Gastrointestinal system	Celiac disease Ulcerative colitis Crohn's disease
	Neurologic system	Multiple sclerosis Myasthenia gravis Narcolepsy
	Thyroid and parathyroid gland	Graves' disease Hashimoto's autoimmune thyroiditis Autoimmune hypoparathyroidism
	Connective tissue	Rheumatoid arthritis Scleroderma Ankylosing spondylitis
Systemic (organ nonspecific) autoimmune diseases	Lungs, liver, kidneys, central nervous system, salivary, and lacrimal glands	Sjögren's syndrome
	Heart, joints, skin, lungs, blood vessels, liver, kidneys, and nervous system	Systemic lupus erythematosus

B. Systemic Autoimmune Diseases

- Autoimmune disease is considered systemic when immune cells react to self-antigens throughout the body and in various tissues.[5]
  - Examples of systemic autoimmune diseases include systemic lupus erythematosus (SLE) and Sjögren syndrome (SS). Both these conditions can affect several organ systems, including the lungs, liver, and nervous system.

V. Treatment Modalities

- There is a wide range of treatment options classified into the following categories:
  - Nonsteroidal anti-inflammatory drugs (NSAIDs).
  - **Glucocorticosteroid** medications.
  - Immunosuppressive medications.
  - Therapeutic monoclonal antibodies.
  - Immunoglobulin replacement therapy.
  - Medications to replace hormones secreted by the target organ, such as thyroxine in autoimmune thyroid disease.

Connective Tissue Autoimmune Diseases

- Connective tissue autoimmune diseases are a diverse group of conditions affecting a variety of organs.[7]
- Most connective tissue diseases have significant genetic risk factors.
- A few connective tissue autoimmune diseases will be reviewed, here including oral lichen planus (OLP), RA, and scleroderma.

Oral Lichen Planus

- OLP is a chronic or recurrent inflammatory disease that affects the inside of the oral cavity on any mucosal surface, such as the cheeks, tongue, and gingiva.[8]
  - Buccal mucosa is the mostly commonly affected site.
- OLP is at risk of malignant transformation to oral squamous cell carcinoma in 1.1% of cases.[9]

I. Prevalence

- Global prevalence is 1.01%.[8]
- OLP risk increases after age 40.[8]

II. Etiology

- Etiology is unknown, but considered to be multifactorial and may include[10]:
  - Genetic susceptibility.
  - Other systemic diseases such as diabetes.
  - Frequently associated with hepatitis B and hepatitis C virus (HCV).

III. Clinical Presentation

- Six types of OLP[10]:
  - Reticular: characteristic **Wickham striae**: mossy, lacy white threads that are slightly raised found on the buccal mucosa (**Figure 63-2**).
  - Plaque-like white lesions: occurs more frequently on the dorsal surface of the tongue and may look like oral leukoplakia.
  - Papular: appear as papules on the oral mucosa, especially the buccal mucosa.
  - Atrophic/erosive: may resemble an oral erythroleukoplakia lesion, but is typically bilateral and symmetric.
  - Ulcerative: similar to erosive OLP, but there is central ulceration in the lesion.
  - Bullous: bulla or a separation of the oral epithelium from the underlying connective tissue is present.
- The condition tends to have periods of remission and flare-ups.

IV. Treatment

- OLP can be definitively diagnosed with a biopsy, which will also rule out the possibility of malignancy.

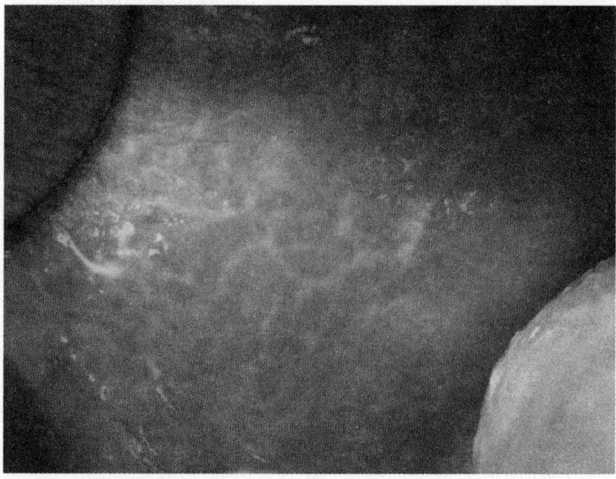

Figure 63-2 Wickham Striae of Oral Lichen Planus. A white, lacy network of lesions and erosions is present on the buccal mucosa.

    - OLP must be carefully monitored as there is a small risk of transformation to oral squamous cell carcinoma.[9]
- There is no definitive treatment for OLP and management of symptoms is the usual approach to care.[11]
- When erosive or ulcerative lesions are present, pain is possible when eating or drinking with temperature extremes and acidic, coarse, or spicy foods.
- Symptoms may be managed by topical **corticosteroids** for mild and moderate symptomatic lesions.[12]
    - Systemic corticosteroids, such as prednisolone, may also be needed for those with a severe outbreak of lesions.
- A healthy lifestyle of a well-balanced diet, exercise, and stress reduction may help with flare-ups.
    - Many OLP patients have deficiencies of iron, vitamin B_{12}, and folic acid, so ensuring an adequate intake and possibly supplementation may help in management.[10]

V. Dental Hygiene Care

- Avoid food and drink that aggravate OLP.
- Painful lesions may limit a patient's ability to adequately remove dental biofilm.
- **Palliative** care for painful lesions may be required and include viscous lidocaine mouthrinses.
- For erosive or ulcerated lesions, it may be best to avoid toothpastes with pyrophosphates and mouthrinses with alcohol.

Rheumatoid Arthritis

- RA is an autoimmune disease resulting in joint inflammation and ultimately destruction of the joint and loss of cartilage.[13]
- Systematic reviews of the literature suggest an association between periodontal disease and RA, possibly due to commonalities in the inflammatory processes.[14]

I. Prevalence

- The global prevalence is 0.46% and the highest prevalence is in North America (0.70%).[15]
    - Prevalence in the United States is 0.53 to 0.55% with 1.28–1.36 million people affected by RA.[16]
    - American Indigenous populations such as Pima and Chippewa communities have the highest prevalence (5.3 to 6.8%).[15]
- More than twice as many women (0.73 to 0.78%) are affected with RA when compared to men (0.29 to 0.31%).[13,16]
- Peak incidence is at age 50 years.[13]

II. Etiology

- RA is a multifactorial disease with complex interactions between the host and environment.
- Host factors:
    - Genetic risk factors determine 50 to 65% of the risk for RA.[17]
        - Family history of RA increases the risk two to five times for developing RA.[17]
    - Endocrine imbalances such as estrogen have proinflammatory properties.[17]
    - Comorbid conditions such as other autoimmune diseases increase risk for RA.[17]
- Environmental factors:
    - Cigarette smoking has the strongest association with development of RA and may predict 20 to 25% of risk.[17]
    - Socioeconomic and other environmental factors.[17]
        - Low socioeconomic status increases RA risk.
        - Exposure to pollutants such as pesticides.
        - Higher levels of recreational physical activity may decrease risk of RA by 33 to 35%.
    - Infectious agents such as periodontal disease.[17]
        - Periodontal bacteria, such as *Porphyromonas gingivalis*, may contribute to RA autoantibody production.
    - Diet.[17]
        - Low to moderate alcohol intake may be protective against RA development.
        - Healthy eating patterns high in fruits vegetables and omega-3 and -6 fatty acids are associated with a decreased risk for RA.

III. Clinical Presentation

- **Arthralgia** is a nonspecific symptom that may be suggestive of RA.[18]
- Swelling and pain in multiple joints for 6 weeks or more with morning stiffness lasting 1 hour or more.[18]

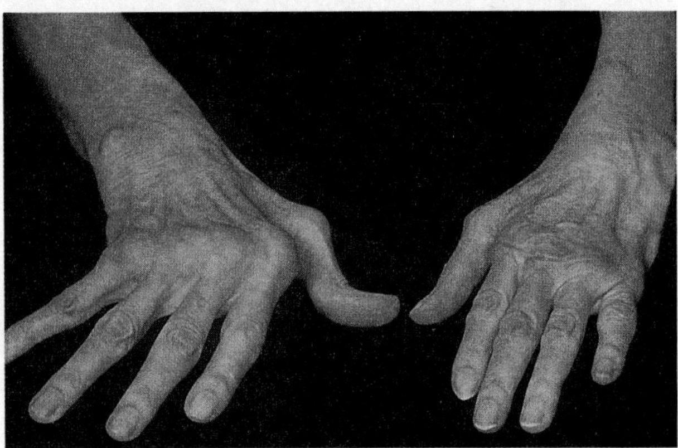

Figure 63-3 Rheumatoid Arthritis. Deformity to the hands caused by rheumatoid arthritis.

- As joint destruction progresses, deformity with limited motion and muscle atrophy occurs in severely involved joints (**Figure 63-3**).
- May experience weakness, loss of motor control, or difficulty making a fist.[18]
- There is an association between RA and bone changes in the temporomandibular joint (TMJ) resulting in pain, stiffness, joint sounds, and limitations in opening.[19]

IV. Treatment

- Early intervention is essential to limit destruction and progression of the disease.[20]
- Pharmacologic management includes[20]:
  - Disease modifying antirheumatic drugs (DMARDs) are the cornerstone of RA treatment and methotrexate is a **first-line** DMARD.
  - Corticosteroids may be used early in the disease along with DMARDs to reduce progression.
- Nonpharmacologic management includes[21]:
  - Consumption of a Mediterranean diet has been shown to reduce pain and improve quality of life in those with RA.
  - Physical activity including cardio, muscle strength, flexibility, and neuromotor exercise is recommended and may reduce pain and improve function.[22]
  - Weight loss for those who are overweight or obese.
  - Adequate sleep.
  - Smoking cessation.

V. Dental Hygiene Care

- Nonsurgical periodontal therapy to eliminate periodontal inflammation may reduce severity of RA in addition to standard medical care.[23]
- Adaptations for the patient's decreased manual dexterity may include:
  - Power toothbrushes.
  - Floss holders or interdental brushes.
  - Modification of the toothbrush handle to make it larger for easier grasp.
- Dental professionals also need to support healthy eating, weight management, and tobacco cessation.

Scleroderma

- Systemic scleroderma, also called systemic sclerosis, is an autoimmune disease affecting connective tissue associated with the skin, blood vessels, heart, lungs, kidneys, GI tract, and musculoskeletal system.
  - **Fibrosis**, or hardening, of the skin and internal organs, and **vasculopathy**, may occur.[24]
- There are three types of systemic scleroderma[19]:
  - Limited cutaneous systemic scleroderma, also known as CREST syndrome (see **Box 63-1**), is the milder form of scleroderma and usually involves thick skin on the fingers and/or face.
  - Diffuse cutaneous systemic scleroderma involves large areas of the skin on the arms, legs, and trunk that are thick and tight.
  - Diffuse scleroderma affects internal organs and worsens more quickly than the other types.

I. Prevalence

- Prevalence of systemic sclerosis in the United States is estimated to be 0.03 to 0.05% and is similar in Canada (0.033 to 0.047%).[25]
- Women are 4 to 17 times more likely than men to develop scleroderma.[25]

II. Etiology

- Genetic factors leading to the production of autoantibodies increase the risk for development of systemic scleroderma.[26]

Box 63-1 CREST Syndrome[24]

- C—calcium deposits under the skin and in tissues (calcinosis).
- R—Raynaud's phenomenon.
- E—esophageal dysfunction resulting in reflux, which is very common in CREST patients.
- S—sclerodactyly or thick skin on the fingers.
- T—telangiectasias appear as red spots on the face and other parts of the body.

- Environmental factors include[26,27]:
  - Infectious agents.
  - Drugs.
  - Chemicals, silica, and solvents.

III. Clinical Presentation

- Raynaud's phenomenon is one of the first clinical signs of scleroderma.[26]
  - Loss of blood supply to the fingers characterized by sensitivity to cold and change of skin color (white or clear) on fingers (**Figure 63-4**).
- GI manifestations may include[26]:
  - Gastroesophageal reflux disease (GERD) occurs in the majority of patients.
  - Severe weight loss and nutrient deficiencies due to malabsorption.
- Skin manifestations include[26]:
  - Thickening and tightening of the skin (**sclerodactyly**) on the fingers and possible fingertip lesions (**Figure 63-5**).
  - Nails may become smaller, curl, and sometimes disappear.
  - Skin on the face becomes waxy and the nose and lips thin.

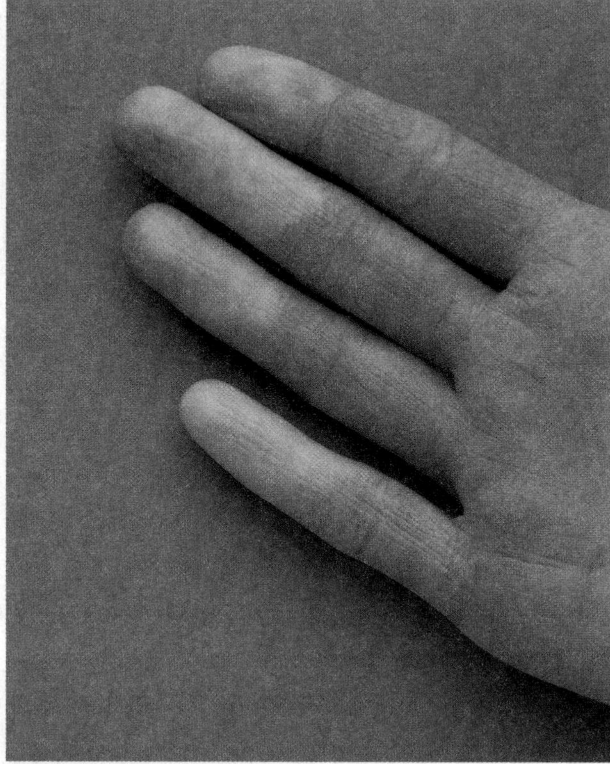

Figure 63-4 Raynaud's Phenomenon. Hands of a young woman suffering from Raynaud's phenomenon showing the white due to loss of blood supply as a result of cold or stress.

- Organ-based manifestations may include[26]:
  - Lung fibrosis.
  - Pulmonary arterial hypertension.
  - Renal failure.
  - Cardiac issues such as arrhythmias and myocardial disease.
- More than 80% of those with systemic sclerosis experience orofacial manifestations, which may include[28]:
  - Fibrosis of the facial skin results in a mask-like appearance.
  - Hypo- or hyperpigmentation.
  - **Microstomia** from sclerosis of the lips and skin around the mouth reduces the mouth opening (**Figure 63-6**).
  - Intraoral **telangiectases** result from dilation of small blood vessels in the skin and appear as small red macular areas. They may appear on the cheeks, nose, lips, and the oral mucosa.

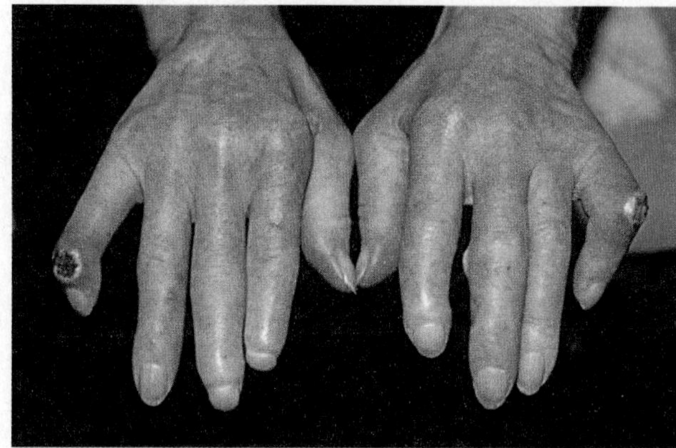

Figure 63-5 Scleroderma. Hard, tight skin with ulcerations.

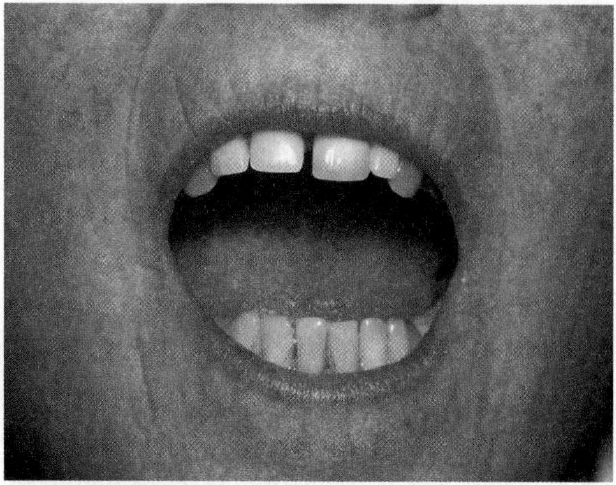

Figure 63-6 Oral Manifestation of Scleroderma. Linear furrows on the lips and decreased mouth opening are common.

- Gingiva may appear pale and sclerotic.
- Burning mouth syndrome.[29]
- Impaired tongue mobility due to tongue fibrosis.
- Xerostomia due to salivary gland involvement appears in 25 to 71% of cases, increasing caries risk.
- TMJ involvement.
- Individuals with systemic sclerosis have an increased odds of tooth loss and worse measures of periodontal health including clinical attachment loss, probing depths, bleeding on probing, and plaque index.[29]
- Widening of the periodontal ligament is a common radiographic finding.[29]
- Trigeminal neuropathy.

IV. Treatment

- Early diagnosis and risk assessment to determine those who may develop new organ complications is ideal to manage progression of systemic sclerosis.[30]
- Treatment will depend on the organ involved, so it can be quite variable.
- Pharmacologic management includes[30]:
  - Raynaud's phenomenon: calcium channel blockers such as nifedipine.
  - Ulcers on fingers or toes: intravenous (IV) iloprost, phosphodiesterase type 5 inhibitors, and bosentan.
  - Renal: angiotensin-converting enzyme inhibitors.
  - GI: proton pump inhibitors.
  - Skin and lung disease: methotrexate, cyclophosphamide (in progressive disease), hematopoietic stem cell transplantation in severe disease.
- Nonpharmacologic recommendations have extremely limited evidence and include[31]:
  - Physical therapy and regular physical activity, including stretching and cardio, may help keep joints flexible, including orofacial exercises to maintain and possibly improve mouth opening.
  - Dietary modifications to minimize GERD may also be helpful.
  - Protect skin from excessive dryness and cold by using multiple layers to cover skin and a humidifier to keep air moist. Creams and soaps designed for dry skin are recommended.

V. Dental Hygiene Care

- Tight facial skin, microstomia, and TMJ involvement may make oral self-care as well as professional care difficult due to limited mouth opening and access.
  - Due to the challenges in providing restorative or surgical dental care, prevention of oral disease is crucial.[32]
  - Due to microstomia, alternatives for interdental cleaning must be explored.[32,33]
- Xerostomia increases the risk of dental caries and management may include[32]:
  - Office and home fluorides. (See Chapter 34.)
  - Keep the mouth moist with saliva substitute sprays, water, saliva stimulants such as sugar-free candy and gum, and medications such as pilocarpine.
  - Recommend xylitol products sparingly as they may irritate the GI tract.
  - Avoid dental products with alcohol.
- Finger lesions and tight skin resulting in hand weakness and reduced grip strength may make oral self-care challenging; a power toothbrush or other modifications may be needed along with more frequent continuing care.[32] (See Chapter 51.)

Gastrointestinal Tract Autoimmune Diseases

- Several autoimmune diseases have effects on the GI tract, but several primarily affect the GI tract through an organ-specific autoantibody.[34]
- As in other autoimmune diseases, these also have a significant genetic component moderated by environmental factors.
- A few GI tract autoimmune diseases will be reviewed in this section, including celiac disease (CD) and the inflammatory bowel diseases (IBDs): Crohn's disease and ulcerative colitis (UC).

Celiac Disease

- CD results in damage to the villi of the small intestine with exposure to dietary gluten (**Figure 63-7**).
- Inflammation and destruction of the intestinal villi result in chronic malabsorption of nutrients such as iron, folic acid, fat-soluble vitamins, and vitamin B_{12}.[26]

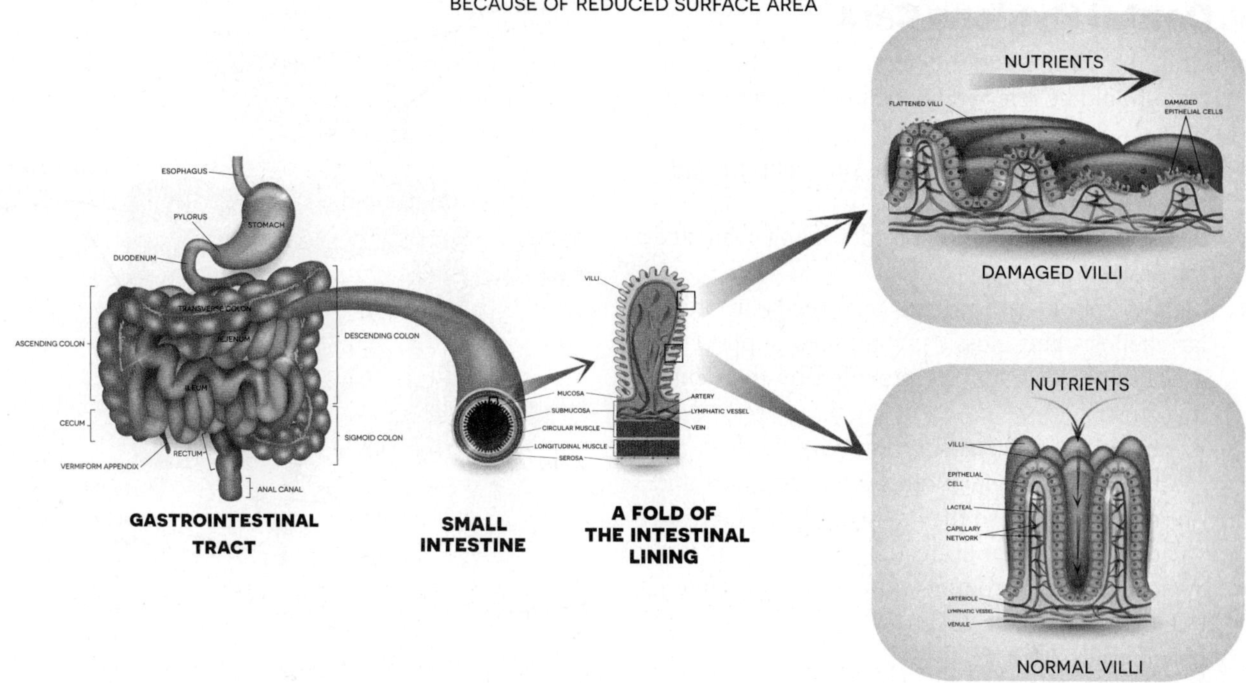

Figure 63-7 Celiac Disease Affecting the Villi of the Small Intestine. In celiac disease, the villi are damaged and nutrients are not absorbed because of reduced surface area.

I. Prevalence

- Global prevalence is 1.4 and 0.7% in the United States.[35,36]
- Occurs more frequently in women and non-Hispanic whites.[35]
- CD is five times more common in individuals living in northern latitudes of 35°–39° of the United States versus southern latitudes.[36]
  - This could be related to differences in levels of vitamin D, which is involved in modulating the immune response in CD.

II. Etiology

- Genetic predisposition.[37]
  - A first-degree family member increases the risk of CD as does having more than one family member with CD.[38]
- Environmental factors[37]:
  - Gluten is the primary trigger and early introduction of gluten before 3 months of age.
  - Perinatal factors such as elective cesarean and small for gestational age.
  - Higher maternal education level.

III. Clinical Presentation

- Some individuals may have no symptoms.
- GI symptoms include diarrhea, **steatorrhea**, weight loss, bloating, flatulence, and abdominal pain.[37,38]
  - Oral symptoms may include oral aphthous ulcers and discolored teeth or developmental enamel abnormalities.[38]
- Non-GI abnormalities may include abnormal liver function tests, iron deficiency anemia, bone disease, skin disorders, fatigue, and delayed puberty.[37,38]
- Often associated with other autoimmune diseases such as type 1 diabetes and autoimmune thyroid disease.[37]

IV. Treatment

- The only effective treatment is a gluten-free diet.[38]
  - Dietary sources of gluten include wheat, barley, rye, and sometimes oats, dependent on processing.
  - Referral to a registered dietitian/nutritionist specializing in CD is recommended.[38]

- Management of nutrient deficiencies is essential to minimize long-term consequences such as low bone mass.[38]

V. Dental Hygiene Care

- Children with enamel defects and aphthous ulcers should be referred for evaluation for possible undiagnosed CD.[39,40]
- Little research has been done on recurrent aphthous ulcers (RAU) in adults with CD, but patients with RAU should consider being evaluated for possible CD.
- Malabsorption of nutrients may result in angular cheilosis and glossitis; continued support for a healthy diet should be provided by the dental hygienist.[40]
    - In children, malabsorption may result in delayed growth, including tooth eruption and malocclusion, so they may need referral to an orthodontist for evaluation.
- Typically, dental products do not contain gluten, but care should be taken to ensure gluten-free products are used.
- Palliative treatment of oral lesions with mouthrinse containing lidocaine and possibly topical steroids.
- Assist the patient in tobacco cessation. (See Chapter 32.)

Crohn's Disease

- Crohn's disease is a chronic, progressive, destructive inflammatory condition impacting any part of the GI tract from the mouth to the anus (**Figure 63-8**).

I. Prevalence

- Prevalence estimates in the United States are that 1.3%, or about 3 million individuals, have a diagnosis of Crohn's disease.[41]
- Slightly higher prevalence in women.[41]
- More common in those of Ashkenazi Jewish origin.

II. Etiology

- Genetic predisposition:
    - 10 to 25% of those with Crohn's disease have a first-degree relative diagnosed with the disease.[41]
- Environmental triggers include[41]:
    - Smoking not only doubles the risk of Crohn's disease, but may also lead to a more aggressive form of the disease.

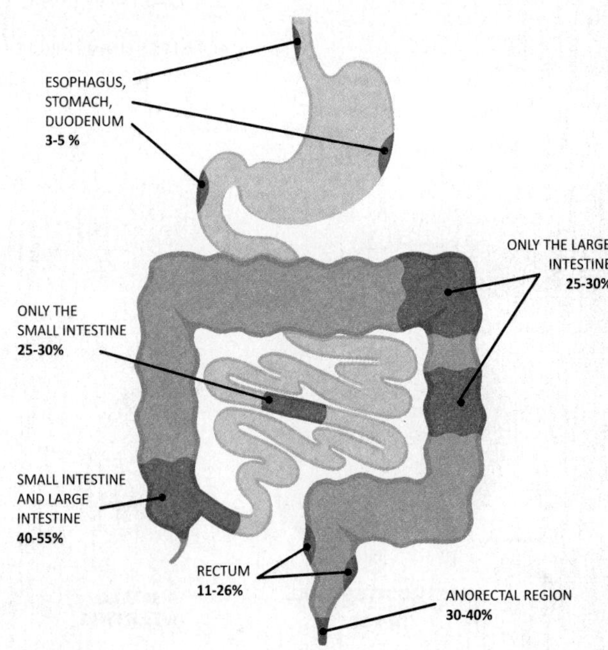

Figure 63-8 Crohn's Disease. Crohn's disease may affect any part of the gastrointestinal tract, but most commonly affects the small and large intestine.

    - Antibiotic use increases the odds nearly three-fold of developing Crohn's disease.
    - Oral contraceptives.
    - Diet triggers seem to include high animal protein intake and high linoleic acid intake which may impact the gut microbiome.
- Protective factors include:
    - Breastfeeding for at least 12 months seems to provide a protective effect.[42]
    - High dietary fiber and fruit intake.[41]

III. Clinical Presentation

- Hallmark symptoms include[41,43]:
    - Abdominal pain.
    - Chronic diarrhea.
    - Nausea and vomiting.
    - Weight loss.
    - Growth failure in children/adolescents.
    - Fever.
    - Fatigue: may be a result of anemia or other nutrient deficiencies along with the effect from the body of trying to manage the inflammation.
    - Iron deficiency.
- Extraintestinal manifestations may include osteonecrosis, metabolic bone disease, and ankylosing spondylitis.[43]

- Orofacial manifestations[44]:
    - Diffuse labial and buccal swelling.
    - Hyperplastic plaques on the buccal mucosa with a cobblestone appearance.
    - Mucosal tissue tags.
    - Deep linear ulcerations.
    - Aphthous ulcers, which are shallow round or oval as compared to the linear ulcerations previously mentioned.
    - Prevalence of periodontitis may be higher, but more research is needed.
    - Xerostomia.
    - Higher caries risk.
    - Angular cheilitis and/or glossitis due to nutritional deficiencies.
- Crohn's disease may be associated with other autoimmune conditions such as celiac disease, rheumatoid artrithis, psoriatic arthritis, and type 1 diabetes.[45]
- Bowel obstructions may also occur and require surgical intervention.[41]

IV. Treatment

- Treatment depends on the severity, location, and subtype of Crohn's disease and can be complex.[41]
    - Remission and maintenance of remission without surgery is a goal of the treatment.
- Pharmacologic therapies may include[41,43]:
    - Corticosteroids or methotrexate may be used to induce remission.
    - Methotrexate, azathioprine, and 6-mercaptopurine may be used to maintain remission of Crohn's disease.
- Biologic therapies like antitumor necrosis factor (anti-TNF) have been most effective in moderate-to-severe Crohn's disease and in maintenance.[41,43]
- Surgical intervention:
    - Eighty percent of those with long-term Crohn's disease will require surgery and many may require multiple surgeries over their lifetime.[41]

V. Dental Hygiene Care

- Avoid use of NSAIDs as they may exacerbate disease activity.
- Encourage and assist with tobacco cessation. (See Chapter 32.)
- Quality of life may be impacted by stress, anxiety, and depression in those with IBD and referral to a mental health specialist may be necessary.[43]
- Working closely with the interprofessional team providing care is important to manage oral health given the complexity of the disease.
- Dietary assessment and counseling may be indicated if frequency of sugar intake impacts caries risk and to support adequate intake of nutrients. (See Chapter 33.)
- Palliative treatment of oral lesions as needed to relieve pain which may include a topical agent or mouthrinse with lidocaine and/or topical steroids.
- Management of dental biofilm is essential to manage caries and periodontal risk.
- Optimal use of home and office fluorides to manage caries risk. (See Chapter 34.)

Ulcerative Colitis

- UC is an autoimmune IBD affecting primarily the colon (**Figure 63-9**).

I. Prevalence

- More common in industrialized countries, particularly North America and Western Europe.[46]
- Prevalence in the United States is 150 cases per 100,000 per year.[47]
- Tends to occur between the ages 15 and 30 years and again from age 50 to 70 years.[48]

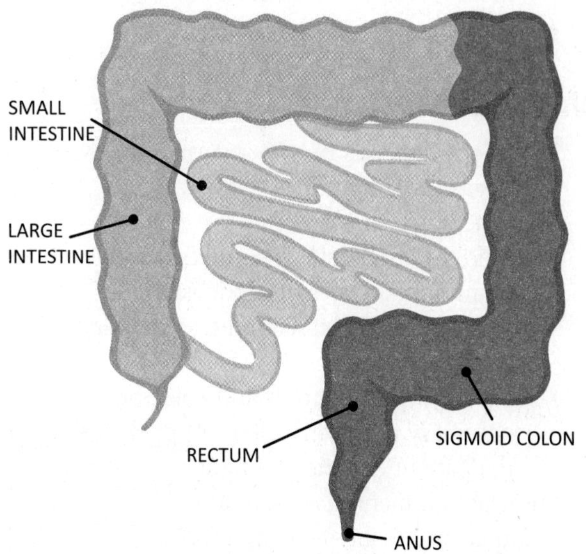

Figure 63-9 Ulcerative Colitis. Ulcerative colitis affects the mucosa of the large intestine.

II. Etiology

- Genetic disposition[48,49]:
  - Family history increases risk 8 to 14%.
  - More common in those of Jewish origin.
- Environmental risk triggers may include[49]:
  - Alterations of the gut microbiome.
  - Possible infectious agent.
  - Being a former smoker.
  - Increased intake of dietary fat.
- Protective factors include[49]:
  - Appendectomy before age 20 reduced risk of UC by 55%.

III. Clinical Presentation

- Intestinal symptoms include[49]:
  - Bloody diarrhea.
  - Abdominal pain/cramps.
- Extraintestinal manifestations may include[49]:
  - Acute or chronic pancreatitis.
  - Colitis-associated arthritis is the most common.
  - Skin lesions.
  - Optic **neuritis**.
  - Increased risk for colorectal cancer and leukemia.
- Orofacial manifestations can be the first manifestation of UC (and Crohn's disease) and include[50]:
  - Pyostomatitis vegetans, which consists of multiple small yellow and white pustules on an erythematous and edematous mucosal base.
  - Aphthous ulcers.
  - The risk of periodontitis may be higher, but more research is needed.
  - Glossitis.

IV. Treatment

- Treatment depends on the severity and extent of the disease and continues to evolve.
- Pharmacologic therapy[51]:
  - Mild to moderate UC: medication such as 5-aminosalicylates or corticosteroids.
  - With more extensive mild to moderate UC: corticosteroids and anti-TNF.
  - Severe UC: IV steroids and colectomy may be necessary if pharmacologic approaches fail or the patient experiences toxicity.
- Surgical treatment may be required.
- Nonpharmacologic recommendations[52]:
  - Monitor for depression and anxiety.
  - Increased risk for cancers including colon, cervical, melanoma, and nonmelanoma requires regular screening.
  - Monitor bone health for steroid-induced osteoporosis.
  - It is important for an individual with UC to keep their vaccinations current due to immunosuppression.

V. Dental Hygiene Care

- Palliative treatment for oral lesions to help reduce discomfort such as 2% viscous lidocaine or a steroid gel.[53]
- Avoid prescribing NSAIDs as they may trigger a flare-up of the UC.[53]
- Education to enhance dental biofilm removal along with regular preventive services and periodontal maintenance are essential due to the increased risk for oral infections.

Neurologic System Autoimmune Diseases

- Autoimmune conditions affect the central nervous system, which may include the brain, spinal cord, and/or peripheral nervous system.

Multiple Sclerosis

- MS is a chronic demyelinating disease of the central nervous system characterized by progressive disability with motor, sensory, cognitive, and emotional changes.[54]

I. Prevalence

- Globally the prevalence is 35.9 per 100,000 and has increased 30% since 2013.[55]
  - Prevalence tends to be highest in North America (117 per 100,000) and northern European countries (143 per 100,000).
- The mean age of diagnosis globally is 32 years.[55]
  - Pediatric MS in children younger than 18 years has increased globally four fold since 2013.
- Females are two to three times as likely as males to have MS.[54,55]

II. Etiology

- Genetic predisposition has a significant role in the development of MS.[54]

- Environmental factors include[54]:
  - Vitamin D deficiency.
  - Childhood obesity results in a two-fold increase in risk.
  - Smoking.
  - Infectious agents (i.e., Epstein-Barr virus).

III. Clinical Presentation

A. Clinical Forms of MS

There are four clinical forms of MS and relapsing–remitting accounts for 85% of cases.[56]

- Relapsing–remitting: acute episodes worsening with some recovery over weeks to months with no changes in neurologic functioning between attacks.
- Primary progressive: gradual, nearly continuous neurologic deterioration from the onset of symptoms.
- Secondary progressive: gradual neurologic deterioration with or without superimposed acute relapses in a patient.
- Progressive relapsing: gradual neurologic deterioration from the onset of symptoms but with subsequent superimposed relapses (uncommon).

B. Symptoms

- MS can affect any area of the brain, optic nerve, or spinal cord and cause a wide variety of neurologic signs and symptoms (**Figure 63-10**). Symptoms fluctuate, and several years may elapse between bouts of symptoms.
- Symptoms may include[57]:
  - Initial symptoms often fluctuate: transient difficulty in coordination, tremor, or fatigue.
  - May have a sudden onset with paralysis or marked weakness of one or more extremities.
  - Changes in muscular coordination and gait; loss of balance; spasms.
  - Unilateral optic neuritis with blurred vision and pain.
  - Involuntary motion of eyes (nystagmus); the individual may later become partially or completely blind.
  - Speech disorders; **dysarthria** and possible loss of speech in the advanced stages.
  - Susceptibility to infection, particularly upper respiratory.

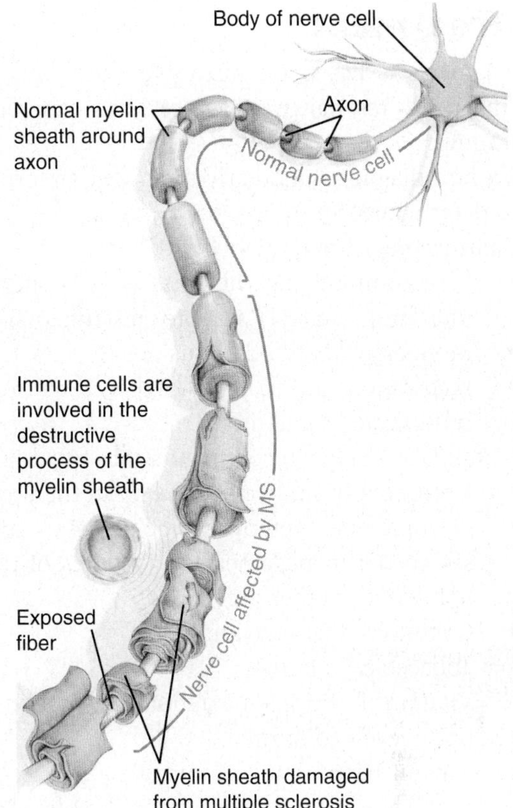

Figure 63-10 Multiple Sclerosis. Nerve cell damage.

  - Cognitive impairment in 65% of MS patients with deficits in memory and attention.
  - Depression.
- Orofacial manifestations[58,59]:
  - TMJ disorder.
  - Motor nerve dysfunction may result in muscle weakness, tremors, and painful spasms of the facial muscles triggered by touch or movement.
  - Trigeminal neuralgia usually is bilateral.
  - Dysphagia.
  - There may be a higher risk for periodontal disease, but more research is needed.
  - Immunosuppressants may result in aphthous ulcers and opportunistic infections such as *Candida*.
- Course of disease:
  - *Relapses and remissions*: an attack may last several days or weeks and be followed by a symptom-free period. The condition worsens with each relapse.
  - *Longevity*: close to normal life span; approximately 80% have functional limitations after 15 years.

IV. Treatment

- Diagnosis is based on history, clinical, imaging (magnetic resonance imaging), and laboratory findings.[54]
- Prompt diagnosis and early treatment are crucial to deter neurologic damage.
- Pharmacologic therapy includes[54]:
  - Disease-modifying therapies (DMT) such as interferons and S1P receptor modulators.
  - Monoclonal antibody infusions.
  - Medications are administered in three ways: self-injected, oral, or IV.
- Nonpharmacologic recommendations include[60]:
  - Exercise, physiotherapy, and hydrotherapy.
  - Occupational therapy may be necessary to assist in the management of activities of daily living as disability progresses.
  - Cognitive and behavioral therapy.
  - Tobacco cessation.
  - Vitamin D supplementation as needed to bring levels to normal.
  - A plant-based, anti-inflammatory diet rich in vegetables, fruit, whole grains, low-fat dairy, high-fiber foods, lean proteins, and omega-3 fatty acids is suggested, although evidence is limited.
  - Maintenance of a healthy weight.
  - Management of mental health and stress.
- Complementary health practices may include yoga, acupuncture, reflexology, magnetic therapy, bee sting therapy, and marijuana (cannabinoids).
  - Some individuals with MS will try alternative medicine approaches and special diets that may not have good evidence of benefit and may cause harm (such as malnutrition).
  - Emerging research suggests cannabinoids may relieve muscle spasticity and pain.[61]

V. Dental Hygiene Care

Factors to consider when planning dental hygiene care for a patient with MS include:

- Medical consultation needs to be the first step to determine patient readiness for dental care.[62,63]
  - Immunosuppressants and other MS medications used may result in neutropenia, so a white blood cell count is essential prior to care.
- Palliative treatment for symptom relief for oral lesions such as mouthrinses with viscous lidocaine or topical steroid agents.
- Orofacial manifestations, such as intermittent headaches, facial pain, parasthesias, palsy, and spasms.
- Oral self-care education needs to be individualized based on patient needs and oral condition.
  - Visual disturbances and changes in motor function may impact the ability to adequately manage dental biofilm.
- Prevention will be recommended based on the risk for oral disease.
  - Home and office fluorides. (See Chapter 34.)
  - Diet counseling. (See Chapter 33.)
- Oral and systemic effects of medications used for treatment may require management, such as candidiasis.
- The possible increased risk for periodontal disease may require more frequent continuing care appointments, particularly if the patient is having issues with motor function.

Systemic Autoimmune Diseases

- In systemic autoimmune diseases, autoantibodies affect various tissues throughout the body causing destruction.

Sjögren's Syndrome

- SS is a chronic, systemic autoimmune disease in which autoantibodies attack healthy cells in the exocrine glands followed by many other organs.[64,65]
  - Exocrine glands are responsible for producing moisture for the mouth, eyes, nose, throat, and skin.

I. Prevalence

- Primary SS prevalence globally is estimated to be 61 per 100,000 individuals.[64]
- The ratio of female to male individuals with SS is 9:1.[65]

II. Etiology

- Genetic predisposition: nearly 20-fold higher risk for SS if a first-degree relative is affected.[66]

- Environmental trigger[64]:
  - Infectious agents may be a trigger for SS such as HCV and Epstein-Barr virus.

III. Clinical Presentation

- Glandular manifestations include[64]:
  - Dry eyes: may result in sensitivity to light, redness, and itching.
  - Dry mouth (xerostomia): reduced quantity and quality of saliva.
  - Glandular swelling of parotid and it may extend to the submandibular and sublingual glands. It begins unilaterally and extends bilaterally.
  - Angular cheilitis.
- Extraglandular manifestations include[64]:
  - Lungs: recurrent bronchitis or pneumonia, pulmonary fibrosis, and chronic dry cough.
  - Kidney: glomerulonephritis.
  - Abnormal liver function tests.
  - Skin: xeroderma (dry skin) and urticaria (rashes).
  - Musculoskeletal involvement: myalgia (muscle pain), arthralgia (joint pain), and Raynaud's phenomenon.
  - Peripheral neuropathy.
  - GI: esophageal dysmotility, dysphagia, and GERD.
  - Fatigue.
  - Lymphoma.
  - Pregnancy complications such as miscarriage and preterm delivery.
- Dental manifestations[64,67-69]:
  - Increased caries risk.
  - Increased biofilm accumulations and gingival inflammation.
  - Periodontal disease risk may be increased, but more research is needed.
  - Oral candidiasis.
  - Dry, erythematous oral mucosa.
  - Stomatitits.

IV. Treatment

- Pharmacologic therapy may include[64]:
  - Artificial tears/saliva, gels, and ointments.
  - DMARDS may include methotrexate, short- or long-term corticosteroids, hydroxychloroquine, and cyclosporine.
  - Biologic therapies such as TNF-α inhibitors.
- Nonpharmacologic recommendations may include[70]:
  - Physical activity to reduce fatigue.

V. Dental Hygiene Care

- An interprofessional approach to care is needed to manage SS and improve the patient's overall quality of life.
- Oral self-care education to aid the patient in developing optimal dental biofilm removal is crucial to manage the risk for oral disease.
- Assess dietary intake and counsel on minimizing intake of fermentable carbohydrates, particularly between meals. (See Chapter 33.)
- Recommend sugar-free chewing gum, mints, or hard candy containing xylitol for salivary stimulation.
- Saliva substitutes with glycerol may help the mouth feel moist.
- Encourage the patient to carry a water bottle to aid in relieving mouth dryness.
- Antifungal rinse or lozenges for oral candidiasis.
- Recommend at-home fluoride therapy, which may include rinses, varnish, and gels. (See Chapter 34.)
- Avoid use of toothpaste with pyrophosphates or sodium laurel sulfate.
- Chlorhexidine as a gel, varnish, or mouthrinse may aid in managing caries risk.[71]
- Nonfluoride remineralizing preparations with calcium phosphate may aid in reducing caries risk.[71]
- More frequent continuing care may be required to maintain oral health.

Systemic Lupus Erythematosus

- SLE is a chronic autoimmune disease causing widespread inflammation, which can affect internal organs and glands by causing tissue damage (**Figure 63-11**).[72]

I. Prevalence

- Prevalence globally varies from 9 to 241 per 100,000 individuals.[73]
- In the United States, prevalence varies from 80 to 103 per 100,000 indivduals.[73]
  - In some populations like American Indian and Alaska Native groups, the prevalence is 178 per 100,000.[74]
  - SLE is two to four times more prevalent in black women than white women.[72]
- The female to male ratio varies across the life span from 9:1.[72]
- Mean age of diagnosis is 35 years.[72]

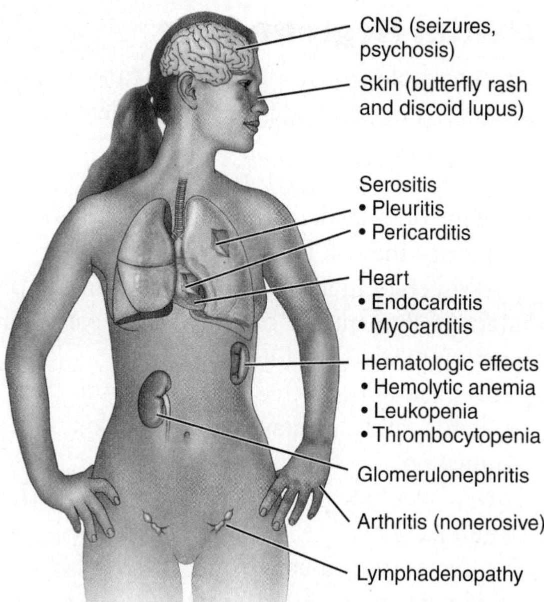

Figure 63-11 Systemic Lupus Erythematosus: Systemic Effects.

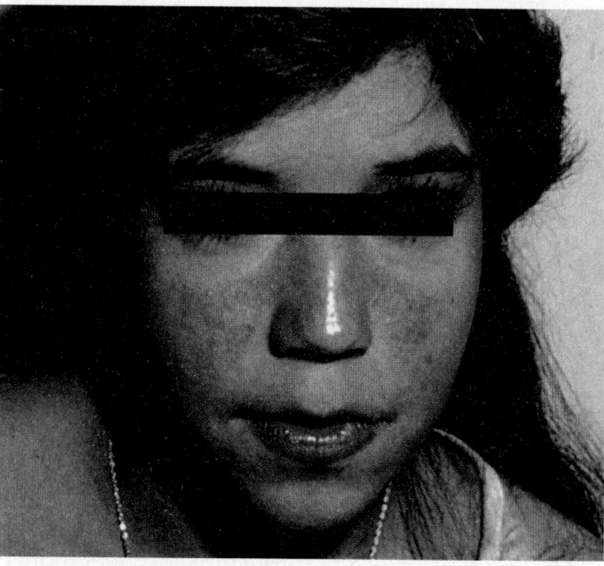

Figure 63-12 Systemic Lupus Erythematosus. This young girl has the classic "butterfly" rash of lupus.

II. Risk Factors

- Genetic predisposition imparts about 40 to 50% of the risk for SLE.[50]
- Environmental risks may include[73,75]:
  - Ultraviolet light exposure.
  - Smoking.
  - About 118 medication are linked to inducing SLE, such as hydralazine and anti-TNFs.
  - Endometriosis.
  - Moderate alcohol consumption (≥ 5 g or half a drink per day).
  - Silica exposure.
- Possible environmental triggers needing more research include[73]:
  - Low vitamin D status.
  - Air pollution.
  - Diet impact on the gut microbiome.
  - Pesticide exposure.
  - Infectious agents such as Epstein-Barr virus.

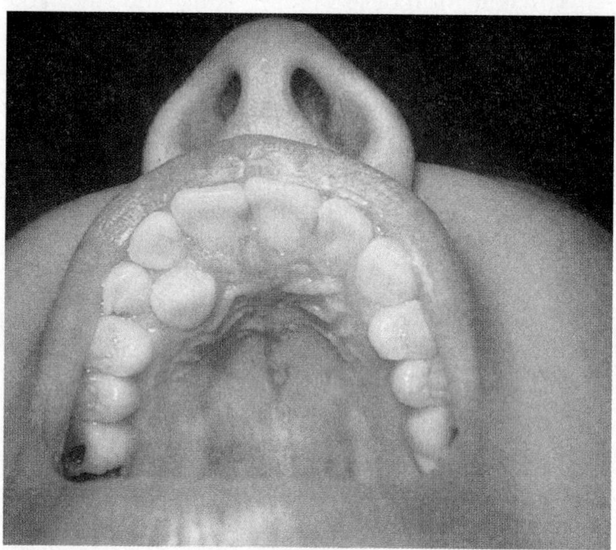

Figure 63-13 Systemic Lupus Erythematosus. The dental professional may be the first to observe the manifestations of some autoimmune disorders because they may present in the oral cavity prior to any cutaneous manifestations. Ulceration is present on the hard palate in this individual with systemic lupus erythematosus.

III. Clinical Presentation

- Skin manifestations include[75]:
  - Butterfly-shaped rash on nose and cheeks (malar rash) (**Figure 63-12**).
  - Erythema on skin exposed to sun (photosensitivity).
  - Alopecia (hair loss).
  - Raynaud's phenomenon.
- Oral lesions may include[75,76]:
  - Oral discoid lesions (**Figure 63-13**).
  - Petechia-like lesions.
  - Gingival bleeding such as desquamative gingivitis.
  - Erosive mucosal lesions in as many as 40% of individuals.
- Arthritis: joint pain, tenderness, swelling, and morning stiffness.[75]
- Lung involvement: pleuritis.

- Renal disorder: high creatinine/protein in urine.[75]
- Neurologic disorders: neuropathy, seizure disorder, etc.[75]
- Hematologic disorder: hemolytic anemia, leukopenia, and thrombocytopenia.[75]
- Immunologic changes: positive blood test for antinuclear antibodies.[75]
- Neuropsychiatric disorders: anxiety, mood disorder, psychosis, cognitive dysfunction.[75]
- Fatigue.

IV. Treatment

- Management is complex and requires an interprofessional team with the goal of controlling disease activity and preventing organ damage.
- Pharmacologic therapy may include[76]:
  - NSAIDs.
  - Antimalarial drugs (e.g., hydroxychloroquine) are believed to help reduce lupus-related symptoms of joint pain, rashes, fatigue, and mouth sores.
  - Corticosteroids.
  - Immunosuppressive therapy such as azathioprine and cyclosporine.
  - Biologic agents such as belimumab.
- Nonpharmacologic recommendations include[77]:
  - Protection from ultraviolet radiation.
  - Stress management such as mindfulness-based meditation.
  - Physical activity.
  - Psychological interventions to improve coping abilities and any mental neuropsychiatric conditions.
  - Acupuncture for pain management.
  - Healthy diet.
  - Achieve and maintain a healthy weight.

V. Dental Hygiene Care

- Consultation with the interprofessional team is crucial to assess the level of immune suppression and any possible risks for dental care.
- Periodontal health must be carefully monitored due to the risk for steroid-induced bone loss with long-term use of corticosteroids.
- Oral self-care education to aid the patient in optimal daily dental biofilm removal for management of gingivitis.
- Preventive services based on oral disease risk and medications.
  - Office/home fluorides. (See Chapter 34.)
  - Diet counseling. (See Chapter 33.)
  - Saliva substitutes.
- For patients with mobility and dexterity issues due to SLE-associated arthritis, modifications to oral self-care techniques and oral health aids may be required. (See Chapter 51.)
- For oral lesions, palliative treatment may be necessary, such as viscous lidocaine.
- Tobacco cessation. (See Chapter 32.)

Documentation

- Record the chief complaint and compare findings with previous recordings, which may include intra and extraoral examinations, intraoral images, and periodontal assessment.
- The patient with an autoimmune disease must provide their thorough health history including any symptoms affecting their oral health.
- Review all medications and document any oral side effects.
- Carefully document the medical providers' patient care recommendations.
- Record recommendations for oral self-care and treatment provided.
- An example documentation may be reviewed in **Box 63-2**.

Box 63-2 Example Documentation: Patient with Autoimmune Disease

- **S**—A 52-year-old female patient arrives in the dental office for an appointment for hygiene care. It has been 3 years since her last prophylaxis and reports her teeth feel "dirty and my gums bleed when I brush."
- **O**—Medical history reveals diagnosis of rheumatoid arthritis 8 years ago. Medications include corticosteroids to help with joint inflammation. Patient states she cannot grasp a toothbrush or floss due to her joint pain. Biofilm scores greater than 50%.
- **A**—A comprehensive periodontal and caries examination including a complete mouth radiographic series indicates generalized stage II grade B periodontitis with heavy calculus, plaque, and bleeding.
- **P**—The dental hygiene care plan includes quadrant NSPT with local anesthetic. Patient education includes a thorough explanation of periodontal disease and why NSPT is recommended. Oral hygiene instruction is reviewed and tailored to help with dexterity. A power brush is recommended with a modification to the handle to make it larger and easier to grasp. Floss holders are also demonstrated to help with interdental care. Patient will return to begin NSPT.

Factors to Teach the Patient

- Maintain recommended continuing care intervals to keep biofilm at a low level.
- The need for interprofessional communication with the autoimmune disease specialists to help optimize management of the autoimmune disease and prevent oral disease.
- Educate the patient about the autoimmune disease specific oral manifestations.
  - For example: Wickham striae, xerostomia, candidiasis, mouth ulcers.
- Discuss options to manage symptoms and optimize overall health.
  - For example: reduce stress, maintain a healthy weight, stop smoking, and be physically active.
- Educate the patient about options for adapting preventive aids to help with dexterity and access.
- Emphasize the dental office is a safe place to share concerns and ask questions.

References

1. Cooper GS, Bynum MLK, Somers EC. Recent insights in the epidemiology of autoimmune diseases: improved prevalence estimates and understanding of clustering of diseases. *J Autoimmun*. 2009;33(3-4):197-207.
2. Lerner A, Patricia W, Matthias T. The world incidence and prevalence of autoimmune diseases is increasing. *Int J Celiac Dis*. 2015;3:151-155.
3. Hayter SM, Cook MC. Updated assessment of the prevalence, spectrum and case definition of autoimmune disease. *Autoimmun Rev*. 2012;11(10):754-765.
4. Desai MK, Brinton RD. Autoimmune disease in women: endocrine transition and risk across the lifespan. *Front Endocrinol*. 2019;10:Article 265.
5. Wang L, Wang FS, Gershwin ME. Human autoimmune diseases: a comprehensive update. *J Intern Med*. 2015; 278(4):369-395.
6. Cárdenas-Roldán J, Rojas-Villarraga A, Anaya JM. How do autoimmune diseases cluster in families? A systematic review and meta-analysis. *BMC Medicine*. 2013;11(1):73.
7. Nevares AM. Overview of autoimmune disorders of connective tissue - bone, joint, and muscle disorders. *Merck Manual*. https://www.merckmanuals.com/home/bone,-joint,-and-muscle-disorders/autoimmune-disorders-of-connective-tissue/overview-of-autoimmune-disorders-of-connective-tissue. Accessed February 8, 2022.
8. González-Moles MÁ, Warnakulasuriya S, González-Ruiz I, et al. Worldwide prevalence of oral lichen planus: a systematic review and meta-analysis. *Oral Dis*. 2021;27(4):813-828.
9. Aghbari SMH, Abushouk AI, Attia A, et al. Malignant transformation of oral lichen planus and oral lichenoid lesions: a meta-analysis of 20095 patient data. *Oral Oncol*. 2017;68:92-102.
10. Nosratzehi T. Oral lichen planus: an overview of potential risk factors, biomarkers and treatments. *Asian Pac J Cancer Prev*. 2018;19(5):1161-1167.
11. Cheng S, Kirtschig G, Cooper S, Thornhill M, Leonardi-Bee J, Murphy R. Interventions for erosive lichen planus affecting mucosal sites. *Cochrane Database Syst Rev*. 2012;(2):CD008092.
12. Lodi G, Manfredi M, Mercadante V, Murphy R, Carrozzo M. Interventions for treating oral lichen planus: corticosteroid therapies. *Cochrane Database Syst Rev*. 2020;2:CD001168.
13. van der Woude D, van der Helm-van Mil AHM. Update on the epidemiology, risk factors, and disease outcomes of rheumatoid arthritis. *Best Pract Res Clin Rheumatol*. 2018;32(2):174-187.
14. Samborska-Mazur J, Sikorska D, Wyganowska-Świątkowska M. The relationship between periodontal status and rheumatoid arthritis - systematic review. *Reumatologia*. 2020;58(4):236-242.
15. Almutairi K, Nossent J, Preen D, Keen H, Inderjeeth C. The global prevalence of rheumatoid arthritis: a meta-analysis based on a systematic review. *Rheumatol Int*. 2021; 41(5):863-877.
16. Hunter TM, Boytsov NN, Zhang X, Schroeder K, Michaud K, Araujo AB. Prevalence of rheumatoid arthritis in the United States adult population in healthcare claims databases, 2004-2014. *Rheumatol Int*. 2017;37(9):1551-1557.
17. Romão VC, Fonseca JE. Etiology and risk factors for rheumatoid arthritis: a state-of-the-art review. *Front Med*. 2021;8:689698.
18. Jutley GS, Latif ZP, Raza K. Symptoms in individuals at risk of rheumatoid arthritis. *Best Pract Res Clin Rheumatol*. 2017;31(1):59-70.
19. Campos DES, de Araújo Ferreira Muniz I, de Souza Villarim NL, et al. Is there an association between rheumatoid arthritis and bone changes in the temporomandibular joint diagnosed by cone-beam computed tomography? A systematic review and meta-analysis. *Clin Oral Investig*. 2021;25(5):2449-2459.
20. Fraenkel L, Bathon JM, England BR, et al. 2021 American College of Rheumatology guideline for the treatment of rheumatoid arthritis. *Arthritis Care Res*. 2021;73(7):924-939.
21. Chehade L, Jaafar ZA, El Masri D, et al. Lifestyle modification in rheumatoid arthritis: dietary and physical activity recommendations based on evidence. *Curr Rheumatol Rev*. 2019;15(3):209-214.
22. Rausch Osthoff AK, Juhl CB, Knittle K, et al. Effects of exercise and physical activity promotion: meta-analysis informing the 2018 EULAR recommendations for physical activity in people with rheumatoid arthritis, spondyloarthritis and hip/knee osteoarthritis. *RMD Open*. 2018;4(2):e000713.
23. Del Rei Daltro Rosa CD, de Luna Gomes JM, Dantas de Moraes SL, et al. Does non-surgical periodontal treatment influence on rheumatoid arthritis? A systematic review and meta-analysis. *Saudi Dent J*. 2021;33(8):795-804.
24. National Library of Medicine. Systemic scleroderma. *Medline Plus*. https://medlineplus.gov/genetics/condition/systemic-scleroderma/. Accessed February 8, 2022.

25. Zhong L, Pope M, Shen Y, Hernandez JJ, Wu L. Prevalence and incidence of systemic sclerosis: a systematic review and meta-analysis. *Int J Rheumat Dis*. 2019;22(12):2096-2107.
26. Odonwodo A, Badri T, Hariz A. Scleroderma. *StatPearls*. Updated August 1, 2022. http://www.ncbi.nlm.nih.gov/books/NBK537335/. Accessed December 15, 2022.
27. Rubio-Rivas M, Moreno R, Corbella X. Occupational and environmental scleroderma. Systematic review and meta-analysis. *Clin Rheumatol*. 2017;36(3):569-582.
28. Benz K, Baulig C, Knippschild S, Strietzel FP, Hunzelmann N, Jackowski J. Prevalence of oral and maxillofacial disorders in patients with systemic scleroderma—a systematic review. *Int J Environ Res Public Health*. 2021;18(10):5238.
29. Isola G, Williams RC, Lo Gullo A, et al. Risk association between scleroderma disease characteristics, periodontitis, and tooth loss. *Clin Rheumatol*. 2017;36(12):2733-2741.
30. Kowal-Bielecka O, Fransen J, Avouac J, et al. Update of EULAR recommendations for the treatment of systemic sclerosis. *Ann Rheum Dis*. 2017;76(8):1327-1339.
31. Willems LM, Vriezekolk JE, Schouffoer AA, et al. Effectiveness of nonpharmacologic interventions in systemic sclerosis: a systematic review. *Arthritis Care Res*. 2015;67(10):1426-1439.
32. Tolle SL. Scleroderma: considerations for dental hygienists. *Int J Dent Hyg*. 2008;6(2):77-83.
33. Yuen HK, Hant FN, Hatfield C, et. al. Factors associated with oral hygiene practices among adults with systemic sclerosis. *Int J Dent Hyg*. 2014;12(3):180-186.
34. Di Sabatino A, Lenti MV, Giuffrida P, Vanoli A, Corazza GR. New insights into immune mechanisms underlying autoimmune diseases of the gastrointestinal tract. *Autoimmun Rev*. 2015;14(12):1161-1169.
35. Singh P, Arora A, Strand TA, et al. Global prevalence of celiac disease: systematic review and meta-analysis. *Clin Gastroenterol Hepatol*. 2018;16(6):823-836.e2.
36. Unalp-Arida A, Ruhl CE, Choung RS, Brantner TL, Murray JA. Lower prevalence of celiac disease and gluten-related disorders in persons living in southern vs northern latitudes of the United States. *Gastroenterology*. 2017;152(8): 1922-1932.e2.
37. Lebwohl B, Rubio-Tapia A. Epidemiology, presentation, and diagnosis of celiac disease. *Gastroenterol*. 2021;160(1):63-75.
38. Rubio-Tapia A, Hill ID, Kelly CP, Calderwood AH, Murray JA, American College of Gastroenterology. ACG clinical guidelines: diagnosis and management of celiac disease. *Am J Gastroenterol*. 2013;108(5):656-676.
39. Alsadat FA, Alamoudi NM, El-Housseiny AA, et al. Oral and dental manifestations of celiac disease in children: a case-control study. *BMC Oral Health*. 2021;21(1):669.
40. Ahmed A, Singh A, Kajal S, et al. Dental enamel defects and oral cavity manifestations in Asian patients with celiac disease. *Indian J Gastroenterol*. 2021;40(4):402-409.
41. Feuerstein JD, Cheifetz AS. Crohn disease: epidemiology, diagnosis, and management. *Mayo Clin Proc*. 2017;92(7): 1088-1103.
42. Xu L, Lochhead P, Ko Y, et al. Systematic review with meta-analysis: breastfeeding and the risk of Crohn's disease and ulcerative colitis. *Aliment Pharmacol Ther*. 2017;46(9):780-789.
43. Lichtenstein GR, Loftus EV, Isaacs KL, et al. ACG clinical guideline: management of Crohn's disease in adults. *Am J Gastroenterol*. 2018;113(4):481-517.
44. Tan CXW, Brand HS, Kalender B, et al. Dental and periodontal disease in patients with inflammatory bowel disease. *Clin Oral Investig*. 2021;25(9):5273-5280.
45. Halling ML, Kjeldsen J, Knudsen T, Nielsen J, Hansen LK. Patients with inflammatory bowel disease have increased risk of autoimmune and inflammatory diseases. *World J Gastroenterol*. 2017;23(33):6137-6146.
46. Alatab S, Sepanlou SG, Ikuta K, et al. The global, regional, and national burden of inflammatory bowel disease in 195 countries and territories, 1990–2017: a systematic analysis for the Global Burden of Disease Study 2017. *Lancet Gastroenterol Hepatol*. 2020;5(1):17-30.
47. Ye Y, Manne S, Bennett D. Prevalence of inflammatory bowel disease in the U.S. adult population: recent estimates from large population-based national databases. *Am J Gastroenterol*. 2018;113:S373.
48. Lynch WD, Hsu R. Ulcerative colitis. *StatPearls*. Updated June 11, 2022. http://www.ncbi.nlm.nih.gov/books/NBK459282/. Accessed December 15, 2022.
49. Gajendran M, Loganathan P, Jimenez G, et al. A comprehensive review and update on ulcerative colitis. *Disease-a-Month*. 2019;65(12):100851.
50. Ribaldone DG, Brigo S, Mangia M, Saracco GM, Astegiano M, Pellicano R. Oral manifestations of inflammatory bowel disease and the role of non-invasive surrogate markers of disease activity. *Medicines*. 2020;7(6):33.
51. Feuerstein JD, Isaacs KL, Schneider Y, et al. AGA clinical practice guidelines on the management of moderate to severe ulcerative colitis. *Gastroenterology*. 2020;158(5):1450-1461.
52. Farraye FA, Melmed GY, Lichtenstein GR, Kane SV. ACG clinical guideline: preventive care in inflammatory bowel disease. *Am J Gastroenterol*. 2017;112(2):241-258.
53. Tan CXW, Brand HS, de Boer NKH, Forouzanfar T. Gastrointestinal diseases and their oro-dental manifestations: Part 2: Ulcerative colitis. *Br Dent J*. 2017;222(1):53-57.
54. McGinley MP, Goldschmidt CH, Rae-Grant AD. Diagnosis and treatment of multiple sclerosis: a review. *JAMA*. 2021; 325(8):765-779.
55. Walton C, King R, Rechtman L, et al. Rising prevalence of multiple sclerosis worldwide: insights from the Atlas of MS, third edition. *Mult Scler*. 2020;26(14):1816-1821.
56. Klineova S, Lublin FD. Clinical course of multiple sclerosis. *Cold Spring Harb Perspect Med*. 2018;8(9):a028928.
57. Papathanasiou A, Saunders L, Sare G. Symptom management of patients with multiple sclerosis in primary care: focus on overlooked symptoms. *Br J Gen Pract*. 2021;71(704):139-141.
58. Covello F, Ruoppolo G, Carissimo C, et al. Multiple sclerosis: impact on oral hygiene, dysphagia, and quality of life. *Int J Environ Res Public Health*. 2020;17(11):3979.
59. Manchery N, Henry JD, Nangle MR. A systematic review of oral health in people with multiple sclerosis. *Community Dent Oral Epidemiol*. 2020;48(2):89-100.
60. Moss BP, Rensel MR, Hersh CM. Wellness and the role of comorbidities in multiple sclerosis. *Neurotherapeutics*. 2017; 14(4):999-1017.
61. Nielsen S, Germanos R, Weier M, et al. The use of cannabis and cannabinoids in treating symptoms of multiple sclerosis: a systematic review of reviews. *Curr Neurol Neurosci Rep*. 2018;18(2):8.
62. Canadian Dental Hygienists Association, Federation of Dental Hygiene Regulatory Authorities, Commission on Dental Accreditation of Canada, National Dental Hygiene Certification Board. *Entry to Practice Competencies and Standards for Canadian Dental Hygienists*. Published January 2010. https://www.cdha.ca/pdfs/Competencies_and_Standards.pdf. Accessed January 25, 2022.

63. American Dental Hygienists' Association. *2016 Revised Standards for Clinical Dental Hygiene Practice*. Published June 2016. https://www.adha.org/resources-docs/2016-Revised-Standards-for-Clinical-Dental-Hygiene-Practice.pdf. Accessed December 11, 2021.
64. Negrini S, Emmi G, Greco M, et al. Sjögren's syndrome: a systemic autoimmune disease. *Clin Exp Med*. 2022;22(1):9-25.
65. Manfrè V, Cafaro G, Riccucci I, et al. One year in review 2020: comorbidities, diagnosis and treatment of primary Sjögren's syndrome. *Clin Exp Rheumatol*. 2020;38 Suppl 126(4):10-22.
66. Kuo CF, Grainge MJ, Valdes AM, et al. Familial risk of Sjögren's syndrome and co-aggregation of autoimmune diseases in affected families: a nationwide population study. *Arthritis Rheumatol*. 2015;67(7):1904-1912.
67. Berman N, Vivino F, Baker J, Dunham J, Pinto A. Risk factors for caries development in primary Sjogren syndrome. *Oral Surg Oral Med Oral Pathol Oral Radiol*. 2019;128(2):117-122.
68. Wu SY, Wu CY, Chen MH, et al. Periodontal conditions in patients with Sjögren's syndrome: a meta-analysis. *J Dent Sci*. 2021;16(4):1222-1232.
69. Chuang CJ, Hsu CW, Lu MC, Koo M. Increased risk of developing dental diseases in patients with primary Sjögren's syndrome-a secondary cohort analysis of population-based claims data. *PLoS One*. 2020;15(9):e0239442.
70. Miyamoto ST, Lendrem DW, Ng WF, Hackett KL, Valim V. Managing fatigue in patients with primary Sjögren's syndrome: challenges and solutions. *Open Access Rheumatol*. 2019;11:77-88.
71. Zero DT, Brennan MT, Daniels TE, et al. Clinical practice guidelines for oral management of Sjögren disease: dental caries prevention. *J Am Dent Assoc*. 2016;147(4):295-305.
72. Nusbaum JS, Mirza I, Shum J, et al. Sex differences in systemic lupus erythematosus: epidemiology, clinical considerations, and disease pathogenesis. *Mayo Clin Proc*. 2020;95(2): 384-394.
73. Gergianaki I, Bortoluzzi A, Bertsias G. Update on the epidemiology, risk factors, and disease outcomes of systemic lupus erythematosus. *Best Pract Res Clin Rheumatol*. 2018;32(2): 188-205.
74. Ferucci ED, Johnston JM, Gaddy JR, et al. Prevalence and incidence of systemic lupus erythematosus in a population-based registry of American Indian and Alaska Native people, 2007-2009. *Arthritis Rheumatol*. 2014;66(9):2494-2502.
75. Fanouriakis A, Tziolos N, Bertsias G, Boumpas DT. Update on the diagnosis and management of systemic lupus erythematosus. *Ann Rheum Dis*. 2021;80(1):14-25.
76. Saccucci M, Di Carlo G, Bossù M, et al. Autoimmune diseases and their manifestations on oral cavity: diagnosis and clinical management. *J Immunol Res*. 2018;2018:6061825.
77. Fangtham M, Kasturi S, Bannuru RR, Nash JL, Wang C. Non-pharmacologic therapies for systemic lupus erythematosus. *Lupus*. 2019;28(6):703-712.

Glossary

#BeThe1To Be The One to Help Save A Life is an organization that recommends a five-step action plan to communicate with someone who may be suicidal that includes: ask, be there, help keep them safe, help them connect and follow up.

1.23% APF gel Acidulated phosphate fluoride (APF) gels, containing 12 300 ppm F– (1.23% APF) consist of a mixture of sodium fluoride, hydrofluoric acid and orthophosphoric acid.

5% NaF varnish active ingredient of fluoride varnish (22,600 ppm fluoride) used to treat hypersensitivity.

A

A1c (A One C) common abbreviation for glycosylated hemoglobin (HbA1c)

AAPD American Association of Pediatric Dentistry.

Abfraction wedge- or V-shaped cervical lesion created by the stresses of lateral or eccentric tooth movements during occlusal function, bruxing, or parafunctional activity, resulting in enamel microfractures.

Abrasion wearing away of surface material by friction.

Abrasion (gingiva) lesion of the gingiva resulting from mechanical removal of the surface epithelium.

Abrasion (tooth) loss of tooth structure produced by a mechanical cause (such as a hard-bristled toothbrush used with excessive pressure and an abrasive dentifrice); abrasion contrasts with erosion, which involves a chemical process.

Abrasive a material composed of particles of sufficient hardness and sharpness to cut or scratch a softer material when drawn across its surface; available in various particle sizes.

Abrasive system cleaning or polishing substances used in dentifrice; best when compatible with fluoride compounds and other ingredients, and does not alter the tooth structure unfavorably.

Absence seizure a type of generalized onset seizure, most often affecting children, producing lapses in awareness, sometimes mistaken for day dreaming.

Absolute contraindication under no circumstances should the local anesthetic or vasoconstrictor be administered.

Absorbed dose the amount of energy imparted by ionizing radiation to a unit mass of irradiated material at a specific exposure point; the unit of absorbed dose is the Gray (Gy).

Abstinence refraining from an activity that is known to be harmful and addictive. Abstinence involves not taking a particular substance, avoiding areas where this is likely to be offered or adopting a healthier lifestyle.

Abuse the nonaccidental physical, emotional (psychological), or sexual acts against a child.

Abutment a tooth or an implant used for the support or retention of a fixed or removable prosthesis.

Accreditation a quality assurance process that colleges, universities and education institutions or programs undergo to confirm that they meet a strict and recognized set of service and operational standards. CODA is the dental accreditation association that accredits programs and colleges for offering dental and dental-related education programs

Acellular not made up of or containing cells.

Acid etch in sealant placement, the enamel surface is prepared by the application of phosphoric acid, which etches the surface to provide mechanical retention for the sealant.

Acidogenic bacteria bacteria in dental biofilm capable of metabolizing fermentable carbohydrates into acids.

Aciduric bacteria bacteria in dental biofilm capable of thriving in an acidic oral environment.

Acoustic turbulence agitation in the fluids surrounding a rapidly vibrating ultrasonic tip; has potential to disrupt the bacterial matrix.

Activation the action of an instrument in the performance of the task for which it was designed; consists of a series of strokes.

Acute (of a disease or disease symptom) beginning abruptly with marked intensity or sharpness, then subsiding after a relatively short time; opposite of **chronic**.

ADA American Dental Association.

Adaptation relationship between the working end of an instrument and the tooth surface being treated.

Adaptive behavior conceptual, social, and practical skills learned by individuals to support the ability to function in everyday life.

Addiction habitual psychological and physiologic dependence on a substance or practice that is beyond voluntary control.

ADHA American Dental Hygienists' Association.

ADHP Advanced Dental Hygiene Practitioner. The dental hygiene–based, alternative workforce model, proposed by the American Dental Hygienists' Association, would be a registered dental hygienist with additional training who could autonomously provide additional oral health services.

ADL/IADL (activities of daily living/instrumental activities of daily living) a measure of ability to carry out the basic tasks needed for self-care.

Adolescence the period extending from the time the secondary sex characteristics appear to the end of somatic growth, when the individual is mature.

Adolescent child from 12 years of age to 18 years of age; considered teen or young adult.

Adrenal crisis also known as Addisonian crisis and acute adrenal insufficiency. A medical emergency and potentially life-threatening situation requiring immediate emergency treatment. It is a constellation of symptoms that indicate severe adrenal insufficiency caused by insufficient levels of the hormone cortisol.

Adsorption attachment of one substance to the surface of another; the action of a substance in attracting and holding other materials or particles on its surface.

Aeroallergen Inhalation of the allergen when the powder (or cornstarch) from the gloves becomes airborne.

Aerobe heterotrophic microorganism that can live and grow in the presence of free oxygen; some are obligate, others facultative; *adj.* aerobic.

Aerosol generating procedures (AGPs) any procedure carried out on a patient that creates aerosols or droplets resulting in risk of airborne transmission of pathogens.

AFB acid-fast bacilli.

Affect as used by mental health professionals, refers to an expressed or observed emotional response or lack of expression or emotional response (flat or restricted affect).

Affirmation to validate or confirm; commending a patient's efforts toward change.

Aging the continuous process (biologic, psychological, social) beginning with conception and ending with death, in which the organ systems age.

Aguesia loss of sense of taste

Air-powder polisher air-powered device using air and water pressure to deliver a controlled stream of specially processed sodium bicarbonate slurry through the handpiece nozzle; also called air abrasive, airpolishing, air-powered abrasive, or airbrasive.

AIs (adequate intakes) the recommended nutrient intake utilized when there is not enough information to establish an EAR.

Akinesia loss or impairment in the ability to move muscles voluntarily.

Alcohol overdose (intoxication) results from recent ingestion of excessive amounts of alcohol; characterized by behavioral changes that alter the usual behavior of the individual.

Alcohol use disorder (AUD) also known as alcoholism, is a pattern of alcohol use in which one has difficulty controlling his or her drinking, being preoccupied with alcohol, continuing to use alcohol even when it causes problems, having to drink more to get the same effect, or having withdrawal symptoms when blood alcohol levels decrease or if one ceases to drink.

Aligner system a series of customized transparent and removable aligners utilized in orthodontic therapy to align or straighten teeth.

Alimentation providing nutrition.

Allergen substance, protein or nonprotein, capable of inducing allergy or specific hypersensitivity; can enter the body by being inhaled, swallowed, touched, or injected.

Alloplast an inert foreign body used for implantation within tissue.

Alopecia a loss of hair.

ALS atropic lateral sclerosis.

Alternative tobacco products (ATPs) tobacco products besides cigarettes, including e-cigarettes, vape pens, water pipe/hookah, and smokeless tobacco.

Alveolectomy surgical removal of a portion of the alveolar bone to allow for fitting of a prosthesis.

Alveolitis infection and inflammation after extraction of a tooth due to the loss of the blood clot.

Alzheimer's disease a form of irreversible dementia, usually occurring in older adulthood, characterized by gradual deterioration of memory, disorientation, and other features of dementia.

Ambient air atmospheric air in its natural state.

Ambivalence simultaneous conflict or uncertainty toward making a change.

Amelogenesis imperfecta imperfect formation of enamel; hereditary condition in which the ameloblasts fail to lay down the enamel matrix properly or at all.

American sign language is a visual/gestural language with a unique grammar and syntax.

Americans with Disabilities Act (ADA) or (AwDA) prohibits discrimination on the basis of a disability and requires public and commercial facilities to meet standards of accessibility by removing architectural, transportation, and communication barriers.

Amnesia impairment of long-term and/or short-term memory.

Amorphous without definite shape or visible differentiation in structure.

Amorphous calcium phosphate a compound used on the teeth as an artificial hydroxyapatite.

Amplitude the distance of power scaler tip movement measured in micrometers.

Anaerobe heterotrophic microorganism that lives and grows in complete (or almost complete) absence of oxygen; some are obligate, others facultative; *adj.* anaerobic.

Analgesia loss of sensibility to pain without loss of consciousness.

Analgesic relieving pain.

Analgesics any member of the group of drugs used to achieve relief from pain. Act on the peripheral and central nervous systems.

Analog continuous and variable representation of an image as opposed to digital, which is a binary representation (0's and 1's) of an image. An analog image will include all levels of clarity and will not be enhanced as the digital representation.

Anaphylaxis a severe, potentially life-threatening allergic reaction. It can occur within seconds or minutes of exposure to an allergen. Anaphylaxis causes your immune system to release a flood of chemicals that may lead to shock—your blood pressure drops suddenly and your airways narrow, blocking breathing. Signs and symptoms include a rapid, weak pulse; a skin rash; and nausea and vomiting.

Anaplasia an irreversible alteration in adult cells toward more primitive (embryonic) cell types; characteristic of tumor cells.

Anesthesia loss of feeling or sensation, especially loss of tactile sensitivity, with or without loss of consciousness.

Angina pectoris (stable angina) Chest pain or discomfort due to coronary heart disease. It occurs when the heart muscle is lacking blood, usually because of blocked arteries (ischemia).

Angioedema swelling of the lower layer of skin and tissue just under the skin or mucous membranes. It may occur in the face, tongue, larynx, abdomen, or arms and legs. Often associated with hives and onset is over minutes to hours.

Angular cheilitis inflammation on the corners of the mouth typically affecting the vermillion border and perioral skin. The cause may be nutrient deficiency, fungal or yeast infection, and overclosure or loss of vertical dimension.

Angulation the angle formed by the working end of an instrument with the surface to which the instrument is applied for treatment.

Ankylosis immobility due to direct union between parts.

Anodontia a rare condition characterized by congenital absence of all teeth, primary and permanent.

Anosmia loss of sense of smell

Anoxemia deficiency of oxygen in arterial blood.

Anoxia oxygen deficiency; a reduction of oxygen in the tissues can lead to deep respirations, cyanosis, increased pulse rate, and impairment of coordination.

Antabuse brand name of the generic drug disulfiram; used to deter consumption of alcohol by persons being treated for alcohol dependency by inducing vomiting.

Antibiotic a form of antimicrobial agent produced by or obtained from microorganisms that can kill other microorganisms or inhibit their growth; may be specific for certain organisms or may cover a broad spectrum.

Antibiotic premedication provision of an effective antibiotic before invasive clinical procedures that can create a transient bacteremia, which, in turn, can cause IE or other serious infection.

Antibody a soluble protein molecule produced and secreted by body cells in response to an antigen; it is capable of binding to that specific antigen.

Anticariogenic substance in foods that inhibits or arrests dental caries formation.

Anticipatory anhedonia lower feelings of reward for use of nicotine.

Anticipatory guidance anticipatory guidance is the process of providing practical, developmentally appropriate information about children's health to prepare parents for the significant physical, emotional, and psychological milestones.

Anticipatory guidance patient education and oral hygiene instructions that anticipate potential oral and systemic health problems associated with risk factors identified during patient assessment.

Anticoagulant a substance that suppresses, delays, or nullifies coagulation of the blood.

Antiepileptic/antiseizure a remedy for epilepsy and/or seizures.

Antigen a toxin or other foreign substance capable, under appropriate conditions, of inducing a specific immune response and of reacting with the products of that specific antibody.

Antimicrobial agent chemical that is bacteriostatic or bactericidal.

Antimicrobial soap a soap containing an active ingredient against skin microorganisms.

Antimicrobial therapy use of specific chemical or pharmaceutical agents for the control or destruction of microorganisms, either systemically or at specific sites.

Antioxidant a compound that stops the damaging effects of reactive substances seeking an electron (oxidizing agent).

Antiseptic a substance that prevents or arrests the growth or action of microorganisms either by inhibiting their activity or by destroying them; term used especially for preparation applied topically to living tissue.

Anxiety a negative, emotional response to an anticipated event, the outcome of which is unknown. This is a learned response from personal experience or the stories of others.

Anxiolytics medication used to relieve anxiety or emotional tension, also called antianxiety agent.

Apatite crystalline mineral component of bones and teeth that contains calcium and phosphate.

APF acidulated phosphate fluoride.

Aphasia defect in, or loss of power of, expression by speech, writing, or signs, or of comprehension of spoken or written language.

Aphtha a little white or reddish ulcer.

Apnea temporary cessation of breathing; absence of spontaneous respirations.

Apoptosis cell death activated by a biochemical reaction; sometimes referred to as "programmed cell death."

Appliance any device designed to influence the shape and/or function of the mouth/jaw system.

Applied behavior analysis (ABA) an evidence-based behavioral approach in ASD that is shown to be effective to improve basic communication, social engagement, activities of daily living, and ability to adapt to change.

Arch wire curved wire positioned in the brackets around the dental arch and held in place by elastomers or ligatures.

Ariboflavinosis a condition resulting from a lack of riboflavin.

Arkansas stone fine-grained sharpening stone quarried from natural mineral deposits.

Arrhythmia variation from the normal rhythm, especially with reference to the heart.

Arterial blood oxygenated blood carried by an artery away from the heart to nourish the body tissues.

Arterial blood pressure pressure within large arteries in the systemic circulation.

Arthralgia joint pain.

Articulating paper paper treated with dye or wax used to mark points of contact (occlusion) between the maxillary and mandibular teeth.

ASA American Society of Anesthesiologists; originally developed the ASA classifications to determine modifications necessary to provide general anesthetic to patients during surgical procedures.

ASA classification developed by the American Society of Anesthesiologists, is a grading system to assess the patient's medical and physical state prior to receiving anesthesia or undergoing surgery.

Asepsis free from contamination with microorganisms; includes sterile conditions in tissues and on materials, as obtained by exclusion, removing, or killing organisms.

Aspiration recommended technique for preventing injection of local anesthetic directly into circulatory system. Negative pressure is created in anesthetic cartridge. If needle tip is in artery or vein, blood will be visible in cartridge.

Assessment the critical analysis and evaluation or judgment of a particular condition, situation, or other subject of appraisal.

Astringent a substance that causes contraction or shrinkage and arrests discharges.

Asymptomatic carrier an individual who harbors pathogenic organisms without clinically recognizable symptoms; a carrier may infect those contacted.

Ataxia problems with coordination and balance due to defects in the cerebellum of the brain.

Atheroma lipid (cholesterol) deposit on the intima (lining) of an artery; also called atheromatous plaque.

Atherosclerosis disease process caused by the deposit of atheromas on the inner lining of arteries that results in the obstruction of blood flow.

Atonic seizure muscles suddenly become limp, eyelids drop, head may nod forward, and person may drop things. Also called drop-attacks or drop seizures, lasting less than 15 seconds.

Atopic form of allergy in which a hypersensitivity reaction may occur in a part of the body not in contact with the allergen.

Atrophy wasting; decrease in size; occurs when muscle fibers are not used or are deprived of their blood supply, or when the nerve connection is interrupted.

Attached gingiva gingiva attached to the underlying alveolar bone.

Attachment apparatus the cementum, periodontal ligament (PDL), and the alveolar bone.

Atypical different, unusual, and not typical.

Augmentation to increase the size beyond the existing size; in alveolar ridge or maxillary sinus augmentation, to increase the bone to accommodate a dental implant.

Aura is a sensory warning that precedes a seizure; may involve flashing lights, dizziness, peculiar taste or tingling and numbness.

Auscultation listening for sounds produced within the body; may be performed directly or with a stethoscope.

Autism spectrum disorder a developmental disorder, generally evident before age 3, affecting verbal and nonverbal communications and social interaction.

Autoantibodies an antibody produced by the immune system against the individual's own body proteins/tissues.

Automatism repetitive tapping, lip smacking, picking at clothes, chewing, mumbling, or spitting.

Autonomic symptoms pale appearance, sweating, pupil dilation, heart arrhythmia, and bladder incontinence.

Autonomy individual's right to make their own decisions.

Avulsion the tearing away or forcible separation of a structure or part. Tooth avulsion is the traumatic separation of a tooth from the alveolus.

B

Backscatter radiation deflected by scattering processes at angles greater than 90° to the original direction of the beam of radiation.

Bacteremia presence of microorganisms in the bloodstream.

Band preformed stainless-steel ring fitted around a tooth and cemented in place; available in shapes for each tooth form; each band has a bracket attached on the facial side, which is the mode of attachment for the arch wire.

Barrier free area freely accessible to all without discrimination on the basis of a disability; obstacles to passage or communication have been removed.

Barrier protection refers to placing a physical barrier between the patient's body fluids (such as blood and saliva) and the healthcare personnel (HCP) to prevent disease transmission.

Baseline an initial known value that is used for comparison with later data.

Behavior manner in which an individual acts or manages himself or herself.

Behavior arrest lack of movement.

Behavior change transition in the way a patient acts or manages himself or herself.

Bell's palsy paralysis of the facial muscles innervated by the facial or seventh cranial nerve.

Benign not malignant.

Best practice a procedure or treatment intervention that has been shown by research and experience to produce optimal results and is established as a standard suitable for widespread adoption.

Beta cells insulin-producing cells of the islets of Langerhans in the pancreas.

Bevel a sloping surface; for an instrument, it refers to reducing the share angle of the cutting edge to a sloping surface.

Bibulous pad absorbent; a flat bibulous pad, placed in the cheek over the opening of Stensen duct, is used to aid in maintaining a dry field while placing sealants.

Bifid uvula cleft of the uvula of the soft palate that divides the uvula into two parts (Figure 49-1, Class 2).

Binge drinking occurs when an individual excessively drinks in a short period, typically 4 drinks for women and 5 drinks for men in about a 2-hour period, increasing blood alcohol concentration (BAC) levels to 0.08 g/dL.

Biodegradable susceptible of degradation by biologic processes, either by bacterial or other enzymatic action.

Biofilm the surface film that contains microorganisms and other biologic substances.

Biohazard a substance that poses a biologic risk because it is contaminated with biomaterial that has a potential for transmitting infection.

Biologic age the anatomic or physiologic age of a person as determined by changes in organismic structure and function; takes into account features such as posture, skin texture, strength, speed, and sensory acuity.

Biologic monitor a preparation of nonpathogenic microorganisms, usually bacterial spores, carried by an ampule or a specially impregnated paper enclosed within a package during sterilization and subsequently incubated to verify that the sterilizer is functioning properly.

Biologic or permucosal seal functional soft-tissue barrier at the base of the peri-implant sulcus; characterized by adhesion of junctional epithelium in the absence of Sharpey fibers, making it more susceptible to bacterial invasion by periodontal pathogens.

Biologic width the distance from the base of the sulcus to the alveolar bone.

Biomedical database organized collection of medically related journal articles, systematic reviews, research reports, theses, and/or dissertations typically in digital form.

Biopsy sample of tissue taken from the body to determine extent, cause, or presence of disease.

Incisional biopsy surgeon removes a part of the lesion along with some normal tissue.

Excisional biopsy surgeon removes the entire lesion along with some normal tissue.

Exfoliative biopsy surgeon removes surface epithelial cells; commonly known as oral brush biopsy.

Biostatistics a branch of statistics directed toward application in the discipline of health sciences.

Biotherapy use of biologic agents to treat cancer.

Bis-GMA (bisphenol A glycidyl methylacrylate) plastic material used for dental sealants.

Blade working end of an instrument with special design for a particular clinical treatment.

Bleaching a cosmetic dental procedure that uses free radicals and breakdown of pigments to whiten teeth.

Bleaching trays synonym for night guard vital bleaching, which requires development of a custom tray that allows for administration and containment of tooth bleaching material such as carbamide peroxide or hydrogen peroxide.

Blind no perception of visual stimuli; lack or loss of ability to see.

Block anesthesia induced by injecting the anesthetic close to a nerve trunk; may be at some distance from the area to be treated; involves multiple teeth and surrounding hard and soft tissues.

Block-out resin light-cured resin materials that can be used as a rubber dam substitute during bleaching procedure or on study models to create space to hold bleaching material on custom trays.

Blood alcohol concentration (BAC) refers to the percent of alcohol in a person's blood stream. A BAC of 0.10% means that an individual's blood supply contains one-part alcohol for every 1,000 parts blood. In most states, an individual is legally intoxicated if he or she has a BAC of 0.08% or higher.

Body mass index (BMI) a measure of body fat based on height in centimeters (cm) and weight in kilograms (kg).

Bond strength expression of the degree of adherence between the tooth surface and the sealant.

Bonded brackets orthodontic appliance used widely in orthodontic treatment that involves resin-bonded brackets.

Bonding (mechanical) physical adherence of one substance to another; the adherence of a sealant to the enamel surface is accomplished by an acid-etching technique that leaves microspaces between the enamel rods; the sealant becomes mechanically locked (bonded) in these microspaces.

Bonding process by which orthodontic brackets are affixed to the tooth surface; a fluoride-releasing, light-activated resin is frequently used.

Border mold the shaping of the edges of a dressing by manual manipulation of the tissue adjacent to the borders (e.g., lips, cheeks) to duplicate the contour and size of the vestibule.

Bracket attachment that is bonded to the enamel for the purpose of holding the arch wire.

Bradycardia unusually slow heartbeat evidenced by slowing of the pulse rate.

Bradykinesia abnormal slowness of movement; sluggish physical and mental responses.

Braille a system of writing and printing by means of raised points representing letters; enables people with a visual disability to read by touch.

Bristle stiffness the reaction force exerted per unit area of the brush during deflection; the term stiffness is used interchangeably with firmness of toothbrush bristles or filaments; the stiffness depends primarily on the length and diameter of the filaments.

Bristle individual short stiff, natural hair of an animal; historically, toothbrush bristles were taken from hog or wild boar, but current toothbrush bristles are made of nylon and are called filaments.

Bronchodilator a drug that relaxes contractions of the smooth muscle of the bronchioles to improve ventilation of the lungs.

Bruxism an oral habit of grinding, clenching, or clamping the teeth; involuntary, rhythmic, or spasmodic movements outside the chewing range; may damage teeth and attachment apparatus.

Buffer a substance that by its presence in solution is capable of neutralizing alkali or acid.

Bulbous bulging or rounded.

Burnish to smooth and polish; an effect that can result when a dull scaler or curet is passed over tenacious calculus in an attempt to remove the deposit.

C

Cachexia ill health, malnutrition, wasting (emaciating).

Calibrate determine accuracy and consistency between examiners in order to standardize procedures and gain reliability of recorded findings.

Calibration determination of the accuracy of an instrument by measurement of its variation from a standard.

CAMBRA (Caries Assessment and Management by Risk Assessment) procedure to assess risk for future dental caries development and identify approaches to managing caries risk.

Cannula tubular instrument placed in a cavity to introduce or withdraw fluid.

Carcinogen substance or chemical that has been known to cause cancer.

Carcinoma a malignant tumor of epithelial origin.

Cariogenic adjective to indicate a conduciveness to the initiation of dental caries, such as a cariogenic biofilm or a cariogenic food.

Cariostatic exerting an inhibitory action on the progress of dental caries.

Carious *adj.* used to define a carious lesion.

Carrier a person who harbors a specific infectious agent in the absence of discernible clinical disease and serves as a potential source of infection. The carrier state may be temporary, transient, or chronic.

Cassette a light-tight plastic, cardboard, or metal container in which x-ray image receptors are placed for exposure to x-radiation; usually backed with lead to reduce the effect of backscatter radiation and contain intensifying screen(s).

Cataract clouding or opacity of the lens of an eye.

Cavitated carious lesion advanced lesion with break through the tooth surface; contrast with noncavitated carious lesion, when a dull probe passed over a white demineralized area detects no roughness or breakthrough.

Cavitated lesion a loss of the integrity of the surface enamel with exposure of dentin.

Cavitation breakthrough of the enamel surface; final stage in the caries process.

CDC Centers for Disease Control and Prevention.

Centric occlusion (or habitual occlusion) the maximum intercuspation or contact of the teeth of the opposing arches; also called habitual occlusion.

Ceramic alumina (Al_2O_3) used as a single-crystal material or as a polycrystalline material.

Cerebrovascular accident (CVA) a focal neurologic disorder caused by destruction of brain substance because of intracerebral hemorrhage, thrombosis, embolism, or vascular insufficiency; also called stroke.

CFU colony-forming unit.

Chain of asepsis a procedure that avoids transfer of infection. The "chain" implies that each step, related to the previous one, continues to be carried out without contamination.

Change talk any self-expressed language that is an argument for change.

Charcot joints a joint that is deprived of any pain or position sense due to severe osteoarthritis or as a result of disease such as diabetic neuropathy.

Chart a form/graphic representation used as a component of a patient's permanent health record.

Charting the process of tabulating clinical information on a graphic form.

Chemical cure mode of self-cure or setting of a dressing in which the ingredients unite in a chemical process that starts as soon as the blending is complete; the setting time is influenced by warm temperature and the addition of an accelerator.

Chemical indicator a color change stripe or other mark, often on autoclave tape or bag, used to monitor the process of sterilization; color change indicates that the package has been brought to a specific temperature, but color change is not an indicator of sterilization.

Chemotherapeutic agent a chemical that is used for therapeutic reasons.

Chemotherapeutic treatment by means of chemical or pharmaceutical agents to treat disease.

Chemotherapy treatment of illness by chemical means, that is, by medication or drugs.

Chief complaint the patient's concern as stated during the initial health history preparation; may be the reason for seeking professional care; a complaint such as pain or discomfort may require emergency dental diagnosis.

Chlorophyll green plant pigment essential to photosynthesis.

Chromogenic producing color or pigment.

Chronic (of a disease or disorder) developing slowly and persisting for a long period, often for the remainder of a person s lifetime; opposite of **acute.**

Chronically ill a condition or disease that persists for a long period of time, usually more than 3 months. Can be maintained, but not often cured.

Chronologic age the actual measure of time elapsed since a person's birth.

Chronologic the order a series of events occurs. Often refers to timing as related to age.

CHX chlorhexidine.

Cleaning agent round, flat nonabrasive particles that do not scratch surface materials.

Clefts flossing injury that occurs primarily on facial and lingual or palatal surfaces directly beside or in the middle of an interdental papilla.

Cleft lip a unilateral or bilateral congenital fissure of the upper lip, usually lateral to the midline; can extend into one nostril or both and may involve the alveolar process; caused by defect in the fusion of the maxillary and globular processes.

Cleft palate a congenital fissure of the palate caused by failure of the palatal shelves to fuse; may extend to connect with unilateral or bilateral cleft lip.

Clinical attachment level (CAL) probing depth (PD) as measured from the cementoenamel junction (CEJ) (or other fixed point) to the location of the probe tip at the coronal level of attached periodontal tissues.

Clinical practice guidelines statements that include recommendations intended to optimize patient care.

Clinical significance practical or observed difference expected in patient care outcomes following a clinical intervention; in research, a clinically observable difference rather than statistical difference.

Clonic sustained rhythmical jerking of parts or the whole body.

Coapt to approximate, as the edges of a wound; bring edge to edge with no overlap.

Cochlear implants is a surgically **implanted** electronic device that provides a sense of sound to a person who is profoundly deaf or severely hard of hearing in both ears.

Cognitive mental process of comprehension, judgment, and memory.

Cognitively impaired difficulty remembering, learning new things, concentrating, or making decisions that affect everyday life. Ranges from mild to severe.

Col a depression between the buccal and lingual interproximal papilla.

Collaborative practice the science of the prevention and treatment of oral disease through the provision of educational, assessment, preventive, clinical, and other therapeutic services in a collaborative working relationship with a consulting dentist, with general supervision.

Collagen white fibers of the connective tissue.

Color a phenomenon of light or visual perception that enables the differentiation of otherwise identical objects. Usually determined visually by measurement of hue, saturation, and luminous reflectance of light.

Colostomy bag a removable, disposable bag that attaches to the exterior opening of a colostomy(stoma) to permit sanitary collection and disposal of bodily wastes.

Communicable an infectious agent may be transferred directly or indirectly from an infected person to another person.

Communicable disease (contagious) any disease transmitted from one person or animal to another. *Direct:* from excreta or other bodily discharges. *Indirect*: from substances or inanimate objects (contaminated drinking glasses, water, insects, or toys).

Communication a process of defining the meaning of a message shared between a sender and one or more intended recipients.

Nonverbal communication sending and receiving wordless messages; usually refers to body language, gestures, facial expressions, eye contact, and verbal elements such as rhythm and intonation.

Verbal communication sending and receiving messages using words; usually defined as spoken or written communication.

Communication disorders any disorder that affects an individual's ability to comprehend, detect, or apply language and speech to engage in discourse effectively with others. The delays and disorders can range from simple sound substitution to the inability to understand or use one's native language.

Communication style attitude and approach to assisting patients, a way of talking with them that describes the clinician's relationship with the patient.

Comorbid medical condition(s) existing simultaneously but independently with another condition.

Comorbidities the simultaneous presence of two chronic diseases or conditions in a patient.

Compensatory behavior behavior meant to relieve guilt or anxiety over eating.

Competency the skills, understanding, and professional values of an individual ready for beginning professional practice.

Complete denture dental prosthesis that replaces the entire dentition and associated structures; may be a complete maxillary denture or a complete mandibular or both.

Compliance action in accordance with request; extent to which a person's health behaviors coincide with dental/medical health advice. Also called *adherence*.

Computer screen reader software programs that allow visually impaired individuals to read data displayed on a computer screen with a speech synthesizer.

Condyloma acuminatum multiple papillary or focal sessile-based lesions caused by the human papilloma virus (HPV6 or HPV11).

Cone-beam computed tomography (CBCT) radiographic technology that produces three-dimensional (3-D) images of teeth, soft tissues, nerve pathways, and bone in a single scan.

Confidence interval a range of values defining a specific probability that the value of a factor lies within it.

Congenital hypothyroidism partial or complete lack of production of thyroid hormone in infants from birth.

Congenital present at and existing since birth.

Conscious sedation the combination of medications to help a patient relax (sedation) and block pain (anesthesia) during a medical or dental procedure.

Consent voluntary agreement to an action proposed by another.

Contamination introduction of microorganisms, blood, or other potentially infectious material or agent onto a surface or into tissue.

Context personal and environmental factors that influence patient care.

Continuing care system of appointments for the long-term maintenance phase of patient care; the system is carried out by computer, telephone, and/or mail. Also called recare or maintenance.

Continuing education Post-licensure short-term educational experiences for refresher, updating, and renewal; continuing education units may be required for relicensure.

Controlled release local delivery of a chemotherapeutic agent to a site-specific area; may be a patch worn on the skin or a polymeric fiber, such as that used to deliver an agent to a periodontal pocket.

Convulsion violent spasm.

Copolymer a substance with a high molecular weight that results from chemically combining two or more monomers.

Core values basic values of a profession; guide to choices or actions by implying a preference for what is deemed to be acceptable in the profession.

Corium the dermis or true skin just beneath the epidermis; well supplied with nerves and blood vessels.

Coronal polishing polishing of the anatomic crowns of the teeth to remove dental biofilm and extrinsic stains; does not involve calculus removal.

Coronary heart disease narrowing of the arteries that supply blood and oxygen to the heart caused by the buildup of plaque in the arteries.

Corticosteroids a type of anti-inflammatory drug used in the treatment of various medical conditions including rheumatoid arthritis, asthma, allergies, and inflammatory bowel disease.

Coryza profuse discharge from mucous membrane of the nose.

Co-therapist term used to describe the relationships between patient, dentist, and dental hygienist when coordinating the efforts to attain and maintain the oral health of the patient.

Cotinine a by-product of nicotine found in body fluids; cotinine levels are used in behavioral research to determine recent use of nicotine-containing products or recent contact with passive smoke and in clinical research to determine correlations between cotinine levels and oral disease.

CRA (caries risk assessment) procedure to predict future dental caries development before the clinical onset of the disease.

Craniofacial pertaining to the cranium, the part of the skull that encloses the brain, and the face.

Crepitation dry crackling sound, such as that produced by the grating of the ends of a fractured bone.

Cricothyrotomy incision through the skin and the cricothyroid membrane to secure a patent airway for emergency relief of upper airway obstruction.

Critically ill patient survival of the patient is at stake. Intensive care or hospitalization is usually required.

Cross-contamination the transfer of microorganisms, blood, or other potentially infectious material or agent onto a surface or into tissue.

Crust outer scablike layer of solid matter formed by drying of a body exudate or secretion.

Cultural competence a set of congruent attitudes, skills, behaviors, and policies that enable effective cross-cultural communication for delivery of oral health services.

Cultural rapport actions that foster understanding, empathy, and enhanced communication between individuals with different cultural backgrounds.

Cultural sensitivity making an effort to understand the language, culture, and behaviors of diverse individuals and groups.

Culturally effective healthcare refers to a dynamic relationship between provider and patient, resulting in culturally relevant and culturally specific healthcare recommendations; delivery of healthcare services in a way respectful of and responsive to the cultural norms and linguistic needs of individual patients.

Culture a learned set of beliefs, values, attitudes, convictions, and behaviors that are common to a group (especially an ethnic group) of people and usually passed down from generation to generation.

Cumulative trauma disorders injuries of the musculoskeletal and nervous systems caused by repetitive tasks, forceful exertions, vibrations, mechanical compression or sustained postures.

Curet a curved, rounded dental instrument utilized primarily for subgingival scaling and root planing.

Area-specific curet a specialized instrument designed with specific angles in the shank for adaptation to a certain group of tooth surfaces.

Universal curet a curet designed for use on any tooth surface where the adaptation, angulation, and other principles of instrumentation can be correctly and effectively accomplished.

Curing the process is used for **polymerization** of resin-based sealant and composites so that the material hardens by which plastic becomes rigid.

Custodial care nonmedical care provided by nonlicensed caregivers. Often at home, but can be in a nursing facility.

Cutting edge the fine line formed where the face and lateral surfaces of a scaler or curet meet when the instrument is sharp; when the instrument is dull, the line has thickness and may even reflect light.

Cyanosis bluish discoloration of the skin and mucous membranes caused by excess concentration of reduced hemoglobin in the blood.

Cyst a closed, epithelial-lined sac, normal or pathologic, that contains fluid or other material.

D

Data collection the process of gathering information (through the use of tools such as dental indices).

Data pieces of information collected using measurements and/or counts.

Debonding removal of brackets and residual adhesive, after which the tooth surface is returned to its normal contour.

Decoding the reverse process of encoding; the receiver takes the words, gestures, or other signs to recreate the thought.

Decompensate appearance or exacerbation of a mental disorder, which may include hallucinations, delusion, violent, or bizarre behavior.

Decubitus ulcer ulcer that usually occurs over a bony prominence as a result of prolonged, excessive pressure from body weight; also called pressure sore or bed sore.

De-densification limiting the number of people in a space at a specific time through strategies like staggering appointments or work hours, etc. to reduce the risk of disease transmission.

Defluoridation lowering the amount of fluoride in fluoridated water to an optimum level for the prevention of dental caries and dental fluorosis.

Delirium extreme mental and usually motor excitement marked by a rapid succession of confused and unconnected ideas; often with illusions and hallucinations; may be accompanied by tremors.

Delirium tremens (DTs) a serious acute condition associated with the last stages of alcohol withdrawal. Usually lasting 2 or 3 days, the individual can experience hallucinations, shaking, shivering, irregular heart rates, sweating, hyperthermia, or seizures that could result in death.

Delusion false belief firmly held, although contradicted by social reality.

Dementia severe mental deterioration involving impairment of mental ability; organic loss of intellectual function.

Demineralization breakdown of the tooth structure with a loss of mineral content, primarily calcium and phosphorus.

Demineralization major stage in the dental caries process in which minerals, primarily calcium and phosphorous, are removed from tooth structure by acids formed by acidogenic bacteria, primarily *mutans streptococci* and lactobacilli.

Dental biofilm a biofilm of microorganisms that grows on surfaces within the mouth, which is a primary risk factor for gingivitis, inflammatory periodontal diseases, and dental caries.

Dental calculus also referred to as "tartar," calculus is dental biofilm that has been mineralized primarily with calcium and phosphorus and occurs on the teeth and prosthetic appliances worn in the mouth.

Dental caries disease of the mineralized structures of the teeth characterized by demineralization of the hard components and dissolution of the organic matrix.

Arrested caries carious lesion that has become stationary and does not show a tendency to progress further; frequently has a hard surface and takes on a dark brown or reddish brown color.

Incipient caries early signs of a carious lesion.

Rampant caries widespread formation of chalky white areas and incipient lesions that may increase in size over a comparatively short time.

Recurrent caries occurs on a surface adjacent to a restoration; may be a continuation of the original lesion; also called secondary caries.

Root caries occurs on root surfaces.

Dental home an ongoing relationship between the dentist and the patient, including all aspects of oral healthcare delivered in a comprehensive, continuously accessible, coordinated, and family-centered way.

Dental hygiene care the science and practice of the prevention of oral diseases; the integrated preventive and treatment services administered for a patient by a dental hygienist.

Dental hygiene care plan the services within the framework of the total treatment plan to be carried out by the dental hygienist, patient, and caregiver.

Dental hygiene diagnosis identification of an existing or a potential oral health problem that a dental hygienist is qualified and licensed to treat.

Dental hygiene process of care an organized, systematic group of activities that provides the framework for delivering quality dental hygiene care.

Dental hygienist oral health specialist whose primary concern is the maintenance of oral health and the prevention of oral disease (see also opening section of Chapter 1).

Dental neglect the willful failure of a parent or guardian to seek and follow through with treatment necessary to ensure a level of oral health essential for adequate function and freedom from pain and infection.

Dental therapist a midlevel oral healthcare provider with expanded training who provides direct patient care under an expanded scope of practice that includes the ability to diagnose and perform restorative services. Dental therapists provide safe, quality dental care in many countries around the world.

Dentinal hypersensitivity transient pain arising from exposed dentin, typically in response to a stimulus, which cannot be explained as arising from any other form of dental defect or pathology and subsides quickly when stimulus is removed.

Dentinogenesis imperfecta hereditary disorder of dentin formation in which the odontoblasts lay down an abnormal matrix; can occur in both primary and permanent dentitions.

Dentition the natural teeth in the dental arch.

- **Primary (deciduous) dentition** the first teeth; normally will be shed and replaced by permanent teeth.
- **Permanent dentition** the natural 32 teeth that serve throughout life.
- **Mixed dentition** combination of primary and permanent teeth between the ages of 6 and 12 when primary teeth are being replaced; starts with the eruption of the first permanent tooth.

Denture adhesive a soft material used to adhere a denture to the underlying mucosa; also referred to as an adherent.

Denture foundation area the surfaces of the oral structures available to support a denture.

Denture insertion the process of directing a prosthesis to a desired oral location; introduction of a prosthesis into a patient's mouth; other terms used are denture delivery or denture placement.

Denture stomatitis an inflammation of the oral mucosa that bears a complete or partial removable dental prosthesis, typically a denture.

Denture artificial substitute for missing natural teeth and adjacent tissues.

Dependence dependence develops when the neurons in the brain adapt to the repeated substance exposure and only function normally in the presence of the substance. When the substance is withdrawn, several physiologic reactions can occur from mild to life-threatening (withdrawal syndrome).

- **Chemical dependence** the use of substances, alters an individual's brain making the brain more dependent on the chemical substance to operate.
- **Physical dependence** occurs when a person requires the substance to function, if the substance is not present in their system, the person could experience physical symptoms ranging from anxiety to seizures.

Depression temporary mental state or chronic disorder characterized by feelings of sadness and low self-esteem.

Descriptive statistics use of numbers to describe the main features or characteristics of a particular person, event, or group; to determine the frequency with which something occurs; or to categorize information.

Desensitization techniques a **technique** used in behavior therapy to treat phobias and other behavior problems involving anxiety desensitization to accept dental treatment might consist, for example, of short exposures to the dental chair, instruments, air syringe, and sound of a handpiece along with building trust in the dental team members.

Desquamation shedding of the outer epithelial layer of the stratified squamous epithelium of skin or mucosa.

Determinant a factor that can influence the outcome of some process. Health determinants include physical and social factors that influence the health outcomes of an individual or in a community.

Detoxification treatment designed to assist in recovery from the toxic effects of a substance; involves withdrawal and may include pharmacologic and/or nonpharmacologic treatment with psychotherapy and counseling.

Developmental disability a substantial handicap of indefinite duration with onset before the age of 18 years. Examples include autism and cerebral palsy.

DHCP dental healthcare personnel.

Diabetic ketoacidosis (DKA) diabetic coma; too little insulin; accumulation of ketone bodies in the blood. Occurs primarily in type 1 diabetes mellitus.

Diagnosis a statement of the problem; a concise technical description of the cause, nature, or manifestations of a condition, situation, or problem; identification of a disease or deviation from normal condition by recognition of characteristic signs and symptoms.

- **Dental hygiene diagnosis** identification of an existing or a potential oral health problem that a dental hygienist is qualified and licensed to treat.
- **Dental hygiene prognosis** a judgment regarding the results (outcomes) expected to be achieved from oral treatment provided by a dental hygienist.

Diastema a space between two adjacent teeth in the same arch.

Diastole the phase of the cardiac cycle in which the heart relaxes between contractions and the two ventricles are dilated by the blood flowing into them; diastolic pressure is the lowest blood pressure.

Diet customary amount and kind of food and drink taken by an individual from day to day.

Dietary assessment assessment of quality of food intake, whether an individual is consuming an adequate diet, and where modifications are needed to promote optimum health.

Differential cell count record of the number of white blood cells, including determination of the percentage of each type of cell present; the "differential" is used in the diagnosis of various blood disorders, infections, and other abnormal conditions of the body.

Differential diagnosis determining the probability of one disease or condition versus another by comparing and contrasting the symptoms.

Diffusion hypoxia lack of adequate amounts of oxygen that can result from the rapid diffusion of nitrous oxide molecules from the bloodstream into the lungs.

Digital sensors include CCD, CMOS, and PSP plates.

Digitize to convert an image into a digital form that can be used by the computer using a grid of pixels.

Diplopia double vision.

Direct access ability to maintain a direct patient provider relationship; allows dental hygienist to deliver care without the specific or previous authorization of a dentist and provide treatment without the presence of a dentist.

Direct access allows a dental hygienist to initiate dental hygiene treatment based on assessment of the patient's needs and without the specific authorization or presence of a dentist.

Disability physical, mental, or functional impairment that restricts a major activity; may be partial or complete.

Disease activity ongoing dynamic process that results in loss of clinical attachment and alveolar supporting bone; an area is quiescent when a diseased site becomes inactive or stable without treatment.

Disinfectant an agent, usually a chemical, but may be a physical agent, such as x-rays or ultraviolet light, that destroys microorganisms but may not kill bacterial spores; refers to substances applied to inanimate objects.

Diversion (in relation to drugs) drugs being used in ways not intended by the prescriber.

DMFT/dmft decayed, missing, and filled teeth (permanent and primary dentition, respectively).

Domestic violence violent or aggressive behavior within the home, typically involving the violent abuse of a spouse or partner.

Dominant hand the hand generally used for performing tasks, such as writing and holding instruments for scaling.

Dorsal back surface; opposite of ventral.

Dose equivalent the product of absorbed dose and modifying factors, such as the quality factor, distribution factor, and any other necessary factors; different types of radiation cause differing biologic effects; the unit of dose equivalence is the Sievert (Sv).

DOT directly observed therapy.

DRIs (Dietary Reference Intakes) a comprehensive term for categories of reference values that concentrate on maintaining a healthy state for the healthy general population to avoid overeating and prevent chronic disease.

Drug Enforcement Administration (DEA) drug schedules drugs, substances, and certain chemicals used to make drugs are classified by the US Drug Enforcement Administration (DEA) into five distinct categories or schedules depending on the drug's acceptable medical use and the drug's abuse or dependency potential.

Drug resistant a microorganism having developed the ability to withstand medications like antibiotics, making it harder to treat.

Dysarthria a motor/speech disorder that weakens or paralyzes the muscles of the face, mouth, larynx, and vocal cords, causing slurred, slow, and difficult-to-understand speech.

Dysbiosis an imbalance in the intestinal microflora, often associated with disease.

Dysgeusia distortion of the sense of taste.

Dysmorphic abnormality in morphologic development.

Dysphagia difficulty in swallowing. Do not confuse with dysphasia loss of ability to understand language as a result of injury or disease to the brain.

Dyspnea labored or difficult breathing; indication of inadequate ventilation or of insufficient oxygen in the circulating blood.

Dystonia muscles contract uncontrollably.

E

Early childhood caries (ECC) the presence of one or more decayed (noncavitated or cavitated lesions), missing (due to caries), or filled tooth surfaces in any primary tooth in a child younger than 6 years.

EARs (Estimated Average Requirements) estimates the nutrient requirements of the average individual.

Ecchymosis discoloration on the skin that is blue-black with irregularly formed hemorrhagic areas. Color changes with time to yellow or greenish brown.

Echocardiography recording of the position and motion of the heart walls and internal structures of the heart and neighboring tissue by the echo obtained from beams of ultrasonic waves directed through the chest wall; used to show valvular and other structural deformities; the record produced is called an echocardiogram.

Edema abnormal accumulation of fluid in the intercellular spaces of the body.

Edematous enlargement caused by fluids in inflamed tissues.

Edentulous without teeth; referred to as partially edentulous when some, but not all, teeth are missing.

Efficacy the benefits of a product or procedure that lead to intended results, such as reduction in gingivitis.

Elastomer elastoplastic ring or latex elastic used to hold an arch wire in a bracket wing.

Electroconvulsive therapy (ECT) electroshock therapy; a form of somatic therapy in which an electric current is used to produce convulsions; primarily used to treat severe depression.

Electroencephalography EEG is an electrophysiologic monitoring method to record electrical activity of the brain.

Electromagnetic ionizing radiation forms of energy propagated by wave motion as photons; the radiations differ widely in wavelength, frequency, and photo energy; examples are infrared waves, visible light, ultraviolet radiation, x-rays, gamma rays, and cosmic radiation.

Electronic cigarette see electronic nicotine delivery system (ENDS).

Electronic nicotine delivery system (ENDS) also called an ENDS, electronic cigarette or e-cigarette, the nicotine liquid is heated to deliver vaporized nicotine through a device that is made to look similar to a regular cigarette but comes in a variety of shapes, including one that looks like a USB jump drive. E-cigarettes come as disposable or rechargeable models with a variety of flavors. May also be called vaping.

Electronic patient record in a computerized database management system, a record is a complete set of information. Records are composed of electronic fields, each of which contains space for one item of information.

Elicit to draw forth or bring out.

EMB ethambutol.

Embolism the sudden blocking of an artery by a clot of foreign material, an embolus, that has been brought to its site of lodgment by the bloodstream; the embolus may be a blood clot (most frequently) or an air bubble, a clump of bacteria, or a fat globule.

Embrasure a triangle-shaped space below the contact area of two adjacent teeth.

Emphysema a lung condition that causes shortness of breath, reducing the amount of oxygen that reaches the bloodstream.

Enamel opacities a mild form of dental fluorosis on the enamel surface.

Enamel organ cellular aggregation in a developing tooth, lying above the dental papilla; also called dental organ.

Encoding the translation of a thought into words, gestures, or other linguistic signs that will allow thoughts to be expressed in some understandable way to another; encoding can be verbal or nonverbal, oral, visual, or tactile.

Encryption translation of computerized data into a secret code; the most effective way to achieve data security; in order to read an encrypted file, the reader needs access to a secret key or password that enables changing the "cipher text" into plain text.

Endemic the constant presence of a disease or an infectious agent within a geographic area.

Endocrine pertaining to secretion of a substance directly into blood or lymph rather than into a duct; the opposite of exocrine.

Endogenous having an internal cause or origin.

Endometrium the lining of the uterus.

Endoscope a minimally invasive diagnostic procedure used in medicine to examine inaccessible tissues by inserting a fiberoptic tube into the body.

Endosseous or root form dental implant tooth root replacement with a cylindrical or conical shape similar to a natural tooth root.

Endotoxin LPS complex found in the cell wall of many gram-negative microorganisms; contained superficially within periodontally involved cementum.

End-rounded characteristic shape of each toothbrush filament; a special manufacturing process removes all sharp edges and provides smooth, rounded ends to prevent injury to gingiva or tooth structure during use.

Environmental Protection Agency (EPA) registered number on a label indicates that the product has the acceptance of EPA.

Environmental tobacco smoke (ETS) or passive smoke tobacco smoke present in room air resulting from ignited tobacco products burning in an ashtray or exhaled by a smoker (people who are currently smoking are also exposed to other smokers' sidestream smoke).

EPA US Environmental Protection Agency.

Epicanthic fold a vertical fold of skin on either side of the nose, sometimes covering the inner canthus; a normal characteristic in persons of certain races.

Epidemiology the study of the relationships of various factors that determine the frequency and distribution of diseases in the human community; study of health and disease in populations.

Epidermis outermost and nonvascular layers of the skin composed of basal layer, spinous layer, granular layer, and horny layer.

Epilepsy a disease of the brain characterized by recurrent unprovoked (or reflex) seizures.

Epileptic spasm a sudden flexion and extension of proximal and truncal muscles.

Epinephrine a catecholamine hormone that causes the "fight-or-flight" response to physical or emotional stress; increased secretion produces marked dilation of bronchioles and increased blood pressure, blood glucose level, and heart rate.

Epithelium specialized single layer (simple) or multiple (stratified) layers of cells that form on the surface of skin, mucosa, or serous membranes.

Oral epithelium the tissue serving as a liner for the intraoral mucosal surfaces.

Squamous epithelium composed of a layer of flat, scale-like cells; or may be stratified.

Ergonomics study of designing and arranging the working environment around the worker for the most efficient and safe function.

Erosion soft-tissue slightly depressed lesion in which the epithelium above the basal layer is denuded.

Erythema redness of the skin or mucous membranes caused by increased blood flow in superficial capillaries. Occurs with injury, infection, or inflammation.

Esthetic pertaining to the study of beauty and the sense of beautiful; objectifies beauty and attractiveness, elicits pleasure.

Ethical dilemma a problem that involves two morally correct choices or courses of action. There may not be a single answer, and, depending on the choice, the outcomes can differ.

Ethical issue a common problem wherein a solution is readily grounded in the governing practice act, recognized laws, or acceptable standards of care. Decisions involving ethical issues are generally more clearly defined than are dilemmas.

Ethics a sense of moral obligation; a system of moral principles that governs the conduct of a professional group, planned by them for the common good of people; principles of morality.

Eugenol constituent of clove oil; used in early periodontal dressings with zinc oxide for its alleged antiseptic and anodyne properties; more recently found to be toxic, to elicit allergic reactions, and to hinder, more than promote, healing.

Euphoria feeling of well-being, elation; without fear or worry.

Evaluation design a description of the purpose, plans, and strategies that will be needed to gather, process, and interpret the data used to determine treatment outcomes.

Evaluation assessment of changes in patient's behavior or oral health status.

Evidence source of information used to support, determine, or demonstrate the truth of a statement.

Evidence-based approach providing oral care based on relevant, scientifically sound research.

Evidence-based decision-making (EBDM) process of making decisions grounded in best available research, professional experience, and contextual factors.

Evidence-based dental hygiene (EBDH) practice a scientific, research-supported approach to decide dental hygiene interventions for each patient.

Evidence-based practice (EBP) the practical application of evidence-based decision-making in diverse professions, including healthcare contexts.

Evocation eliciting or drawing out from patient through open-ended questions.

Exacerbation increase in severity of a disease or any of its symptoms.

Exfoliation loss of primary teeth following physiologic resorption of root structure.

Exodontics branch of dentistry dealing with the surgical removal of teeth.

Exogenosis related to external factors.

Exogenous originating outside or caused by factors outside.

Exogenous insulin insulin delivered from a source outside the body, such as by injection.

Exophytic growing outward.

Exostosis a benign bony growth projecting from the surface of bone.

Expert witness a person licensed to perform treatment in a specific health profession or with specialized knowledge, beyond that of the average person, in an area of treatment; a source for determining legal professional standard of care in a court case.

Expiration release of air from the lungs through the nose or mouth. See **inspiration**.

Explorer an instrument with a fine flexible, sharp point used for examination of the surfaces of the teeth to detect irregularities.

Extracellular polymeric substance (EPS) extracellular polymeric substances are compounds secreted by microorganisms and form a matrix for biofilm.

Extravascular not occurring or contained in body vessels.

Extrinsic stain tooth discoloration or staining on the surface of the tooth surface.

Extrinsic derived from or situated on the outside; external.

Exudate fluid and dead cells produced during inflammation, which can vary in color, thickness, and odor.

F

F.A.S.T acronym used to detect symptoms of stroke. **F:** Face drooping or numb on one side; **A:** Arm weakness; **S:** Speech difficulty (may slur words); **T:** Time to call EMS/911.

Facet a small flattened surface on a hard body, such as a tooth; a wear facet can result from attrition or repeated parafunctional contact.

Fallow period duration of time for which the operatory is left in solitude to allow for any aerosols (and any microorganisms contained in them) to clear or settle before the next patient is brought in.

Family violence (FV) any threatening or abusive behavior perpetrated by any person in a family, domestic or intimate relationship.

Fasting plasma glucose (FPG) measurement of blood glucose taken at least 8 hours after a meal.

Fatigue a state of physical exhaustion triggered by stress, overwork, and other factors.

FDA US Food and Drug Administration; regulates food, drugs, biologic products, medical devices, and radiologic products.

Feedback the receiver's direct response to a communicated message.

Ferromagnetic type of rod with unusually high magnetic permeability used in magnetostrictive ultrasonic unit inserts.

Fetus an unborn offspring, from the embryo stage until birth.

Fibrosis thickening and scarring of connective tissue.

Fibrotic fibroblasts (fiber-producing cells) of the connective tissue produce a change in the texture of the tissue, especially the gingiva, because of chronic inflammation; fibrotic gingiva may appear outwardly healthy and not bleed on probing, thus masking underlying disease.

Fibrous encapsulation layer of fibrous connective tissue between the implant and surrounding bone. Also called fibrous integration; indicative of failed osseointegration.

Filament individual synthetic fiber; a single element of a tuft fixed into a toothbrush head.

Filled sealant contains, in addition to bis-GMA, microparticles of glass, quartz, silica, and other fillers used in composite restorations; fillers make the sealant more resistant to abrasion.

Financial exploitation improper, illegal, or unethical exploitation of resources or assets.

Finger rest for an intraoral rest, the place on a tooth or teeth where the third or ring finger of the hand holding the instrument is placed to provide stabilization and control during activation of the instrument.

First-line refers to a drug or therapy that is the first choice for treatment.

Fissure a narrow slit or cleft in the epidermis where infected ulceration, inflammation, and pain can result.

Fixed appliance a bonded or banded appliance affixed to individual teeth or groups of teeth.

Fixed partial denture a replacement for one or more missing teeth that is securely cemented to natural teeth and/or dental implant abutments that furnish the primary support for the prosthesis; also called a fixed prosthesis or bridge.

Flora the collective organisms of a given locale.

Oral flora the various bacteria and other microorganisms that inhabit the oral cavity. The mouth has an indigenous flora, meaning those organisms that are native to that area of the body. Certain organisms specifically reside in certain parts, for example, on the tongue, on the mucosa, or in the gingival sulcus.

Floss cleft a cleft in the gingival margin usually at a mesial or distal line angle of a tooth where dental floss was repeatedly applied incorrectly. The lining of the cleft can be completely lined with epithelium.

Floss cut unintentional incision at the gingival margin due to incorrect positioning and placement of dental floss.

Fluorapatite the form of hydroxyapatite in which fluoride ions have replaced some of the hydroxyl ions; with fluoride, the apatite is less soluble and, therefore, more resistant to the acids formed from carbohydrate intake.

Fluoride a salt of hydrofluoric acid; the ionized form of fluorine that occurs in many tissues and is stored primarily in bones and teeth.

Fluorosis form of enamel hypomineralization due to excessive ingestion of fluoride during the development and mineralization of the teeth; depending on the length of exposure and the concentration of the fluoride, the fluorosed area may appear as a small white spot or as severe brown staining with pitting.

Focal onset level of awareness a person has when experience a seizure. This seizure originates in one hemisphere of the brain, previously known as partial seizure.

Focal onset aware the patient is awake and aware during the seizure, formally called simple partial seizure.

Food impaction the forceful wedging of food into the periodontium by occlusal forces.

Food pouching trapping of food in the mouth between cheek and teeth, commonly seen in individuals with poor control of facial muscles.

Forensic dentistry aspect of dental science that relates and applies dental facts to legal problems; encompasses dental identification, malpractice litigation, legislation, peer review, and dental licensure.

Forensic pertaining to or used in legal proceedings.

Formative evaluation ongoing evaluation to monitor each step in the dental hygiene process of care; ongoing feedback that determines any needed changes in the dental hygiene care plan prior to the completion of a treatment sequence.

Frail elderly medically and/or physically fragile, delicate, or weak older person; usually refers to those older than 80 years.

Free gingiva the part of the gingiva exposed to the oral cavity that surrounds the tooth and is not attached to the tooth.

Free gingival groove a shallow line or groove that may be visible between the free and attached gingiva.

Fremitus a vibration perceptible by palpation.

Frenum a membrane that supports or restricts movement, that is labial frenum.

Frequency the speed of tip movement, measured in cycles per second (CPS).

Friable gingival tissue may become fragile and easily traumatized during examination and instrumentation.

Fulcrum the support upon which a lever rests while force intended to produce motion is exerted.

Functional age how well an older adult performs.

Functional dependence inability to perform one or more ADL without help; the level of functional dependence is based on the level of assistance needed to perform ADL or the number of activities for which assistance is needed.

G

Gamma radiation short-wavelength electromagnetic radiation of nuclear origin similar to x-rays but usually of higher energy.

Gastroesophageal reflux disease (GERD) backflow of stomach contents into the esophagus where gastric juices produce a burning sensation.

Gastroparesis delayed gastric emptying. Occurs when the vagus nerve is damaged or stops functioning normally and movement of food is slowed or stopped.

GCF (gingival crevicular fluid) fluid secreted from the gingival crevice or sulcus around the tooth.

Gel semisolid or solid phase of a colloidal solution.

General anesthesia the elimination of all sensations, accompanied by the loss of consciousness.

Generalized onset refers to seizures that are generalized from the onset or beginning, can also be described as motor or nonmotor, formerly known as grand mal.

Genetic susceptibility an increased likelihood of developing a particular disease based on a person's genetic makeup.

Gerontology study of the aging process; includes the biologic, psychological, and sociologic sciences.

Gestation gestation is the period of time between conception and birth.

Gestational diabetes diabetes with initial onset or recognition during pregnancy.

Gestational diabetes mellitus (GDM) diabetes that occurs during pregnancy.

Gingival abrasion pathologic wear of the gingiva as a result of a foreign substance.

Gingival sulcus crevice or space between the free gingiva and the tooth extending from the free gingival margin to the JE.

Gingivitis inflammation of the gingival tissues.

Gland organ or structure that secretes or excretes substances.

Glaucoma group of diseases of the eye characterized by intraocular pressure from pathologic.

Glossitis inflammation of the tongue.

Glossodynia pain in the tongue.

Glucocorticosteroid (or corticosteroid) steroids produced by the adrenal gland (or medication) involved in anti-inflammatory activity through metabolism (catabolism) of proteins, carbohydrates, and fat.

Glycated or glycosylated hemoglobin (HbA1c) the primary assay for assessing long-term glycemic control. Indicates blood glucose levels for the previous 2–3 months.

Glycemia presence of glucose in blood.

Glycerin clear, colorless, syrupy fluid used as a vehicle and sweetening agent for drugs and as a solvent and vehicle for abrasive agents.

Glycine an amino acid–based water-soluble powder used for airpolishing.

Goblet cell specialized epithelial cell that secretes mucus.

Gonad sex gland in which reproductive cells form.

Grafting tissue that is transplanted and expected to become a part of the host tissue.

Grand mal former name for a generalized or major seizure as contrasted with petit mal, a minor or relatively mild seizure.

Grit with reference to abrasive agents, grit is the particle size.

H

Half-life the time it takes for the plasma concentration of a drug to reach half of its original concentration; the time it takes for half of the dose to be eliminated from the bloodstream.

Halitosis bad breath or unpleasant odor or smell from the mouth.

Hallucination false sensory perception in the absence of an actual external stimulus.

Halo or diffusion effect occurs when foods and beverages processed in a fluoridated community are imported and consumed in a nonfluoridated community.

Hand hygiene a general term that applies to either handwashing, **antiseptic** handwash, **antiseptic** hand rub, or surgical hand antisepsis.

Hawley retainer a removable plastic and wire appliance used to stabilize teeth; may be modified for special applications during or after orthodontic therapy.

HbA_{1c} see glycated or glycosylated hemoglobin.

Health literacy the ability of a patient to obtain, process, understand, and respond to health messages, and be motivated to make health decisions that promote and maintain good health.

Health promotion the process of enabling people to improve their health through self-care, mutual aid, and the creation of a healthy environment.

Health state of physical, mental, and social well-being, not only the absence of disease.

Hearing aids an electronic device worn in or behind the ear. It amplifies and shapes sound waves that enter the external auditory canal

Hearing impairment a full or partial reduction in the ability to understand or detect any sounds.

Hearing the sense by which sounds are perceived; conversion of sound waves into nerve impulses, which are then interpreted by the brain.

Hemarthrosis blood in a joint cavity.

Hematocrit volume percentage of erythrocytes (red blood cells) in whole blood.

Hematopoiesis formation and development of blood cells.

Hemidesmosome half of a desmosome that forms a site of attachment between junctional epithelial cells and the tooth surface.

Hemiparesis slight or incomplete paralysis of one side of the body.

Hemiplegia paralysis of one side of the body; usually caused by CVA or a brain lesion.

Hemoglobin protein in the erythrocyte that transports molecular oxygen to body cells.

Hemolysis rupture of erythrocytes with the release of hemoglobin into the plasma.

Hemolytic destruction of blood cells, resulting in liberation of hemoglobin.

Hemoptysis spitting of blood because of a lesion in the larynx, trachea, or lower respiratory tract.

Hemostasis the termination of bleeding by mechanical or chemical means or by the complex coagulation process of the body that consists of vasoconstriction, platelet aggregation, and thrombin and fibrin synthesis.

Heparin anticoagulant; prevents platelet agglutination and thrombus formation.

Hirsutism abnormal hair growth on the face or body in women.

HIV human immunodeficiency virus.

Homeostasis the tendency of biologic systems to maintain constant internal stability while continually adjusting to external changes.

Hormone a chemical product of an organ or of certain cells within the organ that has a specific regulatory effect upon cells elsewhere in the body.

Hospice an interprofessional practice program providing a continuum of home and inpatient palliative and supportive care to meet the physical, emotional, spiritual, social, and economic needs experienced by terminally ill individuals and their families during the final stages of illness and during dying and bereavement.

Human subjects living individuals whom an investigator conducts research about and obtains.

Human trafficking human trafficking is the trade of humans for the purpose of forced labor, sexual slavery, or commercial sexual exploitation for the trafficker or others.

Humectant substance contained in a product (such as in a dentifrice) to retain moisture and prevent hardening upon exposure to air.

Hydrodynamic theory currently accepted mechanism for pain impulse transmission to the pulp as a result of fluid movement within the dentinal tubule, which stimulates the nerve endings at the dentinopulpal interface.

Hydrolysis a process in which water slowly penetrates the suture filaments, causing breakdown of the suture's polymer chain. Hydrolyzation yields a lesser degree of tissue reaction.

Hydroxyapatite $Ca_{10}(PO_4)_6(OH)_2$; the form of apatite that is the principal mineral component of teeth, bones, and calculus.

Hyperactivity abnormally increased activity.

Hyperarousal an abnormal state of increased sensitivity or responsiveness to stimuli.

Hypercholesterolemia excess of cholesterol in the blood.

Hyperemesis gravidarum extreme, persistent nausea and vomiting during pregnancy.

Hyperglycemia high blood glucose: opposite of hypoglycemia.

Hyperinsulinemia excess insulin relative to the level of glucose in the blood.

Hyperkalemia a higher-than-normal level of potassium in the bloodstream.

Hyperkeratosis abnormal thickening of the keratin layer (stratum corneum) of the epithelium.

Hypernatremia elevated sodium level in the bloodstream.

Hyperpnea abnormal increase in depth and rate of respiration.

Hypertension systolic blood pressure of 140 mm Hg or greater and diastolic blood pressure of 90 mm Hg or greater.

Hyperthermia higher-than-normal body temperature.

Hypertriglyceridema raised triglyceride blood level.

Hyperventilation greater rate and volume of breathing than metabolically necessary for pulmonary gas exchange; may lead to dizziness and possible syncope.

Hypogeusia abnormally diminished acuteness of the sense of taste.

Hypoglycemia an abnormally low level of glucose in the blood.

Hypoinsulinemia abnormally low levels of insulin he blood.

Hypokalemia a lower-than-normal level of potassium in the bloodstream.

Hypomaturation a defect in the enamel crystal structure as it forms.

Hypomineralization deficiency in mineralization of the tooth enamel.

Hypoplasia incomplete development or underdevelopment of a tissue or an organ.

Enamel hypoplasia incomplete or defective formation of the enamel of either primary or permanent teeth. The result may be an irregularity of tooth form, color, or surface.

Hyposalivation reduced salivary flow rates due to medication or medical-related effect on the salivary gland function.

Hypotension systolic blood pressure of 90 mm Hg or lower and diastolic blood pressure of 60 mm Hg or lower.

Hypothermia lower-than-normal body temperature.

Hypoxia diminished availability of oxygen to body tissues.

I

IADLs (instrumental activities of daily living) a measure of the ability to perform more of the complex tasks necessary to function in our society; tasks that require a combination of physical and cognitive ability.

Iatrogenic resulting from treatment by a professional person.

Iatrosedation reduction of anxiety as a result of the clinician's behavior or actions. A psychosomatic method of pain control.

ICCMS™ (International Caries Classification and Management System) a caries management system based on evidence and a consensus of international experts.

ICDAS™ (International Caries Classification and Management System) a caries classification system created by a consensus of international experts.

Ictal (or Ictus) a psychological state or event such as a seizure, stroke, or headache.

Idiopathic thrombocytopenia purpura hemorrhages on the skin caused by abnormal decrease in the number of blood platelets with unknown etiology.

Idiopathic of unknown etiology.

Idiosyncratic unusual feature of a person; unusual or exaggerated response.

IF (intrinsic factor) produced by the parietal cells in the stomach; aids in vitamin B_{12} absorption.

IGRA interferon-gamma release assay.

Illicit and illegal substance; not authorized, not sanctioned by law.

Image receptors traditional film and digital sensors used to capture and record a radiographic image.

Immediate denture any removable dental prosthesis fabricated for placement immediately following the removal of a natural tooth/teeth.

Immunity the resistance that a person has against disease; it may be natural or acquired.

Immunization the process of rendering a subject immune to a particular disease by stimulation with a specific antigen to promote antibody formation in the body.

Immunocompromised when the immune response is attenuated by administration of immunosuppressive drugs, by irradiation, by malnutrition, or by certain disease processes.

Impact evaluation assesses long-term effectiveness of dental hygiene care in achieving health goals.

Impaction forceful wedging of food, floss, and so on into the periodontium by occlusal forces.

Impaired fasting glucose (IFG) A prediabetes state when the fasting blood glucose level is consistently above normal, but not in the range for a diagnosis of diabetes.

Impaired glucose tolerance (IGT) A prediabetes state of hyperglycemia associated with insulin resistance.

Impairment in health, any loss or abnormality of physiologic, psychological, or anatomic structure or function, whether permanent or temporary.

Implied consent the granting of permission of healthcare without a formal agreement between the patient and the healthcare provider.

Impulse the burst of radiation generated during a half cycle of alternating current (AC); film exposure time is measured in impulses.

Incidence the rate at which a certain event occurs, as the number of new cases of a specific disease occurring during a certain period of time.

Incipient caries early or beginning caries, caries not limited to the enamel.

Incubation period the time interval between the initial contact with an infectious agent and the appearance of the first clinical sign or symptom of the disease.

Index a graduated, numeric scale with upper and lower limits; scores on the scale correspond to a specific criterion for individuals or populations; *pl.* indices or indexes.

- **Dental index** describes oral status by expressing clinical observations as numeric values.

Indicators measurable information used to assess whether a treatment or program is achieving the expected outcomes.

Indurated hardened; abnormally hard.

Induration localized thickening and hardening of soft tissue of the body.

Infant child younger than 1 year.

Infarct localized area of ischemic necrosis produced by occlusion of the arterial supply or venous drainage of the part.

Infection a state caused by the invasion, development, or multiplication of an infectious agent into the body.

- **Latent infection** persistent infection following a primary infection in which the causative agent remains inactive within certain cells.
- **Primary infection** first time; no preexisting antibodies.
- **Recurrent infection** symptomatic reactivation of a latent infection.

Infection control the selection and use of procedures and products to prevent the spread of infectious disease.

Infectious agent organism capable of producing an infection.

Infective endocarditis (IE) infection of the heart lining; previously termed subacute bacterial endocarditis (SBE).

Inferential statistics numerical data designed to allow generalization from a sample to a population.

Infiltration anesthesia induced by injecting the anesthetic directly into or around the area to be anesthetized; anesthetizes the smaller terminal nerve endings of the tooth.

Infiltration the diffusion or accumulation in a tissue or cells of substances not normal to it or in amounts in excess of normal.

Informed consent a patient's voluntary agreement to a treatment plan after details of the proposed treatment have been presented and comprehended by the patient.

Informed refusal of care a patient's decision to refuse recommended treatment after all options, potential risks, and potential benefits have been thoroughly explained.

INH isoniazid.

INR (international normalized ratio) ratio between actual blood coagulation time and the normal coagulation time.

Insoluble incapable of being dissolved.

Insomnia wakefulness; inability to sleep in the absence of noise or other disturbance.

Inspiration inhaling air into the lungs. See **expiration**.

Institutional review board (IRB) an independent ethics committee formally designated to approve, monitor, and review biomedical and behavioral research involving humans.

Instrumentation zone area on tooth where instrumentation is confined; area where calculus and altered cementum are located and treatment is required.

Insulin a powerful hormone secreted by the beta cells in the islets of Langerhans of the pancreas; the major fuel-regulating hormone; enters the blood in response to a rise in concentration of blood glucose and is transported immediately to bind with cell surface receptors throughout the body.

Insulin resistance when the insulin does not adequately absorb blood glucose and thus produces higher quantities of insulin to maintain balance.

Insulin-dependent diabetes mellitus (IDDM) former name for type 1 diabetes mellitus that is no longer used because some people with type 2 diabetes mellitus also use insulin.

Intellectual functioning a broad term that takes adaptive behavior, mental health, opportunities to participate in life activities, and the context in which a life is lived into consideration.

Intelligence quotient (IQ) a score derived from one of several standardized tests used to assess intellectual ability.

Interdental gingiva (interdental papilla) the unattached gingiva found in the space between teeth.

Interdental papilla papilla that occupies the interproximal area between two adjacent teeth that are in contact.

Interdisciplinary two or more disciplines or professions working together as a team to provide care.

Interim denture a fixed or removable dental prosthesis designed to enhance esthetics, stabilization, and/or function for a limited period, after which it is to be replaced by a definitive dental or maxillofacial prosthesis. Also referred to as provisional prosthesis, provisional restoration.

Interim therapeutic restoration (ITR) a provisional placement of a fluoride-releasing glass ionomer restoration without using local anesthesia and utilizing a spoon excavator to remove most—all caries; purpose is to prevent the progression of dental caries in young patients, uncooperative patients, patients with special healthcare needs, and situations in which traditional cavity preparation and/or placement of traditional dental restorations are not feasible. It is necessary to "recharge" the glass ionomer material using fluoridated toothpaste daily and regular 3–6-month professional fluoride applications.

Intermaxillary fixation (IMF) fixation of the maxilla in occlusion with the mandible held in place by means of wires and elastic bands; the healing parts are stabilized following fracture or surgery.

International system two-digit tooth-numbering system known as the by Fédération Dentaire Internationale system. The system uses a unique two number system for the location and naming of each tooth.

Interocclusal record a registration of the positional relationship of the opposing teeth or dental arches made in a plastic material, such as a soft baseplate wax; also called the maxillomandibular relationship record or wax-bite.

Interpersonal violence violent act, such as physical, sexual, domestic and so forth, by one person against another.

Interprofessional collaborative practice comprehensive healthcare delivered by multiple healthcare providers with different professional backgrounds who work together with each other, the patient, the family, and other caregivers to meet the patient's needs.

Interprofessional healthcare teams patient care team consists of specialists from many fields; combines expertise and resources to provide insight into all aspects of the patient's needs.

Interproximal space the triangular region bounded by the proximal surfaces of contacting teeth and the alveolar bone between the teeth, which forms the base of the triangle; the space is normally filled with the interdental papilla; also called the interdental area.

Intervention to happen or take place between other events; to intervene, as with a specific treatment.

Intimate partners marriage partners, partners living together, dating relationships, and former spouses, partners, and boyfriends/girlfriends.

Intratubular or peritubular dentin increased deposition of minerals into tubules that become more mineralized with increasing age, resulting in thicker, sclerotic dentin.

Intrinsic situated entirely within.

Irradiation exposure to radiation; one speaks of radiation therapy and irradiation of a body part.

Irrigant substance used for irrigation.

Irrigation flushing of a specific area or site with a stream of fluid; application of a continuous or pulsated stream of fluid to a part of the body for a cleansing or therapeutic purpose.

Ischemia deficiency of blood to supply oxygen in part resulting from functional constriction or actual obstruction of a blood vessel.

J

Junctional epithelium (JE) epithelium that is at the base or bottom of the sulcus.

K

Keratinized a horny layer of flattened epithelial cells containing keratin.

Keratinized epithelium outer, protective surface of stratified squamous epithelium; covers the masticatory mucosa; interdental col area is not normally keratinized.

Ketones normal metabolic products of lipid (fat) within the liver; excess production leads to urinary excretion of these acidic chemicals.

Kilohertz (kHz) a unit of energy equal to 1,000 cps.

Korotkoff sounds the sounds heard during the determination of blood pressure; sounds originating within the blood passing through the vessel or produced by vibratory motion of the arterial wall.

Kussmaul breathing loud, slow, labored breathing common to patients in diabetic coma.

Kyphosis naturally occurring curve of the back in the thoracic region of spine that, when viewed from the side, is curved outward.

L

Latent image the invisible change produced in an x-ray film emulsion by the action of x-radiation or light from which the visible image is subsequently developed and fixed chemically.

Lateral pressure the minimal pressure that is required of an instrument against the tooth to accomplish the objective of the assessment or treatment.

Latex allergy an acquired hypersensitivity reaction to the proteins found in natural rubber latex (NRL).

Lavage the therapeutic washing of the pocket and root surface to remove endotoxins and loose debris.

LDL (low-density lipoprotein) is a carrier of cholesterol in the body, which leads to buildup of cholesterol in the arteries causing an increased risk for cardiovascular disease. Sometimes called the "bad" cholesterol.

Leakage radiation the radiation that escapes through the protective shielding of the x-ray unit tube head; it may be detected at the sides, top, bottom, or back of the tube head.

Learning acquiring knowledge or skills though study, instruction, or experience.

Legal blindness is less than 20/200 vision with corrective eyeglasses.

Lesion any pathologic or traumatic discontinuity of tissue or loss of function of a part; broad term including wounds, sores, ulcers, tumors, and any other tissue damage.

Leukemia an acute or chronic progressive malignant neoplasm of the blood-forming organs, marked by diffuse proliferation of immature white blood cells (leukocytes); subsequent reduction in erythrocytes and platelets results.

Leukocyte white blood corpuscle capable of amoeboid movement; functions to protect the body against infection and disease.

Leukocytosis increase in the total number of leukocytes.

Leukopenia reduction in total number of leukocytes in the blood; count under 500/mL.

Levels of evidence pyramid visual hierarchy for making clinical judgments related to patient care based on the strength and types of research studies.

Libido sexual urge or desire.

Lichenification area of skin that has thickened and hardened from continuous irritation.

Lifestyle relatively permanent organization of activities, including work, leisure, and associated social activities, characterizing an individual.

Lifestyle factors the habits, attitudes, moral standards, economic status that together constitute a mode of living that are often associated with disease. Examples would be physical inactivity, obesity, unhealthy diet, tobacco smoking, risky alcohol consumption.

Ligation application of a wire or thread (suture) to hold or constrict tissue.

Listening to make an attempt to hear what someone is saying.

Active listening a listening style of maintaining focus and remaining engaged with what the patient is saying and reacting by demonstrating you are listening and have understood the patient either through reflection of the main points or summarizing what has been said.

Reflective listening response to what the patient is conveying with a statement or summary that is more than repeating verbatim what the patient has said.

Literature review summary and critical analysis of published sources on a particular topic.

Local anesthesia loss of sensation, especially pain, in a circumscribed area without loss of consciousness; also called regional anesthesia.

Long-term care assistance with physical, mental, and emotional needs for an extended period of time due to terminal condition, disability, illness, injury, or frailness of old age. Can be custodial or skilled care.

Lordosis the normal curvature of the cervical and lumbar regions of the spine that, when viewed from the side, is curved inward.

Low birth weight as weight at birth less than 2,500 g (5.5 lb).

LTBI latent tuberculosis infection.

Lumen the cavity or channel within a tube or tubular organ, such as a blood vessel or the intestine.

Luxation loosening or dislocation of the tooth.

Lymphadenopathy disease of the lymph nodes; regional lymph node enlargement.

M

Macrocephaly head circumference that is greater than 2 standard deviations larger than the average for a given age and sex.

Macroglossia very large tongue.

Macrognathia enlargement or elongation of the jaw.

Magnetostrictive ultrasonic scaling device that generates a magnetic field and produces tip vibrations by the expansion and contraction of a metal stack or rod.

Main caregiver the person who has primary daily care of the child.

Mainstream smoke smoke inhaled directly into the user's lungs.

Malaise a vague uneasy feeling of body weakness, often marking the onset of, and persisting throughout, a disease.

Malignant tending to become progressively worse and to result in death; having the properties of anaplasia, invasiveness, and metastasis; said of tumors

Malnutrition poor nourishment resulting from improper diet or some defect of metabolism that prevents the body from utilizing the intake of food properly.

Malpractice professional negligence; an act or omission by a healthcare provider that causes injury to a patient; a deviation from acceptable standards of care.

Mandibular tori nontender, bony growth in the mandible closer to the tongue.

Mast cell constituent of connective tissue; releases substances in response to injury or infection.

Mastalgia fullness, soreness, or pain in the breast.

Masticatory force created by the action of the masticatory muscles during chewing.

Materia alba white or cream-colored "cheesy" mass that can collect over dental biofilm on unclean, neglected teeth; it is composed of food debris, mucin, and bacteria sloughed epithelial cells.

Matrix a surrounding framework, enabling development in a structured manner.

Maturation stage or process of attaining maximal development; become mature.

Maxillofacial pertaining to the jaws and the face.

Maxillofacial prosthetics the branch of prosthodontics concerned with the restoration of the mouth and jaws and associated facial structures that have been affected by disease, injury, surgery, or a congenital defect.

Maximum recommended dose (MRD) the highest amount of an anesthetic agent that can be given safely and without complication to a patient.

MDR-TB multidrug-resistant tuberculosis.

Meal plan a selectively planned or prescribed regimen of food to meet certain needs of the individual.

Mechanical dental biofilm control oral hygiene methods for removal of dental biofilm from tooth surfaces using a toothbrush and selected devices for interdental cleaning; contrasts with chemotherapeutic biofilm control in which an antimicrobial agent is used.

Media communication the use of tools or technology to convey information.

Mediator a substance that effects a change in a disease state.

Menarche onset of menstruation; may occur from ages 9 to 17 years.

Menopause the time of life when a woman ceases menstruation; defined as a period of 12 months of amenorrhea in a woman over 45 years of age.

Menses menstruation.

Metastasis transfer of disease from one organ or part to another not directly connected with it; for example, regional or distant spread of cancer cells from the site primarily involved.

MGJ (mucogingival junction) the line where mucosa from the cheeks or floor of the mouth and attached gingiva come together.

Microabrasion a proven method for treating tooth discolorations by microreduction of superficial enamel through various methods of mechanical and/or chemical actions.

Microcephalus abnormally small head size in relation to the rest of the body.

Microorganism minute living organisms, usually microscopic; includes bacteria, rickettsiae, viruses, fungi, and protozoa.

Micropores tiny openings.

Microstomia small mouth opening.

Mineralization addition of mineral elements, such as calcium and phosphorus, to the body or a part thereof with resulting hardening of the tissue.

Miniplate osteosynthesis a method of internal fixation of mandibular fractures utilizing miniaturized metal plates and screws formerly made of titanium or stainless steel and currently made primarily of biodegradable or resorbable synthetic materials.

Moral a principle or habit with respect to right or wrong behavior.

Morphology science that deals with form and structure.

Motivation internal driving force that prompts an individual to act to satisfy a need or desire or to accomplish a particular goal.

Motivational interviewing (MI) a patient-centered communication approach to changing health behaviors (see Chapter 24).

Mucositis painful inflammation with ulcerations of mucous membranes found in the gastrointestinal tract including the mouth. Oral mucositis is a debilitating complication of cancer therapies including chemotherapy and radiotherapy and can lead to increased morbidity and mortality.

Mucus *n.* viscous, slippery secretion of mucous membranes and glands. Contains mucin, white blood cells, inorganic salts, and exfoliated cells.

Multidisciplinary team professional individuals from different backgrounds/specialties working together for the benefit of the patient.

Multifactorial pertaining to, or arising through the action of, many factors.

Munchausen syndrome by proxy (MSBP) a form of child abuse and mental health problem in which a caregiver makes up or causes an illness or injury in a person under his or her care, such as a child, an elderly adult, or a person who has a disability.

Murmur irregularity of heartbeat caused by a turbulent flow of blood through a valve that has failed to close.

Musculoskeletal disability are conditions that can affect your muscles, bones, and joints. They include conditions such as tendinitis and carpal tunnel syndrome.

Musculoskeletal disorder, cumulative trauma disorder, repetitive stress injury terms used to describe disorders of the musculoskeletal, autonomic, and peripheral nervous system caused by repeated, forceful, and awkward movements of the human body, as well as by exposure to mechanical stress, vibration, and cold temperatures; often work related.

Mutation the change in a gene because of alteration of units of the DNA.

Myalgia muscle pain accompanied by malaise.

Mycoplasma bacteria without a cell wall, more resistant to antibiotics.

Myocardial infarction irreversible necrosis of heart muscle secondary to prolonged lack of oxygen supply (ischemia). Commonly known as heart attack.

Myocardium the middle and thickest layer of the heart wall, composed of cardiac muscle.

Myoclonic seizures with brief shocklike jerks of an individual or multiple muscles.

Myoclonus isolated or repetitive shocklike contractions of a muscle or groups of muscles, myoclonic.

Myxedema a disease caused by decreased activity of the thyroid gland characterized by dry skin, swellings around the lips and nose.

Myxedema coma blunting of the senses and intellect, labored speech, swelling all over the body associated with hypothyroidism. Condition is life-threatening.

N

NaF neutral sodium fluoride.

Nasal cannula a semicircle of plastic tubing with two plastic tips that fit into the patient's nostrils.

Nasoalveolar molding appliance (NAM) treatment used for unilateral and bilateral cleft palate to reduce the severity of the cleft in the maxillary gingiva or alveolar ridges and to reduce the deformity of the nose.

Neglect the intentional or unintentional failure to provide basic physical, emotional, educational, and medical/dental needs.

Neoplasm any new and abnormal growth, specifically one in which cell multiplication is controlled and progressive; may be benign or malignant.

Neural depolarization mechanism (sodium/potassium pump) reduction of the resting potential of the nerve membrane so that a nerve impulse is fired. At rest, the inner surface of the nerve fiber is negatively charged and impermeable to sodium ions. A stimulus temporarily alters the membrane, making it permeable so that potassium leaks out and sodium rushes into the nerve fiber. This mechanism is known as the sodium–potassium pump. The reversal of electrical charge, or depolarization, creates the nerve impulse. The process then reverses, and the membrane potential is restored, or repolarized.

Neuritis inflammation of a peripheral nerve, causing pain and loss of function.

Neurodevelopmental disability physical, behavioral, and/or ID, that first manifests symptoms during developmental period (before age 21) and leads to intellectual, social, and/or physical impairment in everyday life activities.

Neurologic disabilities are caused by damage to the nervous system (including the brain and spinal cord) that results in the loss of some bodily or mental functions. Heart attacks, infections, genetic **disorders**, and lack of oxygen to the brain may also result in a **neurologic disability**.

Neurologist a doctor who has special training in disorders of the brain, including epilepsy.

Neutral working position the position of the body in which the normal curvatures of the spine are maintained and the muscles and joints are naturally aligned to allow for reduction of muscles and joints fatigue during work activities.

Neutropenia diminished number of neutrophils (polymorphonuclear leukocytes or PMNs).

New attachment the union of connective tissue or epithelium with a root surface that has been deprived of its original attachment apparatus; the new attachment may be epithelial adhesion and/or connective-tissue adaptation or attachment, and it may include new cementum.

Nicotine a poisonous, addictive stimulant that is the chief psychoactive ingredient in tobacco.

NIDDM (noninsulin-dependent diabetes mellitus) former name for type 2 diabetes mellitus, but it is no longer used since people with type 2 diabetes may use insulin.

Nidus nucleus, focus, point of origin.

Nitroglycerin sublingual, extended-release vasodilator used to treat angina in people with coronary artery disease.

Nitrosamines cancer-causing chemicals found in tobacco.

Nocturia waking at night one or more times to urinate.

Nonambulatory inability to walk or move about freely.

Noncariogenic does not support or promote bacterial growth responsible for caries formation.

Nondominant hand the hand that is often times used for essential supplementary functions to assist the dominant hand.

Nonkeratinized mucosa lining mucosa in which the stratified squamous epithelial cells retain their nuclei and cytoplasm.

Nonnutritive sucking sucking fingers, thumb, pacifiers, or other objects for comfort.

Nonsurgical periodontal therapy NSPT includes dental biofilm removal and biofilm control (by patient); supragingival and subgingival scaling; root planing; and the adjunctive use of chemotherapeutic agents for control of bacterial infection, desensitizing hypersensitive exposed root surfaces, and dental caries prevention as related to the health of the periodontium.

Nonvocal a type of cue, such as body position, movement of body parts, eye movements, and facial expression, that occurs during communication.

Norepinephrine a catecholamine that functions as a neurotransmitter, sending signals from one neuron to another neuron or to a muscle cell.

Normotensive normal tension or tone; of or pertaining to having normal blood pressure.

Nosocomial pertaining to, or originating in, a healthcare facility.

Nosocomial pneumonia pneumonia contracted during confinement in a healthcare facility.

Nurse practitioner (NP) a licensed registered nurse who has had advanced preparation for practice that includes clinical experience in diagnosis and treatment of illness; NPs may work in collaborative practice with physicians or independently in private practice or nursing clinics; in some states, NPs can prescribe medications.

Nutrient a chemical substance in foods needed by the body for growth and repair; the six classes of nutrients are proteins, fats, carbohydrates, minerals, vitamins, and water.

- **Macronutrients** energy-yielding nutrients needed in larger amounts in the diet: carbohydrate, protein, and fat.
- **Micronutrients** nutrients needed in small amounts in the diet and are not energy yielding: vitamins and minerals.

Nutrient or Nutritional Deficiency inadequacy of nutrients in the tissues; the result of inadequate dietary intake or impairment of digestion, absorption, transport, or metabolism.

Nutrient-dense food with high content of vitamins and minerals, but comparatively low in calories.

Nutrition sum of processes involved in taking nutrients into the body, assimilating and utilizing them; includes ingestion, digestion, absorption, transport, utilization of nutrients, and excretion of waste products.

Nystagmus involuntary, rapid, rhythmic movements of the eyeball.

Obstructive sleep apnea (OSA) occurs when the muscles in the back of the throat relax, causing the airway to narrow on inspiration that lowers the oxygen levels in the blood and triggers the brain to wake the person. This causes disruptive sleep patterns and possible intermittent periods of suspended breathing.

Obturator a prosthesis designed to close a congenital or an acquired opening, such as a cleft of the hard palate.

Occlusal plane the average plane established by the incisal and occlusal surfaces of the teeth; generally not actually a plane, but the planar mean of the curvature of those surfaces

Occlusal trauma injury to the periodontium that results from occlusal forces in excess of the reparative capacity of the attachment apparatus; also called occlusal traumatism.

Occlusal vertical dimension the distance measured between two points when the occluding members are in contact.

Occlusion blockage; state of being closed.

Occupational exposure reasonably anticipated skin, eye, mucous membrane, or parenteral contact with blood or other potentially infectious materials that may result from the performance of one's usual duties.

Occupational exposure subject to an action or influence, usually negative, as a result of one's occupation or work environment.

Odontogram a graphic representation of the patient's hard and soft tissues.

Offset blade the blade of an area-specific Gracey curet in which the lower shank is at a 70° angle to the face of the blade; contrasts with a universal curet blade, which is at a 90° angle with the lower shank.

Oncology the study of tumors; the sum of knowledge regarding tumors.

Opiate antagonist examples include naltrexone and naloxone. These drugs have a high affinity for opiate receptors but do not activate them and block the effect of exogenously administered opioids (e.g., morphine, heroin, and methadone) or of endogenously released endorphins.

Opioid synthetic narcotic that has opiate-like activities but is not derived from opium.

Opportunistic infectious agent capable of causing disease only when the host's resistance is lowered.

Oral glucose tolerance test (OGTT) a test of the body's ability to utilize carbohydrates; aid to the diagnosis of diabetes mellitus. After ingestion of a specific amount of glucose solution, the fasting blood glucose rises promptly in a nondiabetic person, then falls to normal within an hour. In diabetes mellitus, the blood glucose rise is greater, and the return to normal is prolonged.

Oral microbiome the complex community of microbes composed of bacteria, fungi, and so on, inhabiting the oral cavity.

Oral mucositis/stomatitis inflammation and ulceration of the oral mucous membranes; can increase the risk for pain, oral and systemic infection, and nutritional compromise.

Orthodontic appliance device used to influence growth and/or position of teeth and jaws.

Orthognathic surgery surgery to alter relationships of the dental arches and/or supporting bone; usually coordinated with orthodontic therapy.

Orthopedics branch of surgery dealing with the preservation and restoration of function of the skeletal system, its articulations, and associated structures.

Orthosis orthopedic appliance or apparatus used to support, align, prevent, or correct deformities or to improve the function of a movable part of the body.

Orthostatic hypotension a drop in systolic and diastolic blood pressure due to change in body position, usually from lying back or sitting to a standing position. The resulting reduction in blood flow can cause temporary shortage of oxygen to the brain and a feeling of lightheadedness or syncope.

Osmotic alteration of pressure in dentinal tubules through a selective membrane.

Osseointegration the direct attachment or connection of osseous tissue to an inert alloplastic material without intervening connective tissue.

Osteonecrosis of the jaw (ONJ) occurs when the jaw bone is exposed and begins to starve from a lack of blood.

Antiresorptive drug-related osteonecrosis of the jaw (ARONJ) is exposed bone in maxilla or mandible that can occur when a patient is treated with a bisphosphonate or other antiresorptive drug with no history of radiation to the head/neck tissues.

Medication-related osteonecrosis of the jaw (MRONJ) equivalent term for exposed bone in maxilla or mandible that can occur when a patient is taking other antiresorptive or antiangenic medications that are not bisphosphonates.

Osteoporosis low bone mass resulting from an excess of bone resorption over bone formation, with resultant bone fragility and increased risk of fracture.

Osteoradionecrosis blood vessel compromise and necrosis of bone exposed to high-dose radiation therapy, resulting in decreased ability to heal if traumatized and in extreme susceptibility to infection.

Osteosynthesis internal fixation of a fracture by mechanical means, such as metal plates, pins, or screws.

OTC over-the-counter.

Outcome evaluation a measure of the effectiveness of dental hygiene clinical and educational interventions in meeting oral health goals identified in the patient care plan.

Overclosure the vertical relationship between the jaws is impaired due to missing teeth.

Overdenture a removable denture that covers and is partially supported by one or more remaining natural teeth, roots, and/or dental implants and the soft tissue of the residual alveolar ridge; also called overlay denture.

P

Pain threshold point at which a sensation starts to be painful and a response results. Varies between individuals based on interpretation of sensation. May be altered by some drugs.

Palliative that which minimize or relieve pain without dealing with the cause of the pain.

Palliative care affording relief, but not cure.

Pallidotomy surgical excision or destruction of part of the globus pallidus in the basal ganglia to prevent symptoms of Parkinsonism, including tremor, muscular rigidity, and bradykinesia.

Palpation perceiving by sense of touch.

Pancytopenia abnormal depression of all cellular elements of the blood.

Pandemic widespread epidemic usually affecting the population of an extensive region, several countries, or sometimes the entire globe.

Papillae small, raised protrusive structures on the upper surface of the tongue.

Papillary small, nipple-shaped projection or elevation (papillary: adjective).

Parafunctional abnormal or deviated function, as in bruxism.

Paralysis a symptom of the loss or impairment of motor function in a body part caused by a lesion of the neural or muscular mechanism.

Parenteral injection by a route other than the alimentary tract, such as subcutaneous, intramuscular, or intravenous.

Paresthesia abnormal sensation such as tingling, tickling, prickling, numbness, or burning of a person's skin with no apparent physical cause. May be transient or chronic. Multiple possible causes.

Paroxysm or paroxysmal sharp spasm or convulsion; sudden recurrence or intensification of symptoms.

Paroxysmal a sudden, violent recurrence or intensification of symptoms, such as a spasm or seizure.

Patch circumscribed flat lesion larger than a macule; differentiated from surrounding epidermis by color and/or texture.

Patent open, unobstructed; a patent dentinal tubule allows fluid flow to signal pain; many desensitizing agents work by decreasing the patency of the tubule.

Pathogen a virus, microorganism, or other substance that causes disease.

Pathogenic of or related to a pathogen such as bacterium, virus, or other microorganism causing disease.

Pathognomonic (of a sign or symptom) specifically characteristic or indicative of a particular disease.

Pathognomonic sign or symptom A sign or symptom specific to a disease which is used for diagnosis.

Pathologic migration the movement of a tooth out of its natural position as a result of periodontal infection; contrasts with mesial migration, which is the physiologic process maintained by tooth proximal contacts in the normal dental arches.

Pathophysiology disruption of bodily functions due to disease.

Patient record a written document that contains information identifying an individual patient, such as a patient's name, address, and phone number, as well as information related to that particular patient's care, such as health history information, dental charting items, treatment dates, and treatment codes.

Pediatric obstructive sleep apnea (POSA) a disorder of breathing characterized by prolonged, partial upper airway obstruction and/or intermittent/complete obstruction (obstructive apnea) that disrupts normal ventilation during sleep and normal sleep patterns.

Pedunculated elevated lesion attached by a thin stalk.

Peer review review of a journal article by a panel of experts prior to publication.

Penumbra the secondary shadow that surrounds the periphery of the primary shadow; in radiography, it is the blurred margin of an image detail (geometric unsharpness).

Percutaneous by way of, or through, the skin.

Peri-implant mucositis reversible inflammation of the periodontal tissues around an implant with no subsequent bone loss; similar to gingivitis in a natural tooth.

Peri-implantitis destructive inflammatory process of the periodontal tissues around an implant characterized by progressive bone loss in addition to soft-tissue inflammation with hemorrhage and/or exudate; similar to periodontitis in a natural tooth.

Perimolysis erosion of enamel and dentin as a result of chemical and mechanical effects.

Periodontal debridement disruption and removal of dental biofilm and associated endotoxins along with calculus from the root.

Periodontal ligament (PDL) connective tissue connecting the cementum covering the root to the alveolar bone.

periodontal maintenance (PM) also called preventive maintenance, supportive periodontal therapy (SPT); procedures performed at selected intervals as an extension of periodontal therapy to assist the patient in maintaining oral health; includes complete assessment, review of and/or additional instruction in dental biofilm control, and such clinical procedures as scaling and root planing.

Periodontal probe instrument with a rounded tip calibrated in millimeter increments to facilitate measurement of the pocket depth.

Periodontal risk assessment (PRA) periodontal risk assessment web-based tool based on tooth loss, and genetic and systemic conditions to predict risk for disease.

Periodontal risk calculator (PRC) periodontal risk calculator is a web-based periodontal risk assessment tool based on factors such as smoking, diabetes, and periodontal history to predict risk for disease.

periodontal screening and recording (PSR) used as a screening procedure to determine the need for comprehensive periodontal evaluation; described in Chapter 21.

Periodontitis inflammation in the periodontium, affecting gingival tissues, periodontal ligament, cementum, and supporting bone.

Periodontium tissues surrounding and supporting the teeth are divided into two sections the gingival unit, composed of the free and attached gingiva and the alveolar mucosa, and the attachment apparatus, which includes the cementum, PDL, and alveolar process.

Permeable permitting passage of a fluid.

Pervasive throughout entire individual, entire development is severely and markedly impaired, as in ASD.

Petechia hemorrhagic nonraised spot of pinpoint to pinhead size.

Petit mal attack or brief impairment of consciousness often associated with flickering of the eyelids and mild twitching of the mouth.

Phagocytosis engulfing of microorganisms and foreign particles by phagocytes, such as macrophages.

Photon a finite bundle of energy of visible light or electromagnetic radiation.

Physical abuse the intentional use of force resulting in bodily injury, pain, or anguish.

Physical neglect the failure to provide basic necessities such as food, clothing, water, shelter, medicine, dental care, and personal hygiene.

Piezoelectric ultrasonic scaling device activated by dimensional changes in crystals housed in the handpiece.

Pixel the smallest discrete component of an image or a picture on a screen that makes up the overall picture; usually dots arranged in rows and columns.

Plain language verbal or written health information provided using simplified terminology, clear and to the point sentence structure, pictures, or any other method that can enhance understanding for patients with limited language proficiency or health literacy.

Planktonic free floating single bacteria such as in saliva gingival crevicular fluid.

Pleura delicate membrane enclosing the lungs.

Pneumothorax collection of air or gas causing the lungs to collapse.

Polishing the production, especially by friction, of a smooth, glossy, mirror-like surface that reflects light.

Polishing agent an abrasive used to achieve a smooth, lustrous finish to a tooth surface.

Polyautoimmunity presence of more than one autoimmune disease in the same patient.

Polycystic ovarian syndrome (PCOS) Hormonal disorder where the ovaries or adrenal glands produce more male hormones than normal. Women with PCOS are at risk for diabetes, metabolic syndrome, cardiovascular disease, and hypertension.

Polydipsia excessive thirst.

Polymer a compound of high molecular weight formed by a combination of a chain of simpler molecules (monomers).

Polymeric repeating molecular structures; in biofilms, the polymers are glycoprotein polysaccharides.

Polymerization a reaction in which a high-molecular-weight product is produced by successive additions of a simpler compound.

> **Autopolymerized** self-curing; a reaction in which a high-molecular-weight product is produced by successive additions of a simpler compound; hardening process of pit-and-fissure sealants.
>
> **Photopolymerized** polymerization with the use of an external light source.

Polyp any growth or mass protruding from a mucous membrane.

Polyphagia excessive ingestion of food.

Polypharmacy concurrent use of a large number of drugs.

Polyuria excessive excretion of urine.

Pontic an artificial tooth on a partial denture that replaces a missing natural tooth, restores its function, and usually occupies the space previously filled by the natural crown.

Position-indicating device (PID) a device used to direct the x-ray beam during the exposure of dental radiograph.

Post hoc fallacy understanding that correlation does not mean causation between multiple variables.

Postictal a period of decreased activity of the brain following a seizure, usually lasting less than 48 hours.

Postprandial after a meal.

Postradiation caries (PRC) posttreatment oral complication involving highly destructive dental caries that progresses rapidly.

Postural hypotension also called orthostatic hypotension; a sudden drop in blood pressure often associated with dizziness, syncope, and blurred vision that occurs upon moving from lying down to standing up position.

Potassium nitrate active ingredient in many antisensitivity dentifrices.

Potency strength of a drug. Amount of a medication or drug necessary to achieve a desired effect.

Power toothbrush a brush driven by electricity or battery; also called power-assisted, automatic, or electric.

PPD purified protein derivative.

PPE personal protective equipment.

ppm (parts per million) measure used to designate the amount of fluoride used for optimum level in fluoridated water, dentifrice, and other fluoride-containing preparations (1 ppm is equivalent to 1 mg/L).

Precision attachment a type of connector that consists of a metal receptacle and a close-fitting part; the metal receptacle is usually included within the restoration of an abutment tooth, and the close-fitting part is attached to a pontic or RPD framework.

Prediabetes IFG (impaired fasting glucose) and IGT (impaired glucose tolerance) are risk factors for future diabetes and cardiovascular disease.

Premaxillary anterior part of maxilla that contains the incisor teeth; bilateral cleft lips separate the premaxilla from its normal fusion with the entire maxilla.

Premedication antibiotics prescribed in advance of dental procedures in patients known to be at high risk for an adverse medical outcome.

Premenstrual syndrome a cluster of behavioral, somatic, affective, and cognitive disorders that appear in the premenstrual (luteal) phase of the menstrual cycle and that resolve rapidly with the onset of menses.

Premonitory when symptoms give warning of a more serious attack, such as headache or "funny feeling" shortly before the onset of a seizure.

Presbycusis progressive loss of hearing due to the normal aging process.

Presbyopia a condition of farsightedness (hyperopia) resulting from a loss of elasticity of the lens of the eye due to the normal aging process.

Preschooler child 3–5 years of age; may or may not be attending a preschool program.

Prescription drug monitoring programs (PDMP) is statewide electronic database for healthcare providers to see patients' prescribing histories especially for controlled substances, in attempt to reduce the over prescribing of substances such as opioids.

Prevalence the total number of cases of a specific disease or condition in existence in a given population at a certain time.

Prevented fraction the proportion of disease occurrence in a population that is averted due to an intervention.

Preventive counseling professional guidance and support to assist a patient with acting ahead regarding oral health through the utilization of MI methods.

Primary radiation all radiation coming directly from the target of the anode of an x-ray tube.

Primate space space or gap in the tooth row occasionally observed in the human primary dentition. It is characteristic of nearly all species of primates except man. The maxillary primate spaces accommodate the mandibular canines, and the mandibular primate spaces accommodate the maxillary canines when the teeth are in occlusion. As a reduction in the length of canines accompanied man's evolution, the canines no longer protruded beyond the occlusal level. The diastema (primate space) was no longer functional.

Prioritize to arrange in order of importance.

Probability value (*p* value) calculated probability of finding the observed results when the null hypothesis is true.

Probing depth (PD) the distance from the gingival margin (GM) to the location of the periodontal probe tip at the base of the sulcus.

Process evaluation Ongoing evaluation to determine whether dental hygiene services are being implemented as intended.

Prodrome a premonitory symptom; a symptom indicating the onset of a disease or condition; *adj*., prodromal.

Profession occupation or calling that requires specialized knowledge, methods, and skills; requires preparation, from an institution of higher learning, in the scholarly, scientific, and historic principles underlying such methods and skills; continuously enlarges its body of knowledge; functions autonomously in formulation of policy; and maintains high standards of achievement and conduct.

Prognosis prediction of outcome; a forecast of the probable course and outcome of a disease and the prospects of recovery as expected by the nature of the specific condition and the symptoms of the case.

Prolapse when an organ falls out of its normal position due to lack of support from ligaments and muscles.

Prostaglandin synthesis the process of making lipid compounds that takes place in the cells; chemical messengers that mediate biologic processes, such as inflammation, and are important in the normal function of many different tissues.

Prostheses intraoral device designed restore or reconstruct missing teeth.

Prosthesis an artificial replacement of an absent part of the human body; a therapeutic device to improve or alter function.

pruritus itching.

Pruritus itchy skin.

Pseudomembrane a loose membranous layer of exudate that contains microorganisms, precipitated fibrin, necrotic cells, and inflammatory cells produced during an inflammatory reaction on the surface of a tissue.

Psychoactive drug possessing the ability to alter mood, behavior, cognitive processes, or mental tension.

Psychogenic reaction having an emotional or psychological origin.

Psychological abuse mental anguish and despair caused by ridicule, name-calling, humiliation, harassment, manipulation, threats, and controlling behavior.

Psychological neglect nonverbal anguish caused by the lack of communication and isolation.

Psychotherapy treatment of emotional, behavioral, personality, and psychiatric disorders by means of individual or group verbal or nonverbal communication with the patient.

Ptosis drooping of the upper eyelid due to paralysis or disease.

Puberty period during in which adolescents reach sexual maturity and become capable of reproduction.

Thyroiditis inflammation of the thyroid.

Pulmonary hypertension condition of abnormally high pressure within the pulmonary circulation.

Pulp vitality testing a test to determine whether the nerves in the pulp are healthy.

Pulse pressure the difference between systolic and diastolic blood pressure; normally 40 mm Hg.

Punctate marked with points or punctures differentiated from the surrounding surface by color, elevation, or texture.

Purpura hemorrhage into the tissues, under the skin, and through the mucous membranes; produces petechiae and ecchymoses.

Purulent containing, forming, or discharging pus.

Pyrexia an abnormal elevation of the body temperature above 37.0°C (98.6°F).

Pyrophosphate inhibitor of calcification that occurs in parotid saliva of humans in variable amounts; anticalculus component of "tartar-control" dentifrices.

PZA pyrazinamide.

Q

Quid a portion of a substance, like tobacco, to be chewed, but not swallowed.

Quorum sensing bacteria produce chemical signal molecules, resulting in development of the plaque biofilm.

R

Raccoon sign bilateral periorbital ecchymosis, which can occur as a result of a basilar skull fracture.

Radiation therapy the treatment of disease by ionizing radiation; may be external megavoltage or internal by use of interstitial implantation of an isotope (radium).

Radiation the emission and propagation of energy through space or a material medium in the form of waves or particles.

Radiograph a visible image on a radiation-sensitive film emulsion or a digitized image on a computer monitor after exposure of the image receptor to ionizing radiation that has passed through an area, region, or substance of interest.

Radiography the art and science of making radiographs.

Radiology a branch of science that deals with the use of radiant energy in the diagnosis and treatment of disease.

Radium a highly radioactive chemical element found in uranium minerals; used in the treatment of malignant tumors in the form of needles or pellets for interstitial implantation.

Ramfjord index teeth teeth used for epidemiologic studies of periodontal diseases: the maxillary right and mandibular left first molars, maxillary left and mandibular right first premolars, and maxillary left and mandibular right central incisors.

Randomized clinical trials (RCT) a specific type of scientific experiment that is the gold standard for a clinical trial. RCTs are often used to test the efficacy and/or effectiveness of various types of interventions within a patient population.

Randomized controlled clinical trial controlled experiment where researchers aim to predict and/or test causal relationships.

Rare earth intensifying screen commonly used to refer to intensifying screens containing rare earth elements in the form of a plastic sheet coated with fluorescent material positioned singly or in pairs in a cassette. When the cassette is exposed to x-radiation, the visible light from the fluorescent image on the screen adds to the latent image produced directly by x-radiation.

Receptors refer to both traditional film and digital sensors used to capture a radiographic image.

Recommended Dietary Allowances (RDAs) recommendations for the average amounts of nutrients recommended to be consumed daily by healthy people to achieve adequate nutrient intake to prevent deficiency.

Refractory resistant; not responding to routine therapy.

Registered dietitian or Registered dietitian nutritionist (RD or RDN) a healthcare professional with a minimum of a bachelor's degree in nutrition or dietetics who has attended an internship program or equivalent and passed the registration examination, all under the approval of the American Dietetic Association. Continuing education is required to keep credentials current.

Rehabilitation the process of restoring a person's ability to live and work as normally as possible after a disabling injury or illness; aims to help the individual to achieve maximum possible physical and psychological fitness and to regain ability to carry out personal care.

Relapse the return of a disease weeks or months after its apparent cessation.

Relative contraindication the offending drug (either local anesthetic or vasoconstrictor) can be administered after careful review of the medical history and assessment of risk factors. Use minimal effective amount; stay below the MRD.

Reliability ability of an index or a test procedure to measure consistently at different times and under a variety of conditions, reproducibility, and consistency.

Remineralization restoration of mineral elements in a tooth surface; enhanced by the presence of fluoride; remineralized lesions are more resistant to initiation of dental caries than is normal tooth structure.

Remission diminution or abatement of the symptoms of a disease; the period during which such diminution occurs.

Removable partial denture (RPD) a dental prosthesis that supplies teeth and/or associated structures in a partially edentulous jaw and can be removed and replaced at will.

Repetitive stress injuries painful or uncomfortable conditions of the muscles, tendons, nerves due to overuse and repeated motions.

Research question answerable inquiry into a specific concern or issue.

Residence-bound (homebound) inability to leave home due to illness or injury; leaving requires considerable and taxing effort. Can be temporary or permanent situation.

Residual ridges the portion of the alveolar bone and its soft-tissue covering that remains after the removal of teeth.

Resorption gradual dissolution of the mineralized tissue, that is the root of the tooth; may be internal or external; occurs during exfoliation of a primary tooth and from the pressure of orthodontic treatment.

Respirator personal protective device worn on the face covering the mouth and nose to filter airborne particles like pathogens.

Rest any component of a partial denture on a tooth surface that provides vertical support

Restenosis recurrent stenosis.

Retainer an orthodontic appliance, fixed or removable, used to maintain the position of the teeth following corrective treatment.

Retinopathy of prematurity a condition peculiar to premature infants; characterized by opaque tissue behind the lens resulting from a high concentration of oxygen, which causes spasm of the retinal vessels, leads to retinal detachment, and arrests eye growth and development; prevented by keeping oxygen administration as low as possible and discontinuing the oxygen as soon as possible.

Retinopathy noninflammatory degenerative disease of the retina; called diabetic retinopathy when it occurs with diabetes of long standing.

Rhinoplasty plastic surgery of nose.

RIF rifampin.

Rights expectations by the patient that correlate with the duties of a professional person when providing care.

Risk factor an attribute or exposure that increases the probability of disease, such as an aspect of personal behavior, environmental exposure, or an inherited characteristic associated with health-related conditions.

Modifiable risk factor a determinant that can be modified by intervention, thereby reducing the probability of disease.

Root form endosseous implant shaped in the approximate form of a tooth root.

Rosin/colophony sticky secretion typically made from plants or trees contained in fluoride varnishes (FVs)

rpm revolutions per minute.

Rubefacient reddening of the skin.

Rx prescription.

S

Saddlenose deformity a collapse of the nasal bridge seen in substance users who snort cocaine.

Safe work practice any work practice that improves clinician and patient safety. This includes, but is not limited to, decreased physical demands, improved layout, environmental factors, and work process organization.

Salivary gland hypofunction objective reduction in the production of saliva, often a long-term complication of head/neck radiation.

Sample a portion or subset of an entire population.

Sanitation the process by which the number of organisms on inanimate objects is reduced. It does not imply freedom from microorganisms and generally refers to a cleaning process.

Sarcoma a tumor, often highly malignant, composed of cells derived from connective tissue such as bone and cartilage, muscle, blood vessel, or lymphoid tissue.

Scale photography a method of photography to record bite marks; the use of a metric scale placed directly above or below the injury to indicate scale; use of grid photographic film.

Scaler instrument designed for initial removal of supragingival calculus, prior to finishing with a curet.

Scaling instrumentation of the crown or root surfaces to remove dental biofilm and calculus.

Scar cicatrix; mark remaining after healing of a wound or healing following a surgical intervention.

School-aged children child from 6 to 12 years of age, considered middle childhood.

Scientific evidence evidence repeatedly tested through research with valid and reliable methods.

Sclerodactyly localized thickening and tightening on the skin of the fingers or toes.

Sclerosis induration or hardening.

Screening assessment of characteristics in individuals that indicate need for additional examination or, if performed on many individuals, can disclose the incidence or prevalence of specific diseases in a population.

Sealant organic polymer that bonds to an enamel surface by mechanical retention accommodated by projections of the sealant into micropores created in the enamel by etching; the two types of sealants, filled and unfilled, both are composed of bis-GMA.

Secondary dentin dentin that is secreted slowly over time after root formation to "wall off" the pulp from fluid flow within dentinal tubules following a stimulus; results in narrower pulp chamber and root canals.

Secondary radiation particles or photons produced by the interaction of primary radiation with matter. Scatter radiation is a form of secondary radiation.

Seizure is an event, a transient occurrence due to abnormal excessive synchronous neuronal activity in the brain.

Self-monitoring of blood glucose (SMBG) regular home blood glucose testing for diabetic people to understand diabetes control and possible changes needed to improve blood glucose.

Self-neglect the behavior of an elderly person that threatens his or her own health or safety. This can occur owing to depression from a loss of a loved one. The elder may feel unable to continue living.

Sensor a small detector that is placed intraorally to capture a radiographic image.

Sensory impairment is a disability of the senses (e.g., sight, hearing, smell, touch, taste).

Sequelae a condition that may happen as a result of a previous disease or injury.

Sequence a continuous or related series of things (such as dental hygiene interventions) following in a certain order or succession.

Sequestrum a piece of dead bone tissue.

Seroconversion after exposure to the etiologic agent of a disease, the blood changes from negative ("seronegative") to positive ("seropositive") for the serum marker for that disease; the time interval for conversion is specific for each disease.

Sessile elevated lesion with a broad base.

Severe early childhood caries (S-ECC) the presence of any area of smooth surface decay in a child younger than 3 years.

Sexual abuse sexual contact with an individual who is unable to consent or otherwise nonconsensual sexual contact or exploitation.

Shank the part of the instrument between the handle and the working end.

Sharpey's fibers connective tissue with bundles of fibers that connect bone to the periosteum covering the bone.

Sharpness when a scaler or curet is sharp, the cutting edge is a fine line that does not reflect light.

Shear bond strength (SBS) the amount of force needed for a restoration or bonded material to be broken or fractured from a tooth surface.

Shelf life stability of an item after it has been prepared; length of time a substance or preparation can be kept without changes occurring in its chemical structure or other properties.

Shunt passage between two natural channels; to bypass or drain an area.

Sialadenitis a salivary gland infection from bacteria or viruses.

Sialorrhea excessive secretion of saliva.

Sidestream smoke the aerosol emitted directly into the surrounding air from the lit end of a smoldering tobacco product; may be inhaled by the user; is a major component of environmental smoke.

Sign objective, observable evidence of an illness or disorder; a physical manifestation of a disorder that is apparent to a trained healthcare provider and sometimes to the patient.

Silver diamine fluoride colorless liquid containing silver particles and fluoride ion. Used for the prevention and nonsurgical arrest of caries.

Sinus augmentation (sinus lift) site preparation procedure that elevates the floor of the maxillary sinus to accommodate a dental implant by increasing the vertical height of bone via grafting/augmentation.

Sippy cup a special cup with a lid that may have a straw or a drinking projection to teach a young child to drink.

Sjögren's syndrome an immunologic disorder characterized by insufficient production of the lacrimal gland to produce tears and the salivary glands to produce saliva, resulting in abnormally dry eyes and mouth.

Skilled nursing medically necessary care that can only be provided by or under the supervision of licensed medical professional. Often in a nursing facility, but can be delivered at a home.

Smear layer has been referred to as "grinding debris" from instrumentation or other devices applied to the tooth; consists of microcrystalline particles of cementum, dentin, tissue, and cellular debris; serves to plug tubule orifices.

Smokeless (spit) tobacco term used to define all forms of tobacco that are not ignited or inhaled.

SnF_2 stannous fluoride.

Social determinants of health social, environmental, and physical circumstances that have an effect on health status; these conditions are shaped by the distribution of power, money, and resources at a global, national, or local level.

Sonic scaler type of mechanical power-driven scaler that functions from energy delivered by a vibrating working tip in the frequency of 2,500–7,000 cps; driven by compressed air, the handpiece connects directly to a conventional rotary handpiece tubing.

Sordes foul matter that collects on the lips, teeth, and oral mucosa in patients with low fevers or dehydration; consists of debris, microorganisms, epithelial elements, and food particles; forms a crust.

Spasm sudden involuntary contraction of a muscles; may be tonic or clonic; may vary from small twitches to severe convulsions.

Speech aid prosthesis a prosthetic device with a posterior section to assist with palatopharyngeal closure; also called bulb, speech bulb, or prosthetic speech appliance.

Speech reading recognizing spoken words by watching the speaker's lips, face, and gestures.

Spinal shock immediately after the injury, spinal shock causes a complete loss of reflex activity. The result is a flaccid paralysis below the level of injury that may last from several hours to several months.

Spirit of MI the underlying perspective with which one practices MI.

Spirometer instrument for measuring volume of air entering and leaving the lungs to determine lung function and breathing capacity.

Sputum matter expectorated (coughed up) from the respiratory system, especially the lungs in a diseased state, composed chiefly of mucus and may contain pus, blood, or microorganisms.

Stack magnetostrictive inserts made of flat metal strips stacked, or sandwiched, together; metal in stack acts like an antenna to pick up magnetic field and cause vibration.

Staging the succinct, standardized description of a tumor with regard to origin and spread. This clinical classification is based on physical assessments, biopsy, imaging, and endoscopy. Each stage (I–IV) consists of three components T (size of tumor); N (lymph node involvement); and M (presence or absence of distant metastasis).

Standard of care criteria or protocols that define the minimal quality of care required to defend against a legal dispute against the practice of one's profession; usually established by federal laws, state, and local statutes and codes and/or testimony from an "expert witness" and is supported by guidelines or recommendations documents published by professional associations.

Standard precautions an approach to infection control to protect healthcare providers and patients from pathogens that can be spread by blood or any other body fluid, secretion, or excretion.

Statistical significance identifies the extent to which the results are not due to chance; indicated in research by the "*p* value" notation.

Status epilepticus rapid succession of epileptic seizures without intervals of consciousness; life-threatening; emergency care is urgent.

Status refers to the state or condition of an individual or population.

Steatorrhea excretion of abnormal quantities of fat with the feces as a result of malabsorption.

Stenosis narrowing or contraction of a body passage or opening.

Stereotypes attitudes or judgments (either positive or negative) made about people that are usually not based on personal experience but rather on what has been learned from other sources; seeing individuals from a population group as having no individuality as though all have the same characteristics.

Stereotypic movement disorder repetitive, nonfunctional motor behavior that interferes with normal activities and may result in bodily injury.

Sterilization process by which all forms of life, including bacterial spores, are destroyed by physical or chemical means.

Stethoscope instrument used to hear and amplify the sounds produced by the heart, lungs, and other internal organs.

Stippled the pitted, orange-peel appearance frequently seen on the surface of the attached gingiva.

Strain a variant of something like bacteria or a virus.

Stress a physical, chemical, or emotional factor that causes physical or mental tension and may be a factor in disease causation or fatigue.

Stroke a single unbroken movement made by an instrument against a tooth surface during an examination or treatment procedure to accomplish a particular objective; the motion made for activation of an instrument.

Study model a positive life-size reproduction of the teeth and adjacent tissues usually formed pouring dental plaster or stone into a matrix or impression. Used in the study of a patient's oral condition in preparation for treatment planning and patient education.

Subgingival irrigation the point of the delivery of the irrigation is placed in the sulcus or pocket and may reach the base of the pocket depending on its probing depth.

Subperiosteal the periosteum that is tacked in place on the bone with a few small implant screws to support an overdenture.

Substance abuse refers to the harmful or hazardous use of psychoactive substances, including alcohol and illicit drugs.

Substance use disorder (SUD) continued use of alcohol and/or drugs results in significant impairment such as health, social, and work problems.

Substantivity the ability of an agent to bind to the pellicle, tooth surface, and soft tissue and be released over an extended period of time with the retention of its potency.

Succedaneous the permanent teeth that erupt into the positions of exfoliated primary teeth.

Sulcular brushing a method in which the end-round filament tips are directed into the gingival sulcus at approximately 45° for the purpose of loosening and removing dental biofilm from both the gingival sulcus and the tooth surface just below the gingival margin.

Supererupt a tooth will continue to migrate occlusally if there is no opposing tooth for it to occlude with.

Superinfection a second infection superimposed over a first infection and often resistant to the treatment used for the first infection.

Supernumerary tooth a condition where extra teeth are present.

Supersaturated a solution containing more of an ingredient that can be held in solution permanently.

Supervision term applied to a legal relationship between dentist and dental team members in practice. Each state practice act defines the type of supervision required for dental hygiene practice.

Supine flat face-up position with head and feet on the same level.

Suppuration (or pus) formation of a fluid product or process of discharging pus as a result of inflammation. The fluid contains leukocytes, degenerated tissue elements, tissue fluids, and microorganisms. Color may range vary from blood tinged to white, yellow, or green.

Supragingival irrigation the point of delivery of the irrigation is at, or coronal to, the free gingival margin.

Surfactant a wetting agent.

Surveillance the ongoing systematic collection, analysis, and interpretation of outcome-specific data for use in planning, implementing, and evaluating the effect of public health programs and practices.

Survival rate is the percentage of people in a study or treatment group still alive for a given period of time after diagnosis.

Susceptible host host not possessing resistance against an infectious agent.

Sustain talk the individuals own arguments for not changing.

Suture a stitch or series of stitches made to secure apposition of the edges of a surgical or traumatic wound.

Swaged the fusion of a suture material to the needle, allowing for a smooth eyeless attachment. The suture will then pass through the tissue as smoothly as possible.

Symptom any change in the body or its function that is perceived by the patient; the subjective experience of a disease or disorder.

Syncopal episodes (syncope) temporary loss of consciousness caused by a sudden fall in blood pressure; can have serious consequences, particularly in patients with a cardiovascular disease; commonly referred to as *fainting*.

Syndrome a combination of symptoms either resulting from a single cause or occurring so commonly together as to constitute a distinct clinical picture.

Syngeneic healthy bone marrow stems cells collected from identical twin for hematopoietic stem cell transplantation.

Systole the contraction, or phase of contraction, of the heart, especially the ventricles, during which blood is forced into the aorta and the pulmonary artery; systolic pressure is the highest, or greatest, pressure.

T

Tachycardia abnormally high heart rate (>100 beats/minute) for an adult.

Tachypnea abnormally high respiration rate (>20 breaths/minute) for an adult.

Tactile pertaining to the touch.

Tardive dyskinesia involuntary movements of the mouth, lips, tongue, and jaws, usually associated with long-term use of antipsychotic medication.

TB Tuberculosis.

Telangiectases dilation of capillaries making them appear as small red or purple cluster, which may have a "spidery" appearance.

Telangiectasia dilated or broken veins near the skin surface; also called "spider veins."

Teledentistry a model of healthcare delivery that uses web-based technology to send electronic information such as patient history and digital radiographs, between on-site and off-site practitioners; this model can be used to support collaborative practice between dentists and dental hygienists who are caring for patients in nontraditional settings.

Temporomandibular disorder (TMD) a collective term that includes a wide range of disorders of the masticatory system characterized by one or more of the following pain in the preauricular area, temporomandibular joint (TMJ), and muscles of mastication, with limitation or deviation in mandibular motion and TMJ sounds during mandibular function.

Temporomandibular joint joint on either side of the face connecting the jawbone to the skull.

Tensile strength amount of strength the suture material will retain throughout the healing period. As the wound gains strength, the suture loses strength.

Tension test application of tension at the mucogingival junction (MGJ) by retracting cheek, lip, and tongue to tighten the alveolar mucosa and test for the presence of attached gingiva; area of missing attached gingiva is revealed when the alveolar mucosa and frena are connected directly to the free gingiva.

Terminal (lower) shank the part of the shank next to the blade.

Terminally ill patient a person who is experiencing the end stages of a life-threatening disease and for whom there is no longer hope of a cure.

Tertiary/reparative dentin a type of dentin formed along the pulpal wall or root canal as a protective mechanism in response to trauma or irritation, such as caries or a traumatic cavity preparation.

Testing stick plastic 1/4-inch rod, 3 inches long, used to test the sharpness of a scaler or a curet.

Therapeutic a chemical with therapeutic properties that is delivered by rinsing or irrigation device.

Therapeutic rinses mouthrinses with healing properties that are delivered by rinsing or irrigation device.

Third-hand smoke tobacco smoke residue absorbed by furnishings.

Thixotropic type of gel that sets in a gel-like state but becomes fluid under stress; the fluid form permits the solution to flow into interdental areas.

Three-body abrasion polishing involves loose abrasive particles that move in the interface space between the surface being polished and the polishing application device.

Thrombus blood clot attached to the intima of a blood vessel; may occlude the lumen; contrast with embolus, which is detached and carried by the bloodstream.

Thyrotoxic crisis (thyroid storm) potentially life-threatening condition for people with hyperthyroidism. The thyroid suddenly releases large amounts of thyroid hormone.

Tic an involuntary, sudden, rapid, recurrent, nonrhythmic, stereotyped motor movement or vocal sound.

Tinnitus ringing, buzzing, tinkling, or hissing sounds in the ear.

Titanium a uniquely biocompatible metal used for implants either in the commercially pure form or as an alloy.

Titanium alloy a common titanium alloy (Ti-6A1-4V) used for dental implants that contains 6% aluminum to increase strength and decrease weight and 4% vanadium to prevent corrosion.

Titration a technique for individualization of drug dose. Administration of small, incremental dose of a drug until the desired clinical action is observed.

Toddler child from age 1 year to 3 years of age.

Tolerance is an individual's diminished response to a substance, which occurs when the substance is used repeatedly and the body adapts to the continued presence of the substance, requiring increased amounts to achieve the same effect.

Tomography a three-dimensional image of the internal structures of a solid object like the mandible.

Tongue thrust the infantile pattern of suckle-swallow movement in which the tongue is placed between the incisor teeth or alveolar ridges; may result in an anterior open bite, deformation of the jaws, and abnormal function.

Tonic state of continuous, unremitting action of muscular contraction; patient appears stiff.

Tonic-clonic seizure also known as convulsion or "grand mal." Usually begins on both sides of the brain, but can start in one side and spread to the whole brain. Last 1 to 3 minutes and have a longer recovery period.

Tooth abrasion pathologic, non-carious wear of a tooth.

Toothbrush head the part of the toothbrush composed of the tufts and the stock (extension of the handle where the tufts are attached).

Torus/tori (pl) bony elevation or prominence usually located on the midline of the hard palate (torus palatinus) and the lingual surface of the mandible in the premolar area (torus mandibularis).

Transdermal method of drug delivery by patch on skin; a mode for slow release over extended time.

Transducer a device that converts energy or power from one form to another.

transient ischemic attack (TIA) brief episode of cerebral ischemia that results in no permanent neurologic damage; symptoms are warning signals of impending CVA (stroke).

Translucency having the appearance between complete opacity and complete transparency; partially opaque.

Transmission-based precautions a second-tier beyond standard precautions to help prevent spread of disease from one person to another.

Transmucosal type of drug delivery by infiltration of mucosal lining.

Transosseous dental devices implanted through the bone.

Traumatic alopecia an area of baldness on the head caused by pulling out the hair at the roots.

Trendelenburg position the modified supine position when the head is lower than the heart.

Trendelenburg position the patient is supine with the heart higher than the head on a surface inclined downward about 45°.

Triage screening and classification of individuals in order to make optimal use of treatment resources; sorting and allocating relative priority for patient treatment needs.

Tribiology tribiology incorporates the study and application of the principles of friction, lubrication, and wear as they apply to polishing.

Trigger/signs factor that precipitate a seizure, usually something that may occur prior to a seizure.

Trismus motor disturbance of the trigeminal nerve with spasm of masticatory muscles and difficulty in opening the mouth (lockjaw).

TST tuberculin skin test.

Tuft a cluster of bristles or filaments secured together in one hole in the head of a toothbrush.

Two-body abrasion polishing involves abrasive particles attached to a medium (polishing application device) that move directly against the surface being polished.

U

ULs (Tolerable Upper Intake Levels, or Upper Levels) maximum intake by an individual that is unlikely to create risks of adverse health effects in almost all healthy individuals.

Ultrasonic cleaner a device, in which a denture is placed in water or some type of solvent cleaner, that uses ultrasonic waves to dislodge debris on a denture.

Ultrasonic scaler power-driven scaling instrument that operates in a frequency range between 25,000 and 50,000 cps to convert a high-frequency electrical current into mechanical vibrations.

Ultrasonic sound whose frequency is above the threshold of human hearing, typically above 20 kHz.

Unclassified seizures of unknown onset.

Unknown onset onset was unobserved, or determination of origin is unknown.

Upper-room ultraviolet germicidal irradiation (UVGI) ultraviolet light meant to kill or inactivate airborne pathogens, but remain at a safe level for individuals in the room.

Urticaria vascular reaction of the skin with transient appearance of slightly elevated patches (wheals) that are redder or paler than the surrounding skin; may be accompanied by severe itching; also called hives.

USDA U.S. Department of Agriculture.

USPHS US Public Health Services.

V

Validity ability of an index or a test procedure to measure what it is intended to measure.

Vaporoles a brand of smelling salts or aromatic ammonia in a small capsule-type container that is crushed and put under the syncope victim's nose to stimulate respiration.

Variable factors in a research study that can be manipulated and measured; includes dependent, independent, and extraneous variables.

Variant another form or subtype of a microorganism.

Vasculopathy this term is applied to any disease affecting blood vessels.

Vasoconstrictor a drug that constricts blood vessels. An additive to most local anesthetic solutions to offset the vasodilating actions of the local anesthetic.

Vaso-occlusion blood vessel blockage resulting in organ damage.

Vegan diet a diet consisting of only plant foods. Other varieties of the vegan diet are the fruitarian: fruits, nuts, honey, and vegetable oils; lacto-vegetarian: vegan based with the inclusion of dairy products; lacto-ovo-vegetarian: vegan based with the inclusion of dairy products and eggs.

Venous blood nonoxygenated blood from the tissues; blood pumped from the heart to the lungs for oxygenation.

Ventral inferior surface; opposite of dorsal.

Ventriculoatrial shunt surgical creation of a communication between a cerebral ventricle and a cardiac atrium by means of a plastic tube; for relief of hydrocephalus.

Ventriculoperitoneal shunt communication between a cerebral ventricle and the peritoneum by means of a plastic tube; for relief of hydrocephalus.

Verruca verrucous (verrucose), a wartlike growth.

Verruca vulgaris common warts; a benign lesion of skin and mucous membranes caused by human papillomovirus (HPV).

Vertigo dizziness.

Viral shedding presence of virus in body secretions, in excretions, or in body surface lesions with potential for transmission.

Virus a subcellular genetic entity capable of gaining entrance into a limited range of living cells and capable of replication only within such cells; a virus contains either DNA or RNA, but not both.

Viscosity in general, the resistance to flow or alteration of shape by any substance as a result of molecular cohesion.

Visible light-cure light activation using a photocure system; shorter curing time than self-cure (chemical cure); does not start setting until the light is activated, thereby allowing longer working time for adapting the dressing material.

Vision the faculty or state of being able to see.

Visual impairment a visual condition that impacts a person's abilities to succeed normal everyday activities during life.

Vital signs refers to body temperature, blood pressure, pulse or heart rate, and breathing rate.

Vocal a type of cue, such as accent, loudness, tempo, pitch, cadence, and tone that occurs during communication.

W

Water pipe (or hookah) a water pipe used to smoke specially made flavored tobacco.

Waste

- **Contaminated waste** items that have contacted blood or other body secretions.
- **Hazardous waste** poses a risk to humans or the environment.
- **Infectious waste** capable of causing an infectious disease; contaminated with blood, saliva, or other substances; potentially or actually infected with pathogenic material; officially called "regulated" waste.
- **Regulated waste** liquid blood or saliva, sharps contaminated with blood or saliva, and nonsharp solid waste saturated with or caked with liquid or semisolid blood or saliva or tissue including teeth.

Wheeze breathe with difficulty, usually with a whistling sound.

White spot lesion early stage of the caries process when demineralization causes a change in the enamel to appear chalky white.

White spot term used to describe a small area on the surface of enamel that contrasts in appearance with the rest of the surface and may be visible only when the tooth is dried; two types of white spots can be differentiated: an area of demineralization and an area of fluorosis (also referred to as an "enamel opacity").

White-coat hypertension elevated blood pressure as a result of feeling anxious in a medical environment.

Whitening use of abrasive agents in the dentifrice that results in whitening of teeth. Often used interchangeably with the term bleaching, but not actually the same procedure.

Wickham striae whitish lines visible on oral mucosa giving a lace-like appearance in oral lichen planus.

Withdrawal syndrome a group of signs and symptoms, both physiologic and psychological, that occurs on abrupt discontinuation of a substance use.

Working end the part of an instrument used to carry out the purpose and function of the instrument.

X

XDR-TB extensively drug-resistant tuberculosis.

Xerostomia dry mouth from reduced or absent salivary flow; may be related to medical conditions, head and neck radiation, or medications.

Xylitol a natural sugar-alcohol that is approved for use in food by the US Food and Drug Administration.

Index

Note: Page numbers followed by "*f*", "*t*", and "*b*" refer to figures, tables, and boxes, respectively.

B

C

D

E

F

G

H

I

J

K

L

M

N

P

Q

R

S

T

U

V

W

Z